Quick Reference Problem-Solver

The following guide serves as a quick reference for information needed by students. The expanded table of contents, the list of procedures, and the index will help you find other information.

If you need help with . . .	Refer to . . .
Interviewing	interviewing techniques, p. 349
	interviewing as a data collection method, p. 256
	components of a nursing history, p. 256
	sample interview questions in Chapters 27 through 39
Understanding medical symbols and abbreviations	Table 18-1, Abbreviations and Symbols, p. 311
Converting assessment data into nursing diagnoses	list of 1988 NANDA-approved nursing diagnoses, facing page
	writing nursing diagnoses, p. 279
	how a nursing diagnosis differs from a medical diagnosis, p. 274 and Table 16-1, p. 276
	how to correct common diagnostic errors, Table 16-3, p. 282
Constructing care plans	how to write a nursing diagnosis, p. 279
	establishing priorities, p. 290
	writing goals, p. 290
	developing evaluative strategy, p. 290
	writing nursing orders, p. 295
	writing the nursing care plan, p. 295
	evaluation criteria and standards, p. 322
	work-up of common nursing diagnoses at the end of Chapters 27 through 39 (see expanded table of contents, pp. xiv–xxv)
Constructing teaching plans	planning for teaching, p. 364, and Sample Teaching Plan, Table 21-1, p. 365
Documenting care	guidelines for documenting, p. 310
	legality of documentation, p. 91
Understanding and avoiding legal conflicts	legal safeguards for the nurse, p. 87
Resolving ethical dilemmas	six-step process for resolving ethical problems, p. 72
Strategies for providing care in well clients	Self-Test, p. 27
	Promoting Wellness extracts, Chapters 9, 28, 29, 31, 32, 34, 36
	designing exercise programs, p. 673
Managing pain	Assessment of the Pain Experience, p. 735
	McGill-Melzack Pain Questionnaire, p. 732
	noninvasive nursing relief measures, p. 740
	stress management teaching, p. 140
Administering medications	common abbreviations used in prescribing medications, Table 40-4, p. 1129
	equivalents, Appendix A
	dosage calculations, p. 1130
	3 checks and 5 rights of medication administration, p. 1131
	medication administration procedures in Chapter 40
Managing stress (client's or mine)	stress management skills, p. 140
Protecting yourself and clients against AIDS	Recommendations for Prevention of HIV Transmission in Health Care Settings, p. 520
Meeting needs of grieving and dying individuals	Chapter 13, p. 232
Making admission to a health care setting less traumatic	admitting the client, p. 531
Preparing clients for diagnostic procedures	nursing responsibilities prior to the test, p. 118
Performing a physical examination	Chapter 24

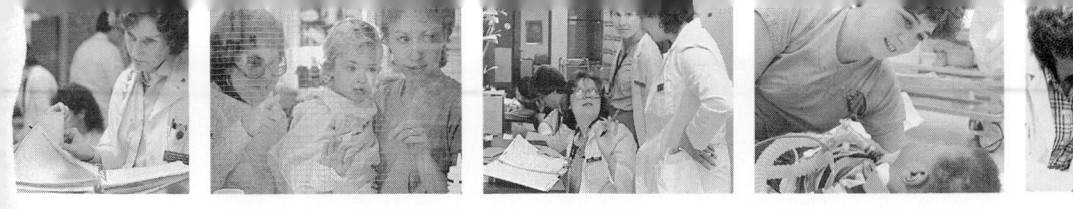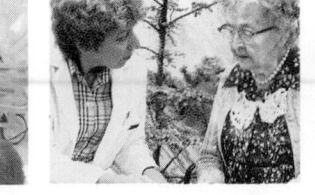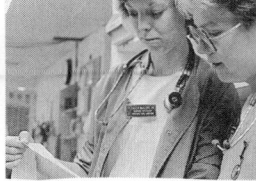

FUNDAMENTALS OF NURSING

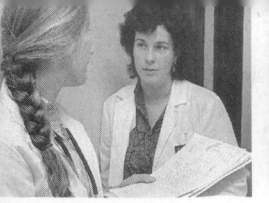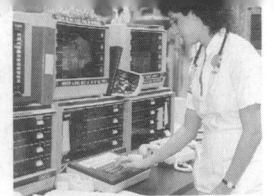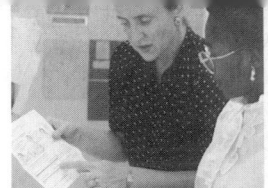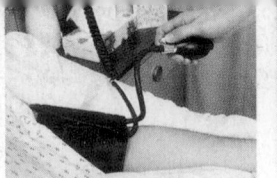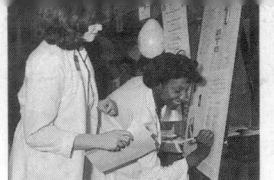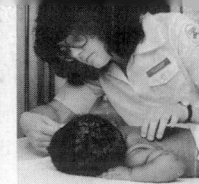

Carol Taylor
CSFN, RN, MSN
Division of Nursing
Holy Family College
Philadelphia, Pennsylvania

Carol Lillis
RN, MSN
Nursing Program
Delaware County Community College
Media, Pennsylvania

Priscilla LeMone
RNC, MA
Department of Nursing
Southeast Missouri State University
Cape Girardeau, Missouri

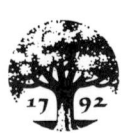

J. B. Lippincott Company
Philadelphia

London   Mexico City   New York
St. Louis   São Paulo   Sydney

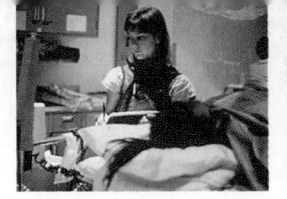
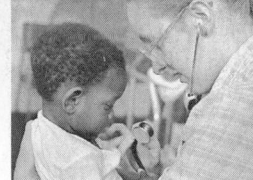

FUNDAMENTALS OF

NURSING

THE ART AND SCIENCE OF NURSING CARE

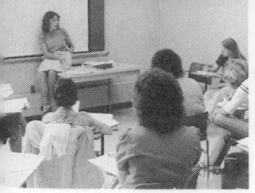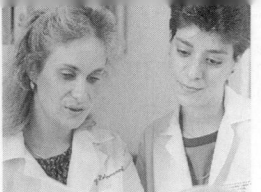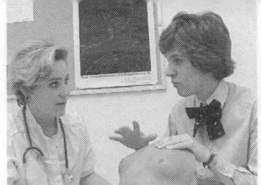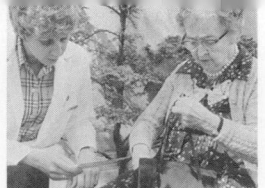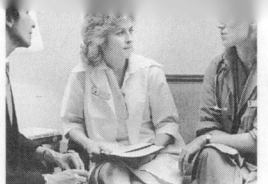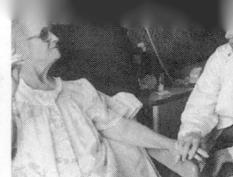

Acquisitions Editor: Patricia L. Cleary
Developmental Editor: Eleanor Faven
Manuscript Editor: Helen Ewan
Indexer: Ann Cassar
Senior Designer: Anita Curry
Illustrator: Bob Jackson
Production Manager: Carol A. Florence
Production Supervisor: Charlene Squibb
Compositor: Tapsco, Inc.
Printer/Binder: R. R. Donnelley and Sons Company

6   5   4   3   2

Library of Congress Cataloging-in-Publication Data
Fundamentals of nursing.
   Includes bibliographies and index.
   1. Nursing.   I. Taylor, Mary Carol.   II. Lillis,
Carol.   III. LeMone, Priscilla.
[DNLM: 1. Health Promotion.   2. Nursing.   3. Nursing
Process.   WY 16 F981]
RT41.F882   1989   610.73   88-8937
ISBN 0-397-54659-9

Any procedure or practice described in this book should be applied by the health-care practitioner under appropriate supervision in accordance with professional standards of care
used with regard to the unique circumstances that apply in each practice situation. Care
has been taken to confirm the accuracy of information presented and to describe generally accepted practices. However, the authors, editors, and publisher cannot accept any responsibility for errors or omissions or for consequences from application of the information in this book and make no warranty, express or implied, with respect to the contents
of the book.

   Every effort has been made to ensure drug selections and dosages are in accordance
with current recommendations and practice. Because of ongoing research, changes in government regulations and the constant flow of information on drug therapy, reactions and
interactions, the reader is cautioned to check the package insert for each drug for indications, dosages, warnings, and precautions, particularly if the drug is new or infrequently used.

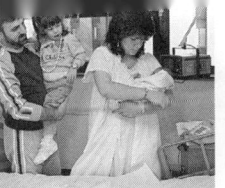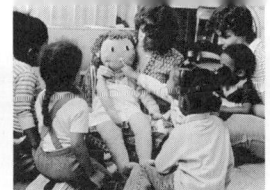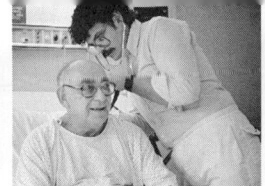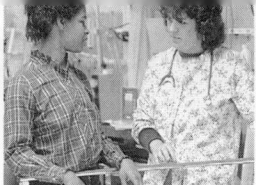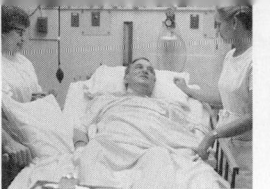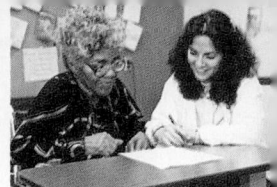

To my parents, Mildred and Ray Taylor, who encourage excellence by their love and example.

Carol Taylor

To my husband, Jack, and my four sons, whose sense of humor and caring kept everything in perspective.

Carol Lillis

To my family, who give me roots, and to my students, who give me wings.

Priscilla LeMone

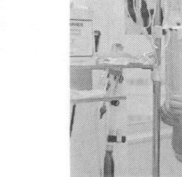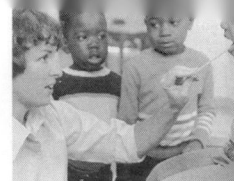

Contributors/ Reviewers

Joan Berends, RN, PhD
Director, Nursing Programs
Grand Rapids Junior College
Grand Rapids, Michigan

Deborah J. Borelli, RN, MSN
Instructor
Nursing Department
St. Petersburg Junior College
Clearwater, Florida

Nancy L. Bradley, BSN, MEd
Coordinator and Assistant Professor
School of Nursing
Kent State
Kent, Ohio

Anne Carlson, BS
Health Consultant—Nutrition
Salvation Army Grace Hospital
Calgary, Alberta, Canada

Anne M. Carty, RN, MA, MSN
Director, Nursing Program
Southwest Missouri State University
West Plains, Missouri

Donita D'Amico, EdM, RN
Assistant Professor
Nursing Department
William Paterson College
Wayne, New Jersey

Susan G. Dudek, RD, BS
Consulting Dietitian
Bertrand Chaffee Hospital
Springville, New York

Vicki V. Earnest, RN, MS
Associate Professor
Health and Human Services
Community College of Denver
Denver, Colorado

Blanca Rosa Garcia, RNC, FNP, MSN
Chair, Department of RN Education
Del Mar College
Corpus Christi, Texas

Ellen B. Gloyd, RN, MSN
Professor
Nursing Department
Montgomery College
Takoma Park, Maryland

Ruth E. Gordon, RNC, MSN
Assistant Professor
Division of Nursing
Holy Family College
Philadelphia, Pennsylvania

Mary Elizabeth Haney, RN, BSN, MAEd
Instructor
Nursing Department
Asheville Buncombe Technical Community College
Asheville, North Carolina

Sharolyn B. Heatwole, RN, MSN
Associate Professor
Nursing Program
Division of Health Technology
J. Sargeant Reynolds Community College
Richmond, Virginia

Daisy Hines, RN, MSN
Professor
Nursing and Health Technologies
Long Beach City College
Long Beach, California

Sylvia Huber, RN, BScN
Former Instructor
Department of Nursing and Allied Health
Mount Royal College
Calgary, Alberta, Canada

June Johnson, MS, RN
Professor, Curriculum Coordinator
Department of Nursing
Sinclair Community College
Dayton, Ohio

Cheryl Kieffer, MSN, RN, CS
Instructor
Department of Nursing
Southeast Missouri State University
Cape Girardeau, Missouri

Jane McCausland Kurz, RN, MSN, CCRN
Nurse Consultant
Department of Mental Retardation, State of Delaware
Newark, Delaware

Monica Kwong, RN, MS
Clinical Nurse Educator
Kaiser Permanente Medical Center
Oakland, California

Kathleen Malic, BSN, MA, RN
Lecturer
Division of Nursing
Holy Family College
Supervisor, Pennsylvania Hospital
Philadelphia, Pennsylvania

Filomela A. Marshall, RN, MSN
Assistant Professor
Division of Nursing
Holy Family College
Philadelphia, Pennsylvania

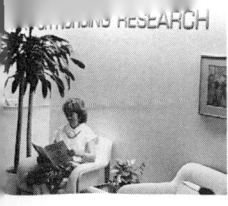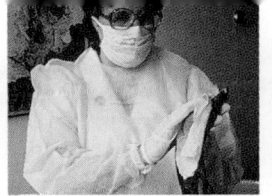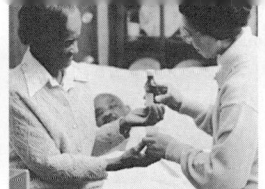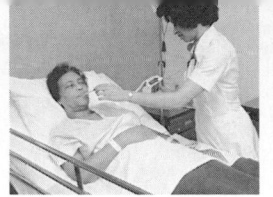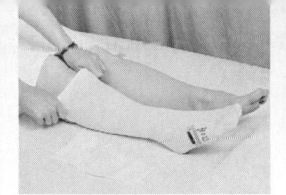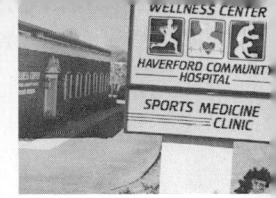

Rosemary Russo Miley, *RN, BSN*
Clinical Supervisor
Mercy Catholic Medical Center
Darby, Pennsylvania

Mary C. Mitchell, *RN, BS, MA*
Associate Professor
Morrisville A&T College, SUNY
Hamilton, New York

Maureen J. Osis, *RN, MN*
Clinical Nurse Specialist, Consultant
Calgary, Alberta, Canada

Paulette LaCava Osterman, *RN,*
BSN, MA, CAGS
Professor
Nursing Department
Community College of Rhode Island
North Kingston, Rhode Island

Gracie H. Perry, *MSN, CRNP*
Nurse Practitioner
School District of Philadelphia
Philadelphia, Pennsylvania

Faith M. Reierson, *RN, MN*
Coordinator, Nursing Programs
Olympic College
Bremerton, Washington

Linda Ann Robinson, *RN, MSN*
Staff Nurse
Presbyterian University of Pennsyl-
vania Medical Center
Philadelphia, Pennsylvania

Eileen M. Roche, *RNC, MSN*
Assistant Professor
School of Nursing
Widener University
Chester, Pennsylvania

Christine M. Rosner, *RN, MSN*
Assistant Professor
Division of Nursing
Holy Family College
Philadelphia, Pennsylvania

Joyce Soehnlen, *RN, MSN*
Assistant Professor
Department of Nursing
Walsh College
Canton, Ohio

Shirley M. Solberg, *RN, MN*
Assistant Professor
School of Nursing
Memorial University of Newfoundland
St. Johns, Newfoundland, Canada

Melissa Spezia, *RN, MSN*
Instructor
Department of Nursing
Southeast Missouri State University
Cape Girardeau, Missouri

Wanda Stephenson, *RN, MS*
Instructor
Nursing Program
Anne Arundel Community College
Arnold, Maryland

Janet L. Storch, *RN, MHSA, PhD*
Associate Professor
Department of Health Services
The University of Alberta
Edmonton, Alberta, Canada

Barbara R. Stright, *RN, MSN*
Assistant Professor
Division of Nursing
Clarion University of Pennsylvania
Oil City, Pennsylvania

Jacqueline Sullivan, *RN, MSN,*
CCRN, CNRN
Clinical Nurse Specialist
Neurosensory Care Program
Thomas Jefferson University Hospital
Philadelphia, Pennsylvania

Barbara Timby, *RN, BSN, MA*
Instructor, Medical–Surgical Nursing
Glen Oaks Community College
Centerville, Michigan

Karen L. Wall, *RN, BScN*
Curriculum Coordinator
Nursing Department
Community College
Winnipeg, Manitoba, Canada

Joyce Welliver, *RN, MSN*
Assistant Professor, Senior Level Co-
ordinator
Division of Nursing
Holy Family College
Philadelphia, Pennsylvania

Eileen M. Williams, *RN, MSN*
Professor
Nursing Program
Mesa College
Grand Junction, Colorado

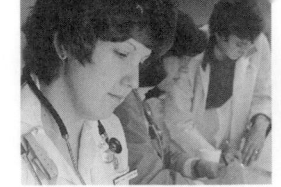
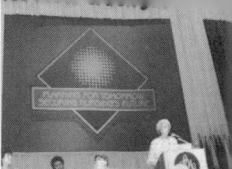

Preface

Never before in the history of modern nursing has the need for nurses been greater and never before has so much been asked of those beginning the study of nursing. Complex health-care demands challenge the nurse's knowledge, technical competence, interpersonal skills, and commitment. Experienced nurses speak and write of nursing as both an art and a science, distinguished by a unique spirit of caring.

Therefore, much care has gone into the selection of both the content of this text and the manner of its presentation. Throughout, the aim was to capture the unique essence of both the art and science of nursing, distilling what the person beginning the study of nursing needs to know and presenting this content in a straightforward manner. The learner is invited to identify with the profession, to share in its pride, and to respond to its challenges.

The authors are sensitive to the different meanings nurses attach to the terms "client" versus "patient." We chose to use the term "client" to emphasize respect for the autonomy (self-determination) of the client and to encourage the nurse to actively involve the client and family as much as possible in care decisions. Care has been taken to communicate that both nurses and clients may be male or female and that they come from every racial and ethnic background and socioeconomic group. Whenever possible we have tried to avoid male/female distinctions in personal pronouns.

Realizing that our textbook is used by a variety of people throughout North America, we have strived to generalize many statements and use references to Canada throughout the book. Other Canadian materials appear in the Appendix and the Instructor's Manual.

Organization

The textbook is organized into nine units. The learner is first introduced to the concepts "nurse," "client," and "nursing process," and then to basic nursing roles and actions common to nursing practice. The remaining units focus specifically on how nurses can work with clients to promote healthy physiologic and psychosocial responses. Although, ideally, the text is followed sequentially, every effort has been made to respect the differing needs of diverse curricula and students. Thus each chapter stands on its own merit and may be read independently of others.

Unit I, The Nurse: Foundations for Nursing Practice, describes contemporary nursing. Chapters focus on the profession of nursing, nursing's role in promoting wellness in health and illness, the changing health-care system, nursing theories, and the ethical and legal dimensions of nursing practice.

Unit II, The Client: Concepts for Holistic Care, offers foundational knowledge about clients, essential to accurate nursing assessments and effective nurse–client interactions. Chapters describe the human needs of individuals, families, and communities and explore the concepts of culture and ethnicity, and stress and adaptation.

Unit III, Promoting Wellness Across the Lifespan, provides a comprehensive picture of growth and development throughout the lifespan and acknowledges the differing needs for nursing arising from different developmental stages and abilities to meet developmental tasks. The unit includes chapters on basic developmental concepts, conception to midlife, the older adult, and the concepts of loss, grief, and death.

Unit IV, The Nursing Process, offers a detailed, step-by-step guide to each component of the nursing process. Practical guidelines and examples are included in each chapter. Separate chapters address the nursing process as a whole, assessing, diagnosing, planning, implementing, and evaluating. Documentation guidelines are discussed in the chapter on implementing and are noted wherever appropriate.

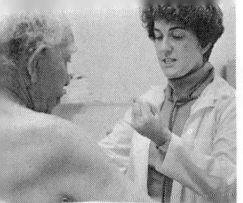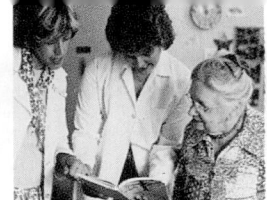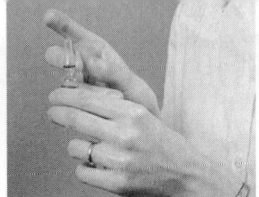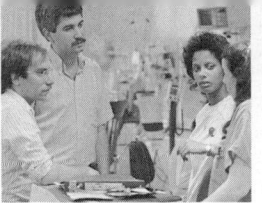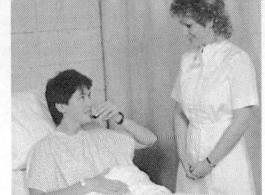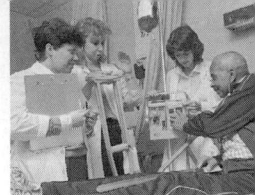

Unit V, Roles Basic to Nursing Practice, describes major roles in which nurses function as they interact holistically with clients. Chapters focus on the communicator, teacher/counselor, and leader/researcher/advocate roles of the nurse as caregiver.

Univ VI, Actions Basic to Nursing Practice, presents the foundational skills used by nurses in most practice settings. Skills are developed in measuring vital signs, performing nursing assessments (physical examination), ensuring client safety, and in admitting and discharging clients and performing home visits.

Unit VII, Promoting Healthy Physiologic Responses, explores the nurse's role in helping clients meet basic physiologic needs: hygiene, activity, rest and sleep, comfort, nutrition, bowel elimination, urinary elimination, oxygenation, and fluid, electrolyte, and acid–base balance. In each chapter guidelines are included for assessing and diagnosing unhealthy responses and for planning, implementing, and evaluating appropriate care strategies. Chapters conclude with a case study illustrating the use of the nursing process to resolve selected nursing diagnoses.

Unit VIII, Promoting Healthy Psychosocial Responses, using the same format as Unit VII, focuses on psychosocial needs of clients: self-concept, sensory stimulation, sexuality, and spirituality.

Unit IX, Promoting Optimal Health in Special Situations, includes chapters describing nursing responsibilities related to medication administration, diagnostic procedures, wound care, and perioperative nursing.

Integrated Nursing Process

After the nursing process is introduced in Unit IV, it provides the organizational framework for successive chapters. Chapters in Units VII and VIII, dealing with physiologic and psychosocial responses, begin with a succinct background discussion of the concept followed by an identification of factors that influence how different individuals respond to these needs. Steps in the nursing process are used to describe related nursing responsibilities.

Assessing. Common elements of both a comprehensive and problem-focused nursing assessment are presented; sample interview questions are included, and specific physical assessment techniques described.

Diagnosing. NANDA-approved nursing diagnoses related to the human need being discussed are identi-

fied, and tables illustrate the relationship between diagnostic cues, contributing factors, and the problem statement.

Planning. Sample client goals are suggested based on client strengths. Each chapter concludes with a care plan designed for the client described in a case study.

Implementing. Nursing measures are clearly explained and are illustrated when this is deemed helpful. Procedures have been streamlined to facilitate mastery. A sufficient variety of nursing interventions is provided to enable the development of a repertoire of nursing actions that makes practicing the art of nursing possible.

Evaluating. Criteria for evaluating the effectiveness of the plan of care are suggested.

Each chapter in Units VII and VIII concludes with the workup of several diagnoses that demonstrate the comprehensive nursing management of common nursing problems. This section and the concluding case studies with a nursing care plan afford the reader ongoing illustrations of the correct use and documentation of nursing process. As the learner progresses through the text, the nursing process becomes an integral part of nursing care.

Key Features

In planning this textbook, we chose to develop the following features:

- **Nursing as an art and science.** As a science, nursing is characterized by a growing body of knowledge and varied technical competencies; as an art, nursing demands of its practitioners creativity in designing individualized strategies that help clients reach personal health goals.
- **Wellness orientation.** A wellness rather than an illness orientation is followed. Wellness promotion display extracts highlight assessment checkpoints for specific components of high-level wellness and include suggestions for designing a self-care prescription. The extracts serve a twofold purpose: a self-care model for the learner and an aid in client instruction.
- **Nurses as role models.** Learners are directed to assess their own health behaviors before attempting to help clients; health goals for the nurse are presented in clinical chapters.

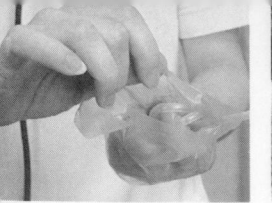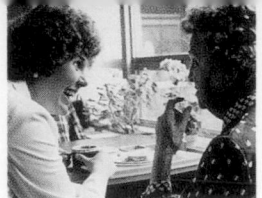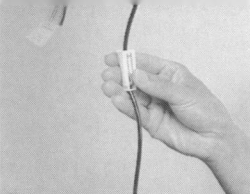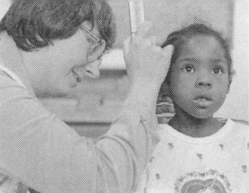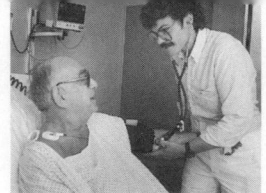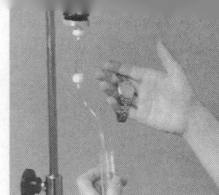

- **Aims of nursing.** Learners are gradually introduced to the theory, interpersonal skills, and nursing procedures that will enable them to work successfully with clients to promote wellness, prevent illness, restore health, and facilitate coping with altered functioning.
- **Basic human needs.** Common to all people and essential to wellness and survival are basic human needs. These human needs provide the foundation for the clinical chapters in Units VII and VIII, as the nurse strives to assist the client and family in meeting those needs.
- **Holistic care across the lifespan.** Holistic orientation to basic human needs exists across the lifespan. Unit III, growth and development factors in Units VII and VIII, and age considerations in many procedures address the lifespan continuum.
- **Respect for client autonomy.** The learner is consistently reminded to actively involve the client and family, according to their ability and motivation, in all aspects of care.
- **Nursing process.** Fundamental to nursing care is the nursing process, discussed earlier in the Preface.
- **Collaborative dimensions of care.** The client's achievement of health goals is related to the efficient functioning of the health-care team; the nurse, as a vital member of the team, possesses unique knowledge of the client. Respect for the contributions of different members of the team is encouraged.
- **Nursing procedures.** Procedures are presented in a concise, straightforward, and simplified format that is intended to facilitate competent performance of nursing skills. Scientific rationales accompany every nursing action, and the many photographs and illustrations further reinforce mastery. Special considerations are included where appropriate.
- **Broad scope of nursing.** The text has been written to encompass learning fundamental skills in a laboratory as well as in actual clinical settings caring for well or ill clients. Numerous examples are given to illustrate nurses interacting with clients of all ages and backgrounds, in traditional and nontraditional settings.

- **Research highlights.** Research display extracts, appearing in many chapters, describe how nursing research is making a difference in clinical practice and assist learners to value nursing research and see its relevance to practice.
- **Computer highlights.** Various computer extracts acquaint the learner with innovative computer applications in nursing and health care.
- **Key terms/glossary.** Key terms precede the text in each chapter. When these terms are defined in the chapter, they are boldfaced for clarity. A Glossary appears at the back of the book for easy studying of terms used in the book.

Teaching/Learning Package

To facilitate mastery of this text's foundational content a comprehensive teaching/learning package has been developed to assist faculty and students.

Two supplemental books are available for the learner. A Procedure Manual provides an easy, portable reference for clinical experience. Foundations of learning developed in the text are augmented in the Student Workbook. Chapter-by-chapter lessons may be followed by the learner as expertise in theory and application is developed.

Supplemental materials for the faculty member include an Instructor's Manual and a computerized test bank. The Instructor's Manual provides theoretical and clinical resources. Chapter objectives and activities encompass a range of cognitive, affective, and psychomotor domains. Another section provides a Student Learning Guide for each chapter for practical application by the student. The guides may be used to complement either practice laboratory or actual clinical nursing experience. Masters for transparencies are included in the Instructor's Manual.

A computerized test bank program assists faculty members in testing knowledge attained by learners during the course. Questions are based on material discussed in **Fundamentals of Nursing**.

Carol Taylor, RN, MSN
Carol Lillis, RN, MSN
Priscilla LeMone, RNC, MA

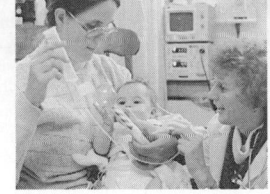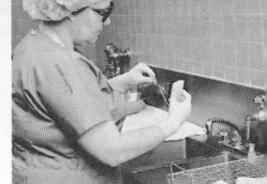

Acknowledgments

*T*his text is truly the creation of many talented and committed individuals, and we wish to acknowledge gratefully the assistance of all who have contributed in any way to the completion of this project. The idea for a fundamentals text that would be different from its contemporaries because of the manner in which it captures and communicates the art and science of nursing was conceived and nurtured by the Nursing Department of J. B. Lippincott Company. Our special thanks to:

Patti Cleary, Senior Editor, simultaneously our friend, chief challenger, encourager, and strongest critic, who continually renewed our faith in the project and ourselves.

Eleanor Faven, Developmental Editor, whose patience, loving care, and meticulous attention to detail made this text a reality.

Diana Intenzo, Editor-in-Chief, offered wise guidance throughout.

Helen Ewan, Charlene Squibb, and Anita Curry, who followed through each step of production with patience and determination.

Tracy Baldwin coordinated the art program and designed the book. Her suggestions and talents give a visual interpretation to the text. She patiently worked through deadlines, shooting schedules, and various drafts of manuscript to perform her craft, for which we express our thanks.

The illustration program seeks to communicate the excitement and spirit of the multi-disciplined and person-centered character of nursing. The energies of many people contributed to that end. We thank all who generously gave their time, ideas, and resources. We gratefully acknowledge the special contributions of the following:

Bob Jackson, illustrator

Ken Kasper, photographer

Maria Zacierka, Media Product Manager, Department of Audio Visual Media, J. B. Lippincott Company

Gates Rhodes and Denise Angelini, School of Nursing, University of Pennsylvania

The faculty and administration of the Career Education Allied Health Department, Delaware County Community College

Enid U. Rosenblatt and Vinnie Guglietti, Department of University Relations, Thomas Jefferson University

Don Walker, photographer

Barbara Proud, photographer

Robert Neroni, photographer

Joan E. Lynaugh, R.N., Ph.D., F.A.A.N., Director, the Center for the Study of the History of Nursing

Robert Koenig, Community Home Health Services of Philadelphia

Marcia Geary, Office of Public Information, University of Pennsylvania Medical Center

Art Siegel and staff, Biomedical Communications, University of Pennsylvania School of Medicine

Judy Robbins, Nursing Archive, Thomas Jefferson University

As for the actual writing of the text, we gratefully acknowledge the influence of our mentors and teachers, each person we have been privileged to care for as nurses, our students who continually challenge us to find more effective means to teach nursing, our professional colleagues, and perhaps most importantly, our friends—whose love sustained us through the lonely hours of research and writing.

We are grateful to our contributors and reviewers, whose expertise has broadened both the scope and depth of the text.

Carol Taylor
Carol Lillis
Priscilla LeMone

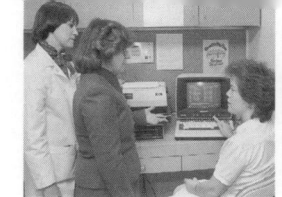
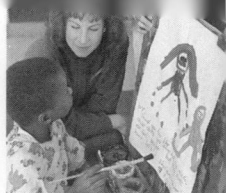

Contents

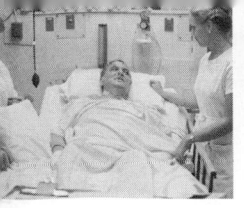
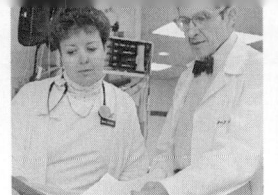
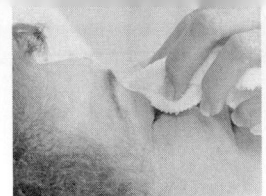
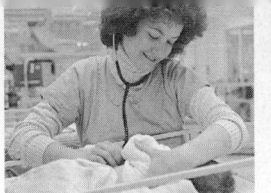
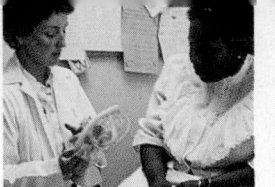
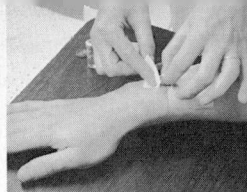

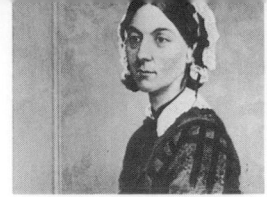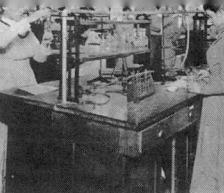

Expanded Contents

UNIT I

The Nurse: Foundations for Nursing Practice 1

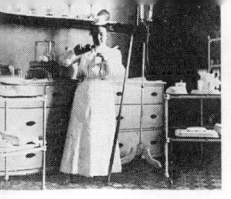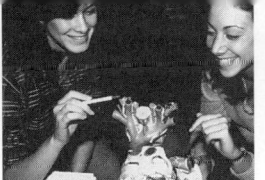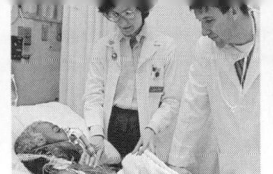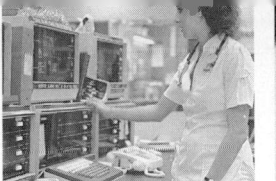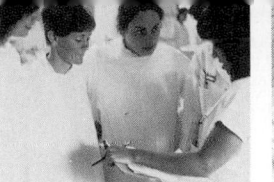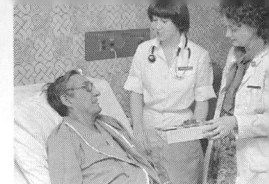

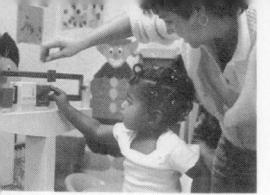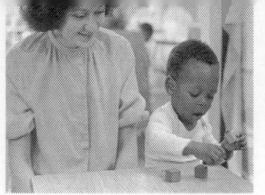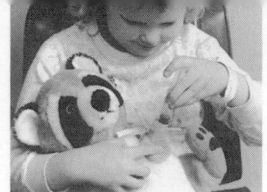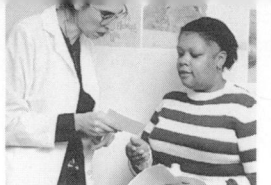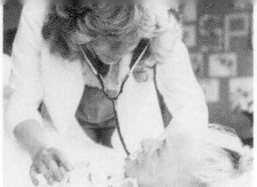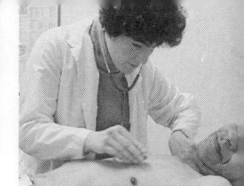

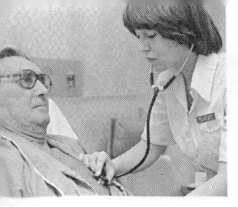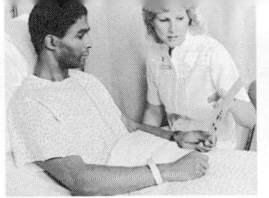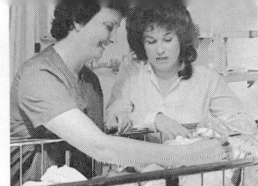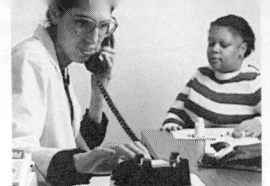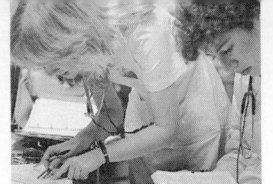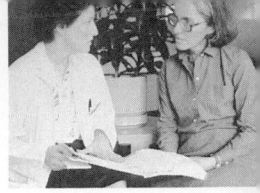

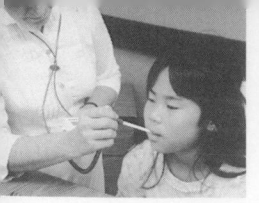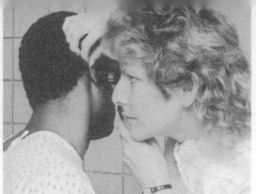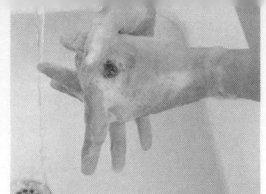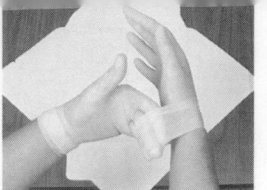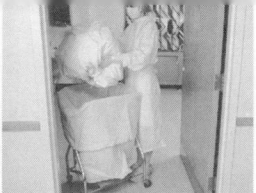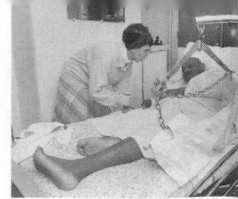

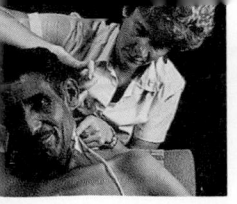
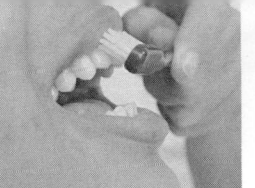
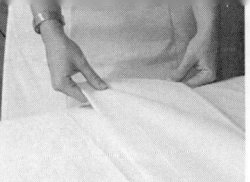
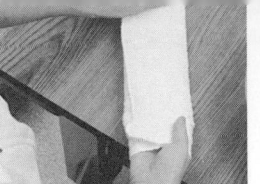
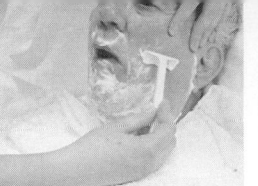
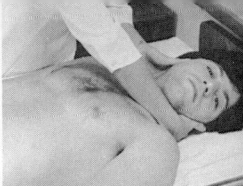

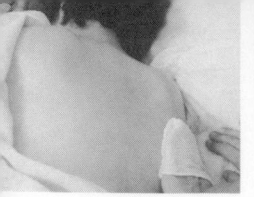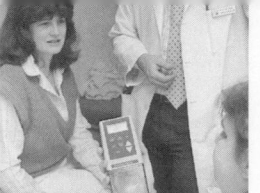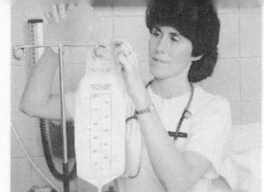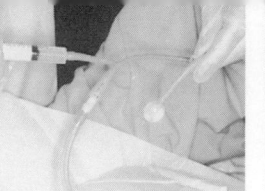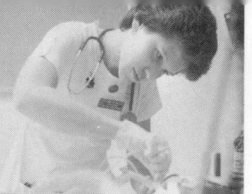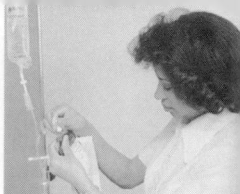

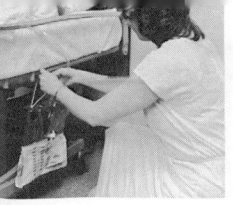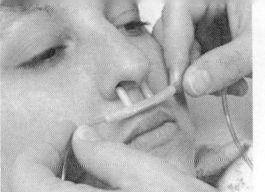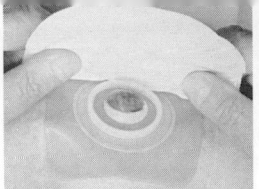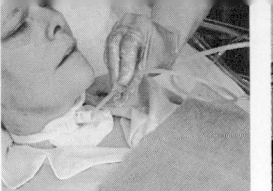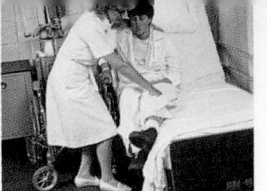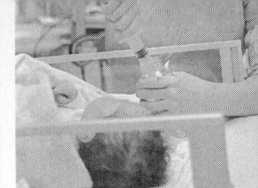

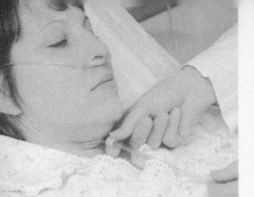
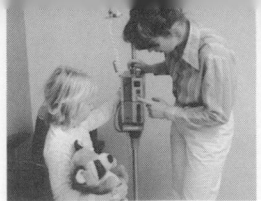
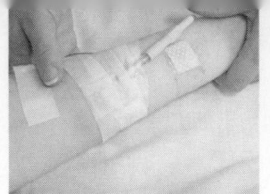
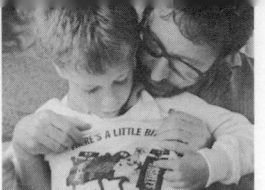
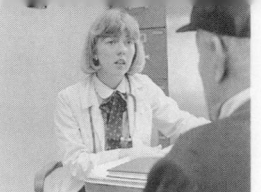
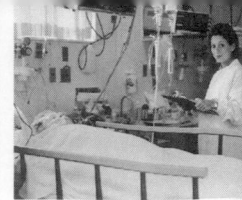

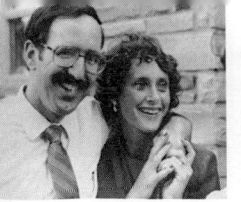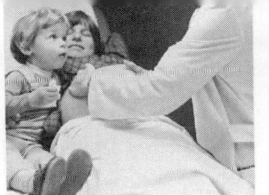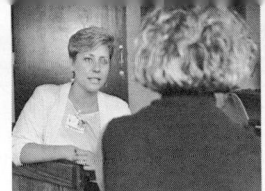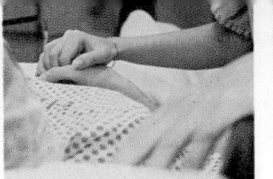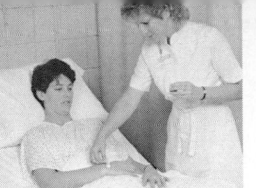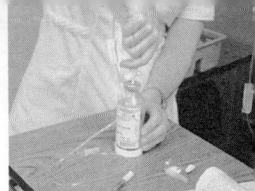

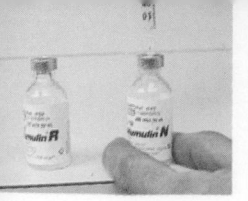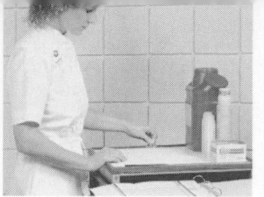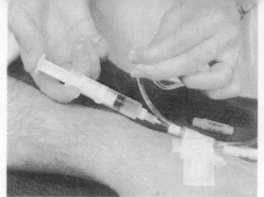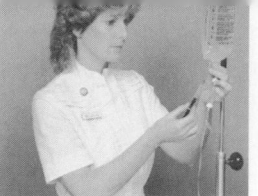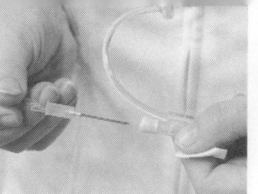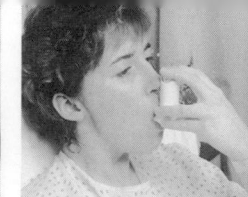

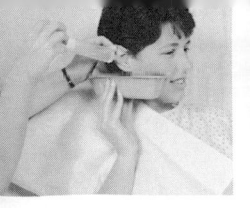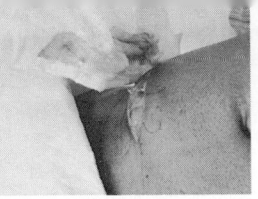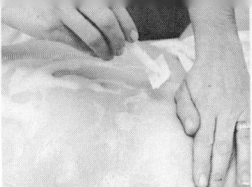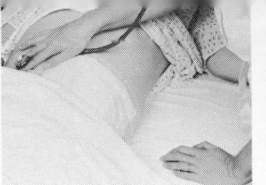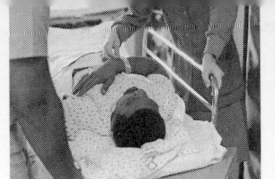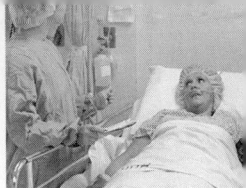

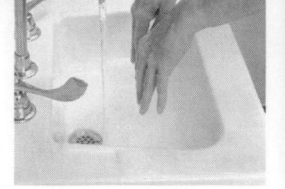
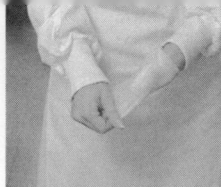

List of Procedures

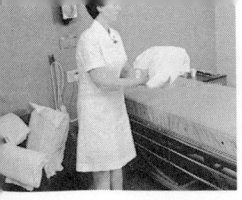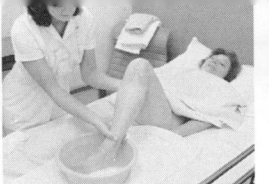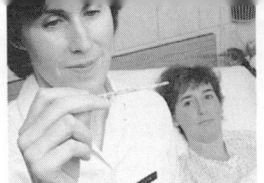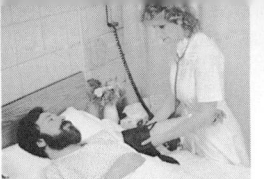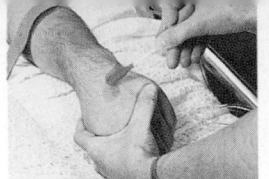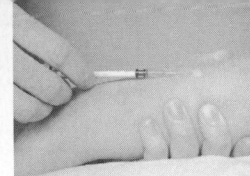

The Nurse: Foundations for Nursing Practice

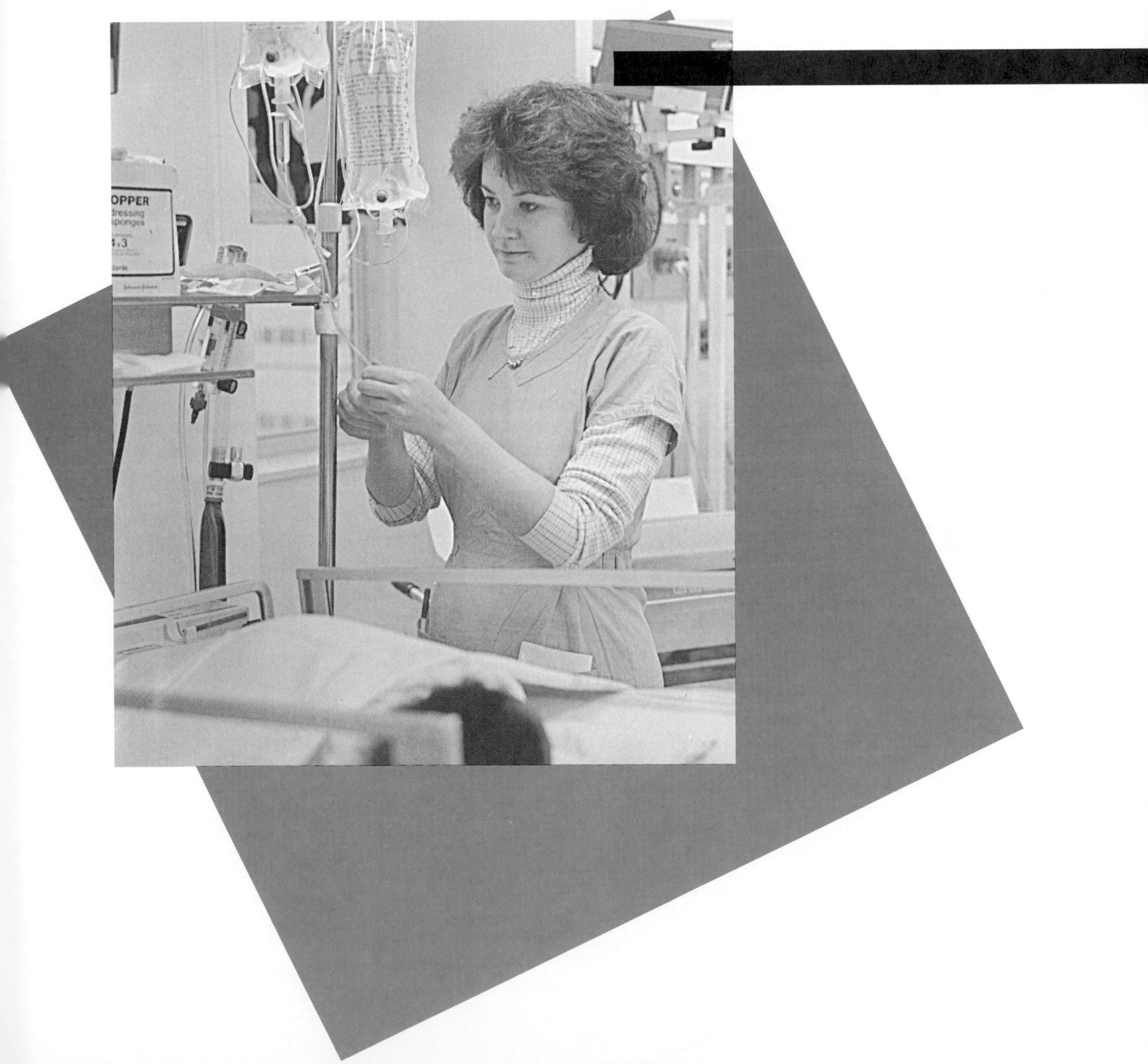

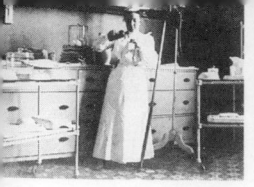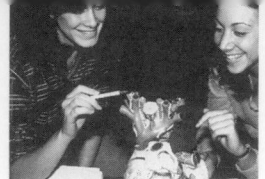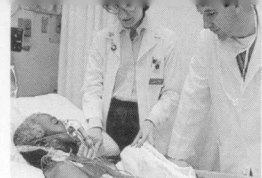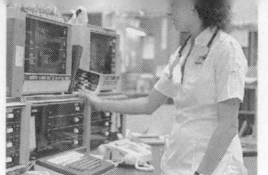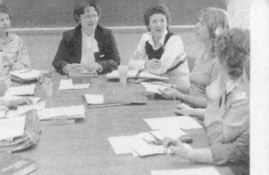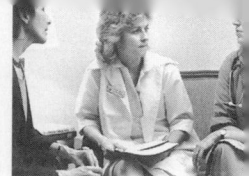

Nursing is both an art and a science. It is a profession that utilizes specialized skills and knowledge to give care to the whole person, in both health and illness and in a variety of settings. Unit I introduces concepts necessary to provide the nurse with the foundations for nursing practice by defining nursing as a whole. Chapters in this unit discuss the profession of nursing, describe the concepts of health and illness, define the health-care system in society today, give an introduction to nursing theory, and provide the necessary knowledge base for ethical and legal implications of nursing actions and relationships.

Historical perspectives, educational preparation, professional organizations, and guidelines for professional nursing practice serve as a base for understanding what nursing is and how it is organized. An understanding of basic human needs and the individualized definitions of wellness and illness prepares the nurse to integrate the human dimensions—the physical, intellectual, emotional, sociocultural, spiritual, and environmental aspects of each person—into the care given to promote wellness, prevent illness, restore health, and facilitate coping with altered function or death. Knowledge of the varied methods of health delivery is necessary in today's complex health-care system.

Nursing theories provide a base for nursing practice, defining the rationale for nursing actions and allowing a focus for nursing care. An understanding of the influence of values on human behavior and of the ethical dimensions of nursing practice is essential to knowledgeable and holistic client care. Lastly, legal responsibility and accountability are integral components of all areas of nursing practice.

Unit I gives the foundations for nursing practice from the perspective of the nurse, providing a knowledge base for the development of nursing actions and skills and nurse–client relationships, as well as growth within the profession of nursing.

Introduction to Nursing

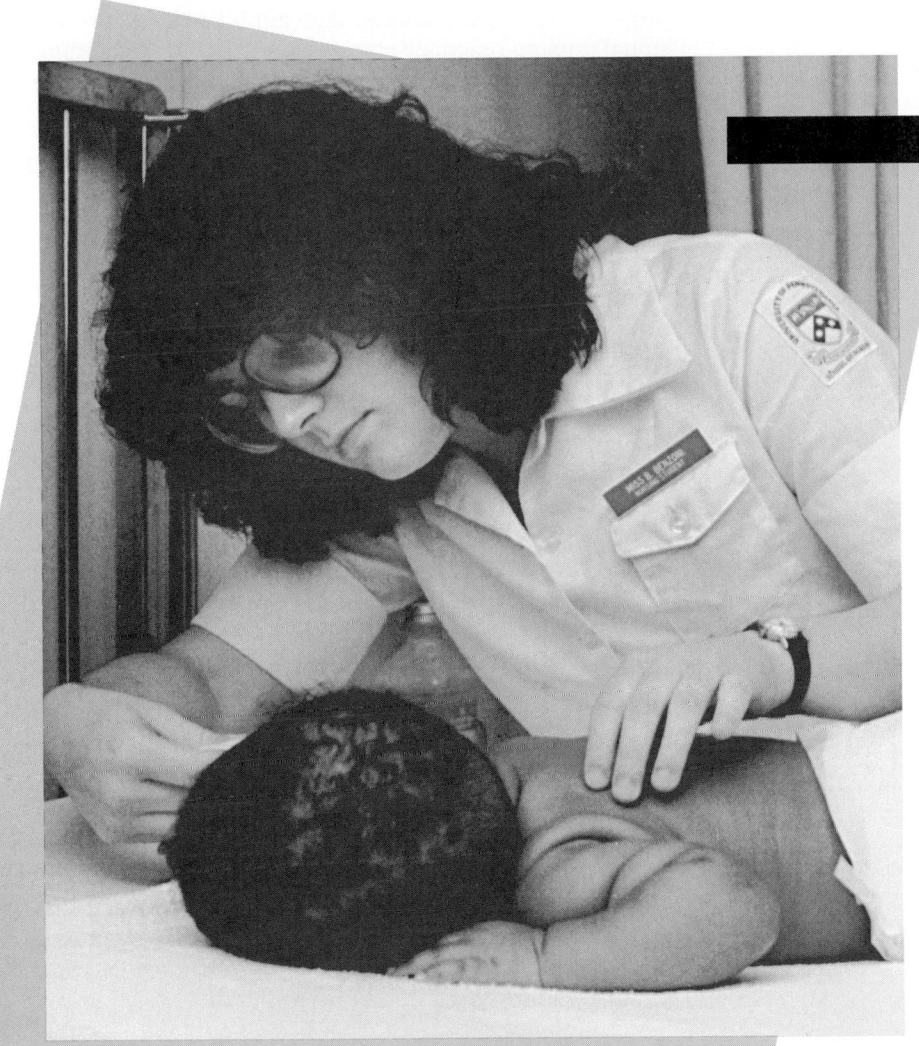

OBJECTIVES

After studying this chapter, the learner should be able to

Define key terms used in the chapter.

Describe the historical background, the definitions, and the professional status of nursing.

Identify the aims of nursing, including nursing activities necessary to promote wellness and prevent illness.

Describe the various levels of educational preparation and offerings in nursing.

Discuss the impact on nursing practice of nursing organizations, standards of nursing practice, nurse practice acts, and the nursing process.

Identify current trends and issues in nursing.

Nursing is a complex and difficult word to define because nurses do so many different things. If your class were asked to complete the sentence "Nursing is _____ ," there would be a number of different responses because each person would answer based on his or her own personal experiences and knowledge. As you progress through your nursing program, your definition of nursing will change, reflecting additional learning and understanding of what nursing is.

This chapter introduces you to nursing as a whole, including definitions of nursing and a brief history of nursing to the present time. Educational preparation, professional organizations, and guidelines for professional nursing practice serve as a base for understanding what nursing is and how it is organized. Because nursing is part of an ever-changing society, a brief summary of trends and issues is also included.

KEY TERMS

continuing education	licensure
dependent nursing actions	nurse practice act
holistic health care	nursing
independent nursing actions	nursing education
in-service education	nursing process
interdependent nursing actions	profession
	standards

NURSING: AN EMERGING PROFESSION

Historical Background

From Early Civilization to the Twentieth Century

Nursing has never existed in isolation. From the beginning of time, the role of the nurse has been defined by the groups and social structure in which people were living. Health care—and nursing—as we know it today is influenced by what happened in the past.

In primitive cultures, humans believed that illness had supernatural causes. To help explain the unknown, the theory of animism described that "everything in nature is alive with invisible forces and endowed with powers: good spirits bring blessings; evil spirits bring sickness and death" (Dolan, 1978). During this time, the roles of the physician and nurse were separate and distinct. The medicine man was a male who "treated" disease through chanting, fear, or, in desperation, opening the skull to let out evil spirits. The nurse was usually the mother who cared for her family when they were sick by providing physical care and herbal remedies. This nurturing or caring role of the nurse has remained constant to the present.

As tribes became civilizations, temples became the centers of medical care because of the belief that illness was caused by sin and the gods' displeasure (*disease* = dis-ease). Priests were highly regarded as physicians, but neither human life nor women were valued by society; the nurse was seen as a slave, carrying out menial tasks based on the orders of the priest-physician. In contrast, during the same time period, the ancient Hebrews proposed rules for ethical human relationships, mental health, and disease control through the Ten Commandments and the Mosaic Health Code. Nurses cared for the sick in the home and the community and also practiced as nurse-midwives (Dolan, 1978).

With the beginning of Christianity, nursing began to have a formal and more clearly defined role. Led by the belief that love and caring for others were important, the first organized visiting of the sick was done by women called *deaconesses,* while male religious orders gave nursing care and buried the dead. During the Crusades, both male and female nursing orders were founded. Hospitals were built to care for the enormous numbers of pilgrims needing health care, and nursing became a respected vocation. The early Middle Ages ended in chaos, but nursing had developed purpose, direction, and leadership.

With the beginning of the 16th century, society changed from one with a religious orientation to one that emphasized warfare, exploration, and expansion of knowledge. Many monasteries and convents closed, leading to a tremendous shortage of people to care for the sick. To meet this need, women who committed a crime were recruited into nursing in lieu of serving jail sentences. From this background evolved a long-held view of society that nurses were disreputable and that respectable women did not work outside the home. Along with a poor reputation, nurses received low pay and worked long hours in bad conditions.

From the middle of the 18th century to the 19th century, social reforms were changing the roles of nurses and of women in general. It was during this time that nursing, based on many of the beliefs and examples of Florence Nightingale, began as we know it today.

Florence Nightingale was born in 1820 to a wealthy family. She grew up in England and was well educated and traveled extensively. Despite strong opposition from her family, Miss Nightingale received nurse's training at the age of 31. The outbreak of the Crimean War and a request by the British to organize nursing care for a military hospital in Turkey gave Miss Nightingale an opportunity for achievement (Kalish and Kalish, 1986). Because she was able to overcome enormous difficulties successfully, Miss Nightingale challenged prejudices against women and elevated the status of all nurses. After the war, she returned to England, where she established a training school for nurses and wrote books about health care and nursing education.

The contributions of Florence Nightingale include
- Recognizing that nutrition is an important part of nursing care
- Instituting occupational and recreational therapy for the sick
- Identifying personal needs of the patient and the role of the nurse in meeting those needs
- Establishing standards for hospital management
- Establishing a respected occupation for women
- Establishing nursing education
- Recognizing the two components of nursing: health and illness

- Believing that nursing is separate and distinct from medicine
- Stressing the need for continuing education for nurses (Dolan, 1978)

Florence Nightingale elevated the status of nursing to a respected occupation, improved the quality of nursing care, and founded modern nursing education.

Nursing in North America

The work of Florence Nightingale and the care provided for battle casualties during the Civil War focused attention on the need for educated nurses in both Canada and the United States. Schools of nursing were founded in connection with hospitals, but although these schools were established on the works of Nightingale, the training they provided was based more on apprenticeship than on educational programs. Hospitals saw an economic advantage in having their own school, and most hospital schools were organized to provide more easily controlled and less expensive staff for the hospital. This resulted in the loss of clear guidelines separating nursing service and nursing education. As students and as graduates, female nurses were under the control of male hospital administrators and physicians. The lack of educational standards, the male dominance of health care, and the pervading Victorian belief that women were dependent on men combined to contribute to several decades of slow progress toward professionalism in nursing (Kalish and Kalish, 1986).

World War II had an enormous impact on nursing. For the first time, large numbers of women worked outside the home. In the process, they also became more independent and assertive. These changes in women and in society resulted in increased emphasis on education. The war itself had identified a need for more nurses and had resulted in a knowledge explosion in medicine and technology, which broadened the role of nurses. Following World War II, efforts were directed at upgrading nursing education. Schools of nursing were based on educational objectives and were increasingly developed in university and college settings, leading to degrees in nursing for both men and women.

Nursing broadened in all areas, including (1) practice in both hospital and community settings, (2) the development of a body of knowledge specific to nursing in nursing models and theories, and (3) the conduct and publication of nursing research. The increased emphasis and awareness of the importance of nursing knowledge and practice led to the growth of nursing as a profession in today's world.

Definitions of Nursing

The word *nurse* originated from the Latin word *nutrix,* which means to nourish. Ellis and Hartley (1984) include this timeless word origin when they describe the most basic definition of a nurse as "a person who nourishes, fosters, and protects, a person prepared to take care of the sick, injured, and aged." This definition is probably one that most people would agree with, but it does not include the expanding roles and functions taking place in nursing today. Although this section gives several definitions, Chapter 4 gives more information about nursing as defined in specific nursing theories. The following definitions of **nursing** have widespread acceptance.

International Council of Nurses (ICN). This definition was written by Virginia Henderson and adopted by the ICN in 1972.

> The unique function of the nurse is to assist the individual, sick or well, in the performance of those activities contributing to health or its recovery (or to peaceful death) that he would perform unaided if he had the necessary strength, will, or knowledge. And to do this in such a way as to help him gain independence as rapidly as possible.

American Nurses' Association (ANA). In 1965, the ANA Committee on Education issued a position paper broadly defining nursing as an independent profession. This statement is

> Nursing is a helping profession and, as such, provides services which contribute to the health and well-being of people. Nursing is a vital consequence to the individual receiving services; it fills needs which cannot be met by the person, by the family, or by other persons in the community.
>
> The essential components of professional nursing are care, cure, and coordination. The care aspect is more than 'to take care of', it is 'caring for' and 'caring about' as well. It is dealing with human beings under stress, frequently over long periods of time. It is providing comfort and support in time of anxiety, loneliness, and helplessness. It is listening, evaluating, and intervening appropriately.
>
> The promotion of health and healing is the

Florence Nightingale, initiator of major reforms in health care and nursing training in England

Clara Barton, founder of the American Red Cross in 1882

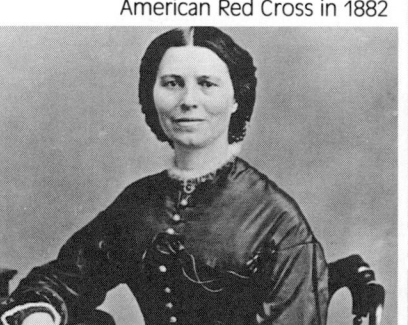

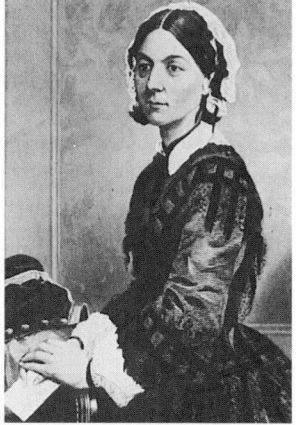

FIGURE 1-1
Images of nurses spanning more than 100 years of service. (Photos courtesy of The Center for the Study of the History of Nursing, University of Pennsylvania)

Vassar training camp classroom, 1918
Vassar training camp faculty, 1918

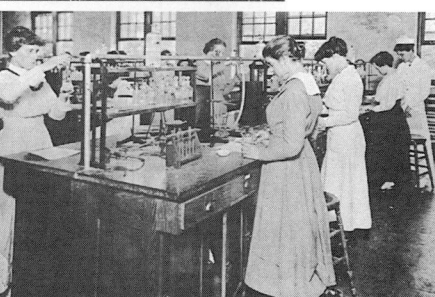

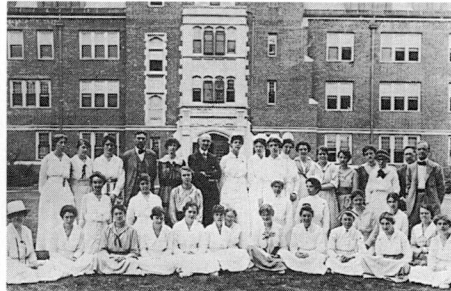

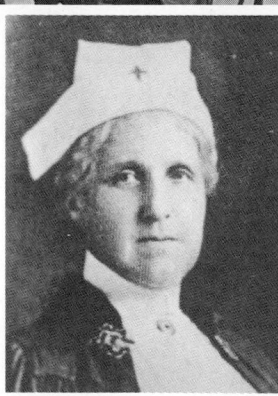

Jane Delano, an Army nurse, instrumental in the organization of the Red Cross Nursing Service in the early 1900 s

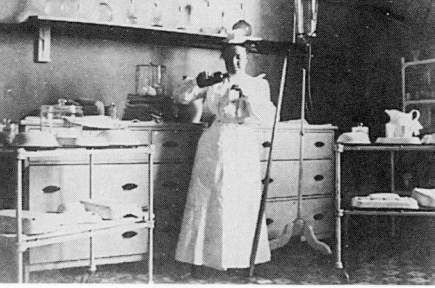

Philadelphia General Hospital nurse, late 1800 s

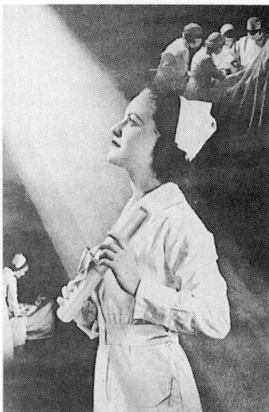

Post-WWII nursing school poster

The Art of Nursing

Nursing is caring: Nurses give care; they also demonstrate nonpossessive caring about and for others.

Nursing is sharing: Nurses share themselves with each other, with other members of the health-care team, and with clients.

Nursing is laughing: Nurses who laugh with others know that humor is a part of feelings of comfort and belonging.

Nursing is crying: Nurses accept tears from others and themselves as a normal response to both happiness and sadness.

Nursing is touching: Nurses touch to comfort, massage, give care—touching says "I care" and "I know what to do to help you."

Nursing is helping: Nurses help others in two broad areas: understanding and taking action.

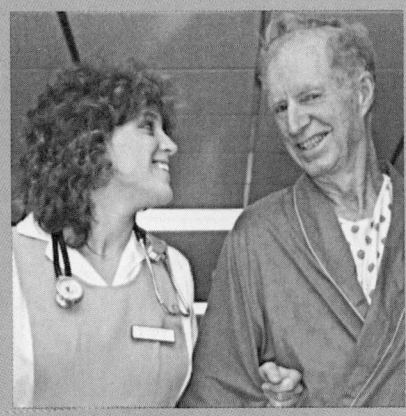

Nursing is believing in others: Nurses believe that others have the desire and ability to reach their individual potential in all areas of human functioning.

Nursing is trusting: Nurses demonstrate trust in others by accepting people as they are and by always expecting positive results from actions.

Nursing is believing in self: Nurses believe they have the knowledge and ability to

help others maintain wellness.

Nursing is learning: Nurses learn new or expanded knowledge and skills throughout their career.

Nursing is respecting: Nurses demonstrate respect for others through unconditional acceptance, ensuring privacy, and individualizing care.

Nursing is listening: Nurses listen to what is said verbally but also are equally attentive to what is not said.

Nursing is doing: Nurses carry out assessments and interventions with knowledge and skill to give safe, comprehensive client care.

Nursing is feeling: Nurses share in the sorrows, joys, frustrations, and satisfactions of others.

Nursing is accepting: Nurses must first accept themselves before they can accept others.

---

cure aspect of professional nursing. It is assisting patients to understand their health problems and helping them to cope. It is the administration of medication and treatments. And it is the use of clinical nursing judgment in determining, on the basis of patients' reactions, whether the plan for care needs to be maintained or changed. It is knowing when and how to use existing and potential resources to help patients toward recovery and adjustment by mobilizing their own resources.

Professional Nursing Practice is this and more. It is sharing responsibility for the health and welfare of all those in the community, and participating in programs designed to prevent illness and maintain health. It is coordinating and synchronizing medical and other professional and technical services as these affect patients. It is supervising, teaching, and directing all those who give nursing care.

These concepts and beliefs were expanded by the ANA in 1980 when the Congress for Nursing Practice defined nursing practice as "the diagnosis and treatment of human responses to actual or potential health problems" (American Nurses' Association, 1980, p 9). This definition further identifies the characteristics of nursing as an independent profession, legitimizing the assessment and identification of human responses, the use of nursing knowledge to understand the responses, and the application and evaluation of nursing actions taken to meet needs for potential or actual health problems.

Canadian Nurses Association (CNA). The CNA makes the following philosophical statement about nursing:

The nursing professional exists in response to a need of society and holds ideals related to man's health throughout his life span. Nurses direct their energies toward the promotion, maintenance, and restoration of health, the prevention of illness, the alleviation of suffering and the ensuring of a peaceful death when life can no longer be sustained. Nurses value a holistic view of man and regard him as a biopsychosocial being who has the capacity to set goals and make decisions and who has the right and responsibility to make informed choices congruent with his own beliefs and values. Nursing, a dynamic and supportive profession guided by its code of ethics, is rooted in caring, a concept evident throughout its four fields of activity: practice, education, administration, and research.

In all of the definitions, the central focus is the person receiving care (patient, client) and includes the physical, emotional, social, and spiritual dimensions of that person. Nursing is no longer considered to be primarily concerned with illness; the concepts and definitions have expanded to include the prevention of illness and the maintenance of health for individuals, families, and communities.

Nursing: A Discipline or a Profession?

As definitions of nursing have expanded to better describe the roles and functions of nurses, increased attention has been focused on the question of nursing as a **profession**. Many nursing leaders believe that nursing is establishing itself as a profession rather than being an occupation or a discipline.

Nursing is certainly an occupation. It is also a discipline, defined as a branch of knowledge. However, acceptance as a profession allows nursing to have more authority and self-governing power (autonomy). There are, as yet, no clear-cut answers to "is nursing a profession?" But as nursing continues to develop in its three primary areas (education, practice, research), it more and more meets the criteria defining a profession.

The seven basic elements, or criteria, defining a profession are that a profession must

- Have a strong scientific base
- Have a strong service orientation
- Be the recognized authority by the professional group with community sanction
- Have a code of ethics
- Have a professional organization that sets standards
- Conduct ongoing research
- Have autonomy
(DeYoung, 1985)

These criteria are focused on nursing by Grippando (1986) as follows:

- Professional status is achieved when an occupation involves a unique practice which carries great individual responsibility and is based upon theoretical knowledge.
- The privilege to practice is granted only after the individual has completed a standardized program of highly specialized education and has demonstrated an ability to meet the standards of practice.
- The body of specialized knowledge is continually developed and evaluated through research.
- The members are self-organized and collectively assume the responsibility of establishing standards for education and practice. They continually evaluate the quality of services provided in order to protect the individual members and the public.

Based on these descriptions, nursing is indeed an emerging profession. Its practice involves specialized skills and application of knowledge, based on an education that includes both theoretical and clinical components. Nursing upholds standards set forth by professional organizations and follows a code of ethics. Nursing carries out research, defining the body of knowledge specific to its own practice. Nurses increasingly assume control and authority to direct and give care to clients, using the nursing process to identify the aspects of care that are unique to nursing.

Aims of Nursing

As previously discussed, there are many definitions of nursing. From these definitions, four main areas of nursing can be identified. These areas describe the broad major aims of nursing:

- Promoting wellness
- Preventing illness
- Restoring health
- Facilitating coping

To meet these goals, the nurse uses knowledge and skills in a variety of traditional and expanding nursing roles. These roles are defined in Tables 1-1 and 1-2, and further described in Unit V. The activities carried out by the nurse take place in many different settings, ranging from the client's home to community agencies, and include the client and his or her family. Health-care settings and specific nursing activities are discussed in Chapter 3.

Promoting Wellness. Activities carried out to promote wellness involve public and individual education, legislation, and direct contact with clients. These activities are aimed at improving health by identifying factors that would put the individual at risk for becoming sick or injured, and in teaching to maintain or improve optimal function. Included here is only a partial list of the many wellness-focused areas in which nursing is involved.

- Encouraging and providing periodic physical examinations and screenings for such disease processes as high blood pressure, diabetes, and cancer
- Conducting community health education through health fairs and mental health programs
- Providing health services and education in nursing homes, university student health services, and public school nursing
- Promoting environmental and occupational safety
- Supporting legislation aimed at maintaining health; for example, the child safety seat program

Preventing Illness. The objectives of illness-prevention activities are to reduce the risk of illness, to promote good health habits, and to maintain the individual's optimal functioning. Health promotion is carried out by organizations and institutions as well as by nurses. Nurses

T A B L E   1-1
Roles and Functions of Nurses

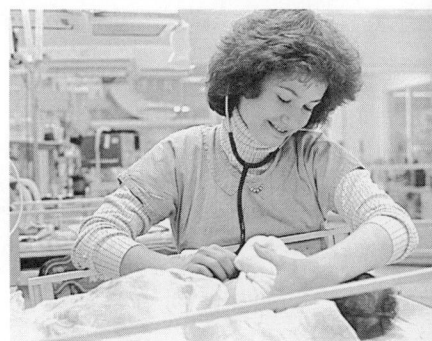

Role	Function
Caregiver	The provision of care to clients based on knowledge and skill and with consideration for physical, emotional, intellectual, sociocultural, and spiritual needs. As caregiver, the nurse integrates all of the other roles and uses the nursing process to promote wellness, prevent illness, maintain health, and facilitate coping.
Communicator	The use of effective interpersonal and therapeutic communication skills to establish and maintain helping relationships with clients of all ages in a wide variety of health-care settings
Teacher	The use of communication and interpersonal skills to meet learning needs of clients and their families. The nursing process is used to develop and carry out individualized teaching plans.
Counselor	Effective use of communication skills enables the nurse to provide information, make appropriate referrals, and facilitate client's problem-solving and decision-making abilities.
Leader	The assertive, self-confident practice of nursing necessary for care of clients, functioning in groups, and effecting change
Researcher	At various levels, nurses conduct or take part in research to improve client care.
Advocate	The protection of human and legal rights based on the belief that clients have the right to make their own decisions about health and life

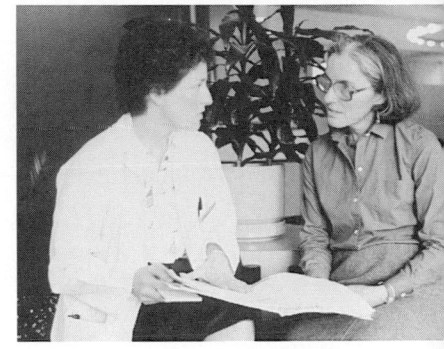

T A B L E   1-2
Expanded Career Roles and Functions of Nurses

Title	Description
Clinical nurse specialist (Examples are enterostomal therapist, geriatrics, infection control, medical–surgical, maternal–child, oncology, quality assurance, nursing process)	A nurse with an advanced degree, education, or experience who is considered to be an expert in a specialized area of nursing; carries out direct client care, consultation, teaching clients, families, and staff, and conducting research
Nurse practitioner	A nurse with an advanced degree, certified for a special area or age of client care; works in a variety of health-care settings or in independent practice to make health assessments and deliver primary care
Nurse anesthetist	A nurse who completes a course of study in an anesthesia school; carries out preoperative visits and assessments, administers and monitors anesthesia during surgery, and evaluates postoperative status of clients
Nurse midwife	A nurse who completes a program in midwifery; provides prenatal and postnatal care and delivers babies to women with uncomplicated pregnancies
Nurse educator	A nurse, usually with an advanced degree, who teaches in educational or clinical settings; teaches theoretical knowledge and clinical skills; conducts research
Nurse administrator	A nurse who functions at various levels of management in health-care settings; responsible for the management and administration of resources and personnel involved in giving client care
Nurse researcher	A nurse with an advanced degree who conducts research relevant to the definition and improvement of nursing practice and education

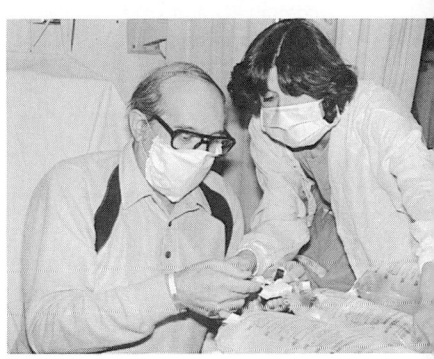

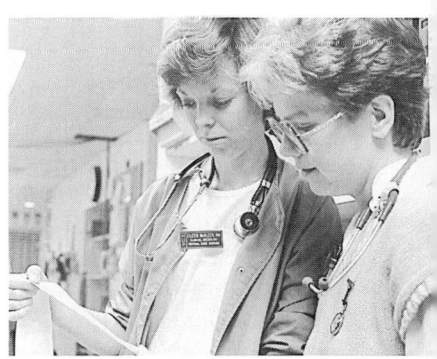

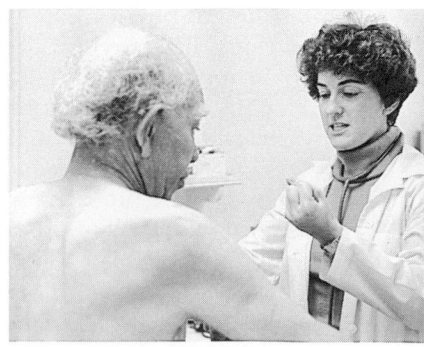

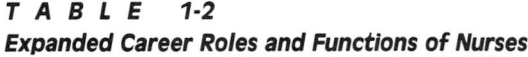

Photos by Gates Rhodes, courtesy of the
School of Nursing, University of Pennsylvania

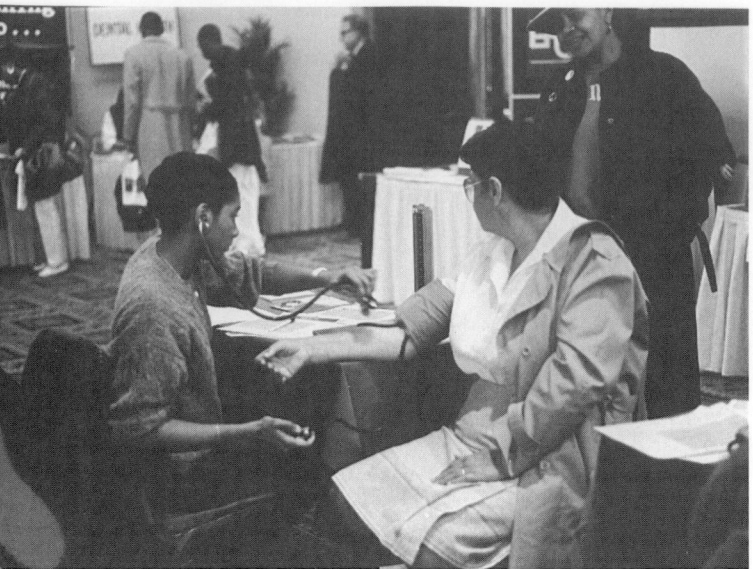

F I G U R E   1-2
Health fairs provide health information and screening tests to the community and are a popular and successful activity to promote wellness. (Photo by Nevin Kishbaugh, courtesy of the Office of Public Information, University of Pennsylvania Medical Center)

primarily promote health by teaching and by personal example. Some such activities are
- Hospital educational programs in areas such as prenatal care for pregnant women, "stop smoking" programs, and stress-reduction seminars
- Community programs and resources that encourage healthy life-styles, including aerobic exercise classes, swimnastics, and physical fitness programs
- Literature and television information on diet, exercise, and the importance of good health habits

Restoring Health.   Activities involving restoring of health encompass those most traditionally considered to be the nurse's responsibility and probably are an area in which the majority of practicing nurses are employed. This area focuses on the individual with an illness but ranges from early detection of a disease to rehabilitation and teaching during recovery. Activities included are
- Direct care of the person who is ill, by such measures as physical care, administration of medications, and carrying out procedures and treatments
- Performing diagnostic measurements and examinations (taking blood pressures, measuring blood sugars) that detect an illness
- Referring questions and abnormal findings to other health-care providers
- Planning, teaching, and carrying out rehabilitation for illnesses such as heart attacks, arthritis, and strokes

- Working in mental health and chemical-dependency programs

Facilitating Coping.   Although the major focus of health care is promoting, maintaining, or restoring health, these goals cannot always be met. Nurses also facilitate client and family coping with altered function and death. Altered function results in a decrease in an individual's ability to carry out activities of daily living and expected roles. Nurses can facilitate an optimal level of function through understanding and acceptance of the individual and family; maximizing strengths and potentials; teaching; and knowledge and referral to community support systems. Nurses provide care to both patients and families during the terminal illness, and they do so in hospitals, long-term nursing facilities, and homes. Nurses are also becoming more active in hospice programs, which are developed to assist individuals and their families in preparing for death and in living as comfortably as possible until death occurs.

EDUCATIONAL PREPARATION FOR NURSING PRACTICE

Levels of Education

The educational preparation for nursing practice currently includes several different methods. The type of preparation varies between states in the United States and provinces in Canada. Students may choose to enter a practical nursing program and be licensed as a licensed practical (or vocational) nurse (LPN, LVN), or they may enter a diploma, an associate degree, or a baccalaureate program to be licensed as a registered nurse (RN). State laws in the United States and some provincial laws in Canada recognize both the LPN and RN as having the proper credentials to practice nursing. Graduate programs are also available in nursing, providing master's and doctoral degrees.

One of the major issues in nursing today involves **nursing education**. The multiple educational systems are confusing to institutions employing nurses, to consumers of health-care services, and to nurses themselves. Nursing organizations are working very hard to answer such questions as "what is technical nursing" and "what is professional nursing," as well as "should graduates of all programs take the same kind of licensing examination and have the same title?" These questions should be resolved during your nursing career.

This section discusses education for LPNs and RNs, as well as graduate nursing education, continuing education for nurses, and in-service education.

Practical/Vocational Nursing Education

Practical nursing was established to provide graduates who give bedside nursing care to clients. Schools for practical nursing programs are located in such varied settings as high schools, technical or vocational schools, community colleges, or independent agencies. Most programs are one year in length and are made up of one-third classroom and two-thirds clinical laboratory hours. Upon completion of the program, graduates are eligible to take the National Council Licensure Examination (NCLEX-PN) for licensure as practical nursing. In Canada, some provinces offer a similar program for practitioners called Registered Nursing Assistants (RNA).

Licensed practical nurses work under the direction of a physician or registered nurse to give direct care to clients, focusing on meeting health-care needs in hospitals, nursing homes, and home health agencies.

Registered Nursing Education

There are three primary types of educational programs leading to **licensure** as a registered nurse. In the United States there are diploma, associate degree, and baccalaureate programs; Canada has two-year community college, three-year hospital-based diploma, and university baccalaureate programs. Graduates of all types of programs take the same registered nurse licensing examination. In the United States, graduates take the NCLEX-RN examination, and graduates of Canadian schools take the Canadian Nurses' Association Testing Service (CNATS) examination. Although both are national examinations, they are administered by, and the nurse is licensed in, each state or province. It is not legal to practice nursing unless one has a license verifying completion of an accredited (by the state or province) program in nursing and has passed the licensing examination. Nurses gain legal rights to practice nursing in another state or province by applying to that state's or province's board of nursing and receiving reciprocal licensure.

Diploma in Nursing

Most nurses practicing in the United States today received their basic nursing education in three-year, hospital-based diploma schools of nursing (Ellis and Hartley, 1988). The first schools of nursing established to educate nurses were diploma programs, and until the 1960s they were the major source of graduates. In recent years, as nursing organizations began to take a stand on the need for education for nursing in institutions of higher education, there has been a decrease in the number of diploma programs.

Graduates of today's diploma programs have a sound foundation of biologic and social sciences. There is a strong emphasis on clinical experience in direct patient care. Graduates work in acute, long-term, and ambulatory health-care facilities (Ellis and Hartley, 1988).

Associate Degree in Nursing

Associate degree nursing education is based on a research project carried out by Dr. Mildred Montag from 1952 to 1957. At that time there was a shortage of nurses, and the project was an attempt to meet the needs of society by preparing nurses in less time then was required in diploma programs. The emphasis of this type of program was education instead of service (Grippando, 1986).

Most associate degree programs are in community junior colleges and universities. These two-year educational programs attract more men, more minorities, and more nontraditional students then do the other types of programs.

Associate degree education prepares nurses to give care to clients in structured settings (acute and long-term facilities). Graduates of these programs are technically skilled and well prepared to carry out the nursing roles and functions previously discussed. Competencies of the associate degree nurse on entry into practice, as defined by the National League for Nursing, are found on page 12.

Baccalaureate in Nursing

The first baccalaureate nursing programs were established in the United States and Canada in the early 1900s. However, the number of programs and the number of enrolling students did not increase markedly until the 1960s. (Most graduates are granted a bachelor of science in nursing [BSN] degree and will be referred to by that degree in this section).

This increase is the result of recommendations made by the American Nurses' Association, the National League for Nursing, and the Canadian Nurses' Association that the entry level for professional practice be at the baccalaureate level. Although nurses with a BSN practice in a wide variety of settings, the four-year degree is required for many administrative and supervisory positions, as well as in community health positions.

In BSN programs, the major in nursing is built on a general education base with concentration on nursing at the upper level. Students acquire knowledge of theory and practice related to nursing and other disciplines, provide nursing care to individuals and groups, work with members of the health-care team, understand research, and have a foundation for graduate study (Grippando, 1986). The box on page 12 describes the characteristics of the graduate of the baccalaureate program in nursing as defined by the National League for Nursing.

Graduate Education in Nursing

The two levels of graduate education in nursing are the master's and doctoral degrees. A master's degree in nursing prepares the graduate to function in educational settings, in managerial roles, and as clinical specialists. Nurses with doctoral degrees meet requirements for academic advancement or tenure and also are prepared to

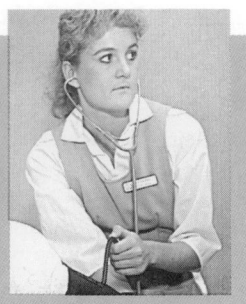

Competencies of the Associate Degree Nurse on Entry into Practice

Assumptions Basic to the Scope of Practice

The practice of graduates of associate degree nursing programs

- Is directed toward clients who need information or support to maintain health
- Is directed toward clients who are in need of medical diagnostic evaluation and/or are experiencing acute or chronic illness
- Is directed toward client's responses to common, well-defined health problems
- Includes the formulation of a nursing diagnosis
- Consists of nursing interventions selected from established nursing protocols where probable outcomes are predictable
- Is concerned with individual clients and is given with consideration of the person's relationship within a family, group, and community
- Includes the safe performance of nursing skills that require cognitive, psychomotor, and affective capabilities
- May be in any structured care setting but primarily occurs within acute- and extended-care facilities
- Is guided directly or indirectly by a more experienced registered nurse
- Includes the direction of peers or other workers in nursing in selected aspects of care within the scope of practice of associate degree nursing
- Involves an understanding of the roles and responsibilities of self and other workers within employment setting

(Competencies of the Associate Degree Nurse on Entry into Practice. Copyright 1978 by the National League for Nursing. Pub No 23-1731)

carry out research necessary to advance nursing theory and practice.

Continuing Education

The American Nurses' Association *Standards for Continuing Education in Nursing* (1974) defines **continuing education** as ''planned learning experiences beyond a basic nursing education program. These experiences are designed to promote the development of knowledge, skills, and attitudes for the enhancement of nursing practice, thus improving health care to the public.'' (p 11)

Formal continuing education offerings in the form of courses, seminars, and workshops are offered by colleges, hospitals, voluntary agencies, and private groups. In some states, continuing education is required to maintain licensure.

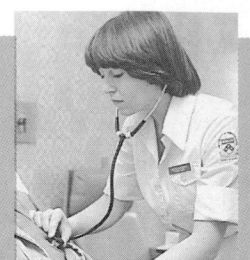

Characteristics of the Graduate of the Baccalaureate Program in Nursing

The graduate of the baccalaureate program in nursing is able to

- Provide professional nursing care, which includes health promotion and maintenance, illness, care, restoration, rehabilitation, health counseling, and education based on knowledge derived from theory and research
- Synthesize theoretical and empirical knowledge from nursing, scientific, and humanistic disciplines with practice
- Use the nursing process to provide nursing care for individuals, families, groups, and communities
- Accept responsibility and accountability for the evaluation of the effectiveness of their own nursing practice
- Enhance the quality of nursing and health practices within practice settings through the use of leadership skills and a knowledge of the political system
- Evaluate research for the applicability of its findings to nursing practice
- Participate with other health-care providers and members of the general public in promoting the health and well-being of people
- Incorporate professional values as well as ethical, moral, and legal aspects of nursing into nursing practice
- Participate in the implementation of nursing roles designed to meet emerging health needs of the general public in a changing society

(Characteristics of Baccalaureate Education in Nursing. Copyright 1987 by the National League for Nursing. Pub No 15-1758. Photo by Gates Rhodes, Courtesy of the School of Nursing, University of Pennsylvania)

In-Service Education

Many hospitals and health-care agencies provide education and training for employees of their institution or organization. This education is called **in-service** and is designed to increased the knowledge and skills of the nursing staff. Programs might include a nursing skill, new equipment use, or an update of knowledge.

PROFESSIONAL NURSING ORGANIZATIONS

When the question "is nursing a profession?" was discussed earlier, one of the elements of a profession outlined was that of "having a professional organization that sets standards." Professional nursing organizations have enormous effects on nursing as they deal with issues, set standards for both practice and education, and influence legislation regulating health care.

Although there are many nursing organizations, only the major ones are discussed here. A selected list of specialty organizations is included in the Appendix so that you can have an idea of the wide variety available to nurses today.

National Nursing Organizations

North America has three major professional organizations for nurses: the American Nurses' Association (ANA), The Canadian Nurses' Association (CNA), and the National League for Nursing (NLN).

The American Nurses' Association is the professional organization for registered nurses in the United States. Founded in the late 1800s, its members are state nurses' associations, with individual nurses belonging to the state organization. The ANA establishes standards of practice, encourages research to advance nursing practice, represents nursing through legislative actions, and supports the National Student Nurses' Association.

The Canadian Nurses' Association is the national nursing association for registered nurses in Canada. The CNA has provincial organizations, supported by local districts. The CNA supports the same goals as the ANA: to improve standards of health, to foster high standards of nursing, and to promote the professional development and welfare of nurses. The CNA has also been active in nursing education, licensing, and registration for nurses.

The National League for Nursing is an organization open to all persons in nursing, including nurses, non-nurses, and agencies. Established in 1952, its objective is to foster the development and improvement of all nursing services and nursing education. The following are the major activities of the NLN:

- Conducts one of the largest professional testing services in the country, including pre-entrance test-

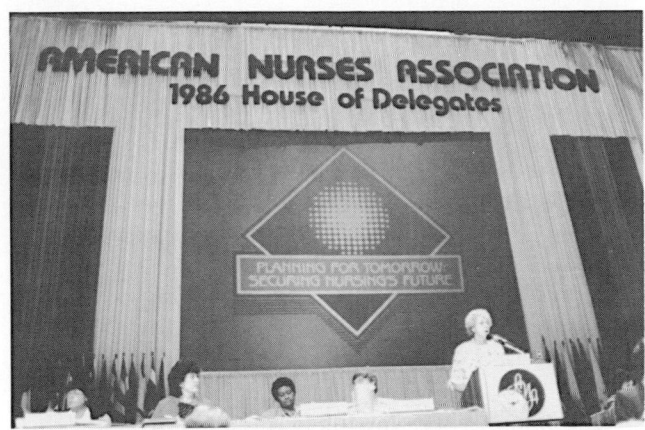

FIGURE 1-3
The American Nurses' Association establishes standards of practice, encourages nursing research, and represents nursing through legislative actions. (American Nurses' Association)

ing for potential students, achievement testing to measure student progress, and conducting state board examinations for licensure
- Sponsors continuing education workshops and seminars nationwide
- Serves as the primary source of research data about nursing education, each year conducting surveys of schools and newly registered nurses
- Provides voluntary accreditation for educational programs in nursing

The national organizations for student nurses are the *National Student Nurses' Association* (NSNA) in the United States and the *Canadian Student Nurses Association* (CSNA) in Canada. These organizations are composed of members who are students actively enrolled in nursing education programs. Programs and activities are focused on professional development and health care.

International Nursing Organization

The International Council of Nurses (ICN) was the first international organization of professional women. The organization was founded in 1899, with nurses from both the United States and Canada among the charter members. The ICN provides a way that national nursing organizations can work together, sharing a commitment to maintaining high standards of nursing service and nursing education and promoting ethics. The ICN's Code for Nurses (1973) states: "The need for nursing is universal. Inherent in nursing is respect for life, dignity and rights of man. It is unrestricted by considerations of nationality, race, creed, color, age, sex, politics, or social status."

Specialty Nursing Organizations

There are specialty nursing organizations for almost every aspect of nursing. A list of names and addresses is included in Appendix C. Students are encouraged to seek additional information on an organization of particular interest.

GUIDELINES FOR NURSING PRACTICE

As you have seen in the brief history included at the beginning of this chapter, nursing is a dynamic process, continuing to evolve and change to meet the needs of society.

The Congress for Nursing Practice (1973) stated that a profession must control its practice to guarantee the quality of its service to the public, and that "a profession that does not maintain the confidence of the public will soon cease to be a social force." Nursing controls and guarantees its practice through standards of practice, nurse practice acts and licensure, and use of the nursing process. Each of these will guide your nursing education as a student and your nursing practice after graduation.

American Nurses' Association Standards of Nursing Practice

1. The collection of data about the health status of the client/patient is systematic and continuous. The data are accessible, communicated, and recorded.
2. Nursing diagnoses are derived from health status data.
3. The plan of nursing care includes goals derived from the nursing diagnoses.
4. The plan of nursing care includes priorities and the prescribed nursing approaches or measures to achieve the goals derived from the nursing diagnoses.
5. Nursing actions provide for client/patient participation in health promotion, maintenance, and restoration.
6. The nursing actions assist the client/patient to maximize his health capabilities.
7. The client/patient's progress or lack of progress toward goal achievement is determined by the client/patient and the nurse.
8. The client/patient's progress or lack of progress toward goal achievement directs reassessment, reordering of priorities, new goal setting, and revision of the plan of nursing care.

(American Nurses' Association: Standards of Nursing Practice. Kansas City, MO, American Nurses' Association, 1973)

Standards of Nursing Practice

The Standards of Nursing Practice, written by the American Nurses' Association in 1973, define the activities of nurses that are specific and unique to nursing. **Standards** allow nurses to carry out professional roles, serving as protection for the nurse, the client, and the institution where health care is given. Each nurse is accountable for his or her own quality of practice and is responsible for the use of these standards to ensure knowledgeable, safe, and comprehensive nursing care. The standards, outlined in the accompanying boxes, apply to the practice of all registered nurses and lay the foundation for the practice of professional nursing in all settings. The Canadian Nurses Association Standards of Nursing Practice provide a parallel purpose in Canada although some provinces have opted to write their own standards.

Nurse Practice Acts and Licensure

Nurse practice acts are laws established in each state (United States) and province (Canada) to regulate the practice of nursing. They are broadly worded and vary among jurisdictions, but all of them have certain elements in common. In general, they

- Are designed to protect the public by defining the legal scope of nursing practice, excluding untrained or unlicensed persons from practicing nursing
- Create a state board of nursing or regulatory body having the authority to make and enforce rules and regulations concerning the nursing profession
- Define important terms and activities in nursing, including legal requirements and titles for registered nurses and licensed practical nurses
- Establish criteria for the education and licensure of nurses

The board of nursing for each state or province is given legal authority to administer the licensing examination to graduates of approved schools of nursing. The individual who successfully meets the requirements for licensure is then given a license to practice nursing in the state or province. The license is valid during the life of the holder and is registered (listing the license) in the state. The license and the right to practice nursing can be denied, revoked, or suspended for professional misconduct (for example, incompetence, negligence, chemical impairment, or criminal actions).

As nursing roles continue to expand, and as issues in nursing are resolved, nurse practice acts will reflect those changes. It is essential that nurses understand and keep up to date on the specific nurse practice act under which they practice.

Nursing Process

The **nursing process** is fully described in Unit IV; it is briefly included here because it is one of the major guidelines for nursing practice and also serves as a foundation for nursing care in health and illness.

The nursing process is, most simply, a method of organizing and giving nursing care. Yura and Walsh (1983) describe the nursing process as follows:

> The nursing process is the core and essence of nursing; it is central to all nursing actions; it is applicable in any setting and within any theoretical conceptual reference. It is flexible and adaptable, adjustable to a number of variables, yet sufficiently structured so as to provide a base from which all systematic nursing actions can proceed.

The five steps of the nursing process are (1) assessing, (2) diagnosing, (3) planning, (4) implementing, and (5) evaluating. By using these steps, the nurse identifies health-care needs, establishes and carries out a plan of care to meet those needs, and evaluates the effectiveness of the plan. The nursing process allows the nurse to focus on the client as an individual and to define those areas of health care that are within the domain of nursing (Carpenito, 1987).

The steps of the nursing process, briefly outlined, are as follows:

Assessing: The systematic and continuous collection, validation, and communication of client data

Diagnosing: Analysis of client data to identify client strengths and health problems that independent nursing intervention can prevent or resolve

Planning: Establishment of client goals that will prevent, reduce, or resolve the problems identified in the nursing diagnoses and determine related nursing interventions

Implementing: Carrying out the plan of care

Evaluating: Measurement of the extent to which the client has achieved the goals specified in the plan of care

Canadian Nurses' Association Standards of Nursing Practice

These four standards are necessarily interdependent and interrelated.

Standard I. Nursing practice requires that a conceptual model(s) for nursing be the basis for that practice.

Nurses are required to have a clear idea, conception, or understanding of (1) goal, (2) client, (3) role of the nurse, (4) source of difficulty, (5) focus and modes of intervention, and (6) consequences.

Standard II. Nursing practice requires the effective use of the nursing process.

Nurses are required in any practice setting to do the following: (1) collection of data, (2) analysis of data, (3) planning of the intervention, (4) implementation of the intervention, and (5) evaluation.

Standard III. Nursing practice requires that the helping relationship be the nature of the client–nurse interaction.

Nurses are required to perform the following parts of the helping relationship: (1) initiation, (2) maintenance, and (3) termination.

Standard IV. Nursing practice requires nurses to fulfill professional responsibilities.

Nurses are expected to respect or comply with the following: (1) legislation, (2) ethics, and (3) collaboration.

(Summarized and adapted from the Canadian Nurses' Association Standards for Nursing Practice. Prepared and revised by a Task Group to Develop a Definition of Nursing Practice and Standards for Nursing Practice. Ottawa, Canadian Nurses Association, 1987)

NURSING IN TRANSITION

As you have seen, nursing is constantly changing in response to the needs and resources of society. Nursing also changes in response to those factors identified in this chapter: definitions, aims, educational levels, and expanding practice roles. Some of the issues and trends in nursing today are briefly described in this section; many are further discussed in the following chapters. Included here are changes in nurses and nursing, changes in client populations, and changes in the provision of care. These are complex trends; the information given is intended to serve only as an introduction.

Changes in Nurses and Nursing. At the present time, there is a critical shortage of nurses. In addition to lesser numbers of practicing nurses, there are fewer students entering nursing education programs. Various factors have been identified as significant to these problems, including changes in health-care needs of clients, economic conditions affecting salaries and client populations, working conditions and status, and career mobility.

Individuals entering the health-care system are more acutely ill but spend fewer days in the hospital. This has resulted in an increased demand for nurses in the hospital setting and also an increased need for nurses to care for clients in the community and home-based settings. Nurses in hospital settings work varied shifts, often believe they have little autonomy, and are not highly paid. With advanced education, experience, and expanding roles, nurses are taking advantage of career mobility to move into management, educational, and community clinical settings. Although these areas are considered to be more rewarding (in terms of autonomy, status, salary, and/or personal satisfaction), the shift from traditional hospital-based nursing care further compounds the problem of nursing shortage.

Changes in Client Populations.   One change in client population has already been addressed: the change, especially in hospital settings, to the more acutely ill. Another change that will continue to have a major impact on nursing is the increasing population of elderly adults. The population as a whole is aging, and this fact has implications for nursing care in both hospital and community settings. The elderly have more chronic illnesses and fewer financial or social support systems, and they often require long-term care. The problems and health-care needs of the elderly have become a national issue, but the day-to-day needs of the individual older adult are nursing care issues.

Changes in Provision of Care.   Three issues will be discussed here that have an impact on nursing: technological changes, the concept of holistic nursing care, and nursing actions.

One cannot visit an acute-care health setting today without being aware of the rapid advances in technology. Diagnostic procedures, surgical procedures, intensive-care units, and patient-care areas are all heavily based on "high-tech" concepts and machines. The nurse must continually update knowledge and skills to use the technology to give individualized client care. One tool that is beneficial in time management for nurses is the computerization of many formerly time-consuming activities.

(Computer applications in nursing are included throughout this text.)

The concept of **holistic health care** is a trend with great implications for nursing. No longer do nurses focus only on the disease or the technical skills needed to care for an individual client. Holistic nursing care considers all aspects of a person: the physical, psychosocial, and spiritual dimensions. Rather than focusing on illness, health care is wellness oriented, directed toward maintaining and improving health, and facilitating optimal potential.

Nursing actions, or the activities nurses carry out, are also in transition. As you saw in the discussion of nursing history, nurses were considered to have only a dependent role for a long time. With changes in nursing (brought about by role changes, advanced and specific education, nursing theory, nursing research, and nursing organizations), three categories of nursing action are now defined. These categories are

Dependent nursing actions: Those activities carried out following orders of other members of the health-care team (*e.g.*, physician, dietitian, physical therapist)

Interdependent nursing actions: Those activities that the nurse carries out in collaboration with other members of the health-care team

Independent nursing actions: Those activities performed by the nurse based on assessments, knowledge, and judgment

Although care of clients is usually a blending of all three nursing actions, nurses are more and more initiating and performing independent actions, defining the unique role of nursing in giving individualized, holistic care.

K E Y   P O I N T S

- The definition of the nursing role has changed and expanded through history in response to the needs of the social and political structure in which nursing existed.

- Nurses have always emphasized caring; this aspect of nursing has been present since early civilizations.

- From early human cultures to the 20th century, nurses were regarded in a variety of ways, ranging from respect as independent practitioners to contempt as disreputable and unacceptable members of society.

- Nursing as we know it today is based on the examples and work of Florence Nightingale, who positively influenced health-care standards, nursing education, nursing practice, and women's rights.

- Nursing education in North America has changed from service-based training schools to educational programs largely based in colleges and universities.

- Definitions of nursing's roles, functions, and professional status have been written by the International Council of Nurses, the American Nurses' Association, and the Canadian Nurses' Association. Regardless of the definition, the central focus of nursing is the client.

- Using the criteria defining a profession, nursing is an emerging profession; it is a practice that involves specialized skills and knowledge, upholds standards developed by professional organizations, develops theories and conducts research, is gaining autonomy, and uses the nursing process to give individualized nursing care.

■ The four major aims of nursing are centered around the promotion of wellness, prevention of illness, restoration of health, and facilitation of coping. Nurses carry out a variety of activities to meet these goals.

■ Education for nursing presents an issue in today's world. Basic educational programs are the LPN and the three different types of programs leading to designation as an RN. Advanced degrees in nursing include the master's and doctoral degrees. Nurses are life-long learners, continuing to gain knowledge and skills through continuing education and in-service programs.

■ Nursing organizations represent and support nurses in areas such as education, legislation, research, and practice. Major organizations are the ANA, CNA, NLN, and ICN.

■ The practice of nursing is guided and legitimized by written standards of practice, state practice acts and licensure, and use of the nursing process.

■ Nursing is in transition, reflecting changes in health-care populations, nurses, and nursing. The central focus of nursing care is the client; the nurse today carries out a wide variety of independent activities to provide holistic, wellness-centered care.

BIBLIOGRAPHY

Abu-Saad H: Nursing: A World View. St Louis, CV Mosby, 1979

Aiken L (ed): Nursing in the 1980's: Crisis, Opportunities, Challenges. American Academy of Nursing. Philadelphia, JB Lippincott, 1982

American Nurses' Association: American Nurses' Association first position on education for nursing. Am J Nurs, pp 106–111, Dec 1965

American Nurses' Association Committee on Education: A Position Paper. New York, American Nurses' Association, 1965

American Nurses' Association: Standards for Continuing Education in Nursing, p 11. Kansas City, MO, American Nurses' Association, 1974

American Nurses' Association: Nursing and Social Policy Statement. Kansas City, MO, American Nurses' Association, 1980

Canadian Nurses' Association: A Definition of Nursing Practice: Standards for Nursing Practice. Ottawa, Canadian Nurses' Association, 1980

Carnevali F: Computers in nursing. Canadian Critical Care Nursing Journal 3(4):22–26, 1986

Carpenito L: Nursing Diagnosis: Application to Clinical Practice, 2nd ed. Philadelphia, JB Lippincott, 1987

Characteristics of Baccalaureate Education in Nursing. National League for Nursing, Pub No 15-1758, 1978

Competencies of the Associate Degree Nurse on Entry into Practice. New York, National League for Nursing, Pub No 23-1731, 1978

DeYoung L: Dynamics of Nursing, 5th ed. St Louis, CV Mosby, 1985

Dolan J: Nursing in Society: A Historical Perspective. Philadelphia, WB Saunders, 1978

Ellis J, Hartley C: Nursing in Today's World: Challenges, Issues, Trends, 3rd ed. Philadelphia, JB Lippincott, 1988

Fitzpatrick M: Prologue to Professionalism. Bowie, MD, Robert J Brady, 1983

Grippando G: Nursing Perspectives and Issues, 3rd ed. Albany, NY, Delmar Publishers, 1986

Hames C, Joseph D: Basic Concepts of Helping: A Wholistic Approach. New York, Appleton-Century-Crofts, 1980

Hood G: At Issue: Titling and licensure. Am J Nurs 5:592, 1985

International Council of Nurses: 1973 Code for Nurses. Geneva, International Council of Nurses, 1973

Kalish P, Kalish B: The Advance of American Nursing, 2nd ed. Boston, Little, Brown & Co, 1986

Lee A, Sandroff R: 1984 and beyond: What's ahead for nursing. RN 1:26–29, 1984

London F: Reflections: Why choose nursing? Am J Nurs 1:114, 1985

McCann/Flynn J, Heffron P: Nursing: From Concept to Practice. Bowie, MD, Robert J Brady, 1984

Nursing is still considered "women's work." RN 6:7–75, 1984

Redman B: Issues and Concepts in Patient Education. New York, Appleton-Century-Crofts, 1981

Standards: Nursing Practice. Developed by the Congress for Nursing Practice. Kansas City, MO, American Nurses' Association, 1973

Westfall N: Standards of practice: Nursing values made visible. Journal of Nursing Quality Assurance 1:21–30, 1987

World Health Organization: Constitution of the World Health Organization. Chronicle of the World Health Organization 1, 1947

Yura H, Walsh M: The Nursing Process: Assessing, Planning, Implementing, Evaluating, 4th ed. E Norwalk, CT, Appleton-Century-Crofts, 1983

Zeidler E: Hospitals in 2005: A rearview mirror prediction. Dimens Health Serv 62(7):18–21, July–August, 1985

2 Promoting Wellness in Health and Illness

OBJECTIVES

After studying this chapter, the learner should be able to

Define key terms used in the chapter.

Define health and illness, using a variety of models.

Explain the influence of the human dimensions, basic human needs, and self-concept on health and illness status, beliefs, and practices.

Compare acute illness with chronic illness.

List the causes of disease and death.

Summarize the activities of the nurse in promoting wellness and preventing illness, incorporating risk factors, illness behaviors, and the effects of illness on the family.

Describe the levels of nursing care in promoting wellness and preventing illness.

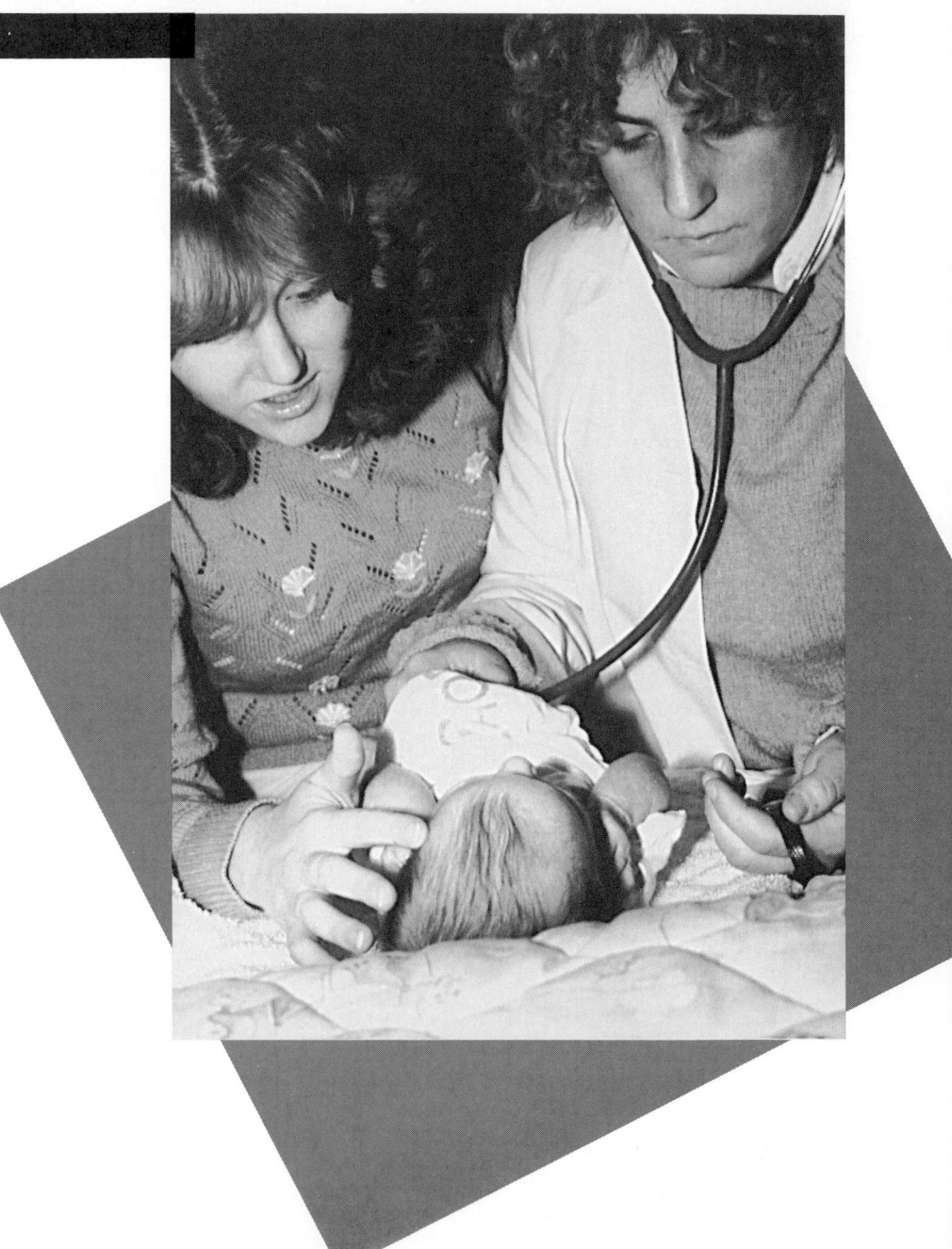

Chapter 1 focused on the broad perspectives of the nursing profession as we know it today. In contrast, this chapter discusses how the practice of nursing is influenced by both the person receiving care and the nurse giving care. To give effective and holistic care, the nurse must understand and accept each person's individual definition of wellness and reaction to illness.

DEFINING HEALTH AND ILLNESS

Health is a relative concept, defined by each person on a personal basis. Consider the following examples:

- Amy Jones, age 7, was born with one arm that ended at the elbow. She is in the second grade, plays soccer in a community children's league, and belongs to the Girl Scouts.
- Tom Bye is the 32-year-old father of three young children. As a teenager, he was involved in an automobile accident and as a result must wear a back brace. In wet weather, his right ankle is "stiff." Tom is an accountant, a member of a drama club, and takes an active role in his church.
- Martha Thyme is 76. She takes medications every day for arthritis and "heart problems." Martha spends two days a week as a volunteer in her local hospital, working in the gift shop.

Would these people be defined as healthy? Although each of them has some physical condition that could define them as ill, they are all productive members of society and would not define themselves as anything but healthy.

Wellness is not simply the absence of illness. Any definition of health must consider the dimensions of the individual, including physical, intellectual, emotional, sociocultural, spiritual, and environmental aspects and influences. Equal consideration of all these interdependent parts of the whole person is the basis for *holistic* health care (Fig 2-1).

Because health cannot be measured and its perception is highly individualized, definitions are difficult. The most widely accepted definition of health is the one given by the World Health Organization, which is "a state of complete physical, mental, and social well-being, not merely the absence of disease or infirmity." Compared to this professional definition, most of your clients will define their state of health according to their feeling state ("I feel good"), the presence or absence of symptoms ("I have a terrible pain in my stomach"), or their ability to carry out activities of daily living ("I'm just too tired to get up and clean the house") (Phipps et al, 1987).

Like health, illness is defined in many ways. Adding to the difficulty in clearly defining illness is that the terms *disease* and *illness* are often used interchangeably. *Disease* indicates a change in the structure or function of a person's body or mind; **illness** is an abnormal process

KEY TERMS

acute illness
agent–host–environment model
basic human needs
chronic illness
health
health-belief model
health–illness continuum
health-risk appraisal

high-level wellness
illness
primary preventive care
risk factor
secondary preventive care
self-concept
tertiary preventive care
wellness

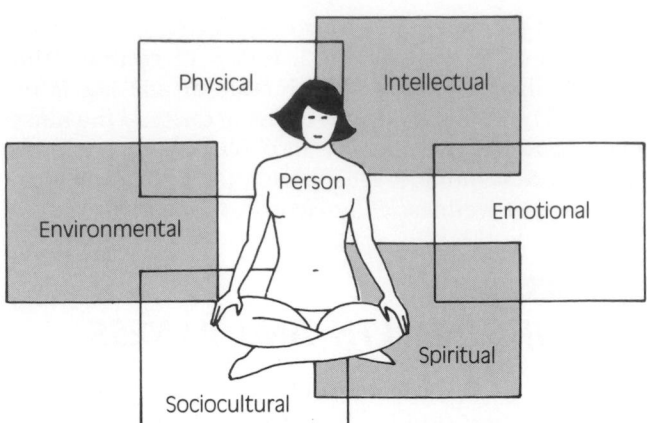

F I G U R E   2-1
The human dimensions. All of these interdependent parts make up the whole person.

in which any aspect of a person's functioning is altered as compared to a previous level. Illness, like health, is defined and described by the individual within his or her personal context. Most people describe themselves as being ill using the same standards that they do for describing themselves as healthy.

MODELS OF HEALTH AND ILLNESS

Because definitions of health and illness are not very specific, health models (examples developed to give a visual impression of something that cannot be observed directly) have been developed to help describe the concepts and relationships involved in health and illness. The models described in this chapter are the health–illness continuum, the high-level wellness model, the agent–host–environment model, and the health-belief model.

The Health–Illness Continuum.   One way to measure a person's level of wellness is to use the **health–illness continuum**. According to this model, health is a constantly changing state, with high-level wellness and death being on opposite ends of a graduated scale, or continuum (Fig. 2-2). The nurse must be aware that a client with a chronic illness may place himself at different points on the continuum at any given time depending on how well he believes himself to be functioning for his illness (McCann/Flynn and Heffron, 1984).

High-Level Wellness Model.   Halbert Dunn (1961) described his model of **high-level wellness** as functioning to one's maximum potential while maintaining balance and purposeful direction in the environment. The concept of high-level wellness can be applied to the individual, family, community, environment, and society. This

discussion focuses on Dunn's model as it applies to the individual.

Dunn differentiates "wellness" from "good health," believing that good health is a passive state wherein the person is not ill. Wellness, on the other hand, is a more complex and active state.

In this model, human beings are viewed as having five aspects:

1. Each individual functions as a total personality.
2. Each person possesses dynamic energy.
3. Each person is at peace with inner and outer worlds.
4. Each person has a relationship between energy use and self-integration (the interweaving of all the aspects of life).
5. Each person has an inner world (cells making up the organized whole) and an outer world (environment).

Combined with these five aspects are processes that help the person know who and what he is. These processes are *being* (recognizing self as separate and individual), *belonging* (being part of a whole), *becoming* (growing and developing), and *befitting* (making personal choices to befit the self for the future).

Dunn's model is holistic, allowing the nurse to care for the total person with regard for all dimensional factors affecting the person's state of being as he or she strives to reach maximum potential. For example, when planning and giving care to a young male college student paralyzed after a diving accident, the nurse would include nursing activities to meet his educational needs (intellectual dimension), incorporate friends and family (social dimension), identify and refer for counseling (emotional dimension), and ask the hospital chaplain to visit (spiritual dimension).

Agent–Host–Environment Model.   The **agent–host–environment model** of health and illness, developed by Leavell (1965), initially concentrated on community

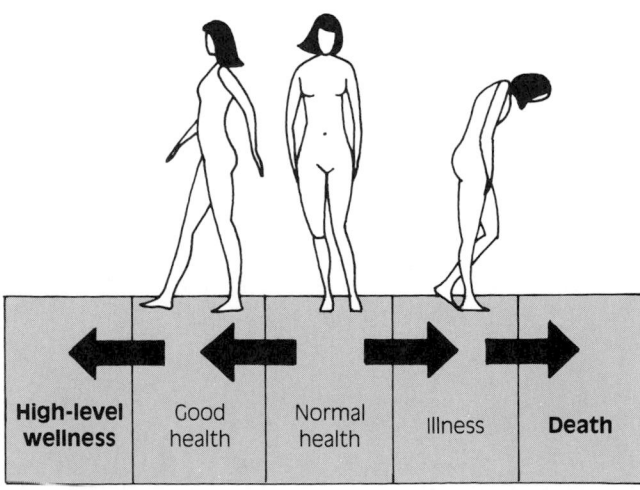

F I G U R E   2-2
The health–illness continuum.

health but is also appropriate when examining the causes of disease in an individual (the "multiple causation" of disease). The model is actually more useful in predicting illness than in promoting wellness, although recognition of risk factors resulting from interaction of agent–host–environment is important in the promotion and maintenance of health.

The three variables involved are defined as follows:

Agent: A factor that must be present or absent for an illness to occur. It may be biologic, chemical, physical, mechanical, or psychosocial.

Host: Living beings (human, animal) capable of being infected or affected by an agent. Host reaction is influenced by family history, age, and health habits.

Environment: Everything external to the host that makes illness more or less likely. Examples of environmental factors are living conditions and sound (noise) levels.

The triangle in Figure 2-3 shows that each of the agent–host–environment factors affects and is affected by the others. The factors are constantly interacting, and a combination of factors increases the possibility of illness. When the variables (agent–host–environment) are balanced, health is maintained; when they are out of balance, disease occurs. Thus, health is an ever-changing state (Clemen et al, 1981).

Health-Belief Model. In the United States and Canada, free or low-cost screenings and information are available to help in the early detection of disease and to educate about healthy living to prevent illness. Why don't more people take advantage of these services or change their life-styles? This can be answered by using the health-belief model, widely employed to describe health behavior.

The **health-belief model** (Rosenstock, 1974) is based on what people perceive, or believe, to be true about themselves in relation to health. This model is based on three components: perceived susceptibility to a disease, perceived seriousness of a disease, and perceived value of action.

Perceived susceptibility to a disease is an individual's belief that he either will or will not contract a disease. Perceived susceptibility may range from being very afraid of contracting a disease to complete denial that certain behaviors will result in illness. For example, the person who smokes cigarettes may believe he is at danger for lung cancer and may stop smoking, or he may believe smoking will pose no serious threat and will continue to smoke.

Perceived seriousness of a disease involves two factors: seriousness of the disease and its perceived effect on the person's life-style. This component is based on how much the person knows about the disease and can result in a change in health behavior. If the person who smokes believes that lung cancer could lead to physical disability or death and would affect his ability to work and care for his family, he is more likely to stop smoking. Both perceived susceptibility to a disease and perceived seriousness of a disease are part of beliefs about the threat of disease.

Perceived value of action is concerned with how effective the individual believes preventive measures will be in preventing illness. It is influenced by two factors: conviction that carrying out a recommended action will prevent or modify the disease, and the person's perception of the cost and unpleasant effects of performing the health behavior (as compared to taking no action at all). Based on this component, the person may believe that stopping smoking will prevent altered respiratory function and that the initial withdrawal symptoms can be overcome, and therefore will stop smoking.

Figure 2-4 illustrates the component health-belief perceptions and modifying factors. This model is useful in teaching individuals about health and illness. The nurse can identify the client's health beliefs and then structure goals to realistically meet client needs. Teaching and wellness-promotion activities are not effective unless the client believes them to be important and necessary.

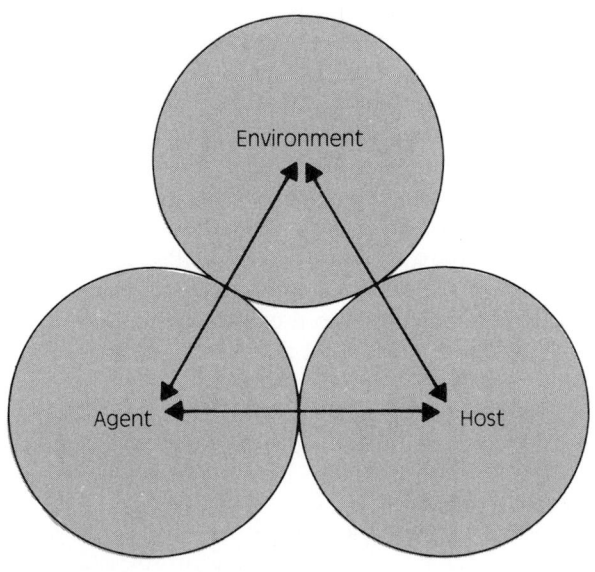

FIGURE 2-3
The agent–host–environment triangle.

FACTORS AFFECTING HEALTH AND ILLNESS

As illustrated in the models of health and illness, there are many internal (such as genetic make-up) and external (such as the environment) influences and factors

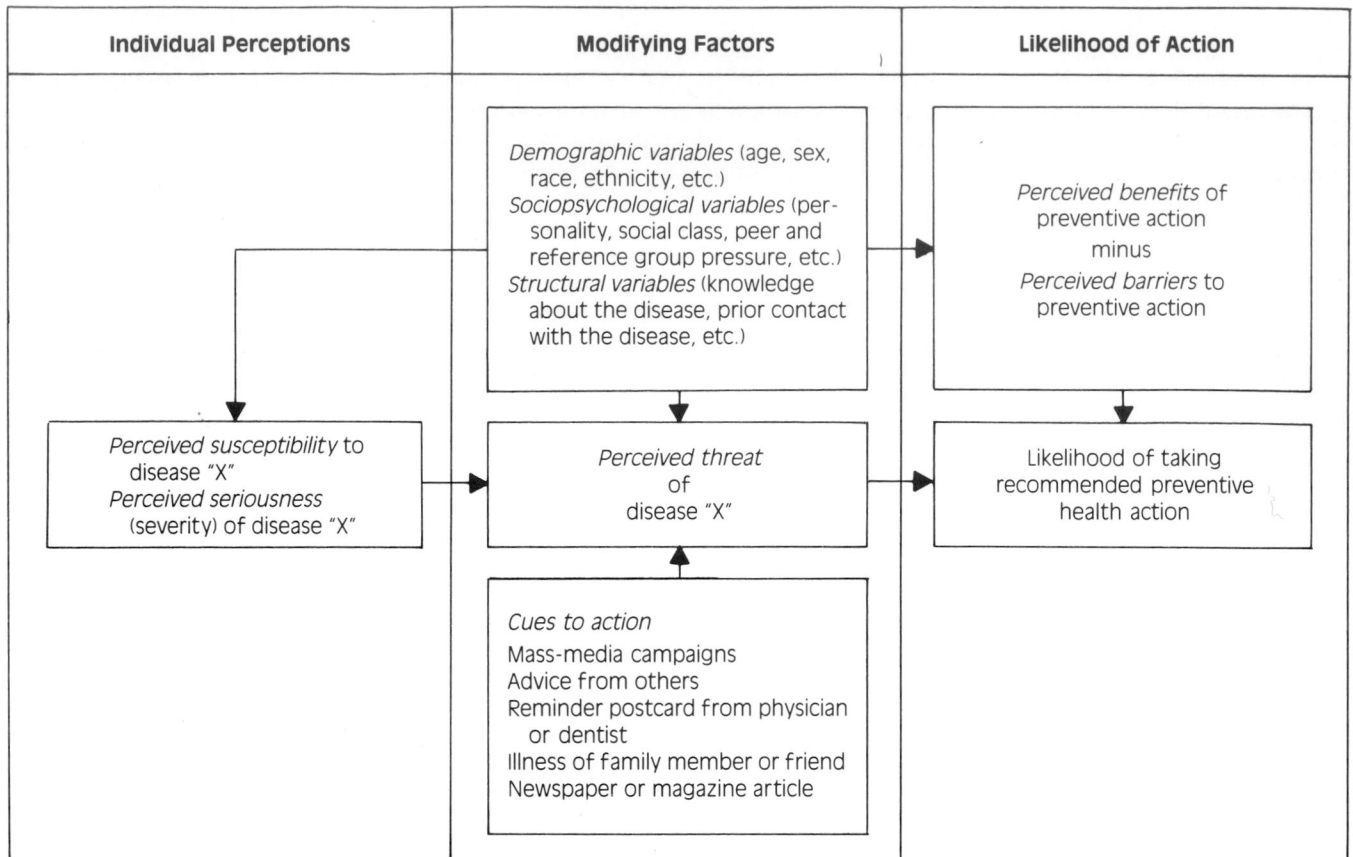

Individual Perceptions	Modifying Factors	Likelihood of Action

FIGURE 2-4

Health belief model. (Redrawn from Becker M [ed]: The Health Belief Model and Personal Health Behavior. Thorofare, NJ, Charles B Slack, 1974. Copyright © 1974, Charles B. Slack. Used with permission)

involved in a person's health status. Although an individual has varying degrees of control over some of these factors, they do affect client reactions to nursing care in both health and illness. To plan and give holistic care, the nurse must understand how these factors influence behavior in both healthy and ill clients.

The factors included in this section are those that influence health–illness status, beliefs, and practices; basic human needs; and self-concept.

Factors Influencing Health–Illness Status, Beliefs, and Practices

The factors influencing health–illness status, beliefs, and practices are described here as they relate to the human dimensions discussed earlier in this chapter (see Fig. 2-1). Many of the factors are also discussed in greater detail in other chapters of this book.

Each person is a composite of these human dimensions, and they all influence the behaviors of the person receiving health care. As you assess, plan, and give nurs-

ing care to clients, these dimensions will be an integral part of the nursing process.

Physical Dimension. Genetic make-up, age, developmental level, race, and sex are all part of an individual's physical dimension and strongly influence health status and health practices. Examples are

- The toddler just learning to walk, who is prone to fall and injure himself
- The young woman who has a family history of breast cancer and diabetes and therefore is at higher risk to develop these conditions
- The middle-aged black man who is more prone to develop high blood pressure
- The elderly person with normal aging changes that result in diminished sight and hearing

Emotional Dimension. How the mind and body interact to affect body function and to respond to body conditions also influences health. Long-term stress affects the body systems and anxiety affects health habits; conversely, calm acceptance and relaxation can actually change body responses to illness. Consider the following:

- Prior to a test, a student always has diarrhea.
- Worried about her teen-age son, a mother chain smokes.
- The adolescent who is not socially outgoing begins to experiment with drugs.
- Extremely nervous about surgery, a man experiences severe pain following his operation.
- Using relaxation techniques, a young woman reduces her pain during the delivery of her baby.
- After learning biofeedback skills, a man reduces his previously elevated blood pressure.

Intellectual Dimension.   The intellectual dimension encompasses cognitive abilities, educational background, and past experiences. These influence a client's responses to teaching about health and reactions to nursing care during illness. They also play a major role in health behaviors. Examples of situations involving this dimension include

- An elderly woman who has only a third-grade education who needs teaching about a complicated diagnostic test
- A young college student with diabetes who follows a diabetic diet but continues to drink beer and eat pizza with friends several times a week
- A young woman who quits taking her high blood pressure medication after developing unpleasant side-effects

Environmental Dimension.   The environment has many influences on health and illness. Housing, sanitation, climate, and pollution of air, food, and water are aspects of the environmental dimension. There are many examples of environmental causes of illness, a selected few of which are

- Deaths, especially among the elderly, resulting from inadequate heating and cooling
- Increased incidence of asthma and respiratory problems in large cities with smog
- Food poisoning
- Drowning

Sociocultural Dimension.   Health practices and beliefs are strongly influenced by a person's economic level, life-style, family, and culture. Low-income groups are less likely to seek medical care to prevent or treat illness; high-income groups are more prone to stress-related habits and illness. The family and the culture to which a person belongs determine patterns of living and values about health and illness that are often unalterable. All of these factors are involved in personal care, patterns of eating, life-styles, and emotional stability. For example

- The adolescent who sees nothing wrong with smoking or drinking because his parents smoke and drink

- The parents of a sick baby who do not seek medical care because they have no money
- The single parent, abused as a child, who in turn physically abuses her own small son
- The person of Asian descent who uses herbal remedies and acupuncture to treat an illness

Spiritual Dimension.   Spiritual and religious beliefs and values are important components of the way a person behaves in health and illness. It is important that the nurse accept these values and understand their importance to the individual client. Included in this dimension, for example, are

- Roman Catholics require baptism for both live births and stillborn babies.
- Orthodox and Conservative Jews may observe kosher laws, prohibiting the intake of pork or shellfish.
- Jehovah's Witnesses are opposed to blood transfusions.
- A person with a strong Fundamentalist belief may accept a serious disease as a punishment from God.

Basic Human Needs

All of us are familiar with the following occurrences:

- A drink of water "goes the wrong way" and you experience a sense of panic until you can take a breath.
- You are too busy to eat breakfast and are "starving to death" by lunchtime.
- As you start your first college class, your thoughts are filled with questions about how you will react to the new experience.
- You plan to spend a part of each weekend with your family.
- A neighbor has emergency surgery and you volunteer to care for her children.

These actions—and many more like them—are the result of needs. A need is something that is *essential* to the emotional and physiologic health and survival of humans. Because they are essential and because they are common to all people, they are called **basic human needs.** All people strive to meet basic needs; at any given time an individual's needs may be met, partially met, or unmet. A person whose needs are met may be considered to be healthy, and a person with one or more unmet needs is at increased risk for illness or health alterations in one or more of the human dimensions.

In nursing, we are concerned with the needs of the client. Abraham Maslow's (1968) hierarchy of needs is useful in understanding the relationships of basic human needs and in establishing priorities of nursing care. Maslow's framework of basic needs is based on the theory that something is a basic need if

- It's absence results in illness.
- It's presence prevents or signals health.
- Meeting an unmet need restores health.

- It, if unmet, is preferred over other satisfactions.
- It is minimally active or not active in a healthy person.
- There is a feeling of something missing when the need is unmet.
- There is a feeling of satisfaction when the need is met.

Maslow arranges basic human needs in a hierarchy, in which certain needs are more basic than others. Although all the needs are present, the individual strives to meet certain of the needs at least to a minimal level before attending to others. The five levels of basic human needs, with physiologic needs being most basic, are

- Level 1—Physiologic needs
- Level 2—Safety and security needs
- Level 3—Love and belonging needs
- Level 4—Self-esteem needs
- Level 5—Self-actualization needs

It is important to understand that needs are an integral part of each person's human dimensions, as follows:

- *Physical needs* involve all of the body's physiologic processes, including breathing, the intake and output of food and fluids, temperature, circulation, and movement.
- *Emotional needs* are concerned with the feelings of a person, such as fear, happiness, sadness, and loneliness.
- *Intellectual needs* are focused on processes such as thinking, learning, problem solving, and decision making.
- *Environmental needs* deal with our physical surroundings as they affect safety and security, and include housing, neighborhood, climate, and atmosphere.
- *Sociocultural needs* relate to the relationships and communications a person has with others, such as friends, a sense of belonging to a group or community, and being loved by others.
- *Spiritual needs* concern a person's values and beliefs as they relate to a higher being and to the performance of activities to help others.

Nursing care is often directed toward clients with unmet needs. Maslow's hierarchy provides a framework for assessing and understanding the needs of all clients and for prioritizing nursing actions. However, nurses also consider needs at all levels and include them in the plan of care. For example, in caring for a person coming to the emergency room with a heart attack, the nurse's immediate concern would be the physical needs (oxygen, pain relief), but at the same time, safety needs (following proper precautions with oxygen use, ensuring the person does not fall off the examining table) and love and belonging needs (letting the family stay with the person) are a major consideration.

The nursing procedures and actions that you will learn as you progress through your education are aimed toward meeting your clients' basic human needs (Fig. 2-5). Chapter 7 describes each level of human needs, as well as family and community influences on basic human needs.

Self-Concept

Another variable influencing health and illness is **self-concept**, or a person's mental self-image. Self-concept has both physical and emotional aspects and is a complete part of the total person.

Luft (1970) describes four parts of each person in terms of self. These are (1) the part known to both self and others; (2) those parts of self that others know, but the self isn't consciously aware of; (3) a private part known to the individual but not shared with others; and (4) parts of self not known by either others or self. Using this description, it is apparent that no one ever totally knows oneself.

A person's self-concept is the product of a variety of past experiences, interpersonal interactions, physical and cultural influences, and education. It includes a person's perceptions of his or her strengths and weaknesses. Illness can alter one's self-concept as it affects roles, independence, and relationships with family members. (Chap. 36 gives additional information about self-concept.)

PROMOTING WELLNESS AND PREVENTING ILLNESS

This section looks at the client at risk for illness and the client who becomes ill. Nurses often work with clients entering the health-care system because of an illness;

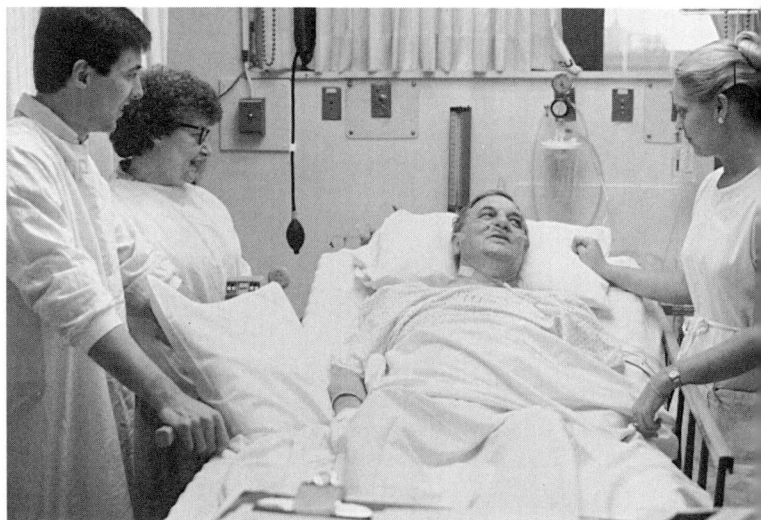

F I G U R E   2-5
Comprehensive nursing care involves using skills and knowledge effectively to meet a variety of needs. (Photo by Gates Rhodes, courtesy of the School of Nursing, University of Pennsylvania)

therefore, illness behavior and the effects of illness on the family will be discussed. Acute and chronic disease are defined to serve as a base for learning about different kinds of illnesses. Lastly, the levels of health-care activities carried out by nurses to promote health and prevent illness are included to illustrate the expanded role of nurses in today's society.

Risk Factors

A **risk factor** is a factor in a person's human dimensions that increases that person's chance for illness or injury. Risk factors can be categorized into six major areas. These areas, with examples, are listed in Table 2-1.

As with other components of health and illness, risk factors are often interrelated; as the number of risk factors increases so does the possibility of disease. For example, the overweight executive, under pressure to increase sales, smokes and drinks alcohol in excess. These factors, combined with a family history of heart disease, place this person at higher risk for illness.

A **health-risk appraisal** is an assessment of the total person. The "picture" of the individual that is made from the assessment indicates areas of risk of disease or injury, as well as areas that support health. There are a variety of forms used to perform the assessment, but all of them take a broad approach to health, focusing on life-style and health behaviors. Following the appraisal, the client can be taught to continue healthy living habits and change unhealthy life-styles.

Certain practices are supportive of health, including
• Sleeping regularly 7 to 8 hours per night
• Eating breakfast
• Eating regular meals, with few snacks
• Maintaining ideal body weight
• Using alcohol in moderation
• No smoking
• Maintaining positive mental health and self-concept
As the number of health practices increases, so does the level of wellness.

Acute and Chronic Illness

An **acute illness** has a rapid onset of symptoms but lasts only a relatively short period of time. Usually an acute illness runs its course (is self-limiting), after which the person's previous level of functioning is resumed. Most acute illnesses respond rapidly to specific medical or surgical treatment; many are self-treated by over-the-counter medications. Examples of acute illness include the common cold, the flu, appendicitis, and pneumonia.

A **chronic illness** is characterized by remissions (during which the disease is present but the individual experiences no symptoms) and exacerbations (the symptoms reappear). Additionally, the following are true of chronic illnesses:

T A B L E   2-1
Major Areas of Risk Factors

Risk Factor	Example
Age	School-age children are at higher risk for communicable diseases.
	After menopause, women are more likely to develop cardiovascular disease.
Genetic	A family history of cancer or diabetes predisposes a person to developing the disease.
Physiologic	Obesity increases the possibility of heart disease.
	Pregnancy places increased risk on both the mother and the developing fetus.
Health habits	Smoking increases the probability of lung cancer.
	Poor nutrition can lead to a variety of health problems.
Life-style	Multiple sexual relationships increase the risk of sexually transmitted diseases (gonorrhea, acquired immunodeficiency syndrome [AIDS])
	Events that increase stress (such as divorce, retirement, work-related) may precipitate accidents or illness.
Environment	Working and living environments (such as hazardous materials and poor sanitation) may contribute to disease.

- They cause irreversible pathologic changes.
- There is permanent impairment or alterations in normal functioning.
- Long-term health care is required.
- Special rehabilitation is necessary.

Some examples of chronic illnesses are diabetes, arthritis, and chronic kidney failure.

Causes of Disease and Death

The accepted causes of disease are outlined in the accompanying box. However, there are many diseases for which the cause is still unknown. Diabetes, which is one of humanity's oldest recorded diseases, is a good example of a disease for which a specific cause is still not known.

The leading causes of death in the United States, as compiled by the National Center for Health Statistics, United States Public Health Services (1983), in order of frequency, are
- Diseases of the heart and blood vessels
- Cancer
- Accidents
- Chronic respiratory diseases
- Pneumonia and influenza

Illness Behaviors

A person who becomes ill progresses through certain identifiable stages. As you read about the behaviors in each of these stages, remember how you felt the last time you had a "bad cold" and were too sick to go to school or to work. An understanding of illness behavior is necessary to give holistic nursing care to clients. These behaviors are seen more readily in the person experiencing an acute illness, but they also occur with the acute exacerbation of any chronic disease process.

Causes of Diseases

- Inherited genetic defects
- Developmental defects resulting from exposure to such factors as virus or chemicals during pregnancy
- Biologic agents or toxins
- Physical agents such as temperature, chemicals, radiation
- Generalized tissue responses to injury or irritation
- Physiologic and emotional reactions to stress
- An excessive or insufficient production of body secretions (hormones, enzymes, etc.)

Stage 1: Experience of Symptoms.   How do we define ourselves as "sick"? The first indication of an illness is usually the recognition of symptoms that are not compatible with our personal definition of health. Although pain is the most significant symptom indicating illness, other common symptoms include a rash, fever, chills, or cough.

The person then defines himself or herself as being sick, seeks validation of this experience from others, gives up normal activities, and assumes a "sick role." At this stage, most people center on their symptoms and bodily functions. Depending on individual health beliefs and practices (and on the variables discussed previously) the person may choose to (1) do nothing, (2) buy over-the-counter medications to relieve symptoms, or (3) seek health care for diagnosis and treatment. In our society, an illness becomes truly legitimate when the diagnosis and prescribed treatment are determined by a physician. When these activities take place, the person becomes a client and enters the next stage.

Stage 2: The Dependent Role.   A major part of accepting the dependent role is the decision to accept the diagnosis and follow the treatment plan. This stage of illness is complex and involves all of the human dimensions and basic human needs.

In the dependent sick role, a person conforms to the opinions of others, often requires assistance in carrying out activities of daily living, and needs emotional support through acceptance, approval, physical closeness, and protection.

It is at this stage that many clients enter the hospital. To facilitate adherence to treatment plans, the hospitalized client needs effective relationships with caregivers, knowledge about the illness, and an individualized plan of care. The client is expected, by both caregivers and family, to get well and resume normal roles.

Stage 3: Recovery and Rehabilitation.   Recovery and rehabilitation may begin in the hospital and conclude at home. As hospitals become increasingly acute-care centered, more and more clients will complete this final stage of illness behavior at a convalescent center or at home.

In this stage, the person is expected to give up the dependent role and resume normal activities and responsibilities. If the plan of care included health education, the individual may return to health at a higher level of functioning (and at a higher level on the health–illness continuum) than was present prior to the illness.

There are no specific timetables for the stages of illness behaviors. The stages may occur rapidly or slowly and are highly individualized. The nursing roles throughout the stages remain constant. In all stages, the nurse accepts the client as an individual, gives nursing care based on priority of needs, and facilitates recovery through physical care, emotional support, and health education.

Healthstyle: a self-test

All of us want good health. But many of us do not know how to be as healthy as possible. Health experts now describe *lifestyle* as one of the most important factors affecting health. In fact, it is estimated that as many as seven of the ten leading causes of death could be reduced through common-sense changes in lifestyle. That's what this brief test, developed by the Public Health Service, is all about. Its purpose is simply to tell you how well you are doing to stay healthy. The behaviors covered in the test are recommended for most Americans. Some of them may not apply to persons with certain chronic diseases or handicaps, or to pregnant women. Such persons may require special instructions from their physicians.

Cigarette smoking

If you <u>never smoke</u>, enter a score of 10 for this section and go to the next section on *Alcohol and Drugs*.

	Almost always	Sometimes	Almost never
1. I avoid smoking cigarettes.	2	1	0
2. I smoke only low tar and nicotine cigarettes *or* I smoke a pipe or cigars.	2	1	0

Smoking score: __10__

Alcohol and drugs

	Almost always	Sometimes	Almost never
1. I avoid drinking alcoholic beverages *or* I drink no more than 1 or 2 drinks a day.	(4)	1	0
2. I avoid using alcohol or other drugs (especially illegal drugs) as a way of handling stressful situations or the problems in my life.	(2)	1	0
3. I am careful not to drink alcohol when taking certain medicines (for example, medicine for sleeping, pain, colds, and allergies), or when pregnant.	(2)	1	0
4. I read and follow the label directions when using prescribed and over-the-counter drugs.	(2)	1	0

Alcohol and drugs score: __10__

Eating habits

	Almost always	Sometimes	Almost never
1. I eat a variety of foods each day, such as fruits and vegetables, whole grain breads and cereals, lean meats, dairy products, dry peas and beans, and nuts and seeds.	(4)	1	0
2. I limit the amount of fat, saturated fat, and cholesterol I eat (including fat on meats, eggs, butter, cream, shortenings, and organ meats such as liver).	2	(1)	0
3. I limit the amount of salt I eat by cooking with only small amounts, not adding salt at the table, and avoiding salty snacks.	2	(1)	0
4. I avoid eating too much sugar (especially frequent snacks of sticky candy or soft drinks).	(2)	1	0

Eating habits score: ____

Exercise/fitness

	Almost always	Sometimes	Almost never
1. I maintain a desired weight, avoiding overweight and underweight.	(3)	1	0
2. I do vigorous exercises for 15-30 minutes at least 3 times a week (examples include running, swimming, brisk walking).	(3)	1	0
3. I do exercises that enhance my muscle tone for 15-30 minutes at least 3 times a week (examples include yoga and calisthenics).	(2)	1	0
4. I use part of my leisure time participating in individual, family, or team activities that increase my level of fitness (such as gardening, bowling, golf, and baseball).	(2)	1	0

Exercise/fitness score: __10__

Stress control

	Almost always	Sometimes	Almost never
1. I have a job or do other work that I enjoy.	(2)	1	0
2. I find it easy to relax and express my feelings freely.	(2)	1	0
3. I recognize early, and prepare for, events or situations likely to be stressful for me.	2	(1)	0
4. I have close friends, relatives, or others whom I can talk to about personal matters and call on for help when needed.	(2)	1	0
5. I participate in group activities (such as church and community organizations) or hobbies that I enjoy.	(2)	1	0

Stress control score: __9__

Safety

	Almost always	Sometimes	Almost never
1. I wear a seat belt while riding in a car.	(2)	1	0
2. I avoid driving while under the influence of alcohol and other drugs.	(2)	1	0
3. I obey traffic rules and the speed limit when driving.	(2)	1	0
4. I am careful when using potentially harmful products or substances (such as household cleaners, poisons, and electrical devices).	(2)	1	0
5. I avoid smoking in bed.	(2)	1	0

Safety score: __10__

(Reprinted with permission of National Health Information Clearing House)

What your scores mean to you

Scores of 9 and 10

Excellent! Your answers show that you are aware of the importance of this area to your health. More important, you are putting your knowledge to work for you by practicing good health habits. As long as you continue to do so, this area should not pose a serious health risk. It's likely that you are setting an example for your family and friends to follow. Since you got a very high test score on this part of the test, you may want to consider other areas where your scores indicate room for improvement.

Scores of 6 to 8

Your health practices in this area are good, but there is room for improvement. Look again at the items you answered with "Sometimes" or "Almost never." What changes can you make to improve your score? Even a small change can often help you achieve better health.

Scores of 3 to 5

Your health risks are showing! Would you like more information about the risks you are facing and about why it is important for you to change these behaviors? Perhaps you need help in deciding how to successfully make the changes you desire. In either case, help is available.

Scores of 0 to 2

Obviously, you were concerned enough about your health to take the test, but your answers show that you may be taking serious and unnecessary risks with your health. Perhaps you are not aware of the risks and what to do about them. You can easily get the information and help you need to improve, if you wish. The next step is up to you.

Where do you go from here

Start by asking yourself a few frank questions: *Am I really doing all I can to be as healthy as possible? What steps can I take to feel better? Am I willing to begin now?* If you scored low in one or more sections of the test, decide what changes you want to make for improvement. You might pick that aspect of your lifestyle where you feel you have the best chance for success and tackle that one first. Once you have improved your score there, go on to other areas.

If you already have tried to change your health habits (to stop smoking or exercise regularly, for example), don't be discouraged if you haven't yet succeeded. The difficulty you have encountered may be due to influences you've never really thought about—such as advertising—or to a lack of support and encouragement. Understanding these influences is an important step toward changing the way they affect you.

There's help available. In addition to personal actions you can take on your own, there are community programs and groups (such as the YMCA or the local chapter of the American Heart Association) that can assist you and your family to make the changes you want to make. If you want to know more about these groups or about health risks, contact your local health department or the National Health Information Clearinghouse. There's a lot you can do to stay healthy or to improve your health—and there are organizations that can help you. Start a new HEALTHSTYLE today!

For assistance in locating specific information on these and other health topics: write to the National Health Information Clearinghouse.

National Health Information Clearinghouse
P.O. Box 1133
Washington, DC 20013

Effects of Illness on the Family

You will rarely give nursing care to a client who does not have some form of support system. The system is usually made up of family members but may also include, or be made up of, significant others, peers, and friends.

When an illness occurs, there are role changes for both the client and the family. Included here are several examples of family reactions to, and influences on, illness of a member. This brief introduction to the family in health and illness serves to demonstrate that consideration of the family is an integral component in nursing care.

- A chronic illness creates stress for the client and family because it may require lifelong alterations in life-style, frequent hospitalizations, economic problems, and decreased social interactions among members.
- Parents of a sick child often react with blame, over-protection, and severe anxiety.
- Family members of clients requiring intensive care often feel alone and frightened. They may also feel guilty and imagine the worst possible outcome.
- The reactions of family members to the hospital experience will vary; some want to be there all the time, whereas others avoid visiting.
- Family members need information about the client's care and health status, both in the hospital and at home. They often rely on the nurse for answers, for emotional support, and for feeling a part of the care given.

Nursing Care as Preventive Care

Levels of Preventive Care

The focus of health care today is on preventive care. Leavell (1965) describes the three levels of preventive care as primary, secondary, and tertiary.

Primary Level. Primary preventive care is directed toward health promotion and specific protection against illness. Activities at this level may focus on individuals or groups. Examples of primary-level activities are immunizations, family planning services, dental care teaching, poison-control information, and accident prevention education.

Secondary Level. Secondary preventive care focuses on health maintenance for clients experiencing health problems or on prevention of complications or disabilities. Examples of activities for this level are the nursing actions carried out for hospitalized clients (*e.g.,* skin care, giving medications, exercising arms and legs), assessing children for normal growth and development, teaching breast self-examination, and encouraging regular medical and dental screenings and care.

Tertiary Level. Tertiary preventive care is aimed at helping rehabilitate clients and restore them to a maximum level of functioning following an illness. Nursing activities on a tertiary level include teaching a diabetic client how to recognize and prevent complications or referring a woman to a support group following removal of a breast for cancer.

The Nurse as Role Model

Nurses who strive to be competent practitioners learn early that they must take care of their own health to be able to give effective nursing care to others. Not only does good personal health enable nurses to practice more efficiently, it also enables them to serve as health models for clients and their families. Nurses can help clients acquire new health behaviors by modeling the very behaviors that are important to the clients' well-being.

It is difficult for nurses to be sincerely attentive to the needs of clients when their own human needs are not being met. Since no one is perfectly healthy or "whole" all of the time, it is important that as nurses prepare for professional practice they spend time getting to know themselves. From this self-knowledge should come a commitment to pursue holistic health actively. To help you begin your self-knowledge, a self-test is given on pages 27 and 28. Take the test and compute your score. As you develop skills as a nurse and work directly with clients, you may want to use this self-test to help your clients learn a new health style.

In summary, the most effective nurse serves as a role model of healthy self-care behaviors. Therefore, in Units VII and VIII, health-care goals for the nurse are listed under the heading Nurse as Role Model before the text explores how nurses can help clients. Taking the time to see how many of these goals you can meet right now will give you some idea of how effective you will be as a role model for your clients. The results may also spur you to develop new health behaviors. The wellness promotion guides highlighted throughout the text may be useful to you as well as to your clients.

K E Y   P O I N T S

■ Health and illness are relative qualities, defined by each person. Wellness is affected by the human dimensions; consideration of the whole person is the basis for holistic health care.

■ Health and illness relationships and interactions can be described by the use of scales and models such as the health–illness continuum, the high-level wellness model, the agent–host–environment model, and the health-belief model.

■ There are many factors affecting health–illness status, beliefs, and practices, including the effects of the human dimensions, basic human needs, and self-concept.

■ Wellness levels are influenced by the physical, emotional, intellectual, environmental, sociocultural, and spiritual dimensions of the individual. These dimensions are interrelated and affect both actual and potential health–illness status and behaviors.

■ The use of Maslow's hierarchy of basic human needs is helpful in understanding the relationships and priorities of client needs. Nursing care is directed toward meeting unmet needs; this hierarchy provides a framework for giving holistic nursing care.

■ Self-concept affects and is affected by the way a person responds to health–illness levels and influences.

■ Persons at risk for illness can be identified using health-risk appraisal. Life-style practices supporting health should be encouraged by the nurse.

■ Acute illnesses have a rapid onset and are of relatively short duration; chronic illnesses result in permanent physical and life-style changes.

■ Illness behavior follows a pattern, proceeding through the stages of (1) experiencing symptoms, (2) assuming a dependent role, and (3) recovery and rehabilitation.

■ Nursing care of a client in health and illness must include the client's family. Illness results in altered expectations and reactions from family members.

■ Nurses carry out wellness promotion activities on primary, secondary, and tertiary levels.

BIBLIOGRAPHY

Birchfield M: Stages of Illness: Guidelines for Nursing Care. Bowie, MD, Brady Communication, 1985

Clemen S et al: Comprehensive Family and Community Health Nursing. St Louis, CV Mosby, 1981

DeYoung L: Dynamics of Nursing, 5th ed. St Louis, CV Mosby, 1985

Dimond M, Jones S: Chronic Illness Across the Life Span. East Norwalk, CT, Appleton-Century-Crofts, 1983

Dunn H: High-Level Wellness. Arlington, VA, RW Beathy, 1961

Eddman C, Mandle C: Health Promotion Throughout the Lifespan. St Louis, CV Mosby, 1986

Hames C, Joseph D: Basic Concepts of Helping: A Wholistic Approach. New York, Appleton-Century-Crofts, 1980

Leavell H et al: Preventive Medicine for the Doctor in His Community, 3rd ed. New York, McGraw-Hill, 1965

Lewis S, Collier I: Medical-Surgical Nursing: Assessment and Management of Clinical Problems, 2nd ed. New York, McGraw-Hill, 1987

Luft J: Group Processes: An Introduction to Group Dynamics, 2nd ed. Palo Alto, CA, National Press Books, 1970

Maslow A: Toward a Psychology of Being, 2nd ed. New York, D Van Nostrand, 1968

McCann/Flynn J, Heffron P: Nursing: From Concept to Practice. Bowie, MD, Robert J Brady, 1984

National Center for Health Statistics: US Public Health Service, Department of Health and Human Services, 1983

Phipps W et al: Medical-Surgical Nursing: Concepts and Clinical Practice. St Louis, CV Mosby, 1987

Redman B: Issues and Concepts in Patient Education. New York, Appleton-Century-Crofts, 1981

Rosenstock I: Historical origin of the health belief model. Health Education Monographs 2:334, 1974

Smitherman C: Nursing Actions for Health Promotion. Philadelphia, FA Davis, 1981

Stickney S, Gardner E: Companions in suffering, Am J Nurs 12:1491–1493, 1984

Suchman E: Stages of illness and medical care. Journal of Health and Human Behavior 6:114, 1965

Wardell S: Acute Intervention: Nursing Process Throughout the Lifespan. Reston, VA, Reston Publishing, 1979

The Health-Care System

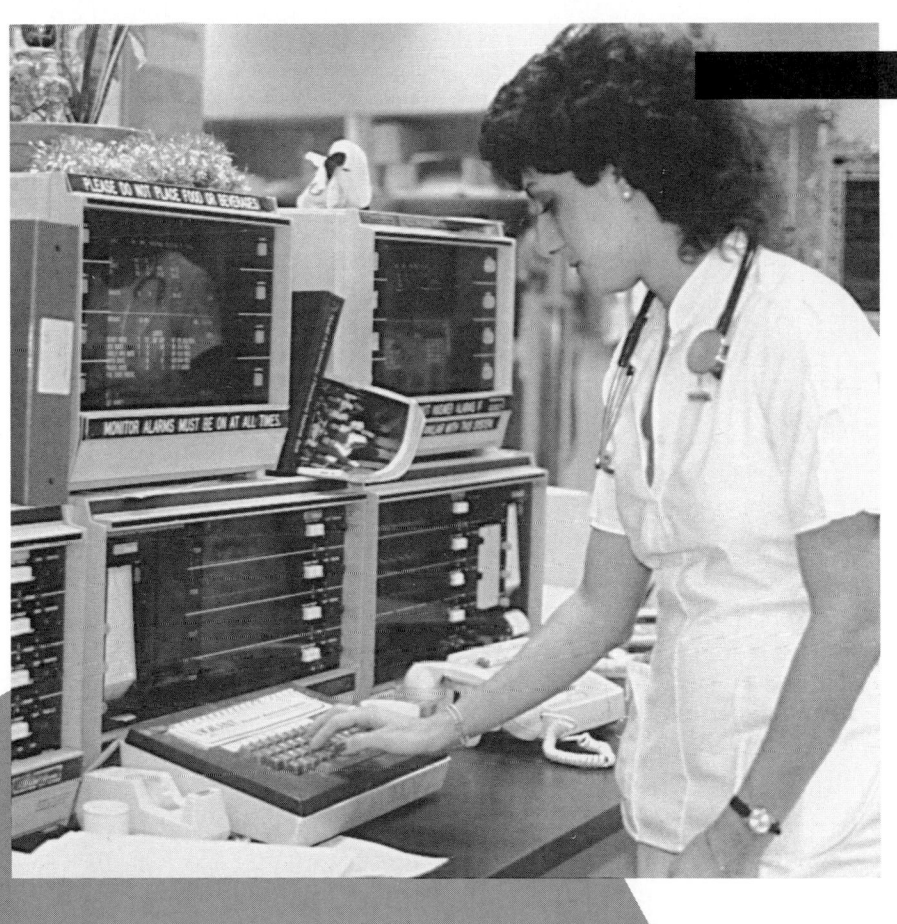

OBJECTIVES

After studying this chapter, the learner should be able to

Define key terms used in the chapter.

Discuss the social and economic trends affecting the health-care delivery system.

Describe the various types of health-care insurance.

Describe several types of alternative health-care delivery.

Compare and contrast the various types of health-care agencies.

Discuss the problems experienced by the health-care system.

List the services provided by various health-care agencies.

The health-care system faces more challenges and changes than ever before. Consumers concerned about the rapidly increasing cost of health care have helped bring about some dramatic financial changes in health insurance and health-care payment plans. Increasing health-care costs and the rising number of elderly and poor are forcing changes in governmentally funded health care.

Some of these changes are having positive effects on the health-care system, others are negatively affecting the system, and the effects of some changes have not yet been determined.

TRENDS IN HEALTH-CARE DELIVERY

Current societal issues influencing health-care delivery focus on promoting wellness, preventing illness, and rehabilitation to increase the independence of clients who are frail or ill. The public's interest in self-care has evolved into a strong force in terms of the education and services provided by the health-care system. Today's clients are more highly educated in health-care matters, prefer more control and decision making over their personal health, and are becoming active participants in planning and implementing health care.

These changes in societal attitude have influenced the health awareness evident in contemporary society. People are becoming increasingly involved in stress-management programs, exercise and physical fitness regimens, weight control, and improved nutrition programs, as well as in anti-smoking and anti–toxic substances campaigns and various other methods to decrease the incidence of illness and promote and maintain wellness.

Consumerism is also having a major effect on the health-care system. Clients are asserting their rights as human beings and consumers of a service by voicing dislike of the sometimes dehumanizing and uncaring treatment they receive in the health-care system. People want to be treated as intelligent individuals in a holistic manner (see Chap. 8). Health-care providers can no longer just treat an illness but must also consider and care for the human responses to illness. As consumers of health care, the public is outraged at its costs. This outrage has led to cost-reduction and cost-containment plans such as prospective payment systems in which fixed rates are assigned to particular procedures. Health maintenance organizations (HMOs), initially developed in California in the 1960s, promote illness prevention and provide health care at a relatively low cost to the consumer.

KEY TERMS

adult day-care centers
ambulatory care centers
continuing-care retirement community
crisis intervention center
diagnostic related groups
governmental agencies
health maintenance organization
home health-care agency
hospice
life-care center
long-term care facilities
Medicaid
Medicare
mutual aid self-help groups
preferred provider arrangement
preferred provider organization
prospective payment plan
psychiatric agency
Public Health Service
rehabilitation center
respite care
voluntary health-care agency

TYPES OF HEALTH-CARE SETTINGS

The following section discusses settings for health-care delivery, as well as the nurse's role in these settings. Table 3-1 defines nursing functions in these settings.

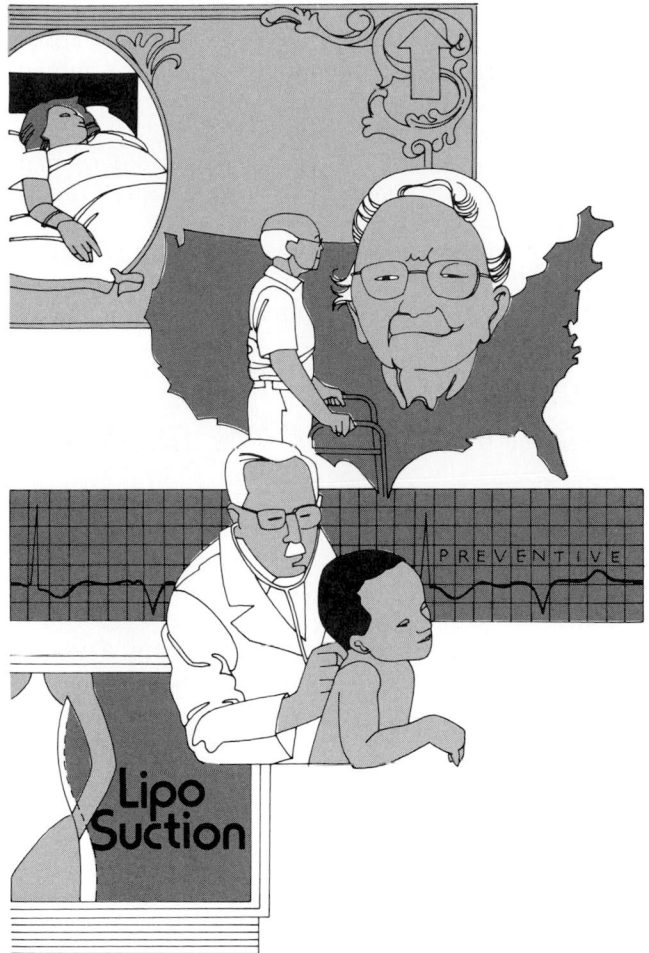

FIGURE 3-1

Key trends influencing health-care delivery include increasing emphasis on preventive medicine, growing consumerism, the "graying of America," and escalating health-care costs.

Hospitals

Traditionally, an ill client was hospitalized and, in most cases, not discharged from the hospital until well or treated with all available resources. This type of long-term hospitalization is no longer considered appropriate or even possible owing to the high cost of hospital care and the limited stays encouraged by prospective payment plans such as diagnostic related groups (discussed later in this chapter). Hospitals are progressively being viewed as acute-care centers for clients who are severely ill, although most hospitals continue to provide various outpatient and support services. In many cases, once the client begins to recover from an illness, traumatic surgical procedure, or injury, transfer is made to a rehabilitation or extended-care facility, or to a home-care program to complete progress toward wellness.

Hospitals come in all sizes and provide a wide range of health-care services to the public. Most provide generalized types of care and services to the consumer: testing and diagnostic procedures, ambulatory care units, surgi-

cal interventions, emergency-care services, inpatient services, and client education. Some hospitals provide only specialized care, such as rehabilitation or mental health care, or care to children and their illnesses.

Hospitals may also be identified as public, private, or community based. Public hospitals are financed and operated by local or national government agencies. In the United States, public hospitals care for the majority of poor and uninsured clients. They commonly maintain an open-door policy, offer unpopular or unprofitable services, and are committed to a not-for-profit philosophy (Gage, 1985). In Canada, the majority of hospitals are publicly funded.

Private hospitals may be for-profit or not-for-profit, depending on their individual philosophy. They may be owned and operated by groups, corporations, churches, or charitable organizations. Community-based hospitals are usually more aware of community needs and wishes than are private hospitals because community members are actively encouraged to become involved in decisions made by the hospital.

There are also government hospitals such as Veterans Administration (VA) hospitals and military hospitals. VA hospitals primarily care for veterans with service- and non–service-related illnesses or disabilities. Military hospitals provide care for military personnel (Armed Forces) and their immediate families.

Many hospitals are promoting and experiencing changes within their health-care system. Some hospitals are updating and expanding certain areas such as pharmacies, laboratories, and skilled long-term care facilities in an effort to develop profit-making units whose services can be used by people outside the hospital environment. Other hospitals are getting involved in occupational health programs, offering illness prevention, health education, disease screening/detection, and rehabilitation services.

Some hospitals have already, or are planning to, add or expand the following:

- Home health services
- Outpatient in-house surgery (short procedure unit, SPU)
- Outpatient in-house diagnosis
- Wellness and health promotion programs
- Rehabilitation units or facilities
- Substance-abuse units or facilities
- Affiliations with HMOs, preferred provider organizations (PPOs), or preferred provider arrangements (PPAs)

Large multihospital firms, such as American Health Care Management, Inc., Hospital Corporation of America (HCH), American Healthcare Systems, Inc. (AHS), and Humana, Inc., have also emerged as a result of changes in the health-care system.

A nurse in a hospital setting is responsible for many and varied direct and indirect client-care activities, including assessing and monitoring the client's physical, emotional, and mental status; educating the client and family about self-care, home care, disease processes, and

T A B L E   3-1
Nursing Functions in Various Health-Care Settings

Health-Care Settings	Nursing Functions
Hospital	
• Inpatient • Outpatient • Rehabilitation • Specialty area	• Assesses and monitors client status • Teaches client and family • Coordinates activities of health team members • Gives direct client care
Physician's Office	
	• Assesses health status • Assists with diagnostic tests and procedures • Teaches client and family • Manages office
Outpatient Facilities	
• Hospital based • Walk-in clinics • Urgent-care facilities	• Assesses health status • Assists with procedures and tests • Teaches clients and families • Gives direct client care • May provide primary care if a nurse practitioner or clinical nurse specialist
Adult Day-Care Centers	
• Hospital based • Long-term facility • Independent	• Involved in meeting nutritional, rehabilitation, occupational therapy, counseling, and medical therapy needs
Respite Care	
• Hospital based • Agency • Home based	• Gives direct client care • Counsels and teaches client and family
Home Health-Care Agencies	
• Hospital based • Agency • Independent	• Gives direct client care • Assesses and monitors health status • Teaches client and family • Makes appropriate referrals
Long-Term Care Facilities	
• Retirement centers • Nursing homes • Convalescent centers • Hospital based	• Gives direct client care • Assesses and monitors health status • Makes appropriate referrals • Directly manages other health-care providers
Specialized Facilities	
• Rehabilitation centers • Psychiatric facilities • Hospice	• Functions as a member of the health-care team to promote optimal level of functioning • Provides counseling and emotional support

(Continued)

TABLE 3-1
Nursing Functions in Various Health-Care Settings
(Continued)

Health-Care Settings	Nursing Functions
Other Agencies and Settings	
• Veterans' hospitals • Military hospitals • Public health • Prisons • Voluntary agencies • Community volunteer agencies • Support groups	• Carries out a variety of functions and nursing roles to meet client needs

prescribed diagnostic or treatment procedures; and coordinating the interaction of other members of the health-care team involved in a client's care. Most hospitals employ nurses in both inpatient and outpatient settings. A nurse may practice in a general-care unit within the hospital or may specialize. The increased technologic growth of the health-care field and the expanding knowledge base often encourage health-care providers to specialize.

Physician's Office

In the spirit of competition and to improve the continuity and quality of care, the traditional physician's office has expanded in size and services provided. Generally, the services provided to a client in the physician's office consist of primary health care in the form of diagnosing illnesses and prescribing appropriate treatments. Some offices include small laboratories where various blood and urine specimens can be collected and analyzed. Electrocardiograms (ECGs), radiographs (x-ray films), and ultrasonograms may also be done in the office. Physicians are becoming more responsive to societal wishes and demands by offering health education services and performing minor surgical procedures in the office setting.

A nurse in a physician's office may be responsible for collecting blood and urine specimens for analysis, taking and documenting vital signs, doing initial client health assessments, teaching clients, organizing client files, arranging client appointments, and dispensing prescribed medications.

Outpatient Facilities

Ambulatory Care Centers.   Ambulatory care centers (ACCs) are dramatically increasing in number and type. ACCs may be hospital sponsored or affiliated, or may be independent facilities. *Walk-in clinics* have been in existence for years; because of their relatively lower costs,

they are frequently used by clients from the lower economic levels. In many instances, clinics supply the same or similar services as the physician's office.

A more recent type of ACC is the *urgent-care center,* which clients may use in lieu of the emergency room of a hospital.

Most ACCs are not open on a 24-hour basis, but hours of availability vary from center to center. Payment policies also vary greatly from center to center, depending on whether the ACC is independent or associated with a hospital.

A nurse in an ACC may fulfill a variety of roles from that of a physician's office nurse to that of an expanded nursing role, such as nurse practitioner or clinical nurse specialist.

Adult Day-Care Centers.   Adult day-care centers offer a variety of services to elderly or physically or mentally challenged adults. Clients who are unable to perform activities of daily living (ADLs) without assistance cannot be left alone for long periods of time. In the past, these clients were usually admitted to a nursing home or extended-care facility, or their families had to adapt to economic and organizational upheavals within the home. Day-care centers can alleviate or reduce these problems by providing care to the client during the hours when family members are at work and thus allow a family to care for a debilitated family member in the home.

Adult day-care centers may be a service offered by a long-term care facility or a hospital, or they may function independently. The services offered vary from center to center but usually include a meal, rehabilitation, occupational therapy, counseling, and the dispensing of prescribed medications and treatments. A nurse employed at an adult day-care center can expect to be involved in any or all of these activities.

Respite Care.   Some institutions, especially agencies affiliated with a hospice program, offer the service of respite care. **Respite care** involves a short-term inpatient stay to give relief to the primary care provider of a client being cared for in the home by family members. In some areas in-house respite care is available where a person comes to the client's residence for a short period of time while the primary caregiver leaves to perform errands or to have a break from the constant responsibility of caring for someone in the home environment. Some health insurances, such as Medicare, have realized the necessity of respite care for a family's well-being and will pay for a limited amount of this type of health care.

As more families are attempting to care for the elderly or physically challenged at home, respite care is becoming an increasingly important resource for helping maintain the health of the entire family involved in a home care situation.

Home Health-Care Agencies.   Home health-care (HHC) **agencies** provide care to the client in the home. HHC agencies offer many services in the home setting. Home care is usually provided on a short-term basis, but it may be long term depending on the client's condition and the number and type of resources available to the client. Community health nursing is a form of home health care.

The prospective payment system, in which predetermined rates are assigned for specific health-care procedures, has resulted in many clients being discharged from the hospital while still requiring care. Home health care is rapidly expanding in an effort to meet the health-care needs of these clients. The nurse's responsibilities as a community health nurse are becoming more complex and may include the care of clients on ventilators

Women's health-care clinics

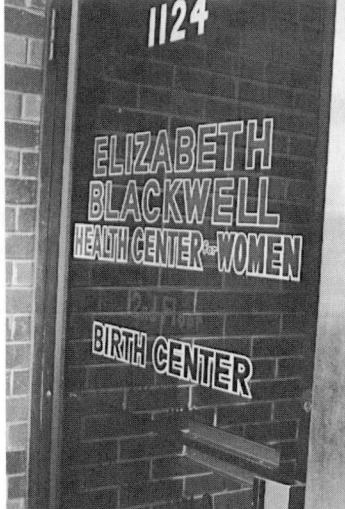

FIGURE   3-2
In recent years, the number and variety of health-care settings has increased dramatically.

Private practice group facilities

Urgent care centers

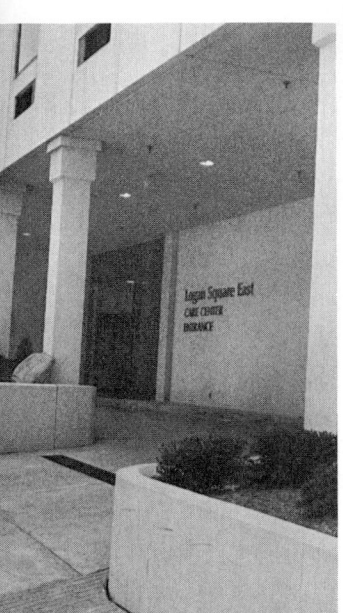

Long-term independent living care facilities

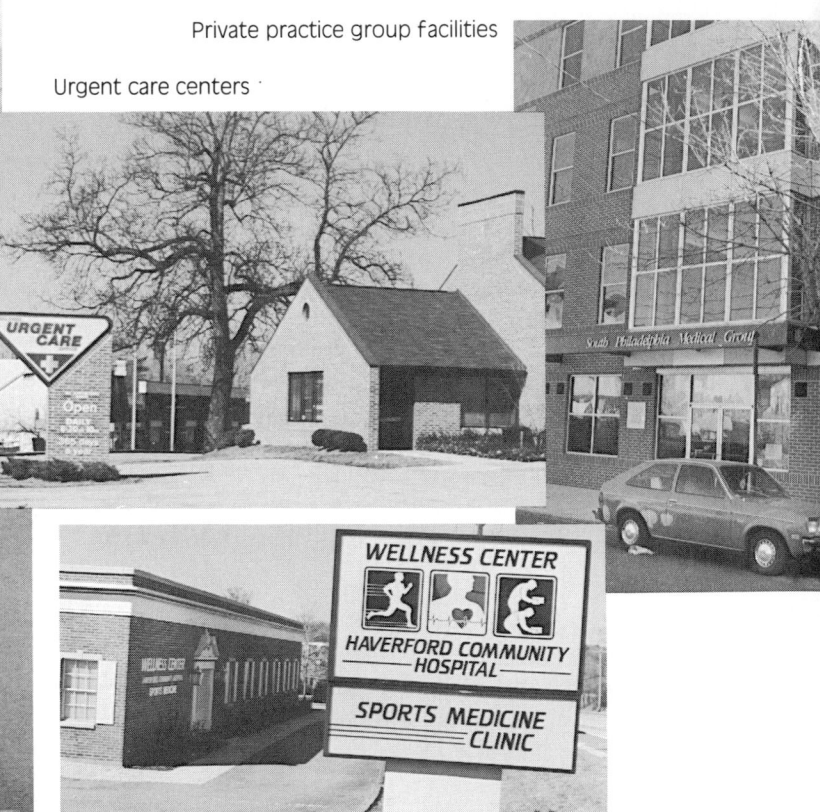

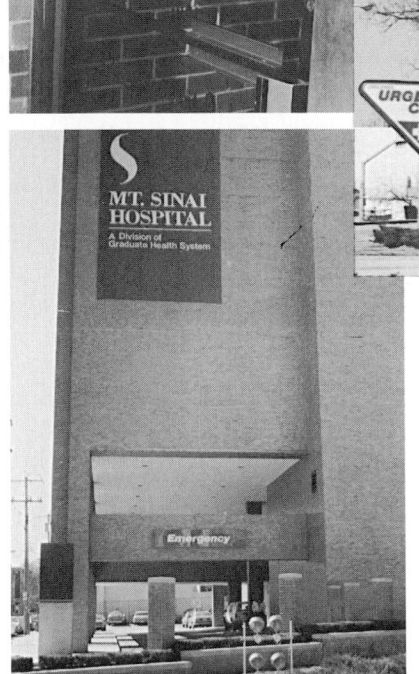

Multi-facility health-care systems

Wellness centers

(assistive respiratory machines), enteral feedings, and intravenous therapies, in addition to providing direct care, teaching, emotional support, and referrals.

Long-Term Care Facilities

Long-term care (LTC) facilities are more commonly known as nursing homes, where the elderly or physically or mentally challenged are cared for. LTC is another rapidly expanding portion of the health-care delivery system. The percentage of the population over the age of 65 is growing rapidly. By the year 2040 the United States Bureau of Census projects that there will be 66 million residents over the age of 65 (Riffer, 1985a). This means that 21% of the United States population will be 65 years of age or older by the year 2040, and a comparable increase in the number of elderly is predicted in Canada.

Prospective payment systems are also having an impact on the growth and development of LTC facilities. Earlier hospital discharges are channeling younger clients with more complex health problems to these facilities. This new mix of clients is resulting in a larger number of discharged clients from LTC facilities to home, after rehabilitative measures have increased their level of functioning and independence.

LTC centers are primarily concerned with three levels of care: independent living, community care, and skilled inpatient nursing care. An LTC facility may offer only one of these options or all three. Various names for LTC centers have evolved depending on the services offered by the center. One of the more recent types of LTC facilities is the continuing-care retirement community (CCRC) or life-care center. This type of center offers the client independent living units similar to apartments or condominiums. Residents are encouraged to bring their personal furnishings when they enter these facilities. The centers provide 24-hour emergency care on the premises, as well as intermediate or skilled nursing care when the need arises. Other services available for the residents may include housekeeping, laundry and food services, transportation, social activities, and assistance with ADLs such as dressing, eating, bathing, and ambulation. Some life-care centers also offer financial counseling, security services, and recreational activities. Many of these centers are affordable to the middle-class elderly.

Another long-term care option is the traditional nursing home, convalescent center, or extended-care facility. Nursing homes may be affiliated with a hospital or may be independent. They usually offer custodial and intermediate care and may offer skilled nursing care. *Skilled nursing care* means that the care given to a client can only be performed by or under the direct supervision of a licensed nurse. In most instances, health insurance will cover only skilled nursing care. Custodial and intermediate care must be paid for by the client or the family.

Nursing homes usually offer rehabilitative services such as physical and occupational therapies. Periodic health check-ups may also be done at the facility by a physician. Residents in a nursing home are most commonly elderly but may include clients of any age with chronic or debilitating illnesses.

Specialized Facilities

Rehabilitation Centers.   The primary focus of **rehabilitation centers** is to return a client to a pre-illness level of functioning or to provide education and training to enable a client to function as independently as possible. Through intensive and well-synchronized team work the client is assisted in reaching full potential. The rehabilitation team is usually composed of nurses; physicians; social workers; counselors; speech, physical, and occupational therapists; and a variety of other health-care professionals. Team membership depends on the client's diagnosis and recommended treatments.

Rehabilitation centers may be a unit within a hospital, a rehabilitation hospital associated with a general hospital, or independent. The centers are specialized to provide support and treatment for chemically dependent clients or for physically challenged individuals following a debilitating illness or injury.

Psychiatric Facilities.   A mental health or **psychiatric agency** provides counseling, support, and treatment for clients experiencing emotional or behavioral illnesses. Services may be supplied on an inpatient or outpatient basis. A psychiatric facility may be a unit within a hospital, an independent clinic, or an independent public or private mental health hospital. The goal of returning the client to pre-illness functioning or reaching full potential may be achieved through a long-term or short-term program. A client's admission into a psychiatric-care facility may be voluntary or involuntary. An involuntary commitment procedure may be necessary if the client is harmful to self or to others.

For the immediate or emergency care of clients experiencing behavioral or emotional illnesses, a **crisis intervention center** may be appropriate. The client may come or be brought to the center, or may contact a counselor by a 24-hour telephone line. A crisis center provides immediate assistance, support, and guidance for further psychiatric care. A client's contact with a crisis center is on a short-term basis only. The client population tends to be violent, self-destructive, suicidal, or drug or alcohol abusers. Once the immediate crisis has been controlled, the client is referred for inpatient treatment or outpatient counseling at a psychiatric center.

Hospice.   A **hospice** is a private or public agency engaged in activities that provide pain relief, symptom management, and supportive services to terminally ill clients and their families. Hospice programs can be developed in a variety of settings. Some programs are offered by a hospital for inpatient and home care. Other hospices function as independent entities or may be community based and offered through a community nursing service. In most programs the majority of client and family care and support is given in the home setting. The hospice team commonly includes nurses, physicians, counselors, therapists, and many specially trained volunteers. The volunteers listen; supply emotional and physical comfort; act as liaisons between client/family and health-care personnel; supply transportation, shopping, and household duties when necessary; and provide short-term respite care for family members who are primary caregivers. The hospice volunteers are frequently the foundation of the hospice program.

Governmental Agencies

VA hospitals, public hospitals, and military hospitals all come under the umbrella of government-supported and -operated health care. **Governmental agencies** are financed by national, state, local, or provincial taxes. City taxes help support city hospitals and public health clinics; state and provincial taxes help support state mental health hospitals; and national taxes aid in financing national health and welfare programs such as the Canadian Department of Health and Welfare.

Public Health Service.   The **Public Health Service** (PHS) in the United States is a federal health agency that falls under the direction of the Department of Health and Human Services. A similar health service is provided by the Department of Health and Welfare in Canada. The PHS is a multifaceted program that covers a wide range of services. It is the medical branch of the United States Coast Guard and the principle source of Native American health care through the Indian Health Services (IHS). The amount of direct client care provided by the PHS is more limited than in the past.

The PHS supplies funds to health centers that provide care to migrant workers and for community agencies that supply health care to the poor or uninsured. The principal budget of the PHS goes to grant programs for the poor and uninsured.

The Centers for Disease Control (CDC) in Atlanta, Georgia, and the National Institutes of Health (NIH) are both part of PHS. The CDC focuses on the epidemiology, prevention, control, and treatment of communicable diseases such as sexually transmitted diseases (STD). The NIH is engaged in various health research activities.

PHS also supplies health-care professionals (*e.g.,* nurses, physicians, dentists, and pharmacists) to the Justice Department to provide care in federal prisons. The service is also involved to varying degrees in drug and alcohol abuse and mental health programs within the state. PHS activities vary from area to area. In most cases they focus on community needs and attempt to meet those needs whenever possible.

Canadian Health Services.   The types of governmental health-care services and agencies available in Canada are similar to those in the United States. The major difference between the two systems is the way that health care is financed.

The Canadian health-care system is composed of health-care plans within each province. These plans cover all Canadian residents for most of their necessary hospital care and physician's fees. These provincial health insurance plans are financed by federal and provincial taxes.

Voluntary Agencies

Voluntary health-care agencies are strictly nonprofit. Their functioning depends on volunteers, although health-care professionals such as nurses and physicians are part of the system as volunteers, coordinators, and resource persons. Voluntary agencies include Lupus Alert, Inc., National Multiple Sclerosis Society, Red Cross, Canadian Lung Association, and the Canadian Heart Foundation. These agencies are actively involved in promoting health through the prevention and detection of specific illnesses such as cancer and lung diseases. They also support research related to the specific illness the agency is concerned about. Some voluntary agencies help people pay for the cost of equipment, respite care, or home nursing care for short periods of time. Financially, these agencies are supported by private donation, fund raising, and federal grants. They can be found at community and national levels.

Community Human Services

A large number of communities offer human services to a variety of clients. Most of these service programs depend on a volunteer work force. They are primarily financed by private donations, grants, or fund raisers, although for further financial support some may charge minimal fees or according to a sliding scale that depends on what a client can afford to pay. Such community programs include Meals on Wheels, supplying hot and cold meals to the home-bound; specialized and regular transportation services for the elderly and physically challenged; hearing contact persons for the deaf (telecommunications devices for the deaf); and shopping, housekeeping, and cooking services.

Support Groups.   Member-organized and -run self-help or support groups are flourishing, aided by society's increased interest in self-care. **Mutual aid self-help groups** (MASH) offer emotional support and education to their members to assist them in coping with personal and health problems. They also offer factual information to members through conferences, workshops, and newsletters. Some groups provide 24-hour support for members through telephone hot lines or buddy systems.

In many cases, a health-care professional such as a nurse or physician is recruited as a member of the organization to act as a liaison or contact person between the group and the health-care system.

Hospital interest in MASH groups is on the rise, and it is a hospital that has published the first national directory of self-help groups. Some states have self-help clearing houses where information about MASH groups is available. In Canada, information about MASH groups can be obtained from the Center for Mutual Aid in Montreal.

MASH groups offer a variety of services and resources to people for thousands of different problems. Some self-help groups, such as RESOLVE, Inc., help couples deal with infertility; Alcoholics Anonymous (AA) aids and supports alcoholics in their recovery and also provides support and counseling for family members (Al-Anon), children of alcoholics (Ala-Teen), and adult children of alcoholics. AA has also been used successfully by other chemically dependent persons. Overeaters Anonymous (OA) functions similarly to AA and also encourages the use of a 24-hour buddy system for members having problems controlling and coping with excessive and sometimes obsessive dietary intake.

Self-help groups offer invaluable services to members, members' families, and the community. They are growing in number and type and being recognized as valuable resources for health promotion and maintenance in the community.

FINANCING HEALTH CARE

Historically, health-care insurance or prepayment began in the United States in 1929, when organizations were created that provided pooling or shared risk programs to finance members' medical expenses. Prepayment of hospital expenses grew rapidly, and by the late 1930s commercial insurers offered health insurance plans (O'Connor, 1984).

The public's interest in health insurance continues to grow for various reasons, but primarily as an attempt to fend off the expensive costs of health care. The purchasers of health insurance are usually employed and have a dependable source of income. Most employers offer a variety of health insurance plans for their employees. In many instances the employer will pay all or part of the employees' health insurance premiums as part of employee benefits. Some clients may be able to pay for hospital and medical costs out-of-pocket, although this is a rare occurrence.

Since the inception of health insurance, a variety of programs have been developed to help finance the increasing costs of health care. These programs vary greatly and specific programs require meeting strict criteria for membership.

Group Health Plans

Group plans for financing health care include **health maintenance organizations** (HMOs), **preferred provider organizations** (PPOs), and **preferred provider arrangements** (PPAs). Enrollment in these plans is voluntary. An individual pays a fixed rate on either a monthly or annual plan and, in turn, receives financial coverage for all the health care necessary to maintain wellness and prevent illness. HMOs are especially interested and active in preventive health care and the maintenance of health.

Health Maintenance Organizations.

HMOs were developed as alternative health-care systems. In an effort to help control spiraling health costs, the United States Congress passed the Health Maintenance Organization Act in 1973. This act helped finance the development of HMOs such as the Kaiser-Permanente Medical Program, which began in California. Kaiser-Permanente is expanding into other states and more private agencies are developing HMOs.

Some HMOs offer almost unlimited resources to the client. They own and operate hospitals, clinics, physicians' offices, laboratories, and various other facilities. A person insured by an HMO plan is restricted to using the HMO's facilities and member physicians, except in some emergency situations. To maintain and increase cost effectiveness, HMOs may also place further limitations on a client's use of the system. Second opinions may be required for elective surgical procedures and a physician specialist may be consulted only if the client's primary HMO physician agrees and recommends the appointment. These limitations are effective methods for improving cost containment and keeping health-care expenditures lower than average.

An HMO subscriber pays monthly or annual premiums and generally receives all health care free as long as it is obtained through the HMO. Some services, such as a physician's office visit, may require a minimal fee in addition to the premiums.

A more recent development in HMOs is the use of an independent practice association (IPA) model. The IPA model permits HMOs to contract individually with local, independently practicing physicians. This allows the HMO to expand its client base by adding physicians to an approved provider list.

Preferred Provider Organizations and Preferred Provider Arrangements.

PPOs and PPAs are almost synonymous, the primary difference being that PPOs involve organizations of health-care providers and PPAs can be arranged with individual health-care providers.

According to Fox (cited in Powills and Weinberg, 1985, p 43), the term *PPA* may be used to describe "any arrangement whereby patients are channeled to specific providers." A PPA is a system in which the subscriber receives more extensive benefits if a designated preferred provider, either hospital or physician, is used. Unlike an HMO, a PPA subscriber is not necessarily limited to the use of preferred providers.

A PPA plan may be based on limited or unlimited participation. A limited PPA plan restricts subscribers to the use of only preferred providers of health care. An unlimited PPA plan allows all providers in the area who accept a contractual agreement to participate in the PPA. The payer, usually an insurance company, makes the decision whether to base the PPA plan on a limited or unlimited agreement.

In general, PPAs establish lower health-care prices. They also utilize cost controls such as preadmission certification, second surgical opinion, and client length-of-stay reviews. An increasing number of commercial insurance companies and Blue Cross and Blue Shield are offering PPA plans to subscribers.

Because HMOs, PPAs, and PPOs assume the financial loss or gain of the health-care services used by their clients they encourage preventive health care to avoid the higher costs of illness and hospitalization. For the same reason, these plans carefully monitor the quality and quantity of the health care delivered to clients. They also place limitations on the use of high-cost procedures and require certain guidelines to be followed when a higher-cost procedure is recommended by a physician. Some people do not like these plans because they use a selective contracting approach, mandating subscriber use of specific institutions and health-care providers. Some consumers dislike this lack of control of decisions relating to personal or family health.

Long-Term Care Insurance.   A recent development in the health-care insurance market is the growing interest in long-term care (LTC) insurance. In general, a minimal amount of long-term care is paid for by private insurance. The majority of LTC (approximately 90%) is paid for by Medicaid and out-of-pocket spending (Firshein, 1986b). Medicare pays for a very small percentage of LTC. The "graying of America," the steady increase in the population of persons 65 years of age and older, has become a major concern within the health-care financing area.

Some commercial insurance companies are now offering LTC benefits. Promoters of LTC insurance have developed models of plans that would cover a variety of services such as nursing home care, home care, and other services that would help prevent the institutionalization of the elderly, debilitated, and chronically ill. Adult day-care centers and respite care would also fall under these types of services and would be covered by benefits.

Government Financing: United States.   As health insurance programs grew and prospered, it soon became apparent that a portion of the population (the poor, elderly, and physically or mentally challenged) did not have access to health insurance and ultimately to health care. In 1965 the United States federal government became involved in health insurance when it enacted legislation creating Medicare for the elderly and physically challenged and Medicaid for the poor.

Medicare.   Medicare is a United States federal health insurance program for persons 65 years of age or older, people of any age with permanent kidney failure, and certain physically challenged individuals. It is run by the Health Care Financing Administration. Local Social Security Administration offices can supply all the necessary information about the program. It is financed partly through the Social Security (FICA) Tax.

C O M P U T E R   A P P L I C A T I O N S   I N   N U R S I N G

COMPUTER USE TO REDUCE HEALTH-CARE COSTS

Nursing computer systems can be used to provide a variety of automated services of benefit to consumers of health care. One such service, developed at the Washington Hospital Center, Washington, DC, provides the following:

- An automated patient classification system, capable of analyzing patient acuity data related to DRGs
- Automated staff scheduling and needs, care planning, and charting capabilities

- Complex analysis of finance, budget, and position control as related to patient acuity

The system, based on the slogan "humanizing patient care," improved the accuracy of patient classifications, automated record keeping and nursing documentation, saved time for nurses and administrators, provided data for research, and—by saving time—reduced the costs of hospitalization for patients.

(From Hylton R, Johnson J, Moran M: Automating a patient classification system: Nurse-vendor collaboration. Computers in Nursing 4(1):27–31, 1986)

Medicare has been set up in two parts: hospital insurance and medical insurance.

Hospital insurance helps pay for inpatient hospital and skilled nursing facility care, home health care, and hospice care. It is financed partly through the FICA tax.

Medical insurance helps pay for necessary physician's services, outpatient hospital and home health services, and a variety of other medical supplies and services. Applying for the medical insurance portion of the plan is voluntary. It is financed from the monthly premiums paid by the people who have enrolled in it and from general federal revenues.

The full cost of some services is not covered by Medicare; it is recommended that clients subscribe to supplemental insurance policies offered by private insurance companies. Also, because Medicare is federally funded, benefits may change from year to year according to decisions made concerning the federal budget.

Physicians and facilities are voluntary Medicare providers. Therefore, no physician or health institution is forced to care for Medicare clients. This voluntary agreement process may be jeopardized since some states are considering denying licensure renewal to physicians who do not care for Medicare clients.

To remain financially viable Medicare depends on FICA taxes. A relative decrease in the number of working adults who pay FICA taxes has put a definite strain on the federally supported insurance plans. At the same time, there has been an increase in the elderly and chronic illness populations and a progressive rise in health-care costs. Some believe that the Social Security system will collapse within the next decade and the Medicare Trust Fund will become financially insolvent during the early 1990s (cited in O'Connor, 1984, p 12).

Diagnostic Related Groups. In 1983, Medicare converted to a prospective payment plan referred to as **diagnostic related groups** (DRGs). A **prospective payment plan** pays the hospital a predetermined, fixed rate determined by the diagnosis or specific procedure involved regardless of the actual cost of the hospitalization. DRG payment rates are based on analyses of recent charges for care in various diagnosis categories plus an adjustment for inflation. These rates are updated annually.

Although there are 467 DRG categories, they cannot possibly cover all admissions accurately or comprehensively. Therefore, the program does allow for unusually long hospital stays, unusually costly cases (called outliers), and other extenuating circumstances. To qualify for these exceptions it is necessary that the hospital submit comprehensive documentation and support for the circumstances surrounding each outlier case.

DRGs were implemented by the federal government in an effort to control rising health-care costs. Theoretically, the DRG system is projected to save Medicare hundreds of thousands of dollars. Medicare will pay only the amount of money preassigned to the client's DRG category (*e.g.,* gallbladder surgery). If the cost of the client's hospitalization is above the assigned cost, the hospital must absorb the loss. On the other hand, if hospital costs are below the assigned payment, the hospital makes a profit. The prospective payment system essentially rewards efficiency for the least cost and punishes inefficiency and high costs.

At present, DRGs apply only to inpatient hospital care for Medicare clients. Alternative health-care delivery systems and possibly insurance companies will probably develop similar programs.

Medicaid. Medicaid is the federally funded health insurance program for persons with very low incomes. Current budgetary considerations are forcing state and federal agencies to trim Medicaid expenditures. The rapid growth of an aging population and an increase in the number of poor, many of whom are women and children, are draining the Medicaid budget. For survival, the Medicaid programs are implementing reforms such as reduced benefits or placing clients into utilization-control systems such as PPAs.

Government Financing: Canada

The Canada Health Act became law in 1984. It clarifies and defines the conditions of Canadian health insurance: universality, accessibility, comprehensiveness, and portability among provinces. The organization and services vary from province to province. However, "the health and physician insurance services exist to finance, administer, and regulate the provisions of federal and provincial legislation regarding hospital and medical care" (Storch, 1985). The general areas of involvement of provincial governments are approval of hospitals and budgets, approval of claims and payments, data collection, inspection and consultation, and licensing and financial assistance for hospital and nursing home construction. Other benefits supplemental to medical insurance may be administered by the particular provincial government.

Private Health Insurance

Subscription to private health insurance plans may be done on an individual basis or through a group plan at a person's place of employment. Private health insurance coverage varies from one insurance company to another. Some insurance policies cover all medical and hospital expenses, and others pay only part of the costs. This type of medical insurance payment is referred to as *third-party reimbursement* because a third party, the insurance company, pays the bills.

Charitable Financing

The uninsured may seek health care through charitable agencies. These agencies often provide a budgeted amount of free health care to the indigent or uninsured.

The bulk of charity care is usually offered by public hospitals and hospitals with a religious affiliation. Other hospitals may offer charity care on a very limited basis.

Catastrophic Health Insurance

Catastrophic health insurance exists in theory only, but its promoters feel that it will soon become an actuality. This insurance is an attempt to protect the elderly and their families against financial ruin by a long-term illness. Since Medicare does not cover all hospital and medical expenses, some families are suffering financial ruin. Clients with chronic illnesses are the most frequently affected group.

ISSUES IN THE HEALTH-CARE DELIVERY SYSTEM

Economic Issues

The health-care system is experiencing a financial crisis. Health costs have increased dramatically, and some feel that cost-containment measures have been implemented too late to effectively reverse the current upward swing in health costs. The actual short-term and long-term results of these cost-containment measures remain to be seen. The health-care industry has functioned in a specific manner for many years and has become big business. The process of change can often be difficult.

Historically, the health-care system and the financial arrangements for paying for health care encouraged the use of expensive and sometimes inappropriate or ineffective health services. Many insurance plans paid for inpatient hospital care but not for ambulatory outpatient care. Therefore, to receive payment, clients were often hospitalized unnecessarily. Health care has also focused on the treatment of illnesses instead of on their prevention because preventive strategies often were not covered by a client's health insurance policy.

Third-party reimbursement effectively insulated clients from the actual cost of their health care. Because the insurance company was responsible for paying the incurred bills, the client was often bypassed in this process and seldom saw the bills for the cost of the care received.

The increased competition among hospitals further fueled the rise in health costs. Technologically, we have made amazing advances in health care, but as new machines and more advanced and expensive procedures are developed and utilized, clients' expectations of hospital resources also increase. The media is constantly informing the public of new and innovative treatment modalities. As a result, consumers expect these services to be available in "their" hospital. To attract clients, hos-

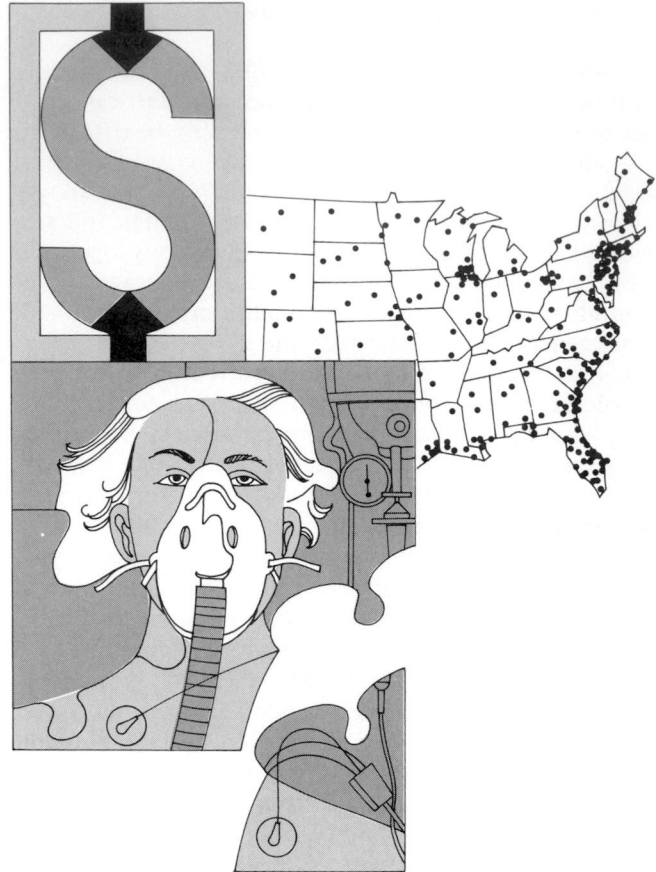

F I G U R E   3-3

Issues in health care requiring resolution in the 1990s include cost containment, adequate distribution geographically, and correction of the negative effects of fragmentation of care.

pitals invest huge sums of money in technologically advanced equipment. Supporters of cost-containment measures are encouraging hospitals to cooperate with each other and to share resources rather than compete with each other.

The decreased number of clients in many hospitals is encouraging or forcing the facilities to become dependent on HMOs and PPAs for a supply of clients to fill hospital beds. Because HMOs and PPAs are interested in keeping health-care costs as low as possible, the hospitals that show the lowest costs are the institutions the HMO or PPA will choose as its contractor.

Some businesses that pay part or all of its employees' insurance premiums as an employee benefit have started hospital bill audit programs. One such program gives a checklist to employees going into the hospital. As services and treatments are received by the employee, they are checked off and then compared to the list of services billed for by the hospital.

Nurses can aid in the war against rising health costs. As the largest group of professionals within the healthcare system, nurses are in a position to ensure correct use of medical equipment and supplies and avoid needless waste. Nurses should also become politically active in promoting legislative changes that will bring down health-care costs and still maintain a high quality of care.

Since health-care costs are being so carefully monitored, it is very important that nurses begin evaluating their worth to the health-care delivery system. Historically, nursing costs have been buried in the general room charges of the hospital. Therefore, nurses have not been able to prove their worth to the hospital in terms of client outcomes. To determine the actual value of nursing, some hospitals are developing nurse-costing methodologies that give more accurate information on nursing costs. Some early results of these studies support the idea that nursing is a bargain (McCormick, 1986).

Fragmentation of Care

Increased research has resulted in an excessive amount of information related to health care. It has become impossible for health-care providers to effectively keep up with the enormous amount of new knowledge, resulting in an increased tendency to specialize within one area of health care.

A family physician diagnoses and treats a variety of minor or common illnesses, but a client who presents with a more complex problem is usually referred to a specialist in that area. For example, a diabetic client with a heart condition may be cared for by a family physician, a cardiologist, and an endocrinologist. A hospitalized client may come in contact with a variety of health-care providers, including physicians, nurses, physical therapists, respiratory therapists, and others. It is no wonder that clients may become confused about their care and treatment. It can also make one wonder how everyone knows what everyone else is doing. Many agree that this fragmentation results in a loss of continuity of care, imposing further problems on the consumer, such as confusing or conflicting plans of care, over- or undermedication, and higher health-care costs.

Fragmented care offers advanced knowledge for the treatment of illnesses, but it can also be confusing, disruptive, and potentially dangerous to the client. Nurses can use a variety of strategies to reduce the number of problems resulting from fragmented care. A nurse can encourage the client to obtain all medication prescriptions from a single pharmacy. The majority of pharmacists keep a running file of medications used by a client and can quickly determine any potential problems with drug interaction or overmedication. The nurse can also encourage the client to communicate changes in treatment plans to each physician to keep them updated on other care the client may be receiving. The nurse can also limit further problems by effectively meeting responsibilities as client advocate and care coordinator in the hospital and community setting. Nurses frequently participate in updating a facility's policies and procedures and can therefore help initiate or support the idea of integrating inpatient and outpatient records to improve the clients' continuity of care upon discharge.

THE HEALTH-CARE TEAM

The professional nurse is not the only health-care provider involved in a client's care. In many situations a collaborative effort among many health-care professionals is necessary to promote or restore a client to health. There is a variety of health-care team members who provide necessary and specialized services to clients and their families.

Physician.   The physician is primarily responsible for diagnosing and treating clients medically. The nurse is responsible for following physician's orders or prescriptions in relation to client care. The nurse is also responsible for assessing the client for any physical and behavioral changes and relaying that information to the physician. In most situations the working relationship between physicians and nurses is collaborative.

An individual becomes a physician after many years of intensive training and education and passing a licensing examination. Depending on the curriculum completed, a physician obtains a degree of doctor of medicine (MD) or doctor of osteopathy (DO). A physician may be a generalist, such as a family practitioner, or a specialist, such as a neurologist or cardiologist.

Physicians' Assistant.   A physicians' assistant (PA) has completed specific courses of study as preparation for providing support to the physician. The PA's responsibilities usually depend on the physician supervising the activities.

In most states a nurse is not legally bound to follow a PA's orders unless they are cosigned by a physician. This is an important aspect to investigate if PAs are employed by hospitals in your area. PAs do not practice in Canada.

Physical Therapist.   A physical therapist (PT) seeks to restore function or prevent disability or further disability in the mobility of a client following an injury or an illness. The PT uses various techniques to treat clients, including massage, heat, cold, water, sonar waves, exercises, and electricity. Most PTs are also educated in the use of psychologic strategies to motivate clients.

To become a physical therapist, the individual must complete four years of college and obtain a baccalaureate degree in physical therapy. A state licensing examination must also be passed. In some areas a college graduate with a degree in another area may enroll in a 6- to 12-month certificate program to become a candidate for taking the state licensing examination for PTs.

Respiratory Therapist. A respiratory therapist (RT) has been trained and educated to administer techniques that will improve ·pulmonary (lung) function and oxygenation. RTs may also be responsible for administering a variety of tests that measure lung functioning, and for educating the client about the use of various devices and machines prescribed by the physician.

Occupational Therapist. An occupational therapist (OT) is licensed to assist the physically challenged (handicapped) client to adapt to limitations. The OT may use a variety of adaptive devices and strategies to aid a client in carrying out activities of daily living (ADL). Four years of college in the field of occupational therapy is required before a person can take the licensing examination for OTs.

Speech Therapist. A speech therapist is trained to help the deaf speak more clearly, a stroke victim to relearn how to speak, and correct or modify a variety of speech disturbances in children and adults. Four years of college study in speech therapy is required to become a speech therapist.

Dietitian. Generally, a registered dietitian (RD) is responsible for managing and planning for the dietary needs of clients. The RD is knowledgeable about all aspects of nutrition and its effects on the body. An RD can adapt specialized diets for the individual needs of clients, counsel and educate individual clients, and supervise the dietary services of the entire facility. Dietitians are a valuable resource for nurses.

A dietitian's education includes four years of college in an approved, coordinated undergraduate program in dietetics. After completing four years of education, the person takes a registration examination to become an RD. Another educational option is four years of college with an approved dietetics major and one year of a dietetics internship, followed by the registration examination.

Pharmacist. A pharmacist is licensed to formulate and dispense medications. The pharmacist is also responsible for keeping a running file of all client medications and for informing the physician when a potential or actual medication error in prescribing has occurred or when prescribed drugs may interact adversely. The pharmacist is an excellent resource for both clients and nurses for any information related to medications. A pharmacist must complete at least four years of college with a major in pharmacology before taking the licensing examination.

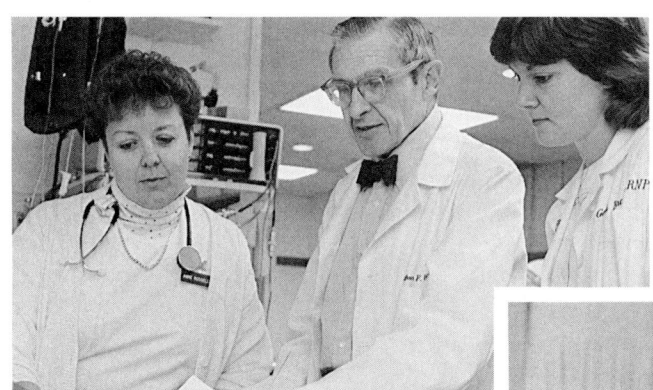

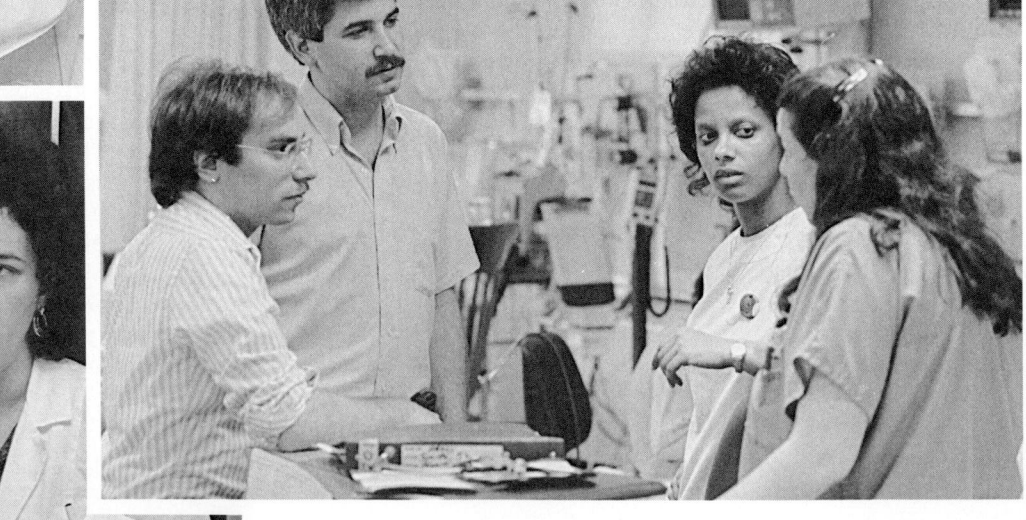

F I G U R E 3-4
Quality health-care results from the collaborative efforts of a team of professionals, many fulfilling specialized functions.

Social Worker.   A social worker counsels clients and family members and also informs them of and refers them to various community resources. A social worker has usually obtained a baccalaureate or master's degree in social work.

Chaplain.   Most agencies employ a chaplain to give spiritual support and guidance to clients and their families. The chaplain can also refer a client to a priest, minister, or rabbi of the client's own religious denomination.

KEY POINTS

- Current societal issues influencing health-care delivery focus on promoting wellness, preventing illness, rehabilitation, cost containment, and consumerism. Today's clients are more highly educated in health matters, prefer more control and decision making over personal health, and are becoming active participants in planning and implementing health care.

- The physician's office provides primary health care to the client in the form of diagnosing illnesses and prescribing appropriate treatments.

- Urgent-care centers, adult day-care centers, and home health-care agencies are growing in number and services provided.

- Long-term care centers are primarily concerned with three levels of care: independent living, community care, and skilled inpatient nursing care.

- The primary focus of rehabilitation centers and psychiatric or mental health agencies is to return the client to a pre-illness level of functioning or to provide education and training to function as independently as possible.

- A hospice is a private or public agency that engages in activities that provide pain relief, symptom management, and supportive services to terminally ill clients and their families.

- Health maintenance organizations are especially interested and active in preventive health care and the maintenance of health.

- Medicare is a federal health insurance program in the United States for persons 65 years of age or older, people of any age with permanent kidney failure, and certain physically challenged individuals. Medicaid is the federally funded health insurance program for those with very low incomes.

- In 1983, Medicare converted to a prospective payment plan, referred to as *diagnostic related groups* (DRGs), that pays a predetermined, fixed rate regardless of actual hospitalization costs. Private health insurance is referred to as *third-party reimbursement* because a third party, the insurance company, pays the bills.

- Nurses can have a powerful effect on the health-care system by initiating and supporting positive changes and by protesting changes that would jeopardize the health of individuals, families, communities, and nations.

BIBLIOGRAPHY

The ABCs of DRGs. RN June: 55–58, 1985

Aday LA, Fleming GV, Anderson R: Access to Medical Care in the U.S.: Who Has It, Who Doesn't. Chicago, Pluribus Press, 1984

Bowen OR: Cost control key to Medicare's future. Provider 12(6):9–10, 1986

Brickfield CF: Long term care financing solutions are needed now. American Health Care Association Journal 11(6):11–15, 1985

Brucker MC, MacMullen NJ: Understanding health insurance (Making it work for the patient and you). Nursing Success Today 2(12):7–9, 1985

Deane RT: Looking at Medicare after the promise. Provider 12(6):25–27, 1986

Evans R: Strained Mercy: The Economics of Canadian Health Care. Toronto, Butterworth, 1984

Fine J: Physicians group plans to expand national campaign against HMOs. Modern Healthcare 16(22):92, 1986

Friedman E: The health lifeline: Out of the reach of women and children. 60(20):46–51, 1986

Friedman E: Increasing numbers of Americans lack health insurance. Hospitals 59(5):21, 1985

Gage L: Interview: Public hospitals in a private market. Hospitals 59(4):114–116, 1985

Heinz J: The DRG challenge is to ensure quality. Provider 12(6):11–12, 1986

Kickbusch I: Health promotion: A global perspective. Can J Public Health 77:321–326, 1986

Last JM: Editorial: Achieving health for all. Can J Public Health 77:384–385, 1986

LeClair M: The Canadian health care system. In Andreopoulous S (ed): National Health Insurance: Can We Learn from Canada? pp 11–92. New York, John Wiley & Sons, 1975

LTC insurance needs increased awareness. Contemporary Long-Term Care June: 26–30, 63, 1986

McCormick B: What's the cost of nursing care? Hospitals 60(21):48–52, 1986

Millenson ML: Managed care: Will it push providers against the wall? Hospitals 60(19):66–71, 1986

Newman HN: Medicare at '21': History can teach. Provider 12(6):4–8, 1986

O'Connor P: Health care financing policy: Impact on nursing. Nursing Administration Quarterly Summer:11–20, 1984

Powills SE, Weinberg W: PPAs: A new payment system evolves. Hospitals 59(9):43–46, 1985

Richman D: Drug abuse may present growth opportunity for nation's hospitals. Modern Healthcare 16(21):46–47, 1986

Riffer J: Elderly 21 percent of the population by 2040. Hospitals 59(5):41–44, 1985a

Riffer J: Diversification push drives day care rise. Hospitals 59(5):68, 1985b

Rozovsky L: The Canadian Patients Book of Rights. Toronto, Doubleday Canada, 1980

Rozovsky L: Canadian Hospital Law, 2nd ed. Ottawa, Canadian Hospital Association, 1979

Ruderman A: Editorial: Marketing health promotion in Canada. An idea whose time has come. Can J Public Health 77:315–317, 1986

Shannon K: Swing-bed program's success spurs proposals to expand eligibility. Hospitals 59(5):78, 1985

Storch J: The Canadian health care delivery system. Policies, programs, services. In Stewart M et al: Community Health Nursing in Canada, pp 33–48. Toronto, Gage, 1985

Storch J: Patients Rights: Ethical and Legal Issues in Health Care and Nursing. Toronto, McGraw-Hill, 1982

Traska MR: Physicians' groups in uphill battle against HMOs. Hospitals 60(21):70, 1986

US Department of Health and Human Services: Health Care Financing Administration. Your Medicare Handbook 1986. Publication No. HCFA-10050 ICN-461250.

Williams DL: Providers talk the Medicare realities: Maximizing quality care and revenues. Provider 12(6):16–19, 1986

Theoretical Base for Nursing Practice

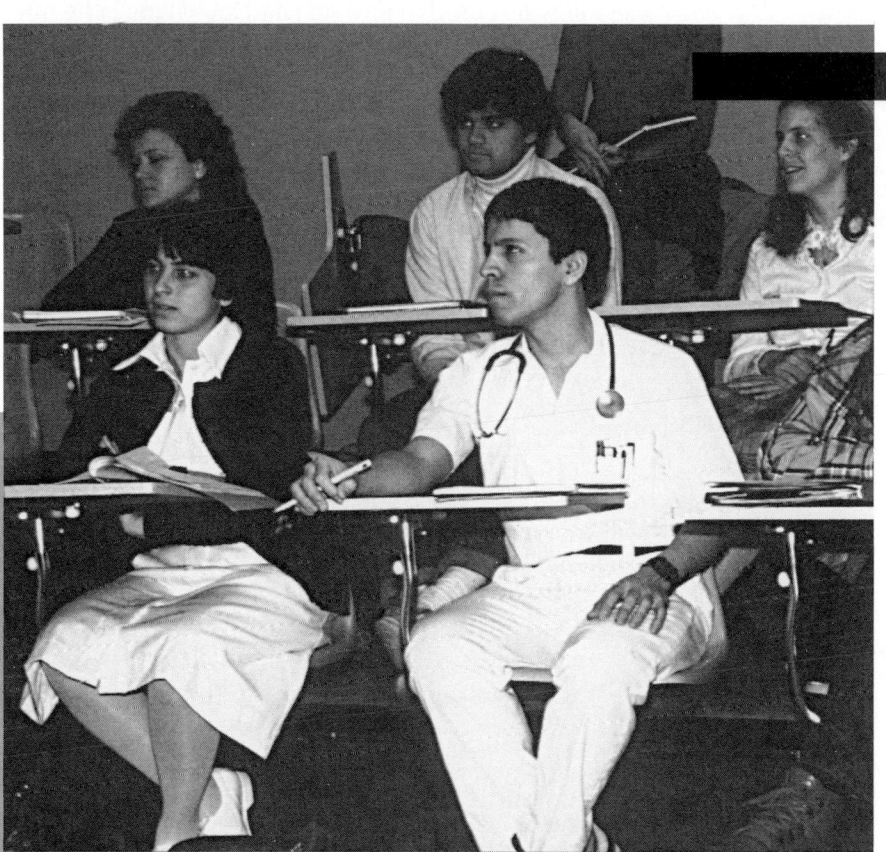

After studying this chapter, the learner should be able to

Define key terms used in the chapter.

Describe the underlying processes and characteristics of nursing theory.

Define the four common components of nursing theory.

Summarize the historical background, cultural influences, and value of nursing theory.

Discuss selected nursing theories, including definitions, assumptions, beliefs, and applications to nursing practice.

Nursing is a unique health-care discipline in which a service, based on knowledge and skill, is provided to others. Nursing therefore has two parts: (1) a body of knowledge and (2) the application of that knowledge through nursing practice. The body of knowledge, called a *knowledge base,* provides a rationale for everything that a nurse does. As you learn and practice nursing, you will use rationales from many different areas, such as anatomy, physiology, chemistry, nutrition, psychology, and sociology. You will also use a knowledge base and rationale developed *specifically for nurses,* allowing you to know what nursing care is and why and how it is given. This chapter discusses how the nursing knowledge base —also known as *nursing theory*—has been developed and how it is used to give safe and knowledgeable nursing care.

KEY TERMS

adaptation theory
concept
conceptual framework or
    model
developmental theory
environment
general systems theory
health
nursing
nursing theory
person
philosophy
process
theory

AN INTRODUCTION TO THEORY

Definitions

Each individual collects, organizes, and arranges facts to build a knowledge base that defines his or her personal reality. A similar organization and a structure of facts and events are present in large bodies of knowledge, through philosophies, concepts, theories, and processes.

Philosophy is the study of wisdom, fundamental knowledge, and the processes used to develop and construct our perceptions of life. Philosophy both provides a viewpoint and implies a system of values and beliefs. Each individual develops a personal philosophy to give meaning to experiences and to direct behavior and attitudes. A personal philosophy may be developed through learning from interpersonal relationships, formal and informal educational experiences, religious and cultural backgrounds, and from the environment.

The philosophy of each nurse and the philosophies of schools of nursing and of health-care institutions form the basis of giving nursing care. As nurses give care, teach, and work with others, they reflect both a personal and a professional philosophy through values and beliefs about concepts such as goodness, wellness, health, illness, accountability, and ethics. In the same way, nursing education and nursing practice settings provide education or client care based on philosophical beliefs about humans, health, teaching and learning, and standards of client care.

Concepts can be compared to ideas: they are abstract impressions from the environment organized into symbols of reality. Concepts describe objects, properties, and events, and the relationships among them. A group of concepts that follows an understandable pattern makes up a **conceptual framework** or **model.** Concepts can be thought of as the individual bricks and boards used to build a house, with the blueprint that specifies where each brick and board should go being the conceptual framework.

A **theory** is a group of concepts that form a pattern of reality. A theory is a statement that explains or characterizes a process, an occurrence, or an event, and is based on observed facts but lacks absolute or direct proof. Theories arrange a group of related statements or concepts in such a way as to give meaning to a series of events. Theories can be tested, changed, or used to guide research or to provide a base for evaluation. They are derived through two principal methods: *deductive reasoning,* in which a general idea is examined, after which specific actions or ideas are considered; or *inductive reasoning,* where the reverse process is used—a specific idea or action is identified, and then conclusions are made about general ideas. Nursing theorists use both of these methods.

A **process,** which is the action phase of a conceptual framework or a theory, is a series of actions, changes, or functions that bring about a desired result. During a process, systematic and continuous steps are taken to meet a goal, and both assessments and feedback are used to direct actions to meet the goal. A particular theory or conceptual framework with its own specific definitions directs the way in which these actions are carried out.

The nursing process consists of applied nursing theories and concepts. The delivery of nursing care within the nursing process is directed in an institution by specific conceptual frameworks and theories.

Nursing Theory

Nursing theory, as defined by Stevens (1984), "attempts to describe or explain the phenomenon (process, occurrence, or event) called nursing." Nursing theory differentiates nursing from other disciplines and activities in that it serves the purposes of describing, explaining, predicting, and controlling desired outcomes of nursing care practices.

Basic Processes in the Development of Nursing Theories

Nursing theories are often based on and influenced by other broadly applicable processes and theories. The ideas and principles of the theories that follow are basic to many nursing concepts and are a part of the nursing literature. It is important that nurses have an understanding of these theories and their terminologies in order to develop their own knowledge base in nursing. The following is a brief description of the major points of each theory.

General Systems Theory
General systems theory has been used by a wide range of disciplines since it emerged in the 1920s. Its primary theorist, Ludwig von Bertalanffy, developed the theory so that it could be universally applied. This theory explains the breaking of whole things into parts and then learning how the parts work together in "systems." It includes the relationship between the whole and the parts and defines concepts about how the parts will function and behave. These concepts may be applied to different kinds of systems, for example, to molecules in chemistry, cultures in sociology, organs in anatomy, and health in nursing.

Key points in general systems theory are

- A system is a set of interacting elements, all serving the common purpose of contributing to the overall goal of the system; the whole system is always greater than the sum of its parts.
- Systems are hierarchical in nature and are composed of interrelated subsystems that work together in such a way that a change in one element could affect other subsystems as well as the whole.
- *Boundaries* separate systems both from each other and from their environments.
- A system communicates with and reacts to its environment through processes that enter the system (input) or are transferred to the environment (output).
- An *open system* allows energy, matter, and information to move freely between systems and boundaries, whereas a *closed system* does not allow input from or output to the environment (no known closed systems exist in reality).
- To survive, open systems maintain balance through feedback.

Stress/Adaptation Theory
Adaptation theory defines adaptation as the adjustment of living matter to other living things and to environmental conditions. Adaptation is a dynamic or continuously changing process that effects change and involves interaction and response. Human adaptation occurs on three levels: the internal (self), the social (others), and the physical (biochemical reactions). See Chapter 9 for more information on stress and adaptation.

Developmental Theory
Developmental theory states that the process of growth and development of humans is orderly and predictable, beginning with conception and ending with death. Although the pattern is one of definite stages, the progress and behaviors of an individual within each stage are unique. The growth and development of an individual are influenced by heredity, temperament, emotional and physical environment, life experiences, and health status.

There are several theorists important to developmental theory, but two deserve brief mention here because their work is often used to develop nursing theory and to organize nursing practice. Eric Erikson based his *theory of psychosocial development* on the process of socialization, emphasizing how individuals learn to interact with the world. Erikson recognized the role of social, biologic, and environmental factors in development and defined specific tasks or conflicts to be accomplished or overcome during what he defined as the *eight stages of life*. More information on developmental theory is given in Chapter 10.

Abraham Maslow divided his *theory of human needs* by the physical and psychosocial needs considered essential to human life, rather than by chronologic age, as Erikson did. Maslow defined five levels of need (physiologic well-being; physical safety; affection, love, and relationships; self-esteem; and self-actualization) existing in a hierarchy, with several needs being able to exist simultaneously. More information on the theory of human needs is given in Chapter 7.

As you continue in your nursing education and practice, you will learn how systems, adaptation, and developmental theories are used in planning and giving holistic care to clients. The discussion of specific nursing theories will enable you to better understand the knowledge base used to develop the concepts unique to nursing.

Basic Characteristics of Nursing Theory

Although many authors have discussed nursing theory, materials by Torres (1985) and Chinn and Jacobs (1983) best define its basic characteristics. The five basic characteristics are described briefly below.

Nursing theories identify and define *interrelated concepts* specific to nursing and clearly state the relationship between these concepts. Nursing theories must be *logical in nature;* they should use orderly reasoning and describe relationships that are developed using a logical sequence. Theories must also be consistent with the basic assumptions used in their development. Nursing theories should be *simple and general;* simple terminology and broadly applicable concepts ensure their usefulness in a wide variety of nursing practice situations. Nursing theories should also *increase nursing's body of knowledge* by generating research. Finally, nursing theory should *guide and improve practice*. Theory in nursing is valuable in research, education, and practice, and guides nurses by providing a knowledge base, organizing concepts, providing guidelines for practice, and identifying nursing care goals.

Common Components in Theories of Nursing

There are four concepts common to nursing theory that influence and determine nursing practice: **person, environment, health,** and **nursing**. These concepts are defined and described by each nursing theorist, and although these concepts are common to all nursing theories, both the definitions and the relationships among them may differ greatly from one theory to an-

other (these are discussed in the second half of this chapter). Of the four concepts, the most important is that of the person. The focus of nursing, regardless of definition or theory, is the person.

NURSING THEORY AND NURSING PRACTICE

Why Do We Need Nursing Theories?

Historical Perspectives and Influences

Nightingale's Definition and Belief

Florence Nightingale, the nurse who established the theoretic base of nursing, developed and published a philosophy and a theory of health and nursing that has served as a solid foundation for the nursing profession. Her contributions to nursing theory (Dolan, 1978) include identifying the role of the nurse in meeting the client's personal needs; recognizing the importance of environmental influences on the care of the sick; elevating the standards and acceptance of nursing by developing sound principles of nursing education, as well as by demonstrating efficient and knowledgeable nursing care; defining nursing practice as separate and distinct from medical practice; and differentiating between health nursing and illness nursing.

Cultural Influences on Nursing

Certain cultural influences have affected nursing as we know it today. At various stages of history, nursing has been regarded with attitudes ranging from religious awe to complete contempt. Although since the beginning of time both men and women have given comfort and assistance to the sick, until the last two decades, nursing essentially had been considered "women's work." In the 18th and 19th centuries, women were viewed as subservient and inferior to men, but after Nightingale established an occupation for educated women and facilitated improved attitudes toward nursing, the role of the woman as nurse became more favorably accepted.

It must be remembered, however, that despite Nightingale's belief in the uniqueness of nursing, the training of nurses was carried out primarily under the direction and control of the medical profession (Kalish and Kalish, 1978). Because the basis for nursing practice came from outside the profession, nursing has struggled for years to establish its own identity and to receive recognition for its significant contributions to health care.

Nursing in the United States

Influences of Educational Frameworks on Nursing Practice

Most schools of nursing established in the United States were adapted from Nightingale's model. There was no planned educational curriculum; rather, learning came from lectures by physicians and by practical experience acquired through caring for the sick in the hospital (Dolan, 1978). This service orientation for nursing education remained the strongest influence on nursing practice until the 1950s. Rather than developing a body of knowledge specific to nursing, nursing care was carried out under the control and direction of the hospital administration and the physicians practicing in that hospital. Nursing care was based on traditional ideas about following orders, as well as on common wisdom about caring for others based on either "common sense" or widely accepted scientific principles (Chinn and Jacobs, 1983). It is no wonder that nursing knowledge remained undeveloped and fragmented for so long.

Developing a Scientific Base for Nursing

During the first half of the 20th century, a change in the structure of society resulted in a change of roles for women and in turn in nursing. As a result of the First and Second World Wars, women increasingly entered the work force, became more independent, and sought higher education. At the same time, nursing education began to focus on education instead of on training, and nursing research was performed and published. As women became more assertive, nursing's need for a clearly defined identity of unique contributions to the health-care system emerged. In the 1950s, the idea of nursing as a science became more generally accepted, and philosophical beliefs and a knowledge base for nursing practice began to evolve. The nursing practice used by nurses today is one that focuses more and more on giving effective client care based on sound rationales from nursing knowledge.

Evolution of Nursing Theory

Research and Publishing in Nursing

Beginning in the 1950s, as great advances were made in technology and medical research, nursing leaders realized that research into the practice of nursing was necessary to meet the health needs of modern society. Increasing numbers of nurses began to do nursing research and write articles telling other nurses how to carry out nursing research. The 1950s saw two major developments in nursing theory: the first research journal, *Nursing Research,* began publishing in 1950, and as ideas were published, they served as a basis for theory development (Kalish and Kalish, 1978; Chinn and Jacobs, 1983).

Educational Advances in Nursing

Beginning in the 1960s, college- and university-based baccalaureate programs in nursing began to increase in both number and enrollment. At the same time, master's and doctoral programs in nursing were established. This upward trend in education for nurses was reflected in the nursing literature, with more attention being given to the consideration and formulation of knowledge specific to nursing.

Value of Nursing Theory

Broad Goals of Nursing Theory. Nursing theory provides a rational and knowledgeable reason for nursing actions, based on organized, written descriptions of the reality of nursing. Additionally, nursing theory gives nurses the knowledge base necessary to act and react appropriately in nursing care situations; provides a base for discussion and, ideally, resolution of the issues in nursing today; allows the nurse who knows and practices theory to have better problem-solving skills, so that nursing actions are organized, considered, and purposeful; and prepares the nurse to question assumptions and values in nursing, thus further defining nursing and increasing the knowledge base.

Application to Practice. Nurses have difficulty agreeing on what nursing really is; however, if theory-based nursing is practiced, directions are provided that allow nurses to work toward a common goal, with the ultimate outcome being improved client care.

Improving and Facilitating Communication. Nursing is based on communication with others—clients, other members of the health-care team, members of the community— as well as with nurses practicing in a variety of specialty settings. Because concepts are both abstract and highly individualized, words used in communicating with others can be interpreted in many different ways. As ideas are developed and words are defined, nurses build a knowledge base and a common terminology to use in communicating with other professionals.

Improving Autonomy of Nursing. The term *autonomy* means being independent and self-governing. As a discipline, nursing is in the process of defining its own independent functions and contributions to health care. The development and use of nursing theory provide autonomy in several interdependent ways:

- Having a body of knowledge specific to the discipline allows members of that discipline to be viewed by others as experts; this, in turn, gives nurses authority to carry out actions.
- Actions carried out and based on sound rationale are trusted and respected.
- Nursing theory makes nursing care visible, leading to increased internal control by nurses.
- As nurses demonstrate that nursing care does indeed make a difference, and that nursing services are valuable, the discipline becomes more independent.

CONCEPTUAL AND THEORETICAL FRAMEWORKS FOR NURSING

Theorists and Their Models

The theories and conceptual models included here have been selected because they represent different approaches to defining the reality of nursing, and because they are used in a variety of educational, research, and practice settings. For each theory or model, a brief summary is given of its central theme, basic assumptions, definitions, and basic applications in nursing practice. Students who find a particular framework relevant and useful are encouraged to explore the literature to learn more about both the theorist and the theory.

Sister Calista Roy: Roy's Adaptation Model

Sister Calista Roy developed the adaptation model of nursing in 1964. This model is widely used as a philosophical base and conceptual model in nursing education. The adaptation model is essentially a systems model. The assumptions basic to this model are

- Each person is a biophysical being and an integrated whole. All body systems are balanced to produce a functioning person with biologic, psychosocial, and social needs. Constant interaction with the changing environment of the modern world subjects the person to continual changes and stressors.
- Each person uses both innate and acquired mechanisms to cope with changes and adapt individually, with either positive or negative responses. The adaptation level reached is the result of three classes of stimuli: the primary cause of the change, other situational factors, and beliefs and past experiences shaping the response.
- Each person responds to needs (requirements within the individual stimulating a response to maintain integrity) in one or more of four modes: physiologic, self-concept, role-function, and interdependent behaviors.
- Each person's position on the health–illness continuum changes in relation to the effectiveness of coping to maintain an adaptive state.

As defined by Roy, response to a decrease in body integrity creates a need state, and the individual responds with an act or behavior. The *physiologic* mode involves oxygenation and circulation, fluid and electrolyte balance, nutrition, rest and activity, and regulation of temperature, hormones, and sensory function. The *self-concept* mode is concerned with the perception of one's physical self and personal self, including personality, moral and ethical beliefs, and values. The *interdependence* mode involves social relationships, including both the need to be interdependent and the need for support by others. The *role-function* mode involves the behaviors of a person in each role taken on in life (Rambo, 1984).

In Roy's model, all nursing activity is aimed at promoting the individual's adaptation to health and illness in all four adaptive modes. This model guides the nurse in using observation and interviewing skills to make an individualized assessment of each person, and serves as a guide in planning and carrying out nursing actions.

Martha E. Rogers: Nursing—A Science of Unitary Man

Martha Rogers has written a complex theory of nursing. The goal of this theory is to develop a science of nursing that would provide a growing body of theoretical knowledge applicable in nursing practice to the achievement of meaningful service to humanity.

Rogers' theory is built on a knowledge base of the history of humanity and of the universe (anthropology, sociology, astronomy, religion, philosophy, history, and mythology). Based on the belief that human beings are the center of nursing's purpose, Rogers' theory considers the total individual, describing the human life process and explaining and predicting the nature and direction of human development. Both systems and developmental theories are a part of Rogers' theory.

Rogers' basic assumptions about humans are
- Humans are unified wholes that are more than a sum of their parts.
- Humans are constantly interacting with their environment.
- Anything that occurs in life is unique because no two things in life can ever be repeated in an identical manner or under identical circumstances.
- Humans develop patterns of behaving, and their behavior becomes predictable.
- Humans are distinctive in their capacity for abstract thought, imagery, and emotion.

Nursing concepts are derived and nursing science principles are identified from these five basic assumptions. Based on these assumptions, Rogers identifies "four building blocks":
- *Energy fields*—Both the human and the environment are viewed as energy fields; there is a constant exchange of energy between the two that is essential to life.
- *Openness*—This is based on the belief that the universe consists of open systems.
- *Pattern and organization*—These are identifying characteristics of the energy field that is undergoing continuous change.
- *Four-dimensionality*—This is a characteristic of both human and environmental fields.

Dorothy E. Johnson: Behavioral Systems Model

Dorothy Johnson believes that nursing care is directed toward caring for the whole patient to facilitate effective and efficient behaviors necessary to prevent illness. Her behavioral systems model integrates systems, developmental, and needs theories into a specific nursing focus. Johnson believes the four goals of nursing are to assist the person

- Whose behavior is commensurate with social demands
- Who is able to modify his behavior in ways that support biologic imperatives
- Who is able to benefit, to the fullest extent during illness, from the physician's knowledge and skill
- Whose behavior does not give evidence of unnecessary trauma as a result of illness

Johnson views nursing as being separate from medicine in that medicine focuses on pathologic changes in the ill person, whereas nursing focuses on the behaviors of the person. She sees nursing's role as being complementary to the medical role. Nurses, giving care, supply functional requirements to the patient through protection, nurturance, and stimulation. Humans are seen as individuals who act in ways that make up a behavioral system specific to each person. Within this behavioral system are seven interrelated subsystems. Changes in one subsystem affect all the others. The seven subsystems are

- *Attachment or affiliative:* This is the first behavioral subsystem to develop, initially allowing the infant to attach (bond) to a significant caregiver and continuing through life with other individuals. These attachments provide a sense of security.
- *Dependency:* These behaviors precipitate nurturing by others and result in approval, attention, and physical assistance.
- *Ingestive:* Behaviors surrounding the intake of food belong in this subsystem, including social and cultural factors.
- *Eliminative:* These behaviors are involved with the execretion of waste products from the body and also relate to physical control and social situations.
- *Sexual:* These are cultural and gender behaviors related to procreation and gratification.
- *Aggressive:* These behaviors are concerned with protection and self-preservation.
- *Achievement:* Behaviors that attempt to control the environment, including intellectual, physical, creative, mechanical, and social skills, belong in this subsystem.

Johnson believes that both the internal and external environments of the system need to be orderly and predictable to maintain homeostasis. If the subsystems are out of balance, "tension" and disequilibrium result. Nursing, as part of the external environment, can help the patient return to a state of balance.

Dorothea E. Orem: Self-Care Model

The nursing model of Dorothea Orem is based on the belief that the individual has a need for self-care actions and that nursing can assist in meeting that need to maintain life, health, and well-being. The model is widely used in all areas of nursing. Self-care, as defined by Orem, consists of the activities that individuals carry out on their own behalf. These actions are deliberate, having pattern and sequence, developed from day-to-day living. The ability of the individual to perform self-care is called *self-care agency* and is normally carried out by adults. Infants, children, the aged, the ill, and the disabled require complete care or help with self-care activities. Three categories of self-care requisites (the purposes of actions directed toward the provision of self-care) are

- *Universal self-care requisites:* These are common to all humans and are associated with maintaining life, health, and well-being. They include air, water, food, elimination, activity and rest, solitude and social interaction, prevention of hazards, and promotion of human functioning.
- *Developmental self-care requisites:* These include maintaining conditions to support life and human development.
- *Health deviation self-care:* This is required in illness, injury, or as a result of medical tests or treatments to correct the condition.

Orem defines the need for nursing as when a person has a health-related self-care deficit. The areas of nursing practice are

- Entering into and maintaining nurse–client relationships with individuals, families, or groups
- Determining if and how clients can be helped through nursing
- Responding to clients' requests and needs
- Giving direct help to clients and families.
- Coordinating and integrating nursing with the client's daily living, other health-care activities, and social or educational services required.

Orem has defined three nursing systems on the premise that the nursing system is dependent on the self-care needs and abilities of the client. In the first, the nurse gives total care to meet all needs. In the second, both the nurse and the client perform care measures. In the third, the client can carry out self-care activities but requires assistance.

Imogene M. King: Open Systems Framework

Imogene King developed both a conceptual framework (open systems) and a theory of goal attainment derived from the framework. Many sources were used to develop these bodies of knowledge.

Open Systems Framework

Assumptions basic to this framework are

- The focus of nursing is the care of human beings.
- Nursing's goal is the health of individuals and health care for groups.
- Human beings are in constant interaction with their environment.

Within the framework are three interacting systems, each of which is defined and has relevant concepts, as follows:

- *Personal systems:* Each individual is a personal system. The concepts defined in personal systems are perception, self, growth and development, body image, space, and time.
- *Interpersonal systems:* Interpersonal systems are formed as humans interact. The concepts are interaction, communication, transaction, role, and stress.
- *Social systems:* Social systems include families, religious groups, educational systems, work systems, and peer groups. The concepts are organization, authority, power, status, and decision making.

King developed the conceptual framework and defined the concepts based on the belief that the individual actively interacts with others and objects in the environment and is changed as a result of the experiences.

Theory of Goal Attainment

King describes her theory of goal attainment as the interpersonal system in which two people come together in a health-care organization to help or be helped to maintain a state of health that permits functioning in roles. A nurse (having special knowledge and skills) and a client (with knowledge of self and personal problems) interact to identify problems and to establish and achieve goals. Based on this theory, several propositions are given, including

1. If perceptual accuracy is present in nurse–client interactions, transactions will occur.
2. If nurse and client make transactions, goals are attained.
3. If goals are attained, effective nursing care will occur.
4. If nurses with special knowledge and skills communicate appropriate information to clients, mutual goal setting and goal attainment will occur.

Betty Neuman: Health-Care Systems Model

Neuman's model, called the *total person approach,* can be used to provide an organized approach to a variety of nursing problems and for understanding humans and their environment. The model focuses on the client system's reaction to stress and the factors of reconstitution or adaptation. The person is defined as an open system interacting with the environment. Surrounding each person are internal and external factors that are stressors. Over a lifetime, the person becomes a "normal line of defense" made of biologic, psychological, sociocultural, and developmental skills to deal with stressors. Stressors cause the line of defense to react or respond as the total person. The stressors may be extrapersonal, interpersonal, or intrapersonal. The effect of the stressors on the system is individualized and depends on such variables as the number of stressors, how long they last, and the system's coping skills.

Nursing interventions can be carried out on three preventive levels. When the stressor is identified but no reaction has occurred, interventions can decrease the degree of reaction or increase the line of defense. This is called *primary prevention.* When the reaction has already happened, *secondary prevention* is carried out, with interventions aimed at treating symptoms and reducing reactions. Following active treatment, *tertiary prevention* strengthens the lines of defense through education and uses the system's total resources to prevent further occurrences.

Myra E. Levine: Theory of Nursing

Myra Levine based her theory of nursing on the belief that the essence of nursing is human interaction. Assumptions that define the theory are

- *Condition:* Clients entering the health-care system are in a state of illness or altered health.
- *Responsibilities:* The nurse is responsible for recognizing the client's organismic response (changes in behavior or level of body function) as the client adapts or attempts to adapt to the environment (environment equals illness and nurse). The four levels of response are fear, stress, inflammatory, and sensory.
- *Functions:* Nursing functions include interventions to promote adaptation to illness and evaluation of interventions as supportive or therapeutic. Supportive interventions help maintain the present health state and prevent further illness. Therapeutic interventions promote healing and restore health.

The foundation for all nursing intervention, as defined by Levine, consists of four conservation (meaning to maintain balance) principles that support the goal of nursing, which is to maintain or restore a person to a state of health. The principles are

- *Conservation of energy*—Balancing energy intake and output to avoid excessive fatigue (rest, nutrition, exercise)
- *Conservation of structural integrity*—Maintaining or restoring the structure of the body (promoting healing)
- *Conservation of personal integrity*—Maintaining or restoring a sense of identity and self-worth (recognition of unique qualities)
- *Conservation of social integrity*—Recognizing the patient as a social being (especially with significant others)

Levine's theory is focused on one person—the client. This theory has major implications in acute-care settings, where nursing interventions are supportive or therapeutic.

Application of Conceptual and Theoretical Frameworks

The aims of nursing (described in Chap. 1) are the same for all the nursing theorists, but the values, assumptions, and beliefs individualize each theory's framework for giving nursing care. Table 4-1 summarizes the central theme and definitions of each of the nursing theories included in this chapter. A brief case study is given on page 56 to illustrate the application of these conceptual and theoretical frameworks in the practice of nursing; the nursing care focus of each of the theories as it would apply in this case study is then summarized.

TABLE 4-1
Theorists and Their Conceptual Models

Theorist	Central Theme	Definitions			
		Person	Environment	Health	Nursing
Roy's adaptation model	The person in constant interaction with a changing environment	A biopsychosocial being that is basically good	All the conditions, circumstances, and influences surrounding and affecting the development of organism(s)	A state or process of being or becoming an integrated and whole person	A theoretical system in which knowledge prescribes a process of analysis and action related to the care of the ill or potentially ill person
Rogers' science of unitary man	Unitary man and his life processes; nursing science	Human beings who are unified beings with individuality, in continuous exchange of energy with the environment	All of the patterns that exist external to the individual	Not specifically defined	An art and a science directed toward the unitary human and concerned with the nature and direction of human development
Johnson's behavioral systems model	The human as a behavioral system	Human beings with two major systems, biologic and behavioral	Society as the environment in which an individual exists, influencing the individual's behavior	Purposeful, adaptive responses (physical, mental, emotional, social) to internal and external stimuli in order to maintain balance and comfort	Primary goal is to foster balance within an individual, specific to the behavioral system, when illness occurs.
Orem's self-care model	Nursing and self-care activities	Human beings with physical, psychologic, interpersonal, and social components, meeting self-care needs through learned behavior	Modern society's values and expectations	Wellness in the integrity of the individual; illness results in the person's inability to maintain self-care.	The giving of direct assistance to a person who is unable to meet his own self-care needs, developed through nursing education and experiences
King's open systems framework and theory of goal attainment	Interrelationships of concepts and the process of human interactions	Human beings are open systems who are social, rational, perceiving, controlling, purposeful, and action and time oriented.	Not specifically defined	Dynamic life experience of a human being, implying continuous adjustment to stressors in the internal and external environment through optimal use of one's resources to achieve maximum potential for daily living	A process of human interactions between nurse and client whereby each perceives the other and the situation, and, through communication, together set goals, explore means, and agree on means to achieve goals
Neuman's health-care systems model	A health-care systems model for a total person approach to client problems	Each human is a total person as a client system and is a composite of biologic, psychologic, sociocultural, and developmental variables.	Those internal and external forces that surround humans and with which they constantly interact	Views health as levels of wellness or stable lines of defense	A unique profession, concerning itself with all the variables affecting human response to stressors, with a primary concern for the total person
Levine's theory of nursing	Conservation, the holistic person	A living being who continually interacts with his environments and adapts to change	The health-care system, including the nurse	Maintenance of the unity and integrity of the client	A discipline that focuses on the human being and the complexity of his relationships with the environment; the essence of nursing is human interaction.

C A S E   S T U D Y

Julie Smith is an 18-year-old college freshman. She has an academic scholarship and is active in music and art activities. When Julie came home for the winter vacation, her parents were alarmed to see her so thin. Her mother cooked all of Julie's favorite food, but Julie refused to eat more than a few bites, saying that she was "too fat."

Mrs. Smith finally convinced Julie to go to the doctor. The examination showed that Julie weighed only 85 pounds; she had lost more than 20 pounds in 4 months. After tests showed no disease process, Julie was diagnosed as having anorexia nervosa.

Using *Roy's model,* the nurse will focus on promoting Julie's adaptive responses to improve health. A nursing process will be utilized first to assess behaviors affecting Julie's health and then to make a nursing diagnosis, stating the desired adaptive behaviors. The goals of the nursing care plan are derived through mutual agreement with Julie. The nursing interventions planned and carried out are aimed at altering the environmental stimuli so that an adaptive response can be made or at increasing Julie's coping ability to make healthy adaptive responses.

When planning and giving nursing care to Julie using *Roger's theory,* the nurse must become an integral part of the environment that is focused on Julie as a whole person, working toward achieving optimal health. The plan of care is based on an analysis of Julie's interactions with the environment, including past and present experiences as well as behavioral patterns and developmental level. Nursing activities are directed toward modifying variations in the behavior patterns and life processes so that Julie can reach her total potential as a human being.

Based on *Johnson's model,* nursing care for Julie will initially focus on ineffective functioning within or between the behavioral subsystems. Planning and implementation are carried out by the nurse to give Julie external support necessary to modify her behaviors, return to a state of equilibrium, and regain effective functioning of her whole system.

Using *Orem's framework,* the nurse must first assess and analyze Julie's inability to maintain therapeutic self-care through her own self-care agency. Self-care deficits are identified to determine why nursing is needed. Based on this information, the nurse designs a system that will be most effective in overcoming the self-care deficits. The nurse then implements the system to help Julie change conditions in herself or in her environment, and meet her self-care requirements.

Based on *King's theory,* nursing care for Julie utilizes communications and mutual participation in the plan of care. The nurse and Julie mutually interact to identify problems, set goals, and carry out planned activities. An effective plan of care will result in Julie's self-fulfillment and health maintenance.

Using *Neuman's model,* the plan of care for Julie is based on a total person approach. Assessments and interventions will focus on Julie's perceptions, responses, and resources relative to stressors in her environment and to the variables affecting her responses. Goals and interventions are mutually designed for all three levels of preventive nursing care: strengthening the flexible line of defense, facilitating wellness, and maintaining a maximum level of wellness. Nursing interventions should reduce the degree of Julie's reaction to stressors.

Levine's theory emphasizes the nurse's interventions necessary to help Julie adapt to and reach a state of health. A holistic assessment of Julie will provide information about strengths and weaknesses and allow a nursing diagnosis. The plan of care includes supportive or therapeutic interventions that are evaluated in terms of their effect on Julie's health status.

In conclusion, the application of conceptual and theoretical frameworks of nursing provides a focus for nursing care activities. The person receiving care is the central theme, but the way each theorist defines that person, the environment, health, and nursing gives the methodology of nursing a unique focus specific to a particular theory or model. The ultimate goal of each, however, is holistic client care, individualized to meet needs, prevent illness, and promote wellness.

K E Y   P O I N T S

■ Nursing is both a body of knowledge and the application of that knowledge through nursing practice.

■ Large bodies of knowledge organize and structure facts and events into philosophies, concepts, and theories. These bodies of knowledge are put into action by a process. In nursing, this is the nursing process.

■ Nursing theory describes or explains nursing and usually includes the concepts of person, environment, health, and nursing.

■ Nursing theories are often based on other processes and theories, including general systems, adaptation, and human development.

- Nursing theories define concepts and relationships specific to nursing, using orderly reasoning and logical sequence. They should be both understandable and widely applicable.

- Nursing theories provide for the improvement of nursing practice through nursing research.

- Florence Nightingale's philosophy and theory of nursing provided the base for modern nursing.

- Changes in society during the 20th century led to improvement and advances in nursing education, nursing research, and nursing practice.

- Nursing theory provides rationale for nursing actions, gives direction to all aspects of nursing, improves communications, and provides autonomy for the profession of nursing.

- Individual theories and conceptual models provide an organizing framework that can be applied to nursing practice.

BIBLIOGRAPHY

Chinn P, Jacobs M: Theory and Nursing: A Systematic Approach. St Louis, CV Mosby, 1983

Dolan J: Nursing in Society: A Historical Perspective, 14th ed. Philadelphia, WB Saunders, 1978

Fawcett J: Analysis and Evaluation of Conceptual Models of Nursing. Philadelphia, FA Davis, 1984

George J (ed): Nursing Theories: The Base for Professional Practice. (The Nursing Theories Conference Group). Englewood Cliffs, NJ, Prentice-Hall, 1985

Kalish P, Kalish B: The Advance of American Nursing. Boston, Little, Brown & Co, 1978

Kim H: The Nature of Theoretical Thinking in Nursing. Norwalk, CT, Appleton-Century-Crofts, 1983

McCann/Flynn J, Heffron P: Nursing from Concept to Practice. Bowie, MD, Robert J Brady, 1984

Orem D (ed): Concept Formalization in Nursing: Process and Product, 2nd ed. (The Nursing Development Conference Group). Boston, Little, Brown & Co, 1979

Rambo B: Adaptation Nursing: Assessment and Intervention. Philadelphia, WB Saunders, 1984

Riehl J, Roy C: Conceptual Models for Nursing Practice, 2nd ed. Norwalk, CT, Appleton-Century-Crofts, 1980

Stevens B: Nursing Theory: Analysis, Application, Evaluation, 2nd ed. Boston, Little, Brown & Co, 1984

Stevens B: Theory Development: What, Why, How? New York, National League for Nursing, 1978

Thibodeau J: Nursing Models: Analysis and Evaluation. Monterey, CA, Wadsworth Health Sciences Division, 1983

Torres G: In George J (ed): Nursing Theories: The Base for Professional Practice. (The Nursing Theories Conference Group). Englewood Cliffs, NJ, Prentice-Hall, 1985

Whaley L, Wong D: Nursing Care of Infants and Children. St Louis, CV Mosby, 1987

SUGGESTED READINGS

Johnson D: The nature of a science of nursing. Nurs Outlook 7(5), May, 1959

King I: Toward a Theory for Nursing: General Concepts of Human Behavior. New York, John Wiley & Sons, 1971

King I: A Theory of Nursing Systems, Concepts, Process. New York, John Wiley & Sons, 1981

LeVine M: Introduction to Clinical Nursing, 2nd ed. Philadelphia, FA Davis, 1973

Neuman B: The Neuman Systems Model: Application to Nursing Education and Practice. East Norwalk, CT, Appleton-Century-Crofts, 1982

Orem D: Nursing: Concepts of Practice, 2nd ed. New York, McGraw-Hill, 1980

Rogers M: The Theoretical Basis of Nursing. Philadelphia, FA Davis, 1970

Roy Sr C: Introduction to Nursing: An Adaptation Model, 2nd ed. Englewood Cliffs, NJ, Prentice-Hall, 1984

5 Values and Ethics in Nursing

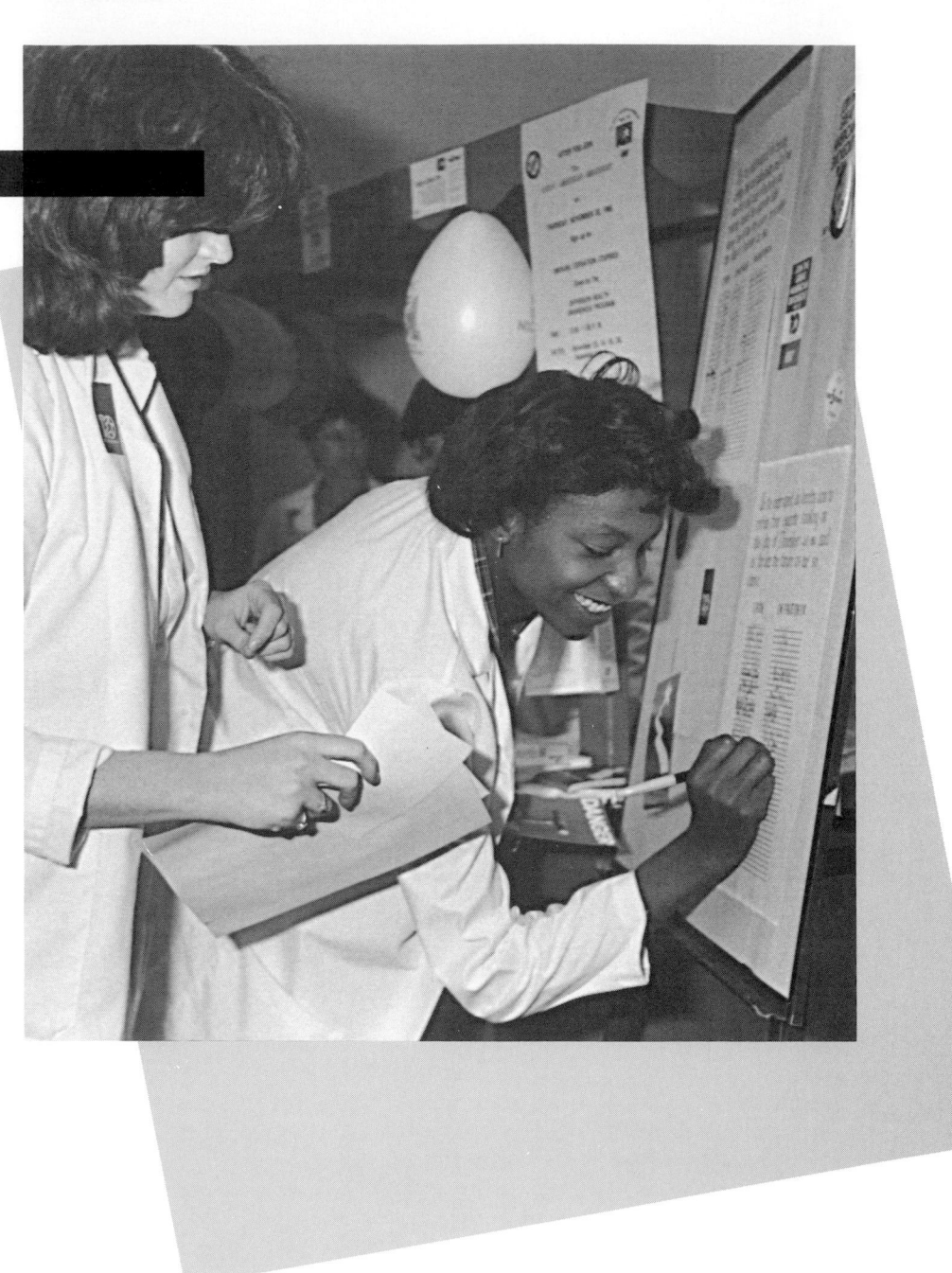

OBJECTIVES

After studying this chapter the learner will be able to

Define key terms used in the chapter.

Explain how the six basic value orientations can result in persons in the same situation responding differently.

Identify five common modes of value transmission.

Identify the seven basic values essential in the practice of nursing.

Describe the seven steps in the valuing process.

Utilize values clarification strategies in clinical practice.

Describe professional ethical conduct.

Describe how different sources of moral authority may reach different decisions regarding ethical problems.

Recognize ethical issues as they arise in nursing practice.

Utilize a nursing code of ethics to guide nursing actions.

Utilize an ethical framework/model to assist in the assessment and resolution of ethical dilemmas.

Respect valid alternatives for solving the ethical problems that arise in clinical practice.

The unique nature of nursing places nurses at the bedside and in groups of professionals where sensitive decisions are made about the best way to treat illness and solve health-care problems. Often the question confronting the nurse is not "how to" but rather "should I?" The more science and technology increase the options available to clients and health-care professionals, the more frequently nurses will find themselves asking "just because we can do this, *should we,* here and now, for this client?" The answer to this and other ethical questions is too important for the nurse to base on some intuitive, opinionated, or self-imposed sense of right and wrong.

This chapter explores the influence of values on human behavior and the ethical dimensions of nursing practice. Nurses who understand how clients' values and their own values shape nurse–client interactions and who continually develop sensitivity to the ethical dimensions of nursing practice are best able to provide quality care.

VALUES

A **value** may be defined as a personal belief about worth that acts as a standard to guide one's behavior. A **value system** is an organization of values in which each value is ranked along a continuum of importance; a value system often operates as a personal code of conduct.

Since attitudes and beliefs also influence human behavior, it is important to distinguish them from values. An **attitude** is a feeling or an emotion, generally including positive or negative judgment, toward persons, objects, or ideas. **Beliefs** refer to a special class of intellectual attitudes based primarily on faith as opposed to fact.

A person's values influence beliefs about human needs, health, and illness; the practice of health behaviors; and human responses to illness. Nurses who work effectively with clients are sensitive to how a client's values and their own values influence their interactions.

Types of Values

There are six basic types of values underlying a person's interests and motives (Feldman and Newcomb, 1969):

- *Theoretical:* The theoretical person values truth and tends to be empirical, critical, and rational.
- *Economic:* The economic person is interested in what is practical and useful.
- *Aesthetic:* The aesthetic person values beauty, form, and harmony.
- *Social:* The social person values human beings in terms of love and is kind, sympathetic, and unselfish.
- *Political:* The political person values power.
- *Religious:* The religious person values unity.

Although each person's value orientation is a unique blend of these six types of values, one of the types

KEY TERMS

advocacy

attitude

autonomy

beliefs

beneficence

confidentiality

ethics

fidelity

justice

morals

nonmaleficence

utilitarianism

value

value system

values clarification

veracity

usually predominates. Table 5-1 illustrates different nursing responses to the problem of understaffing based on these value types. Identifying one's own orientation as well as that of others helps the nurse understand how people perceive situations differently and choose different courses of action.

Development of Values

An individual is not born with values. Rather, values are formed over a lifetime from information from environment, family, and culture. As a child observes actions he quickly learns what has high and low value for family

T A B L E 5-1

Basic Value Types and Related Interest and Motives

Situation: Nurses on a 21-bed surgical unit are upset because at the present time nursing management has no plans to replace two full-time nurses who transferred out of the unit. Understaffing has resulted in the other nurses frequently being asked to work extra shifts.

Nurse/Value Orientation	Interests/Motives
Nurse 1	
Theoretical orientation	"Let's begin keeping some data . . . how many clients, what level of nursing care they need, how many nurses are on duty each shift, how often we work doubles. . . . If we've got the figures to prove we can't give quality care while understaffed this way (that clients are actually at risk), management will have to listen!"
Nurse 2	
Economic orientation	Leaves work promptly at the end of the shift: "I do the best I can and then I go home and forget about this place. It's just a job. If it gets much worse I'll find a better job somewhere else."
Nurse 3	
Aesthetic orientation	Lives one day at a time and judges each day on its own merit; responsible for many environmental improvements at the nurse's station and lounge.
Nurse 4	
Social orientation	Consistently stays overtime, without pay, to complete what hasn't been finished during shift; will agree to work extra shifts, even when too tired, because of perceived client need; excellent candidate for burnout. "We've just got to find a way to give better care or die trying. The clients should be getting better care."
Nurse 5	
Political orientation	"The longer we put up with these working conditions, the longer we'll have them. I say we need action and we need it now. If we could just unite we'd make them listen to us fast!"
Nurse 6	
Religious orientation	Quiet source of strength and encouragement for both colleagues and clients. "There seems to be an awful lot wrong with the system and no one is happy. Let's each see what we can do, as individuals and together, to improve things."

members. If mother spends a good portion of each day cooking and the family sits around the table eating and talking for a long time, the child learns to value food and the good times it represents. Similarly, the child learns helpfulness is a good and respected quality if praised when helping parents, grandparents, and siblings.

Common modes of value transmission are

- *Modeling:* The child learns what is of high or low value by observing parents, peers, and significant others. Thus, modeling may lead to socially acceptable or unacceptable behavior.
- *Moralizing:* The child is taught a complete value system by parents or an institution (church, school) that allows little opportunity for the child to weigh different values.
- *Laissez-faire:* The child is left to explore values (no one set of values is presented as best for all) and to develop a personal value system. This approach is often accompanied by little or no guidance and can lead to confusion and conflict.
- *Rewarding and punishing:* The child is rewarded when demonstrating values held by parents and punished when demonstrating unacceptable values.
- *Responsible choice:* The child is encouraged to explore different values and to weigh their consequences. Support and guidance are offered as the child develops a personal value system.

Values Essential to the Professional Nurse

In 1985 the American Association of Colleges of Nursing undertook a project that included the identification of values essential to the practice of professional nursing. The group identified seven values (altruism, aesthetics, equality, freedom, human dignity, justice, truth) and related attitudes and personal qualities. These are defined, along with examples, in Table 5-2.

Several researchers have studied the values of nursing students. One study comparing selected values of students entering nursing in 1982 with those of students who entered nursing in 1972 discovered that the three highest value scales for both groups were social (highest in both groups), religious (ranked second in 1982 and third in 1972), and aesthetic. The 1982 students also scored significantly higher on economic values than did the 1972 students (Garvin and Boyle, 1985).

Many values underlie a person's selection of nursing as a career, including serving others, respect, glamour, drama, autonomy, independence–dependence, authority, creativity, financial security, status, education, work, traditions, health, physicians, marriage, responsibility (Steele and Harmon, 1983). To a large extent a nurse's satisfaction with nursing is based on the degree to which the experience of nursing matches expectations. The nurse who values independence and feels qualified to direct many aspects of client care may become discouraged quickly if practicing in a setting that is heavily physician dominated.

Value Neutrality

In an effort to encourage health-care professionals to respect and accept the individuality of clients, some educators have advised that professionals be "value-neutral" and "nonjudgmental" in their professional roles. Thus the nurse has a "commitment to clients whether or not the nurse and the clients hold the same values. The nurse does not assume that personal values are right and should not judge the client's values as right or wrong depending on their congruence with the nurse's personal value system" (Steel and Harmon, 1983, p 27). This kind of thinking enables a nurse to care for a client with different values. For example, a nurse who strongly believes that any premarital or extramarital sex is wrong may offer competent and compassionate nursing care to a young prostitute with active herpes lesions. On the other hand, if the same client, following education, indicates that she is unconcerned about whom she might infect in future sexual encounters, the nurse is in no way bound to be nonjudgmental about this response. In this case, it would not be morally permissible for the nurse to view this behavior with indifference. Because not all values are equal, nurses may have a moral obligation to respond to a client's value that may cause harm to the client or others.

Values Clarification

Values clarification is a process by which persons come to understand their own values and value system. "It is a process of discovery and allows the person to discover through feelings and analysis of behavior what choices to make when alternatives are presented, and to identify whether or not these choices are rationally made or are the result of previous conditioning" (Steele and Harmon, 1983, p 13). Values clarification has a beneficial application to nursing.

Values theorists most often describe the process of valuing as having seven steps centered on three main activities: choosing, prizing, and acting (Raths et al, 1978; Simon, 1972). When one values something, one

Chooses:
  (1) freely
  (2) from alternatives
  (3) after careful consideration of the consequences of each alternative

Prizes:
  (4) with pride and happiness
  (5) with public affirmation

Acts:
  (6) with incorporation of the choice into one's behavior
  (7) with consistency and regularity on the value

Values Clarification by the Nurse

For example, if respect for human dignity is a value that characterizes your nursing practice, you

TABLE 5-2
Essential Values, Attitudes, and Personal Qualities of the Professional Nurse

Essential Values*	Examples of Attitudes and Personal Qualities	Examples of Professional Behaviors
1. Aesthetics		
Qualities of objects, events, and persons that provide satisfaction	Appreciation Creativity Imagination Sensitivity	Adapts the environment so it is pleasing to the patient/client Creates a pleasant work environment for self and others Presents self in a manner that promotes a positive image of nursing
2. Altruism		
Concern for the welfare of others	Caring Commitment Compassion Generosity Perseverance	Gives full attention to the patient/client when giving care Assists other personnel in providing care when they are unable to do so Expresses concern about social trends and issues that have implications for health care
3. Equality		
Having the same rights, privileges, or status	Acceptance Assertiveness Fairness Self-esteem Tolerance	Provides nursing care based on the individual's needs irrespective of personal characteristics† Interacts with other providers in a nondiscriminatory manner Expresses ideas about the improvement of access to nursing and health care
4. Freedom		
Capacity to exercise choice	Confidence Hope Independence Openness Self-direction Self-discipline	Honors individual's right to refuse treatment Supports the rights of other providers to suggest alternatives to the plan of care Encourages open discussion of controversial issues in the profession
5. Human dignity		
Inherent worth and uniqueness of an individual	Consideration Empathy Humaneness Kindness Respectfulness Trust	Safeguards the individual's right to privacy Addresses individuals as they prefer to be addressed Maintains confidentiality of patients/clients and staff Treats others with respect regardless of background

(Continued)

TABLE 5-2
Essential Values, Attitudes, and Personal Qualities of the Professional Nurse (Continued)

Essential Values*	Examples of Attitudes and Personal Qualities	Examples of Professional Behaviors
6. Justice		
Upholding moral and legal principles	Courage Integrity Morality Objectivity	Acts as a health-care advocate Allocates resources fairly Reports incompetent, unethical, and illegal practice objectively and factually*
7. Truth		
Faithfulness to fact or reality	Accountability Authenticity Honesty Inquisitiveness Rationality Reflectiveness	Documents nursing care accurately and honestly Obtains sufficient data to make sound judgments before reporting infractions of organizational policies Participates in professional efforts to protect the public from misinformation about nursing

* The values are listed in alphabetic rather than priority order.

† From Code for Nurses, American Nurses' Association, 1976.

(Printed with permission from Essentials of College and University Education for Professional Nursing. Washington, DC, American Association of Colleges of Nursing, 1986)

1. Freely choose to believe in the worth and uniqueness of each individual
2. Realize that you have other options (that you could treat with human dignity only those persons who are most like you)
3. Believe that respecting each person's human dignity yields the best consequences for you and for all of society
4. Feel proud and happy with your choice (you especially enjoy when clients let you know they appreciate your care and when nursing colleagues and supervisors compliment you on interpersonal skills)
5. Are able to defend this value when someone's human dignity is being ignored
6. Incorporate this value into your practice
7. Attempt consistently to respect human dignity in both your personal and professional life

As you become more conscious of this value you will be sensitive to those of your actions that are not consistent with it. You may feel uncomfortable after gossiping with other nurses during break about a client no one likes; you realize that this behavior contradicts your basic respect for human dignity. Thus, values clarification is a "process by which we increase the likelihood that our living in general, and a decision in particular [to respect human dignity], will, first, have a positive value for us, and, second, for the society we serve" (Kirschbaum, 1977).

The nurse interested in values clarification strategies is referred to the book by Steele and Harmon (1983), who offer numerous exercises for nurses seeking to clarify their personal and professional values, and to the article by Uustal (1978), who offers ten strategies "designed to increase your awareness and appreciation of yourself, and to explore selected values conflicts and ethical dilemmas in nursing."

Clinical Applications

Unless the nurse is comfortable with change and believes that health is important enough to merit learning a new treatment regimen, client education is doomed to failure. Table 5-3 illustrates how the steps in the valuing process can be used to assist a client with high blood pressure take charge of his health and manage his medications. Other clinical examples follow.

Client Places Low Value on Health and Health Behaviors. You become frustrated when repeated attempts to teach/counsel a 26-year-old pharmaceutical salesman

T A B L E   5-3
Examples of the Valuing Process

Steps in the Valuing Process	Examples
Chooses	
1. Choosing freely	Client, rehospitalized for high blood pressure after he abruptly stopped taking his antihypertensive medication, decides from now on to take his medication as prescribed.
2. Choosing from alternatives	After teaching–learning session with the nurse the client understands he has basically three options: 1. Comply with prescribed treatment regimen 2. Refuse to take medication but try harder to control his pressure through diet, exercise, stress management 3. Refuse to take medication and assume a "we'll see" attitude
3. Choosing after consideration of the consequences	Client understands that the *probable* consequences of the above options are 1. Compliance with treatment regimen will yield best control of high blood pressure (may cause some annoying side-effects). 2. Diet, exercise, and stress management may reduce his blood pressure somewhat but did not yield sufficient control in the past. 3. High blood pressure may result in serious complications, such as stroke, kidney disease, or impaired vision.
Prizes	
4. With pride and happiness	Client states "now that I understand high blood pressure better and know what I can do to control it, I feel more in charge of my life—and I like that!"
5. With public affirmation	Client states to wife "I guess I was wrong to stop taking that medicine when I blamed it for how lousy I was feeling. You can bet that won't happen again. If you ever hear me complaining about my pills, remind me to see my doctor right away."
Acts	
6. With incorporation of the choice into one's behavior	Client takes medication as prescribed following discharge from hospital.
7. With consistency and regularity on the value	Client seeks to understand any new medication he is prescribed (reason for the medication, possible side-effects, consequences of noncompliance) and successfully manages treatment regimen; he feels proud of his new knowledge and self-care abilities.

(Steps in the valuing process are adapted from Raths, LE: Values and Teaching. Columbus, Ohio, Charles E Merrill Books, 1966.)

meet with failure. Although hospitalized with a serious duodenal ulcer, all he can talk about is his job and meeting his sales quota.

Values Clarification. First help this client identify his basic life values. Ask him "What three things are most important to you in life?" or have him rank the following behaviors in terms of how he would most likely spend an unexpected free day:

____ Enjoy some quiet time alone (thinking, reading, listening to music)

____ Spend time with family, friends

____ Do something active (hiking, play ball, swimming)

____ Watch television

____ Volunteer time and energy to help someone else

____ Use time for my job

____ Other _____

Discuss what these rankings indicate about his values. Determine whether his rankings would be different if he were asked how he *wished* he would spend the free day versus how he would most *likely* spend it.

Choosing. After exploring with this client how values might affect other aspects in his life (*e.g.,* long-term effects of stress related to his present preoccupation with job performance), counsel him to choose his key values freely. It would be a positive sign if health were among these values, but it might not be.

Prizing. Use affirmation to reinforce the client's wellness-promoting values and when possible enlist the support of family members. "Your wife seemed so happy yesterday when you told her you decided to quit smoking. You can see how much she loves you and values your health."

Acting. Assist the client to *plan* new behaviors consistent with the values he has chosen and to think of ways they can be incorporated into his life. "Once you get home, how will your life be different?" "You said you wanted to begin to take time for yourself—how are you going to do this?"

Values of Client and Family Members Conflict. You sense a growing tension while counseling the young parents of a child with asthma. Questioning ("You seem uncomfortable with what I'm saying now. Is there something wrong?") reveals that the wife is a confirmed smoker and cat lover who has told her husband that even if these behaviors are hurting their child, she is unwilling to give them up.

Values Clarification. Suggest that both parents complete the "values voting" exercise below and then share with one another what factors influence their behavior.

Where do you stand on the following issues? (Indicate your responses in the following manner: **SA,** strongly agree; **A,** agree; **D,** disagree; **SD,** strongly disagree; **U,** undecided.)

____ A parent's primary obligation is to meet the needs of his/her child.

____ Each member of a family is entitled to pursue personal pleasures—even if these are not in the best interest of all.

____ Pleasure is more important than health.

____ The choices one family member makes can dramatically affect other family members (positively and negatively).
(Format adapted from Uustal, 1978)

This exercise will help the parents to evaluate their basic values, explore areas of conflict, and, it is hoped, move toward joint *choosing, prizing,* and *acting on* several health-promoting values.

ETHICS

Ethics is a system dealing with professional standards of behavior related to what is right and wrong. **Morals,** although similar in meaning to ethics, usually refers to personal standards. Ethical conduct, then, is behavior conforming to accepted professional standards of conduct.

In a national study of baccalaureate nursing students prior to graduation and one year after graduation (Cassells et al, 1986), 72% of respondents reported having been involved in an ethical issue in clinical practice. In order of frequency, these issues were

- Clients refusing treatment (73%)
- Moral dilemmas in caring for clients with a poor prognosis (72%)
- Issues regarding resuscitation or discontinuation of lifesaving treatment (67%)
- Issues of informed consent (54%)
- Evaluation of client's competency to make own decisions (50%)
- Issues regarding withholding information from clients (46%)
- Allocation of care resources (12%)

Rather than providing clear-cut answers for resolving ethical problems, ethics offers the nurse a means of evaluating alternative courses of action using basic moral principles. The more complex the dilemma, the more likely it is that several courses of action can be justified as being morally right.

Professional Ethical Conduct

Nurses, in their quest for high-quality care of clients, determine and clarify their values, develop ethical behavior, and learn ethical decision-making skills. Where do nurses learn these ethical standards? The study of ethical behavior begins in nursing school, and ethical conduct is further developed in group discussions with colleagues and peers. Other sources are codes of ethics and various bills of rights that have emerged over the last decade or so. Some of the sources for developing ethical nursing conduct are discussed here.

Sources of Moral Authority

Today's society recognizes and respects many sources of moral authority: clients, family members, physicians and other health-care providers, institutions, ethics committees, and the public. Problems arise when different sources of moral authority reach different decisions about the course of right action. For example, if an alert client with a terminal illness decides that he has suffered long enough and requests his physician to administer a lethal dose of narcotic, the following sources may be involved:

- Sole moral authority for decision making may be placed in the hands of *either* the client or the physician.
- Family members may become involved in the decision-making process.
- Other health-care professionals (nurses, spiritual counselors, social workers, etc.) may become involved.
- The institution might decide the course of right action based on institutional policy.
- An institutional ethics committee could become involved as a consulting or decision-making body.

The President's Commission for the Study of Ethical Problems in Medicine and Biomedical and Behavioral Research (1982) rejects placing absolute authority for decisions in the hands of either the client or physician and calls instead for mutual participation, respect, and shared decision-making by clients and professionals. Nurses can contribute much to the decision-making process because the nature of the nurse–client relationship often gives them more intimate knowledge of the client than any other health-care professional.

Nursing Codes of Ethics

A professional code of ethics provides a framework for making ethical decisions and sets forth professional expectations. Nursing codes of ethics inform both nurses and society of the primary goals and values of the profession. Reflected in the codes are universal moral principles such as **respect for persons, autonomy** (self-determination), **beneficence** (doing good), **nonmaleficence** (avoiding harm), **veracity** (truth-telling), **confidentiality** (respecting privileged information), **fidelity** (keeping promises), and **justice** (treating people fairly). These principles should be compatible with the nurse's personal value system and moral code. Other functions of professional nursing codes include

- Indicating nursing's acceptance of the responsibility and trust with which it has been invested by society
- Providing guidance for conduct and relationships in carrying out nursing responsibilities consistent with the ethical obligations of the profession and with high quality in nursing care
- Providing a means for the exercise of professional self-regulation

(American Nurses' Association, 1985)

Codes are effective in accomplishing their goals only to the extent that they are upheld by members of the profession. Code requirements may exceed legal requirements. While violations of the law subject a nurse to civil or criminal liability (see Chap. 6), violations of the code of ethics may result in reprimands, censure, suspension, and expulsion.

Codes of ethics for nursing include the International Council of Nurses (ICN) Code for Nurses (adopted in 1953 and revised in 1965 and 1973), the American Nurses' Association (ANA) Code for Nurses (adopted in 1950 and revised in 1968, 1976, and 1985), and the Canadian Nurses' Association (CNA) Code of Ethics for Nursing (adopted in 1980 and revised in 1985). Ethical statements in the codes are given on pages 68 and 69.

The Patient's Bill of Rights

The American Hospital Association described A Patient's Bill of Rights (see p 70) in 1973. The bill of rights includes the rights and responsibilities of the client while receiving care in the hospital. A number of other bills of rights have emerged in recent years, such as the Pregnant Patient's Bill of Rights, the Indian Patient's Bill of Rights, a Nursing Home Bill of Rights, and the Veterans Administration Code of Patient Concern. Each of these emphasizes a specific aspect of client rights within a particular health agency. These bills of rights imply a code of ethics the nurse observes professionally.

Advocacy

Nursing has traditionally held that its primary commitment is to the client and more recently has claimed client advocacy as a legitimate nursing role. **Advocacy** is the protection and support of another's rights (it is discussed in Chap. 22). Nurses who wish to practice in this tradition

- Ensure that their loyalty to an employing institution or to a physician does not compromise their primary commitment to the client
- When making an ethical decision, place more weight on the good to be produced for the *individual client* than on the greatest good for the greatest number (**utilitarianism**)
- In each situation, carefully evaluate the competing claims of autonomy (self-determination) and client well-being

When respecting autonomy, the nurse respects and supports the client's right to make decisions. When promoting client well-being, the nurse acts in the best interests of the client. Ideally both autonomy and client well-being are promoted in each nurse–client interaction but conflicts sometimes arise. For instance, if an elderly male client with a serious chronic lung disease, who understands full well the danger of smoking asks the nurse to get him a pack of cigarettes, the nurse must decide whether to respect his autonomy and follow his wishes or to promote his well-being. Nurses sensitive to the need to promote both client autonomy and well-being may often experience conflict, but they are more likely than other nurses to succeed in securing the client's genuine best interests.

Types of Moral and Ethical Problems

As mentioned at the beginning of this discussion on ethics, the nurse in clinical practice is actively involved in resolving ethical issues. Jameton (1984) describes three types of moral and ethical problems faced by nurses (see Table 5-4):

- *Moral uncertainty,* where the nurse is unsure of which moral principles or values apply
- *Moral dilemmas,* where two (or more) clear moral principles apply but support mutually inconsistent courses of action
- *Moral distress,* where the nurse knows the right thing to do but institutional constraints make it nearly impossible to pursue the right actions

Moral and ethical problems may arise between nurses and clients, nurses and physicians, and nurses and other nurses.

Nurses and Clients

Troublesome nurse–client situations that can result in ethical distress for nurses include difficulty identifying the nurse's primary client, paternalism (supplying needs or regulating conduct of clients), deception, confidentiality, allocation of scarce nursing resources, informed consent, and conflicts between the client's and nurse's interests.

Difficulty Identifying Primary Client.   When admission of a child with acquired immunodeficiency syndrome (AIDS) to a large elementary school results in furor, the school nurse has obligations to the child with AIDS, to the other children in the school, and to teachers and staff. If the interests of these groups conflict, the nurse must decide whose interests take precedence.

Paternalism.   An alert elderly client who is at high risk of falling refuses to call the nurse for assistance getting out of bed. The nurse must decide whether to obtain an order to restrain the client. Does preventing potential harm justify violating the client's right to autonomy (self-determination) and make it acceptable for the nurse to act as a "parent" and choose an action the client does not want because it is believed to be in the client's best interest?

Deception.   A postoperative client asks the student nurse who is about to administer an intramuscular injection for pain "Is this your first shot?" It is the student's first injection and the student is anxious. Would the student's intent to decrease the client's anxiety justify telling the client "No, I've given several before"?

Confidentiality.   A nurse asks a middle-aged woman who is crying quietly "Would you like to share what's troubling you?" The woman tells the nurse she has no idea how she will pay for this hospitalization because she entered the country illegally two months ago and is trying to earn enough money to help her family back home. She begs the nurse not to tell anyone. If the nurse believes this anxiety is interfering with the client's recovery, would it be ethical to break the woman's confidence to obtain help for her?

Allocation of Scarce Nursing Resources.   A nurse has just been pulled from your unit, leaving it understaffed. Among your clients are a 33-year-old man recovering from a serious heart attack who is being discharged in the morning (he tells you he still has many questions), an elderly client who is close to death, and a woman with cancer who has been vomiting all day and who is in severe pain. You know you can't meet everyone's needs well. How do you "distribute" your nursing care? (You really *like* the client who is going home in the morning.)

Informed Consent.   A resident is attempting to perform a spinal tap on an adolescent who you know dislikes the resident. After one failed attempt the adolescent tells the resident to stop. The resident asks you to administer an antianxiety medication to the client so the resident can get the spinal tap done quickly. Should you administer the medication knowing the client no longer consents to the procedure?

Conflicts Between the Client's and Nurse's Interests.   Nurses are taking turns caring for a client with a highly contagious disease. One nurse, who is nursing her 8-month-old infant, refuses to take her turn, fearing to transmit the disease to her baby. The other nurses tell her she must take care of the client because none of them are willing to take her turn.

Nurses and Physicians

Nurse–physician situations can also result in ethical distress for nurses. Common problems include disagree-

Three Codes of Ethics for Nurses

International Council of Nurses Code for Nurses*

The fundamental responsibility of the nurse is four-fold: to promote health, to prevent illness, to restore health, and to alleviate suffering.

The need for nursing is universal. Inherent in nursing is respect for life, dignity, and rights of man. It is unrestricted by considerations of nationality, race, creed, color, age, sex, politics or social status.

Nurses render health services to the individual, the family and the community and coordinate their services with those of related groups.

Nurses and People

The nurse's primary responsibility is to those people who require nursing care.

The nurse, in providing care, promotes an environment in which the values, customs and spiritual beliefs of the individual are respected.

The nurse holds in confidence personal information and uses judgment in sharing this information.

Nurses and Practice

The nurse carries personal responsibility for nursing practice and for maintaining competence by continual learning. The nurse maintains the highest standards of nursing care possible within the reality of a specific situation.

The nurse uses judgment in relation to individual competence when accepting and delegating responsibilities.

The nurse when acting in a professional capacity should at all times maintain standards of personal conduct which reflect credit upon the profession.

Nurses and Society

The nurse shares with other citizens the responsibility for initiating and supporting action to meet the health and social needs of the public.

Nurses and Co-workers

The nurse sustains a cooperative relationship with co-workers in nursing and other fields. The nurse takes appropriate action to safeguard the individual when his care is endangered by a co-worker or any other person.

Nurses and the Profession

The nurse plays the major role in determining and implementing desirable standards of nursing practice and nursing education.

The nurse is active in developing a core of professional knowledge.

The nurse, acting through the professional organization, participates in establishing and maintaining equitable social and economic working conditions in nursing.

American Nurses' Association Code for Nurses†

1. The nurse provides services with respect for human dignity and the uniqueness of the client unrestricted by considerations of social or economic status, personal attributes, or the nature of health problems.
2. The nurse safeguards the client's right to privacy by judiciously protecting information of a confidential nature.
3. The nurse acts to safeguard the client and the public when health care and safety are affected by the incompetent, unethical, or illegal practice of any person.
4. The nurse assumes responsibility and accountability for individual nursing judgments and actions.
5. The nurse maintains competence in nursing.
6. The nurse exercises informed judgment and uses individual competence and qualifications as criteria in seeking consultation, accepting responsibilities, and delegating nursing activities to others.

(continued)

---

ments about the proposed medical regimen, conflicts regarding the scope of the nurse's role, and physician incompetence.

Disagreements About the Proposed Medical Regimen.   In the nursing home where you work, any client who loses a significant amount of weight (more than 10% of usual body weight) is automatically subjected to an exhaustive battery of tests (including a complete gas-trointestinal series) to determine whether there are any physical causes for the weight loss (*e.g.,* tumor). You strongly object to one client being put through these tests because she has made it clear that she wants to die and is willing to starve herself to death if that is the only way she can do it. The medical director insists that the client undergo the diagnostic studies because there is a long history of the client's family being dissatisfied with the medical care and the director wants to avoid causing

Three Codes of Ethics for Nurses (Continued)

7. The nurse participates in activities that contribute to the ongoing development of the profession's body of knowledge.
8. The nurse participates in the profession's efforts to implement and improve standards of nursing.
9. The nurse participates in the profession's efforts to establish and maintain conditions of employment conducive to high quality nursing care.
10. The nurse participates in the profession's effort to protect the public from misinformation and misrepresentation and to maintain the integrity of nursing.
11. The nurse collaborates with members of the health professions and other citizens in promoting community and national efforts to meet the health needs of the public.

Canadian Nurses' Association Code of Ethics for Nursing‡**

Clients

I. A nurse is obliged to treat clients with respect for their individual needs and values.
II. Based upon respect for clients and regard for their right to control their own care, nursing care should reflect respect for the right of choice held by clients.
III. The nurse is obliged to hold confidential all information regarding a client learned in the health care setting.
IV. The nurse has an obligation to be guided by consideration for the dignity of clients.
V. The nurse is obligated to provide competent care to clients.

VI. The nurse is obliged to represent the ethics of nursing before colleagues and others.
VII. The nurse is obligated to advocate the client's interest.
VIII. In all professional settings, including education, research and administration, the nurse retains a commitment to the welfare of clients. The nurse bears an obligation to act in such a fashion as will maintain trust in nurses and nursing.

Health Team

IX. Client care should represent a cooperative effort, drawing upon the expertise of nursing and other health professions. Acknowledging personal or professional limitations, the nurse recognizes the perspective and expertise of colleagues from other disciplines.
X. The nurse, as a member of the health care team, is obliged to take steps to ensure that the client receives competent and ethical care.

The Social Context of Nursing

XI. Conditions of employment should contribute to client care and to the professional satisfaction of nurses. Nurses are obliged to work towards securing and maintaining conditions of employment that satisfy these connected goals.

Responsibilities of the Profession

XII. Professional nurses' organizations recognize a responsibility to clarify, secure and sustain ethical nursing conduct. The fulfillment of these tasks requires that professional organizations remain responsive to the rights, needs and legitimate interests of clients and nurses.

* From International Council of Nurses: ICN Code for Nurses: Ethical Concepts Applied to Nursing. Geneva, Imprimeries Populaires, 1973. Reprinted with permission of the ICN.
† From American Nurses' Association: Code for Nurses. Kansas City, MO, American Nurses' Association, 1985. Reprinted with permission.
‡ This represents only one element of the code—*values. Standards,* which provide more specific directions for conduct than values, and *limitations,* which describe exceptional circumstances in which a value or standard cannot receive its usual application, are provided with each value in the publication.
** Canadian Nurses' Association: Code of Ethics for Nursing. Ottawa, Ontario, Canadian Nurses' Association, 1985. Reprinted with permission.

further dissatisfaction. Are you responsible for preparing the client for these diagnostic studies and scheduling them? Are there grounds for refusing to participate?

Conflicts Regarding the Scope of the Nurse's Role. A young woman needing surgery that will result in a permanent colostomy tells the nurse how afraid she is and how much she dreads getting used to "the thing." The nurse is certain this client would benefit greatly from the help of the young staff enterostomal therapist (ET), who also has a colostomy, but when this is mentioned to the surgeon, the surgeon tells the nurse that he does his own teaching and counseling for all his clients and does not "believe" in ETs. He points out that the nurse's duty here is to carry out his orders. Does it fall within the scope of nursing to recommend the ET to the woman? Is the nurse morally obligated to make this recommendation to the client?

A Patient's Bill of Rights

1. The patient has the right to considerate and respectful care.
2. The patient has the right to obtain from his physician complete current information concerning his diagnosis, treatment, and prognosis in terms the patient can be reasonably expected to understand. When it is not medically advisable to give such information to the patient, the information should be made available to an appropriate person in his behalf. He has the right to know by name the physician responsible for coordinating his care.
3. The patient has the right to receive from his physician information necessary to give informed consent prior to the start of any procedure and/or treatment. Except in emergencies, such information for informed consent should include but not necessarily be limited to the specific procedure and/or treatment, the medically significant risks involved, and the probable duration of incapacitation. Where medically significant alternatives for care or treatment exist, or when the patient requests information concerning medical alternatives, the patient has the right to such information. The patient also has the right to know the name of the person responsible for the procedures and/or treatment.
4. The patient has the right to refuse treatment to the extent permitted by law, and to be informed of the medical consequences of his action.
5. The patient has the right to every consideration of his privacy concerning his own medical care program. Case discussion, consultation, examination, and treatment are confidential and should be conducted discreetly. Those not directly involved in his care must have the permission of the patient to be present.
6. The patient has the right to expect that all communications and records pertaining to his care should be treated as confidential.
7. The patient has the right to expect that within its capacity a hospital must make reasonable response to the request of a patient for services. The hospital must provide evaluation, service, and/or referral as indicated by the urgency of the case. When medically permissible, a patient may be transferred to another facility only after he has received complete information and explanation concerning the needs for and alternatives to such a transfer. The institution to which the patient is to be transferred must first have accepted the patient for transfer.
8. The patient has the right to obtain information as to any relationship of his hospital to other health care and educational institutions insofar as his care is concerned. The patient has the right to obtain information as to the existence of any professional relationships among individuals, by name, who are treating him.
9. The patient has the right to be advised if the hospital proposes to engage in or perform human experimentation affecting his care or treatment. The patient has the right to refuse to participate in such research projects.
10. The patient has the right to expect reasonable continuity of care. He has the right to know in advance what appointment times and physicians are available and where. The patient has the right to expect that the hospital will provide a mechanism whereby he is informed by his physician or a delegate of the physician of the patient's continuing health care requirements following discharge.
11. The patient has the right to examine and receive an explanation of his bill regardless of source of payment.
12. The patient has the right to know what hospital rules and regulations apply to his conduct as a patient.

No catalogue of rights can guarantee for the patient the kind of treatment he has a right to expect. A hospital has many functions to perform, including the prevention and treatment of disease, the education of both health professionals and patients, and the conduct of clinical research. All these activities must be conducted with an overriding concern for the patient and, above all, the recognition of his dignity as a human being. Success in achieving this recognition assures success in the defense of the rights of the patient.

(A Patient's Bill of Rights. Chicago, American Hospital Association, 1973. Reprinted with the permission of the American Hospital Association.)

Physician Incompetence.   A nurse who works in the operating room notices that a pediatric surgeon who has been on the staff for several years and done excellent work seems all of a sudden not to be concentrating during surgery and to be making more mistakes than usual. There are rumors of a problem with cocaine abuse following the surgeon's divorce. The parents of one pediatric client dissatisfied with the progress the client is making come back to the nurse and ask for an opinion about the surgeon. Should the nurse voice personal concerns?

T A B L E 5-4
Types of Moral and Ethical Problems in Nursing

Problem	Description	Example
Moral uncertainty	One is unsure what moral principles or values apply, or even what the moral problem is.	A nurse notices that the clients of a particular surgeon seem to have more postoperative complications and slower recoveries than usual; the nurse feels uncomfortable about the situation but is unsure of the nature and cause of the problem and the best course of action.
Moral dilemmas	Two (or more) clear moral principles apply but they support mutually inconsistent courses of action.	An alert client who has cancer and is on a ventilator repeatedly attempts to remove the tube; the nurse can (1) *respect the client's autonomy* (self-determination) even if this results in death or (2) *respect the sanctity of life* by restraining the client so tubes cannot be removed.
Moral distress	One knows the right thing to do but institutional constraints make it nearly impossible to pursue the right course of action.	A nurse believes that clients on a cancer unit are being subtly forced to participate in cancer research studies; to speak up and question what is being done could easily mean job jeopardy.

(Adapted from Jameton A: *Nursing Practice: The Ethical Issues,* p 6. Englewood Cliffs, NJ, Prentice-Hall, 1984)

Is the nurse morally obligated to report the physician to the proper hospital authority for investigation?

Nurses and Other Nurses

Some of the most difficult ethical problems nurses encounter result from nurse–nurse interactions and may be complicated by obligations of friendship. Problems include claims of loyalty and nurse incompetence.

Claims of Loyalty. A nurse working the 11 PM to 7 AM shift tells the other nurse on the unit, "I just made rounds and everyone is OK. Please cover for me while I catch an hour of sleep. I had an awful day." She neglects to tell the nurse who is covering that it was mentioned in report that one client needed special monitoring. This client dies unexpectedly while the nurse sleeps. When she wakes up and discovers the death she begs the other nurse, her friend, not to ever tell anyone she was sleeping. "The client could have died anyway between my rounds."

Nurse Incompetence. Because of change in behavior of a nurse who started working the same time you did,

you strongly suspect a problem with chemical dependency. Recently you notice that several clients who were medicated for pain by that nurse complain about not getting relief and tell you that "Your shots are better." This nurse happens to be extremely popular, although not someone with whom you get along. Should you notify the proper hospital authority about your suspicions regarding this nurse?

Ethical Decision Making

This section on developing analytical skills may be helpful to you in working out your response to the ethical problems listed above.

Decision making cannot be based on emotional content; rather, it requires intellectual problem solving. Several models of ethical decision making are available in the literature, most of which have similar steps. The model described here is a six-step process proposed by Jameton (1984):

- Identify the problem.
- Gather data.
- Identify options.

(Text continues on p. 74.)

A Case Study Using a Six-Step Process for Resolving the Ethical Problem

Case: Jean W. is a labor and delivery room nurse in a small community hospital that serves both private clients and clinic clients. Jean has always felt that certain members of the obstetrics–gynecology medical staff have treated these two groups of clients differently. On this particular morning Jean is caring for a woman who is scheduled for an elective cesarean delivery. The woman (who is a clinic client) has made it very clear that she wants to be awake for the delivery and has requested epidural or spinal anesthesia. Jean is dismayed when the anesthesiologist enters the delivery room because the anesthesiologist's success rate with epidural anesthesia is poor. The anesthesiologist unsuccessfully attempts to perform an epidural block. After waiting 20 minutes for results the obstetrician is growing impatient and instructs the anesthesiologist to put the client to sleep. Jean feels the rights of this client are being violated but is unsure of what her response should be.

Step 1: Identify the Problem

State the problem clearly: unsure of ethical issue; two or more moral principles are in conflict; object to proposed course of action.

Jean W. objects to the obstetrician's intent to disregard the client's wish to be awake for her delivery; she is aware of no good reasons justifying this course of action.

Identify your relationship to the decision.

The nurse will be a participant in carrying out the decision.

Identify time parameters.

The decision for this case must be made immediately; it would be helpful to plan to avoid situations like this in the future.

Step 2: Gather Data

Describe the situation that gives rise to the problem: main people involved (their views and interests); client's overall nursing, medical, and social situation; relevant legal, administrative, and staff considerations.

The client is in stable medical condition (elective cesarean delivery, not an emergency) and has made it very clear that she wishes to be awake for the delivery. The client is not a private paying client of the obstetrician. The nurse believes her role is to promote/protect the client's interests; she knows of no reason in this case why the client's preferences should be disregarded.

The anesthesiologist has a poor success record with epidural anesthesia.

The obstetrician seems to want to complete delivery quickly. In the past he has seemed to give more weight to following wishes of private clients as opposed to clinic clients. He is the head of the obstetrics–gynecology department; he believes nurses should obey physicians unquestioningly.

Nurses have in the past informally expressed dissatisfaction with the different levels of care being provided private and clinic clients but no one to date has formally addressed the concern.

Step 3: Identify Options

Identify all the possible courses of action open to you and weigh the outcomes of each; consider immediate consequences to the people involved as well as long-term consequences to institution/society.

The nurse can say nothing to the obstetrician and help with the delivery. If asked by the client later why she needed to be put to sleep, the nurse can (1) tell the truth, (2) refer her to the obstetrician, (3) express

(Continued)

A Case Study Using a Six-Step Process for Resolving the Ethical Problem
(Continued)

sympathy that she could not be awake, or (4) say nothing. *Outcome:* The client's wishes are disregarded; delivery occurs in record time and the obstetrician is happy; the nurse fulfills obligation to physician and hospital but feels she has betrayed the client's trust. *Long-term outcome:* There is a good probability the same problem will happen again.

Or

The nurse can remind the obstetrician that the client was adamant about wanting to be awake and suggest that a different anesthesiologist be called in. If the obstetrician agrees, the client may get her wish and everyone is satisfied with the outcome (the nurse must still decide how to prevent recurrence of this dilemma). If the obstetrician refuses and insists that the client be put to sleep, the nurse can (1) refuse to participate (if another nurse is not available and willing to replace her, the nurse has abandoned the client and harm may ensue), or (2) participate and proceed as above or resolve to speak to the obstetrician in a "cool moment" after the delivery to see how to avoid this problem in the future. If the nurse does not get satisfaction with the obstetrician, then she must decide whether or not to move through the proper administrative channels. Depending on the institution and people involved, the nurse may be affirmed or censored for this move. *Long-term outcome:* Future clients may be helped by the nurse following through with her concerns.

Or

The nurse can say nothing and assist with this delivery believing it to be the wisest course of action for the time being, but resolve to take the steps above to correct the perceived injustice. *Outcome:* There is no benefit for the present client but potential benefit to future clients.

Step 4: Think the Ethical Problem Through

See if conventional principles of professional ethics address and resolve the problem; if not, see if broader ethical principles and theories clarify and resolve the problem. Rely on those principles you judge most important and of which you feel most sure.

Basic conventional principle: The good of clients should be the nurse's primary concern strongly suggests that the nurse should act, but it does not address the nurse's obligation to do so if she feels it would jeopardize her own good (job security).

Basic moral principle: Respect for persons would suggest that the client's autonomy (right to self-determination) should be respected unless there is strong justification for not doing so. *Equality* would suggest that whether or not a client pays the obstetrician privately should have no bearing on the quality of care received.

(Continued)

A Case Study Using a Six-Step Process for Resolving the Ethical Problem (Continued)

Step 5: Make a Decision

Choose a course of action that best reflects your considered judgment; consultation with an institutional ethics committee or other staff may be helpful.

Jean W. feels from past interactions with this obstetrician that her speaking up will not influence his decision to have the client put to sleep. She decides to speak with the obstetrician after the delivery and follow up with whatever approach is necessary to avoid recurrence.

Step 6: Act and Assess

Act and compare the actual outcome with what you considered and hoped for in advance. How can you improve the decision process next time?

Jean W. will never know if speaking up would have resulted in the client's wishes being respected. Although she is not satisfied with the outcome of this case, she hopes to prevent this from happening to other clinic clients in the future. In this instance a hospital committee was formed to study the problem and make recommendations. If Jean W. had been told to "mind her own business" unless she wanted trouble, she would have to make a decision weighing client benefit on one hand with potential personal risk/harm on the other.

(Adapted from Jameton A: Nursing Practice: The Ethical Issues. Englewood Cliffs, NJ, Prentice-Hall, 1984)

- Think the ethical problem through: (1) consider basic *conventional principles* of professional ethics and determine whether they address the issue and resolve the problem; if this fails, (2) see if any reflective ethical considerations clarify and resolve the problem.
- Make a decision.
- Act and assess.

These steps are illustrated on pages 72 to 74. However, the following text will help you understand the fourth step.

Conventional Principles and Values

Conventional principles are "rules for action, related principles, ideals, standards, and values, . . . commonly used as standards . . . and followed in practice" (Jameton, 1984, p 71). Examples of conventional principles of nursing practice include the following:

- Nurses have an obligation to be competent.
- The good of clients should be the nurse's primary concern.
- Nurses should not use their positions to exploit others.
- Nurses should be loyal to each other.

Unfortunately, many nurses find themselves in situations where conventional principles conflict or are otherwise deficient in resolving ethical dilemmas. The staff nurse who suspects that her charge nurse is both stealing and abusing narcotics will need to report the charge nurse even if this is being disloyal to a colleague.

Basic Moral Concepts

When conventional principles fail to provide nurses with a guide to action, the nurse needs to explore ethical values and principles in a deeper and broader way. Jameton (1984) identified five basic moral concepts:

1. *Respect for persons*—This involves having empathy for others (listening and understanding) and not using people as a means to an end.
2. *Justice*—Distributive justice of the allocation of goods and services is the type of justice most relevant to health care, including how much of our national resources should be devoted to health care, which aspects of health care should receive the most resources, and which clients should have access to these resources. Models for distributing the burdens and benefits of society include
   - To each equally
   - To each according to merit

COMPUTER APPLICATIONS IN NURSING

Computer-Generated Ethical Decisions in Medicine

Acknowledging the great difficulty many physicians experience in resolving ethical dilemmas about consent, Dr. John Dawson and Mr. Paul Sieghart, a lawyer, have written some moral software for the British Medical Association. This software consists of a personal-computer program dealing with consent to medical treatment, called *COMET,* and incorporates more than 100 generally accepted ethical rules and legal judgments. The user follows a question-and-answer routine that leads either to a clear conclusion or to a recommendation that the

(The Economist, p 84, July 18, 1987)

issue needs further examination. The print-out shows the logic behind the final decision. The purpose of the software is not to make ethical decisions for physicians but rather to place pertinent ethical and legal principles literally at their fingertips. The British Medical Association says that COMET is the world's first computer program dealing with medical ethics. It will soon be followed by a program on the disclosure of medical information to third parties, which AIDS has made a pressing dilemma.

- To each according to past or future social contribution
- To each according to what can be acquired in a free market
- To each according to need
- To each according to need, from each according to ability

3. *Values*—These underlie the goods and purposes sought in life; relevant to health care is whether there are some values that take precedence over others and the role values play in shaping client decisions and professional behavior.

4. *Rights*—These are justified claims on others not to interfere with what we have or are doing (negative rights) or to provide something (positive rights). Associated with rights are responsibilities. In health care the issue of rights most often focuses on identifying what clients are entitled to but do not always receive.

5. *Responsibility*—Before making moral judgments it is necessary to identify who is responsible for what; as the nurse's professional role is expanding, nurses are becoming both morally and legally responsible for more aspects of client care.
(Jameton, 1984, pp 124–145)

KEY POINTS

■ Knowing whether or not to perform a nursing action ("should I?") is often as important as knowing how to perform the action.

■ A value is a belief about worth that acts as a standard to guide behavior. Values influence beliefs about human needs, health and illness, the practice of health behaviors, and human responses to health and illness.

■ Values are formed over a lifetime from information a person receives from the environment and from the family and culture. Common modes of value transmission are modeling, moralizing, laissez-faire, rewarding and punishing, and responsible choice.

■ The American Association of Colleges of Nursing identified altruism, aesthetics, equality, freedom, human dignity, justice, and truth as essential values for the practicing nurse.

■ While it is important for nurses to respect the value orientations of others, not all values are equal. Nurses may find themselves morally obligated to respond to client values likely to cause harm to the client or others.

■ Values clarification is a process by which persons come to understand their own values and value system. The process of valuing is centered on choosing, prizing, and acting.

■ The President's Commission for the Study of Ethical Problems rejects polarized models of decision making that place absolute authority for decisions in the hands of either the client or physician, and call instead for a relationship between clients and professionals characterized by mutual participation, respect, and shared decision making.

■ Nurses who are sensitive to the need to promote both client autonomy (self-determination) and client well-being may experience ethical conflict but are more likely than other nurses to be successful in securing the client's genuine best interests.

■ The nursing codes of ethics (ICN, ANA, CNA) provide a framework for making ethical decisions and set forth professional expectations. They inform both nurses and society of the profession's primary goals and values. Codes are effective only when upheld by members of the profession.

■ Ethical problems faced by nurses include moral uncertainty, moral dilemmas, and moral distress.

■ One of several processes for resolving ethical problems in nursing is the following six-step process: identify the problem, gather data, identify options, think the ethical problem through (explore conventional principles and basic moral concepts), make a decision, and act and assess.

■ Rather than offering clear-cut answers, ethics offers the nurse a means to look at and evaluate alternative courses of right action using basic moral concepts and principles. It reduces the likelihood that nursing actions to resolve ethical problems will be based solely on intuition, opinions, and self-interest.

BIBLIOGRAPHY

American Association of Colleges of Nursing: Essentials of College and University Education for Professional Nursing. Washington, DC, American Association of Colleges of Nursing, 1986

American Hospital Association: A patient's bill of rights. Nurs Outlook 24(1):29, 1976

American Nurses' Association: Code for Nurses with Interpretive Statements. Kansas City, MO, American Nurses' Association, 1985

Aroskar MA: Are nurses' mind sets compatible with ethical practice? Topics in Clinical Nursing 4(1):22–32, 1982

Aroskar M: Anatomy of an ethical dilemma: The theory. Am J Nurs 80(4):658–660, 1980

Aroskar M: Anatomy of an ethical dilemma: The practice. Am J Nurs 80(4):661–663, 1980

Beauchamp TL, Childress JF: Principles of Biomedical Ethics, 2nd ed. New York, Oxford University Press, 1983

Benjamin M, Curtis J: Ethics in Nursing, 2nd ed. New York, Oxford University Press, 1987

Bernal EW, Bush EG: Values clarification: A critique. J Nurs Educ 24(4):174–175, 1985

Callahan D, Bok S (eds): Ethics Teaching in Higher Education. New York, Plenum Press, 1980

Canadian Nurses' Association: Code of Ethics for Nursing. Ottawa, Ontario, Canadian Nurses' Association, 1985

Cassells JM, Redman BK, Jackson SS: Generic baccalaureate student satisfaction regarding professional and personal development prior to graduation and one year post graduation. Journal of Professional Nursing 2(2):114–127, 1986

Chinn PL (ed): Ethical Issues in Nursing. Rockville, MD, Aspen, 1986

Coletta SS: Values clarification in nursing. Am J Nurs 78(12):2057, 1978

Curtin L, Flaherty MJ: Nursing Ethics: Theory and Pragmatics. Bowie, MD, Brady, 1982

Feldman KA, Newcomb TM: Impact of College on Students. San Francisco, Jossey-Bass, 1969

Felton GM, Parsons MA: The impact of nursing education on ethical/moral decision making. J Nurs Educ 26(1):7–11, 1987

Fenner KM: Ethics and Law in Nursing. New York, D Van Nostrand, 1980

Fowler M, Levine-Areff J: Ethics at the Bedside: A Source Book for the Critical Care Nurse. Philadelphia, JB Lippincott, 1987

Garvin BJ, Boyle KK: Values of entering nursing students: Changes over 10 years. Res Nurs Health 8(3):235–241, 1985

International Council of Nurses: ICN Code for Nurses: Ethical Concepts Applied to Nursing. Geneva, Imprimeries Populaires, 1973

Jameton A: Nursing Practice: The Ethical Issues. Englewood Cliffs, NJ, Prentice-Hall, 1984

Ketefian S: A case study of theory development: Moral behavior in nursing. Advances in Nursing Science 9(2):10–19, 1987

Kirschbaum H: Advanced Values Clarification. La Jolla, CA, University Associates, 1977

Mitchell C, Smith L: If it's AIDS, please don't tell. Am J Nurs 87(7):911–914, 1987

Murphy CP, Hunter H: Ethical Problems in the Nurse-Patient Relationship. Boston, Allyn & Bacon, 1983

Muyskens JL: No easy choice resolving everyday ethical dilemmas. Nursing Life 4(4):29–32, 1984

Ozimek D: Rights and responsibilities of students and faculty. Imprint 29(2):50–51, 63–64, 68–69, 72–76, 78–79, 1982

President's Commission for the Study of Ethical Problems in Medicine and Biomedical and Behavioral Research: Making Health Care Decisions, vol 1, A Report. Washington, DC. US Government Printing Office, 1982

Quinn CA, Smith MD: The Professional Commitment: Issues and Ethics in Nursing. Philadelphia, JB Lippincott, 1987

Raths LE, Simon SB, Harmin M: Values and Teaching, 2nd ed. Columbus, Ohio, Charles E Merrill, 1978

Royal College of Nursing of the United Kingdom: Guidelines on Confidentiality in Nursing. London, Royal College of Nursing of the United Kingdom, 1980

Rozovsky LE: The Canadian Patient's Book of Rights. Toronto, Doubleday Canada, 1980

Silva MC: The American Nurses' Association's code for nurses: Purposes, content, and enforceability. Health Matrix 2(2):55–63, 1984

Simon SB: Values Clarification: A Handbook of Practical Strategies for Teachers and Students. New York, Hart, 1972

Spicker SF, Gadow S (eds): Nursing: Images and Ideals. New York, Springer-Verlag, 1980

Steele SM: AIDS: Clarifying values to close in on ethical questions. Nursing and Health Care 7(5):247–248, 1987

Steele SM, Harmon VM: Values Clarification in Nursing, 2nd ed. Norwalk, CT, Appleton-Century-Crofts, 1983

Storch J: Patients Rights: Ethical and Legal Issues in Health Care and Nursing. Toronto, McGraw-Hill Ryerson, 1982

Taylor SG: Rights and responsibilities: Nurse-patient relationships. Image 17(1):9–13, 1985

Taylor Sr C, Hobaugh R: The role of the critical care nurse in developing informed consent. Dimensions of Critical Care Nursing 5(2):98–106, 1986

Travelbee J: Interpersonal Aspects of Nursing. Philadelphia, FA Davis, 1971

Uustal DB: Values clarification in nursing: Application to practice. Am J Nurs 78(12):2058–2063, 1978

Veatch RM, Fry ST: Case Studies in Nursing Ethics. Philadelphia, JB Lippincott, 1987

Wilson J: A new code of ethics for nursing. Can Med Assoc J 130(7):920–921, 1984

Yarling R, McElmurry B: The moral foundation of nursing. Advances in Nursing Science 8(1):63–73, 1986

Yeaworth RC: The ANA code: A comparative perspective. Image 17(3):94–98, 1985

6 Legal Implications of Nursing

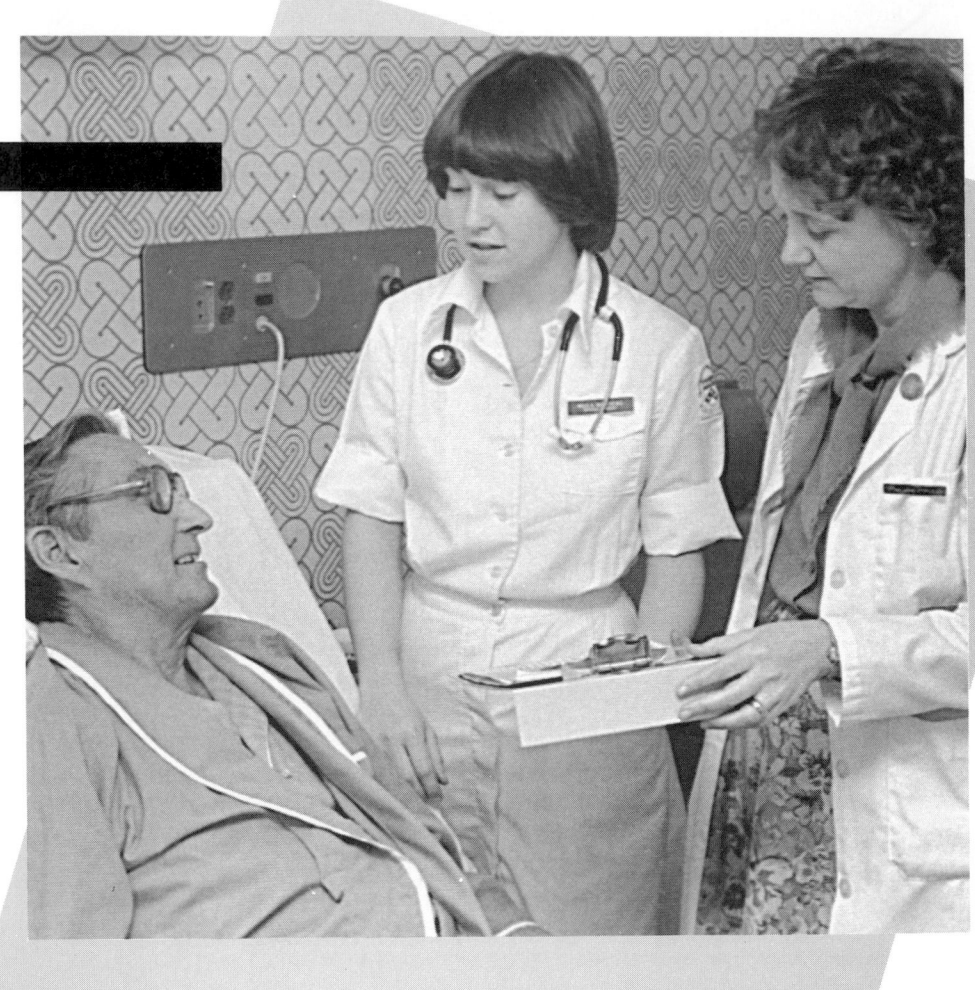

OBJECTIVES

After studying this chapter, the learner should be able to

Define key terms used in the chapter.

Define law, describing its four sources.

Describe the professional and legal regulation of nursing practice.

Identify the purpose of credentialing; using as examples accreditation, licensure/registration, and certification.

Identify grounds for suspending or revoking a license or registration.

Differentiate intentional torts (assault and battery, defamation, invasion of privacy, false imprisonment, fraud) and unintentional torts (negligence).

Evaluate personal areas of potential liability in nursing.

Describe the legal procedure once a plaintiff files a complaint against a nurse for negligence.

Describe the roles of the nurse as defendent, fact witness, and expert witness.

Understand the need for use of appropriate legal safeguards in nursing practice (competent practice within scope defined by nurse practice act, careful documentation, participation in risk management programs, use of professional liability insurance)

Explain the purpose of incident reports.

Describe laws affecting nursing practice.

As the roles and duties of nurses have expanded in the present health-care system, so too has their legal accountability. In the not so distant past many nurses worked under the supervision of a physician, few carried liability insurance, and even if a nurse's actions were the direct cause of harm to a client, primary liability for the nursing action fell on the employing agency or physician. Today, nurses independently assess and diagnose clients and plan, implement, and evaluate nursing care. Full legal responsibility and accountability for these nursing actions rest with the nurse. A steadily increasing number of nurses are being named as litigants in negligence cases and being brought to court to defend their practice.

Nurses wishing to avoid legal conflicts

- Know the law and incorporate it into their practice
- Maintain good nurse–client relationships (satisfied clients rarely sue)
- Incorporate the rights of clients into their health care
- Practice within the bounds of their competence (Klein, 1986)

LEGAL CONCEPTS

Definition of Law

A **law** is a standard or rule of conduct established and enforced by the government of a society. Laws are intended chiefly to protect the rights of the public. **Public law** is a law in which the government is directly involved. It regulates the relationships between individuals and the government. Also, an important body of public law describes the powers of the government in authority. Private law, also called **civil law**, regulates the relationships among people. Civil law includes laws relating to contracts, ownership of property, and the practice of nursing, medicine, pharmacy, and dentistry.

Sources of Laws

There are four sources of law existing at both the federal and state (provincial) level: constitutions, statutes, administrative law, and common law.

Constitutions.   Federal and state constitutions indicate how their governments are created and given authority and state the principles and provisions for establishing specific laws. Although they contain relatively few laws (called *constitutional laws*), they serve as guides to legislative bodies.

Statutes.   A **statutory law** is enacted by a legislative body. In the United States, statutory laws must be in

KEY TERMS

assault	law
battery	liability
civil law	licensure
common law	litigation
credentialing	living will
crime	malpractice
defamation of character	misdemeanor
defendant	negligence
false imprisonment	plaintiff
felony	public law
fraud	risk management
incident report	standard of care
informed consent	statutory law
invasion of privacy	tort

keeping with the federal constitution and with the constitution of the state as well. Nurse practice acts are an example of statutory laws.

Administrative Law.

Executive officers (the president of the United States or prime minister of Canada, state governors or provincial premiers, city mayors) administer various agencies that, among other functions, are responsible for law enforcement. These agencies have power to make administrative rules and regulations, in conformity with enacted law, which act as laws and are enforceable. Boards of nursing are administrative agencies at the state level. Rules and regulations they adopt are administrative laws. One example of a municipal administrative agency is a city's board of health.

Common Law.

The government provides for a judiciary system, which is responsible for reconciling controversies. It interprets legislation at the local, state (province), and national level as it has been applied in specific instances and makes decisions concerning law enforcement. A body of law known as **common law** has grown out of these accumulated judiciary decisions. Common law is thus court-made law. Most law in the area of malpractice is court-made law. The exception to this is the province of Quebec, where a civil law system is in effect.

Common law is based on the principle of *stare decisis,* or "let the decision stand." In other words, after a decision has been made in a court of law, that decision becomes the rule to follow when other cases involving similar circumstances and facts arise. The case that first sets down the rule by decision is called a *precedent.* Court decisions can be changed, but only when strong justification exists. Common law helps prevent one set of rules from being used to judge one person and another set to judge another person in similar circumstances.

Litigation

A lawsuit is a legal action in a court. **Litigation** is the process of a lawsuit. The person or government bringing suit against another is called the **plaintiff**. The one being accused of a crime or tort (defined later) is called the **defendant**. The defendant is assumed innocent until proven guilty of a crime or tort. Being accused does not necessarily imply guilt.

The two levels of courts in the United States are trial court and appellate court. The *trial court* is the first-level court and hears all the evidence in a case and makes decisions as to facts, usually through a jury. The *appellate court* only hears cases questioning a point of law decided by the trial court. No witnesses testify at the appellate court level. The opinions of appellate judges are published and become common law (Fiesta, 1983).

PROFESSIONAL AND LEGAL REGULATION OF NURSING PRACTICE

Nurses who engage in the safe practice of their profession respect both the voluntary and legal controls that map the boundaries of nursing practice. Both these controls are designed to provide quality health care and to protect society from unsafe nursing practice (Fig 6-1).

Voluntary standards, developed and implemented by the nursing profession itself, are not mandatory but are used as guidelines for peer review. Professional nursing organizations continually reassess the functions, standards, and qualifications of their members. The organizations are guided by their own assessment of society's need for nursing and by the public's expectations of nursing. Examples of voluntary standards include the American Nurses' Association and Canadian Nurses' Association standards of practice (see Chap 1), professional standards for the accreditation of education programs and service organizations, and standards for the certification of individual nurses in general and specialty areas of practice.

Legal standards are developed by legislative action and are implemented by authority granted by the state or province to determine minimum standards for the education of nurses, set requirements for licensure/registration, and decide when a nurse's license may be suspended or revoked. Examples of legal standards include state and province nurse practice acts and rules and regulations of nursing.

Credentialing

Nursing has taken several steps to ensure the competence of its practitioners, one of them being through the process of credentialing. **Credentialing** is a general term that refers to ways in which professional competence is ensured and maintained.

Three processes are used for credentialing in nursing. The first is *accreditation,* which is the process by which an educational program is evaluated and then recognized as having met certain predetermined standards of education. A second is **licensure**, which is the process by which a state determines that a candidate meets certain minimum requirements to practice in the profession of his or her choice and grants a license to do so. A third is *certification,* which is the process by which a person who has met certain criteria established by a nongovernmental association is granted recognition.

Accreditation

Constitutions in the United States provide governments with the responsibility of securing the public welfare.

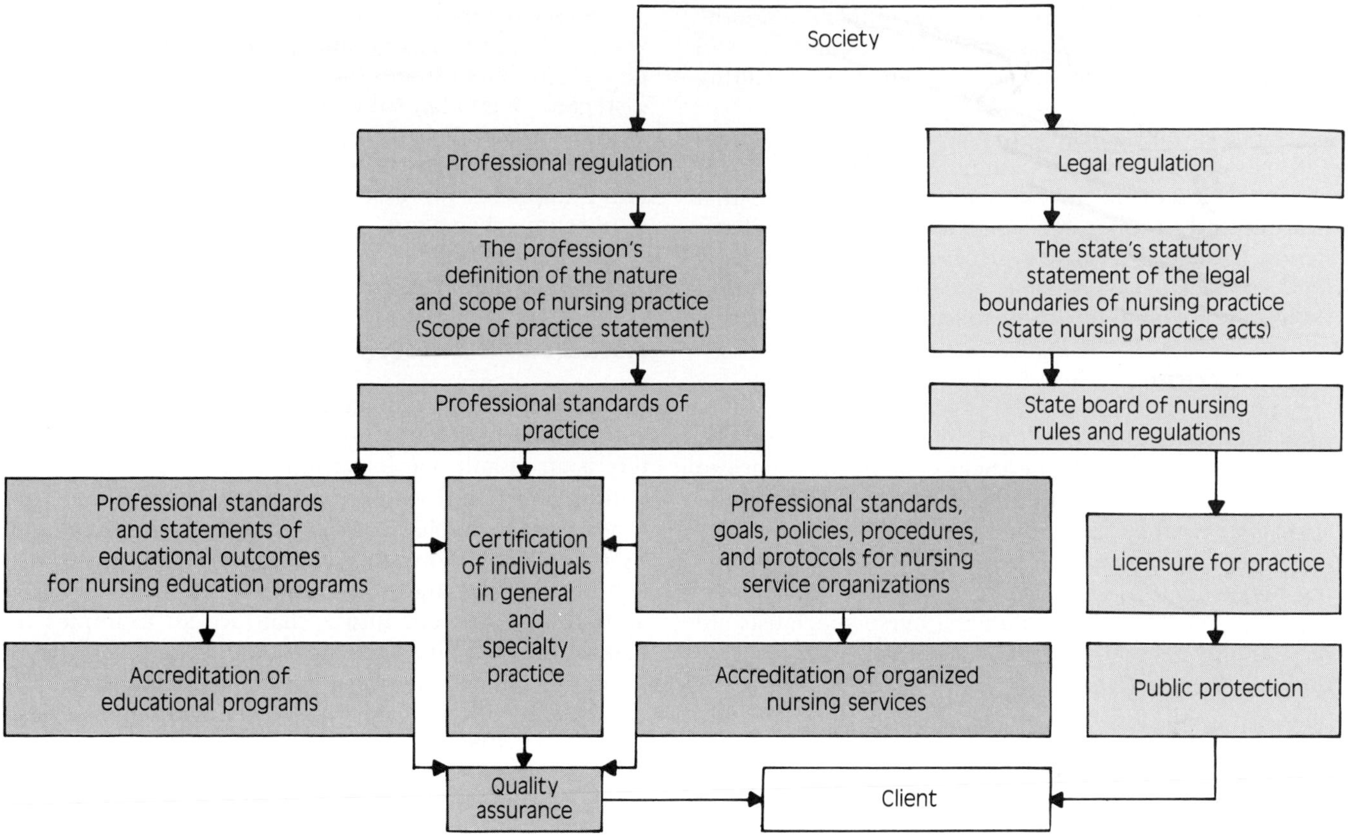

FIGURE 6-1

Diagram of proposed professional and legal regulation of nursing practice showing the separation of and parallels between professional and legal regulatory processes. (Redrawn from American Nurses' Association: The Scope of Nursing Practice. Kansas City, The Association, 1987)

Legislative bodies have used this principle to enact laws that provide certain controls on occupational and professional groups. One function of these laws is to see to it that schools preparing practitioners maintain certain minimum standards of education. Nursing is one group operating under state laws that aim to promote the general welfare by determining minimum standards of education through accreditation of schools of nursing. In each Canadian province there is in place an approval mechanism to certify schools of nursing. In the United States, state-approved, or accredited, educational programs in nursing include practical/vocational, associate-degree, diploma, baccalaureate, and graduate programs in nursing.

Legal accreditation of a school preparing nursing personnel should not be confused with voluntary accreditation. The National League for Nursing is a voluntary agency that accredits schools when they meet certain criteria established by the League. Most schools choose to seek this voluntary accreditation, and many prospective students prefer selecting a school that has been accredited by the League. Accreditation by the National

League for Nursing of educational programs to prepare nurses is not a legal requirement for a school to exist. State accreditation is a legal requirement.

Licensure and Registration

Licensure is a specialized form of credentialing that has a legal basis in laws passed by a legislative body. A *license* is a "legal document that permits a person to offer to the public his skills and knowledge in a particular jurisdiction, where such practice would otherwise be unlawful without a license" (Creighton, 1986a, p 9). Licensure and registration are discussed in Chapter 1.

Licensure and registration are mandatory in Canada. Both must be renewed periodically.

Licensure or Registration Revocation

The State Board of Nurse Examiners (or the registering body in Canada) may revoke or suspend a nurse's license/registration for drug or alcohol abuse (currently the most frequent reason) as well as for many other acts of unprofessional conduct, including fraud, deceptive practices, criminal acts, previous disciplinary action by other state boards, gross or ordinary negligence, and physical or mental impairments, even those resulting from aging (Northrop, 1986).

Once earned, a license to practice is a property right and may not be revoked without *due process.* This includes notice of the investigation, a fair and impartial hearing, and a proper decision based on substantial evidence. Critical to a nurse's successful defense are early legal counsel, use of character and expert witnesses, and thorough preparation for all proceedings.

Certification

As of July 1987, 21 professional organizations offer nursing certification in the United States, led by the American Association of Critical-Care Nurses, which represents the specialty with the largest number of certified nurses, and the American Nurses' Association, which began certifying nurses in 1974 and today certifies in 17 specialties. Although certification is voluntary, nurse specialists are increasingly becoming certified. There also are certification programs in Canada.

CRIMES AND TORTS

A **crime** is a wrong against a person or his property, but the act is considered to be against the public as well. In a criminal case, the government, called "the people," prosecutes the offender. When a crime is committed, the factor of intent to commit wrong is present in most cases. However, persons who break certain laws are guilty of a crime, whether there was intent or not. For example, failure to observe the Federal Food, Drug, and Cosmetic Act may constitute a crime.

In most cases, criminal law is statutory law and only infrequently, common law. Crimes are classified as *felonies* or *misdemeanors.* A **misdemeanor** is a less serious crime than a felony. A **felony** is punishable by imprisonment in a state or federal penitentiary for more than 1 year. Misdemeanors are commonly punishable with fines or with imprisonment for less than 1 year, or with both, or with parole.

A **tort** is also a wrong committed by a person against another person or his property. Torts generally result in civil trials. In most instances, the court in a civil case will settle damages with money but rarely by imprisonment. Torts may be intentional or unintentional acts of wrongdoing. Some of the intentional torts for which nurses may be held liable include assault and battery, defamation of character, invasion of privacy, false imprisonment, and fraud. A person committing an intentional tort is considered to have knowledge of the permitted legal limits of his words or acts. Violating these limits is grounds for prosecution. Unintentional torts are referred to as *negligence.*

An act generally considered a tort may, because of its severity, be classed as a crime. For example, gross negligence that demonstrates the offender guilty of complete disregard for another's life may be tried as both civil and criminal action. It is then prosecuted under criminal as well as civil law. By its very nature, a wrong tried as a crime implies a more serious offense with more legal implications than a tort.

Intentional Torts

Assault and Battery

Assault is a threat or an attempt to make bodily contact with another person without that person's consent. **Battery** is an assault that is carried out and includes every willful, angry, and violent or negligent touching of another's person or clothes or anything attached to or held by that person. Forcibly removing a client's clothing, administering an injection following the client's refusal, and shoving a client into a chair are all examples of battery. When a nurse needs to defend herself from an assaultive client, only those actions necessary for self-protection or the aid of another are permitted (Creighton, 1986c).

Every individual has the right to be free from invasion of his person, and the adult client who is alert and oriented has the right to refuse any aspect of treatment. The fact that treatment is desirable does not allow the nurse or physician to proceed without the consent of the client or to go beyond the limits to which the person has consented.

Informed Consent

Every person is granted freedom from bodily contact by another unless consent has been granted. In hospitals and other health-care settings, a signed informed consent form is needed (1) on admission (for routine treatment), (2) for each specialized diagnostic procedure or medical or surgical treatment, and (3) for experimentation involving clients. The central values underlying **informed consent** include the promotion of a client's well-being and respect for the client's self-determination (President's Commission for the Study of Ethical Problems in Medicine and Biomedical and Behavioral Research, 1982), although informed consent also protects against lawsuits. Elements of informed consent include disclosure, comprehension, competence, and voluntariness (see also the box entitled Checklist to Ensure Informed Consent).

Obtaining an informed consent is the responsibility of the person who will execute the diagnostic or treatment procedure or conduct the research study. The nurse's role is to double check that a signed consent is in the client's chart and to respond to any questions the client has about the consent. In some instances the nurse may be responsible for having the client sign the consent form after the physician has explained to the client the

Checklist to Ensure Informed Consent

Disclosure

1. Patient has been informed of his current medical status and course of treatment.
2. Patient has been informed of the risks and benefits of various treatment alternatives.
3. Patient has been told that no outcomes can be guaranteed.
4. Patient has been given a professional opinion as to the best alternative.

Comprehension

5. The nurse has been innovative in transmitting information to aid understanding.
6. Interior impediments to comprehension, such as anxiety, pain, and medication, have been assessed.
7. Exterior impediments to comprehension, such as transcultural barriers, terminology, and speed of presentation, have been assessed.

Competence

8. The nurse has assessed competence in terms of the abilities of the patient considering age, education, and emotional stability.
9. The nurse has assessed the requirements of the task.
10. The nurse has assessed the possible deleterious effects of the patient's decision.
11. The patient possesses a set of values and goals which make possible reasonably consistent choices.
12. The patient is able to communicate and understand the information presented.
13. The patient has the ability to reason and deliberate.

Voluntariness

14. The nurse has determined that the patient has not been forced to consent.
15. The nurse has been careful to avoid coercive influences by herself/himself or others.
16. The nurse has been careful to avoid subtle manipulation of the patient by herself/himself or others.

(Taylor C, Hobaugh R: The role of the critical care nurse in developing informed consent. Dimens Crit Care Nurs 5(2):98–105, 1986)

procedure, its risks and benefits, and alternative treatments. The documentation of the consent process through the use of a printed consent form should not be confused with the actual explanation given to the client and the informed consent itself. When documenting consent the nurse should assess if the client understands what he is signing and report to the physician any problems. Nurses often find themselves in a position where they question the client's understanding of the proposed procedure and its risks, or the client's ability to voluntarily consent to the procedure. Impediments include effects of anxiety, pain, medication, depression, and temporary or permanent states of disorientation and confusion. The nurse signs the consent form as a witness to having seen the client sign the form, not to having obtained the consent (Fig. 6-2).

Guidelines for informed consent follow (Springer, 1970):

- Informed consent is required for all routine health-care services and for nonroutine diagnostic, treatment, or research procedures.
- A signed consent is not needed in an emergency *if* (1) there is an immediate threat to life or health, (2) experts agree that it is an emergency, and (3) the client is unable to consent and the legally authorized person cannot be reached.
- A signed consent is not needed for action taken in response to an unanticipated complication during surgery when the legally authorized person cannot be reached.
- Elements of a valid consent include disclosure, comprehension, competence, and voluntariness. The consent must (1) be written, (2) be signed by the client or person legally responsible for the client, and (3) be for the procedure performed.
- The client signs the consent whenever able. Exceptions include a client who is physically unable to sign, legally incompetent, or a minor (unless married or self-supporting).
- Consequences of not obtaining a valid consent include charges of battery against the nurse, doctor, and hospital (hospital has a duty to protect clients and is responsible for its employees' actions).
- A client's refusal to sign a consent should be documented and the client should be informed of the possible consequences of the refusal. The client should sign a release form indicating his refusal to consent and releasing the nurse, physician, and hospital from responsibility for outcomes of this act. This statement should be witnessed.

Defamation

Defamation of character is an intentional tort in which one party makes derogatory remarks about another, diminishing the other party's reputation. *Slander* is an untruthful, oral statement about a person that subjects that person to ridicule or contempt. *Libel* is written defama-

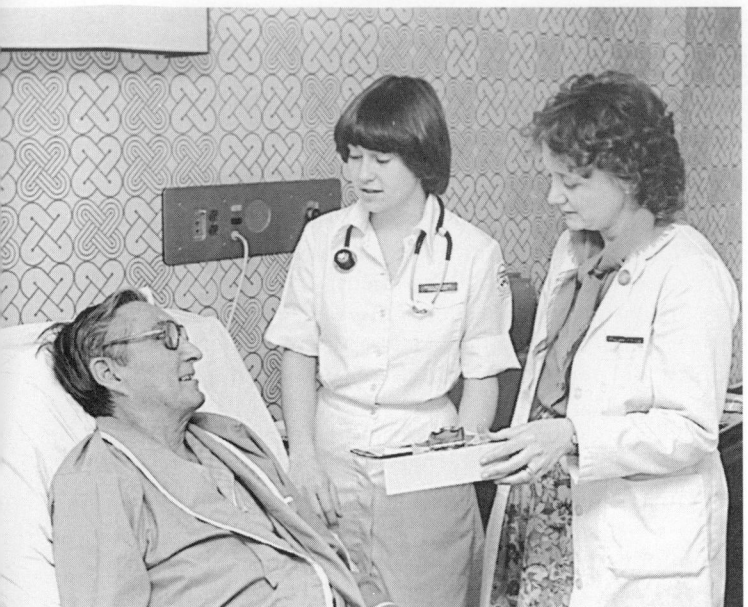

F I G U R E   6-2

Elements of informed consent include disclosure, comprehension, competence, and voluntariness. The documentation of the consent process through the use of a printed consent form does not substitute for the actual explanation given to the client and the informed consent itself. (Photo by Gates Rhodes, courtesy of the School of Nursing, University of Pennsylvania)

tion. Defamation of character is grounds for an award of civil damages. Damages are awarded on the basis of the degree of harm done to the plaintiff. Nurses who make false statements about their clients or co-workers run the risk of being sued for slander or libel. A person charged with slander or libel may not be liable if it can be proved that his statement was made not to injure another but for a nonmalicious, justifiable purpose (*e.g.,* proof of consent, truth, privilege, or fair comment).

Invasion of Privacy

In the United States, the Supreme Court has interpreted the right against **invasion of privacy** as inherent in the federal constitution. It holds that the Fourth Amendment protects citizens by giving them the right of privacy and the right to be left alone. Disclosure of confidential information whenever a client's problem is inappropriately discussed with a third party may be construed as invasion of privacy and may subject the nurse to liability. The nurse's intimate knowledge of the client increases legal risk in this regard.

There is as yet no uniformity in the Canadian laws dealing with the right to privacy, although two provinces have statutory laws protecting the right to privacy (Storch, 1982).

Certain acts by nurses could constitute invasion of privacy, as the following examples illustrate:

- Unnecessary exposure of clients while moving them through health-agency corridors or while caring for them in rooms they share with others
- Talking with clients in rooms that are not sound-proof
- Discussing information concerning clients with persons not entitled to the information (*e.g.,* with the client's employer or the press)
- Pressing the client for information not necessary in care planning
- Interacting with the client's family in ways not authorized by the client
- Using tape recorders, dictaphones, computer banks, and the like, without taking precautions to ensure the client's confidentiality
- Preparing written or oral class assignments about clients without concealing their identity
- Carrying out research without taking proper precautions to ensure the anonymity of clients

At times an individual's right to privacy may conflict with other rights such as the public's right to information. For example, although the client with acquired immunodeficiency syndrome (AIDS) has the right not to publicize the diagnosis, health-care professionals caring for the client have the right to know that the client has AIDS so that they can protect themselves and other clients. When in doubt about disclosing confidential information, the nurse should consult the nursing supervisor, ethics committee, or public relations department of the institution.

False Imprisonment

Unjustified retention or prevention of the movement of another person without proper consent can constitute **false imprisonment.** For example, only a reasonable amount of restraint should be used in circumstances that warrant it. The indiscriminate and thoughtless use of restraints on a patient can constitute the act of false imprisonment.

A person cannot be legally forced to remain in a health agency, such as a hospital, if he is of sound mind, even when health practitioners believe the person should remain for additional care. Health agencies have special forms to use when a client insists on being discharged "against medical orders." The person's signature indicates that the agency cannot be held responsible for any harm that may result from the client's leaving. Persons who are mentally ill may be committed to a psychiatric institution for treatment without their consent (involuntary commitment) only when it can be proved that they are harmful to themselves or others.

Fraud

Fraud is willful and purposeful misrepresentation that could cause, or has caused, loss or harm to a person or property. Misrepresentation of a product is a common fraudulent act. In nursing, persons fraudulently misrepresenting themselves to obtain a license to practice may be prosecuted under nurse practice acts. Also, misrepresenting the outcome of a procedure or treatment may constitute fraud.

Unintentional Torts

Negligence and Malpractice

Negligence is defined as performing an act that a reasonably prudent person under similar circumstances would not do, or conversely, failing to perform an act that a reasonably prudent person under similar circumstances would do. As the definition implies, an act of negligence may be an act of omission or commission. Malpractice is the term generally used to describe negligence of professional personnel.

Elements of Liability

Liability consists of four elements that must be established to prove that malpractice or negligence has occurred: duty, breach of duty, causation, and damages. *Duty* refers to an obligation to use due care (what a reasonably prudent nurse would do) and is defined by the standard of care appropriate for the nurse–client relationship. *Breach of duty* is the failure to meet the standard of care. *Causation,* the most difficult element of liability to prove, refers to the failure to meet the standard of care (breach), which actually *causes* the injury. *Damages* are the actual harm or injury resulting to the client. Examples of these four elements are presented in Table 6-1.

Common Negligent Acts

The areas in which health-care providers run the greatest risks of being negligent include (1) foreign objects left in clients; (2) burns; (3) falls; (4) failure to observe and take appropriate action; (5) medication errors; (6) drug administration and drug distribution errors; (7) mistaken identity; (8) administration of blood; (9) failure to communicate; (10) failure to exercise reasonable judgment; (11) defects in apparatus; (12) errors due to family assistance in patient care; (13) abandonment; (14) loss of or damage to patients' property; (15) elopement; and (16) infections (Creighton, 1986a, pp 157–190).

Standards of Care

To determine negligence, a standard of care is devised by deciding what a reasonably prudent person would or would not have done under similar circumstances.

Each nurse is responsible for following the standards of care for her particular area of practice. For example, the labor and delivery nurse must understand how standards for nursing practice differ from those for medical obstetric practice (nurse practice act), be familiar with specific standards for obstetric nursing (NAACOG Standards, Nurses' Association of the American College of Obstetricians and Gynecologists), and execute the nursing responsibilities detailed in the hospital's policies and procedures and in the job description. If hospital policy dictates an assessment of each woman in the early stages of labor every 30 minutes, this standard must be adhered to unless the nurse documents a reason for doing otherwise.

Malpractice Litigation

When a client believes that he has been injured through the negligence of a nurse or other health-care professional and pursues legal action, one of three outcomes usually ensues:

T A B L E   6-1
Examples of Elements of Liability

Element	Example
Duty	Hospital staff nurses are responsible for • Accurate assessment of clients assigned to their care • Alerting responsible health-care professionals to changes in a client's condition • Competent execution of safety measures for clients
Breach of duty	• Failure to note and report that an elderly client assessed as alert on admission is exhibiting periods of confusion • Failure to execute and document use of appropriate safety measures (*e.g.,* upper and lower bedside rails, use of restraints if necessary, assisted ambulation)
Causation	• Failure to utilize appropriate safety measures, which causes the client to fall while attempting to get out of bed and to fracture left hip
Damages	• Fractured left hip, pain and suffering, lengthened hospital stay, and need for rehabilitation

- All parties concerned work toward a fair settlement.
- Case is presented to a malpractice arbitration panel (in the United States).
- Case is brought to trial court.

The steps involved in malpractice litigation where the case is brought to the trial court are shown in Figure 6-3. The nurse may be involved in legal proceedings as a defendant, a fact witness, or an expert witness.

The Nurse as Defendant

When a nurse is named a defendant it is important to work closely with an attorney while preparing the defense. The attorney representing the nurse's interests will be secured either by the nurse (if carrying personal liability insurance) or by the employing hospital or institution. Recommendations for the nurse defendant include the following:

- Don't discuss the case with anyone at your hospital (in the United States the case may be discussed with the risk manager).
- Don't discuss the case with the plaintiff.
- Don't discuss the case with the plaintiff's lawyer.
- Don't discuss the case with anyone testifying for the plaintiff.
- Don't discuss the case with reporters.

- Don't alter the patient's records. *Tampering with a chart is the worst mistake you can make*—you may well ruin your defense.
- Don't hide any information from your lawyer.
- Don't go to the witness stand unprepared.
- Don't be discourteous on the witness stand.
- Don't volunteer any information.

(Mandell, 1987a)

The Nurse as a Fact Witness

A nurse who has knowledge of the actual incident prompting the legal case may be called on by either attorney to testify as a *fact witness*. It is critical that fact witnesses, who are placed under oath, base their testimony only on *first-hand knowledge* of the incident and not on assumptions. The nurse will be asked if the testimony is based on independent recollection of the incident or on documentation in the client record. The nurse may testify "I do not remember Mrs. Jones but I see from review of her record that I cared for her on the evenings of June 10, 13, 14, and 17." When in doubt about the facts of the incident the nurse should simply testify "I do not remember that." New research into memory is showing that people often remember things differently from the way they were and challenges the value of the eye-wit-

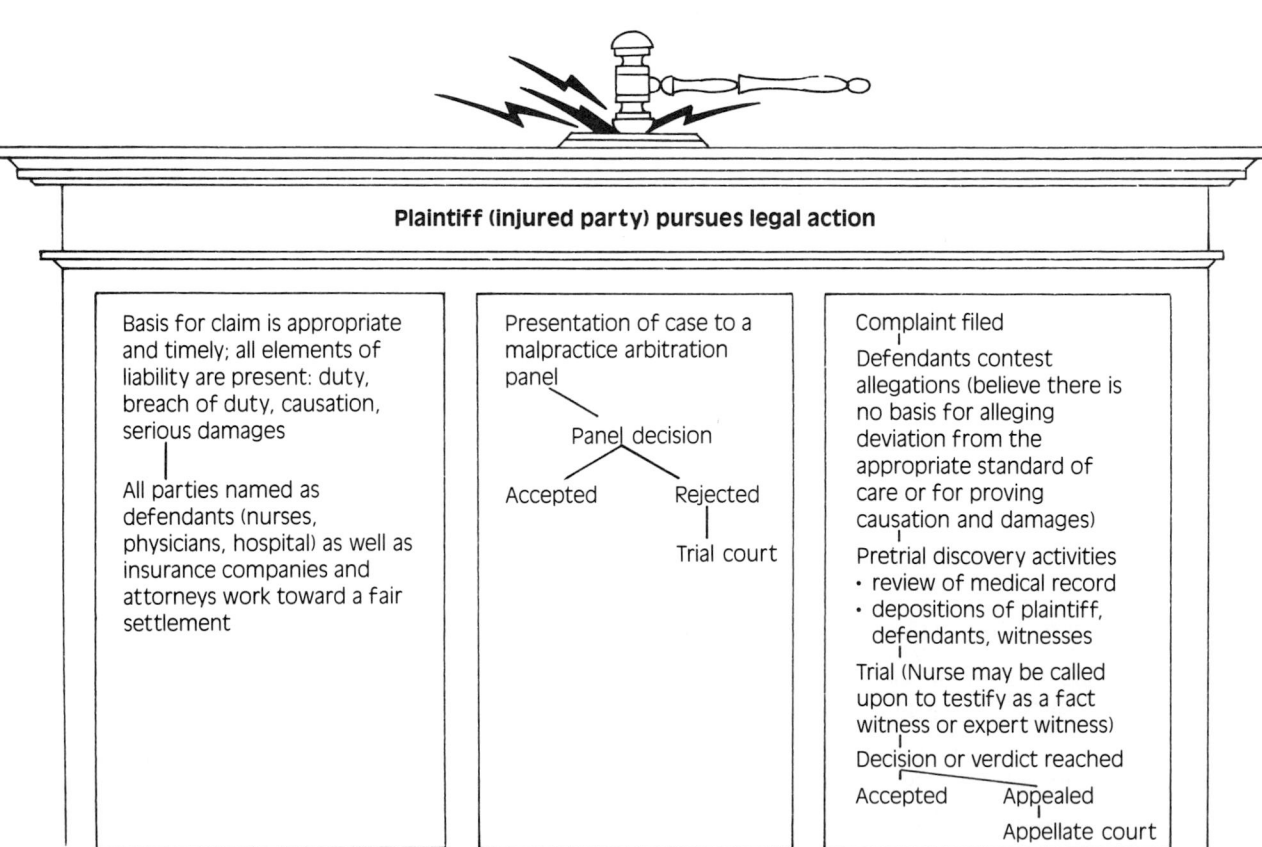

Plaintiff (injured party) pursues legal action

Basis for claim is appropriate and timely; all elements of liability are present: duty, breach of duty, causation, serious damages All parties named as defendants (nurses, physicians, hospital) as well as insurance companies and attorneys work toward a fair settlement	Presentation of case to a malpractice arbitration panel Panel decision Accepted Rejected Trial court	Complaint filed Defendants contest allegations (believe there is no basis for alleging deviation from the appropriate standard of care or for proving causation and damages) Pretrial discovery activities • review of medical record • depositions of plaintiff, defendants, witnesses Trial (Nurse may be called upon to testify as a fact witness or expert witness) Decision or verdict reached Accepted Appealed Appellate court

F I G U R E   6-3
Civil legal procedure in malpractice litigation.

ness memory. Thus, accurate documentation remains the nurse's best defense.

The Nurse as an Expert Witness

The role of a nurse called on by either attorney to testify as an *expert witness* is to explain to the judge and jury what happened based on the client's record and to offer an opinion as to whether or not the nursing care met acceptable standards. Nurse expert witnesses need a solid educational background and strong clinical experience comparable to the nurse defendant's. An understanding of the legal aspects of nursing and malpractice liability and knowledge of the state or province nurse practice act and the standard of nursing care where the incident occurred are also necessary.

LEGAL SAFEGUARDS FOR THE NURSE

Contracts

A *contract* may be defined as the exchange of promises between two parties. The law of contracts provides a remedy for a breach of contract so that the person who suffers from a broken contract may be compensated for any resulting loss. For a contract to be legally enforceable, it must contain (1) real consent of the parties, (2) a valid consideration, (3) a lawful purpose, (4) competent parties, and (5) the form required by law (Creighton, 1986a, p 35).

Practicing nurses enter into legally valid and binding contracts with both their employers and their clients. It is thus important that they understand and are able to fulfill the terms of their agreement before giving consent.

Competent Practice

Competent practice remains the nurse's most important and best legal safeguard (Fig 6-4). Each nurse is responsible for making sure that educational background and clinical experience are adequate to fulfill the nursing responsibilities described in the job description. Legal safeguards include

- Respecting legal boundaries of practice
- Following institutional procedures and policies
- "Owning" personal strengths and weaknesses; seeking means of growth, education, supervised experience, discussions with colleagues
- Evaluating proposed assignments; refusing to accept responsibilities for which one is not prepared
- Keeping current
- Respecting client rights and developing rapport with clients
- Keeping careful documentation
- Working within the institution to develop and support management policies

Table 6-2 lists areas of potential liability associated with each of the American Nurses' Association Standards of Practice. Although any nurse can make an error, nursing errors can result in serious outcomes for the client, as is illustrated in the examples.

Competent practice includes developing sensitivity to common sources of client injury, such as falls, use of restraints, and malfunctioning equipment, and then taking specific measures to prevent client injury. Table 6-3 illustrates guidelines for nursing interventions to reduce legal risks.

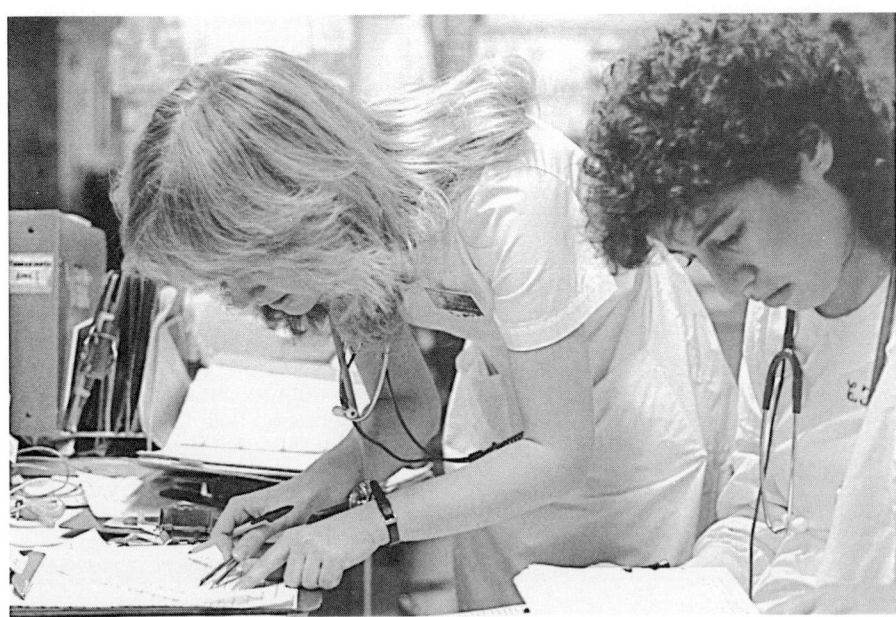

FIGURE 6-4

Competent practice is the nurse's most important legal safeguard. Careful documentation is the key to competent practice. (Photo by Gates Rhodes, courtesy of the School of Nursing, University of Pennsylvania)

T A B L E   6-2
Areas of Potential Liability for Nurses

Standards of Practice*	Areas of Potential Liability	Examples
1. The collection of data about the health status of the client is systematic and continuous. The data are accessible, communicated, and recorded.	• Incomplete database obtained (occurs frequently when client is too ill at admission to respond to questions) • Significant omissions or errors in recording database • Failure to note in the client's plan of care (and to execute) need for more frequent nursing assessments • Failure to recognize and to report significant changes in the client's condition	• Child too weak to be weighed on admission; chart contains no record of client's weight; dosage of postoperative antibiotic therapy (which should be calculated on child's weight) too small to prevent infection; abscess develops • No record of client's allergies on chart; medication administered, which led to anaphylactic shock • Previously alert client was exhibiting periods of confusion; found beating roommate with a hairbrush • Mother's labor is failing to progress, nurses unaware of signs of fetal distress; obstetrician not informed; irreversible cerebral damage to fetus • Healthy client is making slower than usual postanesthesia recovery; signs of developing cerebrovascular accident (slurred speech, difficulty moving extremities (falling to one side) are present and unnoted.
2. Nursing diagnoses are derived from health status data.	• Failure to identify priority nursing diagnosis critical to the client's care • Nursing diagnosis incorrectly developed and "labels" the client negatively	• Nowhere in the client's plan of care was it noted that the client had a history of choking on food ("impaired swallowing") and that close supervision was indicated during meals; client aspirated brussel sprout and died. • Homosexual client without AIDS admitted for gallbladder surgery questions the few interactions he has with staff. Nursing diagnosis on cardex reads "Potential for violence to others (AIDS) related to homosexuality."
3. The plan of nursing care includes goals derived from the nursing diagnoses.	• Nursing care plan contains no indication that nurses were aware of and sensitive to the client's health-care priorities.	• Obese client with a history of impaired circulation continually refuses to ambulate after major abdominal surgery; client dies following a massive pulmonary embolism. Plan of care showed no concern or attempt to compensate for client's lack of mobility.
4. The plan of nursing care includes priorities and the prescribed nursing approaches or measures to achieve the goals derived from the nursing diagnosis		
5. Nursing actions provide for client participation in health promotion, maintenance, and restoration.	• The client's record contains no documentation of attempts to teach the client and family appropriate self-care measures.	• Client discharged from short-procedure unit on crutches; falls first day home, refracturing leg; alleges his not receiving instructions for crutch-walking caused fall; client record contains no documentation of client education.

(Continued)

TABLE 6-2
Areas of Potential Liability for Nurses
(Continued)

Standards of Practice*	Areas of Potential Liability	Examples
6. The nursing actions assist the client to maximize his health capabilities.	• Nursing interventions deviate from usual standard of care (understaffing, indifference on part of nurse, inexperience of nurse, faulty or scarce equipment/resources).	• Skin breakdown on frail, elderly client worsens with eventual muscle deterioration; sepsis; nurses seem confused about treatment regimen for pressure ulcers and treatment is inconsistent.
7. The client's progress or lack of progress toward goal achievement is determined by the client and the nurse.	• Plan of care and nursing notes show no evidence that nurses evaluated whether the client achieved target goals. • Client discharged before key goals are met with no follow-up instructions.	• Client newly started on insulin therapy is discharged without understanding the relationship among food, exercise, and insulin and after giving himself the insulin only once—no referral made to visiting nurse; client readmitted after two weeks with dangerously *low* blood sugar following overdose with insulin.
8. The client's progress or lack of progress toward goal achievement directs reassessment, reordering of priorities, new goal setting, and revision of the plan of nursing care.		

* American Nurses' Association: Standards of Nursing Practice. Kansas City, The Association, 1973

Client Education

United States courts affirm the client's right to know and view client education as the legal duty of the nurse. Standards for client education are derived from national professional standards and from state nurse practice acts in the United States and provincial nurse practice acts in Canada, as well as the local standards described in hospital policies, procedure manuals, and job descriptions. Special forms for documenting the nurse's assessment of the client's learning needs and for subsequent teaching are available at some agencies. Failure to conduct or document the assessment of learning needs and teaching may later be construed as negligence.

Smith (1987) describes typical nursing responsibilities for client education:
- Discuss nursing care plan and interventions with client and family.
- Identify client's and family's learning needs.
- Assess client's and family's learning readiness.
- Document teaching plan as part of the nursing care plan.
- Teach the client and family, and help other staff members teach them as needed.
- Evaluate and document results of client teaching.

General guidelines for the nurse wishing to execute client education responsibilities competently include the following:
- Determine in your practice setting what specific aspects of client education are the responsibility of nursing. Consult your job description and be familiar with agency policies regarding client education and its documentation.
- Remember that an important aim of nursing is to assist clients in managing their own care. Document all nursing efforts to educate the client and family about health-care management and also document the client's response. If a client refuses health education or refers the nurse to a family member ("Talk to my wife about my pills, she'll be giving them to me at home"), document this on the client's record. If client education greatly increases the client's anxiety and he requests not to be given any more information, the nurse should document the client's initial response to teaching, the request that it be stopped, and, if the nurse complied, the reason for doing so.
- Since lack of time is a frequently offered reason for failing to document client education, nurses should assess what type of client documentation is rou-

T A B L E   6-3
Nursing Interventions to Reduce Three Common Legal Risks
You can reduce the frequency and severity of client injuries and your risk of liability by following these guidelines. Remember that the client's record should evidence ample documentation of your implementation of these measures.

Falls	Use of Restraints	Malfunctioning Equipment
• Assess *every* patient carefully to determine his risk of falling; if he's at high risk, follow these guidelines: • Write your nursing diagnoses and care plan to reflect his risk of falling. • Monitor him regularly, following your hospital's policy. • Keep his bed side rails raised, as indicated. • As always, provide adequate lighting and a clean, uncluttered environment. • Help him when he gets out of bed, and make sure he wears proper shoes when walking. • Have adequate staff available if he needs help getting in or out of bed. • Take special precautions with an elderly or medicated patient, especially if the doctor's orders include having him sit in a chair several times a day. If you can't supervise him, assign someone else. • Keep the patient oriented to time and place, especially if he's elderly or confused.	• Use restraints only as a last resort or as ordered; use minimal restraints when possible. • Check your hospital's written protocol: Besides reflecting state laws, it should specify when you can use restraints and who may order their use. A doctor's order may be required. • In an emergency—such as when you believe a patient's condition will lead to violent behavior —you may need to apply restraints without an order, but be sure to get a written order afterward. • Assess and document the reason for restraining the patient, and record what type of restraints you use, how you supervise their use, and what time you apply or remove them. • Once you've applied restraints, you may be liable for any injuries they cause. Check at least every half hour to make sure that the patient doesn't work his way out of them (or strangle himself) and that they're still properly placed. • Reassess him frequently for signs of impaired circulation and skin irritation. Loosen the restraints every 2 hours: If he's awake, be sure to take proper precautions. • Place the patient in an upright position for eating to help keep him from aspirating food or choking. • Don't ever use restraints as punishment or as a substitute for treatment.	• Follow the manufacturers' instructions for operation and maintenance of all equipment. • Know your hospital's policy on equipment checks and maintenance. Nurses routinely check some equipment (for example, intubation equipment, monitors, and defibrillators); the maintenance department or a biomedical specialist checks the rest. Be sure you know what equipment you're responsible for checking and whom to call if you find a malfunction or if the equipment needs to be serviced. • Fix or report any defective equipment immediately. And ask that it be removed from the unit before someone else tries to use it. • When equipment fails while you're using it, document the entire incident, including the actions you took, and advise your hospital's risk manager. • Urge your hospital to hold continuing education classes (if it's not already doing so) to review proper use of new equipment and equipment already in use.

(Nursing Life 6(6):26–30, 1986)

tinely offered on their unit and, where possible, develop forms or checklists facilitating rapid documentation. For example, preoperative checklists have greatly facilitated the recording of preoperative teaching and are often introduced as evidence in court that preoperative teaching was done. Other successful models include forms for documenting (1) diabetic teaching, (2) teaching following a myocardial infarction, and (3) teaching postpartal and baby care to mothers.

Executing Physician's Orders

Nurses are legally responsible to carry out the orders of the physician in charge of a client unless an order is one that would lead a reasonable person to anticipate injury

if it were carried out. Guidelines when executing orders follow:
1. Be familiar with the parties, designated in your nurse practice act, who can legally write orders for the nurse to execute (in many states this does not include a physician's assistant).
2. Attempt to have all physician's orders in writing. Verbal and telephone orders should be countersigned within 24 hours. To eliminate errors caused by telephone orders
   • Limit telephone orders to true emergency situations in which there is no alternative.
   • Designate the nurses who may take telephone orders (those who have more education and experience, a primary nurse).
   • Repeat a telephone order back to the physician.

- Document the order, its time and date, the situation necessitating the order, the physician prescribing and reconfirming the order as it is read back, and your name; indicate if the order is a VO (verbal order) or TO (telephone order).
- When telephone extensions make this possible, have two nurses listen to a questionable telephone order, with both nurses countersigning the order.

3. Question any physician order that is
   - Ambiguous
   - Contraindicated by normal practice (*e.g.,* dose of medication that is abnormally high)
   - Contraindicated by the client's present condition (*e.g.,* as a client's present condition improves, he may no longer need aggressive forms of treatment)

It is good practice for the nurse to check any order a client questions.

Documentation

Documentation is discussed in Chapter 18, and thus only the legality of documentation is discussed here. Although most nurses prefer to spend their time interacting with clients rather than writing in a client's record, careful documentation is a critical legal safeguard for the nurse. The presumption of the law is that if something was not documented, it was not done. This includes even routine acts such as taking vital signs, repositioning clients, and using side rails.

Nurses should be sure their institutions have flow sheets or some type of documentation form that enables them to check off routine aspects of care rapidly and completely. A comprehensive nursing note should be written for each client problem addressed by the nurse during her time of duty. The note should include the current nature of the problem, how the nurse intervened, the client's response, and, when appropriate, future priorities for care. Once a problem is noted nursing documentation should evidence continuity of care until the problem is resolved.

A common problem reported by nurses is not knowing how to document an incident, for example, when the nurse believes the client needs medical attention and intervention but the responsible physicians are not responding to calls for assistance. In this case, the best legal safeguard for the nurse is to document the *facts* of the incident, being careful not to make incriminatory statements like "anyone could see we were losing this client rapidly" or "once again Dr. Jones was unavailable when his client needed him." The note should document the time the physician was called and the time of his response. Such a note documents that the nurse is carefully assessing the client, recognizing significant cues, and reporting them appropriately. The nursing supervisor should write the next note after reviewing the case and choosing a course of action. Client noncom-

pliance with the therapeutic regimen should also be documented along with the nurse's attempts to increase compliance.

Understaffing

Understaffing is a problem that results in reduced quality of nursing care and may jeopardize client safety. Temporary management solutions to understaffing, such as "floating" nurses from one unit to another or asking nurses to work overtime or "doubles" (back-to-back shifts), are ineffective because they further jeopardize client safety. A nurse on an understaffed hospital unit will be held to a professional standard of judgment with respect to accepting responsibility for work and for delegating nursing responsibilities to others. If client injury results, the hospital employer and nurse employee will most likely be named as codefendants (Creighton, 1986b).

Professional Liability Insurance

Although a nurse's best legal safeguard is always competent practice, the increasing number of malpractice claims naming nurses as defendants make it wise for nurses to carry their own liability insurance. This insurance may be obtained through the American Nurses' Association, through provincial nursing associations in Canada, and through other sources.

Risk Management Programs

In the hope of reducing malpractice claims, many health-care institutions have initiated **risk management** programs designed to identify, analyze, and treat risks. Elements of a comprehensive risk management program include
- *Safety program:* The aim is to provide a safe environment in which the basic safety needs of clients, employees, and visitors are met.
- *Products safety program:* The aim is to ensure safe and adequate equipment; this involves ongoing equipment evaluation and maintenance.
- *Quality assurance program:* The aim is to provide quality health care to clients; this involves ongoing evaluation of all systems used in the care of the client.

Incident Reports

An **incident report** is a tool used by health-care institutions to document the occurrence of anything "out of the ordinary" that results in or has the potential to result in harm to a client, employee, or visitor. It is the chief means of identifying risks. More harm than good results from ignoring mistakes. Incident reports improve the management and treatment of clients by identifying high-risk patterns and initiating inservice programs to prevent future problems. These forms also make all the facts about an incident available to the institution in case of litigation.

The nurse responsible for a potentially or actually harmful incident or who witnesses an injury is the one who fills in the incident form. This form should contain (1) the complete name of the person or persons involved and the names of all witnesses; (2) a complete *factual* account of the incident; (3) the date, time, and place of the incident; (4) pertinent characteristics of the person or persons involved (alert, ambulatory, asleep) and of any equipment or resources being used; and (5) any other variables believed to be important to the incident. A physician completes the incident form with documentation of the medical examination when there has been actual or potential injury to a client, employee, or visitor.

In some states the incident report may be used in court as evidence. The nurse documenting a client incident should include a complete account of what happened in the client's record as well as preparing the incident report. However, documentation on the client record should not include the fact that an incident report was filed. In Canada incident reports are on file in the institution.

Good Samaritan Laws

Good Samaritan laws are designed to protect health practitioners when they give aid to persons in emergency situations. For example, a physician at the scene of an auto accident may give emergency care if it appears necessary without fear of legal suit, unless care is given in a grossly negligent manner.

Forty-eight states and the District of Columbia have good Samaritan laws, although the laws vary considerably. Nurses are covered in some states, while in others they are not. Good Samaritan legislation exists in four Canadian provinces and covers both physicians and nurses. So far, there appears to be no common law resulting from decisions based on these statutes.

No person has a legal obligation to help another, and a health practitioner, as any other person, may choose to help or to leave the scene of an emergency. However, in many situations, there would appear to be an ethical responsibility to assist. When health practitioners assist a person in an emergency situation and consent for the care is not possible, they are expected to use good judgment in determining whether an emergency exists and to give care that a reasonably prudent person with a similar background and in a similar circumstance would give.

STUDENT LIABILITY

Student nurses are responsible for their own acts of negligence if these result in client injury. Moreover, they are held to the *same standard of care* that would be used to evaluate the actions of a registered nurse. Legal responsibilities of student nurses include (1) careful preparation for each new clinical experience and (2) a duty to notify their clinical instructor if they feel in any way unprepared to execute a nursing procedure. For no reason should a student attempt a clinical procedure if unsure of the correct steps involved in its application. The student nurse is responsible for being familiar with agency policies and procedures.

A hospital may also be held liable for the negligence of a student nurse enrolled in a hospital-controlled program since the student is considered an employee of the hospital. The status of students enrolled in college and university programs is less clear, as is the liability of the educational institution in which they are enrolled and the health-care institution offering a site for clinical practice.

Nursing instructors may share a student's responsibility for damages in the event of client injury if (1) the student's assignment called for clinical skills beyond the student's competency or (2) the instructor failed to provide reasonable and prudent clinical supervision. Since the status of clients can change rapidly, especially in an acute-care setting, students should notify their instructor or a staff member of any significant changes in the client's condition, even if they are unsure of the meaning of these changes.

Most nursing programs require students to carry personal professional liability insurance. School policies provide coverage only for clinical nursing done for educational purposes. Moreover, student nurses who work as nursing assistants or in some other health-care role are legally permitted to offer only the services contained in their job description. Even if they feel confident with medication administration, catheter insertion, and other professional nursing acts, they risk disciplinary action when they perform these procedures outside the supervised clinical practice setting.

LAWS AFFECTING NURSING PRACTICE

Occupational Safety and Health

The Occupational Safety and Health Act of 1970, commonly known as OSHA, set legal standards in the United States in an effort to ensure safe and healthful working conditions for men and women. The act is intended to reduce work-related injuries and illnesses. It has had an impact on health agencies and has increased certain responsibilities for many nurses. Occupational health and safety acts are provincial statutes in Canada. The following examples illustrate situations that could violate standards, if care is not taken, because of the potential threat to worker safety:

- The use of electrical equipment
- The use of isolation techniques for patients with infectious diseases and the management of contaminated equipment and supplies
- The use of radiation, such as infrared or ultraviolet radiation; sound or radio waves; and laser beams
- The use of chemicals, such as those that are toxic or flammable

The law is specific concerning its applications, and fines can be severe when infractions are noted. Nurses can assist in implementing this law by promoting health and safety precautions wherever they work. Nurses employed in industrial settings have a particularly important role in conforming to the law's requirements.

Reporting Obligations

The unique nature of nurse–client interactions frequently results in the nurse's having knowledge of something (child abuse, rape, communicable disease) that a state or province requires to be reported. Legislation varies in this regard and the nurse is responsible for knowing what needs to be reported in the local area and to what authority.

Controlled Substances

Both the United States and Canada have special laws governing the distribution and use of controlled substances (drugs with abuse potential) such as narcotics, depressants, stimulants, and hallucinogens. Drug abuse laws are specific and violations are considered criminal acts. Nursing responsibilities for controlled substances include their storage in special locked compartments and documentation responsibilities.

Wills

State and provincial laws regulate requirements for a will. The person who makes a will is called the *testator*. A will describes intentions a testator wishes carried out upon his death. A person who receives money or property from a will is called a *beneficiary*. Nurses are occasionally asked to witness a testator's signing of his will.

There are certain guidelines concerning a will and witnessing the testator's signature with which the nurse should be familiar:

- The witness should feel sure that the testator is of sound mind, that is, he knows what he is doing and is free of the influence of drugs that could likely distort his thinking.
- The witness should feel sure that the testator is acting voluntarily and is not being coerced in any way concerning the terms of his will.

- Witnesses should see the testator sign his will and they should sign in the presence of each other. State law indicates how many witnesses must acknowledge the testator's signature on a will. Two or three witnesses are most commonly required.
- Witnesses to the signature on a will need not read it, but they should be sure that the document being signed is a will and not some other type of document.
- In most states, a person who is a beneficiary in a will is disqualified to act as a witness to the testator's signature.

Legal Issues Related to Dying and Death

Legal responsibilities for the dying or deceased client are discussed in Chapter 13. Prolonging life, living wills, and no-code orders are discussed here.

Prolonging Life and the Living Will. Family members of terminally ill patients are often asked to participate in making a decision about sustaining life when many artificial means are being used. The physician usually initiates this discussion with the family, but relatives often involve the nurse in their decision-making process. The nurse's role may be one of providing information, helping relatives explore their feelings and ideas, and offering support. If called upon, the nurse may offer advice but should not attempt to persuade family members to follow a particular course of action. There are no clear-cut guidelines on prolonging life; each case is handled on an individual basis. The tendency is to respect the wishes of the closest relatives in relation to prolonging life by artificial means.

Many persons are now planning ahead before trauma or terminal illness occurs by seeking an alternative to prolonging life unnecessarily. One method for facilitating an objective personal decision on prolonging life is for the person to prepare a living will. A **living will** describes a person's wishes with regard to being kept alive by artificial means or heroic measures when there is no reasonable expectation of recovery from a physical or mental disability. The Euthanasia Educational Council has prepared a form for a living will and offers it to anyone upon request (Fig. 6-5). The physician notes on the client's chart when resuscitation and life-prolonging measures are not to be used. Questions about living wills may be directed to the Society for the Right to Die, Department NL, 250 W. 57th Street, New York, NY 10107. Natural death act legislation exempts the physician and other health professionals from liability when they act on living wills. There is no such legislation in Canada. The dying patient's bill of rights is shown in Chapter 13.

No-Code and Slow-Code Orders. To prevent the improper use of cardiopulmonary resuscitation (CPR),

TO MY FAMILY, MY PHYSICIAN, MY LAWYER, MY CLERGYMAN
TO ANY MEDICAL FACILITY IN WHOSE CARE I HAPPEN TO BE
TO ANY INDIVIDUAL WHO MAY BECOME RESPONSIBLE FOR MY HEALTH, WELFARE OR AFFAIRS

Death is as much a reality as birth, growth, maturity and old age—it is the one certainty of life. If the time comes when I, _____ can no longer take part in decisions for my own future, let this statement stand as an expression of my wishes, while I am still of sound mind.

If the situation should arise in which there is no reasonable expectation of my recovery from physical or mental disability, I request that I be allowed to die and not be kept alive by artificial means or "heroic measures". I do not fear death itself as much as the indignities of deterioration, dependence and hopeless pain. I, therefore, ask that medication be mercifully administered to me to alleviate suffering even though this may hasten the moment of death.

This request is made after careful consideration. I hope you who care for me will feel morally bound to follow its mandate. I recognize that this appears to place a heavy responsibility upon you, but it is with the intention of relieving you of such responsibility and of placing it upon myself in accordance with my strong convictions, that this statement is made.

Signed _____

Date _____

Witness _____

Witness _____

Copies of this request have been given to _____

TO MAKE BEST USE OF YOUR LIVING WILL

1. Sign and date before two witnesses. (This is to insure that you signed of your own free will and not under any pressure.)

2. If you have a doctor, give him a copy for your medical file and discuss it with him to make sure he is in agreement.

   Give copies to those most likely to be concerned "if the time comes when you can no longer take part in decisions for your own future". Enter their names on bottom line of the Living Will. Keep the original nearby, easily and readily available.

3. Above all discuss your intentions with those closest to you, NOW.

4. It is a good idea to look over your Living Will once a year and redate it and initial the new date to make it clear that your wishes are unchanged.

Prepared by the
EUTHANASIA EDUCATIONAL COUNCIL
250 West 57th Street, New York, N.Y. 10019

F I G U R E   6-5
This is a living will prepared by the Euthanasia Education Council.

which is designed to prevent *unexpected death,* some physicians will write "do not resuscitate" (DNR) or "no-code" orders on the chart of a terminally ill client if the client or family has expressed their wish for a peaceful death without heroic measures. Many physicians are reluctant to write these orders, especially when this issue is a source of conflict between the client and family or between individual family members. In these cases a physician who believes the client will not benefit from resuscitative measures may verbally indicate to the nurse that only a "slow-code" should be called, that is, in the case of cardiopulmonary or respiratory arrest, calling a code and resuscitating the client are to be delayed until these measures will be ineffectual. The legality of no-code and slow-code orders is not well established and is generally decided on a case-by-case basis. It is very likely that a nurse could be charged negligent in the event of a slow-code and resultant client death.

K E Y   P O I N T S

■ As the roles and duties of the nurse have expanded, so too has the legal accountability of the nurse.

■ Laws are standards or rules of conduct established and enforced by the government of a society to protect the rights of the public. Laws may be constitutional, statutory, administrative, or common.

■ Voluntary standards regulating nursing practice are developed and implemented by the nursing profession itself. These standards include the American Nurses' Association and Canadian Nurses' Association standards of practice, professional standards for the accreditation of education and service programs, and certification standards.

■ Legal standards are mandatory and are developed by legislative action controlling professional conduct. They include the nurse practice acts and rules and regulations of nursing.

■ Credentialing is the process of ensuring and maintaining professional competence. Credentialing involves accreditation, licensure/registration, and certification.

■ A nurse whose license is suspended or revoked for drug and alcohol abuse or for other acts of unprofessional conduct is entitled to due process of law.

■ Intentional torts for which the nurse may be liable include assault and battery, defamation of character, invasion of privacy, false imprisonment, and fraud.

■ Every individual has the right to be free from invasion of person, and thus consent is needed for all diagnostic, treatment, or research procedures. The person performing the procedure is responsible for obtaining informed consent. Documenting the informed consent may be delegated to nursing.

■ Negligence is defined as performing an act that a reasonably prudent person under similar circumstances would not do or failing to perform an act.

■ Legal safeguards for the nurse include (1) understanding and fulfilling the terms of contracts with employers and employees, (2) competent practice, (3) thorough client education, (4) safe execution of physician orders, (5) careful documentation, (6) professional liability insurance, and (7) participation in risk management programs.

■ The client's record should never be tampered with in an attempt to prepare a better defense.

■ Competent practice includes (1) respecting legal boundaries of nursing, (2) following institutional procedures and policies, (3) owning personal strengths and being aware of weaknesses, (4) evaluating proposed assignments, (5) keeping current, (6) respecting client rights and developing rapport with clients, (7) careful documentation, and (8) working with nursing management to develop and implement programs to improve quality care and decrease risks of client injury.

■ Student nurses are legally responsible for their own acts of negligence resulting in client injury. They are held to the *same standard of care* that would be used to evaluate the actions of a registered nurse.

■ Nurses need to be knowledgeable about specific laws affecting nursing practice. These include laws regulating occupational health and safety, reporting obligations, controlled substances, wills, and legislation related to dying and death.

BIBLIOGRAPHY

Arbeiter J: A buyer's guide to malpractice insurance. RN May: 22–26, 1986

Becker M: Five orders you must question to protect yourself legally. Nursing Life 3(1):21–23, 1983

Cazalas MW: Nursing and the Law, 3rd ed. Germantown, MD, Aspen, 1978

Collins HL: Certification: Is the payoff worth the price? RN July: 36–44, 1987

Cournoyer CP: Protecting yourself legally after a patient's injured. Nursing Life 5(2):18–22, 1985

Creighton H: Law Every Nurse Should Know, 5th ed. Philadelphia, WB Saunders, 1986a

Creighton H: Understaffing. Nursing Management 17(4):24, 27–28; 17(5):14, 16, 1986b

Creighton H: When can a nurse refuse to give care? Nursing Management 17(3):16, 18–20, 1986c

Cushing M: When the courts define nursing: What it is, what it does. Am J Nurs 87(6):773–774, 1987

Cushing M: Incident reports: For your eyes only? Am J Nurs 85(8):873–874, 1985

Cushing M: Malpractice: Are you covered? Am J Nurs 84(8):985–986, 1984

DeMilliano M: 8 common charting mistakes to avoid. Nursing Life 4(3):30–32, 1984

Ferrari MR: Avoiding legal risks in pediatrics. Nursing Life 6(2):24–25, 1986

Ficsta J: The Law and Liability. New York, John Wiley & Sons, 1983

Fine ERJ: What to do when the doctor's wrong. Nursing Life 2(6):22–24, 1982

Forkner DJ: Expert advice on becoming an expert witness. Nursing 17(6):69–71, 1987

Hogue E: 5 lessons you can learn from court decisions. Nursing 16(4):45–47, 1986

Kadzielskie MA: Legal implications for health care providers. Health Progress 67(4):48–52, May, 1986

Klein CA: Preventing malpractice suits. Nurse Pract 11(3):78, 80, 82, 1986

Mancini M: Charting: Keeping it professional so your care can't be faulted. Nursing Life 4(5):50–51, 1984

Mandell M: How to defend yourself against lawyer's attacks. Nursing Life 7(3):25–29, 1987a

Mandell M: Preventing patient injury. What you don't do can land you in court. Nursing Life 7(1):26–28, 1987b

Mandell M: Ten legal commandments for nurses who get sued. Nursing Life 6(3):18–21, 1986

Murchison I, Nichols TS, Hanson R: Legal Accountability in the Nursing Process, 2nd ed. St Louis, CV Mosby, 1982

Northrop CE: Unprofessional conduct and licensure revocation. Nurs Outlook 34(1):48, 1986

Northrop CE: Student nurses and legal accountabilities. Imprint 32(4):16, 18–20, 1985

Northrop CE: Status of recent nursing litigation. Nursing Economics 2(6):423–427, 1984

Parsons MS: 5 common legal risks. Nursing Life 6(6):26–31, 1986

President's Commission for the Study of Ethical Problems in Medicine and Biomedical and Behavioral Research: Making Health Care Decisions, vol 1, A Report. Washington, DC, US Government Printing Office, 1982

Rabinow J: Avoiding legal trouble when you and the doctor disagree. Nursing Life 4(4):41–44, 1984

Rehm M: Lessons learned from a lawsuit. Nursing 17(12):62–63, 1987

Report to house outlines scope of nursing practice. The American Nurse June: 13–14, 1987

Rocerto LR, Maleski CM: All about rights to medical records. Nursing Life 4(4):50–51, 1984

Rozovsky LE, Rozovsky FA: The legal dilemma: Getting caught between a rock and a hard place. Canadian Critical Care Nursing Journal 3(1):15–16, 19, 1986

Smith CE: Patient teaching: It's the law. Nursing 17(7):67–68, 1987

Springer EW (ed): Nursing and the Law. Pittsburgh, Aspen, 1970

Storch J: Patients' Rights: Ethical and Legal Issues in Health Care and Nursing. Toronto, McGraw-Hill Ryerson, 1982

Strader MK: Malpractice and nurse educators: Defining legal responsibilities. J Nurs Educ 24(9):363–367, 1985

Taylor C, Hobaugh R: The role of the critical care nurse in developing informed consent. Dimensions of Critical Care Nursing 5(2):98–105, 1986

Tobin BK: Living wills. Nursing Life 6(5):44–45, 1986

The Client: Concepts for Holistic Care

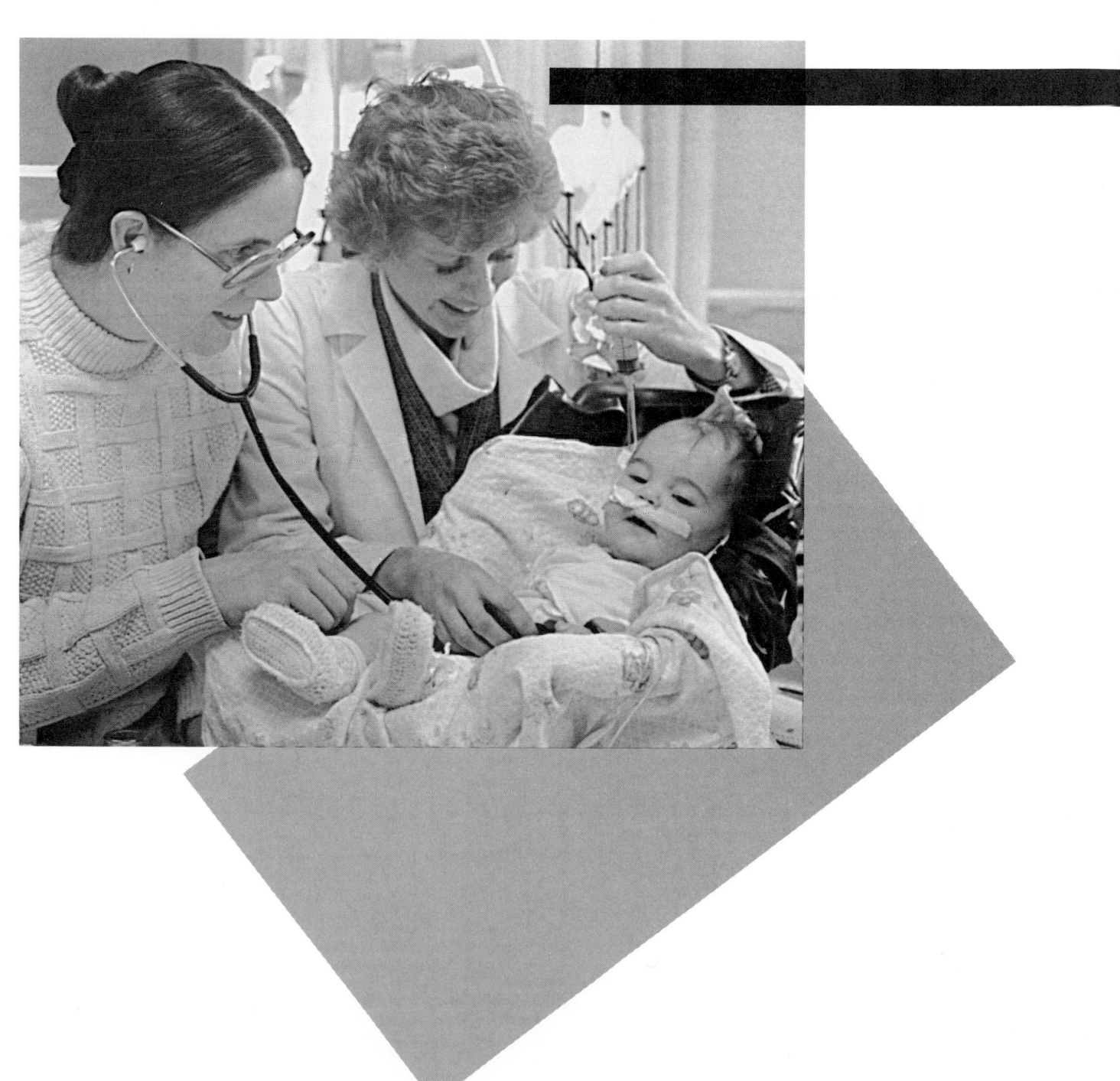

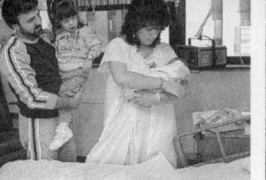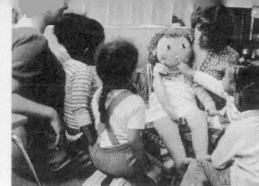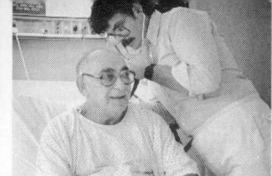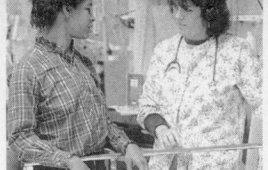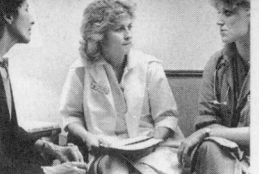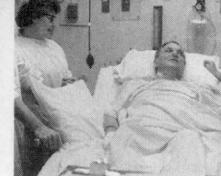

U N I T I I   *The Client: Concepts for Holistic Care*

*T*he chapters in Unit II focus on the client—the person receiving health care from the nurse. Concepts necessary in providing holistic care for the client as an individual and as a member of a family and community include basic human needs, culture and ethnicity, and stress and adaptation. By considering all aspects of the individual, a nurse can provide health care oriented toward wellness and maximizing the client's strengths to reach his or her potential.

In Unit II Maslow's hierarchy of basic human needs provides a framework for prioritizing nursing actions and for understanding the relationship between the ability to meet needs and the social environment. Family structures and functions are examined; the influence of the family and the community on health and illness is described. Consideration of cultural and ethnic factors in client care expands the nurse's holistic perspective of the client.

Stress and adaptation have great importance for nurses who are themselves subject to stress and who care for clients experiencing physiologic and psychologic stressors. Stress affects basic need attainment, is in-fluenced by sociocultural environments, and may either promote health or precipitate illness. Nursing actions to reduce stress, facilitate wellness, and promote coping must be individualized and holistic.

Unit II provides the knowledge necessary to understand the integration of basic human needs, sociocultural influences, and stress and adaptation—factors that make up the composite whole of each individual client—into nursing care, which will make that care holistic and individualized.

Human Needs: Person, Family, and Community

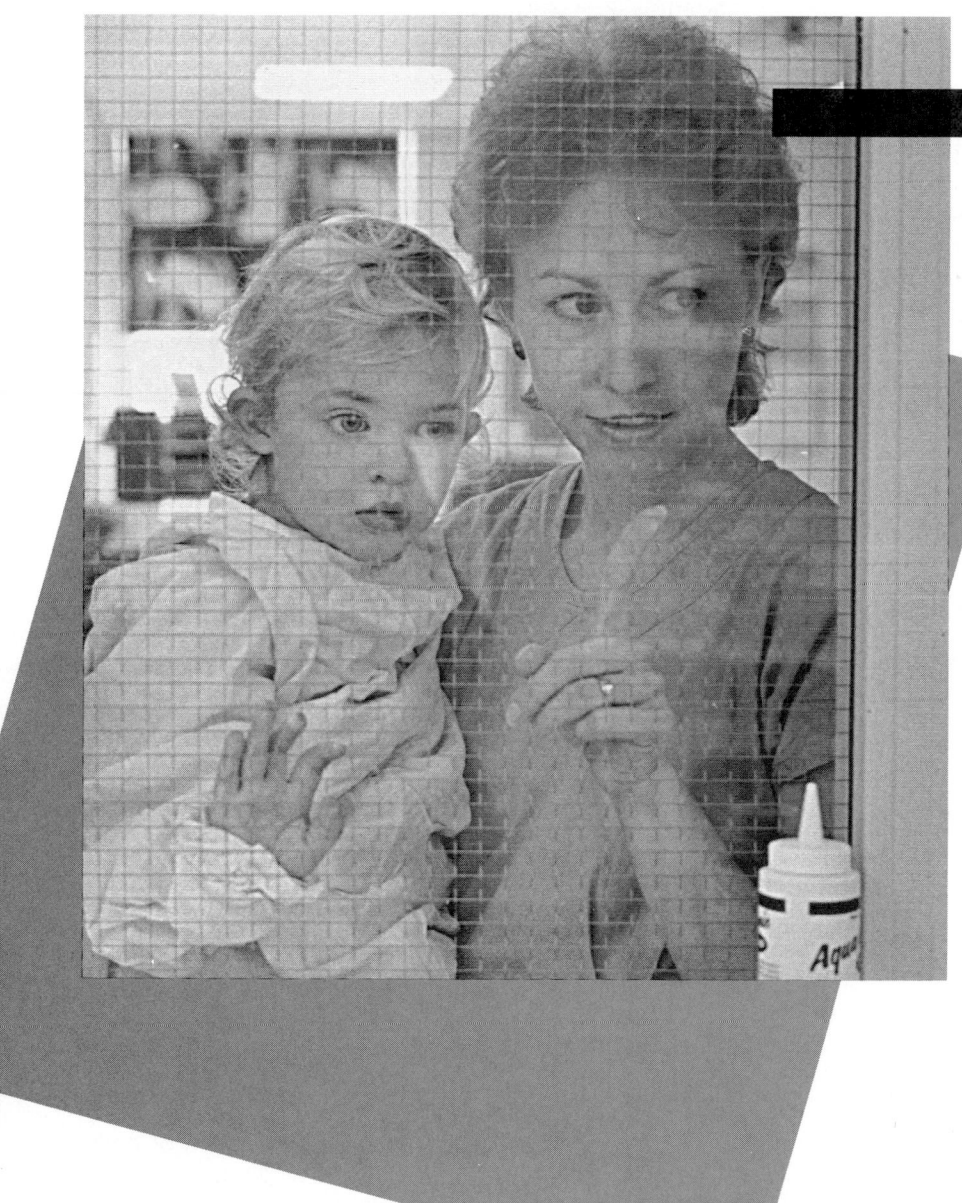

OBJECTIVES

After studying this chapter, the learner should be able to

Define key terms used in the chapter.

Describe each level of Maslow's hierarchy of basic human needs.

Discuss nursing actions necessary to meet needs for each level of the hierarchy.

Define family concepts, including family role, structures, functions, developmental stages/tasks, and risk factors.

Identify aspects of the community that impact individual and family health.

Describe nursing interventions to promote and maintain health in the individual, the family, and the community.

Human beings are complex organisms, shaped and influenced by both internal and external environments. The way we act, the way we feel, the things we value, and the priorities we set for ourselves are all the result of physiologic and psychosocial needs. These needs are common to all people, are essential to the health and survival of all people, and so are called **basic human needs**. Maslow's **hierarchy of needs** (described in Chap 2) prioritizes and helps us understand the interrelated nature of basic human needs.

Basic human needs are met (or unmet) in many ways. Some needs are met independently, but most require relationships with others for partial or complete fulfillment. Need satisfaction is largely dependent on a person's social environment, specifically family and community.

Holistic nursing care is based on the consideration of all the dimensions affecting human needs in health and illness. This chapter will discuss how basic human needs affect the individual, the family, and the community.

KEY TERMS

basic human needs
blended family
cohabiting family
community
extended family
hierarchy of needs
human sexuality
love and belonging needs

nuclear family
physiologic needs
safety and security needs
self-actualization needs
self-esteem needs
single-parent family
traditional family

THE INDIVIDUAL

Certain needs are more basic than others and must be at least minimally met before other needs can be considered. Because of this, needs are arranged in a hierarchy (Maslow, 1968). Although the hierarchy was outlined in Chapter 2, it is reviewed again so that you can identify each level as you read the descriptions and related nursing actions. The levels of the basic human needs hierarchy are illustrated in Figure 7-1.

Levels of Needs

Physiologic Needs

Physiologic needs, located at the base of the hierarchy of needs, have the highest priority. **Physiologic needs**—oxygen, food, water, temperature, elimination, sexuality, physical activity, and rest—must be minimally met to maintain life.

Most healthy children and adults meet their physiologic needs, but physiologic needs are often a major part of the nursing care plan for very young, very old, handicapped, and ill persons who require assistance in meeting these needs.

Oxygen is the most essential of all needs; all body cells require oxygen for survival. Oxygenation of body cells is carried out primarily by the respiratory and cardiovascular systems, and any alteration in their structure and function can result in increased need for oxygen. This need may be acute (necessitating cardiopulmonary resuscitation [CPR]) or chronic (requiring special positioning, treatments, and teaching). Nurses evaluate oxygen needs by continual assessment of skin color, vital signs, and responsiveness.

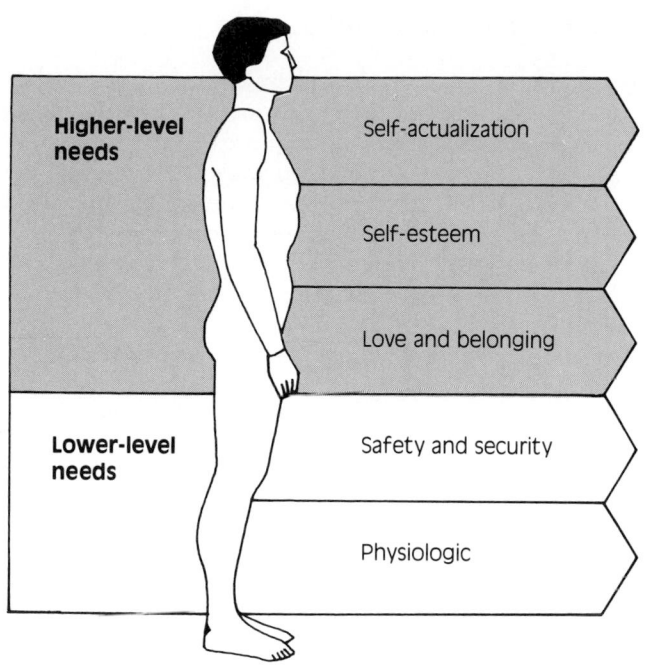

FIGURE 7-1
Maslow's hierarchy of basic human needs.

Taking in a balance of *food and fluids* and *eliminating* waste are also vital to human life. The body can survive longer without food or elimination than without water. Many of the body's structures are involved when meeting these needs: the gastrointestinal system, the urinary system, the skin, the lungs, and metabolic processes in cells. These processes are often interrelated; for example, the person with severe diarrhea loses excessive amounts of water. Nursing assessments common to these needs are (in part) excess fluid loss (dehydration) or gain (edema), weight loss or gain, and urinary and bowel elimination. Nursing actions to meet needs for food, fluid, and elimination include special procedures and teaching about normal nutrition and elimination.

Body *temperature* must remain in a fairly narrow range (approximately 97°F to 106°F [36°C to 41°C]) for the body to function normally. The body, under normal conditions, maintains body temperature by homeostatic mechanisms such as shivering and sweating. Prolonged exposure to heat or cold can lead to tissue damage and even death. The primary nursing role in meeting temperature needs is assessing the client's environment and teaching preventive measures.

Human sexuality is a component of health, just as sexual needs are physiologically basic. Sexuality involves human relationships, touch, and belonging as much as it does sexual activity. Without sexual needs, the human race would not continue. This area of human functioning is influenced by age, culture, values, and the presence of illness. Nurses are becoming more comfortable with assessing sexual needs and planning interventions to meet those needs.

Physical activity and *rest* are also basic physiologic needs. Physical activity is accomplished by intact and functioning neuromuscular and bony systems. Immobility, with disuse of muscles and bones, affects all other basic needs. *Rest and sleep* allow time for the body to rejuvenate and be free of stress. Individual requirements for rest and sleep vary widely, but the effects of deprivation have been well documented. Factors that influence sleep are age, environment, exercise, stress, and drugs. Clients entering the health-care setting often need increased rest and sleep but are unable to meet these needs without or because of the nurse's interventions.

Safety and Security Needs

Safety and security needs come next in priority and involve both physical and emotional components.

Physical safety means protecting a person from potential or actual harm. Nurses carry out a wide variety of activities to meet client's physical safety needs, for example,

- Handwashing and using sterile techniques to prevent infection
- Using electrical equipment properly
- Giving medications knowledgeably
- Using skill and rationale to transfer and ambulate clients
- Teaching parents about household chemicals that are dangerous to children

Emotional safety and security involves trusting others and being free of fear, anxiety, and apprehension. Clients entering the hospital may have increased emotional security needs; often they fear the unknown and become dependent on others through no fault of their own. Needs in this area can be met through such nursing actions as encouraging religious practices that give peace, allowing as much independent decision making and control as possible, and carefully explaining new and unfamiliar procedures and treatments.

Love and Belonging Needs

All humans have a basic need for love and belonging. Following physiologic and safety/security needs, this is the next priority of need and is often called a higher level need. **Love and belonging needs** include the understanding and acceptance of others in both giving and receiving love and the feeling of belonging to others: friends, peers, families, neighborhoods, communities.

Persons who perceive that their love and belonging needs are unmet often have a sense of loneliness and isolation. They may withdraw physically and emotionally, or they may become overly demanding and critical. Often these behaviors are a signal (or cue) that unmet needs are present. Nurses should always consider love and belonging needs in their plan of care. Some nursing interventions to meet this need are

- Including family and friends in the care of the client (Fig. 7-2)

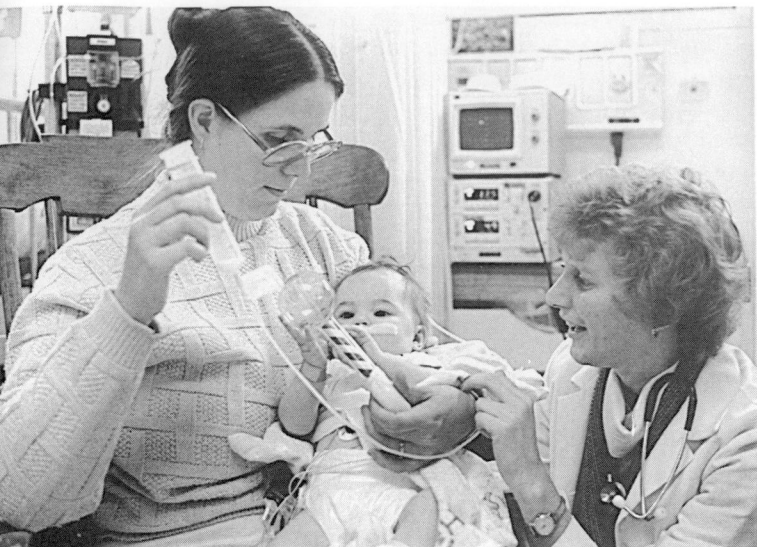

F I G U R E   7-2
By teaching the mother to feed her infant by gavage, the nurse is helping to fulfill the need for love and belonging of both mother and child. (Photo by Gates Rhodes, courtesy of the School of Nursing, University of Pennsylvania)

- Establishing a nurse–client relationship based on mutual understanding and trust (through demonstration of caring, communication, and respect for privacy)
- Referring patients to groups that focus on problems (such as cancer support groups or Alcoholics Anonymous)

Self-Esteem Needs

The next highest priority on the hierarchy is **self-esteem need**—the need to feel good about oneself, to feel pride and a sense of accomplishment in what one does, and to believe that others also hold one in high regard. Self-esteem gives the individual confidence and independence.

Self-esteem is affected by many factors. When a person's role changes (such as loss of job, or the parent whose last child just left home), self-esteem can be seriously altered because responsibilities and relationships have also changed. Other changes that may impact self-esteem are a change in body image, such as a gain or loss of weight, an injury, or a growth spurt during puberty.

It is important to remember that the perception of the person about the change—rather than the actual change itself—is what affects one's self-esteem.

Nurses can meet clients' self-esteem needs by accepting values and beliefs, encouraging clients to set attainable goals, and facilitating support by family or significant others. These actions will promote a sense of worth and self-acceptance.

Self-Actualization Needs

The highest level on the hierarchy of needs is **self-actualization need**—the need to reach one's potential through full development of one's unique capabilities. In general, each lower level of need must be met to some degree before this need can be satisfied. The process of self-actualization is one that continues throughout life. Maslow lists the following qualities that indicate achievement of one's potential:

- Acceptance of self and others as they are
- Focus of interest on problems outside of self
- Ability to be objective
- Feelings of happiness and affection for others
- Respect for all persons
- Ability to discriminate between good and evil
- Creativity as a guideline for solving problems and carrying out interests

To meet clients' self-actualization needs, the nurse must focus on strengths and possibilities, rather than on problems. Nursing interventions are aimed at caring for the total person (holistic care), providing a sense of direction and hope, and teaching aimed at maximizing potentials.

Applying Maslow's Theory

Maslow's hierarchy of basic needs is applicable in assessing, planning, implementing, and evaluating client care. Several nursing diagnoses, approved by the North American Nursing Diagnosis Association, are based on the levels of needs. (The five steps of the nursing process are discussed in Chap 1 and Unit IV.) The hierarchy can be used with all ages, in all health-care settings, and in both health and illness. It provides a vehicle for holistic nursing care—identifying unmet needs as they become health-care needs and considering all dimensions.

The hierarchy of basic needs allows the nurse to place the client on the health–illness continuum and to incorporate the health models into meeting needs.

As the nurse identifies and carries out interventions to meet needs, he or she must remember that this is only a framework or guideline, and that in actuality each individual person sets priorities and meets needs on the level most important to *that* person. Additionally, basic human needs are related and may require nursing actions at more than one level at a given time.

THE FAMILY

With rare exceptions, each person is a part of a number of groups. An individual probably has a group of friends, belongs to a church group, goes to school with a class group, and works with another group. Each of these groups is concerned with a specific part of the individual's life and is important. However, only one group is concerned with all parts of an individual's life and all his or her physical, personal, and social needs. That group is the family.

Family Concepts

Role

The family is the basic unit of society. Families exist in all sizes and configurations and are essential to the health and survival of the individual members, and to society as a whole. As *the* primary group for the individual, the family serves as a buffer between the needs of that individual and the demands and expectations of society. The role of the family is to meet the needs of its members while also meeting the needs of society (Friedman, 1981).

Definitions

Duvall (1971) defines the family as "a unity of interacting persons related by ties of marriage, birth, or adoption, whose central purpose is to create and maintain a common culture which promotes the physical, mental, emotional, and social development of each of its members." In today's society, that definition is still broadly applicable, but is expanded by Friedman (1981, p 8), who defines the family as "composed of two or more people who are emotionally involved with each other and live in close geographical proximity."

These are only two of the many ways of defining the family, but regardless of the definition, there are three essential criteria: structure (or form), functions, and common residence.

Family Structure

In today's society, there is no one commonly accepted family structure. The following narrative briefly discusses different family forms.

Traditional Family

The **traditional family** is composed of a father, a mother, and their children. These people, married and living together in one house, make up the **nuclear family** (Fig. 7-3). The nuclear family represents 73% of all households (U.S. National Center for Health Statistics, 1982). Relatives, such as aunts, uncles, cousins, and grandparents, who may or may not live with the nuclear family, are part of the **extended family**. For years, the traditional family was characterized by a father who worked (providing economic resources) and a mother who stayed at home to provide physical and emotional safety and security. This family group usually lived in close geographic proximity to members of the extended family, who provided a sense of stability and belonging.

Although the traditional family unit still has the same form (father, mother, children), the roles of the members have changed significantly. Two major factors impacting this change are (1) increased education and career opportunities for women and (2) an unstable economy, making additional income necessary to maintaining a desired standard of living.

As a result, the two-career family, in which both parents work, has become the norm instead of an uncommon occurrence. In the family in which both parents work, there is usually a blending of tasks. The father has a more active part in child care and household chores, and the mother assists in economic support.

It is important to remember that the traditional family (as previously defined) is no longer the dominant form. With changes in the traditional family come other influences on the needs of individual members. Considerations for the family, and for nursing care, include support systems (in our mobile society, members of the extended family are often not geographically nearby), availability of child care, time for leisure and recreation, and changing role models.

Other family structures are childless couples, couples with children no longer living at home, and the **blended family** made up of family units who join together to form a new family structure.

Single-Parent Families

Single parents may be never-married, separated, divorced, or widowed. Most often, the single parent is divorced or widowed, but increasing numbers of never-married men and women are choosing to become parents. The **single-parent family**, however, is most often headed by women. Nearly 95% of all single parents are women; single parents make up over 16% of North American families (U.S. Bureau of the Census, 1984).

Single parents have many special problems and needs, including financial concerns, role shifts (being both father and mother, remarriage or relationships with the opposite sex), and social stigma (divorce, unmarried, other). All of these problems are important considerations when planning and implementing nursing care (Friedman, 1981).

Alternate Family Structures

Some families do not meet the definition of traditional or single-parent, but meet the criteria previously outlined. As nurses, it is critical to remember that there are no absolute "rights" or "wrongs," and that one's own values must not be imposed on others. Acceptance of family members and relationships is essential to holistic, individualized client care. Alternate family structures include the following:

- *Cohabiting families:* This form includes those individuals who choose to live together for a variety of reasons: relationships, financial need, changing values. **Cohabiting families** include unmarried adults living together, communal or group marriages, and gay/lesbian families.

R E S E A R C H   I N   N U R S I N G   *Making a Difference*

Basic Human Needs—The Family

The family is the base of civilization and the continuity of society. Nursing has always recognized the impact of the family in planning and giving care to individual clients. Nursing research seeks to improve the assessment, intervention, and management of clients as individuals and as families who seek care from the health-care delivery system.

Related Research

Duffy M: Primary prevention behaviors: The female-headed, one parent family. Res Nurs Health 9: 115–122, 1986

Duffy's study was the first to investigate primary prevention practices in the female-headed, one-parent family. Health maintenance practices of the families included a balanced diet, rest, exercise, and personal hygiene. These health behaviors originated in the women's childhood and were practiced without conscious thought of their health effect. The major barriers to health promotion practices were lack of time, laziness, limited finances, and lack of support. The research shows the need for assessment of primary prevention behaviors practiced by the family and acknowledgment of those behaviors as strengths.

Hathaway D et al: Health promotion and disease prevention for the hospitalized patient's family. Nursing Administration Quarterly 11(3): 1–7, 1987

This study investigated the health of families of hospitalized clients to determine how hospitalization of a family member alters the other members' health-related activities and health status; it sought to identify what health-promotion activities could be provided. A significant number of family members experienced alterations in physical and emotional health, and changes in their usual health practices. Those practices most severely altered were exercise, sleep, nutrition, and relaxation. It was further found that the alterations stemmed from knowledge deficits related to the client and the client's care, resulting in stress and anxiety. The re-searchers suggest that family needs must be considered when client care plans are developed, and emphasize that providing information is basic nursing care.

Phillips L, Rempusheski V: Caring for the frail elderly at home: Toward a theoretical explanation of the dynamics of poor quality family caregiving. Advances in Nursing Science 8(4): 62–84, 1986

This research study, conducted to describe the dynamics involved when care is provided to the frail elderly by family caregivers in the home, found several factors influence the quality of care: (1) the caregiver's expectations and perceptions of the elderly person's behavior is directly related to the management strategies selected by the caregiver; (2) the caregiver's perception of the reality of the situation compared to the caregiver's perception of appropriate living impact on how the caregiver's role is carried out; (3) whether the caregiving is positive, neutral, or negative is related to the caregiver's belief about the role and the elderly person's behavior; and (4) the quality of family caregiving is related to the caregiver's self-esteem and ongoing performance evaluation. Findings indicate that the nurses who provide care to elderly persons in the home must understand and assess the family dynamics associated with home caregiving. Early identification and intervention to meet the needs of family members will decrease high-risk caregiving situations.

Summary

Health behaviors are integrated into each individual family member's health values, beliefs, and practices. These behaviors affect family members of all ages and at all levels of wellness. Nurses must remember that each person is part of a family whole and that the health status of one member of the family affects all the other members. Nursing research can clarify how health and illness affect the needs, structure, and functions of the family and how nursing care can best meet those needs.

Although this functional model of the family is more focused on society, it also interrelates with individual human needs. Physical and economic functions are essential to meeting many physiologic and safety/security needs, especially in infants and children. The affective and coping functions help satisfy love and belonging and self-esteem needs, as does socialization. Lastly, socialization provides cognitive and adaptive abilities to meet self-actualization needs.

Developmental Tasks of Families

Duvall (1977) has identified stages of the family life cycle and critical family developmental tasks. Duvall's Theory, based on Erikson's theory of psychosocial development (defined in Chap 10), states that all families have certain basic tasks for survival and continuity, and also have specific tasks related to each stage of development throughout the life of the family.

The basic tasks defined in the box entitled Tasks for Family Survival and Continuity are closely related to the functions of the family. They are included here because they expand those functions previously discussed.

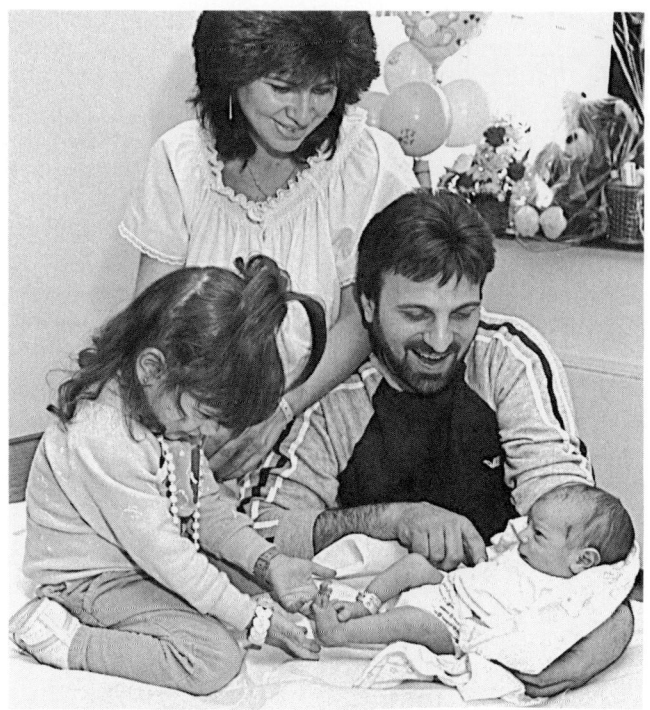

FIGURE 7-3
The members of this nuclear family—mother, father, and child— celebrate the new addition to their family. (Photo by Don Walker, courtesy of Thomas Jefferson University Hospital)

- *Single adults:* Although the single person is not living with others, he or she is part of a family of origin, usually has a social network with significant others, or may even regard a pet as family. The majority of single adults living alone are found in two age groups: the young adult who has achieved independence and enters the work force, and the elderly person, left alone through death of a spouse.

Family Functions

The family provides a set of functions important to the needs of the individual members and to society as a whole. The family provides the individual with the necessary environment for development and interactions; it also provides new and socialized members for society.

There are six major functions of the family. The *physical* function is carried out by providing a safe, comfortable environment necessary to growth, development, and rest/recuperation. The family's *economic* function is to provide financial aid for members, as well as meeting monetary needs of society. The *reproductive* function is met by the birth of children. Through the *affective/coping* functions families provide emotional comfort and help members establish an identity and maintain that identity in times of stress. The *socialization* function is of major importance and includes teaching; transmitting beliefs, values, attitudes, and coping mechanisms; providing feedback; and guiding problem solving (Friedman, 1981; Jones et al, 1982).

Tasks for Family Survival and Continuity

Providing shelter, food, clothing, and health care

Allocating resources (money, time, space) according to each member's needs

Determining individual roles and responsibilities in the support, management, and care of the home and family members

Ensuring socialization of members through the internalization of increasingly mature roles in the family and in society

Establishing socially acceptable ways of interacting, communicating, and expressing feelings (*e.g.,* affection, aggression, sexuality)

Rearing children (natural, adopted) and then releasing them appropriately

Relating to the community (school, church, work, neighborhood) and establishing rules for relatives, guests, friends

Maintaining morale and motivation, rewarding achievement, meeting personal and family crises, setting attainable goals, and developing family loyalties and values

(Duvall E: Marriage and Family Development, 5th ed. Philadelphia, JB Lippincott, 1977)

The developmental tasks of the family are related to sequential stages in the life of a family. Seven stages and related developmental tasks are identified in Table 7-1.

If developmental tasks are not met, societal disapproval and intervention may occur in areas such as child abuse, police actions, welfare agencies, or health departments (Edelman and Mandle, 1986). The successful mastery of each developmental stage is important to adaptation and family growth through successive stages.

The Family in Health and Illness

Family-Centered Nursing

Health-care activities, health beliefs, and health values are learned as part of a family. In health and illness, as well as in other areas of human life, the individual reflects behaviors learned as a family member. When a person enters the health-care system, he brings his own personal behaviors and needs, but he also brings (in a sense) his family too. Friedman (1981) has clearly identified the importance of family-centered nursing care, based on the following rationale:

- The family is made up of interdependent members who affect each other. If some form of illness occurs in one or more members, all other members become a part of the illness. Nursing assessment and interventions must consider the whole family to be holistic.
- There is a strong relationship between the family and the health status of its members; therefore the role of the family is essential in every level of nursing care.
- The level of wellness of the family, and in turn in each member, can be significantly improved through health promotion activities.
- Illness or disease in one family member may be indicative of the same problem in other members;

T A B L E   7-1
Family Stages and Tasks

Stage	Task
Beginning family	Establishing a mutually satisfying marriage Planning to have or not have children
Childbearing family (see Fig 7-3)	Having and adjusting to infant Supporting needs of all three members Renegotiating marital relationship
Family with preschool children	Adjusting to costs of family life Adapting to needs of preschool children to stimulate growth and development Coping with parental loss of energy and privacy
Family with school-age children	Adjusting to the activity of growing children Promoting joint decision making between children and parents Encouraging and supporting children's educational achievements
Family with teenagers and young adults	Maintaining open communication among members Supporting ethical and moral values within the family Balancing freedom with responsibility for teenagers Releasing young adults with appropriate ritual and assistance Strengthening marital relationship Maintaining supportive home base
Postparental family	Preparing for retirement Maintaining ties with older and younger generations
Aging family	Adjusting to retirement Adjusting to loss of spouse Closing family home

(Data from Duvall E: Marriage and Family Development, 5th ed. Philadelphia, JB Lippincott, 1977 and Aldous J: The Developmental Approach to Family Analysis. Minneapolis, University of Minnesota Press, 1975) through assessment and intervention, the nurse can assist in improving the health status of all family members.

Risk Factors

Family patterns of behavior and the environment provided by the family are critical to the health of individual members. Many health problems are the result of family habits (*e.g.,* diet, smoking, lack of exercise, alcohol abuse, and stress) and could be substantially reduced (U.S. Department of Health and Human Services, 1982).

Family-related risks include the following:

Life-style
- Lack of knowledge about sexual and marital roles, leading to teenage marriage, divorce, sexually transmitted diseases, and lack of prenatal or infant/child care
- Inadequate nutrition, either more or less than body requirements at any age
- Chemical dependency, including smoking, alcohol, and drug dependency
- Unsafe or unstimulating home environment

Biologic Factors
- Birth defects
- Mental retardation

T A B L E 7-2
Nursing Interventions to Promote Family Health and Wellness

Family Developmental Level	Nursing Interventions and Referrals
Couple and child-bearing family	Family planning clinics Prenatal classes Immunization information Poison-prevention programs
Family with school-age children	Vision and hearing screenings Dental health information Parent support groups Communicable disease control
Family with adolescents	Alcohol and drug abuse information Accident prevention programs Sex education Nutrition support groups Mental health programs
Family with middle-aged adults	Blood pressure screenings Exercise classes Stress reduction programs Specific support groups (stop smoking, Alcoholics Anonymous, coping with grief)
Family with older adults	Screening for chronic diseases (hypertension, glaucoma, diabetes) Retirement information Home safety programs Pharmacology information

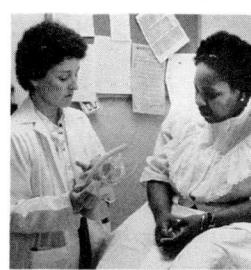 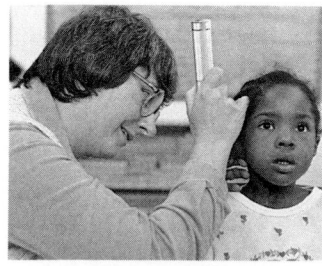 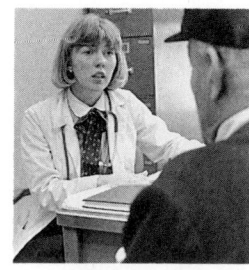

Photos by Gates Rhodes, courtesy of the School of Nursing, University of Pennsylvania

- Genetic predisposition to certain diseases, including cardiovascular diseases and cancer

Environmental Factors

- Lack of knowledge or finances to provide clean, safe home
- Work or social pressures leading to increased stress
- Air, water, or food pollution

Social/Psychological Factors

- Working parents with inadequate child-care resources
- Abuse or neglect of children, adults
- Inadequate health-care measures
- Crowded, low-income living conditions
- Conflict between family members

Nursing Interventions to Promote Health

The role of the nurse in reducing risk factors is primarily focused on activities that promote health for all family members at any level of development. Each person has a personal definition of health, based on family beliefs and values about health and illness. By providing interventions that emphasize wellness, the nurse can assist both the individual and the family meet basic human needs. Examples of nursing interventions to promote wellness in the family are shown in Table 7-2. Nurses may carry out the activities or may refer the individual or family to groups for additional education.

In conclusion, the family is the primary educational and support structure for the individual. The family, as a social unit, provides the environment and relationships necessary to meet physiologic and psychosocial individual basic human needs. Health beliefs and practices are learned within the family context and are strongly influenced by the family's developmental level. Health promotion activities and nursing interventions can reduce the risk of illness and facilitate healthy behaviors at any age within the family life cycle.

THE COMMUNITY

A person, as an individual and as a member of a family, belongs to the community. The community environment affects the ability of the individual to meet basic human needs. This section of the chapter will briefly discuss the community as it relates to basic human needs, including influences on health and illness.

A community can be defined in a variety of ways, but the most basic definition is that a **community** is a specific population (or group of people) living in a specified geographic area under similar regulations and having common values, interests, and needs. Within a community, people interact and share resources.

The community has a strong influence on the health promotion and illness prevention of its individuals and families (Fig. 7-4). Just as the family has risk factors for the health of individual members, so does the community have risk factors involving resources, economics, and services. Nursing assessments and interventions would not be comprehensive and individualized if the community influence were not also considered.

Community Risk Factors

It is not within the scope of this book to discuss community health nursing as a whole. However, as the community provides the environment affecting health and illness, it is important to discuss environmental factors influencing the safety and security of the individuals within that community. Listed below are community factors affecting health:

- Number and availability of health-care institutions and services
- Housing codes, police and fire departments
- Nutritional services for low-income infants, mothers, school lunch programs, and the elderly
- Zoning regulations separating residential and industrial areas

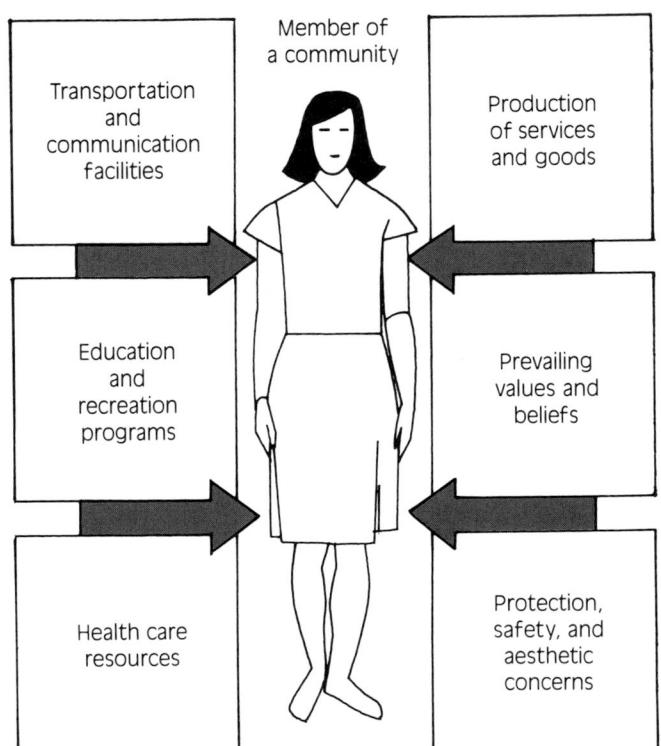

F I G U R E   7-4
Many characteristics of a community influence the health of its members. This diagram shows six categories of characteristics that influence the health of a member of a community.

• Waste disposal services and locations
• Air and water pollution regulations
• Food sanitation guidelines
• Health education services and dissemination
Consider the different community environments of the following two women:

• Mary, at the age of 21, already has two small children. She is an unmarried single parent, living in a housing project in the middle of a major North American city. Her only source of income is public assistance. Her two-room apartment lacks adequate heat and sanitation. Because she speaks only Spanish, she is unaware of health-care services, and she rarely leaves her apartment because of her fear of street gangs.

• Ann, also age 21, lives in a small town in the western United States. She too is a single parent of one small child, but she has a job providing adequate income. She lives close to her family, her apartment is within walking distance of her family doctor, and she takes part in monthly classes on parenting.

These two very opposite examples are given to demonstrate that the community plays a major role in the health of those people who live within it. Mary and her children are subject to a far greater risk of physical and mental illness than are Ann and her child. Even if the two women had identical health-care needs, the nursing care plan would reflect very different interventions because of their community environments.

Nursing in the Community

Nurses carry out a variety of activities that involve community health, designed to promote wellness and prevent illness. Nurses promote wellness as individuals, as caregivers within institutional settings, and as community-based health-care providers.

As individuals, nurses provide community services as volunteers in health-related activities (screenings, educational programs, blood drives, and so forth), and as role-models for healthy practices and life-styles.

Nurses working in health-care institutions include community influences in developing individualized nursing care plans, and in making referrals to community agencies and support groups.

Community-based nurses are employed in many different kinds of health-related practice settings, including home health care, community health centers, school nursing, occupational nursing, and independent nursing practice.

KEY POINTS

■ Basic human needs are common to all people and are essential to health and survival.

■ Maslow's hierarchy of basic human needs describes relationships and priorities of needs.

■ Many human needs are met through social environment, specifically the family and community.

■ Physiologic needs have the highest priority and are the base of the hierarchy. These needs include oxygen, food, water, temperature, elimination, sexuality, physical activity, and rest.

■ Safety and security needs include a physical component, involving protection from potential or actual harm, and an emotional component, including trust and freedom from fear.

■ Love and belonging needs include both giving and receiving love, and having a sense of belonging to others.

■ Self-esteem needs focus on feeling good about oneself and believing that others also hold one in high regard.

■ Self-actualization needs are the highest level of need and are met when one achieves one's potential.

■ The family, the basic social unit of society, serves as a buffer between the needs of society and the needs of individual members. There are many different family structures (or forms), but all families carry out the same functions: physical, economic, reproductive, affective/coping, and socialization.

■ The family life cycle has definite stages and developmental tasks.

■ Family-centered nursing care incorporates basic human needs, family concepts, and risk factors into nursing actions to promote and maintain health.

■ The community provides an environment that is an integral component of individual needs and family functions. Holistic nursing care integrates community risk factors and influences in all types of health-care settings.

BIBLIOGRAPHY

Aldous J: The Developmental Approach to Family Analysis. Minneapolis, University of Minnesota Press, 1975

Duvall E: Family Development, 4th ed. Philadelphia, JB Lippincott, 1971

Duvall E: Marriage and Family Development, 5th ed. Philadelphia, JB Lippincott, 1977

Edelman C, Mandle C: Health Promotion Throughout the Lifespan. St Louis, CV Mosby, 1986

Friedman M: Family Nursing: Theory and Assessment. New York, Appleton-Century-Crofts, 1981

Johnson S: Nursing Assessment and Strategies for the Family at Risk: High-Risk Parenting, 2nd ed. Philadelphia, JB Lippincott, 1986

Jones S et al: Family theory and family therapy models: Comparative review with implications for nursing practice. J Psychosoc Nurs Ment Health Serv 20(10): 12–19, 1982

Lewis S, Collier I: Medical-Surgical Nursing: Assessment and Management of Clinical Problems, 2nd ed. St Louis, McGraw-Hill, 1987

Maslow A: Toward a Psychology of Being, 2nd ed. New York, D Van Nostrand, 1968

Pender N: Health Promotion in Nursing Practice. Norwalk, CT, Appleton-Century-Crofts, 1982

Smitherman C: Nursing Actions for Health Promotion. Philadelphia, FA Davis, 1981

U.S. Bureau of the Census: Household and family characteristics, Popular Report's Series P-20, No. 398. Washington, DC, U.S. Government Printing Office, March 1984

U.S. Department of Health and Human Services: Healthy People: The Surgeon General's Report on Health Promotion and Disease Prevention. Health and Human Services Publication No. 79-55071, Washington, DC, U.S. Government Printing Office, 1982

U.S. National Center for Health Statistics, U.S. Bureau of the Census, U.S. Department of Commerce: Washington, DC, The Center, 1982

Culture and Ethnicity

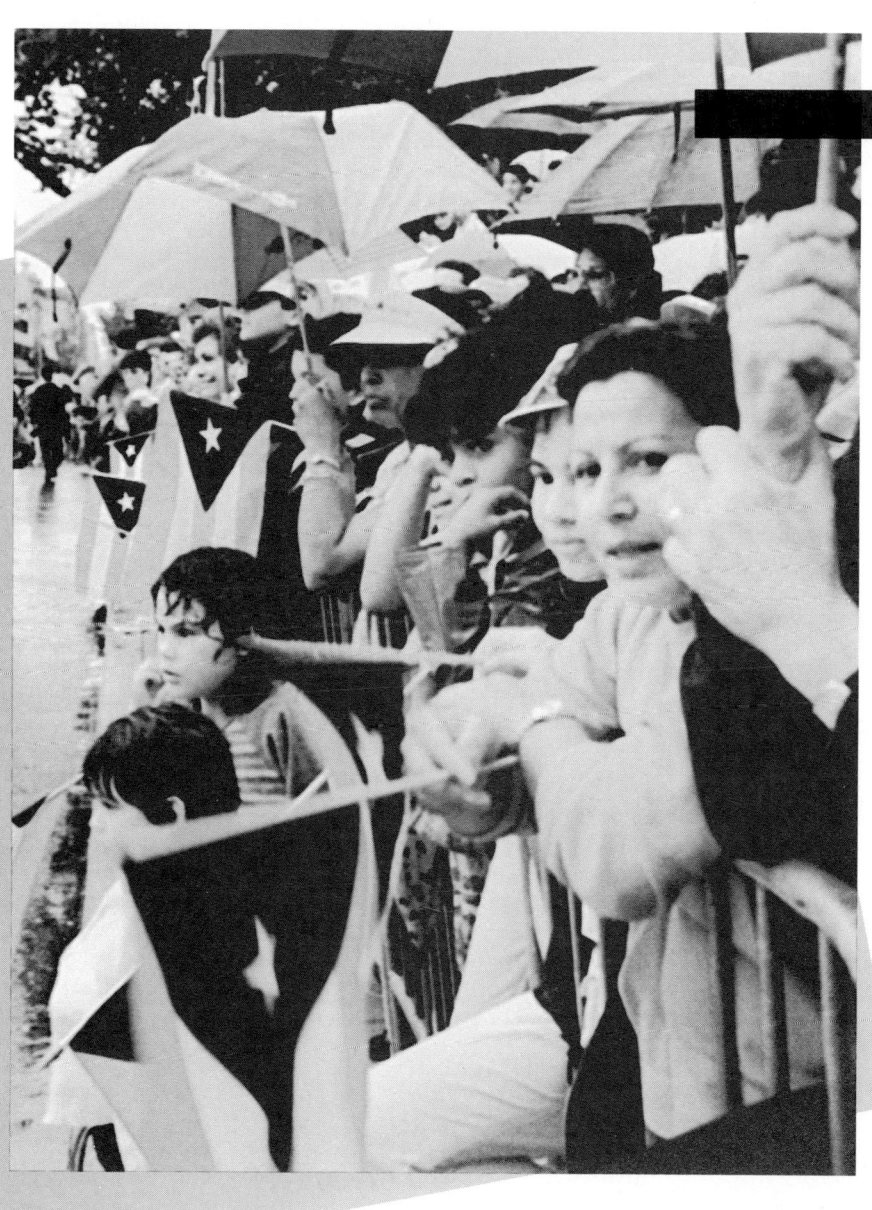

OBJECTIVES

After studying this chapter, the learner should be able to

Define key terms used in the chapter.

Describe the concepts of stereotyping and ethnocentrism.

Identify cultural norms of the health-care system.

Discuss the importance of culture in holistic nursing care, incorporating socioeconomic, psychosocial, and ethnic/racial factors.

Define the "culture of poverty" as it specifically relates to the issues of power and health care.

List physiologic and psychosocial health risks common to certain ethnic/racial populations.

Discuss the significance of cultural health beliefs and traditional folk medicine for clients entering the health-care system.

Describe key concepts and specific guidelines for giving transcultural nursing care.

Throughout the history of North America, economically, religiously, and politically oppressed individuals have come to this continent seeking freedom. Each decade, war, or regional problem brought an influx of immigrants and refugees. They arrived as minorities and, in many cases, became part of the melting pot of North America. This is especially true of the various European nationalities.

In the last four decades the number of Hispanics (people of Spanish-speaking origin in the United States) has increased significantly. In the last two decades the number of Southeast Asian refugees has also grown as a result of unsettled conditions in that part of the world. Currently in Canada, Asia has replaced Britain and Europe as the principal source of immigrants, with the greatest numbers coming from Hong Kong, India, and Southeast Asia. The number of Latin American immigrants to Canada, particularly from Chile, Argentina, and El Salvador, is growing steadily (MacQueen, 1986).

In addition to immigration to this country, there has been significant emigration within the country and its territories. For instance, many southern blacks have moved northward, many Puerto Ricans have moved back and forth between the mainland and Puerto Rico, many northerners have moved to the Sunbelt, and many native Americans have moved from reservations to urban areas.

The concept of the "melting pot," where everyone becomes alike, has become a concept of "vegetable soup" or "tossed salad." This contemporary concept indicates that people become part of the whole but still retain their individual characteristics. This has been a positive step for the self-image of minority groups.

Many nurses must function in cross-cultural settings with clients with different values or styles of behavior. The modern health-care system is based primarily on white, middle-class standards, beliefs, values, and practices, many of which are different from those of other cultures. Some nurses are members of minority groups and must deal with a culture that is in the majority. This chapter is presented to help nursing students learn to function in cross-cultural care settings.

KEY TERMS

culture	humanism
culture shock	race
ethnic group	stereotyping
ethnocentrism	subculture
holism	Yin and Yang
holistic health care	

CONCEPTS IN CULTURAL AND ETHNIC CHARACTERISTICS

Nurses must be aware of the diversity of people and must understand the terminology and concepts pertaining to race, culture, and ethnicity. This section of the chapter deals with general concepts; application of these concepts is discussed later in the chapter.

Humanism and Holism

Humanism attests to the dignity and worth of all individuals through concern for and understanding of their network of attitudes, values, behavior patterns, and way of life. All humans share certain common values, behaviors, and needs. Humanism means that all individuals have the right to meet those needs. Not every society views the individual as the primary receiver of rights. In some societies the family, country, or intangibles such as pride or dignity is valued above the individual's needs and rights. Human rights is an issue currently being promoted by humanitarian groups all over the world.

The concept of holism arises logically from humanism. **Holism** views an individual as more than the total sum of parts and shows concern and interest in all aspects of the individual. Although human beings are composed of organs, muscles, blood vessels, and bones, these structural components alone do not make the individual. An individual exists as a biopsychosocial and spiritual being with interacting cultural, racial, and ethnic factors. Modern health care is based on humanism and holism.

Race and Ethnicity

Sometimes the terms race, ethnic group, and culture are used interchangeably, but technically there is a difference. **Race** refers to the divisions of humans based on distinct physical characteristics such as skin color, eye color, hair color and texture, and body proportions transmitted by heredity. Most ethnologists (scientists concerned with distinguishing and categorizing the various types of humans) recognize three races: white, black, and yellow.

Within each of the three primary races there are a variety of **ethnic groups**—minority groups that retain distinctive customs, language, or social values as a result of their common heritage and traditions. These groups usually form in accordance with such factors as language, nationality, ancestry, religion, or geographic location. Examples of ethnic groups are Irish, Italian, Inuit (Eskimo), Vietnamese, Jamaican, and Chinese.

Culture and Folkways

Culture can be defined as the sum total of human behavior or social characteristics peculiar to a specific group and passed from generation to generation or from one to another within the group. The body of characteristics may include beliefs, values, traditions, experiences, practices or customs, rituals, diet, speech, or artifacts developed by the group. It may also be described as a blueprint for social living, a way of life, or an adaptation to the rules that have to be known if a person is to act appropriately within a particular group. Culture is learned behavior. Its survival depends on its ability to transmit its values to succeeding generations. People may change or add cultures and use them as means of meeting basic human needs.

The following illustrates the differences in race, ethnic group, and culture. Russians are an ethnic group. They may be of the white or yellow race. Within the Russian ethnic group there are many cultures, such as the Jewish culture. On the other hand, communism could be considered a culture and many races and ethnic groups fall under that culture. In North America there are many members of the black race and, although one can say there is a black culture, it is evident that there are many cultures (or subcultures) within the black culture. For instance, cultures of middle class and poor blacks are different, as are the cultures of those living in rural and urban areas.

Subculture

Subcultures may form within a culture. A **subculture** is formed by a group of persons who have developed interests or goals different from the primary culture, based on such things as occupation (Hollywood culture), sex (gay culture), age (youth culture), social class (middle class), or religion (fundamentalism). The United States and Canada have many diverse subcultures formed for a variety of reasons and purposes.

Two prevalent subcultures in our society are the drug culture and street people. The drug culture is composed of individuals involved in receiving, selling, or using illegal drugs. Members of the drug subculture have a language and life-style decidedly different from those of the general public. Larger cities have residents commonly referred to as "street people" or "bag ladies"—homeless people who carry all their belongings with them in a bag or shopping cart. Many of them have been released from mental institutions. The life-style of the members of these subcultures is very different from what the majority of the population would consider appropriate or desirable.

Stereotyping and Ethnocentricism

Stereotyping involves assigning characteristics to a group of people without considering specific individuality. Most people use stereotyping on an almost daily basis in varying degrees. It allows an individual to classify and retain large amounts of information. It is commonly and unconsciously used as a ready aid in recognizing objects and events in our environment. However, stereotypical interpretations and perceptions are superficial. Although they may provide comfort and direction to an individual in a strange environment, they should never be used to guide an interpretation of another human being as an individual.

The determination of a person's ethnic background does not form a solid basis for assessing cultural practices, values, or needs. Each generation in a family tends to move further away from traditional cultural practices as they are assimilated into the culture surrounding them. Newly immigrated individuals may uphold their traditional practices more consistently and rigidly than individuals who are second-generation citizens. Older family members who have lived in their adopted country for many years may still cling to traditional practices. This may result in some degree of conflict within the family, especially in health-care practices.

Stereotypes, like attitudes, are learned and can

therefore be unlearned. An individual can actively attempt to unlearn negative or rigid stereotypical thinking (Fig. 8-1). Learning about a person's cultural background and the history behind the development of that culture can help eliminate stereotypical thinking. Taking the time to know a client as an individual rather than as a member of a particular cultural group may also discourage stereotyping and encourage acceptance. Learning to accept people as they are is an important step in providing the best care possible to clients of all ethnic and cultural backgrounds.

It is a natural inclination for all individuals to assume that their culture is better or superior to another. This is called **ethnocentrism**. An ethnocentric individual judges other people by the standards and practices of his own culture. Health-care professionals may sometimes engage in ethnocentric thinking because they feel comfortable with the fact that their way—modern technology and health practices based on scientific research—has been proven to be the "right way." This type of thinking is judgmental, condescending, and insulting to others. The following is an example of ethnocentricity:

An elderly Chinese client is admitted to the hospital for various diagnostic procedures, including the drawing of many vials of blood. Some Chinese people believe that blood is not regenerated or replaced by the body. The client is horrified at the amount of blood being withdrawn from his body and refuses to have any further blood work done. In response to his refusal the nurse informs him that his concerns are ridiculous because his body will replace the blood he has lost and that a person does not become ill or die as a result of diagnostic blood studies.

Although the nurse in this situation may have been attempting to convince the client that his beliefs were incorrect in an effort to encourage him to cooperate, the approach is ethnocentric.

THE HEALTH-CARE SYSTEM AS A CULTURE

As nursing students, and as practicing nurses in the future, you are socialized into the health-care society. Through this process, you are developing and acquiring skills that allow you to participate effectively as an active member of the nursing profession; you are being socialized into the culture of modern-day health care. You are

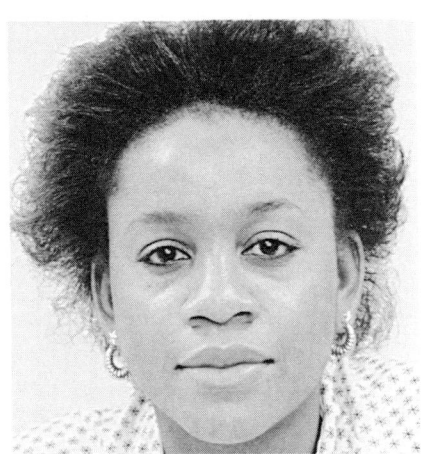
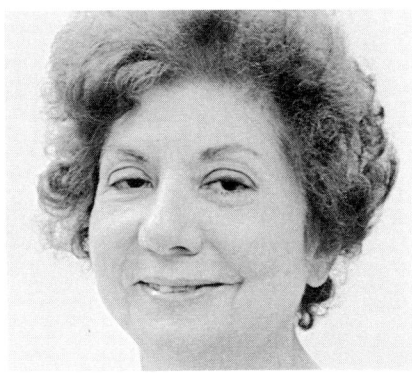
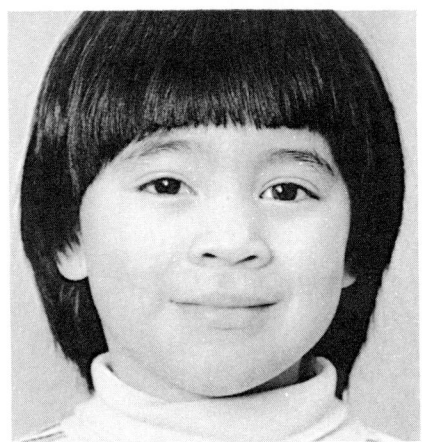
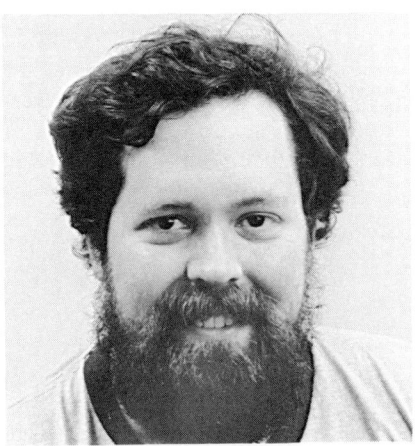
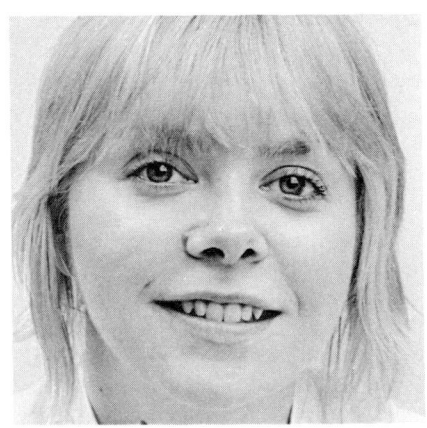

F I G U R E   8-1
Identifying one's own prejudices is the first step toward eliminating them. Think about the assumptions you make about the people in these images.

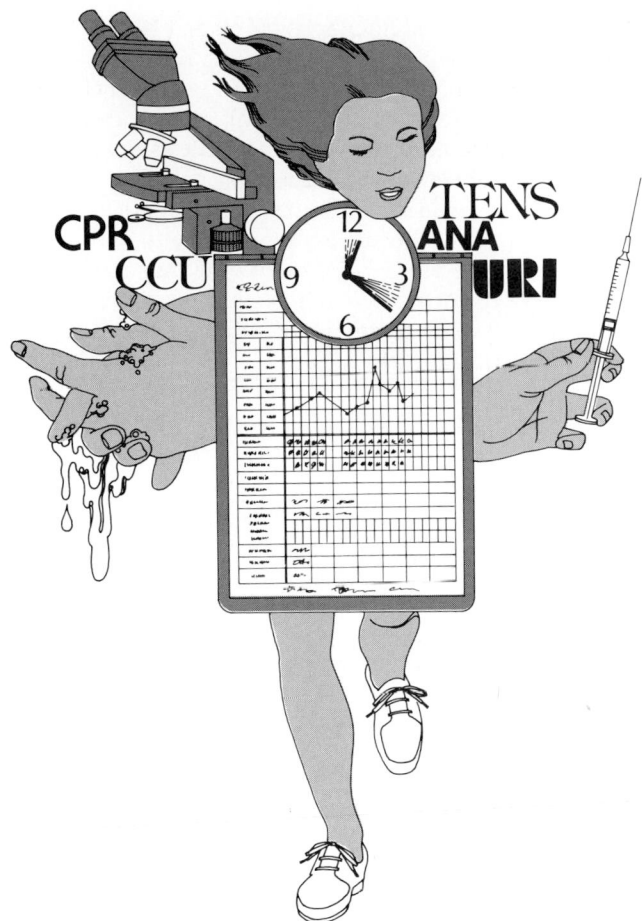

F I G U R E 8-2
Symbols of the health-care culture.

slowly internalizing a set of beliefs, practices, habits, likes, dislikes, customs, and rituals that may be different from your own primary culture. Cultural norms learned by most modern health-care providers are listed in the box on page 116.

Although it is advantageous to have an established culture within which to work, adaptations must sometimes be made in order to adjust to the many variables that occur when providing care for individuals.

FACTORS AFFECTING THE PROVISION OF HEALTH CARE

Major factors in the provision of health care are related to the socioeconomic culture and the ethnic/racial make-up of the client. The latter involves biologic, psychological, spiritual, and social characteristics of the client's background. These factors are important in giving holistic and individualized nursing care.

Socioeconomic Cultures

How much money a person does or does not have has a major impact on that person's life. The economic well-being of an individual depends on factors such as education, health, personal skills or abilities, family heritage, area in which the person lives, and the economic status of the community or country. North America is primarily made up of a large middle class and smaller upper- and lower-class economic groups. It is projected that this will eventually evolve into large lower and upper classes with a progressively dwindling middle class, similar to many of the third world countries. The cause of this projected fluctuation is primarily changing economics. Product competition from other industrialized nations is having an effect on general economics, and will eventually affect individual citizens.

Poverty

In many societies, including North America, poverty is often taken for granted or accepted as a fact of life. This commonly leads to apathy. Recently several northern hemisphere countries began to realize the consequences and their social responsibilities. In 1985 a worldwide music concert sparked a universal interest in supplying food and medical assistance to the starving in Ethiopia, and, in 1986, the "Hands Across America" campaign collected vast sums of money for the homeless in the United States. Large-scale efforts such as these, with enormous media coverage, have made it more and more difficult to ignore poverty.

Poverty as a Power Issue

There is much debate concerning the true definition of poverty. Economically, an individual whose income falls below the poverty line is considered poor. The United States Bureau of Census states, "A family is poor if it falls short of the pretax money income needed to purchase a minimum amount of goods and services, whose overall level, if not precise composition, is regarded as fixed" (Moccia and Mason, 1986). On the other hand, it has been stated that poverty is "a relative term that reflects a judgment made on the basis of standards prevailing in the community. The standards change in time and place; what is judged poverty in one community might be regarded as wealth in another" (Spector, 1979). The first definition is based on income; the second definition focuses on attitudes of individuals or communities. A more recent view says poverty is a power issue—"It is the relative lack of an individual's access to and control over environmental resources" (Moccia and Mason, 1986). No matter how poverty is defined, it is an increasingly devastating epidemic. According to the 1983 statistics from the United States Bureau of Census, over 35 million people (15.2% of the population) are poor in terms of financial income (U.S. Bureau of the Census, 1984).

Cultural Norms of the Health Care System

Beliefs
- Standardized definitions of health and illness
- Omnipotence of technology

Practices
- Maintenance of health and prevention of illness
- Annual physical examinations and diagnostic procedures

Habits
- Charting
- Frequent use of jargon
- Use of a systematic approach and problem-solving methodology

Likes
- Promptness
- Neatness and organization
- Compliance

Dislikes
- Tardiness
- Disorderliness and disorganization

Customs
- Professional deference and adherence to the "pecking order" found in autocratic and bureaucratic systems
- Use of certain procedures attending birth and death

Rituals
- Physical examination
- Surgical procedure
- Limiting visitors and visiting hours

(Spector 1979, pp. 79–80)

The "feminization of poverty" threatens to continue the increase in poverty level individuals. Female-headed households are increasing as a result of divorce, abandonment, and unmarried motherhood. Because many present-day households depend on two incomes for economic survival, a single woman supporting a household is at a decided financial disadvantage. In fact, many of the newly "homeless" are single-mother families.

The "graying of America" has resulted in the largest number of elderly persons the country has ever experienced, and a continual increase in the elderly population is projected well into the next century. Most elderly people depend on fixed incomes, which frequently do not keep up with inflation, and many are on the borderline of poverty or have already slipped into the poverty culture.

Nearly 30% of Hispanics and 36% of blacks are attempting to live on insufficient incomes (U.S. Bureau of the Census, 1984). The existence of these increasing numbers of poor, combined with the decreasing availability of resources to help them, has become a source of concern.

Some individuals believe that the subculture of poverty is passed from generation to generation, as are other cultures. This seems to be true when one observes certain segments of society. Migrant workers, for instance, seem to be caught in a web of poverty passed on from generation to generation. Cultural pockets of mountain people who do not venture out to seek employment

elsewhere seem to be destined to remain in a poverty culture also. Characteristics of these poverty cultures are:
- Feelings of despair, resignation, and fatalism
- Day-to-day attitude toward life with no hope for the future
- Unemployment and need for financial or government aid
- Use of "escape valves" such as alcohol and drugs
- Unstable family structure with abusiveness and abandonment
- Decline in self-respect and retreat from involvement with the community

Moccia and Mason (1986) assert that viewing poverty as a power issue can aid nurses in approaching a poor client's care in a more effective and productive manner. They recommend an emphasis on social factors that will encourage the client to gain more control over the environment. Such factors may include teaching clients how to deal with landlords and work supervisors, and how to access the health-care system, social services, and community self-help agencies.

Poverty as a Health Issue

Poverty has long been considered a barrier to health care. Poverty prevents many individuals from adequately meeting their basic human needs. Lack of affordable or adequate housing is a problem frequently experienced by the poor. When low-income housing is available, it is often associated with low-cost maintenance, sometimes resulting in the lack of such necessities as running water, heat, and electricity. To stretch their available money and to pool resources, many poor people live in crowded conditions, with several families living in one household.

Close living quarters pose a variety of problems because research has demonstrated that high-density living conditions foster impersonalization, correlate with higher crime rates, and lead to psychological problems such as schizophrenia, alienation, and feelings of personal worthlessness (Spector, 1979). Crowded living conditions also contribute to increased incidences of illness and disease because of the close proximity of people, the sharing of utensils and belongings, poor sanitation, and other poor health habits. The health effects of these various living conditions are numerous:

- Poor people get sick more often than people in higher income groups.
- When poor people are ill they usually experience more and greater complications.
- The poor take longer to recover from an illness.
- The poor are less likely to regain their pre-illness level of functioning (Kotelchuck, 1985).

Access to health-care facilities frequently requires transportation, many times neither affordable nor available to the poor. The poor's access to health insurance is also frequently limited, and a choice between food or health care is a common occurrence. In 1968, Canada introduced a medicare program aimed at ensuring equal access to health care for Canadian people regardless of age, economic status, creed, or ethnic origin. Despite this national health insurance program and a high-quality health-care system, people's health remains directly related to their economic status. Members of the upper income group live longer and are freer of disability than those with a low income (Storch, 1982). Other barriers to health care include isolation, language or communication difficulties, seasonal work occupations, migration patterns, depersonalization, and institutional prejudice (Spector, 1979).

In many situations, a poor person will choose to have an illness treated by a traditional folk healer. Folk healers are frequently less expensive, more accessible, and seen as more understanding of the clients' needs than modern health-care professionals.

Wealth

To varying degrees, the wealthy are affected by their money. Much depends on the length of time the family has been wealthy (how many generations), the means by which the family attained wealth, the ethnic or cultural background of the family prior to becoming wealthy, the resultant material gains, and the way in which the wealth is used. The appreciation of the work ethic may change from generation to generation.

Generally, the wealthy make effective use of the health-care system. They usually expect and are able to afford amenities not usually available to low-income clients. Occasionally, they may be perceived as demanding by hospital staff.

Physiologic Characteristics

It is theorized by researchers that past generations of peoples slowly adapted to their surrounding environment. Darker skinned people gradually developed lighter skin as early populations moved to colder, northern climates where there is less sunlight throughout the year compared to equatorial climates. Lighter skin is better able to utilize the vitamin D from sunlight than darker skin. It is also theorized that nose shapes and sizes evolved according to the climate in which an individual lived (Henderson and Primeaux, 1981). From a scientific and anthropologic point of view, these adaptations were logical changes necessary for improving the lives and the well-being of human beings. Some of these biologic variations were effective adaptations for a particular period of time or for living in a certain environment. However, once an individual has been removed from the environment that encouraged the biologic variation to occur, the variation could have a detrimental effect on health and well-being. Various research studies have concluded that certain ethnic groups have particular characteristics that make them more prone to the development of specific diseases or conditions. These conditions may be acquired as a result of environmental factors, or may be inherited. Some of the variations are discussed in the following section.

Keloid Formation. This occurs as the result of the overgrowth of connective tissue during the healing process following an injury. Individuals with an African heritage have a much stronger tendency toward the development of keloids following cuts, surgery, and other types of connective tissue damage. Rather than healing flush with the surrounding skin tissue an individual with a tendency toward keloid formation will heal with a rough, lumpy, or elevated scar.

Lactase Deficiency. Milk and many milk products contain lactose, a sugar. For lactose to be broken down during digestion the enzyme lactase must be present in the body. Without lactase the milk ferments in the intestines, resulting in gas (flatus) formation, diarrhea, and abdominal bloating, pain and cramping. Approximately 90% of Afro-Americans, Asians, and Native Americans have a lactase deficiency. About 10% of the white population lack the lactase enzyme (Henderson and Primeaux, 1981). These individuals will frequently have to get their calcium and protein requirements from alternative sources because they are not able to tolerate milk products. There are some special milks available for individuals with this enzyme deficiency. Also, these individuals may tolerate the ingestion of sharp cheeses (aged over 60 days) and/or fermented milk products such as yogurt, buttermilk, and sour cream. (Henderson and Primeaux, 1981)

Sickle Cell Anemia. The sickle cell trait originally served as a protective mechanism against malaria. Sickle cell anemia is most commonly found in people with African or Mediterannean ethnic backgrounds. Individuals with sickle cell anemia have sickle-shaped red blood cells which break down more rapidly than normal-shaped red blood cells. The sickle shape can also prevent the red blood cells from moving easily through the smaller vessels in the body. This factor can lead to a "clogging" of the red blood cells in these smaller vessels, which can cause many potentially serious problems. Carriers of this disease can be identified by a blood test.

Tay-Sachs Disease. Individuals of Eastern European Jewish descent may be carrying a gene for a hereditary disorder called Tay-Sachs disease. A child born with this progressive disease has a very short life span, usually less than 2 years. At present, there is no cure or treatment for this devastating disease. However, carriers of the disease can be identified by blood serum analysis.

G-6-PD Deficiency. Glucose-6-phosphate dehydrogenase is an enzyme normally found in the red blood cells. G-6-PD deficiency affects approximately 10% of the black population. The deficiency is sex-linked and carried on the X female chromosome. A person with this deficiency will have red blood cells that are unable to maintain a cell membrane. Without this protective membrane the red blood cell is easily destroyed (hemolyzed) by a variety of oxidant drugs, such as aspirin, ascorbic acid, probenecid, sulfa drugs, and vitamin K, and fava beans (also called horse or broad beans). The destruction of the red blood cells results in anemia which may be severe and life threatening, and elevated bilirubin levels (a result of the hemolyzed red blood cells) which will result in jaundice (yellowing of the skin and eye sclera).

Thalassemia. This is a genetic disorder affecting the hemoglobin in the red blood cells. The production of the alpha or beta globin chains is defective and disrupts red blood cell function. This disorder is most commonly found in people of Mediterranean, Asian (especially Chinese), and African origin.

Sarcoidosis. This condition is much more prevalent in the black population. It involves the formation of multiple tubercles or nodules on various parts of the body, most commonly the lymph nodes, liver, spleen, lungs, skin, eyes, and the small bones of the feet and hands. Eventually these nodules form into fibrous tissue. Skeletal muscle involvement can result in muscle atrophy

(wasting), and if the myocardium is involved major cardiac problems can result.

Gout. This disease is most commonly found in men, especially of Puerto Rican or Filipino descent. Excessive quantities of uric acid are found in the blood and may be deposited in joints and cartilage. The deposition of uric acid results in swelling, inflammation, and pain in the affected area. Eventually the uric acid crystals may cause permanent damage to the joints. These crystals also predispose the person to the formation of renal calculi (kidney stones).

Research continues to be done in an effort to further identify illness tendencies in relation to ethnic background and high-risk groups of individuals so a more concentrated effort can be made in controlling, preventing, and eventually eradicating many of these diseases.

Psychological Characteristics

Mental Health Norms

In most situations, an individual will relate the behaviors of another person to the individual's own familiar culture. This process is usually multidirectional; for example, in a health-care setting, the client is evaluating the attitudes and actions of the health-care provider at the same time the health-care provider is gathering perceptions about the behavior of the client. It is important to remember that what may seem perfectly reasonable and important to a client may seem ridiculous and irrelevent to a nurse. The reverse perception is also apparent in that practices the nurse perceives as logical and effective may seem senseless, incompetent, or even dangerous to the client.

Most mental health "norms" have been based on research and observations made of the white, middle-class people. Many ethnic groups have their own "norms" or acceptable patterns of behavior concerning psychologic well-being and psychologic reactions to certain situations. For example, members of the Puerto Rican culture may be very close mouthed about personal and family affairs, making effective psychotherapy difficult to achieve. Many traditional Chinese people consider mental illness a stigma and, therefore, seeking psychiatric help is a disgrace to the family. Traditionally, Chinese people prefer to avoid or minimize any type of conflict so the use of any direct confrontation during psychotherapy may not work as well as expected. Also, Chinese people have traditionally been taught that the expression of strong emotions will result in disharmony and imbalance between the body's energy forces (**Yin and Yang**) and is considered a sign of weakness. As a result of this belief, therapy involving the venting of strong feelings and emotions may be unacceptable to the client. In situations of extreme stress or high anxiety, some Puerto Ricans may demonstrate hyperkinetic seizure activity known as *ataques*. This behavior is a culturally accepted reaction.

Culture Shock. Culture shock, or the feelings an individual experiences when placed in a different and often strange culture, may result in psychologic discomfort or disturbances. Often, the patterns of behavior that an individual found acceptable and effective in his own culture are not adequate in the new one. The individual may then feel foolish, fearful, incompetent, inadequate, embarrassed, humiliated, and inferior. These feelings can eventually lead to frustration and anxiety.

As a reaction to these perceptions of inadequacy and inferiority, an individual experiencing culture shock may become angry. If supressed, the anger may build up and may eventually result in hostility. Hostility may be overt (openly expressed) or covert (hidden). Covert hostility may be expressed in a variety of ways. The hostile person may be categorized by health professionals as "uncooperative."

Reaction to Pain. Health-care researchers maintain that the expressions and behaviors exhibited by individuals in pain are culturally prescribed. Some cultures allow and even encourage the open expression of emotions experienced by a person in pain, while other cultures frown on the open and free expression of emotions. The main concern of nurses in this area of cultural expression is the categorization of clients as the "ideal" client. A client who quietly and stoically deals with pain may have pain reduction needs ignored by nurses. It is often assumed that a client who does not complain of pain is not experiencing any great degree of pain. Nurses should be sensitive to other signals of discomfort such as holding or applying pressure to the painful area, self-restriction of activities that intensify the pain, or uncontrollable, spontaneous expressions of discomfort such as facial grimacing or moaning. Clients who freely express their discomfort should not be classified as constant complainers whose requests for pain relief sometimes seem excessive. Pain is a warning from the body that something is wrong, and every complaint of pain should be carefully assessed.

Spiritual Characteristics

Some Puerto Ricans, as well as other Hispanics, may consider evil spirits or forces to be the cause of mental illness. Traditionally, Hispanic individuals prefer to be treated by a "spiritualist medium" rather than a psychiatric professional. Physical illnesses may be thought of as a punishment from God by some cultural groups, and religious intervention may be necessary to help treat a disorder. Other religious sects believe in the treatment of illnesses by "laying on" of hands and faith healing. Individuals from the West Indies or Caribbean may firmly believe in the powers of voodoo. Voodoo, a mixture of African rites and Christian beliefs, frequently attributes the cause of illness to a "fix" or "hex." The symbols of voodoo, called gris-gris, are used to place or remove fixes or illnesses. There are both good and bad gris-gris, commonly composed of oils, powders, candles, or relics. The subject of spirituality is more comprehensively discussed in Chapter 39.

Social Characteristics

Language. Language can often be a barrier to receiving adequate health care. Obtaining pertinent information, explaining procedures, and teaching clients is often very difficult, if not impossible, when the health-care professional and the client do not speak the same language. Even with English-speaking clients the nurse should avoid the use of unfamiliar medical jargon. All directions given to a client should be repeated back to the nurse to validate the client's understanding of the content. If the client does not speak or understand the English language, an interpreter should be made available. For more information on communicating with non-English speaking clients see Chapter 20.

Diet. Many cultures have specific food preferences which may not be available in the hospital. If the client is not on a dietary restriction, family members can bring home-prepared foods into the hospital. When a client is on a restricted diet, the agency's dietitian can be used as a resource person to evaluate the appropriateness of the foods being brought to the client from home. People from cultures who practice a hot–cold theory of illness may avoid certain foods and ingest large quantities of other foods. In general, **hot–cold theories** assert that many diseases, foods, and herbs can be categorized as either hot or cold. To treat an illness, thought to be caused by an imbalance within the body, the proper foods must be taken in to rebalance the body. Therefore, if the disease is classified as cold the person will avoid all foods classified as cold and will ingest foods categorized as hot.

Orientation to Time. The health-care system in North America places great value on promptness. Clients are expected to be on time for appointments and to take medications according to the prescribed schedule. These expectations are not of equal value in all other cultures. Many cultures have a different time orientation that frequently conflicts with the value of punctuality. Some cultures, such as Hispanic, are not concerned with the exact time of day. The appointment for Thursday is the important issue, not that the appointment is scheduled for 9:00 AM on Thursday. Hispanics may be late for appointments or fail to appear at all. Native Americans are another cultural group that often follows a different time orientation. A Native American will often finish what he is doing before moving on to another goal even if finishing one project will make him late for another, such as an appointment. These people are not being irresponsible; rather they just do not allow the clock to direct their lives as much as other people do.

Orientation to Family. Usually, hospitals place restrictions on visiting hours, how many people may visit at one time, and age of visitors. Because of age limitations some of the client's children may not be able to visit while the client is hospitalized. In some cultures, having a large extended family around during an illness is important. Some cultures prefer to have personal care such as bathing and feeding done by family members rather than the nurse. Some cultures are very family oriented and may expect various members of their extended family to be included in the nurse's plan of care. In other cultures the nuclear or immediate family may be most important.

Orientation to Sex Roles. In some cultures the male is considered to be stronger and more intelligent. Males may refuse to display signs of weakness such as crying or admitting that they are in pain. They may also be looked on as the primary decision maker for all situations. In other cultures decisions are the responsibility of the eldest family member regardless of gender. Some cultures require that females be cared for only by other females.

Perceptions of Illness/Wellness

An individual's ideas or perceptions of illness, wellness, and care are developed as a direct result of their personal cultural influences. For example, some Mexican-Americans perceive illness as a disability. Therefore, if a condition is not disabling, the client may not believe that an illness exists. In a situation such as this it may be difficult for the nurse to convince the client that treatment or health-care interventions are necessary. In other cultures illness may be considered to be a punishment from God, the results of a hex, or an imbalance within the body. Cultural explanations of illness and traditional folk methods for treatment are listed in Table 8-1.

Folk Healers. Some cultures believe that healing is a gift from God and that the healer "knows" what is wrong with a client through divine intervention and experience. A client familiar with these healers may perceive modern health-care providers as incompetent because they have to ask many questions before they are able to treat the illness. Other folk healers may prescribe one dose of a boiled herb tea to treat illnesses. A person accustomed to this type of treatment will find it difficult to have to take a succession of pills that are not even steeped in hot water. Traditionally, folk healers are less expensive, are usually more accessible, and more understanding of the client's cultural and personal needs, and speak the client's language.

Traditional Folk Medicine. Having knowledge and understanding of traditional folk remedies used by culturally different clients will greatly improve and enhance effective nursing care and facilitate a safe return of the client to a state of wellness or health.

A common mode of treatment in many cultures is

T A B L E   8-1
Cultural Explanations of Illness and Related Treatments

Cause of Illness	Treatment of Illness
Evil spirits	Root doctors, spiritualists, exorcism of evil spirits
Witchcraft (black), "fixes" (voodoo), hexes, spells	Witchcraft (white), good gris-gris (symbols of voodoo to remove hexes)
Germs and viruses	Antibiotics and "aseptic" techniques, antiviral medications
Too many hot foods } too many cold foods } imbalance of body energy	Eat cold foods } eat hot foods } balance of body energy
Disruption of bodily systems	Herbs
Punishment from God	Forgiveness/absolution of sins, atonement
Spinal misalignments	Realignment of spinal vertebrae and disks (chiropractic)
Body imbalances	Herbs, acupuncture, acupressure, massage, application of hot/cold packs to various parts of the body

the use of herbs. In fact, many medications used today have a basis in herbs or other plant sources that have been used for centuries to cure illnesses. However, a problem may arise when a client is being cared for both by a herbalist and a physician. The herbalist may be prescribing an herb and the physician a drug, both of which have the same actions on a body. The client may be overmedicated or undermedicated because of the double prescription.

In most instances, the nurse should not discourage the client's use of traditional folk medicine unless it is harmful to the client's health and well-being or it will decrease the effectiveness of the nursing and medical care planned. Incorporating the client's traditional health-care beliefs into the care plan is an effective way to gain his trust and cooperation. For example, if a client would traditionally drink an herbal tea to alleviate symptoms of an illness, there is no reason why both the herbal tea and the medications prescribed by the physician cannot be used as long as the tea is safe to drink and the ingredients will not interfere with or exaggerate the actions of the medication.

PRACTICING CROSS-CULTURAL NURSING

Health care can become complicated when the client and nurse are operating from distinctly different norms. A nurse sometimes is placed in a cultural bind—the nurse's cultural upbringing influences values and beliefs and the nurse is expected to adopt the customs of the nursing profession while also accommodating the folkways and norms of individual clients. A careful merging of modern and traditional cultural beliefs is a necessary prerequisite for safe, considerate and successful nursing care of all clients.

A major theme of cross-cultural nursing is to focus on the caring practices of various cultures. Caring is a universal phenomenon, however, the forms and manifestations of caring vary among cultures. Caring practices are the protecting and assisting activities related to health and performed as a part of a culture. In cross-cultural research, efforts are being made to explain caring practices in order to provide a sound rationale for intelligent and therapeutic nursing care.

Once a nurse has attained cultural awareness and sensitivity in planning client care, it is easier to recognize the client's use of traditional folk medicine and its importance. When caring for a client who subscribes to such a practice, the nurse will take this circumstance into account during assessment and planning.

Cultural Assessment. Logically, the most effective way to identify specific factors that influence behavior is to do a cultural assessment of the client. The primary informant should be the client, if possible. If the client is not able to respond to the questions, a family member or a friend can be consulted.

Client differences in values, religion, dietary practices, family lines of authority, family life patterns, and beliefs and practices related to health and illness can be anticipated. Research has made it possible to obtain this anticipatory information before initiating contact with the client, with the reminder that information about specific cultures is general in content and must be individualized according to each client once interaction has begun.

Holistic Health Care. Rationale for cultural nursing is the fact that the nursing profession values holistic and comprehensive approaches to providing care. **Holistic health care** takes into consideration the whole person interacting in his environment. With the philosophy of holistic health care, the knowledge and use of cultural factors cannot be ignored, because a person's culture is an integral part of his life and, therefore, of holistic nursing care. Clients can be placed in jeopardy if a health professional lacks cultural awareness or sensitivity.

Guidelines for Care

The following guidelines will be useful for the nurse in practicing cross-cultural nursing. Table 8-2 lists key concepts for specific cultural groups.

- Become conscious of the role of cultural influences in your own life. Objectively examine your own beliefs, values, practices, and family experiences. As you become more sensitive to the importance of these factors, you will also become more sensitive to cultural influences in others' lives.
- Identify biases in your own life. How do they affect your feelings about others? How could they affect your nursing care of others?
- Learn about the varieties of cultures and some general observations about variables in their health care.
- Learn as much as possible about the belief system and practices of people in your community and, specifically, about clients in the area where you work. Cultural practices and beliefs are generally deeply rooted and must be considered in planning health care in order for it to be successful.
- Display an accepting, nonjudgmental, objective attitude about clients' cultural beliefs.
- Practice techniques of observation and listening to acquire knowledge of beliefs and values of clients to whom care is being given. Some persons, especially those of minority cultures, may have been belittled and subjected to ridicule and insults and may be hesitant to discuss their beliefs and practices. The topic must be approached carefully. If the nurse is motivated by sincerity, respect, and concern for the client, his or her attitude will generally convey this and the person will usually respond positively. On the other hand, if the motivation is mere curiosity and the nurse's attitude is

R E S E A R C H   I N   N U R S I N G   *Making a Difference*

Culture

Nurses must recognize and understand cultural differences existing in this pluralistic culture. The way a person responds to stressors in the environment is greatly influenced by his or her cultural background. Assessment of a client's values, beliefs, and methods of coping helps the nurse assist the client to reach the goal of wellness.

Related Research

Brink P: Value orientation as an assessment tool in cultural diversity. Nurs Res 33(4):198–203, 1984

Brink conducted this research to test the theory that "when people are faced with problems, solutions are found; the way in which the solutions are found creates the shape of a culture." The five problems isolated were Human–Nature, Man–Nature, Time–Orientation, Activity, and Relational Orientation. Results of the study include (1) an emphasis on responsibility to the group, (2) belief in the extended family, (3) women are more positive about the future than men, and (4) indecision in

Man–Nature orientation was evidence of change occurring in a culture.

Morgan B: A semantic differential measure of attitudes toward black American patients. Res Nurs Health 7:155–162, 1984

This study was conducted to measure nursing students' attitudes toward black Americans and black American clients. Results demonstrated differential attitudes toward black and white Americans by white students (more positive attitudes toward white Americans) and more favorable student perceptions of black American clients as compared to black Americans.

Nursing research focusing on culture indicates numerous implications for nursing practice; differences among clients need to be accepted and respected, students need to be taught various cultural differences, and recruitment of varied ethnic groups into nursing should be encouraged.

---

one of condescension, there will likely be little or no response.

- Incorporate factors from the client's cultural background into health care whenever possible and when the practices are not considered harmful to health. To ignore or contradict the client's background may result in refusal of care or noncompliance with prescribed therapy.
- Keep in mind that health practices are a part of the overall culture and that changing them may have widespread implications for the person. An accurate understanding of these implications is essential before such a change is encouraged. The nurse also needs to be prepared to put forth sufficient time and effort to provide the necessary support and reinforcement for the client if a change in a health practice with a cultural basis is considered necessary.
- Do not force the client to participate in care that is in conflict with the client's values. If the client is forced to accept it, the care may even be harmful, because resulting feelings of guilt and alienation from a religious and cultural group are likely to threaten the client's well-being.
- Accommodate the cultural dietary practices of

clients as much as possible. Dietary departments in many hospitals supply clients with meals consistent with special dietary practices. Families may be encouraged to bring food from home for clients with particular preferences when this practice does not violate hospital policy. Teaching clients and families about therapeutic diets can also be done within the framework of particular cultural practices.
- Take into consideration the cultural role of the family member who makes most of the important decisions. In some cultures, it is the husband or father, while in others, it is the grandmother or other respected elder. To disregard this fact or to proceed with nursing care that is not approved by this person can result in conflict or ignoring what has been taught. The nurse should be certain this person is involved in the nursing care planning.
- Seek assistance of a respected family member, member of the clergy, or folk medicine practitioner as indicated so the client is more likely to accept familiar health-care services. Acknowledging the role of the person's folk medicine practitioner can be an important way of building trust. If invited, folk medicine practitioners can work closely with professional health practitioners in the

(Text continues on p. 126.)

T A B L E 8-2
Cultural Factors Affecting Nursing Care

Culture—white middle class

Family
- Nuclear family is highly valued.
- Elderly family members may live in a nursing home when they can no longer care for themselves.

Folk/Traditional Health Care
- Self-diagnosis of illnesses
- Use of over-the-counter drugs (especially vitamins and analgesics)
- Dieting (especially fad diets)
- Extensive use of exercise and exercise facilities

Values and Beliefs
- Youth is valued over age
- Cleanliness
- Orderliness
- Attractiveness
- Individualism
- Achievement
- Punctuality

Common Health Problems
As a result of the high value placed on achievement:
- Cardiovascular diseases
- Gastrointestinal diseases
- Some forms of cancer
- Auto accidents
- Suicides
- Mental illness
- Chemical abuses

Nursing Considerations
- Careful assessment of client's use of over-the-counter medications (observe for signs and symptoms of toxic medication levels, especially fat-soluble vitamins)
- Nutritional assessments of dietary habits

Culture—black

Family
- Close and supportive extended family relationships
- Develop strong kinship ties with non-blood relatives from church or organizational and/or social groups
- Family unity, loyalty, and cooperation are important
- Usually matriarchal

Folk/Traditional Health Care
- Varies extensively and may include spiritualists, herb doctors, root doctors, conjurers, skilled elder family members, voodoo, faith healing

Values and Beliefs
- Present oriented
- Members of the black clergy are highly respected in the black community
- Frequently highly religious

Common Health Problems
- Hypertension (precise cause unknown, may be related to diet)
- Sickle cell anemia
- Skin disorders; inflammation of hair follicles, various types of dermatitis and excessive growth of scar tissue (keloids)
- Lactose enzyme deficiency resulting in poor toleration of milk products
- Higher rate of tuberculosis
- Diabetes mellitus
- Higher infant mortality rate than in the white population

Nursing Considerations
- Many black families may still use a variety of folk healing practices and home remedies for treating particular illnesses.
- Special care may be necessary for the hair and skin.
- Special consideration should be given to the sometimes extensive and frequently informal support networks of black clients (*i.e.,* religious and community group members who offer assistance in a time of need).

(Continued)

Culture—Asian (beliefs and practices vary but most Asian cultures share some characteristics)

Family
- Welfare of the family is generally valued above the person.
- Extended families are common.
- Respect for a person's lineage (ancestors)
- Sharing among family members is expected.

Folk/Traditional Health Care
- Theoretical basis in Taoism which seeks a balance in all things
- Good health is achieved through the proper balance of Yin (feminine, negative, dark, cold) and Yang (masculine, positive, light, warm).
- An imbalance in energy is caused by an improper diet or strong emotions.
- Diseases and foods are classified as hot or cold and a proper balance between them will promote wellness (*e.g.,* treat a cold disease with hot foods).
- Many Asian health-care systems use herbs, diet, and the application of hot or cold therapy. Also, many Asians believe that there are points on the body that are located on the meridians or energy pathways. If the energy flow is out of balance, treatment of the pathways may be necessary to restore the energy equilibrium.

> *Acumassage*—Technique of manipulating points along the energy pathways
> *Acupressure*—Technique for compressing the energy pathway points
> *Acupuncture*—Technique by which fine needles are inserted into the body at energy pathway points

Values and Beliefs
- Strong sense of self-respect and self-control
- High respect for age
- Respect for authority
- Respect for hard work
- Praise of self or others may be considered poor manners.
- Strong emphasis on harmony and the avoidance of conflict

Common Health Problems
- Tuberculosis
- Communicable diseases
- Malnutrition
- Suicide
- Various forms of mental ilness
- Lactose enzyme deficiency

Nursing Considerations
- Some members of Asian cultures may be upset by the drawing of blood for laboratory tests. They consider blood to be the body's life force and some do not believe that it can be regenerated.
- Some members believe that it is best to die with the body intact, so they may refuse surgery except in dire circumstances.
- Members of many Asian cultures seldom complain about what is bothering them. Therefore, the nurse must carefully assess the client for pain or discomfort by observing for nonverbal signs of discomfort such as facial grimacing or wincing or holding of the painful area.
- Some Asians consider it polite to give a person the responses the person is expecting. Therefore, misinformation may sometimes be transmitted to the questioner in an effort on the client's part to be respectful.
- Some members may move from physician to physician in an attempt to be cured of an illness but, in order to avoid insulting or embarassing a physician, they will not inform him or her that they are going to another physician. This can result in confusion, inaccuracies, and overmedication.
- Some Asians may refuse to have diagnostic studies done because they believe that a skilled and competent physician can diagnose an illness solely through a physical examination.

(Continued)

TABLE 8-2
Cultural Factors Affecting Nursing Care   (Continued)

Culture—Asian (continued)

- Some members may have a difficult time understanding the importance of taking a regimen of medications because many of their folk treatments involve the ingestion of one dose of herbal mixtures.
- Dietary counseling may be necessary if the client is on a salt-restricted diet because many Asian foods have a high salt content related to the use of soy sauce.

Culture—Hispanic, Mexican-American

Family
- Familial role is very important.
- *Compadrazgo:* special bond between a child's parents and his/her grandparents
- Family is the primary unit of society.

Folk/Traditional Health Care
- *Curanderas (os):* frequently folk healers who base treatments on humoral pathology—basic functions of the body are controlled by four body fluids or "humors"
     blood—hot and wet
     yellow bile—hot and dry
     black bile—cold and dry
     phlegm—cold and wet
- The secret of good health is to balance hot and cold within the body, therefore most foods, beverages, herbs, and medications are classified as hot (*caliente*) or cold (*fresco, frio*) (a cold disease will be cured with a hot treatment).

Values and Beliefs
- Respect is given according to age (older) and sex (male).
- Roman Catholic church may be very influential.
- God gives health and allows illnes for a reason, therefore may perceive illness as a punishment from God. An illness of this type can be cured through atonement and forgiveness.

Common Health Problems
- Diabetes mellitus and its complications
- Poverty and resultant problems such as: poor nutrition, inadequate medical care, poor prenatal care
- Many have lactose enzyme deficiency

Nursing Considerations
- May be difficult to convince an asymptomatic client that he is ill
- Special diet considerations if the client believes in the hot/cold theory of treating illnesses
- Diet counseling may be necessary at times because many members have a normal diet that is high in starch.

Culture—Hispanic, Puerto Ricans (since the Jones Act of 1917 all Puerto Ricans are American citizens)

Family
- Compadrazgo—same as in Mexican-American culture

Folk/Traditional Health Care
- Similar to other Spanish-speaking cultures

Common Health Problems
- Parasitic diseases, such as dysentery, malaria, filariasis, and hookworms, are particularly common among Puerto Ricans.
- May also have lactose enzyme deficiency

Values and Beliefs
- Place a high value on safe-guarding against group pressure to violate an individual's integrity (may be difficult for Puerto Ricans to accept team work at times)
- Very close-mouthed about personal and family affairs (psychotherapy may be difficult to achieve at times because of this belief)
- Proper consideration is given to cultural rituals such as shaking hands and standing up to greet and say goodbye to people.
- Time is a relative phenomenon, and little attention may be given to the exact time of day.
- *Ataques*—a culturally acceptable reaction to situations of extreme stress, characterized by hyperkinetic seizure activity

(Continued)

T A B L E   8-2
Cultural Factors Affecting Nursing Care   (Continued)

Culture—Hispanic, Puerto Ricans (continued)

Nursing Considerations
• May be difficult to teach Puerto Rican clients to follow time-oriented actions
  (*e.g.,* taking medications, keeping appointments)

Culture—Native Americans (each tribe's beliefs and practices vary to some degree)

Family
• Large extended families
• Grandparents are official and symbolic leaders and decision makers.
• A child's namesake may become the same as another parent to the child.

Folk/Traditional Health Care
• Medicine men (shaman) are still used heavily.
• Heavy use of herbs and psychologic treatments, ceremonies, fasting, meditation, heat, and massages

Common health problems
• Alcoholism
• Suicide
• Tuberculosis
• Malnutrition
• Communicable diseases
• Higher maternal and infant mortality rates than in the majority of the population
• Diabetes mellitus
• Hypertension
• Gallbladder disease

Values and Beliefs
• Present oriented. Taught to live in the present and not to be concerned about the future. This time consciousness emphasizes finishing present business before doing something else.
• High respect for age
• Great value is placed on working together and sharing resources.
• Failure to achieve a personal goal is frequently believed to be the result of competition.
• A person who gives to others is highly respected. The accumulation of money and goods is often frowned upon.
• Some Native Americans practice the Peyotist religion in which the consumption of peyote, an intoxicating drug derived from mescal cacti, is part of the service. Peyote is legal if used for this purpose. It is classified as a hallucinogenic drug.

Nursing Considerations
• The family is expected to be part of the nursing care plan.
• Note taking is often taboo because it is considered to be an insult to the speaker because the listener is not paying full attention to the conversation. Good memory skills are often required by the nurse.
• Indirect eye contact is acceptable and sometimes preferred.
• It is often considered rude or impolite to indicate that a conversation has not been heard.
• A low tone of voice is often considered respectful.
• A Native American client may expect the caregiver to deduce the problem through instinct and not through asking many questions and history taking. If this is the case it may help to use declarative sentences rather than direct questioning.

interest of the client and family. Such efforts promote mutual understanding, respect, and cooperation.
• Use past transcultural experiences as a guide, but never as the solution to all transcultural solutions.
• Learn from your mistakes and do not repeat them. All nurses will make mistakes at some time caring for culturally different clients. Inadvertent mistakes

are just that, but repeated mistakes are careless and disrespectful; they adversely affect the nurse's interaction with clients and coworkers.
• Treat each person as an individual. What was true of one person will not be true of another, even if they are from the same cultural background. View each person as an individual with rights, and help the client retain dignity.

KEY POINTS

- The population of the United States and Canada is a composite of cultures, made up of a wide variety of races and ethnic groups.

- Culture is a learned behavior, encompassing the social characteristics of a specific group of people. Within a culture are divisions by physical characteristics (race), minority groups retaining distinctive traditions (ethnic groups), and subcultures.

- Stereotyping on the basis of culture, race, and ethnic group decreases individualization of nursing care and diminishes the values, rights, and dignity of others.

- The health-care system is a culture, and members are socialized to its norms.

- Cultural factors influencing health care include socioeconomic background and ethnic/racial characteristics.

- Poverty has a major influence on health and illness and affects health-seeking and health-giving behaviors. As a universal concern, the issue of poverty is made even more complex by trends toward single-parent families headed by women, an increasingly elderly population, and minority issues.

- Certain physiologic and psychosocial characteristics within cultures are risk factors for illness and strongly influence health care. Nursing assessments and interventions must adapt to specific and individualized needs involving culture shock, pain responses, spiritual characteristics, language, diet, time orientation, family structures, and health/illness beliefs.

- Folk healers and traditional folk medicine are important components in transcultural nursing care.

- Guidelines for transcultural nursing help the nurse accept the values, beliefs, and behaviors of others. Holistic nursing care requires that cultural influences and factors become a part of an individualized plan of care.

BIBLIOGRAPHY

Ailinger RL: Beliefs about treatment of hypertension among Hispanic older persons. Top Clin Nurs 7(3):26–31, Oct 1985

Andrews MM, Ludwig PA (eds): Nursing Practice in a Kaleidoscope of Cultures. Salt Lake City, University of Utah College of Nursing, 1984

Brink PJ: Value orientations as a cultural assessment tool in cultural diversity. Nurs Res 33(4):198–203, July/Aug 1984

Capers CF: Nursing and the Afro-American client. Top Clin Nurs 7(3):11–17, Oct 1985

Elliott JL (ed): Two Nations, Many Cultures: Ethnic Groups in Canada, 2nd ed. Scarborough, Ontario, Prentice-Hall of Canada Ltd, 1983

Epp J: Achieving health for all: A framework for health promotions. Discussion paper. Can J Public Health 77(6):Nov-Dec 1986

Fong CM: Ethnicity and nursing practice. Top Clin Nurs 7(3):1–10, Oct 1985

Henderson G, Primeaux M: Transcultural Health Care. Menlo Park, CA, Addison-Wesley, 1981

Hodgson C: Transcultural nursing—The Canadian experience. Can Nurse 76(6):23–25, June 1980

Kotelchuck R: Poor diagnosis, poor treatment. Health PAC Bulletin 16(1):8, Jan/Feb 1985

LaFargue JP: Mediating between two views of illness. Top Clin Nurs 7(3): 70–77, Oct 1985

Leininger M (ed): Transcultural Nursing. New York, Masson International Nursing Publications, 1979

Lipson JG, Meleis AI: Culturally appropriate care: The case of immigrants. Top Clin Nurs 7(3):48–56, Oct 1985

Louie KB: Providing health care to Chinese clients. Top Clin Nurs 7(3):18–25, Oct 1985

Louie KB: Transcending cultural bias: The literature speaks. Top Clin Nurs 7(3):78–84, Oct 1985

Low SM: The cultural basis of health, illness and disease. Soc Work Health Care 9(3):13–23, 1984

MacQueen K: Opening the doors. Maclean's 99(41):12–15, Oct 13, 1986

Moccia P, Mason DJ: Poverty trends: Implications for nursing. Nurs Outlook 34(1):20–24, Jan/Feb 1986

Muecke MA: Caring for Southeast Asian refugee patients in the USA. Am J Public Health 73(4):431–438, Apr 1983

Orque MS et al: Ethnic Nursing Care: A Multicultural approach. St Louis, CV Mosby, 1983

Sobralske MC: Perceptions of health: Navajo Indians. Top Clin Nurs 7(3):32–39, Oct 1985

Spector E: Cultural Diversity in Health and Illness. New York, Appleton-Century-Crofts, 1979

Storch, J: Patients' Rights: Ethical and Legal Issues in Health Care and Nursing. Toronto, McGraw-Hill Ryerson Ltd, 1982

U.S. Bureau of the Census: Current Population Reports, Series P-60, No. 145, Money income and poverty status of families and persons in the United States: 1983 Table B, p 3, Aug 1984

U.S. Commission on Civil Rights: A growing crisis: Disadvantaged women and their children. Washington, DC, The Commission, May 1983

9 Stress and Adaptation

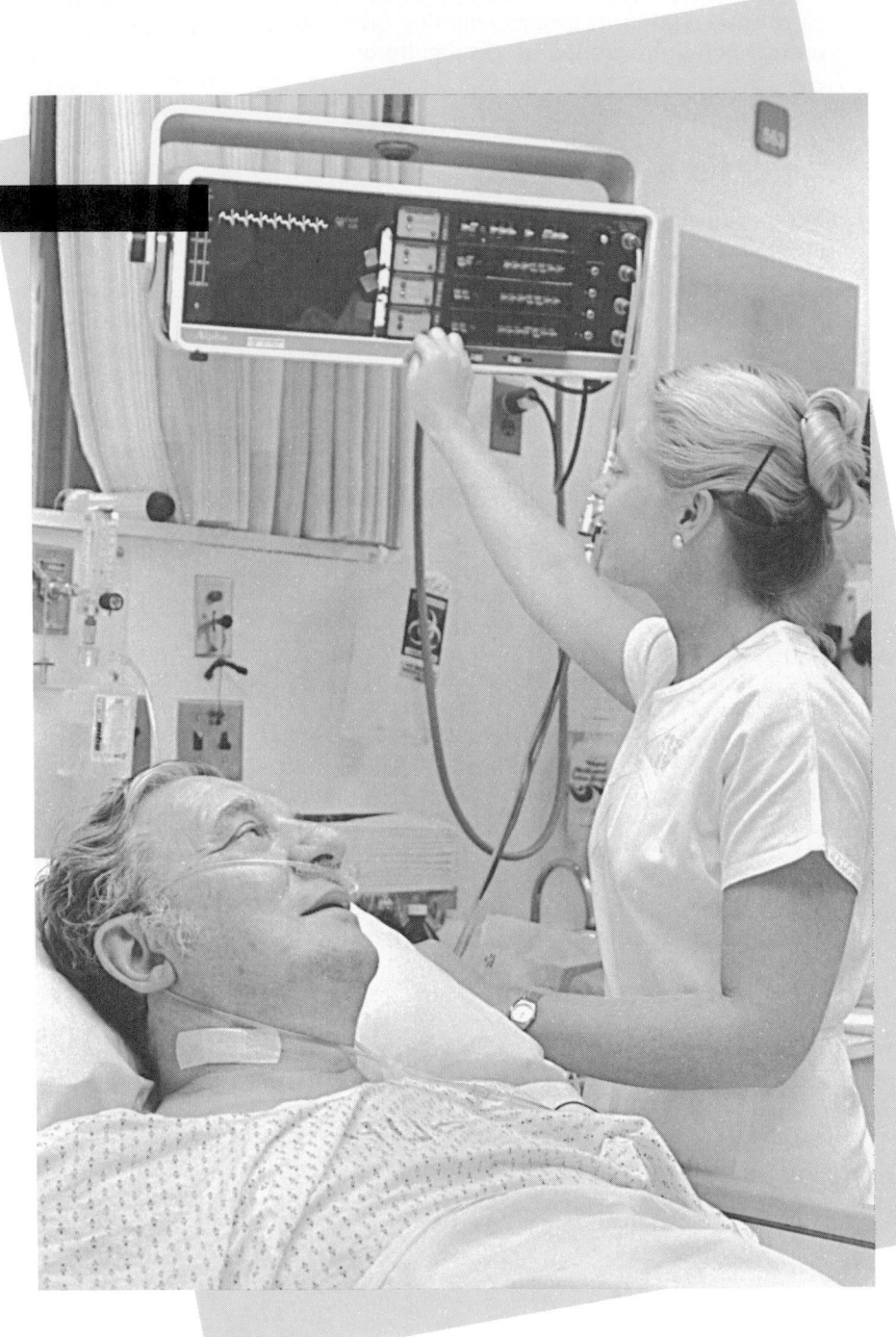

OBJECTIVES

After studying this chapter, the learner should be able to

Define key terms used in the chapter.

Describe the mechanisms involved in maintaining physiologic homeostasis.

Explain the interdependent nature of stressors, stress, and adaptation.

Compare and contrast developmental and situational stress, incorporating the concepts of physiologic and psychosocial stressors.

Describe the physical and emotional responses to stress, including mind–body interaction, local adaptation syndrome, general adaptation syndrome, and coping/defense mechanisms.

Discuss the effects of short- and long-term stress on basic human needs, health and illness, and the family.

Integrate knowledge of healthy lifestyle, support systems, stress management techniques, and crisis intervention into nursing care plans.

Recognize and effectively cope with stress unique to the nursing profession.

Stress, as a part of daily life, is a concept that is used and understood by most people. Magazines and books are filled with the causes of stress and methods to reduce it. Advertisements promise stress relief through a wide variety of products. Stress is blamed for overweight, high blood pressure, smoking, and chemical dependency. Some people do their best work "under stress"; others say "I just can't get everything done under all this stress!"

Knowledge of the concepts and dimensions of stress is important to nurses. Health-care settings are filled with clients who require nursing care to prevent or promote the reduction of stress. Nurses, too, are subject to increased stress and need to know healthy ways of responding. This chapter will discuss homeostasis, stress and adaptation, and nursing actions to promote stress reduction.

KEY TERMS

adaptation
anxiety
burnout
coping mechanisms
crisis
crisis intervention
defense mechanisms
developmental crisis
"fight or flight" response

general adaptation syndrome (GAS)
homeostasis
inflammatory response
local adaptation syndrome (LAS)
psychosomatic disorders
reflex pain response
situational stress
stress
stressor

HOMEOSTASIS

To maintain life, the internal environment of the human body must remain balanced within a fairly narrow range. Various physiologic mechanisms within the body respond to changes to maintain this essential balance, in a process named **homeostasis**.

The concept of homeostasis was first introduced by W. B. Cannon in 1939, but throughout history the belief that health is the result of a balanced state has been present. This belief was written about and discussed by some of the most important people in medical history, including Hippocrates (the father of medicine) and Claude Bernard (the father of physiology). The knowledge that the human body responds to an ever-changing environment originally focused on life processes within the body, such as heart rate, blood pressure, and water balance. The definition of homeostasis has now been expanded to include both internal and external environments and to include physiologic *and* psychologic balance.

Physiologic Homeostasis

Long before you entered nursing you knew that sweating when you were hot and shivering when you were cold were ways to maintain a stable body temperature. This part of the chapter will summarize the homeostatic mechanisms that regulate our internal environment.

Regulation of the homeostatic mechanisms is primarily controlled by the autonomic nervous system and the endocrine system (Fig. 9-1). Other body systems involved to a lesser degree are respiratory, cardiovascular, gastrointestinal, and renal. These mechanisms are self-regulating, come into action without conscious thought, and usually function to correct abnormal conditions.

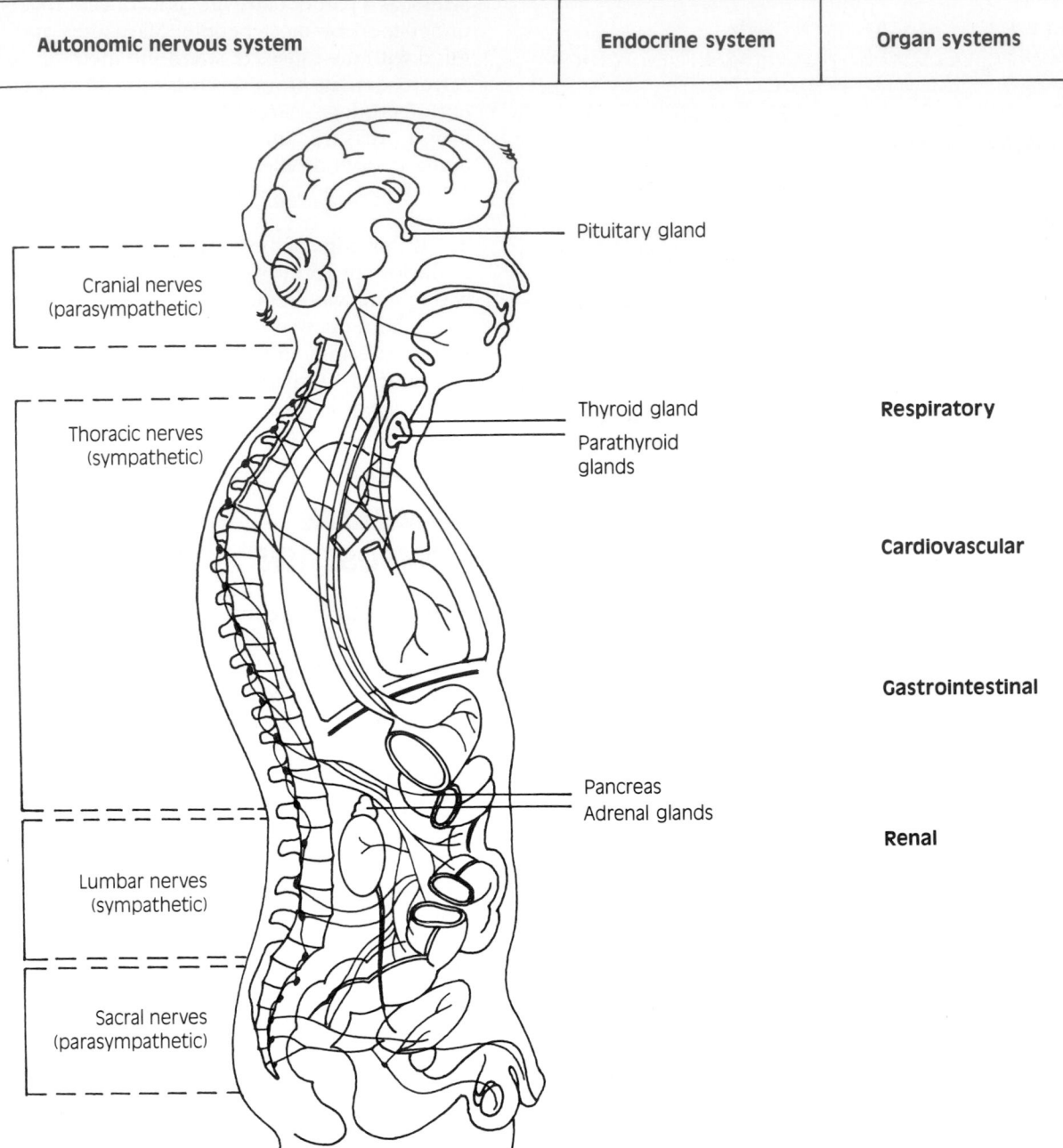

Autonomic nervous system	Endocrine system	Organ systems

FIGURE 9-1
Homeostatic regulators of the body.

They can be compared, on a very simple level, to the thermostat of a furnace. When the temperature of the house falls below a set number of degrees, the furnace is automatically turned on to return the house to the desired temperature.

The regulatory mechanisms of the body are constantly reacting to change to maintain health. When a person is ill, injured, or subjected to long-term stress, the mechanisms continue to try to restore balance, but they may either become ineffective or lose their normal control. The result is increased illness or death.

The body systems, with homeostatic mechanisms, are summarized in Table 9-1. The actions and effects are only briefly included, and are actually much more complex than is shown. They are important in understanding the effects of both short- and long-term stress and will make material included later in this chapter much more meaningful.

TABLE 9-1
Homeostatic Regulators of the Body

System	Action	Effect
Autonomic Nervous		
Parasympathetic—Functions under normal conditions and at rest		
(Cranial and sacral nerves)	• Regulates heart rate • Stimulates secretion of digestive juices and digestive tract smooth muscle • Stimulates insulin secretion	• Slows rate • Improved digestion, increased peristalsis • Increased uptake of glucose by cells
Sympathetic—Functions under stress conditions to bring about the fight-or-flight response		
	• Stimulates heart rate and force • Dilates skeletal muscle blood vessels • Dilates blood vessels to the brain • Stimulates release of glycogen stores	• Increased rate, stronger contractions, increased cardiac output • Increased muscle strength • Increased mental alertness • Increased levels of blood glucose
Endocrine		

Pituitary	• Secretes hormones:
	  Adrenocorticotropic hormone (ACTH)
	  Thyroid-stimulating hormone (TSH)
		• Stimulates the adrenal cortex
		• Stimulates the thyroid

Adrenals	• Medulla produces epinephrine and norepinephrine. • Cortex secretes mineralocorticoids, glucocorticoids, and androgens.	• Prepare the person for emergencies; support the sympathetic system • The mineralocorticoid, aldosterone, regulates fluid and electrolytes. • Glucocorticoids raise glucose levels (for energy) and increase resistance to physical stress.
Thyroid	• Secretes thyroid hormone and calcitonin	• Regulates metabolic rate and growth
Other		
Cardiovascular	• Serves as transport system and pump	• Provides oxygen and nutrients/removes carbon dioxide and wastes from cells
Renal	• Filters, excretes, and reabsorbs metabolic products and water	• Maintains fluid, electrolyte, and acid–base balance
Respiratory	• Intake and output of oxygen and carbon dioxide	• Necessary for metabolism, helps maintain acid–base balance.
Gastrointestinal	• Takes in food and fluids • Eliminates waste products	• Energy sources, maintains fluids and electrolytes

Psychologic Homeostasis

To remain healthy, humans must also maintain psychologic homeostasis, or a state of mental well-being. As was discussed in Chapter 7, each person needs to have love and belonging, safety and security, and self-esteem. When the needs are not met, or a threat to need attainment occurs, homeostatic measures in the form of coping or defense mechanisms are utilized to return to emotional balance. Additional information about psychologic homeostasis is included later in this chapter.

BASIC CONCEPTS OF STRESS AND ADAPTATION

As with any concept or process, one must first understand the meaning of the terms used. Although the concepts are discussed in greater detail in the next section, it is important to first know the definitions of stress, stressors, and adaptation.

Definitions

Stress.   All of us experience stress, of varying levels, everyday. In fact, the responses of the individual to stress are necessary to life (as was seen in homeostasis). Stress has both positive and negative effects and is produced by a change in the environment that is perceived as a challenge, a threat, or a danger (Brunner and Suddarth, 1988). Stress has a holistic effect—it affects the whole person in all the human dimensions (physical, emotional, intellectual, social, and spiritual). The perception of stress as well as the responses to stress are highly individualized, not only from person to person, but also from one time to another in the same person. Because stress is individualized and holistic, there is no commonly accepted definition or measurement. Most simply, **stress** is a condition in which the human system responds to changes in its normal balanced state.

Stressor.   A **stressor** is anything that causes an individual to experience stress. It is the change in the balanced state of the person. Stressors may be either internal (such as an illness, a hormonal change, or fear) or external (such as loud noise or cold temperature). As with stress, the perception and effects of the stressor are holistic and

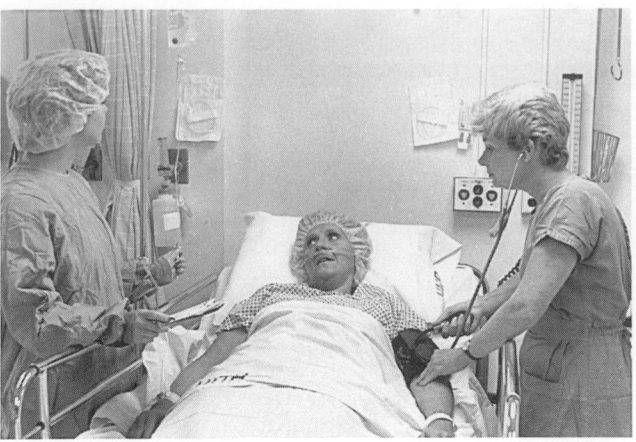

F I G U R E   9-2
Preoperative preparation of the client can represent situational stress for the nurse as well as the client. What stressors can you imagine might affect the preoperative client and the nursing staff preparing the client for surgery? (Photo by Denise Angelini, courtesy of the School of Nursing, University of Pennsylvania)

highly individualized. Stressors are neither positive nor negative, but rather have positive or negative effects as the person responds to change.

Adaptation.   **Adaptation** is the series of responses made by the individual in reaction to stressors. These

---

R E S E A R C H   I N   N U R S I N G   *Making a Difference*

Stress and Adaptation

During the past two decades, stress and adaptation have been widely discussed and researched. Research has examined a variety of maladaptive and adaptive human responses to stress in both health and illness. The study of the relationship between behavioral and biologic responses to stress continues to have important implications for nursing.

Related Research

MacDonald-Ross S, McKay R: Postoperative stress: Do nurses accurately assess their patients? J Psychosoc Nurs 24(4)
       MacDonald and McKay compared client's perceptions of psychosocial stress in hospitals with nurses' estimates of the client's stress. It was found that nurses perceived client stress to be higher than the self-reported by the client. The researchers suggest that nurses may tend to make global assessments of stress from one observation.

Mishel M: Perceived uncertainty and stress in illness. Res Nurs Health 7:163–171, 1984
       This study examined how nurses actually cope with stress and the mechanisms recommended by nurses to reduce stress. Nurses in general-care areas were compared with intensive care nurses and were found to have greater environmental stress and to use different coping strategies.

Summary

       Nurses need to determine their own causes of stress and means of coping. Management of stress through awareness and workshops has been indicated to be valuable. Assessment of clients' stress levels must be a priority for nurses to better promote adaptation to hospitalization and illness. Finally, a health-promoting life-style should be considered for all persons.

responses are constant as the individual strives to maintain balance in both the internal and external environments (Fig. 9-3). Although it is simpler to describe adaptation in terms of individual responses, adaptation also occurs in families and groups.

The end results of adaptation are optimal functioning in all dimensions, normal growth and development, and the ability to meet new or changing situations.

To summarize, stress, stressors, and adaptation are individualized and holistic. The process is constant and dynamic, and is essential to physical, emotional, and social well-being. Stress and adaptation are major components in health and illness, and strongly influence nursing care.

Dimensions of Stress and Adaptation

Sources of Stress

Although there are an infinite number of sources of stress, they can be categorized into two broad areas that create major demands for adaptive responses. The areas are (1) developmental and (2) situational.

Developmental stress or a **developmental crisis** occurs as an individual progresses through the normal growth and development stages from birth to old age. Developmental crises are fully described in the next unit. Within each stage, certain tasks must be satisfactorily met to resolve that crisis and reduce the stress.

Selected examples of developmental stress include
- The infant learns to trust others.
- The toddler learns to control elimination.
- The school-age child socializes with peers.
- The adolescent strives for independence.
- The middle adult accepts physical signs of aging.

Situational stress is different from developmental stress. It does not occur in predictable patterns as one progresses through life. Rather, **situational stress** can occur at any time, although the ability to adapt may be strongly influenced by the development level of the individual (Phipps et al., 1987). Examples of situational stress (or crises), which may be either positive or negative, include
- Illness or accidents
- Marriage or divorce
- Loss (belongings, relationships, family member)
- A new job
- A change in roles

To further illustrate the positive or negative aspects of situational stress, consider pregnancy as an example. A young married couple may be overjoyed at the prospect of becoming parents, while an unmarried teenager may be panic-stricken to find that she is pregnant. In this case, the situations and the development levels of both the young couple and the teenager will have major impact on the adaptations made. The physical and psychosocial capacities to cope with the demands of the situa-

Factors influencing stress management

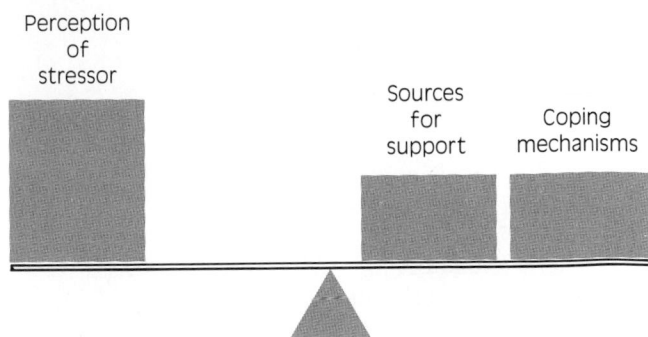

A balance is achieved when the perception of the stressful event is realistic and support and coping mechanisms are adequate

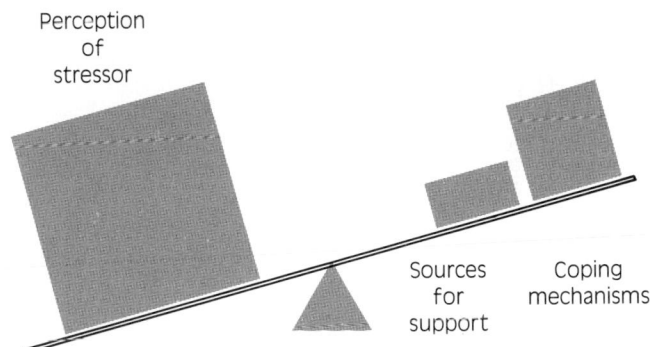

An imbalance can occur if the perception of the event is exaggerated or if sources for support or coping mechanisms are inadequate

FIGURE 9-3
A realistic perception of a stressful event, sources for emotional support, and appropriate coping mechanisms are components of a system of balances during stress.

tion depend not only on the stage of maturation, but also on the support systems available (Phipps et al., 1987).

Stressors

We are constantly bombarded with stressors, and we adapt to the changes to maintain a normal or healthy state. However, if stressors are increased in number or intensity, the physical or psychologic balance of the individual is impaired and illness may result.

Physiologic stressors have both a specific effect and a general effect. The specific effect is seen in alteration of normal body structure and function. The general effect is the stress response, discussed in the next section. The box on page 134 lists the agents considered to be primary physiologic stressors.

Psychosocial stressors are many and varied, and are often so much a part of daily living that we overlook

Primary Physiologic Stressors

Chemical agents
  • Drugs
  • Poisons
  • Toxins
Physical agents
  • Heat
  • Cold
  • Radiation
  • Electrical shock
  • Trauma
Infectious agents
  • Viruses
  • Bacteria
  • Fungi
Faulty immune systems
Genetic disorders
Nutritional imbalances
Hypoxia

them. Antonovsky (1979) has described 11 categories of psychosocial stressors, summarized as follows:
  • Accidents and their survivors: Stress is present for the victim, the person causing the accident, and the families of both.
  • The experience of others in our social relationships: Whatever happens to our friends and families also affects us.
  • Horrors of history: Concentration camps, Hiroshima, Biafra
  • Unconscious conflicts and anxieties: Included are hunger, thirst, sex (biologic drives) and other Freudian concepts (*e.g.,* the Oedipus complex)
  • Fear of aggression, mutilation, and destruction: Common fears in our society are muggings, rape, terrorist attacks, and atomic wars.
  • Events of history are brought into our homes: Through world communication systems and live coverage of events, we vicariously experience and are threatened by violent and frightening events which would otherwise be unknown.
  • Changes of the world in which we live: Society today experiences rapid changes in demographics, economy, and technology.
  • Phase-specific psychosocial crises: The developmental crises previously described.
  • Other life crises: Includes all events that occur as the individual encounters new social roles (*e.g.,* parent, student)
  • The inherent conflicts in all social relations: Within every sociocultural group of every society are conflicts of everyday existence as we interact with others.

  • The gap between culturally imposed goals and society structured means: Within any given group, only a few have both the wisdom and the means to reach the goal. The gap between goals and means is a potential stressor.

Psychosocial stressors may be actual or may be perceived by the individual as a threat. Adaptation is an ongoing process and includes **coping mechanisms**—all the ways we react to anxiety, fear, guilt, frustration, and loss. These serve to maintain psychologic balance or homeostasis (Pasquali et al., 1985).

Adaptation: Responses to Stress

Each person constantly encounters changes in the internal and external environment; these include physical, psychologic, or social changes. Perception of the change may be made consciously or unconsciously. If the individual has the necessary resources, adjustments are made, and balance is maintained. If, however, the resources are not able to handle the change, a state of stress will result. The degree of stress produced and the responses made depend on the nature, intensity, and duration of the stressor.

This section of the chapter will examine adaptive responses to stress and will include the mind–body interaction, the local adaptation syndrome, the general adaptation syndrome, and coping/defense mechanisms.

Mind–Body Interaction

Consider the following situations:
  • You are having a final examination tomorrow, and a passing grade for the course is dependent on a score of at least 86. You feel uneasy and can't sleep, your heart is beating rapidly, and you have diarrhea. As the time for the test grows close, you are pale, shaking, and perspiring. Even though you know you need to eat breakfast, you can't swallow food.
  • Sally Jones is the mother of a five-year-old retarded son. She is his sole support and has devoted all her time to him since he was born. Sally has been coming to the health clinic with increasing frequency for the past 6 months, having symptoms of headaches, weight loss, and gastric pain.

These two examples illustrate the relationship between physiologic and psychologic stress, and reinforce the holistic nature of stress. In the first example, the symptoms of stress rapidly disappear as you begin the test and find you know most of the answers. However, in Sally's situation, the cause of stress is always present and long-term. Sally is at risk for developing an illness.

Why does this happen? Although the actual cause is not well understood, it is believed that humans react to threats of danger as if they were actual stressors. The person perceives the threat on an emotional level, and the body prepares itself to either resist or to run away and avoid the danger (the "fight-or-flight" response). Each person reacts on an individual basis. For example, some may have chronic diarrhea, and others may develop asthma. These illnesses are real, but are often called **psychosomatic disorders**, because the physiologic alterations are thought to be at least partially due to psychologic influences (Lewis and Collier, 1987).

Another component of mind–body interaction is the impact of life change on an individual. Research has demonstrated that the number of changes in one's life (both positive and negative) has a positive correlation with the onset of illness. A life change can be defined as an event in one's life that requires energy for adaptation. When energy is expended to adapt to the event, the person has a lowered resistance to illness. Table 9-2 illustrates the Social Readjustment Rating Scale, a tool used to measure the stress of life changes. A high score does not mean one is ill, but it does indicate the risk of illness.

Physiologic Responses to Stress

As we have seen, there are both physical and emotional components in the response—or adaptation—to stress. The physiologic responses are the local adaptation syndrome (LAS) and the general adaptation syndrome (GAS).

Local Adaptation Syndrome (LAS)

The **local adaptation syndrome** is a localized response of the body to stress. It does not involve the entire body, but rather involves a body part (tissue, organ) only. The stress precipitating the LAS may be traumatic or pathologic. LAS is an adaptive response, primarily homeostatic, and short-term. Although there are many localized stress responses in the body, two of the most common that influence nursing care are the reflex pain response and the inflammatory response.

The **reflex pain response** is a response of the central nervous system when pain is the stimulus. This response is rapid and automatic, serving as a protective mechanism to prevent injury. The reflex depends on an intact and functioning neurologic reflex arc and involves both sensory and motor neurons. For example, if you step into a bathtub of overly hot water, your skin senses the heat and immediately sends a message to the spinal cord. In turn, the message is sent to a motor nerve, activating the muscles of your leg, and you quickly withdraw your foot. All of this happens before you consciously realize the water was too hot to be safe.

The **inflammatory response** is a localized response to injury or infection. This response serves to localize and prevent the spread of infection and so promote wound healing. When you cut your finger, you often develop the symptoms of the inflammatory response: pain, swelling, heat, redness, and changes in function. There are three phases in the inflammatory response. They are

1. In the first phase, bleeding is initially controlled by vasoconstriction (or narrowing) of blood vessels at the site of the injury. Following control of bleeding, histamines are released and capillary permeability increases, allowing increased blood flow and white blood cells to the area. The blood flow then returns to normal, but the white blood cells remain to help resist infection.

2. During the second stage, exudate (made up of fluid, cells, and inflammatory by-products) is released from the wound. The amount of exudate depends on the size, location, and severity of the wound.

3. During the third and final stage, damaged cells are repaired by either regeneration (replacement with identical cells) or formation of scar tissue. Some body tissues (skin, bone) are easily reproduced and regain their former function; others (nervous system, intestines) do not regenerate, but rather form nonfunctional scar tissue.

General Adaptation Syndrome (GAS)

The **general adaptation syndrome** is a biochemical model of stress developed by Hans Selye. The concept of stressors as factors causing stress was also made by Selye (1976). The GAS describes the body's general response to stress and serves as a part of the knowledge base essential to all areas of nursing care.

There are three stages in the GAS. They are described in the following narrative and illustrated in Figure 9-4.

1. In the first stage, the *alarm reaction,* the person perceives a specific stressor, and various defense mechanisms are activated. The perception of threat may be conscious or unconscious. The autonomic nervous system initiates the fight-or-flight response, and hormone levels rise to fully prepare the body to react. This phase of the alarm reaction, called the *shock phase,* is characterized by increases in energy levels, oxygen intake, cardiac output, blood pressure, and mental alertness. (If you think of the last time you narrowly missed having a car wreck, you will easily identify these body reactions!) During the second phase of the alarm reaction, *countershock,* there is a reversal of body changes.

2. The second stage of the GAS is *resistance.* Having perceived the threat and mobilized its resources, the body now attempts to adapt to the stressor. Vital signs, hormone levels, and energy production return to normal. If the stress can be managed or confined to a small area (LAS), the body regains homeostasis. However, if the damage to the body is too great (for example, severe injury and bleeding or a major illness such as cancer or a heart attack), the adaptive mechanisms fail, and the third phase of the GAS begins.

3. The third stage, *exhaustion,* is the result of exhaustion of the adaptive mechanisms. Without defense against the stressor, the body may either rest and

T A B L E   9-2
Social Readjustment Rating Scale

Rank	Life Event	LCU Value
1	Death of spouse	100
2	Divorce	73
3	Marital separation	65
4	Jail term	63
5	Death of close family member	63
6	Personal injury or illness	53
7	Marriage	50
8	Fired at work	47
9	Marital reconciliation	45
10	Retirement	45
11	Change in health of family member	44
12	Pregnancy	40
13	Sex difficulties	39
14	Gain of new family member	39
15	Business readjustment	39
16	Change in financial state	38
17	Death of close friend	37
18	Change to different line of work	36
19	Change in number of arguments with spouse	35
20	Mortgage over $10,000	31
21	Foreclosure of mortgage or loan	30
22	Change in responsibilities at work	29
23	Son or daughter leaving home	29
24	Trouble with in-laws	29
25	Outstanding personal achievement	28
26	Wife begin or stop work	26
27	Begin or end school	26
28	Change in living conditions	25
29	Revision of personal habits	24
30	Trouble with boss	23
31	Change in work hours or conditions	20
32	Change in residence	20
33	Change in schools	20
34	Change in recreation	19
35	Change in church activities	19
36	Change in social activities	18
37	Mortgage or loan less than $10,000	17
38	Change in sleeping habits	16
39	Change in number of family get-togethers	15
40	Change in eating habits	15
41	Vacation	13
42	Christmas	12
43	Minor violations of the law	11

The Social Readjustment Rating Scale is an example of a tool used by health practitioners for identifying persons at risk for developing health problems. The scale is based on the premise that change requires adjustment, and excessive adjusting is a causative factor in illness. A value has been assigned to common changes in one's life, called life change units or LCUs. The LCU values are an indication of the amount of adjusting required by each change. The sum of the LCUs is an indication of the total amount of adjusting required of an individual at a particular time. The higher the cumulative score, the greater the amount of adjustment required, and the greater the likelihood of life crisis within 1 to 2 years, including health problems. An LCU score of 150 to 199 is felt to be an indicator of probable mild life crisis. A score of 200 to 299 is predictive of moderate life crisis, and a score of 300 or more is a predictor of major life crisis.

(Holmes TH, Rahe RH: The Social Adjustment Rating Scale. J Psychosom Res 11:216. August 1967. Copyright © 1967, Pergamon Press, Ltd.)

mobilize its defenses to return to normal or may reach total exhaustion and die.

Although the alarm stage is short-term (from minutes to hours), the length of the resistance and exhaustion stages varies greatly, depending on such variables as the severity and duration of the stressor, the previous health of the individual, and the immediacy and effectiveness of health-care interventions.

The GAS is a physiologic response to stress, but it is important to remember that the response is the result of physical and emotional stressors. The stages occur in both physical and psychosocial damage to the human body. Obvious examples are seen in clients following severe injury, or who have an illness, but GAS is a factor in mental illness, social isolation, and loss (or lack) of human relationships.

Psychosocial Responses to Stress

Humans respond to threat—and stress—psychologically as well as physically. A variety of emotional responses may be made, but the response most common in the human experience is anxiety. Anxiety is experienced from birth to death by all persons, and involves one's body, self-perceptions, and social relationships (Stuart and Sundeen, 1987). **Anxiety** is a vague sense of impending doom or apprehension which appears to have no reason. (In contrast, fear is a response to a real stressor.) It is precipitated by the unknown and comes before all new experiences, serving as a threat to one's identity and self-esteem.

There are four levels of anxiety, each having different effects. The levels are

- *Mild anxiety:* Present in day-to-day living, mild anxiety increases alertness and perceptual fields. It motivates learning and growth.
- *Moderate anxiety:* Narrows the person's perceptual fields so that the focus is on immediate concerns, with inattention to other communications and details.
- *Severe anxiety:* Creates a very narrow focus on specific detail. All behavior is geared toward getting relief.
- *Panic:* The person has loss of control and experiences dread and terror. The resulting disorganized state results in increased physical activity, distortion of perceptions and relationships, and loss of rational thought. This level of anxiety can lead to exhaustion and death.

Anxiety, at a mild level, can have a positive effect. For example, mild anxiety about an upcoming examination can motivate you to do the required reading and review. However, anxiety beyond that level is regarded almost universally as negative, with unpleasant effects. In an attempt to neutralize, deny, or counteract the anxiety, a person develops individualized patterns of coping (Stuart and Sundeen, 1987).

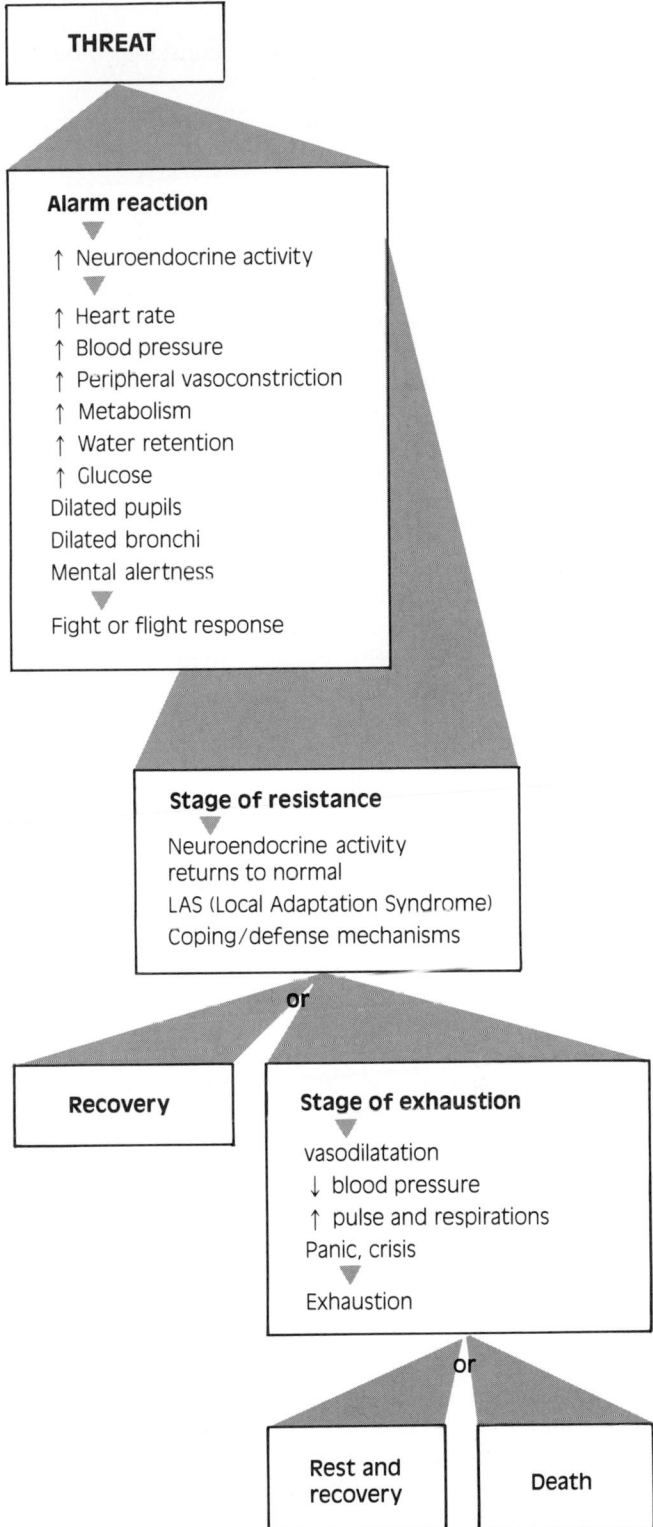

F I G U R E 9-4
The general adaptation syndrome (general response to stress).

Coping Mechanisms

Mild anxiety is often handled without conscious thought. Coping mechanisms include

- Crying, laughing, sleeping, cursing
- Physical activity and exercise
- Smoking, drinking
- Lack of eye contact and withdrawal
- Limiting relationships to those with similar values and interests

Moderate, severe, and panic levels of anxiety are greater threats and involve more complex coping mechanisms as the person strives to reduce the stress and anxiety. Coping mechanisms are categorized as task-oriented reactions or defense mechanisms.

Task-oriented reactions involve consciously thinking about the stress situation and then taking action to solve problems, resolve conflicts, or satisfy needs. These reactions, as defined by Stuart and Sundeen (1987) are

- *Attack behavior,* when a person attempts to overcome obstacles to attack a problem. The behavior may be constructive, with assertive problem solving, or destructive, with feelings and actions of aggressive anger and hostility.
- *Withdrawal behavior,* involving physical withdrawal from the threat or emotional reactions such as admitting defeat, becoming apathetic, or feeling guilty and isolated
- *Compromise behaviors* are usually constructive, involving the substitution of goals or negotiation to partially fulfill one's needs.

These behaviors are often learned behaviors and are based on past experiences and sociocultural influences and expectations.

Defense Mechanisms. If the mechanisms used to cope with stress are not successful, other reactions, called **defense mechanisms**, are often used to protect the self. These mechanisms serve to protect one's self-esteem, and are useful in mild to moderate anxiety. They do, if used to extreme, distort reality and create problems with relationships. At that point, the mechanisms become maladaptive instead of adaptive.

Defense mechanisms are summarized here. You will learn more about them later in your curriculum component focusing on mental health and illness.

Compensation occurs when an individual substitutes what is perceived as a good or a strength for a perceived weakness. A person may compensate for blindness by perfecting other senses.

Denial occurs when an individual refuses to acknowledge the presence of a condition that is disturbing. An ill person uses denial when refusing to accept a diagnosis or prognosis.

Displacement occurs when an individual can satisfy a need, blocked by one type of behavior, by using another type of behavior. For example, the person angry with a coworker displaces anger by kicking a chair.

Introjection occurs when an individual internalizes some part of the external world and keeps it intact in the psyche. Following the death of a loved one, for instance, an individual may internalize the deceased person or some attribute of the deceased person.

Projection occurs when an individual's own undesirable impulses are attributed to another person or object. For example, a person carelessly trips over an article on the floor and blames the article for the accident.

Rationalization occurs when a person gives questionable behavior a logical or socially acceptable explanation. It amounts to behavior justification. A person may be rationalizing when an appointment with a health-care practitioner is forgotten and the client explains that the practitioner is incompetent and the client does not want to continue seeing such a person.

Reaction formation occurs when an individual gives a reason for behavior that is opposite from its true cause. A common example is the parent of an unwanted child who overindulges the child.

Regression occurs when an individual returns to an earlier method of behaving. Children often demonstrate regressive behavior when ill, such as soiling diapers and demanding a bottle.

Repression occurs when the individual excludes an anxiety-producing event from the conscious awareness. There is a tendency for humans to forget the unpleasantness of the past and remember only the good times.

Sublimation occurs when an individual consciously expresses an unacceptable or impossible impulse or feeling in a more acceptable way. A woman who has chosen to be celibate and forgo motherhood may sublimate her maternal drives by working with children, by breeding pets, or by nurturing plants.

Suppression occurs when an individual consciously turns attention away from a perceived threat. "If I let myself give into this headache I'll never accomplish what I must do today."

Effects of Stress

Stress affects all of the human dimensions. Stress has a strong influence on attainment of basic human needs, is a factor in health and illness, and becomes a component in family reactions to illness. Long-term or prolonged stress, as well as crisis situations, have serious effects on the physical and emotional health of an individual. Each of these areas will be discussed in this section.

Interactions with Basic Human Needs

Basic human needs, described in Chapter 7, are common to all people. Stress, too, is common to all people. Both need attainment and the adaptation to stress require energy, respond to internal and external environments, and motivate behaviors. As the person strives to meet basic human needs at each level, stress can serve as either a stimulus or a barrier.

Basic human needs and responses to stress are individualized; both are modified by sociocultural backgrounds, priorities, and past experiences. In all persons, however, the failure to meet needs results in imbalance in homeostatic mechanisms and eventual illness.

Following are only a few of the ways stress affects basic human needs:

Physiologic needs
- Changes in appetite
- Changes in activity patterns
- Changes in sleep patterns
- Changes in elimination

Safety and security needs
- Feeling threatened and nervous
- Focus on stressor results in inattention, resulting in accidents
- Ineffective coping mechanisms (smoking, drinking) are harmful to physical and emotional health.

Love and belonging needs
- Is withdrawn and isolated
- Blames others for own faults
- Becomes overly dependent on others
- Demonstrates physical or emotional violence toward family members

Self-esteem needs
- Becomes a ''workaholic''
- Exhibits behaviors that draw attention to oneself
- Has increasing complaints of physical illness

Self-actualization needs
- Refuses to accept reality
- Centers on own problems
- Demonstrates lack of control

Stress in Health and Illness

The health–illness continuum (described in Chap. 2) also integrates the process of stress. Wellness and homeostatic balance are at one extreme of the continuum; exhaustion and death are at the other extreme.

Stress, in the healthy person, may serve to promote health and prevent illness. For example, the fear of lung cancer may motivate an individual to stop smoking, or anxiety about baby care will result in prospective parents attending prenatal classes and reading child care books. Stressors in health also facilitate normal growth and development, provide the stimulus for learning constructive adaptive behaviors, stimulate problem-solving abilities, encourage social relationships, and help develop spiritual strength.

The effects of stress on the person who is sick or injured are, in contrast, usually negative. Stress can cause illness; illness causes stress. The presence of an illness or disability demands new coping skills at a time when homeostasis is out of balance. Additionally, persons who enter the health-care setting are subjected to stressors unique to the situation.

Adaptation to acute and chronic illness involves two sets of adaptive tasks: (1) *general tasks* (as in any situational stress situation) involving maintaining self-esteem and personal relationships and preparing for an uncertain future; and (2) *illness-related tasks,* including the following (Moos, 1985):
- Losing independence and control
- Handling pain and incapacitation
- Facilitating body function recovery
- Dealing with the hospital environment
- Developing relationships with caregivers
- Controlling symptoms
- Carrying out medical treatment
- Confronting economic and family problems

Nursing interventions designed to reduce stress and promote coping must be individualized and holistic. Considerations include the person's major concern, specific illness, sociocultural background, and resources available. For example, one elderly woman may be anxious about the cost involved in repairing her hip fracture, while her roommate, with the same injury, is seriously concerned about the care of her cats while she is in the hospital. Or, as another example, two women (Mary and Jane) have entered the hospital with the medical diagnosis of cancer of the breast. Mary is worried about possible disfigurement and death but believes surgery and chemotherapy can overcome the malignancy. Jane, on the other hand, comes from a community that has strong fundamental religious beliefs. She believes that the cancer is a punishment from God and refuses any form of medical treatment.

As nurses, it is important to remember that each situation is different, that each person perceives and reacts to stressors in an individual manner, and that there is no one best way to cope with any given situation.

Family Reactions to the Stress of Illness

The stress that affects the person who is ill also affects the family members or significant others of that person. Viewing the family as a system, the behavior of the individual is influenced by the family, and any alterations in behavior by the individual in turn affects the family. The family thus is an integral part in the assessment, planning, and nursing interventions for stress.

The family of a person with an acute or chronic illness is subjected to a variety of stressors, including
- Changes in family structure and roles
- Isolation from the loved person
- Loss of control over normal routines
- Feelings of helplessness, guilt, or anger
- Lack of information about care
- Concern for future economic stability

The family, both as individuals and as a unit, uses many of the same coping and defense mechanisms previously described. They may be overly protective, deny the seriousness of an illness, or blame the hospital staff for the client's condition or behaviors. On the other hand, the family can provide important social support necessary to help the client handle and adapt to stress. Emotional support from family members allows open expression of feelings and meets love and belonging needs. The inclusion of family members in problem solving, teaching–learning activities, and physical care helps maintain self-esteem and feeling of worth by both the client and the family.

Prolonged Stress

Prolonged or long-term stress is a serious threat to physical and emotional health. As the duration, intensity, or number of stressors increases, a person's ability to adapt is lessened. The failure of adaptive mechanisms is also influenced by a person's level of wellness and past experiences with stress.

Long-term stress affects physical status, increasing the risk of disease or injury; recovery and return to normal function are also compromised by prolonged stress. High levels of stress are associated with cardiovascular disease, gastrointestinal disorders, and cancer. It is believed that these diseases are the result of a variety of factors including the effects of the fight-or-flight response, eating patterns, life-style, and coping mechanisms. A person who reacts to stress by overeating, smoking, becoming chemically dependent, or becoming hyperactive puts additional strain on a body prepared to react to threat. Homeostasis cannot be maintained, and illness results.

Prolonged stress can also serve as a serious threat to mental health. As coping or defense mechanisms become ineffective, the person may try less effective coping patterns or maladaptive defense mechanisms. As anxiety increases despite these measures, the person may experience difficulties on the job, with personal relationships, and with self-esteem. These problems in turn serve as stressors, and mental illness may result.

Crisis

A **crisis** occurs when coping and defense mechanisms, used to solve problems and adapt to change, are no longer effective. This failure produces high levels of anxiety, disorganized behavior, and an inability to function adequately. A crisis situation is the result of a person's perception and emotional response to a loss of self-esteem (or threat of a loss) from events such as illness, a change in status, a failure in school, or a verbal put-down.

The acute period of a crisis is self-limiting, lasting from 4 to 6 weeks. By that time, the threat is reduced, and the person has found some method of coping to reduce the emotional imbalance (Rambo, 1984). A person in crisis needs immediate help. Crisis intervention will be discussed in the next section.

NURSING ACTIONS TO PROMOTE STRESS REDUCTION

Stress is a fact of life and must be integrated into plans of care in health promotion and maintenance for clients of all ages. A variety of stress reduction methods are included in this part of the chapter, but you must remember the individualized nature of stressors and stress. The methods used should be carefully selected based on each person's physical and emotional characteristics, family and social structure, and previously used coping mechanisms.

Activities of Daily Living

An individual's normal life-style will greatly influence perceptions and reactions to stressors. The person who is overweight, sedentary, and chronically tired is at increased risk to develop an illness as a result of stress. (Those factors also serve as stressors, increasing the risk even more.) Exercise, rest, and nutrition are important components in stress reduction.

Regular *exercise* helps maintain physical and emotional health. The benefits of exercise include an improved musculoskeletal system, more effective cardiovascular function, weight control, and relaxation. Exercise improves one's general sense of well-being, allowing a person to relieve feelings of tension and to better cope with day-to-day stressors. General health guidelines recommend that an exercise program include 30 to 45 minutes of activity three to four times a week. Persons who are overweight, chronically ill, or over 35 should first have a thorough physical examination before beginning a program. The type of exercise can be individualized to what one enjoys most and includes walking, jogging, bicycling, swimming, or participation in sports, such as golf or tennis.

Rest and sleep allow the body to maintain homeostasis and restore energy levels. Adequate rest serves as "insulation" against stress, but stress may interfere with one's ability to sleep. Relaxation techniques can be helpful in health and illness in facilitating rest and sleep. However, hospitalized clients may require additional nursing interventions to relieve pain and promote comfort to get needed rest.

Nutrition plays an active role in maintaining the body's homeostatic mechanisms and in increasing resistance to stress. Both obesity and malnutrition are major stressors and greatly increase the risk of illness. Individuals of all ages are encouraged to maintain a normal body weight and to follow guidelines established by the U. S. Senate Committee on Nutrition and Human Needs to

- Reduce levels of salt, refined sugar, animal fat, and cholesterol

- Eat more fruit, vegetables, and whole grains
- Eat less red meat and more fish and poultry

Support Systems

As has previously been discussed, the family has an important role in helping a client cope with stress. This support can also be provided by other social support systems.

Support systems provide emotional support which helps the individual identify and verbalize feelings associated with stress. Other valuable contributions are the provision of information and services, maintaining positive self-concept, and establishing an avenue for new relationships and social roles. Additionally, families and support groups provide an accepting environment, allowing the individual to explore problem-solving methods and try out new coping skills.

There are support groups for almost every situation, for example,

Alcoholics Anonymous
Overeaters Anonymous
Weight Watchers
Parents Without Partners
Reach to Recovery (Cancer)
Ostomy clubs
Child abuse support groups
Sudden infant death support groups
Stroke clubs
Assertiveness training groups

Stress Management Techniques

Stress creates emotional distress, often having outward symptoms. All of us have had experiences with stress and know how we feel and how we react. One person may have tension headaches, another becomes irritable, another clenches his fists. Often people take drugs (legal and illegal), drink or smoke to excess, or eat compulsively. These behaviors can be modified and adaptive mechanisms strengthened through specific techniques aimed at managing stress. Only a few techniques are included here, but the literature is filled with stress reduction methods. Students are encouraged to learn a variety of methods useful for themselves and for varied clinical situations.

Relaxation. Relaxation techniques are useful in many situations: childbirth, pain, anxiety, sleeplessness, illness, anger (and other uses are being discovered). Relaxation promotes a body reaction opposite to the fight-or-flight response—decreasing respirations, blood pressure, pulse, metabolic rate, and energy use.

Relaxation can be taught to individuals or groups and is especially helpful because it allows the individual to control feelings and behaviors. Various techniques are used, but each involves rhythmic breathing, reduced

Relaxation Activities

Deep Breathing
- Sit comfortably and place your hands on your stomach. Inhale slowly and deeply, letting your stomach expand as much as possible. Hold your breath for a few seconds.
- Exhale slowly through your mouth, blowing the air out through pursed lips. When your stomach feels empty, repeat the cycle.
- Repeat three to four times each session.

Progressive Muscular Relaxation
- Tighten your hand into a fist and notice how it feels; hold the tension for a few seconds.
- Loosen the grip on your muscles, relax your muscles, and let the tension slip away.
- Continue through each muscle group—hands, arms, shoulders, face, chest, back, stomach, legs, feet.

muscle tension, and an altered state of consciousness (Stuart and Sundeen, 1987). Two relaxation activities are discussed in the box. Relaxation is also discussed as a pain relief measure in Chapter 30.

Meditation. Meditation also facilitates relaxation and involves four components: (1) quiet surroundings, (2) a passive attitude, (3) a comfortable position, and (4) a word or mental image to focus on. The person practicing meditation closes his/her eyes, relaxes each of the major muscle groups, and repeats the selected word silently with each exhalation. Alternately, the person may focus on a pleasant scene and mentally place himself in it as he slowly breathes in and out. This process should be carried out for 20–30 minutes, twice a day.

Anticipatory Guidance. Anticipatory guidance is a method of stress reduction that focuses on the psychologic preparation of a person for an unfamiliar or painful event. Nurses use this technique to teach clients about procedures and the surgical experience. By knowing what to expect, anxiety is reduced and coping is more effective. For example, before changing a dressing, teaching would include all the information about the pain involved—onset, severity, cause, methods of relief. With this knowledge, the client feels less threat and tolerates the procedure more easily.

Guided Imagery. In guided imagery, the individual creates an image in his mind, concentrates on the image, and becomes less responsive to stimuli (including pain). The nurse sits by the client and uses a scene or experience the client has described as happy, pleasant, or peaceful. The client is then "guided" through the image. For example, using a soothing, soft voice, the nurse might start as follows:

"You are floating in your swimming pool. The water is cool and comfortable. Birds are singing in the trees. The roses are perfuming the air."

As the client becomes more and more focused on the scene, the nurse will only need to verbally "paint the picture" at intervals.

Biofeedback.   Biofeedback is a method of gaining mental control of the autonomic nervous systems, and thus regulating body responses, such as blood pressure, heart rate, and headaches.

A measurement device (for example, skin temperature sensors) is used, and the client tries to voluntarily control the readings through relaxation and conscious thought. The feedback from the change in readings teaches the person to control physiologic functions normally considered to be involuntary responses. The process is long-term and still being researched.

Crisis Intervention

As defined previously in this chapter, a crisis is a situation that cannot be resolved by usual coping mechanisms. As a result, a person is unable to function normally and requires interventions to regain equilibrium. **Crisis intervention** is a five-step problem-solving tech-

nique designed to promote a more adaptive outcome, including improved abilities to cope with future crisis. The steps are

1. *Identifying the problem:* This may be more difficult than it appears; often the cause of the crisis is difficult for the person to accurately identify. Until it is clear, a solution is impossible.
2. *Listing alternatives:* Any and all possible solutions to the problem need to be listed. An appropriate solution to a problem is much more likely if a substantial number of options are considered.
3. *Choosing from among alternatives:* Each option needs to be carefully considered, using a "what would happen if I _____" approach. The alternative chosen will be highly individualized, based on priorities and values.
4. *Implementing a plan:* The alternative chosen is put into action. It may be necessary to provide support and encouragement so that action is taken.
5. *Evaluation:* In this final step, the effectiveness of the plan needs to be carefully considered. If it did not work as well as expected, another alternative needs to be chosen. If it did work, it has the positive benefit of improving self-confidence and future problem solving.

The major factor in helping clients adapt to high levels of stress is to identify and plan for the individuality of each situation. The following list of suggestions is useful:

- Help the individual recognize his own stress level and specific responses to stress.
- Encourage a philosophy of accepting what can't be changed, and changing what can't be accepted.
- Encourage the individual to accept help from others—and to give support to others when needed.
- Encourage active but deliberate involvement in problem solving and decision making.
- Be an active listener, increasing therapeutic relationships and communications.
- Provide health teaching about developmental crises and threatening events.

Stress Management for Nurses

A discussion of stress would not be complete without including a section on the stress in nursing. Nursing is an occupation involving activities and interpersonal relationships that create stress and anxiety.

Nurses carry out tasks regarded by non-nurses as embarrassing, disagreeable, or painful. Rapid changes in staffing patterns and technology result in an environment that is rarely stable. In addition, nurses must constantly learn new knowledge to give care safely.

The interpersonal relationships in the health-care setting are complex and often unpredictable. Clients may be in a period of crisis and may require intensive physical and emotional support. Demands are made by families, physicians, administration, and staff.

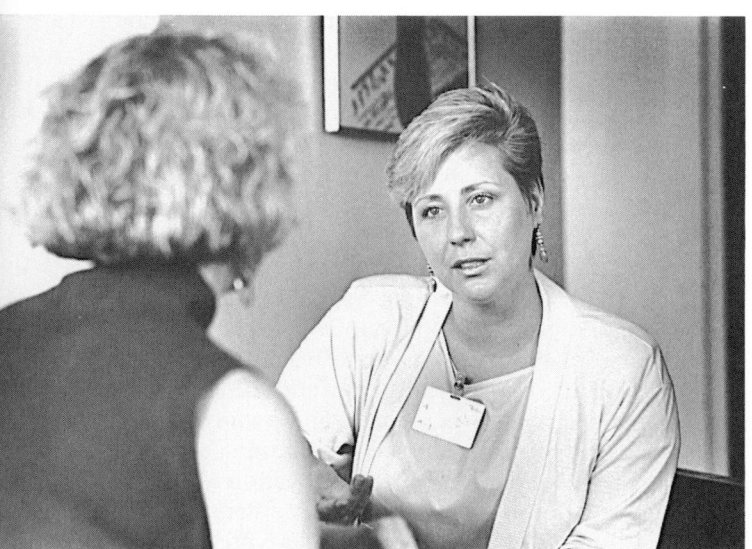

F I G U R E   9-5
In crisis intervention, it is important for the nurse to help clients recognize their own stress levels and to encourage accepting what cannot be changed and changing what cannot be accepted.
(Photo by Robert Neroni, courtesy of Thomas Jefferson University)

PROMOTING WELLNESS

Stress and Adaptation

Use the assessment checklist to determine how well you are adapting to stress. Then develop a prescription for self-care by choosing appropriate behaviors from the list of suggestions.

Assessment Checklist

almost always	some-times	almost never	
☐	☐	☐	1. I have realistic perceptions of new situations, self, and others.
☐	☐	☐	2. I understand my own personal physical and emotional responses to stress.
☐	☐	☐	3. I anticipate and prepare for change.
☐	☐	☐	4. I have the ability to satisfactorily solve problems and make decisions.

Self-Care Behaviors

1. Accept as positive indicators of growth the changes that come with different parts and stages of life.
2. Maintain an open mind about change—change what you can, and accept what you can't.
3. Avoid self-defeating behaviors to cope with stress, such as smoking, alcohol, and drugs.
4. Practice methods of stress management that work best for you: relaxation techniques, exercise, hobbies.
5. Set realistic goals.
6. Develop problem-solving strategies for use in stressful situations.
7. Accept help from others.
8. Take life one day at a time.

The stress has been shown to be even greater for two groups: the new graduate, faced with an environment different than was experienced as a student, and nurses working in areas such as intensive care and emergency care.

The anxiety is further complicated by the expected behavior of nurses—even though they may have strong negative feelings and reactions, their role does not include behaviors and verbal expressions that are less than positive and supportive.

Most nurses thoroughly enjoy their work and cope with the physical and emotional demands effectively. Some, however, are overwhelmed and develop symptoms of anxiety and stress. The complex of behaviors exhibited is called professional burnout. **Burnout** can be compared to the exhaustion stage of anxiety and is characterized by a wide range of behaviors. Some nurses may try to become "super nurses," expecting perfection in themselves and others. Some may withdraw and do only minimal work; still others may resort to drugs or alcohol. A large number of nurses, unable to handle the stress, leave the profession entirely.

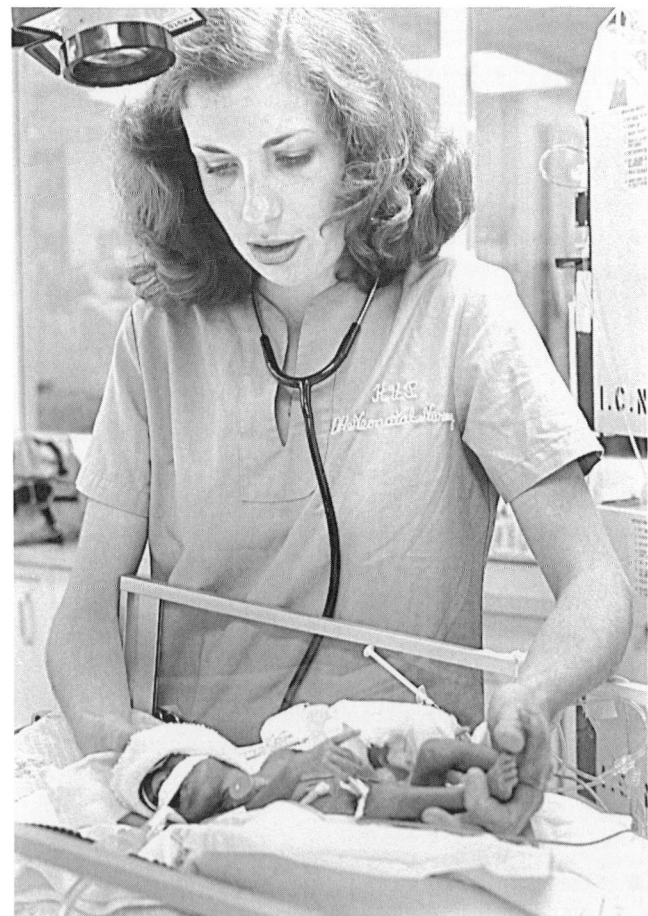

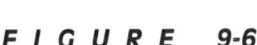

FIGURE 9-6

Some nursing specialities can be more stressful than others. To prevent burnout and alleviate stress, a nurse may need to work in another area of nursing, temporarily or permanently. (Photo by Robert Neroni, courtesy of Thomas Jefferson University Hospital)

What can be done? The first step in preventing a stress level high enough to cause burnout is to identify and accept the stress. It may be necessary to work in another area of nursing; the wide variety of settings available today provides opportunities for jobs that are less stressful in general, or to the individual nurse.

The stress reduction methods used to help clients have the same benefit for nurses. By recognizing the early signs of stress and taking steps to reduce the anxiety, nurses will continue to be effective, productive, and self-satisfied in the profession.

Some useful measures are (Rambo, 1984)

- Take time for relaxation—use break time for a relaxation technique that works, eat lunch away from the unit.

- Include physical coping mechanisms in your daily routine—join an aerobic dance class, play tennis, mow the yard.
- Allow some time each day to "wind down" and relax—soak in a bubble bath, listen to music, read.
- Develop assertive skills—learn to say "No" to additional tasks, accept the fact that no one person is perfect or indispensable.
- Learn something new that develops another part of yourself—learn to knit, take a class, join a gourmet food group.

Nurses need to accept that they are as individual as their clients. Nurses have the same needs and frustrations, but also have the knowledge and skill to recognize and cope with stress—in themselves as well as in others.

KEY POINTS

- Homeostasis, or a healthy balanced state, is maintained by various physiologic and psychologic mechanisms. Physiologic mechanisms are largely involuntary responses of the autonomic and endocrine systems, necessary to health maintenance. Psychologic balance is maintained through the use of coping or defense mechanisms.

- Stress, stressors, and adaptation are all interrelated parts of a process. *Stressors* (a challenge, a danger, or a threat) cause *stress* (a change in the balanced state). The person *adapts* through a series of responses. Each component is highly individualized and holistic in effect.

- Stress may be developmental or situational; stressors may be physiologic or psychosocial. Physiologic stressors have both a general and a specific effect. Psychosocial stressors affect us constantly in day-to-day living.

- The relationship between physical and emotional stress is illustrated by the mind–body interaction, in which the perception of a threat on an emotional level results in the fight-or-flight response by the body. Resulting illnesses are often called psychosomatic disorders.

- The impact (and stress) of life-changing events have an impact on health. The Social Readjustment Rating Scale can be used to predict risk of illness.

- The LAS is a localized body response to traumatic or pathologic stress which serves to maintain homeostasis and adaptation. Two examples of the LAS are the reflex pain response and the inflammatory response.

- The inflammatory response occurs in response to injury or infection, serving to prevent the spread of infection and promote wound healing through regeneration of tissue or formation of scar.

- The GAS is a biochemical model describing the body's general response to stress. There are three stages to the GAS: alarm reaction, stage of resistance, and stage of exhaustion. The stages occur in response to both physical and emotional stress.

- The most common psychologic response to stress is anxiety. Anxiety, precipitated by new experiences and the unknown, serves as a threat to self-esteem and identity. Anxiety has four levels: mild, moderate, severe, and panic.

- Coping mechanisms are largely unconscious methods of attempting to adapt to stress.

- Higher levels of stress may require psychologic adaptation by coping with task-oriented reactions (attack, withdrawal, or compromise behavior) or defense mechanisms. Many of these behaviors are learned, based on past experiences and sociocultural environment.

- Stress can interfere with basic need attainment, disrupting homeostasis and causing illness.

- Stress can promote health and learning, but the stress of illness imposes additional burdens on an individual who is out of balance. Adaptation to illness involves general tasks and illness-related tasks. Nursing interventions to reduce the stress of illness must be individualized and holistic.

- Stress affects the family as well as the individual. Families use varied coping methods and provide an important support system for the ill person.

- Prolonged stress affects physical and mental health.

■ Crisis results from ineffective coping, leading to severe anxiety, disorganized behavior, and malfunction.

■ Nurses can promote health through the use of stress reduction teaching and methods, including healthy life-style, support groups, stress management techniques, and crisis intervention.

■ Nursing is a stressful occupation. Nurses may become overwhelmed by the demands made and may develop symptoms of burnout. Nurses can practice stress management techniques both on and off the job to help prevent stress and improve career satisfaction.

BIBLIOGRAPHY

Antonovsky A: Health, Stress, and Coping. San Francisco, Jossey-Bass, 1979

Brunner L, Suddarth D: Textbook of Medical-Surgical Nursing, 6th ed. Philadelphia, JB Lippincott, 1988

DiMotto J: Relaxation. Am J Nurs 6:754, 1984

Donovan M: Relaxation with guided imagery: A useful technique. Cancer Nurs 2:27–32, 1980

Hames C, Joseph D: Basic Concepts of Helping: A Wholistic Approach. New York, Appleton-Century-Crofts, 1980

Johnson B: Psychiatric-Mental Health Nursing: Adaptation and Growth. Philadelphia, JB Lippincott, 1986

Lewis S, Collier I: Medical-Surgical Nursing: Assessment and Management of Clinical Problems, 2nd ed. New York, McGraw-Hill, 1987

Miller J: Inspiring hope. Am J Nurs 1:22–25, 1985

Moos R: Coping with Physical Illness, 2nd ed. New York, Plenum Publishing, 1985

Pasquali E et al: Mental Health Nursing: A Holistic Approach, 2nd ed. St Louis, CV Mosby, 1985

Phipps W, Long B, Wood N: Medical-Surgical Nursing: Concepts and Clinical Practice, 3rd ed. St Louis, CV Mosby, 1987

Rambo B: Adaptation Nursing: Assessment and Intervention. Philadelphia, WB Saunders, 1984

Richter J, Sloan R: The relaxation technique. Am J Nurs November 11:1960–1964, 1979

Ryan J: The neglected crisis. Am J Nurs 10:1257–1258, 1984

Selye H: *The Stress of Life*. New York, McGraw-Hill, 1976

Sparacino J: Blood pressure, stress, and mental health. Nurs Res 1:89–94, Jan/Feb 1982

Stuart G, Sundeen S: Principles and Practices of Psychiatric Nursing, 3rd ed. St Louis, CV Mosby, 1987

Taylor C: Mereness' Essentials of Psychiatric Nursing, 12th ed. St Louis, CV Mosby, 1986

Wyka G, Caraulia S: Crisis intervention: Stopping push before it comes to shove. Nursing 86, Nov 16:44–45, 1986

UNIT

III

Promoting Wellness Across the Lifespan

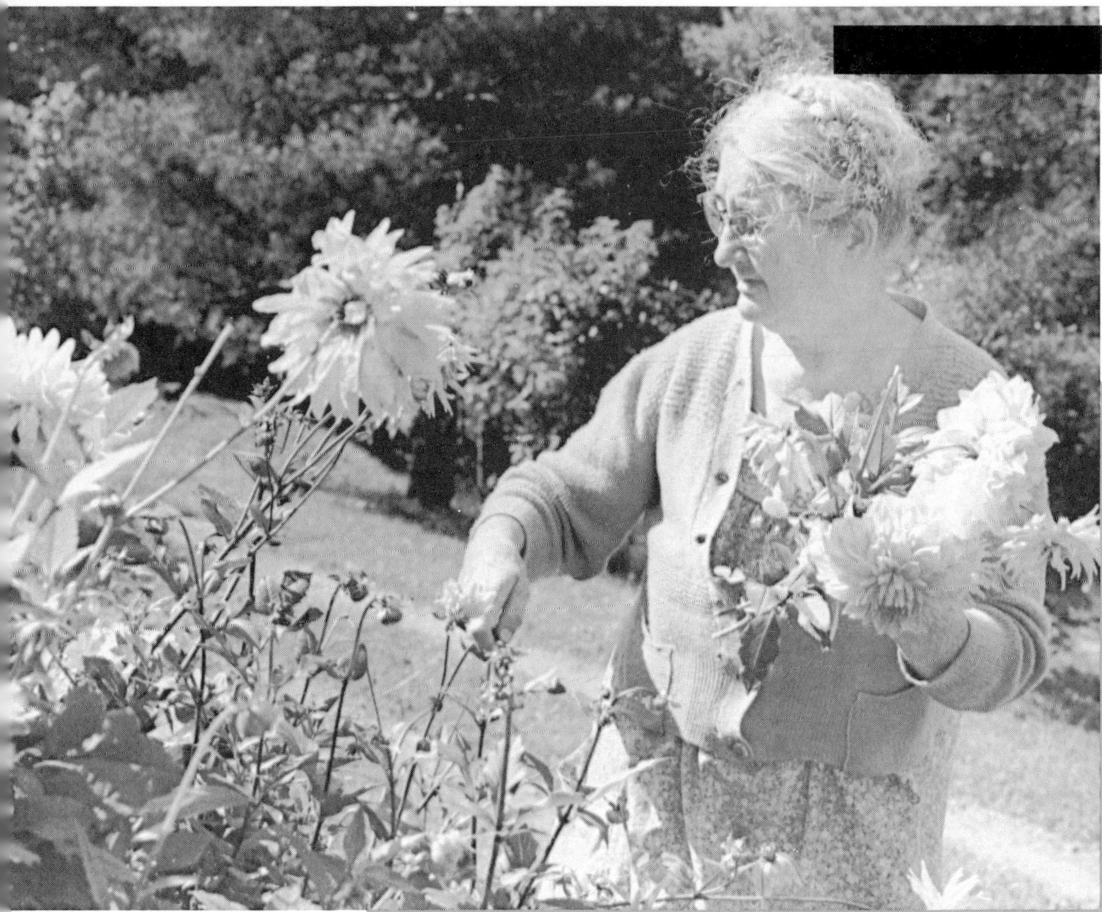

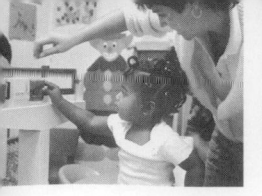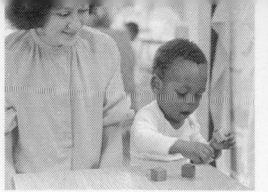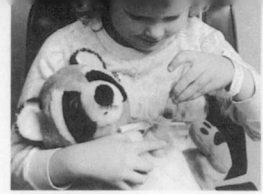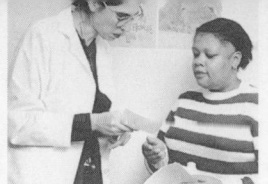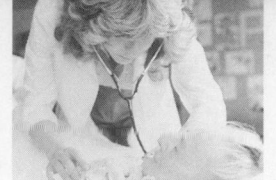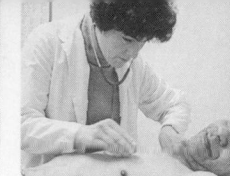

*N*urses give care to clients of all ages, and at all stages of growth and development. Unit III discusses the impact of developmental stages and tasks on nursing care for clients and families throughout the entire lifespan from conception to death.

Developmental theories provide guidelines for giving individualized client care, with consideration for physiologic, cognitive, psychosocial, moral, spiritual, and family components of each individual person. Each person progresses through life in well-defined stages, with critical tasks and common health needs and problems. The chapters in this unit follow the sequential stages of growth and development, describing factors that influence normal development, common age-related health problems, and the role of the nurse in preventing illness and promoting health.

With increasing numbers of the population over the age of 65, the health needs of the older adult are a major nursing concern today, and will continue to be so in the future. Chapter 12 discusses normal age-related changes, common myths and realities of the older age group, and the nurse's role in promoting wellness and coping with change.

Death, as the final stage of life, requires nursing interventions to meet individual and family needs, and to facilitate coping with loss and grief.

Unit III provides a comprehensive picture of growth and development throughout life, enabling the nurse to individualize care and meet needs for clients in all stages of life.

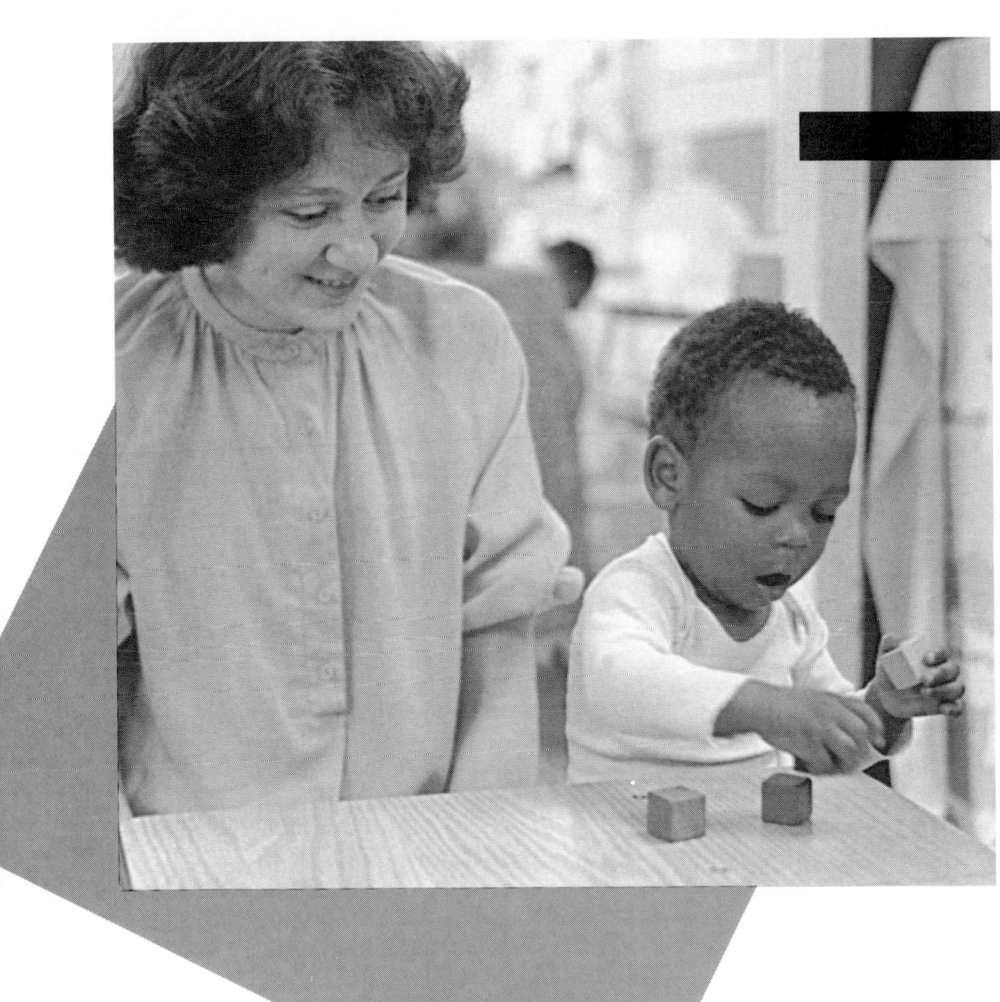

Developmental Concepts

OBJECTIVES

After studying this chapter, the learner should be able to

Define key terms used in the chapter.

Summarize basic principles of growth and development.

Discuss the theories of Freud, Piaget, Havighurst, Erikson, Kolberg, and Fowler.

Describe the importance of incorporating multiple theories of growth and development in assessing and planning nursing care for an individual client.

Describe the dynamics of family in providing nursing care.

List implications for nursing practice that derive from a knowledge of growth and development.

Nurses provide care to people of all ages, whether individual clients or families. Each person brings a unique set of health-care needs or concerns to the nurse–client relationship. These needs result from physical, emotional, intellectual, social, spiritual, and cultural aspects of development. The nurse must understand typical behavior for each developmental level to evaluate normal versus abnormal responses and to plan age-appropriate care. For example, when collecting health information the nurse may relate an adolescent's unexplained weight loss to body image concerns or family problems. The cause of the weight loss is important in relation to the developmental approach to be initiated by the nurse.

Physical development has a predetermined genetic base due to inheritance patterns carried on chromosomes. Thus, the unborn child begins life with specific physical attributes, either properly formed or malformed. Environmental factors from birth through the early years of growth provide initial psychologic and social contact through positive or negative parenting experiences. As environmental influences expand beyond the immediate caregivers or family, psychosocial experiences increase and affect development. Cognitive, moral, and spiritual growth is fostered through contact within families, schools, and communities. Information derived from multiple theories of human and family development assist the nurse in perceiving these interrelated variables at designated stages throughout life.

This chapter presents basic principles of growth and development to serve as a foundation for understanding the human being at various life stages. Major theories examining cognitive, psychosocial, spiritual, and moral development are discussed. In addition to reviewing theories specific to the individual's development, the family and its influence on personal development are discussed briefly.

KEY TERMS

accommodation	growth
assimilation	maturation
cognitive development	moral development
developmental task	psychosocial theory
faith	sexuality

THE NATURE OF HUMAN GROWTH AND DEVELOPMENT

There still are debates regarding "nature versus nurture" and research investigating to what extent behaviors are part of an inherited nature and to what extent they are the result of experiences during childhood. However, the interplay of heredity and environment guides the human processes of growth and development. Although most theories present only one aspect of growth and development, individuals proceed in all areas of growth and development not independent of one another.

The human organism evolves in physical, cognitive, psychosocial, moral, and spiritual dimensions simultaneously. The product of the whole being is always greater than the sum of its individual dimensions.

Growing older, a life experience common to all living beings, consists of more than rapid physical and cognitive growth during childhood, achievement of multiple psychosocial tasks during adulthood, and a decline in later years. Development is a continuous dynamic process affecting each person with a series of ascents, plateaus, and declines for each age.

Each phase of development has not only the previously mentioned traits, but also a period of equilibrium when the individual adjusts more easily to internal and environmental demands, and a period of disequilibrium when adjustment is more difficult (Erikson, 1963; Mussen, Conger, and Kagan, 1974). If developmental tasks are not accomplished or they are delayed, difficulties may arise at later stages.

PRINCIPLES OF GROWTH AND DEVELOPMENT

From knowledge of the biologic and behavioral sciences, certain generalizations about the nature of human development can be made. These generalizations form the basic principles for interpreting the complex processes underlying **growth** and **development**. The principles serve only as guidelines, because each individual's profile is the outcome of genetic potential and environment.

Principle 1: Growth and Development are Orderly and Sequential. As a child grows, maturation is predictable and follows a general timetable. Developmental milestones give indications of the average time that the child will maintain head control, attempt to roll over, crawl, walk, and say his first words. The occurrence of each milestone typically follows a universal pattern.

Principle 2: Growth and Development are Continuous and Complex. Although it is an ongoing process, there are varying rates of physical growth, resulting in growth spurts during infancy and adolescence. Intellectual curiosity increases markedly during the preschool years as language and motor skills advance. This continuous process of growth and development is multifaceted, influenced by biophysical, psychologic, and environmental factors which contribute to the whole being. Genetic potential is determined with conception and stimulated by the environment.

Principle 3: The Pace of Growth and Development is Specific for Each Individual. Although growth and development are continuous, they do not occur simultaneously. Acquisition of skills and changes in physical appearance or behaviors may vary with each individual. Thus, physiologic and psychologic maturation varies among people. For example, as the child is learning locomotion skills, he may be exerting all of his energies on this task, while language skills may not be heightened during this brief period. Because of this variation, most developmental assessment guides list a wide span for

norms according to age. Cultural variations can also be observed, for example, Oriental or Asian children tend to be smaller than Caucasian children of the same age.

Principle 4: Psychosocial Development is Influenced by Many Environmental Factors. Socialization and emotional behavior are learned from family, friends, church, and community. Values, roles, rules, and regulations are determined in different cultural or social groups. The task of clarifying one's own value system proceeds throughout life.

Principle 5: There are Regular Trends in the Direction of Human Development. Some unifying directions give order to growth and development. Three rudimentary trends can be easily observed. The first trend is that development is cephalocaudal, meaning that areas such as the brain and head develop first, followed by the trunk, legs, and feet. Pictures of an embryo in utero demonstrate the large size of the head in comparison to body size (Fig. 10-1).

The second trend is proximodistal development, which means that growth progresses from the central axis of the body toward the periphery. Gross motor movements, such as learning to roll over, are developed earlier than fine motor movements, such as picking up small objects with the fingers. Psychologically, a child focuses on himself (egocentric) before developing an appreciation for others' viewpoints.

The third trend is that growth and development are symmetric so that what occurs on one side of the body tends to occur on the other, unless there is a physical handicap.

Nurses can use knowledge of these trends as they assess their patients at all ages. For example, in determining muscle strength of the upper extremity, the nurse can compare the patient's hand grips bilaterally.

Principle 6: Growth and Development are Both Quantitative and Qualitative. During the formative years, the body size of the individual increases continuously. As size increases, differentiation occurs to support refinement of quality functioning. As the nerve pathways form in the neonate, they become more and more specialized for transmitting certain impulses in the growing child.

Another example of differentiation refers to the behavioral changes manifested from a painful stimulus. The newborn responds to pain with his whole body, kicking arms and legs, while grimacing and crying. The older child and adult express pain in more specific mannerisms, seen predominantly in the face.

Principle 7: Growth and Development Become Gradually Integrated. Behavior and function progress from simple to complex as the child builds on previously learned skills to achieve more difficult tasks. The acquisition of more complex skills proceeds into and throughout the adult years. The young toddler learning

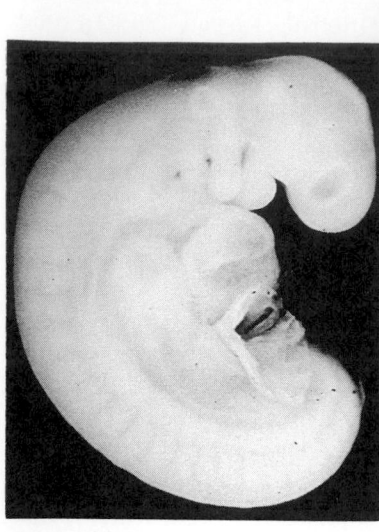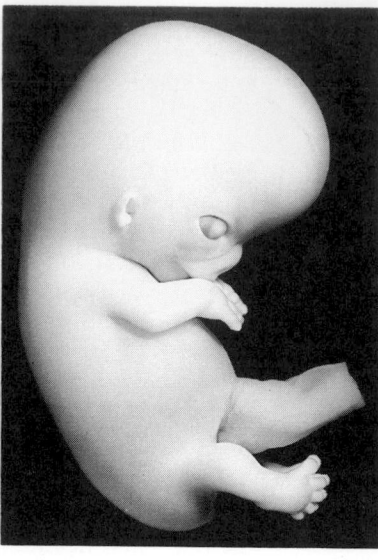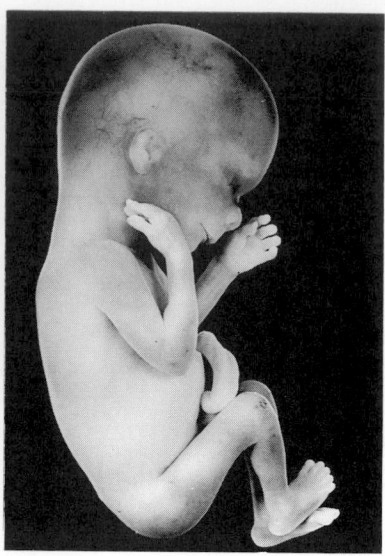

F I G U R E   10-1
Three stages of human development in utero—at approximately 4, 8, and 16 weeks—showing the development first of the head and then the trunk and limbs. (Carnegie Institute, Washington, D.C.)

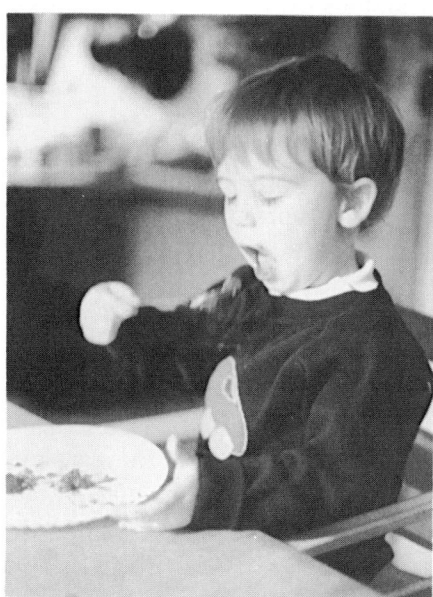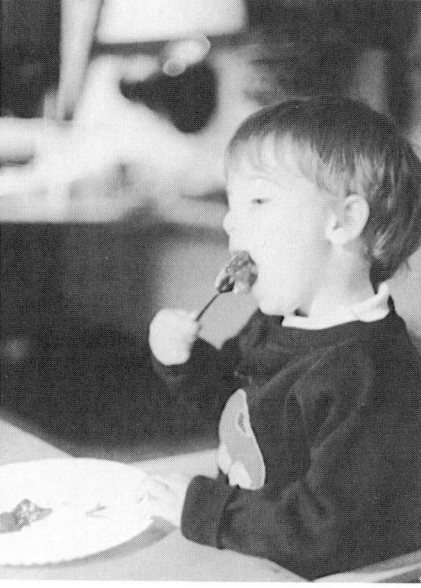

F I G U R E   10-2
The toddler learning to use a spoon is integrating hand–eye coordination, cognitive patterning, and social imitation in mastering the task. (Photo by Tracy Baldwin)

to use a spoon combines motor skills from hand–eye coordination, cognitive patterning to repeat the act when appropriate, and social imitation from observing others (Fig. 10-2). As toddlers grow and develop, the task of using a spoon becomes basic, forming the foundation to learning more advanced skills requiring manual dexterity.

Principle 8: There are Vulnerable Periods in Development. The susceptibility of the human organism to certain effects during critical periods has been proposed.

Research has verified that during the time of rapid cellular growth of the fetus in the first 3 months, the organism is more prone to insults from viruses, chemicals, or drugs, leading to congenital defects. Early malnutrition, such as poor nutrition in infancy, can lead to delayed brain development and resulting learning deficits.

Klaus and Kennell (1982) defined a sensitive period during the first hour after birth when the initiation of parent–infant bonding is optimal. The infant is found to be in a reactive phase at this time, alert and responding to the appearance, smell, and voices of his parents. Many researchers have questioned the potential negative effects on personality development when parent–infant bonding and attachment are impaired. Kempe and Helfer (1968) referred to this phenomenon when studying predisposition to child abuse and the link of parents who abuse their children to personal abuse as children themselves.

Principle 9: The Rate and Pattern of Growth and Development Can Be Modified. Nutrition is one factor which can affect physiologic development at any age. Both positive and negative effects are seen. The child with malabsorption may be small for age on growth charts for height or weight. The adult with chronic ulcerative colitis may appear emaciated and dehydrated. An opposite response occurs when the infant is able to progress from bottle or breast milk to baby foods or soft table foods and gains weight appropriately. Adult body weight, size, and tone are best maintained through regular exercise and daily meals prepared from the four basic food groups.

Principle 10: Different Aspects of Growth and Development Occur at Different Stages and at Different Rates. Muscle and bone growth both occur most rapidly during the first year of life, increasing the integration of neuromuscular function. During the toddler and preschool years, muscle fibers increase in strength and size, whereas bone growth slows.

Primary dentition begins by approximately 5 months and is completed by 30 months. Dentition slows during the toddler and early preschool years. By age 6, permanent teeth development begins to occur.

The most intense period for speech development is between ages 3 and 5. By age 4, the child has a vocabulary of 1000 words and has figured out the basic rules for communicating past plural, possessive, and conditional forms of words (Newman and Newman, 1975).

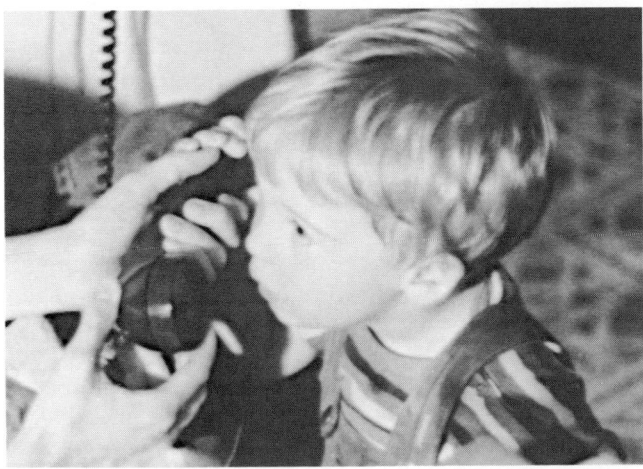

F I G U R E 10-3
The most intense period for speech development is between the ages of 3 and 5 years. (Photo by Patrick O'Kane)

Physical sexual maturity first begins during the preadolescent years, often occurring earlier in females than males. The rate varies tremendously from person to person. The concept of sexuality progresses into the adult years and has its first impressions formed as early as preschool years during sex-role identification.

OVERVIEW OF DEVELOPMENTAL THEORIES

Human behavior has been studied by researchers since the early part of the twentieth century. From these studies, some classic theories of development have been formed in an attempt to explain human responses usually expected at certain ages during life. Approaches to these explanations have varied, depending on the individual researcher's perspective. A psychologic approach is common to all developmental theories, with some theories focusing more on cognitive influences, social influences, or instinctual influences. The theories to be discussed in this chapter include those developed by Sigmund Freud, Jean Piaget, Robert Havighurst, Erik Erikson, Lawrence Kohlberg, and James Fowler.

Psychoanalytic Theory of Sigmund Freud

One of the earliest developmental theories that has influenced nursing and the behavioral sciences is the psychoanalytic theory by the Viennese physician Sigmund Freud (1856–1939). Out of an interest in identifying possible causes for some perplexing physical symptoms in his patients that had no medical etiology, he tried to connect influences between the mind and the body. He stressed the impact of instinctual human drives on determining behavior.

Freud is well-known for the concepts of the unconscious mind; the id, ego, and superego; and the stages of development based on sexual motivation (Freud, 1923). Freud identified the underlying stimulus for human behavior at all ages to be **sexuality**, which he called libido. His concept of sexuality was much broader than the context in which it is used today, which has led to some confusion and misinterpretation of his theory. *Libido* was meant to refer to pleasure-seeking instincts in more general terms than solely to genital gratification.

The unconscious mind, according to Freud, contains memories, motives, fantasies, and fears usually not accessible to recall, but directly affecting behavior. Freudian theory stresses that all behavior is meaningful if unconscious motives can be discovered. Analyzing a person's dreams could determine possible underlying meaning to thought patterns and behavior.

Freud viewed the mind in three separate dimensions: the id, the ego, and the superego. The *id* is the part

R E S E A R C H   I N   N U R S I N G   *Making a Difference*

Growth and Development

Quality care of children is based on knowledge of growth and development. Nurses must anticipate and explain normal behavior and identify variations from normal. Both normal and delayed development require nursing support if children are to reach their optimum potential. Several nursing research studies in this area have facilitated continued improvement in parent–child nursing care.

Related Research

Acuilino M, Ely J: Parents and the sexuality of preschool children. Pediatr Nurs 11:41–46, 1985

Aquilino and Ely investigated parents' ability to handle normal sexual behavior of preschool children and found that most parents are knowledgeable and positive about the sexual curiosity and activity of their children. Based on these findings, it is recommended that nurses use an assessment tool to elicit parental concerns and then coordinate discussions and offer support as parents deal with the sexual development of their children.

Moller J: Relationships between temperament and development in preschool children. Res Nurs Health 6:25–32, 1983

This study was the first to examine the relationship between temperament and development in preschool children. A correlation between several categories of temperament to developmental levels was found. Children who were mildly active, rhythmic, approachable, adaptable, and persistent had higher levels of development than did children who were withdrawn and nonadaptive. Moller urges the use of clinical assessment tools to measure temperament and to individualize interventions to promote optimum development in preschool children.

Strauss S, Munton M: Common concerns of parents with disabled children. Pediatr Nurs 11:371–375, 1985

This research was conducted to assess the problems and concerns of parents of children with developmental delay. Conclusions of the study were (1) all parents grieved, although the expression and intensity of the grief was individualized; (2) parents had varying degrees of problems obtaining adequate services for their children; and (3) all parents worried about the future of their children. Based on these conclusions, nurses must make assessments of parents' coping skills; give information in an objective, sensitive, and positive manner; and provide ongoing support and assistance.

Nurses, utilizing knowledge of growth and development and nursing research findings, are in a unique position to facilitate optimum development in young children. Research studies have indicated the importance of meaningful anticipatory guidance, health counseling, and parental support.

---

of the psyche concerned with self-gratification by the easiest and quickest available means. Newborn behavior is an example of reaction to instinctual needs, determined by the id. The hungry, wet, or uncomfortable newborn will cry until needs are met. Freud noted that with interaction and repetition of a familiar response, the demand for such immediate gratification is lessened. As a person grows older, the desire of need gratification based on the id is modified with ego development.

The *ego* is the conscious part of the psyche which serves as a mediator between the desires of the id and the constraints of reality producing behaviors that are compatible with others and the environment. It includes the functions of intelligence, memory, problem solving, separation of reality from fantasy, and incorporation of experiences and learning into future behavior. Collectively, the functions of the ego assist the individual to live effectively within his actual social psychologic and physical environment. Ego development begins during the first year of life so that by 6 months of age the infant views himself as a separate part from his mother or primary caregiver and alters behaviors in response to cues received from her. Ego development continues throughout childhood and to a lesser degree throughout the adult years.

The *superego* is the part of the mind representing one's conscience, which develops from the ego beginning in the first year of life as the child learns praise versus punishment for actions. The superego represents the internalization of socially acceptable behavior based on rules and values adapted from ethical or moral standards.

A major contribution from Freud's theory is the description of *defense mechanisms,* which are means of unconscious coping when the id's impulses cannot be satisfied so as to reduce stress in the conscious mind.

These defense mechanisms include repression, displacement, projection, and reaction formation. Defense mechanisms are discussed in Chapter 9.

Stages of Development

Freud's theory presents a series of stages through which all persons must pass. These stages all have predictable id–superego conflicts which must be resolved by the ego through the use of defense mechanisms. As conflicts are resolved at each stage, enough psychologic energy remains to advance to future stages. Poorly resolved conflicts result in less available energy (Billingham, 1982).

The five stages of psychoanalytic theory are oral, anal, phallic, latency, and adult sexuality. The infant's pleasures are believed to center around gratification from using his mouth for sucking and satisfying hunger. Feelings and activities are focused on and expressed by the mouth and are orally dominated.

The anal phase begins with attainment of neuromuscular control of the anal sphincter. Toilet training is the crucial issue causing conflict and requiring delayed gratification in compromising between enjoyment of bowel function and limitations set by social expectations for the toddler.

By age 4, the child becomes interested in gender differences, identification of one's own gender, and conflict and then resolution with the parent of the same sex. The phallic phase constitutes increased curiosity regarding the genitals, questioning, and self-stimulation or masturbation.

Preschool males demonstrate an intimate sexual possessiveness of their mothers called the Oedipus complex. Preschool females show preference for their fathers, seen as coy or seductive behavior toward them and jealousy or fear toward their mothers. This corresponding phenomenon is called the Electra complex.

The latency stage marks the transition from the phallic period to the beginning of adult sexuality (genital stage) during adolescence. Usually around the age of 6, the school-age child realizes that desires directed to the parent of the opposite sex are not feasible, and becomes occupied with socializing with peers, refining roles and relationships. There is increasing sex-role identification with the parent of the same sex in preparation for adulthood.

Adolescence represents an emergence of sexual interest which can now be expressed in an overt heterosexual relationship. Sexual pressures and conflicts instill turmoil as the adolescent makes adaptations in the progress to mature adult adjustment in relationships. Refer to Table 10-1 for summarization of Freud's theory.

Theory of Erik Erikson

The developmental theory of Erik Erikson (1963) was based on Freud's work. Erikson expanded Freud's theory to include cultural and social influences in addition to

TABLE 10-1
Freud's Stages of Psychosexual Development

Stage	Age	Sexual Activity
Oral	0–18 months	Sucking, swallowing, chewing, biting
Anal	8 months–4 years	Expulsion and retention of waste products
Phallic	3–7 years	Masturbation
Latent	5–12 years	———
Genital (Adult sexuality)	12–20 years	Masturbation, sexual intercourse, feelings for others

(Adapted from Fong C, Resnick R: The Child: Development Through Adolescence. Menlo Park, CA, Benjamin/Cummings, 1980)

biologic processes. He believed there was an interrelationship between such variables that impact the psychosocial development of an individual throughout life.

Psychosocial theory is based on four major organizing concepts: (1) stages of development, (2) developmental goals or tasks, (3) psychosocial crises, and (4) the process of coping (Newman and Newman, 1975).

Erikson (1963) believed that development is a continuous process consisting of distinct phases characterized by the achievement of developmental goals. He emphasized that certain tasks progressed in a definite order, but were affected by the social environment and significant others.

Stages of Development

Erikson identified eight stages of development from birth through old age and death. He was one of the first theorists who acknowledged the continuation of personality development into the adult years. At each stage, Erikson presented a developmental crisis which had to be mastered. Each crises is a set of normal stresses imposed on a person by the demands of society. The internal ego identity and the external expectations of an individual's behavior by society are in conflict. These demands vary from one stage to the next and must be resolved or at least the tension must be reduced to successfully advance to the next stage.

Erikson expressed each stage in polarities to indicate the possibility of successful or unsuccessful resolution of the crisis. As the person actively attempts to cope with certain stressors, ego adjustment occurs with successful resolution as societal demands are incorporated into personal viewpoints. Unsuccessful resolution at any one stage may delay progress through the next stage, but mastery can occur later. Erikson believed that complete unsuccessful resolution rarely happened, but that some negative aspects of coping could influence preparation for future crisis and difficulty in coping with the next crisis.

Trust Versus Mistrust.   The first stage is the period of infancy. As the infant learns to rely on caregivers so that basic needs of warmth, food, and comfort are met, he begins to believe and trust in his caregivers. Mistrust may occur if care is inconsistent or inadequate. The infant may view the environment as being unsafe or chaotic.

Autonomy Versus Shame and Doubt.   During the toddler years from about age 1 to 3, the child begins to learn more about his environment through newly learned motor and language skills. He is gaining independence through parental encouragement with activities of daily life, such as eating, toileting, and dressing. Shame and doubt result if the parents are overprotective and do not allow the child a chance to attempt new skills. Expectations that are too high for the developmental age of the child can produce feelings of inadequacy in the child.

Initiative Versus Guilt.   The preschool period, from age 4 to 6 years, is a time for seeking new experiences

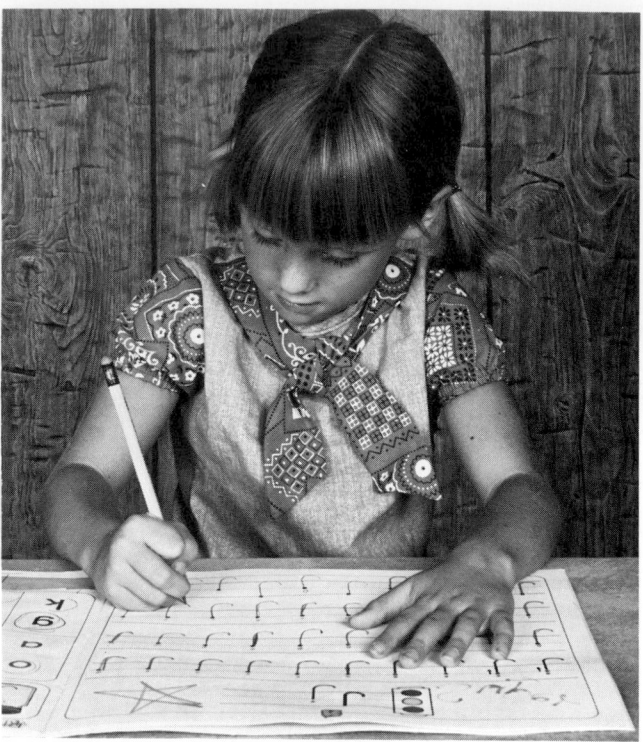

F I G U R E   10-5
The school-age child focuses on the end results of accomplishments—recognition and praise from family, teachers, and peers—developing a sense of competition and industry.

and imagining the "how" and "why" of surrounding activities. Confidence gained as a toddler now allows the preschooler a sense of initiative in learning. Guilt is the negative result of restrictions or reprimands for their many questions and explorations. Guilt can be seen as a hesitancy to attempt more challenging skills in motor or language development.

Industry Versus Inferiority.   The school-age child focuses on the end results of his accomplishments. He gains much pleasure in finishing projects and receiving recognition from family, teacher, and schoolmates. This sense of industry is benefited by rewards, such as good grades or winning games. A sense of competition develops through peer interaction and also assists in development of a sense of industry.

If the child is not accepted by his peers or cannot meet expectations of adults, a feeling of inferiority and lack of self-worth may occur. However, the school-age child receives feedback from many persons at this time due to increased social interaction from the home. This increased interpersonal exchange allows for negative influences to be counteracted with support from more positive influences.

Identity Versus Role Confusion.   The adolescent is faced with the many changes occurring in his own body.

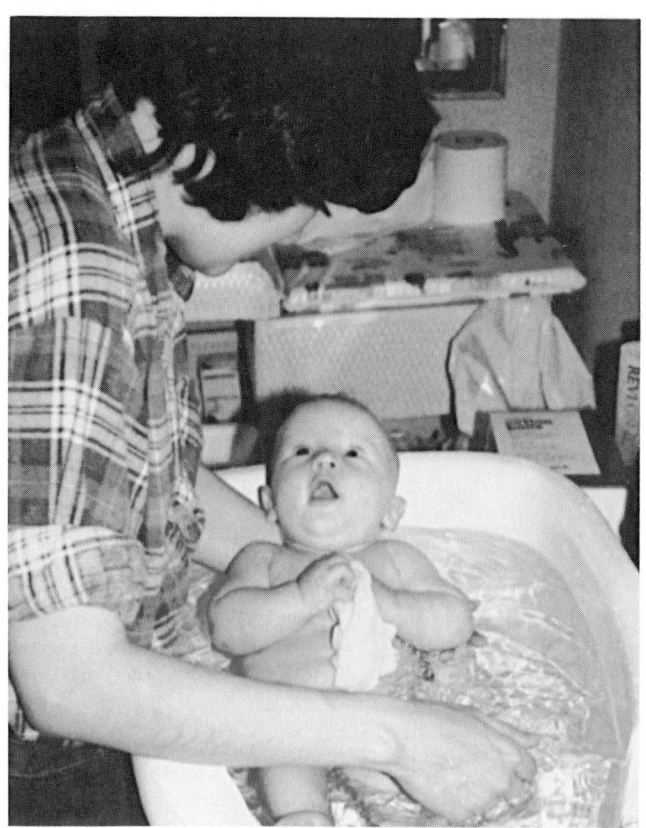

F I G U R E   10-4
The infant develops a sense of trust and security as he learns that he can rely on his caregivers to fulfill his needs. (Photo by Patrick O'Kane)

Hormonal changes cause physiologic growth of secondary sex characteristics and labile mood swings. The transition from childhood to adulthood requires many decisions based on the teenager's perception of self. Achieving a stable sense of identity is the major task for the adolescent. Attempting various roles enables one to acquire an idea of self from personal observations and from peers, parents, or other role models. Occasionally, rebellion and resistance to conformity are the norm.

Role confusion may occur if the adolescent is unable to obtain a sense of who he really is, or the direction in which he plans to take in his life. This fluctuation between identity and role confusion makes adolescence a period of turmoil for many.

Intimacy Versus Isolation. The task of the young adult is intimacy, which involves uniting self-identity with identities of friends for social or career endeavors. It includes the development of close personal relationships based on commitment to others, which necessitates self-sacrifice and compromise. Fear of such commitments can predispose the young adult to isolation and loneliness.

Generativity Versus Stagnation. The middle adult years are a time of concern for the next generation and guiding one's own children or those of friends, relatives, or community groups. This sense of guidance is exhibited in a variety of creative approaches to one's work or life experiences. There is an intense desire to leave a contribution to the world. If generativity does not occur,

TABLE 10-2
Erikson's Stages of Psychosocial Development

		Developmental Crisis	Stage
Stage	I	Trust vs mistrust	Infancy
Stage	II	Autonomy vs shame and doubt	Toddler years
Stage	III	Initiative vs guilt	Preschool years
Stage	IV	Industry vs inferiority	School-age years
Stage	V	Identity vs role confusion	Adolescence
Stage	VI	Intimacy vs isolation	Young adulthood
Stage	VII	Generativity vs stagnation	Middle adulthood
Stage	VIII	Ego integrity vs despair	Later adulthood

stagnation results. The person becomes self-absorbed, is obsessed with his own health needs, or regresses to earlier means of coping.

Ego Integrity Versus Despair. Later adulthood or old age allows for the reminiscence of life events with the attainment of purpose and fulfillment. Positive feelings present a sense of ego integrity. When the aging adult believes his life was a series of failures or missed directions, a sense of despair may prevail. During this final stage of development a final attempt to resolve the cumulative conflicts throughout life should occur.

Erikson (1963) recognized that personality development is dynamic and constantly changing. Crises at one stage can reappear at subsequent stages if not completely resolved, only to be met with better resolutions at some point later in life. See Table 10-2 for a summary of Erikson's theory.

Theory of Robert J. Havighurst: Developmental Tasks

Havighurst's theory postulates that living and growing are based on learning and that to understand human development, one must understand learning. An individual must continually learn to adjust to changing societal conditions. Learning throughout life is a series of inclines and plateaus, which pattern an individual's behavior.

Havighurst (1972) describes learned behaviors as **developmental tasks** derived from biologic, social and psychologic origins at certain periods in life. Successful achievement of these tasks leads to happiness and success with later tasks. Failure leads to unhappiness, disapproval by society, and difficulty with later tasks.

A combination of factors leads to the formation of developmental tasks. These factors arise from physical **maturation**, such as the neuromuscular growth of an infant's legs which enables him to walk, or from cultural pressures of society, such as the importance of learning to read and write. Personal motives and values of an

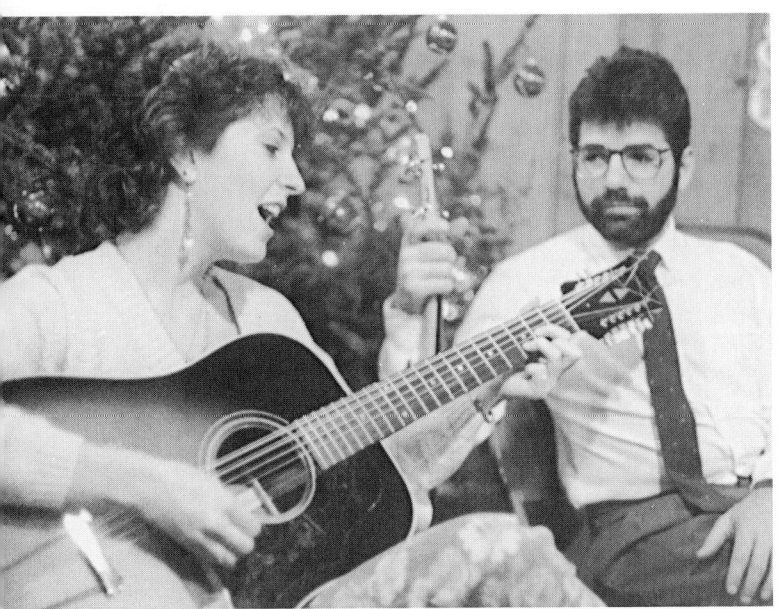

FIGURE 10-6
Establishing intimacy in young adulthood involves integrating self-identity and identities of others, and establishing relationships based on commitment, which necessitates self-sacrifice and compromise. (Photo by Tracy Baldwin)

T A B L E   10-3
Developmental Tasks Described by Robert J. Havighurst

Infancy and Early Childhood

Learning to walk

Learning to take solid foods

Learning to talk

Learning to control the elimination of body wastes

Learning sex differences and sexual modesty

Forming concepts and learning to describe social and physical reality

Getting ready to read

Middle Childhood

Learning physical skills necessary for ordinary games

Building wholesome attitudes toward oneself as a growing organism

Learning to get along with age-mates

Learning an appropriate masculine or feminine social role

Developing fundamental skills in reading, writing, and calculating

Developing concepts necessary for everyday living

Developing conscience, morality, and a scale of values

Achieving personal independence

Developing attitudes toward social groups and institutions

Adolescence

Achieving new and more mature relations with age-mates of both sexes

Achieving a masculine or feminine social role

Accepting one's physique and using the body effectively

Achieving emotional independence from parents and other adults

Preparing for marriage and family life

Preparing for an economic career

Acquiring a set of values and an ethical system as guide to behavior—developing an ideology

Desiring and achieving socially responsible behavior

Early Adulthood

Selecting a mate

Learning to live with a marriage partner

Starting a family

Rearing children

Managing a home

Getting started in an occupation

Taking on civic responsibility

Finding a congenial social group

Middle Age

Assisting teen-age children to become responsible and happy adults

Achieving adult social and civic responsibility

Reaching and maintaining satisfactory performance in one's occupational career

Developing adult leisure-time activities

Relating oneself to one's spouse as a person

Accepting and adjusting to the physiologic changes of middle age

Adjusting to aging parents

Later Maturity

Adjusting to decreasing physical strength and health

Adjusting to retirement and reduced income

Adjusting to death of a spouse

Establishing an explicit affiliation with one's age group

Adopting and adapting social roles in a flexible way

Establishing satisfactory physical living arrangements

(From Developmental Tasks and Education by Robert J. Havighurst, 3rd Edition. Copyright © 1972 by Longman Inc. All rights reserved.)

individual determine choices made regarding an occupation, marriage and family, and civic responsibility. The appearance of the developmental tasks is believed to be due to the existence of a sensitive period for learning the specific tasks. Timing for teaching is very important according to Havighurst. For example, teaching an infant to take food from a spoon during the first few months of life is not appropriate because the extrusion reflex, the tendency to push the tongue outward when stimulated, does not disappear until the infant is 4 or 5 months old. Wide age ranges are presented in each stage of development so that the detail of more restrictive stages is lost to more generalized categories. Refer to Table 10-3 for a review of Havighurst's stages and primary tasks.

Theory of Jean Piaget: Cognitive Development

Jean Piaget (1896–1980), a Swiss psychologist, is well known for his theory of cognitive development from infancy through adolescence, focusing on the intellectual processes at each stage of development. The quality of thinking of the adolescent according to Piaget approaches the acuity of the adult mind. Piaget's theory resulted from research on children of various countries and cultural backgrounds. He believed that learning was a part of development that occurs as a result of the internal organization of an event, a sort of mental representation or scheme. Series of such memory traces are called schemata (Piaget and Inhelder, 1969). Development schemes of an adult are built on those developed in childhood.

Intellectual growth is more than an accumulation of facts and information. It is a continued restructuring of knowledge to progress to higher levels of problem solving and critical thinking. A child's cognitive development expands through interaction with the environment and discovery of new objects and problems. Cognitive behavior increases as a child adjusts and adapts to new experiences. Two continual processes, assimilation and accommodation, stimulate the intellectual growth of the young child. **Assimilation** is the continuous process of integrating new experiences into existing schemata. If new information does not fit the present way of thinking, a disequilibrium results causing confusion. Adaptation and equilibrium occur through **accommodation**, an alteration of thought processes (schemata) to correlate more complex data (Piaget and Inhelder, 1969).

The quality of a child's thought patterns change gradually as adaptation to the environment through higher levels of reasoning occurs. Piaget emphasized that children of similar age groups respond to problem-solving tasks in similar ways, and can be somewhat predictable.

Cognitive Developmental Stages

Four stages of **cognitive development** have been identified by Piaget: (1) the *sensorimotor stage*—from birth to 24 months; (2) the *preoperational stage*—from 2 to 7 years of age; (3) the *concrete operational stage*—from 7 to 11 years of age; and (4) the *formal operational stage* —from 11 years of age through adulthood. The stages are sequential, but the ages listed for each stage are only estimations of average ages because each child progresses through them at his own pace. An overlap of characteristics between two stages can be observed during transition from one stage to the next.

Sensorimotor Stage

The *sensorimotor stage* of development is divided into six substages, demonstrating the rapid advances in intellectual functioning that formulate during the first 2 years of life. Piaget's substages of sensorimotor development include

- The *reflective stage* occurs during the first month of life, controlled by exercising basic reflexes such as sucking for needs attainment (Fig. 10-7). There is no understanding of the environment at this time beyond having physiologic needs being met.
- The *primary circular reaction stage* occurs from approximately 1 to 4 months of age. The infant discovers that random behaviors bring on a sense of enjoyment and are therefore repeated. These behaviors tend to focus on the infant's own body such as sucking the thumb or smiling.
- The *secondary circular reaction stage* occurs from about 4 to 8 months of age. The infant is now able to relate his own behavior to a change in his environment. An example would be kicking a mobile to see it move or shaking a rattle to hear a new sound.

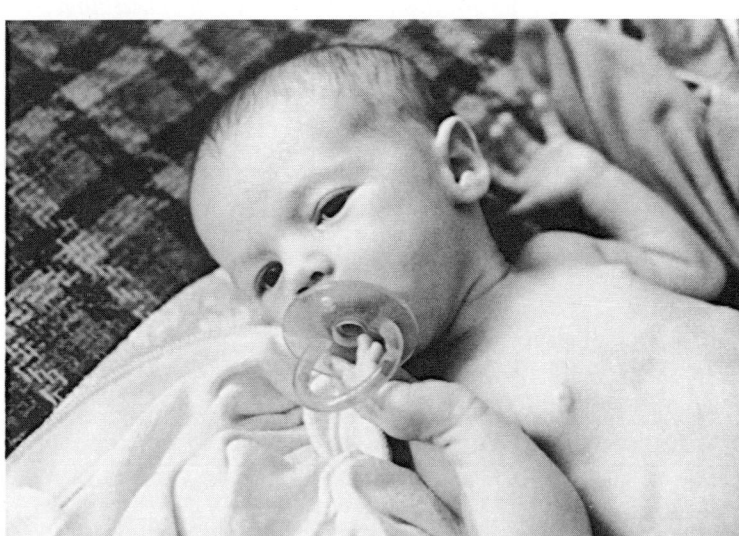

F I G U R E   10-7
During the first month of life, the infant has no understanding of the environment and can respond only by exercising basic reflexes such as sucking. (Photo by Tracy Baldwin)

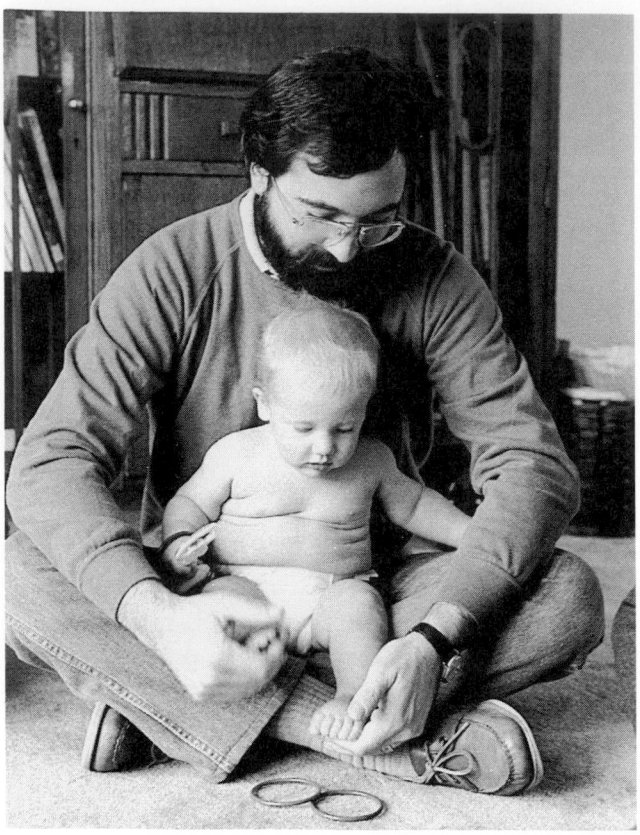

F I G U R E 10-8
From about the 4th month of age, the infant can begin to relate his own behavior as causing a change in the environment and, from about the 8th month, can integrate more than one thought pattern to obtain a purposeful goal. (Reeder SJ, Martin LL: Maternity Nursing, 16th ed. Philadelphia, JB Lippincott, 1987)

- The *coordination of secondary schemata stage,* from about 8 to 12 months of age, is a time when the infant coordinates more than one thought pattern (scheme) to obtain a purposeful goal. For example, the infant may throw a toy onto the floor, looking for it to be retrieved by a familiar person, and repeat the action once again. The infant can only familiarize himself with objects that are in sight and is not yet able to understand object permanence.
- The *tertiary circular reaction stage,* from about 12 to 18 months of age, allows the child to recognize the continued existence or permanence of objects so that he will look for objects placed out of his sight. The beginning use of accommodation broadens the child's ability to modify behaviors beyond repetitions to produce desired results. The child is able to understand simple commands and requests.
- The *mental combinations stage,* from about 18 to 24 months of age, is a transitional period from sensorimotor to preoperational thought. Reasoning

begins to develop as the child can anticipate events over the previous trial-and-error level of understanding.

Preoperational Thought

Piaget's (1969) *preoperational stage* of development is characterized by the beginning use of symbols, through increasing language skills and pictures, to represent the preschooler's world. Limited in their ability to generalize information, children in this stage are now able to learn sequences to routine tasks and basic means to categorizing objects. For example, they may be able to select all objects which are round from a group of objects because that trait is easily observable.

A primary aspect of preoperational thought is the concept of irreversibility, or the inability to reverse a thought process and belief that the end result is the final identity of an object or event. They are not yet able to understand that a lump of clay can be changed to another shape and then once again be reversed to the original shape. This experience has been called a lack of conservation. Conservation is the ability of certain properties such as mass or volume to remain constant.

Piaget subdivided the preoperational stage into two substages, the *preconceptual phase,* from about 2 to 4 years of age, and the *intuitive phase,* from about 4 to 7 years of age. Language skills become more sophisticated in the intuitive phase and allow for the incessant questioning typical for this age group. There is a transition

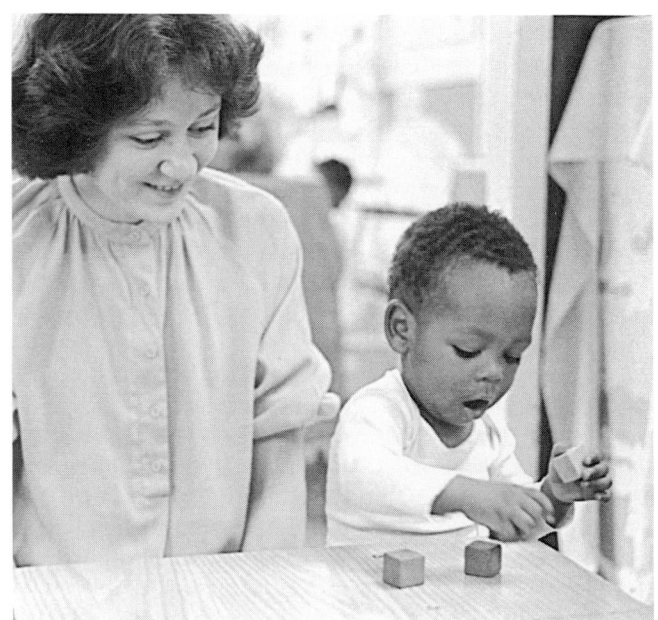

F I G U R E 10-9
The preschool child's development is characterized by the beginning use of symbols through language and pictures, an ability to learn simple sequences, and a basic ability to categorize objects. (Photo by Gates Rhodes, courtesy of the School of Nursing, University of Pennsylvania)

from symbolic play based predominantly on fantasy in the preconceptual phase to symbolic play derived mostly from reality in the intuitive phase. Egocentricity, or the inability to comprehend the viewpoint of another person and focusing on self, is characteristic and strongest in the preconceptual stage of development.

Through play activities, the preschooler and early school-age child are better able to understand life events and relationships among family members and playmates. Their play reflects magical thinking in the preconceptual stage as noted by evidence of animism. Animism is the belief that inanimate objects have human characteristics and feelings. For example, a 3-year-old could be heard saying "The sun gets up early in the morning and sleeps when the moon is up!" As the child gets older and progresses to the intuitive stage, less magical thinking takes place and an increasing use of accommodation occurs.

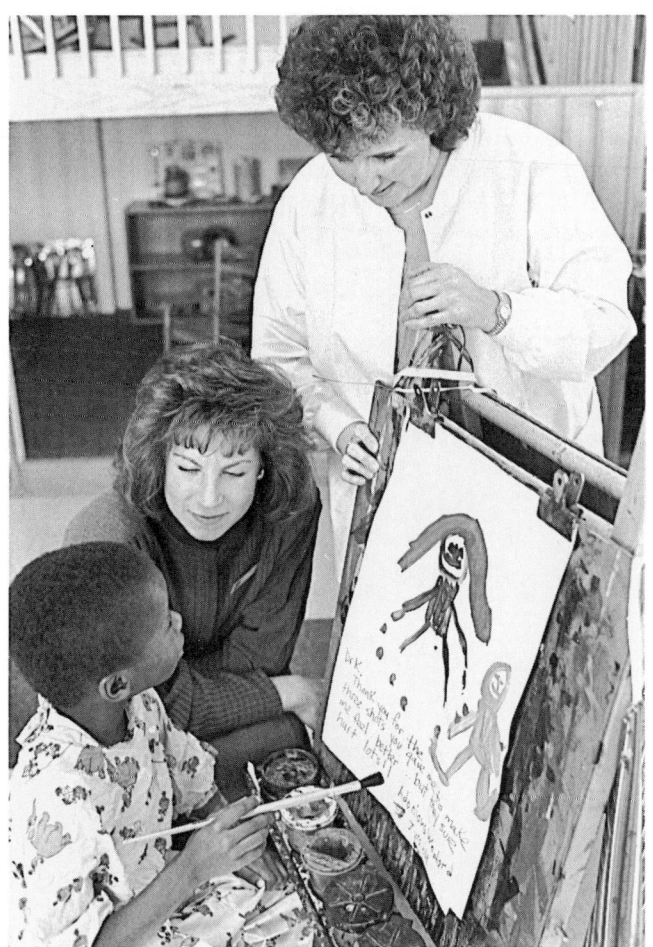

FIGURE 10-10
Abstract reasoning is required for a child to understand that painful medical treatments given now will make him feel better later. A child who is not old enough to have reached the formal operational stage, in which abstract reasoning develops, may require special attention from the health-care staff to understand the uncomfortable experiences of his hospital stay. (Photo by Don Walker, courtesy of Thomas Jefferson University Hospital)

TABLE 10-4
Jean Piaget's Theory of Cognitive Development

Stage	Age
Sensorimotor	0–24 months
Reflective	0–1 month
Primary circular reactions	1–4 months
Secondary circular reactions	4–8 months
Coordination of secondary schemata	8–12 months
Tertiary circular reactions	12–18 months
Invention of new means through mental combinations	18–24 months
Preoperational	2–7 years
Preconceptual	2–4 years
Intuitive	4–7 years
Concrete operational	7–11 years
Formal operational	11 years+

Concrete Operational Stage

Children in the *concrete operational stage* learn through manipulation of concrete or tangible objects. They are able to classify articles according to two or more characteristics, and order items based on deviation, such as arranging according to size from smallest to largest. Logical thinking is developing, as they show an understanding of reversibility, relationship between numbers, and loss of egocentricity. They comprehend basic explanations and are able to incorporate another's perspective.

Formal Operational Stage

The *formal operational stage* of development is represented by the use of abstract thinking and deductive reasoning. Children can now relate general concepts to specific situations or consequences and consider alternatives. They evaluate their world through the ability to test beliefs in an attempt to establish values and meaning in their lives. Increased scientific problem solving typically occurs. A continual building of the cognitive pattern initiated in the formal operational stage proceeds throughout the adult years. See Table 10-4 for a summary of Piaget's stages of development.

Theory of Lawrence Kohlberg: Moral Development

Lawrence Kohlberg (1969) studied the moral judgment and reasoning of individuals at different ages. From his research three successive levels of **moral development** emerged. The levels identified closely follow Piaget's theory of cognitive development. Each level is further subdivided into two separate stages (Kohlberg, 1969).

The *preconventional level* follows intuitive thought and is based on external control as the child learns to conform to rules imposed by authority figures. At stage 1, *punishment and obedience orientation,* the motivation for choices of action is fear of physical consequences of authority's disapproval. As a result of the consequences a perception of goodness or badness develops. At stage 2, *instrumental relativist orientation,* the thought of receiving a reward will overcome fear of punishment, so actions which satisfy this desire are selected.

The *conventional level* is when the individual becomes concerned with identification with significant others and shows conformity to their expectations. Values and ideals supported by family and friends are respected, regardless of consequences. Stage 3, *"good boy–good girl" orientation,* is when the person strives for approval in an attempt to being viewed as "good." Stage 4, *"law and order" orientation,* is when behavior focuses on following social or religious rules as a respect for authority. In his later work, Kohlberg maintained that many adults are at this stage because they think abstractly and view themselves as members of society (Duska and Whelan, 1975).

The *postconventional level* is associated with moral judgment that is rational and internalized into one's standards or values. Stage 5, *social contract, utilitarian orientation,* supports that correct behavior is defined by the legal rights of society. However, laws can be changed to meet society's needs, while maintaining respect for self and others. Stage 6, *universal ethical principle orientation,* represents the individual's concern for equality for all human beings, which is guided by personal opinions and standards regardless of those set by society or laws. Justice may be internalized at an even higher level than society. Few adults ever reach this stage of development.

Kohlberg recognized that moral development is influenced by cultural effects on perceptions of justice in interpersonal relationships. The beginnings of moral development are witnessed in parent and child communications during the early childhood years, as the young child tries to please his parents. The concept of morality emerges as a subset of an individual's beliefs or values, which governs choices made throughout life. Rules and regulations established by society are eventually challenged and evaluated as a person accepts or rejects societal rules into his own internal set of values.

Theory of James-Fowler: Faith Development

The spiritual identity of humans, a development theory contributed by James Fowler, is essential for holistic care. Fowler's work was influenced by the previous theories of Piaget, Kohlberg, and Erikson. Research was compiled from interviews of people of all ages, from 4 to 88, and from a variety of religious backgrounds, including agnostics and atheists. Fowler (1981, p 4) explained that

faith is not always religious in its content or context. . . . **Faith** is a person's or group's way of moving into the force field of life. It is our way of finding coherence in and giving meaning to the multiple forces and relations that make up our lives. Faith is a person's way of seeing him or herself in relation to others against a background of shared meaning and purpose.

Faith, therefore, is not necessarily religious, but it comprises the reasons one finds life worth living.

Fowler's theory is composed of prestage and six separate stages of faith development. The age when a certain stage exists varies among individuals, but the sequence does not. Equilibrium or the plateau of faith development can occur at any stage, beginning with stage 2.

In the organization of the stages of faith development, Fowler explained a triadic relationship between self, shared causes or values, and others which is the unifying factor in all stages and is based on trust. During the prestage, called *undifferentiated faith,* trust, courage, hope, and love compete with threats of abandonment or inconsistencies in the infant's environment. The strength of faith in this stage is based on the relationship with the primary caregiver.

Stage 1, *intuitive-projective faith,* is most typical of the 3- to 7-year-old child. Children imitate religious gestures and behaviors of others, primarily parents. They

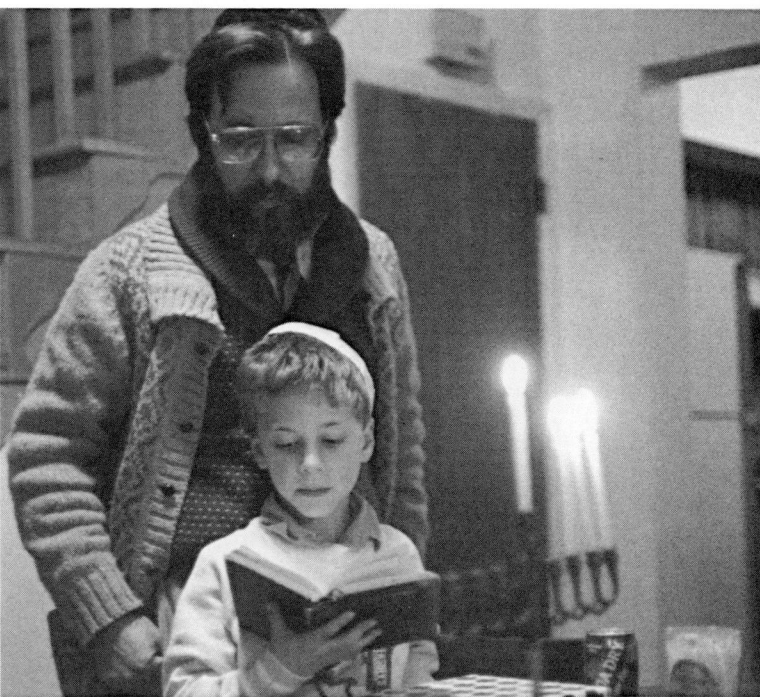

F I G U R E   10-11

In the earliest stage of faith development, the child imitates religious gestures and behaviors of his parents and others. Images and feelings experienced in early years will be reevaluated and reintegrated in later stages. (Photo by Tracy Baldwin)

follow parental attitudes toward religious or moral beliefs without a thorough understanding of them. Imagination in this stage leads to longlasting images and feelings which must be questioned and reintegrated in the later stages.

Stage 2, *mythical-literal faith,* predominates in the school-age child with increased social interaction. Stories represent religious and moral beliefs, and existence of a deity is accepted. Perspectives of others can be appreciated as well as the concept of reciprocal fairness.

Stage 3, *synthetic-conventional faith,* is characteristic for many adolescents. As the person experiences increasing demands from work, school, family, and peers, the basis for identity is very complex. An ideology has emerged but has not been closely examined until now. The person begins to question some of the life-guiding values or religious practices in an attempt to stabilize his own identity.

Stage 4, *individuative reflective faith,* is a very critical stage for the late adolescent or young adult as the responsibility for his or her own commitments, beliefs, and attitudes becomes his or her own. Many adults do not construct this stage and at times it does not emerge until they are in their thirties or forties. Searching for self-identity no longer defined by the boundaries of faith compositions of significant others is a primary concern.

Stage 5, *conjunctive faith,* integrates other viewpoints about faith into one's understanding of truth. One is able to see the paradoxical nature of the reality of his own beliefs. Along with this realization, the divisions of faith development among people become apparent.

Stage 6, *universalizing faith,* involves overcoming paradoxes noted in stage 5 and makes tangible the values of absolute love and justice for mankind. The faith relationship noted in stage 6 is characterized by total trust in the principle of being and the existence of the future, whether derived from the Judeo-Christian image of faith or otherwise. Table 10-5 compares Erikson's psychosocial stages to Fowler's faith stages.

APPLYING GROWTH AND DEVELOPMENT PRINCIPLES AND THEORIES TO NURSING

In review, the complex and interrelated influences that contribute to the total phenomenon of human development comprise not only biophysical factors, but also factors of personality development. The theories presented from Freud, Piaget, Havighurst, Erikson, Kohlberg, and Fowler give knowledge of the evolution of cognitive, psychosocial, moral, and spiritual development. In relating to the whole person, all of the components of development need to be evaluated to understand certain life events or concerns.

Although these theorists have brought a great deal of insight into the process of human development, some limitations exist in each theory. Therefore, in planning holistic nursing care for clients with diverse needs, backgrounds, and ages, nurses should assess the client and support decisions for interventions on rationale from multiple theories of development so as to provide comprehensive health promotion. A few examples are discussed here.

While interviewing a young mother with her first child, the nurse senses a frustrated single parent as the mother reviews the task of rearing her 14-month-old child alone. Based on Freud, the nurse can relate the behaviors typical of the oral stage of development for the infant. Havighurst and Erikson support the stage of gaining independence in learning to walk for the toddler. Recognizing that the mother may be limited in her sup-

TABLE 10-5
A Comparison of Psychosocial and Faith Stages

Erikson's Psychosocial Stages	Fowler's Faith Stages
Trust vs mistrust	Undifferentiated (infancy)
Autonomy vs shame and doubt Initiative vs guilt	Intuitive-projective (early childhood)
Industry vs inferiority	Mythical-literal (school years)
Identity vs role confusion	Synthetic-conventional (adolescence)
Intimacy vs isolation	Individuative-reflective (young adulthood)
Generativity vs stagnation	Conjunctive (midlife)
Integrity vs despair	Universalizing faith

(Data from Fowler JW: Stages of Faith: The Psychology of Human Development and the Quest for Meaning. New York, Harper & Row, 1981)

port system, the nurse may need to assess further to identify problems with intimacy and a feeling of generativity. In planning care for this young mother, the nurse anticipates needed emotional support and health teaching about the normal toddler years. The mother's anxiety level and the child's attempts to investigate the environment through locomotion and oral exploration place them at risk for injury from falls or aspiration. The nurse has a primary role in prevention through client education based on astute observation and knowledge of child development.

A 16-year-old girl is admitted to the nursing unit having sustained multiple injuries in a motor vehicle accident. The injuries include several deep facial lacerations and a fractured femur. The young woman is stabilized, medicated for pain, and placed in traction. The nurse notices the girl crying quietly in her room. Realizing the importance of self-identity for the adolescent (Erikson), the nurse approaches the girl and asks if she would like to talk. Initially seeming very hesitant, the girl is able to discuss her fears of scar formation on her face and comments from her friends. The nurse can assist by allowing her feelings to be shared and encouraging her to talk with her physician to find out the possible outcome after healing occurs.

A 70-year-old man fell and fractured his hip while repairing the exterior of his home. Having been the traditional head of his household, he now is troubled by needing others, including his wife, to care for him. He appears withdrawn, refusing to talk and eating poorly. Reflecting on Havighurst and Erikson's theories, the nurse knows that he is possibly fluctuating between feelings of nonadjustment and acceptance of declining health and a sense of ego integrity.

These are only a few situations used to demonstrate the application of the growth and development theories to the practice of nursing. Health-care needs change quickly as an individual grows and passes through the life span. These needs are individual for each person, but include certain similarities at specific periods in one's life. The nurse is faced with the dynamic task of planning care based on both general and unique health needs of a client and continually revising aspects of care in the evolution of the growth process or alteration in health status.

FAMILY DYNAMICS

The functions, structures, and developmental tasks of the family are discussed with human needs in Chapter 7, while Chapter 11, under the young adult, discusses establishing a family. The family is mentioned in this chapter because the study of growth and development would not be complete without mentioning the interrelationship between an individual and the family. Family dynamics, a major environmental influence, begins with conception and continues throughout life.

Along with structural variety, families are the product of cross-cultural principles. Due to the many different ethnic groups who have immigrated to the United States, the nurse is exposed to different perspectives on the management of health and illness. Religious practices, dietary restrictions, childrearing, and care of the elderly are affected by certain cultural beliefs. Friedman (1981, p 271) stated that culture "circumscribes and guides the ways in which societies and ethnic groups solve their problems and derive meaning from their lives." (Culture and ethnicity are discussed in Chap 8, and spirituality is discussed in Chap 39.)

The family plays a vital role in wellness promotion and illness prevention. The family inflicts values and cultural influences on decisions regarding interpretation of illness. Health problems or a developmental crisis of any one member can affect the remainder of the family unit. Health practices, whether positive or negative, are often shared in the family, being learned by younger members. Family at times may even be the cause of illness of individual members. It is well known that heart disease, arthritis, alcoholism, and emotional disorders, to list only a few examples, run in families. Alterations in coping and communication patterns may predispose families to dysfunctional means of relating to one another.

Applying Family Dynamics to Nursing

The nurse has a responsibility to assess not only the health needs of individual members of the family but also the demands placed on the total family in meeting every member's needs. The nurse can then function as a catalyst in planning appropriate interventions and teaching, and as a collaborator with other health professionals (social workers, psychologists, physicians, clergy) in achieving optimal family wellness.

Marilyn M. Friedman (1981) described the family using a structural-functional approach. They include (1) the affective function, meeting psychosocial needs of the family; (2) socialization; (3) reproduction; (4) family coping; (5) economic function; and (6) the provision of physical necessities. Through four basic structural components the family strives to obtain these goals. Friedman has devised a family assessment tool comprised of these four components to information to plan family nursing care. These components include role structure, value systems, communication patterns, and power or decision-making structure.

With a thorough family assessment, the nurse can identify or assist families in identifying the priorities of their health-care needs. Analysis of data collected can lead to the development of nursing diagnoses to systematically organize a plan of care with selected interventions. Through mutual goal setting with family members, the nurse guides the evaluation process in helping the family meet developmental needs and quality levels of health for its members.

IMPLICATIONS FOR NURSES

Some general guidelines for incorporating principles and theories of growth and development and family dynamics into daily practice of nursing care are listed below. They are given as suggestions for working with all ages.

- Be knowledgeable concerning the various stages of cognitive, psychosocial, moral, and spiritual development. Be prepared to support developmental stages typical of certain ages.
- Maintain flexibility in assessing individuals, and respect the uniqueness of each person. Although the literature describes development typical of a particular age, not all persons fit into an exact mold.
- Although development follows an order of succession, the rate of progress differs among people in certain life stages. Anticipate possible regression during difficult times or crisis, accepting and supporting the individual's return to a forward progression in development.
- Become cognizant of environmental and cultural influences because of their strong effect on development, especially psychosocial development. A deprived environment can be detrimental while an enriched one enhances development.
- Assess each person with an awareness that within each stage of development a person may retain some behaviors of a previous stage, attain goals of the present stage, and begin to exhibit behaviors of the next stage. There is a time of transition to the next stage with no definite beginning or ending to the particular stage of development.
- Remember that clients are members of families and that the family unit can have both positive and negative influences on development of individual members. Attempt to support good family relationships and healthy environments that assist members to reach their greatest potential for growth.
- Provide client teaching to individuals and their families to aid in their understanding of periods of development.
- Aid clients in setting priorities for family health. Conflicts can occur when trying to meet their own needs, their children's needs, and those of aging parents.
- Be ready to provide health care to clients suffering from illnesses or failure to meet developmental goals. Collaborate with other members of the health team in providing care to prevent or minimize disruption of development and promote optimal wellness throughout life.

KEY POINTS

■ Nurses provide care to all ages in the life continuum, and this care involves both individuals and their families.

■ Growth and development theories, taken together, involve all aspects of life: physiologic, cognitive, psychosocial, moral, spiritual, and family dimensions.

■ Principles of growth and development state that the processes (1) are orderly and sequential; (2) are continuous and complex; (3) are specific for each person; (4) are influenced by environmental factors; (5) are directed by regular trends; (6) are quantitative and qualitative; (7) become integrated; (8) have vulnerable periods; (9) have rates and patterns that can be modified; and (10) occur at different stages and at different rates.

■ Freud's psychosexual theory explains ego development through predictable id–superego conflicts.

■ Erikson identifies personality development in a series of stages from birth to later adult years, where critical tasks must be mastered.

■ Havighurst focuses on the concept of learning in order to understand growth and development.

■ Piaget's theory describes cognitive development from infancy through adolescence based on assimilation, accommodation, and formation of schemata.

■ Kohlberg presents a theory of moral judgment of reasoning which begins in early childhood years.

■ Fowler defines faith or spirituality as comprising meaning for life, which includes values, beliefs, and possibly religious affiliation.

■ Each developmental theory explains a portion of the process of development and provides a part of the nurse's understanding of the total being and coping abilities. Such theories are limited by their specific focus and the theorist's beliefs about growth and development.

■ The family plays a vital role in promoting wellness and preventing illness. Both positive and negative health practices are shared in the family and learned by younger members. Health problems affect the family unit.

BIBLIOGRAPHY

Billingham KA: Developmental Psychology for the Health Care Professions. Boulder, CO, Westview Press, 1982

Duska R, Whelan M: Moral Development: A Guide to Piaget and Kohlberg. New York, Paulist Press, 1975

Erikson EH: Childhood and Society, 2nd ed. New York, Norton, 1963

Fong BC, Resnick MR: The Child: Development Through Adolescence. Menlo Park, CA, Benjamin/Cummings, 1980

Fowler JW: Stages of Faith: The Psychology of Human Development and the Quest for Meaning. New York, Harper and Row, 1981

Freud S: The Ego and the Id. London, Hogarth Press, 1923 (1974 translation)

Friedman MM: Family Nursing: Theory and Assessment. New York, Appleton-Century-Crofts, 1981

Havighurst RJ: Developmental Tasks and Education. New York, David McKay, 1972

Kempe H, Helfer RE: The Battered Child. Chicago, University of Chicago Press, 1968

Klaus MH, Kennell JH: Parent–Infant Bonding. St Louis, CV Mosby, 1982

Kohlberg L: Stage and sequence: The cognitive-development approach to socialization. In Gaslin D (ed): Handbook of Socialization: Theory and Research, pp 347–380. Chicago, Rand McNally, 1969

Mott SR, Fazekas NF, James SR: Nursing Care of Children and Families: A Holistic Approach. Menlo Park, CA, Addison-Wesley, 1985

Mussen PH, Conger JJ, Kagan J: Child Development and Personality, 4th ed. New York, Harper and Row, 1974

Newman BM, Newman PR: Development Through Life: A Psychosocial Approach. Homewood, IL, Dorsey Press, 1975

Piaget J, Inhelder B: The Psychology of the Child. New York, Basic Books, 1969

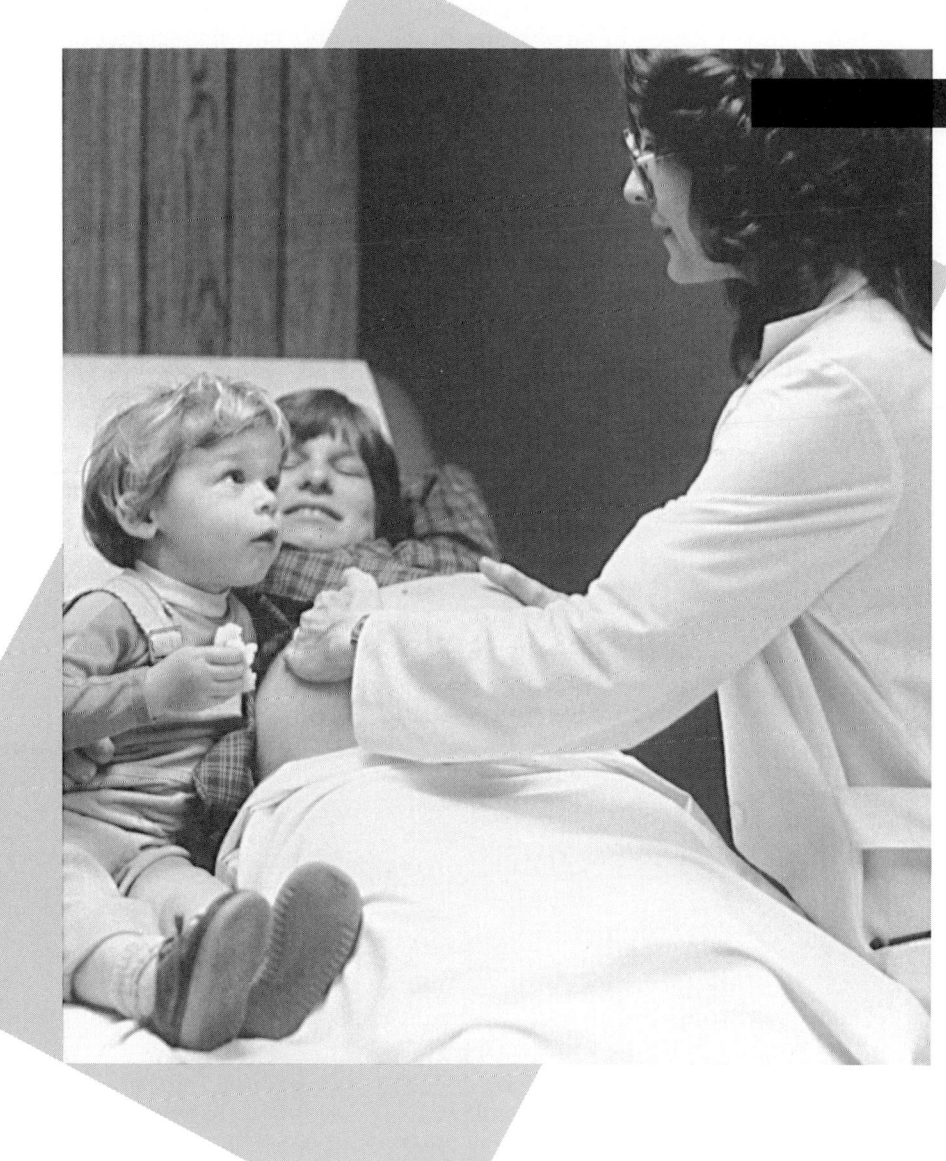

Conception to Midlife

OBJECTIVES

After studying this chapter, the learner should be able to

Define key terms used in the chapter.

Summarize major physiologic, cognitive, psychosocial, moral and spiritual development for each age period from conception through adolescence.

Describe the influences of play and recreation on development at specific ages.

List common health problems of each age period through childhood requiring intervention by health practitioners.

Identify major nursing roles specific to each period of development.

Identify the major developmental tasks of the young and middle-adult as described by Erikson, Levinson, and Gould.

Describe the physical, psychosocial, intellectual, moral, and spiritual development of the young adult and middle adult.

Discuss the common health problems and nursing interventions to promote health in the adult from age 20 to 60.

Current theorists believe that knowledge of childhood development provides key information for understanding the significance of development in later life. The current preponderance of literature and research relating to child development might suggest that it is a more significant growth period than others. It seems more likely, however, that it is the speed of childhood development that makes it an attractive research area. Developmental researchers must look at occurrences as they relate to the passage of time, and no time passes more quickly than childhood.

Chapter 10 gives an overview and introduction to developmental theories. This chapter continues the discussion with specific discussion relating to the various stages of growth and development. The first section of this chapter lays the foundation for understanding the similarities and differences in the growth of the human child, in sequential developmental stages, from conception through adolescence. The last section of the chapter discusses adult development theories and then follows the development of the young adult and middle adult. The development of the older adult is discussed in Chapter 12.

CHILDHOOD

Childhood, by its nature, should be a physically and psychosocially healthy experience, with chronic physical and emotional problems being the rare exception rather than the norm. Because of the nature of childhood, the primary focus of nursing should be wellness promotion and illness prevention, especially through education. Nursing aims should include the promotion of physical growth, psychologic integrity, self-esteem, self-identity, role function, and interpersonal/social relationships. These goals should be accomplished within the context of family relationships, being ever mindful of the uniqueness of each child.

Heredity, Environment, and Nutrition

Heredity and environmental and nutritional factors influence all stages of development. The influence of each can occur independently, but is more likely to occur interrelatedly. The several examples which follow illustrate this interrelatedness:

- Infants who are malnourished in utero develop fewer brain cells in total than infants who have been adequately nourished prenatally (Winick, Brasel, and Rosso, 1972).
- Smoking in pregnancy increases the risk of congenital anomalies, low birth weight, and prematurity in newborns (Papilia and Olds, 1986, p 66).
- Federally sponsored school lunch programs attest to the belief that learning is enhanced if nutrition is adequate (Papilia and Olds, 1986, p 90).

KEY TERMS

accommodation
acquired immune deficiency
   syndrome (AIDS)
active transport
andropause
anorexia nervosa
anterior fontanelle
caput succedaneum
cleft lip
cleft palate
congenital anomaly
congenital syphilis
dentition
Down's syndrome
empty-nest syndrome
failure to thrive (FTT)
fertilization
gonorrhea
herpes simplex II (genital
   herpes)
hypospadias
immunization
immunoglobulin
inguinal hernia
intellectualization
lanugo
linguistic
meconium
menopause

midlife crisis
milia
molding
mongolian spots
monilial infection
myelination
ossification
ovulation
physiologic jaundice
posterior fontanelle
pregnancy
prelinguistic
pseudomenstruation
puberty
quickening
reflex
school phobia
sebaceous gland
sexually transmitted disease
spermatogenesis
sphincter
spina bifida
subconjunctival hemorrhage
syphilis
temperament
trichomonal infection
trimester
vernix caseosa
visual recognition memory
widowhood

- Failure to thrive, a condition of early infancy, has been clearly linked to both nutritional and emotional deprivation (Waechter, Phillips, and Holaday, 1985, pp 628, 1132).
- Child abuse is an extreme example of physical and emotional harm/deprivation in the environment, leading to disturbed physical and psychosocial development (see the box below).

These examples show clearly that adequate physical growth and healthy psychosocial development are intimately linked with heredity, balanced nutrition, and positive environmental influences.

Conception and Prenatal Development

Human growth and development begin at the moment of **fertilization**. The fertilized ovum, or *zygote,* contains the full complement of genetic information provided from each parent. This genetic legacy determines the gender of the developing individual and profoundly influences physical and psychologic traits, intellect, and personality. Development within the womb proceeds in an orderly manner according to the genetic blueprint. The process whereby a human being develops from a single cell to a complex organism with billions of specialized cells takes place in three stages: *pre-embryonic, embryonic, and fetal.*

Pre-Embryonic Stage (0 to 3 Weeks). The pre-embryonic stage lasts for approximately 3 weeks after conception. During this period the fertilized ovum divides at regular intervals, becomes increasingly more complex, and implants in the uterine wall. Cellular division begins

Child Abuse

Child abuse has reached epidemic proportions and is a major, worldwide concern. Child abuse is a complex phenomenon usually symptomatic of severe family dysfunction. It involves the interaction of several variables, the major ones including the following:
- Personality and upbringing of the caregiver(s)
- Personality, age, gender, temperament, and physical status of the child
- Social conditions of the family
- Stress on individual caregiver(s) or family as a whole

A multidisciplinary approach to the problem involves the expertise of police, social workers, lawyers, clergy, and health-care personnel.

almost immediately after fertilization. Even at this early period (approximately 5–6 days), a cluster of cells called the embryonic disk is differentiating into two distinct germ layers. The *ectoderm,* or outer germ layer, will eventually form the brain, spinal cord, nervous system, and some of the outer body parts (*i.e.,* skin, nails, hair). The *endoderm,* or inner germ layer, will develop into the respiratory and digestive systems and several accessory digestive organs such as the liver and pancreas. By the end of the pre-embryonic stage the ectoderm and endoderm will begin to differentiate, and the third germ layer, the *mesoderm,* will appear. The mesoderm will develop into the body's supportive structures: the skeleton, connective tissue, cartilage, and muscular layer. It is also the precursor of the circulatory, lymphoid, urinary, and reproductive systems.

Embryonic Stage (4 to 8 Weeks). The primary activity of this period is the rapid growth and differentiation of the three germ layers into the respective body organs and systems for which they are responsible. This differentiation process is called *organogenesis.* Because of the rapid transformation and growth which occurs during the embryonic stage, it is during this phase that the developing human is most vulnerable to the influences (either within its own genetic structure or from the outside) that cause congenital anomalies. By the end of the embryonic stage all basic organs are established, and some human features are clearly recognizable. In addition, the ossification of bones has begun (Santrock and Yussen, 1987, p 74).

Fetal Stage (9 Weeks to Birth). In the fetal stage definite development and functioning of organs progresses (Table 11-1). The length of a pregnancy may vary from 240 to 300 days, the average being 266 days or 9½ lunar months (Reeder and Martin, 1987, p 161).

The Neonate (Birth to 28 Days)

At birth the neonate is required to make several significant physiologic adjustments to adapt to extrauterine life. These adjustments occur in all body systems, but most profoundly in the circulatory and respiratory systems. With the completion of these adjustments the neonate becomes an independent human being. The average newborn is about 20 inches (50.8 cm) long and weighs approximately 7.5 pounds (3400 g). A number of measurement tests are available for neonatal assessment. Two of the most common are The Apgar Rating Scale and The Brazelton Neonatal Behavioral Assessment Scale.

The *Apgar Rating Scale* was developed in 1953 by Dr. Virginia Apgar. It is routinely applied to newborns at 1 minute and 5 minutes after birth (Table 11-2). Each category is rated individually as 0, 1, or 2. The scores for each category are then totaled to a maximum of 10. Normal, healthy infants will score between 7 and 10. Infants scoring between 4 and 6 will require special assistance,

TABLE 11-1
Development in the Fetal Stage

Age	Development
3 months	Weight 1 oz (28 g) Length 3 in. (7.5 cm) Fingers and toes are distinct. Sex can easily be determined. Breathing movements are made.
4 months	Weight 7 oz (196 g) Length 6–10 in. (15–25 cm) External features are easily discernable. Placenta is fully developed. Mother can feel fetal movements (**quickening**)
5 months	Weight 1 lb (454 g) Length 1 ft (30.5 cm) **Lanugo** covers body. Fetal heartbeat is clearly audible with a fetoscope.
6 months	Weight 1 1/4 lb (625 g) Length 14 in. (35.5 cm) Fetus cries and can make a fist. If born, fetus would have a slim, although not impossible, chance of survival. The relative immaturity of the lungs results in a high mortality rate for infants born this prematurely.
7 months	Weight 3–5 lb (1360–2270 g) Length 16 in. (39.5 cm) Although body fat is inadequate, survival chances, in an intensive care setting, are good.
8 months	The major fetal activity from the 8th month until birth is the accumulation of sufficient body fat to promote insulation against varying environmental temperatures encountered outside the womb.
9 months	Skull is fully formed. Average weight 7 1/2 lb (3400 g) Average length 20 in. (50.8 cm) Boys tend to be heavier and longer than girls. Birth occurs.

and those scoring below 4 are in need of immediate, life-saving support (Bee and Mitchell, 1984, pp 71–72; Mott, Fazekas, and James, 1985, p 181; Reeder and Martin, 1987, pp 551–552).

The *Brazelton Neonatal Behavioral Assessment Scale* was developed in 1973 by Dr. T. B. Brazelton and colleagues. The scale was designed to identify, through neurologic and behavioral assessment, subtle differences in the way infants respond to their surroundings. It involves a complex performance of activities on the part of the infant and, as such, measures behaviors like alertness, muscle tone, sleep–wake patterns, reflexes, hand–mouth activity, response to startling, and self-calming abilities.

Because of the nature of the Brazelton test, future developmental expectations of the infant are more predictable than with less specific assessment tools. In addition, the activities involved in performing the test can be used by trained parents to stimulate a reserved infant (Bee and Mitchell, 1984, p 52; Papilia and Olds, 1986, p 86; Santrock and Yussen, 1987, p 83).

Physical Characteristics

The healthy neonate has an amazingly competent level of physical ability as Table 11-3 illustrates.

Common Health Problems

Particular difficulties related to the birth process, the transition to extrauterine life or **congenital anomalies** may require intervention by health personnel. Breathing difficulties are common, especially if the infant has been sedated by drugs given to the mother during labor and delivery. The premature infant is vulnerable to *respiratory distress syndrome* because of the relative immaturity of lung function. The infant delivered by cesarean birth is at risk for respiratory difficulties because of excess mucus in the lungs. Therefore, frequent suctioning is common in the cesarean-delivered neonate.

Incompatability between the blood group of the mother and the infant requires prompt care at the time of birth. *Congenital malformations,* such as **cleft palate** and

TABLE 11-2
The Apgar Scoring Chart

Sign	0	1	2
Heart rate	Absent	Slow (less than 100)	Over 100
Respiratory effort	Absent	Slow, irregular	Good, crying
Muscle tone	Flaccid	Some flexion of extremities	Active motion
Reflex irritability	No response	Weak cry or grimace	Vigorous cry
Color	Blue, pale	Body pink, extremities blue	Completely pink

cleft lip, spina bifida, and Down's syndrome, present profound and long-term health problems. Newborns with congenital syphilis and drug addiction require special care. Birth traumas, which ordinarily have temporary symptoms, are of concern because the parents need reassurance that symptoms disappear with interference. Examples include caput succedaneum, molding, bruises from the use of forceps during delivery, and subconjunctival hemorrhage. Parents also need help to understand the nonthreatening nature of physiologic jaundice, which is frequently present during the newborn's first days.

Infancy: 1 Month to 1 Year

At the end of 28 days the newborn "officially" enters the infancy period which lasts until the end of the first year of life.

Physiologic Development

Normal physiologic development during the infancy period is described in Table 11-4.

General Immunity. A newborn will have acquired a transient immunity from immunoglobulins which have crossed the placenta by active transport. Between the ages of 3 and 6 months the infant begins to manufacture his own immunoglobulins. This production ability gradually increases over childhood, with levels comparable to adulthood being reached by adolescence (Waechter, Phillips, Holaday, 1985, p 1178).

Immunity and Breastfeeding. Breastfeeding provides an infant with protection against both bacterial and viral infections. Breast milk has several components that offer protection against bacterial infection: immunoglob-

(Text continues on p. 174.)

FIGURE 11-1
Reflexes and behaviors of the newborn.
(Reeder SJ, Martin LL: Maternity Nursing, 16th ed. Philadelphia, JB Lippincott, 1987)

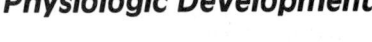

Stepping reflex

Active crying state

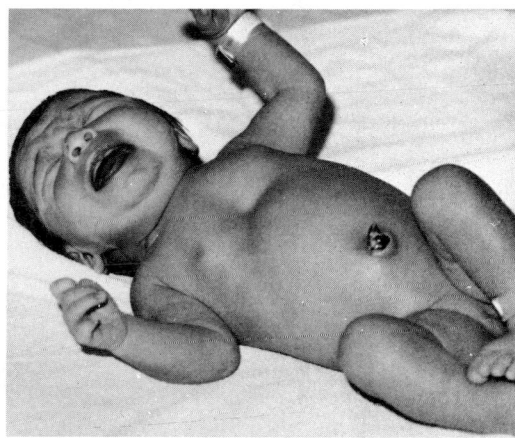

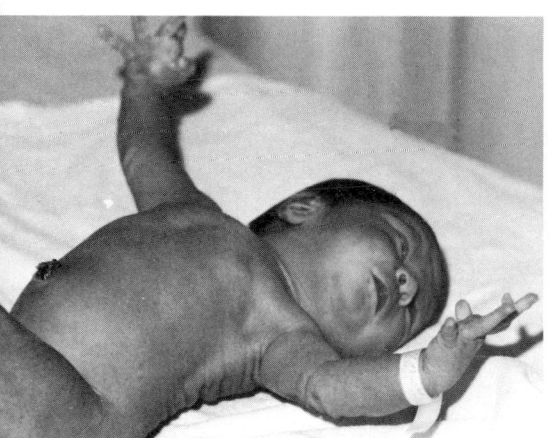

Moro reflex

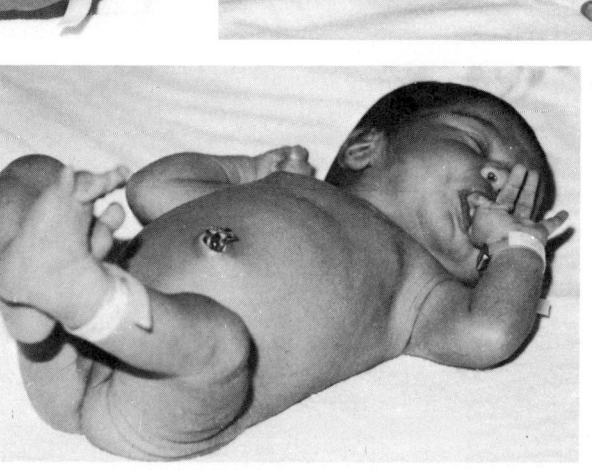

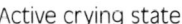

Quiet alert state

Hand-to-mouth and sucking activity

T A B L E   11-3
Physical Characteristics of the Newborn

Category	Normal Characteristics
Nervous, muscular, and skeletal systems	• Immature neurologic integration causes uncoordinated movements and tremors of the extremities and chin. • Many **reflexes** are present: *Rooting reflex:* The newborn turns his mouth in the direction of the cheek being touched. *Grasp reflex:* The newborn grasps an object placed in his hands, clings to it momentarily, and then lets go. This may be followed by a hand-to-mouth movement and sucking. *Sucking, swallowing, and gag reflexes:* Although the sucking reflex is strong, the three are poorly coordinated. *Moro reflex:* A sudden stimulus causes the newborn to draw up his legs and bring his arms forward as if to embrace, and he usually cries. The thumb and forefinger form a C. The movements are symmetric. *Tonic neck reflex:* The newborn lies on his back with his head turned to one side; the arm and leg on the side he is facing extend, and the opposite arm and leg flex. *Stepping reflex:* The newborn makes walking motions when the soles of his feet touch a solid surface. This is sometimes called the dancing reflex. *Protective reflexes:* blinking occurs in the presence of a bright light. Coughing and sneezing occur to clear the respiratory passages. Yawning increases oxygen intake. • The newborn pulls an extremity away from a painful stimulus, cries when uncomfortable, and resists restraint. He tends to open his eyes when held up and to close them when lying down, which is called "baby doll" activity. • Muscle tone is good, but responses to stimuli are random, purposeless, and global. • The **anterior fontanelle** is between the parietal bones and is diamond shaped. • The **posterior fontanelle** is between the occipital and parietal bones and is triangular in shape. The posterior fontanelle may be closed already at birth. • There is little true ossification of bones, except for the skull and face. • Arms and legs are proportionately shorter than an adult's extremities.
Endocrine/Thermoregulation	• Normal temperature is 97.5° to 99°F (36.4°C–37.2°C) • Temperature control is labile, and body temperature responds quickly to environmental temperatures.
Sensory organs	• The newborn is very alert to the environment, as Figure 11-1 illustrates. He shows a preference to certain stimuli and avoids unpleasant stimuli. This is logical as it is now known that all the senses are functional at 6–7 months gestation. • *Eyes:* The newborn's eyes are slate blue. They can fixate briefly and follow an object. The newborn sees color and form and prefers patterned items to unpatterned.

(Continued)

TABLE 11-3
Physical Characteristics of the Newborn   (Continued)

Category	Normal Characteristics
	• He can see with good acuity 10–12 in. (25–30 cm) from his face. From an evolutionary point this is interesting, as that is about the distance from the mother's breast to the mother's face. • **Accommodation** is poor beyond a few feet. • *Hearing:* The newborn hears and turns his head to noise. He selectively prefers the human voice, particularly the high-pitched, female voice. • *Taste:* All four tastes are present, with a preference for a sweet taste. • *Smell:* Smell is present. Experts indicate that infants can distinguish their own mother's breast milk (Santrock and Yussen, 1987, p 130). • *Touch:* The newborn is very sensitive to touch and pain.
Gastrointestinal tract	• The intestinal tract is proportionately longer than an adult's intestinal tract. • The newborn is able to handle breast milk, glucose water, and plain water at birth. • The first stool is **meconium**, which is dark green, sticky, and odorless. This is followed by a transitional stool which is greenish brown. Breastfed babies then have bright yellow, soft, sweet-smelling stool. Formula-fed babies have yellow-gray, pasty, and pungent stool. • The newborn regurgitates easily, owing to an immature cardiac sphincter. • Hepatic functioning is present during intrauterine life, but independent functioning to sustain life begins at birth. • The newborn's water and caloric requirements are high in relation to his size. • Intestinal elimination is involuntary.
Respiratory system	• Respirations are initiated at birth by physical, chemical, and sensory stimuli. • Considerable mucus is present in the newborn's respiratory passageways. • Respirations are diaphragmatic. • The respiratory rate varies between 50 and 80 per minute.
Cardiovascular system	• Peripheral circulation is sluggish which accounts for the cyanosis often observed in the newborn's hands and feet. • The pulse rate varies from 100, while sleeping, to as high as 180, when crying. The average normal range is between 120 and 160. • Blood pressure at birth is about 80/46 mm Hg. • The newborn has high red blood cell, hemoglobin, and hematocrit values, probably owing to the hypoxic environment during intrauterine life. • Total body fluids comprise about 75% of the newborn's body weight. • Circulatory functioning is present during intrauterine life, but independent functioning is initiated at birth.

(Continued)

T A B L E **11-3**
Physical Characteristics of the Newborn *(Continued)*

Category	Normal Characteristics
Genitourinary system	• Labia majora are large. May be a transient blood tinged discharge called **pseudomenstruation**. Hymen tag may be visible. • Testicles are palpable, unless they have not descended, in which case they normally descend within 3 months. Scrotum is large due to transient edema. Foreskin covers the glans. • There is limited reabsorption from kidney tubules. • The newborn voids involuntarily two to six times in the first 24 hours. • Uric-acid crystals in the urine may cause a reddish stain on the diaper. • Renal functions are present during intrauterine life but reach sufficient maturity to support independent life at birth.
Integumentary system	• Skin is smooth, turgor is good. • **Vernix caseosa** in body creases only • Nails are soft, pliant, and well-formed. • Skin pink in whites or incomplete pigmentation in dark-skinned races • Jaundice after 24 hr, which subsides with adequate liver function • **Milia** over nose and chin • **Mongolian spots** in dark-skinned races and Native Americans.
Sleep/activity	• The newborn is alert and may cry at birth. This alertness decreases after about 1/2 hr. • The newborn sleeps as much as 22 hr every 24 hr.

Size	• The head of a newborn is about 1 in. (2 1/2 cm) larger than the chest.
	• *Head circumference:* This is usually 13 to 14 1/2 in. (32 1/2 cm–35 1/2 cm) the average being 13 1/2 in. (33 cm)
	• *Weight:* the newborn weighs between 5 1/2 and 9 1/2 lb (2500 g and 4300 g).
	  The average female newborn weighs 7 lb (3200 g).
	  The average male newborn weighs 7 1/2 lb (3400 g).
	• *Length:* The average newborn is between 18 and 22 in. (45 cm and 55 cm), the average being 20 in. (50 cm).

ulins and leukocytes. High lactose content in breast milk, combined with limited protein and a low buffering capacity, allows for the creation of an acid environment unsuitable for the growth of pathogenic bacteria (Scipien, et al 1986, pp 79–80). Antibodies secreted in breast milk assist in controlling some viral infections.

Immunization of Infants. The infant under 1 year of age is susceptable to many communicable diseases. This is the rationale for recommending that **immunization** against common communicable diseases begin in in-

fancy. Diphtheria, tetanus, pertussis (whooping cough and DPT), and polio (OPV) vaccines are usually recommended at 2, 4, and 6 months. Tuberculin skin tests are commonly used on infants exposed to tuberculosis.

Growth Patterns During the First Year. The prevalent approach for assessing the adequacy of rate and totality of growth in a child is by comparison to a standardized growth chart. There are several such charts available. As well, each standardized chart is gender specific because the growth rates of boys and girls differ. By

TABLE 11-4
Physiologic Development During Infancy

Category	Normal Characteristics
Nervous, muscular, and skeletal systems	• The brain grows to about half its adult size during infancy, most occurring in the cerebral cortex. After 1 year all brain tissue cells are present. Further tissue growth will occur. • The brain stem reaches most of its maturity by 1 year of age. • **Myelination**, which begins before birth, continues. • Posterior fontanelle closes at 2–3 months of age, although it may be closed at birth. • Anterior fontanelle closes at about 18 months of age, but may begin to close at 9–10 months. • Body temperature is less influenced by environmental conditions and becomes stable by late infancy. • The Moro reflex disappears by about 3 months of age. and the stepping reflex fades. • Ossification of bones progresses. • There is an increase in interneural connections and in the complexity of axon and dendrite structure. • Conductive time becomes more rapid as nerve fibers and cellular membranes mature, resulting in increased sensitivity to stimuli. • Concurrent development of the neurons, musculature, and skeletal systems results in motor functions that become more specific and less random. Using building blocks, scribbling with crayons, and trying to feed oneself are examples. • Development of the musculoskeletal system progresses from the head downward and from the center of the body outward. • Crawling begins, followed by walking, during this period.
Sensory organs	• The eyes begin to focus and fixate together by about 6 to 8 months of age. By 1 year eye muscle movements are functionally mature. • Hearing and smell become more discriminating than they were at birth. • Salivary glands increase activity at 3–4 months so sense of taste becomes more discriminatory.
Gastrointestinal system	• Solid food can be handled in the mouth at about 5–6 months of age, and chewing begins at about 6–8 months. • There is rapid growth in the size of the stomach. • There is improved absorption of water from the large intestine, which causes stools to change from soft to formed. • Regurgitation ceases as the cardiac sphincter matures.
Respiratory system	• The alveoli increase in number and complexity. • The weight of the lungs triples in the first year • The respiratory rate at 12 months is between about 20 and 40 per minute.
Cardiovascular system	• The heart doubles in weight in the first year. • The left ventricle becomes more muscular in order to pump blood more effectively in the growing body. • The heart rate slows, and blood pressure rises as the heart becomes more efficient.

(Continued)

T A B L E   11-4
Physiologic Development During Infancy   (Continued)

Category	Normal Characteristics
	• The pulse rate is between about 80 and 160 beats per minute and can be labile during first year. • The blood pressure is about 80/60 mm Hg at 1 year of age. • Total body fluids in relation to body weight begin to approximate adult levels. Fluid intake remains critical, because water turnover is greater and the proportion of body surface in relation to body size is larger when compared with older children and adults. • The red blood cells, hemoglobin, and hematocrit values drop. • The white blood cell value reaches the adult level by as early as late infancy.
Genitourinary system	• The reproductive organs remain immature and dormant. An erect penis and clitoris may be observed but are without sexual significance. • Tubular reabsorption in the kidneys slowly improves, so that proportionately large amounts of fluid are necessary to prevent dehydration. Overhydration will occur easily because of the immaturity of kidney functioning.
Integumentary system	• Skin gradually becomes less sensitive to topical irritants. • Hair at birth is lost, and new hair growth occurs. • Perspiration is possible by about 2 months, and this assists with thermoregulation.
Dentition	• The deciduous teeth begin to erupt, beginning at about 4–6 months of age. Girls tend to get teeth earlier than boys.
Sleep/activity	• The infant sleeps about 16–18 hours a day at 6 months, and about 12–14 hours a day by about 1 year of age. • Napping is necessary to prevent undue fatigue during infancy, first twice a day and eventually once a day.
Size	• The infant may gain as much as 1 oz (28 g) a day during early weeks and will double birth weight by about 4–5 months. • The infant triples his birth weight by about 1 year of age. At 1 year average male is 22 lb (10 kg) and average female is 21 lb (9.5 kg). • The infant's length increases by 50% during the first year. • The head grows slowly in comparison with the rest of the body, resulting in a change in head and trunk proportions. • Weight gain gradually changes from fat to muscle production.

measuring the specific growth statistics of one individual child against the norms for his or her age and gender, some useful comparisons can be made (Fig. 11-2).

Care must be taken, however, to use the results of such comparisons cautiously for several reasons:

- Each child has individual variations and short-term spurts and lags in growth.
- Atypical infants such as premature or low-birth-weight infants are not addressed.
- Growth charts may be ethnically and socio-economically weighted in favor of the white middle class.

The *Denver Developmental Screening Test* (DDST) is a commonly used screening test for determining, quickly and inexpensively, infants and children with atypical developmental (behavioral) patterns. The test involves assessment of the child's behavior in four critical developmental areas:

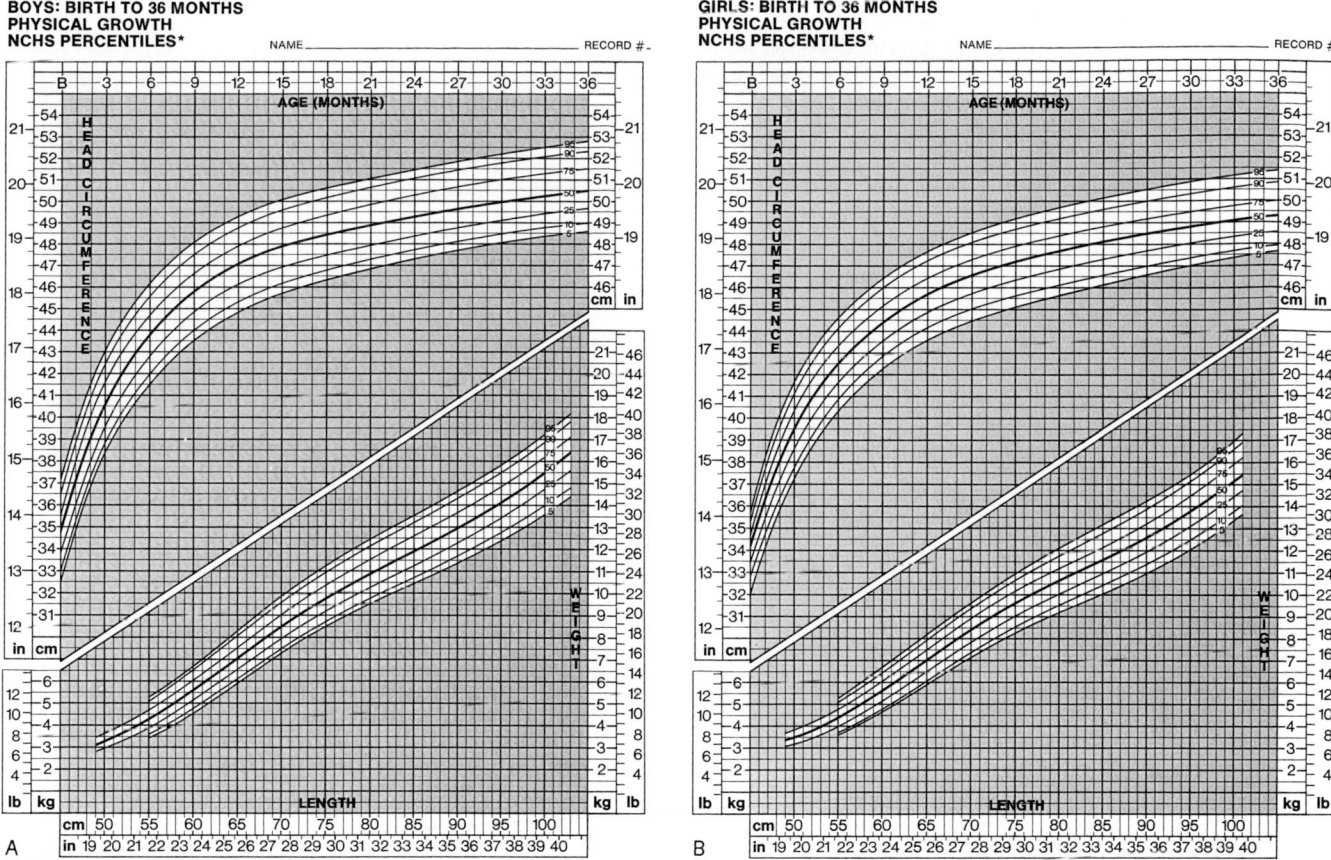

F I G U R E 11-2
Average relationships between the head circumference or occipital–frontal circumference (OFC) and the age, and between the weight and length in (A) the normal male infant (B) the normal female infant. (Adapted from Hamill PVV, Drizd TA, Johnson CL, Reed RB, Roche AF, Moore WM: Physical Growth: National Center for Health Statistics percentiles. Am J Clin Nutr 32:607–629, 1979. Data from the Fels Research Institute, Wright State University School of Medicine, Yellow Springs, Ohio. © 1982 Ross Laboratories)

- Gross motor behavior/skills
- Fine motor behavior/skills
- Language acquisition
- Personal/social interaction

The test is not diagnostic in and of itself, but does isolate problem areas requiring more precise assessment and diagnosis. The test is discussed in many pediatric textbooks.

Cognitive Development

Sensorimotor Stage. The infant from birth to 1 year of age is in the sensorimotor stage of development according to Piaget. There are six substages in the sensorimotor stage of development; substages one to four occur during the first year of life. These substages are described in Chapter 10.

Language Development. The infant begins language development in what is referred to as the **prelinguistic**

phase. Babies begin to coo and make pleasurable sounds very soon after birth. By 12 months of age they are able to use a few key words to deliberately convey their wishes. The acquisition of speech skill has several consistent characteristics which transcend the specific language being learned. Three of these characteristics are

- The use of syllable repetition (*e.g.,* ma-ma, choo-choo, bye-bye)
- Identical early phonetic expressions (*i.e.,* babbling sounds)
- Imitation, by the infant, of sounds and intonations spoken to him (Salkind and Ambron, 1987, p 154)

Engel (1973) believes that babbling, which occurs readily in the second 6 months of life, is the first true attempt at **linguistic** expression. From that point onward, as infantile speech patterns are abandoned, speech mastery slowly develops.

Memory. Assessing memory ability in infancy is difficult. Papilia and Olds (1986, p 126) describe infant memory as "visual recognition memory" and use techniques to clearly substantiate that infants do have memory capacity.

Psychosocial Development

Oral Stage. Freud believes that the younger the infant, the more likely he is to be governed by the id. The newborn strives for immediate gratification of his needs and is totally egocentric in his approach to life. The newborn is in the oral stage of development and, thus, has a strong sucking need. Breastfeeding, bottle feeding, soothers, and even the infant's own fingers will be used to satisfy the need to suck.

Trust Versus Mistrust Theory. Erikson describes the stage of psychosocial development most prominent in infancy as trust versus mistrust. While there are several situations involving the infant and the primary caregiver in which basic trust is tested, the feeding situation pro-

vides the ideal circumstance. While Freud viewed feeding from the oral gratification perspective, Erikson saw it more as a potential opportunity for intense primary caregiver–infant interaction. The critical element in this interaction is whether or not the infant feels the caregiver can be counted on to provide food when the infant is hungry. This inner certainty can also be fueled through diaper-changing, comfort provision when distressed, and so forth. Without inner trust, the infant has difficulty forging on to stages involving independence.

Developmental Tasks. Havighurst emphasized that development involved learned, goal-oriented behavior. This learned behavior is influenced by maturing physical and psychosocial resources. In infancy, then, the baby learns to

- Take solid food
- Walk
- Talk

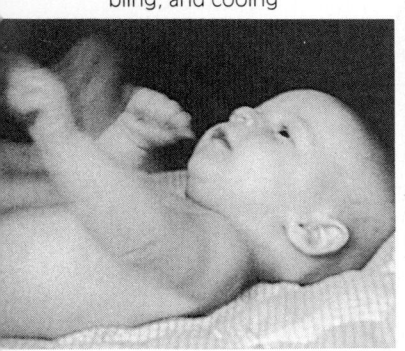

Initial play behavior by infants is centered on self: repetitive hand play, babbling, and cooing

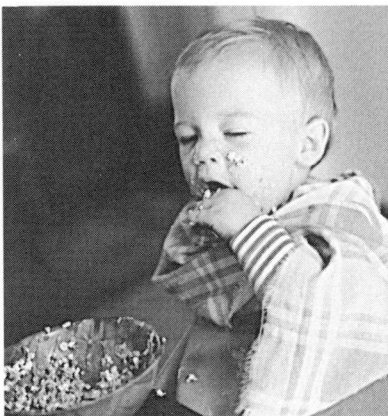

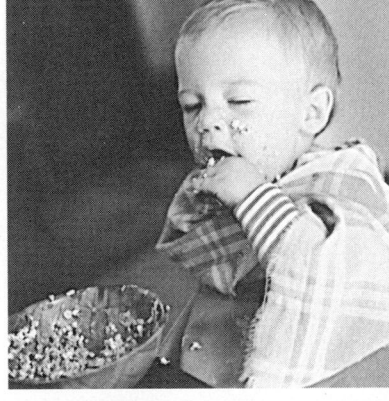

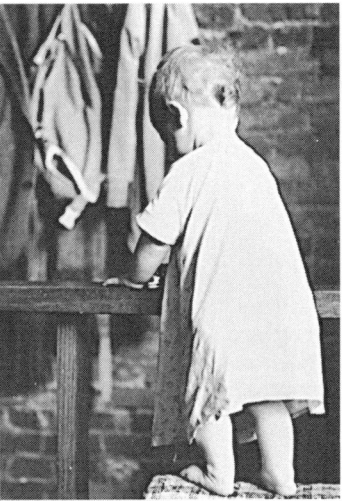

Developmental tasks of the first year include: taking solid food, learning to walk and talk

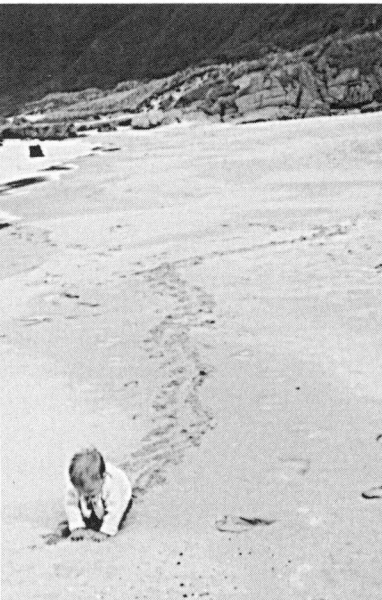

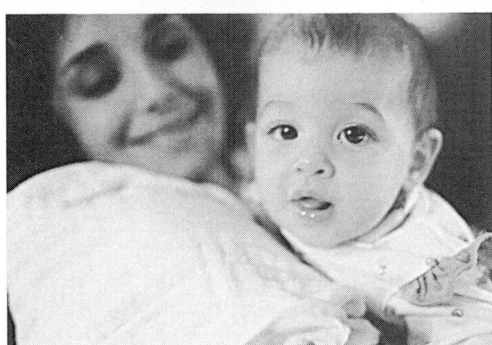

Erikson describes the psychosocial development prominent in infancy as "Trust vs Mistrust"

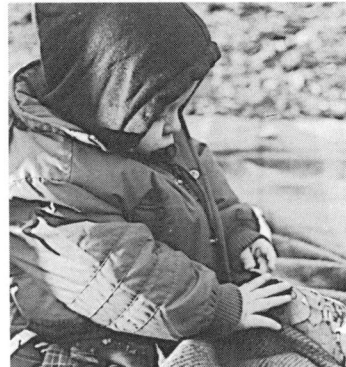

As the infant enters the second half of his first year, play will begin to involve manipulation of objects and the environment

F I G U R E **11-3**
Development during the first year of life.

Attachment. Papilia and Olds (1986, p 154) describes attachment as "an active, affectionate, reciprocal relationship between two people." *Attachment* can be differentiated from *bonding* by describing bonding as the "initial fusing" of two individuals and attachment as the long-term maintenance and strengthening of the "fused" state. Attachment behavior in infancy has been the focus of considerable current research because of the popular belief that the success of mature, adult relationships hinges on the quality of infant–primary caregiver relationships. Of the considerable work done in this area that of Mary Ainsworth and colleagues is notable.

Play. A discussion of the theoretical aspects of play are useful prior to looking at age-specific play patterns. Papilia and Olds (1986, pp 233–234) identify two general dimensions to play: *Social play* is motivated by a desire for fun, pleasure, and relationships with others, while *cognitive play* is motivated by a need or desire in the child to learn. These two general dimensions of play are shown in Table 11-5. Each level in one dimension complements its equivalent level in the other dimension.

Play allows the infant to discover the environment and to begin to control it to some degree. Play begins as soon as the baby becomes aware of sensations and the

T A B L E   11-5
Two Dimensions to Play

Social Play	Cognitive Play
Level 1—Solitary play Child plays alone	*Level 1—Functional/sensorimotor play* Purpose of the play is pleasure, environmental manipulation, and perfecting developmental skills.
Level 2—Parallel play Child plays in close proximity to another but no significant interaction takes place.	*Level 2—Constructive Play* Play is for the purpose of creating something.
Level 3—Associative play Play involves associating with others, some give and take, but no common purpose is present.	*Level 3—Pretend play* Imagination is used to satisfy needs and work out feelings.
Level 4—Cooperative play Play occurs in a pair or group, and the common goals of the pair or group supercede individual goals.	*Level 4—Games with rules* Group play occurs with an end motivation like winning and pre-agreed upon rules.

(Adapted from Papilia D, Olds S: Human Development. New York, McGraw-Hill, 1986)

pleasure they produce. Initial play behavior by infants is centered on the self. Hand play, babbling, and cooing are repeated over and over because they produce self-pleasure.

As the infant begins to see himself as separate from the environment and other persons, play begins to take on some interactive qualities. Touching and vocalizing with the primary caregiver in various ways produces enjoyment. As the infant enters the second half of his first year, play activities will begin to involve objects he can manipulate and simple games like "peek-a-boo." As well, improved mobility will tend to encourage exploratory gross motor play.

Temperament. Research clearly indicates that **temperament** is primarily inborn, although environment does influence the degree to which specific temperament traits will be displayed. In a major study by Thomas, Chess, and Birch (1968), nine characteristics of temperament were isolated. These traits are visible in infancy and remain fairly consistent into adulthood. The range of characteristics from positive to negative isolates three basic temperaments. The most positive range of the traits belongs to the "easy" child, the most negative to the "difficult" child and variability in the range belongs to the "slow to warm" child.

The behavior of the caregiver(s), however, and their handling of the child can influence (both positively and negatively) the degree to which temperament will dictate behavioral style.

The "easy" infant's style will be clearly rhythmic; sleeping, eating, and elimination will be conducted with ease, smiling will occur spontaneously, and crying will be limited to significant need states. The "slow to warm" infant will be more passive, perhaps distant, and may need gentle encouragement and attention before responsiveness is evident. The style of the "difficult" infant may be described as volatile or labile. Most responses, both positive and negative, will be intense. These infants will likely be restless sleepers, highly sensitive to noise, and will eat poorly. They are likely to be the colicky babies.

Common Health Problems in Infancy

Various health problems in infancy may require the intervention of health personnel. Gastroenteritis and food allergies are common. Skin disorders such as diaper dermititis (diaper rash), seborrheic dermatitis (infant dandruff), prickly heat rash, and thrush (infection of the oral mucus membrane by the fungus *Candida albicans*) are also common.

There are several safety concerns which must be addressed during infancy. The relative immobility of the young infant makes susceptibility to suffocation a concern. The swallowing reflex matures progressively from birth, but until such time as it becomes refined, the risk of aspiration must be addressed. As the infant becomes more mobile the risk of falling increases. Preventive measures against such safety hazards must often be taught and emphasized to new parents.

Three particular health problems in infancy are significant enough to warrant some elaboration.

Infant Colic. *Colic* can best be described as "acute, paroxysmal abdominal pain caused by spasmodic contractions of the intestine during the first 3 months of life" (Miller and Keane, 1987, p 275). Its exact cause is not known, but the following factors have been isolated as possibly contributing to its occurrence: excessive swallowing of air, too rapid feeding, overfeeding, excessive carbohydrate ingestion, overexcitement, allergy to formula, emotional distress in the infant, and anxiety in the primary caregiver (Miller and Keane, 1987, p 275).

Failure to Thrive. Failure to thrive (FTT) can be described as a condition resulting in severely inadequate physiologic development (particularly height and weight) in an infant. This condition is believed to be related to disturbed infant–primary caregiver interaction. While this appears to be true in most instances, underlying physical causes must first be ruled out. If the cause is deemed to be psychosocial, then the dynamics usually involve inadequate nutritional intake related to caregiver ignorance and lack of concern for emotional nurturing. Specialized health intervention is usually warranted.

Sudden Infant Death Syndrome (SIDS). "SIDS" or "crib death" is the leading cause of death in infants between 1 week and 1 year of age, with a peak incidence between 2 and 4 months (Waechter, Phillips, and Holaday, 1985, p 774). Although the exact cause of SIDS is not yet known two hypotheses (described in Whaley and Wong, 1987, p 578) are gaining credence.

- *Hypoxemia hypothesis*—SIDS is caused by damage to the respiratory control center in the brain-stem as a result of chronic hypoxemia.
- *Apnea hypothesis*—SIDS victims have long periods of prolonged apnea during sleep and die during one of these episodes.

Nurses' Role in Infant Health Care

The most essential role assumed by the nurse working with families of infants is that of preventive teacher. The primary areas in which preventive teaching is required and examples of information the nurse may provide are shown in Table 11-6. Care activities may range from providing basic information about treatment for skin rashes to facilitating grieving in parents who have lost a baby to SIDS.

The nurse caring for a new family on the postpartum unit may make a referral to the community health nurse if there are indicators for such a follow-up. As well, specific community groups are available to parents with special needs. Some examples are Parents Without Partners, The Society of Compassionate Friends, and SIDS support groups. Facilitating role transition from nonparent to parent and facilitating and supporting attachment behaviors in both parents and infant lay the groundwork for healthy functioning of the new family unit.

Toddlerhood: 1 to 3 Years

Physiologic Development

Physiologic development continues steadily during toddlerhood, but the pace slows considerably from infancy. The physiologic development of the toddler is described in Table 11-7.

Immunity. The tonsils, adenoids, and lymph nodes of the toddler enlarge in response to general growth and infections. The short, straight eustachian tubes of toddlers make them highly susceptible to middle ear infections, particularly otitis media. Recommended immunizations in toddlerhood include the MMR (measles, mumps, rubella) vaccine at age 15 months and at age 18 months, completion of DTP (diphtheria, tetanus, and pertussis), and OPV (polio) vaccine series begun in infancy.

Cognitive Development

Sensorimotor and Preoperational Stages. Piaget purports that toddlerhood is primarily represented by the last two substages of the sensorimotor stage. As the child is leaving toddlerhood for the preschool period there is a transition to the preconceptual phase of the pre-operation stage. The various substages and phases of Piaget's theories that apply to toddlerhood are discussed in Chapter 10.

Language Development. Linguist speech, as opposed to prelinguistic speech, begins at approximately 1 year of age (Bee and Mitchell, 1984, p 178). Although there are variations of time on either side of age 1, this appears to be the average time when children begin to use single or bisyllabic sounds. These sounds may represent a single meaning such as identifying mother by saying "mama" or may represent a whole thought such as "ta" meaning "give me that toy." Papilia and Olds (1986, p 130) refer to a single word which represents a whole thought as a "*holophrase.*" Nelson (1973) suggests that language acquisition has a lag time in toddlerhood. The author believes that these lag times represent storage periods for acquiring and understanding new words before expressing them.

Around the age of 2, children begin to use short sentences and become quite adept at this as they enter the preschool period. This adeptness at making sentences, however, does not include an ability to use grammatic structure correctly.

TABLE 11-6
Promoting Wellness in Infancy

Areas of Concern	Preventive Teaching
Accident prevention	• Associate common accidents to developmental abilities of the infant • Encourage relaxed, slow feeding and regular "bubbling" (burping) to prevent aspiration • Emphasize that bottles should not be propped and left with an unattended infant • Emphasize the use of bumper pads and keeping crib sides up at all times to prevent injury related to bumping or falling • Teach the correct usage of infant car seats • Emphasize never leaving an infant unattended on a table • Teach proper positioning of infant for sleeping and discourage the use of pillows to prevent suffocation
Nutrition and feeding methods	• Assist the mother with the initiation and maintenance of breastfeeding • If bottle feeding, provide information on the preparation of formula at feeding, expulsion of air from the bottle, nipple type and hole size and positioning for an effective feeding experience • Emphasize the significance of emotional nurturing during feeding • Discuss the age at which solid foods are needed (*i.e.,* 5–6 months) • Discuss the sequence of solid foods. (*i.e.,* cereals, vegetables, fruits, meats and protein products)
Infections	• Encourage prompt attention for infections • Encourage completion of required immunizations of infancy
Hygiene and skin care	• Teach proper infant bathing techniques (*i.e.,* washing eye from inner to outer canthus, washing genitals last, cord care) • Discuss the proper use of creams, oils, powders • Describe the nature of infant skin and its susceptibility to disturbance • Teach diapering and hygienic practices related to the disposal of products of elimination • Teach care related to hair, nails, and genitals (particularly circumcised males)
Developmental performance	• Provide accurate information about development norms. This can prevent unrealistic expectations in caregivers and assist in isolating and treating developmental delays earlier
Emotional attachment	• Encourage intimate child—caregiver contact in the crucial period immediately after birth • Provide information about the sequence of normal attachment behaviors in infants • Reassure concerned caregivers that attachment feelings occur at different rates for different caregivers and infants

F I G U R E   11-4
Some characteristics of toddler-development years.

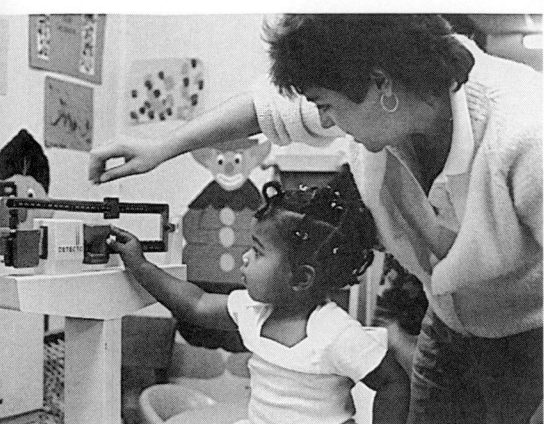

Cognitive abilities in toddlerhood include mastery of seeing oneself as separate from others and perception of body image

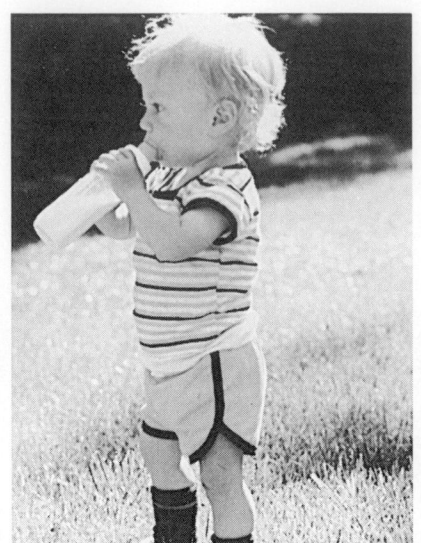

A broad stance and protruding abdomen are characteristic of the physical development of the toddler

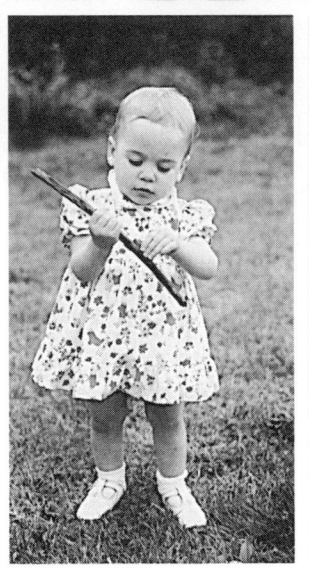

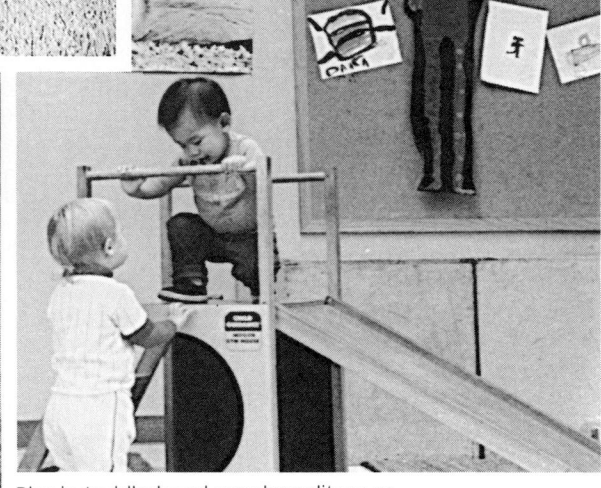

Play in toddlerhood may be solitary or parallel

Gross motor skills are prominent in toddlerhood

Memory.   Memory ability in toddlerhood continues to have a visual recognition focus. As life experience expands, the toddler approaching age 3 is occasionally able to recall or name an item he has seen, but which is now out of view.

Body Image.   Because cognitive abilities in toddlerhood include the mastery of seeing oneself as separate from others, primary perception of body image begins at this stage. The focus of body image in toddlerhood is self-discovery through self-exploration. As toddlerhood ends, the child is able to name several body parts, identify the function of some and can state whether they are a girl or a boy (based primarily on what the child has been told and not on a understanding of physical differences).

Psychosocial Development

Anal Stage.   In keeping with his belief that behavior has an essentially biologic focus, Freud describes tod-

dlerhood as the "anal stage." Increased muscular development and **sphincter** control encourage the child to focus on the pleasure of sphincter tension and relaxation, particularly the anal sphincter. Because Freud believed that the child's personality was anally fixated in toddlerhood, he felt that the manner in which toilet training occurred was the most significant determinant in how this stage affected later life. Freud identified two focuses of toilet training which he believed resulted in distinctly negative behavior patterns in later life. If the caregiver focused too heavily on cleanliness and an emphasis that bowel contents were dirty, Freud suggested that an unresolved anal personality could result in adulthood. Such an individual would become either obsessed with cleanliness or, as a means of defiance, excessively messy. If, on the other hand, toilet training focused too heavily on the fecal matter itself being an item of great value given as a means of expressing love for the caregiver, the unresolved anal personality in adulthood may be selfish. Such an individual could become obsessed

TABLE 11-7
Physiologic Development During Toddlerhood

Category	Normal Characteristics
Nervous, muscular, and skeletal systems	• Rapid brain growth leads to a top-heavy appearance. • Stance is broad, abdomen is protruding. • Myelination continues. • Body proportions change, neck elongates. • Long bones of arms and legs increase in length in relation to the torso. • Right- or left-handedness becomes apparent. • By age 1, pincer grasp is present. • By age 2, length has increased 60–76% from infancy. • Walking skill completed • General muscle production increases and muscle fibers grow rapidly. • Ossification and calcification of bone continues. • Spine takes on more "S"-like adult characteristics. • Smaller bones joint together to form larger bone units. • New bones form from cartilage in wrist and ankles. • Anterior fontanelle closes by 18 months.
Gross motor skills	• Gross motor activities are prominent. • Walks forward and backward with a broad stance • Can run, jump, kick, ride a tricycle • Climbs stairs
Fine motor skills	• Uses a spoon fairly adeptly • Can pile blocks • Drinks from a cup • Can turn pages of a book • Scribbles and by age 3 may be able to draw "stick" people
Sensory organs	• Hearing is adultlike but short, straight eustachian tube increases susceptibility to infection. • Smell and taste are more or less at full capacity. • *Sight:* farsightedness is fairly normal. Vision is about 20/70 at age 2 and about 20/50 at age 3.
Gastrointestinal system and nutrition	• Food intake decreases as growth rate decreases. • Appetite waxes and wanes. • Finger foods allow maintenance of nutrition while constantly on the move. • Diet high in protein and calories needed. • Drooling stops. • Swallowing ability improves. • Toilet training can begin at 2–2 1/2 years.
Respiratory system	• Breathing is primarily diaphragmatic. • Rate is approximately 24 breaths/minute.
Cardiovascular system	• Growth of the cardiovascular system increases the overall activity capacity of the toddler • By age 3 the blood pressure is approximately 100/60 mm Hg. • Pulse ranges from 90–100 beats per minute.
Genitourinary system	• Genitals increase in size but remain functionally dormant. • Bladder control during the day and some at night occurs by 2 1/2 to 3 years of age.

(Continued)

T A B L E   **11-7**
Physiologic Development During Toddlerhood   (Continued)

Category	Normal Characteristics
Integumentary system	• Epithelium toughens and becomes more resilient. • Skin tenderness occurs primarily in genital area related to elimination.
Dentition	• Growth of deciduous teeth continues. • *"Bottle mouth caries"* may result from extended bottle feeding at bedtime.
Sleep/activity	• Intense activity level requires that toddlers have one to two naps per day. • Total daily sleep requirements are approximately 12 hours/day
Size	• Toddler is characteristically chubby and pot-bellied. • At age 2 child is approximately four times his birth weight. • At age 2 weight is approximately 30–35 lb (18–32 kg) on average. • Height at 2 averages 23–37 inches (80–92.5 cm).

with possessions, seeing them as a measure of his own personal worth. Regardless of the validity of Freud's beliefs, behavior in toddlerhood is certainly focused on body function in general and elimination functions in particular.

Autonomy Versus Shame and Doubt.   The infant who enters toddlerhood with the right balance of trust for security and mistrust for self-protection, will be ready to enter Erickson's second stage: autonomy versus shame and doubt. Increased physical mobility and a recognition of a separate self are the premises on which Erickson bases his beliefs about this second stage. If the right equilibrium is struck, the psychologically healthy child will gain independence in some basic activities of daily living such as feeding, walking, dressing, and toileting. The toddler becomes more adept at expressing wishes as language proficiency increases. This new found autonomy will have to be balanced with a healthy respect for potentially dangerous activities such as hot stoves and electric outlets. If an imbalance occurs in favor of the negative side of this stage, the child becomes excessively reticent to explore and unnecessarily fearful of activities and people.

Developmental Tasks.   According to Havighurst, the major developmental task of toddlerhood is
• Learn to control the elimination of body wastes
Havighurst also indicates that *beginning* efforts at mastering three other developmental tasks occur in toddlerhood:

• Learn sex differences
• Form concepts and learn language
• Learn to distinguish right and wrong

Separation Anxiety.   A child's fear of being away from those individuals who are his love objects and security base is called *separation anxiety*. Although this difficulty has its roots in infancy during the process of trust development, it blossoms as a common difficulty in toddlerhood. The absence of the caregiver, coupled with a limited understanding of time and reason, make separation anxiety such a prominent difficulty in these years. As the toddler becomes more secure in his own autonomy and in his knowledge that the caregiver will return, separation anxiety becomes increasingly less traumatic.

Negativism.   Testing the notion that they have some measure of control over their environment (autonomy) results in the toddler's favorite response to any controlling effort by the caregiver being "No!". This phenomenon is universal and is called negativism. Once the child has developed a good measure of environmental mastery, the need for unrelinquished control diminishes.

Regression.   Regression can be described as behaving in a manner more characteristic of a younger age. Regression can occur at any time in childhood and is usually a temporary response to stressful circumstances.

The three most common behavioral expressions of regression are excessive clinging to the primary caregiver, reduction of control over elimination, and reverting to more infantile speech patterns. With patience and help from the primary caregiver, the toddler can find new ways to cope with stress and return to more mature behavior patterns.

Toilet Training. By combining the beliefs of all the theorists discussed so far, certain prerequisites for successful toilet training can be delineated: physiologic, cognitive, and psychosocial readiness. Combining these prerequisites with a relaxed, confident caregiver will help assure that toilet training occurs with little difficulty.

Play. Social play in toddlerhood is likely to fall into levels 1 and 2: solitary and parallel play (Table 11-5). The toddler begins by playing with items that interest him, oblivious of those around. As he matures, he may play close to other children or even with the same toys but rarely attempts to socialize with the other children.

Cognitive play in toddlerhood is primarily at level 2: constructive play (Table 11-5). Building blocks, simple puzzles, and finger painting can all be enjoyable and creative activities. As the child's imaginative abilities improve in toddlerhood the desire to use cognitive level 3: pretend play will increase.

Threaded through toddler play as well should be a combination of activities that allow the toddler to refine gross motor skills and begin to perfect fine motor skills and language ability.

Temperament. By reflecting back to the theory of temperament referred to in infancy, some assumptions can be made about the expression of the three personality styles in toddlerhood. It is likely that toilet training will be undramatic for the "easy" child, take longer for the "slow to warm" child and be a battle of wills for the "difficult" child. As well, the desire for autonomy may be a smoother transition for the "easy" child, require gentle pushing and patience for the "slow to warm" child, and necessitate extreme patience and limit-setting for the "difficult" child.

Common Health Problems in Toddlerhood

Accidents, such as motor vehicle accidents, poisonings, burns, drownings, aspiration, and falls, remain the number one cause of mortality in toddlerhood (Mott, Fazekas, and James, 1984, p 4). Dental problems can occur, especially if a toddler is allowed to bottle feed longer than is physiologically and psychosocially necessary (Waechter, Phillips, and Holaday, 1985, p 416). Respiratory infections and otitis media are common infections. Some surgeries, such as repair of a cleft lip and palate, may begin in the toddler years. Often, however, reparative surgery for congenital anomalies requires significant physiologic growth of the organ or tissue involved. Thus, later childhood is often a more optimum time for many such surgeries.

Nurses' Role in Toddler Health Care

The role of the nurse as preventive teacher continues. The major areas of concern for preventive teaching and examples of specific information the nurse might provide are described in Table 11-8. Because of some of the inherent frustrations in raising toddlers, community outlets for both caregivers and toddlers are useful. Perhaps the most significant role the nurse can play during toddlerhood is helping the caregivers find the means to provide their toddler with the right balance of healthy independence and firm limits.

Preschooler: 3 to 6 Years

The chubby toddler begins to give way to the leaner and more coordinated preschooler around 3 years of age. Preschool development is slower than in both infancy and toddlerhood, but nonetheless, steady.

Physiologic Development

The physical characteristics of the normal preschooler are described in Table 11-9.

Immunity. The preschooler's tonsils reach peak growth by age 6. The susceptibility to respiratory infections and otitis media is still present, especially if the preschooler is in a nursery school or day care environment. DPT (diphtheria, tetanus, and pertussis) and OPV (polio) boosters are required between ages 4 and 6 years.

Cognitive Development

Preoperational Stage. Piaget's analysis of cognitive development places the preschooler in the preoperational stage of development. The major characteristics of this stage are discussed in Chapter 10. As the preschooler gains experience, improves language skills, socializes, and plays, he passes through two phases of the preoperational stage: the preconceptual phase followed by the intuitive phase. As the child passes through these two phases, some transitional changes can be seen.

- Egocentrism decreases as the child's socialization with other children increases and his ability to express himself through language improves.
- Symbolic play gradually becomes more related to real-life events and less fantasy-related.
- Basic curiosity results in constant questioning and an improvement in reasoning ability.
- Increasing multidimensional perception skills allow the preschooler to move into the next cognitive stage at about age 6.

Language Development. The speech patterns of preschoolers become more elaborate and grammatically sound than those of the toddler. Sentence length in-

T A B L E   11-8
Wellness Promotion in Toddlerhood

Areas of Concern	Preventive Teaching
Accident prevention	• Explain how the autonomy needs of the toddler need to be met with an eye to safety • Suggest locking poisons out of child's reach • Suggest safety plugs for electric outlets • Advise to block stairs with a gate, then help the child learn how to maneuver stairs. • Advise not allowing toddler to have small, hard food items like popcorn, peanuts, raw carrots which may cause aspiration • Discourage toddler from running with food in his mouth • Encourage proper use of carseats • Advise never to leave child unattended near water • Suggest teaching toddler of dangers in clear, simple terms (*e.g.,* stove hot)
Toilet training	• Explain developmental tasks necessary for toilet training • Correct misconceptions about mastery of this task • Suggest some helpful literature for caregivers
Negativism	• Help caregivers understand the normality of negativism in toddlerhood and its meaning from the child's point of view
Feeding and nutrition	• Suggest that food be provided in forms the toddler can manipulate independently • Advise caregivers to not be concerned about the messiness of toddler eating habits because the independence gained by the child is more important • Provide soft finger foods which child can eat while playing • Reassure caregivers that short anorexic periods are common in toddlerhood
Hygiene and dental care	• Emphasize the teaching of good hygiene habits (*e.g.,* handwashing after toileting or before eating) • Suggest teaching the toddler how to brush his teeth (with assistance) • Encourage caregivers to take toddler with them for dental appointments as an observer. Many dentists encourage this.
Infections	• Encourage caregivers to attend to respiratory infections promptly because of the high correlation between such infections and otitis media • Encourage completion of initial immunization schedule and any necessary boosters
Play habits	• Encourage the selection of toys that emphasize gross motor skill and creativity • Advise parents that sharing is not likely to occur and that parallel play is an important precursor to interactive play

creases until 6 to 18 word sentences become common by age 6 (Papilia and Olds, 1986, p 192). The incessant use of "Why?" allows the preschooler to increase knowledge, encourage continued conversation, and further language development. As the child passes through the preoperational stage, egocentric monologues give way to more social dialogue.

Memory.   Experiments by Myers and Perlmutter (1978) indicate that an increase in general knowledge and cognitive ability allows the preschooler to improve the ability to: (1) recognize objects that have been shown before; (2) recall objects shown previously but are currently out of view. Recognition (as in toddlerhood) is still the better developed memory skill.

Basic curiosity results in questioning and an improved reasoning ability in the preschooler

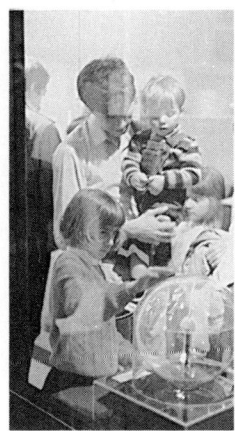 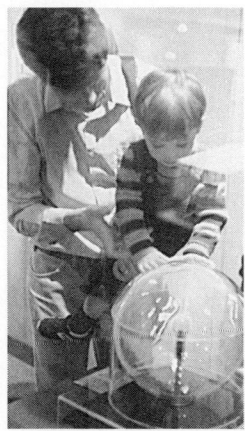 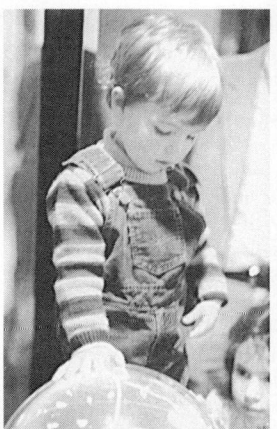

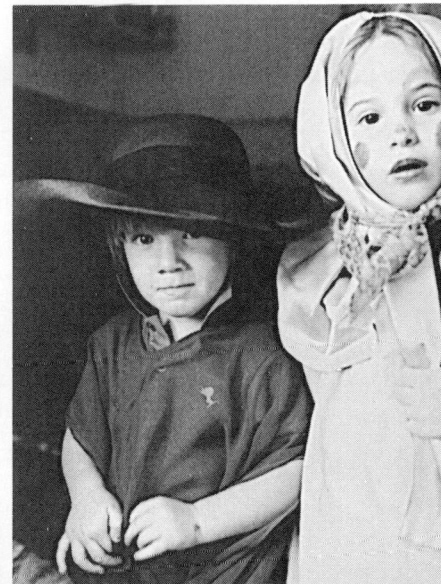

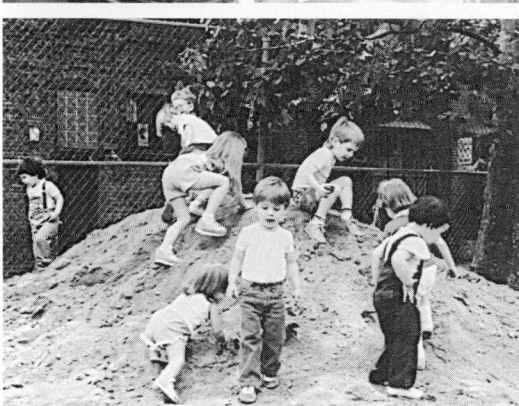

Preschooler play is associative and cooperative in its social dimension and cognitive development is demonstrated in constructive and pretend play

Symbolic play gradually becomes more related to real life events

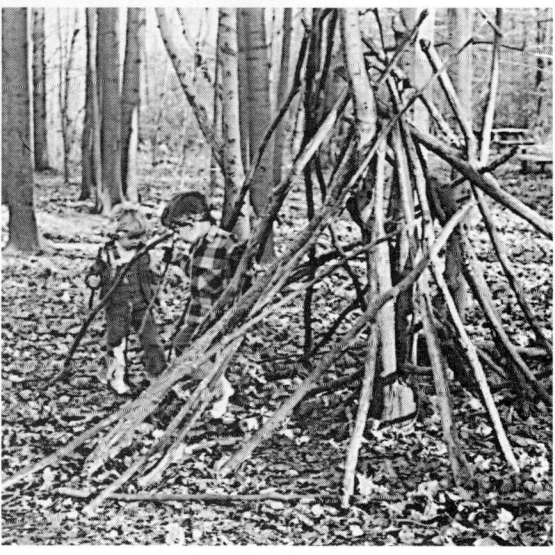

FIGURE 11-5
Some characteristics of preschool development.

Body Image. Preschoolers have a clear perception of themselves as male or female. Children of this age are competent at understanding basic body functions and are clearly able to distinguish the physical characteristics that separate the two sexes. Curiosity about sex differences leads to "playing doctor." This is a normal behavioral expression of a basic curiosity.

It is not uncommon at this time for a child to desire to "look nice" or wear something "special." There is a sense of increased self-esteem coming from compliments about appearance, although these compliments are often accepted awkwardly.

Psychosocial Development

Phallic Stage. Freud theorized that preschoolers were in the phallic stage of development, the biologic focus being primarily genital. The awareness of sexual differences sets up some psychologic conflicts for the child. Freud described the nature of these conflicts as parent-related. The basic premises is that the child has a sexual desire for opposite-sexed parent. Finding this psychologically unacceptable, the child, as a means of defense, makes a strong identification with the same-sexed parent. In the process of resolving these conflicts at about age 6, the child begins to develop the superego or conscience.

More current social theorists see sex-role identification as psychologically less complex and more a matter of observation and modeling (Salkind and Ambron, 1987, p 414).

Initiative Versus Guilt. Erickson places the preschooler in the stage of initiative versus guilt. A preschooler has developed a level of cognitive and psychosocial maturity that allows for the planning and executing of actions with some competence. The conscience at this stage, however, is fairly inflexible. The

T A B L E   11-9
Physiologic Development of the Pre-Schooler

Category	Normal Characteristics
Nervous, muscular, and skeletal systems	• Head approaches adult size by age 6. • Chest is adultlike in shape by age 6. • Musculature improves. • Pot belly is replaced by a flat, firm abdomen. • Walking becomes less wide-stanced. • Ossification and calcification of bones continue. • Running, hopping, going up and down stairs are done with ease. • Red bone marrow is replaced by fatty tissue in most bones except the sternum, pelvis, and vertebrae.
Gross motor skills	• Gross motor skills are conducted with considerable finesse. • Can skip, throw and catch a ball • Balance improves.
Fine motor skills	• Copying figures becomes easier (*e.g.,* circles, squares). • Is able to trace • Printing of letters and numbers is a common ability.
Sensory organs	• By age 5 20/20 vision is probable. • All other senses are essentially at full functioning capacity.
Gastrointestinal system and nutrition	• Bowel control is complete. • Food habits and diet become more adultlike. • Stomach acidity increases.
Respiratory system	• Toward the end of the preschool years, diaphragmatic breathing patterns give way to more adultlike chest breathing. • Respiratory rate is 22–24/minute.
Cardiovascular system	• Pulse rate is 90–95 beats/minute. • Blood pressure is approximately 100/60 mm Hg. • Heart is four times larger than at birth. • Hematopoietic and lymphatic systems mature markedly.
Genitourinary system	• Bladder control is completed. • Kidney is approaching adult capacity. • Sexual organs grow steadily but are functionally dormant.
Integumentary system	• Skin is approaching adult resilience.
Dentition	• Twenty deciduous teeth are present. • Some ''baby'' teeth may begin to fall out and be replaced by permanent teeth.
Sleep/activity	• Napping continues but needs to taper off in preparation for the school years. • 10–12 hours sleep per day required on average.
Size	• Weight at age 6 is double the weight at 1 year. • Weight increases at a rate of about 5 lb (2.3 kg) per year. • Average weight at 5–6 years is 45 lb (20.9 kg). • Boys are slightly heavier than girls. • Height increases less than 1 inch (2.5 cm) per year. • Birth length doubles by age 6 to about 40–45 in. (100–113 cm). • Genetic influences in height and weight are discernable.

child creates inner turmoil by pitting natural curiosity and a sense of personal power against the constant examination of the propriety of his actions by a rigid conscience. The preschooler must learn to set realistic self-limits as an offshoot of social interaction.

Developmental Tasks. According to Havighurst, the preschool years present four developmental tasks based on physical growth and cognitive awareness:

- Learn sex differences and sexual modesty
- Form concepts and learn language to describe social and physical reality
- Get ready to read
- Learn to distinguish right and wrong and begin to develop a conscience (It is this awakening of a conscience that forms a basis on which values and morals in later life are built.)

Fears and Fantasies. Because one of the primary tasks of the preschooler is to become more socially oriented, many fears relate to socialization. Shyness toward new people and fear of new places are common. Observation of a parent's anxious reaction to a situation is a frightening experience for a child. The parent's fear is assumed by the child because he believes that something which can cause his parent (his stable support base) to be afraid must be evil.

Two common fears during the preschool years are fear of darkness and of nightmares. As the ability to fantasize becomes more developed, the child's own fertile imagination becomes his worst enemy. These fears, however unfounded, are still frightening to the child. Support and validation of these feelings by caregivers are essential.

Play. By identifying the developmental highlights of the preschool years, common play activities can be deduced. The preschooler is sexually curious, imaginative, and social. Using the classifications of play described in Table 11-5, preschoolers use levels 3 and 4 of social play: associative and cooperative play. In the cognitive dimension, levels 2 and 3 are prominent: constructive and pretend play. Puzzles, coloring, cutting, and painting are enjoyable activities. Dress-up play is especially attractive. Simple games involving some interaction with others are pleasing. Most of the play of preschoolers involves considerable imagination and a degree of interaction with others. Most child experts consider the preschool years the most relevant time for nursery school experience. It is important to note, however, that the emphasis in nursery school should be play and socialization, not academic learning.

Temperament. Using the temperament classifications described earlier, some assumptions can be made about the effect of temperament on preschool development. The "easy" child manages with the least difficulty. Socialization is welcomed by the "easy" child, and he is likely to be popular. The "slow to warm" child might find the preschool years especially difficult as socialization is such an important task. Much gentle encouragement will likely be required from caregivers. The frustrations of the preschool years may cause the "difficult" child to act aggressively and have difficulty with self-control. Again, patience and firm guidance from caregivers are important.

Moral Development

The pre-school years are dominated by Kohlberg's first phase of moral reasoning: the preconventional phase. This phase has two focuses of orientation: punishment and obedience orientation (rules are obeyed to avoid punishment) and instrumental-relativist orientation (rules are obeyed because it is in one's own self-interest to do so, for example, some reward will be forthcoming).

Spiritual Development

The cognitive, social, and moral development of the preschooler provide clear indications as to what the spiritual development is likely to be as described by Fowler. The preschooler will attend church and Sunday school if the family does. Lessons in Sunday school for the young preschooler often involve coloring religious pictures or singing religious songs. The religious concepts implied in either the pictures or songs are usually lost on the child. The older preschooler may hear stories illustrating a religious principle but the interpretation of the meaning of the story is likely beyond reasoning ability. The concept of a deity will be based on what is known and literal. Four to five year olds will draw God like a human male. Imagination at this age can be a powerful influence. Concepts like heaven, hell, or holy spirits are incomprehensible and provide fuel for a vivid imagination.

Common Health Problems in the Preschool Child

Preschoolers continue to have some of the health problems common in the toddler years. Communicable diseases and respiratory infections are frequent, especially with increased socialization at nursery schools and day care. Preschoolers are prone to accidents because of their increased curiosity about the world.

Some congenital disorders such as **hypospadias, inguinal hernias,** and cardiac anomalies will require surgery at this time. Dental caries become common if teeth are neglected. As language becomes more sophisticated, speech disorders may become apparent.

Nurses' Role in Preschool Health Care

Continuing with a preventive teaching focus for the nurse, areas of concern and examples of useful information the nurse might provide are described in Table 11-10.

T A B L E   11-10
Promoting Wellness in Preschoolers

Area of Concern	Preventive Teaching
Accident prevention and safety	• Advise that preschoolers, now out of carseats, need to learn how to use seat belts • Advise that clear boundaries regarding where tricycles or bicycles can be ridden need to be given • Teach simple road safety (*e.g.,* looking both ways before crossing the street) • Encourage education of children regarding strangers and block parent programs • Encourage education about sexual abuse (*i.e.,* explaining to child what is and is not appropriate touching by an adult) • Swimming lessons can begin and basic water safety taught • Teach the dangers of matches and practice home fire safety drills
Infections	• Advise that these are an inevitable result of increased socialization • Advise teaching children sound hygiene practices such as handwashing after toileting, correct disposal of tissues after use, nonsharing of items like eating utensils • Keep immunizations current
Sleep disorders	• Explain to caregivers the commonality of this problem among preschoolers • Suggest that relaxed bedtime rituals and a night light can help • Advise that a comforting and warm reassurance is needed when child is awakened by nightmares
Dental hygiene	• Teach that preschoolers should be brushing their teeth and flossing with caregiver assistance • Advise that a dental visit at this time is useful for teaching dental hygiene and overcoming fear of the unknown
Play habits	• Advise caregivers that make-believe play and imaginary friends are common and normal in the preschool years • Encourage caregivers to promote socialization through neighborhood play groups and nursery school

Surgery or Hospitalization.   Most preschoolers have two common concerns if hospitalization or surgery is required. The concerns are fear of pain or body mutilation and, to a lesser degree, separation anxiety. The nurse can allay some of the child's fears by explaining procedures clearly in language the child understands. Honest explanation of the amount of pain a procedure will cause is most helpful. Sanctioning of the child's feelings can be done by allowing the child to practice procedures on a doll and encouraging the child to express feelings openly. Separation anxiety can be reduced by encouraging caregivers to take an active role in the child's care.

Speech Disorders.   Some peculiarities of speech are an element of immaturity and will correct themselves

with time. If there is a genuine concern about a child's speech development, caregivers should be referred to a speech specialist for assessment and guidance.

School-Age Child: 6 to 12 Years

The child is sturdy, strong, and usually lean by the time he reaches school age. His physical growth during middle childhood is relatively slow but steady. Physiologic stability is well developed by age 12.

Physiologic Development

Table 11-11 summarizes physiologic development during middle childhood. It will be noted that while there is

T A B L E   11-11
Physiologic Development of the School-Age Child

Category	Normal Characteristics
Nervous, muscular, and skeletal systems	• The brain reaches 90%–95% of the adult size. • Myelination of nerve fibers continues. • By age 12, maturation of the nervous system is almost complete, making fine motor and manipulative skills well perfected and coordinated. • There is a slight increase in skull size, and individual facial characteristics develop. • Centers of bone ossification are established. • The body is well coordinated, and strength and resistance to fatigue increase. • Boys tend to be stronger than girls, owing to the fact that boys have more muscle cells. • Growth of bones, which is rapid, often exceeds growth of muscles, leading to gangliness, "growing pains," and swayback late in this period. • Overall posture is more perfect.
Gross motor skills	• Child has increasing control over body movements. • Can participate in games requiring many coordinated muscle movements
Fine motor skills	• A 6 year old can hold a pencil and print words. • A 12 year old can write in script and in sentences. • Enjoys making models • Use of scissors, rulers, and mathematical equipment becomes refined.
Sensory organs	• Sensory organs are fully developed and discriminating.
Gastrointestinal system	• The gastrointestinal tract reaches maturity. • Appetite and caloric needs decrease owing to a drop in activity and growth rate. • The diet is similar to an adult's diet. Definite food preferences become noticeable, and eating is more social than simply satisfying hunger.
Respiratory system	• Adultlike in function • Respiratory rate is 18–20 breaths/minute.
Cardiovascular system	• Functioning of the cardiovascular system is similar to that of an adult. • The pulse rate is about 85–100 at 6 years of age and slows to about 60–80 by 12 years of age. • Blood pressure is about 100/60 mm Hg at 6 years of age and rises to 110/70 by age 12. • There is cardiac growth with increased cardiac functioning to meet the needs of physical activity and the growing body. Heart is six times birth size. • Blood values and proportion of body fluids approach adult levels by age 12.
Genitourinary system	• The urinary system reaches maturity. • The sexual organs grow but are still dormant until late in this period, when hormonal changes influence them.
Integumentary system	• Has adult characteristics except for the absence of perspiration activity in axilla

(Continued)

T A B L E   11-11
Physiologic Development of the School-Age Child   (Continued)

Category	Normal Characteristics
Dentition	• Deciduous teeth are replaced by permanent teeth. All permanent teeth are present by age 12, except for the second and third molars.
Sleep/activity	• The average 6 year old requires about 10–12 hours sleep in every 24 hours. By age 12, the need for sleep is about 10 hours.
Size	• Between ages 6 and 12, the youngster grows about 2–3 in. (5–7.5 cm) each year and gains 3–6 lb (1.4–2.8 kg) each year. Hereditary factors influence size to a large extent. • Boys are taller and heavier than girls until about age 10. Between ages 10 and 12 the reverse occurs.

a definite lull in physiologic development, refinement and changes continue on a subtle and gradual basis.

Immunity.   Body immune systems are maturing steadily and the school-age child is less susceptible to common infections than the preschooler. Childhood immunization should be complete by this time. Many schools require accurate immunization records prior to the child entering school. If records are lost, booster immunization or assessment of titre levels in the blood may be required.

Cognitive Development

Concrete Operational Stage.   Continuing the theme of restructuring knowledge through intellectual growth, Piaget places the school-age child at the *concrete operational stage* of development.

Piaget refers to an operation as the process of organizing facts about the environment to be used for problem solving:

• The mind operates logically, and concepts of mass, volume, weight, and measurement develop.
• The child deals best with actual objects and people, but he discovers how concepts are related and how events can be compared through multiple relations.
• The child learns to perform concrete operations by dealing with properties of the present environment to solve new problems. Reasoning is inductive.
• With the development of relativism, specific encounters in the environment lead to generalizations about persons, places, and things.
• Numerous classification systems develop. The child likes to collect things of one category.

• Egocentric thought gives way to social cognition ability. This allows the child to become aware of and understand others' feelings and points of view.
• The understanding of transformation and reversal of events becomes clear.

Language Development.   School-age children have well-developed language skills. Their increased experience and cognitive ability allow them to use language in a more sophisticated manner than the preschooler. An interesting perspective on language development is offered by Vygotsky (1962), who believes that the egocentric speech of the preschooler is a means of problem solving out loud. As the child matures, vocal problem solving gives way to "silent inner speech." The school-age child, then, expresses only the solution to a problem and not the entire process of arriving at the solution.

Memory.   The school-age child's memory is considerably improved from the preschool years. The ability to store information in long-term memory and retrieve it in the remembering process (recall) is much more efficient in the middle years. Advancing cognitive abilities are likely the most influential factor in this improvement.

Body Image.   Body image, self-concept, and sexuality are clearly intertwined in the school-age child. These children identify with parental and other role models. Sexual development, while not observable until late in this period, produces a strong need for these children to clearly understand body function and have questions about sexuality answered correctly and honestly. Menstruation may begin as young as age 9, and girls and boys need sound knowledge of sexual functioning and emotions well before becoming sexually mature.

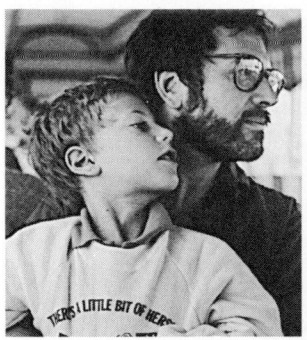
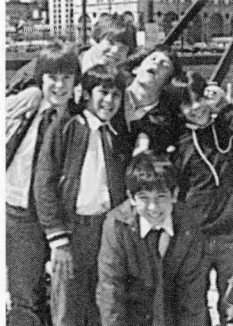

The school-age child has limited interest in members of the opposite sex and strong identification with one's own sex is dominant

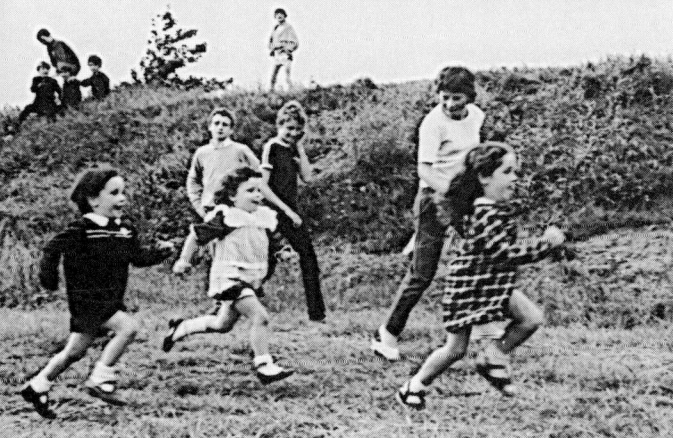

Play involves development of skills, games with rules, and competitive activities

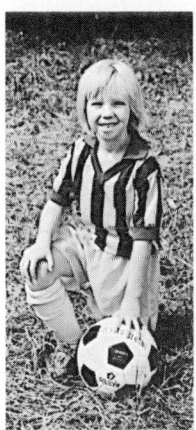

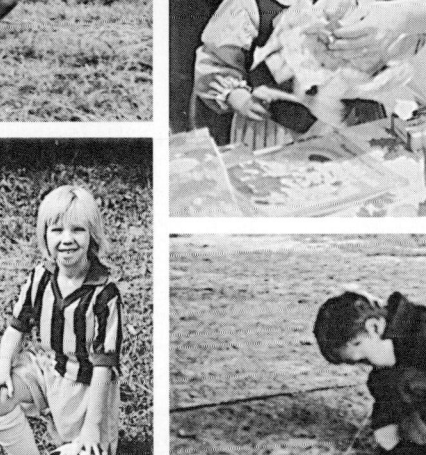

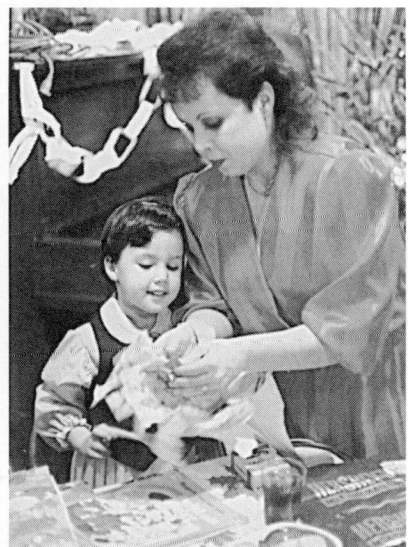

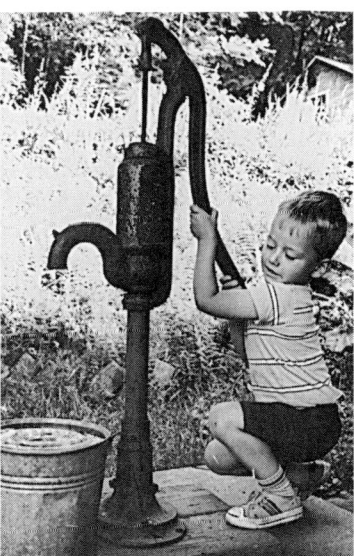

Total play gives way to productivity in the school-age child

Fine motor coordination develops

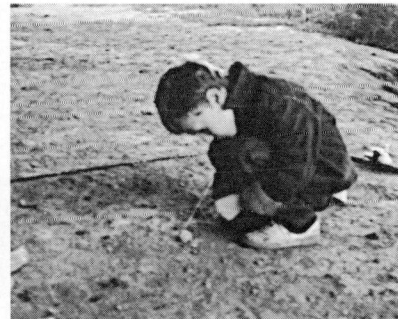

Psychosocial Development

Latency Stage. Freud describes middle childhood as the *latency stage.* The psychosexual energies of the school-age period are channeled in other directions. Interest in the opposite sex is limited, and strong identification with one's own sex is dominant. This does not preclude the fact that information about sex is wanted. In fact, in efforts to put order in the world, the school-age child needs answers to many questions, including those of a sexual nature.

Industry Versus Inferiority. The emotional and sexual calm of this particular period allows children to concentrate on cognitive growth. This sets the stage for the *industry versus inferiority* phase of Erikson's developmental theories. Total play begins to give way to productivity. By becoming adept at learning useful skills in society positive self-esteem is developed. If a child feels his productivity is inferior to what is expected by caregivers or what peers are accomplishing, he may view himself as inferior. The other extreme is, of course, the child who gives productivity too high a status and neglects social needs. Such a child may become a "workaholic" in adulthood.

This period of development is critical in terms of a social attitude and the child's own social worth. A sense of identity begins to appear, and a scale of values develops as the youngster becomes aware of origins, including such factors as race, religion, ethnic background, and the family's economic status. There is rapid movement to outerworld interest, with emphasis on doing, succeeding, and accomplishing.

Developmental Tasks. Havighurst describes developmental tasks that typically occur during middle childhood as being characterized by three outward thrusts: thrust from home to peer groups; physical thrust into games and activity requiring neuromuscular skills; and mental thrust toward adulthood with the use of concepts, communication, symbols, and logic. Tasks are the following:

- Learn physical skills necessary for ordinary games. (Skills such as throwing, kicking, catching, swimming, and using simple tools become important.)
- Build wholesome attitudes toward oneself as a growing organism (There is little sexual behavior from a physiologic point of view. However, curiosity, experimentation, and talk of sex are present. If sexual education at home and school is not provided, the child satisfies curiosity elsewhere. There is emphasis and value on cleanliness, eating properly, being healthy, having good health habits, and being physically fit.)
- Learn an appropriate masculine or feminine social role (Different behaviors between the sexes is les⸃ sharply defined today with the move toward equality between the sexes.)
- Develop fundamental skills in reading, writing, and calculating
- Develop concepts necessary for everyday living (The child can think effectively about such matters as an occupation and civic and social responsibilities. Several thousand concepts are developed during middle childhood.)
- Develop conscience, morality, and a scale of values
- Achieve personal independence
- Develop attitudes towards social groups and institutions (In the North American culture, this task involves developing democratic attitudes and includes the development of attitudes in relation to school, church, and political and economic groups.)

Peer Relationships. By middle childhood the peer group becomes the major gauge for determining status, skill, and personableness. This group acts as a strong influence in making alterations and adjustments in the values learned from caregivers. Peer groups in middle childhood help prepare the child for getting along in the larger world to come, as well as assisting in teaching appropriate sex-role behavior. While it is clear that much positive behavior can be gleaned from peer interaction, peer pressure can also push children to act or think in a manner that, as an individual, may go against sound judgment. Peer groups act as transition modes for the child in leaving total caregiver influence and heading toward adult independence.

Play. Because the nature of development in the school-age child is both cognitively and socially important, the direction of play patterns in middle childhood are social—level 4, co-operative play; and cognitive—level 4, games with rules (see Table 11-5). In combination, these two aspects of play allow for

- Learning to abide by rules
- A degree of competitiveness
- Cooperation in the process of rule agreement
- An ability to socialize in groups
- An ability to see positive group function as an important precursor to understanding societal functioning as a whole

This is the age period when organized activities become most meaningful: church groups, sports teams, scouting, community and club programs.

Temperament. In middle childhood the "easy" child is likely to fit in with peers quickly and probably be well liked. The "slow to warm" child will likely need a measure of gentle encouragement to prevent becoming a loner. The "difficult" child has two possibilities. If efforts are positive, his strong-willed nature gives him leadership potential. If his approach is hostile and aggressive, he is likely to be shunned by the group.

Moral Development

Although the school-age child begins middle childhood in the *preconventional phase* of moral development, the majority of this developmental age is spent in the *conventional phase.* Behavior is based on familial and peer group beliefs, and conformity is the norm. The conventional phase has two focuses of orientation: *the "good boy–good girl" orientation* (behaving in a manner that pleases others of importance makes the child "good," for example, sharing, not using foul language, giving up seat on the bus to an elderly person) and *the "law and order" orientation* (inherent in this is respect for authority as a means of social order. Following school regulations and traffic laws and respecting teachers and police officers are characteristic).

Justice as a means of fair play is extremely important to the school-age child.

Spiritual Development

Consistent with the moral focus at this time, Fowler's theories indicate that school-age children view religious faith as a relationship involving reciprocal fairness. In the Christian and Jewish faiths biblical stories and parables with morals are particularly appealing because of the emphasis on justice. Children of this age may belong to organizations for the young within their own faith (*e.g.,* junior choir). They are able to participate in the rituals of their faith with a basic understanding of their significance. The concept of a spiritual dimension to humanity and the possibility of life after death is believed, even if not entirely understood.

Common Health Problems in the School-Age Child

Accidents continue to be frequent in middle childhood. Because of the increased interaction involved with school, communicable conditions such as scabies, impetigo, and pediculosis are common. **School phobia**, an uncommon but severe anxiety state, requires psychiatric assistance if persistent. Drug and alcohol abuse, while not as common as in adolescence, has been documented in children as young as age 8 (Salkind and Ambron, 1987, p 533). Suicide statistics for children under age 10 have risen also (Papilia and Olds, 1986, p 559).

Nurses' Role in School-Age Health Care

While the role of the nurse continues to emphasize preventive teaching, it is likely that the school nurse will fill this role. The health concerns of middle childhood, with some examples of teaching by the nurse, are described in Table 11-12.

Hospitalization. The school-age child may be hospitalized for many reasons. Treatment measures aside, hospitalized school-age children need assistance with maintaining family and peer relationships and school progress, as much as is reasonably possible.

Adolescence: 12 to 18 Years

Of life's many transitional phases, adolescence has generated the most attention, concern, controversy, and confusion (Lerner and Spanier, 1980, p xix). Rapid physiologic growth, reproductive maturity, and emotional development are only three of several growth activities that give credence to the fact that adolescence is one of the most turbulent and profoundly influential phases of life.

Physiologic Development

The body changes in adolescence transform the individual from child to adult. The major physiologic changes of adolescence are described in Table 11-13.

Immunity. Body immune systems reach full capacity in adolescence. If childhood immunization schedules

T A B L E   11-12
Promoting Wellness in School-Age Children

Area of Concern	Preventive Teaching
Accident prevention	• Emphasize traffic safety • Encourage the use of seatbelts • Emphasize bicycle, skateboard, scooter safety • Teach children to take water safety programs
Communicable conditions	• Encourage proper hygiene habits, including not sharing personal items like combs • Home visit may be required to discuss home health practices if a child has a communicable condition like pediculosis • Advise of common treatment methods for conditions like scabies, impetigo, pediculosis
Substance abuse	• Early preventive teaching which includes guidance for families is essential.
Sexuality	• Sex education needs to begin as early as age 7 or 8 years. • Families need encouragement to talk about sex at home. • Caregivers need encouragement to answer questions honestly and correctly. • Menstruation needs to be discussed by at least age 8 because some girls menstruate as young as age 9.
Mental health concerns: School phobia Depression/suicide	• Nurse needs to work with teachers and families so that they learn to recognize behavior indicating mental health difficulties. • Nurse can provide referral for specialized assistance.

T A B L E 11-13
Physiologic Development During Adolescence

Category	Normal characteristics
Nervous, muscular, and skeletal systems	• The central nervous system is essentially mature by the end of childhood. Myelination and reticular formation continue into adulthood. • Maturation of the skeletal system occurs after a period of rapid growth. The feet, hands, and long bones grow rapidly. • The growth of the trunk in relation to the legs is responsible for most growth influencing height. • The rapid growth spurt during adolescence requires learning how to handle the body again. Until the adolescent does, stumbling, dropping articles, and running into things is likely. • When the adolescent becomes accustomed to the larger body frame, agility returns and the individual moves about with grace and litheness. • Muscle growth continues, and by about 17 uears of age, a boy's muscle mass is twice that of a girl, on average. • Girls broaden at the hip, boys at the shoulder. • Waist narrows. • Face grows in length. Head circumference increases approximately 1 inch (2.5 cm).
Gross motor skills	• Clumsiness common until growth spurt ceases
Fine motor skills	• Adultlike in finesse
Sensory organs	• Adultlike in functioning
Gastrointestinal system	• The gastrointestinal tract matures and becomes able to take in and digest large quantities of various foods. • Gastric acidity increases to aid digestion. It may cause abdominal pain and ulcer symptoms in some adolescents. • Food/caloric requirements are high owing to rapid growth and marked physical activity of this age.
Respiratory system	• There is an increase in vital capacity owing to the increase in the size of the structural body frame. • The boy's respiratory rate is slower than the girl's on average.
Cardiovascular system	• The cardiovascular system matures to adult levels. • The pulse rate is about 10% faster in girls than in boys. • Blood volume increases more fapidly in boys than in girls because the boy is heavier than the girl. • Blood pressure and blood values reach adult levels.
Genitourinary system	• The urinary system reaches full maturity • Reproductive maturity arrives as primary and secondary sexual development occurs. Primary development includes maturation of the sexual organs. Secondary development includes changes in other parts of the body as a result of hormonal changes; examples include the presence of axilla and pubic hair, and in males, facial hair and voice changes. Breast development in females. • Hormonal changes are primarily responsible for the maturity of the genital system.

(Continued)

TABLE   11-13
Physiologic Development During Adolescence
(Continued)

Category	Normal characteristics
	• Menstruation and spermatogenesis begin. • Puberty begins at about 10 or 11 for girls and at about age 12 or 13 for boys. Menstruation begins, on average between ages 11 and 14.
Integumentary system	• The skin becomes coarser and thicker, and pores enlarge. • **Sebaceous glands** become active and produce oily secretions often leading to acne. • Sweat glands in the axilla begin to function.
Dentition	• Permanent teeth are ordinarily all present by the end of this period.
Sleep/activity	• Adolescence is marked by overactivity, with fatigue being a common symptom when sleep or nutritional needs are not being met adequately.
Size	• Full adult size is reached, although some males may continue to grow in their 20s.

have been followed as recommended, a booster of tetanus and diphtheria vaccine (Td) is all that is required.

Growth Patterns and Reproductive Maturity

A true assessment of adolescent development would be incomplete without an expansion of the profound changes in reproductive functioning. **Puberty** can be divided into three stages:

- *Prepubescence*—The stage at which secondary sex characteristics begin to develop but the reproductive organs do not yet function
- *Pubescence*—The stage at which the secondary sex characteristics continue to develop and ova and sperm begin to be produced by the reproductive organs
- *Postpubescence*—Reproductive functioning and the development of secondary sex characteristics reach adult maturity.

The developmental occurrences at each stage are described in Table 11-14. Examples of normal female breast and pubic hair development and male pubic hair and exterior genital development are shown in Figures 11-7 through 11-9.

Cognitive Development

Formal Operations Stage. According to Piaget, adolescence is when the *formal operations stage* of cognitive development is formed. Important for this stage of development is the approaching acuity of the adult mind. The adolescent mind becomes capable of using deductive, reflective, and hypothetical reasoning. The culmination of logical thought occurs, and sophisticated and abstract concepts can be handled. Abstract universals such as justice and freedom can be grasped. The adolescent is able to conceive of terms outside his own realm of experience and knowledge. The concepts of time, its passage, and the future become realistic, resulting in the adolescent's ability to set long-term goals, an improbable task for a younger individual (Salkind and Ambron, 1987, p 525).

Because of the increasing ability to form and test hypotheses, problem solving can be difficult for the adolescent. The omniscience of adults is clearly seen as illogical, and challenging adult decision making becomes common. Interest in theoretical ideas allows the adolescent to construct idealistic solutions to societal problems without being hampered by the realities of adult experience.

Egocentrism returns in adolescence. Its re-emergence appears to be related to the ability to hypothesize and use abstract thinking. Because these newly acquired skills are attractive to the adolescent, much time is spent using them. Personal thought processes become a major focus of cognitive concern. Use of imaginary audiences and day dreaming are the observable behaviors (so irritating to adults) that illustrate this need to be introspective.

Memory and Language. The ability to classify and understand one's own memory style is usually accomplished during adolescence. In fact, adolescence is likely the time of peak memory function. Abstract thinking and scientific reasoning combined with increasing

T A B L E   11-14
Adolescent Sexual Development

Stage	Males	Females
Prepubescence	• Progressive enlargement of testicles, seminal ducts, prostate gland • Enlargement and reddening of the scrotal sac • Increase in length and circumference of penis • Appearace of downy pubic hair	• Progressive enlargement of the ovaries • Ripening of graafian follicles • Rounding of the hips • Appearance of breast buds • Enlargement of the fallopian tubes, vagina, and uterus • Appearance of downy pubic hair
Pubescence	• Increase in amount, pigmentation, and curling of pubic hair • Growth spurt involving peak pace of height and weight increase • Deepening of the voice due to growth of larynx • Testes enlarge • Scrotum grows and its pigmentation increases • Penis grows in length and circumference • **Spermatogenesis** begins	• Increase in amount, pigmentation, and curling of pubic hair • Growth spurt involving peak pace of height and weight increase • Menarche • Axillary hair appears • Vulva and clitoris enlarge • Breast tissue develops • **Ovulation** begins
Postpubescence	• Completion of sexual growth and development • Fertility	• Completion of sexual growth and development • Fertility

(Data from Lerner R, Spanier G: Adolescent Development: A Lifespan Approach, pp 193–199. New York, McGraw-Hill, 1980)

knowledge of word meanings, allow for a sophisticated level of language development.

Psychosocial Development

Genital Stage.   In keeping with Freud's theories, at puberty the libido re-emerges. The libido is genital in nature, but, contrary to the phallic stage, it takes a mature adult form. Freud's perception of adolescence as an imbalanced or disturbed state comes from his belief that the newly acquired adult genital drive upsets the delicate balance of the id, ego, and superego. As the adolescent attempts to deal with this new drive, old defense mechanisms seem inefficient. New ones are formed using simultaneously acquired new cognitive abilities. **Intellectualization** becomes a common mechanism used to justify behavior.

Freud further postulates that if new and old defense mechanisms appear inadequate, the potential for interacting with "old love objects" (*i.e.,* caregivers) in a genital manner reappears. As this is an unacceptable state, the only solution for the adolescent is the abandonment of the "old love objects" in favor of new, acceptable love objects. These new love objects are usually peers who provide a less threatening means of dealing with libidinal drives.

Identity Versus Role Confusion.   The "trying out" of different roles, personal choices, and beliefs is part of the adolescent developmental phase Erikson refers to as *identity versus role confusion.* Erikson indicates that the basic developmental goals of adolescence can be isolated in two questions: "Who am I?" "What do I want to be?"

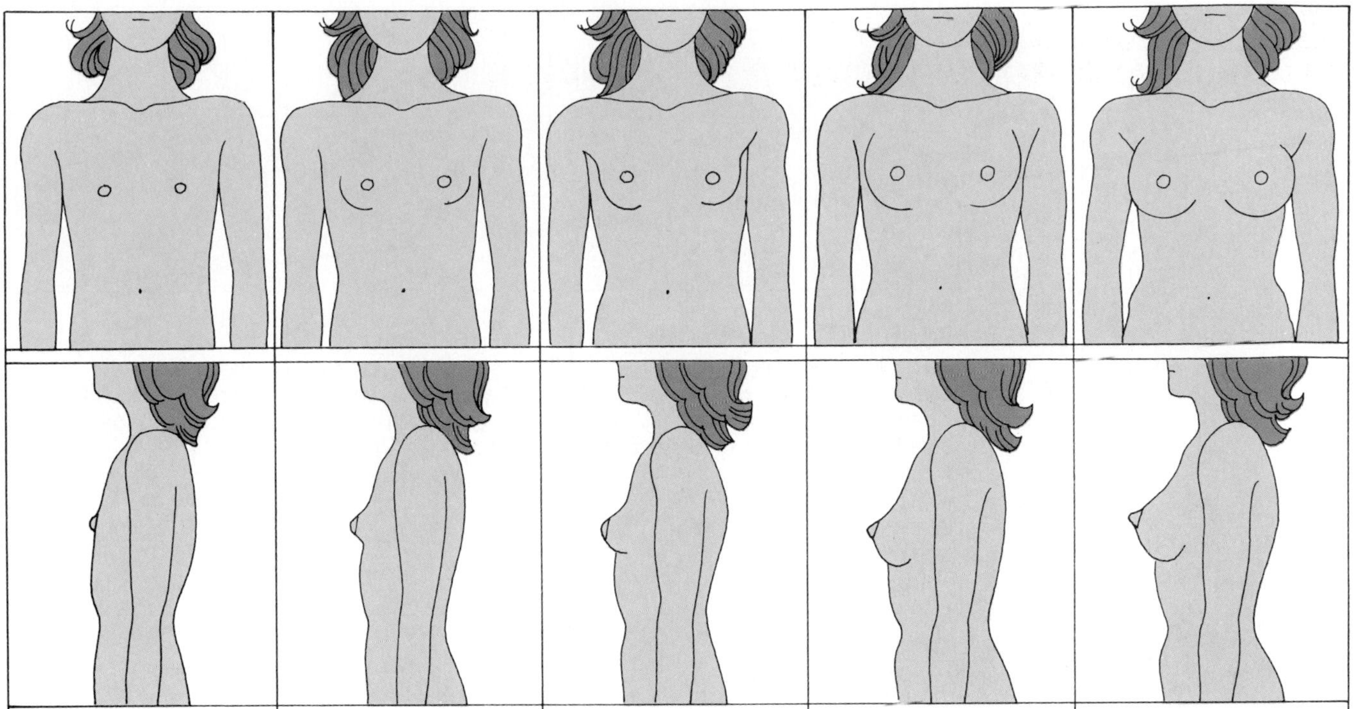

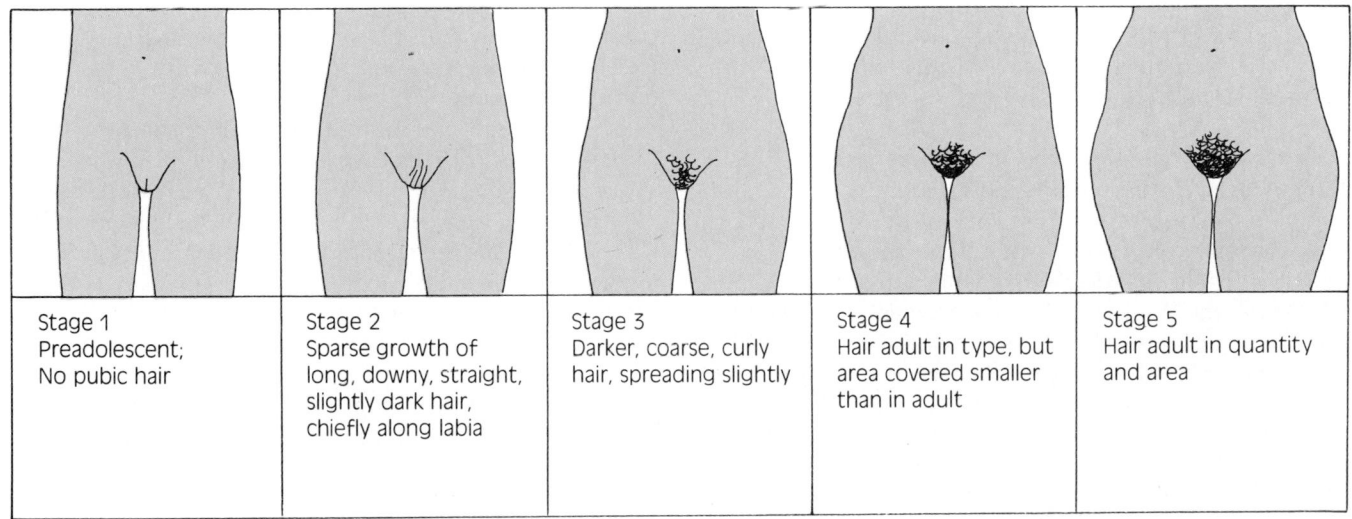

Stage 1 Preadolescent; elevation of papilla only	Stage 2 Breast bud stage; elevation of breast and papilla as small mound; enlargement of areolar diameter	Stage 3 Further enlargement of breast and areola with no separation of their contours	Stage 4 Projection of areola and papilla to form secondary mound above level of breast	Stage 5 Mature; projection of papillae only; recession of areola into contour of breast

FIGURE 11-7
Maturational stages of female breast development.

Stage 1 Preadolescent; No pubic hair	Stage 2 Sparse growth of long, downy, straight, slightly dark hair, chiefly along labia	Stage 3 Darker, coarse, curly hair, spreading slightly	Stage 4 Hair adult in type, but area covered smaller than in adult	Stage 5 Hair adult in quantity and area

FIGURE 11-8
Maturation stages of female pubic-hair development.

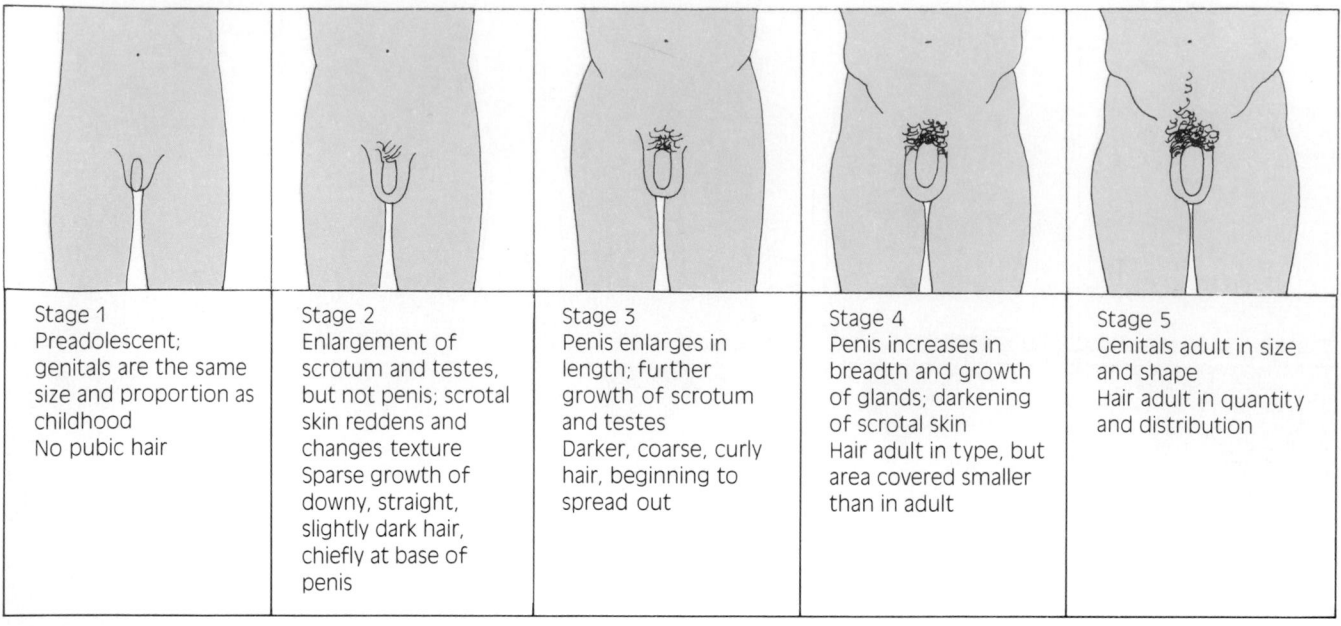

Stage 1 Preadolescent; genitals are the same size and proportion as childhood No pubic hair	Stage 2 Enlargement of scrotum and testes, but not penis; scrotal skin reddens and changes texture Sparse growth of downy, straight, slightly dark hair, chiefly at base of penis	Stage 3 Penis enlarges in length; further growth of scrotum and testes Darker, coarse, curly hair, beginning to spread out	Stage 4 Penis increases in breadth and growth of glands; darkening of scrotal skin Hair adult in type, but area covered smaller than in adult	Stage 5 Genitals adult in size and shape Hair adult in quantity and distribution

F I G U R E   11-9
Maturational stages of male genital development.

Because their physical, and particularly sexual, development is so rapid and unstable and because their social roles, particularly in North America, are so ambivalent, adolescents become preoccupied with self-identity. By clinging to peer groups, emulating and idolizing heroes, and forming idealistic viewpoints, young people attempt to stabilize emerging self-concepts. The peer group acts as an influential body in developing and evaluating new ideas, views, and values. As extremes are tested and retested and new experiences provide insight, the adolescent will begin to see himself as a unified whole. Once this process is complete (and it is not uncommon for this to last into the adult years), the adolescent is then able to make a mature emotional commitment to another.

Identity Crisis/Diffusion in Adolescence.   Adolescents typically experience ongoing identity crises. Two common examples in current society are:
- *Sex-object preference*—At a time when gender identity is at its most sensitive developmental phase, the discovery that one's sexual preference is not that of the societal norm disrupts self-identity.
- *Sex-role behavior*—At no other time in history have role behavior options for males and females been so limitless. Many believe that the reduction of sexual stereotyping is beneficial to both men and women. This reduction in stereotyping does, however, pose identity difficulties for adolescents of both sexes. Often a clear sex-role identity is not defined until well into adulthood.

If adolescent identity crises are not resolved, identity diffusion may result. Erikson describes identity diffusion as the failure to integrate various childhood identifications into a harmonious adult psychosocial identity. Adolescents who lack a clear sense of self may "play act" or copy the behaviors of associates. They are as chameleons and take on the characteristics of those around them in different situations.

Developmental Tasks.   Consistent with his beliefs that development is based on learning, Havighurst points out that development during adolescence is concerned primarily with physical and emotional maturing. He supports this with observations of typical tasks seen during this period.
- Achieve new and more mature relationships with age-mates of both sexes (Adolescents begin learning the techniques of dating as a precursor to establishing long-term relationships. A characteristic of this age is the strong desire for sameness and group approval by peers.)
- Achieve a masculine or feminine social role (Appropriate gender behavior in North America is currently in a state of flux.)
- Accept one's physique and use the body effectively (Adolescents are interested in their changing bodies and are preoccupied with personal appearance, body image, and being normal.)
- Acquire a set of values and an ethical system as a guide to behavior (This task, described by Havighurst, resembles Erikson's emphasis on the adoles-

FIGURE 11-10
Some characteristics of adolescent development.

Athletic activities and skills are important to both sexes in adolescence

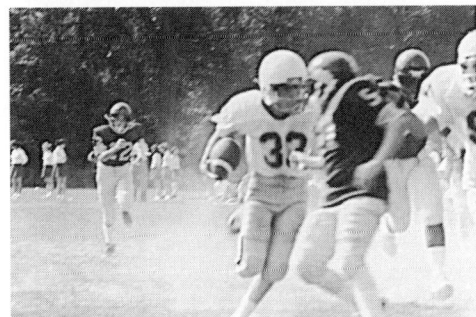

A primary developmental task of adolescence is to achieve new and more mature relationships with peers of both sexes

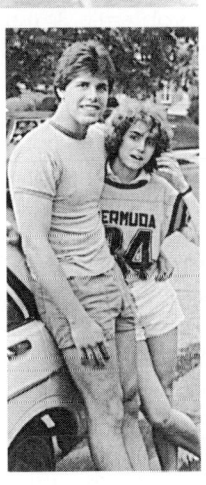

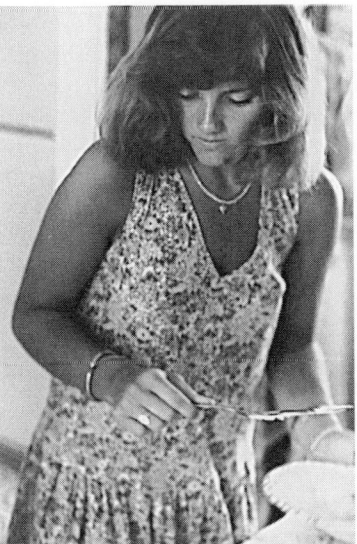

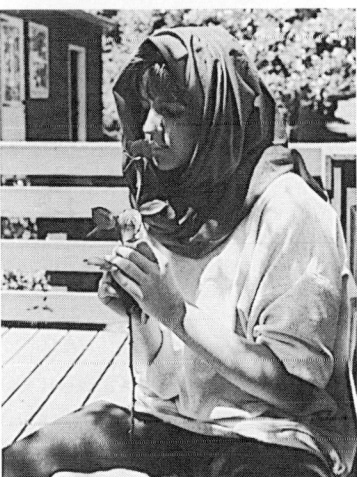

Physical appearance is extremely important to the adolescent

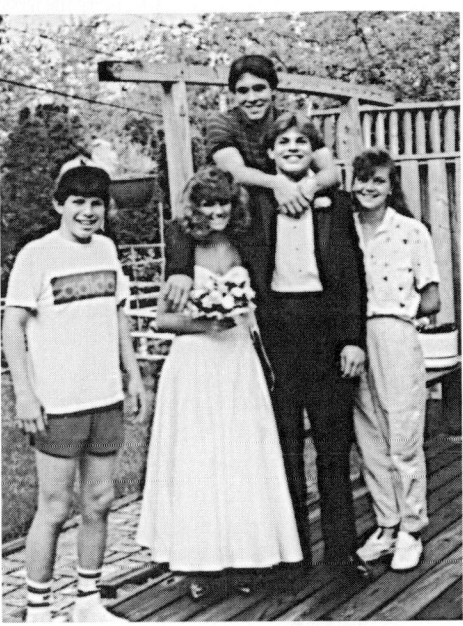

The prom is an opportunity to practice formal adult social skills among one's peers

The development of self-identity in adolescence involves "trying out" different roles and self-images, even if only in play

cent's need to achieve identity. Both theorists imply a need during adolescence for forming an ideology encompassing social, political, philosophical, and ethical values.)

- Desire and achieve socially responsible behavior
- Achieve emotional independence from significant adults (This period is characterized by ambivalence with a desire to be independent of adults yet with a lingering desire to be dependent. This ambivalence often results in rebellion against adults and in estrangement.)
- Prepare for long-term heterosexual relationships
- Prepare for a career

Temperament.   Remaining consistent with previous assumptions about temperament, the "easy" adolescent is likely to have the least difficult passage to adulthood. The "slow to warm" adolescent may have some under-

standable difficulties with developing significant heterosexual relationships. Such relationships may in fact be delayed until some adult confidence is gained. Turbulent adolescence will likely be the norm for the "difficult" individual. If the turbulence is purposeful and leads to the development of a secure self-concept in young adulthood, the possibilities are limitless for the headstrong adolescent.

Self-Esteem/Body Image.   Although not necessarily related, *self-esteem* and *body image* tend to be linked in these years because of the adolescent's preoccupation with physical appearance being a measure of personal worth. Considerable research abounds that gender and body type directly influence body image, self-concept, and self-esteem (Lerner and Spanier, 1980, p 217). Maturation allows for the inclusion of characteristics other than physical to influence self-concept.

Sexual Behavior. Rosemary Hogan (1985) has researched adolescent sexual behavior. While 62% of adolescents feel that premarital sex is acceptable, paradoxically, 51% feel that virginity is important to a marriage partner (p 250). Sexual intercourse among adolescent females living in cities was 50% in 1979, with the male percentage assumed to be higher (p 249). Masturbation and some homosexual activity in the form of mutual *masturbation* is quite common among males, less common in females (p 249). It is estimated that 1 million unwanted teenage pregnancies occur in the United States yearly, with 300,000 of these being terminated by abortion (pp 250, 252). While sexual activity is frequent in adolescence, accurate knowledge about sexual function and birth control is not.

Activities. Adolescent activity centers around the peer group. The activity may be purposeful such as watching a movie or sports event, or seemingly aimless, like driving around in a car "cruising" or "hanging around" a shopping center. The importance of the activity itself is secondary; with whom the activity is shared is of primary concern.

Athletic activity and skill are important to both sexes, both as a means of gaining prestige and maintaining general fitness. School clubs and activities, church groups, and community organizations and programs offer the necessary blend of activity and peer group opportunities.

Moral Development. Although Kohlberg's stages of moral development do not necessarily coincide with chronologic age, it can be assumed that the child enters adolescence at the "law and order orientation." It is possible that an individual can pass through adolescence and into adulthood remaining at that orientation. Because social order as an end in itself is the focus of the "law and order orientation," it is not entirely uncommon for individuals *never* to progress to a higher level of moral reasoning.

If, however, an individual begins to assess society itself as having moral obligations, a transition can be made to the next level of moral reasoning: *The postconventional level.* This level involves the presumption that society's rules are subjective and, therefore, relative. Because such moral reasoning requires formal operational thinking abilities, adolescence is the first developmental age at which such reasoning can occur.

Postconventional moral reasoning often places adolescents in conflict with their families. This conflict is a reaction to the adolescent's efforts to develop the process of making moral judgments on the basis of universal beliefs extracted from self-conscience.

Spiritual Development. The child enters adolescence with an accepted belief in a deity and literal interpretations of religious stories illustrating justice and righteousness. The ability to think in the abstract and the profound changes occurring in self-identity allow the adolescent to question beliefs and practices which may no longer stabilize identity or purpose. It is not uncommon for adolescents to temporarily abandon traditional religious practices. This abandonment is often disturbing to the adolescent's family. Some adolescents may find comfort in holding on to traditional beliefs as a means of maintaining some constancy to their lives. Questioning and reworking traditional beliefs, however, is more the norm.

At some time between late adolescence and adulthood, if the individual is able to take personal responsibility for self beliefs, a return to traditional practices, with a deeper understanding, may occur. Perhaps, however, the adolescent's search will produce a new set of beliefs entirely different from earlier traditions.

Common Health Problems in Adolescence

Many health problems occur in adolescence. It is not within the parameters of this book to elaborate on adolescent health problems. A pediatric or mental health nursing text can provide that information. The mention of a few common facts is prudent.

Acne. Although acne can be linked to the development of secondary sex characteristics, there are probably other compounding causes not yet proven. There are several factors linked to the development of acne: hormones, sensitivity to androgen levels, sebaceous gland hyperactivity, genetic factors, immunologic aberrations, and bacterial irritation (Waechter, Phillips, and Holaday, 1985). Poor hygienic practices are not seen as significantly influential in acne development. Overall self-esteem and body image are clearly affected in most adolescents with severe acne.

Substance Abuse. The use of illicit drugs and alcohol remains widespread in North America. Johnston, Bachman, and O'Malley (1984) indicated that nearly two-thirds of high school students in the United States had used illicit drugs in 1980. Similar information appears to be true of alcohol use.

Accidents. Accidents, particularly motor vehicle accidents, were the number one killer of adolescents in America in 1980 (Salkind and Ambron, 1987, p 562). A further disturbing feature of these statistics is that there is a high correlation between alcohol use and motor vehicle accidents involving adolescents.

Homocide. Homocide was the number two killer of adolescents in America in 1980 (Salkind and Ambron, 1987, p 562). The psychologic and sociologic dimensions involved in adolescent homocides are too complex to address in detail. The statistic itself, however, is disturbing.

Suicide. In 1980, suicide was the third leading cause of death in the age group 15 to 24 years (Salkind and Ambron, 1987, p 562).

Nutritional Difficulties. Fad dieting and socialization involving fast foods are common among adolescents. In the short run, such nutritional imbalances are harmless. For those adolescents who are obsessed with body image (particularly females), severe nutritional disorders can result. The two most common are **anorexia nervosa** (compulsive dieting to the point of self-starvation) and *bulimia* (a destructive cycle of binge eating followed by self-induced vomiting in an effort to prevent weight gain). The psychodynamics of these conditions are complex, but almost always involve severe family dysfunction. While these disorders were once considered rare, they now affect approximately 10% to 15% of young women between the ages of 12 and 25 years (Salkind and Ambron, 1987, p 510).

Adolescent Pregnancy. "If current trends are not reversed, 4 out of 10 teenaged girls will become pregnant before leaving their teens" (Papilia and Olds, 1986, p 252). Of these young women, the majority terminate their pregnancies by abortion. Of those who choose to maintain their pregnancy, 55% choose to keep their infants (Hogan, 1985, p 251). The economic, social, physical, and psychologic consequences of teenage parenthood are profound for the mother, the child, the father, and society as a whole.

Sexually Transmitted Diseases (STD). Adolescents engaging in sexual intercourse are at a higher risk for sexually transmitted diseases and their complications than are adults (Waechter, Phillips, and Holaday, 1985, p 593). Ignorance, lack of psychosexual maturity, and embarrassment are the most common reasons for this increased risk. **Gonorrhea** is the most prevalent STD among adolescents of both sexes. **Trichomonal** and **monilial infections** are very common in adolescent girls. *Chlamydial* infections occur in both sexes, as does **syphilis. Herpes simplex II (genital herpes)** occurs in both sexes and is considered one of the most serious STDs because it is incurable.

None of the current STDs, however, possess the serious implications for individuals and society as a whole that **Acquired Immune Deficiency Syndrome (AIDS)** does. Although AIDS can be transmitted by means other than sexual contact (*e.g.,* blood transfusions), the vast majority of transmission occurs through sexual relations. If current predictions are accurate, hundreds of thousands will die from AIDS and related complexes before the turn of the century. While initially thought to be unique to the homosexual population, its spread to the heterosexual population means that sexually active adolescents are at risk.

Nurses' Role in Adolescent Health Care

The emphasis on preventive teaching by the nurse (particularly the school nurse) continues in the adolescent years. Because of the nature of adolescence, a collaborative approach to teaching and planning is likely to be most effective. Areas of concern in adolescence and examples of teaching by the nurse are described in Table 11-15.

If required, nursing intervention may focus on care for acne, menstrual difficulties, prenatal care for a pregnant adolescent, or in hospital care for a drug abuser or adolescent diagnosed with anorexia nervosa. Perhaps one of the more significant roles the nurse may have during this crucial developmental phase is that of facilitator of healthy family relationships. Mutual respect, open communication, and accurate information exchange within families paves the road for a healthy transition from adolescent to adult.

YOUNG AND MIDDLE ADULTHOOD

Growth and development continue as a sequence of predictable patterns throughout life. As long as a person lives, he or she learns, adapts, and changes. The theorists discussed in Chapter 10 defined growth and developmental stages and tasks in all dimensions of the individual across the life span. Theories have also been developed to describe adult growth and development. Briefly included here is a summary of the theories most commonly used for the young and middle adult.

Adult Development Theories

Erikson's Developmental Crises. Erikson (1963) describes two major crises, with related tasks, for the young and middle adult. They are described in Table 11-16. If the developmental tasks are not accomplished and the crisis not resolved, the young adult becomes isolated and self-absorbed; the middle adult feels a sense of stagnation and loss. Adults who do not achieve the tasks satisfactorily tend to focus on themselves, becoming overly concerned with their physical and emotional health needs.

Levinson's Individual Life Structure. Levinson (1978) based his theory on what he calls "individual life structure," centered around the belief that the pattern of life at any point in time is formed by the interaction of three components—the self (values, motives), the social and cultural aspects of one's life (family, religion, career, ethnic background), and the particular set of roles in which one participates (*e.g.,* husband, daughter, friend, student). When anything changes in one component, the whole life structure must then reorganize. According to

T A B L E   11-15
Promoting Wellness in Adolescents

Area of Concern	Teaching
Substance abuse	• Advise adolescents of statistics, re: substance abuse • Discuss the risks of substance abuse • Discuss the physical consequences of substance abuse • Discuss the psychosocial consequences of substance abuse • Assist in preparing strategies for saying "no" to substance use
Motor vehicle accidents	• Encourage driver education classes for adolescents • Discuss the relationship of alcohol consumption and motor vehicle accidents
Suicide	• Assist teachers and caregivers to identify risk factors and data indicative of suicide risk (*e.g.,* decreased school performance, social withdrawal) • Advise adolescents with depression where to seek help (*e.g.,* psychiatrist, community clinics, crisis centers)
Nutrition	• Discuss healthy eating habits • Discuss dangers of excessive or nutritionally unsound dieting • Help caregivers and teachers recognize "risk" students • Advise adolescents who legitimately need to lose weight to consult a physician or respected weight loss organization (*e.g.,* Weight Watchers)

Sex education	• Provide factual information about physical and psychosexual development
	• Discuss the nature and prevention of STDs
	• Discuss "safe sex" pracites in relation to STDs, particularly AIDs
	• Assist with developing strategies for saying "no" to sexual activity for those who wish
	• If adolescent is or intends to become sexually active discuss responsible sexual behavior and birth control
	• Provide assistance to pregnant adolescents by
	  1. Discussing options
	  2. Encouraging medical care
	  3. Encouraging psychosocial counseling

Levinson, the major periods in young and middle adult life are

1. *Early adult transition* (age 18–22)—The major concerns are to break away from one's family, make initial career choices, establish intimate relationships, and select personal values, goals, and life-style.
2. *Entering the adult world* (age 22–28)—The person now builds on previous choices; there may be a transient quality to occupational choices and friendships.
3. *Settling down* (age 30–40)—The person invests energies in those areas of life most personally important (family, work, community) and strives to gain status, respect from others, and a sense of authority.
4. *Midlife transition* (age 40–45)—At this time of life, there is a reappraisal of goals and values. The indi-

vidual may choose to either continue, or reorganize and change, the established life-style.

5. *The pay-off years* (age 45–65)—This is a time of maximum influence, self-direction, and self-approval.

Gould's Transformation.   Gould (1972) believes that a central theme for the adult years is "transformation," with specific beliefs and developmental phases. These are that adults

- Age 18–22: Believe they have established control of themselves, but could be pulled back into the family
- Age 22–28: Feel established as adults and separate from their family, but believe they must demonstrate their competence as independent adults to their parents. They want to enjoy the present, but also build for the future.

TABLE 11-16
Developmental Tasks of Young and Middle Adulthood

Young Adult (20–30 years)	Middle Adult (40–60 years)
Stage/Crisis	
Intimacy versus isolation	Generativity versus stagnation
Tasks	
• Selecting a life partner • Choosing an occupation or career • Establishing independence from parents • Establishing intimate relationships • Establishing a social network • Forming a personal philosophical and ethical structure	• Establishing and guiding the next generation • Accepting middle-age changes • Adjusting to the needs of aging parents • Being comfortable with spouse • Reevaluating goals and accomplishments

- Age 29–34: There is no longer the preceived need to "prove" oneself, and self-acceptance increases. Marriage and careers are well-established, but questions about life in general are present.
- Age 35–43: Continually look inward and question self, values, and life. See time as having an end, and believe there is little time left to shape the behavior of adolescent children.
- Age 43–50: Believe personalities are set. Accept life span as having definite boundaries. Have a special interest in spouse, friends, and community.
- Age 50–60: Have decreased negativism and increased feelings of self-satisfaction. Spouse becomes a valued companion. There is a realization of mortality and a concern for health.

Although theorists divide adult life into various age groups by developmental stages and tasks, it is fairly common to use two major adult age groups. The remainder of the chapter will discuss the young adult (age 20–40) and the middle adult (age 40–60). Chapter 12 will focus on the changes and special needs of older adults.

Young Adulthood: The 20s and 30s

The young adult is considered to have reached maturity —to have completed physical growth and to have developed internal and external controls and values acceptable to society. There are no specific measurements of maturity of the average adult person. Each person is an individual, and a wide range of normal values and behaviors is considered to be healthy.

Physiologic Development

The young adult has well developed and coordinated organ systems, functioning at peak efficiency. Although some normal changes begin to take place during the latter part of the time period, for the most part physical changes are minimal. The major exception is in the pregnant woman. Table 11-17 illustrates the physical development of the young adult (as compared to the middle adult).

Psychosocial Development

Although physical growth and development are minimal, there are major psychosocial developmental requirements for the young adult. Included in the discussion of psychosocial development will be the major tasks of vocational and relationship choices.

Choosing a Vocation. The decision to enter the world of work is strongly influenced initially by the need to become independent of one's family and to be self-sufficient. Other factors influencing the choice of an occupation or career are the desire to get married, raise a family, and become a part of the community.

Occupational and career choices are largely tied to educational choices. Many careers necessitate education beyond high-school level. Adults learn from both informal and formal learning experiences, and are largely goal-directed learners. If the identified goals are to increase career opportunities, maintain financial stability, and pursue upward mobility, the adult will be motivated to learn and change. The major factor in achieving satisfaction with one's vocational choice is the belief that one is functioning to capacity and making a contribution to society.

Choosing Relationships. The developmental tasks of the young adult are centered around choosing a mate and establishing a family. In today's society, increasing numbers of young adults choose to remain single or to live together in heterosexual or homosexual relation-

T A B L E   11-17
Physiologic Development: Young and Middle Adult

Assessment	Young Adult	Middle Adult
General body structure	• Weight evenly distributed (wide normal individual variations)	• Fatty tissue is redistributed; men tend to develop abdominal fat, women thicken through the middle. • Weight gain
Skin and hair	• Skin smooth with decreased acne • Hair resilient and evenly distributed	• Dry skin • Wrinkle lines appear on the face. • Gray hair appears. • Men may begin to lose hair on the head.
Cardiovascular	• Well-developed with peak efficiency	• Cardiac output starts to decrease. • Increased fatigue
Musculoskeletal	• Maximum tone, strength, coordination	• Gradual decrease in muscle mass, strength, and agility • Loss of calcium from bones, especially in postmenopausal women
Sensory	• Normally full visual and hearing acuity	• Changes in visual acuity, especially for near vision (presbyopia) • Diminished hearing acuity, especially for high-pitched sounds
Reproductive	• Fully developed • Females have regular menstrual cycles • Males' sexual maturity remains at a peak.	• Decreasing hormone production resulting in menopause/andropause

ships. However, the accepted societal norm is still to fall in love with a member of the opposite sex, get married, and establish a family.

Establishing a Family.   The child-bearing family is a whole entity even though the physiologic changes take place in the woman. A brief description of the physiologic and psychologic adaptations and needs of pregnancy are included here because they are a major area in the life of the young adult.

Physiologic and Psychosocial Adaptations of Pregnancy.   The physiologic adaptations of pregnancy are summarized in Table 11-18; psychosocial adaptations and tasks are included in the following narrative.

Pregnancy may be considered a period of developmental crisis during which certain tasks must be completed for acceptance and coping by the expanding fam-
ily. The completion of the tasks is influenced by the psychosocial, cultural, and educational dimensions of the prospective parents. The gestational period can be considered to be 9 months in length, with each 3-month period called a **trimester**. Psychosocial needs of the pregnant woman, by trimester follow.

• *First trimester:* The verification of pregnancy may raise conflicting emotions in the woman. Her reactions will be influenced by factors such as whether the pregnancy was planned or unplanned, how the baby will affect career goals, and acceptance of her pregnancy by significant others. The tasks to be achieved are acknowledgement and acceptance of the pregnancy by self and others. If these tasks are met satisfactorily, the woman will have increased self-esteem and accept her new role as a mother.

• *Second trimester:* During the second trimester, body changes and fetal movement actualize the

FIGURE 11-11

The developmental tasks of the young adult center around establishing intimate relationships and a home, and getting started in an occupation.

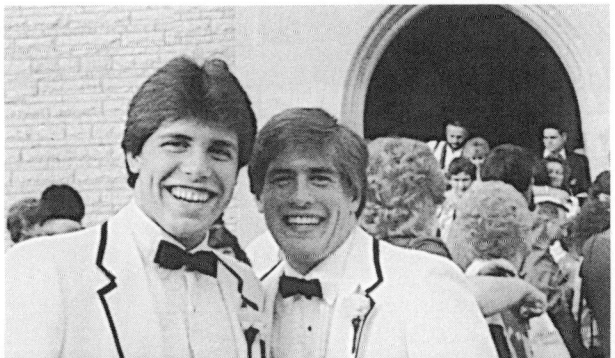

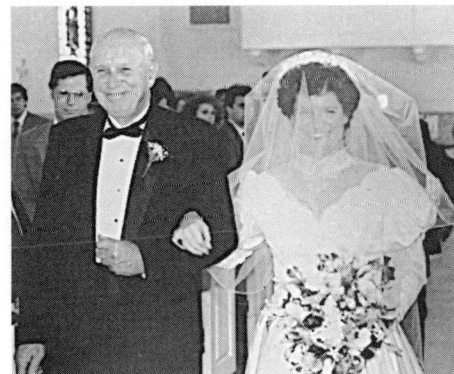

The primary tasks of young adulthood involve establishing intimate relationships and a social network, choosing an occupation or career, establishing a home, parenting, and forming a personal philosophical and ethical structure

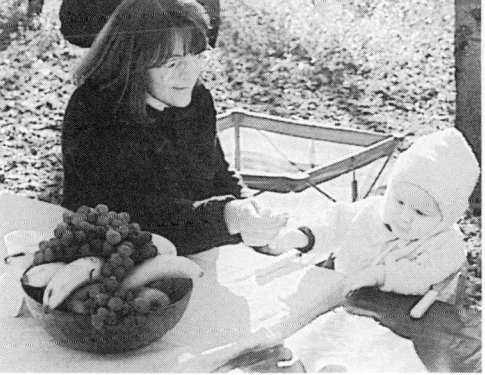

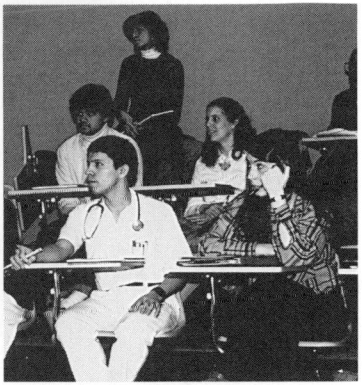

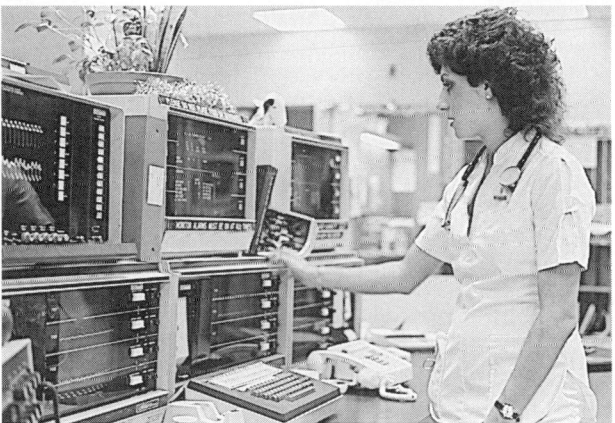

baby's presence. The woman can visualize herself as a mother, and the tasks to be achieved are to focus attention on her pregnancy and to assume responsibility for fetal well-being.

During this time period, visible body changes can result in altered body image, with either positive or negative effects. The woman commonly has mood swings. Concerns during the second trimester include normal development and health of both the baby and self, mothering capabilities, family acceptance, adjustments to the addition of a new baby, and labor and delivery of the baby. These concerns often lead to participation in prenatal classes by both parents.

• *Third trimester:* During the third trimester, physical and emotional changes, combined with altered body image and fatigue, can cause lowered self-esteem and irritability. The woman now centers on maternal tasks and the maternal role. She makes plans for the baby (room, clothes) and prepares herself for the labor and delivery process. During the latter months of pregnancy, the woman has increased needs for love and attention.

Psychosocial Needs of the Prospective Father.
The needs of the prospective father must be assessed too. Considerations for the father include

• Learning the physical and psychologic changes of pregnancy
• Accepting his supportive role in meeting maternal dependency needs
• Understanding alterations in sexual need and activity during pregnancy
• Exploring feelings about the developing infant

T A B L E   11-18
Physiologic Adaptations of Pregnancy

System	Normal Changes
Reproductive system	• Uterus enlarges to result in a 500–1000-fold increase in capacity. • Cervis has increased vascularity and mucous production. • Ovaries stop producing ovum, but produce hormones to maintain pregnancy. • Vagina increases in size, vascularity, and secretions. • Breasts increase in size and nodularity and begin to secrete colostrum.
Respiratory system	• Increase in oxygen consumption and tidal volume. Breathing changes from abdominal to thoracic as pregnancy advances
Cardiovascular system	• Blood volume increases to 30–50% above pregestational level. Blood flow to kidneys and uterus increases.
Gastrointestinal system	• May have nausea and vomiting during first trimester. Intestines and stomach are displaced by the growing baby; gastric emptying time and intestinal motility are decreased.
Urinary tract	• Enlarging uterus puts pressure on kidneys, ureters, and bladder.
Skin	• Changings in skin pigmentation are common, especially on the face and abdomen.
Skeletal system	• Accentuated lumbosacral spinal curve and postural changes accommodate the increased size and weight of the uterus.
Metabolic changes	• Average weight gain of 25–30 lb • Increased water retention • Increased protein, carbohydrate, and iron needs

• Learning about the birthing process
• Accepting his own feelings about the actual birth

In today's world, both parents are active participants in child care. They may share a leave of absence from work so that both can take turns in caring for the baby and in continuing in their respective careers. No longer is love and caring for children considered "women's work"; the result is stronger family unity and a greater acceptance of individual needs and goals.

Cognitive, Moral, and Spiritual Development

The young adult has the ability to solve problems and carry out logical reasoning. The ability to learn is enhanced throughout adult life by educational and life experiences. The young adult, as compared to the adolescent, is creative in thought, objective, realistic, and less centered on self. Although learning takes place in a variety of settings, the young adult often actively seeks formal educational opportunities, both as a post-high-school choice and as a means of changing directions in careers.

Young adults who have satisfactorily mastered previous levels of moral development (as defined by Kohlberg in Chap 10) enter the conventional level. At the conventional level, the person is concerned with maintaining expectations and values conformity, loyalty, and social order. It is estimated that 80% of adults do not move beyond this stage, or only do so as middle adults (Murray and Zentner, 1985).

Spiritually, the young adult focuses on reality and may ask questions about spirituality. This individuating–reflective period (as defined by Fowler) brings discovery of the meaning of values as they relate to the achievement of social purposes and to the acceptance of the value systems of others.

Common Health Problems of the Young Adult

The twenties and thirties are normally a time of generally good health, but physical and emotional health problems can result from life-style, developmental, or situational crises, family history, and the environment. Even if an illness does not appear at this age, the person is at increased risk later in life.

Life-style. There are a variety of risk factors present in the way a young adult chooses to live. Actual and potential health hazards of life-style are

- *Violent death:* Accidents are the leading cause of death in young adults, and suicide ranks third. Alcohol is associated with a major number of vehicular accidents.
- *Relationships:* Sexual experimentation and changing social values may result in unwanted pregnancy or sexually transmitted diseases (STD). STD include genital herpes, gonorrhea, syphilis, and acquired immune deficiency syndrome (AIDS).
- *Drug abuse:* Drug abuse is a major threat to the health of young adults. Prolonged use of a variety of substances can cause death, physical and emotional problems, and disease. Commonly abused substances are nicotine, alcohol, marijuana, amphetamines, and cocaine.
- *Diet and exercise:* Young adults require fewer calories than during adolescence (as growth is completed). Fast foods and busy life-styles often are a way of life, resulting in increased caloric intake and little exercise. As a result, obesity can become a health problem.

Developmental or Situational Crises. Throughout this period of life, stress is a factor in maintaining physical and emotional health. Increased stress may be job-related or family-centered. Family-centered problems include both positive and negative aspects: marriage, divorce, parenthood, death of a parent. The increased stress may precipitate mental or physical health problems, aggravated by ineffective coping mechanisms such as substance abuse, decreased nutrition and rest, and risk-taking behavior.

Family History. A family history of chronic diseases such as hypertension, heart disease, and diabetes increases the risk of the individual developing the disease.

Environmental. The young adult may be exposed to environmental pollutants at work. He or she may be at increased risk for illness or injury because of economic difficulties, poor housing and hygiene, and increased probability of accidents. Additionally, the young adult, actively spending leisure and work time in contact with others, increases exposure to acute infectious diseases.

Nurses' Role in Health Care

Many activities that promote health were discussed in Chapter 2. As with any client, the nurse must consider each young adult as an individual, taking a holistic view of special needs and influences on health maintenance. Nursing considerations specific to the young adult are

- Teaching the need for regular physical examinations and dental care, including screenings for diseases most common for this age
- Teaching preventive health practices related to nutrition, rest, substance use, and stress-related illnesses
- Providing information about sexuality, pregnancy, and health of the reproductive system through self breast and testicular examination, birth control and prevention of STD
- Providing and supporting safety education in the work place and in activities of daily living

Acute illness in the young adult is more of an annoyance that of serious consequence. If the young adult is hospitalized, he or she is usually strongly motivated to recover and regain normal activities. The nurse must remember that independence and self-sufficiency are important to the young adult; the dependent sick role is not easily accepted. Health care will be facilitated if the young adult is informed and involved in decisions about care.

Although chronic illnesses are less common, their occurrence in the young adult can lead to delayed development, loss of independence, and permanent changes in personal and career goals.

Middle Adulthood: The 40s and 50s

The middle adult years are a time of change in both physical and psychosocial dimensions. However, the changes are gradual and individualized. As the normal life span increases, most people in this age group still consider themselves young in relation to the older population. However, visible signs of aging and an awareness of time left to live make the middle adult evaluate achievement of goals and influence adaptation to older age.

Physiologic Development

The beginning of this period of life is one of maximum physical development and functioning. As the years progress, gradual physiologic changes—both internal and external—occur. These are not pathologic changes, but are rather normal changes resulting from aging. Self-image and self-concept must be altered to successfully adapt to and accept these normal changes. Physical development of the middle adult is illustrated in Table 11-17.

The hormonal changes that take place in midlife affect men and women differently. Women undergo a change called **menopause**, a gradual decrease in ovarian function, with subsequent depletion of estrogen and progesterone. This change usually occurs between ages 40 and 55. With the cessation of ovulation, menstrual periods stop (either gradually or abruptly); the woman usually also experiences "hot flashes," mood swings, and fatigue. The whole process lasts for several years, and on completion, the woman is no longer able to become pregnant. Men, however, do not have physical symptoms from the decreased levels of hormones, called **andropause**. Androgen levels diminish very slowly; the male may have some loss of sexual potency, but is still capable of reproduction.

Psychosocial Development

The middle adult years are a time of increased personal freedom, economic stability, and social relationships. Over 40 million Americans are in this age group; as a group they strongly influence government, education, business, and industry through earning power, payment of taxes, and decision making (Murray and Zentner, 1985). Two of the major developmental crisis faced by the middle adult are role transition and midlife crisis.

Role Transition.   A variety of changes can take place during the middle years. These changes may include marital relationship changes, as well as changes in relationships with both aging parents and independence-seeking children.

Relationships with one's spouse may go through contrasting changes during the 40s and 50s. Although this is usually a time of security and stability, with stronger emotional commitment and sharing, it may also be a time of disenchantment. The husband or wife may develop negative, critical feelings and attitudes as a result of changes in physical appearance, energy levels, and sexual needs and abilities. Dissatisfaction with achievement of career and family goals also contributes to the stresses placed on the marriage. Extramarital affairs and divorce may be the result.

Widowhood (the status change resulting from the death of a husband or wife) may take place in the middle years. The loss of a spouse is a major crisis and a threat to self-concept as well as a major role change. A multitude of changes may occur, including reduced income, changes in life-style and social relationships, and the need for help to work through the loss and grief.

The middle-aged adult is also caught in the middle of a "generation sandwich." Children are often independent, married, and have children of their own. Although much has been written about the "**empty-nest syndrome**" (resulting from the last child leaving home), most middle-age parents welcome the space, time, and independence when freedom from parenting occurs. However, as involvement and responsibility for children are decreasing, there may be increasing needs for care of and involvement with aging parents and other family members. The physical aging or death of a parent makes one's own aging and inevitable death a reality.

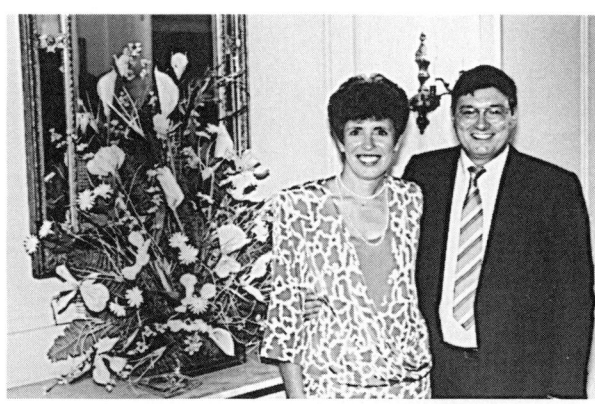

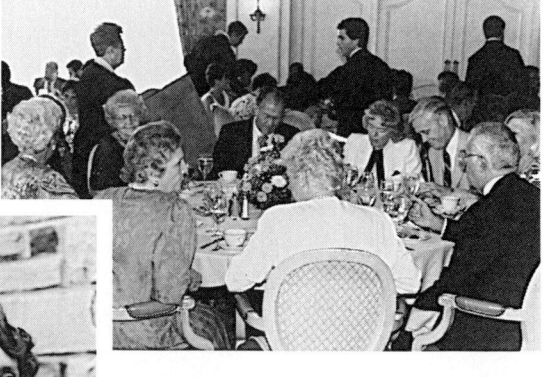

F I G U R E   11-12
The middle adult years are a time of increased personal freedom, economic stability, and social relationships.

The middle adult years are generally characterized by greater expendable wealth, renewed relationship with spouse, and expanded social relationships

Midlife Crisis. Gail Sheehy (1976) describes the ages of 35 to 45 as the "deadline decade" in which a midlife crisis occurs. The crisis results from the realization that the halfway point in life has been reached, and youthful goals may not have been achieved. Both men and women feel a sense of urgency to accomplish those things they have always wanted to do but have set aside to meet other responsibilities.

Women often respond to the crisis by getting a job or returning to school to prepare for a long-desired career. Men, on the other hand, may change jobs, seek upward promotions, or become involved in social and community activities. The successful resolution of the midlife crisis results in personality growth and increased self-satisfaction, as well as an acceptance and renewed enjoyment of the remaining years of one's life.

Cognitive, Moral, and Spiritual Development

Cognitive and intellectual abilities of the middle adult change very little from the young adult. There often is increased motivation to learn, especially if the knowledge gained can be immediately applied and has personal relevance. Problem-solving abilities remain throughout adulthood, although the time of response may be slightly longer. This is not due to a decrease in ability, but rather due to a longer memory search of increased amounts of material and to a desire to think a problem through before responding.

Morally, the middle adult may remain at the conventional level or may move to the postconventional level, especially if the person has had sustained responsibility for the welfare of others and has consistently applied ethical principles developed in adolescence. At this level, the adult believes that the rights of others take precedence and takes steps to support those rights.

As with moral development, not all adults progress to Fowler's paradoxical–consolidative state of spiritual development. Fowler believes that only some individuals reach this stage, and only after the age of 30. The middle adult usually is less rigid in beliefs and has increased faith and trust in spiritual strength.

Common Health Problems of the Middle Adult

The middle adult, like the young adult, is subject to physical and emotional health problems from life-style, developmental or situational crisis, family history, and the environment. Both acute and chronic illnesses may occur, but with increased age recovery time is lengthened. This is a result of slower and more prolonged responses to stressors, more pronounced reactions to an illness, and the possibility of more than one illness being present at a time (Schuster and Ashburn, 1986).

The leading causes of death in the middle adult years are motor vehicular accidents, occupational accidents, suicide, and chronic disease (cancer in women and heart attacks in men). Major health problems are cardiovascular and pulmonary diseases, cancer, rheumatoid arthritis, diabetes mellitus, obesity, alcoholism, and depression.

The risk of developing these common health problems is often a result of the combination of life-style and aging. As one gets older, energy requirements decrease. The middle adult tends to maintain eating patterns and caloric intake while, at the same time, having less physical activity. This trend can result in obesity and atherosclerosis, with increased risk for high blood pressure, coronary artery disease, renal failure, and diabetes. Additionally, smoking and alcohol consumption put the person at greater risk for lung cancer, chronic respiratory problems, liver disease, and peptic ulcers.

Chronic illness in the middle adult has a major impact on self-concept and may precipitate changes in life structure. For example, following a serious heart attack, a man may face changes in his family role, his earning capacity, and his social relationships. All of these changes are a source of great stress.

It is important to remember that middle age does not automatically result in physical and emotional health problems. The majority of men and women remain healthy throughout their lives, but knowledge of proper preventive health care and the special needs of this age group can lead to improved quality and quantity of life.

Nurses' Role in Health Care

Nurses have a major role in promoting health in the middle adult by teaching, serving as role models, and encouraging self-care responsibilities.

The following health promotion activities are recommended for the healthy middle adult:

- Complete physical examination every 2 years
- Annual dental examination
- Eye examination every 1 to 2 years; to include a test for glaucoma
- Maintain current immunizations
- Annual examination of fecal material for the presence of blood
- Women should
    Continue monthly breast self-examinations
    Have a baseline mammogram at 40 (especially if a family history of breast cancer is present) and periodically thereafter
    Have a Pap smear every 3 years (more often if estrogens or oral contraceptives are taken)
- Men should carry out regular testicular self-examinations and have regular prostate examinations.

The middle adult also should be taught the importance of proper nutrition, rest, and exercise, as well as the dangers of substance abuse. Referrals to support groups and individual counseling may be necessary in strengthening coping mechanisms and acceptance of personal and family changes.

Although the young and middle adult years are a

time of change, they are also the period of life when a person is at optimal physical and psychosocial functioning. Having successfully met developmental tasks, the adult is ready to enjoy the rest of life. A sense of continuity and adaptability, achieved from the beginning of the 20s to the end of the 50s, is essential to satisfactorily meeting developmental tasks of aging and to the enjoyment of one's remaining years.

KEY POINTS

- Heredity dictates an individual child's growth potential, while environment and nutrition influence the degree to which that potential will be reached.

- Growth and development in childhood begin rapidly, increase at a slower steady pace in the middle, and end rapidly.

- The development of higher levels of moral and spiritual reasoning is directly related to higher levels of cognitive ability.

- The family is an integral part of the growth and development of a child.

- Healthy development occurs if the tasks of each stage are completed prior to entering the next stage.

- The nurse's role in child health care is primarily focused on preventive teaching.

- An understanding of childhood development is essential to understanding adulthood.

- Growth and development continue as a sequence of predictable patterns throughout the adult life span.

- Erikson, Levinson, and Gould have described major developmental stages and tasks for the young and middle adult.

- The young adult has reached optimal physical development, but major psychosocial adaptation centers around choosing a vocation and defining relationship choices.

- Establishing a family (and the expanding family group) creates special tasks and needs of the young adult.

- During the middle adult years, visible signs of aging and an awareness of mortality appear. A variety of role changes may occur, and ''midlife crisis'' may precipitate changes in life-style.

- Young and middle adults are generally healthy, but increased risk for illness results from life-style, developmental or situational crises, family history, and the environment.

- Nursing considerations to promote health and prevent illness in adulthood focus on teaching self-care activities and the importance of regular physical examinations.

BIBLIOGRAPHY

Ainsworth MDS, Bleher MC, Waters E et al: Patterns of Attachment: A Psychological Study of a Strange Situation. Hillsdale, NJ, Erlbaum, 1978

Bee H, Mitchell S: The Developing Person: A Lifespan Approach. New York, Harper and Row, 1984

Engel W: The development from sound to phenome in child language. In Ferguson CA, Slobin DI (eds): Studies of Child Language Development. New York, Holt, Rinehart and Winston, 1973

Erikson E: Childhood and Society. New York, WW Norton & Co., 1963

Gould R: The phases of adult life: A study in developmental psychology. Am Psychiatry 129:33–43, November 1972

Hogan R: Human Sexuality: A Nursing Perspective. Norwalk, CN, Appleton-Century-Crofts, 1985

Johnston L, Bachman J, O'Malley P: Student Drug Use in America 1975–1980. Rockville, MD, National Institute on Drug Abuse, 1984

Lambs ME: The development of father–infant relationships. In Lamb ME (ed): The Role of the Father in Child Development. New York, Wiley, 1981

Lerner R, Spanier G: Adolescent Development: A Lifespan Approach. New York, McGraw-Hill, 1980

Levinson D et al: The Season's of a Man's Life. New York, Alfred A. Knopf, 1978

Miller B, Keane C: Encyclopedia and Dictionary of Medicine, Nursing and Allied Health. Philadelphia, WB Saunders, 1987

Mott S, Fazekas N, James S: Nursing Care of Children and Families. Menlo Park, CA, Addison-Wesley, 1985

Murray R, Zentner J: Nursing Assessment & Health Promotion Through the Life-Span, 3rd ed. Englewood Cliffs, NJ, Prentice-Hall, 1985

Myers N, Perlmutter M: Memory in the years from 2 to 5. In Ornstein P (ed): Memory Development in Children. Hillsdale, NJ, Erlbaum, 1978

Neeson J, May K: Comprehensive Maternity Nursing. Philadelphia, JB Lippincott, 1986

Nelson K: Structure and strategy in learning to talk. Monographs of the Society for Research in Child Development, 38, 1973

Papilia D, Olds S: Human Development. New York, McGraw-Hill, 1986

Reeder S, Martin L: Maternity Nursing: Family, newborn and women's health. Philadelphia, JB Lippincott, 1987

Salkind N, Ambron S: Child Development. New York, Holt, Rinehart and Winston, 1987

Santrock J, Yussen S: Child Development: An Introduction. Dubuque, IA, WC Brown, 1987

Schuster C, Ashburn S: The Process of Human Development: A Holistic Life-Span Approach, 2nd ed. Boston, Little, Brown, & Co, 1986

Scipien G et al: Comprehensive Pediatric Nursing. New York, McGraw-Hill, 1986

Sheehy G: Passages: Predictable Crisis of Adult Life. New York, EP Dutton, 1976

Thomas A, Chess S, Birch HG: Temperament and Behavior Disorders in Children. New York, New York University Press, 1968

Vygotsky L: Thought and Language. Cambridge, MA, MIT Press, 1962

Waechter E, Phillips J, Holaday B: Nursing Care of Children. Philadelphia, JB Lippincott, 1985

Whaley L, Wong D: Nursing Care of Infants and Children. St Louis, CV Mosby, 1987

Winick M, Brasel J, Rosso P: Nutrition and cell growth. In Winick M (ed): Nutrition and Development. New York, Wiley, 1972

12 The Older Adult

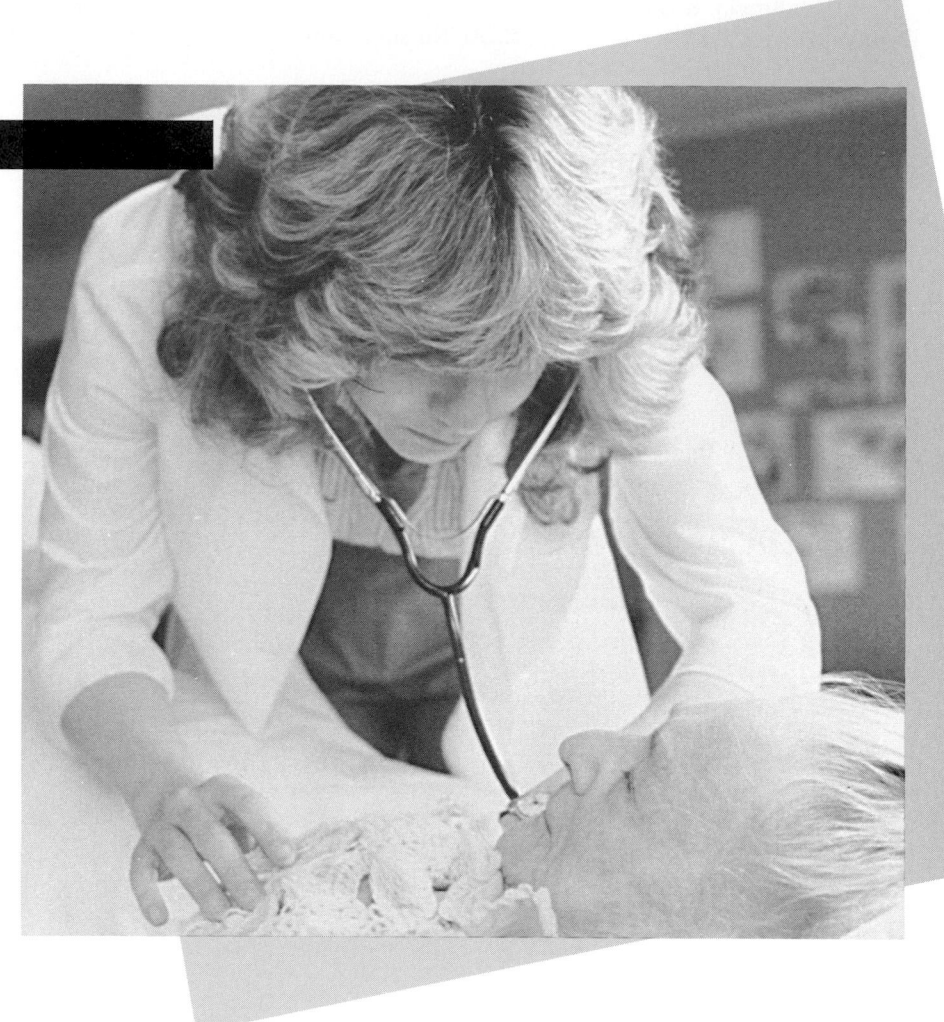

OBJECTIVES

After studying this chapter, the learner should be able to

Define key terms used in the chapter.

Describe common myths and stereotypes that perpetuate ageism.

Gain awareness of own feelings and attitudes toward the aging process and the older adult.

Compare physiologic and functional changes that occur with normal aging.

Discuss developmental tasks of the older adult, as described by Erikson and Havighurst.

Identify socioenvironmental factors in our society that may inhibit the older adult from meeting needs and realizing potentials.

Discuss nursing implications concerning the continued growth and development of the elderly client.

List family and community resources that can be utilized to maintain the health and independence of the elderly client.

The growth and development process continues as one ages, with no specific time or experience that causes a person to feel old versus young. Rather, aging is gradual and characterized by continued development, maturation, and ongoing adaptation in all areas of life. Our society has arbitrarily identified the **older adult** as someone over the age of 65 years. Those over age 65 are often grouped together and the same characteristics are applied to all of them. However, these individuals represent a diverse group, with a wealth of socioeconomic and cultural backgrounds and varied life experiences.

The population of the United States and Canada is growing older, and approximately 35% of the acute-care beds are now occupied by persons over 65 years old (Dychtwald, 1986). As the health-care system changes to accommodate the needs of the elderly, the nurse will increasingly care for both well and ill older adults in a variety of settings and therefore must understand the concepts of growth and development as they relate to older adults. Illness, functional disabilities, and hospitalization may cause major disruptions in the growth and development of any individual, but they can be particularly devastating to the elderly.

The nurse recognizes that these disruptions are small in relationship to the whole of life experiences. It is within the nurse's role to promote wellness, prevent illness, restore health, and facilitate coping with life experiences and to assist the client to continue to challenge and complete developmental tasks successfully to reach individual potentials as a unique human being.

AGING—A PARADOX IN SOCIETY

The older adult population is the most unique and diversified group in today's society because its members have lived the longest and have participated in and adapted to complex societal changes. Within the life span of the older adult, society has developed largely from a rural agricultural base, through industrialization, into a service-oriented high-technology base. Consider that in 1900, a 20-mile trip meant an all-day undertaking —probably in a horse-drawn wagon. Today a person can fly across the continent in less time and with considerably less effort. Most older adults have lived through the trauma of one or two world wars. Most had parents with strong ethnic ties to another country and many were immigrants themselves. The older adult has lived through the Great Depression of the 1930s and developed self-sufficiency. Major societal changes such as the enactment of Social Security and Medicare necessitated adaptations and helped shape the values and life-styles of older adults.

With advancing age, further adaptations become necessary because of physical or mental limitations, retirement, loss of a spouse or family members, or changing income. The older adult is faced with numerous role

KEY TERMS

ageism
alternative care
Alzheimer's disease
cognition
dementia
ego-integrity versus despair
frail-old
functional health
gerontic nursing
gerontology
iatrogenic
life review or reminiscence
old-old
older adult
reality orientation
social isolation
sundowning syndrome

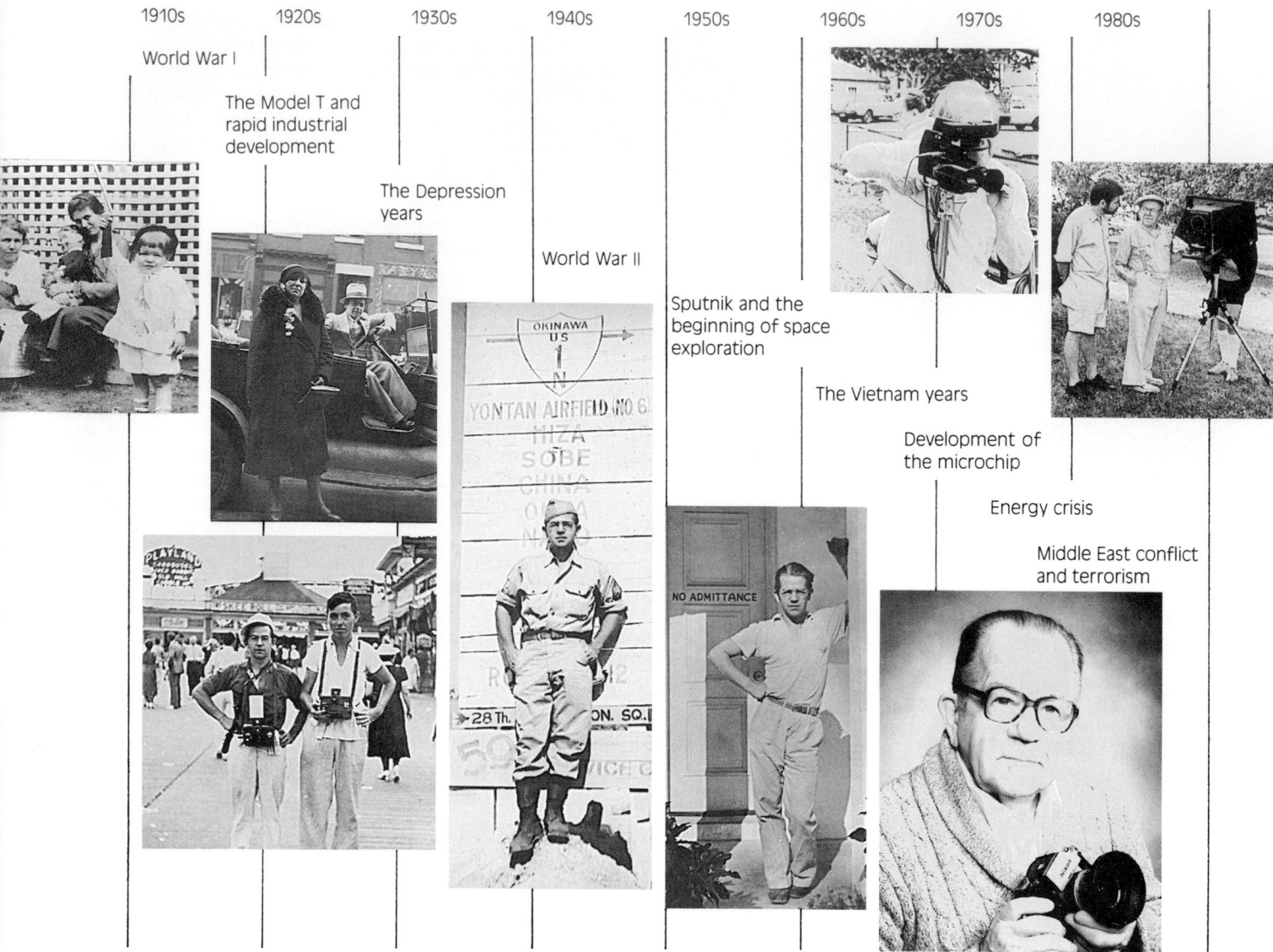

F I G U R E   12-1
The older adult population is a unique group with vast and diverse experience. Images from one man's life highlight some of the social events and change that this population group has experienced.

changes that may be directly related to chronologic age or health status. Lost roles must be replaced with new roles and activities that are acceptable and satisfying to the individual.

The elderly are thus facing a world that has necessitated both slow and abrupt adaptations. It is a time to reach one's potential and to satisfy long-range goals that may have been delayed because of other responsibilities. Willingly or unwillingly, it can also be a time to turn over to others "productive" tasks such as career or community leadership. Research has shown that the vast majority of older adults do adjust and adapt to new roles (Costa et al, 1981), and most are satisfied with their lives

and what they have. Depending on the older adult's adaptability and supportive resources, older adulthood may promote feelings of happiness, peace, and understanding, or of sorrow, conflict, and confusion.

Ageism—Common Stereotypes

The older adult has been the victim of ageism. **Ageism** is a form of prejudice, like racism, in which older adults are stereotyped by characteristics found in only a few of the members of this group. Fundamental to ageism is the view that the elderly are different from "me" now and will remain different from "me" in the future; they there-

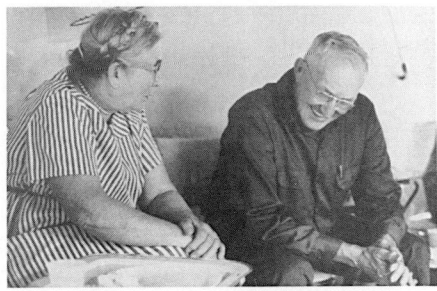 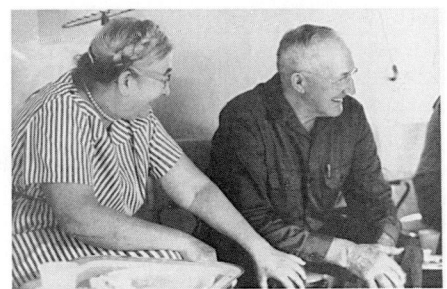
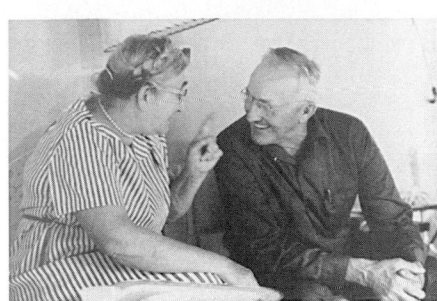 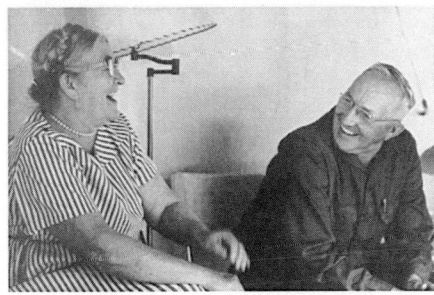

F I G U R E 12-2
Stereotypical images of the older adult as narrow-minded, forgetful, sexless, and dependent are untrue for most of the older adult population. This couple exhibits the vitality, sensuality, joy, and playfulness of a young couple. (Photos by Karen Baldwin)

fore do not experience the same desires, needs, and concerns (Hendricks and Hendricks, 1986). Perhaps this viewpoint developed with the post–World War II baby boom and the emphasis on a youth-oriented society, along with a tendency to deny our own aging and mortality. Industrialism and technologic advancements have placed a high priority on productivity so that retired individuals may be said to have "outlived their usefulness." Along with this, the younger generations have often lost ties to the older generation because of increased mobility of the nuclear family and thus lack experiences with older relatives and their friends.

The elderly may be *incorrectly* depicted as rigid or narrow minded, unable to learn, unreliable because of memory loss, too old for sex, or child-like and dependent. People often fear advancing age because of the pervasive views that the elderly are very poor, lonely, in frail health, and able to look forward only to institutionalization in a nursing home. The above descriptors, each of which is discussed in this chapter, are not true for the large majority of older adults.

Changing Values With a Graying Population

A man reaching his sixty-fifth birthday can expect to live approximately 14 more years; a woman of the same age can expect 18.5 years (Hendricks and Hendricks, 1986). Because of declining birth rates and longer life spans, the percentage of the population over age 65 is growing rapidly. It is estimated that by the year 2030, one in five persons in the United States and Canada will be over 65 years of age. (AARP, 1987). Not only are people living longer, but they are healthier at older ages than ever before. Medical advances have played a major role in the decline of morbidity and mortality, as have a variety of other factors, including improved nutrition, environmental and sanitation controls, and a growing emphasis on exercise and healthy life-styles.

This shift in the age of the population is influencing all of society and helping to shape social, political, and health-care issues. Older adults are emerging as a strong social and political force. Consider organizations such as the American Association of Retired Persons (AARP), which provides educational and community service programs for those over 50 and lobbies for legislative change in issues regarding the older adult at both state and federal levels. Other examples include the proliferation of retirement planning magazines, media advertisements for health and life insurance, and retirement centers.

Who Is the Older Adult?

Contrary to myth, most older adults adjust well and continue to live active, independent, and productive lives. The majority are satisfied with their lives, finding retirement and old age more enjoyable than they had anticipated. Three fourths live in their own homes and one third of these live alone. Because of their longer life span, there are 1.5 times as many older women as men. The great majority of older adults continue to maintain close ties with their families and have incomes above the poverty level (AARP, 1987; Kovar, 1986).

Functional Health Versus Disease

The majority of older adults regard themselves as healthy, and most deny severe limitations in activities.

The vast majority will never be institutionalized, nor will they suffer effects of senility. *Healthy,* however, does not necessarily mean the absence of disease. Over 80% of older adults suffer from at least one chronic illness. Like younger adults, older adults tend to define their health in relation to how well they function, that is, whether or not they are able to engage in their usual and desired daily activities. This functional health definition includes the individual's ability to remain self-reliant, to "make do," and to maintain a sense of control and independence over self and environment.

It is important to note that *older adulthood* is a general term encompassing everyone over 65 years old. **Old-old** or **frail-old** are terms used increasingly to identify individuals over 75 years old. This group is the fastest growing segment in our population. In 1984, there were two million people over 85 years of age still living in the community (Kovar, 1986). In fact, only 5% of all older adults live in nursing homes, but 40% of those who do are over the age of 85 (Ebersole and Hess, 1985). The old-old have special significance for nursing care because they are more likely to need help with mobility and basic activities of daily living. They may need increasing assistance to maintain a safe and comfortable living environment. The older the individual, the more likely that he or she will need family and community support to maintain functional health.

Family and Reverse Roles

Spouse and other family members are natural support systems who help the older adult maintain functional health and independence and meet developmental tasks of old age. Supportive assistance may include the provision of transportation, food, shelter, ongoing social interactions, and even complex medical and nursing treatments. It should be remembered that significant others, such as close friends or neighbors, may also take on tasks formerly assumed to be the responsibilities of the traditional family. Contrary to common stereotypes, families do feel a responsibility toward their elders; most live within an hour of each other and have visited within the last week (Hendricks and Hendricks, 1986).

Not all families are able to assist an aged member satisfactorily because of factors such as geographic distance, low income, poor health, strained marital relationships, or infringement on career or life-style. Adult children may feel "sandwiched" between responsibilities for their own children and careers and the needs of elderly parents. It can be a very guilt-ridden and emotionally draining time for all involved when physical or emotional illness reverses roles and strains family resources.

The nurse must recognize that the whole family is the client and assess the family for capabilities and limitations in assisting the aged member. The nurse can help ease the strain by listening to client and family concerns and by validating the importance of family needs. The nurse assists the client and family to find workable solutions and may refer the family to community support services.

GROWTH AND DEVELOPMENT THROUGHOUT THE LIFESPAN

The principles of growth and development apply to people of all ages. As discussed in Chapter 10, the process of growth and development involves a series of changes that usually occur in an orderly and predictable sequence but at variable rates. The onset and the effect of those changes are influenced by numerous biologic, psychosocial, and environmental factors. Each individual is therefore unique. In old age, growth hastens the process of physiologic decline first encountered in middle adulthood. However, development and maturation continue throughout older adulthood, depending to a great extent on the individual's sense of self-concept and prior ability to adapt.

Physiologic Theories

Growth refers to biologic processes that result in physical change. In older adulthood, the process of aging becomes progressively more rapid. There are numerous theories describing how and why aging occurs, but none are universally accepted. The genetic theory of aging explains that life span depends to a great extent on genetic factors. Genes within the organism control "genetic clocks" that determine the occurrence and rate of metabolic processes, including cell division. The wear-and-tear theory explains that organisms "wear-out" from increased metabolic functioning, and that cells become exhausted from continual energy depletion in adapting to stressors (Schuster and Ashburn, 1986). There is no agreement as to why some people, even within families or similar environments, age much more rapidly than others. Although internal processes may in part predetermine aging, other factors such as drugs, nutrition, and smoking may also play a role.

Physiologic Status

In the older adult, all organ systems experience some degree of decline in overall functioning and the body becomes less efficient (see the box entitled Normal Physiologic Changes of Older Adulthood). Body functions that require integrated activity of several organ systems are the most affected. For example, renal function, which is dependent on cardiac output and condition of the vascular system, declines by about 50% from age 30 to age 80 (Schuster and Ashburn, 1986). The most frequently encountered chronic disorders are cardiovascular disorders such as hypertension or coronary artery dis-

Normal Physiologic Changes of Older Adulthood

General Status
- Progressively decreasing efficiency of physiologic processes results in a fragile balance and hinders the body's ability to maintain homeostasis.
- Physical or emotional stressors cause the older adult to be more vulnerable because of decreased physiologic reserves.
- The older adult may continue to engage in all activities of middle age but intuitively adjusts to a modified pace and more frequent rest periods.

Integumentary
- Wrinkling and sagging of skin occur with decreased skin elasticity; dryness and scaling are common.
- Balding becomes common in men, and women experience thinning of hair also; hair loses pigmentation.
- Skin pigmentation and moles are common, although the skin may become pale because of loss of melanocytes.
- Nails typically thicken and become brittle and yellowed.

Musculoskeletal
- Decreases in subcutaneous tissue and weight are frequently found in the old-old.
- Muscle mass and strength decrease.
- Bone demineralization occurs and bones become somewhat porous and brittle.
- Joints tend to stiffen and lose flexibility and range of motion may decrease.
- Overall mobility commonly slows and posture tends to "stoop." Height decreases slightly.

Neurologic
- The central nervous system responds more slowly to multiple stimuli. Hence, the cognitive and behavioral response of the older adult may be delayed somewhat.
- Rate of reflex response decreases.
- Temperature regulation and pain perception become less efficient.
- The sense of balance declines, and fine movements may become more difficult.
- Sleep at night typically shortens and the older adult may awaken more easily. Cat naps become common.

Special Senses
- Diminished visual acuity (**presbyopia**) occurs, with increased sensitivity to glare and decreased ability to adjust to darkness. Cataracts may further obscure vision.
- Diminished hearing acuity (**presbycusis**) occurs, particularly diminished pitch discrimination in the presence of environmental noises.
- The senses of taste and smell are decreased.

Cardiopulmonary
- Blood vessels become less elastic and often rigid and tortuous. Venous return becomes less efficient. Fatty plaque deposits continue to occur in the linings of the blood vessels. Lower extremity edema and cooling may occur, particularly with decreased mobility.
- The body is less able to increase heart rate and cardiac output with activity.
- Pulmonary elasticity and ciliary action decrease so clearing of the lungs becomes less efficient. Respiratory rate may increase, accompanied by diminished depth.

Gastrointestinal
- Digestive juices continue to diminish and nutrient absorption decreases.
- Malnutrition and anemia become more frequent.
- With reduced muscle tone and decreased peristalsis, constipation and indigestion are common complaints.

Dentition
- Tooth decay and loss continue for the majority of older adults.
- Eating habits may change, particularly if the older adult lacks teeth or has ill-fitting dentures.

Genitourinary
- Blood flow to the kidneys decreases with diminished cardiac output.
- The number of functioning nephron units decreases by 50%; waste products may be filtered and excreted more slowly.
- Fluids and electrolytes remain within normal ranges, but the balance is fragile.
- Bladder capacity decreases by 50%. Voiding becomes more frequent; two to three times a night is usual. A decrease in bladder and sphincter muscle control may result in stress incontinence or incomplete bladder emptying.
- About 75% of men over 65 years old experience hypertrophy of the prostate gland; surgery may be required if urinary retention occurs.
- There is atrophy, decrease of secretions, and thinning of the older woman's genital tract.

ease, cancers, and skeletal disorders such as arthritis and osteoporosis.

Functional Status

There is growing evidence that aging is not synonymous with disease or disability. Although 80% of older adults experience one or more chronic disorders, their ability to adapt determines whether they are ill or healthy. Most continue their activities from middle age and adapt intuitively to gradual limitations of aging. It may take longer to complete any given activity, or the activity may need to be modified. An older adult with arthritis may need to use an electric rather than a manual can opener; an individual with coronary artery disease may need three hours, with intermittent rest periods, rather than one hour to mow the lawn.

The greatest threat to the health of older adults is that the physiologic reserve of the various organ systems is gone. When illness occurs, increased physical and emotional stress places the older adult at risk for complex reactions. The older adult is more likely to develop complications and to require longer to recover. For instance, an elderly client with a hip fracture is at high risk for pneumonia and skin breakdown because of immobility, decreased ability to expel pulmonary secretions, and thinner and more fragile skin. The nurse knows that the older client has less reserve and works to maintain normal functioning. Complications are prevented by careful assessment of the symptoms and by assisting the client to cough and deep breathe, turn, and carry out personal hygiene.

Cognitive Development

The term **cognition** is used to indicate cerebral functioning, including the ability to perceive and understand

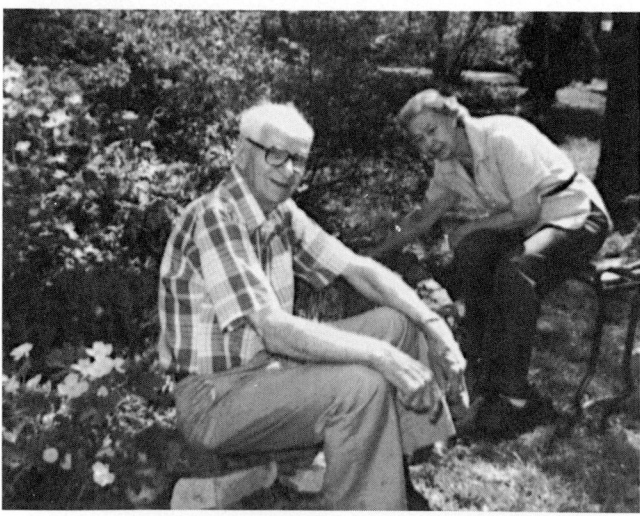

F I G U R E   12-3
This couple, married 61 years, enjoy gardening together. They've found that they can continue most activities of middle age with only minor adjustments.

Cognitive Status of the Older Adult

- Intelligence increases into the 60s, and learning continues throughout life.
- Cognitive functioning is related to use. Reasoning ability and abstract thought remain astute, particularly for usual situations and familiar experiences.
- Processing and reaction times increase and may be evident in slower and seemingly more deliberate responses.
- There is a decreased capacity for adaptation, especially in stressful or unfamiliar environments and with impaired senses.
- Recent memory loss may occur but long-term memory remains intact.

---

one's world. Cognition does not change appreciably with aging. The older adult continues to learn and problem solve, and intelligence and personality remain consistent (see the box entitled Cognitive Status of the Older Adult). It is normal, however, for the older adult to take longer to respond and react, particularly in new or unfamiliar surroundings. Knowing this, the nurse should slow the pace of care and allow the older client extra time to ask questions or complete activities. In the United States, of the 25 million persons over the age of 65, only 5% suffer from a serious mental impairment, and only 10% will experience a moderate loss of memory (Dychtwald, 1986). Mild short-term memory loss occurs commonly, but can be remedied by the older adult with the use of notes, schedules, and calendars.

When serious mental impairment occurs, the effect on the client and family can be devastating. **Dementia** is a term used to describe a variety of organically caused disorders that progressively affect cognitive functioning. Of the dementias affecting older adults, **Alzheimer's disease** is the most common. Alzheimer's disease affects brain cells and is characterized by patchy areas of the brain that degenerate, or break down. The person with Alzheimer's faces a progressively serious and ultimately fatal disease. At first, forgetfulness and impaired judgment may be evident. Over a period of several years, the person becomes progressively more confused, forgetting family and becoming disoriented in familiar surroundings. When the ability to care for even simple activities of daily living is lost, the person will require constant supervision and care, often in a nursing home. Currently, there is no effective medical treatment for Alzheimer's disease. Comprehensive and empathetic nursing care, however, is important for any of the dementias. The nurse directs nursing care to ensure the client's safety and to meet basic needs of nutrition and fluids, elimination, and hygiene. Both the client and family need emotional support and teaching and may benefit from community resources that can ease the family's burden.

In the health-care field, confusion and depression in the older adult are sometimes mistaken for permanent dementias. However, drug interactions, circulatory or metabolic problems, or even nutritional deficiencies are likely to be the real cause. The older adult may also become confused when too many changes or losses occur at one time or when moved to a radically different environment. A type of confusion called **sundowning syndrome** sometimes occurs, where the older adult habitually becomes confused with darkness. The nurse can assist other members of the health team in determining the cause of the client's confusion and in helping to reorient the client. For example, the nurse uses **reality orientation** to redirect the client's attention to what is real in the environment. Nursing interventions include the use of calendars and clocks, calling the client by name, and talking about the client's family and the season. The client is also encouraged to make decisions to promote a sense of control over the environment. The nurse must remember that frequently older adults have hearing and visual impairments. These impairments can be counteracted by speaking clearly and slowly, looking directly at the client, and repeating instructions. The environment should be well lighted but without glare.

Developmental Theories

Development continues throughout the life span; new tasks associated with older adulthood are identified, and new behavioral patterns emerge. An early controversial psychosocial theory, called *the disengagement theory,* maintained that older adults withdraw from societal interactions because it is mutually desired and satisfying for both the individual and society (Schuster and Ashburn, 1986). However, later studies have shown that isolation is not desired or acceptable, and that as societal interactions decrease, the healthy older adult increases close relationships with family and friends (Berkman, 1983). According to the *activity theory,* successful aging involves the ability to maintain high levels of activity and functioning. The older adult may substitute activities but does not slow down or disengage from society. The *identity–continuity theory* assumes that healthy aging is related to the ability of the older adult to continue similar patterns of behavior that existed in young to middle adulthood (Schuster and Ashburn, 1986).

Most theorists agree that a person's self-concept is relatively stable throughout adult life. The older adult who has developed a strong sense of self-identify and has successfully met challenges in earlier life will probably continue to do so. This person will substitute new roles for old roles and perhaps continue former roles in a new context. For example, the business manager, on retirement, may continue to use leadership talents in community organizations. Older adults with a strong self-concept typically describe themselves as being healthier than others or "young for my years." On the other hand,

events that accompany aging can threaten a person's self-concept. Depending on the person's outlook on life and past ability to cope, events such as retirement, loss of health or income, or isolation can be devastating. For example, the retired teacher whose sense of identity was closely tied to career may suddenly find that friends, income, and sense of accomplishment are lost and consequently may feel a great loss of control and self-identity.

Psychosocial Development—Erikson

Erikson identifies **ego-integrity versus despair** and disgust (Erikson, 1980) as the last stage of human development, which begins around the age of 60. The older adult continues to look forward, but now also looks backward, and begins to reflect upon his or her life. It is a time for realization of a "wholeness" perspective, with an inner search for meaning and order of the life cycle. The older adult searches for emotional integration and acceptance of the past and present, as well as acceptance of physiologic decline without fear of death. The nurse is familiar with older adults who like to retell stories or past

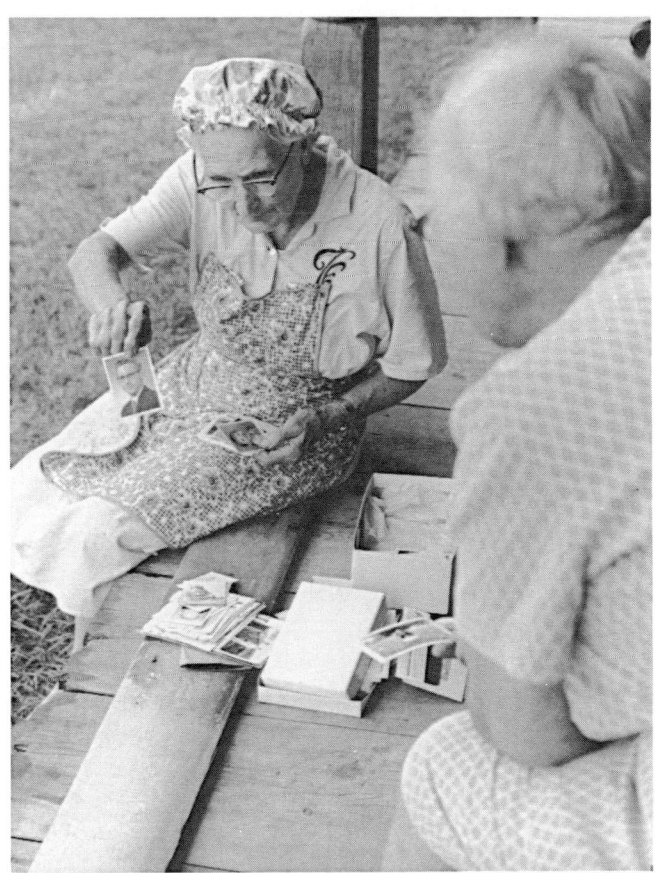

F I G U R E **12-4**
Reminiscing is a culturally universal phenomenon of aging. It is a way for the older adult to reassess life experiences and further develop a sense of accomplishment, fulfillment, and reward in life. (Photo by Karen Baldwin)

events. This phenomenon is called **life review** or **reminiscence** and has been identified worldwide. In a sense, it is a way for the older adult to relive and restructure life experiences, and is a part of achieving ego-integrity.

As with other developmental stages identified by Erikson, ego-integrity is facilitated when the older adult has successfully accomplished tasks earlier in life. It can be a time to look backward with pride and without regrets and forward with optimism and enthusiasm. However, the individual who regrets the past and sees the problems of the present as insurmountable may despair. This person may view life as a series of unresolved problems and missed opportunities, and feel worthless or hopeless. The despairing individual may wish to do things over but fears the lack of time before death.

Tasks of midlife continue or resurface. The older adult still strives to guide the coming generations and to leave something behind (generativity vs stagnation). The need for love and closeness continues (intimacy vs isolation), as does a strong sense of who one is in relation to family and community (identity vs role diffusion). Because of physical and social changes associated with aging, the older adult is repeatedly faced with the need to adapt and to again face already completed tasks.

Developmental Tasks—Havighurst

According to Havighurst, the major tasks of old age are primarily concerned with the maintenance of social contacts and relationships. Successful aging depends on the individual's ability to be flexible and adapt to new age-related roles. The individual must "find new and meaningful roles in old age while maintaining reasonable comfort within the social customs of our times" (Ebersole and Hess, 1985, p 131). The developmental tasks that according to Havighurst are associated with "later maturity" (Havighurst, 1972) are listed in the accompanying box. Each task is further discussed below.

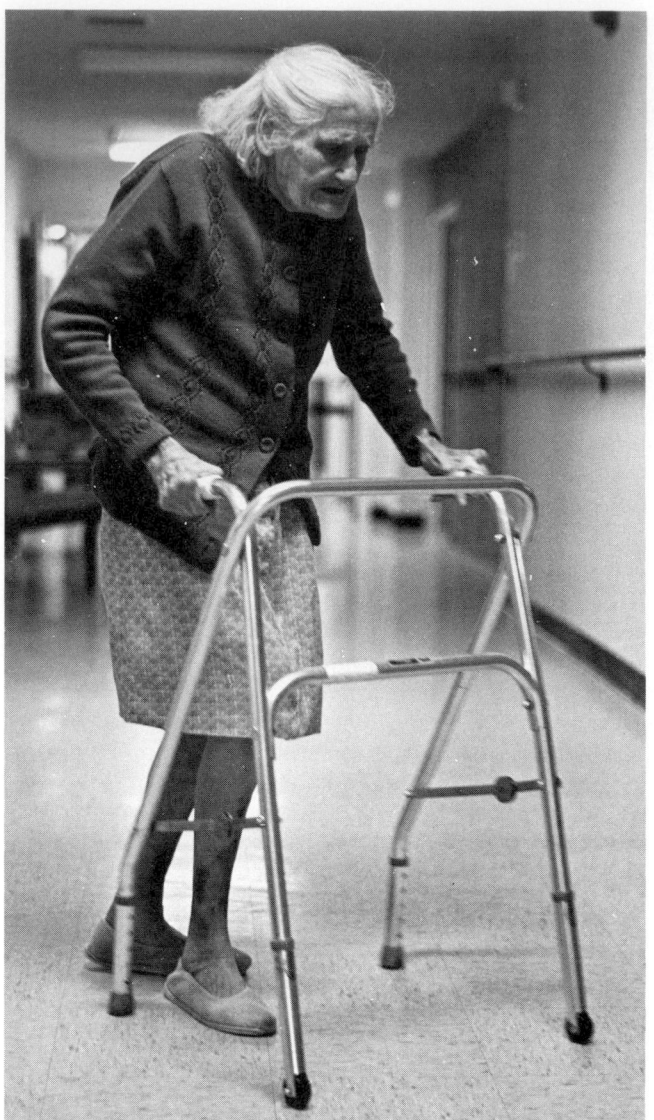

F I G U R E   12-5
This resident of an extended-care facility illustrates some of the characteristics found in the old-old: chronic disease such as arthritis, stooped body posture, gray hair, wrinkled, pigmented skin, circulation changes, and loss of teeth. Yet she maintains her functional health and independence with the assistance of her walker.

Havighurst's Developmental Tasks of Later Maturity

- Adjusting to declining physical strength and health
- Adjusting to retirement and reduced income
- Adjusting to changes in health of one's spouse
- Establishing an explicit affiliation with one's age group
- Adopting and adapting social roles in a flexible way
- Establishing satisfactory physical living arrangements

Adjusting to Declining Physical Strength and Health. As stated earlier, most older adults gradually modify their life-styles to accommodate for declining vigor and strength. Rest periods become more frequent; at the same time, continued activity is very important for maintaining all physiologic functions. The older adult is at high risk for accidents and falls and may need to curtail driving or use a cane or other aid to remain mobile. Modification in diet and prescribed medications may be necessary, and because of chronic illness, the older adult may need to adjust to living with pain. With severe illness, loss of independence over oneself and one's environment can occur. The loss of health is difficult to adjust to because it affects every aspect of life.

Adjusting to Retirement and Reduced Income.

Retirement brings a change in a person's concept of time. The older adult must learn to occupy leisure time in a way that maintains self-esteem and is personally satisfying. Retirement is considered to be the hallmark of old age, and satisfaction with retirement is closely tied to income and the relationships one has outside of work. Most older adults manage on smaller incomes after retirement, but about 21% live at or near the poverty level (AARP, 1985). Lack of finances can affect the older adult's ability to meet all needs, from adequate medical care and housing to social and creative interests.

Adjusting to Changes in the Health of One's Spouse.

When one's spouse becomes ill or dies, numerous and difficult adjustments must be made. The older adult may face new roles for the first time. The husband may begin to cook meals; the wife may learn to handle family finances. These role changes come at a time when stress is already very high. Physical care can be overwhelming if the other spouse is also in poor health. Adaptations may occur in living conditions and life-style, and the spouse may need to plan social and recreational events alone.

The need for love and belonging does not diminish with age and may become acute with the loss of one's spouse. We are sexual beings and our sexual behavior does not necessarily stop in old age. Sexuality encompasses who we are and the older adult is no exception. Like younger adults, the older adult needs to express intimacy physically by touching and emotionally by sharing joys, sorrows, ideas, and values.

Establishing an Explicit Affiliation With One's Age Group.

With an aging population, social organizations for older adults are becoming more numerous. For example, most communities have senior citizens' centers that offer meals, social and informational programs, and other activities for a nominal fee. Other organizations offer the opportunity for travel, cultural events, and political involvement. Affiliation with other people of the same age allows older adults to share common interests and concerns and find status among their own age group. It should not be assumed, however, that older adults want to associate only with others of the same age.

Adapting and Adopting Social Roles in a Flexible Way.

Social roles change with the developmental tasks and adjustments of older adulthood, but the need to feel valued, useful, and productive continues. The older adult may develop new hobbies or increase involvement in community, church, or family affairs. He or she may do volunteer work or even launch into a new career. If the older adult is unable to adjust and form new relationships, social isolation can become a real problem. **Social isolation** is a sense of being alone and lonely because of fewer meaningful relationships. It may occur because of declining health or income, transportation problems, or ageism. Whatever the cause, prolonged social isolation has been correlated to declining health and higher mortality rates (Berkman, 1983).

Establishing Satisfactory Physical Living Arrangements.

The ability to function safely and independently at home depends a great deal on functional health, transportation, income, and family. The older adult, for example, may need assistance with home repairs, house cleaning, or grocery shopping. Architectural barriers such as steps may need to be modified. Easy community access to medical and recreational facilities and churches may become more important. In urban areas, fear of crime may necessitate changes in living arrangements. Many older adults in poor health may be able to continue to live at home with some assistance from visiting community nurses or with the aid of other services such as home-delivered meals or senior transportation.

Most older adults prefer to live in their own homes. It is very difficult to move from one's home. Moving in with adult children creates changes in roles and author-

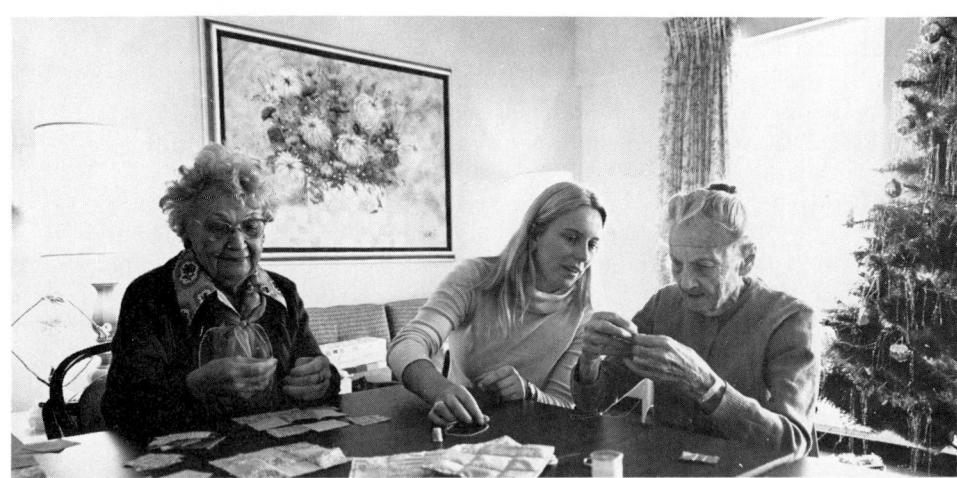

FIGURE 12-6
Social relationships and satisfying leisure activities remain important throughout life. These women are making holiday gifts to help support their community nutrition center.

ity. When moving to an extended-care facility such as a nursing home, the loss of one's home and sometimes possessions and the need to conform to the routines of institutional living can be very traumatic for the client and family. However, some people choose to move for convenience, social relationships, and needed health care.

In recent years, retirement centers and senior citizens' housing have flourished. For those needing health care, alternative methods of care have become available. Examples of **alternative care** are respite care facilities that allow the family a needed rest by temporarily housing and caring for an ailing older family member and day-care centers that provide a safe and stimulating environment during the day when family members must work. The nurse must be knowledgeable as to what health care and social services are available in the client's community so the client and family can be in-

formed. Thus, the nurse can effectively work with other members of the health-care team to ensure that the client gets needed services.

GERONTOLOGY AND THE HEALTH-CARE SYSTEM

Knowledge of aging has increased dramatically in the last 40 years. **Gerontology** is the scientific and behavioral study of all aspects of aging and its consequences. Normal changes that occur with aging are the result of complex interactions between genetics, biologic systems, and physical and social environments. Disease complicates a person's ability to adapt and maintain **functional health** (the ability to carry out usual and desired daily activities). Often, mental or physical decline in the older

R E S E A R C H   I N   N U R S I N G   *Making a Difference*

Older Adult

Demographic trends project that the number of older adults in our society will continue to rise. The health concerns of older adults are unique and often poorly understood. Nurses have begun to research the elderly from such varied perspectives as risk management, physiologic changes occurring with aging, and nursing care systems to best meet the health-care needs of this population.

Related Research

Franz R, Kinney C: Variables associated with skin dryness in the elderly. Nurs Res 35:98–100, 1985

Franz and Kinney's study compares sebum secretion rates and dry skin in the older adult. Although decreased sebum secretion was found, there was no significant correlation with the presence of dry skin. They concluded that variables such as hygiene, nutrition, medications, and medical conditions contribute to dry skin, and that more research needs to be done to learn the causes and effective treatment methods to combat skin dryness in the elderly.

Lund C, Sheafor M: Is your patient about to fall? Journal of Gerontological Nursing 11(4):37–41, 1985

This study examined the question "Could a profile of risk elements [for the elderly] for falling be identified?" High-risk indicators identified were (1) hospitalization during September, October, or

November; (2) three or more unit transfers; (3) use of assistive ambulatory devices; (4) certain medications (vitamins, iron, diuretics, hypotensives, anticonvulsants); and (5) having a cognitive impairment. Implications for nursing include assessments of high-risk elderly clients and protection from falling by implementing safety measures.

Miller A: Nurse/patient dependency—Is it iatrogenic? J Adv Nurs 10:63–69, 1985

In this study, Miller investigated the effects of nursing care on client dependency levels. No significant differences in dependency were found in short-stay clients who received either task-oriented or individualized (based on nursing process) care. However, the provision of the two types of nursing care for long-stay clients resulted in higher levels of dependency being associated with task-oriented care. The conclusion was that dependency levels of geriatric inpatients often result from the type of nursing care given and are therefore iatrogenic.

Nursing research in this area has important implications for nursing practice. As the elderly population increases, it becomes more and more important to determine how to best maintain optimal functioning. Implications include (1) implementing safety strategies to prevent falls, (2) individualizing care based on age-related needs, and (3) evaluating the impact of nursing care delivery systems on the elderly.

adult may not be directly related to the aging process but rather results from the absence of supportive care and services that could prevent disease and maintain the older adult's ability to function.

The aging population has greatly strained a health-care system that has traditionally focused on "cures" and acute disease processes. For the older client with chronic disorders, the focus of care should include the client's and family's goals and emphasize the promotion of functional health and independent living to the greatest extent possible. Gerontologic or gerontic nursing does just that. **Gerontic nursing** combines basic knowledge and skills of nursing with a specialized knowledge of aging in both illness and health.

Nursing Implications

Although specific nursing care adapted to the needs of the elderly client is described throughout this text, general implications for care are included here. The nurse must recognize physiologic and psychosocial interrelationships and view the older client holistically.

Illness can severely disrupt an older adult's ability to function independently. The ill client is under increased physical and emotional stress, which increases the risk for complications because of the lack of physiologic reserves. When a client is hospitalized or institutionalized, family and community interactions are severely inhibited. The acute-care environment itself adds new stressors, such as diagnostic tests, treatments, or surgery. In the face of new and unfamiliar routines and sensory stimulation, prior coping skills may not work, and the older client will likely feel a decrease in the ability to understand and control the new environment. The elderly client is more likely than a younger client to suffer multisystem dysfunctions, **iatrogenic** complications caused by medications or treatments, accidents such as falls, and increasing dependence and confusion.

Major nursing care goals are to assist the elderly client to function as independently as possible and to continue to develop individual potentials. The nurse works with the family and other disciplines to prevent complications of illness, to secure a safe and comfortable environment, and to promote the client's return to wellness. General guidelines for nursing care follow:

- Maintain the client's physiologic reserves. Closely assess the client so that complications caused by the stress on other body systems are discovered early.
- Prevent multisystem complications. Include nursing care that maintains physical integrity and function, such as skin care and planned rest and activity times.
- Provide a safe and uncluttered environment with comfortable temperatures and good lighting. If the environment is new or unfamiliar, orient the client to routines and equipment. Closely observe the client for his or her ability to protect against falls and other accidents.
- Slow your pace of care. Allow the client extra time to carry out activities, particularly those requiring physical coordination, such as grooming and eating.
- Encourage independence. Do not help the client if your assistance will benefit a "time factor" only. Keep your client and family informed and involved as much as possible.
- Beware of the stereotype of ageism. Treat each client as a unique individual. Although many older clients have similar needs, factors such as background, interests, capabilities, values, and life-style may differ greatly.
- Promote continued development. Assist the client and family to accept physical limitations. Work with them to adapt the environment so that functional health is maintained. Ask yourself the following questions:

  Does the client have obvious developmental lags that need to be further identified?

  Is the client/family deprived of normal needs or activities because of institutionalization?

  Is the client deprived of normal learning experiences because of physical or sensory limitations?

  How can we help the client/family to find creative alternatives to accomplish developmental tasks?

- Know resources available in your facility and community. Work with the health-care team to provide assistance needed and desired by the client and family.

KEY POINTS

- Aging is a gradual process. Older adulthood is characterized by continued development and adaptation. The older adult population is the most unique and diversified group in our society.

- Ageism is a form of prejudice in which the older adult is incorrectly stereotyped as "different" from other members of society. Also, aging is not synonymous with disease.

- The aging population shift is helping to shape social, political, and health-care issues.

- Most older adults adjust well to aging and continue to live active, independent, and productive lives. The majority of older adults regard themselves as healthy, although 80% have one or more chronic disorders.

■ The old-old (those over 75) are most likely to need assistance with carrying out activities of daily living.

■ The spouse and family are natural support systems who typically help the older adult maintain health and independence.

■ Gerontic nursing is a specialty field within the nursing profession, with specialized knowledge of aging in both health and illness that can benefit all nurses.

■ In older adulthood, physiologic aging becomes more rapid, with all organ systems showing decline in efficiency. The lack of physiologic reserves places the elderly client at risk for multisystem complications.

■ The older adult continues to learn and problem solve; intelligence and personality remain consistent after middle age.

■ According to Erikson, ego-integrity versus despair is the last stage of human development. The older adult continues to look forward but also reflects back on life experiences to find meaning and acceptance.

■ Havighurst views the major tasks of older adulthood to be primarily concerned with social relationships and roles.

■ A major goal of nursing care is to help the client promote functional health; the nurse does this by working with the client, family, and health-care team.

BIBLIOGRAPHY

American Association of Retired Persons: A Profile of Older Americans: 1987. Washington, DC, Program Resources Dept. AARP. Publ. #PF3049 (1187). D996, 1987

American Nurses' Association: A Statement on the Scope of Gerontological Nursing Practice. Kansas City, MO, American Nurses Association, 1981

American Nurses' Association: Standards for Gerontological Nursing Practice. Kansas City, MO, American Nurses' Association, 1976

Beam IM: Alzheimer's disease: Helping families survive. Am J Nurs 84:228–232, 1984

Berkman LF: The assessment of social networks and social support in the elderly. J Am Geriatr Soc 31:743–749, 1983

Boettcher EG: Linking the aged to support systems. J Gerontol Nurs 11(3):27–33, 1985

Burggraf V, Dolan B: Assessing the elderly: System by system. Am J Nurs 85:974–984, 1985

Costa PT, McCrae RR, Norris AH: Personal adjustment to aging: Longitudinal prediction from neuroticism to extraversion. J Gerontol 36:78–85, 1981

Delapp TD: Helping the elderly live longer and better. Nursing '83 13(11):61–63, 1983

Dychtwald K: Wellness and Health Promotion for the Elderly. Rockville, MD, Aspen, 1986

Ebersole P, Hess P: Toward Health Aging—Human Needs and Nursing Response, 2nd ed. St Louis, CV Mosby, 1985

Eliopoulos C: Gerontological Nursing, 2nd ed. Philadelphia, JB Lippincott, 1987

Erikson E: Identity and the Life Cycle. New York, WW Norton & Co, 1980

Fulmer TT et al: Assessing elder abuse. Journal of Gerontological Nursing 10(12):16–20, 1984

Gerontological Nursing Special Interest Group: Statement on Gerontological Nursing in Missouri—MoNA. The Missouri Nurse 55(2):6–7, 1986

Golightly CD et al: Planning to meet the needs of the hospitalized elderly. J Nurs Adm 14(5):29–39, 1984

Havighurst RJ: Developmental Tasks and Education, 3rd ed. New York, Longman, 1972

Hawranik P, Kondratuk B: Depression in the elderly. The Canadian Nurse L'infirmiere 82(9):30–34, October, 1986

Hazard MP, Kemp RE: Keeping the well elderly well. Am J Nurs 83:567–569, 1983

Hendricks J, Hendricks CD: Aging in Mass Society—Myths and Realities, 3rd ed. Boston, Little, Brown & Co, 1986

Kovar MG: Aging in the Eighties: Preliminary data from the supplement on aging to the national health interview survey. Vital and Health Statistics of the National Center for Health Statistics, number 115, Jan–June 1984. United States, 1986

Nagley SJ: Predicting and preventing confusion in your patients. Journal of Gerontological Nursing 12(3):27–31, 1986

National League for Nursing: Overcoming the Bias of Ageism in Long Term Care. NLN Publication #20-1975, 1–147. New York, National League for Nursing, 1985

Picariello A: A guide for teaching elders. Geriatric Nursing 7(1):38–39, 1986

Ravish T: Prevent social isolation before it starts. Journal of Gerontological Nursing 11(10):10–13, 1985

Schuster CS, Ashburn SS: The Process of Human Development—A Holistic Life-Span Approach, 2nd ed. Boston, Little, Brown & Co, 1986

Sherwood S et al: Alternative paths to long-term care: Nursing home, geriatric day care hospital, senior center, and domiciliary care options. Am J Public Health 76(1):38–44, 1986

Shine MS: Discharge planning for the elderly patient in the acute care setting. Nurs Clin North Am 18:403–410, 1983

Yurick AG, Spier BE, Robb SS, Ebert NJ: The Aged Person and the Nursing Process, 2nd ed. Norwalk, CT, Appleton-Century-Crofts, 1984

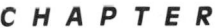

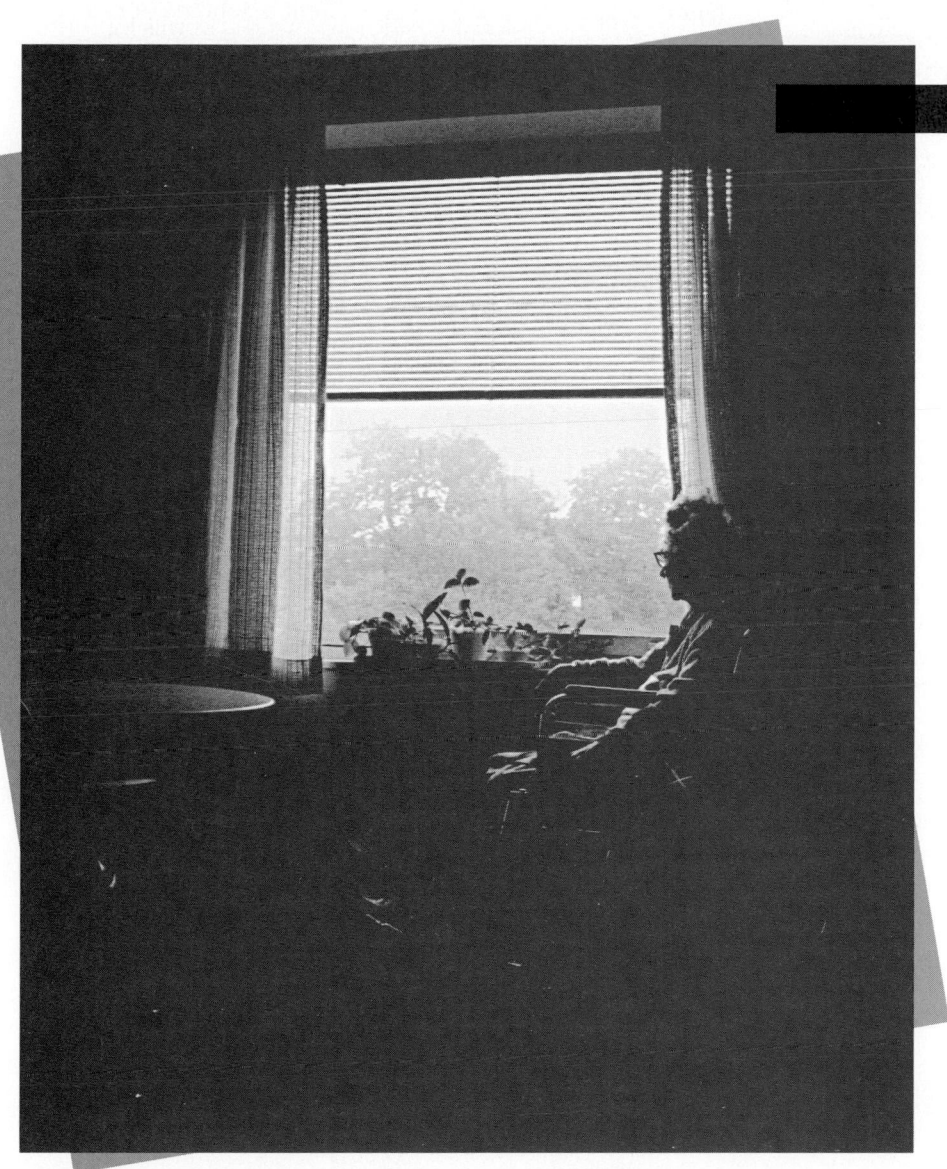

Loss, Grief, and Death

OBJECTIVES

After studying this chapter, the learner should be able to

Define key terms used in the chapter.

Differentiate the types of loss.

Describe the grief process and the stages of grief.

Outline physiologic and psychologic care of a dying client.

Identify ethical/legal issues concerning death.

List the clinical signs of approaching death.

Outline nursing responsibilities following death.

Discuss the role of the nurse in caring for a client's family.

The life continuum begins with birth and ends with death. As a member of a family, a person may experience the death of a loved one at any point in the continuum. This chapter appears in the section on human development because at some point in each individual's life, he or she will experience loss and grief, which can impact on the developmental stages of life. The concept of death is difficult to accept for many individuals.

Because the goals of health-care personnel and agencies are cure, health maintenance, and health restoration, a client's death is often viewed as a personal failure on the part of health personnel. The nurse is a key person in the care of both the client who is dying and the family, regardless of whether the client is at home or in a health care agency. Both the client and family turn to the nurse for support and assistance. To provide effective care, the nurse must have reconciled his or her own feelings about death and must understand the phases of grieving and dying and be able to recognize their manifestations.

KEY TERMS

actual loss	hospice
anticipatory loss	loss
bereavement	mourning
death	perceived loss
dysfunctional grief	physical loss
grief	psychologic loss
grieving	terminal illness

LOSS AND GRIEVING

Loss

Loss occurs when a valued person, object, or situation is changed or made inaccessible so that its value is diminished or removed. There are several types of loss, all of which may be experienced at some time by every individual. **Actual loss** can be recognized by others as well as by the person sustaining the loss; loss of a limb, of a spouse, of a valued object such as money, or of a job are all examples of actual loss. **Perceived loss** is perceived by the individual but is intangible to others; loss of youth, of financial independence, or of a valued environment are examples of perceived loss. Directly related to actual and perceived loss are **physical loss** and **psychologic loss**. An individual who loses an arm in an automobile accident suffers from both the physical loss of the arm and the psychologic loss that may be caused by an altered self-image and the inability to return to his or her occupation. These losses are simultaneously physical, psychologic, and actual. An individual who is scarred but does not lose a limb may suffer a perceived and psychologic loss of self-image.

Another type of loss is **anticipatory loss**, where the individual displays loss and grief behaviors for a loss that has yet to take place. Anticipatory loss is often seen in families of terminally ill clients and serves to lessen the impact of the actual loss of a family member.

Loss can have a tremendous impact on the development of an individual, and age affects an individual's reaction to loss (see Factors Affecting Grief, later in this chapter). Although adults can often accept death on an intellectual level, they may have trouble dealing with it on an emotional one. The loss of a friend, a pet, or a job often helps adults anticipate and cope with the loss of a spouse or other loved one.

Grieving

Grieving is the emotional reaction to loss and occurs with loss due to separation as well as loss due to death. Individuals who divorce often experience grief, and loss of a body part, a job, a house, or a pet may cause grief. **Bereavement** is the state of grieving during which an individual goes through grief reaction. **Mourning** is the period of acceptance of loss and grief during which the individual learns to deal with the loss.

Bereavement, which is experienced by both the client and the family, may have profound health consequences, requiring additional care. Bereaved persons often neglect their health to an extreme, whereas mourning is characterized by a return to more normal living habits.

Grief Reactions

Grief is the emotional pain caused by a loss. Reactions to both grief and dying are similar. The stages of these reactions overlap and vary among individuals. One individual may skip a reaction stage, while another may repeat an earlier stage; each individual is different, and clients and family members may be at different reaction stages.

Engel (1964) was among the first to define stages of grief. Engel's six stages are (1) shock and disbelief, (2) developing awareness, (3) restitution, (4) resolving the loss, (5) idealization, and (6) outcome. *Shock and disbelief* are usually defined as refusal to accept the fact of loss, followed by a stunned or numb response: "No, not me." *Developing awareness* is characterized by physical and emotional responses such as anger, feeling empty, or crying: "Why me?" *Restitution* involves the rituals surrounding loss, and with death includes religious, cultural, or social expressions of mourning such as funeral services. *Resolving the loss* is dealing with the void left by the loss, and *idealization* is the exaggeration of the good qualities of the person or object lost, followed by acceptance of the loss and a lessened need to focus on it.

Outcome is the final resolution of the grief process, including dealing with loss as a common life occurrence.

Kübler-Ross (1969), considered a pioneer in the study of grief and death reactions, defined five stages of reaction similar to those of Engel: (1) denial and isolation, (2) anger, (3) bargaining, (4) depression, and (5) acceptance. Kübler-Ross's work is discussed in greater depth under Stages of Dying, later in this chapter. Other works in the grief process literature include that of Clark (1984), who describes three stages of grief, and Martocchio (1985), who describes five grief groupings. More important than the actual stages of any given grief reaction is the idea that grief *is* a process and that it varies from individual to individual.

Normal Versus Dysfunctional Grief

Both normal and dysfunctional grief may be delayed, and normal grief may be either abbreviated or anticipatory. *Abbreviated grief* is of short duration but is genuine; *anticipatory grief* is grief that occurs before the actual loss, as in the extended terminal illness of a family member. **Dysfunctional grief** is abnormal or distorted; it may be either unresolved or inhibited. In *unresolved grief,* the individual may have trouble expressing feelings of loss or may deny them; unresolved grief also describes a state of bereavement that extends over a lengthy period of time. In *inhibited grief,* the individual suppresses feelings of grief and may manifest somatic symptoms instead.

FACTORS AFFECTING GRIEF AND DEATH

Many factors, including age, family relationships, socioeconomic position, and cultural and religious influences, affect an individual's reaction to and expression of grief, and like the stages of grief reaction, vary from individual to individual.

Developmental Considerations. Children do not understand death on the same level as adults do, but their

---

Grief and Death Reactions

Engel's Six Stages of Grief Reactions
1. Shock and disbelief
2. Developing awareness
3. Restitution
4. Resolving the loss
5. Idealization
6. Outcome

Five Stages of Kübler-Ross' Grief and Death Reactions
1. Denial and isolation
2. Anger
3. Bargaining
4. Depression
5. Acceptance

sense of loss is just as great. Both terminally ill children and their siblings are more likely to talk and ask questions about death in an attempt to understand it (Waechter et al, 1985). Terminally ill children of all ages require parental love and support, as well as social interaction with other children. Death of a parent or another significant person can retard a child's development or may cause the child to regress developmentally; children need to go through the same grief reactions that adults do in order to accept such a loss and maintain emotional well-being.

The loss of a parent by a middle-aged adult often helps to prepare the adult for the loss of a spouse or significant other, as well as to accept his or her own eventual death. The elderly may lose a spouse or have friends and relatives their own age die. As this happens they reminisce about life, put their lives and the purpose of living in perspective, and prepare themselves for their own inevitable death.

Family. Roles within families are important factors affecting reactions to and expressions of grief. For example, the eldest sibling may feel a need to "be strong" and therefore may not grieve openly; an individual who loses a spouse will often display the same type of behavior in order to "protect the children."

The death of a child is usually a devastating experience for the family. The family of a child needs time to accept the reality of the situation, opportunities to talk and to be listened to, and the experience of expressing themselves behaviorally in a nonjudgmental environment. The family of a terminally ill child may express feelings of guilt for wondering if they were responsible for the impending death. A sibling may suppress a guilt feeling for having wished the ill child (or a parent) dead.

Socioeconomic Factors. A bereaved family may suffer more acutely if there is no health or life insurance or pension after the death of the family provider. Such families face not only the loss of a loved one, but an economic loss that may further disrupt family life. The elderly especially may be placed in a difficult position, since the death of a spouse may result in a source of retirement income being either diminished or cut off for the surviving spouse, leading to loss of home, community, and support systems.

Cultural Influences. Both the physical and emotional manifestations of grief may be influenced culturally. Schulz (1978) defined the clinical symptoms of grief as repeated somatic distress, tightness in the chest, choking or shortness of breath, sighing, empty feeling in the abdomen, loss of muscular power, and intense subjective distress. Other symptoms include vomiting, dizziness, fainting, fatigue, weight loss, headaches, and chest pains (Gonda and Ruark, 1984).

Culture also influences an individual's expression of grief. In many families in the Western culture, grief is a private matter shared only with the family. As such, many individuals internalize their feelings of grief and may not express grief or feelings of loss to others. On the other hand, cultural background may necessitate the client's and family's public display to be emotional and distressed, with loud weeping and moaning.

Although sex roles have become more unified in the last few decades, male and female reaction to death may differ. The widow who has a job may not be as emotionally distraught as the woman who has needed her husband for support. Likewise, the widower who has not taken care of the children or the house may view the future more bleakly than the man who has cooked meals and changed diapers. Some ethnic traditions may be ingrained in certain persons and the woman may be expected to be weak and need support, whereas the man may be expected to be emotionally supportive. This varies from culture to culture and from person to person.

Religious Influences. Faith and religious practices play an important role in the expression of grief and provide comfort and solace to the individual experiencing loss. Often, persons who have put spiritual matters in the background of their lives have found death to be an impetus for a return to earlier practices of religion. At the same time, others may blame God for the death of their loved one and turn away from God.

Cause of Death. Death may result from a variety of causes, and the grief response often depends on the cause. Many deaths are sudden and involve shock as well as normal grieving in the survivors. *Death from disease* brings with it a variety of responses, including belief that the death is a punishment (for example, when AIDS was first diagnosed in homosexuals and drug users), terror and panic (when people are reminded of the devastation caused by plagues of earlier centuries), and guilt (when family and friends feel they could have prevented the death). *Accidental death* is often associated with feelings of bad luck. The guilt response can be enormous, especially when children die as the result of an accident. *Death while defending a country* usually is viewed by most of society as honorable and necessary. *Violent deaths* occur daily, especially in the bigger cities of North America. Suicide accounts for a great number of violent deaths, and in fact, among teenagers has become a major concern. It is also believed that many accidental deaths are actually suicides.

DYING

Needs of the Dying

A dying client has a variety of options concerning death, and the client's wishes should, if possible, be followed. Clients may choose to die at home, in a hospital or nursing home, or in a hospice. It is important that the client, if able, and the client's family take an active role in planning for care. Such planning ensures that the client's preferences are taken into consideration and also aids the client and the family in the acceptance of death. It also recognizes psychologic as well as physical needs of the client.

Impact of Terminal Illness

The Diagnosis. In the case of a **terminal illness**, the physician is usually responsible for deciding what and how much the client should be told. These decisions are usually made after consulting with the client's family and assessing the client. The nurse, social worker, clergyman, or others in the service professions may also be involved with this decision and in discussing the client's condition with him or her. Most clients want to know their prognosis as soon as possible so that they can both come to grips with it and take care of business and personal affairs. It is important for all involved with the client's care to know exactly what the client and the family have been told, and it is also important for members of the client's health team to communicate among themselves.

Impact on Client. Many clients realize without being told that they are suffering from a terminal illness; this is often picked up from nonverbal communication by the client's family and by health-care professionals. The client must be allowed to go through the stages of the grieving process, permitted to make decisions about care, and supported in all decisions. The adult client has the right to refuse treatment and should be offered this option.

Impact on Family. The family of a terminally ill client should be encouraged to participate in planning the client's care. Health-care personnel should be available to discuss the client's condition with family members and should offer support and care as the family begins the grieving process. The family may want to make arrangements with the client for funeral or memorial services; this is contingent on which stage of grief both client and family members have progressed to.

Stages of Dying

Although each person reacts to the knowledge of impending death or to loss in his or her own unique way, there are similarities in the psychosocial responses to the situation. The world-renowned authority, Dr. Elisabeth Kübler-Ross, has studied the emotional responses to death and dying in depth, and her findings have been used extensively by nursing and other helping professions.

The stages of dying, much like the stages of grief, may overlap, and the duration of any stage may vary from as little as a few hours to as long as a period of months. The process varies from individual to individual. Some individuals may be in one stage for such a short time it seems a stage was skipped. Sometimes an individual returns to a previous stage.

According to Kübler-Ross, the stages of dying are (1) denial and isolation, (2) anger, (3) bargaining, (4) depression, and (5) acceptance.

Denial and Isolation. In the denial and isolation stage, the client denies that he or she will die, may repress what is discussed, and may isolate self from reality. The client may think, "They made a mistake in the diagnosis. Maybe they mixed my records with someone else's."

Anger. The client expresses rage and hostility in the anger stage and adopts a "why me" attitude. "Why me? I quit smoking and I watched what I ate. Why did this happen to me?"

Bargaining. The client tries to barter for more time. "If I can just make it to my son's graduation I will be satisfied. Just let me live til then." Many clients will put their personal affairs in order, make wills, and fulfill last wishes such as trips, visiting relatives, and so forth. It is important to meet these wishes, if possible, because bargaining helps clients move into later stages of dying.

Depression. In the depression stage, the client goes through a period of grief before death. The grief is characterized by crying and not speaking much. "I waited all these years to see my daughter get married. And now I may not be here to see her walk down the aisle. I can't bear the thought of not being there for the wedding—and to see my grandchildren."

Acceptance. When the stage of acceptance is reached, the client feels a state of tranquility and peace. The client has accepted death and is prepared to die. The client may think, "I've tied up all the loose ends—made the will, made arrangements for my daughter to live with her grandparents. Now I can go in peace knowing everyone will be fine."

Hospice Care

A **hospice** offers the same type of care as a hospital, but specific for the terminally ill. Hospices are designed for clients whose therapy has been discontinued because cure is considered unlikely, because the client wants no further treatment, or because the client wants to die at home. The goal of the hospice is to allow the client to die a natural death with dignity and as free of pain as possible.

Hospices may be located in special sections of the hospital or in a separate building, or they may offer programs of care in the client's home. In the past it was customary for persons to die at home with family support. With increased specialization of hospitals, the care of terminally ill clients moved to the hospital. Now, the pendulum has swung again and more terminally ill clients are remaining in their homes as long as possible or dying at home. The family assumes responsibility for the client's care in such situations, although various health agencies offer services. The nurse in the hospital may anticipate this need and assist the family in obtaining such services. Discharge planning, using the nursing process, is a vital factor in giving quality home care. Some hospitals permit nursing-staff members to make home visits between hospitalizations to provide support and continuity of care. The community health nurse may provide some aspects of care, teach necessary skills to family members, promote the use of other community services, and provide support and guidance to the client and family.

MEETING THE NEEDS OF GRIEVING AND DYING INDIVIDUALS

The nurse's aims in caring for the dying client and grieving family include facilitating coping of the dying person and family and promoting wellness and preventing illness of the family. Nursing care to facilitate coping and promote wellness is outlined and summarized in the box entitled Nursing Care to Facilitate Coping in Grief and Death.

Clarifying One's Own Feelings

Holistic care of the terminally ill client and family almost always involves some personal emotional investment. It is unrealistic and unfair to expect nurses to handle circumstances surrounding death without feelings. The best policy seems to be taking the time to explore one's own feelings and express them. The nurse who neglects to deal with personal feelings about life, dying, and death is in a questionable position to analyze and consider the needs of clients facing death. Therefore, a nurse's own feelings play a major role in determining how he or she cares for a client with a terminal illness. The following are some personal questions the nurse should use to help clarify feelings about finiteness of self:

- If I could control the events that result in my own death, where would I want to be? What cause of death would I choose? Whom would I want to have present during my terminal illness?
- What fears do I have about death?
- How would I answer these same questions for a client for whom I have been caring?
- How could I improve the quality of care for a terminally ill client for whom I am caring?
- If I were a member of the client's family, what things would I want a nurse to do for me?

Assessing Needs

The nursing process, discussed in Unit IV, is a helpful tool in the nursing care of a dying client and the grieving family. Before client and family needs are met, the nurse must assess for strengths and weaknesses in coping and relationships.

The nurse assesses the knowledge base of the client and family. If this is a chronic illness, how have they dealt with its problems in the past? What do they know about the disease process, the treatment, and the prognosis? Each family member is assessed for reactions to the illness or death, recognizing the individual differences mentioned earlier. What stage of grieving is each in?

Each person can be cared for according to the individual stage, remembering that all stages are normal and acceptable for a period of time. The reaction process is a highly individual one, and the nurse should not try to force movement from one stage to another.

The nurse determines if the client and family have developed good coping behaviors. Is the coping functional or dysfunctional? Coping mechanisms are discussed in Chapter 9.

Explaining the Client's Condition and Treatment

All involved health-care personnel should know exactly what the client and family have been told. Telling different things puts the nurse and other team members at cross purposes and sets up distrust in the family. Because clients and families often direct questions about prognosis to the nurse, it is up to the nurse to take the initiative in determining a means to be consistent in terminology, prognosis, and description of progress.

The client's condition and treatment should be explained to both the client and the family. Patience is required during explanations. Clients and family may be so grieved by the diagnosis they do not hear all the information that is shared with them. The nurse can question them to learn how much they have retained. Then the information they missed can be repeated. Any care options, as well as the expected outcomes of each option, should be fully explained.

Providing Open Communication

Communication, which is essential for persons to continue self-concept, is a lifelong need up to the moment of death and should be maintained at all times with the client and family.

To develop meaningful communications, the nurse must develop a trusting relationship with the client. This relationship is explored throughout this text. The nurse needs skills in listening and the ability to pick up both verbal and nonverbal cues given by the client and family. These skills are discussed in Chapter 20.

Nursing Care to Facilitate Coping in Grief and Death

- Assess the knowledge base of the client/family pertaining to the client's illness and previous care. Determine their perception of the present situation, strengths, and weaknesses.
- Assess the client/family for strengths and weaknesses and use these in planning care.
- Assess coping behaviors and priorities of needs.
- Use information gathered during family assessment to plan client care and anticipate potential family concerns.
- Encourage the client/family to take an active role in planning and providing care.
- Let your genuine concern and caring show. Do not be afraid to cry with the client/family.
- Encourage questions and respond positively.
- Meet with the family before the client arrives in the unit. Describe the environment and equipment being used for other clients as well. Reinforce that equipment is present for prevention and early detection of problems.
- Remain with the family during the first visit to provide additional information and support.
- Plan with the health-care team to be consistent in discussions with client/family as to terminology and what and how much is being said.
- Use simple terminology in explaining care, treatment, and progress. Do not use generalizations.
- Maintain good communications at all times. Use both verbal and nonverbal communication in assessing and giving care and be an understanding listener.
- Develop a trusting relationship between the client/family and self.
- Be patient in explaining the condition, treatment, and progress of the client. Sometimes information must be repeated or information sessions must be divided.
- Be as realistic as possible, being aware of coping mechanisms and needs for hope.
- Encourage independence as long as possible. Be creative in finding self-care activities for the client.
- Encourage the family to bring pictures and other familiar and favorite items from home.
- Support the client psychologically by being present, by listening, and by touching.
- Arrange for visits by the client/family's spiritual advisor, if desired. Pray with the client, if asked, and discuss faith and beliefs if appropriate.
- Consider the client as a unique individual and special to the family when discussing issues.
- Assure the family that the best possible care is being given to the client. Emphasize that the health-care personnel are experienced and have special training to provide expert care.

- Give regular progress reports to family and notify them of changes in the client's condition.
- Review the agency's policy for visiting hours to determine if it is adequate for the family.
- Suggest simple things the family can do to provide care for the client.
- Remind family members to take care of themselves: eat, rest, and exercise. Tell them where the chapel is, if appropriate.
- Indicate a place where family members may relax if they must leave the client's room during nursing care or so the client can sleep.
- Help the family to understand the needs and emotions of the dying person.
- Prepare the family for the client's death by discussing the normalcy of the grieving process.
- Allow the client to go through the stages of dying and the family to go through the stages of grief. Accept these stages and do not be judgmental. Offer support where needed.
- Support the family as adjustments in roles are made. Be prepared to make referrals and suggest support groups when needed.
- If the prognosis is poor, allow adequate time to be with the family. Establish time to meet again.
- Meet with family and physician to discuss extraordinary measures and advanced life-support systems.
- Speak to the client (including the comatose client) when performing care.
- Encourage the family to discuss among themselves or with the client ethical and legal concerns, organ donations, support systems, the will, and the funeral arrangements.
- Discuss follow-up visits with the family prior to the death. Set a date for such visits after the death.
- Encourage the family upon the client's death to express their feelings but do not tell them what they should feel and do.
- Perform nursing responsibilities: care of the body, ensuring the attending physician's signature is on the death certificate, placing identification tags on the body and shroud. Tags are also placed on dentures and eyeglasses.
- Provide sympathetic support to the family. Do not rush them out of the hospital. Provide a private place for them to begin their grieving, especially in sudden deaths.
- Allow the family to talk about the person as much as they want to. Encourage them to discuss special qualities and memories.
- Reassure them they did everything they could and that the medical care was the best. State other true and positive things about care.

(These interventions have been assembled and adapted from a variety of sources, including Bouman C: Identifying priority concerns of families of ICU patients. DCCN 3(5):316–317, 1984; Schmidt L: Parent Bereavement Outreach. Santa Monica, CA, 1979.)

The nurse should be willing to discuss the client's fears and doubts openly and to serve as a nonjudgmental listener. A caring nurse feels at ease in crying with the grieving person and sharing experiences with fears, loneliness, and death. This allows the griever the freedom to express his or her deepest concerns. Nonverbal communication is equally important. A smile, a touching hand or stroke, and eye-to-eye contact are all meaningful. The warmth behind the gesture and the honest concern of the nurse are what counts.

It is believed that the sense of hearing is the last sense to leave the body; many clients retain a sense of hearing almost to the moment of death. It is kind and thoughtful of the nurse to speak to the comatose client and to encourage family members to do likewise. The nurse should explain to the client the nursing care being given and the noises in the unit.

Promoting Self-Care and Self-Esteem

The client should be encouraged to retain independence and decision making as long as possible. If strong enough, the client should be allowed to help with light housekeeping and kitchen duties early in the course of care. Personal hygiene practices and self-feeding should also be managed by the client as long as possible. Once the client is confined to bed, the creative nurse and family should attempt to find self-care activities the client can perform. When physical abilities fail, determining when to take medication, for example, may be all the control the client can retain.

Having familiar objects in view can help make the client feel more comfortable and secure. Whether the client is at home or in a health-care agency, it is desirable to have the environment reflect personal preferences. This gives the client some degree of control when health and other activities of daily living have slipped out of the client's control and supports self-esteem.

Allowing Family Members to Assist in Care

Allowing family members to assist in nursing care can be beneficial to both the client and the family members: the client is comforted by having loved ones near, and family members are comforted by knowing that they helped comfort the client. Family members providing nursing care to the client must be supervised by the nurse.

Family members may not want to provide care themselves but may want to know what to expect and how they can psychologically aid the client. The nurse can help by explaining the client's condition, what treatment he or she is undergoing, and what result the family can expect from the treatment. Knowing the facts can often help family members to cope better with impending loss.

Meeting Client Needs

Physiologic Needs. *Physiologic care* of the client involves meeting physical needs such as personal hygiene, pain control, nutritional and fluid needs, movement, elimination, and respiratory care. Briefly, *personal hygiene* includes cleanliness of the skin, hair, mouth, nose, and eyes. Frequent baths and linen changes may be necessary. The mouth and nose should be kept free of mucus, and secretions should be wiped from the eyes. The physician will determine the medication and dosage needed for *pain control,* but the client's wishes should be considered. Some clients prefer and are able to control their own medication. Many dying clients suffer from malnutrition and dehydration, so *nutritional and fluid needs* must be addressed. The client may require intravenous feeding but should be encouraged to take sips of water if still able to swallow. Periodic *movement* should also be allowed; regular changes of position help prevent decubitus ulcers. Problems with *elimination* include the development of incontinence, constipation, or urinary retention. Absorbent pads or a nearby bedpan may be used for incontinent clients; laxatives or enemas may be used for relieving constipation; and catheterization may be required for urinary retention. Bed linens should be changed often. *Respiratory care* can be provided by repositioning the conscious client in semi-Fowler's position; the unconscious client should be positioned in a semiprone position that allows drainage of saliva and mucus. Oxygen therapy may be necessary for some clients.

Psychologic Needs. When persons speak of their fears of death, responses typically include fear of the unknown, pain, separation, leaving loved ones, loss of dignity, unfinished business, and so on. However, Kübler-Ross believes there is still another more overwhelming and more significant fear that is often repressed and unconscious—that of the catastrophic destructive force that has befallen a person and that the person cannot change. Kübler-Ross points out that terminally ill persons communicate this fear of a destructive force but do so largely through symbolic language. The person may use nonverbal language, such as a facial expression, a particular kind of hand clasp, or, in the case of children, through drawings and manner of play with toys. Verbal communication may also be used symbolically.

A fear of isolation, of having to face death alone, is a primary fear of the dying client. The nurse supports the client by indicating his or her presence, giving full attention, and showing concern. The presence of family members in the room should be encouraged. Reminiscences should be shared.

Spiritual Needs. Many terminally ill patients find great comfort in the support they receive from their religious faiths. It is important to aid in obtaining the services of a clergyman as each situation indicates.

Although not all clients follow specific spiritual or religious beliefs, most require some form of *spiritual care*. Most clients need to feel that their lives have meaning; many feel a need for hope in the face of death. Nurses should not impose their own beliefs on the client, but should let the client know that his or her beliefs are important. The nurse should arrange for visits from a spiritual advisor if this is desired. Spiritual needs are discussed more fully in Chapter 39.

Meeting Family Needs

The nurse can provide care for the *family facing loss* by listening to the family's concerns. Family members need to verbalize their worries and fears, and nurses and other health-care personnel can provide support by being nonjudgmental listeners. Likewise, nursing care of the *grieving family* involves communication and listening. Application of communication skills discussed in Chapter 20 and earlier in this section aids the nurse in being a nonjudgmental listener; feedback to the family can be provided by summarizing or paraphrasing, without questioning the validity of the family's emotions. All family members, including children, should be part of the grieving process.

There are instances when the nurse spends more time with the relatives than with the client, such as may occur when the client becomes comatose. Family members may need to be reminded to get rest and to eat. Too many visitors may tire the client, and when explanations are offered, relatives usually understand this readily. When they wish to remain at the hospital, they should be directed to a place where it is quiet and where they may relax.

The reality of death can be made less painful by preparing the family ahead of time. When the process has been explained to the family, they are better prepared to understand the needs of and support the dying person.

The steps of the grieving process should be explained to all members of the family ahead of time so they will recognize the specific stages as they experience them and understand the process is normal. They will be able to recognize that other members of the family are going through the same stages, perhaps at different times. This preparation allows for better understanding and communication within the family.

Death creates a change in family roles. As one person (the dying person) leaves a role, adjustments must be made within the family to compensate. Each member plays a part in that compensation. The nurse can help in these adjustments.

Meeting Self Needs

The nurse who cares for a client for an extended period of time will undergo a grief reaction when the client dies. Grief following the death of a client is natural, and the nurse should allow himself or herself to go through the grieving process, rather than shutting off grief. The nurse should also address personal health needs.

DEATH

Before death occurs, the client and family should have the opportunity to discuss what will happen following death, review the client's will, and discuss ethical and legal issues of concern.

Ethical and Legal Dimensions

Ethical and legal implications of nursing are discussed in Chapters 5 and 6. Religious beliefs and practices concerning spiritual beliefs and medical procedures are summarized in Chapter 39. The following issues and their implications should be discussed with the family and their wishes made known to the physician.

Euthanasia and Living Wills

A bill of rights for the dying person may be discussed with the client and family (see the box entitled The Dying Person's Bill of Rights). Euthanasia and living wills are discussed in Chapter 6.

Organ Donations

Clients who express a wish to donate functional organs, such as hearts, corneas, livers, lungs, and kidneys, can fill out an organ donor consent card (Fig. 13-1). The family of a deceased client may also decide to donate the client's functional organs. The nurse should be able to review options and provide consent forms to interested clients and their families.

The Autopsy

An *autopsy* is an examination of the organs and tissues of a human body following death. Consent of autopsy is a legal requirement. Generally the closest surviving family member or members have the authority to determine whether or not an autopsy is performed. Some religious groups prohibit autopsies except for legal purposes.

It is generally the physician's responsibility to obtain permission for an autopsy. Sometimes the client may grant this permission before death. The nurse often can assist by helping to explain the reasons for an autopsy. Many relatives will find comfort when they are told that an autopsy may help to further the development of medical science as well as establish proof of the exact cause of death.

If death is caused by accident, suicide, homicide, or illegal therapeutic practice, the coroner must be notified according to law. The coroner may decide that an au-

The Dying Person's Bill of Rights

I have the right to be treated as a living human being until I die.

I have the right to maintain a sense of hopefulness however changing its focus may be.

I have the right to be cared for by those who can maintain a sense of hopefulness, however changing this might be.

I have the right to express my feelings and emotions about my approaching death in my own way.

I have the right to participate in decisions concerning my care.

I have the right to expect continuing medical and nursing attention even though "cure" goals must be changed to "comfort" goals.

I have the right not to die alone.

I have the right to be free from pain.

I have the right to have my questions answered honestly.

I have the right not to be deceived.

I have the right to have help from and for my family in accepting my death.

I have the right to die in peace and dignity.

I have a right to retain my individuality and not be judged for my decisions which may be contrary to beliefs of others.

I have the right to discuss and enlarge my religious and/or spiritual experiences, whatever these may mean to others.

I have the right to expect that the sanctity of the human body will be respected after death.

I have the right to be cared for by caring, sensitive, knowledgeable people who will attempt to understand my needs and will be able to gain some satisfaction in helping me face my death.

(This Bill of Rights was created at a workshop on The Terminally Ill Patient and the Helping Person, in Lansing, Michigan, sponsored by the Southwestern Michigan Inservice Education Council and conducted by Amelia J. Barbus, associate professor of nursing, Wayne State University, Detroit.)

topsy is advisable and can order that one be performed, even though the family of the patient has refused to consent. In many cases, a death occurring within 24 hours of admission to the hospital must be reported to the coroner.

Clinical Signs of Death

The clinical signs of *impending or approaching* death include failure to swallow; pitting edema; decreased gastrointestinal and urinary tract activity; bowel and bladder incontinence; loss of motion, sensation, and reflexes; elevated temperature but cold or clammy skin; cyanosis; lowered blood pressure; noisey or irregular respiration; and Cheyne-Stokes respirations. The client may or may not lose consciousness.

Death was defined in 1981 by the President's Commission for the Study of Ethical Problems in Medicine and Biomedical and Behavioral Research as follows:

Death is present when an individual has sustained either (1) irreversible cessation of circulatory and respiratory functions, or (2) irreversible cessation of all functions of the entire brain, including the brain stem.

Another definition of *death* proposed by a Harvard University committee states that the following character-istics must be present for at least 24 hours before death can be declared:

- Lack of receptivity and responsiveness
- Lack of movement or breathing
- Lack of reflexes
- Flat encephalogram

Nursing Responsibilities

When a client dies, the nurse's responsibilities include care of the client's body, care of the family, and discharging specific legal responsibilities. The latter involve ensuring that a death certificate is issued and signed by a physician, labeling the body, and reviewing organ donation arrangements (if any).

The Death Certificate

Laws in the United States and Canada require that a death certificate be prepared for each patient who has died. The laws specify needed information. Death certificates are sent to local health departments, which compile many statistics from the information. The mortician assumes responsibility for handling and filing the death certificate with proper authorities. However, the physician's signature is required on the certificate, as well as that of the pathologist, the coroner, and others in special

RESEARCH IN NURSING *Making a Difference*

Death and Dying

Even though death and dying are more readily discussed now than in the past, levels of anxiety about the topic have not necessarily decreased. In many cases, a person dies in an institutional setting, without the support of family or friends. Too often, the survivors are also isolated and left to face the death of a loved one surrounded by strangers. It has been demonstrated that many health professionals try to cope with death by avoidance and withdrawal, as well as with high levels of anxiety.

Related Research

Finkelmeier B, Kenwood N, Summers C: Psychologic ramifications of survival from sudden cardiac death. Critical Care Quarterly 7(2):71–79, 1984

This study of the recollections of clients surviving sudden cardiac death was done to better define the emotional sequelae of that experience, so that improved psychologic support could be provided. The study found that significant numbers of persons had memories of the actual events occurring during the cardiac arrest, especially of the people around them and conversations of caregivers.

Murphy P: Reduction in nurses' death anxiety following a death awareness workshop. The Journal of Continuing Education in Nursing 17(4):115–118, 1986

Murphy carried out this study to examine the effects on nurses of a workshop specifically designed to lower death anxiety levels. Levels of anxiety about death were found to be significantly decreased in nurses participating in the workshop.

Williams M: Use of a concluding process to assist grieving families. Journal of Emergency Nursing 10(5):254–258, 1984

The purpose of this study was to determine whether the use of a concluding process at the time of sudden death would help survivors with grieving. Although results were not conclusive, the study focuses on the needs of families at the time of a member's death and gives guidelines for effective communications at this time of crisis and loss.

The implications of nursing research in this area focus on increasing an awareness of both the nurse's and client/family's feelings and anxieties about death. Once aware of these feelings, the nurse is better able to support clients and families experiencing this phenomenon.

cases. The nurse's responsibility is to ensure that a death certificate has been signed by the physician.

Care of the Body

After the client has been pronounced dead by a physician, the nurse is responsible for preparing the body for discharge. The body is placed in normal anatomic position to avoid pooling of blood, and soiled dressings are replaced and tubes are removed. It is usually unnecessary to wash the body; the mortician generally attends to this. Some religions strictly forbid the washing, while others must have it performed by a special person. In cultures in which the family's washing the body of the deceased is considered the last service a family can give a loved one, the family should be given the supplies needed and allowed to be alone in the room with the body. If an autopsy is to be performed, tubes should not be removed. Procedures for the care of the body, in this case, should be verified with hospital policy.

It is the nurse's legal responsibility to place identification tags on both the shroud or garment the body is clothed in and on the ankle to ensure that the body can be identified even if it is separated from the shroud. The nurse should also place an identification tag on the client's dentures or other prosthesis to ensure that these are received by the mortician. The client's body may have to be placed in the hospital's morgue refrigerator if mortuary arrangements were not made before the client's death. *The importance of proper and complete identification cannot be overstressed.*

If the client died following certain communicable diseases, the body may require special handling to prevent the spread of the disease. Requirements for such handling are usually specified by local law and are contingent on the disease-causing organism, mode of transmission, and other characteristics.

Care of the Family

After a client has died, the nurse provides support and care to the client's family. In most cases, this involves listening to the family's expressions of grief, loss, and helplessness. Because comforting words are often diffi-

Signed by the donor and the following two witnesses in the presence of each other:

_____   _____
Signature of Donor   Date of Birth of Donor

_____   _____
Date Signed   City and State

_____   _____
Witness   Witness

This is a legal document under the Uniform Anatomical Gift Act or similar laws in all 50 states.

For further information call

Delaware Valley TRANSPLANT PROGRAM

800 KIDNEY-1
2401 Walnut St., Suite 404
Philadelphia, PA 19103

UNIFORM DONOR CARD

_____
Print or type name of donor

In the hope that I may help others, I hereby make this anatomical gift, if medically acceptable, to take effect upon my death. The words and marks below indicate my desires.
I give: a)_____any needed organs or parts
         b)_____only the following organs or parts

_____
Specify the organ(s) or part(s)

for the purpose of transplantation, therapy, medical research or education;
         c)_____my body for anatomical study if needed

_____
Limitations or special wishes, if any

F I G U R E   13-1
Organ donor card.

cult to find, the nurse should offer solace and support by being an attentive listener. Often it is necessary for family members to see the body of the client in order to fully accept the death; in such cases, the nurse should arrange for family members to view the body before it is discharged to the mortician.

Sudden death creates unique problems for the family. In the case of sudden injury or illness, the physical needs of the client are paramount to the health-care team. This means that family members are not provided as much emotional support or information as they are in a prolonged illness, nor are they permitted to exercise as many options regarding the client's care. The family that loses a member unexpectedly has not had the opportunity to begin the grieving process or to share in grieving with the deceased person. It is important that family members be allowed to express grief and given emotional support. Most often the family is in the emergency waiting room when death is confirmed. They are stunned, bewildered, and numb. They should not be rushed from the waiting room but rather provided a private place to begin grief. The nurse should acknowledge their shock and listen to their grief. The family needs guidance in making plans and help in making decisions.

It is proper for the nurse who was caregiver or who took care of the client for a prolonged period to attend the funeral. It is also appropriate for the nurse to make a follow-up call to the client's family after the funeral or memorial service to offer both concern and care for the family's well-being. Follow-up visits are important to give support to the family. If the nurse assesses that the family is not coping well (dysfunctional grief), appropriate referral should be made.

Care of Other Clients

Because it is not unusual for a nurse to provide care to more than one client at a time, after the death of one client the nurse must continue to provide care to the other clients. Other clients are often aware of a death and may need consoling; this is particularly true of a client who has shared a room with the deceased client. Other clients may have grief reactions and should be supported through the grief process by the nurse. Death of a client often causes depression in other clients and makes them more aware of their own future deaths.

K E Y   P O I N T S

■ Every individual experiences some sort of loss at some point in the life continuum. Such losses can be actual, perceived, physical, psychologic, or anticipatory. Loss can impact on the developmental stages of the human life span, especially in children.

■ Grief is the emotional response to loss, and grief reactions can be divided into identifiable stages. Grief can be manifested both emotionally or physically, and grief reactions are influenced by development, family and socioeconomic factors, and religious and cultural influences.

■ Distorted or abnormal grief is considered dysfunctional; dysfunctional grief often does not fall into grieving process stages.

■ Dying clients have a variety of needs, ranging from the need for open communication to physiologic, psychologic, and spiritual needs. They should maintain self-care as long as possible.

■ Families of dying clients also need open communication and may want to assist the nurse in providing care. This is considered a healthy experience for both client and family members.

- Like grief, dying can be broken into identifiable and overlapping stages.

- Hospices provide several alternatives to hospital or nursing home care for the incurable, terminally ill clients: clients can be nursed at home by hospice personnel or can be given care with fewer behavioral restrictions in the hospice.

- Legal and ethical issues, including euthanasia, organ donation, and living wills, should be discussed with the client and the family.

- Although there is no exact definition for death, the clinical signs of approaching or impending death can be recognized.

- The nurse should provide emotional support for the grieving family by being an attentive, nonjudgmental listener and a good communicator.

- The nurse has specific responsibilities at the time of a client's death, including ensuring that a death certificate is issued, caring for the body, placing identification tags on the shroud and body, ensuring that the body is discharged to the proper party, and caring for the family.

- The nurse should provide care to other clients who are affected by the loss.

BIBLIOGRAPHY

Carpenito LJ: Nursing Diagnosis—Application to Clinical Practice, 2nd ed. Philadelphia, JB Lippincott, 1987

Clark MD: Healthy and unhealthy grief behaviors. Occupational Health Nursing 32(12):633–635, 1984

Corr CA, Corr DM (eds): Hospice Care: Principles and Practice. New York, Springer-Verlag, 1983

Engel GL: Grief and grieving. Am J Nurs 64:93–98, 1964

Gonda TA, Ruark JE: Dying Dignified: The Health Professional's Guide to Care. Menlo Park, CA, Addison-Wesley, 1984

Johnson SH: Nursing Assessment and Strategies for the Family at Risk: High-Risk Parenting, 2nd ed. Philadelphia, JB Lippincott, 1986

Kübler-Ross E: On Death and Dying. New York, Macmillan, 1969

Martocchio BC: Grief and bereavement: Healing through hurt. Nurs Clin North Am 20(2):327–341, 1985

Pennington EA: Post mortem care: More than ritual. Am J Nurs 78:846–847, 1978

President's Commission for the Study of Ethical Problems in Medicine and Biomedical and Behavioral Research: Defining Death. Publication No. 81-600150. Washington, DC, US Government Printing Office, 1981

Schulz R: The Psychology of Death, Dying and Bereavement. Reading, MA, Addison-Wesley, 1978

Waechter EH, Phillips J, Holaday B: Nursing Care of Children, 10th ed. Philadelphia, JB Lippincott, 1985

The Nursing Process

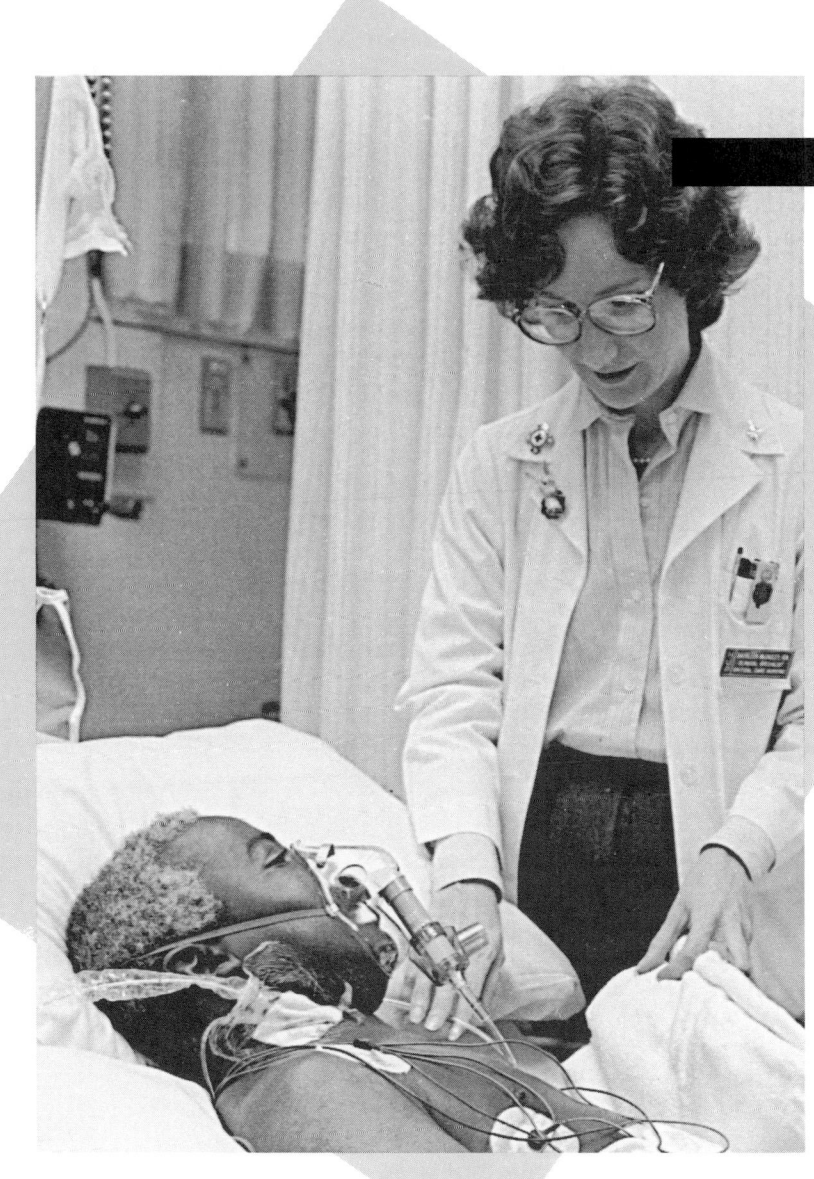

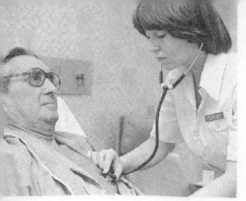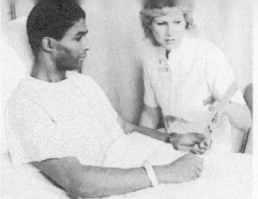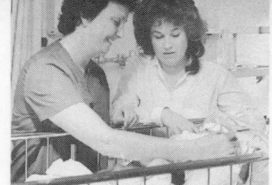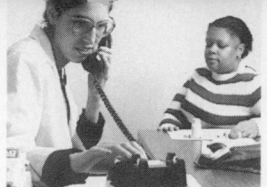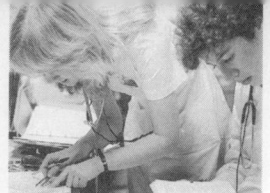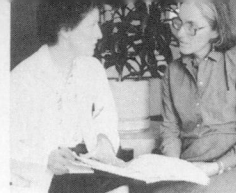

*T*he nursing process is a systematic, client-centered, goal-oriented method of caring that provides a framework for nursing practice. Unit IV discusses each of the five steps of the nursing process: assessing, diagnosing, planning, implementing, and evaluating. The use of the nursing process allows the nurse to apply knowledge and skills in meeting client needs while giving holistic, individualized care.

The steps are not actually separate items, but are rather parts of a whole, used to identify needs, establish priorities of care, maximize strengths, and resolve actual or potential alterations in human responses, thereby promoting wellness to the highest level possible for each individual client.

Assessment, the systematic and continuous collection and communication of data, allows analysis of data to identify problems and strengths of clients. During planning, the nurse and client mutually set goals and agree on nursing interventions necessary to meet the established goals. The nurse implements the plan of care, adapting actions to each individual, and documents nursing actions and client responses. Following implementation, the nurse and client evaluate the effectiveness of the plan, based on achievement of goals, and determine if the plan should be continued, modified, or terminated.

The nursing process is nursing practice in action. Unit IV provides the information necessary for the beginning application of the nursing process; as knowledge and skills are learned and practiced (both as students and as nurses), the process becomes an integral component of each nurse–client interaction. The outcome is comprehensive and individualized client care.

CHAPTER

14

Introduction to Nursing Process

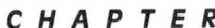

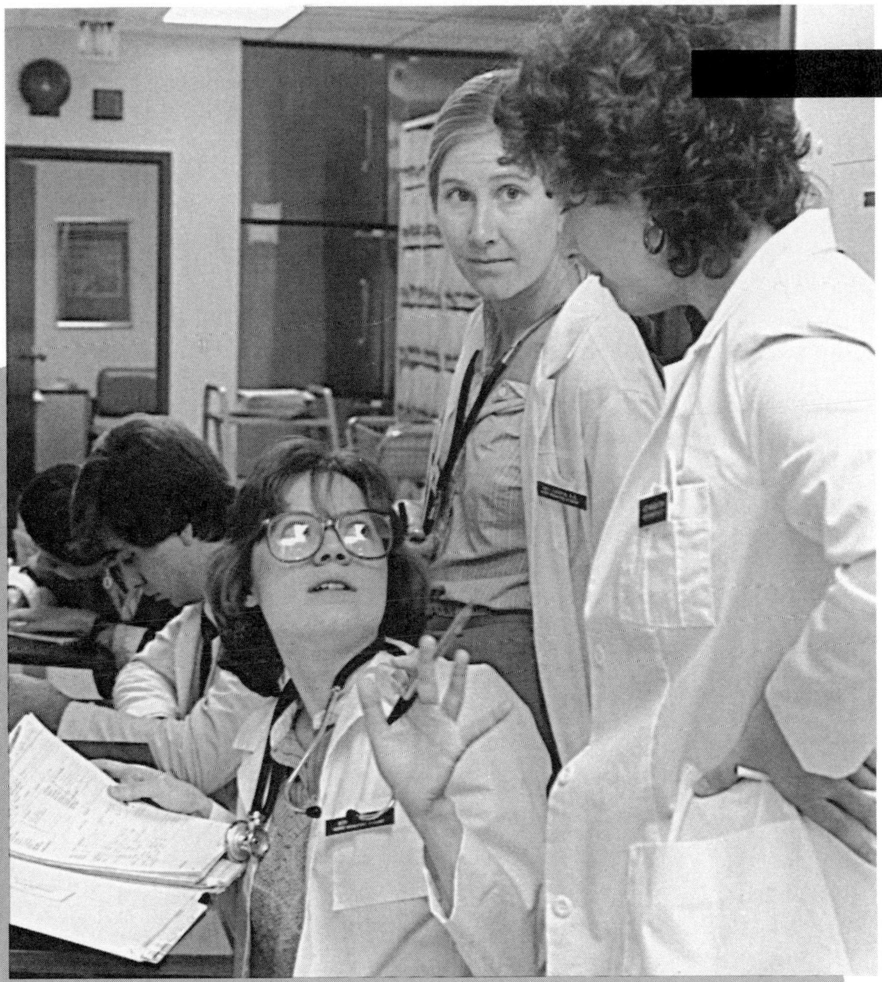

OBJECTIVES

After studying this chapter, the learner should be able to

Define key terms used in the chapter.

Describe the historic evolution of the nursing process.

Describe the nursing process and each of its five steps.

List five characteristics of the nursing process.

List three client and three nursing benefits of using the nursing process correctly.

Traditionally, nurses have prided themselves on comforting the ill and on executing with precision tasks such as dressing wounds, administering medications, and bathing, feeding, and ambulating the ill. Many of these tasks were ordered specifically by physicians, and few nurses would have characterized their "work" as being independent, scientifically based, or creative.

The health-care delivery system has changed, and nursing has changed with it. Nurses now work with both well and ill clients in both private and institutional settings. In addition to their roles as caregivers, nurses also fill roles as care managers/coordinators, teachers, counselors, advocates, and researchers. Nurses are responsible for a unique dimension of health care, "the diagnosis and treatment of human response to actual or potential health problems" (American Nurses' Association, 1980), and as such are knowledgeable, competent, and independent professionals who work collaboratively with other health-care professionals to design and deliver holistic care.

As the practice of nursing became more complex, nurses began to study the *process* of nursing to both understand and improve the means nurses use to accomplish their aims.

KEY TERMS

assessing
diagnosing
evaluating
implementing
intuitive problem solving

nursing process
planning
scientific method
trial-and-error problem
   solving

HISTORIC PERSPECTIVE

Since the term "nursing process" was first used by Hall in 1955 (Hall, 1955), many nurses have struggled to define exactly what constitutes the "work of nursing" and what makes nurses successful. In the 1960s nursing theorists began to describe nursing as a distinct entity among the health-care professions, and also delineated specific steps in a process approach to nursing practice. In 1967 Yura and Walsh published the first comprehensive book on nursing process, in which they described four steps in nursing process: assessment, planning, intervention, and evaluation. They viewed the element of nursing diagnosis as the logical conclusion of the assessment phase, whereas Gebbie and Lavin (1974) made nursing diagnosis an individual step in the process. These and other studies led to the development of the five-step nursing process commonly used today: assessment, diagnosis, planning, implementation, and evaluation.

The steps of the nursing process were legitimized in 1973, when the American Nurses' Association Congress for Nursing Practice developed *Standards of Practice* to guide nursing performance (American Nurses' Association Congress for Practice, 1973) (see Chap 1). These standards for nursing practice were quickly reflected in revised nursing practice acts in many states. In 1982 the state board examinations for professional nursing practice underwent major revisions, and one of the organizing concepts used in the revisions was nursing process. The revised examinations are specifically structured to test the practitioner's ability to assess clients; to diagnose health problems amenable to nursing therapy; and to plan, implement, and evaluate nursing care. The examinations had previously organized content on a medical model, structured according to medical specialties: medicine, surgery, maternity, pediatrics, and psychiatry.

Evolution of Nursing Diagnosis

The term "nursing diagnosis" first appeared in the literature in the 1950s. In 1976 Aspinall described nursing diagnosis as "the weak link" in nursing process (Aspinall, 1976). As early as 1966, Hammond wrote that the nurses need both to be competent in information-seeking strategies and to have a good background of theoretical knowledge with which to conduct the search for cues and evaluate evidence, all resulting in accurate diagnosing (Hammond, 1966). Key elements in the evolution of nursing diagnosis as an integral component of nursing process include:

- In 1972 the New York State Nurse Practice Act identified diagnosing as belonging to the legal domain of professional nursing; practice acts in many other states have been revised similarly since then.
- In 1973 the American Nurses' Association's *Standards of Practice* included diagnosing as a function of professional nursing.
- Also in 1973, Gebbie and Lavin of St. Louis University called the First National Conference on Classification of Nursing Diagnoses, beginning a national effort to identify, standardize, and classify health problems treated by nurses. Conferences are held every 2 years, and much progress has been made in defining, classifying, and describing nursing diagnoses.

At its first meeting in 1973, the National Group, since renamed the North American Nursing Diagnosis Association (NANDA), appointed a task force to

- Gather information and disseminate it through the Clearinghouse for Nursing Diagnosis.
- Encourage educational activities at regional and state levels to promote the implementation of nursing diagnoses. These activities include conferences to organize nurses to identify additional diagnostic labels and workshops to teach nurses about nursing diagnoses.
- Promote and organize activities to continue the development, classification, and scientific testing of nursing diagnosis. These activities include planning national conferences, identifying criteria for accepting diagnoses, surveying current research activities, and exploring varied methods for classification.

DESCRIPTION OF NURSING PROCESS

The **nursing process** is a systematic method that directs the nurse and client as they together (1) determine the need for nursing care, (2) plan and implement the care, and (3) evaluate the results. The steps in this client-centered, goal-oriented process are interrelated; each of the five steps depends on the accuracy of the step before it. The process provides a framework that enables the nurse and client to

- Systematically collect client data (assessing)
- Clearly identify client strengths and problems (diagnosing)
- Develop a holistic plan of individualized care which specifies both the desired client goals and the nursing actions most likely to assist the client to meet those goals (planning)
- Execute the plan of care (implementing)
- Evaluate the effectiveness of the plan of care in terms of client goal achievement (evaluating)

In each step of the process, the nurse and client work together as partners; the client's health state and resources will influence the client's level of participation. When the client is an infant, unconscious, or uncooperative, the steps of the process are worked through with the help of a family member or support person.

The primary purpose of the nursing process is to help the nurse manage each client's care scientifically, holistically, and creatively. To do this successfully, the nurse needs many intellectual, interpersonal, and psychomotor skills, as well as the willingness to use these skills creatively when working with clients to promote wellness, to prevent disease/illness, to restore health, and to facilitate coping with altered functioning. Many of these skills are described in the units that follow.

Steps of the Nursing Process

The five steps of the nursing process are illustrated in Figure 14-1. A brief description of each step follows, and each step is discussed in greater detail in the individual chapters that follow. Those who wish to study nursing process or any of its steps in greater detail should consult one of the nursing texts that deals exclusively with nursing process (Alfaro, 1986; Atkinson and Murray, 1986; Griffith-Kenney and Christensen, 1986; Iyer, Taptich, and Bernocchi-Losey, 1986; LaMonica, 1985; Marriner, 1983; Pinnell and de Meneses, 1986; and Yura and Walsh, 1983).

Assessing

The first step in the nursing process, **assessing**, is the systematic and continuous collection, validation, and communication of client data. Data are collected reflecting the nursing theory of the particular institution.

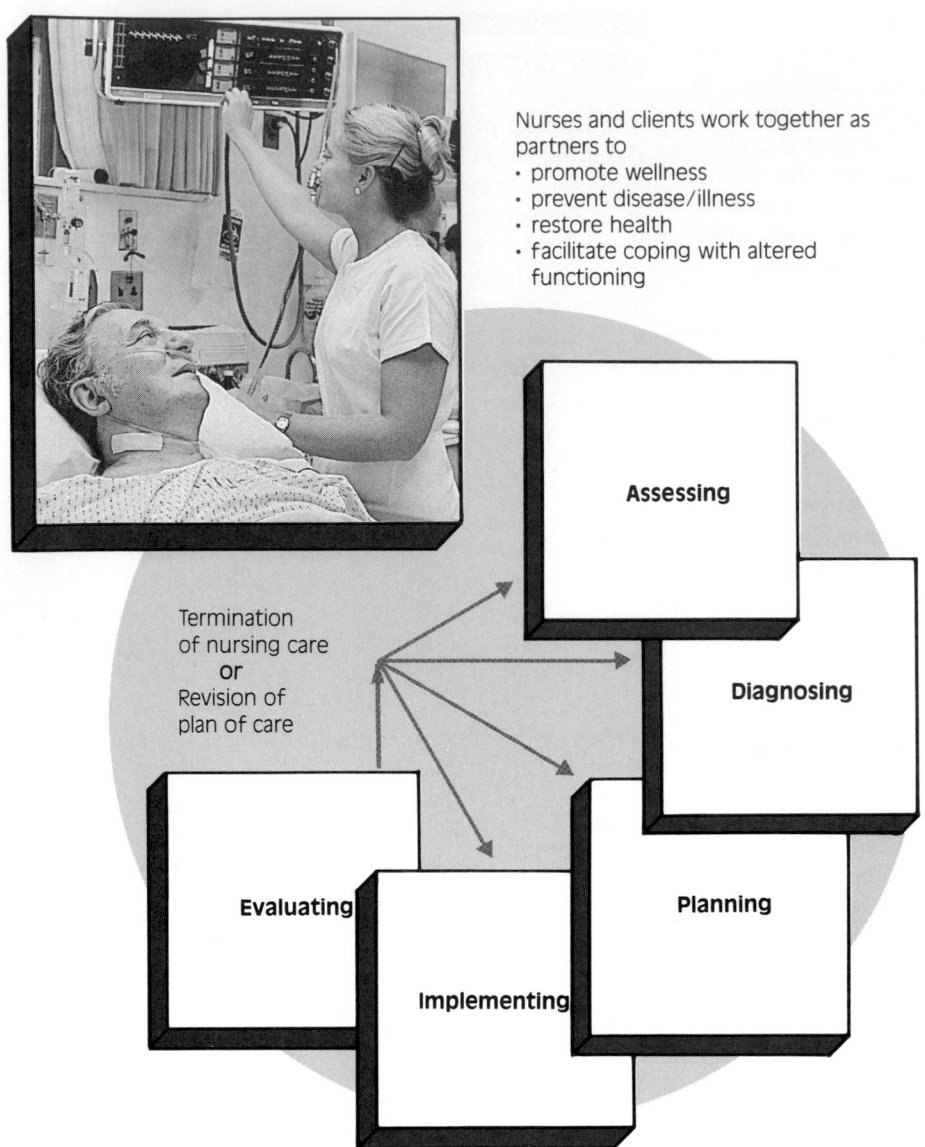

Nurses and clients work together as partners to
• promote wellness
• prevent disease/illness
• restore health
• facilitate coping with altered functioning

Assessing

Diagnosing

Termination of nursing care **or** Revision of plan of care

Evaluating

Planning

Implementing

F I G U R E   14-1

The nursing process. The nursing process is a systematic method that directs the nurse and client as, together, they determine the need for nursing care (assessing and diagnosing), and then plan, implement, and evaluate care. The steps in this client-centered, goal-oriented process are interrelated, and each of the five steps depends on the accuracy of the step before it. Evaluation, the fifth step in the process, leads either to the termination of nursing care or to revision of the plan of care after each preceding step in the process has been evaluated. (Photo by Gates Rhodes, courtesy of the School of Nursing, University of Pennsylvania)

(Nursing theory is discussed in Chap 4.) In general, nurses are concerned with how human functioning is enhanced by health promotion or compromised by illness and suffering. The remaining steps of the nursing process depend on complete, accurate, and relevant data.

During the assessment step of the nursing process the nurse

• Establishes the data base, which includes nursing history, nursing examination, review of the client record and nursing literature, and consultation with the client's support persons and health-care professionals
• Continuously updates the data base
• Validates data
• Communicates data

Diagnosing

Diagnosing is analysis of client data to identify client strengths and health problems which independent nursing intervention can prevent or resolve. Following the collection of client data, the nurse analyzes the data to identify data clusters (discussed in Chap 16) indicating actual or potential problems; factors contributing to or causing these problems; and coping patterns or strengths of the client.

The nurse next determines if each health problem is best treated by nursing or by another health discipline. When data analysis reveals an actual or potential health problem that nursing intervention can prevent or resolve, it is termed a *nursing diagnosis*. During the diagnosis step of the nursing process, the nurse

- Interprets and analyzes client data
- Identifies client strengths and client health problems
- Formulates and validates nursing diagnoses
- Develops a prioritized list of nursing diagnoses

Planning

Planning is the establishment of client goals by the nurse, working with the client, to prevent, reduce, or resolve problems identified in the nursing diagnoses and the determining of related nursing interventions most likely to assist the client in achieving these goals. In addition, a comprehensive plan of care also specifies (1) the nursing assistance needed by the client to meet human needs, and (2) the nursing interventions dictated by the plan of medical care. During the planning step of the nursing process, the nurse

- Establishes priorities
- Writes goals and develops an evaluative strategy
- Selects nursing measures
- Writes the nursing care plan

Implementing

Implementing is simply the carrying out of the plan of care. It includes all actions performed by nurses to promote wellness, prevent disease/illness, restore health, and facilitate coping with altered functioning. During the implementing step of the nursing process, the nurse

- Carries out the plan of nursing care
- Continues data collection and modifies the plan of care as needed
- Documents care

Evaluating

Evaluating is the process of measuring the extent to which client goals have been met. The nurse and the client together measure how well the client has achieved goals specified in the plan of care, and nurse and client identify factors that either positively or negatively in-

fluenced goal achievement. Client response to the plan of care determines whether nursing care should be continued as is, modified, or terminated. If evaluation points to a need to modify nursing care, then the accuracy, completeness, and relevance of the assessment data, as well as the appropriateness of client diagnoses, goals, and nursing interventions should all be carefully reviewed and modified. During the evaluation step of the nursing process, the nurse

- Measures the client's achievement of desired goals
- Identifies factors contributing to the client's success or failure
- Modifies the plan of care, if indicated

An overview of the steps of the nursing process is presented in Table 14-1; the box on page 249 gives examples of each of the steps.

Documenting the Nursing Process

More than ever before, nurses are aware of the need to document nursing care. Legally speaking, a nursing action not documented is a nursing action not performed. Each of the chapters in this unit offers specific documentation guidelines for nursing process activities. It is helpful to practice documentation while learning any given nursing activity; like any other nursing skill, documentation improves with practice. Examples of nursing documentation, nursing assessments, care plans, and notes can be found throughout this text.

PROBLEM SOLVING AND THE NURSING PROCESS

One of the strengths of the nursing process is that it is based on a methodology familiar to most nursing students: problem solving. Problem solving is a basic life skill; identifying a problem and then taking steps to resolve it is a matter of common sense. Different approaches to problem solving yield different results, some of which are more successful than others.

The **trial-and-error method** of problem solving involves testing any number of solutions until one is found that works for that particular problem. This method is obviously not efficient for the nurse and can be dangerous to the client; it is therefore not recommended as a guide for nursing practice.

The **scientific method** of problem solving is a systematic, seven-step, problem-solving process that involves (1) problem identification, (2) data collection, (3) hypothesis formulation, (4) plan of action, (5) hypothesis testing, (6) interpretation of results, and (7) evaluation, resulting in conclusion or revision of the study. The scientific method is used most correctly in a controlled laboratory setting, but is closely related to the more general six-step, problem-solving process com-

T A B L E   14-1
Overview of the Nursing Process

Component	Description	Purpose	Activities
Assessing	Collection, validation, and communication of client data	Make a judgment about the client's health status, ability to manage his own health care, and need for nursing Plan individualized holistic care which draws on client strengths and is responsive to changes in the client's condition	1. Establish the data base • Nursing history • Nursing examination • Review of client record and nursing literature • Consultation with client's support persons and health-care professionals 2. Continuously update the data base 3. Validate data 4. Communicate data
Diagnosing	Analysis of client data to identify client strengths and health problems that independent nursing intervention can prevent or resolve	Develop a prioritized list of nursing diagnoses	1. Interpret and analyze client data 2. Identify client strengths and health problems 3. Formulate and validate nursing diagnoses 4. Develop prioritized list of nursing diagnoses
Planning	Specification of (1) client goals to prevent, reduce, or resolve the problems identified in the nursing diagnoses and (2) related nursing interventions	Develop an individualized plan of nursing care	1. Establish priorities 2. Write goals and develop an evaluative strategy 3. Select nursing measures 4. Write nursing care plan
Implementing	Carrying out the plan of care	Assist clients to achieve desired goals: promote wellness, prevent disease/illness, restore health, facilitate coping with altered functioning	1. Carry out the plan of care 2. Continue data collection and modify the plan of care as needed 3. Document care
Evaluating	Measure the extent to which the client has achieved the goals specified in the plan of care, identifying factors that positively or negatively influenced goal achievement; revise the plan of care if necessary	Continue, modify, or terminate nursing care	1. Measure how well the client has achieved desired goals 2. Identify factors contributing to the client's success or failure 3. Modify the plan of care (if indicated)

monly used by health-care professionals as they work with clients. The relationship between both of these methods and the nursing process is illustrated in Table 14-2.

Intuitive Problem Solving. For years nurse theorists and educators have argued that clinical judgments should be based on data alone (the scientific method), in an attempt to establish nursing as a science, worthy of the respect of other professions. Controversy has recently been sparked by nurses both studying and writing about the role of **intuitive problem solving** in clinical decision making. Many veteran nurses can describe situations in which an "inner prompting" led to a quick nursing intervention that saved a client's life. Benner (1984, p 295) describes intuition as "direct apprehen-

sion of a situation based upon a background of similar and dissimilar situations and embodied intelligence or skill." Schraeder and Fischer (1986, p 161) credit to intuitive perception "a wide range of experience, from the sudden, inexplicable feeling that 'something is wrong,' to recognizing the teaching moment, when to offer encouragement, and when it is most helpful simply to listen."

Advocates of intuition recommend
• Welcoming flashes of intuition as additions to logical reasoning, rather than disruptions
• Validating intuitions—when an intuition cannot be validated (e.g., when the nurse senses something is wrong with the client although there are no clinical signs), careful monitoring of the client should be initiated

Illustration of the Steps of the Nursing Process

Assessing

You are checking on a client who had abdominal surgery yesterday and hear that the client has considerable pain, "It kept me up all night." The client has been reluctant to ask for any pain medication fearing effect of the drug, "I don't want to become a junkie." The client's blood pressure and pulse are slightly elevated.

Diagnosing

You analyze the above data and decide the client probably has an *Alteration in comfort: Acute pain related to a fear of taking pain-relieving medications.* The client agrees that this is becoming a problem.

Planning

You decide to work with the client to achieve the goal: *By 3:00 PM client reports sufficient relief of pain to enable him to rest and to get out of bed to go to the bathroom.* The client wants to accomplish the goal. You identify teaching as the primary nursing intervention.

Implementing

After asking the client about his experiences with pain-relieving medications, you explain that while many of these drugs are addictive when abused, there is no harm if they are taken as prescribed postoperatively. You also explain that it is important for him to experience enough pain relief to be able to cough and deep breathe, ambulate, and do other things important to his recovery. You suggest that the medication will be most effective if taken before his pain peaks and becomes intense. You administer the prescribed medication for pain when the client indicates he is willing to give it a try.

Evaluating

After enough time has elapsed for the medication to take effect, you check back with the client to evaluate whether or not he has obtained relief and met his goal. If the client is satisfied and you both feel comfort is no longer a problem, you terminate the plan of care for this diagnosis. If the client still feels pain or is dissatisfied with the medication, then each of the above steps of the nursing process is reevaluated and necessary changes are made in the plan of care.

- Furthering nursing research to help find ways (1) to cultivate intuition and its typical results (accurate, early diagnosis; vigilant monitoring; better client care), and (2) documenting the information intuition supplies (Rew, 1987).

Beginning nurses must use nursing knowledge and scientific problem solving as the basis of care they give; intuitive problems solving comes with years of practice and observation. However, if the beginning nurse has an intuition about a client, the information should be discussed with the supervisor.

CHARACTERISTICS OF NURSING PROCESS

Many different words and phrases have been used to describe the nursing process; key descriptors include systematic, dynamic, interpersonal, goal-oriented, and universally applicable.

Systematic

A quick look at the many and varied activities of any nurse on a busy day might lead one to conclude that nursing is little more than the execution of countless haphazard tasks. A closer look, however, will reveal that each nursing task is part of an ordered sequence of activities. Moreover, each activity is dependent on the accuracy of the activity that went before it, and will influence the actions that follow it. Without a complete and accurate data base, the nurse cannot identify client strengths and problems; not knowing these, it is impossible for the nurse and client to develop a plan of care based on realistic and valued client goals. And unless the goals are well written, nursing actions and evaluation will be meaningless. The nursing process directs each step of nursing care in a sequential, ordered fashion.

Dynamic

While the nursing process is presented as an orderly progression of steps, in reality there is great interaction and overlapping among the five steps. No one individual step in the nursing process is a one-time phenomenon; each step is fluid and flows into the next step. In some nursing situations, all five stages occur almost simultaneously. When a nurse discovers that a client is choking on food and cannot speak or breathe, the nurse identifies the problem quickly and takes rapid steps to dislodge the food particle blocking the airway—all the while evaluating the effectiveness of the intervention. In other instances, for example, child abuse, the nursing team may labor over each step of the nursing process as nurses work with the family to resolve complex problems. As well as being dynamic, the nursing process is continually open to change: at any point new client data may cause the plan of care to take an entirely different direction.

T A B L E   14-2
Comparison of Steps in the Problem-solving Process, the Nursing Process, and the Scientific Method

Problem-solving Process	Scientific Method	Nursing Process
1. Problem encountered	1. Problem identification	1. Assessing
2. Data collection	2. Data collection	
3. Exact nature of problem specified	3. Hypothesis formulation	2. Diagnosing
4. Plan of action determined	4. Plan of action developed to test hypothesis	3. Planning
5. Plan of action carried out	5. Hypothesis testing	4. Implementing
6. Outcomes of the plan evaluated and the plan continued, modified, or terminated	6. Interpretation of results	5. Evaluating
	7. Evaluation resulting in conclusion or revision of the study	

Interpersonal

Always at the heart of nursing is the human being. Nursing exists as a profession because some individuals require assistance as they respond to health and illness. The nursing process ensures that nurses are client-centered rather than task-centered. Rather than simply walking into a client's room to take vital signs, the nurse thinks: "How is Mr. Warner today? Any new data that indicate a need to modify his plan of care? Are our nursing actions helping him to achieve his goals? How can we better help him?"

The nursing process encourages nurses to help clients to use their strengths to meet all of their human needs. This is very different from viewing the client as a "problem to be solved" and interacting mechanically to provide the solution. Working intimately with clients helps nurses to explore their own strengths and limitations and to develop themselves personally and professionally.

Goal-Oriented

Countless good things can be accomplished for most clients, ranging from improving oral hygiene to helping people cope with the demands of being a new parent, recovering from an acute medical illness, living with chronic pain, or preparing for death. Likewise, it would take hundreds of pages to list and describe all the nursing actions a nurse might perform for a client. Moreover, nurses and clients often differ in the importance they attach to selected goals. The nursing process offers nurses a means for nurses and clients to work together to identify specific goals related to wellness promotion, disease/illness prevention, health restoration, and coping with altered functioning: which are most important to the client, and to match them with the appropriate nursing actions. Once these are recorded in the plan of care, each nurse can quickly determine the client's priorities and begin nursing with a clear sense of how to proceed. The client benefits from continuity of care, and each nurse's care moves the client a little further toward goal achievement.

Universally Applicable

Once nurses have a working knowledge of the nursing process, they find they can practice nursing with well or ill individuals, young or old, in any type of practice setting. Efforts made by the student nurse to master nursing process will result in the student's possession of a valu-

F I G U R E   14-2
One characteristic of the nursing process is that it ensures that nursing is client-centered rather than task-oriented. (Photo by Robert Neroni, courtesy Thomas Jefferson University)

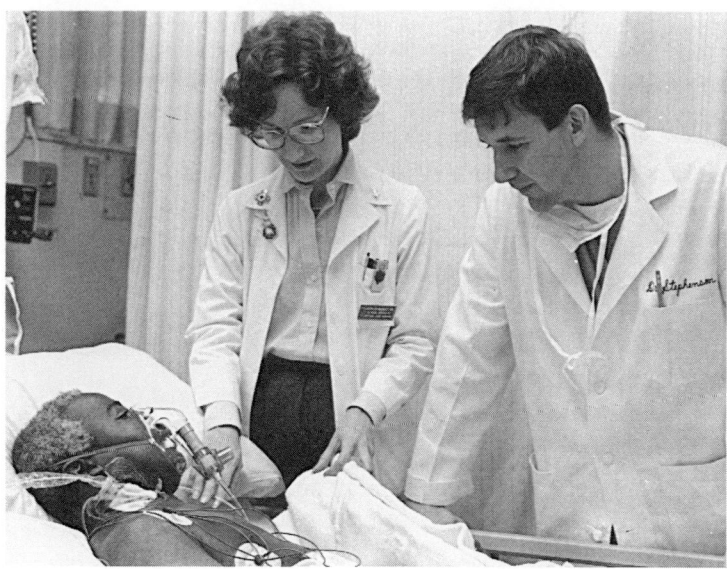

F I G U R E   14-3
The nursing process offers direction for all activities carried out by the nurse, whether they are independent, interdependent, or dependent functions. (Photo by Gates Rhodes, courtesy of the School of Nursing, University of Pennsylvania)

able tool which can be used with ease in any nursing situation.

When caring for clients, nurses act independently, interdependently with other health-care professionals, and dependently, as when they carry out the orders of a physician. (These distinctions will be clarified in Chap 18.) Some nurses mistakenly believe that the nursing process is only applicable in the independent dimension of their practice—that if they are not writing a nursing diagnosis the nursing process has no bearing on what they are doing. This may be especially true for nurses who practice on busy hospital units and find that much of their time is spent carrying out physician orders for clients (preparing clients for diagnostic studies, administering medications, performing treatments, and so forth). What should be clear from the preceding discussion on nursing process is that it provides a framework for all the activities of the nurse. Whether the nurse is carrying out an independent, interdependent, or dependent function, it is important to assess the client, note any significant alterations in health status, determine if the nursing action is helping the client to achieve his or her goals, and modify the plan of care as necessary. Thus, the nurse who feeds a pediatric client through a special tube as ordered by a physician continually assesses how the child is responding to the feeding and if the child or family will be able to manage the feedings independently when the child is discharged. Depending on the results of the nursing assessment, new nursing diagnoses may be needed, as may additions to the plan of care. The nursing process offers direction for *all* the activities carried out by the nurse when caring for clients.

BENEFITS OF THE NURSING PROCESS

When used properly, the nursing process achieves for the client scientifically based, holistic, individualized care; the opportunity to work collaboratively with nurses; and continuity of care. Nurses who use the nursing process in a thoughtful and systematic way achieve a clear and efficient plan of action by which the entire nursing team can get results for clients; the satisfaction that they are making an important "difference" in the lives of their clients; and the opportunity to grow professionally as the nurse evaluates the effectiveness of interventions and variables that contribute positively or negatively to the client's goal achievement.

K E Y   P O I N T S

■ The nursing process is a systematic method that directs the nurse and client as they together determine the need for nursing care (assessing and diagnosing) and then plan, implement, and evaluate care.

■ The primary purpose of the nursing process is to help the nurse manage each client's nursing care scientifically, holistically, and creatively.

■ In each step of the nursing process the nurse and client work together as partners. The client's health state and resources will influence the client's level of participation.

■ Assessment is the systematic and continuous collection, validation, and communication of client data.

- Diagnosing is the analysis of client data to identify (1) data clusters that indicate actual or potential problems in the way the client is responding to health or illness, (2) factors contributing to or causing these problems, and (3) coping patterns or other strengths the client can draw on to prevent or resolve the problem(s).

- During the planning step of the nursing process, the nurse, working with the client, (1) develops client goals which if achieved prevent, reduce, or eliminate the problems specified in the nursing diagnoses; and (2) identifies the nursing interventions most likely to achieve these goals.

- Implementation is simply the carrying out of the plan of nursing care. It includes all the actions performed by the nurse to promote wellness, prevent disease/illness, restore health, and facilitate coping with altered functioning.

- During evaluation the nurse and client measure how well the client has achieved the goals specified in the plan of care and identify factors that positively or negatively influenced goal achieve-ment. Client responses to the plan of care determine if nursing care is to be continued without change, modified, or terminated.

- Underlying the science and art of nursing is a successful blend of the scientific problem-solving method and the intuitive method.

- The nursing process is systematic, each step dependent on the accuracy of the previous step and influencing the steps that follow. The steps of the nursing process are interrelated; each step is fluid and moves into the next.

- The nursing process is an interpersonal process that is always client-centered rather than task-centered. As nurses help clients to use their strengths to meet all their human needs, nurses themselves grow personally and professionally.

- A goal-oriented process, the nursing process offers a means for nurses and clients to work together to identify the specific health goals that are most important to the client—and to match these with the appropriate nursing interventions.

BIBLIOGRAPHY

Alfaro R: Application of Nursing Process: A Step-by-Step Guide. Philadelphia, JB Lippincott, 1986

American Association of Colleges of Nursing: Essentials of College and University Education for Nursing. Washington, DC, The Association, 1986

American Nurses' Association: Nursing: A Social policy statement. Kansas City, American Nurses' Association, 1980

American Nurses' Association Congress for Practice: Standards of Practice. Kansas City, MO: American Nurses' Association, 1973

Aspinall MJ: Nursing diagnosis: The weak link. Nurs Outlook 24(7):433–436, 1976

Atkinson J, Murray ME: Understanding the Nursing Process, 3rd ed. New York, Macmillan, 1986

Benner P: From Novice to Expert. Menlo Park, CA, Addison-Wesley, 1984

Gebbie K, Lavin MA: Classification of nursing diagnosis. Am J Nurs 74:250–253, 1974

Griffith-Kenney JW, Christensen PJ: Nursing Process: Application of Theories, Frameworks, and Models, 2nd ed. St Louis, CV Mosby, 1986

Hall LE: Quality of nursing care. Address given at the Department of Baccalaureate and Higher Degree Programs of the New Jersey League for Nursing, Public Health News, New Jersey State Department of Health, June 1955

Hammond KR: Clinical inference in nursing: A psychologist's view point. Nurs Res 15:27–38, 1966

Hill L, Smith N: Self-Care Nursing. Englewood Cliffs, NJ, Prentice-Hall, 1985

Iyer P, Taptich B, Bernocchi-Losey D: Nursing Process and Nursing Diagnosis. Philadelphia, WB Saunders, 1986

LaMonica E: The Humanistic Nursing Process. Monterey, CA, Wadsworth, 1985

Marriner A: The Nursing Process: A Scientific Approach to Nursing, 3rd ed. St Louis, CV Mosby, 1983

Mauksch A, David M: Prescription for survival. Am J Nurs 72:2189–2193, 1972

McHugh MK: Has nursing outgrown the nursing process? Nursing 17(8):50–51, 1987

McHugh MK (ed): Nursing process. Holistic Nursing Practice 1(3):entire issue, 1987

Pinnell N, de Meneses M: The Nursing Process. Norwalk, CT, Appleton-Century-Crofts, 1986

Rew L: Nursing intuition: Too powerful—and too valuable —to ignore. Nursing 17(7):43–45, 1987

Schraeder BD, Fischer DK: Using knowledge to make clinical decisions. MCN 11:161–163, 1986

Valega TM: It's time for nurses to begin nursing nurses. Nursing and Health Care 5(6):331–335, 1984

Yura H, Walsh MB: The Nursing Process: Assessing, Planning, Implementing, Evaluating. Norwalk, CT, Appleton-Century-Crofts, 1967

Yura H, Walsh M: The Nursing Process, 4th ed. Norwalk, CT, Appleton-Century-Crofts, 1983

Assessing

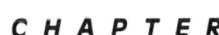

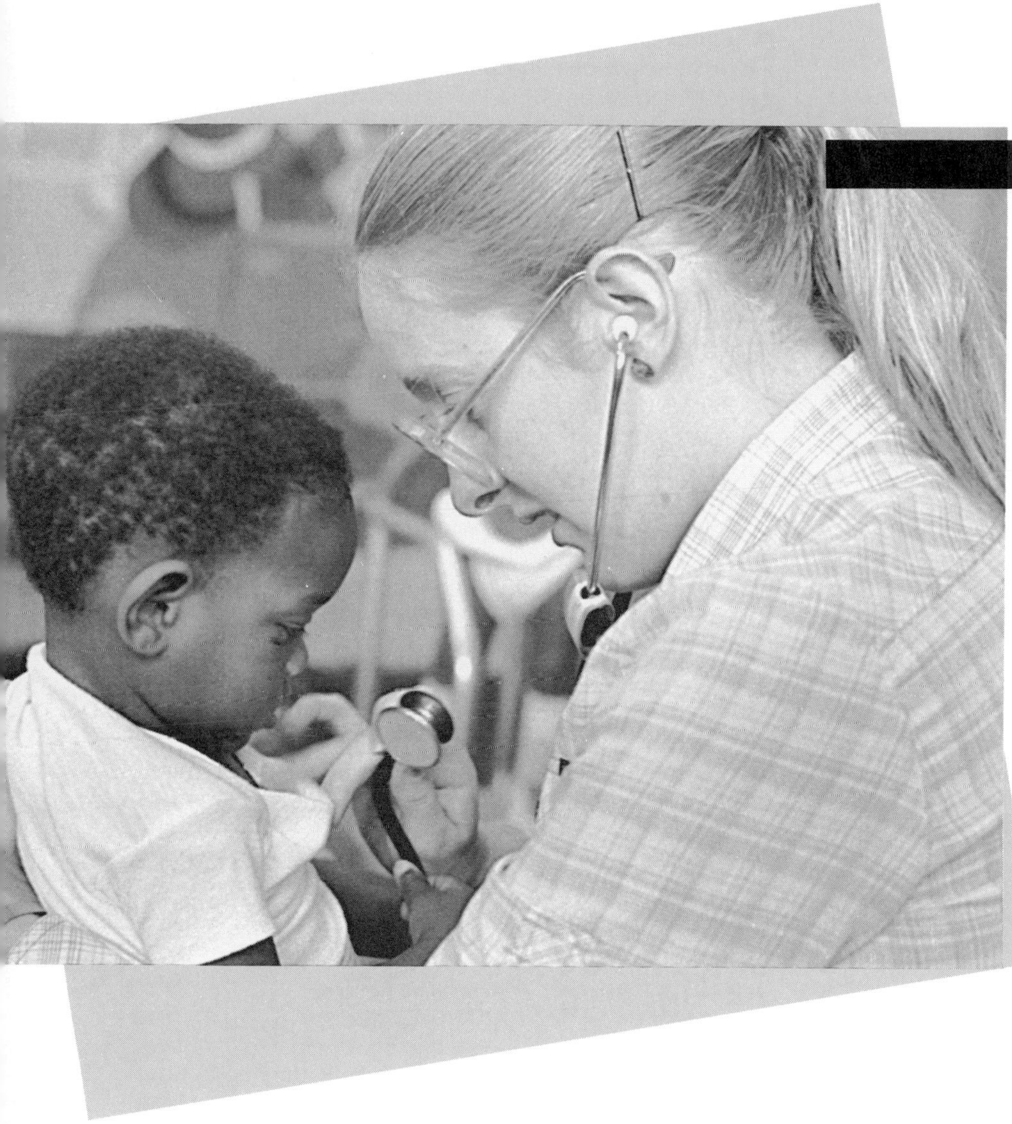

After studying this chapter, the learner should be able to

Define key terms used in the chapter.

Describe the purposes of the initial comprehensive nursing assessment and of ongoing nursing assessments.

Differentiate a nursing assessment from a medical assessment.

Differentiate objective and subjective data.

Describe the purposes of nursing observation, interview, and examination.

Obtain a nursing history using effective interviewing techniques.

Identify five sources of client data useful to the nurse.

Differentiate comprehensive admission assessments from focused assessments.

Plan client assessments by identifying assessment priorities and structuring the data to be collected systematically.

Identify common problems encountered in data collection noting their possible cause and etiology.

Explain when data need to be validated and several ways to accomplish this.

Describe the importance of knowing when to report significant client data and the importance of proper documentation.

Obtain complete, accurate, relevant, and factual client data.

Assessing is the systematic and continuous collection, validation, and communication of client data; these data involve information about the client. A data base (or baseline data) includes all of the pertinent client information collected by the nurse and other health-care professionals; as such, it enables a comprehensive and effective plan of care to be designed and implemented for the client. The collection of client data is a vital step in the nursing process because the remaining steps depend on complete, accurate, relevant, and factual data.

The initial comprehensive nursing assessment results in a data base which enables the nurse to make a judgment about a client's health status, ability to manage his or her own health care, and need for nursing; refer the client to a physician or other health-care professional, if indicated; and plan and deliver individualized, holistic nursing care that draws on the client's strengths. In addition to an initial assessment of the client, ongoing assessments are made by the nurse. Ongoing nursing assessment alerts the nurse to changes in the client's responses to health and illness, and suggests necessary changes in the plan of nursing care or care offered by other health-care professionals.

During the assessment step of the nursing process, the nurse establishes the data base by interviewing the client to obtain a nursing history; the nurse may also perform a nursing examination to collect data. Other sources of client information used by the nurse include the client's support persons, the client record, the client's health-care professionals, and nursing and other health-care literature. After the nurse has established the data base, data about the client are collected continuously because the client's health status can change quickly. Questionable data are verified (validated) as part of the assessment step of the nursing process. All pertinent data are recorded and, when appropriate, verbally communicated to the responsible person, so that it can best benefit the client (see Fig 15-1).

KEY TERMS

assessing	nursing history
data	objective data
data base	observation
interview	subjective data
nursing examination	validation

UNIQUE FOCUS OF NURSING ASSESSMENT

When nurses make nursing assessments, they do not duplicate medical assessments. The primary purpose of the nursing assessment is not to gather data that define underlying pathology and medical problems; rather, nursing assessments focus on client responses to health problems. Is there, for example, interference with basic human needs? Can the client perform activities of daily living? While the findings of a nursing assessment do sometimes contribute to the identification of a medical diagnosis, the unique focus of nursing assessments is on the client's responses to actual or potential problems.

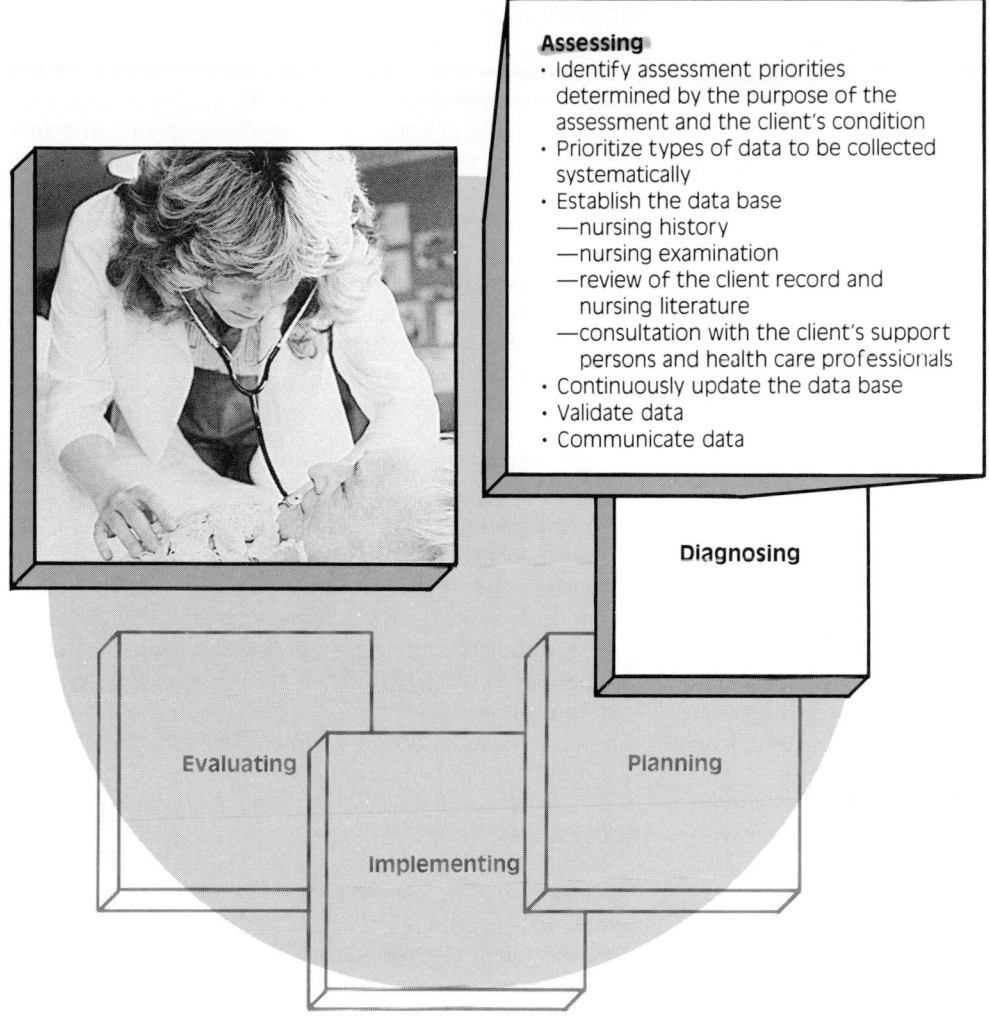

Assessing
- Identify assessment priorities determined by the purpose of the assessment and the client's condition
- Prioritize types of data to be collected systematically
- Establish the data base
  —nursing history
  —nursing examination
  —review of the client record and nursing literature
  —consultation with the client's support persons and health care professionals
- Continuously update the data base
- Validate data
- Communicate data

Diagnosing

Evaluating

Planning

Implementing

FIGURE 15-1

Assessing. The primary source of client information is the client. Resources include the client's support persons, the client record, information from other health-care professionals, and information from nursing and health-care literature. (Photo by Gates Rhodes, courtesy of the School of Nursing, University of Pennsylvania)

DATA COLLECTION

Types of Data

There are two types of data: objective and subjective. **Objective data** is information perceived by the senses; data observed by one person can be verified by another person observing the same client. Examples of objective data are an elevated temperature reading (101°F), skin that is moist to the touch, and the act of refusing to look at or eat food. Objective data are also called signs or overt data.

Subjective data is information perceived only by the affected person; these data cannot be perceived or veri-

fied by another person. Examples of subjective data are feeling nervous, nauseated, chilly, or experiencing pain. Subjective data are also called symptoms or covert data (see Table 15-1).

When collecting and recording client data, it is important to be complete, accurate and factual, and relevant.

Complete. To the extent that it is possible, all the client data necessary to understand a client health problem and develop a plan of care to maximize wellness need to be identified. For example, knowing that a client has lost weight is meaningless until the nurse discovers (1) if the weight loss was either intentional or unintentional, (2) if it was related to a change in eating or exercise patterns or to some underlying pathology, and (3)

Observation

Observation is the conscious and deliberate use of the five physical senses to gather data. The skilled nurse uses each nurse–client interaction to observe and interpret meaningful stimuli (data). Student nurses can develop such observation skills by training themselves to observe carefully the following each time they encounter a client:

- What are the client's current responses (physical and emotional) to his or her situation? Be alert to signs of distress—difficulty in breathing, bleeding, pain, heightened anxiety—as well as to anything out of the ordinary—sudden eruption of skin rash, changes in levels of consciousness, and so forth.
- What is the client's current ability to manage his or her care (need for additional information or nursing assistance)?
- What is the immediate environment? Consider the safety of the environment—side rails, spills on floor—as well as the functioning of equipment (intravenous therapy, oxygen, drains). Who are the people in the room? What are the temperature and odor of the room?
- What is the larger environment (hospital or community)?

Interview

Nursing History.   An interview is a planned communication. During the assessment step of the nursing process, the nurse interviews the client to obtain a nursing

T A B L E   15-1
A Comparison of Objective and Subjective Data

Objective data	Subjective data

32-year-old male
Height: 5'8"
Weight:
  9/18/88—224 lb
  2/4/89—202 lb
	"I'm beginning to feel better about myself now that I'm losing weight and I seem to have more energy."

Posterior, left midcalf feels warm and is red.	"My leg hurts when I walk."
Client observed fidgeting with bed covers; facial features are tightly drawn.	"I'm so afraid of what they might find when they cut me open tomorrow."

how the client views and is responding to the weight loss.

Accurate and Factual.   Both the client and the nurse may intentionally or unintentionally misrepresent or distort client information. For example, a client who values being thin may describe a weight gain of several pounds as the onset of obesity. Nurses concerned with accuracy and fact continually verify what they hear with what they observe using other senses, and validate all questionable data. When nurses suspect that personal bias or stereotyping is influencing their data collection, it is appropriate to consult with another nurse. It is also best to describe observed behaviors rather than the interpretation of the behavior. Such a description may read: "Client is frequently observed lying with his face to the wall. Attempts to engage him in conversation fail. He refused lunch today and ate only soup for dinner." "Client is depressed," conversely, is the nurse's interpretation of the client's behavior; it is not a factual statement. Recording the client's behaviors factually allows other health-care professionals to explore causes of the behavior with the client.

Relevant.   Because recording comprehensive data can become an endless task, one challenge facing nurses is to determine *what type* of data and *how much* data to collect for each individual client. This chapter describes ways to do this. The aim is to record concisely all pertinent data. Often, only experience teaches nurses what data are needed in specific cases.

Learning how to collect, validate, and communicate data that are complete, accurate and factual, and relevant is the focus of the remainder of this chapter.

Data Collection Methods

Common methods used in the collection of data in nursing include observation, interview, and examination.

Components of a Nursing History

- Client's profile: name, age, sex, marital status, religion, occupation, education
- Client's reason for seeking health care
- Client's normal health habits and patterns and any need for nursing assistance
- Client's present state of health, functioning of body systems, and past medical and surgical history
- Meaning client attributes to health and illness and characteristic response/coping patterns
- Client's developmental history, family history, environmental history, and psychosocial history
- Client and family's expectations of nursing and of the health-care team
- Client and family's ability and willingness to participate in the plan of care
- Client's personal resources and deficits

history. Ideally, the nursing history captures the uniqueness of the client and records this, so that care planning may be patterned to meet the client's individual needs. The nursing history should therefore be obtained as soon as possible after a client presents for care, and should be followed by the nursing examination. The **nursing history** should clearly identify client strengths and weaknesses, health risks such as hereditary and environmental factors, and potential and existing health problems. The focus of the nursing history is always on getting to know the *person*. Data included in the nursing history are listed in the box on page 256.

Strong interviewing skills are needed to obtain the necessary client data and to communicate concern for the client. A brief discussion of the work of each phase of the interview follows; specific interviewing techniques are presented in Chapter 20.

Phases of the Interview.

The four phases in the nurse–client interview are: preparatory phase, introduction, working phase, and termination. More detailed information on interviewing techniques can be found in Chapter 20.

Preparatory Phase.

Prior to initiating the interview, the nurse prepares to meet the client by reading present and past records and reports, when available. During this phase it is important not to let stereotypes and prejudices predetermine the nurse–client relationship. If the nurse is aware of personal prejudices, those prejudices can be dealt with constructively. Professional nurses learn to approach clients with open minds and to be sensitive to the human needs that underlie diverse behaviors.

During the preparatory phase, the nurse should ensure that the environment in which the interview is to be conducted will be private and relaxed. Unless the client

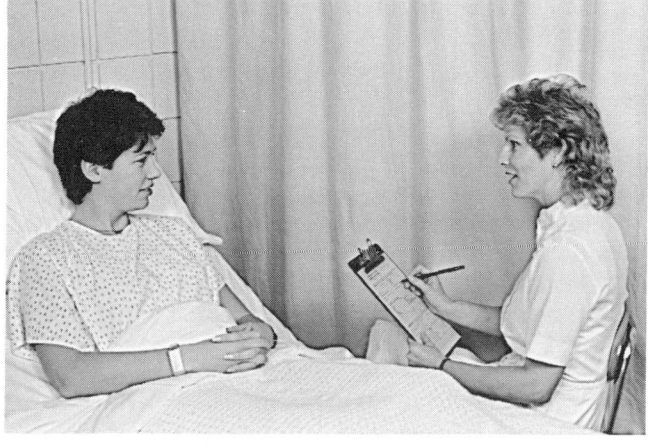

F I G U R E   15-2
In the interview, both the seating arrangement and the distance from the client are important in establishing a relaxed and comfortable environment for data collection. (Photo © Ken Kasper)

wishes to have family members or friends present during the interview, the nurse should interview the client alone, either in the client's room or in a quiet office.

Both the seating arrangement and the distance between nurse and client are important. Chairs placed at right angles to each other and about 1 to 1.2 m (3 to 4 ft) apart facilitate an easy exchange of information. If the client is in bed, placing a chair at a 45-degree angle to the bed is helpful. If the nurse stands at the foot or side of the client's bed and physically talks or looks down at the client, a superior–inferior relationship is communicated and can defeat the interview. Whenever possible, it is best to communicate with clients at eye level.

The interview should be scheduled when both the nurse and the client are free of concerns and distractions, so they can concentrate on the task. Ten to 15 minutes may be all that is necessary in some circumstances, while an hour or more may be required in others. Information can be gathered in several meetings, especially if the nurse notices the client is tiring or is in pain.

Introduction.

The interview's introduction is critical because it sets the tone not only for the remainder of the interview, but also for every nurse–client interaction that follows. At the end of this phase of the interview, the client should know the name of his or her primary nurse and what he or she can expect of nursing; should sense that the nurse is competent and cares about him or her; and should know what is expected of the client in terms of developing the plan of care and participating in its execution.

The nurse initiates the interview by stating his or her name and status, identifying the purpose of the interview, and clarifying the roles of nurse and client. A typical introduction might run like this: "Good afternoon, Mr. Komer. My name is Lisa Gray and I'll be your primary nurse while you are in the hospital. Right now I'd like to ask you a few questions about yourself so that we can plan your nursing care together. Feel free to respond only to those questions you feel comfortable answering, and know your responses will be treated confidentially by the staff. This will take about 20 minutes. Is this time convenient for you?"

The initial impression the nurse creates is critical, especially with clients who are new to the health-care environment. All nurses the client encounters in the future may be judged in light of this first impression. When the nurse communicates respect and genuine concern for the client, the client is then encouraged to discuss health concerns and problems freely. The interpersonal qualities of a respectful presence, professionalism, and caring invite the client's confidence and inspire hope that help is available.

During the introduction, it is important for the nurse to assess the client's comfort and ability to participate in the interview. It is also appropriate to discuss confidentiality. The client should know where the data being recorded are stored, how they will be used, and who has access to them. Some nurses record data on the appropriate form while with the client, while other nurses take notes and complete the form later. Writing should not interfere with the process of sharing information during the interview. If a contractual agreement clearly identifying the responsibilities of both client and nurse is indicated, terms are discussed at this time (see also Chap 6).

Working Phase.　During the working phase of the interview, the nurse gathers all the information needed to form the subjective data base. The accuracy, completeness, and relevancy of the data base are dependent on the nurse's use of the interviewing and basic communication techniques discussed in Chapter 20. The communication techniques highlighted below are important ingredients of a successful interview.

- Focus on the client during the interview, demonstrating interest and concern: use the client's name, use eye contact appropriately, avoid rushing the client.

- Listen to the client attentively, using reflection and paraphrase to communicate to the client that he or she is being understood.
- Ask about the client's main problem first, using terminology the client understands; save personal or delicate questions for when a rapport is established. Defer less important questions until a later interview if the client is too ill or upset to communicate easily.
- Pose questions and comments to the client in the manner best suited to produce the desired communication (see Chap 20).

  Closed questions elicit very specific information.

  Open-ended questions allow the client to verbalize freely.

  Reflective questions encourage the client to elaborate on thoughts and feelings.

  Direct questioning may be used to validate information, to clarify information, or to place events into a meaningful sequence.

T A B L E　15-2

Client Variables that can Negatively Influence an Interview and Suggested Nursing Responses

Client Variables	Effect on Interview	Nursing Response
High anxiety	Client may speak rapidly or incoherently and may jump from one topic to another; client may deny or misrepresent what he is experiencing.	Normalize anxiety: "Many persons find it difficult to talk about their health and become anxious"; approach client gently, speak slowly and softly; underscore importance of the client sharing what he is experiencing so nurses can help
Pain	Client offers clipped responses and yes or no answers whenever possible; overriding concern is pain relief.	Do everything possible to make client comfortable prior to the interview, including obtaining an order for and administering pain medication; if pain persists, obtain only vital data and defer remainder of interview until client is more comfortable.
Language difficulty (client not fluent in nurse's language because of limited education or fears saying the "wrong thing"	Vital client data will not be communicated; client may mistakenly be labeled "indifferent" or "noncommunicative."	Speak clearly (do not raise voice) using simple language; whenever possible obtain the assistance of an interpreter (family member may help but if client data are confidential a stranger may be preferable).
Previous negative experience with nurses and/or health-care delivery system	Client is aloof, unwilling to participate in interview; general attitude: "Why should I waste my time telling you anything . . . it won't do me any good."	"I know other people who have had a tough time with nurses or the system . . . life isn't perfect . . . but how about giving us a chance this time to show you what nurses can do?" Communicate respect for the client and competence.
Unrealistic expectations of health-care professionals	Client expects nurses and other health-care professionals to magically know everything about him and to "take care of him"; "surrenders" himself to the system—"you know best" attitude.	Communicate clearly that no one knows/ understands the client like himself and invite him to become involved in his care; "No two persons are alike and unless you tell me a little more about yourself and how you are feeling there is no way we'll be able to plan good care."

- Avoid comments and questions that impede communication (see Chap 20): cliches, questions that require a "yes" or "no" answer only, intimidating "why" or "how" questions, probing questions, giving advice, using judgmental comments, changing the subject, giving false assurance.
- Use silence and touch appropriately.

Many client variables can positively or negatively affect the outcome of an interview. Table 15-2 identifies selected client variables that can negatively influence an interview unless the nurse responds appropriately.

Termination. The successful interview is concluded carefully. Clients should be advised that the interview is coming to an end. It is helpful to recapitulate the interview, highlighting key points. Both the client and the nurse should be satisfied that the important data is recorded. A helpful strategy is to ask the client after the summary: "Is there anything else you would like us to know that will help us to plan your care?" This gives the client the opportunity to add data the nurse did not think to include.

Before leaving the client, it is helpful to alert the client as to what to expect in the next 24 hours. The client should also know when the nurse will re-establish contact: "Thank you for answering these questions, Mr. Komer. Please feel free to keep us informed of anything you think we should know. I will be leaving soon, but when I return tomorrow morning, I will be back to discuss your plan of care. This afternoon will be busy for you—blood work has been ordered, as has a chest x-ray. Your evening will most likely be quiet. Do you have any questions? Is there anything else I can do for you before I leave?"

Nursing Examination

The **nursing examination** is the assessment of the client for *objective data* that may help to better define the client's condition and help the nurse in planning care. The nursing examination generally follows the nursing history/interview, and may verify data gathered during the history or yield new data. There has been a great deal of controversy about nursing's role in the physical examination of the client, caused by concern that this is a duplication of medicine's role. Traditionally, physicians have performed the intake physical examination, which frequently is the mechanism of entry into the health-care delivery system, as well as the basis for medical treatment. Some nurses in expanded roles are performing comprehensive intake physical examinations, which identify health and illness states, and are then recommending/prescribing the appropriate follow-up care. In any case, all nurses conduct select aspects of physical examination for nursing purposes.

Unlike the physical assessment performed by the physician to identify pathology and its etiology, the nursing examination is focused primarily on the functional abilities of the client. If a neurologic deficit is

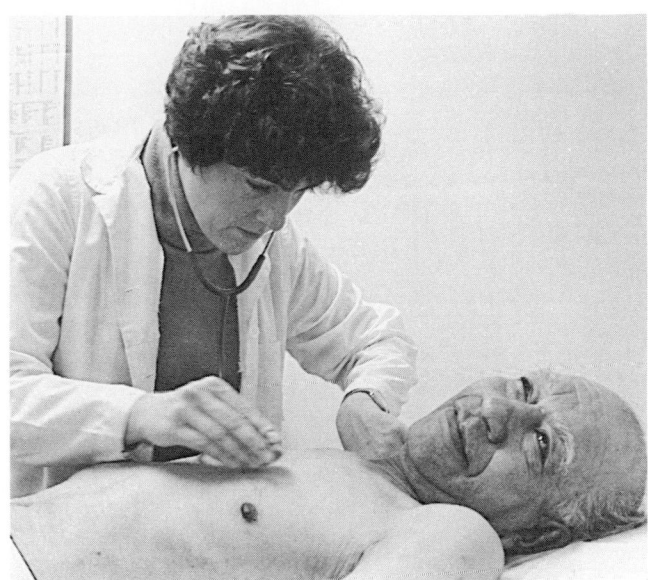

FIGURE 15-3
The nursing examination should include appraisal of health status, identification of health problems, and the establishment of a data base for nursing intervention. (Photo by Gates Rhodes, courtesy of the School of Nursing, University of Pennsylvania)

present, the nurse is concerned with identifying how this deficit affects the reasoning of the client, as well as his or her sensory-motor abilities. For example, the client with a cerebrovascular accident (stroke) will be examined to determine his or her ability to comprehend and communicate information; his or her ability to execute the tasks of everyday life should also be examined.

Purposes of the nursing examination include the appraisal of health status, the identification of health problems, and the establishment of a data base for nursing intervention. Nurses practicing in different settings may use different physical assessment techniques for different purposes. In the coronary care unit, nurses use sophisticated assessment techniques, while in a rehabilitation center, nurses use a wide range of physical assessment skills, which focus clearly on identifying functional and nonfunctional response patterns to disabilities.

The nursing examination involves assessment of all body systems in a systematic manner; often, a head-to-toe format is used. These data may be documented on a separate nursing examination tool or may be incorporated into a combined data base assessment form, as illustrated here. Nurses may also employ physical assessment skills to evaluate selected systems.

Techniques. Four methods are commonly used to collect data during a physical assessment: inspection, palpation, percussion, and auscultation. These techniques and the basic skills the student must learn to perform the nursing examination are described in Chapter 24.

(Text continues on p. 265.)

BRONSON METHODIST HOSPITAL
Kalamazoo, Michigan

Medical/Surgical-Critical Care Admission Assessment

A. Name: *Margaret Tembra*

Prefers to be called: *Mrs. Tembra*   Age: *72*

Date: *9/2/89*   Time of arrival to unit: *2:00 pm*

Mode of admission: *wheelchair*

I.D. bracelet on and coincides with addressograph: ☑Yes ☐ No Information given by: *patient and her daughter Lisa*

If unable to reach next of kin/legal guardian, contact: *Barbara Tembra*   Phone: *634-5221*

Valuables (list and state disposition): *eye glasses (at bedside); purse taken home by daughter Lisa; no other valuables*

Admitted from: ☑Home ☐ Nursing Home ☐ Assisted Living ☐ Foster Care ☐ Senior Citizens' Apartments ☐ Other

Facility Name: ___   Adm. Medical Diagnosis: *T.I.A.*

DEMOGRAPHIC DATA

B. Ht: *5'2"*   Wt: *63.6* Kg

Temp: *98.2°F*   ☑Oral ☐ Ax. ☐ Rectal

Pulse: *88*   ☐ Reg. ☑Irreg.

Resp.: *18*   ☑Reg. ☐ Irreg.

BP: Left: *184/120*
☑Lying ☐ Sitting ☐ Standing

Right: *180/120*
☑Lying ☐ Sitting ☐ Standing

VITAL SIGNS

C. (The following have been explained):

ORIENTATION TO UNIT

Call system/bed-bathroom	☑Yes ☐ N/A	Floor restrictions ☑Yes ☐ N/A
Bed operation/siderails	☑Yes ☐ N/A	Visitation Policy ☑Yes ☐ N/A
Bathroom/bedpan–urinal	☑Yes ☐ N/A	Lounge ☑Yes ☐ N/A
TV/CH2/telephone	☑Yes ☐ N/A	Newspaper/mail ☑Yes ☐ N/A
Meal/cafeteria hours	☑Yes ☐ N/A	Siderails policy ☑Yes ☐ N/A
Smoking policy	☑Yes ☐ N/A	Chaplain services ☑Yes ☐ N/A

Signature: *Margaret Tembra*

D. Health Patterns Assessment: Complete information, **including patient's words.** Indicate N/A if non-applicable. Circle, code, or check all other findings as appropriate.

HEALTH PERCEPTION/HEALTH MANAGEMENT

1. Reason for hospitalization/chief complaint: *"I fell in the kitchen this morning and couldn't move my left leg for awhile; I've also been having headaches"*

Recent illness/exposure to communicable disease: ___

Previous hospitalizations/surgeries: *about 1965 gall bladder surgery; hospitalized for high blood pressure 1985*

What other health problems have you had? ___

Things done to manage health: *"I drink lots of water, eat fruit and avoid fried foods. I try not to worry so much."*

Statement of patient's general appearance (include condition of hair, skin, nails): *Alert, medium-built, well-nourished female; appears anxious about hospitalization: voice low, grabs daughter's hand; neat appearance; skin pale, cool and dry; gray hair-thin; scalp clean; thick nails; adequate cappillairy refill.*

Tobacco use: ☐ Yes ☑No ☐ Used to smoke: ___

EtOH use: *none*

Allergies: ☐ Yes (list with reaction experienced) ☑No

Food: ___

Medications/anesthetics: ___

Other (e.g., wool, tape, pollens): *regular soaps cause skin to be excessively dry*

Patient's Name: *Tembra, Margaret*   Hospital No.: *4629 F*   Date: *9/2/89*

Medications: (e.g., prescript., non-prescript.) ☑Yes ☐No Did you bring? ☐Yes ☑No Taken home? ☐Yes ☐No ☐N/A

NAME	DOSE	SCHEDULE	REASON	PRESCRIBING PHYSICIAN
hydralazine	*?*	*OD*	*high blood pressure*	*Dr. Skomar*
aspirin	*ii*	*PRN*	*headaches*	*—*
metamucil	*1 Tbsp*	*PRN*	*constipation*	*—*

Have you been taking your medication(s) as prescribed? *yes*

OTHER PERTINENT DATA: *—*

| | *SCT* | initials |

2. Special diet? *—*   Supplements: *—*

Pattern of daily food/fluid intake: *Drinks at least 5-6 glasses H₂O daily + juices + tea; ↓ fried, fatty foods; likes baked or broiled meat, vegetables + fruit, "sweet tooth."*

Appetite: *"very good"*   Wt. loss/gain: *—*

Nausea/Vomiting: *—*

GI pain: *—*

Condition of oral mucous membranes: *pink, moist*

Dental condition: *dentures clean*   Dentures: ☑Upper ☑Lower ☐Partial ☐N/A

Skin: ☐Warm ☑Dry ☑Cool ☐Moist ☐Other: *pale*

Turgor: ☑Supple ☐Firm ☐Fragile ☐Dehydrated ☐Other:

Color: ☐Pink ☑Pale ☐Dusky ☐Cyanotic ☐Jaundiced ☐Mottled ☐Other:

Edema: *+ 1 ankles*

Wounds/drains/dressings: *—*

Skin problems (description and location): *skin on legs and upper arms dry + scaley; scratch marks; reddened area under left breast — skin intact.*

I.V.'s: *—*   ☐N/A

OTHER PERTINENT DATA: *—*

| | *SCT* | initials |

NUTRITION/METABOLIC

3. Abd. tenderness/guarding/distention: *—*

Bowel sounds: *present all 4 quadrants*   Stoma (type): *—*

Any problems with hemorrhoids/involuntary stool? *hx hemorrhoid 2° straining/constipation*

Usual bowel pattern (frequency, character, consistency, etc.): *Stools tend to be hard and dry -- q 2-3 days*   Date of last BM: *9/1/89*

If problem, describe: *occasional (1x/wk) constipation*

Use of anything to manage bowels (e.g., laxatives, enemas, suppositories, "home remedies", anti-diarrheals): *↑ fluids, ↑ fruit, metamucil; dislikes bran*

Usual urinary pattern (frequency, character, amount, incontinence, nocturia, etc.): *5-6 x per day; up once at night to void*

Last void (time): *"this AM"*

If problem, describe:

Perspiration/nocturnal sweats: *—*

OTHER PERTINENT DATA: *—*

| | *SCT* | initials |

ELIMINATION

FORM 102 (Revised 10/84) — Page 2

4.

CARDIO-VASCULAR STATUS

Peripheral pulses: _palpable, strong_ ☐ N/A

Neurovascular check (e.g., capillary refill): _↓ sensation (hot/cold sharp/dull) L leg; rapid capillary refill_

Chest pain/radiation: _—_

Jugular vein distention: ☐ Yes ☑ No
Hx of murmur: ☐ Yes ☑ No
Pacemaker: ☐ Yes ☑ No
Presence of A-V Shunt: _—_ ☑ No
Arterio-venous bruit: _____ ☑ N/A
Monitor/rhythm: _____ ☑ N/A
Hemodynamic monitoring: _—_ ☑ N/A

Tembra, M., 4269 F

RESPIRATORY STATUS

Respiratory pattern: ☑ No problem ☐ Dyspnea ☐ Nocturnal Dyspnea ☐ S.O.B. at rest
☐ S.O.B. on exertion: _—_ ☐ Other: _—_
Lung sounds: _clear_ Use of accessory muscles? ☐ Yes ☑ No
Cough/production: _—_ O₂ supplement: _—_ ☑ N/A
Resp. tubes (e.g., ET, trach, chest/describe secretions/drainage): _—_ ☑ N/A
Ventilatory assistance: _____ ☑ N/A

ACTIVITY / EXERCISE

ACTIVITIES OF DAILY LIVING/MOBILITY STATUS

Use the **Activity Level Code** below to assess admission statuses:

	ADL Status		**Mobility Status**	
0–total independence	Feeding _set up tray_	Meal Preparation _—_	Bed mobility _2_	
1–assist with device	Bathing _2_	Cleaning _—_	Cart transfer _bedrest_	
2–assist with person	Dressing _0_	Shopping _—_	Chair/toilet transfer _bedrest_	
3–assist with device & person	Grooming _0_	Laundry _—_	Ambulation _bedrest_	
4–total dependence	Toileting _1_	Other _—_	R.O.M. _2_	

Handedness: ☑ Right ☐ Left
Able to use? ☑ Yes ☐ No
Reasons for ADL/Mobility limitations: _Bedrest ordered during diagnostic work-up; At present able to move all 4 extremities_ ☐ N/A
Devices used for assist: _Bed pan_ ☐ N/A
Do you need assistance with transportation? ☐ Yes ☐ No If "Yes", specify: _—_
Where do you plan to be discharged? _home_ Will you need assistance? ☐ Yes ☑ No
If "Yes", describe: _____
OTHER PERTINENT DATA: _—_

| _SCT_ | initials |

5.

REFLEXES

Level of consciousness: _Alert_ Oriented to: ☑ Person ☑ Place ☑ Time
Behaviors (describe): _Face reflects concern about 's morning's paralysis + hospitalization_
Hx of epilepsy/seizures/Parkinson's, etc.. _—_

Reflexes: ☑ No problem ☐ Problem (If "No problem", do not complete this section.)
Eyes: Pupil size: r _O_ l _O_ Equal? ☑ Yes ☐ No Reaction to light: r _✓_ l _✓_
Accommodation: r _✓_ l _✓_ Deviation: _____
Handgrasp: r _✓_ l _✓_ Gag: _✓_ Swallow: _✓_
Movement of extremities: _↓ strength and ↓ movement left lower extremity_

COGNITIVE / PERCEPTUAL

SENSORIUM

Eyes/sight: ☐ No problem ☑ Deficit: _"blurry vision" at times_ Aid: _eyeglasses_
Ears/hearing: ☐ No problem ☑ Deficit: _"hard of hearing" L ear_ Aid: _none_
Nose/smell: ☑ No problem ☐ Deficit: _____
Tongue/taste: ☑ No problem ☐ Deficit: _____
Skin/touch: ☑ No problem ☐ Deficit: _____
Numbness/tingling: ☐ No problem ☑ Deficit: _left leg "feels queer — pins and needles"_
Dizziness: ☐ No problem ☑ Deficit: _feels "slightly dizzy — unsteady"_

Patient's Name: _Tembra, M._ Hospital No.: _4269 F_ Date: _9/2/89_

COGNITIVE / PERCEPTUAL

PAIN

Pain: ☐ No problem ☑ Problem (If "No problem", do not complete this section.)

If "Problem", describe location, type, intensity, onset, duration: _headaches — began about 6 months ago — of increasing frequency and severity; at present occur 1-2×/wk, last 1-2 days_

Methods of pain management: _Asprin, other OTC extra strength pain relievers only helps "a little."_

COGNITION

Primary language: _English_ Speech deficit: _—_ Aid: _—_

Any learning difficulties? _—_

OTHER PERTINENT DATA: _—_

SCT | initials

---

6. SLEEP / REST

Usual sleep/rest pattern: _11 pm – 7 am_

Adequate? ☑ Yes ☐ No Factors affecting sleep/rest: _gets up to void once during night_

Methods to promote sleep: _—_

Hx of sleep disturbances: _—_

OTHER PERTINENT DATA: _—_

SCT | initials

---

7. SELF-PERCEPTION SELF-CONCEPT

Are there any ways you feel differently about yourself since you've been ill/hospitalized? _____

"never questioned my health" expresses fear

Description of non-verbal behaviors: _quiet speech, wrinkled brow, wants daughter near_

OTHER PERTINENT DATA: _daughter reports mother has been very independent, strong woman - rarely ill_

SCT | initials

---

8. ROLE / RELATIONSHIP

Marital status: _Widowed_ Children: _3_

Do you live? ☐ Alone ☑ With family ☐ Other: _lives with daughter Lisa & her family_

Family feelings regarding hospitalization: _Concern_

Who are the people that will help you most at this time? _2 daughters: Lisa, Barbara_

Are you presently employed? ☐ Yes ☑ No Occupation: _____ ☐ N/A

Are you presently in school? ☐ Yes ☑ No Will illness/hospitalization interfere? _____ ☐ N/A

Upon discharge, if necessary, will you be able to afford?

Medications: ☑ Yes ☐ No Supplies: ☑ Yes ☐ No Medical Care: ☑ Yes ☐ No

OTHER PERTINENT DATA: _Husband died 8 months ago - moved in with daughter 6 months ago after selling family home - High Stress_

SCT | initials

---

9. SEXUALITY / REPRODUCTIVE

Female: ☐ N/A Menopausal: ☑ Yes ☐ No Menstrual pattern: _____ ☐ N/A

Problems/changes: _—_

Date of L.N.M.P. _____ ☑ N/A Possibly pregnant? ☐ Yes ☐ No ☐ N/A

Pregnancy history: _G 3 P 3_

Use of birth control measure ☐ Yes ☐ No ☑ N/A Type: _____

Any problems with use? _____

Monthly self-breast exam? ☐ Yes ☑ No ☐ N/A

Vaginal discharge/bleeding/lesions: _—_

Receiving medical attention? ☐ Yes ☑ No ☐ N/A

OTHER PERTINENT DATA: _—_

SCT | initials

Male: ☑ N/A Prostate problems? _____

Monthly self-testicular exam? ☐ Yes ☐ No ☐ N/A

Penile discharge/bleeding/lesions: _____

Receiving medical attention? ☐ Yes ☐ No ☐ N/A

OTHER PERTINENT DATA: _____

initials

10. Have you experienced any recent stressful situations in addition to your illness/hospitalization? ☑Yes ☐ No

If "Yes", please describe briefly: *In past year :*
death of husband
Sale of family home
relocation with daughter

Are there any ways we can be of assistance? *" can't think of any "*

How do you usually manage stresses? *talk with friends, pray*
" I used to share everything with my husband "

What do you do for relaxation? *used to crochet, watch TV*

Tembra, M. 4269F

Support groups/counselling resources used: ___

Were they helpful? ☐ N/A

OTHER PERTINENT DATA: *misses husband very much*

COPING/STRESS

| SCT | initials |

11. Will illness/hospitalization interfere with any of the following?

Spiritual or religious practices? ☐ Yes ☑No

Cultural beliefs or practices? ☐ Yes ☑No

Familial traditions? ☐ Yes ☑No

If "Yes", to any of the above, please describe briefly: _____

Would you like your clergy or hospital chaplain to be contacted? ☑Yes ☐ No ☐ N/A *daughter will contact minister*

OTHER PERTINENT DATA: _____

VALUE/BELIEF

| SCT | initials |

E. Include: a. Possible nursing diagnostic concept labels to consider for care planning.

b. Possible referral resources to consider for discharge planning needs.

c. Other pertinent information

a. Diagnostic labels : Impaired, altered bowel elimination :
constipation, potential impaired physical mobility,
potential self care deficit related to knowledge deficit :
TIA → stroke management, disturbance in self- concept,
skin integrity impairment

b. Social Service Referral
referral to home Minister

IMPRESSIONS

| SCT | initials |

DATE	TIME	INITIALS	SIGNATURES	
9/2/89	2:00 pm	SCT	S. Carol Taylor RN	(1st Adm. R.N.)
				(2nd Adm. R.N.)
				(3rd Adm. R.N.)
				(4th Adm. R.N.)

Sources of Data

The Client. The client is the primary and generally the best source of information. Unless specified otherwise, it is assumed that the data recorded in the nursing history has been collected from the client. Most clients are willing to share information when they know it will be helpful in planning their care. Although data collected from the client are usually accurate, the nurse should be alert to certain difficulties. For example, a client who is acutely ill may not be able to communicate adequately either if pain is severe or when consciousness is altered in any way. An emotionally upset client may distort information: a client who is fearful because he or she thinks the illness may threaten his or her work or life may deny certain symptoms or deliberately give misleading facts. If the nurse becomes aware that the client's report of symptoms differs from physical findings or data obtained from other sources, it is important to note this and to explore the cause of the discrepancy. The client with limited mental capacity or a very young client cannot be relied on to report accurately. Nevertheless, children, the elderly, and those with decreased mental capacity or impaired verbal abilities should be encouraged to respond to interview questions according to their ability. Bypassing these clients and automatically turning to a family member, friend, or caregiver for information communicates powerfully that the nurse either has no time for the client to express his or her needs, or that the nurse doubts the client's ability to communicate these needs.

Support Persons. Family members, friends, and caregivers are especially helpful sources of data when the client has limited capacity to share information with the nurse or when the client is a child. Husbands and wives often help supply information concerning their spouses. Friends frequently accompany a client to a health agency, and often can supply useful information. Care must be taken to determine that the client does not object to data being gathered from friends, and that these persons wish to participate. Also, the nurse is cautioned that there should be a clear understanding by the client, family, and friends of the confidentiality of the data collected. Whenever data are gathered from support persons, this should be indicated in the nursing history.

The Client Record. Records prepared by different members of the health-care team provide information essential to comprehensive nursing care. The nurse should review records early when gathering data—in some instances, before the first contact with the client. Such a review helps to focus the nursing assessment and to confirm and amplify information obtained from other sources.

The client's hospital record or chart, which lists such information as age, sex, occupation, religious preference, next of kin, and financial status is one type of record. The hospital record includes information entered by various health-care professionals, such as the physician, social worker, dietitian, physiotherapist, and laboratory technicians. Nurses who want their care to be supportive of the client as he or she responds to changes in health status must be familiar with the many sections of the client record other than the documentation of the nursing care plan and nursing notes. Important sources of data for the nurse include the following:

Medical History, Physical Examination, and Progress Notes. These record the findings of physicians as they assess and treat the client; they focus on identifying pathology, its etiology, and on determining the medical regimen that will best treat the problem.

Consultations. The client's physicians may invite specialists to assess and work with the client; focus is on documenting findings helpful in establishing a medical diagnosis or in planning and executing the medical regimen.

Reports of Diagnostic Studies. Reports of laboratory studies and other diagnostic tests, such as x-rays, offer the nurse objective data which can either confirm or conflict with data the nurse has collected during the nursing history or examination. Results of diagnostic studies are helpful to physicians in establishing a diagnosis and in monitoring the client's response to treatment. Results of these same studies may also be helpful to nurses in evaluating the success of nursing interventions.

Reports of Therapies by Other Health-Care Professionals. Other health-care professionals who interact with the client will also record their findings and note any progress the client is making in their specific areas, for example, nutrition, physical therapy, and speech therapy. These reports help the nurse to better assess the client's progress in general and are useful when determining the client's ability to return home and manage care independently.

Records of previous admissions for health care and records from other health agencies, such as a social agency or a visiting nurse agency, are also valuable sources of data. They contain information about the client's previous medical or surgical problems and response patterns, which may be important determinants of the present plan of care.

Health-Care Professionals. Nurses can learn a great deal about a client's normal health habits and patterns and response to illness by talking with other nurses, physicians, social workers, and other members of the health-care team. Although such communication is always important, it can be critical when clients are transferred between home and institution, institution and institution, or from one hospital to another. The only

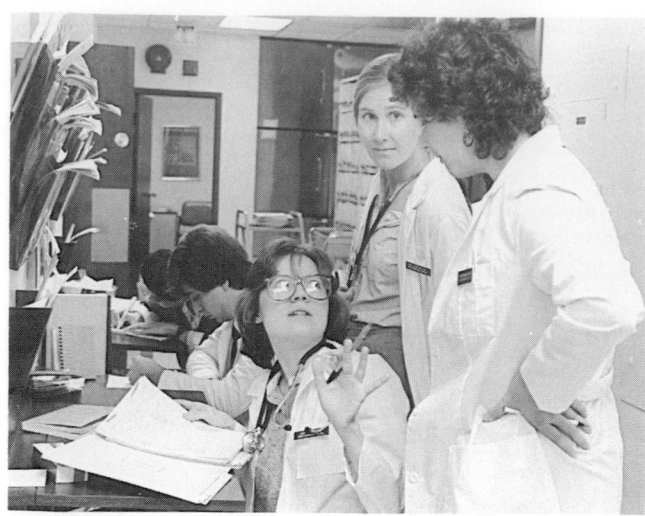

FIGURE 15-4
The client's hospital record and other members of the health-care team are two sources of information for a comprehensive client assessment. (Photo by Gates Rhodes, courtesy of the School of Nursing, University of Pennsylvania)

way to ensure continuity of care is to make special efforts to share pertinent information.

Nursing and Other Health-Care Literature. To obtain a comprehensive client data base, it may be necessary to consult the nursing and related literature on specific health problems. For example, if a nurse has not cared for a client with Paget's disease before, it will be important to read about the clinical manifestations of the disease and its usual progression in order to know what to look for when assessing the client. In addition to information concerning medical diagnoses, treatment, and prognosis, a literature review offers the nurse important information about nursing diagnoses, developmental norms, and psychosocial and spiritual practices that are helpful when assessing clients.

PLANNING DATA COLLECTION

Comprehensive Versus Focused Data Collection

Nursing assessments include both the comprehensive admission assessment (**data base** assessment) and the focused assessment. *Data base assessment* is usually performed during the nurse's initial contact with the client. The nurse collects data concerning *all aspects* of the client's health, establishing priorities for ongoing focused assessments. A data base nursing assessment structured according to Gordon's 11 functional health

patterns appears on pages 260 to 264. *Focused assessment* may be done during the initial assessment if client health problems surface, but it is routinely part of ongoing data collection. The focus is on gathering data about a *specific problem* that has already been identified (Alfaro, 1986, p 20).

Assessment Priorities

Before beginning to collect data on any client, the nurse should have a good sense of the type of data needed to best develop a satisfactory plan of care. Client data of interest to the nurse include
- Client profile (name, address, age, sex, race, culture, religion, education, occupation)
- Client's developmental stage and ability to meet developmental tasks
- Family, psychosocial, and environmental histories
- Health beliefs, habits, patterns (how client meets basic human needs)
- Client's responses (physical and emotional) to health and illness (functioning of each major body system)
- Meaning client attaches to health and illness
- Presence of risk factors
- Client resources: internal (*e.g.,* coping strengths) and external (*e.g.,* support persons, adequate finances, availability of health care)
- Client's expected and preferred modes of treatment (past experiences with health-care professionals)

The purpose for which the assessment is being performed offers the best guidelines as to what type and how much data to collect.

Assessment priorities will be influenced by the health orientation of the client, the developmental stage of the client, and by the client's need for nursing.

Health Orientation. Wellness assessments such as the *Health-style* self-test in Chapter 2, may be used by nurses to assist clients to identify potential and actual health risks and to explore habits, behaviors, beliefs, attitudes, and values that influence levels of wellness (Pinnell and deMeneses, 1986). Hill and Smith (1985) offer nurses interested in wellness a variety of specialized assessment tools that focus on relationships, psychologic self-care, relaxation, spirituality, humor and play, movement and exercise, sleep and dreams, nutrition, sexuality, environmental self-care, and physical self-care. These assessments are very different from comprehensive admission assessments of clients being hospitalized for treatment in terms of the type of client data gathered.

Developmental Stage. Nursing assessments are modified according to the developmental needs of clients. For example, when assessing an infant, special attention is given to weight gain and physical growth, feeding and elimination problems, sleep–activity cycles, and to the parenting skills of caregivers. When children are hospitalized, it is similarly important to note how independent the child is with basic care measures (toileting, hygiene, dressing, eating), what words the child uses to indicate the need to void and defecate, play preferences, and so forth.

Need for Nursing. Whether or not nurses will be interacting with the client for a short or a long period of time (same-day surgery versus surgery necessitating long recovery in an intensive care unit) and the nature of nursing care needed by the client (assistance with the birth of a baby versus support and care throughout a terminal illness) powerfully influence the type of data the nurse collects. A general guideline when assessing clients is to gather only data that will be helpful when planning and delivering care. Thus it would be inappropriate to collect a detailed sexual history on a client admitted to the hospital overnight following a slight concussion. Conversely, the nurse who fails to ask a pregnant woman admitted to the hospital for observation because of bleeding during her first trimester if she has any questions about resuming sexual activity once she gets home is doing the client a great disservice.

Practical Considerations. Data already collected from the client and communicated in the client record should not be repeatedly sought from the client unless there is a need to validate this data. Repetitious questioning can be annoying to the client and may cause the client to wonder about the lack of communication among health-care professionals. A careful review of the client record prior to interviewing the client will avoid this problem.

Before meeting a new client, it is helpful to take a minute to carefully think about the type of data needed to plan quality care. After the comprehensive nursing assessment has been completed, client health problems will dictate assessment priorities for future nurse–client interactions.

Structuring the Assessment

Having now studied the different types of data nurses collect about clients, it is easy to see the need to structure data collection systematically. Developing and using systematic guidelines specifically developed for a nursing assessment ensures that comprehensive, holistic data will be collected for each client and will lead easily to the development of nursing diagnoses. Once the nurse internalizes the assessment guidelines, it is easier to focus on the client during the assessment rather than worrying about what to assess next.

Most schools of nursing and health-care institutions have developed their own structured assessment guide-

---

Functional Health Patterns

Health-perception–health-management pattern Describes client's perceived pattern of health and well-being and how health is managed

Nutritional-metabolic pattern Describes pattern of food and fluid consumption relative to metabolic need and pattern indicators of local nutrient supply

Elimination pattern Describes patterns of excretory function (bowel, bladder, and skin)

Activity-exercise pattern Describes pattern of exercise, activity, leisure, and recreation

Cognitive-perceptual pattern Describes sensory-perceptual and cognitive pattern

Sleep-rest pattern Describes patterns of sleep, rest, and relaxation

Self-perception–self-concept pattern Describes self-concept pattern and perceptions of self (*e.g.,* body comfort, body image, feeling state)

Role-relationship pattern Describes pattern of role-engagements and relationships

Sexuality-reproductive pattern Describes client's patterns of satisfaction and dissatisfaction with sexuality pattern; describes reproductive patterns

Coping–stress-tolerance pattern Describes general coping pattern and effectiveness of the pattern in terms of stress tolerance

Value-belief pattern Describes patterns of values, beliefs (including spiritual), or goals that guide choices or decisions

(Reprinted with permission. Gordon M: Nursing Diagnosis: Process and Application, 2nd ed. New York, McGraw-Hill, 1987, p 93)

---

lines, many of which are based on a selected nursing theory. Gordon (1987) proposes a standardized structure for delineating the basic areas of assessment applicable to all clients and compatible with all nursing theories. This framework (see box) identifies 11 functional health patterns and organizes client data into these patterns.

What all assessment guides offer the nurse is a special way to "look at" the client; this simplifies the assess-

Assessment Priorities Using Orem's Self-care Deficit Theory

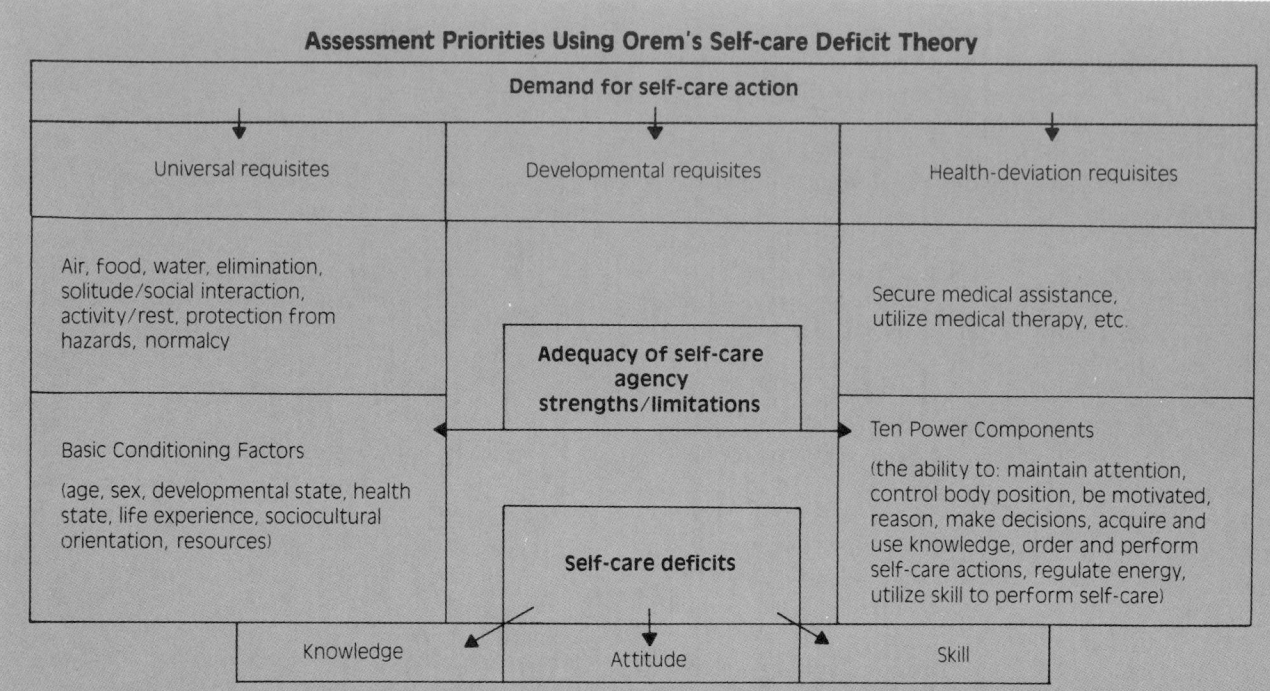

Demand for self-care action

Universal requisites	Developmental requisites	Health-deviation requisites
Air, food, water, elimination, solitude/social interaction, activity/rest, protection from hazards, normalcy		Secure medical assistance, utilize medical therapy, etc.

Adequacy of self-care agency strengths/limitations

| Basic Conditioning Factors (age, sex, developmental state, health state, life experience, sociocultural orientation, resources) | | Ten Power Components (the ability to: maintain attention, control body position, be motivated, reason, make decisions, acquire and use knowledge, order and perform self-care actions, regulate energy, utilize skill to perform self-care) |

Self-care deficits

| Knowledge | Attitude | Skill |

Assessment Priorities Using Gordon's Functional Health Patterns

- Health-perception—health management pattern
- Elimination pattern
- Role-relationship pattern
- Cognitive-perceptual pattern
- Coping-stress tolerance pattern
- Value-belief pattern
- Self-perception self-concept pattern
- Nutritional-metabolic pattern
- Sleep-rest pattern
- Activity-exercise pattern

Assessment Priorities Using Roy's Adaptation Theory

Adaptive Modes

1. Physiologic needs
   - exercise and rest
   - nutrition
   - elimination
   - fluid and electrolytes
   - oxygen and circulation
   - regulation: temperature
   - regulation: the senses
   - regulation: endocrine system

2. Self-concept
   - physical self
   - moral-ethical self
   - self-ideal
   - self-esteem

3. Role function

4. Interdependence

ment. Internalizing this "picture" makes the task of assessment much easier. The display on page 268 shows how the person is viewed by Gordon as compared to two nursing theorists, Orem and Roy. Orem directs the nurse's attention to the client's self-care abilities, while Roy focuses on the client's adaptive responses.

Problems Related to Data Collection

Problems frequently encountered during data collection include an inappropriately organized data base, pertinent data omitted, irrelevant or duplicate data collected, erroneous or misinterpreted data collected, too little data acquired from client, interpretation of data recorded rather than observed behavior, and failure to update data base. Table 15-3 lists these problems and describes possible causes and remedies.

DATA VALIDATION

Validation is the act of confirming or verifying. The purpose of validating is to keep data as free from error, bias, and misinterpretation as possible. Validation is an important part of assessment because invalid information can lead to inappropriate nursing care.

Validation of all data is neither possible nor necessary; the nurse needs to decide which items need verifying. For example, data needs to be verified when there are discrepancies: A client tells the nurse he is fine and has no concerns, but the nurse notes that he demonstrates tense body musculature and seems curt in his responses. There is a discrepancy between what the person is saying and what the nurse is observing, and so

T A B L E **15-3**
Common Problems of Data Collection, Possible Causes, and Suggested Remedies

Problem	Possible Causes	Suggested Remedies
Data base inappropriately organized	Failure to plan for the assessment by identifying needed data; use of inappropriate tools for data collection	Review the guidelines for specifying pertinent data. Consider modifying tool for data collection or select an alternative tool.
Pertinent data omitted	Not following up on clues during data collection; inappropriate guidelines	Identify potentially relevant factors in advance of collection. Practice interview strategies.
Irrelevant or duplicate data collected	Failure to identify specific purpose of data collection; failure to review available client records; use of inappropriate tools for data collection	Determine specific purpose of data collection for each client. Consider existing data before initiating collection. Consider modifying data collection tool or selecting alternative.
Erroneous or misinterpreted data collected	Failure to observe carefully or validate during data collection; interviewer prejudices or stereotypes	Sharpen observation skills by independently observing the same situation with a peer and compare notes afterward. Role play several validation techniques.
Too little data acquired from client	Failure to establish sufficient rapport or use appropriate communication techniques with client; failure to know what information is wanted	Review and practice communication techniques discussed in Chapter 20. Role play several explanations of purpose of data collection. Identify general data desired before collection.
Interpretation of data is recorded rather than the observed behavior	Nurse jumps to hasty conclusion about client's behavior and deprives others of exploring with the client possible causes of the behavior; deficient validation.	Review the distinction between data and interpretation of data. Practice documenting observed client behavior concisely.
Failure to update the data base	Erroneous belief that assessment is concluded once the initial data base is recorded; low priority attached to ongoing data collection	Recollect that it is impossible to give quality individualized care without knowledge of changes in the client's status. Ongoing data collection is critical to the deletion or modification of old problems and the identification of new problems.

validation is necessary to determine accuracy. Validation in this instance may simply take the form of the nurse saying, "You tell me you feel fine but right now your body and behaviors are telling me something else. I wonder why this is?"

Data also need verifying when there is lack of objectivity in the data. For example, a nurse suspects that the patient hears from one ear but does not seem to hear well from the other. The nurse should validate the data before proceeding and should determine whether the patient does indeed have a hearing problem. Suspicions are not objective. In this instance the nurse needs to test the hearing in both ears. Speaking toward the ear that is suspected to hear well, the nurse explains, "It seems to me that you hear better out of one ear than the other. I would like to test this. I'll bring a watch slowly toward your right ear first, and then your left. Please look straight ahead and tell me when you first hear the watch ticking." The nurse then records the distance from each ear at which the client first heard the ticking watch.

The nurse may validate data as they are collected, or may wish to do so at the end of the data-gathering process. When it is clear that the data are correct, the nurse is ready to analyze the data and formulate nursing diagnoses—the next step of the nursing process.

DATA COMMUNICATION

The client data collected by the nurse both initially and as client contact continues is of no benefit to the client and the health care team unless it is appropriately communicated. Appropriate communication involves correct timing and proper documentation.

Timing

Immediate verbal communication of data is indicated whenever assessment findings reveal a critical change in the client's health status that necessitates the involvement of other nurses or health-care professionals. The nurse who observes an elevated temperature of 103.2°F in a client scheduled for surgery that morning must report this to the charge nurse and to the surgeon, who will most likely cancel surgery. Failure to communicate this finding could result in the client's receiving preoperative sedation, being taken to the operating room, and even having the surgery performed. Similarly, a nurse who hears a client making suicidal remarks must communicate this information to the health-care team, so that all are alerted to the client's danger and so that suicide precautions may be taken immediately.

The nurse who is unsure of the significance of a particular finding is well advised to consult with another nurse. In some situations, years of experience are needed to accurately distinguish significant from nonsignificant findings. Neither ignorance nor the fear of ap-

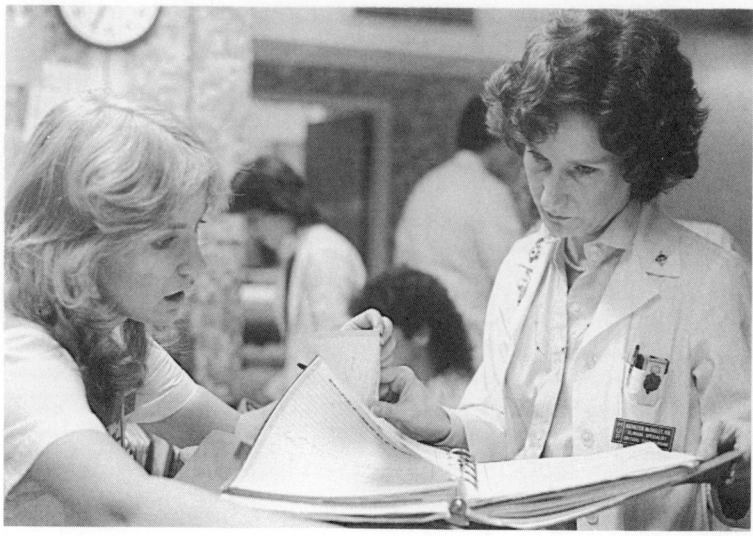

F I G U R E   15-5
Immediate verbal communication of data is indicated whenever assessment findings reveal a critical change in the client's health status. (Photo by Gates Rhodes, courtesy of the School of Nursing, University of Pennsylvania)

pearing "less than competent" justifies failure to report critical data.

Documentation

The initial data base should be recorded in ink, using the designated agency forms, the same day the client is admitted to the agency. If for any reason important data cannot be obtained during the initial assessment, this needs to be documented so that it will be obtained as soon as possible. Objective and subjective client data should be summarized and written, so that data communicate a unique sense of the client and are comprehensive, concise, and easily retrievable. The data should be written legibly, good grammar should be used, and only standard medical abbreviations should be used. To facilitate quick data retrieval, data should be presented under clearly marked headings.

Whenever possible, subjective data should be recorded using the client's own words. Quotation marks should be used: "I feel tired from the moment I first get up in the morning. Any more it seems I have no energy at all." Client reports may also be paraphrased: Client reports feeling dyspneic, "hard to catch my breath" when walking one flight of stairs.

The tendency to record data using nonspecific terms which are subject to individual definition or interpretation—adequate, good, average, normal, poor, small, large—should be avoided. One nurse's sense of what constitutes an "average fluid intake" may be very different from that of another nurse. It is important to be specific.

KEY POINTS

■ Assessing is the systematic and continuous collection, validation, and communication of client data. A data base is all the pertinent client information collected by the nurse and other health-care professionals which enables a comprehensive and effective plan of care to be designed and implemented for the client.

■ Ongoing nursing assessment alerts the nurse to changes in the client's responses to health and illness and suggests necessary changes in the plan of care.

■ Unlike medical assessments whose primary purpose is to define the existence of medical problems and identify the underlying pathology, nursing assessments are focused primarily on client responses to health problems.

■ Objective data are perceptible to the senses and able to be verified by another person observing the same data. Subjective data can only be perceived by the affected person and cannot be perceived or verified experientially by another.

■ Common methods used for collecting data in nursing are observation, interview, and examination. Observation is the conscious and deliberate use of the five senses to gather data. Skilled nurses observe clients for significant data during each nurse–client interaction.

■ Strong interviewing skills are needed by the nurse to obtain a comprehensive nursing history which captures the unique qualities and characteristics of the client in a way that makes individualized care planning possible.

■ During the nursing examination the nurse assesses the client for objective data to better define the client's condition and help the nurse in planning care. The nursing examination is focused primarily on the functional abilities of the client.

■ The primary source of client data is the client. Unless specified otherwise it is assumed that the data recorded in the nursing history are from the client. Other important sources of client data are the client's support persons, the client record, other health-care professionals, and the nursing and related health-care literature.

■ A data base nursing assessment is done during the nurse's initial contact with the client and involves collecting data about all aspects of the client's health. A focused assessment may be done during any nurse–client interaction. Its purpose is to gather data about a specific problem.

■ Before beginning to collect data the nurse should have a good sense of the type of data needed to best develop a satisfactory plan of care. Assessment priorities will be influenced by the health orientation of the client, the developmental stage of the client, and by the client's need for nursing.

■ Using systematic assessment guidelines specifically developed for a nursing assessment ensures that comprehensive, holistic data will be collected for each client which easily lead to the development of nursing diagnoses.

■ Problems related to data collection include data base inappropriately organized, pertinent data omitted, irrelevant or duplicate data collected, erroneous or misinterpreted data collected, too little data acquired from the client, interpretation of data rather than observed behavior is recorded, and failure to update data base.

■ Validation is the act of confirming or verifying. The purpose of validating is to keep data as free from error, bias, and misinterpretation as possible. Common instances when data need validating are when there are discrepancies in the data collected and when there is a lack of objectivity in the data.

■ The client data collected by the nurse, both initially and as client contact continues, are of no benefit to the client and the nursing and health-care teams unless it is appropriately communicated. It is important to learn when significant data need to be communicated verbally immediately and how to document data.

■ Client data should be summarized and written so that they communicate a unique sense of the client and are comprehensive, concise, and easily retrievable.

BIBLIOGRAPHY

Alfaro R: Application of Nursing Process: A Step-by-Step Guide. Philadelphia, JB Lippincott, 1986

American Nurses' Association: Nursing: A Social Policy Statement. Kansas City, MO, The Association, 1980

Bates B: A Guide to Physical Examination, 4th ed. Philadelphia, JB Lippincott, 1987

Cormier LS, Cormier WH, Weisse RJ: Interviewing and Helping Skills for Health Professionals. Monterey, CA, Wadsworth, 1984

Davis AJ: Listening and Responding. St Louis, CV Mosby, 1984

Eggland ET: How to take a meaningful nursing history. Nursing 7(7):22–30, 1977

Farrell J: The human side of assessment. Nursing 10(4):74–75, 1980

Fields WL, McGinn-Campbell KM: Introduction to Health Assessment. Englewood Cliffs, NJ, Reston, 1983

Gordon M: Nursing Diagnosis: Process and Application, 2nd ed. New York, McGraw-Hill, 1987

Hill L, Smith N: Self-Care Nursing. Englewood Cliffs, NJ, Prentice-Hall, 1985

Malasanos L, Barkauskas V, Moss M, Stoltenberg-Allen K: Health Assessment, 3rd ed. St Louis, CV Mosby, 1985

McPhetridge LM: Nursing history: One means to personalize care. Am J Nurs 68(1):68–75, 1968

Orem D: Nursing: Concepts of Practice, 3rd ed. New York, McGraw-Hill, 1985

Parish L: Communicating with hospitalized children. Canadian Nurse 82(1):21–24, 1986

Parker K: Health works: An adolescent assessment tool. Canadian Nurse 82(1):28–31, 1986

Pinnell N, deMeneses M: The Nursing Process. Norwalk, CT, Appleton-Century-Crofts, 1986

Roy, Sr C: Introduction to Nursing: An Adaptation Model. Englewood Cliffs, NJ, Prentice-Hall, 1976

Smith CE: With good assessment skills you can conduct a solid framework for patient care. Nursing 14(12):26–31, 1984

Stewart CJ, Cash WB: Interviewing Principles and Practice, 4th ed. Dubuque, IA, Wm C Brown Publishing Co, 1985

Wolff H, Erickson R: The assessment man. Nurs Outlook 25:103–107, 1977

Diagnosing

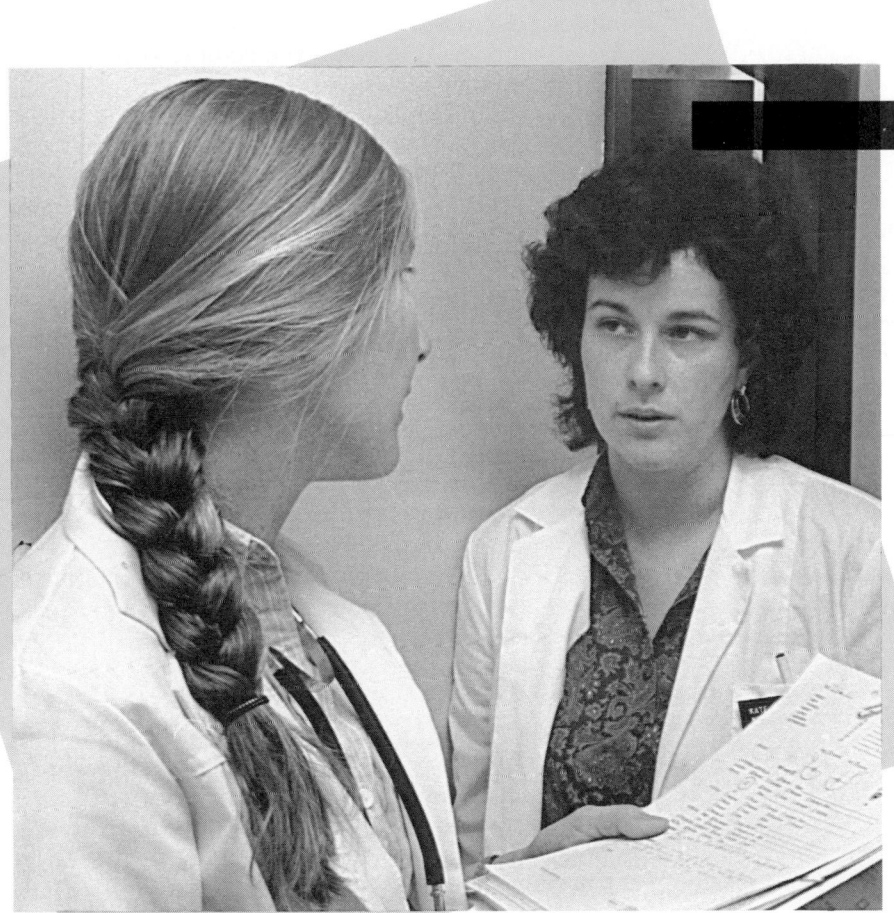

After studying this chapter, the learner should be able to

Define key terms used in the chapter.

Describe the term nursing diagnosis, distinguishing it from a collaborative problem and a medical diagnosis.

Describe the four steps involved in data interpretation and analysis.

Use the guidelines for writing nursing diagnoses when developing diagnostic statements.

List four advantages of using the NANDA approved list of nursing diagnoses.

Describe means to validate nursing diagnoses.

Develop a prioritized list of nursing diagnoses using identifiable criteria.

Describe the benefits and limitations of nursing diagnoses.

Once the nurse has collected and recorded the client data, the work of diagnosing begins—the second step in the nursing process. The purpose of diagnosing is to identify (1) actual and potential problems in the way the client responds to health or illness, (2) factors contributing to or causing the above problems (etiologies), and (3) strengths the client can draw on to prevent or resolve the problems.

During the diagnosing step of the nursing process, the nurse interprets and analyzes data gathered from the client and through the nursing examination and results of tests. These data help the nurse identify client strengths and health problems. A **health problem** is a condition related to health which requires intervention if disease or illness is to be prevented or resolved, and if coping and wellness are to be promoted.

When health problems are identified, the nurse must decide which health-care professional can best treat the problem. Actual or potential health problems that can be prevented or resolved by independent nursing intervention are termed **nursing diagnoses**. The nurse formulates and validates nursing diagnoses, and lists these nursing diagnoses by priority (see Fig 16-1).

A brief history of the evolution of nursing diagnosis may be found in Chapter 14. Now an accepted and essential step in the nursing process, nursing diagnosis was initially confused with medical diagnosis and sparked great controversy. Although this confusion has been clarified, many nurses have been slow to understand and describe the "work" of diagnosing. Several books have been written to describe the relationship of diagnosing to the other steps in the nursing process (see Bibliography).

UNIQUE FOCUS OF NURSING DIAGNOSIS

During the diagnosing step of the nursing process, the nurse identifies what it is about the client that is nursing's unique concern (*i.e.,* what it is about the client that gives rise to the need for nursing as opposed to the need for medicine or for physical therapy). Nursing diagnoses are therefore written to describe client problems that nurses can treat independently. As nurses interpret and analyze client data, they may identify health problems that are better treated by physicians (medical diagnoses) or by nurses working with other health-care professionals (collaborative problems). In such a case, the nurse reports the findings to the physician or health-care professional and works collaboratively with them on resolving the problem (see Fig 16-2).

Nursing Diagnosis Versus Medical Diagnosis

Medical diagnoses identify diseases, whereas nursing diagnoses focus on identifying unhealthy responses to health and illness. Medical diagnoses describe problems

KEY TERMS

collaborative problem
cue
data cluster
diagnosing
health problem

medical diagnosis
nursing diagnosis
actual problems
possible problems
potential problems

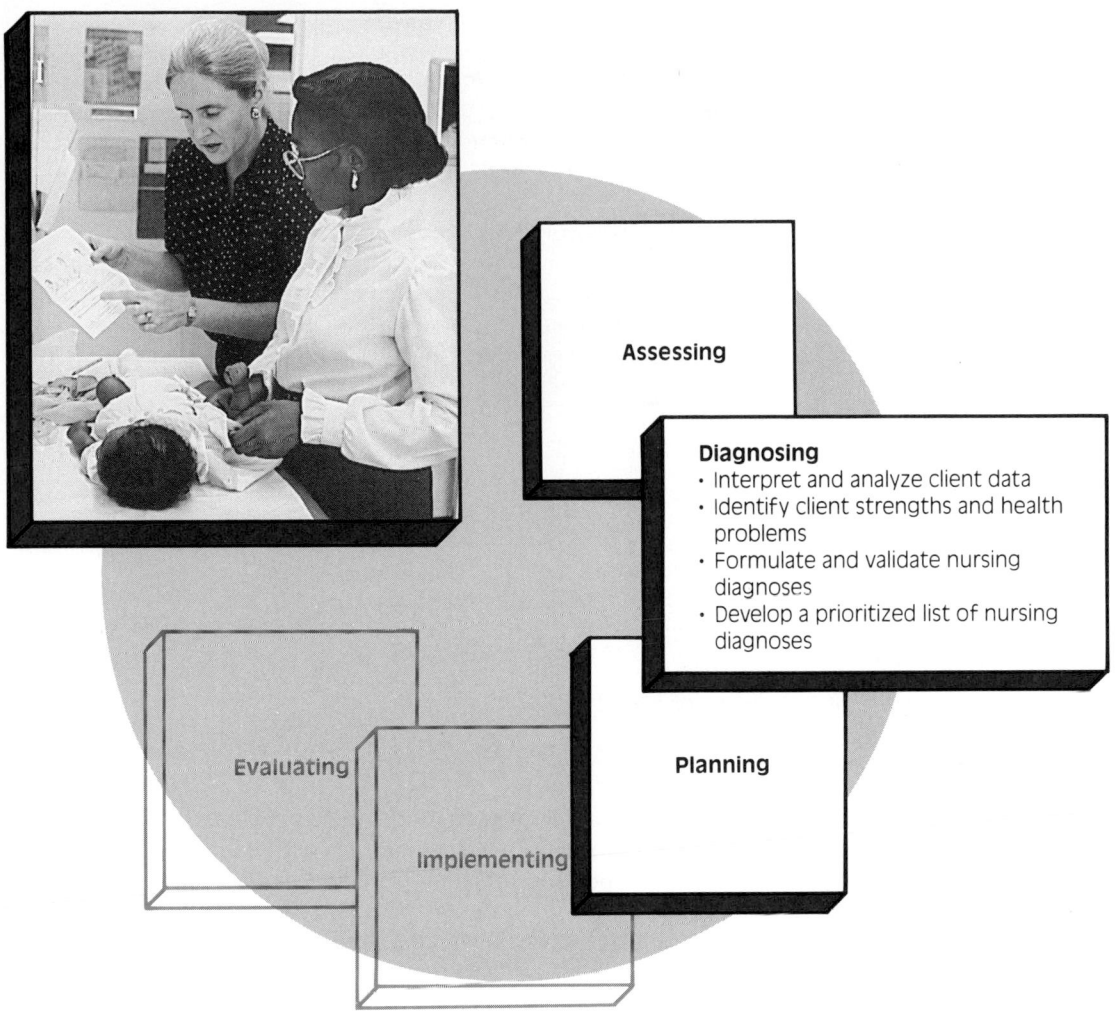

F I G U R E **16-1**

Diagnosing. Diagnosing is the interpretation and analysis of client data to identify client strengths and health problems that independent nursing intervention can prevent or resolve. Nursing diagnoses may change from day to day as the client's responses to health and illness change. (Photo by Gates Rhodes, courtesy of the School of Nursing, University of Pennsylvania)

for which the physician directs the primary treatment, as opposed to nursing diagnoses, which describe problems treated by nurses within the scope of independent nursing practice. A medical diagnosis remains the same for as long as the disease is present; a nursing diagnosis may change from day to day as the client's responses change. These distinctions are in keeping with the differing foci of medical and nursing practices (see Table 16-1).

Nursing Diagnosis Versus Collaborative Problems

Nursing diagnoses should also be distinguished from collaborative problems (see Table 16-1). Alfaro (1986, p 60) defines a **collaborative problem** as "an actual or potential problem that may occur from complications of disease, diagnostic studies, or medical or surgical treatment, and that can be prevented, resolved, or reduced through collaborative nursing intervention." Once a collaborative problem has been identified, the nurse consults with the appropriate health-care professional(s). Because collaborative problems deal with potential complications, it is important that they be identified so that the related nursing care, which is preventive in nature, can be instituted early.

DATA INTERPRETATION AND ANALYSIS

Experienced nurses generally begin the work of interpreting and analyzing data while they are still collecting (assessing) it. The term **cue** is often used to denote significant data or data that influence decisions. Such significant data should raise a red flag for the nurse, who then

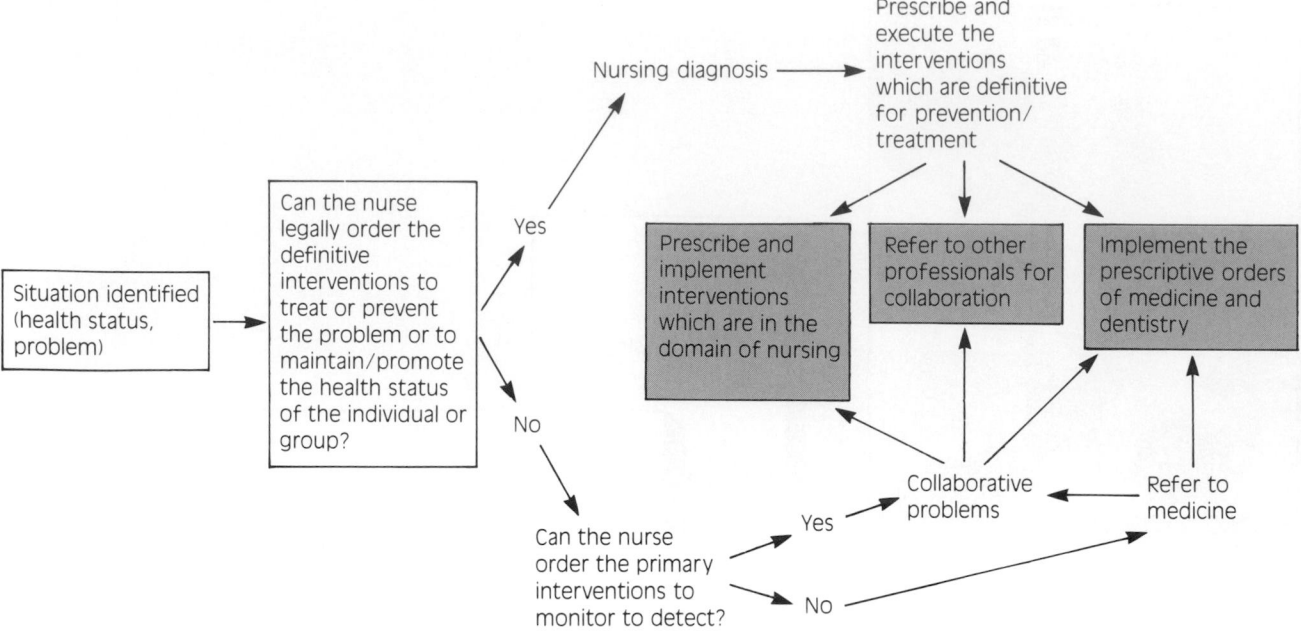

FIGURE 16-2
Differentiation of nursing diagnoses from collaborative problems. (© 1985, Lynda Juall Carpenito; used with permission)

looks for patterns or clusters of data that signal an actual, potential, or possible nursing diagnosis.

Recognizing Significant Data

Sorting out *healthy* client responses from those that are *not healthy* is not as clear-cut as it may seem. To avoid erroneously labeling selected client health patterns as unhealthy while failing to detect actual unhealthy behavior, nurses must be familiar with comparative standards to be used in data interpretation and analysis.

Comparing Data to Standards.   A standard or a norm is a generally accepted rule, measure, pattern, or model which can be used for comparing data in the same class or category. For example, when determining the signifi-

T A B L E   16-1
Comparison of Nursing Diagnoses with Medical Diagnoses and Collaborative Problems

Medical Diagnosis	Nursing Diagnosis	Collaborative Problem
Describes a disease	Describes a human response	Describes an act or potential problem that may result from complications of disease, diagnostic studies, or medical or surgical treatment
Stays the same as long as the disease is present	May change from day to day as human reactions change	May change from day to day as human responses change
Treatable by physicians within the scope of medical practice	Treatable by nurses within the scope of nursing practice	Treatable by nurses and other health-care professionals working collaboratively
Often deals with actual pathophysiologic changes within the body	Often deals with the *patient's perception* of his own health state	Often deals with a potential complication which if left untreated can become serious
Applies to diseases in individuals only	May apply to alterations in individuals or groups	May apply to problems in individuals or groups

(Adapted from Alfaro R: Application of Nursing Process. Philadelphia, JB Lippincott, 1986, p 67.)

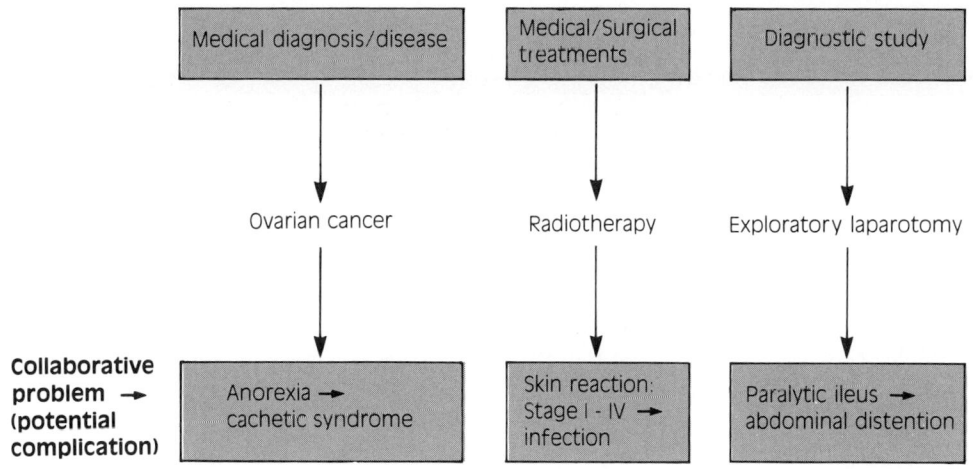

```
Medical diagnosis/disease        Medical/Surgical          Diagnostic study
                                 treatments

         |                            |                          |
         v                            v                          v

    Ovarian cancer              Radiotherapy          Exploratory laparotomy

         |                            |                          |
         v                            v                          v
Collaborative
problem  →      Anorexia →          Skin reaction:          Paralytic ileus →
(potential      cachetic syndrome   Stage I - IV →          abdominal distention
complication)                       infection
```

FIGURE 16-3
Collaborative problems.

cance of a client's blood pressure reading, appropriate standards include normative values for the client's age group, race, and illness category. The client's own normal range, if known, is an important standard. A pressure of 150/90 may be high for someone whose pressure is normally 120/70, but may be normal for an individual with hypertension. Examples of how standards may be used to identify significant cues follow below (Gordon, 1987, p 191):

- Changes in a client's usual health patterns that are unexplained by expected norms for growth and development
- Deviation from an appropriate population norm
- Behavior that is nonproductive in the whole-person context
- Behavior indicating a developmental lag or evolving dysfunctional pattern

Recognizing Patterns or Clusters

A **data cluster** is a grouping of client data or cues that points to the existence of a client health problem. Nursing diagnoses should always be derived from clusters of significant data, rather than from a single cue. The danger of deriving a nursing diagnosis from a single cue is illustrated in the following example. The nurse who diagnoses a woman recovering from gallbladder surgery with ineffective coping may have misinterpreted the client's use of tears as a healthy release of emotion. If, however, the same client begins to exhibit a cluster of significant cues, such as refusing to eat, preferring bed rest to scheduled ambulation, and reporting increasing discomfort, then an unhealthy pattern is emerging. Table 16-2 offers examples of how clusters of significant data lead to accurate nursing diagnoses.

Identifying Strengths and Problems

The next step in analyzing data is to determine client strengths and problems.

Determining the client's strengths. If a client appears to meet a standard, the nurse then concludes that the client has a strength in that particular area, and that this strength contributes to the client's level of wellness. For example, the individual who has a history of maintaining a well-balanced diet is usually better able to cope with illness than the individual who has a history of eating poorly.

Client strengths may include healthy physiologic functioning, emotional health, cognitive abilities, coping skills, interpersonal strengths, and spiritual strengths. Resources such as the presence of support persons, adequate finances, or a healthy environment may all contribute to client strengths. Many individuals take their strengths for granted and may not know how to use them effectively when responding to illness. Discussing observed strengths with clients and counseling clients about ways to develop and use their strengths are important nursing measures.

Determining the client's problem areas. An individual who does not meet a certain health standard most probably has a limitation in this aspect of health status and may profit from professional services. For example, the individual who has a long history of constipation is most likely in need of care to help overcome this problem. As stated previously, the nurse makes a decision concerning whether or not the data represent a nursing diagnosis or a collaborative problem, or whether it should be reported to the physician because it might contribute to the identification of a medical diagnosis.

Determining problems the client is likely to experience. It is also important for the nurse to identify potential health problems. For example, the nurse notes that a client has signs of a wound infection, but laboratory results show that the white blood cell count has not increased, as is usual when such an infection is present. The nurse concludes that the body apparently is not building up normal defenses to combat the infection. The nurse then predicts the problems this client is likely to encounter, such as a longer healing period than is

T A B L E   16-2
Diagnosing

Data Interpretation and Analysis		Formulation of Tentative Nursing Diagnosis	Validation of Nursing Diagnosis
Significant Cues	Sample Data Clusters		
Change in a client's usual health patterns that is unexplained by expected norms for growth and development	• "I guess I lost about 20 to 30 pounds over the last 6 months—I think I've just been too busy to eat." • Ht: 5'8" Wt: 102 lb • 35-year-old mother of 4-year-old twin boys; returned to work (executive secretary) for first time since delivery of twins 7 months ago	Nutritional alteration: less than body requirements related to stress of new job; role conflict/demands	Accurate diagnosis: Client validates this diagnosis, agreeing with contributing factors
Deviation from an appropriate population norm	• Teacher notices and reports frequency of bruises on third-grade boy who is repeatedly observed alone during recess periods and who is withdrawn in classroom • In conversation with the school nurse one parent remarks: "That boy brings out the worst in me! I don't know why but I often have to smack him hard to make him listen."	Potential violence (child abuse) related to ? etiology (deficient parenting skills?)	Incomplete diagnosis: Additional data collection yields new information: • Father out of work for last 18 months • Father was abused as a child Diagnosis restated: Potential for violence (child abuse) related to increased family stress and father's history of being abused
Behavior that is nonproductive in the whole-person context	• Fiance abruptly terminated relationship 3 months prior to established wedding date • Noticeable change in physical appearance; frequently wears same clothes; make-up, jewelry, hair-styling are absent; strong body odors present • No desire to be with others; goes home (lives alone) immediately after work • Stopped attending aerobics classes	Disturbance in self-esteem related to feeling rejected by fiance	Premature diagnosis resulting from incomplete data collection. Client has a long history of major depressive states one of which may have resulted in the break-up of this relationship. Medical disgnosis and treatment indicated. Changes in appearance are indicative of depressive state. Need to explore related nursing diagnoses.
Behavior indicating developmental lags or evolving dysfunctional patterns	• Admitted to nursing home 2 months ago • "I have nothing to live for anymore . . . why don't I die?" • Wishes to remain in room seated in chair—will only ambulate with great urging • Anything requiring movement has become "too much bother." • Decreased muscle mass, tone, and strength; reduced joint mobility	Impaired physical mobility related to difficult transition to nursing home	Accurate but routinized diagnosis which may result in staff's acceptance of status quo unless a more specific etiology is identified

normal. This prediction has implications for nursing care, such as measures related to the client's diet, fluid intake, urinary output, and mobility.

When determining strengths and problems, it is helpful to determine if the client agrees with the nurse's identification of a problem and is motivated to work toward its resolution.

Reaching Conclusions

The nurse reaches one of four basic conclusions after interpreting and analyzing the client data. Each conclusion has different nursing responses possible.

1. No problem
   - No nursing response indicated
   - Reinforce client's health habits and patterns
   - Initiate health promotion activities to prevent disease/illness or to promote a higher level of wellness
2. Possible problem
   - Collect more data to confirm or disconfirm suspected problem
3. Actual or potential nursing diagnosis
   - Unable to treat because client denies problem and refuses treatment (make sure client understands possible outcomes of this stance)
   - Begin planning, implementing, and evaluating care designed to prevent, reduce, or resolve the problem
4. Clinical problem other than nursing diagnosis
   - Consult with appropriate health-care professional and work collaboratively on problem

FORMULATING AND VALIDATING NURSING DIAGNOSES

Writing Nursing Diagnoses

Once the nurse recognizes a cluster of significant client data indicating a health problem that can be treated by independent nursing intervention, it is time to write the nursing diagnosis. Nursing diagnoses are written either as two-part statements listing the client's problem and its etiology, or as three-part statements which also include the problem's defining characteristics.

Problem. The purpose of the problem statement is to describe the health state or health problem of the client as clearly and concisely as possible. Because this section of the nursing diagnosis identifies what is unhealthy about the client and what the client would like to change in his or her health status, it should also suggest client goals. Using the list of health problems accepted by the North American Nursing Diagnosis Association

(NANDA) for testing and study (see p. 280) has several significant advantages when writing nursing diagnoses.

First, using a nationally accepted list of diagnoses will help nurses communicate with each other using common terminology. Nursing knowledge will be easier to teach and learn if authors, faculty, and clinicians all use the same terminology. Second, using common terminology will facilitate the use of computers in nursing, because nurses will be able to retrieve records according to nursing diagnoses rather than by medical diagnoses, and therefore will be able to collect data to further nursing research. Third, using a nationally accepted list of diagnostic categories provides a method for reimbursement according to nursing activities related to nursing diagnoses rather than to those related to medical diagnoses only. Fourth, all nurses can work together toward testing and refining the diagnostic categories to identify assessment criteria and nursing interventions to improve nursing care (Alfaro, 1986, p 67).

Pocket-sized handbooks of NANDA-approved nursing diagnoses are available and may be of great help to the student who is unfamiliar with this grouping of problem statements. Nurses who encounter different health problems within the scope of their practices which they believe to be nursing diagnoses may submit these to the NANDA Diagnosis Review Committee.

Etiology. The etiology identifies the physiologic, psychologic, sociologic, spiritual, and environmental factors believed to be related to the problem as either a cause or a contributing factor. Because the etiology identifies the factors that are maintaining the unhealthy client state and preventing the desired change, the etiology directs nursing intervention. Unless the etiology is correctly identified, nursing actions may be inefficient and ineffective. For example, a diabetic client who is frequently admitted to the hospital with hyperglycemia and who has a poor history of dietary and pharmacologic management is diagnosed to be noncompliant. Assuming that the noncompliance is related to a knowledge deficit and then channeling all nursing activities and energies into teaching the client how to manage the diabetes is useless if the noncompliance is actually a result of the client's decreased will to live.

Defining characteristics. The subjective and objective data that signaled the existence of the actual or potential health problem are the third component of the nursing diagnosis. NANDA has identified defining characteristics for each accepted nursing diagnosis, and familiarity with these characteristics assists nurses in recognizing clusters of significant data. The boxed material on page 281 shows the three components of a nursing diagnosis statement and their relationship to client goals, nursing measures, and evaluation. Other examples of nursing diagnosis statements are found throughout the book.

Approved Nursing Diagnoses, North American Nursing Diagnosis Association, June 1988

Activity intolerance
Activity intolerance, potential
Adjustment, impaired
Airway clearance, ineffective
Anxiety
Aspiration, potential for
Body temperature, altered, potential
Bowel elimination, altered: Constipation
   Colonic constipation
   Perceived constipation
Bowel elimination, altered: Diarrhea
Bowel elimination, altered: Incontinence
Breastfeeding, ineffective
Breathing pattern, ineffective
Cardiac output, altered: Decreased
Comfort, altered: Pain
Comfort, altered: Chronic pain
Communication, impaired: Verbal
Coping, family: Potential for growth
Coping, ineffective family: Compromised
Coping, ineffective family: Disabling
Coping, ineffective individual
   Defensive coping
   Ineffective denial
Decisional conflict (specify)
Disuse syndrome, potential for
Diversional activity, deficit
Dysreflexia
Family process, altered
Fatigue
Fear
Fluid volume altered: excess
Fluid volume deficit, actual
Fluid volume deficit, potential
Gas exchange, impaired
Grieving, anticipatory
Grieving, dysfunctional
Growth and development, altered
Health maintenance, altered
Health-seeking behaviors (specify)
Home maintenance management, impaired
Hopelessness
Hyperthermia
Hypothermia
Incontinence, functional
Incontinence, reflex
Incontinence, stress
Incontinence, total

Incontinence, urge
Infection, potential for
Injury, potential for: (specify) suffocation, poisoning, trauma
Knowledge deficit (specify)
Mobility, impaired physical
Noncompliance (specify)
Nutrition, altered: Less than body requirements
Nutrition, altered: More than body requirements
Nutrition, altered: Potential for more than body requirements
Oral mucous membrane, altered
Parental role conflict
Parenting, altered: Actual
Parenting, altered: Potential
Post trauma response
Powerlessness
Rape trauma syndrome
Role performance, altered
Self-care deficit: Feeding, bathing/hygiene, dressing/grooming, toileting
Self-concept, disturbance in body image, self-esteem, role performance, personal identity
Self-esteem disturbance
   Chronic low self-esteem
   Situational low self-esteem
Sensory perceptual alteration: Visual, auditory, kinesthetic, gustatory, tactile, olfactory
Sexual dysfunction
Sexuality patterns, altered
Skin integrity, impaired: Actual
Skin integrity, impaired: Potential
Sleep pattern disturbance
Social interaction, impaired
Social isolation
Spiritual distress (distress of the human spirit)
Swallowing, impaired
Thermoregulation, ineffective
Thought processes, altered
Tissue integrity, impaired
Tissue perfusion, altered: Cerebral, cardiopulmonary, renal, gastrointestinal, peripheral
Unilateral neglect
Urinary elimination, altered patterns
Urinary retention
Violence, potential for: Self-directed or directed at others

Formulation of Nursing Diagnoses Statement

Problem	Identifies what is unhealthy about the client indicating the need for change	Suggests the client goals (expectations for change)
Etiology	Identifies the factors that are maintaining the unhealthy state or response	Suggests the appropriate nursing measures
Defining characteristics	Identify the subjective and objective data which signal the existence of the problem	Suggest evaluative criteria
Problem	Clear, concise statement of the client health problem	Self-care deficit: bathing ↓ related to ↓
Etiology	Contributing or causative factors	Fear of falling in the tub and obesity ↓ as manifested by ↓
Defining characteristics	Defining characteristics (cues that reflect the existence of a pattern)	Strong body and urine odor, unshampooed hair: "I'm afraid I'll fall in the tub and break something." (5'4", 170 lb)

Two-part diagnostic statement: Self-care deficit: Bathing related to fear of falling in tub and obesity

Three-part diagnostic statement: Self-care deficit: Bathing related to fear of falling in tub and obesity, as manifested by strong body and urine odor, unshampooed hair, statement of fearing falling in tub, and height/weight: 5'4", 170 lb

Guidelines for Writing Nursing Diagnoses

1. Phrase the nursing diagnosis as a client problem or alteration in health state rather than as a client need.
2. Check to make sure that the client problem precedes the etiology and that the two are linked by the phrase "related to."
3. Defining characteristics, when included in the nursing diagnosis, should follow the etiology and be linked by the phrase "as manifested by."
4. Write in legally advisable terms.
5. Use nonjudgmental language.
6. Be sure the problem statement indicates what is unhealthy about the client or what the client wishes to change.
7. Avoid using defining characteristics, medical diagnoses, or something that cannot be changed in the problem statement.
8. Reread the diagnosis to make sure that the problem statement suggests client goals and that the etiology will direct the selection of nursing measures.

Common errors in writing nursing diagnoses are illustrated in Table 16-3, along with corrections.

What is Not a Nursing Diagnosis

The nursing diagnosis statement is written in terms of a client problem, alteration in health state, or client strength *for which nursing provides the primary therapy.* None of the following are nursing diagnoses: medical diagnoses, medical pathology, diagnostic tests, treatments, or equipment. Similarly, while all the following need to be considered when identifying nursing diagnoses, they do not belong as such in the diagnosis statement: therapeutic client needs, therapeutic client goals, a single sign or symptom, nor an *unvalidated* nursing inference. Examples of items frequently and erroneously placed in nursing diagnoses may be found in Table 16-4. Illustrations are derived from clients with diabetes mellitus.

Actual, Potential, and Possible Nursing Diagnoses

Client health problems may be **actual** (problem is present), **potential** (problem *may* occur), and **possible** (problem *may be* present). A *potential nursing diag-*

T A B L E   16-3
Common Errors in Writing Nursing Diagnoses with Recommended Corrections

Error	Example	Correction	Example
Writing the diagnosis in terms of needs and not response	Needs assistance with bathing related to bed rest	Write the diagnosis in terms of response rather than need	Self-care deficit: Bathing related to immobility
Making legally inadvisable statements	Noncompliance due to hostility toward nursing staff (the words "due to" imply a direct cause-and-effect relationship)	Use "related to" rather than "due to" or "caused by" to link the etiology to the problem statement	Noncompliance related to hostility toward nursing staff (denotes a relationship between the problem and etiology but not necessarily a causal relationship)
	Spouse abuse related to husband's immaturity and violent temper	Write the diagnosis in legally advisable terms: statements that may be interpreted as libel or that imply nursing negligence are legally hazardous to all the nurses caring for the client	Potential for violence: Spouse abuse related to husband's reported inability to control behavior
	Impaired skin integrity related to client's lying on back all night		Impaired skin integrity related to mobility deficit
Identifying as a problem a client response that is not necessarily unhealthy	Mild anxiety related to impending surgery	Include in the problem statement of the nursing diagnosis only client responses which are unhealthy or which the client wants to change	No need for nursing diagnosis: Mild anxiety prior to surgery is a healthy response which motivates preoperative self-care behavior
Identifying as a problem signs and symptoms of illness	Cough related to long history of smoking	Avoid including signs and symptoms of illness in the problem statement of the nursing diagnosis	Ineffective airway clearance related to 20-year history of smoking
Identifying as a client problem or etiology what cannot be changed	Alterations in bowel elimination: Permanent colostomy related to cancer of bowel	Express the problem statement and etiologic factors in terms that can be changed; otherwise, nursing energies are being directed to a hopeless task	Self-care deficit: Care of colostomy related to severe anxiety about cancer and feelings of powerlessness
	Grieving related to death of spouse		Dysfunctional grieving related to inability to accept death of spouse
Identifying environmental factors rather than client factors as a problem	Cluttered home related to inability to discard anything	Express the problem statement in terms of unhealthy client responses rather than environmental conditions	Potential for injury related to cluttered home (inability to discard anything)
Reversing clauses	Knowledge deficit related to alteration in parenting	Avoid reversing the problem statement and etiologic statement	Alteration in parenting related to knowledge deficit: Child growth and development, discipline
Having both clauses say the same thing	Alteration in comfort related to pain (pain *is* the comfort alteration—what is contributing to the pain?)	Be sure that the *two* parts of the diagnosis do not mean the same thing	Alteration in comfort: Unrelieved incisional pain related to fear of addiction

(Continued)

T A B L E **16-3**
Common Errors in Writing Nursing Diagnoses with Recommended Corrections **(Continued)**

Error	Example	Correction	Example
Including value judgments in the nursing diagnosis	Poor human maintenance management related to laziness	Write the diagnosis without value judgments; avoid words such as poor, inadequate, abnormal, unhealthy	Impaired home maintenance management related to low value ascribed to home safety and cleanliness
Including the medical diagnosis in the diagnostic statement	Impaired home maintenance management related to arthritis	Do not include the medical diagnosis in the nursing diagnosis statement	Impaired home maintenance management related to mobility, endurance, and comfort alterations

(Common errors adapted from Mundinger MO, Jauron GD: Developing a nursing diagnosis. Nurs Outlook 23(2): 94–98, 1975. Guidelines for writing nursing diagnoses adapted from Iyer P, Taptich B, Bernocchi-Losey D: Nursing Process and Nursing Diagnoses. Philadelphia, WB Saunders, 1986)

nosis is written when the health problem is likely to occur unless the nurse intervenes in a particular way. Defining characteristics are present as risk factors. A *possible nursing diagnosis* is written when the nurse suspects that a health problem exists but needs to gather more data to confirm the diagnosis (Carpenito, 1987, p 30).

An actual nursing diagnosis for a client who has experienced vomiting, diarrhea, and excessive diaphoresis for 3 days is *fluid volume deficit related to abnormal fluid loss.* If the condition persists and weakness interferes with the client's perineal hygiene, he or she may be at risk for skin breakdown. This is then written as the potential diagnosis: *potential impairment of skin integrity.* If the nurse suspects that a disturbance of self-concept is also present but lacks the necessary data (defining characteristics) to confirm this, it can be listed as a possible nursing diagnosis: *possible disturbance in self-concept.* This alerts nurses to the need to collect more data about the client's self-concept.

Validating Nursing Diagnoses

Once a tentative nursing diagnosis is formulated, it should be validated. Price (1980, p 670) indicates that an affirmative response to each of the questions below validates a tentative diagnosis:
- Is my data base sufficient, accurate, and derived from some concept of nursing?
- Does my synthesis of data (significant cues) demonstrate the existence of a pattern?
- Are the subjective and objective data I used to determine the existence of a pattern characteristic of the health problem I defined?
- Is my tentative nursing diagnosis based on scientific nursing knowledge and clinical expertise?

- Is my tentative nursing diagnosis able to be prevented, reduced, or resolved by independent nursing action?
- Is my degree of confidence above 50% that other qualified practitioners would formulate the same nursing diagnosis based on my data?

In addition, clients who are able to participate in decision making should be encouraged to validate the diagnosis. "It seems to me that bathing has become a problem now that you are afraid of falling in the tub. What's your sense of this?" Table 16-2 lists possible outcomes of validating tentative nursing diagnoses.

DOCUMENTING THE PRIORITIZED LIST OF NURSING DIAGNOSES

To develop a prioritized list of nursing diagnoses, the nurse needs guidelines for ranking diagnoses as high, medium, or low priorities. High priority diagnoses pose the greatest threat to the client's well-being; non-life-threatening diagnoses are ranked as medium priorities; other diagnoses not specifically related to the current illness and prognosis are of low priority. At all priority levels, psychosocial needs must be considered as well as physiologic needs. Atkinson and Murray (1986) suggest three helpful guides for prioritizing client problems: Maslow's hierarchy of human needs, client preference, and anticipation of future problems.

Once the prioritized list of nursing diagnoses is developed, the nurse documents this on the nursing care plan. Depending on the documentation system in use, nursing diagnoses may also be recorded on the multidisciplinary problem list at the front of the client record.

T A B L E 16-4

What a Nursing Diagnosis is Not	Example	Rationale
Medical diagnosis	Diabetes mellitus	Although there is nursing care associated with medical illnesses, the illness is not primarily amenable to nursing intervention. Nursing's concern is the *person* who has the illness and the effect of the illness on human functioning.
Medical pathology	Hypoglycemia	Nurses need to understand the pathology underlying disease states to plan appropriate nursing care, but, once again, nursing's focus is the person, not the pathology. The person's response to hypoglycemia, how hypoglycemia affects human functioning—these are the domain of *nursing* diagnoses.
Diagnostic tests, treatments, equipment	Fasting blood sugar Insulin therapy Insulin syringe Infusion pump	Nursing's concern is the individual's response to the diagnostic study, treatment, or equipment. If the need for insulin therapy reveals a knowledge deficit or self-care deficit, this becomes the nursing diagnosis, not insulin therapy in and of itself.
Therapeutic client needs	Needs to learn the relationship among diet, exercise, and insulin	The diagnosis should be written as a client health problem rather than a client need. *Example:* Alteration in health maintenance (diabetic care) related to lack of knowledge of relationship among diet, exercise, and insulin
Therapeutic nursing goals	To develop therapeutic diabetic self-care behaviors	The diagnosis should be written from the client perspective rather than the nursing perspective and phrased as a client health problem. *Example:* Self-care deficit: Diabetic self-care behaviors related to decreased value on life and decreased motivation to learn
A single sign or symptom	After successfully administering own insulin for 3 days client tells nurse, "You give me my shot today."	A nursing diagnosis is not developed until a pattern or cluster of significant cues is detected. The signs and symptoms lead to the identification of the problem statement but are not the problem statement. In this situation no nursing diagnosis is indicated until further data collection, interpretation, and analysis take place.
An *unvalidated* nursing inference	Above incident leads to the nursing inference: Noncompliance related to depression	This is a premature nursing diagnosis which may not accurately reflect a client problem. More data and the validation of the tentative nursing diagnosis (nursing inference) are needed before the diagnoses can be recorded.

NURSING DIAGNOSIS: A CRITIQUE

When reading the current nursing diagnosis literature, one finds many nurses writing about how using nursing diagnosis has improved their clinical practice; one also finds articles detailing the many benefits nursing diagnosis brings to the profession. Conversely, there are also articles listing the limitations of nursing diagnosis and urging nurses to be cautious, so an uncritical use of nursing diagnosis does not restrict their practices.

The primary benefit nursing diagnosis offers the client is the individualization of client care. For example, nurses may be caring simultaneously for three women who have had a modified radical mastectomy because of breast cancer. While the postoperative nursing management of these women will be similar, priorities of care may differ. A prioritized list of nursing diagnoses will enable nurses to direct their energies toward these differing client priorities:

Client A: Body image disturbance
        Ineffective individual coping
Client B: Alteration in comfort: acute pain
        Self-care deficit
Client C: Potential sexual dysfunction related to
        body-image disturbance
        Powerlessness

The use of nursing diagnosis also allows clients to be informed and willing participants in their care as they validate their diagnoses and assist in their prioritization.

Improved communication among nurses and other health-care professionals is probably the most important benefit that accurate, up-to-date diagnoses, expressed in well-defined and standardized terminology, offer nurses. This communication aids in planning, charting, client data retrieval, health team conferences, change-of-shift reports, and health care follow-up. It also promotes nursing accountability for the problems nurses diagnose.

Among the other benefits nursing diagnoses offer the profession is help in defining the domain of nursing to health-care administrators, legislators, and other health-care providers; this is important when seeking funding for nursing and reimbursement for nursing services. Nursing diagnoses are also used to define curriculum content and to direct specialization and advancement in nursing and nursing research.

When the diagnostic process is used incorrectly, a client may be "misdiagnosed." Premature diagnoses based on an incomplete data base, erroneous diagnoses resulting from an inaccurate data base or faulty data analysis, and routinized diagnoses resulting from the nurse's failure to tailor data collection and analysis to the unique needs of the client are common sources of error. Failure to modify diagnoses and to identify new diagnoses as the client's status changes may also be a problem. Failures in diagnosis will lead to failures in nursing care. All of the above, however, are not so much limitations of nursing diagnosis as they are limitations of the nurses who are diagnosing incorrectly.

Nurses inexperienced in working with diagnoses may become frustrated because attempts to standardize nursing diagnoses are still in early stages and confusion still exists about the need to standardize and about the best way to do it. Individual nurses working together at any one time may have very different exposures to nursing diagnoses and may differ widely in their commitment to the use of nursing diagnoses in practice. Once nurses master skills in developing nursing diagnoses and begin to use them to direct care, it is believed that these difficulties will be minimized.

More serious criticisms of nursing diagnosis are raised by nurses who claim that a classification of standardized nursing diagnoses limits nursing, curbing nurses' originality and ability to think things through.

While some nurses believe that diagnosis offers a valued shortcut to practice, critics find this offensive and respond that rather than invest nursing's energies in perfecting a shortcut, nurses need to change the working conditions that interfere with in-depth problem solving and thoughtful nursing care.

Critics of diagnostic labeling point out that instead of identifying what is unique and positive about nursing, nursing diagnoses make a clear statement that nurses are concerned about what is deviant, wrong, or pathologic (Hagey and McDonough, 1984). The everchanging and dynamic human person with a need for nursing care becomes objectified (Gebbie, 1984).

In conclusion, nursing diagnosis has become a valued and essential step in the nursing process. Used correctly, it is a powerful tool for individualized client care and ensures that nursing's energies are being used in the most efficient way to meet client needs. Nurses who are as concerned about the art and spirit of nursing as they are about its science will be careful to avoid labeling clients in a way that objectifies them or limits the potential range of nurse–client interactions.

KEY POINTS

- The purpose of diagnosing is the identification of (1) problems in the way the client is responding to health or illness, (2) factors contributing to or causing these problems (etiologies), and (3) strengths the client can draw on to prevent or resolve the problem(s).

- Actual or potential health problems that independent nursing intervention can prevent or resolve are termed nursing diagnoses.

- Once significant client data are detected, the nurse looks for data clusters signaling a client strength or problem, and checks out these findings with the client.

- The interpretation and analysis of client data may lead to the identification of nursing diagnoses on collaborative problems (best treated by nurses working together with other health-care professionals), or, when shared with a physician, may contribute to medical diagnoses.

- Nursing diagnoses are written as either two-part statements containing the client problem and its etiology connected by the words "related to," or as three-part statements which include the problem's defining characteristics.

- The problem identifies what is unhealthy about the client, indicating the need for change. It suggests the client goals. The etiology identifies the factors that are maintaining the unhealthy state or response and suggests the appropriate nursing intervention. The defining characteristics are the subjective and objective data that initially signaled the existence of the problem. They suggest evaluative criteria.

- Although nursing care may be related to the following, they are not nursing diagnoses and should not appear in the diagnostic statement: medical diagnosis, medical pathology, diagnostic tests, treatments, equipment, therapeutic client needs, therapeutic client goals, a single sign or symptom, and *unvalidated* nursing inferences.

■ Other sources of error when writing nursing diagnoses include: making legally inadvisable statements, reversing the clauses, identifying environmental factors rather than client factors as the problem, identifying as a client response what is

not necessarily unhealthful, having both clauses say the same thing, and identifying as a client problem what cannot be changed.

■ Three helpful guides for prioritizing client problems are Maslow's hierarchy of human needs, client preference, and anticipation of future problems.

BIBLIOGRAPHY

Alfaro R: Application of Nursing Process: A Step-by-Step Guide. Philadelphia, JB Lippincott, 1986

American Nurses' Association: Nursing: A Social Policy Statement. Kansas City, MO, The Association, 1980

Aspinall MJ: Nursing diagnosis—the weak link. Nursing Outlook 24(7):433–436, 1976

Atkinson J, Murray ME: Understanding the Nursing Process, 3rd ed. New York, Macmillan, 1986

Carlson J, Craft C, McGuire A: Nursing Diagnosis. Philadelphia, WB Saunders, 1982

Carnevali DL, Mitchell PH, Woods NF, Tanner CA: Diagnostic Reasoning in Nursing. Philadelphia, JB Lippincott, 1984

Carpenito LJ: Nursing Diagnosis: Application to Clinical Practice, 2nd ed. Philadelphia, JB Lippincott, 1987

Carpenito LJ: Diagnostics: Actual, potential, or possible? Am J Nurs 85(4):458, 1985

Doenges ME, Jeffries MF, Moorehouse MF: Nursing Care Plans: Nursing Diagnoses in Planning Patient Care. Philadelphia, FA Davis, 1984

Dossey B, Guzzetta CE: Nursing diagnosis. Nursing 11(6):34–38, 1981

Dougherty CM (ed): Symposium on nursing diagnosis. Nurs Clin North Am 20(4):1985

Gebbie KM: Nursing diagnosis: What is it and why does it exist? Top Clin Nurs 5(4):1–9, 1984

Gebbie K (ed): Summary of the Second National Conference. St Louis, Clearinghouse for Nursing Diagnoses, 1975

Gebbie K, Lavin MA: Summary of the First National Conference. St Louis, CV Mosby, 1973

Gordon M: Nursing Diagnosis: Process and Application, 2nd ed. New York, McGraw-Hill, 1987

Gordon M: Nursing diagnosis and the diagnostic process. Am J Nurs 76(8):1298–1300, 1976

Hagey RS, McDonough P: The problem of professional labeling. Nurs Outlook 32(3):151–157, 1984

Hammond KR: Clinical inference in nursing: A psychologist's view point. Nurs Res 15(1):27–38, 1966

Hardy E: The diagnostic wheel: Identifying care that is unique to nursing. Canadian Nurse 79(3):38–40, 1983

Hurley M (ed): Classification of Nursing Diagnoses: Proceedings of the Sixth Conference. St Louis, CV Mosby, 1986

Iyer P, Taptich B, Bernocchi-losey D: Nursing Process and Nursing Diagnosis. Philadelphia, WB Saunders, 1986

Kelly MA: Nursing Diagnosis Source Book. Norwalk, CT, Appleton-Century-Crofts, 1985

Kim MJ, McFarland GK, McLane AM (eds): Classification of Nursing Diagnoses: Proceedings of the Fifth National Conference. St Louis, CV Mosby, 1984

Kim MJ, Moritz D (eds): Classification of Nursing Diagnoses: Proceedings of the Third and Fourth National Conferences. New York, McGraw-Hill, 1982

Kritek PB: Nursing diagnosis in perspective: Response to a critique. Image 17(1):3–8, Winter 1985

Lunney M: Nursing diagnosis: Refining the system. Am J Nurs 82(3):456–459, 1982

Martens K: Let's diagnose strengths, not just problems. Am J Nurs 86(2):192–193, 1986

McLane AM (ed): Classification of Nursing Diagnoses: Proceedings of the Seventh Conference. St Louis, CV Mosby, 1987

Mundinger MO, Jauron GD: Developing a nursing diagnosis. Nurs Outlook 23:94–98, 1975

Nursing diagnosis [Special issue]. Top Clin Nurs 5(4):1984

Nursing Diagnosis Newsletter, North American Nursing Diagnosis Association

Orem D: Nursing: Concepts of Practice. New York, McGraw-Hill, 1985

Popkess S: Diagnosing your patient's strengths. Nursing 11(7):34–37, 1981

Porter EJ: Critical analysis of NANDA nursing diagnosis taxonomy I. Image 18(4):136–139, 1986

Price MR: Nursing diagnosis: Making a concept come alive. Am J Nurs 80(4):668–674, 1980

Rogers M: An Introduction to the Theoretical Basis of Nursing. Philadelphia, FA Davis, 1970

Roy C: Introduction to Nursing: An Adaptation Model. Englewood Cliffs, NJ, Prentice-Hall, 1976

Shamansky SL, Yanni CR: In opposition to nursing diagnosis: A minority opinion. Image 15(2):47–50, 1983

Stolte KM: Nursing diagnosis and the childbearing woman. MCN 11:13–15, 1986

Tartaglia MJ: Nursing diagnosis: keystone of your care plan. Nursing 15(3):34–37, 1985

Taylor CM, Cress SS: Nursing 87 Nursing Diagnosis Cards. Springhouse, PA, Springhouse Corporation, 1987

Planning

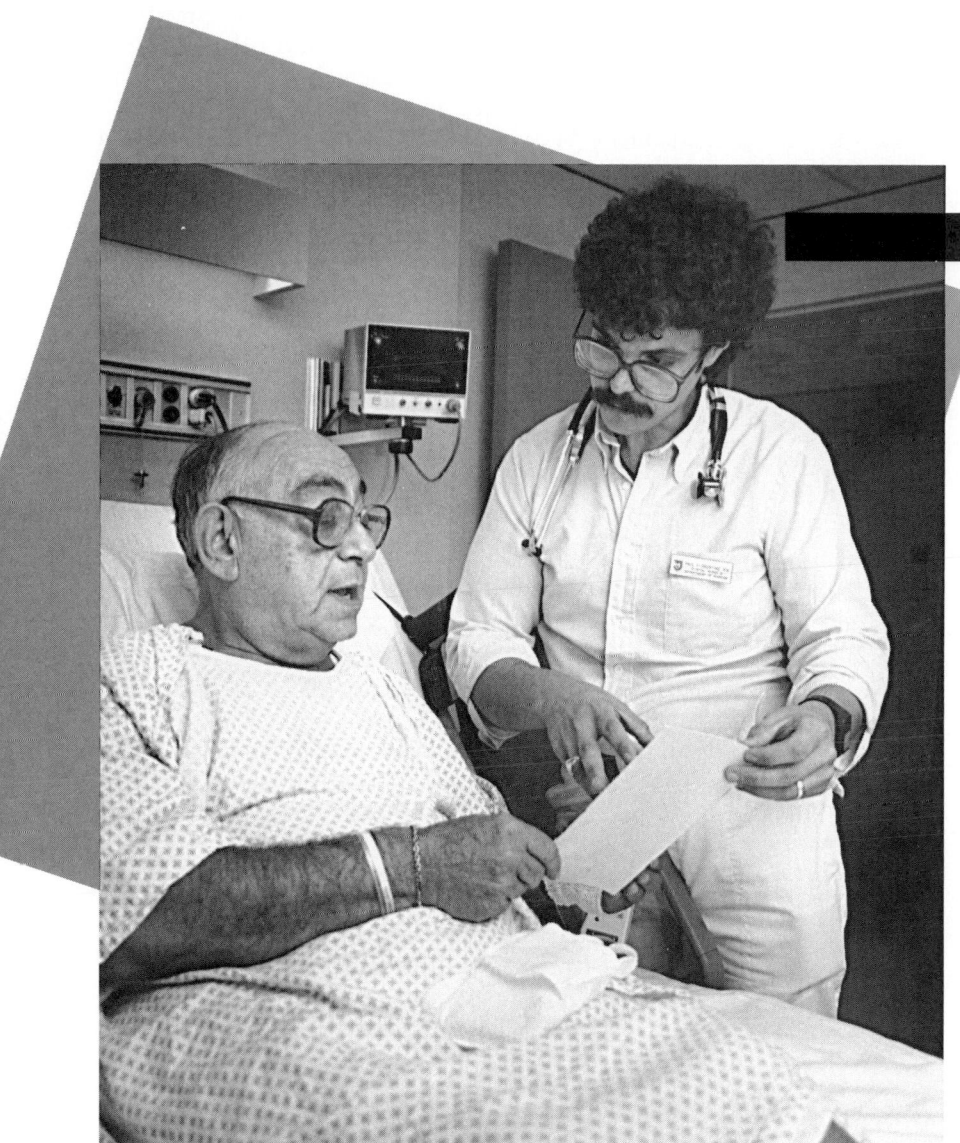

OBJECTIVES

After studying this chapter the learner should be able to

Define key terms used in the chapter.

Describe the purpose and benefits of planning.

Identify three elements of comprehensive planning.

Prioritize client health problems and nursing responses.

Describe how client goals and nursing orders are derived from nursing diagnoses.

Develop a plan of nursing care with properly constructed goals and related nursing orders.

Use criteria to evaluate planning skills.

Describe five common problems related to planning, their possible causes, and remedies.

KEY TERMS

client goal
   (objective,
   outcome)
criteria
discharge planning
goal
Kardex care plan

nursing care plan
nursing measure
nursing order
planning
priority setting
standardized care plan

The purpose of the planning step of the nursing process is the development of a holistic, individualized plan of nursing care acceptable to both the client and the nurse. After client data have been collected and interpreted, client strengths and health problems have been identified, and a prioritized list of nursing diagnoses has been developed, it is time to plan a guide for nursing action. During the planning step of the nursing process the nurse works with the client and the family (1) to develop goals to prevent, reduce, or eliminate the problems specified in the nursing diagnoses; and (2) to identify those nursing interventions most likely to assist the client in achieving these goals.

Elements of planning (outlined in Fig. 17-1) include establishing priorities, writing goals and developing an evaluative strategy, selecting nursing measures, and writing the nursing care plan. It is important that the nurse, client, and family work together as much as possible during planning. If the goals specified in the plan of care are not valued by the client or do not contribute to the prevention, resolution, or reduction of the client's problems, then the plan of care may be meaningless. Goal writing can therefore be a critical skill for the nurse who hopes to successfully intervene with clients.

In this chapter planning is explored as a conscious, deliberate step in the nursing process. Informal planning, however, is such an integral component of nursing practice that it often "happens" without nurses being aware that they are planning. It is the link between the identification of a client strength or problem and the appropriate nursing response. When a nurse on a busy surgical unit learns that a postoperative client is complaining of incisional pain and quickly reshuffles priorities to allow time to assess the course and qualities of the pain and what nursing measures can be implemented to reduce discomfort, planning has occurred. When the 3–11 postpartum nurse realizes that he or she has not seen a particular father hold his new baby daughter and that it is now the evening prior to discharge, if he or she makes a mental note to observe the father–daughter interactions that evening and facilitate their bonding, planning has occurred. When a nurse in a geriatric day-care center hears a client choking and rushes to his side to perform the Heimlich maneuver should it be needed, planning has occurred. Informal planning on a more conscious level is illustrated by the hospice nurse who ponders how to best support a client with terminal cancer who is gradually relinquishing her hold on life. When nurses find formal planning burdensome and are satisfied with this type of informal planning, they are depriving themselves and their clients of the benefits related to formal planning.

Some of the reasons for developing a formal plan of care are to individualize care, to set priorities, to help communication among nursing personnel, to promote continuity of care, to coordinate care, to evaluate the client's responses to nursing care, and to promote the nurse's professional development. Prerequisite skills for

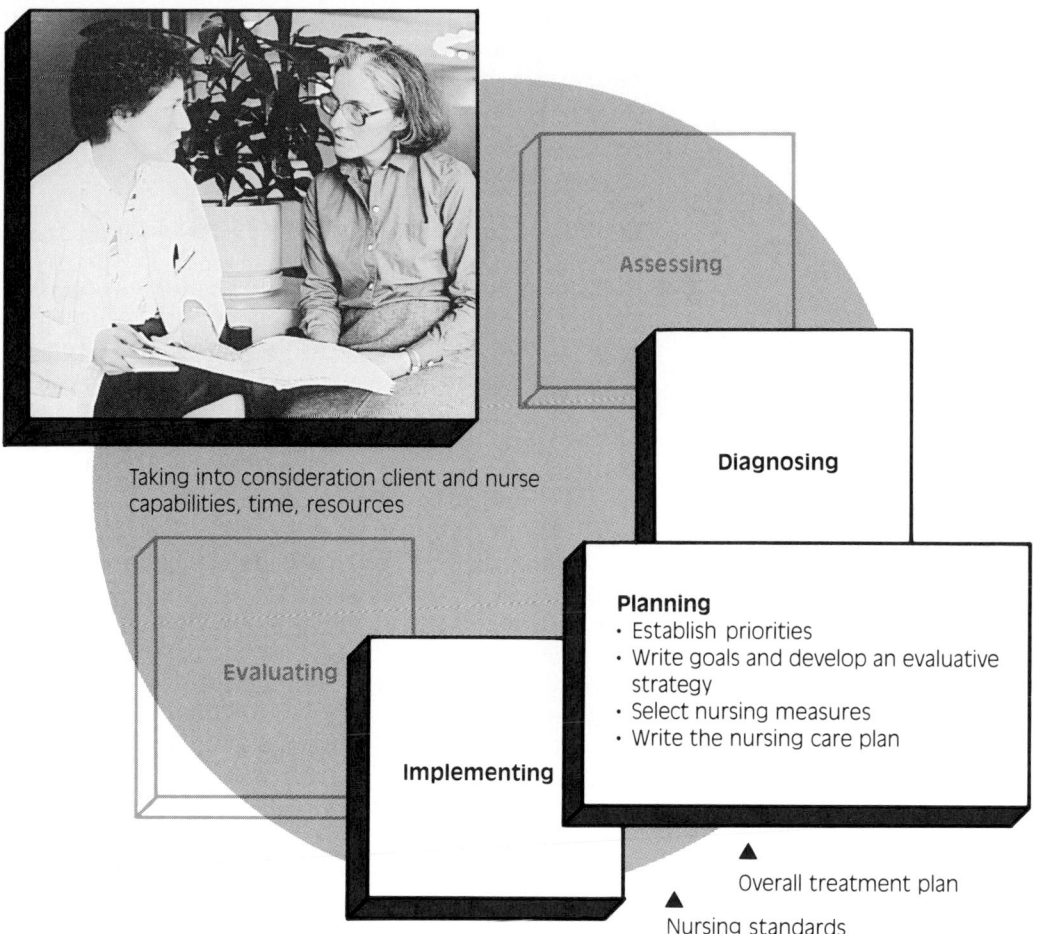

Taking into consideration client and nurse
capabilities, time, resources

Assessing

Diagnosing

Planning
- Establish priorities
- Write goals and develop an evaluative
  strategy
- Select nursing measures
- Write the nursing care plan

Evaluating

Implementing

▲ Overall treatment plan

▲ Nursing standards

F I G U R E   17-1

*Planning. The nurse and client work together to develop client goals and identify the nurs-
ing interventions most likely to assist the client to meet the goals. It is important for the
plan of care to be consistent with nursing standards, congruent with other planned therapies, and realistic in terms of the client and nurses' abilities or resources. (Photo by Gates
Rhodes, courtesy of the School of Nursing, University of Pennsylvania)*

the nurse who designs effective plans of care include a
sound knowledge of nursing (including standards for
professional nursing care); ability to collect, interpret,
and analyze client data, develop nursing diagnoses, construct client goals, and select appropriate nursing interventions; creativity; sensitivity to the unique needs of the
client; and the ability to communicate clearly and concisely in writing.

UNIQUE FOCUS OF NURSING PLANNING

The primary purpose of the planning step of the nursing
process is to design a plan of care for the client which,
once implemented, results in the prevention or resolution of client health problems. A comprehensive plan of
care, however, also specifies any routine nursing assistance the client requires to meet basic human needs
(*e.g.,* assistance with hygiene or nutrition) and describes
appropriate nursing responsibilities for fulfilling the
medical plan of care. For example, physicians may delegate to nurses caring for a surgical client the redressing
of the surgical incision, the administration of prescribed
medications and intravenous therapy, and responsibility
for scheduling laboratory studies. The creative and innovative nurse learns to design a plan of care that incorporates the independent, interdependent, and dependent
responsibilities of the nurse. Because nursing is concerned with the client's responses to health and illness,
the plan of care is always supportive of nursing's broad
aims: to promote wellness, prevent disease/illness, promote recovery, and facilitate coping with altered functioning.

COMPREHENSIVE PLANNING

There are three basic types of planning critical to comprehensive nursing care: initial, ongoing problem-oriented, and discharge. The nurse who develops a comprehensive plan of care on the client's day of admission and then fails to update the plan and to anticipate discharge needs has done the client a great disservice. This is probably the most common problem related to planning.

Initial Planning. The *initial plan* is developed by the nurse who performs the admission nursing history and the nursing examination. Comprehensive in nature, this plan addresses each problem listed in the prioritized nursing diagnoses and identifies appropriate client goals and the related nursing care. Standardized plans can provide an excellent basis for the initial plan *if the nurse tailors them to meet individual client needs.* Resources for standardized plans include computerized plans, textbooks with prepared care plans, and agency-developed plans. By using such standardized plans, the nurse is free to direct time and expertise to individualizing the plan.

Ongoing Planning. *Ongoing, problem-oriented planning* is carried out by any nurse who interacts with the patient. Its chief purpose is to keep the plan up to date. The work of ongoing planning includes stating nursing diagnoses more clearly (both the problem statement and the etiology) and developing new diagnoses as indicated by newly collected and analyzed data; making previously developed client goals more realistic, developing new goals as needed; identifying those nursing actions that will best accomplish the client goals, given a better knowledge of the client; and using and documenting client responses to nursing actions to direct further planning.

At this stage of planning, standardized plans may be useful in "working up" new diagnoses, but the emphasis is clearly on individualizing the plan to meet unique client needs. For example, the standard nursing order "force fluids" would be rewritten as "offer 60 ml cranberry or orange juice between meals, and keep fresh water at bedside." A preliminary order such as "explore with the client existing supports" may be replaced with "keep daughter Barbara informed of mother's progress and coach her in effective support strategies (Barbara Clems, 448-3211)."

Discharge Planning. Discharge planning is best carried out by the nurse who has worked most closely with the client and family, possibly in conjunction with a nurse who has a broad knowledge of existing community resources. Comprehensive discharge planning begins when the client is first admitted for treatment. Careful planning ensures that the teaching and counseling skills of the nurse are used to help the client and family develop sufficient knowledge of the health problem and the therapeutic regimen to competently execute the necessary self-care behaviors at home. Discharge planning is further discussed in Chapter 26.

ESTABLISHING PRIORITIES

Before developing or modifying the plan of care, it is helpful to review the prioritized list of nursing diagnoses to determine if they are correctly ranked as high priority (poses greatest threat to client's well-being), medium priority (non-life threatening), and low priority (not specifically related to current illness and prognosis). Guidelines for establishing these priorities, such as Maslow's hierarchy of human needs, client preferences, and anticipation of future problems, are presented in Chapter 16.

When planning nursing care for each day, it is helpful to consider the following:
- Have changes in the client's health status influenced what are considered the most important threats to the client's well-being? For example, a client who was admitted to the hospital with the tentative medical diagnosis of unexplained weight loss has now been found to have ovarian cancer; this requires a completely new set of priorities for care.
- Have changes in the way the client is responding to health/illness or the plan of care affected those nursing diagnoses that can be realistically addressed? For example, the nurse may have identified ineffective coping as a high priority diagnosis for the client after he or she learned of the medical diagnosis, and planned to initiate counseling. But if the client adamantly requests to be left alone for a day to think things through, the nurse will have to modify priorities of care for that day.
- Are there relationships between problems, such that one must be worked on before another one can be resolved?
- Can several client problems be dealt with together?

After answering these questions, the nurse ranks problems in the order in which they will be worked on. Setting priorities enables the nurse to make sure that time and energy are being directed to the client's most important problems.

WRITING GOALS AND DEVELOPING EVALUATIVE STRATEGIES

A **goal** is an aim or an end. A **client goal** describes an expected client outcome. The words goal, objective, and outcome are often used interchangeably. In some practice settings, the term *goal* or *objective* is used to describe "what is wanted," and the term *outcome* is used to describe the "results achieved."

Deriving Goals from Nursing Diagnoses

Goals are derived from the problem statement of the nursing diagnosis. For each nursing diagnosis in the plan of care at least one goal must be written that, if achieved, demonstrates a *direct resolution* of the problem statement (see Table 17-1).

Other goals that will contribute to the resolution of the problem may be written. For example, for the nursing diagnosis "nutritional alteration: more than body requirements related to excessive snacking and inactivity," in addition to the goal "by 12/6/89 client reaches target weight: 122 lb," the following goals are appropriate: "by 6/6/89 client identifies ten low-calorie snack foods he is willing to try; client's 3-day diet recall is consistent with nutritionally balanced 1500-calorie diet; and client reports incorporating three periods of vigorous exercise into each week." The difference between these goals and the goal that the client reach his target weight is that while the achievement of these goals may contribute to the resolution of the problem, they may also be achieved without the problem being resolved and the client's plan of care mistakenly terminated. Remember, *at least one goal per nursing diagnosis must directly resolve the problem statement in the nursing diagnosis.*

Long-term Versus Short-term Goals

Goals may be either long-term or short-term. Simply defined, long-term goals require a longer period of time (generally more than a week) to be achieved than do short-term goals. Long-term goals may also be used as discharge goals, in which case they are more broadly written and communicate to the entire nursing team the desired end results of nursing care for a particular client.

TABLE 17-1
Examples of Goals to Relieve Problems

Problem Statement of the Nursing Diagnosis	Related Client Goal
Alteration in comfort	By end of shift client reports pain is absent or diminished
Nutritional alteration: More than body requirements	By 12/6/89 client reaches target weight: 122 lb
Impaired mobility	Prior to discharge client ambulates length of hallway independently

For example, two elderly women, both 77 years old, are on a nursing unit after undergoing similar operative procedures for fractured left hips. While one woman has spent the last 2 years in bed in a nursing home, the other woman fractured her hip at the YMCA where she swims daily. Their nursing care should not be the same because it is directed to different long-term goals, although their short-term goals may be similar (see sample goals).

Cognitive, Psychomotor, and Affective Goals

Goals may be categorized according to the type of change they describe for the client. *Cognitive goals* describe increases in client knowledge or intellectual behaviors. *Example:* By 6/12 client lists three benefits of continuing to apply moist compresses to leg ulcer after discharge. *Psychomotor goals* describe the client's

---

Long- and Short-Term Goals

Client from Nursing Home

Long-Term Goal
Mrs. Goldstein returns to the nursing home pain-free with her incision healed and her left leg in good alignment.

Short-term goals
- Whenever observed, client is lying in bed with legs in correct alignment (abductor pillow in place if ordered).
- Prior to discharge Mrs. Goldstein's hip incision demonstrates signs of healing (skin surfaces approximate, free from signs of infection: redness, swelling, heat, purulent drainage).
- Whenever observed, client reports that comfort measures and medication are satisfactorily managing pain.

Client from Private Home

Long-term goal
Mrs. Silverstein returns home to her husband pain-free with incision healed, fully mobile (full weight-bearing on left leg), and capable of independent activities of daily living.

Short-term goals
- By 1/28 client verbalizes willingness to participate in physical therapy program.
- By 2/4 client ambulates (with nursing assistance and walker) to bathroom (full weight-bearing).
- By 2/11 client ambulates with nursing assistance only (no walker) in her room.
- Goals for incision and pain relief same as above.

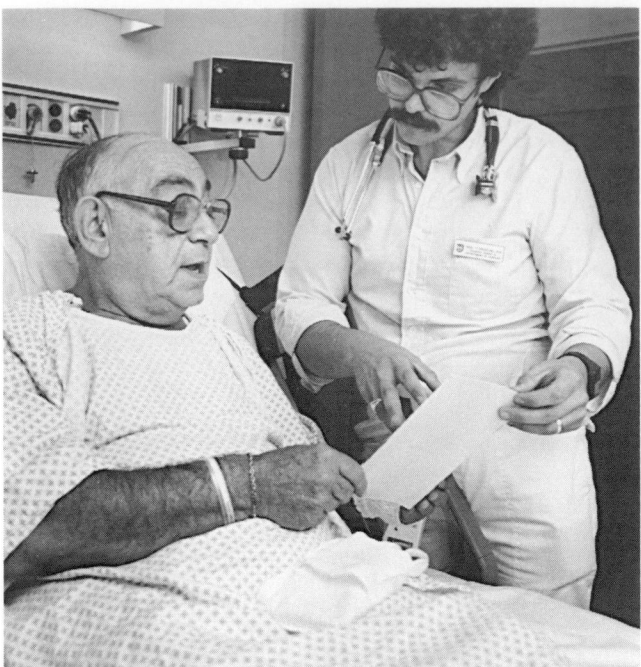

F I G U R E   17-2

What cognitive, psychomotor, and affective goals might be set for a client who must learn new eating patterns following a heart attack? (Photo by Robert Neroni, courtesy of Thomas Jefferson University)

Guidelines for Writing Goals

- Derive each set of goals from only one nursing diagnosis.
- Make sure that at least one of the goals clearly shows a direct resolution of the problem statement in the nursing diagnosis and that other goals contribute to the prevention or resolution of the problem.
- Write goals that are valued by the client and family.
- Check to make sure the goals are supportive of the total treatment plan.
- Write goals that are brief, specific (clearly describe an observable, measurable behavior), and phrased positively.
- Remember that each short-term goal can contain only one client behavior.

achievement of new skills. *Example:* By 6/12 client correctly demonstrates application of wet to dry dressing on leg ulcer. *Affective goals* describe changes in client values, beliefs, and attitudes. Difficult both to write and evaluate, affective goals may be critical to the resolution of a complex client problem. *Example:* By 6/12 client verbalizes valuing health sufficiently to practice new health behaviors to prevent recurrence of leg ulcer. In this example, even if the client intellectually grasps the reasons for taking care of her leg and can competently redress her ulcer, unless she is motivated to take care of herself, her knowledge and skills will not result in healthy outcomes.

Guidelines for Goal Writing

When developing client goals, the nurse and client look at the problem statement of the nursing diagnosis and ask "What client changes or outcomes will result in the prevention or resolution of this problem?" The answer, when carefully worded, becomes the client goal. (See Guidelines for Writing Goals.) One of the most important considerations in goal writing is encouraging the client and family to be as active in goal development as their abilities and interest permit. The more involved they are, the greater chance the goals have of being achieved.

Each client goal must have: a *subject,* which is the client or some part of the client, a *verb,* which indicates

the action the client will perform, and **criteria**, which describe in *observable, measurable terms* the expected client behavior (must include a time criterion, such as 4/6/89, prior to discharge, after viewing film, whenever observed, specifying the targeted time or date by which the goal should be achieved).

Examples of properly constructed client goals follow.

- By end of shift client's 24-hour fluid intake totals at least 1800 ml.
- At next visit (12/23), client correctly demonstrates relaxation exercises.

It may be helpful to include special conditions when writing a goal if this information is important for other nurses (*e.g.,* "Prior to discharge client ambulates independently in hallway, using Philadelphia collar to support cervical vertebrae.").

Common Errors

Common errors when writing client goals include:

- Expressing the *client* goal as a *nursing* goal. *Incorrect:* Offer Mr. Myer 60 ml fluid every 2 hours while awake. *Correct:* Mr. Myer drinks 60 ml fluid every 2 hours while awake, beginning 2/24.
- Using verbs that are not *observable* and *measurable. Incorrect:* Mrs. Gaston will know how to bathe her newborn. *Correct:* After attending the infant care class, Mrs. Gaston correctly demonstrates the procedure for bathing her newborn. Verbs to be avoided when writing goals include know, understand, learn, become aware. Verbs that are helpful when writing goals that are observable and measurable are displayed in the box on page 293.
- Including more than one client behavior in short-term goals. *Incorrect:* Client lists dangers of smok-

---

Verbs Helpful in Writing Goals

define	apply	verbalize
identify	use	choose
list	demonstrate	select
describe	prepare	inject
explain	design	perform

---

ing and stops smoking. *Correct:* By next meeting (3/11/89), client identifies three dangers of smoking. By 3/18/89 client describes a plan he is willing to try to stop smoking. By 6/20/89 client reports that he no longer smokes.

- Writing goals so vaguely that other nurses are unsure of the goal of nursing care. *Incorrect:* Client copes better. *Correct:* After initial interview (10/20), client describes two new coping strategies he is willing to try and demonstrates increased incidence of previously observed noneffective coping behaviors (chain smoking, withdrawal behaviors, heavy alcohol consumption).

Developing Evaluative Strategy

Chapter 19, *Evaluating,* deals specifically with the evaluative component of the nursing process. During the planning step an evaluative strategy must be identified and incorporated into the formal plan of care. Having client goals written on the plan is meaningless unless nurses evaluate whether or not these goals have been achieved. The nurse should record the date the goal was written and the date the goal is achieved. Students learn-

---

Evaluative Statement

Documents that client has met, partially met, or not met the goal.

Goal Statement
Beginning 6/8 client ambulates half length of hallway with assistance three times daily.

Evaluative Statement
6/8 goal partially met; client refused to ambulate in the AM but did walk to the bathroom once in the afternoon with the assistance of one nurse.

Recommendation: Review reason for progressive ambulation with patient; assess motivation to increase independence.

L Gainer, RN

---

ing how to evaluate the effects of nursing care may find it helpful to write an evaluative statement (see box), which includes a statement about the achievement of the desired goal (goal met, goal partially met, goal not met) and lists an actual client behavior as evidence supporting the statement. If indicated, recommendations for revising the plan of care can be included in the evaluative statement (Atkinson and Murray, 1986).

SELECTING NURSING MEASURES

Deriving Nursing Measures from Nursing Diagnoses

Nursing measures, like client goals, are derived from the nursing diagnosis. But while the problem statement of the diagnosis suggests the client goals, it is the etiology of the problem that suggests the nursing measures (see Fig. 17-3). The effective nurse selects nursing measures that specifically address factors causing or contributing to the client's problems.

For example, many factors contribute to obesity: deficient nutritional knowledge, convenience of high-calorie fast foods, lifetime snacking habits, limited food budget, little exercise, and low self-esteem, to name a few. The nurse working with a client who wishes to lose weight could attempt to deal with all these factors, but this approach would be inefficient. However, when a carefully developed nursing diagnosis identifies the specific factors that contributed to a particular client's weight problem, nursing measures can be selected to deal directly with these factors.

For example, nursing measures for the client with the diagnosis *Nutritional alteration: More than body requirements related to lifetime snacking habits and heavy reliance on high-calorie fast foods* might include education about the amount of calories contained in fast foods and an exploration of ways the client could change eating habits in order to eat more nutritionally balanced meals with fewer calories. Thus, not every client with a weight problem is nursed the same way. The art of nursing involves the careful tailoring of select nursing measures to the individual needs of the client.

```
┌─────────────────────────────────┐
│ 1st part of the nursing         │
│ diagnosis                       │
│ (problem statement)             │
│                                 │
│ · identifies the unhealthy      │
│   response                      │
│ · indicates what should         │
│   change                        │
│            │                    │
│            ▼                    │
│ · suggests client goals         │
│   (expectations for             │
│   change)                       │
│                                 │
│      ┌──────────────────────────┴──────┐
│      │ 2nd part of the nursing         │
└──────┤ diagnosis                       │
       │ (etiology)                      │
       │                                 │
       │ · identifies factors            │
       │   causing or contributing       │
       │   to the undesirable            │
       │   response and                  │
       │   preventing desired            │
       │   change                        │
       │            │                    │
       │            ▼                    │
       │ · suggests nursing              │
       │   measures                      │
       └─────────────────────────────────┘
```

F I G U R E   17-3
Deriving client goals and nursing orders from nursing diagnoses.

Identifying Options

After the client goals are written, the nurse identifies various nursing measures to assist the client achieve the goals. The effectiveness of the nurse is directly proportional to his or her command of varied nursing strategies. Consider the nursing options identified by three different nurses when they are told that a woman 2 days postcesarean delivery is complaining of pain in her incisional area:

Nurse A: Check to see what type of pain medication is ordered and give it if the time interval is sufficient.

Nurse B: Assess the quality of the pain and use this time to communicate support via expression and squeeze of hand.
Administer analgesic if indicated.
Assess effectiveness of the analgesic ordered.

Nurse C: Assess quality of the pain and explore the possibility of contributing factors such as the effects of increased gas in the abdominal area

or concern about the newborn, herself, or other family members.
Use empathic listening (possibly touch) to communicate support and to encourage the mother to share her concerns.
Change her position in bed.
Offer a back rub.
Loosen the dressing over the incisional area.
If appropriate, suggest activity that will distract attention from the pain, for example watching a film of newborn care or listening to music).
Give the prescribed medication for pain and observe its effect.
When administering the medication, use the power of positive suggestion to enhance its effectiveness: "This will start taking the pain away in about 10 minutes and will help you relax."

It is possible that the client simply needs her prescribed analgesic to achieve the goal: "Client reports minimal to no pain whenever assessed." In this case, all three nurses would have been effective in meeting the client's need for nursing care. It is also possible, however, that the prescribed medication was not working or that the pain was compounded by the mother's fears about caring for her new baby or by her worries that the baby will ruin her relationship with her husband.

The more varied the options available to the nurse, the more effective the nursing response will be. In different situations, a skilled nursing procedure, an appropriate use of silence, respectful listening, humor, teaching, counseling, and touch can all be effective nursing strategies. The nurse who is "task-oriented" and who is satisfied to meet every client problem with a "procedure" is limiting her effectiveness.

Students who wish to develop a varied repertoire of nursing skills can actively seek assistance from nursing instructors and nurse practitioners. Nurses can learn valuable strategies by watching their successful colleagues and observing and talking with them about what it is they do that is different; by talking with clients and families about the nursing care they find most helpful; and by researching the nursing literature for suggestions to improve care.

Selecting from Options

From the list of options, nurses select those nursing measures that they believe will best assist the client to meet goals. There are broad guidelines the nurse can use when selecting nursing measures. The nursing measures selected must be

- Tailored to the client
- Consistent with standards of care (ANA/CNA standards of practice, nurse practice acts, institutional standards, standards of accrediting agencies (*e.g.,* Joint Commission of Accreditation of Hospitals, JCAH)

- Realistic in terms of the abilities, time, and resources available to the nurse and client
- Compatible with the client's values, beliefs, and psychosocial background
- Valued, whenever possible, by the client and family
- Compatible with other planned therapies

Even if a nursing measure meets the above criteria, there is no guarantee it will result in the client successfully achieving a goal. What may be successful for one client may not work at all for someone else. Nurse researchers are now attempting to establish a statistical pattern for predicting the probability of success of select nursing measures. The competent nurse uses research findings (science of nursing) and knowledge of the client (art of nursing) to select effective nursing measures. Ongoing consultation with nurse colleagues and continuing education are among the best means to explore new and creative nursing approaches to client problems.

Writing Nursing Orders

Nursing orders communicate to the entire nursing staff the specific nursing measures that are to be implemented for the client. Well written nursing orders

- Clearly and concisely describe the nursing action to be performed (answer the questions who? what? where? when? and how?)
- Are dated when the order is written and when the plan of care is reviewed
- Are signed by the nurse prescribing the order
- Use only those abbreviations accepted in the institution. (These may usually be found in the policy manual; a list of commonly accepted abbreviations appears in Chap 18.)
- Refer the nurse to the agency's procedure manual or other literature for the steps of routine, lengthy procedures
  Examples of nursing orders follow:
- Offer client 60 ml water/juice (prefers orange or cranberry juice) every 2 hours while awake.
- Instruct client on necessity of carefully monitoring fluid intake/output; needs to be reminded every shift to report fluid intake.
- Offer assistance with toileting (walk with client to bathroom) every 2 hours while client is awake; client has diminished sensation of full bladder.

The set of nursing orders written to assist a client to meet a goal must be comprehensive. Comprehensive nursing orders specify what *observations* need to be made and how often; what *nursing measures* need to be done and when they must be done; and what *teaching, counseling, and advocacy* needs clients and families have.

Many sets of nursing orders are deficient in that they fail to indicate what the ongoing assessment priority needs to be in relation to a specific problem or goal.

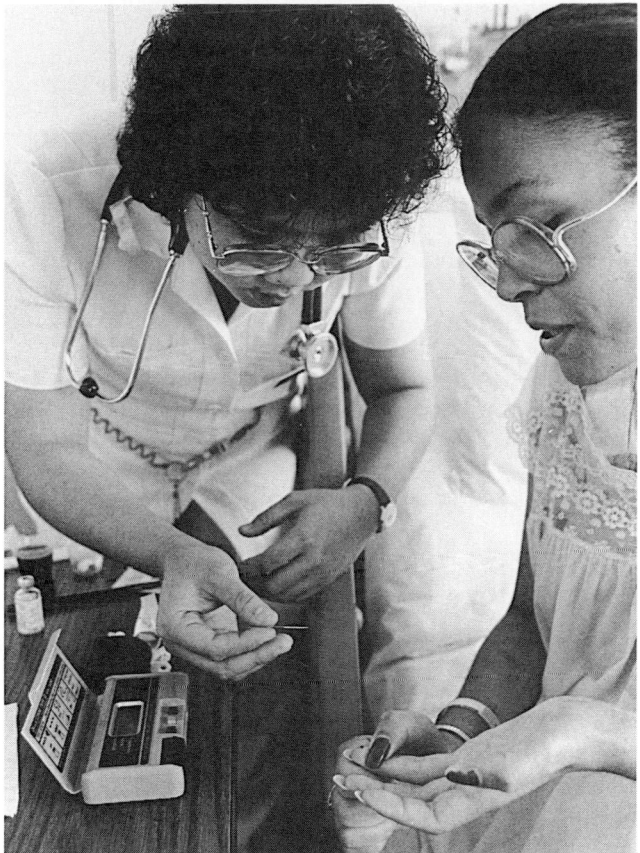

FIGURE 17-4
What comprehensive nursing orders might be written for preparing a client to perform self-testing for blood sugar levels upon discharge from the hospital? (Photo by Kathy Sloane, courtesy of Merritt Hospital)

Clearly noting assessment priorities helps all nurses to be more sensitive to important client data. For example, when assisting a client who wishes to lose weight to reach the target weight, appropriate nursing orders would include: 6/17/89—continue to assess (1) client's motivation to participate in weight loss program, and (2) factors positively or negatively influencing weight loss.

Similarly, it is often assumed that all clients have the same teaching needs. Nothing is farther from the truth. In fact, many clients come to the hospital with an excellent knowledge base (which may be greater than that of the nurse for a particular disease). Their need for nursing may be a need for counseling as they learn to live with a chronic illness. Comprehensive nursing orders relate to individual client needs.

WRITING THE NURSING CARE PLAN

The **nursing care plan** (plan of nursing care, client care plan) is the written guide to direct the efforts of the

Purposes for Nursing Care Plans

For the Client
- Provide quality care
- Monitor progress
- Ensure consistency/continuity

For the nurse
- Communicate information
- Organize care
- Evaluate care

For the clinical unit
- Make assignments
- Organize time-related activities
- Direct shift report
- Evaluate nurse performance

For administration
- Secure resources
- Distribute resources
- Evaluate nursing practice

For nursing
- Educate practitioners
- Develop professionalism
- Define nursing parameters
- Test and develop theory
- Research

(Shea H: The nursing care plan dilemma: Suggestions for resolution. *The Canadian Nurse, 80*(9), 44–46, 1984)

nursing team as they work with clients to meet health goals. Care plans offer many benefits to the client, nurse, nursing unit, nursing administration, and to the nursing profession. These are highlighted in the box. Primarily, nursing care plans ensure that the nursing team works efficiently to deliver holistic, goal-oriented, individualized care to clients.

Guidelines for developing the nursing care plan follow. The nursing care plan
- Is initiated on the day of admission
- Is developed by the nurse who best knows the client (primary nurse) and added to by other members of the nursing team
- Provides for client and family participation as much as possible
- Is signed and dated by the nurse developing the plan
- Is written in ink and kept as a part of the client's permanent record
- Clearly specifies nursing diagnoses, client goals, nursing orders, and evaluation strategies
- Uses standardized symbols, abbreviations, and key phrases specified in the agency's policy manual, as opposed to lengthy descriptions
- Refers nurses to agency procedure manuals for specific steps in routine nursing procedures
- Is updated consistently to reflect changes in client status and related needs for nursing care
Characteristics of a well-written nursing care plan include

COMPUTER APPLICATION IN NURSING

Computer-Generated Nursing Care Plans

Computerized care plans allow nurses to address client care problems at the nurse's station. These programs are set up so that reference texts are edited and individualized before the care plan is saved on the disk and printed. One such program describes the client's medical symptoms, nursing diagnosis, client goals, measurable outcomes, and nursing interventions. There is also space for documenting the care given.

Benefits of the computerized care plans are
- Expanded knowledge base

- Documentation of direct care and independent nursing interventions (*e.g.,* teaching, emotional support)
- Improved record keeping with resultant improvement in audits and quality assurance
- Documentation by all members of the health-care team with printouts for the client's record and for change-of-shift report
- Reduction of time spent on paperwork; in some studies, as much as 2 hours of professional care hours for each new admission

- Represents an adequate philosophy of nursing; advances nursing's four aims: promotes wellness, prevents disease/illness, promotes recovery, facilitates coping with altered functioning
- Is tailored to the individual characteristics and needs of the client
- Clearly identifies (1) any nursing assistance the client needs to meet basic human needs, (2) nursing diagnoses and related client goals and nursing orders, and (3) nursing responsibilities for fulfilling the medical plan of care
- Directs the nurse's assessment priorities, care-giving behaviors, and teaching, counseling, and advocacy behaviors
- Based on scientific principles; incorporates findings of nursing research
- Meets developmental, psychosocial, and spiritual needs of the client, as well as physiologic needs
- Addresses discharge needs of the client and family
- When appropriate, is compatible with the medical plan of care and that of the interdisciplinary team

Formats for Care Plans

Many suggestions for care plans appear in the nursing literature. Each school of nursing and each health-care institution has its own format, which may reflect a particular nursing theory. Common to all formats is a minimum of three columns for documenting nursing diagnoses, client goals, and nursing orders. Formats differ in the way they handle assessment data and nursing evaluation.

Institutional Care Plans

Many health-care institutions use a **Kardex care plan** in which the plan of care for each client is recorded on a 6 × 11-inch card and placed in a central Kardex file. In addition to abbreviated background information on the client, the Kardex file generally contains three types of information: nursing care related to basic human needs, to nursing diagnoses, and to the medical plan of care.

Nursing care related to basic human needs. The plan should be abbreviated and make readily available to caregivers client data concerning health habits and patterns obtained from the nursing history and modified appropriately by current treatment orders. This information is useful to caregivers only if it is kept current as the client's condition changes. Any nurse should be able to find on the nursing Kardex the instructions she needs to confidently and competently provide care.

Nursing care related to nursing diagnoses. The plan contains goals and nursing actions for every nursing diagnosis, as well as a place to note client responses to the plan of care. This section is the heart of the care plan because it represents the independent component of nursing practice. If well developed, it demonstrates the clinical competence of the nurse (knowledge of the science of nursing), sensitivity to the individual needs of the client, and creativity. Development of this portion of the plan is nursing's challenge.

Nursing care related to the medical plan of care. The plan also records medical orders for treatment and diagnostic studies involving nursing care. At one time Kardexes were a bookkeeping system for medical orders.

Student Care Plans

The care plans students are required to develop are often more detailed than those found in practice settings. The aim is to assist students to assimilate each of the five steps of the nursing process. Although care plan formats vary from one nursing program to another, most are designed so that the student can systematically proceed through each interrelated step in the nursing process, and many use a five-column format.

The sample student care plan given here demonstrates a plan developed for the client whose admission assessment form is in Chapter 15. This 72-year-old woman was admitted to the hospital after experiencing a "mini stroke" (transischemic attack, TIA) at home. Her condition is stable and the three prioritized diagnoses developed on the plan address her inability to deal with this new diagnosis and to prevent a major stroke (high priority), ineffective coping (medium priority), and constipation (low priority). In the past year her husband died and she sold her home and moved in with her daughter.

Assessing. In the assessment column the student records the assessment data that led to the establishment of each diagnosis. Recording these data helps to link specific defining characteristics with diagnostic problem statements. On some care plans, pertinent assessment data are recorded in the nursing diagnosis column.

Diagnosing. Priorities are assigned to each diagnosis, and these are recorded in the nursing diagnosis column. For each diagnosis a clear and concise problem statement is followed by an etiology statement which identifies contributing factors.

Planning. The planning column contains the expected changes in client health status or in client behaviors (*i.e.,* the client goals). If achieved, these resolve the problem statement in the nursing diagnosis.

Implementing. Sets of nursing orders are written for each client goal. These specify *what* nursing interventions are to be performed, *how* they are to be performed, *when,* and by *whom.* In many nursing programs, students are asked to document the source of the nursing orders they propose. Although a student may be able to "pull from her head" some nursing strategies, developing the practice of consulting the nursing literature on select client problems is a sure means to increase nursing knowledge. Some programs also require students to

(Text continues on p. 300.)

Student Care Plan

Assessment	Nursing Diagnosis	Goals
Subjective Data: "Will I get a stroke now? I don't think I could handle that." *Objective Data:* Admitting dx: TIA BP: 184/120 *Strengths:* Past pattern of adhering to prescribed health behaviors.	Potential self-care deficit: response to TIA and stroke prevention related to knowledge deficit	Prior to discharge client describes the terms TIA and stroke identifying the underlying disease process, causes, symptoms, and treatment. After discussion with the physician and nurse, the client correctly describes the treatment plan: • medications (drugs, intended effect, dose, time, route) • dietary modifications • exercise prescription • signs and symptoms to report • follow-up appointment date
Subjective Data: Husband died 8 months ago; moved in with daughter 6 months ago after selling family home Daughter reports mother has been a very independent strong woman in the past— seemed to "crumple" after husband's death. History of headaches *Objective Data:* Clutches daughter's hand *Strengths:* Past history of handling life stressors well *Limitations:* In the past, her husband was her primary support.	Ineffective individual coping related to illness, recent death of husband and relocation with daughter	Beginning 9/7 • Client verbalizes her feelings related to the loss of her husband, loss of family home, loss of health. • Client identifies coping patterns that have helped her in the past. • Client identifies three personal strengths and three outside supports which will help her now. Prior to discharge, client verbalizes that she feels "OK" (sufficiently in charge of her life) about returning home.

Nursing Orders	Scientific Rationale	Evaluation
Assess what the client knows about TIA and stroke (correct any misinformation). Assess learning needs, readiness to learn, and factors that will influence learning. Plan teaching/learning sessions to involve family members designated by client. Include in the teaching plan a description of TIA and stroke, the underlying disease process, causes, symptoms, and treatment plan. Once the treatment plan has been developed make sure the client and family understand it (teaching) and *value* the prescribed life-style modification (counseling).	Each person's learning needs different; each person learns in own unique way; learning is dependent on readiness. The more support persons knowledgeable committed to the plan of care, the greater the probability the client will achieve goals. New self-care behaviors are dependent on knowledge. New self-care behaviors are dependent on motivation. Unless the client is committed to stroke prevention and values this outcome, she will not follow the treatment plan.	9/10 Goal not met. Client says her head is "too old" to learn all this stuff. Equates stroke with death. *Revision:* Reteach content in simpler terms. Reassess learning readiness. 9/10 Too early to evaluate.
Once a shift, primary nurse to sit at client's bedside for at least several minutes to communicate caring and to explore with the client her present stressors and the adequacy of her coping response. • Assess factors compounding her losses. • Reinforce her personal strengths and support systems; counsel her to tap into these now. • Suggest local support groups if indicated. Primary nurse to explore with daughter, Lisa, how her mother's moving in with her has affected the family. Recommend support systems.	The nurse's unhurried, attentive, and caring presence will communicate to the client that she is important to the nurse and that the nurse values her well-being = invitation to the client to become actively involved in recovery. Logical to explore adequacy of past and current coping mechanisms before suggesting new approaches Adult children of aging parents are frequently experiencing overwhelming stress as they try to deal with own and their parents' problems. Supporting this family *is* supporting the client indirectly.	9/10 Goal partially met. Client speaks freely about how much she misses her husband and how fearful this hospitalization makes her. When asked about living with her daughter, she becomes uncharacteristically quiet. *C. Taylor, RN* 9/10 Goal met. Client talks about how everything seemed better in the past after she talked it over with her husband and God. *C. Taylor, RN* 9/10 Goal not met. Client couldn't think of anything about herself that is healthy or strong. Says "maybe" her family can help her now. *Revision:* Counsel regarding personal strengths. Help her to experience them. *C. Taylor, RN* 9/11 Too early to evaluate.

(Continued)

Student Care Plan   (Continued)

Assessment	Nursing Diagnosis	Goals
Subjective Data: "I move my bowels every 2–3 days; get constipated at least once a week. Often Metamucil helps." "I drink plenty of fluids and even fruits and vegetables." History of hemorrhoids 2° to straining *Objective Data:* No bowel movement in last 4 days On bed rest since hospitalized	Alteration in elimination: constipation related to decreased physical activity and long-term laxative use (Metamucil)	Beginning 9/7 Client passes soft, formed stool q 1–3 days without use of laxatives. By 9/10, client verbalizes the importance of the following natural aids to bowel elimination: • Daily intake of foods high in bulk • Daily fluid intake of 8–10 glasses • Regular time for elimination • Daily physical exercise: walking

---

provide a scientific rationale for the orders they propose. A succinct rationale statement demonstrates that the student is consciously choosing a nursing intervention because of its high probability to effect the desired change.

Evaluating.   Incorporating evaluative statements on the plan of care communicates clearly the message that nursing care is never complete until client goal achievement is evaluated. Just as some say that teaching has not occurred if learning does not take place, so nursing care is incomplete if the desired client goals are not achieved.

PROBLEMS RELATED TO PLANNING

Some of the common problems student nurses encounter while developing nursing care plans include goals stated too generally, goals not developed from specific nursing diagnoses, nursing orders not written clearly, not involving the client in the planning process, and failure to update the plan of care.

K E Y   P O I N T S

■ During planning, the nurse works with the client and family (1) developing goals which, if achieved, prevent, reduce, or eliminate the problems specified in the nursing diagnoses, and (2) identifying the nursing interventions most likely to assist the client achieve these goals.

■ The purpose of planning is the development of a holistic, individualized plan of nursing care acceptable to both the client and the nurse.

■ Conscious, deliberate planning individualizes care, helps communication among nurses, identifies

Nursing Orders	Scientific Rationale	Evaluation
Monitor bowel elimination patterns; identify causative factors of constipation and successful corrective measures.	*This* client's elimination problems will not be resolved until all the specific etiologies of her constipation and successful corrective measures are identified. Needs to be an ongoing assessment priority.	9/10 Goal met. Soft formed stool q 2–3 days. *C. Taylor, RN*
Explain the importance of adhering to a regular time for defecation (client suggests after breakfast)—adhere to this in the hospital.	Positive use of circadian rhythms	
When given medical clearance, assist client with progressive ambulation. Recommend that she include brisk walking into daily health habits. (build strength to 20–30 minute brisk walk daily).	Peristalsis is stimulated by physical exercise.	9/10 Goal met. Client correctly related value of four natural aids to elimination. Questions whether or not she will be strong enough to walk. *C. Taylor, RN* *Revision:* Encourage assisted ambulation. *C. Taylor, RN*
Explain the long-term effects of laxative abuse on the bowel and discourage their use.	Leads to decreased peristaltic response to food and loss of intestinal tone	
Reinforce the client's adequate fluid intake and ingestion of high bulk foods such as fresh fruits and salad.	Commenting on these positive self-care behaviors reinforces them.	

priorities of care, promotes continuity of care, coordinates care, facilitates evaluating the client's responses to care, and promotes the nurse's professional development.

■ Three types of planning essential to comprehensive nursing care are initial, ongoing problem-oriented, and discharge.

■ When planning care the nurse reviews the prioritized list of nursing diagnoses to see that diagnoses are ranked according to the level of threat they present to client well-being. Any changes in the client's health status or in the way the client is responding to health/illness or the treatment plan may signal the need to reestablish client priorities.

■ A client goal describes an expected client behavior. Client goals are derived from the problem statement of the nursing diagnosis and, once achieved, contribute to the prevention or resolution of this problem.

■ Each client goal must have a subject (the client or some part of the client), a verb (which clearly indicates the action the client is expected to perform), and criteria that describe in observable, measurable terms the expected client behavior.

■ Client goals should be valued by the client, supportive of the total treatment plan, brief, specific, and stated positively.

■ Nursing measures are derived from the etiology of the nursing diagnosis. The effective nurse chooses from a wide variety of possible nursing interventions and nursing measures that specifically address factors causing or contributing to the client's problems.

■ Effective nursing measures are tailored to the client; consistent with standards of care; realistic in terms of the abilities, time, and resources available to the nurse and client; compatible with the client's values, beliefs, and psychosocial background; valued by the client; and compatible with other planned therapies.

■ Nursing orders clearly and concisely describe the nursing action to be performed; are signed by the nurse prescribing the order and dated; use acceptable abbreviations, symbols, and key phrases; and refer nurses to procedure manuals for the steps of lengthy, routine procedures.

■ Comprehensive nursing orders specify what observations need to be made and how often, what nursing measures need to be done (how they are to be done and when), and the teaching, counseling, and advocacy needs of clients and families.

■ The nursing care plan is the written guide that directs the efforts of the nursing team as they work with clients to meet health goals. Primarily, nursing care plans ensure that nursing care is goal-oriented and individualized.

■ The nurse who best knows the client develops the plan of care within 24 hours of the client's admission. The plan is written in ink (a part of the client's permanent record) and signed and dated by the nurse who developed the plan.

■ Many institutions use a Kardex system of care planning, which specifies nursing care related to basic human needs, prioritized nursing diagnoses, and the medical plan of care. Each client's 6 × 11-inch Kardex care plan is placed in a central Kardex file.

■ Most student care plans are designed to help students systematically proceed through each of the five steps of the nursing process. The assessment data establishing and validating nursing diagnoses are often recorded on the plan, scientific rationales and references may be requested for the nursing order chosen, and evaluative statements are documented.

■ Common problems related to planning include stating goals vaguely, failing to develop goals from the problem statement of the nursing diagnosis, writing vague nursing orders, failing to involve the client and family in care planning, and failing to update the plan of care as the client's status and needs change.

BIBLIOGRAPHY

Atkinson LD, Murray ME: Understanding the Nursing Process, 3rd ed. New York, Macmillan, 1986

Boatwright D, Crummette BD: How to plan and conduct a patient care conference. Nursing 17(12):64, 1987

Bower FL: The Process of Planning Nursing Care: A Theoretical Model, 2nd ed. St Louis, CV Mosby, 1981

Carnevali DR: Nursing Care Planning: Diagnosis and Management, 3rd ed. Philadelphia, JB Lippincott, 1983

Carpenito LJ: Nursing Diagnosis: Application to Clinical Practice, 2nd ed. Philadelphia, JB Lippincott, 1987

Lederer J et al: Care Planning Pocket Guide: A Nursing Diagnosis Approach. Menlo Park, CA, Addison-Wesley, 1986

Matthewman J: Combining care plan and Kardex. Am J Nurs 87(6):852–854, 1987

Mayers MG: A Systematic Approach to the Nursing Care Plan. Norwalk, CT, Appleton-Century-Crofts, 1983

Rogers BR: Care planning: A comment on the Canadian experience. Canadian Nurse 77(7):34–35, 1981

Shea H: The nursing care plan dilemma: Suggestions for resolution. Canadian Nurse 80(9):44–46, 1984

Ulrich SP, Canale SW, Wendell SA: Nursing Care Planning Guides: A Nursing Diagnosis Approach. Philadelphia, WB Saunders, 1986

Vasey EK: Writing your patient's care plan . . . efficiently. Nursing 9(4):67–71, 1979

Implementing/ Documenting

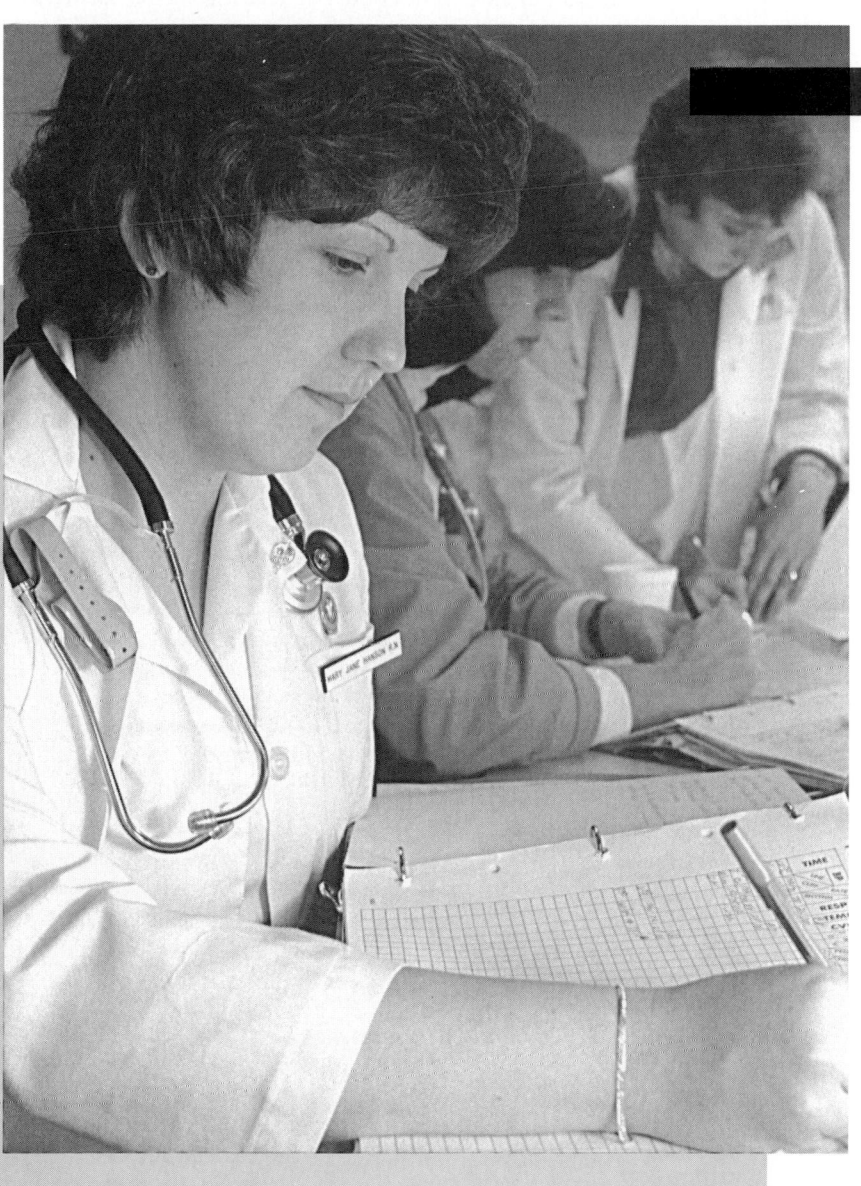

OBJECTIVES

After studying this chapter, the learner should be able to

Define key terms used in the chapter.

Distinguish independent, interdependent or collaborative, and dependent nursing interventions.

Use intellectual, interpersonal, and technical skills to implement a plan of nursing care.

Describe six variables that influence the way a plan of care is implemented.

Use seven guidelines for implementation.

Use ongoing data collection to direct revision of the plan of care.

Compare and contrast different documentation systems: source-oriented record, problem-oriented record, and computer record.

Document nursing interventions completely, accurately, concisely, and factually.

Describe nursing's role in communicating with other health-care professionals by reporting, conferring, and referring.

During the **implementing** step of the nursing process, all of the nursing actions developed during the planning step are carried out. The purpose of implementation is to assist the client in achieving desired health goals: promote wellness, prevent disease/illness, restore health, and facilitate coping with altered functioning. The plan of care is best implemented when clients who are able and willing to participate have maximum opportunities to provide self-care. Family members and other support persons, as well as other health-care professionals, can also become involved in the successful implementation of the plan of care. During the implementation step (Fig 18-1), the nurse continues to collect data and to modify the plan of care as needed. All activities are documented according to the form used in the nurse's institution.

KEY TERMS

change-of-shift report
dependent intervention
discharge summary
flow sheets
implementing
independent intervention
interdependent (collaborative) intervention
narrative notes
nursing actions (interventions, measures, strategies

nursing care conference
nursing care round
problem-oriented record (POR)
progress notes
protocol
record
SOAP format
source-oriented record
standing order

UNIQUE FOCUS OF NURSING IMPLEMENTATION

In all nurse–client interactions, the nurse is concerned with both the client's response to health and illness and the client's ability to meet basic human needs. While other health-care professionals focus on selected aspects of the client's treatment regimen, the nurse is concerned with how the client is responding to the plan of care in general.

Types of Nursing Interventions

When implementing the plan of care, the nurse functions independently, dependently, and collaboratively.

Independent interventions or nursing actions involve carrying out nurse-prescribed orders written on the nursing plan of care, as well as any other actions that nurses initiate without the direction or supervision of another health-care professional and that are the result of their assessment of client needs. Nurses are legally accountable for the assessments they make and for their nursing responses.

Dependent interventions or nursing actions involve carrying out physician orders. Nurse practice acts make it clear from whom nurses can receive orders. Nurses are accountable for the dependent orders they implement and are thus responsible for the clarification of any questionable order.

Collaborative or **interdependent interventions** or nursing actions are those performed jointly by nurses and other members of the health-care team. Because nurses are being increasingly respected as competent colleagues with a unique knowledge of the client, they are becoming more and more involved in collaborative ventures with the health-care team.

All of these actions may be illustrated with reference to the care received by a depressed client with data indicative of a gastrointestinal blockage. If the physician orders a series of GI studies, it is nursing's responsibility

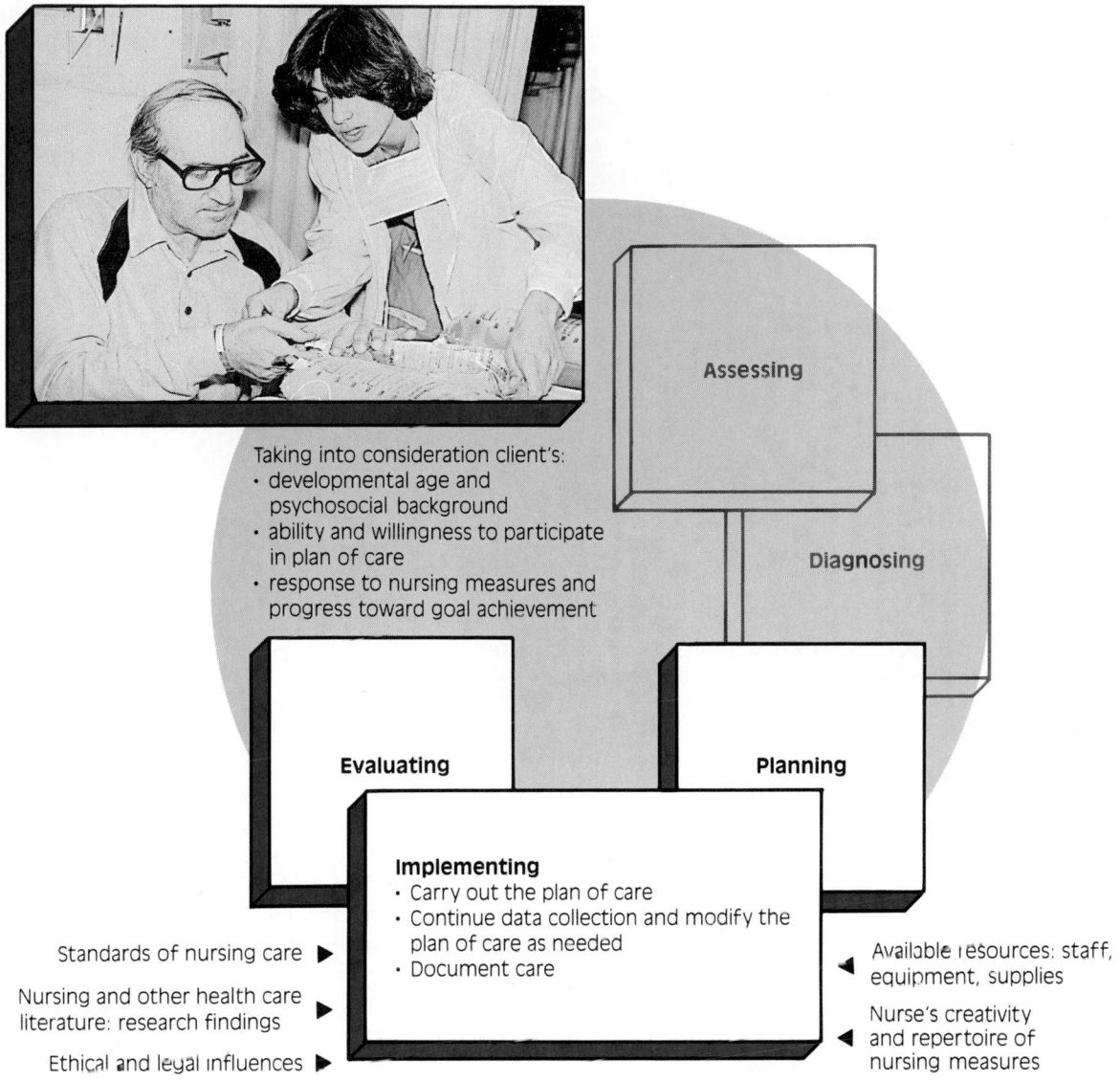

Taking into consideration client's:
- developmental age and psychosocial background
- ability and willingness to participate in plan of care
- response to nursing measures and progress toward goal achievement

Assessing

Diagnosing

Evaluating

Planning

Implementing
- Carry out the plan of care
- Continue data collection and modify the plan of care as needed
- Document care

Standards of nursing care ▶

Nursing and other health care literature: research findings ▶

Ethical and legal influences ▶

◀ Available resources: staff, equipment, supplies

◀ Nurse's creativity and repertoire of nursing measures

F I G U R E   **18-1**

Implementing. Implementing is simply the carrying out of the plan of care, which is modified in response to client changes. Numerous variables influence the way the plan of care is implemented (see arrows). (Photo by Gates Rhodes, courtesy of the School of Nursing, University of Pennsylvania)

to prepare the client by executing the physician's orders for cleansing the bowel. These nursing actions are dependent interventions. If the nurse senses that the client seems unusually fearful of what the outcome of the studies will be and plans to explore the client's fears and follow-up with appropriate teaching and counseling, then the nurse is involved in independent nursing actions. When a multidisciplinary team conference is held to discuss the client's failure to progress, the nurse works collaboratively with the psychiatrist, gastroenterologist, social worker, and pastoral counselor to develop a comprehensive plan of care; these are collaborative or interdependent nursing actions.

Practicing nurses as well as students beginning clinical experience may be surprised when they evaluate how much of their day is devoted to independent nursing practice (care organized by nursing diagnosis) and how much is spent carrying out dependent functions (medically delegated care: disease management, medical orders, and so forth). Using a circle, divide your day into segments illustrating independent nursing practice, dependent nursing practice, collaborative nursing practice, continuing education, and other activities. How your circle is divided will illustrate your priorities, as well as the range of nursing interventions possible in your particular practice setting (see Fig. 18-2).

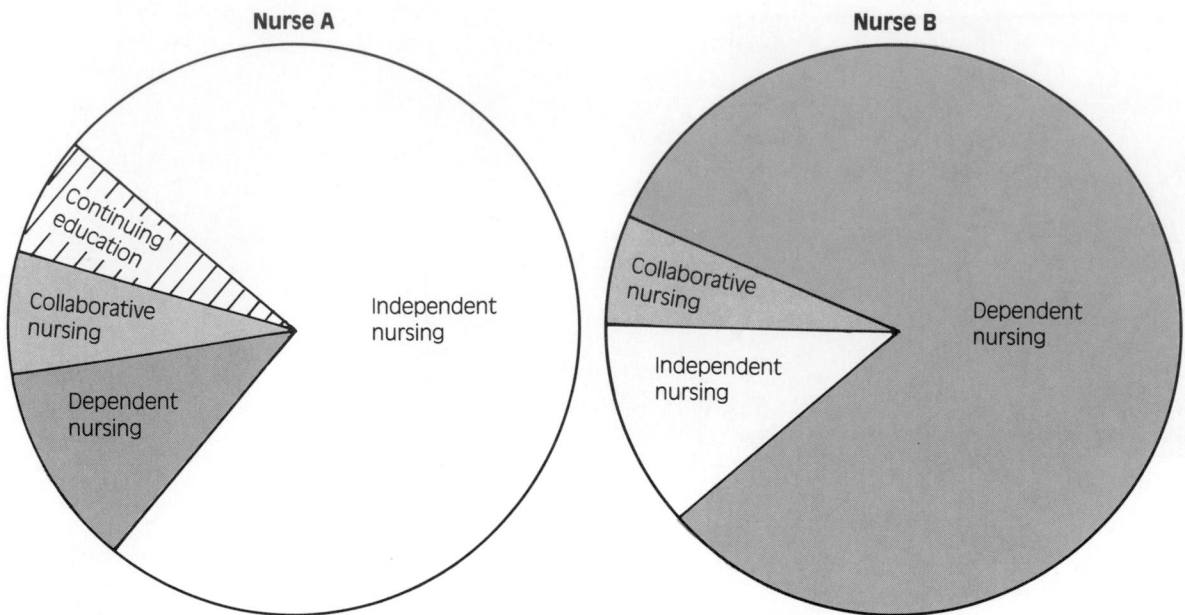

F I G U R E   18-2

Division of nursing time. These circles illustrate the way two nurses in different practice settings spend their work day. This time division quickly indicates the emphasis on independent, dependent, and collaborative nursing.

Protocols and Standing Orders

Protocols and standing orders may expand the scope of nursing practice in certain, clearly defined situations. **Protocols** are written plans that detail the nursing activities to be executed in specific situations. Although some protocols specify routine aspects of nursing care (*e.g.,* protocols describing nursing responsibilities when a client is admitted to or discharged from the institution), other protocols include standing orders that empower the nurse to initiate actions ordinarily requiring the order or supervision of a physician. Examples include admission protocols for OB/GYN clients, protocols for bowel programs that allow the nurse to select and administer necessary bowel interventions, standard orders for narcotic overdoses that specify the agents the nurse is to administer to reverse respiratory depression in an emergency situation, and standard orders for pain management that enable the nurse to select the strength of the medication to be given, within preset ranges.

The Nurse as Coordinator

One of nursing's major contributions to the health-care team is that of the role of coordinator. It is easy for care to become fragmented when clients are seen by numerous specialists—each interested in a different aspect of the client. At best, clients complain that no one person really knows them and can talk with them about what is going on and how it will affect them in the future. At worst, the orders of the different specialists may conflict with one another and be counterproductive. Therefore, it is important for nurses to make rounds with other health-care professionals and to read the results of consultations clients have had with various specialists. The nurse can then interpret the findings of specialists for clients and family members, prepare clients to participate maximally in the plan of care both before and after discharge, and serve as a liaison among the different members of the health-care team.

CARRYING OUT THE PLAN OF CARE

When carrying out the plan of care, nurses use specialized abilities to (1) determine the client's need for nursing assistance, (2) promote self-care, and (3) assist client to achieve health goals.

Prerequisite Nursing Skills

When implementing the plan of nursing care, nurses use intellectual, interpersonal, and technical skills. Each nurse possesses a unique blend of these skills and is effective to the extent that his or her abilities are able to match the client's need for nursing care.

Intellectual Skills. Nurses use cognitive abilities to (1) think critically about nursing situations, bringing to bear pertinent nursing theory; (2) design plans of care that enhance client strengths and resolve problems (problem-solving and decision-making skills and creativity); and (3) develop a work environment that promotes nursing excellence.

Interpersonal Skills. Because nursing generally involves interaction with other individuals, interpersonal skills are essential. These include the ability to communicate competence and caring, eliciting the trust that allows the professional nurse–client relationship to develop; teaching; and counseling. Communication skills are presented in Chapter 20.

Technical Skills. Technical skills include the ability to execute both simple and complex nursing procedures, which often require the skillful use of equipment and supplies. Giving a client a bath, assessing vital signs, administering an injection, irrigating and packing a wound, and suctioning a tracheostomy are all examples of technical skills.

Examples of the nursing skills necessary to implement select plans of nursing care are presented at the end of each clinical chapter in this text.

Determining the Need for Assistance

While most individuals are capable of independently meeting basic human needs, illness and the stress of diagnostic and therapeutic measures may interfere with an individual's usual practice of self-care abilities. A careful nursing assessment of the client's abilities to independently meet human needs is indicated. Nursing has often failed clients by doing too much for them and by encouraging negative, sick role behaviors such as inappropriate dependence. Conversely, there is a time and place for the "tender loving care" that says to a client: "I know you may be able to do this for yourself, but just this once, how about if I do it and we'll talk!" Challenging a client's best self-care effort while meeting the universal human need to feel important and loved is an important component of the art of nursing.

The nursing care plan should include specific instructions for any nursing assistance the client needs to meet basic human needs—including the need for forceful nursing encouragement to promote greater independence in functioning. When routines of self-care are indicated (*e.g.*, colostomy management), instructions should include the time of the procedure, the equipment used, the process, and the level of patient involvement. Continuity of nursing care is essential to the client's development of a comfortable routine.

Promoting Self-care: Teaching, Counseling, and Advocacy

If clients and their families wish to participate actively in seeking wellness, preventing disease/illness, recovering health, and learning to cope with altered functioning, it is important that they possess effective self-care behaviors. Nurses sensitive to the importance of clients learning to direct and manage their own care use nurse–client interactions for both planned and spontaneous teaching, counseling, and advocacy. These nursing roles are described in Chapters 21 and 22. For example, while caring for a child recently diagnosed as having cystic fibrosis, the nurses work continuously with the parents and siblings, helping them to develop the knowledge and skills that will enable them to care for the child upon discharge. Referring families such as this to a community support group or other resources further enhances the self-care behaviors being developed.

Assisting Clients to Meet Health Goals

This is the phase of the implementation process in which the nursing team carries out the nursing orders detailed in the nursing plan of care. If the plan of care is well constructed, carrying out its orders is the nurse's most important task and should receive top priority. The nursing actions planned to promote client goal achievement and the resolution of health problems should be carefully executed.

Because understaffing continues to be a problem in many practice settings, it is important that nurses learn to use time wisely and to maximize each client encounter. A client bath can be simply that, or it can be an opportunity to gather additional focused data, to communicate concern for what the client is experiencing and to offer support, and to teach and counsel as appropriate. How the nurse uses the 30 minutes that he or she is in the client's room for the bath will determine how effective the nurse is in helping the client to his or her goals.

Variables Influencing Implementation. When working with clients to achieve the goals specified in the nursing plan of care, it is important to remember that nothing about the plan of care is fixed. Some of the most important variables that influence the way the plan of care is implemented follow.

Client Variables. Ideally, the client is the primary determinant of how nursing measures are implemented. Successful nurses modify their nursing actions according to the client's (1) changing ability and willingness to participate in the plan of care and (2) previous responses to nursing measures and progress toward goal achievement. Other important client variables are developmental stage and psychosocial background.

Nurses who have studied development often feel they have addressed the developmental needs of a client simply by identifying the client's developmental stage on the plan of care. Exactly what the developmental tasks related to this stage are and how this is related to nursing care are seldom considered. Stereotypes about developmental stages and tasks also influence the care clients receive. For example, the same student nurse who recommends that the parents of a premature infant make a tape of their voices to stimulate the infant in the neonatal intensive care unit also works weekends in a nursing home where the developmental needs of the elderly are routinely violated. This student has never thought to question the staff's selection of a radio station that plays rock music, or other staff actions—humorous comments about "romances" among some of the residents, infantilizing some residents by calling them "cute" names or putting bright, big bows in their hair, or planning childish group activities which many of the clients find demeaning. Perhaps the greatest violation of all is the belief that all the elderly have to do is wait to die, that there are no developmental changes for this age group.

In implementing a comprehensive and holistic plan of care, nurses must find creative ways to meet developmental needs. This is of greatest importance when clients are separated from their families and home environments for long periods of time.

The same is true of the psychosocial needs of clients. While few nurses would claim that individuals from all socioeconomic groups and cultures are the same, some practice nursing as if this were so. When choosing nursing measures, it is important to consider and respect the client's background. Therefore, while it is good to teach a malnourished client to include more protein in his diet, if the client has a marginal income, lives alone in one room, and has little interest in and facilities for cooking, teaching that ends with the above recommendation is terribly inadequate.

Nurse Variables.   Nurse variables that influence the implementation of the plan of care include the nurses' levels of expertise, creativity (ability to match client needs with specific nursing strategies), willingness to provide care, and available time.

Resources.   The most elaborately designed plan of care is doomed to failure on a chronically understaffed or undersupplied nursing unit. Adequate staff, equipment, and supplies are all important determinants of client care.

Current Standards of Care.   All nursing actions that are selected when implementing the plan of care must be consistent with standards for practice. Each nurse is responsible for learning the standards that dictate practice in his or her specialty. Failure to practice according to these standards may result in a charge of negligence.

Research Findings.   Nurses concerned about improving the quality of nursing care use research findings to enhance their nursing practice. Reading professional nursing journals and attending continuing education workshops and conferences are excellent ways to learn about new nursing strategies that have proven effectiveness.

Ethical and Legal Guides to Practice.   It is impossible to practice good nursing today and be ignorant of the laws and regulations affecting health care and the ethical dimensions of clinical practice. As the nurse implements the plan of care, sincere motivation to benefit the client and a conscientious attempt to implement nursing orders well are no longer sufficient. Each nurse is responsible for developing sensitivity to the ethical and legal dimensions of practice, and moral and legal accountability are inherent in the practice of professional nursing. Chapters 5 and 6 deal specifically with the ethical and legal dimensions of practice. Hospital risk managers and ethics committees are increasingly available institutional resources for nurses.

Guidelines for Implementation

1. Before implementing any nursing action, reassess the client to determine if the action is still needed.
2. Approach the client competently. Know how to perform the nursing action, why the action is being performed, and potential adverse responses. Have all equipment and supplies ready.
3. Approach the client caringly. Explain the nursing

Guide for Students

To organize clinical responsibilities check
1. Client profile
2. Name by which client wishes to be addressed
3. Client's current health status
   - Any physical or emotional changes indicating the need to modify the plan or care?
4. Routine assistance client needs to meet basic human needs
   - Note any special safety precautions needed
5. Priorities for nursing care
   - Prioritized nursing diagnoses, client goals, and related nursing interventions
   - Medical orders that need to be implemented
   - Interdependent or collaborative nursing responsibilities
6. Special "events" of the day that may require special observation of the client, teaching, preparation, or after-care
   - Diagnosic tests
   - Consultations with specialists
   - New therapies (physical therapy, medications, surgery, radiotherapy, and so forth
7. Special teaching, counseling, or advocacy needs
8. Special needs of the family

action using language the client understands. Communicate genuine concern for what the client is experiencing.

4. Modify nursing interventions according to the client's (1) developmental and psychosocial background, (2) ability and willingness to participate in the plan of care, and (3) responses to previous nursing measures and progress toward goal achievement.
5. Check to make sure that the nursing actions selected are consistent with standards of care and within legal and ethical guides to practice.
6. Always question that the nursing action selected is the best of all possible alternatives. Consult colleagues and the nursing and related literature to see if other approaches might be more successful. Evaluate the effectiveness of the action selected noting any factors which positively or negatively influenced the outcome.
7. Develop a repertoire of skilled nursing interventions. The more options one can choose from, the greater the likelihood of success.

A Guide for Students

Student nurses trying to organize their nursing care for a particular clinical day in advance may find it helpful to use the headings in the box on page 308 to identify the nursing measures for which they will be responsible. Once these have been identified, working out a time schedule may provide clear direction for the clinical day and ensure that the client's needs are met.

CONTINUING DATA COLLECTION

An important nursing intervention is ongoing data collection. In every client encounter, the nurse needs to be sensitive to both subtle and dramatic changes in the client's condition or response to this condition. These assessment findings are used to update and revise the plan of care. Sensitivity to how the client is responding to nursing measures and to the client's progress toward goal achievement allows the nurse to modify nursing measures appropriately.

COMMUNICATING CARE

The communication process and specific communication techniques are discussed in Chapter 20. This section explores how nurses communicate with other nurses and members of the health-care team about the client. Effective communication among health-care professionals is essential to the coordination and continuity of care. Communicating effectively enables personnel to supplement and complement each other's services and to avoid duplications and omissions in care.

Discussing, reporting, and recording are the primary means of communication used in health care. *Discussion* is a verbal exchange between two or more individuals often used to pool information for the purposes of clearly identifying a problem or developing a strategy for its resolution. For example, one nurse may ask another if he or she has noticed that a client seems to be getting little relief from the prescribed pain medication. If the other nurse concurs, the discussion will proceed to how this can best be remedied.

Reporting is the oral, written, or computer-based communication of client data with the purpose of informing others. A laboratory report, for example, may communicate to the health team that a client's cardiac enzymes are normal or that a biopsy of breast tissue revealed no malignant or atypical cells. A nurse's shift report or nursing note may communicate the progress a client is making toward goal achievement.

Recording is the written, legal documentation of all pertinent interventions with the client: assessing, diagnosing, planning, implementing, and evaluating.

The Joint Commission on Accreditation of Hospitals (1982) specifies that the "nursing process shall be documented for each hospitalized patient from admission through discharge." Each health-care institution has policies specifying the nurse's recording and reporting responsibilities, and each nurse is accountable to practice according to these standards.

The Client Record

The client **record** or chart is a compilation of a client's health-care information. It is the only legal document that provides a comprehensive picture of the nursing care given to the client. This record is composed of various forms on which information pertaining to the client has been recorded by different groups of health-care professionals. The forms are usually placed in a binder or folder and kept where they are easily accessible to health-care practitioners.

Purposes of Client Records. Client records serve many purposes.

Communication. The client record helps health-care professionals from different disciplines and who interact with the client at different times to communicate with one another.

Care Planning. Each professional working with the client has access to the client's baseline and ongoing data and can see how the client is responding to the treatment plan from day to day. Modifications of the plan of care are then based on this data.

Audit. Charts may be reviewed to evaluate retrospectively (after the client's discharge) the quality of care received and the competence of the nurses providing that care. For example, in a nursing audit, a committee decides in advance certain standards of care they wish to evaluate (*e.g.,* pertaining to nursing assessment, nursing documentation, or safety measures). A number of charts are then randomly selected and reviewed to see if the charts give evidence of the nurse meeting the selected standards of care. If deficiencies are found, inservice can be used to remedy them and improve the quality of care.

Research. The record may be studied by researchers hoping to learn from the study of similar cases how best to recognize or treat other clients' health problems.

Education. Health-care professionals reading a client's chart can learn a great deal about the clinical manifestations of particular health problems, effective treatment modalities, and factors affecting client goal achievement.

Legal Document. Client records are legal documents which may be entered into court proceedings as evidence; as such, they play an important role in implicating or absolving health practitioners charged with improper care. The record can also be used in accident or injury claims made by the client.

Historic Document. Because the dates of entries on records are specified, the record has value as a historic document. Years later, information may become pertinent concerning a client's past health care.

Nursing Entries on the Client Record. When the nursing process is fully implemented, nursing documentation on the client's permanent record includes each of the following:

Concise, comprehensive nursing assessment—Initial data base obtained from the nursing history and nursing examinations and ongoing focused assessments.

Up-to-date care plan individualized to the client—Identifies prioritized nursing diagnoses, related client goals and nursing orders, and the status of goal achievement.

Narrative notes—Deal with client problems identified in the plan of care; include a description of the status of the problem, related nursing interventions, client responses, and revisions in the plan of care.

Flow sheets—Record routine nursing interventions.

Graphic sheets—Record, as indicated, the client's vital signs, weight, intake and output, blood sugar, neurologic status, and so forth.

Medication records—Record all medication administered to the client (drug, dosage, route, time), nurse administering the drug, and for some medications (*e.g.,* analgesics) the reason why the drug was administered and its effectiveness.

Discharge summary—Records status of each client problem and the teaching and counseling done to prepare the client for discharge.

Although the client record is the only permanent legal document that details the nurse's interactions with the client, it is not unusual to find critical omissions of nursing documentation, meaningless repetitious entries, and inaccurate entries. While these errors may go undetected and have no effect on the client, they may also seriously affect the care the client receives and cause legal problems for the nurse responsible. Adherence to the following guidelines for documentation will help to prevent errors.

Guidelines for Documentation

Content

- Enter information in a complete, accurate, relevant (concise), and factual manner.
- Record client findings (observations of behavior) rather than your interpretation of these findings.
- Avoid words such as "good," "average," "normal," "sufficient," which may mean different things to different readers.
- Avoid generalizations such as "seems uncomfortable today." A better entry would be "on a scale of 1 to 10, client rates back pain 7 to 9 today as compared to 4 to 5 yesterday; no change in vital signs."
- Note problems as they occur; record the nursing intervention and the client's response; update problems or delete as appropriate.
- Document all medical visits and consultations of which other nurses should be aware, either because of their impact on the client or because of the nursing care the client now requires.
- Carefully document the nursing response to questionable medical orders or treatment (or failure to treat). Factually record the date and time the physician was notified of the concern and the exact physician response. If this occurs by phone, have a second nurse listen to the conversation and co-sign the note. If a nurse administrator was contacted, document this.
- Avoid the use of stereotypes or derogatory terms when charting.

Format

- Chart on the proper form as designated by agency policy.
- Print or write legibly. Use correct grammar and spelling.
- Use only approved abbreviations and symbols (see Table 18-1).
- Date and time each entry.
- Chart nursing entries chronologically on consecutive lines. Never skip lines. Draw a single line through blank spaces.

T A B L E   *18-1*
Abbreviations and Symbols Commonly Used by Health Practitioners

Activities

AMB	ambulatory
BRP	bathroom privileges
CBR	complete bed rest
OOB	out of bed
up ad lib	up as desired

Assessment Data

abd	abdomen
BP	blood pressure
bx	biopsy
C	Celsius (centigrade)
cc	chief complaint
c/o	complains of
dx	diagnosis
F	Fahrenheit
GI	gastrointestinal
GU	genitourinary
h/o	history of
HPI	history of present illness
Imp	Impressions
lt or Ⓛ	left
NAD	no apparent distress
neg	negative
P	pulse
PE	physical examination
PMH	past medical history
R	respirations
R/O	rule out
ROS	review of systems
rt or Ⓡ	right
RX	treatment
Sx	symptoms
T	temperature
WNL	within normal limits
⊕	positive
⊖	negative

Disease

ASHD	arteriosclerotic heart disease
ASCVD	arteriosclerotic cardiovascular disease
BPH	benign prostatic hypertrophy
CA	cancer
CAD	coronary artery disease
CHF	congestive heart failure
COPD	chronic obstructive pulmonary disease
CVA	cerebrovascular accident
DM	diabetes mellitus
HTN (↑ BP)	hypertension
MI	myocardial infarction
PVD	peripheral vascular disease
STD	sexually transmitted disease

Diagnostic Studies

ABG	arterial blood gases
BE	barium enema
CBC	complete blood count
CO_2	carbon dioxide
C&S	culture and sensitivity
CXR	chest x-ray
ECG (EKG)	cardiogram
lytes	electrolytes
RBC	red blood cells
UA	urinalysis
UGI	upper GI
WBC	white blood cells

Symbols

>	greater than
<	less than
↑	increase
↗	increasing
↓	decrease
↙	decreasing
2°	secondary to
=	equal to
≠	unequal
♀	female
♂	male
°	degree

Orders

ā	before
ad lib	as desired
AMA	against medical orders
BM	bowel movement
BP	blood pressure
c̄ (C)	with
CPR	cardiopulmonary resuscitation
dc (disc)	discontinue
dx	diagnosis
DNR (no code)	do not resuscitate
hs	hour of sleep
I&O	intake and output
IV	intravenous
noc	night
NPO	nothing by mouth
NS (NlS)	normal saline
O_2	oxygen
od	daily
p̄	after
O.T.	occupational therapy
post op	postoperative
pre op	preoperative
prep	preparation
PRN	as needed
P.T.	physical therapy
pt	patient
q	every
qs	quantity sufficient
ROM	range of motion
s̄ (S)	without
STAT	immediately
TPR	temperature, pulse, respirations
VS	vital signs
x	times

- Sign your first initial, last name, and title to each entry.
- Do not use dittos, erasures, or correcting fluids. A single line should be drawn through an incorrect entry and the words "mistaken entry" or "error in charting" should be printed above or beside the entry and signed. The entry should then be rewritten correctly.
- Each page of the record should be identified with the client's name and identification number.
- Follow agency policy pertaining to the color of ink or the type of pen or ink to be used.

Timing

- Follow agency policy regarding the frequency of documentation and modify this if changes in the client's status warrant more frequent documentation.
- Indicate in each entry both the time the entry was written and the time of pertinent observations or interventions. This is crucial when a case is being reconstructed for legal purposes.
- Document nursing interventions as close as possible to the time of their execution. The more seriously ill the client, the greater the need to keep documentation current. Never leave the unit for an extended break when caring for a seriously ill client until all significant information is recorded.
- Never document interventions before carrying them out.

Types of Records

Source-Oriented Client Records. A **source-oriented** record is one in which each health-care group keeps data on its own separate form. Sections of the record are designated for nurses, physicians, laboratory and x-ray personnel, and so on. Notations are entered chronologically, with the most recent entry being nearest the front of the record. An advantage of the source-oriented record is that each discipline can easily find and chart pertinent data. The main disadvantage is that data are fragmented, and it is difficult to track problems chronologically with input from different groups of professionals.

While the specifics vary among health agencies, general characteristics of the source-oriented record have remained essentially the same. Types of forms typically used in a source-oriented client record are presented in Table 18-2. Figures 18-3 and 18-4 illustrate various forms used in source-oriented records.

Problem-Oriented Client Records. Another type of record used in many health agencies is the problem-oriented record (POR) or problem-oriented medical record (POMR), which were originated by Dr. Lawrence Weed in the 1960s. The **problem-oriented record** is organized around a client's problems, rather than around sources of information. All health professionals record on the same forms. Advantages of this type of record are that the entire health-care team works together in identifying a master list of client problems and contributes collaboratively to the plan of care. Progress notes are clearly focused on client problems. Some nurses find that the SOAP method (**SOAP** = subjective data, objective data, assessment, plan) of charting focuses too narrowly on selecting problems and are advocating a return to the traditional narrative format. Table 18-3 presents a summary of the four major parts of the problem-oriented record: the defined data base, problem list, care plans, and progress notes.

Computer Records. In more and more health-care institutions, comprehensive computer systems have revolutionized nursing documentation in the client record. Computer capacities are already in operation where the nurse (1) calls up the admission assessment tool on the computer screen and keys in client data which are automatically recorded; (2) develops the care plan using computerized care plans available for each North American Nursing Diagnosis Association approved diagnosis; (3) adds to the client data base as new data are identified and modifies the plan of care accordingly; (4) receives a work list indicating the treatment, procedures, and medications necessary for the client throughout the shift; and (5) documents care immediately using the computer terminal at the client's bedside. Other ways in which computers are being used in health care are highlighted throughout the text.

Agency Policies. Most agencies have specific policies concerning client records. All who have access to the record (direct caregivers) are expected to maintain its confidentiality. At no time may a nurse give a client's chart to a family member or to any person other than an authorized caregiver. State laws differ as to whether or not the client has the legal right to review the chart. Most agencies grant student nurses access to client records for purposes of education. In this instance, the student assumes responsibility to hold the client information in confidence.

Agency policies also indicate which personnel are responsible for recording on each form in the record, and such policies may also describe the order in which the forms are to appear in the record. Additional policies may concern the frequency with which entries are to be made, whether routine care is recorded, the manner in which health personnel identify themselves after making an entry, which types of abbreviations are acceptable, and the manner in which an error in recording is handled.

The storage of client records is a function of the health agency's record department. Many client records are microfilmed for compact storage or are entered into a computer to expedite accessibility of information.

Other Communication Methods

Common methods for communicating among health practitioners other than by the client record include using face-to-face meetings, the telephone, a messenger,

(Text continues on p. 316.)

T A B L E   **18-2**
Examples of Forms and Information in Source-Oriented Client Records

Form	Typical Client Information Entered on the Form
Admission sheet	Legal name, identification number Age, birthdate, sex Marital status Occupation and employer Religious preference Next of kin and person to notify in case of emergency Date, time, reason for admission Name of the attending physician Insurance information Discharge data
Admission nursing assessment	Results of nursing history and nursing examination
Graphic sheet (Fig 18-3)	Daily temperatures, pulse and respiratory rates, blood pressure (vital signs) Daily weight Special measurements, such as the patient's fluid intake and output
Activity flow sheet (Fig 18-4)	Diet and how client has eaten Bathing and skin care Activity level, safety measures Respiratory interventions Elimination Diagnostic measures, treatments Isolation
Nurse's notes (Fig 18-4)	Descriptions of pertinent observations of the client Statements that specify the nursing care, including teaching, received by the client and his responses to nursing care Statements that describe the client's condition and progress, or lack of progress, toward recovery and goal achievement Descriptions of the client's complaints and how the client is coping, or failing to cope, with them and nursing's response
Medication sheet	Name of prescribed medications administered on a regular basis Dosage of the medication administered Route by which the medication was administered, unless given orally Time medication was administered Name or initials of the person administering the medication
Medical history and examination sheet	Results of the physical examination performed by the physician Present medical condition Health history, including previous illnesses Family medical history Confirmed or tentative diagnosis Plan of medical therapy
Physician's order sheet	Orders for medications Orders for treatments Other directives pertinent to a particular client's care
Physician's progress notes	Interpretations of the client's pathology Responses of the client to medical therapy
Miscellaneous forms	Laboratory reports X-ray film reports Consultation reports Dietary requirements Results of social-service consultations Types and results of physical, respiratory, and x-ray therapy

Tembra, M.   4269F

| Nazareth Hospital |
| Graphic Chart |

Date		9/6			9/7			9/8															
Day of Disease		4			5			6															
Day P.O. or P.P.																							
Hour		AM	PM																					

C	F
40.0	104
39.4	103
38.8	102
38.3	101
37.7	100
37.2	99
37.0	98.6
36.6	98
36.1	97
35.5	96

Pulse		72	78	78		70	76	80	88	82	78	76	84	80	80								
Respiration		16	14	18		18	20	20	20	16	18	14	16	16	16								
Blood Pressure		134	130	134	—	138	136	130	140	136	135	136	142	140									
		94	90	92		92	92	90	94	94	90	94	96	96		—							
Weight																							
Height																							
Micturition		bedpan qs			bedpan qs			bedpan qs															
Defecation		+			ō			ō															
Diet: Type		Soft			soft			soft															

How Taken: *G - Good F - Fair P - Poor		B	L	D	B	L	D	B	L	D	B	L	D	B	L	D	B	L	D	B	L	D	B	L	D	B	L	D	B	L	D
		G	P	F	—	G	G	F	—	F	F	P																			

Bath		C (P) Self	C P Self	C (P) Self	C P Self	C (P) Self	C P Self	C P Self	C P Self	C P Self
Activity		CBR		CBR		CBR				
Tolerated		well		wanted to do more →						
Diagnostic Studies & Treatments		CAT Scan IV		ECG IV		IV				

Person Assigned To Patient	11-7	L. Gray RN	L. Gray RN	L. Gray RN					
	7-3	C. Taylor RN	C. Taylor RN	C. Taylor RN					
	3-11	D. Kands RN	C. Pit RN	G. Kearns RN					

F I G U R E 18-3

Sample of graphic client record. (Courtesy of Nazareth Hospital, Philadelphia, PA)

Shift	11-7:30 AM	7-3:30 PM	3-11:30 PM
Diet or NPO	House = Soft	—————————	——————→
Nutrition		BR ☑G ☐F ☐P LU ☐G ☐F ☐P ☐Feed ☑Self	Di ☐G ☑F ☐P HS Snack ☑ ☐Feed ☑Self
Bathing Skin Care	☑Mouth Care ☐Skin Care Keri lotion	☐S ☑P ☐C ☑Mouth Care ☑AM Care	☑PM Care ☑Mouth Care
Activity	☑CBR ☑Pos. q2° ☐BRP ☐BRP č Asst. ☐OOB Chair č Asst. ☐OOB Chair š Asst. ☐AMB č Asst. ☐AMB š Asst.	☑CBR ☑Pos. q2° ☐BRP ☐BRP č Asst. ☐OOB Chair č Asst. ☐OOB Chair š Asst. ☐AMB č Asst. ☐AMB š Asst.	☑CBR ☑Pos. q2° ☐BRP ☐BRP č Asst. ☐OOB Chair č Asst. ☐OOB Chair š Asst. ☐AMB č Asst. ☐AMB š Asst.
Resp. Assessment	☑Cough/D. Breathe q2° ☐Trach Care ☐Suction Freq ____	☑Cough/D. Breathe q2° ☐Trach Care ☐Suction Freq ____	☑Cough/D. Breathe q2° ☐Trach Care ☐Suction Freq ____
Treatments	Assisted ROM	P.T.	——————→
Protective Precautions	☐Full ☑Half	☐Full ☐Half	☐Full ☐Half
Restraints	☐Posey ☐Wrist ☐Ankle ☐None ☑q2° Check ☐Other	☐Posey ☐Wrist ☐Ankle ☑None ☐q2° Check ☐Other	☐Posey ☐Wrist ☐Ankle ☑None ☐q2° Check ☐Other
Elimination Bowel Bladder ☐Foley	bedpan voiding q5 ☐Commode	TBM Voiding q5 bedpan ☐Commode ☐Foley Care	☐Commode ☐Foley Care
Diagnostic Studies +/or Specimens Obtained	—	CAT Scan	—
Isolation Type	—	—	—
Nursing Care Plan	☑Reviewed ☐Revised	☑Reviewed ☐Revised	☑Reviewed ☐Revised
Comments	awake @ 2am did not fall back to sleep	"when can I go home?" napped in pm	—
Signature	L. Gray RN	C Taylor RN	D. Kande RN

Nazareth Hospital
Activity Flowsheet/Patient Care Notes

Date / Time	Notes
9/4/86 7 AM	Pt. awake and alert. Awoke at 2 AM to void — unable to fall back asleep. Refused sedative. Rested quietly. Speech clear, moving all extremities. — L. Gray, RN
9/4/86 10 AM	Prune juice + cup of hot water with breakfast, resulted in soft formed BM — about 1 hour p̄ breakfast (1st stool in 3 days). Keri lotion to dry skin on legs and arms. Strength seems to be increasing in left arm + leg. Performs lt. leg exercises independently. During bath talked about how much she misses her husband and her house. Explored feelings about participating in support group for widows — recommended by her friends. Feels good about babysitting her 2 grandchildren. — C. Taylor, RN
2 pm	Spent 30 min. teaching client + daughter Lisa about T.I.A. and stroke. Strong family history of PVD, CVA and M.I. Reviewed importance of dietary modifications, regular exercise and taking prescribed medication. Excellent motivation for self-care — S Taylor RN
9/4/86	VS 98.8 - 78 - 18 136/92 Quiet this evening. — Napping — Not hungry at dinner: states "Busy day" Moving all extremities; alert. Daughter Barbara says her mother wants to do "too much." Still afraid TIA automatically means stroke & death! — D. Kande RN.

FIGURE 18-4
Sample of an activity flowsheet with patient care notes. (Courtesy of Nazareth Hospital, Philadelphia, PA)

T A B L E   18-3
Organization of the Problem-Oriented Client Record

Part	Information

Data base (Fig 5A)	The data base is a compilation of all initial information about the client and includes the following:
	   Health-state profile prepared by the nurse
	   Medical history and the physical examination, prepared by the physician
	   Social history
	   Initial diagnostic-test results

Problem list (Fig 5B)	The multidisciplinary problem list itemizes major aspects of the client's life requiring health attention and includes the following:
	   Socioeconomic, demographic, psychologic, and physiologic problems
	   Each problem is labeled, numbered, and categorized as active or inactive

Plan of care (Fig 5C)	An initial plan is formulated for each specifically numbered problem on the problem list. The nursing plan, whether *therapeutic, diagnostic,* or *educational,* is expressed through nursing orders.

Progress notes (Fig 5D)
   Narrative
   progress notes
	Progress notes consist of narrative progress notes, flowsheets, and discharge notes, as follows: The narrative progress notes on the client follow the **SOAP format,** as follows:
	   S—Subjective information reported by the client
	   O—Objective observations made by health practitioners
	   A—Assessments drawn from new data
	   P—Goals or plans for action related to the client's problems

Flowsheets	Flowsheets are used for recording information that is monitored over a period of time. This information provides data for making comparisons of a client's status at one time with his status later.

Discharge notes	Discharge notes are the entries made at the time an episode of the client's care is terminated and include the following information:
	   The date of the resolution of each problem, as had been described while using the SOAP format
	   Referrals made for the client
	   Recommendations for unresolved or partially resolved problems

the written message, and the audiotaped message. Each of these methods has certain benefits and limitations, as detailed in Table 18-4. What follows is a brief discussion of three specific communication strategies frequently used by nurses: reporting, conferring, and referring.

Reporting.   To report is to give an account of something that has been seen, heard, done, or considered. For instance, hospital nurses report a summary of a client's condition and care when transferring clients from one unit to another (*e.g.,* from the recovery room to a surgi-

cal floor) and at the conclusion of each shift. Nurses also report to physicians and other health-care professionals. Because the nurse is the one who is "with the client 24 hours a day," the nurse is responsible for determining significant changes in the client's condition and for reporting these findings to the appropriate team member. And finally, nurses are often asked by family members to report on the client's progress.

Change-of-Shift Reports.   A change-of-shift report is ordinarily given by a primary nurse to the nurse replac-

Summary of data base for client
72 year old, white, recently widowed female

brought to hospital after sudden fall caused by temporary paralysis of left leg; admitting diagnosis: transient ischemic attack (TIA), R/O cerebrovascular accident

treated for hypertension since 1985, otherwise in good health; history of headaches—once or twice a week (increasing in severity)—for last six months

ht 5'2"   wt 63.6 kg   98.2 F-88-18   BP L—184/120, R—180/120
↓ strength ↓ movement left lower extremity (LLE)

Problem

XXXX Medical Center   4629F

Date	No.	Problem	Identified	Resolved
9/2/89	#1	transient ischemic attack (TIA) R/O cerebro-vascular accident	J. Gleer MD	
	#1A	impaired physical mobility related to weakness in left lower extremity	D. Kande RN	
9/4/89	#2	impaired adjustment related to major life stressors and decreased supports	D. Kande RN	

Plan of Care

Date	Problem
9/4/89	#2 Impaired adjustment related to major life stressors (including illness) and decreased supports Goal: Prior to discharge client reports feeling able to go home and take one day at a time Plan: *Diagnostic*: explore adequacy of client's usual patterns of coping and motivation to learn new strategies *Therapeutic*: 1) explain all tests/procedures to client who wants to know and understand what is happening to her 2) create a restful environment 3) talk with client's home minister (daughter will contact) *Educative*: Teach client new coping skills, e.g., relaxation exercises. Refer to community support group for widows. —D. Kande RN

Progress Notes

Date	Problem-Oriented Progress Notes
9/6/89	Impaired mobility related to weakness left lower extremity (LLE) S "My left leg still feels queer, pins and needles—but I can move it alright." O Able to lift left leg off bed, positive flexion, positive extension; muscle strength in LLE 3/5 (normal movement against gravity) A recovering mobility as strength returns P *therapeutic*: consult with physician about complete bed rest order; *diagnostic*: continue to monitor muscle strength and movement at least once/shift; be alert for any signs of recurrent TIA; *educative*: instruct not to try to get out of bed without assistance until diagnostic work-up is complete; reinforce need for safety precautions. —D. Kande RN

F I G U R E   **18-5**
Sample of a problem oriented patient record.

ing him or her, or by the charge nurse to the nurse who assumes responsibility for continuing care of the client. The report may be given orally in a meeting or may be audiotaped. Many charge nurses find that using a tape decreases the amount of time spent in report and provides more time for last minute details.

Typical information shared among nurses during a change-of-shift report includes:
• Basic identifying information about each client: name, room number, bed designation, and current diagnosis
• Current appraisal of each client's health status

C O M P U T E R   A P P L I C A T I O N S   I N   N U R S I N G

Computerized Client Care

This story illustrates how often nurses use computer technology on a daily basis in giving client care.

Tom Low, RN, arrives for work at 0645, following the schedule printed by the computer in the staffing office, and is assigned to a general surgery floor based on a computer-generated patient acuity needs assessment. After reading the computer print-out on his assigned patients, he takes vital signs (using computerized equipment), monitors the flow of IV fluids (making sure the computerized flow and amount settings are correct), and gives medications (using a computer-based medication record to check and document administration). Unfamiliar with two medications, he reviews material, before giving them, from the computer medication data base. Tom then changes dressings, entering charges and ordering supplies on the computer.

One of Tom's patients has been having abnormal laboratory test results, so Tom calls up the result of today's tests to monitor changes. At the same time, he looks up the time for a scheduled surgical procedure for another patient, so he will be sure to have time for preoperative teaching, using computer-assisted instruction.

After the morning care is completed, Tom sits down in front of the computer to document care given and to update care plans.

Not all of these computed applications are available in all health-care settings, but the trend in today's high-tech society is toward automated resources to facilitate communications and improve clinical practice. Your career in nursing will definitely be influenced by computers!

Changes in medical condition (results of pertinent diagnostic studies) and client's response to medical therapy
Where the client stands in relationship to identified nursing diagnoses and goal achievement

- Current orders (especially any newly changed orders)
   Independent nursing orders
   Dependent orders (changes in medications, IV fluids, diet, activity level)
- A summary of each newly admitted client, includ-

T A B L E   18-4
Common Methods of Communication

Method	Advantages	Disadvantages
Face-to-face meeting	• Message can be delivered immediately. • Nonverbal messages are readily conveyed. • Message can be clarified; receiver's questions can be raised and answered.	• Both the communicating and receiving persons must be available at the same time, in the same place. • Ordinarily there is no permanent record for later use.
Telephone conversation	• Message can be delivered immediately. • Message can be clarified; receiver's questions can be raised and answered. • Two parties need not be present in same place.	• Only the tone of voice and voice inflections can be communicated—no nonverbal messages. • Ordinarily there is no permanent record.
Written message	• Can be exchanged at times convenient for the people involved • Record is available. • Time-efficient if message is understood	• Message usually cannot be validated with the sender.
Audiotaped message	• Can be exchanged at times convenient for the people involved • Record is available. • Time-efficient if information communicated is complete	• Message usually cannot be validated with the sender.

ing his or her diagnosis, age, plan of therapy, and general condition

- A report of clients who have been transferred or discharged

It is important to avoid unprofessional comments about clients during the shift report that could predispose oncoming nurses to view and respond to clients negatively.

Conferring. To confer is to consult with someone in order to exchange ideas or to seek information, advice, or instructions from another. A nurse may consult with another nurse, as when a team leader consults with a clinical specialist about a particular patient's care. A school nurse may confer with a child's teacher or a psychologist about a behavior problem. A community health nurse and a physician may confer about a client's activity regimen. Health practitioners also confer in order to validate information. Both nurses and other health team members confer in groups to plan and coordinate client care. Often, such conferences are also used for instructing students and practitioners.

Nursing Care Conference. A nursing care conference is a meeting of nurses to discuss some aspect of a client's care. For example, several nurses who have taken care of a generally uncooperative client may initiate a conference. This would allow each nurse an opportunity to offer his or her opinion about the client's problem and its etiology, and then together they could discuss possible solutions to the problem.

Nurses may invite other health-care practitioners to a nursing care conference to gain input concerning a particular client's care. For example, a dietitian may be invited to attend a conference when nurses meet to discuss problems relating to a client's diet.

Nursing Care Round. A nursing care round is a procedure in which a group of nurses visit selected clients individually at each client's bedside. The primary purposes of nursing care rounds are to gather information

that helps to plan nursing care, to evaluate the nursing care the client has received, and to provide the client with an opportunity to discuss his or her care with those administering it. As each client is visited, the nurse assigned provides a short summary of the client's nursing diagnoses, goals, and the care being given. There are two principal advantages of nursing care rounds over a discussion in a meeting room: nursing personnel can actually see the client as a report of care is given, and clients can participate in discussions of their care.

It is important that nursing personnel use language the client can understand when holding discussions at the bedside. Otherwise, the client is likely to feel excluded and cannot intelligently participate in the discussion.

Referring. To refer is to send or direct someone for action or help. The process of sending or guiding someone to another source for assistance is called a referral. A client may be referred by a hospital to a community health nursing service for assistance with home care. A school nurse may refer a student to a hospital emergency room. A community health nurse may refer a problem to the Department of Health. A referral may also be used within a particular agency. For example, a hospital outpatient clinic may refer a client to the hospital's inpatient facilities.

Most health agencies have policies related to referrals. An agency may have a special form that personnel are to use when making referrals. The policies usually indicate who may initiate a referral, how it is to be done, and so on.

Referrals are especially important in providing continuity of care for persons needing a variety of services. It is essential that health practitioners to whom a client is referred are given information that is most useful to the continuity of care. The key question is: What would I want to know about this client if I were the person who had to continue his or her care? The client must know and approve of a referral to another agency or to other health personnel.

KEY POINTS

- Implementing, the fourth step of the nursing process, is the carrying out of the plan of care. Its purpose is to assist clients to achieve desired health goals: to promote wellness, prevent disease/illness, restore health, facilitate coping with altered functioning.

- The plan of care is best implemented when clients who are able and willing to participate have maximal opportunity to do so.

- While other health professionals focus on select aspects of the client's treatment regimen, nursing

is concerned with how the person is responding in general to the plan of care.

- Nurses implement independent, interdependent (collaborative), and dependent nursing actions.

- While carrying out the plan of care, nurses use intellectual, interpersonal, and technical skills. Nursing's first challenge is the determination of how much nursing assistance the client needs to reach desired goals.

- The teaching, counseling, and advocacy skills of the nurse are used to assist clients to develop the self-care behaviors that will enable them to direct and manage their own care.

- Nothing about the care plan or the way it is implemented is fixed. Client and nurse variables, as well as available resources, current standards of care, research findings, and ethical and legal guides to practice, may influence the plan's implementation.

- Ongoing data collection directs the revision of the plan of care.

- Nurses are responsible for documenting each step of the nursing process in the client record. Most health-care institutions have standards for documentation which detail the nurse's responsibilities.

- The client record is the only legal document that provides a comprehensive picture of the nursing care given to the client.

- Each health-care group keeps data on its own separate form in the source-oriented client record. In the problem-oriented record, recording is organized around the client's problems rather than around sources of information. Computer records have simplified nursing documentation in many ways. Use of computer terminals at the client's bedside enables nurses to document care immediately.

- Common methods of communication used by nurses other than the client record include reporting, conferring, and referring.

BIBLIOGRAPHY

Afflerbach D: A flow sheet that saves time and trouble. RN 42–44, January 1986

Allison S, Kinloch K: Problem-oriented recording. Canadian Nurse 77(11):39–40, 1981

Andreoli K, Musser LA: Computers in nursing care: The state of the art. Nurs Outlook 33(1):16–21, 1985

Bailey-Allen AM: Avoid legal pitfalls in charting. Orthopedic Nursing 5(1):21, 1986

Bergerson SR: More about charting with a jury in mind. Nursing 18(4):50–56, 1988.

Black Sr K: Short-Term Counselling: A Humanistic Approach for the Helping Professions. Menlo Park, CA, Addison-Wesley, 1983

Buckley-Womack C, Gidney B: A new dimension in documentation. The PIE method. Journal of Neuroscience Nursing 19(5):256–260, 1987

Bulechek GM, McCloskey JC: Nursing interventions: What they are and how to choose them. Holistic Nursing Practice 1(3):36–44, 1987

Cohen MR: Play it safe: Don't use these abbreviations. Nursing 17(7):46–47, 1987

Cournoyer CP: Protecting yourself legally after a patient's injured. Nursing Life 5(2):18–22, 1985

DeMilliano M: 8 Common charting mistakes to avoid . . . quick review. Nursing Life 4(3):30–32, 1984

Eggland ET: Charting: Document your care daily and fully. Nursing 10(2):38–43, 1980

Fairless PR: 9 ways a computer can make your work easier. Nursing 16(9):55–56, 1986

Hill L, Smith N: Self-Care Nursing. Englewood Cliffs, NJ, Prentice-Hall, 1985

Joint Commission on Accreditation of Hospitals: Accreditation Manual for Hospitals. Chicago, The Commission, 1982

Jones P, Oertel W: Developing patient teaching objectives and techniques: A self-instructional program. Nurse Educator 2(5):3–18, 1977

Keane S, Chastain B, Rudisill K: Caring: Nurse–patient perceptions. Rehabilitation Nursing 12(4):182–184, 1987

Kilpack V, Dobson-Brassard S: Intershift report: Oral communication using the nursing process. Journal of Neuroscience Nursing 19(5):266–270, 1987

Kohnke MF: Advocacy: Risk and Reality. St Louis, CV Mosby, 1982

Kunkel J: Charting: Some pointers for doing it better. Nursing Life 3(2):57–64, 1983

Laing M: Flow sheets—Meeting the charting challenge. Canadian Nurse 77(11):40–42, 1981

Philpott M: Twenty rules for good charting. Nursing 16(8):63, 1986

Redman BK: The Process of Patient Teaching in Nursing, 5th ed. St Louis, CV Mosby, 1984

Rich PL: With this flow sheet less is more. Nursing 15(7):25–29, 1985

Rocerto LR, Maleski CM: All about rights to medical records. Nursing Life 4(4):50–51, 1984

Rutkowski B: How DRG's are changing your charting. Nursing 15(10):49–51, 1985

Siegrist L, Stocks B, Dettor R: The PIE system: Complete planning and documentation of nursing care. QRB 11(6):186–189, 1985

Smith CE: Upgrade your shift reports with the three R's. Nursing 16(2):63–64, 1986

Sundeen SJ, Stuart GW, Rankin ED, Cohen SA: Nurse–Client Interaction: Implementing the Nursing Process. St Louis, CV Mosby, 1985

Valega TM: It's time for nurses to begin nursing nurses. Nursing and Health Care 5(6):331–335, 1984

Vaughan-Wrobel BD, Henderson BS: The Problem-Oriented System in Nursing, 2nd ed. St Louis, CV Mosby, 1982

Zangari ME, Duffy P: Contracting with patients in day-to-day practice. Am J Nurs 80:451–455, 1980

Evaluating

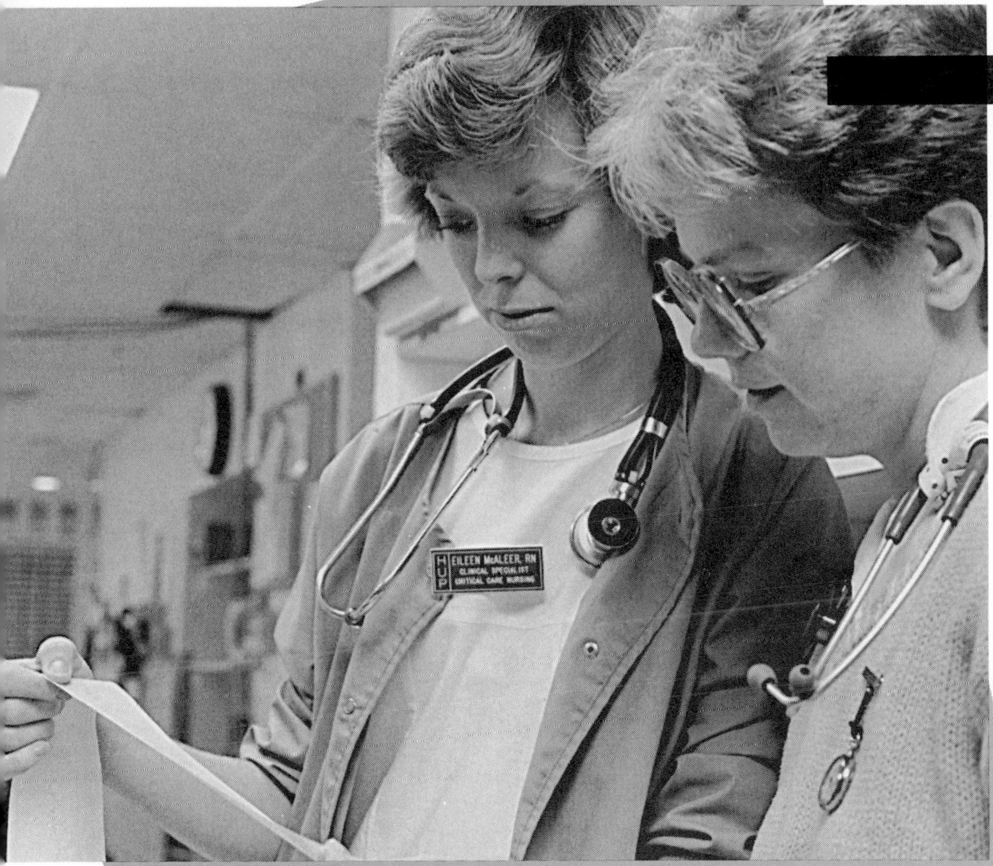

OBJECTIVES

After studying this chapter, the learner should be able to

Define key terms used in the chapter.

Describe evaluation, its purpose, and relationship to other steps in the nursing process.

Evaluate the client's achievement of goals specified in the plan of care.

Manipulate factors contributing to the client's success or failure in goal achievement.

Use the client's responses to the plan of care to modify the plan as needed.

Explain the relationship between quality assurance programs and excellence in health care.

During the fifth step of the nursing process, **evaluating**, the nurse and client together measure how well the client has achieved the goals specified in the plan of care. While evaluating client goal achievement, the nurse identifies factors contributing to the client's success or failure and, when necessary, modifies the plan of care. The purpose of evaluation is to allow client goal achievement to direct future nurse–client interactions. Based on the client's responses to the plan of care, the nurse decides to (1) terminate the plan of care (each client goal is achieved), (2) modify the plan (client is having difficulty achieving goals), or (3) continue the plan of care (client simply needs more time to achieve goals). When evaluation points to the need to modify nursing care, each preceding step of the nursing process (assessing, diagnosing, planning, and implementing) is reviewed.

In summary, during the evaluation step of the nursing process the nurse measures how well the client has achieved desired goals; identifies factors contributing to the client's success or failure; and terminates, continues, or modifies the plan of care as needed (see Fig 19-1).

KEY TERMS

criteria
evaluating
  nursing audit
  concurrent
  retrospective

outcome evaluation
quality assurance program
standard

UNIQUE FOCUS OF NURSING EVALUATION

As members of the health-care team, nurses are involved in many different types of evaluation. Nurses measure how well individual clients have achieved desired goals, how effectively nurses help targeted groups of clients to achieve their specific goals, the competence of individual nurses, and the degree to which external factors, such as different types of health-care services, specialized equipment or procedures, or socioeconomic factors, influence health and wellness. The client, however, is always the nurse's primary concern. A nurse may perform a nursing procedure competently, caringly, creatively, but if this nursing action does not help the client to reach desired goals, it is meaningless. Either directly or indirectly, the aim of all nursing evaluation is quality nursing care that aids client goal achievement. Therefore, the most important act of evaluation performed by the nurse is evaluating the client's goal achievement with the client.

EVALUATION CRITERIA AND STANDARDS

The classic elements of evaluation are identifying evaluative criteria and standards (what you are looking for when you evaluate), collecting data to determine if these criteria and standards are met, interpreting and summarizing findings, and taking appropriate action. In the

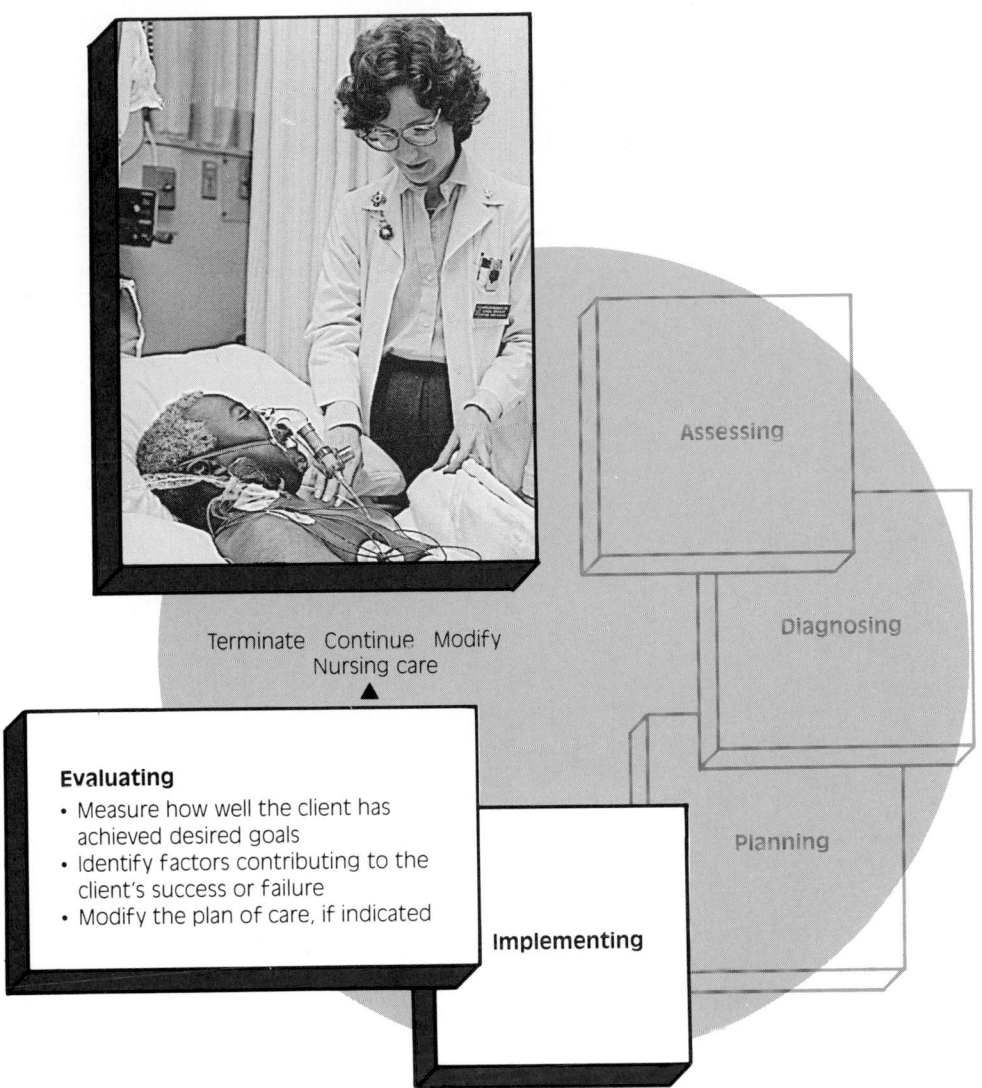

Terminate   Continue   Modify
Nursing care
▲

Evaluating
- Measure how well the client has achieved desired goals
- Identify factors contributing to the client's success or failure
- Modify the plan of care, if indicated

Assessing

Diagnosing

Planning

Implementing

FIGURE 19-1

Evaluating. The nurse and client together measure how well the client has achieved the goals specified in the plan of care. Factors contributing to the client's success or failure are identified, and the plan of care is modified if necessary. Client responses to the plan of care determine if nursing care is to be continued as is, modified, or terminated. (Photo by Gates Rhodes, courtesy of the School of Nursing, University of Pennsylvania)

nursing process, evaluative criteria are the client goals developed during the planning step. Because these goals reflect desired changes or outcomes in client behavior, and because nursing actions are directed toward these goals, it is logical that they be at the core of evaluation. Determining whether or not these goals have been met and then identifying the appropriate nursing response is the function of evaluation.

Although the terms criteria and standard are often used interchangeably in the evaluation step, they have distinct definitions. **Criteria** are measurable qualities, attributes, or characteristics that specify skills, knowledge, or health states. They describe acceptable levels of performance by stating the expected behaviors of the nurse and/or the client.

Standards are acceptable, expected levels of performance by the nursing staff or other health team members. They are established by authority, custom, or consent (Griffith-Kenney and Christensen, 1986, p 223).

MEASURING CLIENT GOAL ACHIEVEMENT

Collecting Evaluative Data

The nurse collects evaluative data to determine whether or not the client has met the desired goals. Whereas the nurse collected data in the nursing assessment to iden-

S A M P L E   C A R E   P L A N

Nursing Diagnosis: Potential alteration in parenting related to no previous experience in child-rearing (fear)

Assessment Data:

Subjective
"My husband and I are both afraid we won't know what to do when we get the baby home."

Both parents are single children, report no childrearing experience

Objective
Healthy newborn son delivered 2/4; first born

Strengths: VIB (very important baby): parents are both 38; history of infertility with one miscarriage; strong motivation to learn and utilize good parenting skills; strong support network

Goals (Expected Outcomes)	**Nursing Orders**	**Evaluative Statement (Actual Outcomes)**

A. Prior to discharge parents demonstrate confidence in:
1. Holding baby
2. Diapering, dressing baby
3. Bathing baby
4. Feeding baby
(Psychomotor objectives)
	1. Assess both parents' knowledge of childrearing practices; identify and reinforce motivation to learn; correct any misinformation
	2. Develop and implement at a time convenient for both parents a teaching plan to include:
	• The primary nurse role-modeling techniques for comfortably and safely holding, talking to, and dressing baby
	• Parents independently viewing video cassettes on:
	    Baby care
	    Baby bath
	    Breastfeeding
	Followed by one-on-one discussion
	• Class for new parents: nurse to demonstrate baby bath and discuss general principles of care
	• Primary nurse observing mother and infant during initial feeding sessions and offering teaching and support as necessary
	3. Answer parents' questions and address related concerns
		A. 2/6 Goal partially met. Both parents have correctly demonstrated safe techniques for holding, dressing and bathing the baby. Mother is still concerned baby is not getting enough milk.
		Revision: Continue to spend time with mother and infant during feeding—provide positive reinforcement.
		
		F. Morales, RN

B. By 2/6 parents report appropriate action to be taken if questions/problems arise following discharge: 1. Name and number of primary nurse 2. Name and number of pediatrician	1. Assess parents' knowledge of infant problems frequently encountered by new parents. 2. Inform parents of available community resources and describe appropriate action to take if questions/problems arise.	B. 2/6 Goal met. Parents discussed some infant problems related to feeding, elimination, illness and reported appropriate community resource to contact. *F. Morales, RN*

(Continued)

SAMPLE CARE PLAN (Continued)

Goals (Expected Outcomes)	Nursing Orders	Evaluative Statement (Actual Outcomes)
3. LaLeche League contact and number (Cognitive objectives)		
C. Prior to discharge parents verbalize decreased anxiety in regards to caring for son. (Affective objective)	1. Assess parents' level of anxiety and potential negative effects on childrearing. Discuss this with parents. 2. Explore adequacy of parents' coping strategies: Increased knowledge, practice in supportive environment, community resources. Counsel as necessary. 3. Compliment parents on new parenting skills. Allow for ventilation of anxiety or specific fears. Respond with teaching or emotional support as necessary.	C. 2/6 Goal partially met. Except for concern about breastfeeding, parents *both* expressed feeling comfortable and eager to care for their son at home. *F. Morales, RN*
D. At 1 month postpartal telephone interview (3/4) the baby's: • Weight gain (birth weight = 7 lb 6 oz) • Sleep–awake patterns • Comfort level (By parents' report) indicates adequate parenting	1. Utilize a 1-month post-delivery telephone interview to assess the adequacy of parenting skills. 2. With positive report of growth and development, compliment (reinforce) the parents. 3. With negative report, teach/ counsel as appropriate.	D. 3/4 Goal met. Parents' report of baby's weight gain and behavior indicates good parenting skills. *F. Morales, RN*

tify client health problems, the nurse collects data in the evaluation step to determine whether or not the identified health problems were resolved through goal achievement.

Types of Goals. The type of client data collected to support the goal achievement evaluation is determined by the nature of the goal. *Cognitive goals* involve increases in client knowledge; these goals may be evaluated simply by having clients repeat information, or, at a higher level of performance, by having clients apply the new knowledge to their everyday situations. For example, having clients describe new dietary restrictions is very different from having them plan a weekly menu compatible with these restrictions. *Psychomotor goals* describe the client's achievement of new skills; they are generally evaluated by having the client demonstrate the new skill. *Affective goals* pertain to changes in client values, beliefs, and attitudes; affective goals are more complex to evaluate. Observation of client behavior and conversation are used to determine whether or not these affective goals have been achieved.

In the final type of goal statement, *physical changes* in the client are the targeted outcome. To evaluate achievement of this type of goal, the nurse uses physical examination skills to collect relevant data and compare these to client data acquired previously.

Samples of these four types of goals are contained in the care plan in the Sample Care Plan. The data collected to determine the degree of goal achievement are recorded in the related evaluative statement.

Time Criteria. In addition to knowing what type of data to collect to determine goal achievement, it is important to know when to collect this data. In properly constructed client goals, a time frame is established for determining whether or not the specified change in client behavior has been achieved. At the designated time, the nurse, in collaboration with the client, the family, and other members of the nursing team, evaluates the client's ability to demonstrate the desired behavior. If goals are developed in observable and measurable terms, the task of collecting data for evaluation becomes clear cut.

Examples of three different types of time criteria follow:
• By 7/8 client walks length of hallway with support of walker.
• Beginning 7/8 client demonstrates a weight loss of 3 lb per month until target weight (135 lb) is achieved. (6/8, weight: 151 lb)

• Prior to discharge parents correctly demonstrate chest physiotherapy procedures for client.

It is important for nurses to evaluate client goal achievement as early as possible. Goal attainment, when celebrated with the client, generally results in the client's encouragement and leads to further goal achievement. When the client's failure to meet designated goals is detected early, the plan of care can be modified to redress the failure. The most common mistake nurses make in evaluation is waiting until the day the client is to be discharged before evaluating goal achievement. It is obviously too late to do anything about the goals the client has not met at discharge.

Documenting Evaluation

Once data have been collected to determine client goal achievement, the nurse writes an evaluative statement to summarize the findings. Atkinson and Murray (1986) have suggested using a two-part evaluative statement on the nursing care plan to underscore the importance of evaluation. The evaluative statement includes a decision on how well the goal was achieved and all client data or behavior that support this decision. The nurse has three decision options: goal met, goal partially met, or goal not met. The nurse signs and dates the evaluative statement (see Sample Care Plan).

FACTORS INFLUENCING GOAL ACHIEVEMENT

Numerous client, nurse, and health-care system variables contribute both positively and negatively to client goal

achievement. Identifying these variables allows the nurse to reinforce positive factors by drawing on them in the future and to deal with those factors that are creating problems. The more sensitive and responsive nurses are to these variables, the more rewarding their practices will be.

Examples of positive factors include a client's strong motivation to learn new health behaviors, a nurse who comes to work well rested and with a new care idea read in a nursing journal, and a health-care institution that offers incentives for quality nursing and that staffs its nursing units well.

Once the nurse understands what is helpful to the client who is trying to reach desired goals, these factors can often be manipulated. For example, if a client is learning to ambulate independently following hip surgery and you notice that he seems to make his best effort when his wife is present, mention this observation to the wife and plan to ambulate the client at least once a day when the wife is present. Conversely, if the client seems more fearful when his wife is present, note in the plan of care that ambulation is best attempted when the client's wife is not on the unit.

Table 19-1 presents common variables individual nurses encounter that can negatively influence client goal achievement. Tentative nursing approaches are suggested. What is important is that nurses become aware of the effects of these variables and respond creatively to them.

MODIFYING THE PLAN OF CARE

When evaluation reveals that the client has made little or no progress toward goal achievement, and attempts to

---

Sample Evaluation Documentation

$$\text{Evaluative statement} = \begin{array}{l}\text{Goal met}\\\text{Goal partially met}\\\text{Goal not met}\end{array} + \begin{array}{l}\text{Actual client}\\\text{behavior as evidence}\end{array}$$

Example

Nursing diagnosis
Diversional activity deficit related to difficult transition to new life in nursing home

Goal statement
Resident participates in a minimum of two planned social activities per week beginning 9/20.

Evaluative statement
9/27 Goal met. Resident attended exercise session, sing-a-long, and trip to greenhouse this week.

L. Davis, RN

***T A B L E* 19-1**

Client, Nurse, and Health-Care System Variables that may Detract from Quality Nursing Care

Variables	Possible Solution
Client Variables	
Client who is physically and cognitively capable of self-care "gives-up"; refuses to cooperate with therapeutic regimen or thwarts the regimen	Identify one nurse who is able to develop a trusting relationship with the client and determine the *reason* underlying the observed behavior: • No longer finds meaning and purpose in life • Overwhelming sense of powerlessness • Previous history of being "hurt," "exploited," "cheated" by the health-care system • Inability to accept illness and related life-style changes Counsel appropriately. Use a team conference to develop a consistent plan of nursing care.
Client who quietly accepts whatever is done or not done for him or her; rarely communicates needs or dissatisfaction	Note on the plan of care the need to assess this client thoroughly because the client will most likely not advocate for himself. Educate the client to become a more assertive health-care consumer.
Nurse Variables	
Nurse who sincerely desires to give 150% all of the time and who becomes quickly frustrated when observing sub-standard care; may feel alienated from other staff; excellent candidate for burnout	Learn to give quality care during designated work period; leave on time; avoid the temptation to do the work of others; leave work concerns at work. After establishing a reputation for delivering quality nursing care, seek creative solutions for nursing problems (strategies to increase nursing resources, motivation, morale) and try them—hopefully with a support network. View concerns as challenges rather than overwhelming obstacles. Develop a realistic sense of how much nursing care and of what quality can be delivered with existing resources. If resources do not permit quality care, explore change strategies within the institution. If administration is not supportive, explore other practice settings.
Nurse with overwhelming outside concerns: • Preparation for marriage, childbirth, divorce • Illness (self or family members) • Role conflict (familial roles, school, work, and so forth) • New apartment, house	During periods of peak demand, may need to accept less than optimal performance at work. If this becomes the norm rather than the exception, carefully evaluate priorities. May need to cut work hours rather than "cheat" patients.
Nurse who is bored	After reflection, write down *personal* objectives related to work. Explore avenues within work setting for professional growth and development: Initiate changes in nursing unit to improve patient care and to stimulate peer development; join institutional committees; participate actively in staff development programs; develop patient/family support groups. Look for new position that offers new challenges within or outside the institution. Join professional organizations and participate actively. Evaluate educational goals and explore possibilities: Continuing education programs and degree work.

(Continued)

T A B L E **19-1**

T A B L E **19-1**
Client, Nurse, and Health-Care System Variables that may Detract from Quality Nursing Care
(Continued)

Variables	Possible Solution
Health-Care System Variables	
Inadequate staffing	Develop and use a patient classification system which incorporates an identification of the kind and amount of nursing services required. Record staffing patterns and relate to needs for nursing care and patient outcomes. Clearly demonstrate/*document* that adequate staffing makes a difference. Present these data to nursing administration with the request for additional staff. If necessary, use professional bargaining unit.
Inadequate supplies	Identify and clearly document problems with obtaining supplies necessary for quality care. Enlist support of as many nursing units in the institution as possible. Talk with nursing administration, if possible, suggesting corrective strategies.
Nursing administration has "sold-out" nursing; insensitivity to nursing demands within the institution	It may be impossible to practice quality, progressive nursing in this environment. If there seems to be no hope for change after appropriate channels have been explored, look for a new practice setting. Evaluate the new setting on the basis of what experience has taught you.

identify the contributing factors point to problems with the plan of care, the nurse needs to reevaluate each preceding step of the nursing process for accuracy. Following this study, new assessment data may need to be collected, diagnoses may be added or altered, goals may need to be modified or completely rewritten, nursing orders may be changed, and evaluation may be targeted more frequently. See the checklist in this chapter for help in evaluating your use of the nursing process. Table 19-2 suggests appropriate nursing responses to common problems encountered during evaluation:

- Inaccurate or incomplete data base
- Vague or missing nursing diagnoses
- Standardized plan of care that offers little direction for individualized care
  - Improperly developed nursing goals
  - Superficial nursing orders
- Plan of care that is unresponsive to changes in the client's condition or that fails to address the discharge needs of the client
- Nurses' lack of knowledge of the client's priority problems: routine care
- Insufficient documentation
- Failure to use evaluation to improve quality of nursing care

Once the nurse has identified the factors contributing to the client's failure to achieve goals, the evaluative statement can be used to suggest the necessary revision in the plan of care.

Using the sample nursing diagnosis and goal given previously, the following evaluative statement might be noted if the client fails to meet the specified behavior: "9/27 Goal not met: Resident refused to participate in any group activities this week." Many courses of action

are then available to the nurse. Possible revision statements to follow the evaluative statement include:

REVISION: This may not be a problem/concern for the resident. Evaluate and validate data pointing to the nursing diagnosis (delete or modify the nursing diagnosis).

REVISION: Carefully determine the resident's need for activities and ability/desire to participate in activities (make the goal statement more realistic).

REVISION: Reevaluate after 3 weeks; resident may need more time to adjust to being institutionalized and more encouragement (adjust time criteria in goal statement).

REVISION: Make special effort to get to know the resident's interests and match these with available programs/activities (change nursing interventions).

EVALUATION PROGRAMS

In addition to each nurse's evaluation of client goal achievement and the subsequent modifications to the plan of care, many formal mechanisms exist to ensure quality nursing care. Since 1972, United States regulatory agencies, such as the State Boards of Nursing, the Joint Commission on Accreditation of Hospitals, Professional Standards Review Organization, and the National Health Planning and Resources Development Act of 1975 have required nurses to document that nursing standards are being implemented and maintained. Each of these agencies is concerned with quality care and quality control.

Checklist for Evaluating Your Use of the Nursing Process

Assessing

☐ The initial data base is obtained by means of a nursing history and nursing examination.

☐ Assessment data are documented:

    ☐ Accurately—Questionnable data are validated.

    ☐ Completely—Use of a systematic guide ensures that recorded data describe (1) the client's functional ability to meet each basic human need and (2) responses to health and illness.

    ☐ Concisely—Irrelevant data and meaningless generalizations are avoided.

    ☐ Factually—Client behaviors are recorded rather than the nurse's interpretation of these behaviors.

☐ The initial data base communicates a "real sense" of the client which makes possible individualized care.

☐ Focused assessment data are recorded for each client problem.

☐ Data collection and documentation are ongoing and responsive to changes in the client's condition.

Diagnosing

☐ A prioritized list of nursing diagnoses is on the plan of care.

☐ Each nursing diagnosis describes an actual or potential client health problem that independent nursing intervention can prevent or resolve. Each nursing diagnosis:

    ☐ Is derived from an accurate and validated interpretation of a cluster of significant client data or "cues"

    ☐ Contains a precise problem statement describing what is unhealthy about the client and what needs to change—suggests client goals

    ☐ Identifies factors contributing to the problem (etiology)—these suggest nursing interventions

    ☐ Uses nonjudgmental language and is written using legally advisable terms

☐ Old nursing diagnoses are deleted from the plan of care once resolved, and new diagnoses are added as soon as identified.

Planning

☐ A comprehensive, individualized, and up-to-date plan of care, which specifies client goals and nursing orders for each nursing diagnosis, is developed with the assistance of the client/family.

☐ Planning is comprehensive:

    ☐ Initial

    ☐ Ongoing

    ☐ Discharge

☐ Long-term goals alert the entire nursing team to realistic client expectations following discharge.

☐ Short-term goals:

    ☐ When achieved, demonstrate a resolution of the problem specified in the nursing diagnosis

    ☐ Describe a single, observable, and measurable client behavior

    ☐ Are valued by the client and family

    ☐ Are realistic in terms of the resources of the client and the nurse

☐ Nursing orders:

    ☐ Clearly and concisely describe the nursing action to be performed (ongoing assessment; nursing treatments and procedures; teaching, counseling, advocacy)

    ☐ Are tailored to the client

    ☐ Are consistent with standards of care and supportive of other therapies

    ☐ Are effective in accomplishing the desired client goals

☐ The plan of care encourages client/family participation.

Implementing

☐ The client record contains daily documentation of the nursing measures used to (1) assist the client to meet basic human needs, (2) resolve health problems, and (3) implement select aspects of the medical plan of care.

☐ The plan of care is implemented:

    ☐ Competently

    ☐ Caringly

    ☐ Creatively

Evaluating

☐ Evaluative statements are recorded on the plan of care to document the client's level of goal achievement at targeted times.

☐ Ongoing evaluation of the client's responses to the plan of care are used to make decisions about terminating, continuing, or modifying nursing care.

The National League for Nursing (NLN), in a public policy bulletin (1986), noted that concerns about the effects of new incentives to control health-care costs under Medicare's prospective payment system (PPS) have made "quality" one of the hottest buzzwords in health policy circles. The NLN advocates greater nursing responsibility for the monitoring and ensuring of quality health care. Client complaints include numerous reports of persons discharged from hospitals before they felt ready to leave, bed shortages in nursing homes, fraud and abuse in home health care, and lack of dependable resources to help coordinate and manage care beyond the acute-care setting. The availability of fewer resources to treat clients in hospitals and the unavailability of sufficient alternative treatment settings pose a strong challenge to the nursing profession to find ways to avoid a compromise in quality of care.

Quality Assurance

Specially designed programs that have as their aim the promotion of excellence in nursing are called **quality assurance programs**. These programs may be as small as one conducted by the nurses on a small nursing unit or may have a scope as broad as that of an entire institution, state, province, or country.

Quality assurance programs enable nursing to be accountable to society for the quality of care it provides. Such programs are also a response to the public mandate for professional accountability and the mandate of professional nursing law. They ensure professional survival, encourage nursing's fidelity to its moral and ethical responsibilities, and assist nursing to comply with other external pressures.

The ANA Quality Assurance Program

The American Nurses' Association in 1975 developed a model quality assurance program consisting of seven steps: (1) identify values; (2) identify structure, process, and outcome standards and criteria; (3) measure the degree of attainment of criteria and standards; (4) make interpretations about strengths and weaknesses based on such measurements; (5) identify possible courses of action; (6) choose a course of action; and (7) take action. The ANA hoped that the model could be used at the local level to develop and implement quality assurance programs.

The ANA model directs attention to three essential components of quality care: structure, process, and outcome. Different types of quality assurance programs may focus exclusively on one component or on a mixture of components.

Structure. This type of evaluation or audit is focused on the environment in which care is provided. Standards describe physical facilities and equipment; organizational characteristics, policies, and procedures; fiscal resources; and personnel resources.

Process. The focus of the process evaluation is the nature and sequence of activities carried out by the nurse implementing the nursing process. Criteria make explicit acceptable levels of performance of nursing actions related to patient assessment, diagnosis, planning, implementation, and evaluation.

Outcome. Outcome evaluations focus on measurable changes in the health status of the client or the end

(Text continues on p. 333.)

C O M P U T E R   A P P L I C A T I O N S   I N   N U R S I N G

Computerized Help in Quality Assurance

In order to perform its job, the hospital quality assurance department has to review large numbers of charts to identify strengths and weaknesses in client care and care documentation. As automated records become more common, the chart review process will change.

Currently, record review may take weeks while mountains of paper are shifted in the medical records department. The data frequently are scattered and incomplete, and trends are hard to detect and develop. In the future nurses in quality assurance departments will be able to look at trends over a period of time and use those trends for forecasting and problem solving.

(Adapted from Walker MB, Schwartz C: What Every Nurse Should Know about Computers. Philadelphia, JB Lippincott, 1984)

(References: McHugh M, Schultz S: Computer technology in hospital nursing departments: Future applications and implications. Proceedings of the Sixth Annual Symposium on Computer Applications in Medical Care, Silver Spring, MD, IEEE Computer Society Press, 1982; Simpson RL: Nursing administrative applications. Proceedings of the Seventh Annual Symposium on Computer Applications in Medical Care. Silver Spring, MD, IEEE Computer Society Press, 1983)

T A B L E 19-2

Common Problems Noted During Evaluation of the Nursing Process

Problem	Effect on Nursing Process	Nursing Response
Assessing		
1. Inaccurate data base	1–3. Inaccurate nursing diagnoses (because the nursing diagnoses establish the client's *need* for *nursing,* inaccuracies here distort and may invalidate the entire plan of care.)	1. a. Identify the client or nurse variable(s) responsible for inaccuracy. b. Revise the recorded data base.
2. Data base does not reflect changes in client condition		2. Inservice the *entire* nursing staff on the importance of making assessment a priority in every client interaction as well as the *recording* of the new data obtained.
3. Data base is superficial: • Fails to communicate uniqueness of client • Lacks sufficient detail on major problems/developments		3. a. Rethink the critical relationship between an adequate data base and quality care. b. Develop interviewing and physical examination skills. c. Begin to identify the key data that need to be collected for specific nursing diagnosis and medical diagnosis and to assess client response to the therapeutic regimen (use of a nursing diagnosis handbook may be helpful).
Diagnosing		
1. General sense that nursing diagnoses are "common sense" and therefore do not need to be put in writing	1. "Common sense" nursing, which fails to address client's real problems, may ensue. Lack of continuity of care.	1. Carefully develop and record priority nursing diagnoses for several clients and fairly evaluate whether or not this makes a difference in terms of the continuity of quality care.
2. General sense that nurses are "too busy" doing treatments, "passing meds," and doing paperwork to carefully develop nursing diagnoses	2. Independent dimension of nursing practice remains underdeveloped; clients experience nurses as busy "doers" who are insensitive to their concerns.	2. Examine practice and see if *independent* nursing has a place; what percentage of everyday is devoted to independent nursing functions? If this percentage is nonexistent or small, there understandably may be *no need* for nursing diagnoses—but a desperate need to revise practice priorities.
3. Nursing diagnoses are too vague to be helpful.	3. Routinized client care results; individualized client problems are overlooked.	3. a. Revise the problem statement to more accurately describe what is *unhealthy* about the client (the behavior that needs to be changed). b. Revise the etiology to more accurately identify what is making the problem a problem—this should be a guide to nursing intervention. c. Check NANDA lists.
4. Nursing diagnoses are not up-to-date.	4. Nurses will not value or use the plan of care, assuming that it does not address the client's ongoing priorities.	4. Have a process for periodically reviewing the plan of care to delete nursing diagnoses when problems have been resolved and to add a new diagnosis as needed.

(Continued)

T A B L E   19-2

Common Problems Noted During Evaluation of the Nursing Process   (Continued)

Problem	Effect on Nursing Process	Nursing Response
Planning		
1. The plan of care contains only the standard knowledge most nurses would know without a written plan.	1. and 2. Lack of personalized care; failure to address client's real problems; nursing staff works haphazardly on different priorities	1. Make use of standardized (computerized) plans as a basis for care planning. Devote nursing energies to *individualizing* this plan.
2. The long-term goal is vague, standard; fails to make clear the discharge goal for this client.		2. Practice writing specific long-term goals that clarify for all nurses the aim toward which all nursing care is directed (*e.g.,* client returns home ambulatory with walker, right hip incision healing, able to manage activities of daily living (ADL) with minimal assistance from spouse).
3. The nursing goals, even if met, do not necessarily guarantee a resolution of the client problem.	3. Client problem(s) are unresolved.	3. When writing goals, it is often helpful to develop short-term goals related to etiologic factors. Because the stated etiology may be incomplete or inaccurate, it is essential that at least *one goal* be written so that if it is achieved, the problem in the nursing diagnosis is resolved.
4. The goals are incorrectly developed.	4. Both the client and nurses may be unsure of the aims of care; progress toward goal achievement will be difficult to evaluate.	4. After writing goals, check them against the following criteria: • Subject is the client or some part of the client. • The client behavior is stated in observable, measurable terms. • Criteria of acceptable performance are specified. • Time criteria are included in notes.
5. Nursing orders are superficial.	5. Client receives routinized care; lack of continuity of care; client goals may never be achieved. Each nurse must figure out a plan of nursing strategies.	5. Review nursing orders to ensure that they indicate the *specific* nursing strategies most likely to result in successful goal achievement *for this client* (*e.g.,* what comfort measures in particular are successful adjuncts to analgesic administration for a particular client?). In specifying the "who, what, when, where, how, and how much" of nursing actions, be sure to list the type of equipment/supplies needed in various treatments. As new client data are obtained, update nursing orders. Delete inappropriate or unnecessary orders.
6. The plan of care initiated on the day of admission fails to be updated.	6. Plan of care will not be consulted by nurses—if used it will be to client's detriment.	6. If personal accountability for updating plan fails, develop a process on the nursing unit to ensure care plan review and revision.

(Continued)

T A B L E **19-2**

Common Problems Noted During Evaluation of the Nursing Process (Continued)

Problem	Effect on Nursing Process	Nursing Response
Planning (continued)		
7. The plan of care addresses the immediate needs of the client but fails to anticipate discharge needs.	7. Client returns home unable to manage self-care activities.	7. Work hard at developing the ability to project yourself into the client's home after discharge. Learn to anticipate problems and concerns and prepare the client/family for these. Use all discharge resources in the institution. Learn from clients what their needs were following previous discharge.
Implementing		
1. Nurses are not aware of client priorities and the plan of care; lack of continuity; inefficient use of nursing resources	1. Client fails to achieve goals.	1. a. Use shift report to update staff on status of priority nursing diagnosis and concomitant nursing care. b. Review plan of care and nursing notes before beginning care.
2. Nursing care becomes routinized and mechanized.	2. Client never has the sense that he or she is personally known by nurses.	2. Explore creative strategies to make quality nursing care on this particular unit a *challenge* rather than a *burden;* use ongoing education, problem-solving strategies by the nursing team, gaming, and other incentives.
3. Inadequate documentation	3. Because there is no complete written record of nursing care, *legally,* this care was never provided.	3. a. Develop the philosophy that quality nursing care *deserves* to be documented. Review legal reasons for careful documentation. b. Become familiar with the flowsheets and note format used within the work setting so that charting can be done quickly and comprehensively.
Evaluating		
1. Not done	1. Mastery of nursing process is stunted; severely limits accomplishment of nursing aims.	1. Develop the belief that quality nursing care does not happen automatically and that only ongoing evaluation will identify needed areas of revision. Devise an evaluative strategy and carry it out. Study its effect on quality of care after 6 months' implementation.

results of nursing care. Whereas the proper environment for care and the right nursing actions are important aspects of quality care, the critical element in evaluating care is demonstrable changes in patient health status.

Nursing Audit

A **nursing audit** is a method of evaluating nursing care which involves a review of client records to assess the outcomes of nursing care or the process by which these outcomes were achieved. Successful nursing audits are dependent on careful nursing documentation.

Concurrent versus Retrospective. The evaluation of nursing care and patient outcomes may be conducted while the patient is receiving care (*i.e.,* a **concurrent** evaluation) or after the patient has been discharged (*i.e.,* a **retrospective** evaluation). Concurrent evaluations are conducted by using direct observation of nursing care, patient interviews, and chart review to determine whether or not the specified evaluative criteria are met.

Retrospective evaluations may use postdischarge questionnaires, patient interviews (telephone or face-to-face), or chart review (nursing audit) to collect data. The type of retrospective audit most familiar to nurses working in hospitals is the Joint Commission of Accreditation of Hospitals (JCAH) retrospective chart review. This accrediting body initially required hospitals to conduct a certain number of audits per year.

SUMMARY

The cultivation of evaluation as a critical component of the nursing process ensures nursing's continued success in achieving desired changes in client health status. Only a firm commitment to evaluation enables nurses to answer the following questions:

- What are nursing's values?
- How can these be formalized in standards and evaluative criteria?
- What data exist to determine whether or not the specified evaluative criteria are being met?
- How can these data best be collected, analyzed, and interpreted?
- To what courses of action do the findings lead?

Nursing actions are far too valuable and costly resources today to be haphazardly implemented. Evaluation, carefully planned and executed, can direct and redirect these actions to maximize client benefit. This is

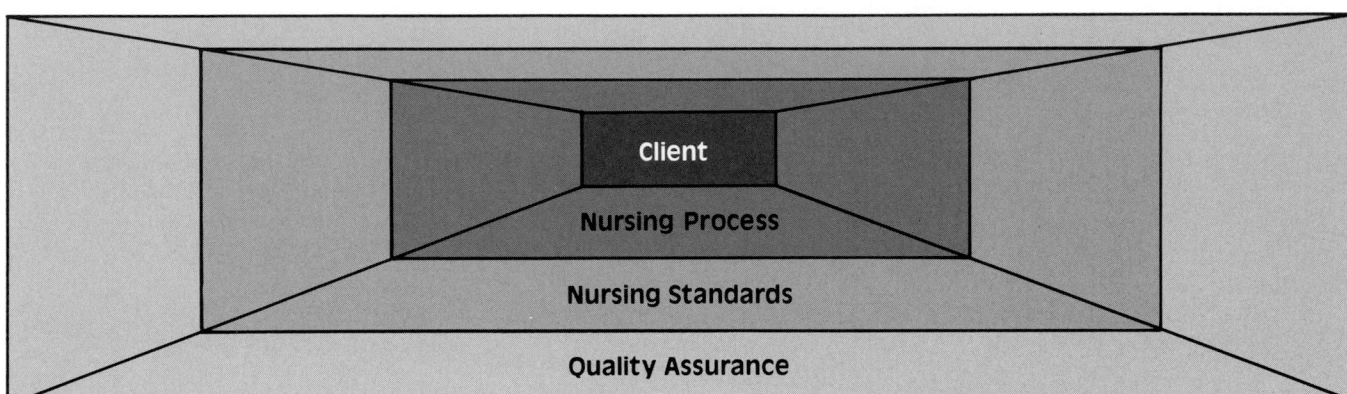

Why evaluate?

- Measure attainment of client goals
- Redirect plan of nursing care
- Enhance nursing's public image
- Ensure nursing's survival: *i.e.,* the selection and funding of nursing services in the competitive health care market

How to evaluate:

- Develop evaluative criteria
- Collect data and compare it to standards
- Summarize findings and make interpretations
- Identify courses of actions
- Take corrective action based on findings

Who is concerned about evaluation of nursing care?

- Nurses
- Clients
- Fiscal intermediaries
- Other health care professionals
- Community that determines allocation of resources to health care delivery

What do they want to know?

- What kinds of health and wellness problems nurses help clients to solve
- What nursing interventions are most successful in achieving desired client outcomes
- What it costs to achieve these results
- Are these the best nursing interventions and client outcomes considering the current status of the science and art of nursing and other health or health-related sciences

Types of evaluation:

- Determination of the client's degree of goal achievement
- Review of the use of nursing process
- Identification of and response to client, nurse, and health care system variables detracting from quality care
- Participation in quality assurance programs
  - structure/process/outcomes
  - concurrent/retrospective
  - institution/nurse/client

F I G U R E   19-2
Overview and summary of the evaluative component of the nursing process.

the goal and challenge of nursing evaluation. Criteria that may be helpful in determining the adequacy of the evaluative component of the nursing process include:

- Evaluation of the client's achievement of desired goals
- Review of how the process is used and revision of the plan of care if necessary
- Participation in quality assurance programs

Figure 19-2 provides a summary and overview of the evaluation step of the nursing process.

KEY POINTS

- During evaluation, the nurse and client measure how well the client has achieved the goals specified in the plan of care. Factors that have positively or negatively influenced goal achievement are identified, and a decision is made to terminate, continue, or modify care.

- When evaluation points to the need to modify nursing care, each preceding step in the nursing process is reviewed for accuracy.

- The type of evaluative data collected to support the decision regarding goal achievement (goal met, partially met, or not met) is determined by the nature of the goal. Goals may be cognitive, psychomotor, affective, or may describe physical changes in the client.

- It is important for nurses to evaluate client goal achievement as early as possible. Achievement, when celebrated with the client, encourages further goal achievement. Failure directs necessary revisions in the plan of care. Waiting until a client is about to be discharged to evaluate goals is the most common mistake nurses make in evaluation.

- Evaluative statements recorded on the plan of care alert the entire nursing staff to the client's level of goal achievement. Each evaluative statement includes a decision about how well the goal was achieved and the client data or behavior that supports the decision. The statement is dated and signed.

- Sensitivity to the client, nurse, and health-care system variables influencing goal achievement enables the nurse to manipulate factors that will help the client reach desired goals.

- Common problems encountered during evaluation that may require a revision of the plan of care include: inaccurate or incomplete data base, vague or missing nursing diagnoses, standardized plan of care, improperly developed nursing goals, superficial nursing orders, plan that is not kept up-to-date, failure to use evaluation to improve quality of nursing care, and insufficient communication among nurses.

- Historically, nursing has been a strong advocate for quality health care. The current availability of fewer resources to treat clients in hospitals and the unavailability of sufficient alternative treatment settings pose a serious challenge to nursing.

- Quality assurance programs are evaluative programs designed to secure and implement excellence in nursing and health care. These programs may include process, structure, or outcome standards and have as their focus the client, the nurse, the institution, or the health-care system.

- Quality assurance programs enable nursing to be accountable to society for the quality of its service. They are also a response to the public mandate for professional accountability and the mandate of professional nursing law. They ensure professional survival, encourage nursing's fidelity to its moral and ethical responsibilities, and assist nursing to comply with other external pressures.

BIBLIOGRAPHY

Allison S, Kinloch K: Four steps to quality assurance. Canadian Nurse 77(11):36–38, 1984

American Nurses' Association: ANA Quality Assurance Workbook. Kansas City, MO, The Association, 1976

American Nurses' Association: A Plan for Implementation of the Standards of Nursing Practice. Kansas City, MO, The Association, 1975

American Nurses' Association: ANA's Eight Standards of Nursing Practice. Kansas City, MO, The Association, 1973

Atkinson LD, Murray ME: Understanding the Nursing Process, 3rd ed. New York, Macmillan, 1986

Barba M, Bennett B, Shaw WJ: The evaluation of patient care through use of ANA's standards of nursing practice. Supervisor Nurse 9(11):42–53, 1978

Bloch D: Evaluation of nursing care in terms of process

and outcome: Issues in research and quality assurance. Nurs Res 24:256–263, 1975

Griffith-Kenney JW, Christensen PJ: Nursing Process: Application of Theories, Frameworks and Models, 2nd ed. St Louis, CV Mosby, 1986

Joint Commission on Accreditation of Hospitals: Manual for Hospitals. Chicago, The Commission, 1983

Joint Commission on Accreditation of Hospitals. Chicago, The Commission, 1975

Laing M, Nish M: Eight steps to quality assurance. Canadian Nurse 77(11):22–25, 1981

Lillesland KM, et al: Nursing process evaluation: A quality assurance tool. Nursing Administration Quarterly 7(3):9–14, 1983

National League for Nursing: The quest for quality. Public Policy Bulletin IV(2):1986

Phaneuf M: The Nursing Audit: Self Regulation in Nursing Practice. New York, Appleton-Century-Crofts, 1976

Phaneuf M: Quality assurance: A nursing view. New Zealand Nursing Journal 69(2):9–11, 1976

Wandelt MA, Ager JW: Quality Patient Care Scale. New York, Appleton-Century-Crofts, 1974

Wandelt MA, Slater SD: Slater Nursing Competencies Rating Scale. New York, Appleton-Century-Crofts, 1975

Wright D: An introduction to the evaluation of nursing care: A review of the literature. Journal of Advanced Nursing 9(5):457–467, 1984

Yura H, Walsh M: The Nursing Process: Assessing, Planning, Implementing, and Evaluation, 4th ed. New York, Appleton-Century-Crofts, 1983

Roles Basic to Nursing Practice

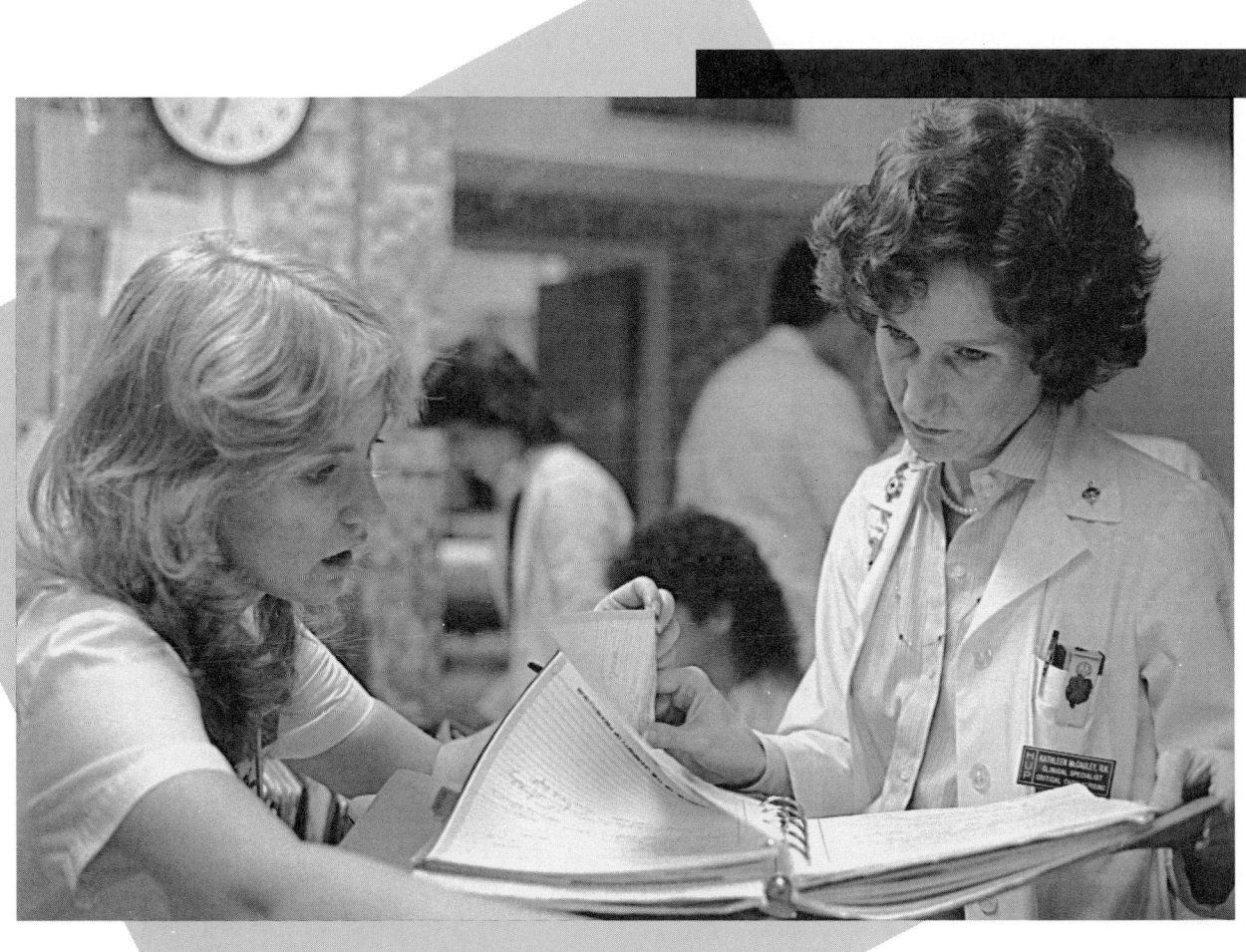

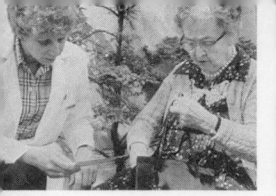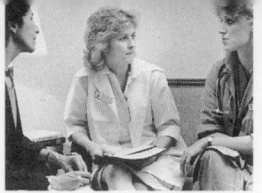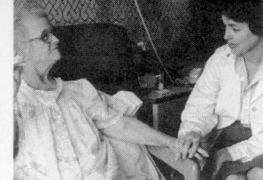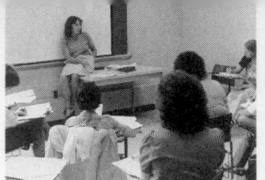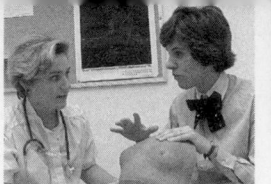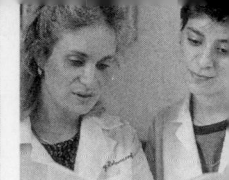

*N*urses, as health-care providers, function in a variety of roles to give holistic client care and to develop as members of the nursing profession. Unit V discusses the nurse's roles of communicator, teacher, counselor, leader, researcher, and advocate. These roles are interdependent and each is an integral part of the broad nursing role of caregiver. The nurse uses these roles to help clients of all ages to meet needs along the health continuum.

To be effective as a caregiver, the nurse must be proficient in both the art and the science of nursing roles. The role of the nurse as communicator is essential to each professional nursing role and is the heart of caring. Nursing is a person-centered service, based on relationships with clients, peers, and other members of the health-care team. By developing effective interpersonal skills and using therapeutic communication skills nurses are able to establish and maintain helping relationships with clients and working relationships with peers.

As a teacher, the nurse uses communication skills to teach individuals and families. Teaching, implemented through the nursing process, is used to meet learning needs. As counselor, the nurse provides information, makes appropriate referrals, and assists the client in developing a systematic approach to problem solving and decision making. The nurse as leader practices assertive, self-directed nursing. Abilities for leadership and bringing about change begin with the student nurse and progress as the nurse develops self-confidence and skill in interpersonal relationships and experience in health-care settings. As researcher, the nurse may conduct research, use research findings to improve client care, or participate in the research done by others. As advocate, the nurse combines all these roles to promote the right of clients to make their own decisions about health and life and to protect human and legal rights.

Unit V provides the content necessary to the caregiver role, integrating each of the defined dimensions in giving holistic care to clients. Nursing practice, as a specialized and unique service to others, is based on the application of knowledge and skills presented in this unit.

Communicator

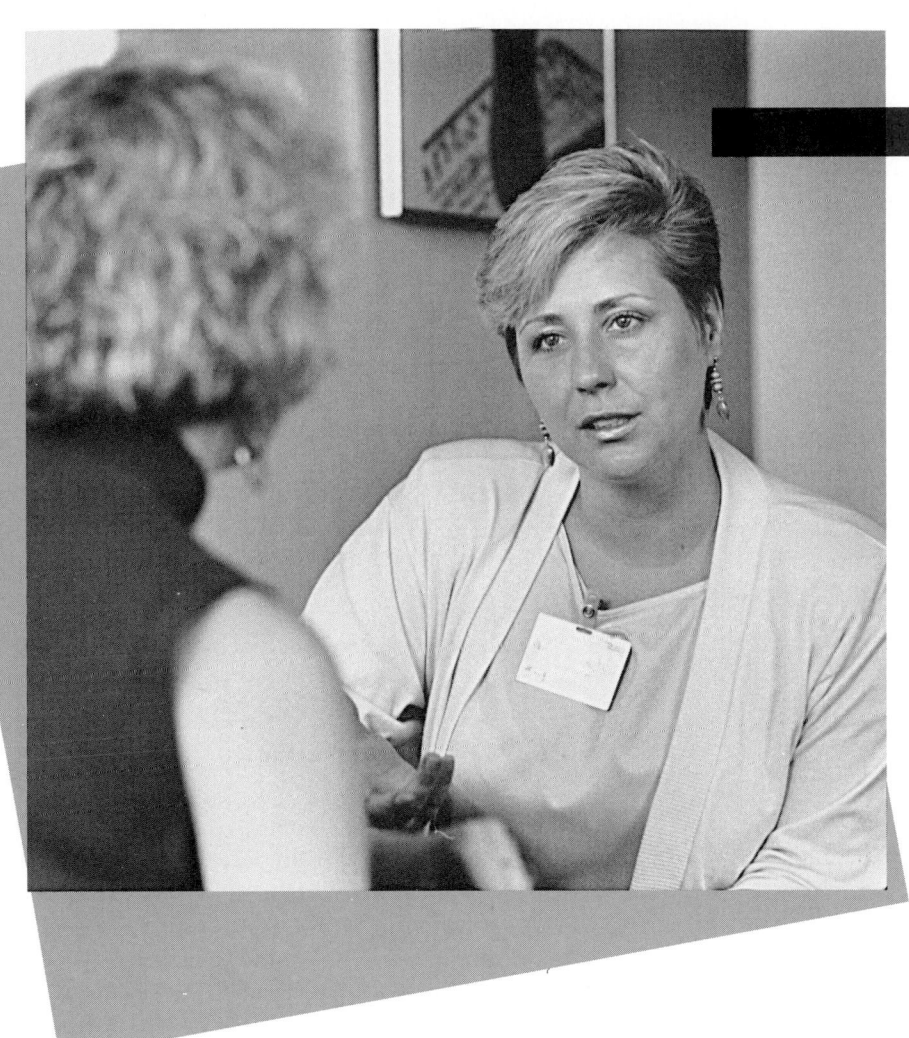

After studying this chapter, the learner should be able to

Define key terms used in the chapter.

Describe the communication process.

List at least eight ways in which people communicate nonverbally.

Describe the interrelationship between communication and the nursing process.

Describe the phases of a helping relationship.

Practice each of the effective communication techniques.

Explain why the development of interpersonal skills is important for a nurse.

Describe each of the ineffective communication techniques.

Explain how to facilitate nurse–client interactions in special circumstances.

An important nursing role in any health-care facility is that of communicator. Whether it be nurse to nurse, nurse to client, nurse to physician (or other health-care worker), or nurse to family, nurses communicate thoughts, ideas, experiences, facts, and a host of other helpful contributions to the client's attainment of wellness.

Communication is one of the most important skills nurses must develop. As a component of therapy, communication can be effective or ineffective in relationships. It addresses human needs and is an integral part of the nursing process.

THE COMMUNICATION PROCESS

Communication can be defined in two ways: the process of sharing information or the process of generating and transmitting meanings. The two definitions are not in conflict since information is produced and has meaning before it can be shared.

Communication is a foundation for our way of life. There could be no way to establish a government, to share family experiences, to run a school, to enjoy most current entertainment, or to practice nursing without communication. Communication is also a requirement for a person's well-being. Social interactions among people are necessary to fulfill some of their most elemental psychosocial needs, such as love, affection, and recognition, discussed earlier in the text.

Basic Characteristics of Communication

There are several basic characteristics of communication, as summarized in the accompanying box and discussed here.

Communication is a reciprocal process in which both the sender and the receiver of messages participate simultaneously, as illustrated in Figure 20-1.

To begin the process, *more than one person must be involved and participants must establish a* **relationship**. A person in isolation does not communicate; isolation may not only be physical, but also may be self-imposed isolation to people and surroundings, as occurs in some mental and emotional illnesses. Also, two or more people next to each other, for instance in a checkout line in a market, do not necessarily communicate with one another. Some kind of relationship must exist between people in order for the process of communication to take place.

Communication is continuous and reciprocal. Communicating persons mutually and continuously send and receive messages. There is not one person who only sends nor is there only one who receives messages.

Messages may be sent through verbal and nonverbal means. Nonverbal communication often helps a person

KEY TERMS

communication	nonverbal communication
empathy	rapport
helping relationship	relationship
interpersonal skills	semantics
interviewing techniques	therapeutic touch
language	verbal communication

Basic Characteristics of Communication

- Communication requires at least two persons who, as a result of communicating, establish a relationship with each other.
- Communication is continuous and reciprocal.
- Communicating persons receive and send messages through verbal and nonverbal means.
- Verbal and nonverbal communications occur simultaneously.
- Communicating persons respond to messages they receive.
- The message cannot always be assumed to mean what the receiver believes it to mean or what the sender intended it to mean.
- Exchanging messages requires knowledge.
- Past experiences influence messages sent, and interpretation by the receiver is based on past experiences.
- Communication is influenced by the way people feel.

understand subtle and hidden meanings in what is being said verbally. For instance, a person may respond to the question "how are you?" by simply answering "fine." However, if this answer is accompanied by a rigid, tense facial expression, the true meaning of the response would need further investigation. (See Figure 20-2.) Verbal and nonverbal communications are discussed in the next section.

Verbal and nonverbal communications occur simultaneously. There is a proverb that says, "What you do

speaks so loud I cannot hear what you say." In other words, one means of communicating may have a positive message while the other is giving a negative message. For instance, the words "hello" and "goodbye" can be said in ways that imply another's presence is either the best or the worst thing that could have happened.

Nonverbal communication is more likely to be involuntary. That is, it tends to be less under the control of the person sending the message than is verbal communication. Hence, nonverbal communication is generally considered as being a more accurate expression of true feelings. For instance, people may say they are well and that everything is fine when obvious appearances and behavior show that all is not well. The latter, the nonverbal expression, more accurately expresses the situation.

Communicating persons respond to messages they receive. This form of feedback is especially important to validate information in order to learn whether a message was received accurately. Even the lack of a verbal response gives feedback to the person sending the message. Failure to respond verbally could be interpreted as inattentiveness, disinterest, or hostility, depending on what nonverbal feedback is received by the sender.

Validation is also necessary to determine the accuracy of not only the message but also the meaning of the message. Things may not always be what they appear to be. True meanings can be camouflaged. For instance, a child may say he does not wish to eat because he has no appetite, whereas the real meaning of his behavior may be that he is seeking attention. The message cannot always be assumed to mean what the receiver believes it to mean or what the sender intended it to mean.

The person sending a message must have knowledge to send, and the person receiving the message must have knowledge to understand what is sent. The levels of knowledge may not always be equal. For example, the nurse who teaches a client about diabetes must have knowledge about the disease and attempts to share that

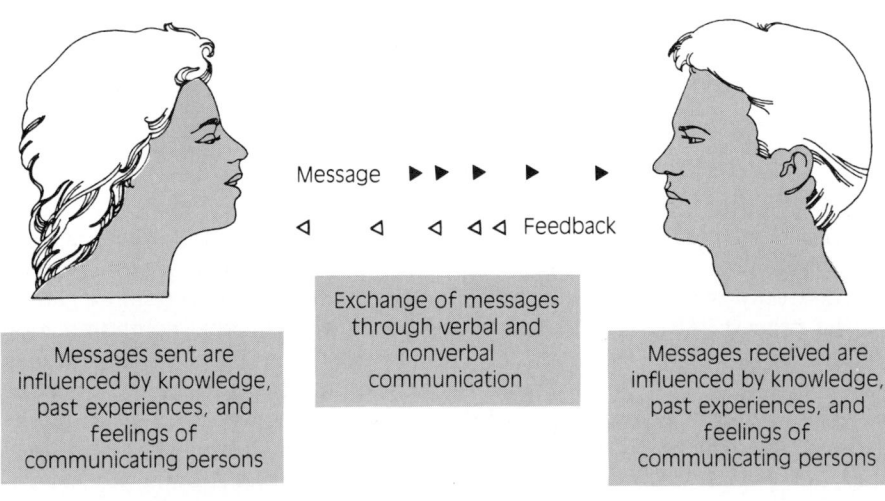

FIGURE 20-1
The various components in the process of communication.

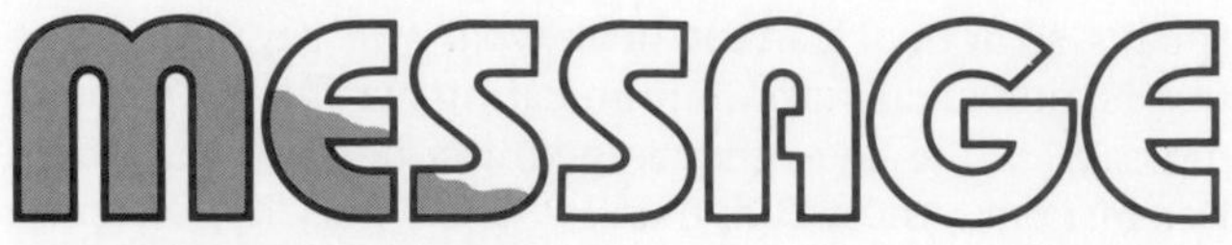

MESSAGE

FIGURE 20-2
Research in communication has shown that words contribute only a small percentage to the communication of a message (the colored area). Nonverbal expression, tone, timing, context, and other characteristics of an exchange complete the message communicated.

knowledge with the client. However, if the client does not understand the disease process or the terminology the nurse uses, the client will not receive the messages the nurse sends.

A person's past experiences influence what is sent, and interpretation by the receiver is based on past experiences as well. For example, what is a big meal, a small child, or a high temperature. Unless the sender's and receiver's past experiences are similar in relation to the manner in which these adjectives are used, effective communication is difficult. Pain may mean one thing to a person who has suffered a great deal but something different to one who has experienced little pain. The grief of death may have a different meaning to a person who has not experienced the loss of a loved one from that of the person who has.

Communication is influenced by the way people feel at the moment or about the subject. The nurse who feels teaching is an important aspect of nursing care will communicate this feeling to patients. In contrast, the nurse who handles teaching as if it were an unimportant and dreary chore is unlikely to share much information with the client. A client motivated to learn will receive the nurse's message but is unlikely to do so if the client feels there is no point in receiving it. Also, an angry or anxious client, because of personal feelings, may not hear what the nurse says.

All of these characteristics comprise the process of communication. Other factors in communication of particular importance to nursing are forms of communications, the use of communication in therapy, and developing communication skills.

Forms of Communication

People communicate in various environments involving a varying number of people.

One-to-one communication occurs when only two people are involved in the communication process. A great deal of nursing situations involve the nurse and client in one-to-one communication.

Communication also occurs in *small groups* of three to ten individuals. Nurses must learn to communicate effectively in small groups because they are often required to be members or leaders of such groups.

Large groups are made up of more than ten persons. Nursing instructors and students frequently experience the communication process in large groups. The nurse's role in teaching large groups is presented in Chapter 21. Attendance at social, religious, or political functions also involves large groups where communication may take place.

As stated earlier, communicating persons *receive and send messages through verbal and nonverbal means,* which *occur simultaneously.* Learning about the two forms of communicating and developing skills in them are important parts of the nurse's education.

Verbal Communication

Verbal communication is an exchange of information using words and includes both the spoken and the written word. Verbal communication depends on language. **Language** is a prescribed way of using words so that people can share information effectively. Language includes a common definition of words as well as a method of arranging the words in a certain order. The development of language is discussed in Chapter 11.

Both written and spoken forms of communication reveal a great deal about a person. The way a person pronounces certain words or uses particular phrases gives clues to such things as geographic or ethnic origins. Vocabulary, sentence structure, and spelling give indications of a person's intellectual development or educational level and may also indicate that English is a second language. Language helps nurses assess what clients know and feel. In turn, nurses must develop their own language skills to aid in reciprocal responses in the communication process.

The verbal form of communication is used extensively by nurses when speaking with clients, giving oral reports to other nurses, writing care plans, and recording in nursing progress notes. Other examples of verbal communication include public speaking, writing for publication, and composing signs and posters. In each of these examples, words and language are communicated to others.

Nonverbal Communication

Nonverbal communication is the exchange of information without the use of words. It is what is *not* said. Nonverbal communication is sometimes referred to as *body language.* There are various ways in which information is exchanged through nonverbal communication. It is generally accepted that nonverbal communication expresses more of the true meaning of a message than does verbal communication. Therefore, nurses must be aware of both the nonverbal messages they send and the nonverbal messages they receive from clients. A great deal of variation exists in nonverbal communication, depending on one's individual or cultural patterns.

The various forms of nonverbal communication include the following.

Touch. Tactile sense has been studied seriously as a form of nonverbal communication only within the last three or four decades. Touch expresses very personal behavior and means different things to different people. Investigations have shown that tactile experiences are largely shaped by familial, regional, class, and cultural influences. Such factors as age and sex also play a role in individualizing meanings associated with touch. Despite its individuality, touch is viewed as one of the most effective nonverbal ways to express feelings such as comfort, love, affection, security, anger, frustration, aggression, excitement, and many others.

Eye Contact. Communication often begins with eye contact. A glance, for example, is often an attention-getting method to open conversation. Eye contact also suggests respect and a willingness to listen and to keep communication open. Lack of it often indicates anxiety or defenselessness or that a person is avoiding communi-cation. However, in some cultures young children and adolescents are taught that it is disrespectful to look an adult "in the eye." In other cultures, women are taught to avoid eye contact, or that out of respect, eye contact should not be made with a superior. In addition, the eyes themselves carry nonverbal messages. For examples, the eyes fix in a stare during anger; they tend to narrow in disgust; and they ordinarily open wide in fear. A blank stare can indicate daydreaming or inattentiveness.

Facial Expressions. The face is the most expressive part of the body. Examples of the various messages facial expressions convey are anger, joy, suspicion, sadness, fear, and contempt. Some people have extremely expressive faces, whereas others mask their feelings, making it more difficult to determine what the person is really thinking. Nurses need to learn some control over their own facial expressions. For instance, a client with extensive burns may watch the nurse's reaction when burn dressings are changed for the first time. Any sign of repulsiveness or disgust would have grave implications for the client's self-image and recovery.

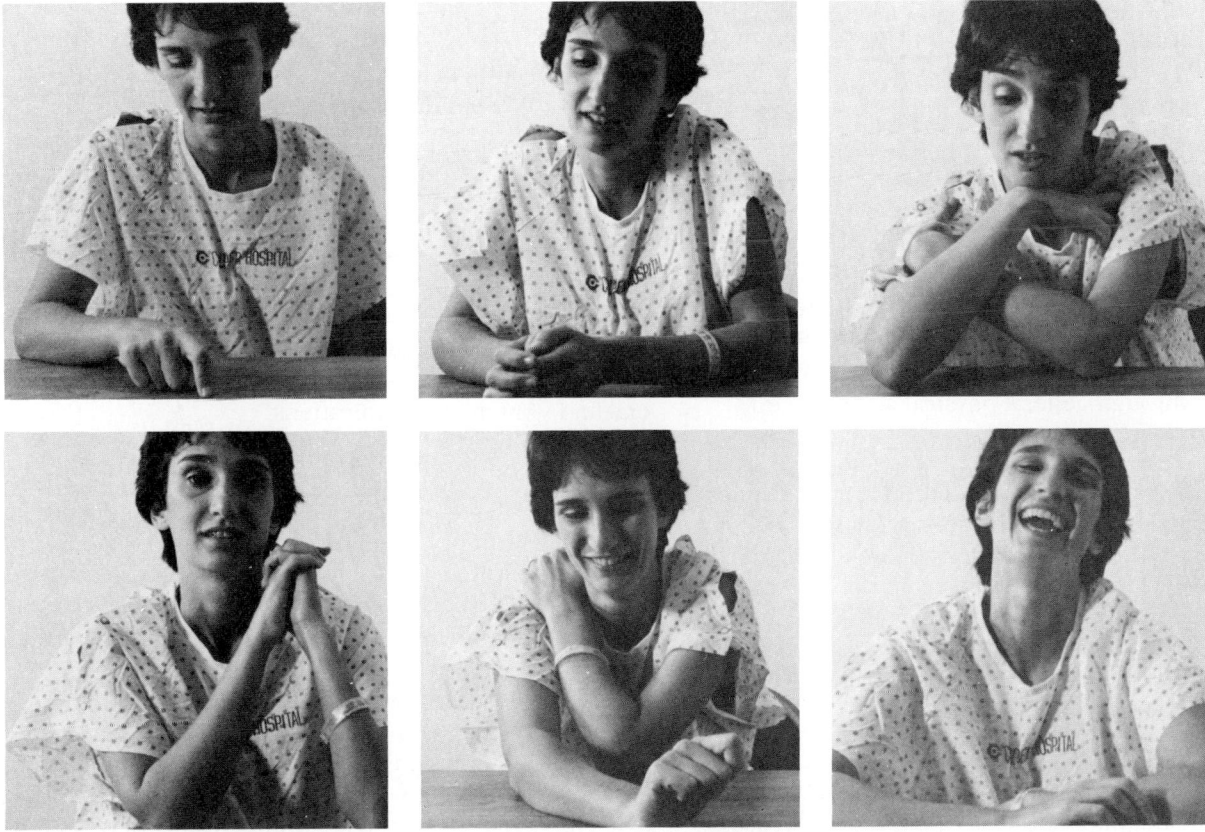

F I G U R E 20-3
Eye contact, the lack of it, facial expression, posture, gesture, and silence send nonverbal messages to the receiver. What messages do you receive from each of these photographs? (Photos by Charles Field, from Patricia Barry, Psychosocial Nursing: Assessment and Intervention. Philadelphia, JB Lippincott, 1984)

Posture.   The way a person holds the body carries non-verbal messages. People in good health and with a positive attitude usually hold their bodies in good alignment. Depressed or tired people are more likely to slouch. Posture also often provides nonverbal clues concerning pain and physical limitations. For instance, a rigid, stiff appearance is a good indication of tension and pain.

Gait.   A bouncy, purposeful walk usually carries a message of well-being. A less purposeful, shuffling gait often means the person is sad or discouraged. Certain gaits are associated with illness. For example, clients recovering from recent abdominal surgery usually walk slightly bent over and very slowly and may need the assistance of hand rails or a helping person.

Gestures.   Gestures using various parts of the body are capable of carrying numerous messages; for example, thumbs up means victory whereas thumbs down carries a negative connotation; kicking an object often expresses anger, as does a clenched fist; wringing of the hands or tapping of the foot usually indicates anxiety or anger; a wave of the hand serves to beckon someone to come, or, if waved in another way, signifies that someone should leave. Gestures are used extensively when two persons speaking different languages attempt to communicate with each other.

General Physical Appearance.   Most illnesses cause at least some alterations in general physical appearance. Observing for changes in appearance is an important nursing responsibility in detecting a particular illness or in evaluating effectiveness of care and therapy. For example, the person with an insufficient intake of fluids has dry skin that wrinkles easily, eyes that may be sunken and dull in appearance, and poor muscle tone. On the other hand, the person in good health tends to radiate health status through general physical appearance.

Mode of Dress and Grooming.   A person's clothing and grooming practices carry significant nonverbal messages. For example, healthy persons with good self-esteem tend to pay attention to details of dress and grooming, whereas those with low self-esteem show much less interest in them. Persons feeling ill often demonstrate little interest in personal appearance, and it is often a sign of returning health when interest in mode of dress and appearance begins.

Sounds.   Crying, moaning, gasping, and sighing are oral but nonverbal forms of communication. Such sounds can be interpreted in numerous ways. For example, a person may cry because of sadness or for joy. Gasping often indicates fear or pain. A sigh may be a sign of reluctant agreement to something or a sign of relief.

Silence.   Periods of silence during communication often carry important nonverbal messages. The silence between two persons may indicate complete understanding of each other or it may mean they are angry with each other. Silence and its possible uses and meanings are discussed further later in this chapter.

COMMUNICATION AS A COMPONENT OF THERAPY

Communication and the Nursing Process

The nurse's ability to communicate with clients and with other nurses is essential to effective use of the nursing process. Knowledge of the communication process and of effective communication techniques is fundamental to all steps of the nursing process. At the same time, the nursing process provides the nurse with the guidance and direction needed to communicate with the client effectively.

Assessing.   Since the major focus of the assessment step is information gathering, verbal and nonverbal communication are essential nursing tools. Nurses use the written word to obtain data concerning their clients. Nurses often read their clients' records or charts before meeting them in person. The spoken word is used to give and receive reports to and from other health personnel. This is a common practice when admitting a client to a hospital unit. Nurses use one-to-one communication to obtain thorough nursing histories and physicals. Effective communication techniques, as well as observational skills, are used extensively during this phase. The data collected verbally and nonverbally are analyzed and then passed on to the appropriate persons through oral and written communications.

Diagnosing.   Once a nurse formulates a nursing diagnosis, it must be communicated through the spoken and written word to other nurses as well as to the client. In many health-care settings, the written diagnosis, as part of the care plan, becomes a permanent part of the client's record.

Planning.   The planning step requires the use of communication to share client objectives/goals and nursing orders with the client and other health-care personnel. Since a nurse is rarely able to implement all parts of a plan alone, oral and written communication is relied on to inform others of what needs to be done to meet the set objectives/goals. Without communication, the nurse's plan would never proceed to the implementation phase.

Implementing and Documenting.   Nurses assume many roles when they implement the plan of care. Verbal and nonverbal communication allows nurses to teach, counsel, and support clients and their families during the implementation phase. Even a simple nursing order such as "encourage to drink 100 ml of fluid every hour while awake" requires countless messages to be sent and received between the nurse and client. The nurse explains why fluids are important, what fluids are beneficial, and how often they are needed. The client, in turn, informs the nurse of his or her ability or inability to comply with the order. The client's verbal and nonverbal messages are assessed during each nurse–client interaction. Then, the implementation of the order is documented in the client's record.

Evaluating. Nurses often rely on the verbal and nonverbal cues they receive from their clients to verify whether or not client objectives/goals have been achieved. Communication also facilitates the revision of parts of the care plan through the exchange of positive and negative messages between the nurse and the client.

The Helping Relationship

One of the basic characteristics of communication listed at the beginning of the chapter stated that persons, *as a result of communicating, establish a relationship with each other.* Another characteristic is that *communication is continuous and reciprocal.* These characteristics work together to establish a helping relationship.

Most people entering the health-care field do so because they want to help people. This is not accomplished through a random method but rather takes preconceived, purposeful paths, as evident in the steps of the nursing process. Another intentional system is the **helping relationship**, sometimes called the *therapeutic relationship,* which uses the nursing process.

A helping relationship sets the climate for the participants to move toward common goals, which arise from human needs. Therefore, need gratification occurs as the result of a successful helping relationship. A helping relationship exists among many persons who provide and receive assistance in meeting human needs in many walks of life, but in this book it refers to the helping relationship between nurses and clients.

When a nurse and client are involved in a helping relationship, the nurse assists the client to achieve goals that allow the client's human needs to be satisfied. In other words, the nurse is the helper and the client is the person being helped. The helping relationship between the nurse and client is sometimes called the *nurse–client* or *nurse–patient relationship.*

The goals of a helping relationship between a nurse and a client are determined cooperatively and are defined in terms of the client's needs. Broadly speaking, common goals might include increased independence for the person, greater feelings of worth, and improved physical well-being. Depending on the goal, the nurse selects nursing care activities that will move the person

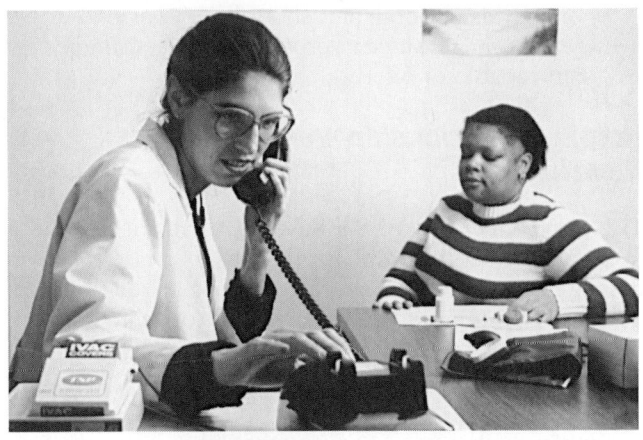

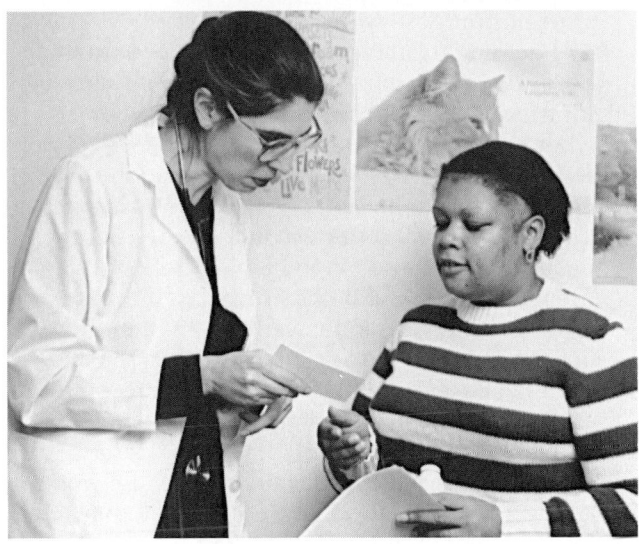

F I G U R E   20-4
The helping relationship is dynamic, purposeful, and focused on achieving client-centered goals.

toward the goal. As the client's needs and goals change, so do the nursing care activities.

The nurse also has many needs to be met, but in the helping relationship between the nurse and the client, the nurse's needs are temporarily set aside and the focus is on the client's needs.

The helping relationship is intangible and therefore difficult to describe, but most authorities agree that it has at least three basic characteristics.

• It is dynamic. Both the person providing the assistance and the person being helped are active participants to the extent each is able.
• It is purposeful and time limited. This means there are specific goals that are intended to be met within a certain period of time.
• The person providing the assistance in a helping relationship assumes the dominant role. The helping person must also assume responsibility for presenting self and his or her helping abilities as

honestly as possible and should not convey the idea that he or she can provide more assistance than capable of offering.

Helping Relationship Versus Social Relationship

The difference between a helping relationship and a friendship must be emphasized. Helping relationships contain many of the qualities of a social relationship. They have in common the components of care, concern, trust, and growth, but they also possess some major differences:

- The helping relationship does not occur spontaneously, as do most social relationships. It occurs for a specific purpose with a specific person.
- The helping relationship is characterized by an unequal sharing of information. The client shares information related to personal health problems while the nurse shares information in terms of professional role. In a friendship, information sharing is more likely to be similar in quantity and type.
- The helping relationship is built on the client's needs, not on those of the helping person. In a friendship, needs of both participants are generally taken into consideration. A friendship may grow out of a helping relationship, but this is separate from the purposeful, time-limited interaction described as a helping relationship.

The helping relationship is ordinarily described as having three phases: the orientation phase, the working phase, and the termination phase. In the helping relationship, the communication process follows the sequence of the nursing process. Both processes are continuous and reciprocal.

Orientation Phase

Ideally, the helping relationship between a nurse and a client is initiated when the nurse starts the data-gathering part of the nursing process. However, it can also be initiated at other times. In the orientation phase, the tone and guidelines for the relationship are established. The nurse and client meet and learn to identify each other by name. It is especially important that the nurse introduce himself or herself to the client. It may even be helpful for the nurse to write his or her name for the client. Failure to do so may result in the client becoming confused and mistrustful because of the number of health-agency personnel with whom most clients come in contact.

The following activities generally take place during the orientation phase of the helping relationship.

- The roles of both persons in the relationship are clarified. It has been observed that a successful relationship is more likely to occur when the responsibilities assigned to each participant are known and accepted and when there is leadership present.

In the nurse–client relationship, the nurse, by virtue of role, generally assumes leadership. Leadership does not mean control in the restrictive or manipulative sense, but here implies taking the initiative to enlist the client's point of view. When cooperative planning occurs with consideration for the client's needs, the relationship between a nurse and a client is more likely to be mutually satisfactory.

- An agreement or contract about the relationship is established. The agreement is usually a simple verbal exchange or, occasionally, a written document, especially if the relationship extends over a long period. Elements in the agreement include the goals of the relationship; location, frequency, and length of the contacts; and the duration of the relationship. Depending on the purpose of the relationship, the agreement may also include the way in which personal information that the client may divulge will be handled.
- An orientation to the health-care agency is provided. The nurse is responsible for seeing that the client is oriented to the health agency, its facilities, admission routines, and so on. The nurse identifies this orientation as one of the goals in the nurse–client helping relationship.

Working Phase

The working phase is usually the longest phase of the helping relationship. Here, the nurse and the client work together to meet the client's needs as identified during the orientation phase. Interaction is the essence of the working phase. The nurse–client interactions that occur at this time are purposeful in that they have been designed to ensure achievement of mutually agreed upon health goals/objectives.

In the working phase, the nurse provides whatever assistance may be needed to achieve each goal. For example, an elderly client has a poor appetite and the goal is to increase food intake. The nurse discusses the idea of small, more frequent meals with the client. With the client's approval, the nurse makes the necessary arrangements. In another instance, a mother explains to a school nurse that she cannot afford dental care recommended for her child, although she would like to have the work done. The nurse asks if a referral to a social agency for financial assistance would be acceptable. With the mother's permission, the nurse contacts the agency.

When sentiments and feelings between persons are unsatisfactory, the persons often cannot work cooperatively toward achieving a common goal. When sentiments and feelings are satisfactory, the persons can usually work together. In the examples in the preceding paragraph, satisfactory sentiments and feelings between the nurse and clients might have been the key aspects. The elderly person's relationship with the nurse may have allowed a positive response to the small, more frequent meals. The mother's feelings about the nurse may have allowed her to accept financial assistance for the dental care without feeling embarassed.

In addition, the nurse as caregiver provides the client with whatever assistance may be needed to perform activities of daily living. For example, if a client with impaired mobility is unable to get out of bed except to a bedside commode, the nurse needs to help with daily hygiene.

The nursing roles of teacher and counselor (see Chap 21) are primarily performed during this phase. These roles involve motivating the client to learn and implement health-promotion activities, to comply with medical treatments such as medication regimens, and to express feelings about health problems, nursing care, any progress or setbacks, and any other areas of concern. This is where the nurse's interpersonal skills are used to their fullest (see the discussions of interpersonal skills and effective communication techniques later in this chapter). A breakdown of the helping relationship on one of these levels could result in serious consequences. For instance, a client began to break clinic appointments, although he had not appeared to lack interest in his health when he began visiting the clinic. When a community health nurse called on the client at home, he said, "The nurse at the clinic seems too busy; she just doesn't seem to care if I come or go. I don't like to go to that clinic." The lack of satisfactory interaction between the nurse and the client discouraged him from continuing the relationship, even at the expense of his health. Had the nurse–client interaction been satisfactory, breaking appointments probably would not have been a problem.

Satisfactory interaction preserves the integrity of persons while promoting an atmosphere characterized by minimal fear, anxiety, distrust, and tension. Persons feel harmonious and contented with each other as they work cooperatively to reach common goals.

Termination Phase

The termination phase occurs when the conclusion of the initial agreement is acknowledged. This may happen at change-of-shift time, when the client is discharged, or when a nurse leaves on vacation or for employment elsewhere. The client and nurse examine the goals of the helping relationship for indications of their attainment or for evidence of progress toward the goals. If the goals have been reached, this fact should be acknowledged. Such acknowledgment generally results in a feeling of satisfaction for both the client and nurse. If the goals have not been reached, the progress can be acknowledged and either the client or the nurse may make suggestions for future efforts.

There ordinarily are feelings associated with the termination of a helping relationship. If the goals have been met, there is often regret about the ending of a satisfying relationship, even though a sense of accom-plishment persists. If the goals have not been completely achieved, the client may experience anxiety and fear about the future. Whatever the feelings, the client should be encouraged to express emotions about the termination.

There are various ways of preparing for the termination of the helping relationship. The thoughtful nurse can set the stage for the client to establish a helping relationship with another nurse, if this is appropriate. The nurse can assist the client transferring from one agency to another or from one unit in an agency to another by offering explanations concerning the transfer. In some instances, the nurse may introduce the client to personnel who will be giving care.

Occasionally, termination of the helping relationship produces emotional reactions. The client may feel angry, rejected by the nurse, or depressed and helpless, or may deny that a relationship ever really existed. Should such reactions occur, the nurse should help and support the client rather than impose feelings of guilt or wrong for having these views. However, emotional reactions of this sort are less likely to occur if the client has been involved in establishing goals and has been helped to anticipate termination of the helping relationship.

Table 20-1 summarizes goals for clients during the three phases of an effective helping relationship.

DEVELOPING SKILLS IN COMMUNICATION

Another basic characteristic of communication is that *exchanging messages requires knowledge*. Part of the knowledge provided by nursing education is developing communication skills. Although humans use communication all of their waking moments, the therapeutic use of communication requires training and practice. As students realize the importance of communication in helping relationships, they may feel awkward at first and feel the relationships are contrived. But as the merits of effective communication become evident through practice, nurses will feel more at ease with the process.

Effective Communication Techniques

Communication takes on many forms depending on the situation in which the communication is taking place. If effective techniques are used appropriately, nurses can enhance the quality and purpose of any communication. At no time, however, should nurses put techniques of communication above the nurse–client relationship itself.

Conversational Skills

A good place to start is with conversation. *Conversation,* or the exchange of verbal communication, is a social

T A B L E   20-1
Summary of Client Goals for the Three Phases of the Helping Relationship

Orientation Phase	Working Phase	Termination

1. The client will call the nurse by name.
2. The client will accurately describe the roles of the participants in the relationship.
3. The client and nurse will establish an agreement about
  a. Goals of the relationship
  b. Location, frequency, and length of the contacts
  c. The duration of the relationship
	1. The client will actively participate in the relationship.
	2. The client will cooperate in activities that work toward achieving mutually acceptable goals.
	3. The client will express feelings and concerns to the nurse.
		1. The client will participate in identifying the goals accomplished or the progress made toward goals.
		2. The client will verbalize feelings about the termination of the relationship.

interaction. As social beings, humans learn as children how to converse with others. Therefore, a person coming into nursing has had years of experience in communicating verbally. Even though this is the case, nurses can improve their communications with clients and achieve a more effective helping relationship by keeping the following points in mind:

- Control the tone of your voice so you are conveying exactly what you mean to say and not a hidden message. Your tone should indicate an interest in your client and not boredom, patience and not anger, acceptance and not hostility, and so forth.
- Be knowledgeable about the topic of conversation and have accurate information. When possible, the nurse should be familiar with the subject of conversation before discussing it with the client. If the topic is not a familiar one, it is best to tell the client so. Convey confidence and honesty.
- Be flexible. The nurse may have selected to discuss a subject but learns the client wishes to discuss something else. It is better to follow the client's lead whenever possible. In due time, the nurse can return to the subject. For example, the nurse arrives at the client's bedside to administer a medication, but the client begins to talk about his diet. It is better to take a little time to allow the client to speak rather than to insist on carrying out a procedure when the time taken for the conversation is not contraindicated.
- Be clear and concise, and state things as simply as possible. Clients are often anxious and will fail to receive the nurse's message unless the conversation is geared to a level the client understands. Stay on one subject at a time and say things concisely.
- Avoid words that may be interpreted differently. The study of the meaning of words is called **semantics**. Even when two persons speak the same language, some words, such as love, hate, freedom, and liberty, may have very different meanings.

- Be truthful. The client will soon distrust the nurse if given false information. Admit not knowing and seek an answer rather than make a comment that is likely to be an error.
- Keep an open mind. An attitude of "I know better than the client" is quickly discerned by the client. Clients can make valuable contributions to their own health care.
- Take advantage of available opportunities. During most caregiving situations, the nurse can facilitate conversation that will make even the most routine task meaningful. For instance, when giving a bed bath to a client, a nurse can introduce the topic of the client's employment. This would allow the client to verbalize any positive or negative feelings about the job and the temporary absence from it. This could reduce the anxiety which often occurs with the loss of work. It is often comforting to know that someone understands and cares.

Listening Skills

Listening is a skill that involves both hearing and interpreting what is said. It requires attention and concentration to sort out, evaluate, and validate clues so that one better understands the true meanings in what is being said. Listening requires concentrating on the client and what is being said. There are various recommended techniques to help improve listening skills:

- Whenever possible, sit when communicating with a client. Do not cross arms or legs; to do so is a type of body language that conveys a message of being closed to the client's comments.
- Be alert but relaxed, and take sufficient time so that the client feels at ease during the conversation. Keep the conversation as natural as possible, and avoid sounding overly eager.
- If culturally appropriate, maintain eye contact with the client, without staring, in a face-to-face pose.

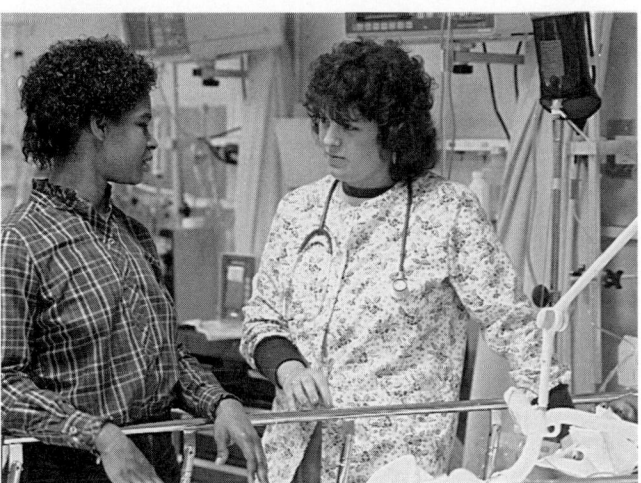

FIGURE 20-5
Listening attentively, with concentration and genuine concern is key to productive communication. (Photo by Gates Rhodes, courtesy of the School of Nursing, University of Pennsylvania)

This technique conveys interest in the conversation and willingness to listen.

- Indicate that you are paying attention to what the client is saying by using appropriate facial expressions and body gestures. Be attentive to both verbal and nonverbal communication.
- Think before responding to the client. Responding impulsively tends to disrupt communication and listening.
- Do not pretend to listen. It is the rare client who is insensitive to an attitude of feigned attention, boredom, and apathy.
- Listen for themes in the client's comments. The following are some questions to keep in mind in helping to detect themes: What are the repeated themes in the person's speech and behavior? What topics does the client tend to avoid? What subjects tend to make the client shift the conversation to other subjects? What inconsistencies and gaps appear in the client's conversation?

Use of Silence

The nurse can use silence appropriately by taking the time to wait for the client to initiate or continue speaking. During periods of silence, the nurse has the opportunity to observe the client without having to concentrate simultaneously on the spoken word.

Periods of silence during communication can carry a variety of meanings:

- The client may be demonstrating comfort and contentment in the nurse–client relationship. Continuous talking is not necessary.
- The patient may be trying to demonstrate stoicism and the ability to cope without help.

- The client may be exploring inner feelings and conversation would disrupt these thoughts. In this situation, the client is really saying "I need some time to think."
- The client may be fearful and use silence as an escape from a threat.

In due time, silence may be discussed with the client, especially if the nurse wishes to validate any speculation about its meaning. Fear of silence sometimes leads to too much talking by the nurse. Also, excessive talking tends to place the focus on the nurse rather than on the client.

Interviewing Techniques

The purpose of any interview is to obtain accurate and thorough information. In nursing, the interview is a major tool for the collection of data during the assessment step of the nursing process (see Chap 15). Consequently, every nurse needs to become proficient in the use of the communication techniques described above, as well as in the following **interviewing techniques**, which are specifically designed to gather and validate information.

All interviews should be started with an explanation of the purpose of the interview. During the interview, the various interviewing techniques are used to obtain the information needed while remaining flexible in approach. The interview itself is a therapeutic interaction and may be an essential part of the orientation phase of the helping relationship. At the end of the interview, plans for further interactions can be made.

The following techniques are useful in nearly all nurse–client interactions, especially the interview.

Open-Ended Question/Comment. When obtaining a nursing history, this technique is used to allow the client a wide range of possible responses. It encourages free verbalization. The greatest advantage of this technique is that it prevents the client from answering with a simple "yes" or "no."

Consider the following example of an open-ended question and the response:

Nurse: What did your doctor tell you about your need for this hospitalization?
Client: He told me that my blood pressure is dangerously high and that I need some special tests done while I am here.

This open-ended question by the nurse allows the client to express what he understands to be true and yet is specific enough to prevent side-tracking from the issue at hand, his hospital admission. The nurse could continue with an open-ended comment such as

Nurse: Yes . . . and . . .
Client: Well, he thinks I could need a change in my blood pressure medicine too.

Now, the nurse has even more information from the client and can continue to seek more information. This should be done in a way that does not make the client feel as though the nurse is prying or probing.

Closed Question/Comment.

This technique allows limited choices in possible responses. It is used to gather specific information from a client and allows the nurse and client to focus on a particular area. The following is an example:

Nurse: What medicines have you been taking at home?

Client: Let me see, my doctor gave me a water pill and a blood pressure pill to take every day.

This technique gives the nurse the exact response that is being sought. Care should be taken to avoid the overuse of closed questions and comments because of the limiting effects they have on the client's responses.

Validating Question/Comment.

This type of question/comment serves to validate what the nurse believes is heard or observed. To continue the example used in the previous technique, the nurse could validate what was said as follows:

Nurse: At home you have been taking both a water pill and a blood pressure pill every day. Did you take them today?

Client: Yes. I took one of each with my breakfast.

The nurse is able to ascertain that the client has been taking the medication regularly, as well as today's dosage. Note, however, that the overuse of questions and comments to validate information may lead the client to suspect that the nurse is not listening.

Clarifying Questions/Comments.

By using this technique, a nurse can try to gain an understanding of a client's comment. An example follows:

Client: I have never needed to take medicine before in my life.

Nurse: Is this the first health problem you have had?

Client: Yes, I've always been healthy.

The overuse of this technique can lead the client to believe that the nurse is not listening or is not knowledgeable. However, when used appropriately, it can prevent possible misconceptions that could lead to inappropriate nursing diagnosis. For instance, by clarifying what the client's (in the example) health has been previously, the nurse can plan for what teaching will be necessary after a thorough assessment of what the client knows about his blood pressure problem (see Chap 21).

Reflective Question/Comment.

This involves repeating what the person has said or describing feelings. It serves to encourage the client to elaborate on thoughts and feelings. An example of this technique follows:

Client: I've been really upset about my blood pressure and having to take these pills.

Nurse: You've been upset . . .

Client: I guess I'm worried about what could happen if my blood pressure gets too bad.

By saying this, the nurse has encouraged the client to expand this topic by expressing a more specific concern. Again, like previous techniques, the overuse of the reflective technique and using it mechanically may lead the client to believe the nurse is not listening or is not interested.

Sequencing Question/Comment.

Sequencing is used to place events in chronologic order or to investigate a possible cause-and-effect relationship between events. This technique is seen in the following example:

Client: I don't feel like myself anymore since I've been taking my blood pressure medicine. I'm tired and don't have any energy.

Nurse: You're tiredness began after you started taking your medicine?

This type of question could lead to a possible contributing factor to the client's problem. Nursing assessment is facilitated when events leading to a problem are placed in sequence.

Directing Question/Comment.

It may become necessary at times to obtain more information about a certain subject brought up earlier in the interview or to introduce a new aspect of the present subject. In such an instance the nurse can attempt to direct the client to the subject by using a technique similar to the following:

Client: Before I knew that I had high blood pressure, I was very active. I felt good at work and at home. I think the medicine is making me tired.

Nurse: When did your doctor start you on your present medication?

Client: I've been on them for six weeks.

Nurse: Have you been told about eating foods high in potassium when on this medication?

Client: My doctor gave me some special diet to follow, but I haven't looked at it. I hate diets.

In this way, the nurse has gained valuable information to consider in assessing the client's health status and educational needs.

Use of Touch

Because of the personal nature of touching, a nurse needs to weigh the beneficial versus the detrimental use of touch for each client. Touch can be a powerful therapeutic tool when used at the right time. However, anxiety or discomfort may result when a client does not understand the meaning of a tactile gesture or when the client simply dislikes being touched.

Touch is the most highly developed sense at birth. Tactile experiences of infants and young children appear essential for the normal development of self and awareness of others. It has also been found that many elderly persons long for touch, especially when isolated from loved ones because of hospitalization or nursing home care. Many older persons have no living family to provide them with the caring touch so necessary for the sense of well-being. In such an instance, a nurse can provide some special care by holding the client's hand (Fig. 20-6).

Many situations require the nurse to touch the client while implementing nursing care. Physical closeness between the client and the nurse is essential and inevitable. Therefore, every nurse needs to become comfortable with the judicious use of this nonverbal communication technique, so that security will be promoted rather than anxiety. Dexterity and sureness in the use of the hands help to assure the client of the nurse's expertise when measuring a blood pressure or giving an injection.

Recently, interest has been growing in the phenomenon known as therapeutic touch. **Therapeutic touch** involves "unruffling" or unblocking congested areas of energy in the body and redirecting this energy. After assessing a person's "energy field," the nurse uses therapeutic touch to promote comfort, relaxation, healing, and a sense of well-being in the client. Many nurses are studying therapeutic touch in nursing educational programs and through special courses or workshops. It is becoming a widely accepted form of therapy as well as a subject for nursing research.

Interpersonal Skills

The skills required for positive relationships between persons are referred to as **interpersonal skills**. In nursing,

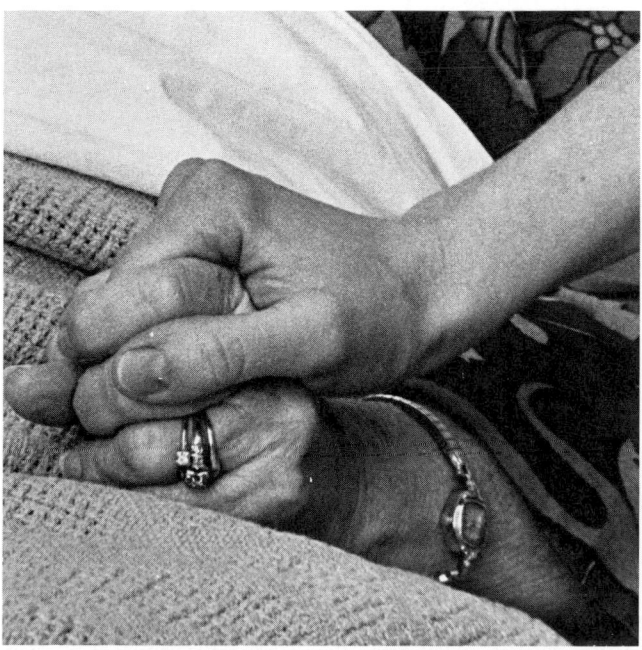

FIGURE 20-6
A reassuring hand clasp uses touch to convey a message. Sometimes touch can be a more effective way of expressing concern and interest than verbal communication.

these skills are essential to the promotion of a nurse–client relationship that will be therapeutic for the client.

Warmth and Friendliness. The helping relationship depends on the nurse's ability to begin the orientation phase successfully. A pleasant greeting accompanied by a smile can facilitate the initiation of this phase and allow the client to relax in the nurse's presence. By maintaining the qualities of warmth and friendliness throughout the helping relationship, the nurse conveys continuous acceptance of the client and interest in discussing the client's feelings and concerns.

Openness. A person who is open conveys an attitude of acceptance, frankness, and lack of prejudice. This is an important quality for a nurse, since a client who feels the nurse is judging could hold back significant information. The nurse must also be open to supporting the client's strengths and promoting the client's growth.

Empathy. **Empathy** can be defined as intellectually identifying with the way that another person feels. An empathic nurse is sensitive to the client's feelings and problems while remaining objective enough to help the client work toward positive outcomes. A nurse who retains this quality can establish successful helping relationships without becoming the cold and stern nurse frequently portrayed in films and television.

Competence. Competent nurses are skilled in all aspects of nursing and are capable of meeting their client's health-care needs through the use of technical, intellectual, and interpersonal skills. Nurses are responsible for evaluating their own strengths and for strengthening any weaknesses so that all clients will receive optimal care. Consequently, the clients develop trust in and respect for their nurses, facilitating helping relationships.

Consideration of Client Variables. Nurses need to develop sensitivity to the variables presented by each client and the effects these factors have on communication. Attention to the following client variables can make the difference between effective and ineffective interactions.

Non–English-Speaking Clients. Caring for non–English-speaking clients is common in many hospital health-care settings. If a particular non–English-speaking group is prominent in the community, nurses should learn some basic phrases in the language of that group (*i.e.,* phrases regarding eating, hygiene, elimination, comfort). Language dictionaries are available that deal with commonly used phrases in health-care settings. Such books should be present on all nursing units. Many hospitals also keep lists of any personnel who speak second languages so that they may be used as translators when needed. This topic is discussed again at the end of this chapter.

Developmental Considerations.   It is imperative for nurses to understand the development of language as well as the intellectual and psychosocial developmental stages so that they can communicate appropriately with clients of all ages. (These stages are presented in Chapts 10 and 11.) Knowing how each age group commonly perceives health, illness, and body functions guides nurses in their interactions with their clients. For instance, a 10-year-old child has a limited understanding of what an infection is and the nurse must explain this in very simple terms so that the child cooperates with the treatment without being frightened. A teenager should be developing abstract thinking, so more detailed and accurate explanations can be given. Being familiar with commonly used slang terminology usually helps nurses when communicating with teens. Communicating with adults can be complicated by many years of negative health-related experiences and inaccurate information. Nurses communicating with elderly clients must assess for any problems with hearing, sight (discussed later in this chapter), confusion, or depression, which could affect nurse–client interactions.

Sociocultural Differences.   Nurses need to develop skills in recognizing "where a person is coming from" in terms of cultural practices and economic influences, as well as personal habits or addictions. As an example, nurses working with expectant mothers must be familiar with street language so that they can determine whether drugs of any kind have been taken during pregnancy since this would have effects on the infant after birth. Also, since women in some cultures may speak of personal things only to their husbands, maternity nurses may have to talk with the client's husband about the postdelivery care that his wife is to receive.

It is best to use lay terminology when speaking with clients unless a client is known to be a health-care professional. Use of medical terminology (*i.e.,* myocardial infarction [MI] for heart attack, cerebrovascular accident [CVA] for stroke, cholecystectomy for gallbladder operation) usually alienates clients and can close the door to further communication.

Occupation.   What a person does for a living gives a nurse a general idea of the person's skills, talents, interests, and economic status. However, stereotyping a person according to occupation can be misleading and should be avoided.

Factors Benefiting Interactions

In addition to the interpersonal and effective communication skills discussed above, it is helpful for the nurse to take into account several other factors that can affect the helping relationship. Controlling these factors helps promote what is referred to as a good **rapport**, which is a feeling of mutual trust experienced by persons in a satisfactory relationship (Fig 20-7).

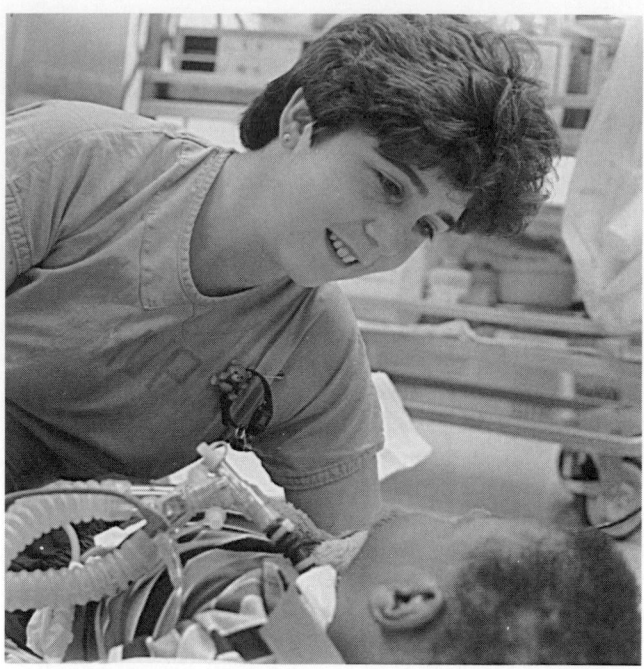

F I G U R E   20-7
This nurse and young client are sharing an enjoyable moment. The nurse has established rapport with the child, and they share a mutual trust. (Photo by Gates Rhodes, courtesy of the School of Nursing, University of Pennsylvania)

Specific Objectives.   Having a purpose for an interaction guides the nurse toward achieving a meaningful encounter with the client. One objective might be to do a quick head-to-toe physical assessment while greeting the client at the beginning of a shift. Another objective might be to discuss a client's feelings about newly diagnosed diabetes. The shortest encounter with a client can have an objective, even if it is as simple as conveying a feeling of friendliness to the client. Flexibility is essential at all times. Cues from the client should be followed to work toward meeting all needs.

Comfortable Environment.   A comfortable environment, in which both the client and the nurse are at ease, helps to promote interactions. Such items as suitable furniture, proper lighting, and a moderate temperature are important. Also, effective relationships are enhanced when the atmosphere is relaxed and unhurried. If the nurse seems preoccupied and "on the run," or if the client is ill at ease for fear of missing visitors or because of another commitment, communications are impaired.

Privacy.   It may not always be possible to carry out conversations with just the client and the nurse in a room. However, every effort should be made to provide sufficient privacy so that conversations cannot be overheard by others. Sometimes merely drawing the curtains around the bed or sitting in a corner of a waiting room or lounge can provide the sense of privacy so necessary for most interactions.

Confidentiality. The confidentiality with which the information is to be treated should be established with the client. The nurse should indicate with whom the information the client gives will be shared. The client should know about the right to specify the persons who may have access to the information. Failure to take this factor into account can be considered a breach of the client's right to privacy.

Client Focus. Communication in the nurse–client relationship should focus on the client and the client's needs, not on the nurse or an activity in which the nurse is engaged. Consider the following example, in which the nurse's comment focuses on the client and the client's needs:

> *Client:* I don't know why these injections scare me, but they do.
> *Nurse:* You are afraid of these injections?

Now consider this example, in which the nurse's comment focuses on a nursing activity:

> *Client:* I don't know why these injections scare me, but they do.
> *Nurse:* Let's hurry and get this shot done. Then you won't have time to worry.

Use of Nursing Observations. Observation, which involves both seeing and interpreting, is especially useful for validating information. For example, a nurse suspected that a client was afraid to hear the results of certain blood tests, but the client kept saying that the tests were not important. However, the nurse observed the client pacing back and forth in the corridor while appearing to be in deep thought. Observing the client's behavior helped validate the nurse's clue that the patient was possibly fearful, and the assertion that he was not concerned appeared to be a cover-up for true feelings.

Observation serves at least three important purposes:

- It helps the nurse become aware of nonverbal messages the client is sending.
- It serves as the primary source of information when a client is unable or unwilling to communicate verbally.
- It demonstrates caring and an interest in the client (Clients often recognize when a nurse is nonobservant and, rightly or wrongly, usually concludes that the nurse does not care).

Optimal Pacing. A nurse must consider the pace of any conversation or encounter with a client. For instance, it would not be very effective if the nurse rushes through a list of questions when obtaining a nursing history. It is more effective to let the client set the pace. The nurse can let the client know at the beginning of the interaction if time is limited. This way, the client will not feel that the nurse is rushing because of a lack of concern or personal interest.

Providing Personal Space. Perceptions of personal space vary from person to person. Nurses must try to determine each client's perception of personal space because invasion of one's personal space can evoke uncomfortable feelings. Nurses can assess a client's personal space through careful observations of nonverbal communication. For example, some persons like to be very close to the person with whom they are speaking. They may also use touch during their conversations and seem comfortable with others in close proximity. Others back away from close encounters or become nervous when their personal space is invaded. It is important for nurses to be sensitive to personal space so that their clients feel comfortable during interactions.

Avoiding Ineffective Techniques

Certain types of comments and questions should be avoided in most situations because they tend to impede effective communications.

Using Cliches. A cliche is a stereotyped, trite, or pat answer. Most cliches tend to indicate that there is no cause for anxiety or concern, or they offer false assurance. Their use tends to be interpreted as a lack of real interest in what has been said. The only purpose a cliche serves is to break the ice when conversation begins. For example, even though the common question, "How are you?" could start a conversation, it can cause a problem if the person has reason to suspect that the nurse is not sincerely interested in how the client feels. The following are some commonly used cliches that are usually best left unsaid, because they tend to impede effective communications:

> Everything will be all right.
> Don't worry. You will be just fine in another day or two.
> Your doctor knows best.
> Cheer up. Tomorrow is another day.

There is another type of cliche that makes a sweeping generalization that does not necessarily apply to a specific patient. It also tends to cut off communications and makes the person feel as though he is just another insignificant being. Consider these examples:

> Men tolerate pain poorly. That must be why you are complaining of such severe pain.
> Everybody is afraid of surgery. Why should you be any different?
> You teenagers are all alike. You aren't being cooperative because you want to defy authority.

Such comments rarely promote communication with clients to whom they are addressed.

Using Questions Requiring Only a "Yes" or "No" Answer. Questions that can be answered by simply saying "yes" or "no" tend to cut off discussion, even when the person might wish to go on. Consider the following question:

Nurse: Did you have a good day?

The question almost begs for a noncommital answer, which tells the nurse very little. A better way to comment is as follows:

Nurse: Tell me about the kind of day you have had.

Another pitfall is to pose a question to which the client can say "no" when his answer could present a problem. Consider the following question which a nurse asks a postoperative client:

Nurse: Are you ready to get out of bed?

By offering the client the chance to say "no," the nurse may have created difficulties if the client is to be out of bed.

There are times when questions that can be answered with "yes" or "no" are legitimate. The following are two examples:

Nurse: Did you take your insulin before breakfast this morning?

Nurse: Do you have pain when I move your arm this way?

The problem arises when the nurse is seeking more detailed information or when the question may create difficulty.

Using Questions Containing the Words "Why" and "How".

Questions using "why" and "how" tend to be intimidating. Consider the following two questions:

Nurse: Why were you not tired enough to sleep?

Nurse: How did you ever decide to go on a crash diet?

These two questions would be better stated as follows:

Nurse: What were you doing while you were unable to sleep?

Nurse: What things prompted you to decide to go on a crash diet?

Questions That Probe for Information.

Questions that appear to probe for information tend to cut off communication. Clients who are made to feel as though they are receiving the "third degree" become resentful and will usually stop talking and try to avoid further conversation. Although the nurse may feel more information is needed, it is better to follow the client's lead. Letting the client take the initiative allows the nurse to delve more deeply at a time when the client is ready. The person who says "Let's get to the bottom of this" is likely to destroy conversation unless the client is ready to face the real cause of the problem.

Using Leading Questions.

A leading question suggests a response that the speaker wishes to hear. Leading questions tend to produce answers that may please the nurse but are unlikely to encourage the client to respond without feeling intimidated. Consider the following two examples:

Nurse: You aren't going to smoke that cigarette, are you?

Nurse: You have been well cared for by your nurses, haven't you?

These questions beg the client to give an answer that pleases the nurse rather than to express thoughts.

Using Comments That Give Advice.

Giving the client advice often implies that the nurse knows what is best for the client and denies the client the right to make decisions and have feelings. Giving advice also tends to increase the client's dependence on health caregivers. However, advice does have a rightful place when it is requested, and the person giving the advice may have expert knowledge that the client does not.

Using Judgmental Comments.

Using judgmental comments tends to impose the nurse's standards on the client. Consider the comment of a nurse who noted that a young woman was crying:

Nurse: You aren't acting very grown-up. How do you think your husband would feel if he saw you crying like this?

The nurse judged the client as being immature, and the apparent hostility could end effective communication. A better comment in this situation might be as follows:

Nurse: I would like to help. Tell me what causes you to cry.

Consider the following exchange between a nurse and a client about to have surgery:

Client: I think I have a right to be afraid of this operation.

Nurse: Tell me what has made you afraid.

This client is likely to feel safe when allowed to express feelings without being judged.

Changing the Subject.

A quick way to stop conversation is by changing the subject. The client may be at a point of readiness to discuss something and can be expected to feel frustrated if put off by a change in the topic of conversation. The following example illustrates:

Client: When can I expect to be told about taking my own insulin?

Nurse: Let's discuss your diet now so that you will know what to eat when you get home. We can discuss your insulin some other time.

A nurse may also change the subject when feeling uncomfortable about the topic of conversation. For example, the client's needs are being met when the nurse allows the client to speak of impending death, thoughts of suicide, or a contemplated abortion. The nurse is ignoring the client when the subject is changed to meet the nurse's own needs.

Giving False Assurance.

It is easier and more pleasant to deal with positive outcomes than with negative ones. Through comments, the nurse may sometimes try to convince the client that things are going to turn out well even when knowing the chances are not good. False assurance leaves many clients with the impression that the nurse is not really interested in their problems. Cliches are very frequently used when a nurse gives a client false assurance.

Unintentionally impeding communication may sometimes occur. Being aware of it and explaining with an apology to the client will help promote a return to effective communication.

Communication in Special Circumstances

There are certain situations where special communication techniques are required for nurse–client interac-

tions. Several special circumstances are discussed in the boxed material entitled Recommended Guidelines for Nurses Communicating in Special Circumstances.

Documenting Communication

Any information required for the continual assessment of the client's needs and condition should be documented in the appropriate place, unless the information is of a confidential nature. This documentation serves to promote the continuity of care given by nurses and other health-care providers. Since one nurse cannot provide 24-hour coverage for clients, significant information must be passed on to others via nursing progress notes and care plans. Documentation is discussed in Chapter 18.

Recommended Guidelines for Nurses Communicating in Special Circumstances

Clients Who Are Visually Impaired
- Acknowledge your presence in the client's room.
- Identify yourself by name.
- Remember that the visually impaired client will be unable to pick up most nonverbal cues during communication. Speak in a normal tone of voice.
- Explain the reason for touching the client before doing so.
- Indicate to the client when the conversation has ended and when you are leaving the room.
- Keep a call light or bell within easy reach of the client.
- Orient the client to the sounds in the environment and to the arrangement of the room and its furnishings.

Clients Who Are Hearing Impaired
- Orient the client to your presence before initiating conversation. This may be done by gently touching the client or moving so you can be seen.
- Talk directly to the client while facing him. If the client is able to lip read, use simple sentences and speak in a quiet, natural manner and pace. Be aware of nonverbal communication.
- Do not chew gum or cover your mouth when talking with the client.
- Demonstrate or pantomime ideas you wish to express, as appropriate.
- Use sign language or finger spelling, as appropriate.

- Write any ideas that you cannot convey to the client in another manner.

An Unconscious Client
- Be careful of what is said in the client's presence. Hearing is believed to be the last sense lost, and therefore the unconscious client is often likely to hear even though there is no apparent response.
- Assume the client can hear you. Talk in a normal tone of voice about things you would ordinarily discuss.
- Speak with the client before touching. Remember that touch can be a very effective means of communication with the unconscious client.
- Keep environmental noises at as low a level as possible. This helps the client focus on the communication.

Clients Who Speak a Foreign Language
- Use an interpreter whenever possible.
- Use a dictionary that translates words from one language to another so that you can speak at least some words in the client's language.
- Speak in simple sentences and in a normal tone of voice.
- Demonstrate or pantomime ideas you wish to convey, as appropriate.
- Be aware of nonverbal communication. Remember that many nonverbal communication cues are universal.

KEY POINTS

- Nurses communicate thoughts, ideas, experiences, and facts to other nurses, clients, physicians and other health-care workers, and families as part of their promotion of wellness and prevention of illness.

- The communication process can be defined two ways: the process of sharing information or the process of generating and transmitting meanings. Communication, as a foundation of life, is a reciprocal process with simultaneous participation.

- People communicate one to one or in small or large groups by verbal and nonverbal communication.

- Nonverbal communication includes touch, eye contact, facial expressions, posture, gait, gestures, physical appearance, sounds, and silence.

- The ability of the nurse to communicate with others is essential to effective use of the nursing process.

- There are three phases to the helping relationship: orientation phase, working phase, and termination phase. A helping relationship is dynamic, purposeful and time limited, and involving one person in a dominant role.

- Effective communication techniques are conversational skills, listening skills, use of silence and touch, and interviewing techniques. The interview is a major tool for the collection of data in the assessment step of the nursing process.

- Interpersonal skills such as warmth and friendliness, openness, empathy, competence, and consideration of client variables are essential to a therapeutic nurse–client relationship.

- In addition to effective communication skills and interpersonal skills, it is helpful for the nurse to consider other factors that benefit the helping relationship. These include having specific objectives, comfortable environment, privacy, confidentiality, client focus, use of nursing observations, optimal pacing, and providing personal space.

- The nurse also needs to learn the ineffective techniques that need to be avoided.

- The nurse must develop communication skills for special circumstances, especially when the client is visually impaired, hearing impaired, unconscious, or speaks a foreign language.

BIBLIOGRAPHY

Carr RM: Sharing perfect communication. Nursing '82 12(3):136, 1982

Chalmers C: Talking to stroke patients. Nursing Times 81:41–42, August 7, 1985

Cormier LS et al: Interviewing and Helping Skills for Health Professionals. Monterey, CA, Wadsworth, 1984

De Blase R et al: Assistive hearing device aids patient-staff communication. Geriatric Nursing 6:223–224, July–August, 1985

Hansen AC: There's a person within! RN 47:31–32, April, 1984

Hein EC: Communication in Nursing Practice. Boston, Little, Brown & Co, 1980

LaMonica EL: Empathy can be learned. Nurse Educator 8:19–23, Summer, 1983

Levenstein A: Emotional versatility: A nursing skill. Nursing Management 17:60–62, February, 1986

Quinn JF: Therapeutic touch as energy exchange: Testing the theory. Advances in Nursing Science 6:42–49, January, 1984

Raucheisen ML: Therapeutic touch: Maybe there's something to it after all. RN 47:49–51, December, 1984

Teacher/Counselor

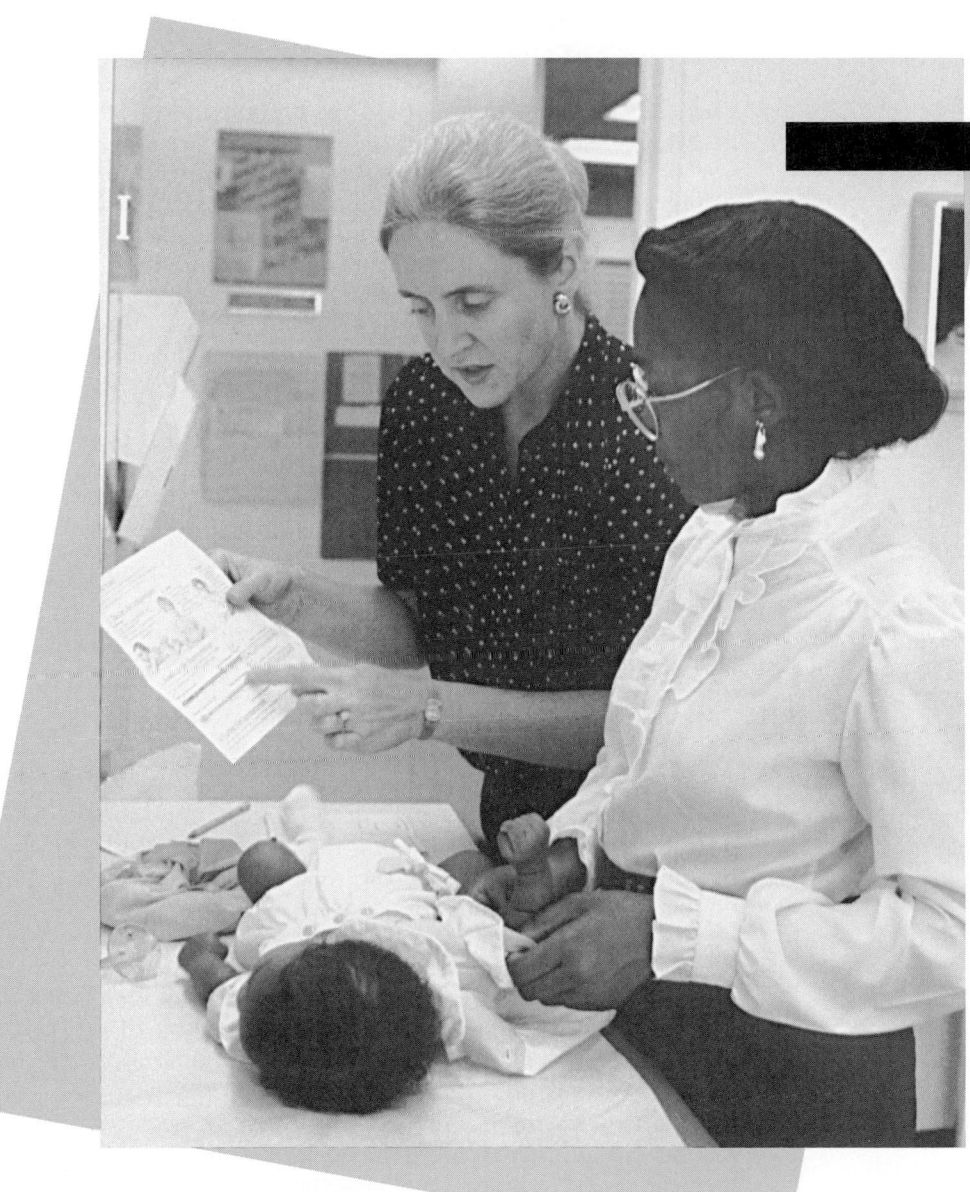

After studying this chapter, the learner should be able to

Define key terms used in the chapter.

Describe the teaching–learning process, including domains, developmental concerns, and specific principles.

Describe what factors should be assessed for the learning process.

Compose diagnoses for identified learning needs.

Explain how to create a teaching plan for a client.

Describe what is involved in implementing a teaching plan.

Name three methods for the evaluation of learning.

Explain what should be included in the documentation of the teaching–learning process.

Discuss the nurse's role as a counselor.

Summarize how the nursing process is used to assist clients in problem solving.

Describe how to use the counseling role to motivate a client toward health promotion.

KEY TERMS

affective learning
cognitive learning
contractual agreement
counseling
developmental crisis

formal teaching
informal teaching
learning
psychomotor learning
situational crisis
teaching

One of the means by which nurses apply communication skills is through the roles of teacher and counselor. They develop nursing skills by learning about the teaching–learning process and adapting the roles of teacher and counselor to nursing care. In fact, the nurse practice acts of most states, as well as the American Nurses' Association's (ANA) Standards of Nursing Practice, specify client teaching as a requirement for acceptable nursing care.

The role of counselor overlaps many other nursing roles. Because nurses have opportunities to counsel clients and their families during various nursing care activities, counseling techniques are a necessary part of each nurse's repertoire of skills.

Nurses alternate between the roles of teacher and learner. Sometimes they themselves are pursuing new knowledge, skills, and values. For example, nurses are encouraged and sometimes required to attend staff development or inservice classes pertaining to current and new practices. More and more nurses are also choosing to pursue further formal education for advanced degrees. At other times, nurses are facilitating learning in others.

Trends in health care have made the roles of teacher and counselor even more important than previously. With the current trend for shorter hospital stays, clients and their families need more extensive instructions for care in the home. Both hospital nurses and home health-care nurses must work together to ensure that clients receive the care they need. With effective methods of client teaching, both hospital care and home recovery are expedited.

Conversely, as the importance of teaching in the hospital increases, the time for teaching decreases. Consequently, the quality of the teaching must be improved. Nurses must learn how to teach effectively and efficiently. As with all skills, teaching skills develop as the nurse matures in professional roles.

The basic purpose of teaching and counseling is the pursuit of wellness. This differs for every client, depending on current status on the wellness–illness continuum. Nurses as teachers and counselors work to direct clients toward the wellness end of the continuum. If a client is in "good health," teaching and counseling are planned to continue present health practices, promoting wellness while also preventing illness. Practices that help prevent heart disease, cancer, and communicable diseases are stressed.

A client who is hospitalized for a disease such as rheumatoid arthritis is counseled on what nursing and medical care is required and how the client's compliance can help restore health. The client is taught how to perform exercises, take medications, and alter unhealthy practices related to the present illness. From there, the nurse works to counsel and teach the client how to cope with the altered functioning brought on by the rheumatoid arthritis.

THE NURSE AS TEACHER

Nurses assume the role of teacher when clients have identifiable learning needs. This teacher–student relationship is enhanced by the continuance of the helping relationship (see Chap 20), where mutual respect and trust have been established. The nurse further builds on this trust by sharing information the nurse and client have mutually identified as important. The client may ask for this information or the nurse may initiate teaching as the result of assessment and diagnostic factors.

Client teaching is approached most effectively by following the steps of the nursing process. The teaching–learning process and the nursing process are interdependent.

The Teaching–Learning Process

How the human brain stores and retrieves information has not yet been determined. However, it is known that the capacity to reason and to learn separates humans from all other creatures. A person plays the role of learner throughout life, although what is learned and the ways learning takes place change according to developmental stages. Basic understanding of the teaching–learning process aids nurses in developing their own teaching and learning skills. The process is summarized in the box entitled Steps in the Teaching–Learning Process.

Teaching can be defined as a planned method or series of methods used to help someone to learn. The person using these methods is referred to as the *teacher*. **Learning** is the process by which a person acquires or increases knowledge or changes behavior in a measureable way as a result of an experience. It is an internal experience that "denotes an integration of thoughts, ideas, theory, and experience—past and present" (La Monica, 1985).

Learning Domains

Learning can be divided into three domains: cognitive, affective, and psychomotor (Bloom, 1956). **Cognitive**

Steps in the Teaching–Learning Process

Assess the client's learning needs.
1. Use all appropriate sources of information.
2. Assess all factors that affect learning.
   - Age and developmental stage
   - Level of education
   - Past experiences with learning
   - Client's physical condition
   - Acuity of senses
   - Emotional health
   - Social and economic stability
   - Responsibility
   - Self-image and body image
   - Attitude toward learning
   - Motivation for learning
   - Culture
   - Communication skills
   - Language spoken
3. Utilize anticipatory guidance.

Diagnose the learning needs.
1. Be realistic.
2. Confirm with client or family, or both.

Compose a teaching plan
1. Formulate learner objectives.
   - Identify short-term and long-term objectives.
   - Prioritize.
   - Determine who should be included (*i.e.,* family members, significant others).
   - Include the client in planning.

2. Create a teaching plan.
   - Match content with appropriate teaching strategies and learner activities.
   - Schedule within limits of time constraints.
   - Decide on group versus individual teaching and formal versus informal.
   - Formulate a verbal or written contract with the client.

Implement the teaching plan.
1. Prepare the physical environment.
2. Gather all AV material and equipment.
3. Deliver content in organized manner using teaching strategies.
4. Be flexible.

Evaluate the teaching–learning.
1. Evaluate completion of learner objectives.
   - Client's comments
   - Direct questioning
   - Observational skills
   - Return demonstration
   - Postdischarge follow-ups
2. Evaluate teaching.
   - Self-evaluation
   - Client questionnaires
3. Revise plan of learner objectives not met.
   - Alter content and teaching strategies.
   - Employ motivational counseling if needed.
   - Reschedule teaching session(s).
4. Document the teaching–learning process.

C O M P U T E R   A P P L I C A T I O N S   I N   N U R S I N G

Computer-Assisted Instruction

Computer-assisted instruction (CAI) has proven to be a valuable tool in the teaching–learning process. Because learners actively interact with the computer, are self-directed, and receive immediate feedback, learning is facilitated and even fun. CAI can be used for all ages and in all types of teaching–learning situations. A brief list of topics, with content, is included as an example.

    The American Heart Association CPR course —Complete CPR course for training and certification

    Measuring blood pressure—Demonstrates the step-by-step procedure for students and the general public; uses animation to illustrate and reinforce material

Healthy living—Risk factor determination; ways to stay healthy; includes individualized testing

Wellness–illness continuum—Wellness–illness continuum and concepts; identifies risk factors

Postoperative care simulation—Experiences in decision making and documenting care of postoperative clients

Introduction to nursing diagnosis—Covers all areas necessary for understanding what a nursing diagnosis is, how to differentiate it from a medical diagnosis, and how to write a correctly formatted nursing diagnosis

learning involves the storing and recalling of new knowledge and information in the brain (example: the client states how salt affects blood pressure) (Flynn and Heffron, 1984). When a physical skill has been acquired, the change that has occurred is called **psychomotor learning** (example: the client demonstrates how to change dressings using clean technique). **Affective learning** includes changes in attitudes, values, and feelings (example: the client expresses her reactions to her mastectomy scar). These three areas of learning give the nurse–teacher a way of categorizing the learning that is planned for the client. This is explained later in this chapter under Planning for Learning.

Developmental Considerations

One of the major learning theories is Piaget's theory of intellectual development (see Chap 10). By understanding the way children and adolescents develop in learning abilities, a nurse can use this knowledge appropriately when teaching clients of all ages. For instance, if an 8-year-old girl must begin to take insulin every day, the nurses who are caring for her must recognize her limitations in understanding diabetes. Information should be simplified to provide only the most basic types of facts with accompanying concrete examples or demonstrations. At no time would discussion of the pathophysiology of diabetes be appropriate. She could be told that she needs a shot every day to keep her from "getting sick" or "feeling funny." She could be allowed to play with the syringes and to give shots to a doll.

    A nurse who is teaching a sexually active 16-year-old girl about contraceptive methods needs to assess whether the young client has reached the stage Piaget

refers to as *formal operations* (the ability to use logical reasoning to solve hypothetical problems). If the client's intellectual development is delayed and is still in the period of concrete operations (use of logical reasoning to solve concrete problems), she may be unable to think abstractly. That is, the adolescent may not perceive pregnancy as a real possibility and therefore may be unable to

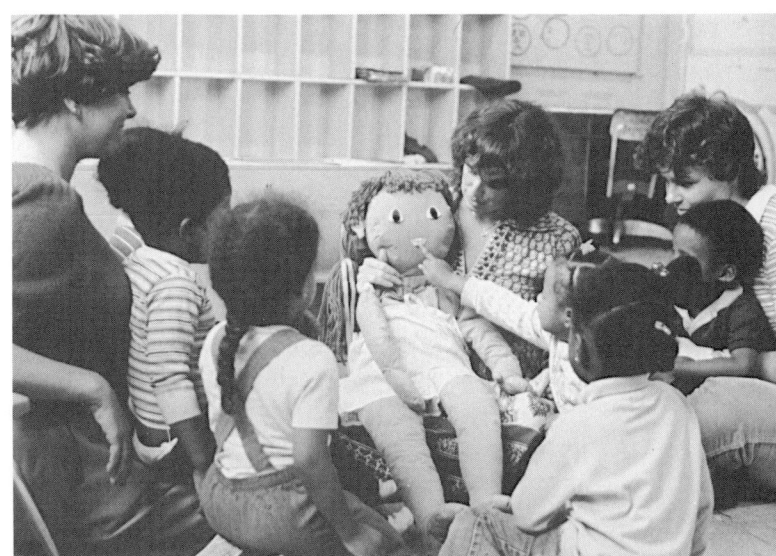

F I G U R E   21-1
The teaching approach must be appropriate to the developmental age of the learner. Small children respond well to teaching strategies that permit them to participate actively. (Photo by Gates Rhodes, courtesy of the School of Nursing, University of Pennsylvania)

understand the need for contraception. If so, the nurse can alter the teaching plan to include audiovisual teaching aids that explain the topic in concrete terms.

Some adults have not attained the formal operations stage. The nurse must be alert to this possibility and teach or re-teach material as needed. For example, an adult taking an antibiotic may not be able to grasp the importance of taking the capsules at the prescribed times to maintain the proper blood level for the best effect. If the nurse sees that the client is not complying with the schedule, the effectiveness of the teaching and learning should be evaluated. Showing a simple diagram of how erratic scheduling affects the body could give the concrete information the client needs to be motivated toward taking the antibiotic as ordered. In this way the teaching is altered to meet the client's intellectual development.

Motor development is also a concern in the teaching–learning process. The 8-year-old girl diagnosed with diabetes cannot be expected to learn to give her own insulin shots because she lacks the fine motor skills needed to manipulate the equipment for insulin injections. On the other hand, a 13-year-old could probably master the technique quickly.

Some other developmental concerns related to the teaching–learning process are emotional maturity and psychosocial development. Chronologic age does not guarantee maturity. It is possible that a 13-year-old client could respond more maturely to health teaching than a 30-year-old client. A great deal depends on how the client has learned to respond to changes and stressful events in the past.

Many of the developmental concerns related to teaching and learning are exaggerated by age. As people age, their personalities as well as their learning abilities change. Most psychologists who have studied the teaching–learning process have based their work on children and adolescents, since a large amount of learning takes place in the early years of life. The science of teaching is referred to as *pedagogy*. It generally refers to the teaching of children and adolescents. In recent years, the study of teaching adults has become popular. This has been given the name *andragogy* to emphasize that adults need to be taught differently. Much of the information taught to children will not be applied until they are older. Andragogy, however, has a problem-centered focus with immediate application of new information (Bille, 1981).

It is generally accepted that adults must believe they need to learn before they are willing to learn. Nurses often use their counseling skills (discussed later in this chapter) to motivate clients to participate in the teaching–learning process. Adults may need to be shown the necessity of learning new information, health practices, or skills.

Many adults are afraid of the teaching–learning process. This may be the result of a fear of failure, since many adults have not participated in formal educational programs since their school days. As aging occurs, adults often express a concern over memory loss, and being required to learn new material can be a threat to their feelings of self-worth. Consequently, the sensitivity and concern of the nurse in the helping relationship are the foundation for a nonthreatening learning environment for the adult client.

Adults may also resist learning because of preconceived ideas about the teaching–learning process and of what is expected of them. Honest and open communication provides the adult learner with a preview of what will be involved. Many adults willingly participate in the process once they have received the reassurance that they are partners in the teaching–learning process. Retaining some control over what is taught and how it is taught gives adult learners the sense of control they are accustomed to in their daily living.

Some elderly clients are especially fearful and threatened by the idea of having to learn new information. They may refer to the old adage, "you can't teach an old dog new tricks," often as a defensive attempt to avoid failure or change. Nurses find that a slower approach is needed when introducing new material so that older clients do not become discouraged or overwhelmed.

Principles of Teaching–Learning

Several basic principles of teaching–learning serve as guidelines for a nurse assuming the role of teacher. They can be applied in situations where the teaching–learning process is used to meet the needs of clients.

- The teaching–learning process is facilitated by the existence of a helping relationship.
- Nurse–teachers need to be able to communicate effectively with individuals, small groups, and, in some instances, large groups.
- Knowledge of the communication process is necessary for the assessment of verbal and nonverbal feedback.
- A thorough assessment of clients and the factors affecting learning helps to diagnose their learning needs accurately.
- The teaching–learning process is more effective when the client is included in the planning of learner objectives.
- The implementation of a teaching plan should include varied strategies for sensory stimulation since this is found to promote learning.
- Relating new learning material to clients' past life experiences is effective in helping to assimilate new knowledge.
- Careful attention should be paid to time constraints, scheduling, and the physical environment.
- Learner objectives provide the basis for evaluating whether learning has taken place.
- When learning objectives have not been met, careful reassessment provides ideas for changing the teaching plan for subsequent implementation.

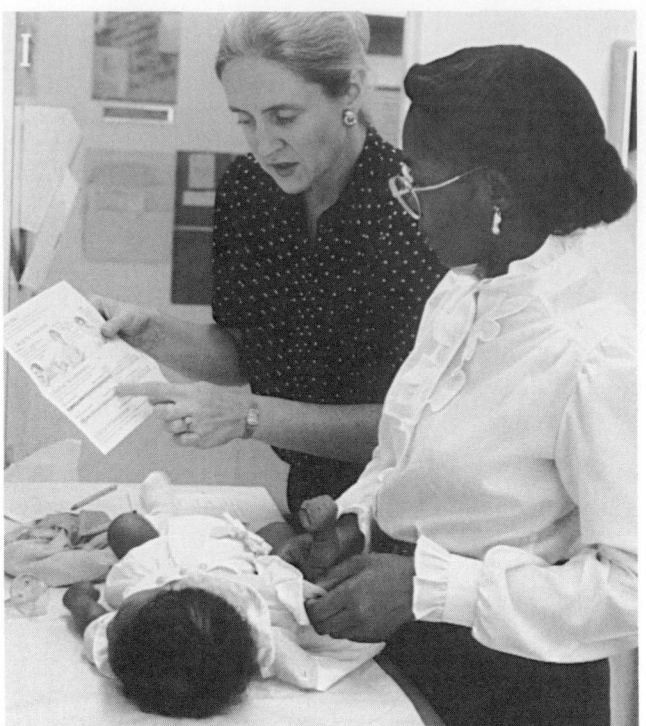

F I G U R E   21-2
The teaching–learning process is facilitated by the existence of a helping relationship and a teaching plan tailored to the client's learning needs. (Photo by Gates Rhodes, courtesy of the School of Nursing, University of Pennsylvania)

The remaining material on assessing, planning, implementing, and evaluating relates to these principles.

Assessing the Client's Learning Needs

Sources of Information

Clients are the best source of assessment information in most instances. By using effective interviewing techniques (see Chap 20) a nurse can obtain the data needed to identify the client's learning needs. Relevant information can be obtained before actually meeting the client by reviewing the client's past and present medical records. These records provide a history of medical problems as well as documentation of the nursing assessments, nursing physical examinations, and nursing interventions that have been performed.

The client's family and significant others are also valuable sources for assessment data. Sometimes the family or significant others are used for assessment data when the client is unable to communicate with the nurse because of health problems, language barriers, or impaired sensory functions. At other times, the family members or significant others may be the most appropriate source for certain information. For example, if seeking information pertaining to the use of salt in cooking, the nurse could speak with the person who prepares the meals in the client's home and then include that person in any teaching pertaining to food preparation for the client.

Assessment Factors Affecting Learning

Many factors influence the teaching–learning process. These factors need to be assessed for every client so that appropriate methods of teaching will be used. They include the following.

Developmental Considerations.   Knowledge of the intellectual, physiologic, and psychosocial developmental stages and tasks of each client is necessary for the selection of age-appropriate teaching methods. Knowing the client's chronologic age will give clues as to whether or not development is as expected. Delayed development in any area should be taken into consideration. Children generally take longer to learn because of their limited past experiences. Adults often learn more quickly because they can use previous knowledge to build upon (Murray and Zentner, 1985).

Level of Education.   Assessment of educational level helps prevent "talking down" to a client or teaching in a manner that is "above his head." A nurse who knows the client's intellectual abilities will effectively promote learning if this information is used.

Past Experiences With Learning.   Past educational experiences influence attitudes toward any future learning. An open-ended comment such as "Tell me about your experience with learning in high school" can encourage a client to express feelings about learning. A nurse needs to know if the client views education negatively so that this can be dealt with before teaching is attempted.

Client's Physical Condition.   It is imperative to consider how the client is feeling physically before teaching is begun. If a client has just had a cesarean section, she will not be ready to attend a class on baby care until she is physically comfortable enough to pay attention to the information presented.

Acuity of Senses.   It is necessary to assess the client's sensory abilities. The senses of sight, hearing, and touch are frequently used to teach the client; therefore, any alteration in these senses needs to be noted so that teaching can be planned appropriately.

Emotional Health.   The client needs to be in an emotional state conducive to learning before any formal teaching is done. If a client is in a state of crisis with a high level of anxiety, teaching would have to wait until the crisis is dealt with (see The Nurse as Counselor, later in this chapter). On the other hand, a moderate amount of anxiety can be a positive motivating factor for learning to take place (Bille, 1981). For example, a client who is

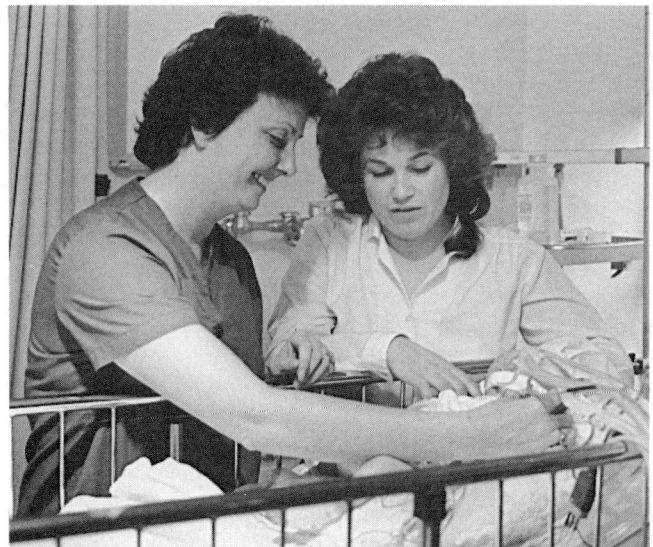

F I G U R E   21-3
Anxiety is sometimes a positive motivating factor for learning. An anxious mother of a sick child may be very receptive to the teaching of special techniques for the care of her child. (Photo by Gates Rhodes, courtesy of the School of Nursing, University of Pennsylvania)

moderately anxious about an elevated blood pressure will probably be attentive to the teaching done for the management of the condition.

Social/Economic Stability.   Hospitalization or absence from work because of illness can cause excessive stress and worry for clients. A nurse sensitive to the client's concerns will help the client deal with any social and economic problems before imposing the additional burden of learning new information and skills.

Responsibility.   A person needs to have a sense of responsibility to learn self-care or to take measures to prevent illness. A nurse can encourage the client to participate in self-care as well as in planning learning experiences. This helps promote the client's feelings of control over the hospital experience and that learning will facilitate recovery.

Self-Image and Body Image.   A person's self-perception has an effect on ability to learn. A poor self-image will carry over into all aspects of the helping relationship. The nurse may need to work on helping the client improve self-image before beginning to focus on learning needs. Body image should also be assessed. Unrealistic perceptions of the body and its functions need attention if effective learning about health problems is to occur.

Attitude Toward Learning.   It is difficult to measure precisely a person's attitude toward learning. However,

the nurse needs to get an idea of how the client feels about learning to improve health. By talking with the client about what types of learning experiences are available, a nurse can detect whether the client is interested in learning. Establishing a helping relationship may be the first step in altering a negative attitude toward learning.

Motivation for Learning.   It is generally accepted that a person must want to learn for teaching to be effective. All of the factors discussed have an effect on one's desire or motivation to learn. If assessment shows that a client is not motivated to learn about a particular topic, the nurse can discuss with the client what information is of interest. It is usually more successful to start with the client's interests and concerns. Then the nurse can continue to assess the client's readiness to learn the material needed for improving health. Maslow's hierarchy of needs (see Chap 7) can be used as a guideline to assess the client's present needs and motivations. The most basic physiologic needs should be met before teaching is attempted.

Culture.   A person's cultural background can have a profound effect on how the teaching–learning process is perceived. Some cultural groups value any type of education that will improve present conditions, whereas others may view any change or new practice as threatening. Stereotyping any person according to cultural background is harmful, and nurses need to recognize that each person comes from a unique family background with its own cultural pattern.

Communication Skills.   Since communication is a basic requirement for the teaching–learning process, any

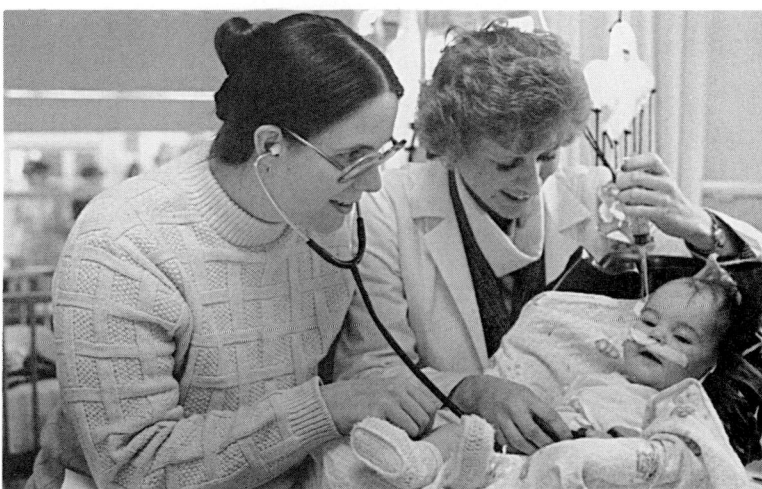

F I G U R E   21-4
A client or family member will have more motivation to learn if the nurse focuses on the learner's interests and concerns. (Photo by Gates Rhodes, courtesy of the School of Nursing, University of Pennsylvania)

problems in this area need to be thoroughly assessed. For instance, reading skills need to be assessed before a client is given a pamphlet on the management of heart disease.

Primary Language. When a client does not speak English as the primary language, the nurse must assess to what degree English is understood and spoken by the client. Hospitals often employ bilingual nurses and staff when many of their clients speak a particular language. Audiovisuals and printed materials are available to meet the needs of the non–English-speaking client.

Diagnosing the Client's Learning Needs

The identification of learning needs is similar to the identification of any health-care need. The learning need is always written as a nursing diagnosis. Diagnoses or problem statements approved by the North American Nursing Diagnosis Association can be used as a guide (see Chap 16). Nursing diagnoses related to learning needs include the following:

Knowledge deficit: low-sodium diet
Knowledge deficit: breastfeeding
Knowledge deficit: insulin administration
Knowledge deficit: normal 2-year-old development
Knowledge deficit: colostomy care
Knowledge deficit: stress management

The assessment data that led to the nursing diagnosis guide the nurse in determining what content needs to be included in the teaching plan.

In addition to identifying the client's learning needs, nurses need to assess their own knowledge base and teaching skills. Nurses cannot teach information and skills to clients if they themselves lack the information and skills to be taught. Often, knowing where to find information or an appropriate resource person is the first step in correcting one's own knowledge deficits.

Planning for Learning

Planning for learning involves the development of a teaching plan. Teaching plans are similar to nursing care plans since both follow the steps of the nursing process. One type of teaching plan is given in Table 21-1 as an example to follow during the remaining steps of the teaching–learning process.

Thoughtful planning for a client's learning experiences maximizes the client's chances for learning, while ensuring the most efficient use of the nurse's time and talents. Planning for teaching is similar to the planning phase of the nursing process. Learner objectives are developed for each diagnosis of a learning need. The nursing orders become the content, teaching strategy, and learner activity columns of the written plan. This phase

requires thought and creativity. The nurse's efforts are rewarded when the client successfully completes objectives at the end of the implementation phase.

When planning for learning, the nurse and client together must decide who should be included in the learning sessions. When the client is a young child, one or both parents may be the primary learners. When the client is an adult, a spouse or close friend who will be giving the care that is to be learned may be included. For instance, the person who does the household cooking is usually asked to be present for any nutritional teaching. If the client is very ill and unable to participate in the teaching–learning process, persons who will provide care at home must be taught procedures. Teaching plans are developed according to the needs of the person being taught.

A teaching plan can be prepared and used by one nurse or by several nurses. When two or more nurses plan and coordinate the implementation of the plan, it is referred to as *team teaching.* An advantage of team teaching is that the talents of more than one nurse are used to promote learning for the client.

The following factors should be considered during the formulation of any teaching plan:

Learner Objectives. Learner objectives are written in the same manner as the client goals of the nursing process (see Chap 17). When planning for the client's learning, it is best to determine first which of the three learning domains (cognitive, psychomotor, or affective) will be utilized when teaching. The nurse can then write learner objectives that reflect what learning is to take place. A well-constructed learner objective serves as a guide for planning evaluation methods.

Choosing the verb for a learner objective is probably the most difficult part when writing objectives. Yet, if chosen carefully, it makes the planning of content, teaching strategies, learner activities, and evaluation methods easier. See the list of verbs commonly used for the three learning domains.

The number of objectives needed for each diagnosis varies. It is better to have several specific objectives than to try to use only one or two broad objectives. Many nurses state one long-term objective for each diagnosis followed by several specific objectives. For example a long-term objective for the sample teaching plan could be "the client will be able to breastfeed her infant as long as desired without sore nipples." This could be met in two weeks or two years! Long-term objectives are general statements. On the other hand, the objectives written in the learner objective column of the sample teaching plan (Table 21-1) are specific behaviors to be accomplished within a short period of time.

Clients and appropriate family members or significant others should be included in the planning of learner objectives. Including them in determining what learning is to take place can usually be effective in assuring compliance.

T A B L E   21-1
Sample Teaching Plan
Diagnosis: Knowledge deficit: Nipple care related to inexperience with breastfeeding
Signs and Symptoms—Complains of sore nipples; first baby; 1 day after delivery; fair skin with freckles; no redness or cracking yet; no prenatal preparation

Learner Objective	Met	Content	Teaching Strategy	Learner Activity
The client		Prevention and care of sore nipples		
[morning session] Begins protective measures immediately (psychomotor)	✓ 8/10/86 L.S.	Protective measures 1. Avoid soap 2. Exposure to air and sunlight 3. Apply lanolin or vegetable oil 4. Avoid plastic liners in bra or bra pads	Lecture with Discussion AV: Flip chart on breastfeeding	Read handout "Nipple Care"
Explains why feedings should be shorter and more frequent (cognitive)	✓ 8/10/86 L.S.	Preparation for breastfeeding 1. Feed baby more frequently. • Every two hours during day • Arrange for rooming in 2. Nipple roll before the feeding.	Discussion AV: Flip chart on breastfeeding	Read handout "Sore Nipples"
Demonstrates nipple roling (psychomotor)	✓ 8/10/86 L.S.			
[10 AM session]			Return demonstration	
Demonstrates correct feeding technique and after care (psychomotor)	✓ 8/10/86 L.S.	Breastfeeding the baby 1. Baby starts on least sore side 2. Holding the breast properly 3. Getting baby onto areolar area 4. Positioning properly 5. Change position for each feeding 6. Removing baby from breast	Discovery: Guide through each step; assist as necessary.	Read handout "Positioning baby for Breastfeeding"
Describes a feeling of improved comfort with each feeding (affective)	✓ 8/10/86 L.S.	After the feeding 1. Air dry 2. Inspect for open or cracked areas 3. Apply lanolin or vegetable oil	Discovery	Borrow book(s) on breastfeeding from client's reference shelf.
[afternoon session]				
Explains the importance of good nutrition and rest at home (affective) Lists the signs of thrush (cognitive)	✓ 8/10/86 L.S.	Considerations for home 1. "Demand" feedings 2. Good nutrition 3. Adequate rest 4. Signs and symptoms of thrush	Lecture with discussion AV: Poster	Refer to handouts at home as needed. Call the maternity department's information number for any questions.

Content. Once the learner objectives are completed, the nurse needs to decide what information the client will need to complete those objectives successfully. This information is the "content" of the teaching plan. It is usually necessary to research the area to be taught to determine what information exists concerning the topic. Books, articles, and manuals are available in many nursing units for the nurse's research needs. It is becoming more common to have preorganized content available for a variety of common health-teaching topics, thus shortening the required research time.

Nurses are concerned about what clients need to know about such topics as illness, procedures, medications, and surgeries. "How much should they know?" is a common topic for debate. It has been found that clients benefit from explanations of the physical sensations they will experience during a procedure. They appreciate advanced knowledge of what they will feel, taste, hear, see,

Verbs That Can Be Used When Writing Learner Objectives

Cognitive Domain	Affective Domain	Psychomotor Domain
categorizes	answers	adapts
compares	chooses	arranges
composes	defends	assembles
defines	discusses	begins
describes	displays	changes
designs	forms	constructs
differentiates	gives	creates
explains	helps	manipulates
gives examples	initiates	moves
identifies	joins	organizes
labels	justifies	rearranges
lists	relates	shows
names	revises	starts
prepares	selects	works
plans	shares	
solves	uses	
states		
summarizes		
writes		

and smell (Redman, 1984). The sample teaching plan in Table 21-1 gives an example of content included for one client's learning needs.

Content explaining *why* certain treatments and medications are needed is included in a teaching plan. Information on the prevention of illness or its complications should also be covered. Compliance with the nursing and medical plans is a major objective for much of the health teaching done; it has been found that persons who have a basic understanding of their illness and its treatment will usually comply with the treatment more readily than those who do not understand their illness (Bille, 1981).

Time Constraints. Time constraints must be considered when planning for the client's learning. A problem for nurses is finding time to meet the client's learning needs. Priorities must be set so that essential content is taught thoroughly. Less important content is taught last so that the more important learner objectives are met within the time available. If time permits, the remaining content can be addressed. Note that in the sample teaching plan in Table 21-1, the client will be taught measures to use immediately.

To meet time constraints, nurses often plan together. Teamwork and cooperation allow deadlines to be met. If teaching must continue beyond the hospitalization, home visit, or clinic visit, the nurse can schedule further learning opportunities through outpatient programs or referrals to community-based programs. Home health-care nurses often receive referrals from hospital

nurses to continue teaching begun during a client's hospitalization. Discharge planning needs to be started early to ensure continuity of teaching.

Scheduling. It is better to plan for shorter, more frequent teaching sessions than for one or two longer sessions. Short sessions allow the client to "digest" the new material and prevent the client from becoming too tired or uncomfortable because of the current health problem. Sessions of 15 to 30 minutes are generally well tolerated. Usually, the more formal classroom programs last for more than an hour. In such cases, breaks should be provided after every 50 minutes of class time. As with all nursing care, the client should be included in planning for the time and frequency of lessons.

Group vs Individual Teaching. There are several factors to consider when choosing the type of setting for the client. Some learner objectives are met more readily in a one-to-one encounter, whereas others are achieved more easily in a group. For example, the objective "the client will change the dressing using sterile technique," would be evaluated during a private session with the nurse. The objective "the client will discuss feelings about returning home after a heart attack" might be met more easily in a group discussion with other clients with similar feelings to express.

The nurse should consult the client concerning preferences for group or individual instruction when such a choice is possible. Some people become extremely anxious in group settings, whereas others prefer to learn with others. In addition, the health status of the client can prevent attendance in a classroom setting, thus requiring bedside instruction. On the other hand, a client who is hospitalized may find the change of scenery beneficial to learning.

Certain topics are learned well in group settings, particularly where a sense of comradeship is beneficial. For instance, persons who are trying to lose weight for health reasons generally find that learning dietary and nutritional information with other overweight clients is less threatening and can actually be enjoyable. Other material, especially information of a personal nature, may be discussed more effectively with the nurse only.

Formal vs Informal Teaching.   Most nurse–client interactions result in **informal teaching** being done by the nurse. These unplanned teaching sessions are often very effective since they deal with the client's immediate learning needs and concerns. Informal teaching often leads to additional, planned, formal sessions. **Formal teaching** refers to the planned teaching done to fulfill learner objectives. Both forms are effective when the nurse uses them appropriately.

Contractual Agreements.   The use of contracts between nurses and clients is becoming a common practice in many health-care settings. Usually the contracts are rather informal and not legally binding. A **contractual agreement** is a pact between two persons made for the achievement of mutually set goals. When teaching a client, such an agreement can serve to motivate both the client and the nurse to do what is necessary to attain the client's learning objectives. The agreement serves to

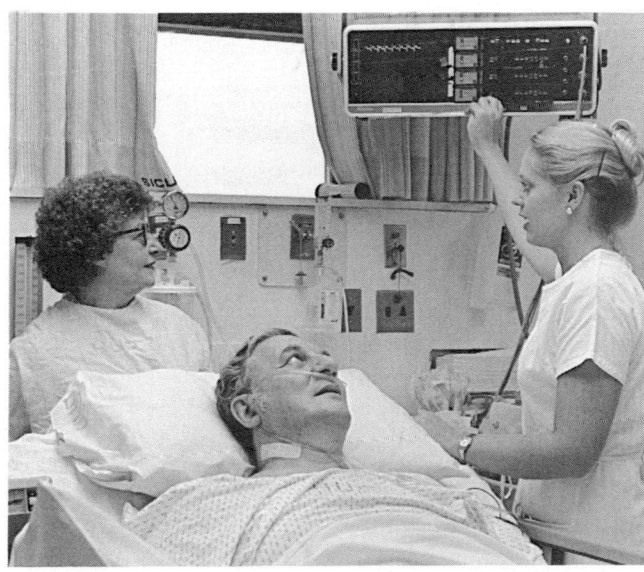

F I G U R E   21-5
Informal teaching occurs in most nursing interactions with the client and family. (Photo by Gates Rhodes, courtesy of the School of Nursing, University of Pennsylvania)

Example of a Contractual Agreement Between a Nurse and a Client

I will participate in the learning activities needed to help me learn about my low-salt diet. During my hospital stay, I will attend the class on low salt diets, read the materials given to me, and ask questions as I need to. I will work with S. Moore, R.N., to plan my meals and food preparation at home. If I need help when I get home, I will contact S. Moore.

Jim Mall

I will provide Jim Mall with the experiences needed for him to follow his low salt-diet accurately.

S. Moore R.N.

point out the responsibilities of both the teacher and the learner, thus emphasizing the importance of the mutual commitment. An example of a contractual agreement is given in the accompanying box. It is not necessary for the contract to be typed; a handwritten agreement is acceptable. Informal oral contracts are also possible. In fact, many teaching–learning contracts are verbal agreements between nurses and their clients regarding how and when learner objectives will be met. Contracts should be viewed as aids to learning and should never be intimidating.

Teaching Strategies.   The techniques used by a teacher to promote learning are referred to as *teaching strategies.* Teaching strategies are planned in advance of the actual teaching sessions so that every content area can be matched with an effective teaching technique. The strategies chosen depend on the teacher's familiarity with the method, the availability of teaching aids such as audiovisuals and printed materials, the facilities for using audiovisuals, and factors in the client's learning, such as, educational level and cultural background. The nurse must also consider age-appropriate methods for her client. For example, a 10-year-old will be receptive to a comic book on personal safety, whereas an adult could learn similar material by discussing the safety measures with the nurse.

Experts in the field of education generally agree that the use of a variety of teaching strategies aids learning. In addition, some methods are better suited to certain learning objectives. Table 21-2 gives suggested teaching strategies for the three learning domains. The sample teaching plan in Table 21-1 shows how teaching strategies are varied for the learner objectives and content of that particular plan. Again, the nurse is free to use creativity in choosing what methods to use. Care should be taken to stimulate as many of the client's senses as possi-

T A B L E   21-2
Suggested Teaching Strategies for the Three Learning Domains

Cognitive Domain	Affective Domain	Psychomotor Domain
Lecture/discussion	Role modeling	Demonstration
Panel discussion	Discussion	Discovery
Discovery	Panel discussion	Audiovisual materials
Audiovisual materials	Audiovisual materials	Printed materials
Printed materials	Role playing	
Programmed instruction	Printed materials	
Computer-instructional programs		

ble when teaching. Seeing, hearing, and touching are superior to hearing alone.

Some common teaching strategies with short descriptions of each follow.

Role Modeling.   The old saying "actions speak louder than words" explains why this strategy is effective. Nurses are watched closely by their clients and this can be used by the nurse to affect a client's behavior positively. For example, nurses who were formerly smokers can be role models for clients trying to quit smoking for health reasons.

Lecture.   In the purest sense, a lecture is a presentation of information by the teacher to the student(s). However, to be more effective, lectures usually include question-and-answer periods to allow for clarification of the material given. This strategy is often used to deliver information to a large group of clients. It is rarely used for individual instruction, without the addition of other strategies.

Discussion.   Discussion involves the two-way exchange of information, ideas, and feelings between the teacher and the student(s). It is a very effective method when used by a nurse who is comfortable with leading a group and knowledgeable in group process (see Chap 22). Also, it can be a very effective method for one-on-one instruction.

Panel Discussion.   This involves the presentation of information by two or more persons. Panel discussions can be used to impart factual material but are also effective for sharing experiences and emotions. Debates are a form of panel discussion and allow for all aspects of a topic to be exposed.

Demonstration.   Demonstration of techniques, procedures, exercises, and the use of special equipment, combined with a lecture and discussion, is an effective strategy. Evaluation of the client's learning can be done by a return demonstration. Practice sessions are often

included for the learner. Models of body parts or practice models such as a resuscitation model are frequently used. When teaching breast self-examinations, the use of a breast model allows the learner actually to feel different types of lumps commonly found in breast tissue. Childbirth educators usually demonstrate the birth of a baby by using a pelvic model, knitted uterus, and a baby doll.

Discovery.   In discovery learning, the nurse presents a problem or situation to the client or group of clients and then guides the client(s) in discovering the solution or approach. Discussion of other possible approaches and solutions can follow the client's own solutions. This is a good method for teaching problem-solving techniques and independent thinking. For instance,

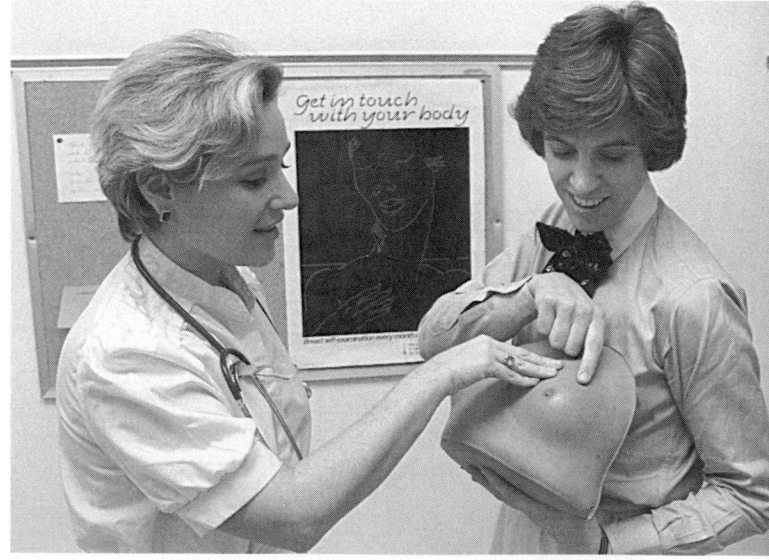

F I G U R E   21-6
Demonstration of techniques using practice models is a very effective teaching strategy. Here, a nurse is increasing her own self-care knowledge and learning use of the model for teaching others self-care. (Photo by Don Walker, courtesy of Thomas Jefferson University)

a nurse could give a group of diabetic clients a short description of a situation that includes signs and symptoms. The clients as a group would decide if the signs and symptoms indicate hypoglycemia (low blood sugar) or hyperglycemia (high blood sugar) and would choose what measures to take. Next, the nurse could discuss the group decision as a further learning experience. Even if the clients chose a poor resolution, the nurse can turn it into an effective learning experience.

Role Playing. This strategy gives the learner a chance to experience, relive, or anticipate an event. The nurse explains the scenerio and then allows the client to play out the scene with the teacher or with one or more clients. Role playing can be used to work through emotional traumas or to plan for possible traumas. For example, a nurse could help a teenage girl prepare herself to tell her mother about her pregnancy by letting the girl play her mother while the nurse plays the girl. This will help the client rehearse what she wants to say and anticipate the emotional atmosphere that she will experience. Role playing is a very good strategy for adults as well as for children. Puppets and dolls can be provided for young children to help express negative feelings that have resulted from hospitalization and traumatic procedures.

Audiovisual Materials. The use of audiovisual (AV) materials can be an effective teaching and learning tool. AVs include films, filmstrips with or without audiotapes, slides, television programs, videotapes, overhead transparencies, flip charts, posters, and diagrams. Their use is a popular and effective teaching strategy when combined with a lecture or discussion. AVs should never be the sole source of learning for the client. It is an accepted practice to allow the client to view an AV alone but to precede and follow it with a discussion of the material.

Printed Material. The use of printed material depends on the nurse's access to it. Many nurses have been involved in the writing of materials for distribution to clients. Writing pamphlets, instruction sheets, books, and comic books for health teaching can be rewarding as well as useful. As with AV materials, printed materials are usually used in conjunction with other strategies. Use of specially prepared games is a popular and fun way for clients to learn. Games can be relatively easy to make. For instance, cards with pictures of foods can be used to develop a nutritional instruction game.

Programmed Instruction. Most programmed instruction books or booklets are prepared so that a student can use them independently of a teacher. However, educators generally agree that the teacher needs to spend time with the student before and after the completion of the program to clarify information, answer questions, and provide the personal touch so needed for a learner's motivation. Since this is a self-paced strategy, it can be beneficial for many learners.

Computer-Instructional Programs. The use of computer programs for teaching is still in its infancy but the future possibilities are unlimited. Perhaps someday individual terminals will be available in each client's room so that instruction will be available at any time. This method can even be personalized by programming the computer to address the learner by name and to give positive feedback when appropriate. Currently, this method is not widely used because of limited access. This technique is only acceptable when personal, human attention is also available.

Learning Activities

While planning teaching strategies, the nurse also decides what learning activities the client is to do independently. There are many ways that the client can preview new material or reinforce what has already been taught. Use of printed material, audiovisual materials, and programmed instructions is often assigned in the learning activity column of the teaching plan. This column is used

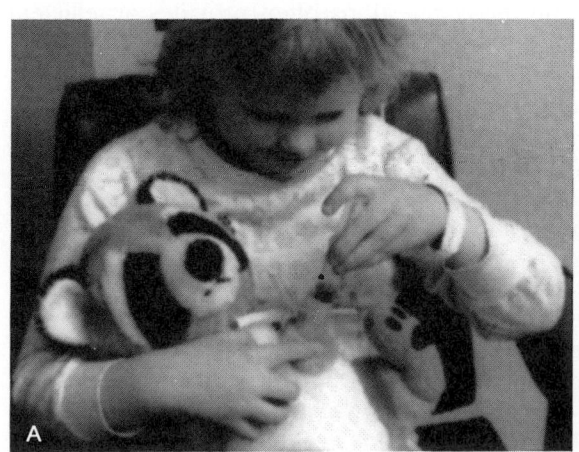
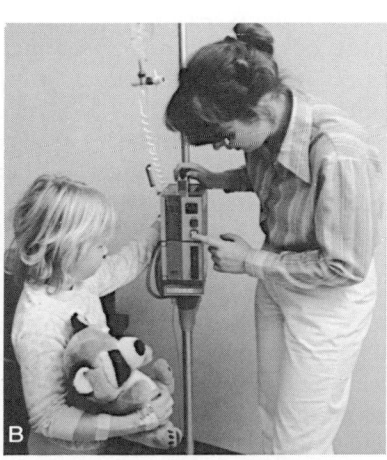

FIGURE 21-7
The nurse preparing a child for an IV allows the child to role play with her stuffed toy and a syringe, and demonstrates how the infusion control monitor works.

to guide the client in learning activities that can be done before, between, and after planned learning sessions.

Implementing the Teaching Plan

Implementing the teaching plan requires use of interpersonal skills as well as effective communication techniques. Teaching the client can be a major part of the working phase of the helping relationship (see Chap 20). The nurse must continually observe the client for additional assessment data that could alter the original teaching plan. This requires skill in adapting and reorganizing the teaching plan.

The nurse can facilitate learning in the client by continuing a warm and accepting approach. The nurse's attitude has more effect on the client than any other factor. A condescending attitude must be avoided. It is always best to avoid technical and medical terms unless the client has a background in this area. A nonthreatening teaching–learning atmosphere allows learning to occur.

The physical environment is another important consideration when implementing the teaching plan. Some preplanning may be needed to ensure adequate space, comfortable chairs, adequate lighting, and good ventilation. Privacy is also important, as is an environment free of distractions and interruptions.

During the implementation phase, the client as a learner must fulfill certain role functions. To avoid any misunderstandings, it is helpful to review the contractual agreement before implementing the teaching plan. The client is expected to listen, observe, and attempt to understand what is being taught.

Some persons are very uncomfortable in the role of learner and the nurse must assess this problem so that the client can be assisted to assume the role more easily. If special techniques or procedures must be learned (*i.e.,* colostomy care, self-injections, or eye medication instillations), the nurse can assure the client that it takes time and practice before anyone can perform new skills confidently.

The implementation phase may be as short as a few minutes, or the sessions may extend over a period of days, weeks, or months, depending on what is being taught and to whom. It can be as simple as learning to check a pulse rate or as complex as cardiopulmonary resuscitation. As with all nursing care activities, teaching involves total concentration on the client.

The nurse needs to be prepared and organized before implementing the teaching plan. All teaching aids (*i.e.,* posters, films, printed materials) should be gathered and organized before the actual teaching session. A disorganized teacher distracts the learner and has negative effect on the learning. If a procedure or skill is being taught, it is important to proceed in the correct sequence so that the client does not become confused.

Finally, an important nursing responsibility is to make each learning session interesting and enjoyable for the client. This is facilitated by an enthusiastic and positive attitude. In addition, the nurse can make learning fun through the creative use of planned teaching strategies. If the nurse approaches teaching positively, the client is more likely to approach learning in a similar way.

Evaluating Teaching–Learning

Evaluating Learning

It cannot be assumed that learning has taken place without some type of proof or feedback. The key to evaluation is the learner objectives written in the teaching plan (see Table 21-1) describing what behaviors to measure. Methods for obtaining feedback of learning are discussed below.

Methods of Evaluation.   Methods of evaluation vary. For instance, cognitive domain learning may be evaluated through oral questioning; affective domain through the client's response; and psychomotor domain by return demonstration. Consider the following learner objective from the cognitive domain: "the client will be able to describe what a blood pressure reading represents." To evaluate this, the nurse could say to the client, "Tell me what this blood pressure reading means to you." The client then has a chance to talk about the current reading while the nurse evaluates the client's understanding of it.

Sometimes the nurse can use observational skills to determine if the client is utilizing the material learned. For example, observing what the client has ordered for lunch tells the nurse if dietary lessons are being put into practice. The nurse depends on observation when evaluating the client's psychomotor skills. The nurse observes any new technique or skill that the client demonstrates to determine if it is performed satisfactorily.

The client's comments can be used to decide whether learner objectives have been met. Sometimes a client verbalizes understanding of information taught, yet avoids further discussion of the topic. In such instances, the use of effective communication techniques when reintroducing the topic at a later time might provide the evaluation data needed.

Using direct questions often provides an efficient method of evaluating learner objectives. The nurse simply asks the client a question to elicit a response that reflects the client's knowledge or lack of knowledge concerning a topic. This can also be used to evaluate the client's affective learning.

A return demonstration is an excellent evaluative method for the psychomotor domain. Letting the client change his own dressing provides the nurse with concrete evidence of satisfactory or unsatisfactory performance of the procedure. Care must be taken to promote a nonstressful environment for the client's return demonstration.

Evaluation of learning may continue once the client has returned home. Home health-care nurses may evalu-

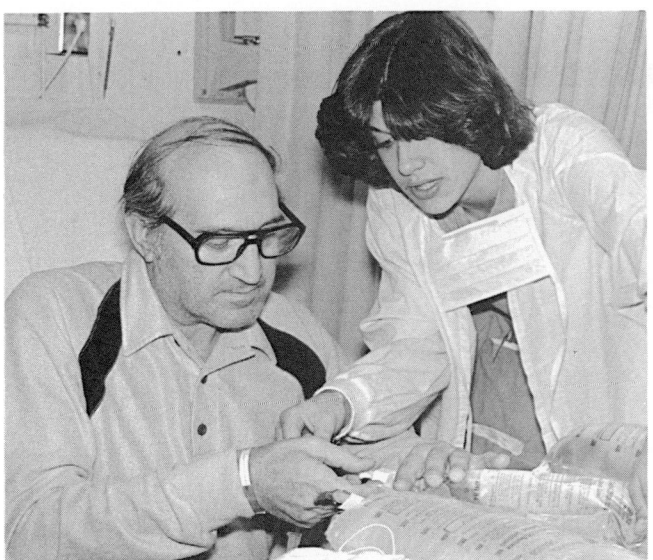

FIGURE 21-8
A return demonstration is an excellent method of evaluating learning. The client is demonstrating to himself and to the nurse that he is prepared to manage his peritoneal dialysis at home. (Photo by Gates Rhodes, courtesy of the School of Nursing, University of Pennsylvania)

ate what was taught to the client in the hospital as well as what is being taught during home visits. Hospital nurses often check with family members or significant others after discharge to evaluate whether or not learner objectives have been met. Short-term objectives are usually evaluated while the client is still hospitalized.

Evaluating Teaching

Nurses need evaluation of their teaching to capitalize on strengths and work on improving weaknesses. As all nursing roles, teaching requires a great deal of practice and experience. Even nurse educators agree that they are always learning better ways to promote learning in students. It is important to avoid becoming discouraged when evaluations of teaching are less than perfect.

It is best to evaluate one's own teaching effectiveness immediately after each session. This involves a quick review of how the nurse/teacher feels the implementation of the plan went. Mentally noting both the strengths and weaknesses of the teaching session helps the nurse when planning for subsequent sessions.

Nurses can also seek feedback from clients. A simple questionnaire can be used at the end of each teaching session or after discharge to evoke the client's perception of the nurse's teaching effectiveness. The questionnaire may be a standardized form used throughout the hospital or agency or a teacher-made questionnaire. If it is an objective format requiring only circles or checkmarks as answers, space should be provided for comments. The most honest and helpful evaluations are

often those that are anonymous. Anonymity, however, is not necessary and can sometimes bring forth harsh and nonproductive evaluations.

Revisions

During evaluation, nurses and clients may establish that revisions are needed in the teaching plan. A reassessment may indicate that there were client factors not considered in the original plan. Adjustments may be made accordingly to meet the client's needs. Often, the selection of a different teaching strategy is all that is needed for a client to achieve learner objectives successfully. Revision is a natural part of the teaching–learning process and should not be viewed negatively.

Neither the nurse nor the client has failed when an objective is not met. Most objectives can be met with a change in approach, but it should be noted that learner objectives are sometimes unrealistic. Further assessment by the nurse may reveal that the content may be too complex or the time too short for successful achievement.

Documenting

Since teaching is such an important nursing responsibility, it must be documented in the client's record. Documentation of the teaching–learning process includes a summary of the learning need, the plan, the implementation of the plan, and the evaluation results. The evaluative statement is crucial and must show whether the client has displayed concrete evidence that learning has taken place. If the desired learning has not taken place, the nurse's notes should include how the problem was resolved. It is not sufficient to document only what was taught. The charting has to show evidence that the client or significant other has learned the material taught (Dobberstein, 1986). See Table 21-3 for an example of documentation.

THE NURSE AS COUNSELOR

Counseling can be defined as giving guidance to a client; it also includes assisting a client in problem solving. Often family members or significant others are included in the counseling sessions. Everyone participating must feel comfortable in the situation and surroundings.

The interpersonal skills of warmth, friendliness, openness, and empathy are necessary ingredients for successful counseling. The effective counselor needs to be a caring individual. Caring is based on humanistic philosophy (Watson, 1979), which is the core of nursing practice. A humanistic approach to counseling utilizes the caring process in helping the client strive toward the greatest health potential. Caring is important to all nursing roles but is fundamental in the counseling role.

T A B L E   21-3
Example of Documentation to Meet a Learning Need

Date	Problem-Oriented Progress Note
8/10/86	#2 New problem—Knowledge deficit: nipple care
	S —Client stated that her nipples were sore during and after her newborn's first feeding.
	O—First day postpartum; client is fair skinned with freckles; no reddened areas, no cracking yet; no nipple preparation prior to delivery
	A —At high risk to develop cracked, open areas. Client lacks experience and knowledge of preventive measures.
	P —Develop teaching plan for nipple care.
	I —Teaching plan implemented
	E —Client was able to meet all of the objectives satisfactorily as recorded on the teaching plan. She is now doing protective and preparatory care for her nipples. When breastfeeding, she is using the correct feeding technique with good after care. She states that her nipples are no longer sore, and she is able to explain what she should do when she goes home.
	R —None needed, but reinforcement of content will be continued.
	L. Sweeney, R.N.

Counseling involves listening carefully to the questions, concerns, demands, and complaints of the client or family and then responding in an effective and facilitative manner. Appropriate responses may be difficult for the nurse to give at first but practice will help to develop these skills. Effective communication techniques (see Chap 20) are utilized during counseling sessions.

The three types of counseling discussed here are short-term, long-term, and motivational. There are times when specialized counseling by other health-care professionals (*i.e.,* psychologist or social worker) is needed for the client. A referral is warranted in such circumstances.

Short-Term Counseling

Short-term counseling focuses on the immediate problem or concern of the client or family. It can be a relatively minor concern or a major crisis, but whatever the situation, it needs immediate attention.

In counseling situations, the nurse does not tell the client what to do to solve the problem but instead assists and guides problem solving or decision making. Many persons lack the knowledge and skills to approach a problem systematically. This is where the teaching and counseling roles can be combined to help the client solve the dilemma successfully.

The nursing process becomes an essential tool for the nurse in guiding and teaching the client. Nurses are educated to approach all nursing situations in a logical, systematic way. In a crisis situation, whether minor or major, the nurse can share problem-solving abilities with the client. The nursing process was used to organize the nurse–client counseling situation described in the accompanying box.

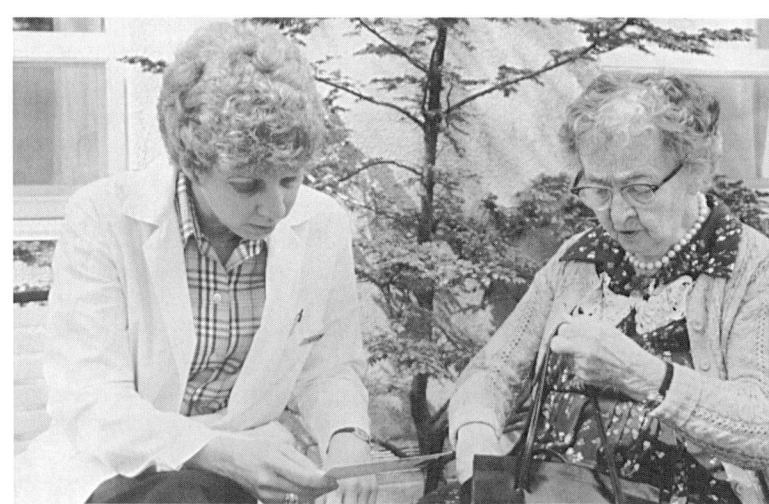

F I G U R E   21-9
Short-term counseling focuses on an immediate concern of the client. (Photo by Gates Rhodes, courtesy of the School of Nursing, University of Pennsylvania)

An example of when short-term counseling could be used is during a **situational crisis**, which occurs when a client faces an event or situation that causes a disruption in life. For example, a client in the hospital finds out that his wife has been involved in a car accident. His wife only received a few scratches but their only car is demolished. His nurse is in an excellent position to help him decide what can be done to solve this situational crisis. The nurse can guide the client in solving the travel, financial, and emotional difficulties that arise as a result of the accident. This holistic approach is especially necessary since the crisis could affect the client's recovery adversely.

Long-Term Counseling

Counseling is considered long-term when it extends over a prolonged period of time. A client may need the counsel of the nurse for daily, weekly, or monthly inter-vals. A client experiencing a developmental crisis may need long-term counseling. A **developmental crisis** can occur when a person is going through a developmental stage or passage. For example, many women going through menopause need the assistance of a nurse when adjusting to the changes they experience. Nurses can lead support groups for the purpose of group counseling.

Another example of long-term counseling occurs when a nurse counsels a client who is breastfeeding. The nurse may give assistance and guidance until the baby is weaned, which could be over a period of 2 to 3 years. This type of counseling is often done over the telephone, which saves the client the inconvenience of traveling to meet with the nurse.

Many hospital specialty units provide clients with a telephone number to call for counseling after discharge. Clients are often relieved to know they can call to talk to a nurse at any time of the day or night. After experiencing the close observation and supervision of hospitalization,

---

An Example of Problem Solving That Follows the Nursing Process

Situation
Monday, 7:30 PM, Amy Purcell has been admitted to the children's unit with dehydration resulting from diarrhea. Amy is responding well to intravenous (IV) fluids. Her mother is visibly distraught.

Assessing
Amy is doing well but will need 24 hours of IV therapy.

Amy and her twin sister Susan have never been separated from their parents or each other. They are 2 years old.

Mrs. Purcell has no idea of who will care for Susan when Mr. Purcell goes to work in the morning.

The Purcells have no regular child-care arrangements and have no family members in the area.

Mrs. Purcell wants to stay with Amy during her hospitalization.

The Purcells' neighbor is home during the day. Sometimes Amy and Susan play at her house.

There is a day-care center near their home, but Susan might be upset about going there. It is also expensive.

Mr. Purcell cannot afford to take Tuesday off but will take Wednesday morning off.

Insurance does not cover a private room, which would allow Susan to come to stay in the hospital too.

Diagnosing
Anxiety related to need for child care for Susan

Planning Goal
Mrs. Purcell will demonstrate decreased anxiety over the care of Susan during Amy's hospitalization.

Together, Mrs. Purcell and the nurse have planned the following:
1. The neighbor will come to the Purcell home to care for Susan when Mr. Purcell leaves for work on Tuesday morning.
2. The neighbor will bring Susan to the hospital for the afternoon visiting hours to be with Mrs. Purcell and Amy.
3. Mr. Purcell will come to the hospital after work to have dinner with the family.
4. Mr. Purcell will take Susan home for bedtime.
5. On Wednesday morning, Mr. Purcell will take off work in the morning. He and Susan will go to the hospital to pick up Mrs. Purcell and Amy.

Implementing
Plan implemented by the Purcells with support of the nursing staff

Evaluating
Mrs. Purcell told the nurse that she feels that both Amy and Susan did well with the care they received from their parents. The family's stress was minimized and she is relieved that everything went so well. The nurse decides that the goals were met.

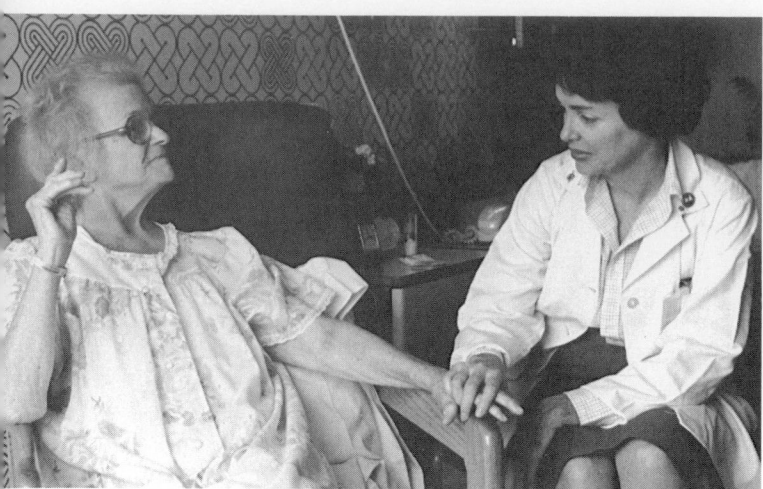

F I G U R E   21-10
Motivation counseling involves discussing feelings and incentives with the client. Having established a helping relationship, the nurse can encourage the client to work through feelings that undermine their motivation. (Photo by Gates Rhodes, courtesy of the School of Nursing, University of Pennsylvania)

this "telephone connection" has helped many clients make the transition from acute care to home care.

Motivational Counseling

Motivational counseling involves discussing feelings and incentives with the client. Nurses often become frustrated because their clients do not seem to want to get better or to learn how to care for themselves. These types of situations may be due to the fact that individual clients may not have the inner drive or motive to cooperate in their own health care. The words "I have nothing to live for" are often expressed by clients. If the nurse has established a helping relationship with the client, these feelings of despair may be worked through. The nurse may be able to get the client to talk about what is generating disinterest in recovery. If a problem is identified, the nurse and client can utilize the problem-solving technique to work toward an acceptable solution.

If a client shows an unwillingness to participate in learning activities, the nurse can assess any factors from the past or present that might be negatively influencing motivation for learning. Sometimes, if the nurse explains why certain knowledge is needed and the consequences of not learning the material, the client will become more receptive to the teaching–learning process. A trial learning session can be suggested to allow the client to see what the sessions will be like. If the nurse uses the nursing process approach for counseling, a satisfactory change in the client's motivation may be achieved.

When a nurse assesses a motivational problem, assessing the client's cultural values is important. Often the way a person feels about something is strongly influenced by cultural background. For instance, if a person has grown up in a family where illness is perceived as an inevitable result of aging, it will be difficult to motivate that person to practice preventive measures for health. These problems seem insurmountable, yet a caring nurse can work toward helping the client become oriented toward promoting self-health. When discouraged, the nurse can seek counsel with a colleague to help solve client-centered problems.

K E Y   P O I N T S

■ Nurses use communication skills in their roles as teachers and counselors. Client teaching is a requirement of acceptable nursing care according to ANA's Standards of Nursing Practice.

■ The nursing roles of teacher and counselor require the use of the nursing process; the teaching–learning process follows the steps of the nursing process.

■ With the trend for shorter hospital stays, clients and families need more extensive instructions for care in the home. But as the importance of teaching increases, the hospital time for teaching decreases. Consequently, the quality of teaching must improve.

■ Learning can be divided into three domains: cognitive learning involves the storing and recalling of new knowledge and information in the brain; psychomotor learning indicates a physical skill has been learned; and affective learning involves changes in attitudes, values, and feelings.

■ A thorough assessment of learning needs involves the client, family, or significant others. Factors influencing learning must be considered also.

■ Planning for the client's learning requires careful consideration to ensure that the nurse's and client's time is used efficently and effectively.

■ Implementing the teaching plan requires use of interpersonal skills as well as effective communication techniques. Teaching is part of the working phase of the helping relationship.

■ The evaluation of learning provides the information needed for revisions and for documenting that learning has taken place.

- Counseling involves the nurse in teaching and assisting the client to learn problem-solving techniques.

- There are three types of counseling: short-term counseling focuses on an immediate problem; long-term counseling extends over a prolonged period of time; and motivational counseling involves discussing feelings and incentives with the client.

- Counseling may be needed for assisting the client through crises or for motivating the client to work toward health promotion.

BIBLIOGRAPHY

American Nurses' Association: Standards of Nursing Practice. Kansas City, American Nurses' Association, 1973

Anthony ML: Patient education: Megatrends reinforce its priority. Nursing Management 16:23–24, January, 1985

Bille D: Practical Approaches to Patient Teaching. Boston, Little, Brown & Co, 1981

Black K: Short-Term Counseling: A Humanistic Approach for the Helping Professions. Menlo Park, CA, Addison-Wesley, 1983

Bloom BS: Taxonomy of Educational Objectives: The Classification of Educational Goals. New York, David McKay, 1956

Cormier LS et al: Interviewing and Helping Skills for Health Professionals. Monterey, CA, Wadsworth, 1984

Dobberstein K: Attacking fuzzy documentation. Am J Nurs 86:599, May, 1986

Du Brey RJ: Promoting Wellness in Nursing Practice: A Step-by-Step Approach in Patient Education. St Louis, CV Mosby, 1982

Flynn J, Heffron P: Nursing: From Concept to Practice. Bowie, MD, Robert J Brady, 1984

Hames C, Doyle J: Basic Concepts of Helping: A Wholistic Approach. New York, Appleton-Century-Crofts, 1980

La Monica EL: The Humanistic Nursing Process. Monterey, CA, Wadsworth, 1985

Magell K et al: Patient education: Progress and problems. Nursing Management 17:44–46, 48–49, February, 1986

Mager RF: Preparing Instructional Objectives, 2nd ed. Palo Alto, CA, Fearon Publishers, 1975

Murray RB, Zentner JP: Nursing Concepts for Health Promotion. Englewood Cliffs, NJ, Prentice-Hall, 1985

Redman BK: The Process of Patient Education, 5th ed. St Louis, CV Mosby, 1984

Stanton MP: Patient and health education lessons from the marketplace. Nursing Management 16:28–30, April, 1985

Streiff LD: Can clients understand our instructions? Image 18:48–52, Summer, 1986

Watson J: Nursing: The Philosophy and Science of Caring. Boston, Little, Brown & Co, 1979

22 Leader/Researcher/ Advocate

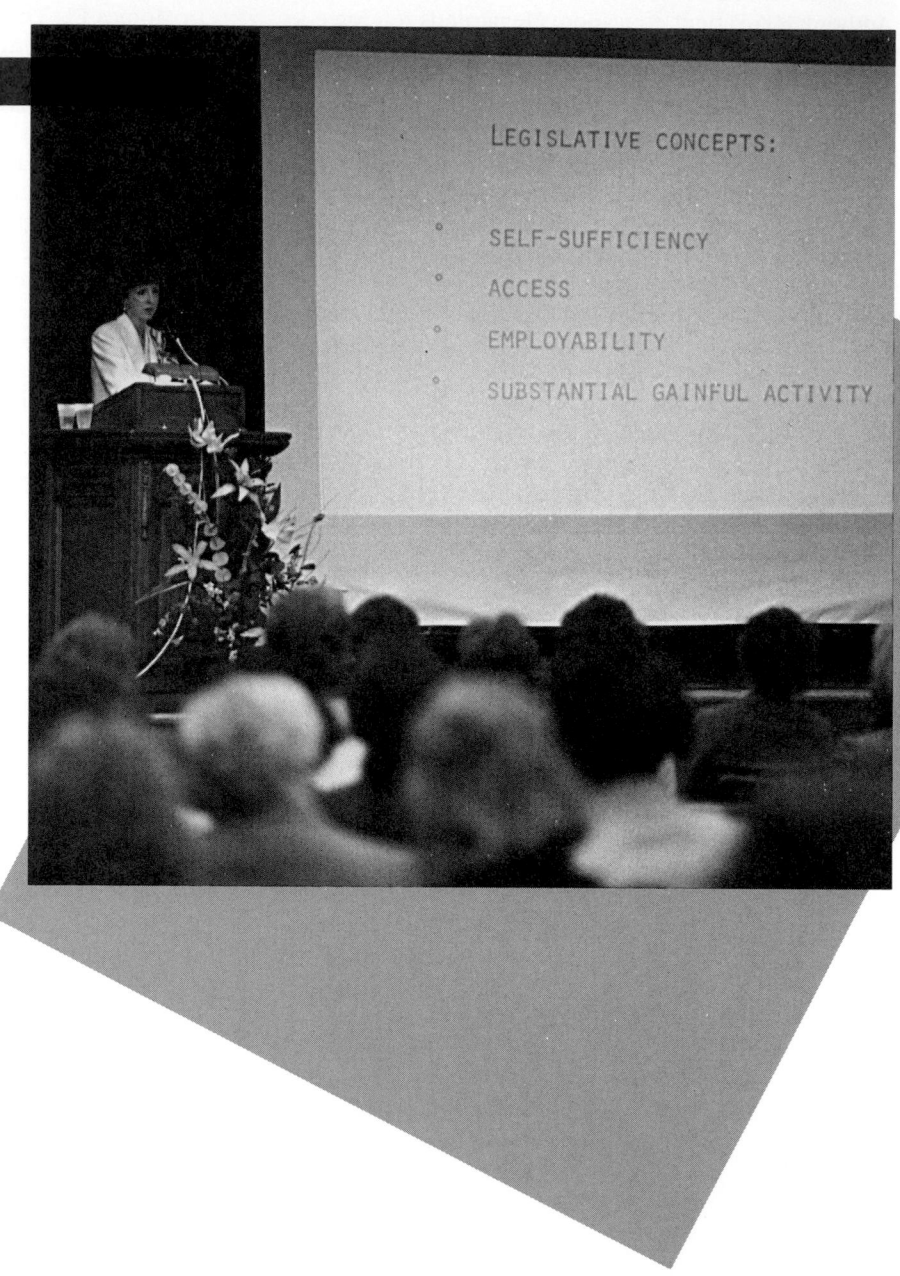

LEGISLATIVE CONCEPTS:

- SELF-SUFFICIENCY
- ACCESS
- EMPLOYABILITY
- SUBSTANTIAL GAINFUL ACTIVITY

OBJECTIVES

After studying this chapter, the learner should be able to

Define key terms used in the chapter.

Identify the qualities of a good leader.

Describe the three styles of leadership.

Summarize the eight steps in the process of change.

List the four functions of a nurse manager.

Describe how the nurse uses leadership abilities for the benefit of the client, the nursing team, the nursing profession, and society.

Give an example of mentorship in nursing.

State one characteristic that differentiates a profession from an occupation.

Describe an example of a nursing intervention based on authoritative knowledge.

Describe a nursing intervention based on scientific knowledge.

Discuss the significance of the Patient's Bill of Rights.

Compare assertive behavior with aggressive behavior.

Describe the nurse advocate's role in situations requiring ethical decisions.

KEY TERMS

advocacy
assertiveness
authoritative knowledge
change
change agent
group process
leadership
    autocratic leadership
    democratic leadership
    laissez-faire leadership
mentorship

objectivity
planned change
professionalism
readiness
scientific knowledge
traditional knowledge
variables
    dependent variables
    extraneous variables
    independent variables

THE NURSE AS LEADER

Good leaders must be advocates of client's rights in order to attain the ultimate goal of improved client care, and good advocates need leadership skills to achieve positive changes for clients. Leadership and advocacy complement each other. Research gives a knowledge base to the leader and advocate. It adds the dignity of professionalism to teaching, counseling, and communication, all nursing skills applied to the leadership role.

Although there have been many great nursing leaders throughout history, the majority of nurses were kept in subordinate positions. This has been diminishing gradually over the last several decades. Today, most nurses feel more self-directed than ever before. This trend is expected to continue and accelerate as more nurses learn to apply their leadership skills in research and advocacy.

Leadership Dynamics

Leadership is the ability to direct or motivate others toward the achievement of predetermined goals; the leader may work toward influencing an individual or a group. Leaders have power, whether it is explicit or implied. Much of this power depends on the style of leadership and how leadership responsibilities are fulfilled. The dynamics of leadership involve applying that power to growth or change. Nurses who use leadership skills can become proficient in bringing about desired changes in many areas, including their clients' health patterns, the health-care agency, the community, and the health-care system in general.

Leadership Qualities

Numerous adjectives can be used to describe the traits or qualities of a leader. It would be impossible for every nurse to excel in each of the qualities. When leaders can accurately identify their own strengths and weaknesses, they are able to capitalize on strengths and work toward improving their weak areas.

Most persons would agree that leaders should be dynamic, enthusiastic, and self-directed. They must present themselves as role models to followers. They need to be comfortable with themselves and have a positive self-image.

Leaders in any given profession must be knowledgeable about that profession. Nursing involves knowledge in countless areas: nursing science, biologic sciences, social sciences, and liberal arts. Because it is impossible to be a master in all of these areas, nurses develop resources; they use each other plus other health-care workers as resource persons. They also learn how to find and use appropriate reference materials quickly and efficiently.

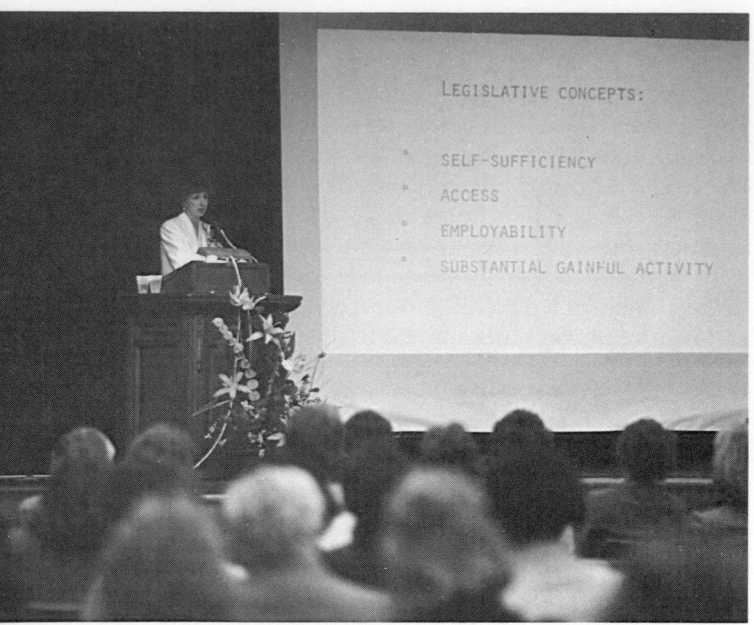

LEGISLATIVE CONCEPTS:

SELF-SUFFICIENCY

ACCESS

EMPLOYABILITY

SUBSTANTIAL GAINFUL ACTIVITY

F I G U R E   22-1

Political awareness is an important component of leadership in nursing. (Photo by Robert Neroni, courtesy of Thomas Jefferson University)

Every nurse must develop and perfect the ability to communicate effectively. This is especially needed in the role of leader. Nurses work on improving their methods of relating with clients, peers, subordinates, and superiors. Interpersonal skills are fundamental qualities for leadership.

Leaders value learning. They continue to keep up with current nursing research. The nurse critiques nursing research for validity, reliability, and applicability. Nurses share this knowledge with their colleagues to improve client care. Political awareness is required of the nurse-leader also (see Fig. 22-1). Knowing how legislation at the local, state, and national levels will affect health care allows the nurse to make informed decisions when voting for and supporting candidates.

Flexibility is a must for leaders. All nursing functions and roles require flexibility. The needs of clients, families, and the nursing team can change from minute to minute. A flexible, knowledgeable nurse is a welcomed team member.

While aggression is rarely suited to the leadership role, leaders need assertiveness in nearly all leadership situations. It is used extensively when effecting change. Assertiveness is a learned quality all nurses can develop. (Assertiveness is discussed again later in this chapter.)

Leadership qualities are present in every nurse. With education and practice, these qualities can be developed to the point where a nurse is skilled in the many behaviors necessary for leadership. A discussion of each of these qualities and skills is beyond the scope of this text; the accompanying box provides an overview of how one might approach the role of leader.

Becoming a Leader

Identify and capitalize on one's present qualities:

Comfortable with self	Intelligent
Creative	Open
Dynamic	Positive self-image
Enthusiastic	Positive thinking
Flexible	Resourceful
Friendly	Self-confident
Honest	Self-directed
Industrious	Values learning
Ingenious	Warm
Innovative	

Acquire and practice these leadership skills:

Assertiveness	Nursing experience
Critical thinking	Political awareness
Effecting change	Problem-solving techniques
Effective communication	Professional knowledge
skills	Role modeling
Group dynamics	
Interpersonal skills	

Gradually and prudently assume leadership responsibilities as a:

Student	Team leader/primary nurse
New graduate nurse	Nurse manager

Leadership Styles

Three styles of leadership are commonly identified in the nurse's work settings: autocratic, democratic, and laissez-faire. Generally speaking, it is best for nurses to use the leadership style with which they are most comfortable if that style is effective for the task at hand and for the groups they are leading. The variables of the nurse's own personality, the group personality, and the tasks or objectives to be accomplished must be considered in each leadership situation.

Autocratic Leadership.

Autocratic leadership occurs when the leader assumes complete control over the decisions and activities of the group. The nurse with an autocratic personality can be described as "firm, insistent, self-assured, and dominating with or without intent, and keeps at the center of attention" (Douglass, 1984). There can be extremes in autocratic leadership, such as a leader who makes all the decisions for the workers or followers without consideration of the followers' ideas or feelings.

Many nurses are used to working under an autocratic leader. This approach has been used in most hospital settings until recent years. It seems to have evolved from the military and religious images that nursing has developed historically. These images and this type of leadership are gradually being replaced by the democratic style of leadership as nurses demand more participation in decision making.

Situation. Nurse A has discovered that one of her clients is bleeding excessively from his surgical incision. She knows that he needs immediate attention so she begins to give specific orders to another team member to attend to the needs of the other clients. She tells the RN on her team to call the surgical resident to come as soon as possible. She implements a nursing plan of care to prevent further blood loss or complications.

Nurse A has chosen the autocratic style of leadership in this situation so that all of the necessary tasks would be accomplished immediately. Although she rarely uses this style, she implemented it effectively in this emergency situation.

Democratic Leadership.

Democratic leadership is characterized by a sense of equality among the leader and the followers. Decisions and activities are shared. The followers are encouraged to develop their skills and strengths within the group. The group and leader strive to work to accomplish mutually set goals. The leader needs to develop skills in group dynamics to apply this type of leadership effectively.

More nurses today are working toward the democratic style of leadership. Nurses, as professionals, tend to respond well to this type when they are the followers and feel more comfortable when they are the leaders of democratic groups. Group satisfaction and motivation can be excellent benefits of this style.

Situation. Nurse B, a head nurse, observes that staff members have not been documenting client teaching and learning in the nurse's progress notes. Nurse B is not sure why this has occurred but feels that this problem must be solved. A staff meeting is called and Nurse B leads a discussion seeking information on possible causes and planning strategies.

Nurse B has decided that staff members need to be included in the problem-solving approach. Nurse B thinks the staff will be more motivated to document their teaching and the clients' learning if they have a say in how the changes will be implemented. The democratic style of leadership has been used.

Laissez-faire Leadership.

In laissez-faire leadership the leader has relinquished all power to the group. This encourages independent activity by the group members (Douglass, 1984). An outsider would not be able to identify the leader in such a group. This style depends on the strengths of the followers to direct the group activities.

This style is rarely seen in the hospital setting because task achievement is difficult when each nurse is working independently. However, it could be used effectively when the leader wants a problem to be solved completely by the group members. It has been successful in cases where there is resistance to a certain policy or change and the leader allows the group to work to achieve an acceptable solution.

Situation. Nurse C, a clinical coordinator, has read an interesting research study which supports a change in the present instructions being given to new mothers who are breastfeeding. The article, with the summary of findings, is posted in all of the nurses' stations in the maternity unit.

Nurse C is using a laissez-faire leadership style and is confident that the individual staff members are capable professionals who are concerned with keeping up with current research findings which can be used to improve their nursing care.

Group Dynamics

A group exists when two or more persons are gathered together. To be functional, the members must communicate with each other for the purpose of achieving a goal or purpose. When functional groups are observed or studied for their effectiveness or ineffectiveness, it is commonly referred to as group dynamics. Group dynamics involves the evaluation of whether a group was effective in making the changes that were planned. If the group was ineffective, the reason for this is investigated. Group dynamics also includes studying how the individual group members relate to each other during the process of working toward group goals. This can be done by the members themselves, the leader, or an outside observer. Much can be gained by the careful assessment of the dynamics or internal life of the group.

Types of Groups

Groups can be categorized by size. One-to-one, small, and large groups were presented in Chapter 21. Nurses, both professionally and personally, commonly belong to each of these types of groups. Many nursing situations involve the nurse and client in a one-to-one group—a collaborative situation in which the nurse maintains a leadership advantage.

Nurses participate in small groups as members and as leaders (see Fig. 22-2). A nurse may lead a group of family members in discussing how they can meet their mother's needs for supervision at home. The same nurse may also belong to the hospital safety committee and work toward achieving committee goals.

Many nurses choose to serve large groups of people through their involvement in community-based programs, such as community health-planning boards, health-promoting organizations (*e.g.,* American Red Cross, American Cancer Society, American Heart Association), or even school board committees.

Groups can also be categorized as formal or informal. Formal groups usually stipulate membership requirements as well as group goals. The local chapter of the American Nurses' Association (ANA) is an example of a formal groups.

Informal groups have fewer rules and regulations; in fact, there may be none at all. A group of nurses gathered together during their lunch break is considered an informal group. A nurse who is discussing the hospital discharge policy with a group of clients in the lounge has formed an informal group.

Purpose of Groups

A group must have a purpose to bind its members together. The purpose may change and grow as the group develops or its membership changes. Most groups are formed for the purpose of effecting change, reflected in the group goals that are set. Some groups dissolve once the goal(s) has been met; other groups may set new goals, thus continuing the group's existence.

The group's purpose may be clearly indicated by the group's name. Many formal groups have names which explain their purpose. Other groups may have more subtle or covert purposes, yet, upon inspection, their mission becomes clear.

Features of Effective Groups

What makes a group effective or ineffective depends on many interrelated features including
- Decision making—The group sees a problem, makes a decision, and plans for follow through.
- Interaction—Members share ideas with each other.
- Flexibility—Members are able to see others' ideas and adjust their own ideas accordingly.

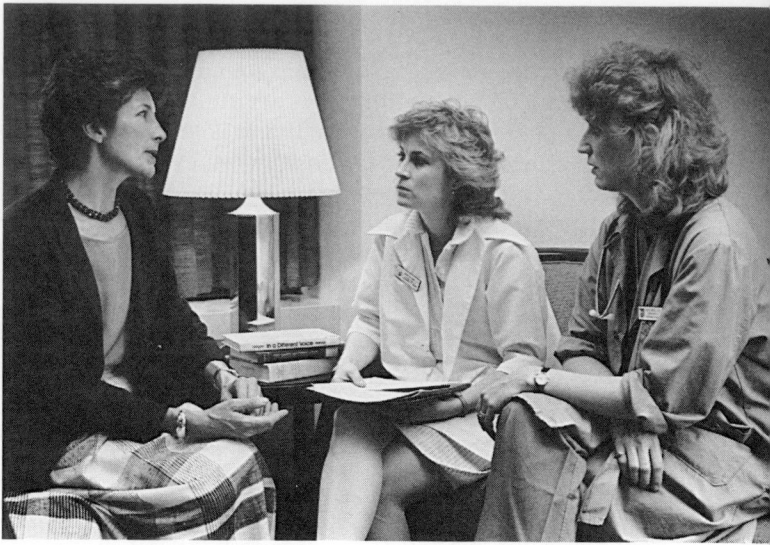

F I G U R E 22-2
Nurses participate in small groups as members and as leaders. (Photo by Robert Neroni, courtesy of Thomas Jefferson University)

- Cooperation—Members are able to use their flexibility to work together.
- Responsibility—Because members have helped to make the decisions, they are expected to follow through with them.
- Effective leadership—A group will fall apart without an effective leader (to be discussed later).
- Power—Once the decision and plan have been made, the group needs the power to effect the change.

If any feature, or ingredient, is missing or weak, it will decrease the group's ability to effect change.

Effecting Change through Leadership

Change is the process of transforming, altering, or modifying something. Nursing and the health-care system are continually changing and evolving. Such factors as the increase in the numbers of chronically ill and elderly persons, the increase in government intervention in health care, the rising cost of health care, and the changing patterns of health-care delivery have helped provoke the need for innovation and change in health care.

Planned change is a purposeful, systematic effort to alter or bring about change through the intervention of a change agent. Basic questions to consider before planning to make changes are highlighted in the box.

The eight steps in the process of change loosely follow the steps of the nursing process.
1. Recognize symptoms that indicate a change is needed and collect data.
2. Identify a problem to be solved through change. Analyze the symptoms, and reach a conclusion.
3. Determine and analyze alternate solutions to the

problem. Consider the advantages, disadvantages, and consequences of each alternative. An analysis of various proposed solutions to a problem may result in using a combination of alternatives.

4. Select a course of action from possible alternatives. It is best to avoid initiating too many courses of action and thereby dissipating resources and energy.

5. Plan for making a change. This step is critical to effect change successfully. Start by stating specific objectives, designing a plan for change, developing timetables, selecting persons to assist with making the change, and anticipating how to stabilize change and how to deal with resistance to change. Unless a plan is clearly designed, effecting change is likely to be a chaotic experience.

6. Implement the selected course of action to effect change. The plan for change is then put into effect. During this period, flexibility is important to adapt to unforeseen problems.

7. Evaluate the effects of change by comparing them with objectives stated in the plan for change. Needed adjustments can be made in the plan as necessary after evaluation. If the results of evaluation indicate that the course of action selected to solve a problem has been unsuccessful, an adjustment or another course of action should be selected.

8. Stabilize the change. When a solution to a problem has been found, take measures to make the change permanent. Continue follow-up until the change is firmly established.

The same steps apply whether dealing with individuals or groups. Figure 22-3 illustrates the process of change.

Resistance to Change

Sometimes there is resistance to change. The leader must decide why there is resistance and what techniques will overcome the resistance.

Factors in Resisting Change. There are various reasons for resisting change.

Threat to Self. People tend to view change in terms of how they are affected personally. Personal threats may include a loss of self-esteem, a belief that more work will be required, and a belief that social relationships will be disrupted. For example, when unit management was instituted in health agencies, many nurses resisted because

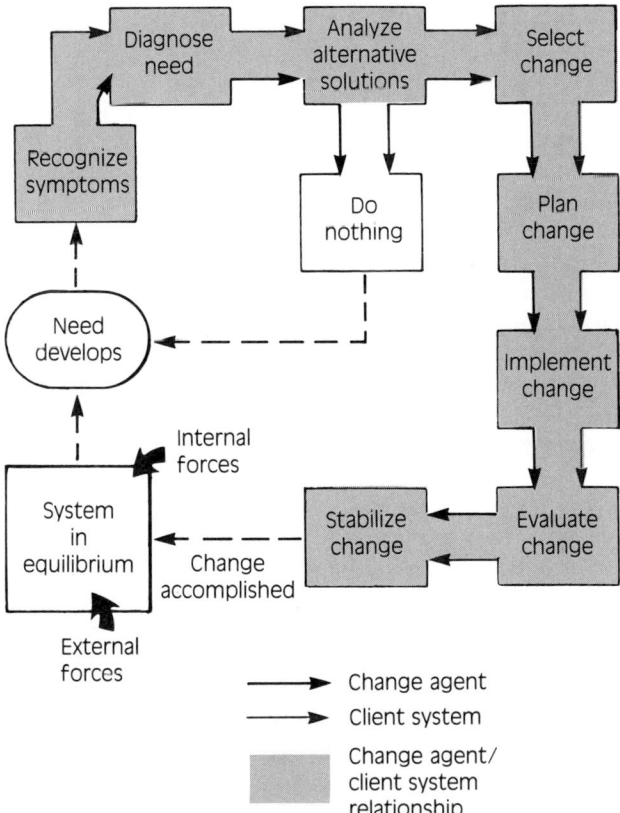

FIGURE 22-3
A planned change model, demonstrating the logical process through which change is planned and implemented. (Redrawn after Spradley BW: Managing change creatively. J Nurs Adm 10(5):33, 1980)

they felt the unit clerks would take away their responsibilities, for example, transcribing physicians' orders.

Lack of Understanding. The person who does not understand the nature of change is likely to resist. The involvement of persons affected by change is important to overcome resistance. For example, nurses who do not realize the effectiveness of nursing care plans tend to resist preparing them because they believe they are not beneficial in providing patient care.

Limited Tolerance for Change. Some people simply do not like to function in a state of flux or disequilibrium. A person may understand the need for change but may be unable to cope emotionally with the change itself. For example, a nurse may resist change because of the confusion a change is likely to cause.

Disagreements about the Benefits of Change. Resistance may occur when the information available to the change agent and those resisting change is different. If the information provided by persons resisting change is more accurate and relevant than information held by the change agent, the resistance may be beneficial. As an example, consider a plan that had been effective in implementing home health care in a middle-class section of a city. The supervisor of community-health services proposed that the plan be implemented in a low-income neighborhood. The nurse in charge of the health program in the low-income area resisted, believing that a plan suitable for a middle-class section of the community could not be used in a financially and educationally disadvantaged neighborhood.

Fear of Increased Responsibility. Many people are worried about having more complex responsibilities placed upon them. This is especially true if they feel unprepared for the planned changes. The changes may seem overwhelming so they respond by resisting.

Overcoming Resistance to Change

Nurses, in their leadership roles, find that they often must work to overcome resistance to change. Assistance can be subtle or distinct, gentle or aggressive. Responding to resistance is a leadership challenge in which one's leadership qualities, leadership style, and knowledge of group dynamics are combined to influence individuals toward a desired outcome. The nurse as an agent of change will find the following guidelines helpful for overcoming resistance to change:

- Explain the proposed change to all affected persons in simple, concise language.
- List the advantages of the proposed change, both for an individual person and for members of a group.
- Relate the proposed change to the existing beliefs and values of the person or group.
- Help overcome resistance by providing opportunities for open communication and feedback.

- Indicate clearly how the change will be evaluated.
- Introduce change gradually. Involve everyone affected by the change in the design and implementation of the process.
- Provide incentives for commitment to change. Incentives may be money, status, time off, or a better working environment.

Developing Leadership Skills as a Nursing Student or Beginning Nurse

No one is born a leader. People develop leadership qualities through observations, knowledge, and experiences. Nurses develop their leadership qualities in the same way, although they may enter nursing with some background in leadership experiences.

Nursing students and beginning practicing nurses have some leadership responsibilities, but they are still working at developing skills and learning where and how to apply them. Fortunately, they have support systems for guidance.

Areas of Leadership

Leadership should be approached as any new role and skill is approached: slowly and carefully. The nursing student and beginning nurse should be prepared with all of the necessary tools/skills before attempting the new role. Initially, a nurse will develop leadership skills in well-defined situations. With each experience, growth occurs and leadership is strengthened. It helps to remember that all nurse managers, nurse administrators, and nursing leaders began as inexperienced nurses too.

Client Care. Even new graduate nurses have leadership responsibilities on the nursing unit where they work. Nursing leadership begins with nursing care of the individual client (Fig. 22-4). Nurses have to take the initiative in helping clients. Although clients are partners in their care planning, they do not have the knowledge base and skills to direct the plan. Through use of interpersonal skills and effective communication techniques, nurses lead their clients in acquiring new knowledge, solving problems, and changing behaviors.

Employee Responsibilities. Nurses have specific tasks or duties to perform. These tasks are determined by the plan and objective of the health-care agency. The nurse is concerned with implementing the plan of the employing agency "in order to meet the predetermined standards for client care through the efficient use of time, equipment and materials, and the capabilities of every worker" (Kron, 1981).

Managerial Responsibilities. New graduate nurses use leadership techniques when they "cover" for the team leader's break. Gradually, new nurses assume increased leadership responsibilities as they become team leaders or primary nurses. The graduate nurse will be responsi-

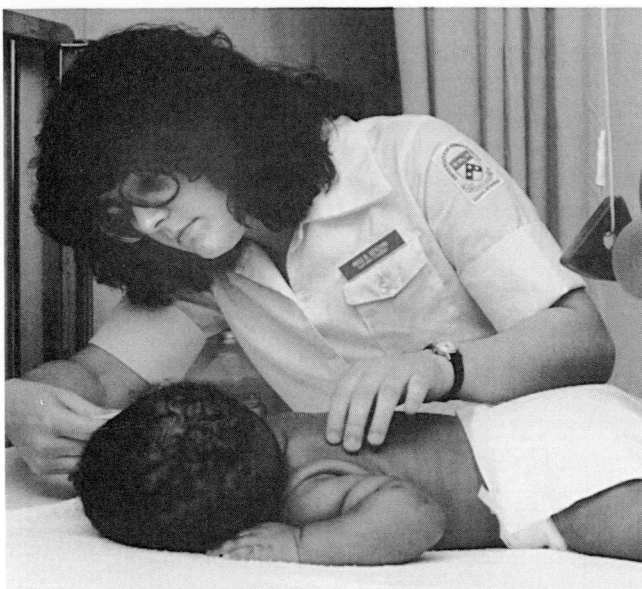

FIGURE 22-4
Nursing leadership begins with nursing care of the individual client. (Photo by Gates Rhodes, courtesy of the School of Nursing, University of Pennsylvania)

ble for one or two auxilliary personnel, and eventually the nurse may be in charge of an entire unit which can include 3 to 10 nursing staff members and up to 60 clients.

Nursing Department. The nursing team can also be viewed in the broader sense of the entire nursing department of a health-care institution or agency. Nurses should have an interest in the functioning of the department. Using this knowledge, nurses can seek information and/or change through appropriate channels. The more nurses understand how the nursing department runs, the better able they are to constructively work toward the objectives of the department.

Employing Institution. Nurses at all levels need to be knowledgeable about the administrative structure and functions of the employing institution. When problems arise concerning professional, unit, departmental, or institutional objectives, nurses must be able to use the proper channels of communication. These channels are structured according to the organization chart of the institution. The organization chart shows the relationships among the various administrative positions, the hospital departments, and the various job titles. Sometimes, the nurse is referred to committees that deal with specific problems or to other hospital departments such as public relations.

Research. Nurses need to be concerned with the advancement of nursing as a profession. Of the many ways to promote nursing's evolution toward greater autonomy and strength, an important facet is nursing research (Fig.

22-5). Nurses have given, and will continue to give, comprehensive and cost-efficient care by utilizing the research findings of their colleagues. Nurse researchers can provide staff nurses with invaluable information to use in client care. On the other hand, staff nurses also contribute to nursing research by

- Observing all nursing care activities to look for any area that needs improvement
- Questioning one's own practice to see if the rationale behind care-giving activities is sound
- Participating in the client-care research done by colleagues or nurse researchers
- Making suggestions for specific topics to be researched

Legislation. Keeping informed concerning local, state, and national legislation allows nurses to write or call legislators before the passage of new laws. Many nursing publications, newsletters, and papers have sections giving nurses specific information and guidelines for writing to elected officials concerning health-related legislation. The ANA has lobbyists in Washington, DC, as well as in the state capitals. The potential influence of nurses in the continued improvement of health care is phenomenal (Fig. 22-6).

Public Image. Nurses create the public's image of nursing whenever they interact with others and are recognized as a nurse. It is critical for beginning practitioners of nursing to understand the power they have to positively or negatively affect nursing's image. Because nurses are often portrayed negatively by the media (*e.g.,* as sex objects, or as uncaring females) it is important that the public experience nurses who are intelligent, competent, and caring to reverse the media's image.

Kalisch and Kalisch (1983) recommend that nurses change negative portrayals of nursing in the media by

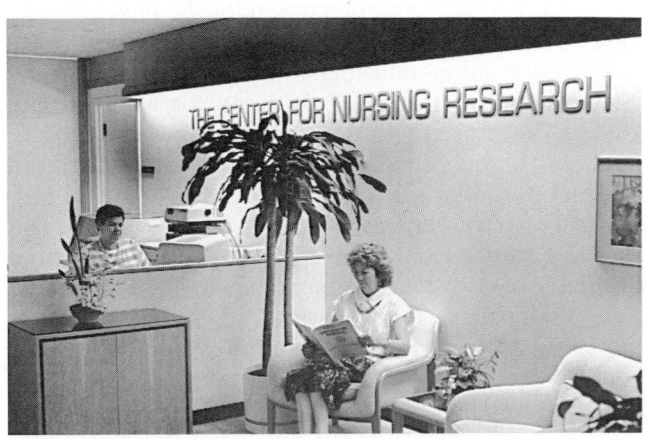

FIGURE 22-5
Research is an important way to promote nursing's evolution toward greater autonomy land strength by contributing to improvement of the quality of health care.

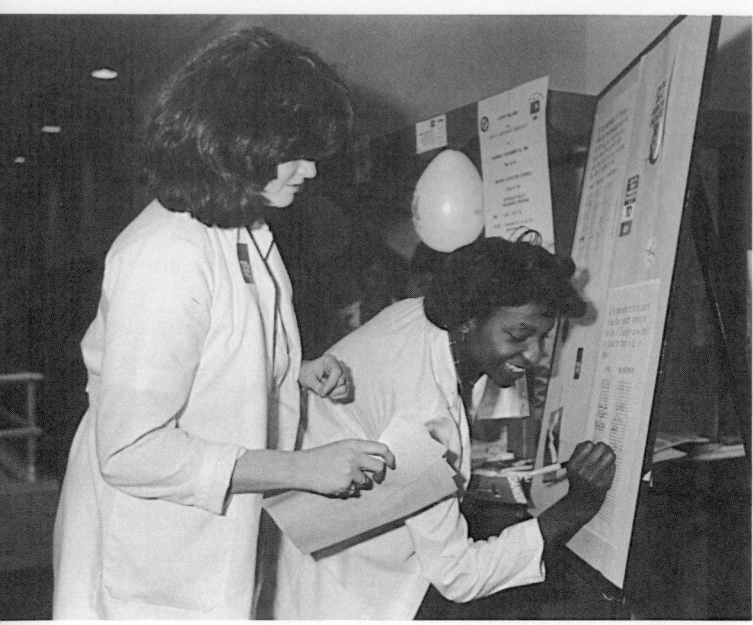

F I G U R E   22-6
If all registered nurses (1.7 million in the U.S. alone) were active in movements for change and improvement in health care, they would command tremendous power and influence. (Photo by Robert Neroni, courtesy of Thomas Jefferson University)

organizing, monitoring the media, reacting to the media, and fostering an improved image. Certainly not all nurses will be interested in joining a "media watch" group, but *all* nurses can practice nursing care in a manner that promotes a positive image of nursing.

Support for Leadership Training

Mentorship.   Mentorship is a relationship in which an experienced individual (the mentor) advises and assists a less experienced individual. This is an effective way of easing a new nurse into the leadership responsibilities that will be expected in the future. The mentor (also called a preceptor) may be chosen for the new nurse by the person responsible for orientation, or the new nurse may choose the mentor, depending on the structure of the orientation program. If no mentor is assigned, the nurse can observe and discuss nursing care with co-workers. The chosen mentor should be a good role model for the new nurse.

Mentorship is employed in all types of nursing positions. As a nurse climbs the ladder of leadership responsibility, a mentor who is experienced in management and administrative functions may be chosen. A mentor can be a critical factor in helping the less experienced nurse to successfully assume added responsibilities and position changes.

When a nurse acts as the mentor, it can be very rewarding. Besides receiving the satisfaction of helping a newer nurse, the mentor is stimulated to further develop his or her own teaching, counseling, and leadership

skills. Sometimes the mentor learns new knowledge and techniques when the newer nurse shares current information learned in school. Many mentorship relationships also become lasting friendships.

Nursing Organizations.   The many nursing organizations at the international, national, state, district, and local levels were discussed in Chapter 1. They are major forces for nursing leadership. These organizations have active groups in the United States and Canada. Membership and participation in a professional organization(s) are important aspects of the nurse's leadership role (Fig. 22-7).

Continuing Education.   Many programs in developing leadership, managerial, and administrative skills are available to nurses. Courses can even be taken by mail correspondence. Periodicals and current books also provide continuing education for the emerging leader. Many of the continuing education programs and methods serve to prepare nurses prior to assuming higher levels of leadership; some are geared to nurses

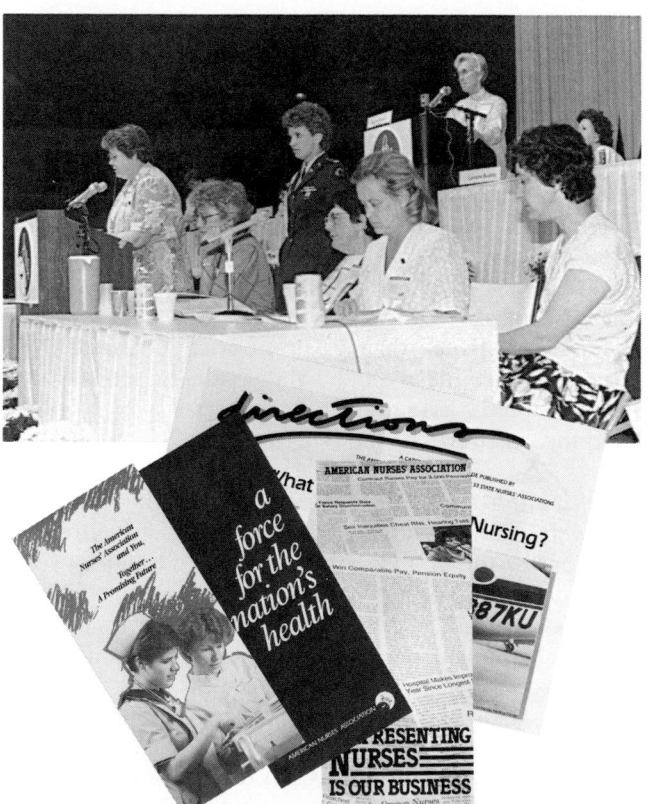

F I G U R E   22-7
Membership and participation in professional nursing organizations help keep the individual nurse up-to-date on issues and recent developments, increase the strength of the group, and are important aspects of the nurse's leadership role. (Courtesy of the American Nurses' Association)

already in such positions. Consequently, it is wise to choose a program carefully so that one's learning needs are correctly met.

THE NURSE AS RESEARCHER

While caring for victims of the Crimean War, Florence Nightingale kept careful and objective records. These records provided baseline data which she later used to determine which nursing interventions were most effective in treating her clients. Since that time nursing research has taken many different pathways.

Nursing research was finally recognized by the public sector when the 1985 session of the United States Congress enacted legislation to establish a National Center for Nursing Research at the National Institute of Health. Today, increasing numbers of health-care institutions are employing postgraduate nurses as researchers.

Studies surrounding nursing education, administration, and practice all impact client care either in a direct or indirect way. Too often practicing nurses mistakenly associate research with professions far removed from caring for clients at the bedside. This false impression has slowed the progress of practice-based nursing research. Yet much of what bedside nurses routinely do constitutes research. The nursing process (assessing, diagnosing, planning, implementing, and evaluating) represents the basic framework of the research process.

Regardless of the specific direction nursing research takes in the future, there will be an increased emphasis on its level of importance. Already schools of nursing have included research principles and methods in the basic curriculum for beginning nurses.

Professionalism of Nursing

Nursing research is fundamental to the recognition of nursing as a profession. As an occupation, nursing has been around since the beginning of time. Many argue however that the *profession* of nursing is still in its infancy. One of the essential elements that differentiates an occupation from a profession is the existence of a unique and distinct knowledge base. The ultimate goal of expanding nursing's body of knowledge is to learn improved ways to promote and maintain health. As health care and illness patterns change, nursing interventions must change. Ongoing practice-based research reflects the nursing profession's commitment to meet the ever-changing demands of health-care consumers.

Roots of Knowledge

How can nursing expand its knowledge base to meet the health-care needs of today's clients? To answer this question one must look to the roots of knowledge. Knowledge comes from a variety of sources. **Traditional knowledge** is that part of nursing practice passed down generation after generation. When questioned about this aspect of nursing practice nurses might reply, "We've always done it this way." Changing of bedclothes provides a practical illustration of how traditional knowledge has impacted nursing practice. It is customary in acute-care settings to change a patient's bedclothes daily whether soiled or not. There are no data to support this, yet virtually millions of hospital beds get changed daily because this practice is accepted as a necessary component of quality patient care. Right or wrong, until this practice is challenged scientifically it will remain a traditional part of patient care.

Authoritative knowledge comes from an expert and is accepted as truth based on a perceived level of expertise, for example when a senior staff nurse teaches a new graduate nurse an easier way of doing a technical procedure such as inserting an intravenous catheter. The senior nurse has gained knowledge through experience, and the new graduate nurse accepts it as truth based on a perceived authority within the experienced nurse. Authoritative knowledge remains unchallenged as long as the presumed authority maintains his or her perceived expertise.

Scientific knowledge is that knowledge arrived at through the scientific method. The term *research* implies the scientific approach to acquiring new knowledge. New ideas are tested and measured systematically using objective criteria. Scientific study implies the presence of control over **variables**—factors that might interfere with results (outcomes). Different types of variables make up a research study. **Dependent variables** are those factors in the study that remain the same. **Independent variables** are those factors that differ. An example of scientific research which might be carried out at the bedside would be to measure the effects of two different skin emollients on opposite limbs of a client over the course of 2 days. The dependent variable in this example would be the client's limbs. The independent variable would be the skin emollients. With careful and objective data collection one might be able to determine which lotion elicited a better client result or outcome. By testing the results of the two emollients on the same client the researcher would have maintained control within the study. Research as simple as this example could have vast implications on practice when results are shared among health-care professionals. Scientific research relies on careful planning. If the emollients were tested on two clients the results of the research might be affected by an unknown factor such as differing skin conditions in the two clients. These factors are called **extraneous variables**. Extraneous variables (*i.e.,* those that are not being studied) can sometimes cause research findings to be considered inaccurate.

Is one source of knowledge better than another? All sources of knowledge are useful to the collective body of knowledge that makes up the nursing profession. While

COMPUTER APPLICATIONS IN NURSING

Computerized literature searches of research

An important element of research is a thorough literature review. Computerized literature searches, once only available through hospitals and libraries (and disadvantageous in terms of cost, travel, and waiting time for search results) can now be easily obtained with a personal computer. The large data bases of interest to most nurses are the Psychological Abstracts (PsycINFO), Medical Literature Analysis and Retrieval System (MEDLARS), Cumulative Index to Nursing and Allied Health Literature (CINAHL), and the Educational Resources Information Center (ERIC) data bases. For information about the number of online data bases available through MEDLARS contact:

Office of Inquiries and Publications Management
National Library of Medicine
8600 Rockville Pike
Bethesda, MD 20209

To access these arsenals of information, five items are needed: (1) a telephone line, (2) a communications card (an RS-232 serial card/adapter), (3) a modem, (4) a cable to connect the modem and the serial card, and (5) communications software. To access the desired data base the user needs to obtain a password and an account number.

(Clark MJ, Clark PE: Personal computers and database access. Image 17(1): 21, 1985; Sinclair VG: Literature searches by computer. Image 19(1): 35–37, 1987; Sparks SM: The National Library of Medicine's bibliographic databases: Tools for nursing research. Image 16(1): 24–27, 1984)

these three methods provide nursing with important contributions, each has inherent strengths and limitations. Traditional and authoritative knowledge are very practical to implement but are often based on subjective data. This limits their usefulness over a wide variety of practice settings. Scientific research is designed to achieve high levels of objectivity, but is often costly, time consuming, and can be impractical given the complexities surrounding client care. Scientific knowledge, because of its control and objectivity, however, can be generalized, making it highly useful in a variety of care settings. Acquiring new knowledge then is one reason why nurses must become more aware and involved in the research process.

Consumerism

The social climate of consumerism surrounding health care has increased the importance of nursing research as well. Today's health-care marketplace is characterized by a rising concern over quality of care while assuring cost containment. Consumers have become dissatisfied with unproven, costly treatments. Today's health-care consumers demand effective methods of treatment at a reasonable cost. Tomorrow's nursing care, therefore, must focus on measureable results to assure the consumer of nursing's committment to improve client care. Unless practice-based research is used to validate the effects of nursing interventions, consumers will not credit nursing for its important contribution.

THE NURSE AS ADVOCATE

Advocacy involves combining the three roles of teacher, counselor, and leader to form a new role where to protect and support the client's rights. Nurses have always been advocates for clients' rights. Today, this role is being emphasized more than ever. Perhaps this is due to clients' changing expectations and demands, as well as to the importance placed on an individual's rights by the nursing profession.

Advocacy requires that nurses inform the clients and then support them in their decisions (Kohnke, 1982). Nurses must recognize that clients have the right to make their own decisions. Through teaching and counseling, the nurse is able to give the client the information needed to make educated decisions about health-care needs.

Many view advocacy as necessary only for those who cannot defend themselves. This is not true when considering the needs and rights of clients. Nearly all clients need a nurse advocate to provide the data needed for making informed decisions. Clients also need nurses to interpret what their rights are in given situations.

The Patient's Bill of Rights

As holism and holistic care became popular, clients began to demand their rights as health-care consumers.

In 1973 the American Hospital Association described A Patient's Bill of Rights which includes the rights and responsibilities of the client while receiving care in the hospital. The bill has been widely disseminated, and in some hospitals, clients receive a copy upon admission. (*The Patient's Bill of Rights* is discussed and printed in Chap 5.)

In the United States, the 1967 Freedom of Information Act and the 1974 Privacy Act were enacted primarily to open personal government records to the persons described in them. Medical records were included in this enactment. Clients in health agencies operated by the United States government (for example, the Veteran's Administration) and clients receiving Medicare are now entitled to see their records. Although some specifics and interpretations of the laws have not been clarified, the trend is apparent: consumers are demanding their right to know about their health care and are seeking legislation to support this right. Nurses are responsible advocates of these client rights.

Persons Requiring Advocacy

Most nurses would agree that a great deal of nursing time is spent representing clients' interests or guiding clients in protecting their own rights. The nurse is often involved as an intermediary between the client and the family, especially when the client and family have conflicting ideas about the management of health-care situations.

For instance, a client with terminal cancer may want to go home to die. He has told this to his nurse. The client's family, however, has told the nurse that they cannot care for him at home. As an advocate, the nurse recognizes the rights of both the client and his family. The nurse then works to assist them in finding a solution that will benefit all concerned. By informing the family of the availability of home care and hospice care, the nurse has given them knowledge that may help satisfy the client's right to a dignified death. Most persons on their own would have no way of getting the financial help needed for such care. The nurse has the resources available to help them and can arrange referrals from other health-care workers, such as social workers, to achieve the desired outcomes.

Persons who need an advocate include persons who are uninformed concerning their rights and opportunities, persons with sensory impairment, persons who do not speak English, the very young, the aged, seriously ill persons, persons who are mentally or emotionally impaired, and persons with physical disabilities or handicaps.

Advocacy Requires Assertiveness

To help clients attain their rights, nurses need to be assertive. Occasionally they need to teach assertive techniques to their clients also. **Assertiveness** means claiming one's rights and defending them; the assertive person gives direct and honest expressions of feelings and confronts strengths and limitations.

Assertive behavior is often confused with aggressive behavior. In contrast to the assertive person, the aggressive person tends to manipulate, humiliate, and dominate others. An aggressive person attacks another person rather than confront his or her own behavior.

There are many situations in which the nurse can use assertive behavior to effect change. For instance, a staff nurse noticed that the charge nurse did not wash hands when visiting clients on a surgical unit. The staff nurse indicated to the charge nurse that all personnel needed to practice handwashing to prevent the spread of infections. The charge nurse subsequently washed hands between visits with clients. The change that occurred because of the nurse's assertiveness positively influenced the type of care the clients received. Sometimes this influence is direct and readily apparent; at other times the client is affected more indirectly. In either case, the nurse has acted as an advocate for the client.

Learning Assertiveness

Many nurses participate in assertiveness training programs so they can help strengthen the position of nursing in the health-care system and increase its influence on client care.

Assertiveness training has been especially useful in helping nurses engaged in independent practice stand up for their rights as health-care practitioners. Also, clients are becoming more assertive about their rights and needs. Assertive behavior helps clients exercise their rights in the best way possible to obtain appropriate health care.

Techniques vary among assertiveness training programs; however, basic activities are the following:

- Assessing present level of assertiveness
- Assessing particular situations and determining rights and responsibilities
- Determining what type of assertive behavior to use in this particular situation
- Practicing the chosen assertive behavior in a safe and comfortable place
- Examining attitudes that may be counterproductive
- Evaluating results of use of assertive behavior, including presentation to others, control of fear and anxieties, and giving and taking criticism

Advocacy and Ethics

Advocacy extends beyond the basic rights of the hospitalized client or ill person to the dilemmas that occur when ethical issues arise. Nurses, as advocates, must realize that they do not make the ethical decisions for their clients. Instead, they facilitate clients' decision making. Nurses interpret findings for their clients, inform them of the various aspects to be considered, let them verbalize and organize their feelings, call in those persons who should be involved in the decision making (*e.g.,* family, physician, clergy), and help clients assess all of their options in relation to their beliefs. In this way, nurses advocate the right of clients to make their own decisions concerning health as well as life. (Values and ethics in nursing are discussed in Chap 5.)

KEY POINTS

- Nurses have the basic qualities for leadership; they need to work toward developing those qualities.

- Nurses choose leadership styles according to their own personality traits, the objectives to be achieved, and the characteristics of the followers.

- Nurse leaders are responsible for effecting positive changes, managing client and staff activities, and using administrative knowledge appropriately.

- Nursing leadership is involved in working for the benefit of the client, the nursing team, the nursing profession, and society.

- Research provides an important step toward expanding the professional role of nursing, acquiring new knowledge to improve client care, and remaining competitive in today's health-care marketplace.

- As an advocate, the nurse informs the client of rights and supports decisions concerning rights and health-care choices.

- Assertiveness is a necessary tool for the nurse to use in both the advocacy and leadership roles.

- Although all persons need an advocate at some time in their lives, certain individuals need advocacy continually.

- The advocate works with the client by supplying the information and support necessary for the client to make ethical decisions.

BIBLIOGRAPHY

American Hospital Association: A Patient's Bill of Rights. Chicago, The Association, 1972

Angel G, Petranko DK: Developing the New Assertive Nurse: Essentials for Advancement. New York, Springer Publishing, 1983

Archer S, Gohner P: Nurses: A Political Force. Monterey, CA, Wadsworth Health Sciences Division, 1982

Cushing M: Wronged rights in nursing homes. Am J Nurs 84:1213, 1216, 1218, Oct 1984

Douglass LM: The Effective Nurse: Leader and Manager, 2nd ed. St Louis, CV Mosby, 1984

Ellis JR, Hartley CL: Nursing in Today's World: Challenges, Issues, and Trends, Philadelphia, JB Lippincott, 1984

Flynn J, Heffron P: Nursing: From Concept to Practice. Bowie, MD, Robert J Brady Co, 1984

Kalisch BJ, Kalisch PA: Improving the image of nursing. Am J Nurs 83:48–52, 1983

Kohnke MF: Advocacy: Risk and Reality. St Louis, CV Mosby, 1982

Kron T: The Management of Patient Care: Putting Leadership Skills to Work. Philadelphia, WB Saunders, 1981

La Monica EL: The Humanistic Nursing Process. Monterey, CA, Wadsworth Inc, 1985

La Monica EL: Nursing Leadership and Management: An Experiential Approach. Monterey, CA, Wadsworth Health Sciences Division, 1983

Lancaster J, Lancaster W: The nurse as a change agent. St Louis, CV Mosby, 1982

Marchewka AE: When is paternalism justifiable? Am J Nurs 83:1072–1073, July 1983

Marriner A: Guide to Nursing Management, 2nd ed. St Louis, CV Mosby, 1984

McGovern W, Rodgers JA: Change theory. Am J Nurs 86:566–567, May 1986

Meissner JE: How autonomous are you? Nursing 81 11:70–71, Oct 1981

Murray RB, Zentner JP: Nursing Concepts for Health Promotion, Englewood Cliffs, NJ, Prentice Hall, 1985

Numerof RE: Assertiveness training. Am J Nurs 80:1796–1799, Oct 1980

Polit D, Hungler B: Nursing Research Principles and Methods, 3rd ed. Philadelphia, JB Lippincott, 1986

Sampson E, Marthas M: Group Process for the Health Professions. New York, John Wiley and Sons, 1981

Shaffer ME et al: Nursing Research and Patient's Rights. Am J Nurs 86:23–24, Jan 1986

Spradley BW: Managing change creatively. J Nurs Admin 10:32–37, May 1980

Wilkinson R: Communication: Learning from the market . . . the "I" world instead of the "you" world. Nursing Management 17:42J, 24L, April 1986

Yura H et al: Nursing Leadership: Theory and Process, 2nd ed. New York, Appleton-Century-Crofts, 1981

Actions Basic to Nursing Practice

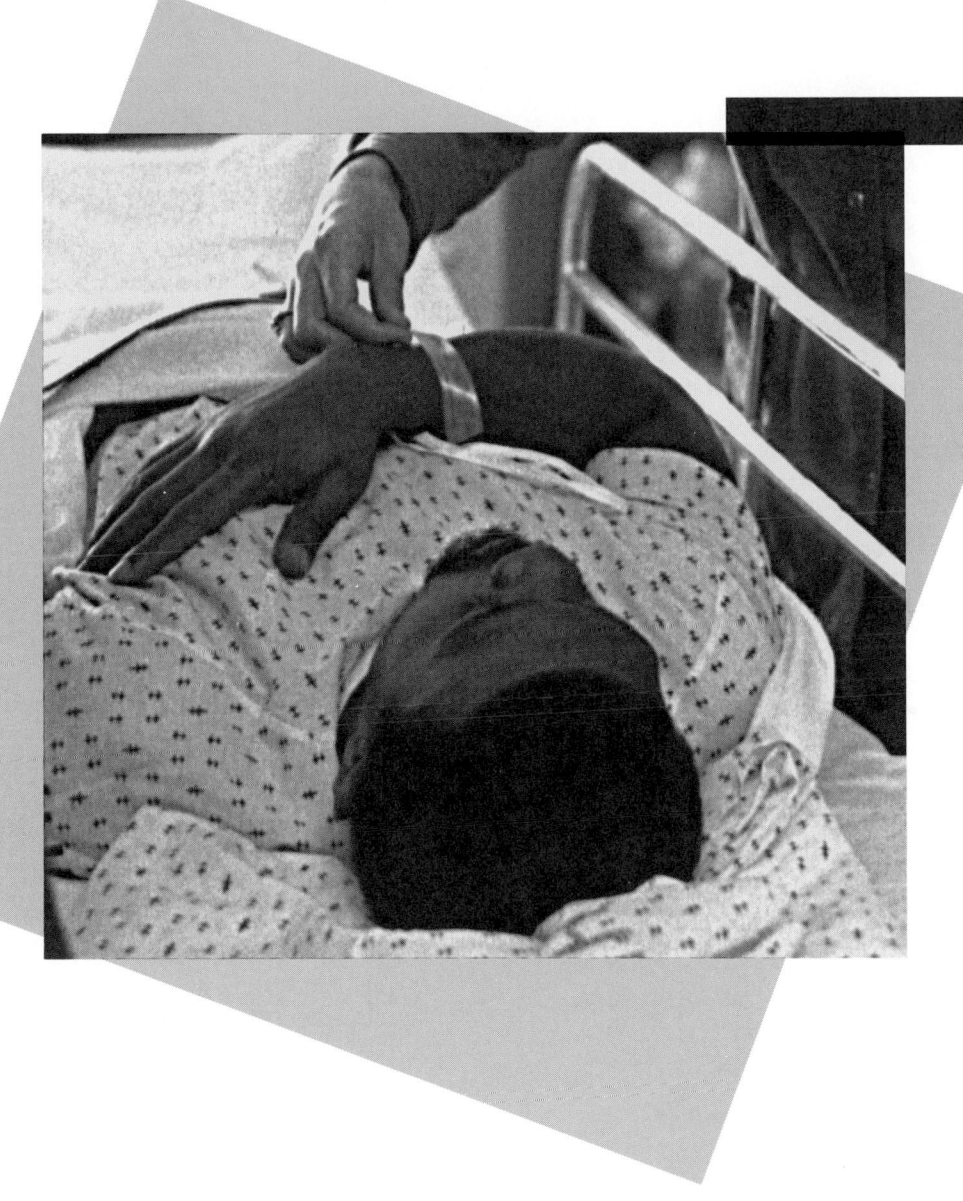

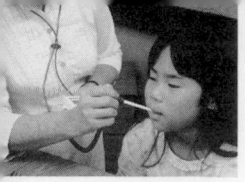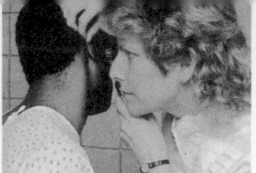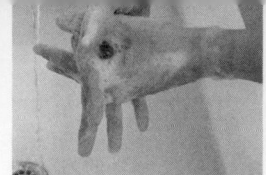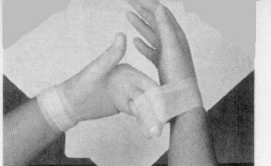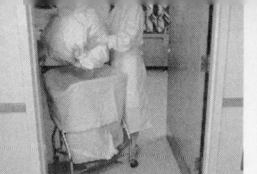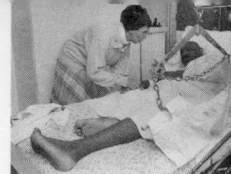

*U*nit VI focuses on the actions basic to nursing practice—those commonly used to meet needs of clients of all ages, at any point on the health–illness continuum, and in both structured and unstructured settings.

Nursing assessment, including a health history and physical assessment, provides a data base necessary to maintaining or restoring health and to promoting wellness. Physical assessment is both an art and a science. The art of performing a skill is integrated into the science of nursing knowledge, so that variations are identified and evaluated and necessary independent and interdependent nursing actions are implemented.

Nurses are responsible for meeting basic human needs for physical safety and security. Chapter 25 discusses environmental safety and the nursing actions necessary to identify risk factors for all age groups, to implement teaching to prevent accidents, and to practice medical and surgical aseptic techniques so that the spread of microorganisms is prevented or controlled.

Many individuals enter the health-care system for in-hospital treatment and care. The person commonly has acute-care needs and is discharged while still requiring skilled nursing care. Nursing care is therefore individualized to meet client needs at home as well as in the hospital; discharge planning literally begins at the time of admission.

Unit VI provides the knowledge and skills basic to nursing practice. Using the nursing process, nurses make accurate assessments, ensure safety, and provide continuity of care in the hospital, the home, and the community.

Vital Signs

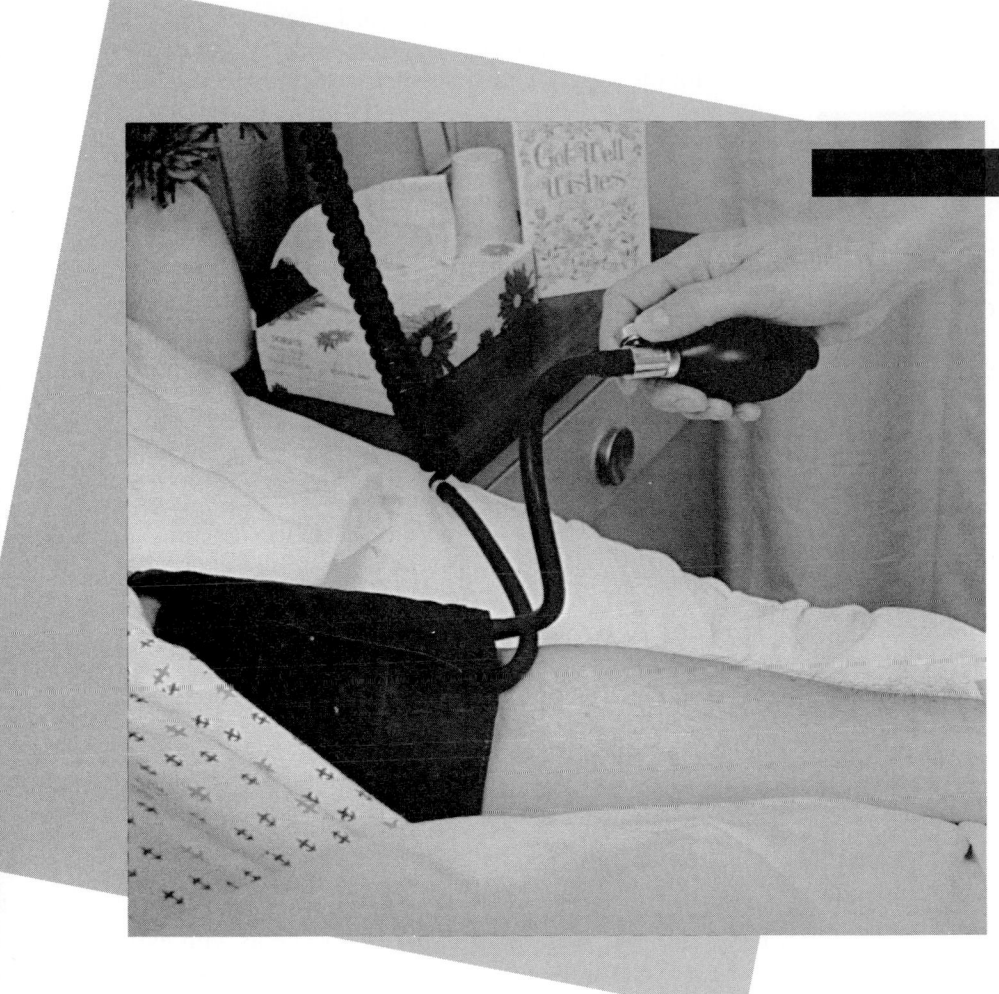

OBJECTIVES

After studying this chapter, the learner should be able to

Define key terms used in the chapter.

Define the phrase vital signs.

Discuss nursing responsibilities in assessing temperature, pulse, respirators, and blood pressure.

Compare normal and abnormal vital sign assessments including causes, effects, and implications of abnormal findings.

Describe the equipment necessary to assess vital signs.

Identify sites for assessing temperature, pulse, and blood pressure.

KEY TERMS

adventitious sounds	intermittent pulse
antipyretic	internal respiration
apical-radial pulse rate	Korotkoff sounds
apnea	lysis
arrhythmia	meniscus
auscultation	orthopnea
blood pressure	orthostatic hypotension
bigeminal pulse	palpitation
biot's respirations	parallax
bradycardia	peripheral resistance
bradypnea	poikilothermic
cardiac output	polypnea
cardinal signs	postural hypotension
Cheyne-Stokes respirations	premature beat
circadian rhythm	primary hypertension
conduction	pulse
constant fever	pulse deficit
convection	pulse pressure
core temperature	pyrexia
crisis	radiation
diastolic pressure	rales
dyspnea	relapsing fever
dysrhythmia	remittent fever
essential hypertension	respiration
eupnea	rhonchi
evaporation	secondary hypertension
exhalation	set point
expiration	sinoatrial node
external respiration	sphygmomanometer
fever	stertorous breathing
friction rub	stridor
homeothermic	stroke volume
hyperpyrexia	systolic pressure
hypertension	tachycardia
hypotension	tachypnea
hypothermia	temperature
inhalation	tissue respiration
inspiration	vital signs
intermittent fever	wheeze

Assessment of the client's temperature, pulse, respiration, and blood pressure, known as **vital signs**, are considered essential when evaluating a client's health status. Obtaining vital signs has been a traditional nursing responsibility. Although these measurements are taken routinely, the nurse must guard against taking their importance for granted. Temperature, pulse, respiration, and blood pressure reflect changes in the functioning of vital organs, such as the heart and lungs. The variations and patterns in these measurements are often critical clinical indicators of a client's condition. Therefore, they must be assessed and interpreted accurately. This chapter describes current techniques and recommendations for the nurse when assessing vital signs.

VITAL SIGNS

Alterations in body function often are reflected in the body temperature, the pulse, respiration, and the blood pressure. Physiologic mechanisms governing vital signs are very sensitive and normally keep them regulated within a narrow range. Any change from normal is considered to be an indication of the person's state of health. Hence, these signs provide excellent clues to the physiologic functioning of the body. That is why they are called *vital signs* or **cardinal signs**.

Frequency of Assessing Vital Signs

Assessing a person's vital signs is part of most agency admission procedures. These data provide part of the baseline information from which a plan of care is developed. It is recommended that upon the person's admission, the nurse assess these signs whenever possible rather than assigning the task to auxilliary nursing personnel who may have less knowledge about measuring these important health-status indicators.

After a client is admitted to a health agency, local policies govern when and how frequently vital signs are to be assessed. It is common policy for clients with elevated temperatures and for those who are in the postoperative period to have vital signs taken every 4 hours. Severely ill clients may have these observations made more frequently. In some self-care and psychiatric units, observations are made on the basis of the nurse's judgment. When a client does not have an elevated temperature or other vital-sign disturbances, there seems to be little justification for taking these signs several times a day. When the nurse visits in the home, the client's condition determines the frequency of obtaining data about vital signs.

The introduction of technologically advanced monitoring devices has made it possible to keep clients' vital signs under constant surveillance in critical care settings. The lives of many patients have been saved because continuous assessment of vital signs provides an accurate means of observing the effects of pathology and therapy.

Auxilliary personnel may obtain vital signs in some situations, but the nurse responsible for the client is ultimately accountable for these observations. If a client has untoward symptoms or demonstrates unexpected changes in vital signs, the nurse should double-check the measurements and further assess the client.

BODY TEMPERATURE

Physiology

Temperature refers to the hotness or coldness of a substance. Some living species are able to self-regulate the temperature of their body while others are warmed and cooled by conditions in the environment. Humans are **homeothermic** that is, they are warm-blooded and maintain body temperature independently of their environment. Cold-blooded animals are **poikilothermic**, meaning their body temperature is the same as their environment. Fish, frogs, and reptiles are poikilothermic animals.

Circadian Rhythm

It has been observed that environmental and physiological processes occur in repeated cycles of time. Some events in humans appear to recur at 24-hour intervals. This cycling pattern is referred to as **circadian** (meaning nearly every 24 hours) **rhythm**. Predictable fluctuations in measurements of body temperature and blood pressure are examples of functions that exhibit a circadian rhythm. For instance, body temperature is usually about 0.6°C (1° to 2°F) lower in the early morning than in the late afternoon and early evening. This variation tends to be somewhat greater in infants and children. Current research indicates that the peak elevation of a person's temperature will occur in late afternoon, between 4 PM and 7 PM.

Temperature Regulation

The body temperature of a healthy person is maintained within a fairly constant range by the hypothalamus in the central nervous system. This structure is located at the base of the brain and plays an important role as the body's thermostat. It normally allows the body temperature to vary only approximately 1 degree throughout the day. This constancy is referred to as the **set point**. The set point can be altered by the body's response to infectious agents, allergens, and inflamed tissue.

The hypothalamus has two parts: the anterior hypothalamus controls heat dissipation, and the posterior hypothalamus governs heat conservation. Thus, the set point is maintained through a balance of mechanisms involving heat production and heat loss. The following are examples of ways in which the body's thermal balance is maintained:

- Heat is produced through the metabolism of food. More heat is produced when metabolism is increased, and less when metabolism is decreased. For example, metabolism is increased when body temperature is elevated.
- Heat production is increased by the body's secretions of epinephrine, norepinephrine, and thyroxin.
- Exercise produces heat through muscle contraction.
- The body's surface, but not its internal structures, gains and loses heat physically from the sun, wind, and humidity in the environment.
- Heat is transferred primarily through physical processes of **radiation**, **convection**, **evaporation**, and **conduction**. These processes are defined and illustrated in Table 23-1.
- Heat is lost in small amounts through the urine, feces, and the process of warming and exhaling inspired air.
- Changes in vascularity of the skin modify body temperature. When blood is directed to the skin through dilated vessels, heat loss is increased; when the skin vessels contract, heat is conserved.
- The contraction of smooth muscles when gooseflesh occurs and the involuntary movement of skeletal muscles when shivering is present produce heat and promote the circulation of blood that has been warmed through this process.

Normal Body Temperature

A thermometer is placed in a person's mouth to obtain an oral temperature, in the anal canal to obtain a rectal temperature, in an axilla (armpit) to obtain an axillary temperature, and in the esophagus to obtain a core temperature. Table 23-2 shows the average normal temperature standards for well adults at various body sites. The body's internal organs require a fairly constant inner or **core temperature** for optimal functioning, whereas the surface and periphery of the body can fluctuate widely while gaining or losing heat.

Variations normally occur in each person, and a range of 0.3°C to 0.6°C (0.5°F to 1.0°F) from the average normal temperature is considered to be within normal limits. However, wider variations from the average temperature have been found to be normal for certain persons. Newborns and young children normally have a higher body temperature than adults.

Elevated Body Temperature

Pyrexia is an elevation of normal body temperature. The lay term is **fever**. **Hyperpyrexia** is a high fever, usually above 41°C (105.8°F), and survival is rare when the temperature reaches 44°C (110°F). Death is probably due to damaging effects to the respiratory center but may be due also to inactivation of body enzymes and destruction of tissue proteins.

Pyrexia is a common symptom of illness, and there is sufficient evidence to indicate that an elevation in tem-

T A B L E   23-1
Mechanisms of Heat Transfer

Process	Definition	Example	Illustration
Radiation	The diffusion or dissemination of heat by electromagnetic waves	The body gives off waves of heat from uncovered surfaces.	
Convection	The dissemination of heat by motion between areas of unequal density	An oscillating fan blows currents of cool air across the surface of a warm body.	
Evaporation	The conversion of a liquid to a vapor	Body fluid in the form of perspiration and insensible loss is vaporized from the skin.	
Conduction	The transfer of heat to another object during direct contact	The body transfers heat to an ice pack, causing the ice to melt.	

TABLE 23-2
Average Normal Temperatures for Well Adults in Various Body Sites

Oral	Rectal	Axillary	Esophageal	Forehead*
37°C	37.5°C	36.5°C	37.3°C	34.4°C
98.6°F	99.5°F	97.6°F	99.2°F	94°F

* The manufacturer of Digitemp® forehead thermometer (Hallcrest Products, 1820 Pickwick Lane, Glenview IL 60025) says, "Most older children and adults have normal forehead temperatures between 93°F and 95°F."

perature helps the body fight disease. In children, this response is often seen quickly. In the elderly person, pyrexia may be one of the later signs of illness, and the temperature may be elevated only 1 or 2 degrees above normal, even when pathologic processes are extensive.

It is generally theorized that when a fever occurs, the set point regulated by the hypothalamus is readjusted to a higher level. As a result, heat loss is decreased or heat production is increased, or both occur through the following mechanisms: shivering, constriction of surface blood vessels, and absence of sweating. After the body temperature rises to the new set point, heat loss mechanisms are again used to control the body temperature from rising to dangerous levels. Most fevers are self-limiting. The body temperature returns to normal range after the disease process is in check. Relieving a moderately elevated body temperature may reduce the body's defenses against disease as well as alter the ability to assess the person's progress.

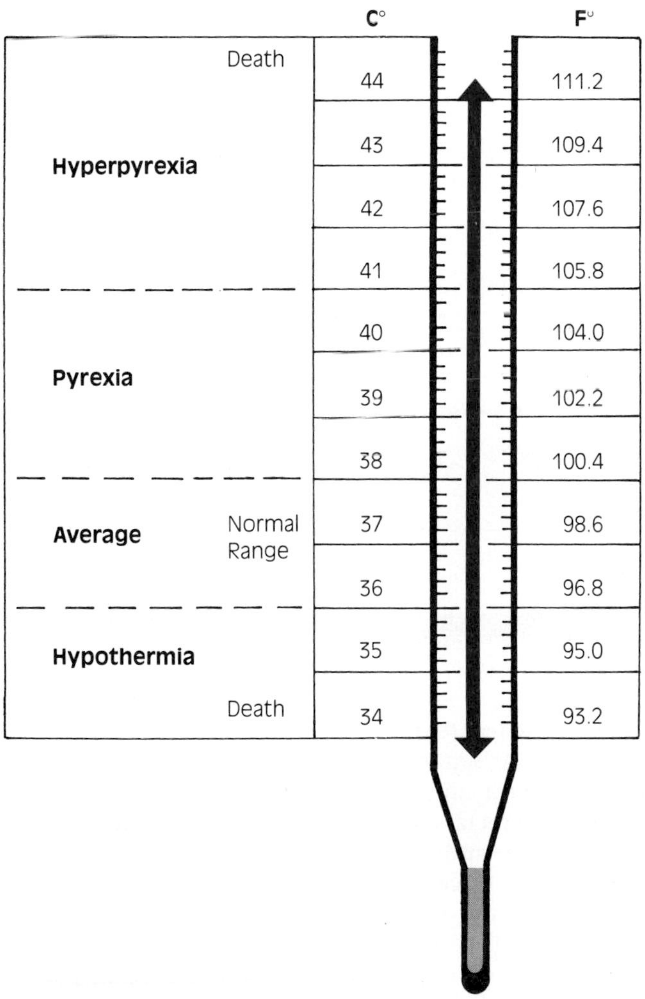

The patient with a fever usually experiences loss of appetite; headache; hot, dry skin; flushed face; thirst; and general malaise. Young children or persons with very high fevers may experience periods of delerium or seizures. Observing for other potential dangerous signs that accompany a fever, such as dehydration, decreased urinary output, and rapid heart rate, are also important nursing assessments.

The onset of an elevated body temperature may be sudden or gradual. Common terms used to describe the course of an elevated body temperature and its resolution are described in Table 23-3.

Antipyretic or fever-reducing drugs, such as aspirin or acetaminophen, may be necessary in certain circumstances. These drugs are believed to lower the elevated set point regulated by the hypothalamus. They do not affect body temperature when it is is within normal range.

Subnormal Body Temperature

A body temperature below the lower limit of normal is called **hypothermia**. Death may occur when the temperature falls below approximately 34°C (93.2°F), but survival has been reported in isolated cases when body temperatures have fallen in the range of severe hypothermia (28°C or 82.4°F). This may happen to a person drowning in cold water or buried by snow. Because body functions are almost imperceptible at this range, health-care personnel should attempt to warm hypothermic patients and continue resuscitation efforts.

Just as an elevated body temperature is a protective device for the body, a lowered body temperature may be

FIGURE 23-1
The range of human body temperature, as measured orally.

T A B L E   23-3

Common Courses of Pyrexia and Its Resolution

Term	Definition	Illustration
Intermittent fever	The body temperature alternates regularly between a period of fever and a period of normal or subnormal temperature.	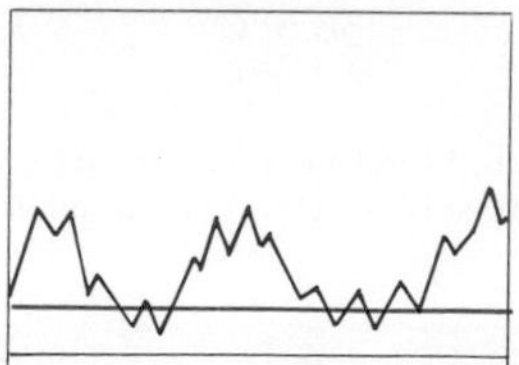
Remittent fever	The body temperature fluctuates several degrees, more than 2°C (3.6°F), above normal but does not reach normal between fluctuations.	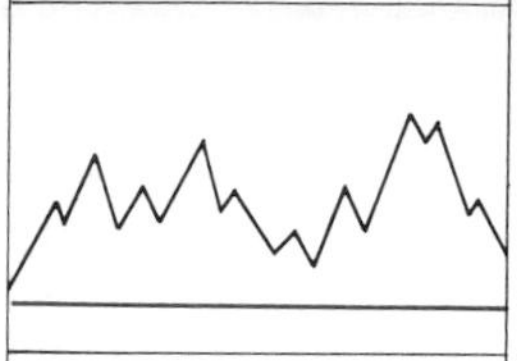
Constant fever	The body temperature remains consistently elevated and fluctuates very little, less than 2°C (3.6°F).	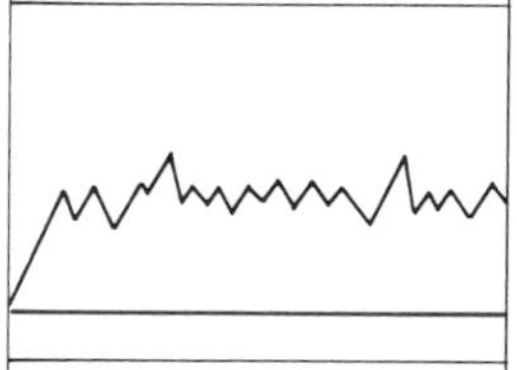
Relapsing fever	The body temperature returns to normal for at least a day, but then fever recurs.	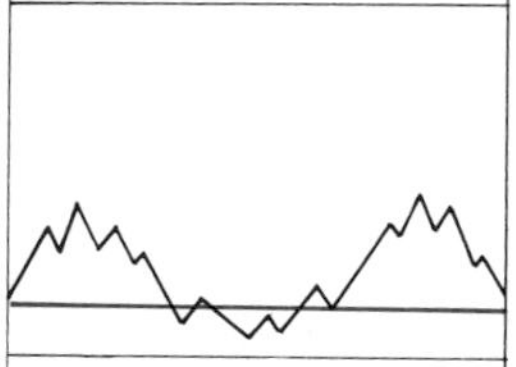
Resolution of pyrexia by **crisis**	An elevated body temperature returns to normal suddenly.	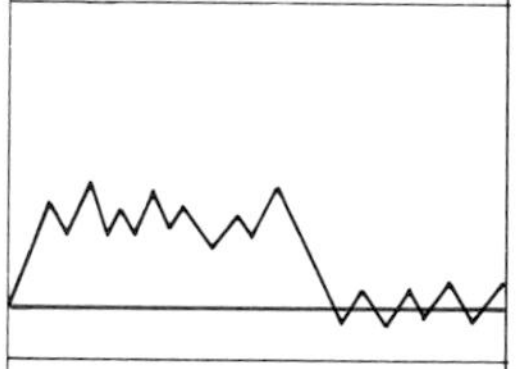
Resolution of pyrexia by **lysis**	An elevated body temperature returns to normal gradually.	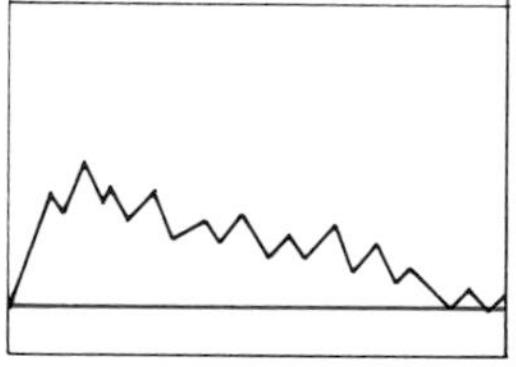

beneficial also. Rates of chemical reactions in the body are slowed, thereby decreasing the metabolic demands for oxygen. Hypothermia as a form of therapy is discussed in clinical texts. Figure 23-1 illustrates the usual ranges of human body temperature.

Assessing Body Temperature

Assessment Methods

Glass Clinical Thermometer. A glass clinical thermometer is most commonly used to measure body temperature. It has two parts, the bulb and the stem. The bulb contains liquid mercury, which expands when exposed to heat and rises within the stem. Figure 23-2 illustrates a rectal and oral clinical thermometer.

Glass thermometers are generally calibrated in either degrees of centigrade (Celsius) or Fahrenheit, abbreviated C and F, respectively. The range is approximately 34°C (94°F) to approximately 42.2°C (108°F). The degrees on a thermometer using the Celsius scale are subdivided into gradients of 0.1; the subdivisions on a thermometer using the Fahrenheit scale are the equivalent of 0.2 degree. It is common practice to report the

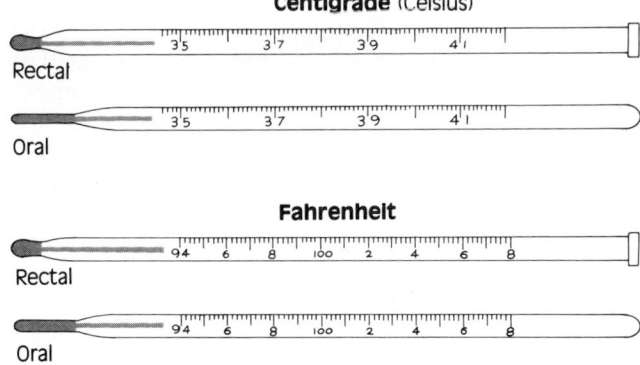

Centigrade (Celsius)

Rectal

Oral

Fahrenheit

Rectal

Oral

F I G U R E   23-2
The two glass thermometers on the top use the centigrade scale to measure temperature; the two on the bottom use the Fahrenheit scale. Note the blunt bulb on the rectal thermometers and the long, thin bulb on the oral thermometers. Either an oral or rectal thermometer may be used to obtain an axillary temperature, although the oral thermometer is generally preferred because of its larger bulb surface.

temperature to the nearest tenth of a degree when the mercury is a bit more or less from a line of calibration. Table 23-4 illustrates comparable centigrade and Farenheit temperatures and explains how temperatures are converted from one scale to the other.

Electronic Thermometer.   Electronic thermometers measure body temperature in 25 to 50 seconds. Most have two nonbreakable temperature probes, one for oral use and one for rectal use. They are equipped with disposable probe covers, a feature that minimizes chances for cross infection and decreases cleaning chores. A sound indicates when the peak temperature has been recorded. This helps the nurse avoid wasting time. Various models are available. The technique for using an electronic thermometer is discussed later in this chapter.

T A B L E   23-4
Equivalent Centigrade and Fahrenheit Temperatures*

Centigrade	Fahrenheit	Centigrade	Fahrenheit
34.0	93.2	38.5	101.3
35.0	95.0	39.0	102.2
36.0	96.8	40.0	104.0
36.5	97.7	41.0	105.8
37.0	98.6	42.0	107.6
37.5	99.5	43.0	109.4
38.0	100.4	44.0	111.2

* To convert Centigrade to Fahrenheit, multiply by 9/5 and add 32. To change Fahrenheit to Centigrade, subtract 32 and multiply by 5/9.

Disposable Single-Use Thermometer.   Disposable single-use thermometers register within seconds, are nonbreakable, and, because they are used only once, eliminate the danger of cross infection.

Temperature-Sensitive Patch or Tape.   The temperature-sensitive tape or patch, commonly applied to the abdomen or forehead, changes color at different temperature ranges. This type of equipment is often used with well infants born at term. Newborns usually are not capable of achieving a fever; assessment of temperature at this age is primarily to determine the infant's ability to regulate body heat. These devices may also be used when it is necessary to check a toddler or young child's temperature who does not appear feverish (Fig. 23-3). A thermometer should be used to check the temperature if the color on the tape or patch indicates that the temperature is either above or below normal average range.

Automated Monitoring Device.   Automated monitoring devices used in hospitals, usually in critical care areas, make it possible to simultaneously measure a patient's body temperature, pulse, and blood pressure. Their use requires less task-oriented nursing time especially when these assessments are obtained frequently.

Assessment Sites

Health agencies specify the site to be used for obtaining clients' temperatures. Most agencies measure temperature by the oral route. However, the nurse will be expected to select and use alternative sites in certain situations. Factors affecting the site selection include such things as age of client, state of consciousness, amount of

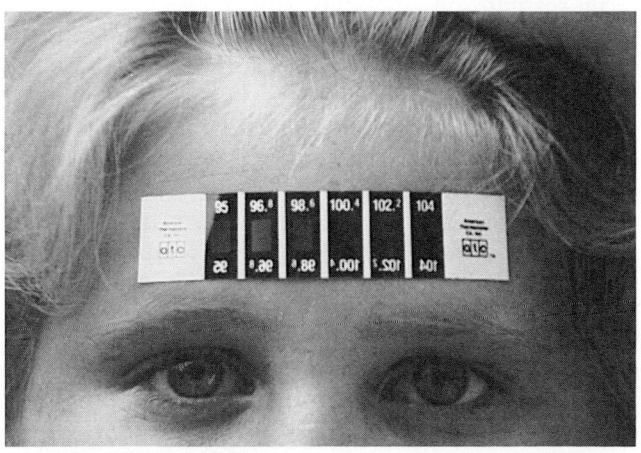

F I G U R E   23-3
This child has a thermometer patch on the forehead. The strip contains liquid crystals, which change colors as the temperature changes. The scale has been adjusted for converting skin-surface temperature to inner-body temperature. Although the calibration is not as detailed as that of a glass thermometer, this type of device is simple to use for a quick assessment. (Photo by Ken Timby)

pain, and other care being provided at the time. It is customary to indicate the site that was used to obtain the temperature when recording the measurement within the client's record.

Obtaining an Oral Temperature.

Obtaining oral temperatures is most common. One criterion for selecting an oral route is that the client must be able to close his mouth around the thermometer. Obtaining an oral temperature using a glass thermometer is contraindicated for unconscious, irrational, and seizure-prone clients, and for infants and young children because of the danger of breaking the glass thermometer in the mouth. Oral temperatures are also contraindicated for persons with diseases of the oral cavity or who have had surgery of the nose or mouth. If a client has had either hot or cold food or fluids or has been smoking or chewing gum, it is generally recommended that a period of approximately 15 minutes elapse before an oral temperature is obtained to allow the oral tissues to return to normal. Traditionally, oral temperatures have not been obtained on clients receiving nasal oxygen because it is believed that the oxygen causes a false low reading. Research is challenging this opinion. However, oral temperatures should not be obtained on clients receiving oxygen by mask, because the time it takes to obtain a reading using a glass thermometer is likely to result in a serious drop in the client's blood level of oxygen. Measures for obtaining an oral temperature are given in Procedures 23-1 and 23-2.

Obtaining a Rectal Temperature.

Obtaining a rectal temperature is a possible alternative whenever obtaining an oral temperature is contraindicated (see Procedure 23-3). It is also recommended practice to check the temperature rectally if the client's oral temperature changes considerably and unexpectedly. Some hospitals require rectal readings on all clients with an elevated temperature. Obtaining a rectal temperature is contraindicated for clients having rectal surgery, diarrhea, and diseases of the rectum. Because the insertion of the thermometer can slow the heart rate by stimulating the vagus nerve, obtaining a rectal temperature is also often not recommended for persons with certain heart diseases.

Using the rectum has been considered by some to be a more accurate way of measuring core temperature than the oral or axillary route. However, this opinion is being challenged by some authorities because studies have shown that the rectal temperature can be influenced by the presence of fecal matter causing a false reading.

Obtaining an Axillary Temperature.

An axillary temperature is generally obtained when both oral and rectal temperatures are contraindicated or when the sites are not accessible. Some hospitals obtain temperatures by the axillary method on normal newborns to avoid the potential for perforating the wall of the rectum with the thermometer. If the axilla has just been washed, obtaining the temperature should be delayed because the tem-

perature of the water and the friction created by drying the skin can influence the temperature. Most authorities believe that when proper procedure is used, axillary temperatures are as accurate as oral or rectal temperatures.

For most clinical purposes, it would appear equally satisfactory to obtain an oral, a rectal, or an axillary temperature *provided proper technique is used* and normal variations among the three methods are taken into account. Figure 23-4 shows the differences in normal body temperature depending on the site selected. Comparing the recordings using two different sites may also be a method for double-checking the validity of an unusual measurement. The procedure for obtaining an axillary temperature is described in Procedure 23-4.

Cleaning a Glass Thermometer

Many health agencies use one thermometer for each client throughout his stay. The thermometer is kept in the client's room, usually in a container of chemical disinfectant. It may be disposed of when the client is discharged, or it may be sent home with the client. It has been recommended that thermometers used for clients having hepatitis be discarded when the client is discharged because of the difficulty of destroying the causative organism. This advice would probably also apply to clients who test positive with the AIDS virus.

It is common practice in some agencies to have thermometers issued from a central supply unit. After being used one time for an individual client, they are returned for cleaning and disinfecting. Procedure 23-5 was prepared for nurses who are expected to clean and disinfect glass clinical thermometers between uses.

(Text continues on p. 407.)

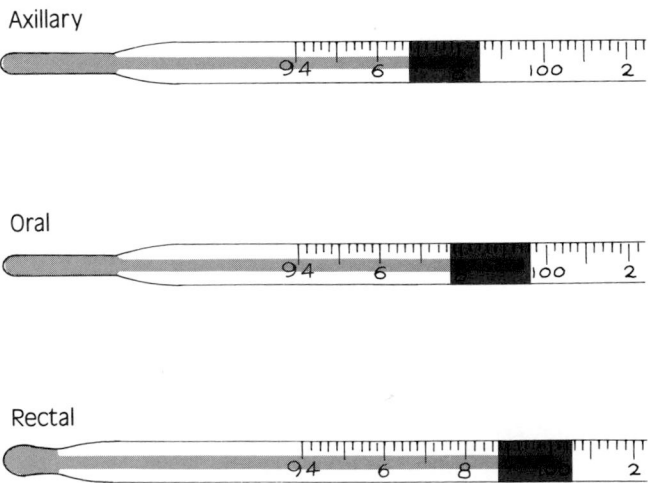

Axillary

Oral

Rectal

F I G U R E 23-4
Comparison of normal adult axillary, oral, and rectal temperature ranges in Fahrenheit.

Assessing Body Temperature by Oral Method/Glass Clinical Thermometer

Equipment

Thermometer   Pencil or pen   Lubricant
Soft tissues   Paper or flow sheet

Action	Rationale
1 Explain the procedure to the client.	An explanation encourages client cooperation and reduces client apprehension.
2 Gather equipment.	Provides for organized approach to task
3 Wash your hands.	Handwashing deters the spread of microorganisms.
4 If the thermometer has been stored in a chemical solution, wipe it dry with a firm, twisting motion, using clean, soft tissue.	Chemical solutions may irritate the mucous membrane and may have an objectionable odor or taste. Soft tissue will approximate the surface, and twisting helps to contact the entire surface.
5 Wipe once from the bulb toward the fingers with each tissue.	Wiping from an area where there are few or no organisms to an area where organisms may be present minimizes the spread of organisms to cleaner areas.
6 Grasp the thermometer firmly with the thumb and forefinger, and with strong wrist movements shake the thermometer until the mercury line reaches at least 36°C (95°F).	Shaking the thermometer moves the mercury back into the bulb below the previously recorded measurement.
7 Read the thermometer by holding it horizontally at eye level, and rotate it between the fingers until the mercury line can be seen clearly.	Holding the thermometer at eye level facilitates reading. Rotating the thermometer will aid in placing the mercury line in a position where it can be read best.
8 Place the mercury bulb of the thermometer well within the back of the right or left pocket under the client's tongue, and instruct him to close his lips around the thermometer.	When the bulb rests deeply in the posterior sublingual pocket it will be in contact with blood vessels lying close to surface and will accurately measure body temperature.

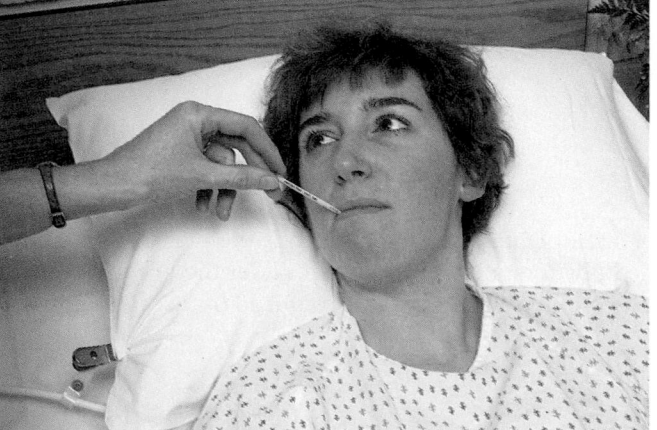

Step 8: Placing the thermometer.

9 Leave the thermometer in place at least 2 minutes. Check agency policy for recommended time interval.	Allowing sufficient time for the mercury to expand ensures an accurate measurement.

(Continued)

Action

10 Remove the thermometer, and wipe it once from the fingers down to the mercury bulb, using a firm, twisting motion.

11 Read the thermometer to the nearest tenth.

Rationale

Cleaning from an area where there are few organisms to an area where there are numerous organisms minimizes their spread to cleaner areas. Friction helps to loosen matter from the surface.

Mercury may rise a bit above or below a calibration on a thermometer.

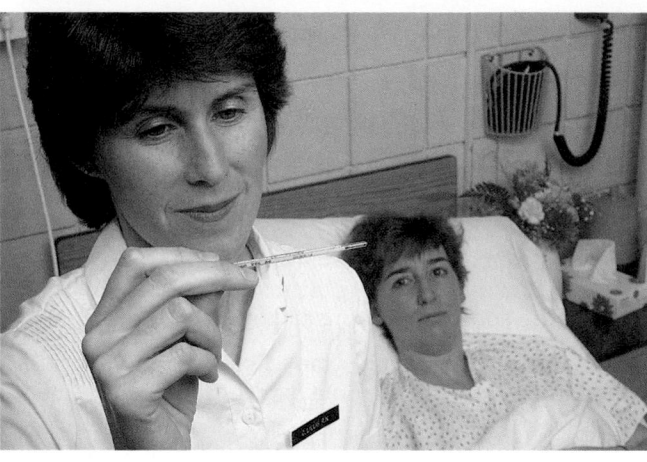

Step 11: Reading the thermometer. (Photos © Ken Kasper)

12 Dispose of the tissue in a receptacle used for contaminated items.

13 Wash thermometer in lukewarm soapy water. Rinse it in cool water. Dry and replace the thermometer in a container at the bedside.

14 Wash your hands.

15 Record temperature on flow sheet or paper. Report any abnormal findings to the appropriate person.

Confining contaminated articles helps to reduce the spread of pathogens.

Mechanical action of washing removes organic material and microorganisms.

Handwashing deters the spread of microorganisms.

Provides accurate documentation.

Age Considerations

The axillary route or a temperature-sensitivity strip is the preferred method of evaluating the body temperature of a child under the age of 6. This should also be the method of choice for a confused or disoriented adult.

Home Care Considerations

Reinforce differences in temperature reading depending on route used. Axillary temperature is generally a degree less than an oral measurement; a rectal temperature is usually a degree higher.

PROCEDURE 23-2
Assessing Body Temperature by Oral Method/Electronic Thermometer

Equipment

Thermometer	Pencil or pen	Lubricant
Soft tissues	Paper or flow sheet	

Action

1 Explain the procedure to the client. Gather equipment.

2 Wash your hands.

3 Release the electronic unit from the charging area.

4 Remove the temperature probe from within the recording unit.

5 Attach a disposable cover over the temperature probe. Make sure it is secure.

6 Place the covered probe in the client's right or left sublingual pocket.

7 Hold the probe in place while it's in the client's mouth.

Rationale

An explanation encourages client cooperation and reduces client apprehension.

Handwashing deters the spread of microorganisms.

Charging sustains the power of the batteries when using the unit as a portable device.

Removal of the probe automatically prepares the machine to measure and record temperature.

A disposable cover prevents the transmission of organisms.

Thermometers placed in the middle area under the tongue have not registered as accurately as those placed in the areas to the sides.

If unsupported, the weight of the probe tends to fall away from the deepest areas under the tongue causing the measurement to be less reliable.

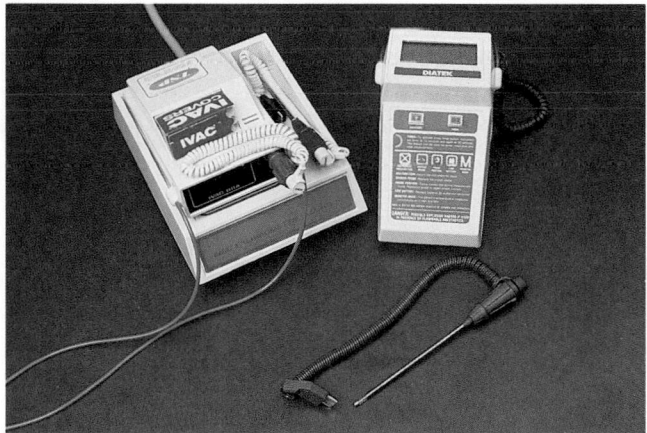

Two types of electronic thermometers and probes.

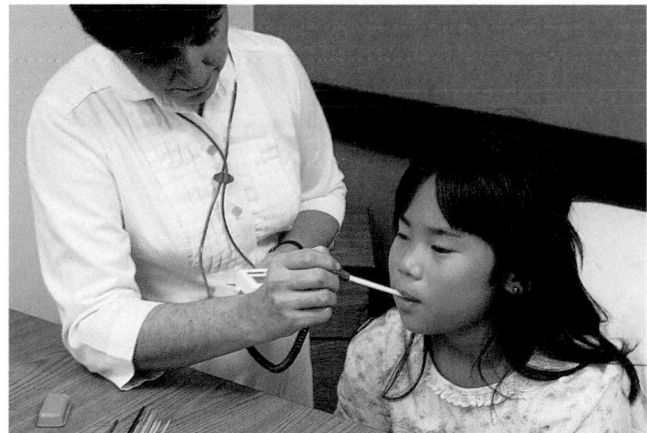

Steps 6 and 7: Placing and supporting the probe in place in the client's mouth.

8 Listen for a sound indicating that a maximum recording has been reached.

9 Remove the probe from the client's mouth, and note the numbers displayed on the electronic unit.

10 Press the probe release button while holding it over a receptacle, such as a wastebasket.

A sound indicates that the unit is no longer sensing any further change in the measurement.

An electronic thermometer is not calibrated with multiple numbers. It displays only the measured temperature.

The release button frees the disposable cover from the probe without being touched by the nurse's hands.

(Continued)

PROCEDURE 23-2

Assessing Body Temperature by Oral Method/Electronic Thermometer (continued)

Action	Rationale
11 Return the probe to its storage location within the electronic unit.	The probe is protected from becoming broken if transported or stored within the recording unit.
12 Wash your hands.	Handwashing deters the spread of microorganisms.
13 Record temperature on flow sheet or paper. Report any abnormal findings to the appropriate person.	Provides accurate documentation.
14 Return the electronic unit, and reconnect it to the source for charging the batteries.	Equipment needed by personnel for multiple patient use should be readily available.

Age Considerations

The axillary route or a temperature-sensitivity strip is the preferred method of evaluating the body temperature of a child under the age of 6. This should also be the method of choice for a confused or disoriented adult.

Home Care Considerations

Reinforce differences in temperature reading depending on route used. Axillary temperature is generally a degree less than an oral measurement; a rectal temperature is usually a degree higher.

PROCEDURE 23-3

Assessing Body Temperature by Rectal Method/Glass Thermometer

Equipment

Thermometer	Pencil or pen	Lubricant
Soft tissues	Paper or flow sheet	Disposable gloves (optional)

Action	Rationale
1 Explain the procedure to the client.	An explanation encourages client cooperation and reduces client apprehension.
2 Gather equipment.	Provides for organized approach to task

(Continued)

3 Wash your hands. Don a disposable glove on your dominant hand or on both hands.

Handwashing deters the spread of microorganisms. Disposable glove protects the nurse from microorganisms in the feces.

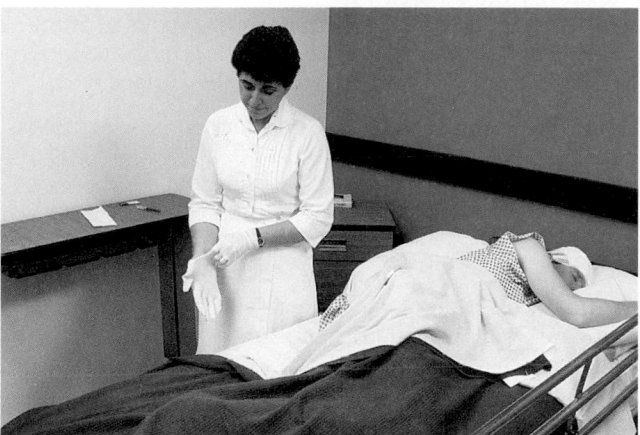

Step 3: Donning clean gloves.

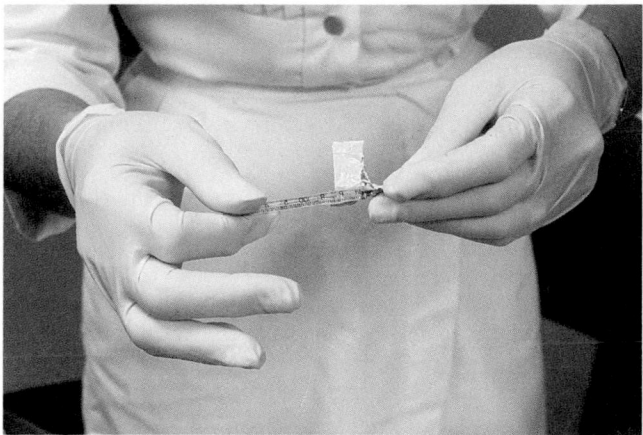

Step 5: Lubricating the mercury bulb.

4 Wipe, shake, and read the rectal thermometer.

A rectal thermometer requires the same preparation as an oral thermometer.

5 Lubricate the mercury bulb and an area approximately 2.5 cm (1 inch) above the bulb.

Lubrication reduces friction and thereby facilitates insertion minimizing irritation or injury to the mucous membrane of the anal canal.

6 Provide for privacy. With the client on his side, fold back the bed linen and separate the buttocks so that the anal sphincter is seen clearly.

If not placed directly through the anal opening, the bulb of the thermometer may injure the adjacent tissue or cause discomfort for the client.

7 Insert the thermometer for approximately 3.8 cm (1½ inches) in an adult, 2.5 cm (1 inch) in a child, and 1.25 cm (½ inch) in an infant.

Insertion length must be adjusted according to the anatomical size of the client's rectum.

8 Permit the client's buttocks to fall in place while holding the thermometer in place for 2 to 3 minutes.

The thermometer may become displaced internally or externally if it is not held in place.

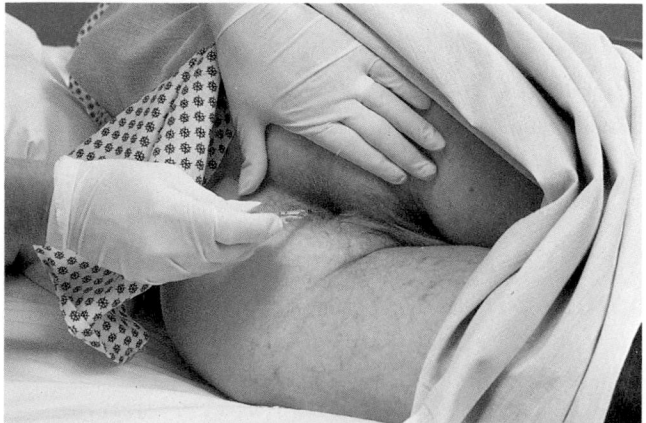

Steps 6 and 7: Separating the buttocks and inserting the thermometer.

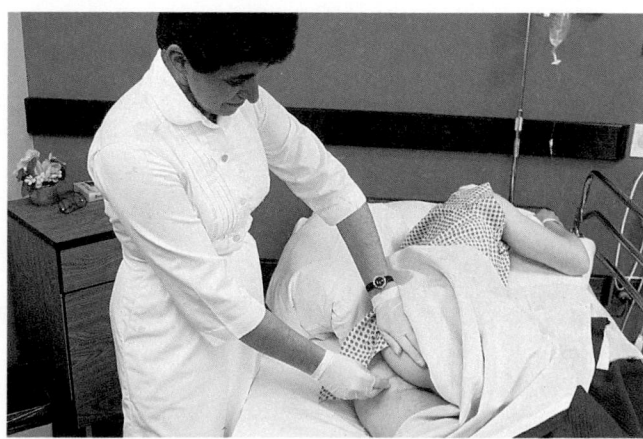

Step 8: Holding the thermometer in place.

(Continued)

Action	**Rationale**
9 Remove the thermometer, and wipe it once with soft tissue from the fingers to the mercury bulb, using a firm, twisting motion.	Cleaning from an area where there are few organisms to an area where there are numerous organisms minimizes the spread of organisms. Friction helps to loosen the lubricant and fecal matter from the surface.
10 Wipe any residue of lubricant or stool remaining about the anus.	Removing lubricant and stool promotes the cleanliness and comfort of the client.
11 Read the thermometer and dispose of the tissue in a receptacle used for contaminated items.	Items containing organisms should be placed in containers for disposal to avoid transmitting them to other persons.
12 Wash thermometer in lukewarm soapy water. Rinse in cool water. Dry and replace the thermometer in container at the bedside. Remove the disposable glove from the inside out and discard the glove.	Mechanical action of washing aids in removal of organic material and microorganisms.
13 Wash your hands.	Handwashing deters the spread of microorganisms.
14 Record temperature on flow sheet or paper. Indicate that rectal route was used. Report any abnormal findings to the appropriate person.	Provides accurate documentation

Age Considerations

The axillary route or a temperature-sensitivity strip is the preferred method of evaluating the body temperature of a child under the age of 6. This should also be the method of choice for a confused or disoriented adult.

Home Care Considerations

Reinforce differences in temperature reading depending on route used. Axillary temperature is generally a degree less than an oral measurement; a rectal temperature is usually a degree higher.

PROCEDURE 23-4

Assessing Body Temperature by Axillary Method/Glass Thermometer

Equipment

Thermometer	Pencil or pen	Lubricant
Soft tissues	Paper or flow sheet	

(Continued)

Action

1 Explain the procedure to the client.

2 Gather equipment.

3 Wash your hands.

4 Provide privacy and move gown to expose axilla.

5 Wipe the thermometer with a clean tissue if it has been stored in a chemical solution. Use a firm, twisting motion to remove the moisture.

6 Shake and read the thermometer as suggested in Procedure 23-1.

7 Place the bulb of the thermometer into the center of the axilla.

8 Bring the client's arm down close to his body, and place his forearm over his chest.

Rationale

An explanation encourages client cooperation and reduces client apprehension.

Provides for organized approach to task.

Handwashing deters the spread of microorganisms.

Ensures accurate placement of thermometer.

Chemical solutions may irritate the skin. The presence of solution may alter skin temperature. Soft tissue and friction help remove the solution.

The mercury must be below the calibrations of the previous recording in order to assess the present temperature accurately.

The deepest area of the axilla will provide the most accurate temperature measurement.

Surrounding the bulb with the skin surfaces of the axilla reduces the amount of surrounding air and ensures a reliable measurement.

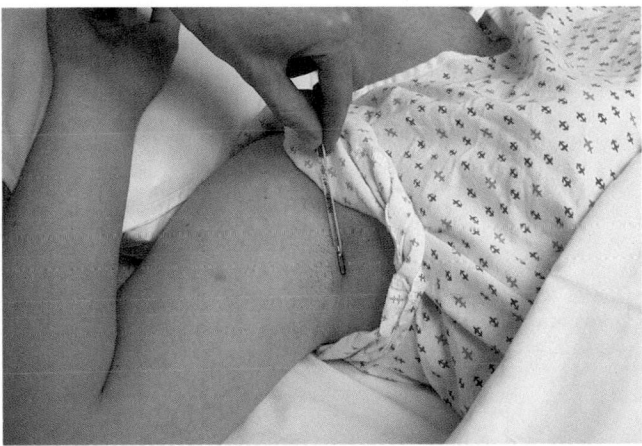

Step 7: Placing the bulb in the center of the axilla.

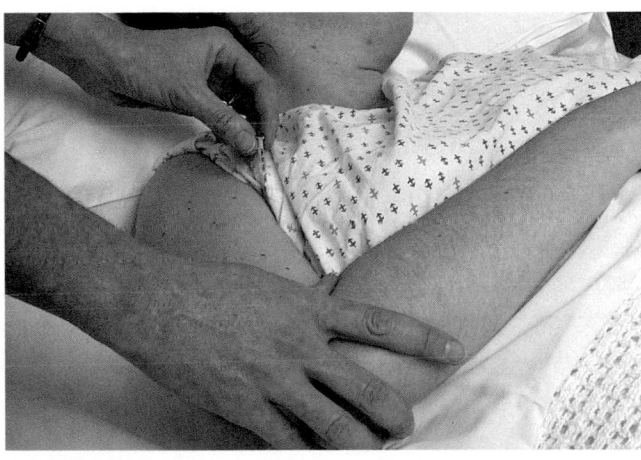

Step 8: Placing the client's arm close to the body. (Photos © Ken Kasper)

9 Remain with the client and leave the thermometer in place for 10 minutes.

10 Remove and read the thermometer. Clean the thermometer and replace it in its location for reuse.

11 Wash your hands.

12 Record temperature on flow sheet or paper. Indicate axillary route. Report any abnormal findings to the appropriate person.

Additional time is required to ensure that the mercury expands to the maximum level of the client's temperature.

A thermometer that has been used for an axillary temperature should be cleaned before using it for another route and vice versa.

Handwashing deters the spread of microorganisms.

Provides accurate documentation.

(Continued)

PROCEDURE 23-4
Assessing Body Temperature by Axillary Method/Glass Thermometer (continued)

Age Considerations

The axillary route or a temperature-sensitivity strip is the preferred method of evaluating the body temperature of a child under the age of 6. This should also be the method of choice for a confused or disoriented adult.

Home Care Considerations

Reinforce differences in temperature reading depending on route used. Axillary temperature is generally a degree less than an oral measurement; a rectal temperature is usually a degree higher.

PROCEDURE 23-5
Cleaning and Disinfecting a Glass Thermometer

Equipment

Glass thermometer	Soap or detergent	Chemical solution
Soft tissues	solution	(if specified)

Action	**Rationale**
1 Use clean, soft tissues for wiping and cleaning the thermometer.	The texture of soft tissues facilitates contact with all surfaces of the thermometer to remove organic matter that interferes with disinfection.
2 Use a fresh tissue each time the thermometer must be wiped.	Using a clean surface prevents redistributing organic matter.
3 Hold the tissue at the stem end, near the fingers holding the thermometer.	Cleaning from an area where there are few organisms to an area where there are numerous organisms minimizes the spread of organisms to cleaner areas.
4 Wipe down toward the bulb, using a twisting motion.	Friction helps to loosen mucus, lubricant, or fecal matter from the surface.
5 After the thermometer has been wiped, clean it with soap or detergent solution, again using friction.	Soap or detergent solutions loosen adhered matter.

(Continued)

Action	Rationale

6 Rinse the thermometer under cold, running water.

Rinsing with water helps to remove organisms and foreign material loosened by washing. Also, certain chemical solutions are rendered ineffective in the presence of soap, for example, benzalkonium chloride (Zephiran Chloride).

7 Dry the thermometer to remove the moisture after it has been rinsed.

The strength of a chemical solution is diluted if a film of water covers the thermometer.

8 Immerse the thermometer in the chemical solution specified.

Chemical solutions must be used in proper strength for the proper length of time to be effective. Heat cannot be used to disinfect a glass clinical thermometer because heat sufficient to kill organisms will cause the mercury to expand beyond the column and ruin the thermometer.

9 Rinse the thermometer with water after disinfection and before reuse.

Chemical solutions may irritate the mucous membrane of the mouth or the rectum. Also, they may have an objectionable odor and taste.

10 Return the thermometer to the storage receptacle.

Covering the thermometer protects it from becoming broken and contaminated with organisms in the general environment.

11 Wash your hands.

Handwashing deters the spread of microorganisms.

In the home, thermometers should be cleaned with soap and water and then stored for reuse. If the thermometer is to be used by more than one person or if the person has a known or suspected infection transmitted by oral secretions, it should be disinfected with an appropriate solution following cleaning. The techniques in Procedure 23-5 may also be used for client or family health teaching.

The nurse should follow manufacturers' recommendations concerning the care and disposal of electronic and other types of thermometers and their sheaths.

PULSE

Physiology

The stimulus for contraction of the heart starts in the **sinoatrial node** (SA node), which is in the upper part of the right atrium. Because this node sets the pace of the beat, it is often called the pacemaker.

Each time the left ventricle of the heart contracts to eject blood into an already full aorta, the arterial walls in the blood system expand or distend to compensate for the increase in pressure. This expansion of the aorta sends a wave through the walls of the arterial system which, on palpation, can be felt as a light tap. This sensation is called the **pulse**.

The quantity of blood forced out of the left ventricle with each contraction is called the **stroke volume**. The average amount of blood per contraction is 70 ml for an adult. The **cardiac output** is the amount of blood pumped per minute. This volume is determined by using the formula

Cardiac Output = Stroke Volume × Pulse Rate

Thus, the cardiac output of an adult with a stroke volume of 70 ml and a pulse rate of 72 beats per minute would be approximately 5000 ml. Many factors can affect both the heart rate, such as exercise, and the volume, such as a person's state of fluid balance. However, the body attempts to maintain a sufficient supply of blood to the cells at all times. For example, when the stroke volume decreases, such as when the blood volume is lowered because of hemorrhage, the contraction rate increases to maintain the same cardiac output. Conversely, in a physically fit athlete whose heart pumps a maximum volume

(Text continues on p. 411.)

PROCEDURE 23-6
Assessing the Radial Pulse Rate

Equipment

Watch with second hand or digital readout

Pencil or pen

Paper or flow sheet

Action

1 Explain the procedure to client.

2 Gather equipment.

3 Wash your hands.

4 Have the client lie down and rest his arm alongside his body with the wrist extended and the palm of the hand downward. Or the client can sit with his forearm at a 90-degree angle to the body resting on a support and with the wrist extended and the palm of the hand downward.

5 Place your first, second, and third fingers along the client's radial artery, and press gently against the radius; rest your thumb in apposition to fingers on the back of the client's wrist.

6 Apply only enough pressure so that the client's pulsating artery can be felt distinctly.

7 Using a watch with a second hand, count the number of pulsations felt for 30 seconds. Multiply this number by two to obtain the rate for 1 minute.

Rationale

An explanation encourages client cooperation and reduces client apprehension.

Provides for organized approach to task

Handwashing deters the spread of microorganisms.

These positions are ordinarily comfortable for the client and convenient for the nurse.

The fingertips, sensitive to touch, will feel pulsation of the client's radial artery. If the thumb is used for palpating the client's pulse, the nurse's own pulse may be felt.

Moderate pressure allows the nurse to feel the superficial radial artery expand with each heartbeat. Too much pressure will obliterate the pulse. If too little pressure is applied, the pulse will be imperceptible.

Sufficient time is necessary to assess the rate, rhythm, and amplitude of the pulse.

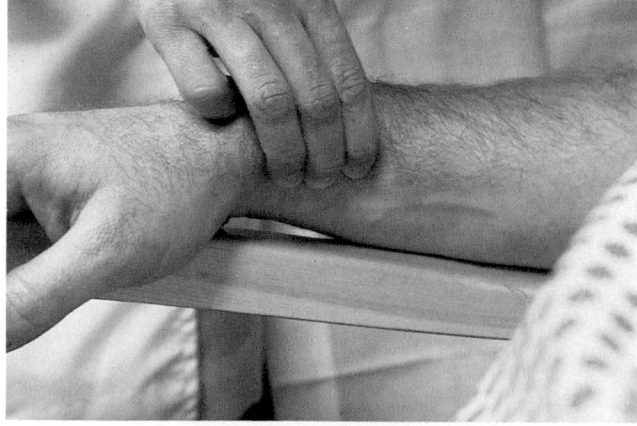

Step 5: Proper placement of the fingers along the radial artery.

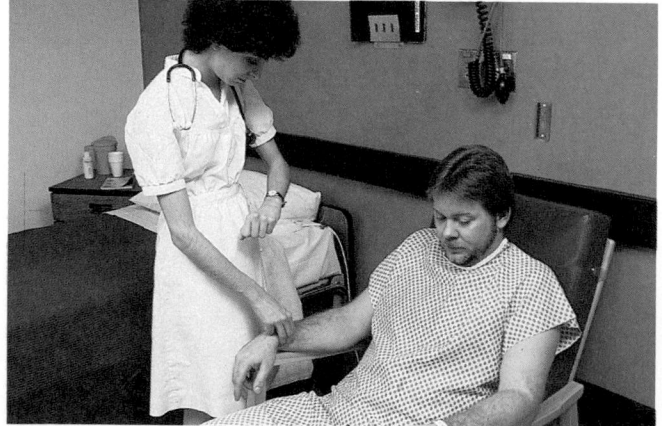

Step 7: Counting the pulsations felt for 30 seconds.

(Continued)

Action	**Rationale**
8 If the pulse rate is abnormal in any way, palpate the pulse for a full minute or longer.	When the pulse is abnormal, longer counting and palpation are necessary to identify most accurately the unusual characteristics of the pulse.
9 Assess rhythm, amplitude, and elasticity of the vessel wall while counting rate.	Irregularity in heart rate may disrupt the cardiac output. Amplitude of pulse indicates the quality of the heart's contraction. Elasticity of blood vessel does not affect the pulse rate but does reflect status of the vascular system.
10 Record pulse on flow sheet or paper. Report any abnormal findings to the appropriate person.	Provides accurate documentation.
11 Wash your hands.	Handwashing deters the spread of microorganisms.

Special Considerations

Inform the client of availability of digital pulse monitoring devices.

Instruct family members about techniques used to locate and monitor other peripheral pulse sites.

P R O C E D U R E   23-7
Assessing the Apical Pulse Rate

Equipment

Watch with second hand or digital readout	Pencil or pen	Alcohol swab
Stethoscope	Paper or flow sheet	

Action	**Rationale**
1 Explain the procedure to the client.	An explanation encourages client cooperation and reduces client apprehension.
2 Gather equipment.	Provides for organized approach to task
3 Wash your hands.	Handwashing deters the spread of microorganisms.
4 Use alcohol swab to cleanse ear pieces and diaphragm of stethoscope if necessary.	Cleansing with alcohol deters transmission of microorganisms.
5 Assist client to sitting position in bed or on a chair if possible.	Eases identification of site for nurse

(Continued)

Action

6 Provide privacy and move gown to expose upper chest area.

7 Hold diaphragm of stethoscope against palm of hand for a few seconds.

8 Palpate fifth intercostal space and move to left midclavicular line. Place diaphragm over apex of heart.

9 Listen for normal heart sounds, identified as "lub dub" beat.

10 Using a watch with a second hand, count the heartbeat for 30 seconds and multiply by two if rhythm is regular. Count for 60 seconds if irregular rhythm is present.

Rationale

Facilitates identification of site for placement of stethoscope.

Warms metal area of stethoscope which may be cold and may startle client.

This is PMI (point of maximal impulse) where heartbeat is easier to hear.

These sounds occur as blood flows through heart valves.

Longer time interval allows for more accurate assessment of heart rate.

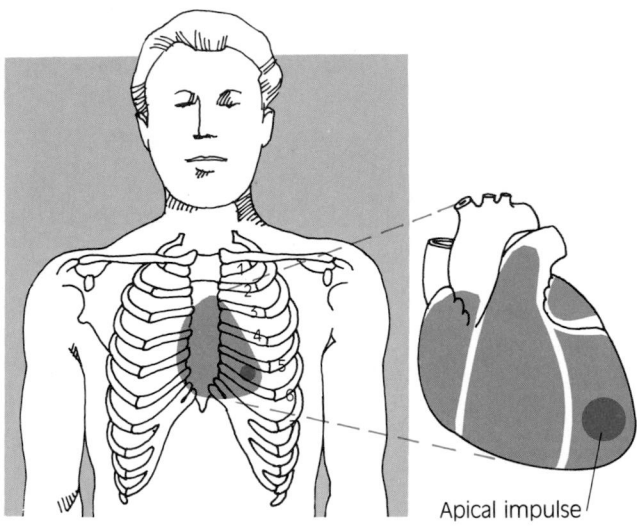

Schematic of the thorax showing location of apical impulse.

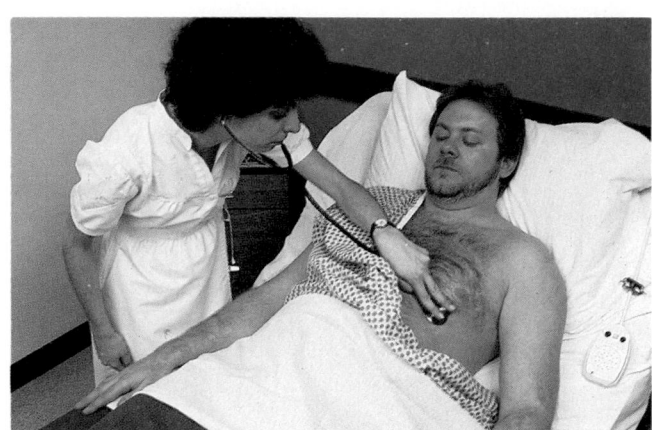

Step 10: Counting the heartbeat for 30 seconds.

11 Assess presence of any irregularity in heart rate and rhythm.

12 Replace the client's gown and assist client to comfortable position.

13 Record pulse on flow sheet or paper. Identify as apical rate. Report any abnormal findings to the appropriate person.

14 Wash your hands.

Indicates adequacy of cardiac function

Provides for privacy and comfort

Provides accurate documentation.

Handwashing deters the spread of microorganisms.

Special Considerations

Inform client of availability of digital pulse monitoring devices.
Instruct family members about techniques used to locate and monitor other peripheral pulse sites.

of blood per stroke, the heart rate may be well at the low range or below the range of normal yet the body cells remain adequately supplied.

Pulse Rate

The pulse rate is the number of pulsations felt in a minute. This ordinarily corresponds to the same rate at which the heart is beating. There are wide ranges for normal pulse rates. Rates differ as individuals age, gradually diminishing from birth to adulthood as shown in Table 23-5.

A rapid heart rate is called **tachycardia**. An adult has tachycardia when the pulse rate is 100 to 180 beats per minute. **Palpitation** means that the person is aware of his own heartbeat without having to feel for it over an artery. The pulse rate is ordinarily unduly rapid when palpitations are noted.

The term used to describe the heart rate when it falls below 60 beats per minute in an adult is called **bradycardia**. A slow pulse rate during illness is less common than a rapid pulse rate, but, when present, bradycardia should be reported promptly.

The pulse rate is generally slower at rest and upon awakening. Females generally have a slightly faster rate, about seven to eight beats per minute, than males. It has been noted that the body size and build of a person may affect the pulse rate. Tall, slender persons often have a slower rate than short, stout ones.

The rate of the heartbeat, and thus the pulse as well, readily responds to impulses conducted along the autonomic nervous system. This system is subdivided into parasympathetic and sympathetic networks of nerves. Stimulation of the parasympathetic system decreases the heart rate. The drug digitalis, commonly used by patients with certain heart ailments, decreases the heart's contractions by stimulating the vagus nerve. Stimulation of the sympathetic system increases the heart rate. The following factors also will contribute to an increase in the pulse rate:

- Pain
- Strong emotions, such as fear, anger, anxiety, and surprise
- Exercise, when the heart's compensatory ability attempts to meet the need for increased blood circulation
- Prolonged application of heat
- A decrease in blood pressure, such as occurs with blood loss, when the heart's compensatory ability attempts to meet the need for increased output of blood from the heart
- An elevated temperature, which usually causes an increase of about seven to ten beats per minute for each 0.6°C (1°F) of elevation above normal
- Any condition resulting in poor oxygenation of blood, for example, chronic pulmonary disease

Rhythm of the Pulse

The pulse rhythm is the pattern of the pulsations and the pauses between them. The pulse rhythm is normally regular (*i.e.*, the beat and the pauses occur similarly throughout the time the pulse is being obtained).

An irregular pattern of heartbeats, and consequently an irregular pulse rhythm, is called a **dysrhythmia** or **arrhythmia**. Any dysrhythmia should be reported promptly. More details about dysrhythmias and their causes can be found in clinical textbooks. Some common pulse rhythm are described and illustrated in Table 23-6.

Amplitude of the Pulse

The pulse amplitude describes the quality of the pulse in terms of its fullness and reflects the strength of the left ventricular contraction. It is noted by the feel of the blood flow through the vessel. Under normal conditions, the amplitude of each pulse beat is strong and feels similarly so at all areas where an artery can be palpated. A strong pulse can be obliterated with relative ease by exerting pressure over the artery, but it remains perceptible with moderate pressure. Table 23-7 presents a scale commonly used to describe pulse amplitude.

Assessing the Pulse

Assessment Sites

The rate, rhythm, and amplitude of the pulse may be assessed by compressing an artery against an underlying bone with the tips of the fingers. The arteries located close to the skin surface are used most often. Most, but not all, are named for the bone to which each is adjacent. Common arteries used for assessment include the temporal, carotid, brachial, radial, femoral, popliteal, posterial tibial, and dorsalis pedis. Collectively they are called peripheral pulses because they are distant from the heart. The location of these sites is illustrated in Figure 23-5.

Radial Pulse Rate. Most commonly, the radial artery at the wrist is used for palpating the pulse because it is

T A B L E 23-5
Normal Pulse Rates per Minute at Various Ages

Age	Approximate Range	Approximate Average
Newborn to 1 month	120–160	140
1 month to 12 months	80–140	120
12 months to 2 years	80–130	110
2 years to 6 years	75–120	100
6 years to 12 years	75–110	95
Adolescence to adult	60–100	80

T A B L E   23-6
Various Pulse Rhythms

Term	Description	Illustration (each vertical line = one heartbeat)
Regular	The pulsations and the pauses occur similarly throughout the entire minute.	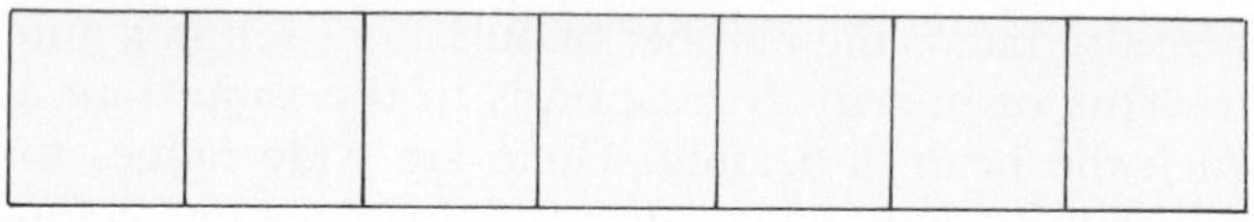 Normal
		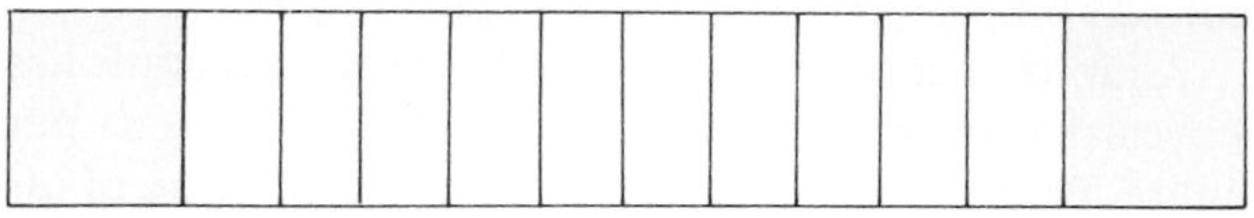 Tachycardia
		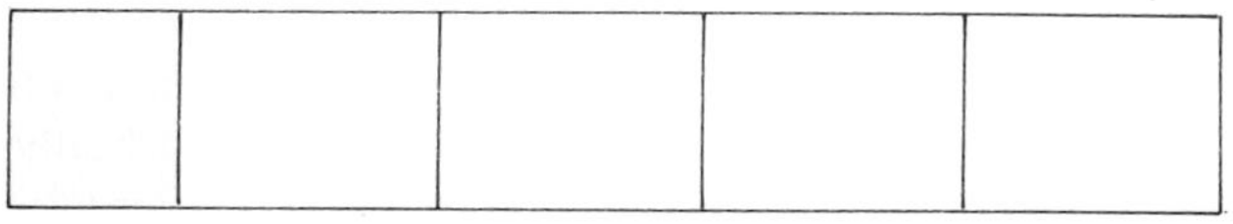 Bradycardia
Dysrhythmia	The pulsations or length of pauses occur with no pattern or predictability.	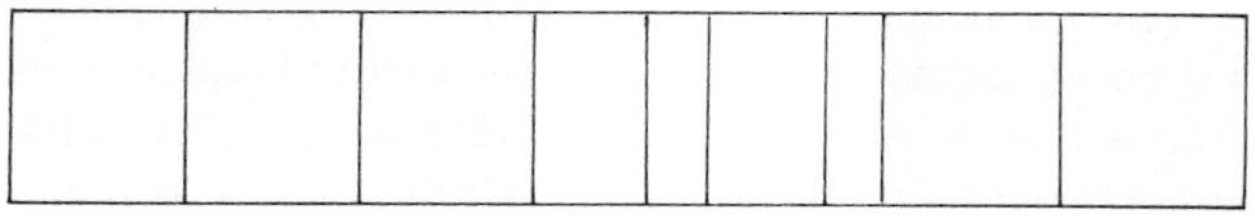 Intermittent — A normal pulse rhythm is broken by periods of irregularity.
		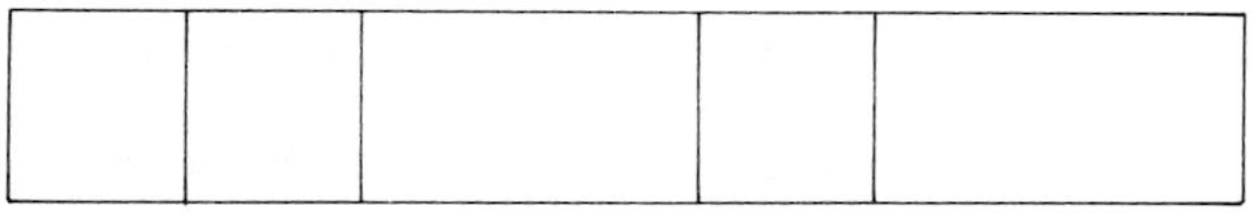 Bigeminal — A normal pulse rhythm of two beats is followed by a pause.
		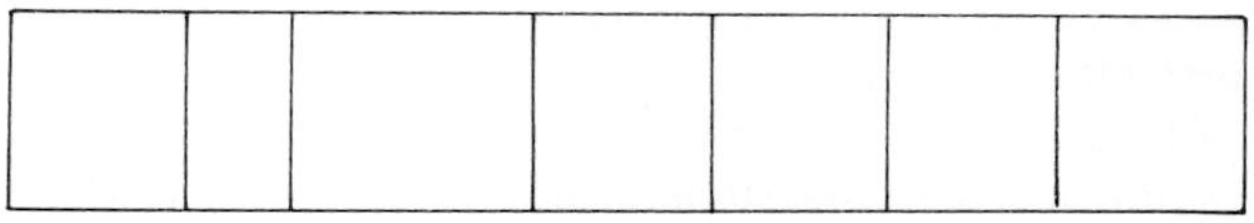 Premature beat — A heartbeat occurs before the normal one.

easily accessible. It is located on the inner, thumb-side of the wrist. Figure 23-6 shows its location and the position of the fingertips during assessment. If this site is not accessible, select an alternative artery that does not require exertion or cause discomfort for the person because this could alter the pulse rate. Procedure 23-6 describes how to obtain the pulse rate using the site of the radial artery.

Apical Pulse Rate.   If a peripheral pulse is irregular, feeble, or extremely rapid causing it to be difficult to assess accurately, the apical rate may be assessed. In the adult, the apical rate is counted by listening with a stethoscope over the apex of the heart. The contraction of the heart can be heard in the space between the fifth and the sixth ribs, about 8 cm (3 inches) to the left of the median line and slightly below the nipple, as illustrated in Fig-

TABLE 23-7
Amplitude of the Pulse

Number	Definition	Description
0	Absent pulse	No pulsation is felt despite extreme pressure.
1+	Thready pulse	Pulsation is not easily felt and slight pressure causes it to disappear.
2+	Weak pulse	Stronger than a thready pulse; light pressure causes it to disappear.
3+	Normal pulse	Pulsation is easily felt, takes moderate pressure to cause it to disappear.
4+	Bounding pulse	The pulsation is strong and does not disappear with moderate pressure.

(Lewis LW, Timby BK: Fundamental Skills and Concepts in Patient Care, 4th ed, p 196. Philadelphia, 1988)

ure 23-7. Nursing actions are given in Procedure 23-7. The apical rate of an infant is easily palpated with the fingertips.

Apical-Radial Pulse Rate. When the radial pulse is irregular, the **apical-radial pulse rate** may be obtained by counting at the apex of the heart and at the radial artery simultaneously. The following techniques are recommended to obtain an apical-radial pulse rate:

- Two nurses are needed; one listens with a stethoscope over the apex of the heart for the heartbeat, and the other counts the rate at the radial artery.
- The client's chest wall is exposed so that the stethoscope can be placed directly on the skin of the chest wall.
- One watch with a sweep second hand is placed so that both nurses can read it conveniently and simultaneously.
- The nurses determine where they can best hear and feel the pulse and decide on a time to start counting, such as when the second hand on the watch is at a specified place.
- Both nurses count for 1 full minute and record their counts.

The difference between the apical and radial pulse rates is called the **pulse deficit.**

RESPIRATION

Respiration, in its broadest sense, begins with the act of breathing and includes the body's use of oxygen and the

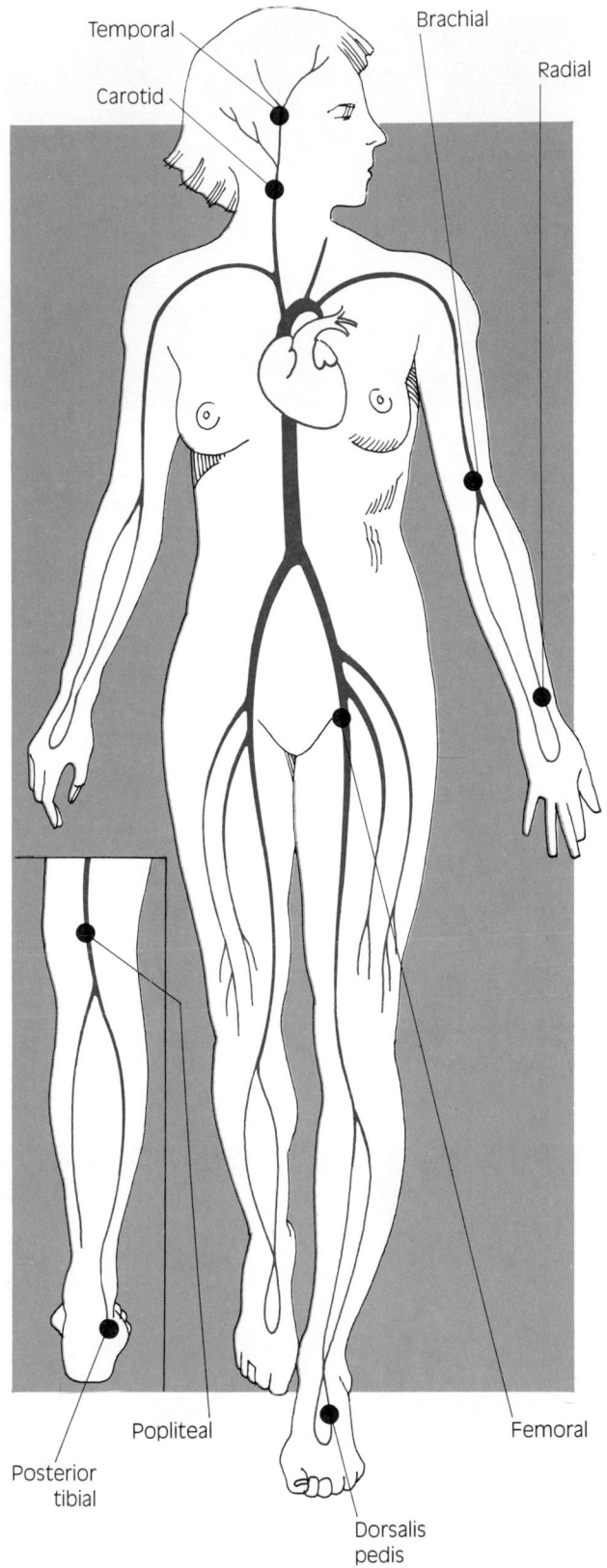

FIGURE 23-5
These arteries are located near the surface of the body. The pulse can be detected in any of these sites by light palpation.

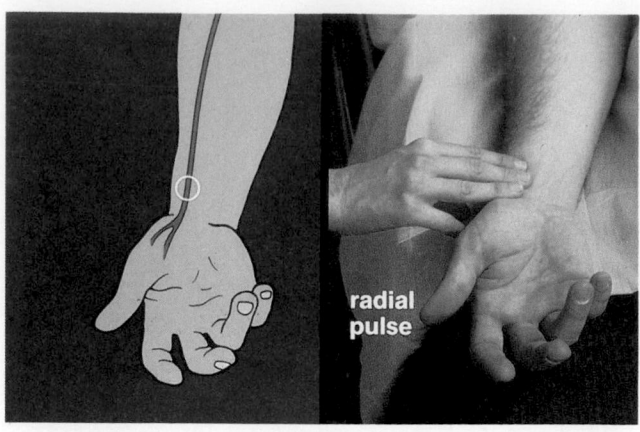

F I G U R E   23-6

The drawing to the left illustrates the location of the radial artery. In the photograph to the right the nurse is shown palpating the artery on a patient.

elimination of carbon dioxide. **Inspiration** or **inhalation** is the act of breathing in, and **expiration** or **exhalation** is the act of breathing out. **External respiration** includes lung ventilation, the absorption of oxygen, and the elimination of carbon dioxide. **Internal respiration**, sometimes called **tissue respiration**, includes the use of oxygen by body cells for the production of heat through oxidation and the liberation of energy from the food we eat.

Physiology

Respirations can be somewhat voluntarily controlled by activating or restricting muscles of the chest and diaphragm. This explains the ability of a person to control breathing when talking and singing. However, chemical

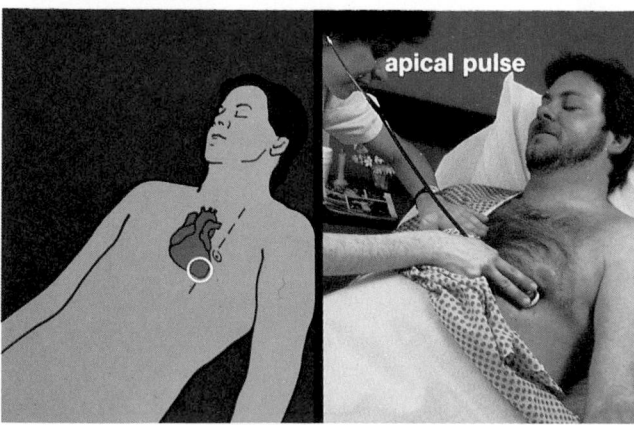

F I G U R E   23-7

The drawing to the left illustrates the site of the apical pulse at the apex of the heart. In the photograph to the right, the nurse listens to the heartbeat using a stethoscope.

receptors act as the primary involuntary regulator for respiration. As carbon dioxide accumulates in the blood, chemoreceptors in the aortic and carotid bodies dispatch impulses to the respiratory center in the medulla oblongata and the rate and depth of respirations are increased. Despite a parent's panic when a child has a temper tantrum and holds his breath, chemical stimulation of respiration eventually overcomes the child's voluntary efforts to control it.

Assessing Respirations

Respiratory Rate

Under normal conditions, healthy adults breathe approximately 16 to 20 times a minute. Wider variations have also been observed in healthy persons. The respiratory rate is more rapid in infants and young children. It has been noted that the relationship between the pulse rate and the respiratory rate is fairly consistent in well persons, the ratio being one respiration to approximately four heartbeats.

During illness, the respiratory rate may vary from normal. When body temperature is elevated, the respiratory rate increases in response to the increased metabolic rate. Cells require more oxygen at this time and have a greater amount of carbon dioxide that must be removed. The rate will increase as much as four breaths per minute with every 0.6°C (1°F) that the temperature rises above normal. Any condition involving an accumulation of carbon dioxide and a decrease in oxygen in the blood will also tend to increase the rate and the depth of respirations.

Some conditions characteristically predispose to slow breathing. An increase in intracranial pressure will depress the respiratory center, resulting in irregular or shallow, slow breathing, or both. Certain drugs also depress the respiratory rate, morphine sulfate being an example.

Respiratory Depth

In a state of rest, the depth of each respiration is approximately the same. The depth of respirations is generally described as ranging from shallow to deep. Periodically, each person automatically inhales deeply, filling the lungs with more air than inhaled with the usual depth of respiration.

Certain terms are used to describe the nature and depth of respirations. **Apnea** refers to periods during which there is no breathing. This is a serious situation in which brain damage and death can occur if it is suppressed for more than 4 to 6 minutes. **Dyspnea** is difficult or labored breathing. A dyspneic client is likely to demonstrate rapid, shallow breathing. Dyspneic patients usually appear to be anxious and worried as they experience the inefficient work of breathing. The nostrils flare (widen) as the client struggles to fill his lungs with air. Dyspneic persons frequently find some relief if they assume an upright position. The condition of being able to breathe easier in this manner is known as **orthopnea**. A sitting or standing position uses gravity to lower organs in the abdominal cavity to fall away from the diaphragm. This gives more room for the lungs to expand within the chest, thus taking in more air with each breath.

Breath Sounds

Ordinarily respirations are relatively noiseless. Several terms are used to describe the nature of sounds that can be heard with the ear as a patient breathes. **Stertorous breathing** is a general term used to refer to noisy respirations. **Stridor** is a harsh, high-pitched sound heard on inspiration when there is narrowing of the upper airway, such as the larynx or trachea. Infants or young children with croup often manifest stridor when breathing.

The nurse may listen to respirations throughout the chest with a stethoscope. The purpose of this assessment is to listen to the sounds of air moving through the large and small air chambers throughout the lobes of the lungs. **Adventitious sounds** are abnormal breath sounds, such as the following:

• **Rales**, also called crackles by some because they sound like air-filled rice breakfast cereal placed in milk, are intermittent sounds caused by moisture in respiratory passages. They are heard more commonly during inspiration and may change in character with coughing. The sound heard as hair is rubbed between the fingers and thumb beside the ear simulates the sound produced by rales.

• **Rhonchi**, also called gurgles by some, are continuous low-pitched sounds produced by air moving across narrowed respiratory passageways often containing an accumulation of secretions. They may occur during inspiration, but are more predominant on expiration, or both, and may change with coughing.

• A **wheeze** is a high-pitched sound repeated during respirations as air is forced through narrow respiratory passages. During an asthma attack, a wheeze is often heard during inspiration. It may even be heard without a stethoscope.

• A **friction rub** is a grating sound made as structures move across one another. Ordinarily a thin layer of moisture helps the pleural membranes glide noiselessly over the lung. When the membranes surrounding the lungs lose their moisture, they produce the characteristic sound referred to as a pleural friction rub.

Table 23-8 presents additional terms used to describe the nature of respirations. Procedure 23-8 describes how to obtain the respiratory rate.

T A B L E 23-8
The Nature of Respirations

Term	Description	Illustration (Each stroke = one respiration and its depth)
Eupnea	Normal respirations; the rate and depth are equal.	
Tachypnea or **polypnea**	A fast respiratory rate	
Bradypnea	A slow respiratory rate	
Cheyne-Stokes	A gradual increase followed by a gradual decrease in the depth of respirations, and then a period of apnea	
Biot's	Respirations of the same depth followed by a period of apnea	

PROCEDURE 23-8
Assessing the Respiratory Rate

Equipment

Watch with second hand or digital readout   Pencil or pen   Paper or flow sheet

Action	Rationale
1 While your fingertips are still in place after counting the pulse rate, observe the client's respirations.	Counting the respirations while presumably still counting the pulse helps to keep the client from becoming conscious of his breathing and possibly altering his usual rate.
2 Note the rise and fall of the client's chest with each inspiration and expiration.	A complete cycle of inspiration and expiration constitutes one act of respiration.
3 Using a watch with a second hand, count the number of respirations for a minimum of 30 seconds. Multiply this number by two to obtain the client's respiratory rate per minute.	Sufficient time is necessary to observe the rate, depth, and other characteristics.
4 If respirations are abnormal in any way, count the respiratory rate for a full minute. Repeat if necessary to determine the rate and characteristics of breathing.	Full minute countings allow for the detection of unequal timing between respirations.
5 Record respiratory rate on flow sheet or paper. Report any abnormal findings to the appropriate person.	Provides accurate documentation
6 Wash your hands.	Handwashing deters the spread of microorganisms.

BLOOD PRESSURE

Physiology

Blood pressure refers to the force of the blood against arterial walls. Maximum blood pressure is exerted on the walls of arteries when the left ventricle of the heart pushes blood through the aortic valve into the aorta during systole. The highest pressure thus is called **systolic pressure**. When the heart rests (diastole) between beats, the pressure drops. The lowest pressure present on arterial walls at this time is called **diastolic pressure**. The difference between the two is called the **pulse pressure**.

Blood pressure is measured in millimeters of mercury, abbreviated mm Hg, and is recorded as a fraction. The numerator is the systolic pressure, and the denominator is the diastolic pressure. For example, if the blood pressure is 120/80, 120 is the systolic pressure, 80 is the diastolic pressure. The pulse pressure, in this case, is 40.

Maintenance of Blood Pressure

The following factors are responsible for maintaining blood pressure. Deviations from normal blood pressure are likely due to alterations in any one or more of these functions.

Peripheral Resistance. Once blood leaves the heart, it is circulated through a continuous loop of blood vessels consisting of arteries, arterioles, capillaries, and veins. Arterioles are fine, elastic tubes with the capacity to contract or dilate to regulate the distribution of blood to various organs, tissues, or cells depending on their moment-by-moment requirements.

Normally, arterioles are in a state of partial contraction; they are neither totally constricted nor fully relaxed. This semicontracted state is referred to as **peripheral resistance**. It creates a relatively constant level of restraint to blood flow. Peripheral resistance is one of the main factors affecting blood pressure.

Pumping Action of the Heart. When increased amounts of blood are pumped into the arteries (*i.e.,* when cardiac output is increased), the arteries will distend more, resulting in an increase in blood pressure. When less blood is pumped into the arteries (*i.e.,* when cardiac output is decreased), blood pressure will fall. Hence a weak pumping action results in a lower blood pressure than a strong pumping action.

Blood Volume. When blood volume is low, as may occur with hemorrhage or dehydration, blood pressure is low because there is decreased fluid within the arteries. Increasing the quantity of blood will increase the pressure because there will be more fluid volume creating pressure within the arteries.

Viscosity of Blood. Viscosity is the state of being sticky or gummy. The viscosity of the blood depends on the proportion of blood cells to plasma. The more viscid the blood, the higher the blood pressure will be. This occurs because the heart requires more force to move the concentrated fluid throughout the circulatory system.

Elasticity of Vessel Walls. Arteries have a considerable quantity of elastic tissue which allows them to stretch. When the heart rests between each beat, the walls of the arteries recoil, although pressure in them does not drop to zero. The state of pressure keeps the blood entering the capillaries and veins in a continuous flow, not in spurts. Simultaneously, the arterioles, normally in a moderate state of contraction, offer certain resistance. Therefore, the elasticity of the walls, in addition to the resistance of the arterioles, helps to maintain normal blood pressure.

With age, the walls of arterioles become less elastic which interferes with their ability to stretch and dilate. This can subsequently limit adequate blood flow and contribute to rising pressure within the vascular system.

Normal Blood Pressure

Studies of healthy persons indicate that blood pressure can be within a wide range and still be normal. Because individual differences are considerable, it is important to know what is the normal blood pressure for a particular person. A rise or fall of 20 mm Hg to 30 mm Hg in a person's blood pressure is significant, even if it is within the generally accepted normal range. Table 23-9 offers a guide for average normal and hypertensive levels of blood pressure measurements for people of various ages.

Various factors will influence blood pressure in the average healthy adult.
- A person's age will influence his blood pressure, as mentioned earlier.
- There are normal fluctuations in the course of a

T A B L E 23-9
Average and Hypertensive Blood Pressures According to Age

Age	Average Blood Pressure	Hypertensive Level*
Newborn	40 mm Hg systolic	Undetermined
1 month	85/54 mm Hg	Undetermined
1 year	95/65 mm Hg	≥110/75 mm Hg
6 years	105/65 mm Hg	≥120/80 mm Hg
10–13 years	110/65 mm Hg	≥125/85 mm Hg
14–17 years	120/80 mm Hg	≥135/90 mm Hg
18+ years	120/80 mm Hg	≥140/90 mm Hg

* Levels determined by the 1984 Joint National Committee on Detection, Evaluation, and Treatment of High Blood Pressure.

day. The blood pressure is usually lowest upon arising in the morning, before breakfast and before activity commences. The blood pressure has been noted to rise as much as 5 mm Hg to 10 mm Hg by late afternoon, and it will gradually fall again during sleeping hours.
- A person's gender also influences blood pressure. Women usually have a lower blood pressure than men of the same age.
- Blood pressure has been observed to rise after the ingestion of food.
- Systolic blood pressure rises during periods of exercise and strenuous activity.
- Emotions, such as anger, fear, excitement, and pain, generally cause the blood pressure to rise, but the pressure falls to normal when the situation passes.
- A person's blood pressure tends to be lower when he is lying down than when he is sitting or standing.

Because of the many factors that influence blood pressure, the measurements of a single blood pressure are not necessarily significant. Persons with a reading near or above the upper limits of normal should be reexamined to determine if the measurement persists. The US Department of Health and Human Services, Public Health Department, has prepared recommended initial action and follow-up guidelines for subsequent blood pressure measurement. These are described in Figure 23-8. The Canadian Heart Fund (Ontario Division) advises that, in adults over 18 years of age not being treated for hypertension, a diastolic pressure less than 95 mmHg is considered normal, diastolic pressure between 95 and 104 mmHg is considered borderline elevation, and diastolic pressure greater than 104 is definitely elevated. Persons found to have a diastolic pressure greater than 104 mmHg are referred for evaluation and care (Ontario Heart Fund Foundation, 1983).

Blood Pressure Classification* and Follow-Up Criteria

Diastolic Blood Pressure (mm Hg)	Systolic Blood Pressure (mm Hg)			
	Less than 140	140 to 159	160 to 199	200 or greater
Less than 85	Normal Blood Pressure	Borderline Isolated Systolic Hypertension	Isolated Systolic Hypertension	
	Recheck within 2 years†	1st occasion: Confirm within 2 months 2nd occasion: Evaluate or refer promptly to a source of care		Evaluate or refer to a source of care within 2 weeks
85 to 89	High Normal Blood Pressure	Borderline Isolated Systolic Hypertension	Isolated Systolic Hypertension	
	Recheck within 1 year	1st occasion: Confirm within 2 months 2nd occasion: Evaluate or refer promptly to a source of care		Evaluate or refer to a source of care within 2 weeks
90 to 104	Mild Hypertension	1st occasion: Confirm within 2 months 2nd occasion: Evaluate or refer promptly to a source of care		
105 to 114	Moderate Hypertension	Evaluate or refer to a source of care within 2 weeks		
115 or greater	Severe Hypertension	Evaluate or refer immediately to a source of care		

*Based on the average of two or more measurements on two or more occasions.
†Rechecking within one year is recommended on 2nd occasion and for individuals at increased risk (i.e., family history, obesity, blacks, oral contraceptive use, and high alcohol intake).
Source: 1984 Report of the Joint National Committee on Detection, Evaluation and Treatment of High Blood Pressure.

F I G U R E   23-8
The recommended actions for various blood pressure readings given here are those of the 1984 Joint National Committee on Detection, Evaluation, and Treatment of High Blood Pressure, published by the US Department of Health and Human Services, Public Health Service, National Institutes of Health, 1984 (Publication Number [NIH] 80-1088) (The Canadian Heart Fund (Ontario division) advises that, in adults over 18 years of age and not being treated for hypertension, a diastolic pressure < 95 mm Hg is considered normal, diastolic pressure between 95 and 104 mm Hg is considered borderline elevation, and diastolic pressure > 104 is definitely elevated. Those individuals found to have a diastolic pressure > 104 mm Hg are referred for evaluation and care. [Source: Proposed Guidelines for Hypertension Screening, Ontario Heart Foundation, June 21, 1983])

Hypertension

A person whose blood pressure is above normal for a sustained period is in a state of **hypertension**. When the cause of hypertension is due to known pathology, it is called **secondary hypertension**. **Primary** or **essential hypertension** is hypertension without a known cause.

Hypertension is a prevalent health problem. The public as well as health practitioners are becoming increasingly aware of the importance of having regular blood pressure measurements because of the many dangers associated with hypertension. Persistent diastolic hypertension is the most serious and most common blood pressure disturbance. It is a major cause of early death and serious disability in millions of people. Although the exact reason has not been determined, hypertension occurs almost twice as frequently in blacks as in whites.

Hypotension

A blood pressure below normal is called **hypotension**. A consistently low blood pressure, for example, a systolic reading of 90 mm Hg to 115 mm Hg in an adult, appears to cause no ill effects. Rather, this is usually associated with longevity.

Orthostatic or **postural hypotension** is a low blood pressure associated with weakness or fainting when rising to an erect position. It is the result of peripheral vasodilation without a compensatory rise in cardiac output. This type of hypotension can usually be prevented by arising and moving about slowly, especially after a

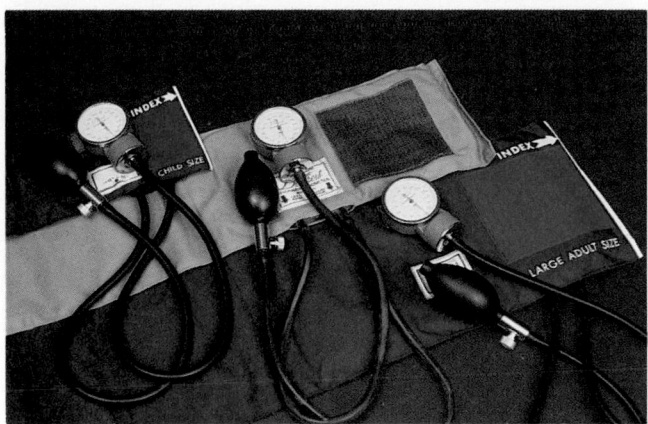

FIGURE 23-9

It is important to select a cuff of an appropriate size to obtain an accurate blood pressure reading. Shown here are three cuff sizes: a small cuff for a child or a small or frail adult, a normal adult size cuff, and a large cuff, called a leg cuff, for measuring blood pressure on a leg or for use on an obese adult.

period of bed rest. Ordinarily it can be corrected by lowering the head, which restores blood flow to the brain.

Some drugs, such as meperidine hydrochloride (Demerol) cause hypotension. There are several illnesses associated with hypotension. For example, the blood pressure will drop when a client is experiencing severe blood loss, burns, severe vomiting and diarrhea, or when cardiac output is impaired following a heart attack.

Assessing Blood Pressure

Sphygmomanometer

A **sphygmomanometer**, consisting of a cuff and a manometer, and a stethoscope are necessary for obtaining an indirect measurement of blood pressure.

Cuff. The sphygmomanometer has a cuff which contains an airtight, flat, rubber bladder covered with cloth. It is important to select a bladder of the proper width to obtain an accurate blood pressure reading. If it is too narrow, the reading could be erroneously high because the pressure is not evenly transmitted to the artery. This occurs, for example, when an average size bladder is used on an obese person. If a bladder is too wide, the reading may be erroneously low because pressure is being directed toward a proportionately large surface area. For example, using an adult cuff on the thin arm of a child may cause this to occur. Recommendations for the selection of an appropriate size cuff are given in Table 23-10.

Cuffs are closed around the limb with contact closures, such as Velcro, or hooks. Some long cuffs are applied by encircling the arm several times.

There are two tubes attached to the bladder within the cuff. One is connected to a manometer. The other is attached to a bulb used to inflate the bladder. The bladder is inflated to the extent necessary to obstruct the flow of blood through the artery. A needle valve on the bulb allows the operator to deflate the cuff while the pressure is being read.

Manometer. A mercury manometer has a mercury-filled cylinder or tube calibrated in millimeters. When mercury rises in the tube, the upper or top surface of the mercury is curved convexly. The topmost point on the curved surface is called the **meniscus**. When determining blood pressure on the mercury manometer, the crest of the meniscus within the calibrated cylinder correlates with the pressure. If the meniscus is observed above eye level, the pressure reading will appear higher than it really is. If the meniscus is lower than eye level, it will appear lower than it really is. The apparent change of position of an object when observed from two different angles is called **parallax**. Figure 23-10 illustrates the me-

TABLE 23-10
Recommended Bladder Sizes for a Blood Pressure Cuff

Arm Circumference at Midpoint* (cm)	Cuff Name	Bladder Width (cm)	Bladder Length (cm)
5–7.5	Newborn	3	5
7.5–13	Infant	5	8
13–20	Child	8	13
24–32	Adult	13	24
32–42	Large adult	17	32
42–50†	Thigh	20	42

* Midpoint of arm is defined as half the distance from the acromion to the olecranon. Use nonstretchable metal tape.

† In persons with very large limbs, the indirect blood pressure should be measured in the leg or forearm.

(Recommendations for Human Blood Pressure Determination by Sphygmomanometers. Copyright © 1987, American Heart Association. Reprinted with permission)

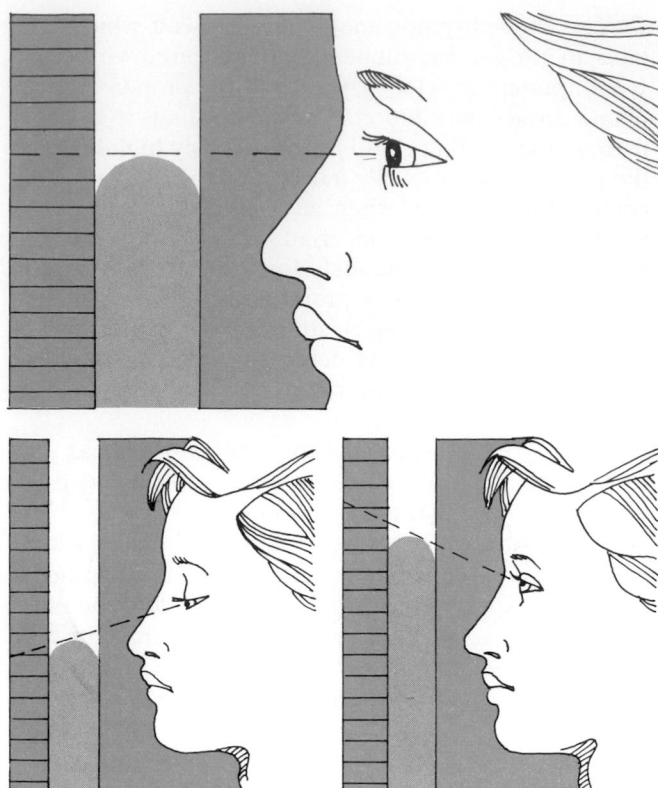

FIGURE 23-10
A blood pressure reading should be made with the eye at the level of the meniscus as shown in the top drawing. The two drawings at the bottom illustrate how parallax can affect the accuracy of a reading when the line of sight is not level with the meniscus.

niscus and how pressure readings may be incorrect when the meniscus is above or below eye level.

Another type of manometer is called the aneroid manometer. It too has a cuff, but it is attached to a round, calibrated dial with a needle that indicates pressure.

Figure 23-11 shows a mercury manometer and an aneroid manometer.

Stethoscope

Auscultation means listening for sounds within the body. The stethoscope is used to auscultate the sound heard directly over the artery as the pressure in the cuff is released and the blood is permitted to flow through the artery. The construction of the stethoscope magnifies the sounds in the artery as they are transmitted to the listener. The blood pressure reading is obtained by listening to the sounds and watching the manometer.

The acoustical stethoscope, the most common type used, has an amplyfying mechanism connected to ear pieces by tubing. Examples of amplifying devices include a diaphragm, which is a large, flat disc, or a bell, which has a hollowed, upright, curved appearance. Some acoustical stethoscopes have both.

The diaphragm is more useful for hearing high-frequency sounds because it is constructed to screen out

low-frequency sounds. For example, the diaphragm is generally used for listening to respiratory sounds. The bell screens out high-frequency sounds and is more useful for hearing low-frequency sounds, such as those commonly made by the heart and the blood within the vessels. Figure 23-12 illustrates the bell and diaphragm of the acoustical stethoscope.

The ear tips of the stethoscope should be selected to fit the ear canals comfortably and snugly for the most effective auscultation. The tips should be sufficiently large to block out extraneous noises in the environment when the stethoscope is being used. The tips should be adjusted to be directed into the ear canal, not against the ear itself. The selection of an appropriate stethoscope for maximum efficiency during auscultation is an individual matter but should be considered carefully.

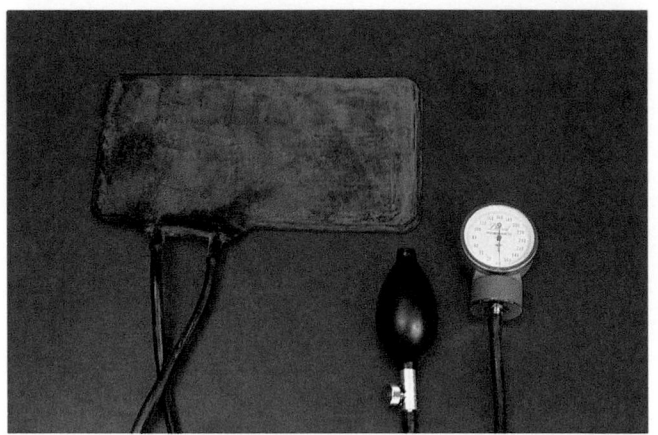

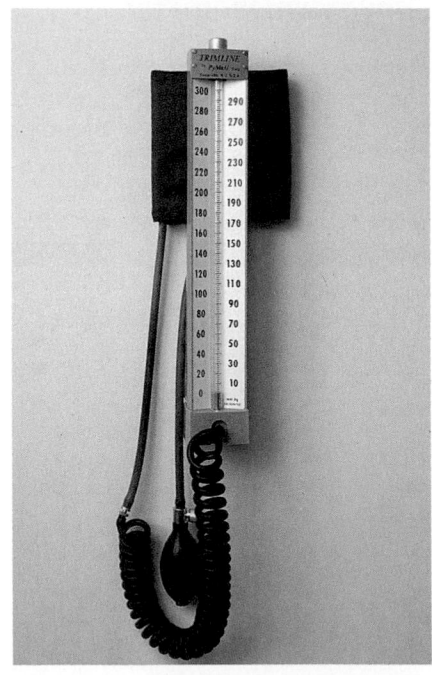

FIGURE 23-11
An aneroid manometer (top) and a mercury manometer (bottom).

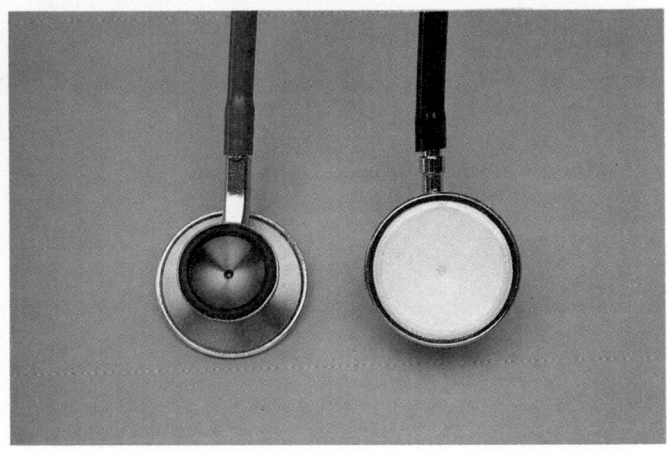

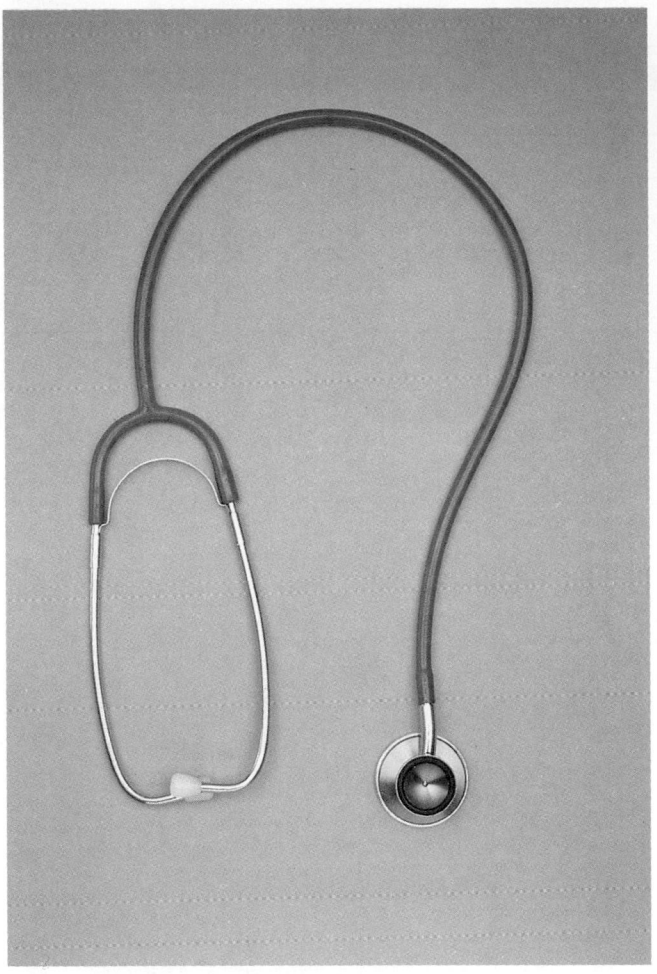

F I G U R E **23-12**
Stethoscope (top); the bell (left) and the diaphragm (right) sides of two stethoscope ampli-fiers (bottom). (Photo © Ken Kasper)

Korotkoff Sounds. The series of sounds for which the nurse listens when measuring the blood pressure, called **Korotkoff sounds**, are described in Table 23-11.

The first sound heard, the onset of phase I, represents the systolic pressure. It is recorded as the first number in the fraction. The second number, the diastolic pressure, is the level at which there is a change in the loud distinct sounds. This marks the onset of phase IV.

Two figures are sometimes used to record the diastolic pressure in adults. The numbers are recorded as, for example, 120/80. When this is the practice, the American Heart Association has recommended that the first diastolic number corresponds with the first changed sound occurring at the onset of phase IV. The second diastolic number is the last sound heard just before a period of continuous silence. This marks the onset of phase V. The numbers are recorded as in this example 120/80/76. If sound is heard down to zero, it would be recorded as 120/80/0. If all sounds disappear with the onst of phase IV, the blood pressure is recorded as 120/80/80.

Assessing at the Brachial Artery

Procedure 23-9 describes how to obtain the blood pressure with a mercury manometer while using the brachial artery. It is important to be conscientious in continuing to follow the recommended techniques to avoid the common errors identified in Table 23-12.

Alternative Techniques

Other types of equipment and other sites may be used as alternatives for measuring blood pressure.

Assessing at the Popliteal Artery. When the client's brachial artery is inaccessible, the nurse can obtain the blood pressure using the client's leg. It can be expected that the systolic blood pressure is likely to be 10 to 40 mm Hg higher using this site. Diastolic pressure will be comparable to that at the brachial site. A cuff of proportionately larger size should be used. The client is best

T A B L E   23-11
Korotkoff Sounds

Phase	Description
Phase I	Characterized by the first appearance of faint but clear tapping sounds which gradually increase in intensity. The first tapping sound is the systolic pressure.
Phase II	Characterized by muffled or swishing sounds. These sounds may temporarily disappear, especially in hypertensive persons. The disappearance of the sound during the latter part of phase I and during phase II is called the auscultatory gap and may cover a range of as much as 40 mm Hg. Failing to recognize this gap may cause serious errors of underestimating systolic pressure or overestimating diastolic pressure.
Phase III	Characterized by distinct, loud sounds as the blood flows relatively freely through an increasingly open artery.
Phase IV	Characterized by a distinct, abrupt, muffling sound with a soft, blowing quality. In adults the onset of this phase is considered to be the first diastolic figure.
Phase V	The last sound heard prior to a period of continuous silence. The pressure at which the last sound is heard is the second diastolic measurement.

positioned on his abdomen or with his knee flexed if lying supine. The technique for assessment is essentially the same as when using the arm.

Palpating Blood Pressure.   Assessing the blood pressure through palpation is sometimes referred to as the sensory detection method. It requires only the use of a sphymomanometer. The cuff is inflated 30 mm Hg above the point at which the pulsation in the artery disappears. As the air in the cuff is released, the nurse feels for the return of a pulse. This corresponds to the systolic pressure. Usually no diastolic pressure is recorded because the artery continues to pulsate as long as blood flows through it. Some home patients assess their blood pressure using this technique. Instead of palpating the artery, the person notes the pressure on the manometer when experiencing the onset and disappearance of the throbbing pulsation. The measurements using this method have been fairly similar to other more sophisticated techniques for assessing blood pressure.

(Text continues on p. 427.)

Assessing Blood Pressure

Equipment

Stethoscope	Blood pressure cuff	Paper or flow sheet
Sphygmomanometer	of appropriate	Alcohol swab
	size	
	Pencil or pen	

Action	**Rationale**
1 Explain the procedure to the client.	An explanation encourages client cooperation and reduces client apprehension.
2 Gather equipment.	Provides for organized approach to task.
3 Use alcohol swab to cleanse ear pieces and diaphragm of stethoscope if necessary.	Cleansing stethoscope deters the transmission of microorganisms.
4 Wash your hands.	Handwashing deters the spread of microorganisms.
5 Select a blood pressure cuff of an appropriate size for the client.	A cuff that is too large or too small will produce a false reading.
6 Delay obtaining the blood pressure if the client is emotionally upset, is in pain, or has just exercised, unless it is urgent to obtain the blood pressure.	Factors such as emotional upset, exercise, and pain will alter usual blood pressure measurements.
7 Select appropriate arm for application of cuff (no IV infusion, breast or axilla surgery on that side, cast, arteriovenous shunt, or injured or diseased limb).	Measurement of blood pressure may temporarily impede circulation to a diseased or compromised extremity.
8 Have the client assume a comfortable lying or sitting position with the forearm supported at the level of the heart and the palm of the hand upward.	This position places the brachial artery on the inner aspect of the elbow so that the bell of the stethoscope can rest on it easily.
9 Expose the area of the brachial artery by removing garments, or move a sleeve, if it is not too tight, above the area where the cuff will be placed.	Clothing over the artery interferes with the ability to hear sounds and may cause inaccurate blood pressure readings. Tight clothing on the arm causes congestion of blood and possibly inaccurate readings.
10 Center the inflatable area of the cuff over the brachial artery, approximately midway on the arm, so that the lower edge of the cuff is about 2.5 to 5 cm (1 to 2 inches) above the inner aspect of the elbow. The tubing should extend from the edge of the cuff nearer the client's elbow.	Pressure in the cuff applied directly to the artery will provide the most accurate readings. If the cuff gets in the way of the stethoscope, readings are likely to be inaccurate. A cuff placed upside down with the tubing toward the client's head, may give a false reading.

(Continued)

Action

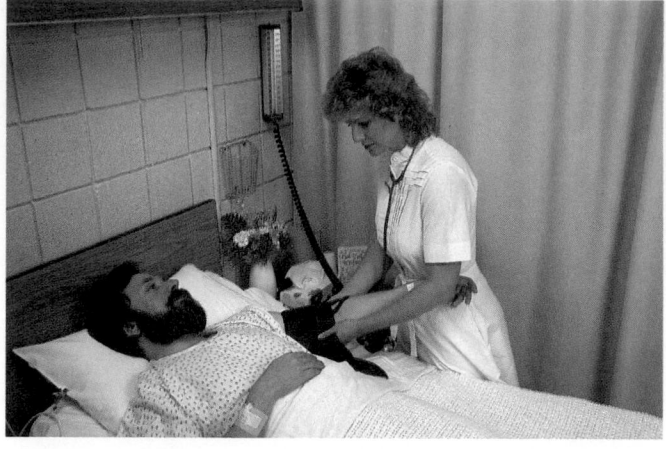

Rationale

Steps 10 and 11: Centering the cuff over the brachial artery and wrapping smoothly and snugly.

11 Wrap the cuff around the arm smoothly and snugly, and fasten it securely or tuck the end of the cuff well under the preceding wrapping. Do not allow any clothing to interfere with the proper placement of the cuff.

A smooth cuff and snug wrapping produce equal pressure and help promote an accurate measurement. A cuff too loosely wrapped will result in an inaccurate reading.

12 Check that a mercury manometer is in a vertical position. The mercury must be within the zero area with the gauge at eye level. If an aneroid gauge is used, the needle should be within the zero mark.

Tilting a mercury manometer, inaccurate calibration, or improper height for reading the gauge can lead to errors in determining the pressure measurements.

13 Palpate the brachial or radial pulse by pressing gently with the fingertips.

Allows for measurement of the approximate systolic reading.

14 Tighten the screw valve on the air pump.

The bladder within the cuff will not inflate with the valve open.

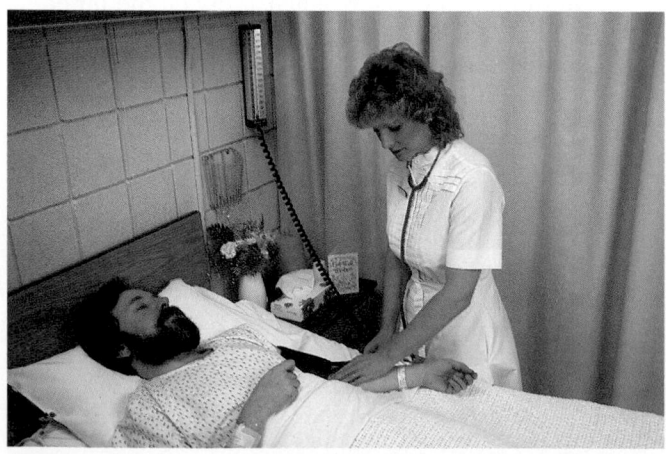

Step 13: Palpating the brachial artery.

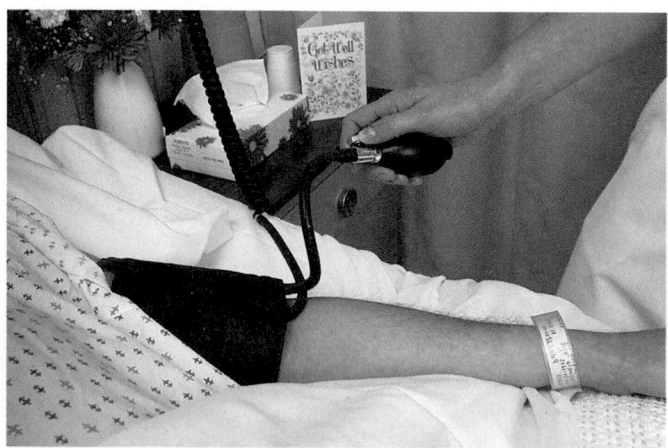

Step 14: Tightening the screw valve on air pump.

(Continued)

Action	Rationale

Action

15 Inflate the cuff while continuing to palpate the artery. Note the point on the gauge where the pulse disappears.

16 Deflate the cuff and wait 15 seconds.

17 Assume a position that is no more than 3 feet away from the gauge.

18 Place the stethoscope earpieces in the ears properly.

19 Place the bell or diaphragm of the stethoscope firmly but with as little pressure as possible over the artery where the pulse is felt. Do not allow the stethoscope to touch clothing or the cuff.

Rationale

To identify the first Korotkoff sound accurately, the cuff must be inflated to a pressure above the point at which the pulse can no longer be felt.

Allowing a brief pause before continuing allows the blood to refill and circulate through the arm.

A distance of more than about 3 feet can interfere with accurate readings of the numbers on the gauge.

The eartips should be directed downward and forward to fit the shape of the ear canal.

Having the bell or diaphragm directly over the artery makes more accurate readings possible. Heavy pressure on the brachial artery distorts the shape of the artery and the sound. Placing the bell or diaphragm away from clothing and the cuff prevents noise which will distract from the sounds made by blood flowing through the artery.

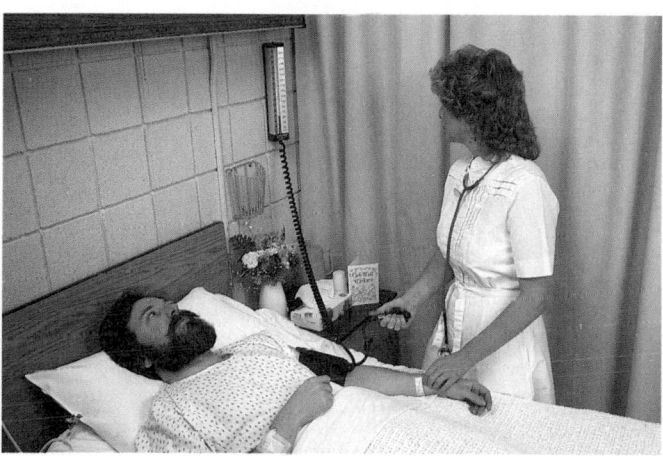

Step 15: Inflating cuff while palpating radial artery.

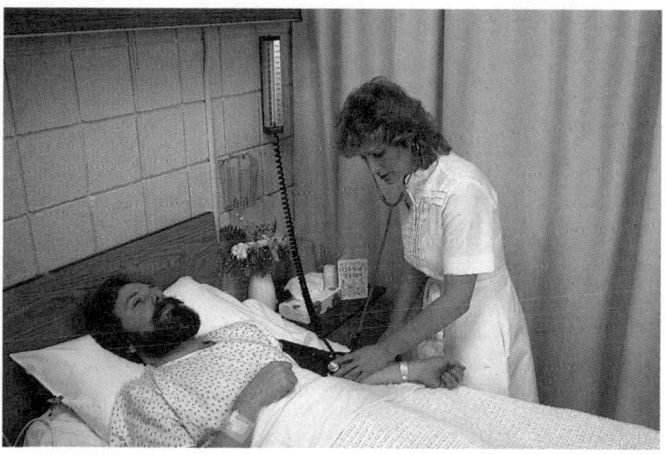

Steps 18 and 19: Placing amplifier of stethoscope over artery, reinflating cuff, and listening for disappearance of sound.

20 Pump the pressure 30 mm Hg above the point at which the pulse disappeared.

21 Note the point on the gauge at which there is an appearance of the first faint, but clear, sound, which slowly increases in intensity. Note this number as the systolic pressure.

22 Read the pressure to the closest even number.

Increasing the pressure above where the pulse disappeared ensures a period of time before hearing the first sound that corresponds with the systolic pressure. It prevents misinterpreting phase II sounds as phase I.

Systolic pressure is the point at which the blood in the artery is first able to force its way through the vessel at a similar pressure exerted by the air bladder in the cuff. The first sound is phase I of Korotkoff sounds.

It is common practice to read blood pressure to the closest even number.

(Continued)

Action

23 Do not reinflate the cuff once the air is being released to recheck the systolic pressure reading.

Rationale

Reinflating the cuff while obtaining the blood pressure is uncomfortable for the client and may cause an inaccurate reading. Reinflating the cuff causes congestion of blood in the lower arm, which lessens the loudness of Korotkoff sounds.

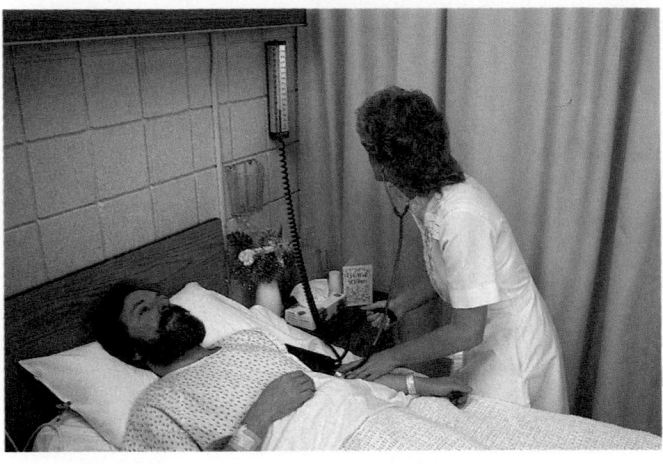

Steps 20, 21, and 23: Listening for Karotkoff sounds and noting systolic and diastolic pressure readings. (Photos © Ken Kasper)

24 Note the pressure at which the sound first becomes muffled. Also observe the point at which the sound completely disappears. These may occur separately or at the same point.

The point at which the sound changes corresponds to phase IV of Korotkoff sounds and is considered the first diastolic pressure reading. According to the American Heart Association, this is used as the diastolic pressure recording in children. The last sound heard is the beginning of phase V and is the second diastolic measurement. The American Heart Association recommends recording the fifth Korotkoff sound as the diastolic pressure in adults.

25 Allow the remaining air to escape quickly. Repeat any suspicious readings but wait 30 to 60 seconds between readings to allow normal circulation to return in the limb. Be sure to deflate the cuff completely between attempts to check the blood pressure.

False readings are likely to occur if there is congestion of blood in the limb while obtaining repeated readings.

26 If it is difficult to hear sounds when checking the blood pressure, raise the client's arm over his head for 15 seconds just before rechecking the blood pressure.

Raising the arm over the head helps relieve congestion of blood in the limb, increases pressure differences, and makes the sounds louder and more distinct when blood enters the lower arm.

27 Inflate the cuff while the arm is elevated and then gently lower the arm while continuing to support it.

Supporting the arm while it is lowered prevents altering the pressure in the manometer by as much as 20 to 30 mm Hg.

(Continued)

28 Position the stethoscope and deflate the cuff at the usual rate while listening for Korotkoff sounds.

29 Remove the cuff, clean and store the equipment.

30 Wash your hands.

31 Record the client's position, the arm that was used to obtain the blood pressure, and the readings that correspond to the systolic and diastolic readings. Compare to previous readings and report any abnormalities to the appropriate person.

The techniques used throughout the remaining assessment of blood pressure do not require any further modification.

Equipment that must be shared among personnel should be left in a manner ready for use.

Handwashing deters the spread of microorganisms.

Circumstances for assessing the blood pressure should be consistent for future comparisons.

Special Considerations

Use cuff size appropriate for limb circumference. Inform client that cuff sizes range from a pediatric cuff to a large thigh cuff and that a poorly fitting cuff may result in an inaccurate measurement.

Inform client about availability of digital blood pressure monitoring equipment. Though costly, most provide an easy-to-read recording of systolic and diastolic measurements.

Electronic Indirect Blood Pressure Meters. Electronic blood pressure meters sense vibrations within the artery wall, record the pressure readings, and display them in digital numbers. These devices are helpful for people who wish to obtain their own blood pressure measurements. They are also advantageous for those who have a hearing deficit because listening for Korotkoff sounds is not necessary. No stethoscope is required. However, because of their delicate instrumentation, electronic machines should be recalibrated when readings are more than a few points different from the person's normal pattern. Clients using these devices at home should also have their blood pressure checked periodically by health personnel.

Direct Electronic Measurement. It is possible to measure blood pressure directly through the insertion of a thin catheter into an artery. This is referred to as an arterial line. The tip of the catheter has the ability to sense pressures and transmit the information to a machine which displays the systolic and diastolic pressure in a waveform. This technique is used exclusively in critical care areas.

Care of Equipment

It is important that equipment used for measuring blood pressure be in good repair and function accurately. Improperly functioning equipment is a major cause of inaccurate measurements. The nurse should check routinely to see that there are no air leaks in the rubber bladder, sphygmomanometer connectors, tubings, or valve. The mercury meniscus and the needle on the aneroid manometer should be checked to see that they are exactly on zero when the cuff is deflated in order for pressure to be measured accurately. The mercury manometer should be cleaned and checked at least annually to see that the mercury is free of foreign matter and air. The aneroid manometer must be checked for accurate calibration frequently against an accurate mercury manometer. Some authorities recommend weekly calibration for the aneroid manometer while others suggest checking it every 6 months. Any time the accuracy of the equipment is questioned, it should be checked and repaired or replaced, as indicated.

TABLE 23-12
Blood Pressure Assessment Errors and Contributing Causes

Error	Contributing Causes	Error	Contributing Causes
Falsely low assessments	• Hearing deficit • Noise in the environment • Viewing the meniscus from above eye level • Applying too wide a cuff • Inserting eartips of stethoscope incorrectly • Using cracked or kinked tubing • Releasing the valve rapidly • Misplacing the bell beyond the direct area of the artery • Failing to pump the cuff 20 to 30 mm Hg above the disappearance of the pulse	Falsely high assessments	• Using a manometer not calibrated at the zero mark • Assessing the blood pressure immediately after exercise • Viewing the meniscus from below eye level • Applying a cuff that is too narrow • Releasing the valve too slowly • Reinflating the bladder during auscultation

KEY POINTS

■ Assessing vital signs, a traditional nursing responsibility, involves obtaining temperature, pulse, respiration, and blood pressure as part of the baseline data from which a plan of care is developed.

■ The frequency of assessing vital signs is governed by the health-care agency's policies and the health status of the client.

■ Humans are warm blooded and maintain body temperature independently of their environment. The hypothalamus in the central nervous system maintains body temperature of the well human, within a fairly constant range, called a set point.

■ Pyrexia or fever, an elevation of normal body temperature, is a common symptom of disease. Most fevers are self-limiting. On the other hand, hypothermia is a temperature below the lower limit of normal. Both may be means by which the body fights disease.

■ Temperature may be assessed by glass clinical thermometer, electronic thermometer, disposable single-use thermometer, temperature-sensitive patch or tape, or automated monitoring device. Although most agencies measure temperature by the oral route, rectal and axillary routes are alternative sites.

■ When the left ventricle of the heart contracts to eject blood into the filled aorta, arterial walls expand or distend; this expansion can be felt as a wave and is called the pulse. Pulse rate is the number of pulsations felt in a minute; pulse rhythm is the pattern of the pulsations and the pauses between them; and pulse amplitude describes the quality of the pulse.

■ Arteries most commonly used for assessment are peripheral pulse or those close to the skin surface (temporal, carotid, brachial, radial, femoral, popliteal, posterior tibial, and dorsalis pedis). Most commonly the radial pulse at the wrist is used.

■ Respiration is the act of breathing and includes the body's use of oxygen and elimination of carbon dioxide. Inspiration or inhalation is the act of breathing in. Expiration or exhalation is the act of breathing out.

■ Healthy adults breathe approximately 16 to 20 times a minute with a fairly consistent relationship of pulse rate to respiratory rate of one respiration to approximately four heartbeats.

■ Apnea refers to periods in which there is no breathing; dyspnea is difficult or labored breathing, demonstrated by rapid and shallow breathing. Dyspneic clients frequently are able to breathe easier in an upright position. Being able to breathe easier in this manner is known as orthopnea.

■ Blood pressure refers to the force of blood against arterial walls. The highest pressure, exerted when the left ventricle of the heart pushes blood through the aortic valve into the aorta during systole, is called systolic pressure. When the heart rests (diastole) between beats the pressure drops and the lowest pressure is called diastolic pressure. They are written as fractions (*e.g.,* 120/80).

■ Deviations from normal blood pressure are likely due to alterations in any one or more of these functions: peripheral resistance, heart's pumping action, blood volume, blood viscosity, and elasticity of vessel walls.

■ Blood pressure can be within a wide range and still be normal. Many factors influence a normal healthy adult's blood pressure.

■ Hypertension is a state in which a person's blood pressure is above normal. Primary or essential hypertension has an unknown cause, while secondary hypertension is due to known pathologic factors. Blood pressure below normal is called hypotension. Orthostatic or postural hypotension is associated with weakness or fainting when rising to an erect position.

■ A sphygmomanometer, consisting of a cuff and manometer, and a stethoscope are necessary for obtaining an indirect measurement of blood pressure. The series of sounds heard in this measurement are called Korotkoff sounds. They are written as fractions (*e.g.,* 120/80).

■ Other equipment and sites for assessing blood pressure are at the popliteal artery or with palpitation, electronic indirect blood pressure meters, or direct electronic measurements.

BIBLIOGRAPHY

Birdsall C: How do you interpret pulses? Am J Nurs 85:785–786, July 1985

Boylan, A, Brown P: Student observations: Temperature. Nurs Times 81:36–40, April 17–23, 1985

Boylan A, Brown P: Student observations: Respiration. Nurs Times 81:35–38, March 13–19, 1985

Boylan A, Brown P: Student observations: More than "doing the obs" . . . the significance of pulse and blood pressure measurement. Nurs Times 81:24–25, February 13–19, 1985

Boylan A, Brown P: Student observations: The pulse and blood pressure. Nurs Times 81:26–29, February 13–19, 1985

Bruya MA, Demand JK: Nursing decision making in critical care: Traditional versus invasive blood pressure monitoring. Nurs Admin Q 9:19–31, Summer 1985

Cashion AK, Cason CL: Accuracy of oral temperatures in intubated patients . . . effectiveness of the electronic thermometer. Dimensions of Critical Care Nursing 3:343–350, November–December 1984

Gurevich I: Fever: When to worry about it. RN 48:14–17, 19, 43, December 1985

King KK, Davis BK: Measuring blood pressure via sensory detection. Journal of Gerontological Nursing 12:8–11, November 1986

Lipsky JG: It's vital! J Pract Nurs 36:26–29, June 1986

Nations LE: Relationship of routine assessment of temperature and febrile illness. Rehabilitation Nursing 11:18–20, September–October 1986

Proposed Guidelines for Hypertension Screening. Ontario Heart Fund Foundation: 1983

Rudy SF: Take a reading on your blood pressure techniques. Nursing 86 16:46–49, August 1986

Samples JF, VanCott ML, Long C: Circadian rhythms: Basis for screening for fever . . . routine temperature assessments in hospitals. Nurs Res 34:377–379, November–December 1985

Siebenaler ME: Taking a baby's temperature: Is it common knowledge? MCN 10:71, January–February 1985

Stone S: A new concept in routine vital signs measurement. Nursing Management 17:28–29, February 1986

Thomas DO: Fever in children. RN 48:18–19, December 1985

US Department of Health and Human Services, Public Health Service, National Institutes of Health: 1984 Report of the Joint Committee on Detection, Evaluation, and Treatment of High Blood Pressure (Publication Number [NIH] 84-1088), 1984

24 Nursing Assessment

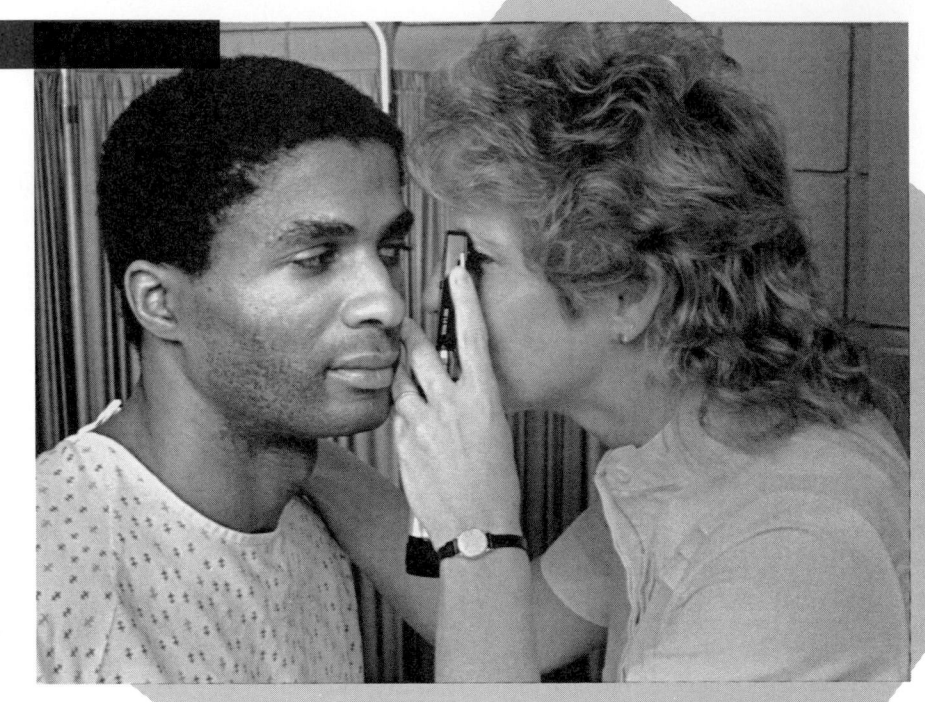

OBJECTIVES

After studying this chapter, the learner should be able to

Define key terms used in the chapter.

Identify the purposes of the nursing assessment.

Describe the techniques used during a nursing examination.

Discuss the importance of client preparation for a nursing assessment.

Identify equipment used in performing a nursing assessment.

Describe positioning used for each body system examination.

Conduct a nursing assessment of each body system in a systematic manner, identifying normal and abnormal findings.

Document significant findings in a concise, descriptive manner.

The nursing assessment of clients is an integral component of holistic care and of the nursing process. Assessments of the dimensions of a person are used to initiate and maintain individualized plans of care to promote wellness, prevent illness, restore health, and facilitate coping, thereby facilitating an optimal level of wellness.

Nursing assessment has two components: a health history and nursing examination (or physical assessment). The health history is usually carried out first, during which the nurse utilizes communication skills and interviewing techniques to elicit primarily subjective data from the client. The nursing examination, a head-to-toe, system-by-system physical assessment, provides objective data. Collectively, the purposes of the nursing assessment are

- To establish a nurse–client relationship
- To gather data about the client's general health status, integrating physiologic, psychologic, cognitive, sociocultural, developmental, and spiritual characteristics
- To identify client strengths and coping abilities
- To identify health problems
- To establish a database for the nursing process

Nursing assessment is a continuous and ongoing component of caring for others. It may be a highly structured information- and data-gathering procedure, as when a client is admitted to a health-care agency, or it may involve selected body systems as the nurse monitors the effectiveness of medical and nursing care. For example, when nurses take vital signs, give physical care, administer medications, or care for clients after surgery, they are carrying out nursing assessment.

This chapter discusses the health history and nursing examination, with the major part of the chapter describing the physical assessment of each body system for the adult client. This is not intended to be a comprehensive discussion of physical assessment. Each chapter that relates to physical care includes more detailed information for specific body systems.

KEY TERMS

accommodation
adventitious breath sounds
apnea
asymmetry
auscultation
bilateral
bounding pulse
bruits
bronchovesicular
clubbing
cyanosis
dorsal recumbent position
dullness
ecchymosis
erect position
flatness
flushing
heaves
hyperperistalsis
hyperresonance
inspection
jaundice
knee–chest position
lifts
lithotomy position
nasal speculum
neurologic hammer
ophthalmoscope
otoscope

pallor
palpation
percussion
percussion hammer
periorbital edema
peristalsis
petechiae
pleural friction rub
polyps
precordium
prone position
rales
rash
resonance
rhonchi
scar
Sims position
stethoscope
striae
supine position
symmetry
thrills
tremor
tuning fork
turgor
tympany
vaginal speculum
vesicular breathing
wound

HEALTH HISTORY

The health history is a collection of data that provides a detailed profile of the client's health status. The information is gathered by interviewing the client. The components of the health history are outlined and briefly described here; more detailed information about collection of data and specific interviewing skills are included in Chapters 15 and 20. A sample health history is included at the end of the chapter to illustrate documentation of data. The components of the health history (Brunner and Suddarth, 1988) are

Biographical data: Included are name, address, sex, age, marital status, occupation, and ethnic origins.

Informant: Although the most reliable source of information about the client *is* the client, other sources of information (*e.g.,* when the client is an infant or child, is unconscious, or is unable to respond appropriately) may be family members, friends, previous records, or other members of the health-care team.

Chief complaint: The chief complaint is the reason the client requires health assessment or care and is stated in the client's own words, usually in quotation marks.

History of present illness: This is a history of the present illness or health concern, recorded in chronologic order. Included are date and manner of onset, specific symptoms, and self-/ medical treatment.

Past health history: Included in the client's past medical history are immunizations, allergies, physical examinations and diagnostic tests, illnesses, surgeries, and injuries. If possible, the client's age and method of treatment for each illness are recorded.

Family history: To determine risk factors for certain disease conditions, the family history records the age and health status (or cause of death) of members of the immediate family (parents, siblings, spouse, children) and extended family (cousins, grandparents).

Review of systems: This part of the interview includes an overview of general health, as well as questions about each body system. This portion of the health history is often documented by use of a checklist.

Patient profile: The patient profile is an assessment of more personal and subjective data and may include

- *Developmental factors:* Place of birth and personal experiences at different ages that were particularly significant
- *Education and occupation:* Job, satisfaction with job or career, past employment, educational level, approximate income, health-care financing
- *Environment:* Type of housing, neighborhood, actual or potential environmental hazards
- *Spiritual factors:* Religious orientation, values, beliefs, and practices important to the client
- *Interpersonal factors:* Cultural and ethnic background (language spoken and understood, foods, values, health habits and beliefs), family relationships, support systems
- *Life-style:* Patterns of rest and sleep, nutrition, social and recreational preferences, the use of alcohol or drugs, activities of daily living
- *Self-concept:* Self-perception of strengths, desired changes, concerns
- *Sexuality:* Developmental level, intimate relationships, values, concerns

- *Stress response:* Coping patterns, support systems, perceptions of current and anticipated stressors

The information collected in the health history may be organized and documented using a variety of formats and organizing frameworks. No matter what format is used, however, the focus is on learning about the client as a unique individual, so that nursing care can be implemented to meet needs and maximize strengths.

NURSING EXAMINATION

The nursing examination is done using a head-to-toe sequence, but it often must be adapted to the needs of the client being examined. This section discusses commonly used positions and techniques for the healthy adult. In the clinical setting, the nurse often modifies and adapts the sequence, positions, and specific assessments to the client's energy level and physiologic status, as well as to time constraints. Even when modified, the nursing examination should be carried out in an organized and knowledgeable manner.

Included in the discussion of the nursing examination are general guidelines and the general survey.

General Guidelines

This section discusses the general guidelines for the nursing examination, including instrumentation, positioning, draping, preparation of the environment, preparation of the client, and techniques of physical assessment.

Instrumentation

The instruments (or equipment) used during a nursing examination should be readily accessible, clean, in proper working order, and organized in the sequence of use (Fig. 24-1). Any equipment that will touch the client should be warmed (either with the examiner's hands or under warm running water) before use. Although all of the instruments described may not be needed in an assessment, they are commonly used in the examination of clients. Additional equipment and supplies are listed in the box on page 434.

Ophthalmoscope. An **ophthalmoscope** is a lighted instrument used for visualization of the interior structures of the eye. It consists of two parts: a body, containing the light source, and a detachable head, containing the magnifying lens used to bring the internal eye structures into focus. The magnification of the lens can be adjusted by a rotating dial. The head is placed into the body and secured. The round black dial located on the head, when depressed and turned, provides illumination. At the beginning of the examination, the lens should be posi-

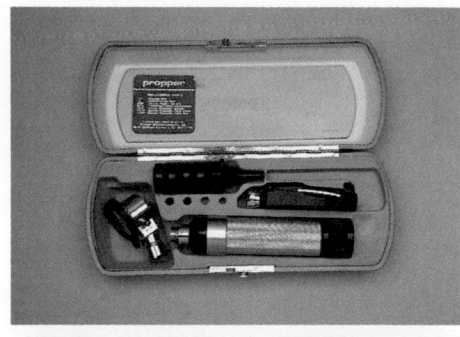

Ophthalmoscope
and otoscope set

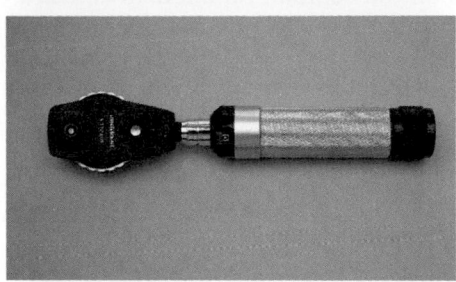

Ophthalmoscope

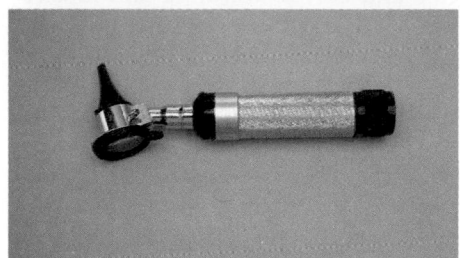

Otoscope

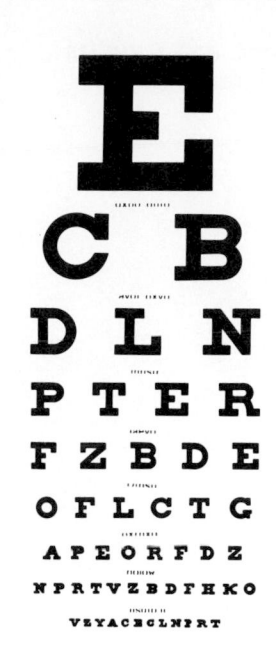

Snellen chart

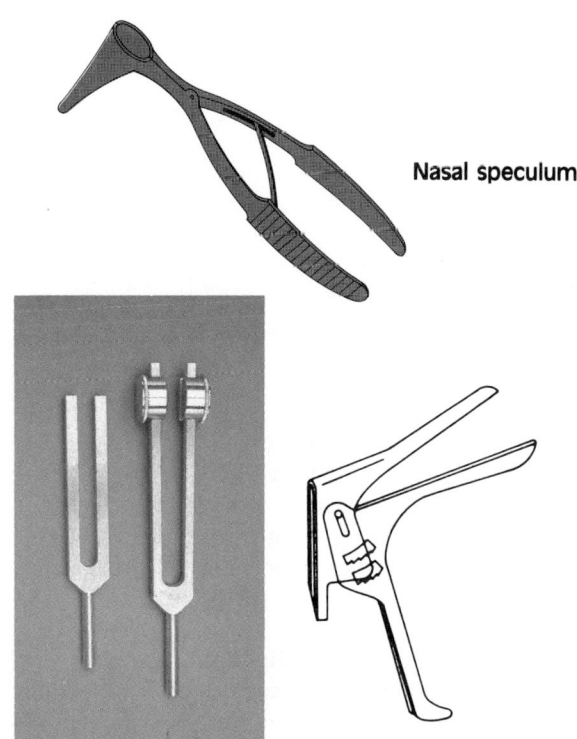

Nasal speculum

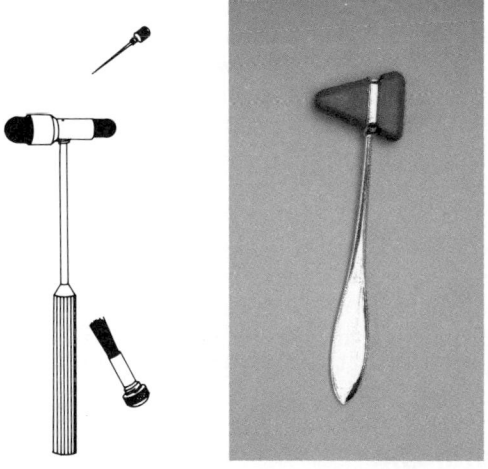

Neurologic hammer   Percussion hammer

Tuning forks   Vaginal speculum

F I G U R E   24-1
Instruments used in the physical examination. (Photos © Ken Kasper)

Instruments, Equipment, and Supplies Needed for a Nursing Examination

Instrumentation
Blood pressure cuff
Stethoscope
Ophthalmoscope
Snellen vision chart
Otoscope
Nasal speculum
Scale
Vaginal speculum
Tuning fork
Percussion hammer
Neurologic hammer

Equipment and Supplies
Alcohol swabs
Cotton applicators
Disposable pad
Drape
Gauze dressing (4 × 4)
Gloves (sterile and nonsterile)
Lubricant
Penlight
Safety pin
Smells (1 or 2 vials for testing sense of smell)
Tape measure
Thermometer
Tongue depressor

tioned at 0 diopters (the 0 magnification power of the lens). The numbers on the rotating dial range from −20 to +40, corresponding to the magnification power of the lens, with the negative numbers shown in red and the positive numbers shown in black. The system of negative and positive numbers compensates for nearsightedness and farsightedness and allows the examiner to visualize structures more distinctly.

Otoscope.   The **otoscope** is a lighted instrument used for examining the external ear canal and the tympanic membrane. The ophthalmoscope and otoscope heads are interchangeable on the same body. An attached speculum directs the light in a narrow beam to improve visualization of structures. The specula come in various sizes; the largest-size speculum that will extend into the client's ear canal is used.

Snellen Eye Chart.   The Snellen eye chart, which is used as a screening test for vision, consists of 11 lines of different size characters arranged with the line of largest characters at the top of the chart and the line of the

smallest characters at the bottom. Scores ranging from 20/10 (the smallest line of characters) to 20/200 (the largest line of characters) are in the left-hand column and distances are in the right-hand column next to the numbers.

Nasal Speculum.   The **nasal speculum** is an instrument that allows visualization of the lower and middle turbinates of the nose. A penlight or flashlight is needed for illumination. The blades of the speculum are inserted about ½ inch (1 cm) into the nares and opened so that they do not press on the septum. An alternative instrument that can be used to visualize the internal nares is the otoscope (described above). The light is provided by the scope, and the shortest, widest speculum that will fit into the client's nares is used.

Vaginal Speculum.   A **vaginal speculum** is a two-bladed instrument used to examine the vaginal canal and cervix. The speculum is inserted into the vagina, and the speculum blades are opened, allowing visualization and examination of the vagina and cervix. Warming and lubrication of the speculum (either with warm water or with a water-soluble agent) are essential prior to insertion.

Tuning Fork.   A **tuning fork** is a two-pronged metal instrument used for testing auditory function and vibratory perception. The fork is activated by gently tapping the prongs of the tuning fork against the palm of the hand. Once activated, the fork is held at the base to avoid diminishing the sound or vibration produced by the prongs.

Percussion Hammer.   The **percussion hammer**, also called the *reflex hammer,* is an instrument with a rubber head used to test reflexes and determine tissue density. The hammer is held between the thumb and index finger to direct a brisk tap on the selected body area. A rapid downward and backward wrist action allows a quick and firm tap to be made (Fig. 24-2). The pointed end of the hammer is used for smaller areas.

Neurologic Hammer.   The **neurologic hammer** is similar to the percussion hammer. It is used to test reflexes during the neurologic assessment and features two additional pieces that unscrew from the base of the instrument: a soft brush and a sharp needle, both used for sensory discrimination.

Positioning

A variety of positions are utilized during a nursing examination. These are illustrated in Figure 24-3 and described below. It is important to consider the client's energy level and privacy; clients who are weak may require assistance with positioning, and uncomfortable or embarrassing positions should not be maintained for long periods of time. The examination should be organized so that several body systems can be assessed with

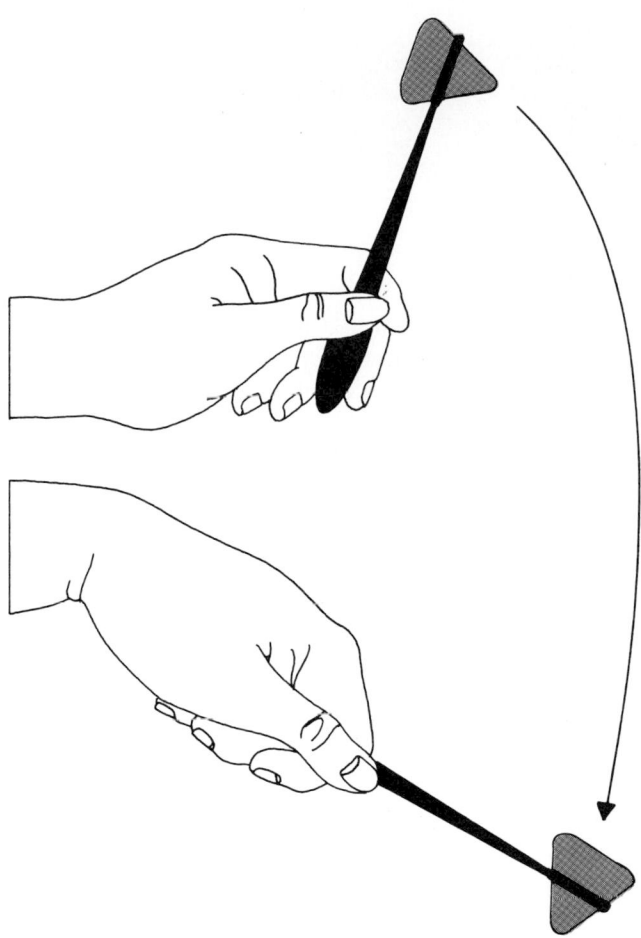

F I G U R E   24-2
The percussion, or reflex, hammer is held between the thumb and index finger to direct a brisk tap on the selected body area.

the client in one position, thus minimizing unneeded and possibly tiring movement.

Sitting Position. The client may sit upright in a chair, on the side of an examining table or bed, or, if physically unable to maintain an upright position, may lie supine in the bed with the head elevated. This position allows visualization of the upper body and facilitates full expansion of the lungs. It is used to assess the head and neck, posterior and anterior thorax and lungs, breasts, heart, and upper extremities, and to take vital signs.

Supine Position. In the **supine position**, the client lies flat on the back with legs together but extended and slightly flexed at the knees. The head may be supported with a small pillow. This position allows relaxation of abdominal muscles and can be used to assess the head and neck, anterior thorax and lungs, breasts, heart, abdomen, extremities, and peripheral pulses.

Dorsal Recumbent Position. The client lies on the back with legs separated, knees bent, and soles of the feet flat on the bed. The **dorsal recumbent position** may be used for clients who have difficulty maintaining the supine position but should not be used for abdominal assessment (because it causes abdominal muscles to contract). Areas that can be assessed in this position are the head and neck, anterior thorax and lungs, breasts, heart, extremities, and peripheral pulse.

Sims Position. The client lies on either the right or left side. The lower arm is behind the body and the upper arm is flexed at the shoulder and elbow. The knees are both flexed, with the uppermost leg more acutely flexed. The **Sims position** is used to assess the rectum or vagina.

Prone Position. In the **prone position**, the client lies on the abdomen, flat on the bed, with the head turned to one side. This position is difficult to assume for many clients. It is used to assess the hip joint and can be used to assess the posterior thorax.

Lithotomy Position. In the **lithotomy position**, the client is in the dorsal recumbent position with the buttocks at the edge of the examining table and the feet supported in stirrups. This position is used for examination of the rectum and female genitalia. It is uncomfortable for older clients and is often embarrassing, so time spent in this position should be minimized.

Knee–Chest Position. In the **knee–chest position**, the client kneels, using the knees and chest to bear the weight of the body. The body is at a 90-degree angle to the hips, with the back straight, the arms above the head, and the head turned to one side. The position is used for examination of the rectal area. The same precautions should be used as with the lithotomy position.

Erect Position. The *standing* or **erect position** is also used in the nursing examination to assess posture, gait, and balance.

Draping

Draping during the physical assessment is primarily used to prevent unnecessary exposure, to provide privacy, and to keep the client warm. Drapes may be paper, cloth, or bed linens (*e.g.,* sheets and bath blankets). As the examination is conducted, only those body parts being assessed are exposed.

Preparing the Environment

An important component in performing a nursing examination is preparing the environment. The nurse should plan time that is appropriate for both the client and the nurse, and, if possible, should confer with the client to set a mutually agreeable time.

Some agencies have a special examination room that provides a quiet, private space for assessment. If such a

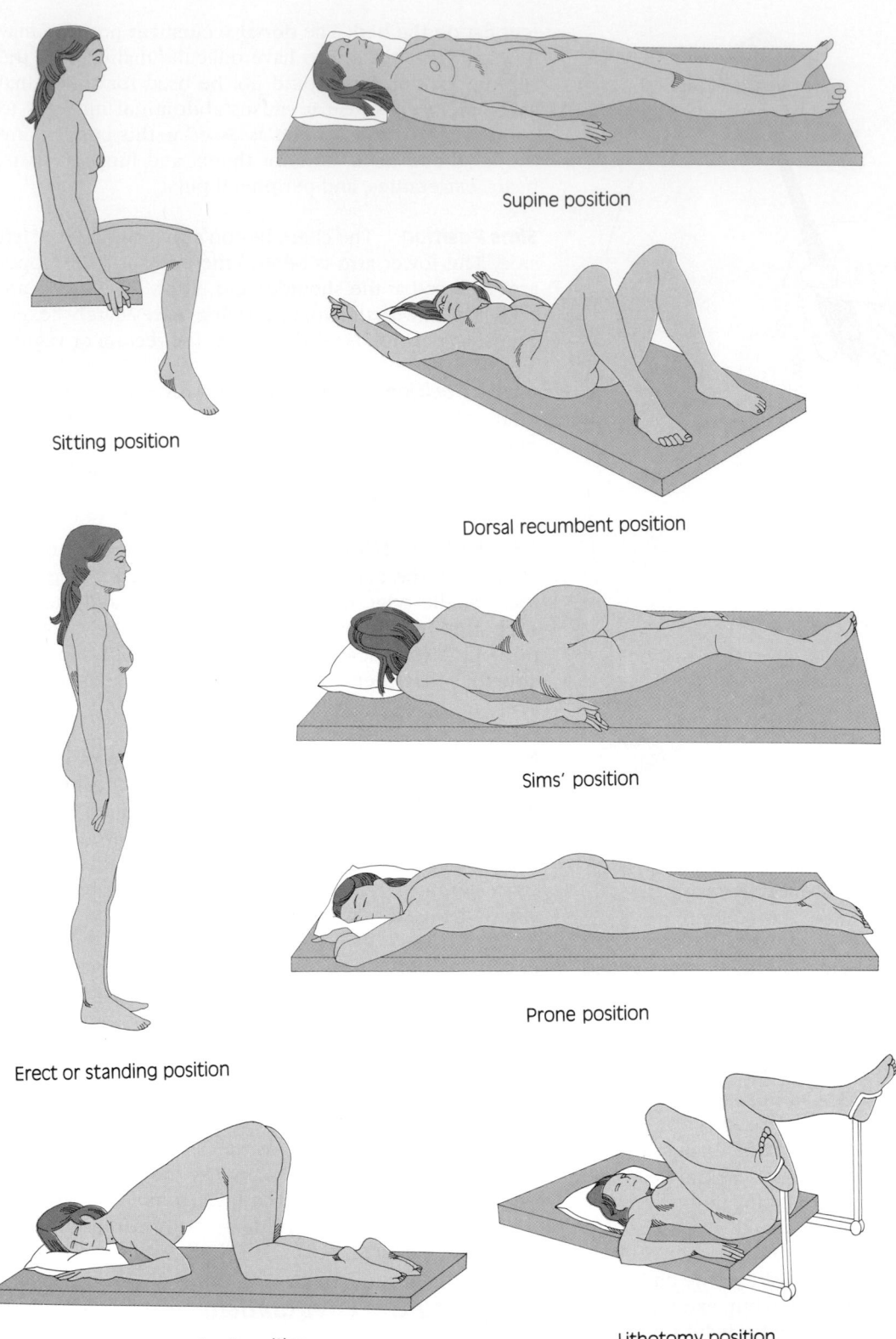

Supine position

Sitting position

Dorsal recumbent position

Sims' position

Prone position

Erect or standing position

Knee-chest position

Lithotomy position

F I G U R E   24-3
Various client positions used during the nursing examination.

room is available, the nurse prepares the examination table, provides a gown and drape for the client, and gathers instruments and special supplies needed for the examination. If the area is accessible to others, an enclosure with a curtain or screen is essential.

Preparing the Client

Physiologic and psychologic needs of the client must be considered when doing a nursing examination (Fig. 24-4). The client is told that a nursing examination will be done, that body structures will be examined, and that the assessments are painless. The client is asked to change into a gown and directed to a private place to change. If necessary, the nurse assists the client with undressing. Once gowned, the client is asked to empty the bladder; this increases comfort during the examination and facilitates assessment of the abdomen. Even though the assessments are painless, the client may be anxious for various reasons. The nurse can help decrease the client's embarrassment, fear of possible abnormal physical findings, or fear of "failing" a test by explaining in general terms how and why the examination will be done and then explaining each assessment in greater detail as it is being done. The nurse should answer any questions asked by the client directly and honestly.

Techniques

There are four primary assessment techniques: inspection, palpation, percussion, and auscultation. These will

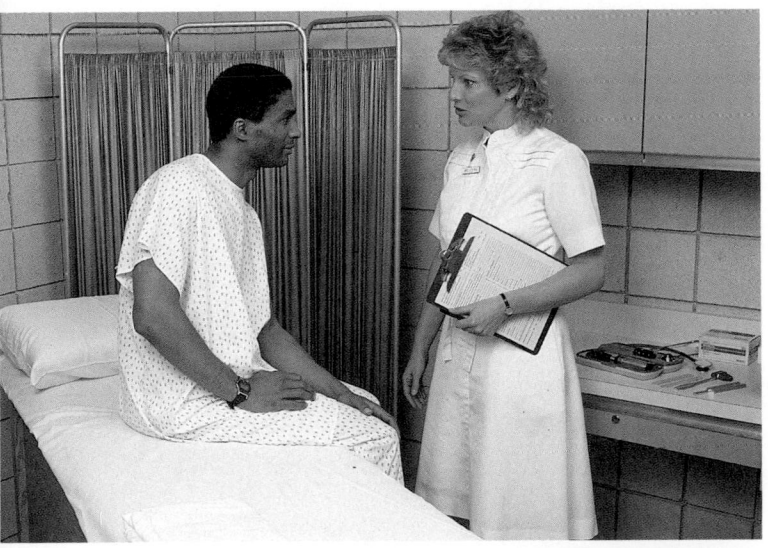

F I G U R E   24-4
The physiological and psychological needs of the client must be considered in preparation for the examination. Care is taken to provide for comfort, warmth, and privacy. A brief explanation of the examination before beginning and just before each stage alleviates client fear and anxiety and improves cooperation. (Photo © Ken Kasper)

be discussed throughout the rest of the chapter as they are used to conduct a nursing examination of various body systems.

Inspection.   Inspection is the process of deliberate, purposeful observations performed in a systematic manner. Observations are made by using visual, auditory, and olfactory senses as tools for gathering data throughout the examination. Inspection begins at the time of initial contact with the client and continues throughout the entire examination. Adequate lighting, either natural or artificial, is essential for distinguishing color, texture, and moisture of body surfaces. A quiet environment eliminates extraneous noises and allows sounds to be heard without interference.

The nurse inspects each area of the body for size, color, shape, position, and symmetry, making observations of normal findings and any deviations from normal. A comparison of **bilateral** body parts during inspection is necessary for recognizing abnormal findings. Inspection may be combined with the palpation phase of the examination.

Palpation.   Palpation is a technique that uses the sense of touch. The hands and fingers are sensitive tools and are used to gather information about temperature, turgor, texture, moisture, vibrations, and shape. The dorsum or back of the hand and fingers is used for gross measure of temperature. When a discriminatory sense is needed for differentiating between texture, shape, fluid, size, consistency, and pulsation, the palmar surface of the fingers and finger pads is used. The sense of vibration is palpated best with the palm of the hand (Fig. 24-5).

General guidelines to use during palpation are the following:

- Provide the client with a warm, comfortable, and relaxed environment.
- The nurse's hands should be warm and fingernails short.
- Any area of tenderness is palpated last.

Light or deep palpation may be used and is controlled by the amount of pressure applied. For light palpation, apply light pressure by placing the fingers together and depressing the skin and underlying structures approximately ½ inch (1 cm) (Fig. 24-6, top). For deep palpation, press inward approximately 1 inch (2 cm) (Fig. 24-6, bottom). Deep palpation, with the risk of possible internal injury, should be used with caution. Applying intermittent pressure to a specific area allows assessment of surface characteristics and underlying structures. Characteristics of masses, as determined by palpation, are described in Table 24-1.

Percussion.   Percussion is the act of striking one object against another for the purpose of producing sound. The sound waves produced by the striking action are known as *percussion tones* and are generated by body tissue.

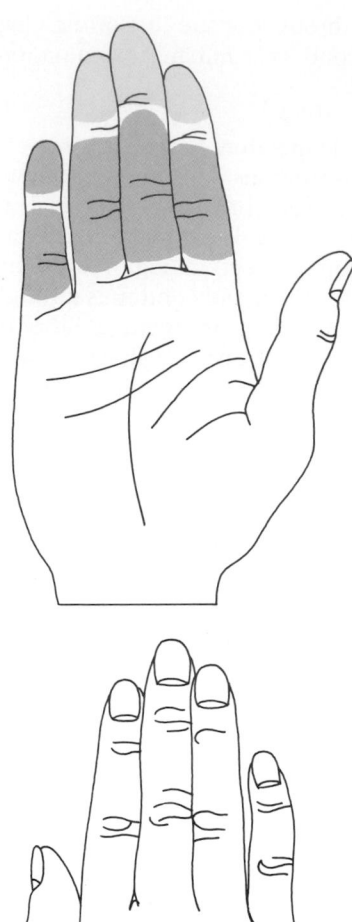

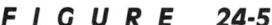

F I G U R E   24-5

(Top) Palmar surfaces of the examiner's fingertips and finger pads
are used for discriminatory sensation, such as texture, presence
of fluid, or size and consistency of a mass. (Bottom) Dorsum, or
back of hand, is used to assess surface temperature.

Percussion is used to assess the location, shape, size, and
density of tissues.

The nurse uses both hands as the tools for producing
sound waves. The nondominant hand is placed directly
on the area to be percussed, with the fingers slightly
separated and the middle finger placed firmly on the
body surface (Fig. 24-7, left). The opposite hand (or
dominant hand) is the striking force, which is initiated
by sharp downward wrist movement with the forearm
stationary and the wrist relaxed. The tip of the middle
finger of the dominant hand strikes the joint of the middle finger of the opposing hand (Fig. 24-7, right). This
action produces a vibration that allows the nurse to discriminate among five different tones. The percussion
tones are

Tympany: A loud drumlike sound that is illustrated
by the sound produced by percussing a puffed-
out cheek. This sound is heard when percussing the stomach, an air-filled organ.

Resonance: A moderate to loud, lower-pitched, hollow sound percussed over lung tissue

Hyperresonance: A very loud, low-pitched sound
with a booming quality. This sound is most
often percussed over the emphysematous lung.

Dullness: A soft to moderate, high-pitched sound
with a thud-like quality. This sound is percussed over the liver.

Flatness: A soft, high-pitched sound that is flat,
usually percussed over muscle tissue

Table 24-2 summarizes percussion tones and their characteristics.

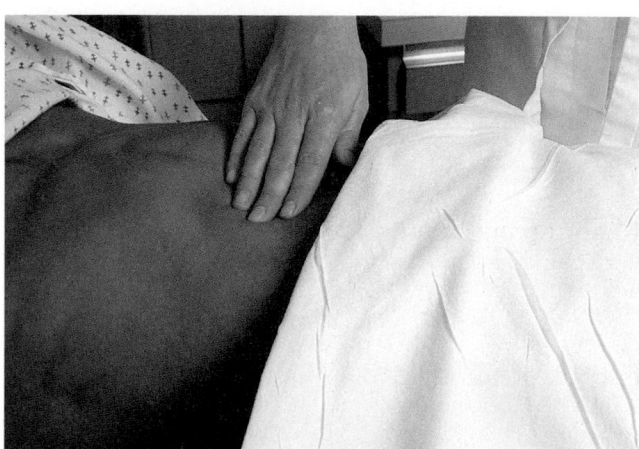

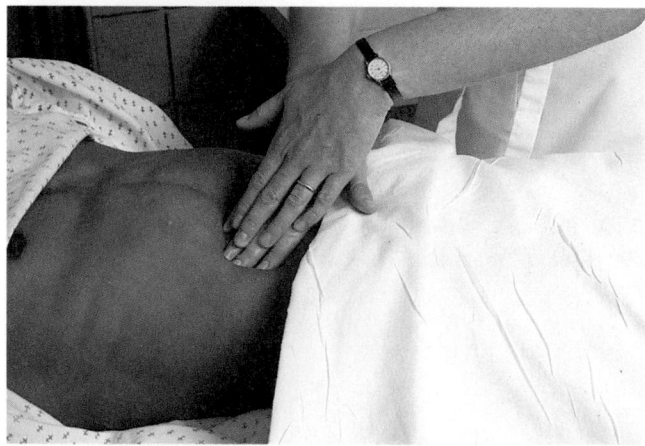

F I G U R E   24-6

(Top) In light palpation, light pressure is applied by placing the
fingers together and depressing the skin and underlying structures approximately 1/2 inch. (Bottom) Deep palpation is used
with caution. The skin and underlying structures are depressed approximately 1 inch. (Photos © Ken Kasper)

T A B L E **24-1**
Characteristics of Masses Determined by Palpation

Quality	Characteristics to Determine
Shape	Round
	Ovoid
	Tubular
	Irregular
Size	Measured in centimeters
Consistency	Firm
	Edematous
	Spongy
	Cystic
Surface	Smooth
	Nodular
	Granular
Mobility	Fixed or nonmobile
	Mobile
Tenderness	Amount of tenderness to touch
Pulsatile	Pulsation can or cannot be felt in the mass

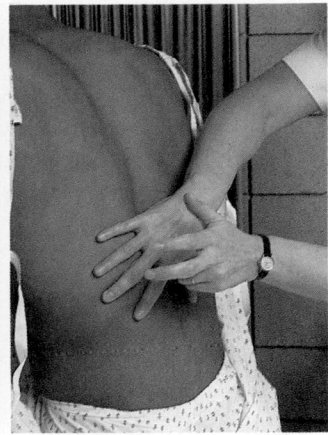

F I G U R E **24-7**
Percussion is used to assess the location, shape, size, and density of tissues. (Left) The nondominant hand is placed directly on the area to be percussed, and the middle finger placed firmly on the body surface. (Right) The tip of the middle finger of the dominant hand strikes the joint of the middle finger of the opposite hand. (Photos © Ken Kasper)

Auscultation. Auscultation is the act of listening to sound produced within the body with a **stethoscope**. Chapter 23 discusses types of stethoscopes, their uses, and specific characteristics.

Auscultation is performed by firmly placing the stethoscope against the body part being assessed. The diaphragm of the stethoscope is used to detect high pitched sounds, such as normal lung and bowel sounds. The bell of the stethoscope is used to detect low-pitched sounds, such as those produced by the heart and vascular system.

There are four characteristics of sound that should be assessed by auscultation. They are *pitch* (ranging from high to low), *loudness* (ranging from soft to loud), *quality* (such as gurgling or swishing), and *duration* (described as short, medium, or long).

General Survey

Some components of the general survey, including self-image and self-concept, are assessed during the health history. Other data assessed in the general survey are the client's general appearance, vital signs, height, and weight.

General Appearance

Assessment of general appearance includes
- Sex and race
- Body build, posture, and gait (Note proportion of height to weight, erect or slumped posture, coordination of movements, pattern of gait.)
- Hygiene, grooming (Note cleanliness, body odors, appropriate dress for age and environment.)

T A B L E **24-2**
Percussion Tones and Their Characteristics

Tone	Relative Intensity	Relative Pitch	Relative Duration	Example Location
Flatness	Soft	High	Short	Thigh
Dullness	Medium	Medium	Medium	Liver
Resonance	Loud	Low	Long	Normal lung
Hyperresonance	Very loud	Lower	Longer	Emphysematous lung
Tympany	Loud	*	*	Gastric air bubble or puffed-out cheek

* Distinguished mainly by its musical timbre

(Bates B: A Guide to Physical Examination, 4th ed., p 237. Philadelphia, JB Lippincott, 1987)

- Signs of illness (Note posture, skin color, respirations, nonverbal communications of pain or distress.)
- Affect, attitude, mood (Note speech, facial expressions, ability to relax, eye contact, behavior.)
- Cognitive processes (Note speech content and patterns, orientation, appropriate verbal responses.)

Vital Signs

Vital signs are measured to establish a database and to detect actual or potential health problems. Vital signs are discussed in Chapter 23.

Height and Weight

In adult clients the correlation (or ratio) of height and weight is an assessment of overall health and nutrition. An indication of body image can be assessed by asking the client his or her height and weight before actually doing the measurements. A large difference in perceived and actual measurements may indicate a potential problem in body image and self-concept. Both height and weight should be measured using accurate scales and measuring devices, and the client should remove shoes and heavy clothing if the measurements are taken before undressing. If the client is unable to stand erect, weight can be obtained by using a chair or bed scales. The client's actual height and weight can be compared to recommended average weights on a standardized chart (Table 24-3) as a general guideline for assessing nutritional status and health.

ASSESSMENT OF BODY SYSTEMS

This section will discuss the assessment of each body system; for each system there is a brief review of normal anatomy and physiology, factors for consideration during assessment, positions, assessment techniques, and common normal and abnormal findings. A completed assessment is included at the end of the chapter to illustrate documentation.

Integument

Skin

The skin is the external covering of the body and consists of three layers: the epidermis, or outer layer; the dermis, or middle layer; and subcutaneous tissue, or the innermost layer. The epidermis protects the body against environmental substances and helps regulate body temperature. The dermis, composed of vascular connective tissue and sensory nerve fibers, supports and separates the epidermis from adipose tissue and provides the sensations of pain, touch, and temperature. The subcutane-

T A B L E   24-3
Desirable Weights for Women and Men*

Height		Weight		
Feet	Inches	Small Frame	Medium Frame	Large Frame
Men of Ages 25 and Over				
5	2	112–120	118–129	126–141
5	3	115–123	121–133	129–144
5	4	118–126	124–136	132–148
5	5	121–129	127–139	135–152
5	6	124–133	130–143	138–156
5	7	128–137	134–147	142–161
5	8	132–141	138–152	147–166
5	9	136–145	142–156	151–170
5	10	140–150	146–160	155–174
5	11	144–154	150–165	159–179
6	0	148–158	154–170	164–184
6	1	152–162	158–175	168–189
6	2	156–167	162–180	173–194
6	3	160–171	167–185	178–199
6	4	164–175	172–190	182–204
Women of Ages 25 and Over†				
4	10	92–98	96–107	104–119
4	11	94–101	98–110	106–122
5	0	96–104	101–113	109–125
5	1	99–107	104–116	112–128
5	2	102–110	107–119	115–131
5	3	105–113	110–122	118–134
5	4	108–116	113–126	121–138
5	5	111–119	116–130	125–142
5	6	114–123	120–135	129–146
5	7	118–127	124–139	133–150
5	8	122–131	128–143	137–154
5	9	126–135	132–147	141–158
5	10	130–140	136–151	145–163
5	11	134–144	140–155	149–168
6	0	138–148	144–159	153–173

* Weight in pounds according to frame (in indoor clothing); height with shoes on—1″ heels for men and 2″ heels for women

† For women between 18 and 25, subtract 1 pound for each year under 25.

(Courtesy of the Metropolitan Life Insurance Company, New York)

ous layer of skin is composed of sweat glands, fat, hair follicles, and blood vessels (see Fig. 27-1).

The skin is a general indicator of a client's health status and provides information that may be significant of an underlying pathology. When assessing the skin, it is helpful to know if the client has been exposed to harmful environmental materials or increased sun exposure, has had recent changes in skin condition, or is currently taking medications.

The skin is assessed by inspection and palpation. The examination begins with an overall assessment of the skin condition; specific areas of the skin can be assessed while performing other body system assessments. Adequate lighting is essential for accurate assessments.

Inspection. The skin is inspected through assessment of color, vascularity, and lesions. Body odors are also included in inspection (Fig. 24-8).

Color. The skin color varies among races and among individuals. Normally, skin color ranges from a pinkish white to various shades of brown, depending on the person's race. The skin areas that are normally exposed, such as the face and hands, may have a somewhat different color from areas that are usually covered by clothing, but generally the color is relatively constant. Special care must be taken to detect color changes in dark-skinned persons, such as blacks, Hispanics, native Americans, persons of Mediterranean extraction, and whites who are deeply suntanned. Some body areas of dark-skinned persons, such as the palms of the hands and the soles of the feet, normally have less pigmentation than other areas of the body.

Various terms used to describe abnormal appearance of the skin are described below and summarized in Table 24-4.

Flushing is redness of the skin, as in sunburn. It is often associated with an elevated body temperature, and the face and the neck are more likely to be affected than

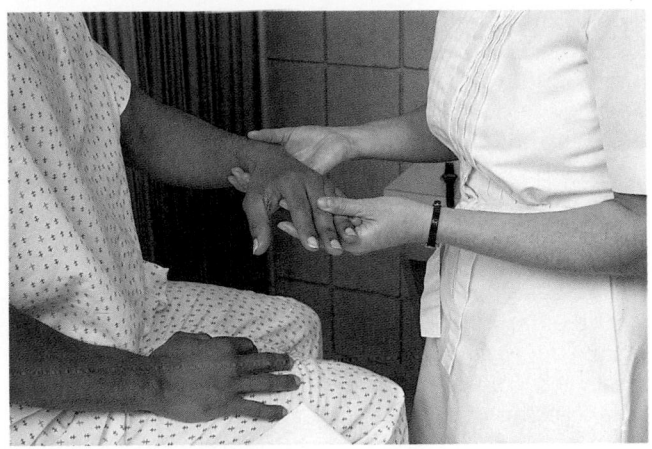

FIGURE 24-8
The skin is inspected for color, vascularity, and lesions.

other parts of the body. **Cyanosis** is a dusky bluish color of the skin and can usually be detected more readily in the conjunctiva, lips, and inside the mouth in dark-skinned persons. **Jaundice** is a yellow color of the skin. In adults it is usually initially seen in the sclera of the eyes and then in the skin and mucous membranes. Jaundice in the dark-skinned person is more difficult to observe because the sclera often has a normal yellowish

TABLE 24-4
Skin Color Assessment

Color Variations	Assessment Areas	Pathologic Causes
Redness, or erythema (flushing)	Facial area, localized areas	Blushing, alcohol intake, fever, injury, trauma, infection
Bluish, or cyanosis	Exposed areas, particularly the ears, lips, inside of the mouth, hands and feet, nailbeds	Cold environment, cardiac or respiratory disease (decreased oxygenation)
Yellowish, or jaundice	Overall skin areas, mucous membranes, and sclera	Liver disease (increase in bilirubin levels)
Paleness, or pallor	Exposed areas, particularly the face and lips, conjunctivae, and mucous membranes	Anemia (decreased hemoglobin)
	Overall skin areas, lips, nailbeds, conjunctivae	Shock (decreased blood volume)
Vitiligo	Whitish patchy areas on the skin	Depigmentation (congenital or autoimmune conditions)
Tanned or brown	Sun-exposed areas	Overexposure (increased melanin production), pregnancy (brown spots?)

color. **Pallor** is paleness of the skin, often resulting from an inadequate amount of circulating blood or hemoglobin, both of which cause inadequate oxygenation of the body tissues. Depending on severity, pallor may be visible over the entire skin surface; locally it is seen in the lips, nailbeds, mucous membranes, and conjunctiva. Pallor may be more difficult to assess in the dark-skinned person.

Vascularity. The skin is also inspected for vascularity, bleeding, or bruising, because these signs may be related to cardiovascular or liver dysfunctions. **Ecchymosis** is a collection of blood in the subcutaneous tissues, causing purplish discoloration. **Petechiae** are very small hemorrhagic spots caused by capillary bleeding. Both of these abnormal findings should be assessed for location, color, and size.

Lesions. The skin is assessed by inspection for the presence of lesions, which are areas of diseased or injured tissue. Normally, the skin is smooth and without breaks in its continuity. Evidence of bruises, scratches, cuts, insect bites, and wounds should be noted. A **wound** is a break in the continuity of the skin and should be assessed and described as to size, shape, depth, location, and presence of drainage or odor (Table 24-5). **Scars** are healed wounds. (Wounds are discussed in Chap 42.) A **rash** is an eruption of the skin. The descriptive details of a rash include the type, size, elevation, coloring, and presence or absence of drainage or itching. The nurse should document the exact body surface areas involved.

Palpation. The temperature, moisture, turgor, and texture of the skin are determined by palpation.

Temperature and Moisture. The skin is normally warm and dry. An increase in skin temperature and moisture can indicate an elevation of body temperature. An excessive amount of perspiration, such as when the entire skin is moist, is called *diaphoresis*. When the body loses excess water, *dehydration,* the depletion of body fluids with dryness and loss of *turgor* occurs.

Turgor. Turgor (Fig. 24-9) is the fullness or elasticity of the skin. Normal turgor results in elasticity of the skin, allowing it to be picked up in a fold and to return to its shape when released. Difficulty in lifting a skin fold may indicate excess fluid in the tissues, or *edema*. Edema is characterized by swelling, with taut and shiny skin over the edematous area. If the area of edema is palpated with the fingers, an indentation may remain after the pressure is released. (Edema is discussed in Chap 35.) Edema may be described on a scale, as follows:

    0 = none
  +1 = trace
  +2 = moderate
  +3 = deep
  +4 = very deep

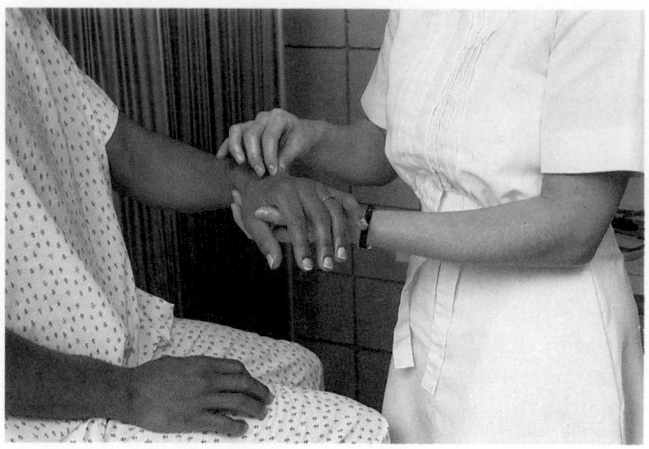

F I G U R E   24-9
To assess skin turgor, a small fold of skin is picked up and then released to return to its normal shape. Difficulty in lifting a skin fold may indicate presence of edema. (Photo © Ken Kasper)

When the client is dehydrated, normal skin elasticity and fullness are decreased and the skin fold returns to normal slowly. (This, however, is a normal finding in the elderly client.)

Texture. The texture of the skin may vary from smooth and soft to rough and dry. In the dehydrated client, the texture is loose and wrinkled and the mucous membranes are cracked and dry.

Nails

The nails are differentiated tissue but continuous extensions of the skin. The nails are inspected for shape, texture, and color. The shape of the nails should normally be somewhat convex and follow the natural curve of the finger. The angle between the nail and its base in the finger should be about 160 degrees. The texture of the nails should be smooth, and the nail base, when palpated, should be firm and nontender. Abnormal findings include indentations, called *Beau's lines,* infection (*Paronychia*), increased brittleness and angulation, changes in the thickness or texture, and **clubbing**. Figure 24-10 illustrates nail abnormalities.

Hair and Scalp

The hair is normally resilient, evenly distributed, and neither excessively dry or oily. Hair is found on all body surfaces except the palms of the hands, the soles of the feet, and parts of the genitalia. Hair has various colors and textures. The hair is examined for color, texture, and distribution. Abnormal findings include unusual balding (*alopecia*) and excessive amounts of hair on the body (*hirsutism*). Decreased oxygenation of peripheral tissues, especially of the lower extremities, may cause the abnormal finding of loss of hair and thickened toenails.

The hair is separated to inspect the scalp for excessive dryness, scaliness, and lumps or lesions. If any

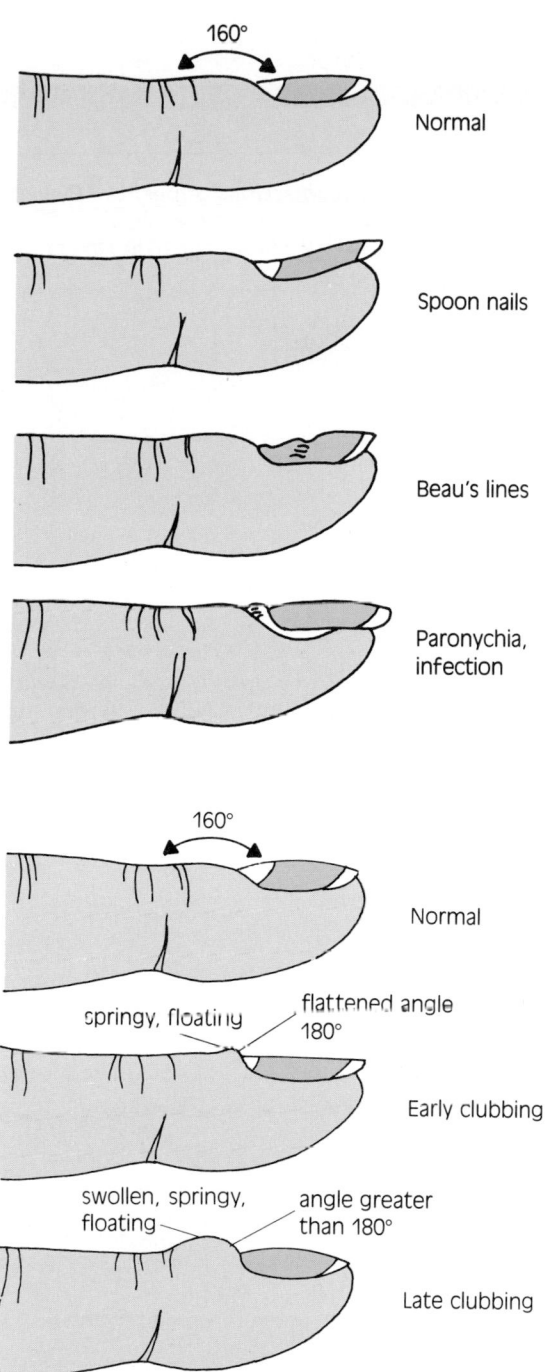

FIGURE 24-10
Examples of nail abnormalities.

lumps or masses are palpated, note location, size, tenderness, and mobility.

Head and Neck

Assessment of the head and neck includes the skull, face, eyes, ears, nose and sinuses, mouth and pharynx, trachea, thyroid gland, and lymph nodes. The skull is composed of bones that protect the brain and neurologic networks, allowing use of sensory and motor functions.

The skull and facial cavities are covered by facial muscles, innervated by cranial nerves V and VII. The neck is composed of vertebrae, ligaments, and muscles to provide support and movement. The trachea and thyroid gland are located in the anterior neck. An extensive arterial network provides the brain with nutrients and oxygen (Fig. 24-11).

Structures of the head and neck are assessed by inspection and palpation, with the client in the sitting position. Factors for consideration while assessing the head and neck are possible head injury, increased levels of stress, and thyroid dysfunction.

(Text continues on p. 446.)

Bones of the Skull

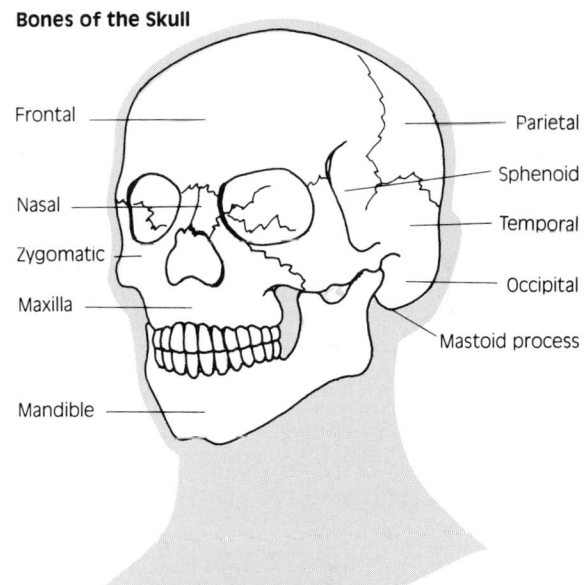

Muscles of the Head and Neck

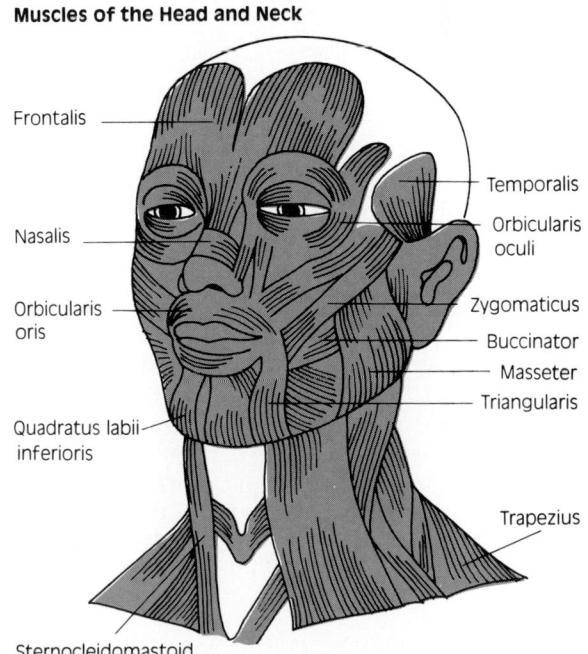

FIGURE 24-11
Structures of the head and neck.

T A B L E   24-5
Basic Types of Skin Lesions

Primary Lesions (May Arise from Previously Normal Skin)

Circumscribed, Flat, Nonpalpable Changes in Skin Color	Palpable Elevated Solid Masses	Circumscribed Superficial Elevations of the Skin Formed by Free Fluid in a Cavity Within the Skin Layers
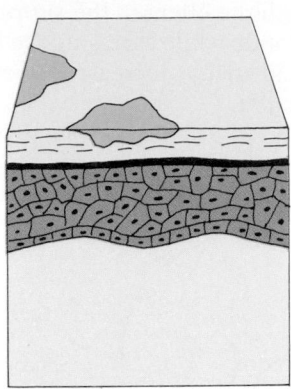	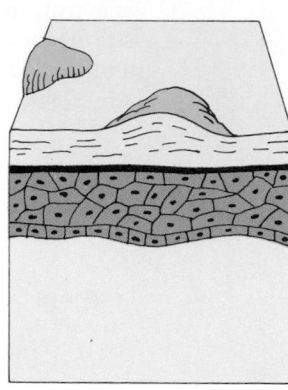	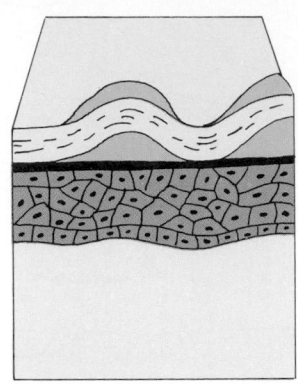

Macule—Small, up to 1 cm.* Example: freckle, petechia

Patch—Larger than 1 cm. Example: vitiligo

Papule—Up to 0.5 cm. Example: an elevated nevus

Plaque—A flat, elevated surface larger than 0.5 cm, often formed by the coalescence of papules

Nodule—0.5 cm to 1 cm–2 cm; often deeper and firmer than a papule

Tumor—Larger than 1 cm–2 cm

Wheal—A somewhat irregular, relatively transient, superficial area of localized skin edema. Example: mosquito bite, hive

Vesicle—Up to 0.5 cm; filled with serous fluid. Example: herpes simplex

Bulla—Greater than 0.5 cm; filled with serous fluid. Example: second degree burn

Pustule—Filled with pus. Examples: acne, impetigo

Secondary Lesions (Result from Changes in Primary Lesions)

Loss of Skin Surface

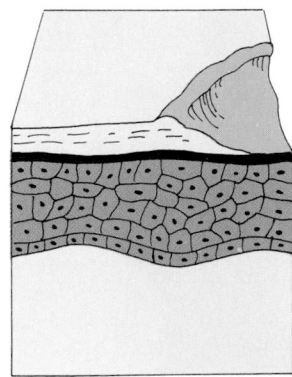	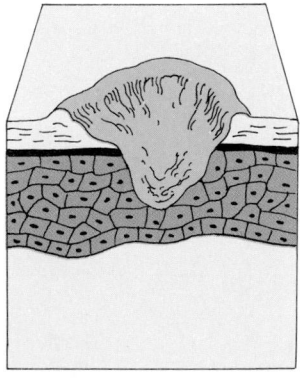	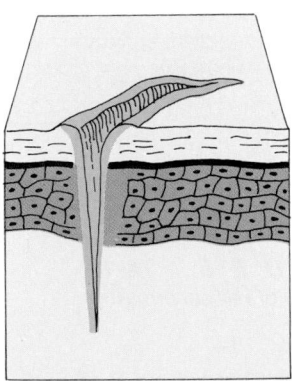

Erosion—Loss of the superficial epidermis; surface is moist but does not bleed. Example: moist area after the rupture of a vesicle, as in chickenpox

Ulcer—A deeper loss of skin surface that involves the epidermis and dermis; may bleed and scar. Examples: stasis ulcer of venous insufficiency, syphilitic chancre

Fissure—A deep linear crack in the skin that extends into the dermis. Example: athlete's foot

* Authorities vary somewhat in their definitions of skin lesions by size. Dimensions given in this table should be considered approximate, not rigid.

(Bates B: A Guide to Physical Examination, 4th ed., pp 142–143. Philadelphia, JB Lippincott, 1987)

Secondary Lesions (Result from Changes in Primary Lesions) (Continued)

Material on the Skin Surface

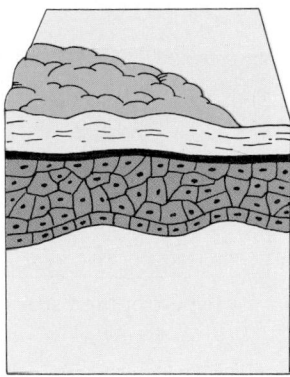

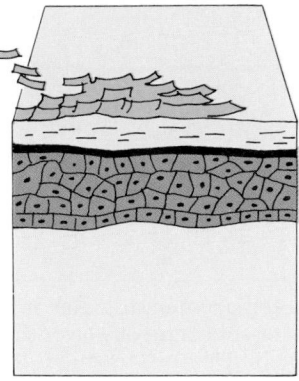

Crust—The dried residue of serum, pus, or blood. Example: impetigo

Scale—A thin flake of exfoliated epidermis. Examples: dandruff, dry skin, psoriasis

Miscellaneous

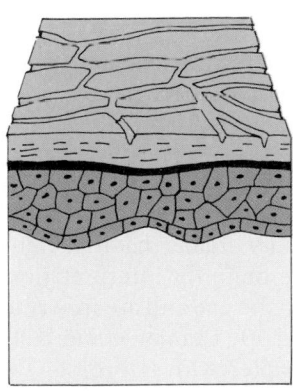

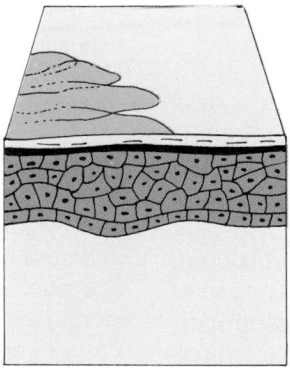

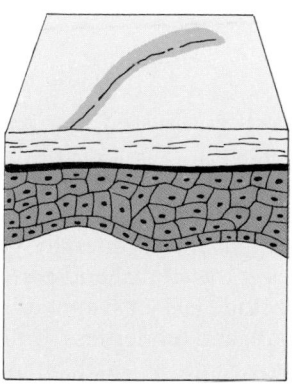

Lichenification—Thickening and roughening of the epidermis with increased visibility of the normal skin furrows. Example: atopic dermatitis

Atrophy—Thinning of the skin with loss of the normal skin furrows; the skin looks shinier and more translucent than normal. Example: arterial insufficiency

Excoriation—A scratch mark involving the epidermis

(Continued)

Secondary Lesions (Result from Changes in Primary Lesions) (Continued)

Miscellaneous (continued)

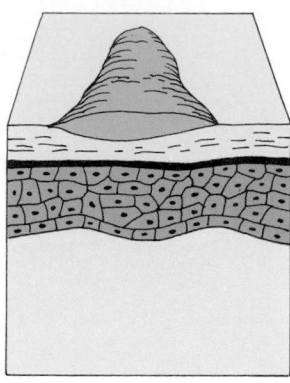

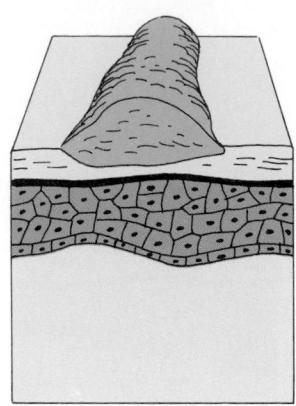

Scar—Replacement of tissue in the dermis or subcutaneous layer that is destroyed by fibrous tissue

Keloid—A hypertrophied scar

Several additional terms, though technically neither primary nor secondary lesions, deserve mention. A *comedo* refers to the common blackhead and marks the plugged opening of a sebaceous gland. Comedones are one of the hallmarks of acne. *Telangiectasias* are dilated small vessels that look either red or bluish. They can appear by themselves or as parts of other lesions such as a basal cell carcinoma or radiodermatitis (skin injury from ionizing radiation). The common mole—a flat to slightly elevated, round, evenly pigmented lesion—is technically called a *nevus,* although there are additional kinds of nevi that look quite different.

Skull

The skull is assessed for size and shape by inspection and palpation. The parts of the head and face should be in proportion to each other and symmetrical. There is considerable variation in the shape of the normal skull, but the shape is generally gently curved with prominences at the frontal and parietal bones. Abnormal findings include lack of symmetry, unusual size or contour of the skull, and tenderness. If the skull appears disproportionately large or small, it is measured for circumference. (Measuring head circumference is a normal part of infant assessment.)

Face

The face is examined for color; **symmetry**; which is a correspondence in contour, size, and position of bilateral sides; and distribution of facial hair. The facial nerve and facial muscles are assessed by asking the client to raise the eyebrows, tightly close the eyes, puff out cheeks, smile, and show the teeth. Edema of the face,

especially around the eye (**periorbital edema**), and involuntary facial movements (*tic* or **tremor**) are abnormal findings.

Eyes and Ears

The eyes and ears are sensory organs that transmit visual and auditory stimuli to the brain for interpretation. The eye muscles are attached to the eye and are innervated by cranial nerves III, IV, and VI. Cranial nerve testing is described later in this chapter with neurologic assessment. The equipment used in assessing the eyes and ears are a penlight, an ophthalmoscope/otoscope, an eye chart, a watch that ticks, and a tuning fork. The eyes and ears are primarily assessed by inspection.

Eye.   Assessments of the eye include external eye structures, pupils and iris, visual acuity, extraocular movements, peripheral vision, and internal eye structures. Factors for consideration while assessing the eye include age, use of corrective lens, artificial eye, allergies, pain, visual disturbances, and health-related factors such as high blood pressure or diabetes.

External Eye Structures.   External eye structures (Fig. 24-12) are assessed for position and alignment of the eyes, eyebrows, eyelids, eyelashes, lacrimal gland, and the pupils and iris. The position of the eyes is inspected for symmetry and parallel alignment. The eyebrows should have equal distribution, with the eyelashes curling outward. The eyelids are examined for color, edema, and equal coverage of the eyeball. The lacrimal glands are inspected and palpated for edema and pain.

Pupil and Iris.   The pupils are normally black, equal in size, round, and smooth, but may be pale and cloudy if the client has cataracts. Injury to the eye, glaucoma, and certain medications may cause the pupil to dilate (*mydriasis*); certain drugs can cause constriction (*miosis*); unequal pupils may result from central nervous system injury or illness. The pupil is assessed for reaction to light and accommodation, and for convergence.

Reaction to light is assessed as follows (Fig. 24-13):
- Ask the client to look straight ahead.
- Bring the penlight from the side of the client's face and shine the light on the pupil.
- Observe the pupil's reaction; normally it will constrict (direct response).

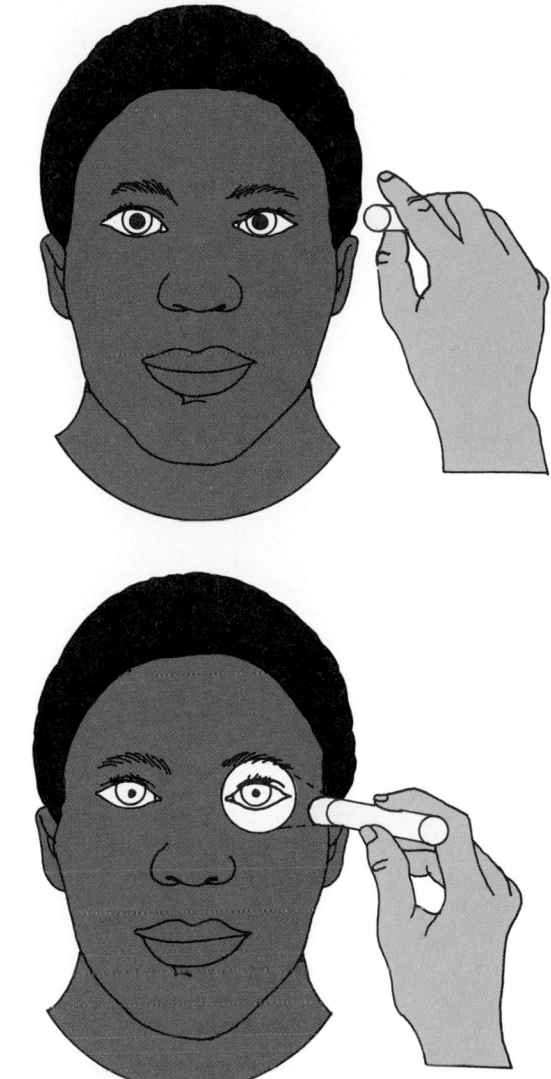

F I G U R E   24-13
To test pupillary reaction to light, a penlight is moved from the side of the client's face to in front of the eye. The pupil should constrict when the light is present. The dilation/constriction shown in the line drawing is exaggerated for clarity.

- Repeat the procedure and observe the other eye; normally it too will constrict (consensual reflex).
- Repeat the procedure with the other eye.

Accommodation is assessed by the following (Fig. 24-14):
- Hold your forefinger about 10 cm to 15 cm (4–6 inches) from the bridge of the client's nose.
- Ask the client to first look at your finger, then at a distant object, then back to your finger.
- Normally the pupil should constrict when looking at a near object and dilate when looking at a distant object.

Convergence is assessed by moving your finger toward the client's nose; the client's eyes should normally converge (assume a cross-eyed appearance).

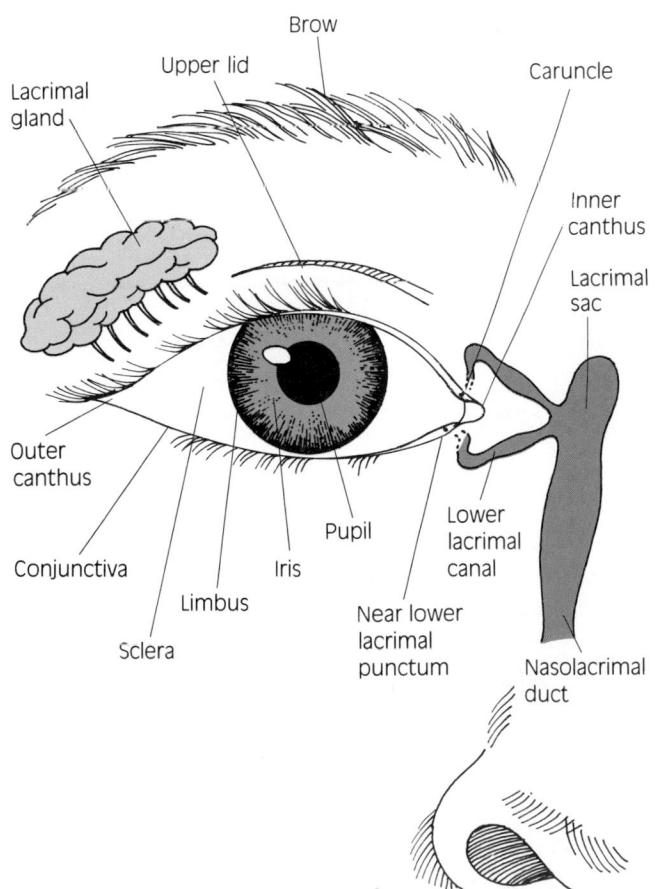

F I G U R E   24-12
The eye and surrounding structures.

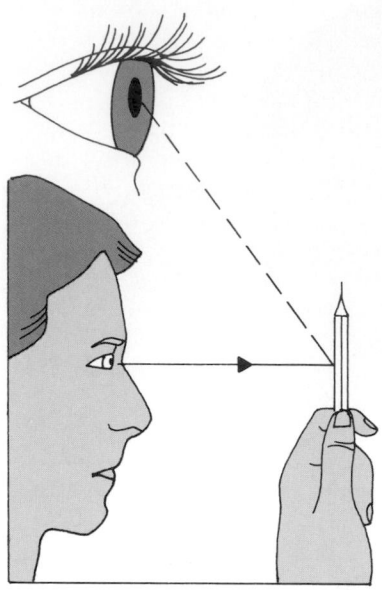

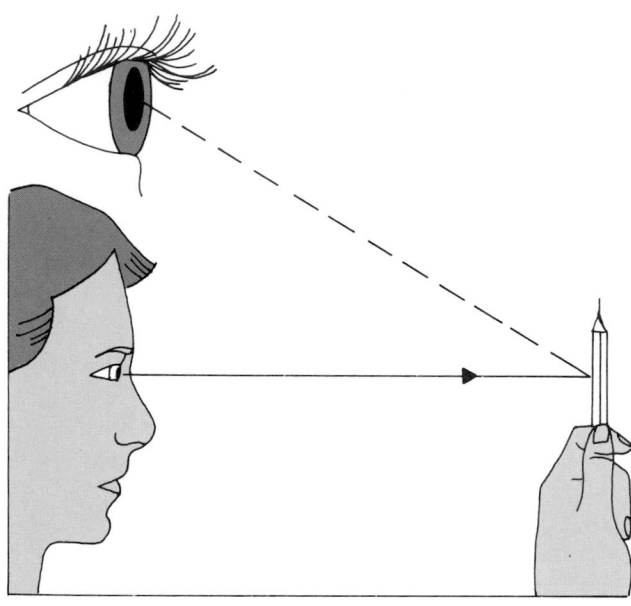

FIGURE 24-14
The normal pupil will constrict when focused on a near object and dilate when focused on a far object. This is called accommodation.

Visual Acuity. Visual acuity is assessed by placing the client 20 feet from the Snellen eye chart and testing each eye. The client is asked to read the smallest possible line of letters, first with both eyes and then with one eye at a time. Visual acuity is measured by standardized numbers listed on the side of the chart. The numerator is 20, representing the distance from which a person with normal vision can read the lettering. The larger the denominator, the poorer the vision. Normal vision is 20/20. Visual acuity is recorded as the smallest line of letters that can be read accurately. If the Snellen chart is not available, the client may read from a newspaper or magazine for an estimate of visual acuity.

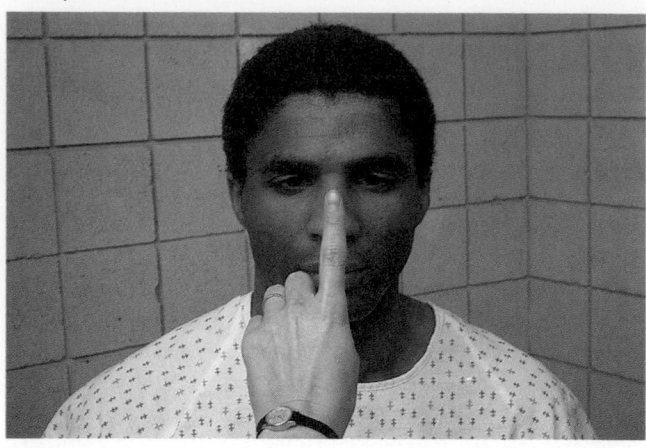

FIGURE 24-15
Convergence is assessed by moving your finger toward the client's nose. (Photo © Ken Kasper)

Extraocular Movements. Extraocular movements (EOM) are tested by assessing the eight cardinal fields of vision (Fig. 24-16) for coordination and alignment. Normally both eyes move together, are coordinated, and are parallel. To assess EOM

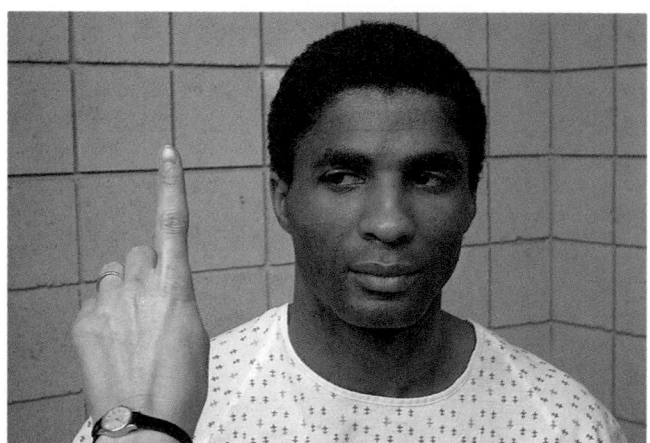

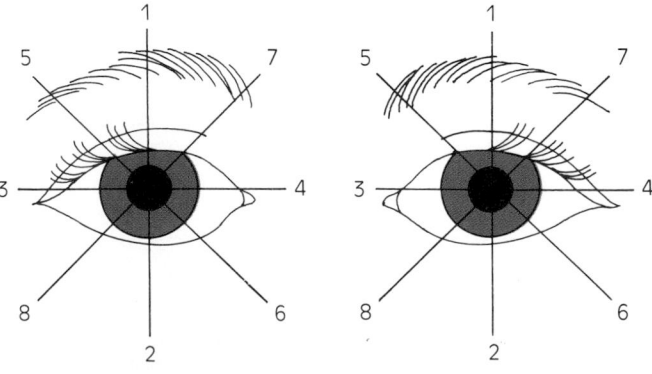

FIGURE 24-16
(Top) Test extraocular movement of the eye by asking the client to hold his head still and follow the movement of your forefinger through the cardinal positions of the eye (bottom). (Photo © Ken Kasper)

- Ask the client to sit or stand about 2 feet away, facing you, as you also sit or stand on eye level with the client.
- Ask the client to hold the head still and follow the movement of your forefinger or a penlight with the eyes.
- Keep your finger about 1 foot from the client's face and move it through the cardinal positions: up and down, left and right, diagonally up and down to the left, diagonally up and down to the right.

Peripheral Vision. Tests for peripheral vision (or visual fields) assess retinal function and optic nerve function. Normally, the client will have full peripheral vision. To assess visual fields

- Have the client stand or sit about 2 feet away, facing you; be sure you are at eye level.
- Ask the client to cover one eye with his hand or an index card.
- Ask the client to look directly at your nose, and fix his or her eyes on that spot.
- Cover your own eye opposite the client's closed eye.
- Hold your hand at arm's length to one side (right or left) and move your fingers into the visual fields from various peripheral points.

- Ask the client to tell you when he or she sees your fingers (both you and the client should see your fingers at the same time).
- Repeat the procedure for the other eye.

Abnormalities of the external eye, pupil and iris, and visual assessment examination include **asymmetry** of position and alignment, inability to open and close the upper lids, scanty eyebrows and eyelashes, edema, redness or drainage, decreased or absent pupillary response, inability of the eyes to accommodate or converge, and alterations in the visual fields.

Internal Eye Structures. The internal eye (Fig. 24-17) is examined with the ophthalmoscope, assessing the eye fundus, including the retina, optic nerve disc, macula, fovea centralis, and retinal vessels. Use of the ophthalmoscope takes practice and may not be a part of the nursing examination in some clinical settings. General guidelines and an outline of the examination are included here. Normal findings are a uniform red reflex; clear, yellow optic nerve disc; reddish retina; and light red arteries and dark red veins with the veins being about 1½ times larger than the arteries (Fig. 24-18).

General guidelines for assessment of the internal eye are as follows:

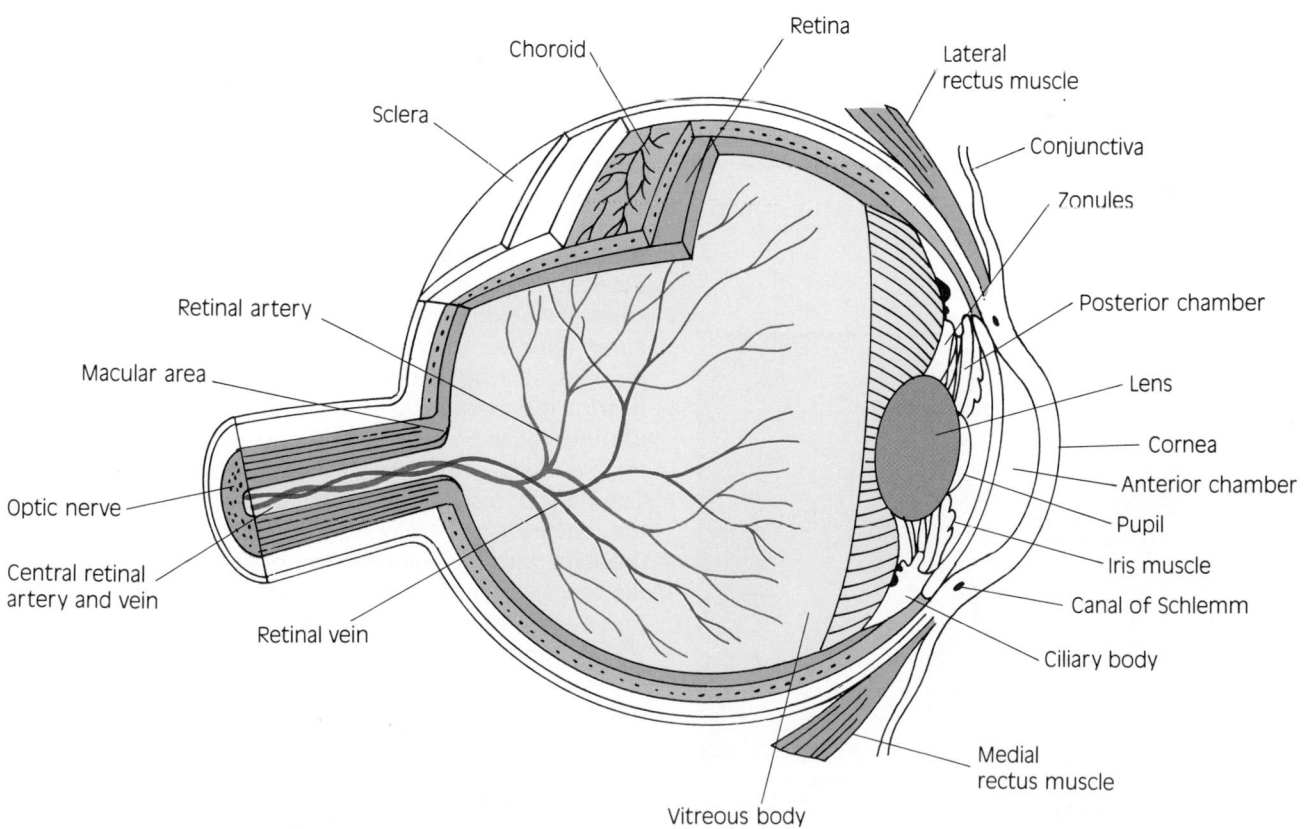

FIGURE 24-17
A cross section of the eye.

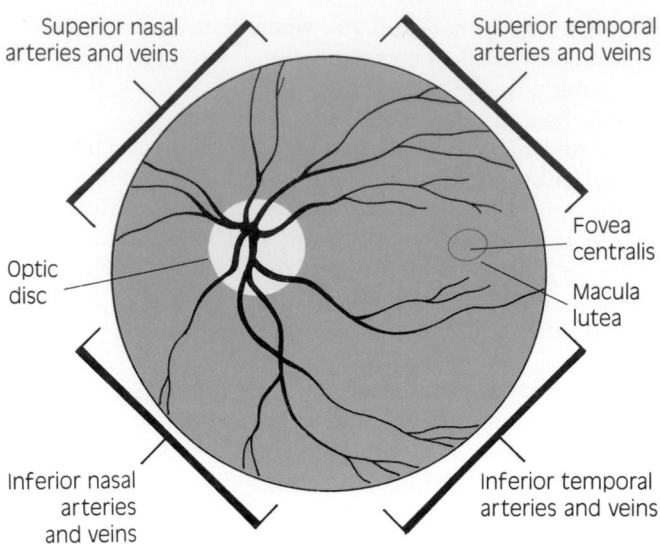

Superior nasal
arteries and veins

Superior temporal
arteries and veins

Optic
disc

Fovea
centralis

Macula
lutea

Inferior nasal
arteries
and veins

Inferior temporal
arteries and veins

F I G U R E   24-18
The normal fundus, as seen through an ophthalmoscope.

- Assemble the ophthalmoscope, beginning with the light setting at the large white light and the lens wheel at 0 setting.
- Darken the room and have the client remove glasses. Allow time for the client's pupils to dilate. The client should be sitting.
- Sit facing the client and ask the client to look straight ahead during the examination.
- Keep both eyes open while looking through the ophthalmoscope viewer.
- Use your right hand and eye to examine the client's right eye, and your left hand and eye for the client's left eye.
- Shine the light on the pupil and observe the round red/orange glow (the red reflex).

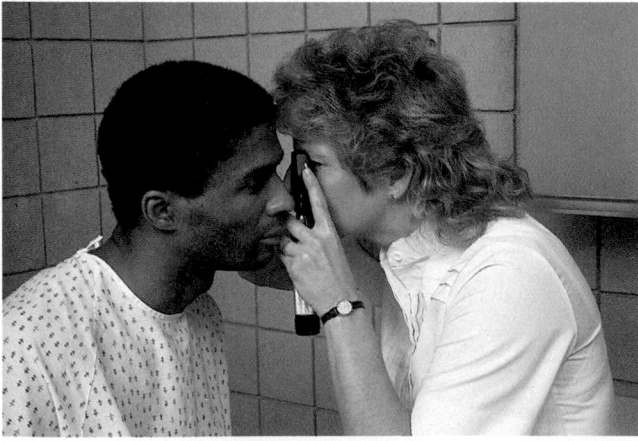

F I G U R E   24-19
Examination of the internal structures of the eye using an oph-thalmoscope. (Photo © Ken Kasper)

- Focusing on the red reflex, slowly move the ophthalmoscope toward the client's eye.
- Rotate the lens wheel until internal eye structures are sharp and clear.
- Follow blood vessels toward the midline to locate the optic disc; note color, size, shape, margins, and central area (physiologic cup).
- Follow blood vessels outward to each of the four quadrants, assessing color, size, and pattern.
- Ask the client to look up, down, and from side to side, assessing the characteristics of the retina.
- Locate the macula by first locating the optic disc and then looking toward the client's temple for a small circular structure near the disc; note color, characteristics, and area of reflected light (fovea centralis).

Abnormal findings include cloudiness of lens, narrowing of blood vessels, and changes in color and surface characteristics.

Ear.   The ear is composed of three major compartments. The external ear is made of cartilage covered with skin. The middle ear is an air-filled cavity that transmits sound from the tympanic membranes to the inner ear. The inner ear transmits sound impulses to cranial nerve VIII (Fig. 24-20).

Risk factors for consideration when assessing the ears are environmental hazards, such as exposure to chemicals, or uncontrolled loud noises. The use of corrective hearing devices should be included in the assessment documentation.

The client remains sitting while the nurse assesses the ears and hearing ability by inspection and palpation. An otoscope with a suitably sized ear speculum may be used to inspect the ear canal; a tuning fork is used in hearing acuity assessment.

Hearing.   Hearing is assessed, one ear at a time, by determining if the client can hear the nurse's whispered voice or a ticking watch from a distance of 1 to 2 feet. The nurse must be certain the client is not lip-reading and assesses hearing acuity out of the line of vision. When hearing loss is found, a tuning fork or audiometer may be used for more precise assessments of hearing; audiometry is not generally used in routine physical assessment. Tuning fork tests are used to assess the type of hearing loss. Hearing loss may be *conductive;* the result of a problem with the transmission of sound waves through the outer and middle ear; *sensorineural,* resulting from inner ear damage; or *mixed,* a combination of both. Weber's and Rinne's tests are used.

Weber's test is used to assess bone conduction. The procedure is

- Hold the tuning fork at its base and strike it against the palm of the opposite hand so the fork vibrates.
- Place the base of the tuning fork on the center of the top of the client's head.
- Ask the client where the sound is heard best.

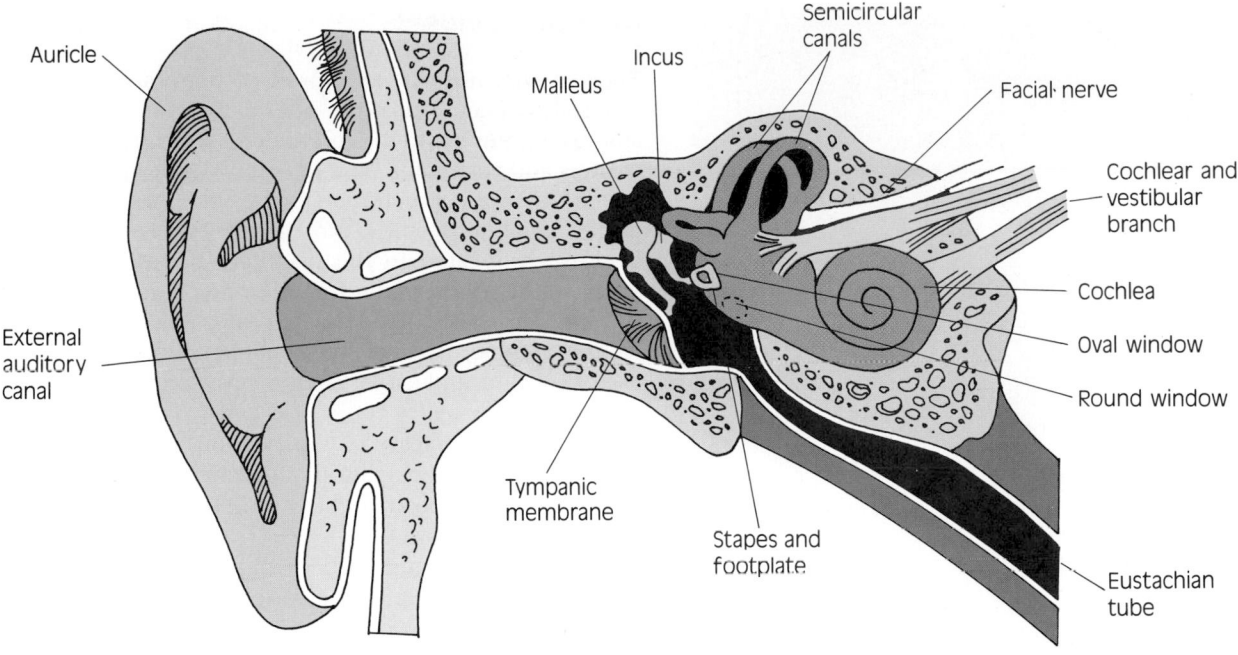

F I G U R E   *24-20*
Internal structures of the ear.

Clients with conductive hearing loss hear the sound better in the affected ear because bone transmits the sound directly to the ear. Normal findings would be sound heard in both ears or in the midline.

Rinne's test compares air conduction (AC) to bone conduction (BC). The test is as follows:

- Activate the tuning fork.
- Hold the base of the tuning fork against the mastoid process of the client and ask the client to tell you when the sound can no longer be heard.
- Immediately place the still-vibrating tuning fork close to the external ear canal and ask if the client can hear the sound; the normal ear will do so.
- Repeat the test with the other ear.

Normally, air conduction is better than bone conduction (positive Rinne with AC > BC). If the hearing loss is conductive, bone conduction will be the same or greater than air conduction.

External Ear.   The external ear is inspected for shape, size, and lesions. The external surfaces of the ear should be smooth, and the shape and size of the ears should be symmetrical and proportionate to the head. The external ear is gently palpated for pain, edema, or presence of lesions (Fig. 24-21). Abnormal findings of the external ear include unequal height and size, uneven color, and lesions.

The otoscope is used to examine the ear canal and the tympanic membrane. The otoscope head is placed on the base, and the largest speculum that will fit into the client's ear comfortably is attached. The otoscope specu-

lum is inserted as the client's head is slightly tilted away from the examiner (Fig. 24-22). The client is in the sitting position. To achieve better visualization, the ear

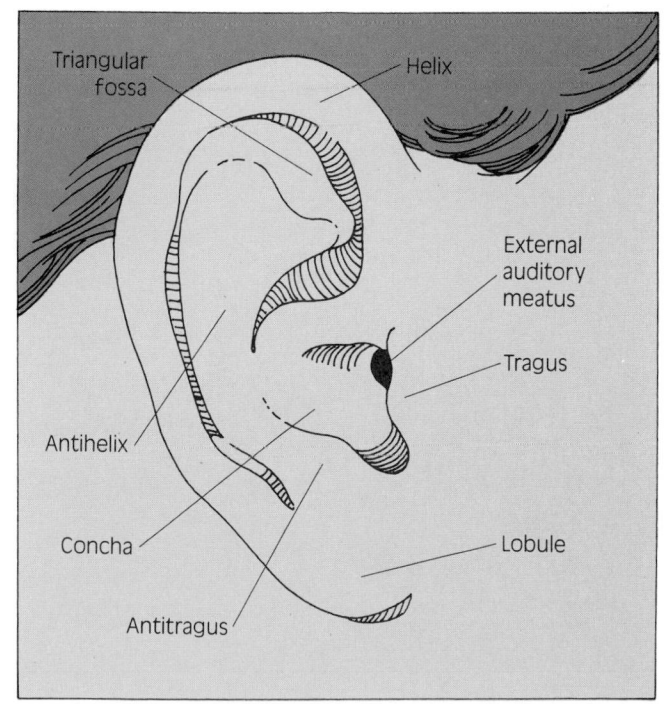

F I G U R E   *24-21*
The external structures of the ear.

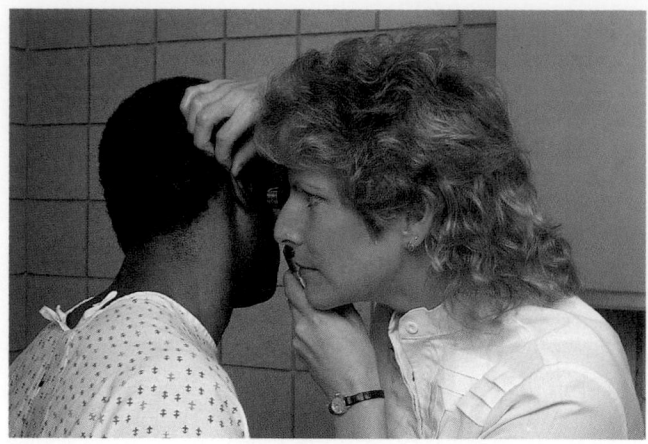

F I G U R E   24-22

Examination of the internal structures of the ear using an otoscope. (Photo © Ken Kasper)

canal of the adult is straightened by gently pulling the pinna up and back (the ear canal is straightened in children under age 3 years by pulling the pinna down and back). The ear canal should be smooth and pinkish in color. It is examined for wax, discharge, and foreign bodies. The tympanic membrane should be intact and without redness or discharge. The membrane is translucent, shiny, and gray in color (Fig. 24-23). Typical abnormal findings include pain when manipulating the pinna, redness of the canal, nodules on the auricle, mastoid tenderness, a red and swollen eardrum, a perforated eardrum, wax plugs in the ear canal, and drainage.

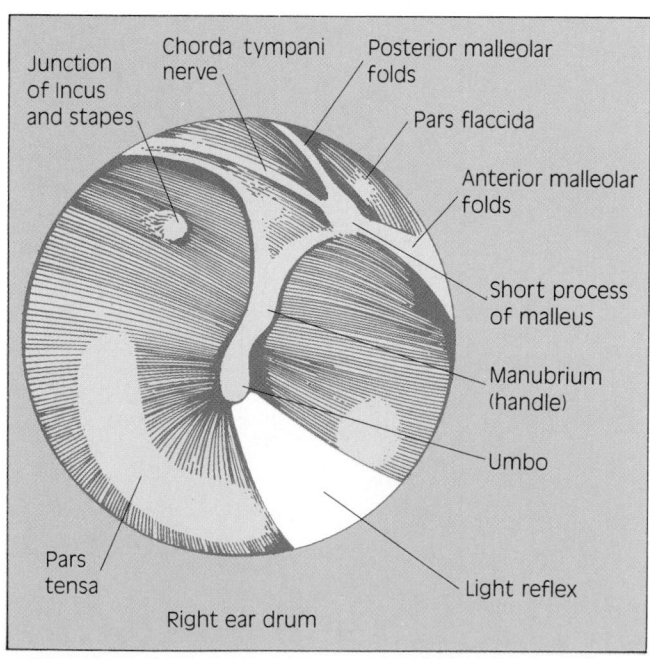

F I G U R E   24-23

Normal tympanic membrane, as seen through an otoscope.

Nose and Sinuses

The external nose is composed of bone and cartilage covered by skin. The nose extends from the nares (or anterior openings) to the internal nose, divided into two cavities and vestibules. The lateral walls of the nose are formed by bony structures (turbinates) that warm, humidify, and filter inspired air (Fig. 24-24). The maxillary sinuses are located in the maxillary bone; the frontal sinuses are located in the frontal bone (Fig. 24-25).

Risk factors to consider when assessing the nose and sinuses include allergies, frequent respiratory infections, use of cocaine, and use of nasal drops, sprays, and medications.

The nose is assessed by inspection, and the sinuses by inspection and palpation. The client is in a sitting position with the head slightly tilted back.

Nose. The nose is tested for nasal patency by occluding one nostril at a time and asking the client to inhale through the nose. Each nostril is inspected, using an otoscope with a short, wide tip or with a nasal speculum and penlight (Fig. 24-26). The mucous membranes are

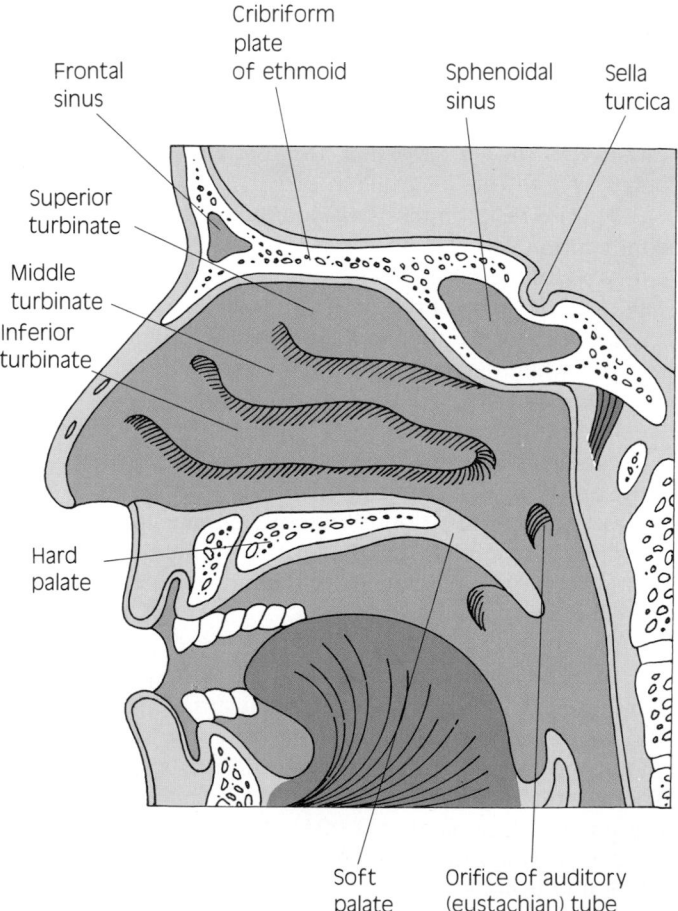

F I G U R E   24-24

Cross section of the nasal cavity.

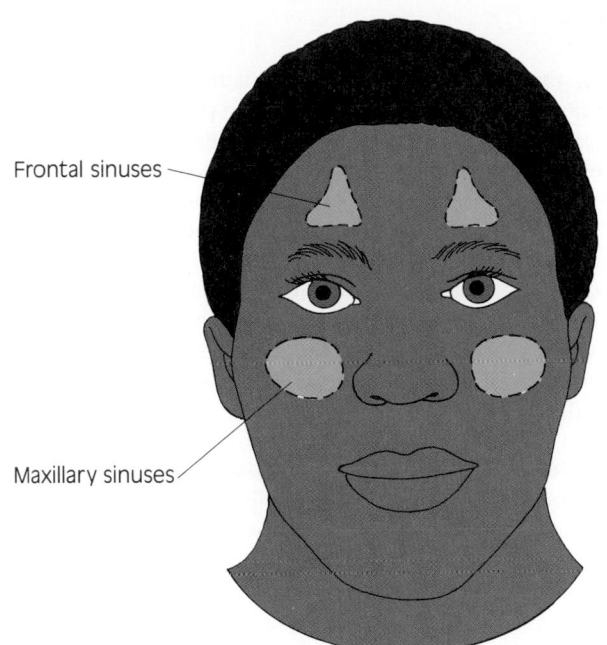

FIGURE 24-25
Location of the frontal and maxillary sinuses.

examined for color and the presence of exudate or growths. The nasal septum is inspected for intactness and deviation. Normally, the nasal mucosa is moist and redder than the oral mucosa. Abnormal findings that should be noted when assessing the nose are swelling of the mucosa, bleeding, discharge, perforation or deviation of the nasal septum, and **polyps**.

Sinuses. The frontal and maxillary sinuses are examined for pain and edema. The frontal sinuses are palpated by gently pressing upward on the bony promi-

nences located above each eye. The maxillary sinuses are palpated by gentle pressure on the bony prominences of the upper cheek (Fig. 24-27). Normally, the sinuses are not painful when palpated. Pain may be a finding if the sinuses are infected or obstructed.

Mouth and Pharynx

The mouth and pharynx are made up of various structures: the lips, tongue, teeth, gums, hard and soft palate, salivary gland, the tonsillar pillars, and the tonsils (Fig. 24-28). The primary function of the mouth and pharynx is to allow passage of air, food, and liquids. Special properties of the mouth aid in digestion and vocalization. Risk factors for consideration during assessment include oral hygiene patterns, eating habits, use of dentures, use of smokeless tobacco, pipe smoking, and medications.

Equipment for assessment of the mouth and pharynx includes a penlight, a tongue blade, and gloves. The mouth and pharynx are assessed by inspection of the

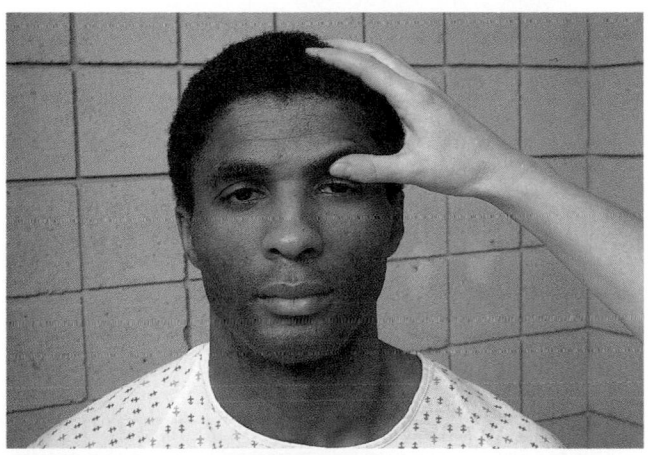

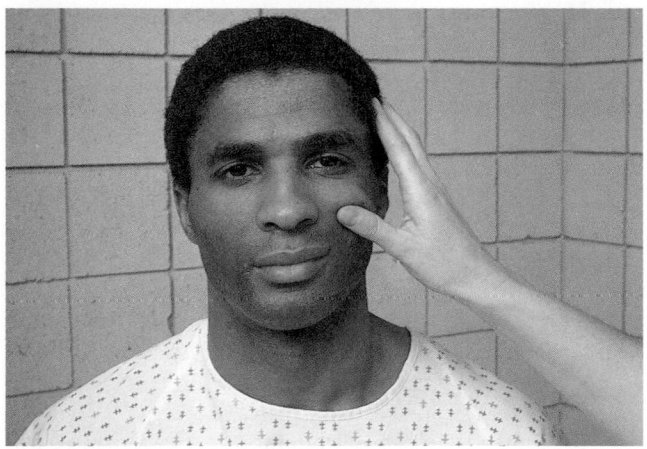

FIGURE 24-27
(Top) The frontal sinuses are palpated by gently pressing upward on the bony prominences above each eye. (Bottom) The maxillary sinuses are palpated by applying gentle pressure on the bony prominences of the upper cheek. (Photos © Ken Kasper)

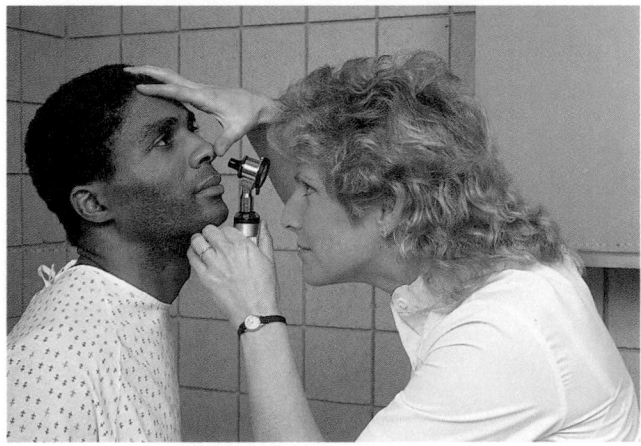

FIGURE 24-26
Examination of the nasal passages using an otoscope with a wide speculum. (Photo © Ken Kasper)

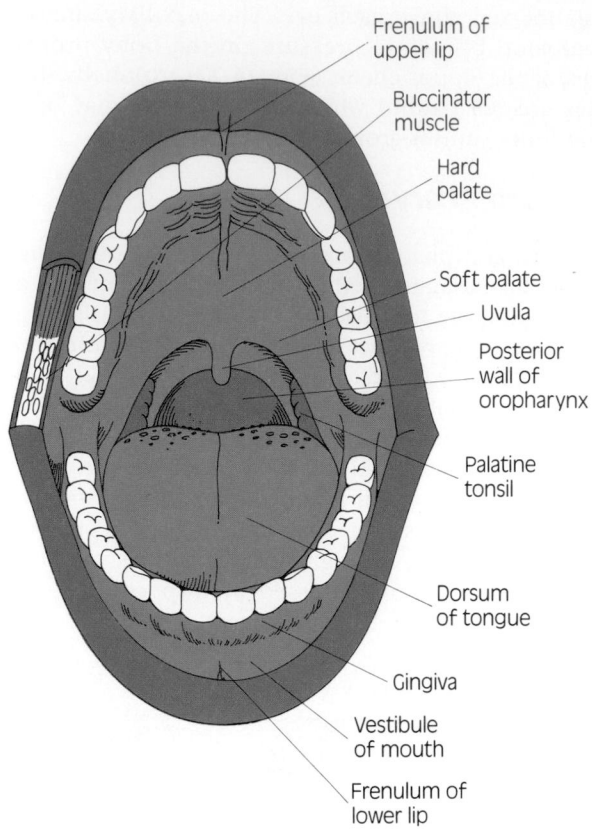

F I G U R E 24-28
Structures of the mouth.

lips, gums and teeth, tongue, and hard and soft palates, using palpation if any abnormalities are noted during inspection. The client is in the sitting position with his head tilted backward and is instructed to open the mouth widely. The nurse should wear gloves when assessing a client's mouth.

The lips should be pink, moist, and smooth. The tongue and mucous membranes are normally pink in color, moist, and free of swelling or lesions. If the client wears dentures, they are removed for inspection of the gums and roof of the mouth. The gums should be pink and smooth. With the tongue relaxed on the floor of the mouth, the mucous membrane of the oropharynx is examined as the base of the tongue is depressed with a tongue depressor. The uvula normally is centered and freely movable. The tonsils, if present, are small, pink, and symmetrical in size. The teeth should be regular and free of cavities or have dental restoration.

Abnormal findings of the mouth and pharynx are redness and swelling of the mucous membranes; lesions of the mucosa and lips; swollen and red tonsils; swollen, red, and bleeding gums; poorly aligned, missing, or carious teeth; a hairy or fissured tongue; and paralysis of the tongue.

Neck

With the client in the sitting position, the neck (Fig. 24-29) is assessed by inspection and palpation. The neck should be slightly hyperextended. Risk factors to consider when assessing the neck include past injury, infections, and evidence or history of thyroid problems.

The neck is assessed for size and position of the trachea and thyroid (Fig. 24-30), range of motion, lymph nodes, and venous distention. Full range of motion is assessed by asking the client to tilt the head backward, forward, and side to side. The neck should be symmetrical with full range of motion. No neck vein distention should be visible.

Trachea.   The trachea is palpated for alignment and position; which is normally midline at the suprasternal notch. Palpate by placing the thumb and forefinger on each side of the trachea at the suprasternal notch; an unequal space between the trachea and the sternocleidomastoid muscle on each side is an abnormal finding indicating tracheal displacement.

Thyroid.   The thyroid gland is assessed by palpation, but in many individuals is normally not palpable. The client is sitting, with the examiner using the posterior

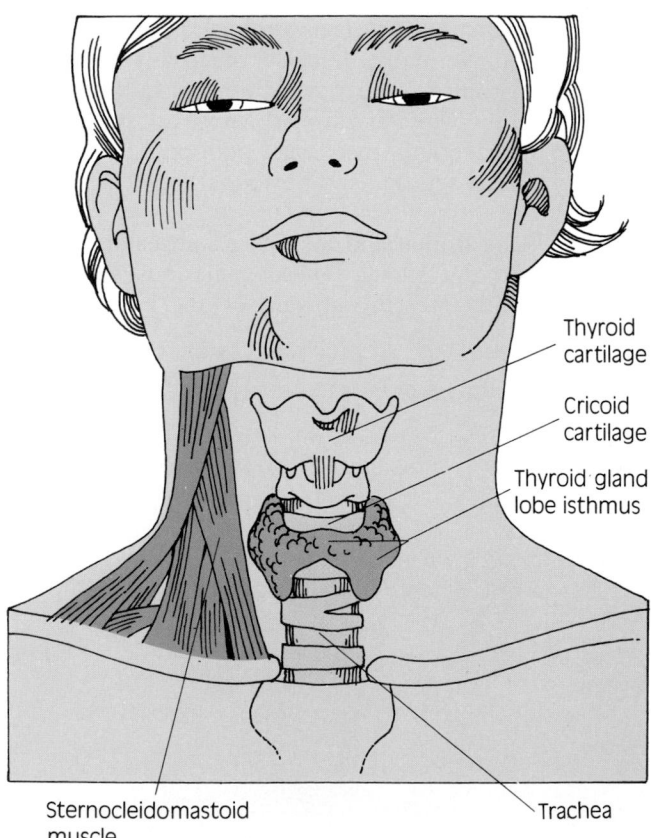

F I G U R E 24-29
Structures of the neck.

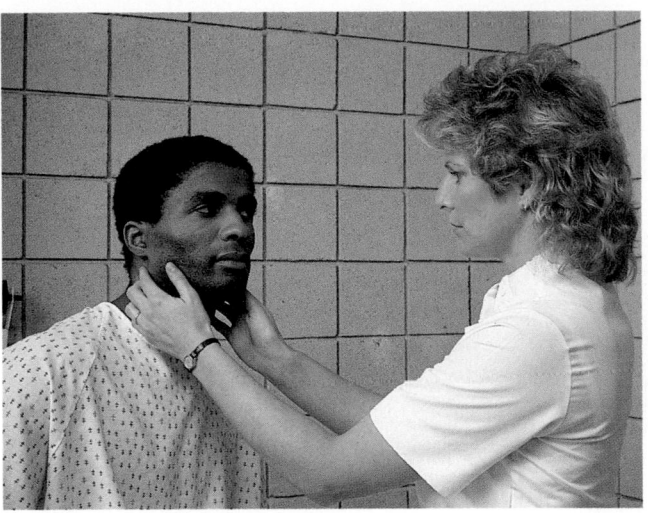

FIGURE 24-30
Palpation of the neck. (Photo © Ken Kasper)

approach (Fig. 24-31). Palpate for size, shape, symmetry, tenderness, and presence of any nodules. To palpate the thyroid gland

- Standing behind the client, place your hands around the client's neck, with your fingertips over the lower half of the neck and trachea.
- Ask the client to swallow, and feel for enlargement of the gland as it rises.
- Palpate each lobe of the thyroid by having the client turn the head slightly toward the side to be examined; then gently displace the trachea with one hand.
- Ask the client to swallow, and palpate the thyroid with your other hand.
- Repeat for the other side.

The thyroid gland should feel soft and should be without tenderness, enlargement, masses, or nodules.

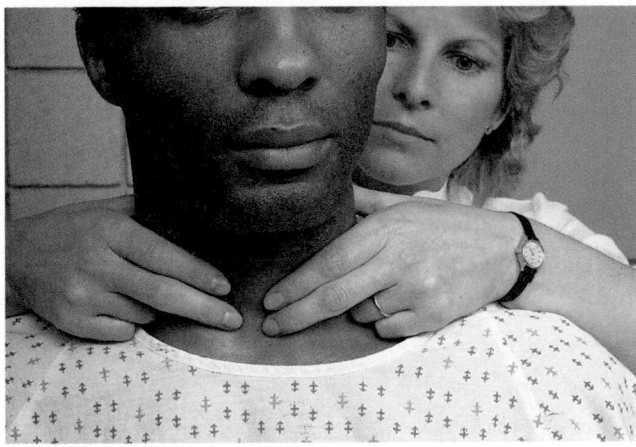

FIGURE 24-31
Examination of the thyroid. (Photo © Ken Kasper)

Lymph Nodes. The lymph nodes are palpated with the pads of the fingers for enlargement, tenderness, and mobility. The nodes form a chain with the preauricular and posterior auricular (located anteriorly and posteriorly to the ear), occipital (base of skull), tonsillar (upper lateral neck), submaxillary and submental (jaw line), superficial cervical and posterior cervical (lateral upper and lower portion of the neck), and supraclavicular (anterior upper to lower neck region) (Fig. 24-32). The nodes are generally not palpable; if palpable, they should be small, mobile, and nontender. If palpable, assess location, size, consistency, mobility, and tenderness.

Abnormal findings of the neck include limited neck movement, enlargement of veins, tracheal deviation, thyroid enlargement, and palpable lymph nodes. Consistent hoarseness should also be documented.

Thorax and Lungs

The thorax (Fig. 24-33) is composed of the rib cage, cartilage, and muscles that enable the respiratory process
(Text continues on p. 457.)

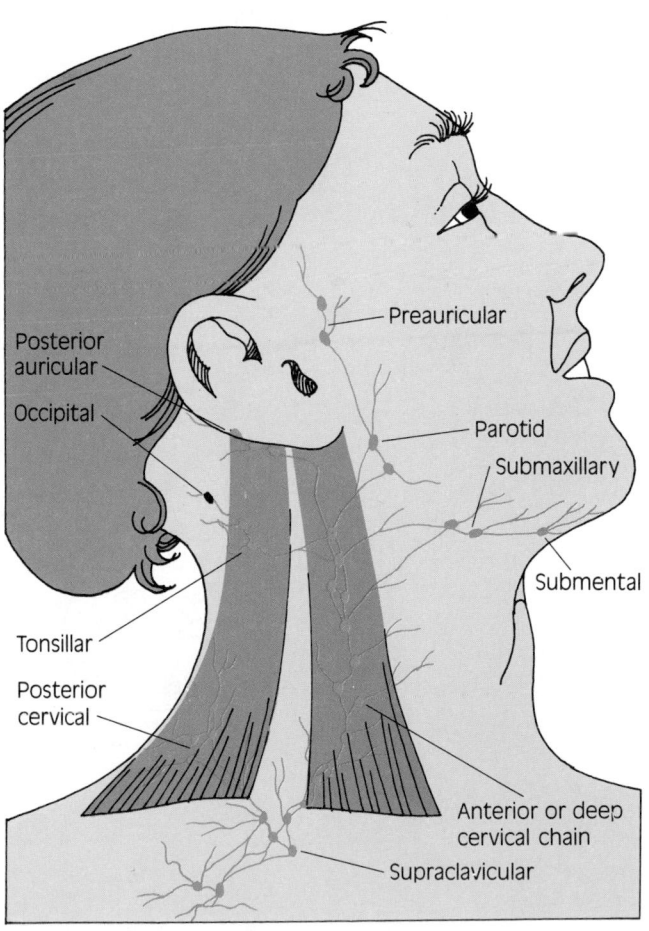

FIGURE 24-32
Location of the lymph nodes of the neck.

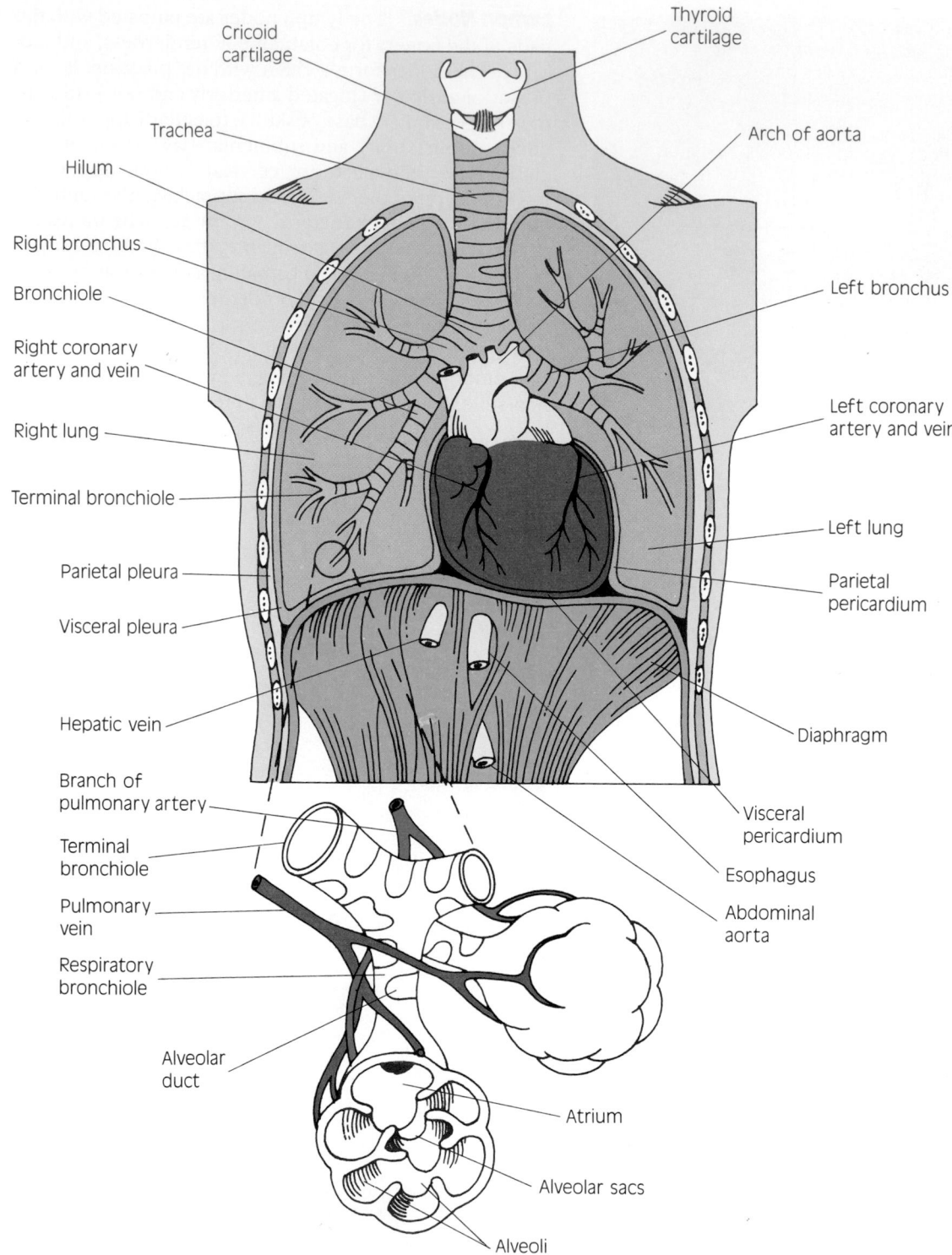

Cricoid cartilage

Thyroid cartilage

Trachea

Arch of aorta

Hilum

Right bronchus

Left bronchus

Bronchiole

Right coronary artery and vein

Left coronary artery and vein

Right lung

Terminal bronchiole

Left lung

Parietal pleura

Parietal pericardium

Visceral pleura

Hepatic vein

Diaphragm

Branch of pulmonary artery

Visceral pericardium

Terminal bronchiole

Esophagus

Pulmonary vein

Abdominal aorta

Respiratory bronchiole

Alveolar duct

Atrium

Alveolar sacs

Alveoli

F I G U R E   24-33
Structures of the thorax, with inset of alveoli.

to occur. The interior chest is divided into the right and left pleural cavities, with three lobes of lung tissue on the right and two lobes on the left. Air is inspired into the tracheobronchial system through the trachea, which branches into the right and left mainstem bronchi. Each bronchus branches into bronchioles, and then into the alveoli, where the exchange of oxygen and carbon dioxide takes place.

Risk factors for consideration when assessing the thorax and lungs include environmental hazards, smoking, nutritional status, and frequent or chronic respiratory infections.

The equipment needed for this examination includes a stethoscope (warmed) and a tape measure. The environment should be warm and have adequate lighting. The techniques for this examination include inspection, palpation, percussion, and auscultation. The client is in a sitting position during the assessment.

Inspection. Inspection begins with observation of the client's chest for color, shape or contour, breathing patterns, and muscle development. The color should be even and consistent with the color of the client's face. The shape or contour should have a downward equal slope at the rib cage. The chest should be symmetrical, with the transverse diameter being greater than the anterior posterior diameter. If the contour of the chest changes, as in chronic lung disease conditions, the contour of the chest wall can be described as *barrel-chest* with noted increase in anterior posterior diameter (Fig. 24-34). The breathing patterns should be smooth and even, ranging from 12 to 20 breaths per minute. Abnormal findings during inspection include an increase in chest size and contour, abnormal breathing patterns with use of accessory muscles, and changes in skin color.

Palpation. Palpation is used to detect areas of sensitivity, chest expansion during respirations, and vibrations (*fremitus*). The examiner uses the palmar surface of the hands to palpate the anterior and posterior thoracic landmarks (Fig. 24-35) in a sequential pattern for temperature, moisture, muscular development, and the presence of tenderness or masses. The same technique and sequence are used to test for tactile (vocal) fremitus, comparing bilateral sides. Normally, equal bilateral mild vibratory sensations will be palpated. The skin should be warm and dry, muscular development symmetrical, and there should be no tenderness or masses. Chest expansion is determined by placing the hands over the anterior and posterior thorax and feeling the amount of movement during shallow and deep respirations. The thorax should expand symmetrically (Fig. 24-36).

Abnormal findings during palpation may be cool, excessively dry or moist skin, muscle asymmetry, tenderness, masses, increased or decreased vibratory sensation, asymmetrical thoracic expansion, and abnormal breathing patterns (Fig. 24-37).

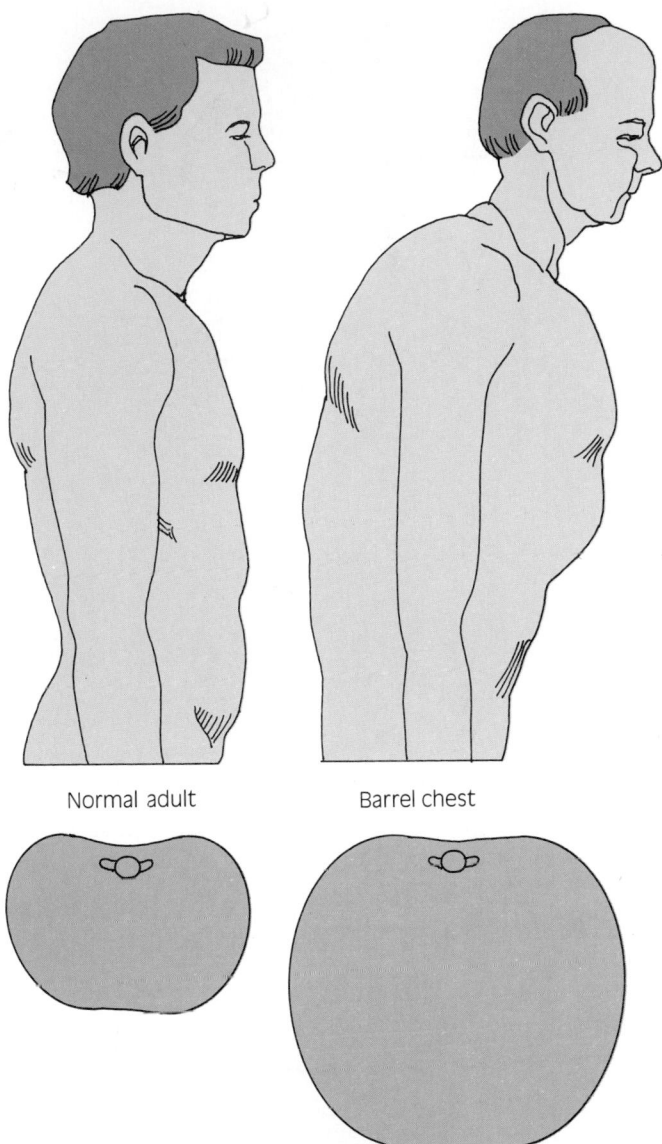

Normal adult   Barrel chest

F I G U R E 24-34
Profile and anteroposterior diameter of normal adult chest and barrel chest.

Percussion. Percussion is used to determine lung position and size and to detect the presence of air, liquids, or solids within the lungs. The shoulder area and anterior and posterior thorax are palpated in a systematic pattern (see Fig. 24-35). The nurse listens for the intensity, pitch, duration, and quality of the sounds produced. When a normal air-filled lung is percussed, the sound is hollow, loud, low-pitched, and of long duration. This percussion tone is known as **resonance.** A *flat* tone will be heard over bony or well-developed muscle tissue. *Tympany,* a hollow sound, is percussed over the stomach. Percussion sounds that are abnormal over lung tissue are *hyperresonance,* heard over emphysematous lung tissue, and *dullness,* heard over fluid or a solid mass.

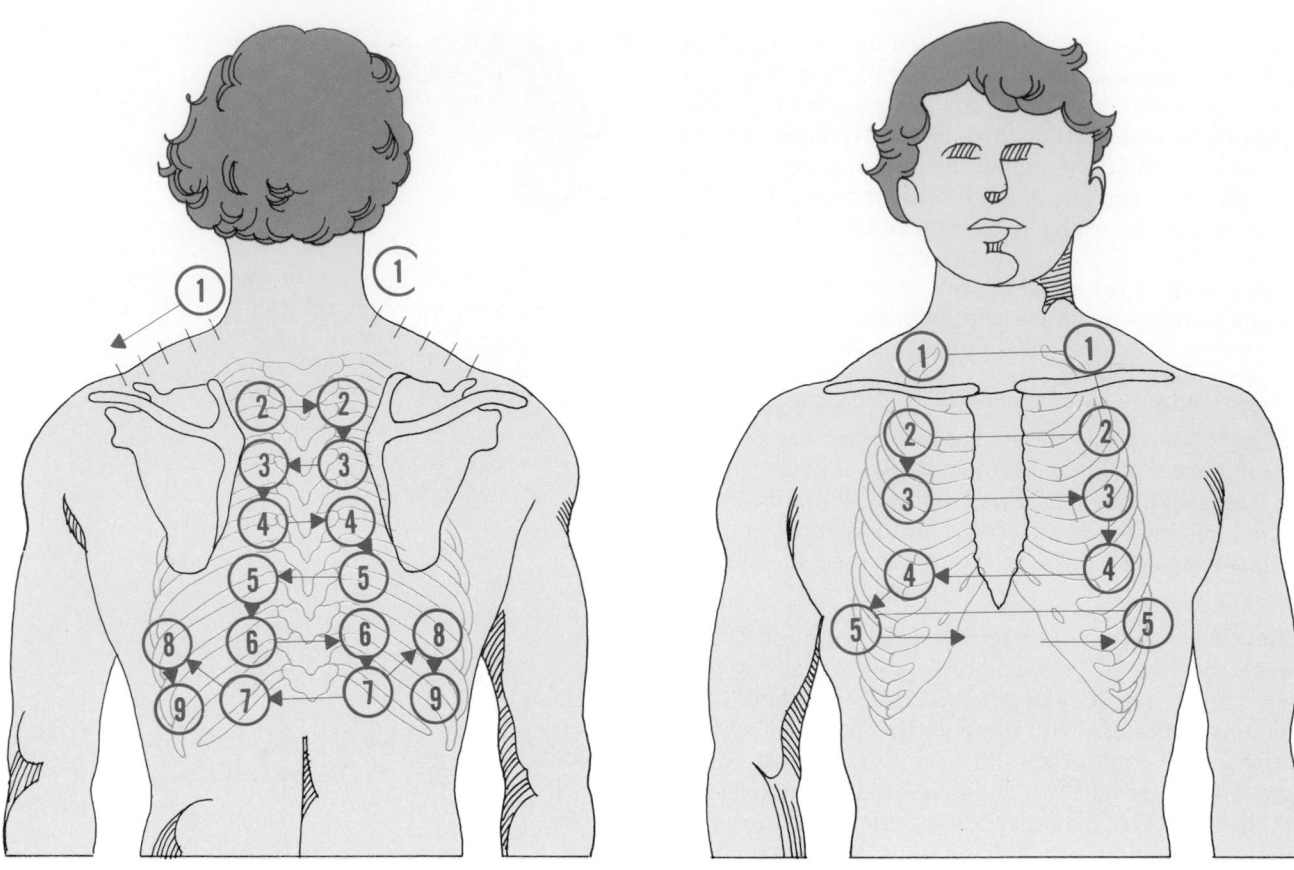

F I G U R E   24-35
Anterior and posterior chest, landmarks and systematic sequence of examination. The pattern is used for palpation, percussion, and auscultation of the chest.

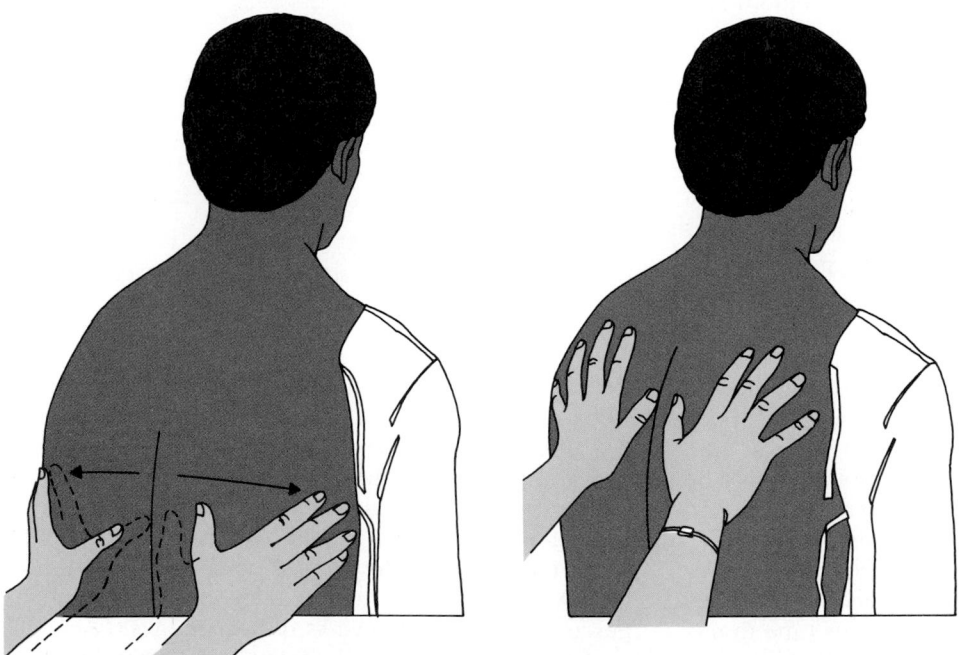

F I G U R E   24-36
(Left) Palpation of the posterior thorax excursion. The examiner's hands are placed symmetrically on client's back. As the client inhales, the examiner's hands should move apart symmetrically. (Right) Palpation of the posterior thorax for vocal or tactile fremitus. The examiner uses the palms of the hands to detect vibrations transmitted through the lung to the chest wall.

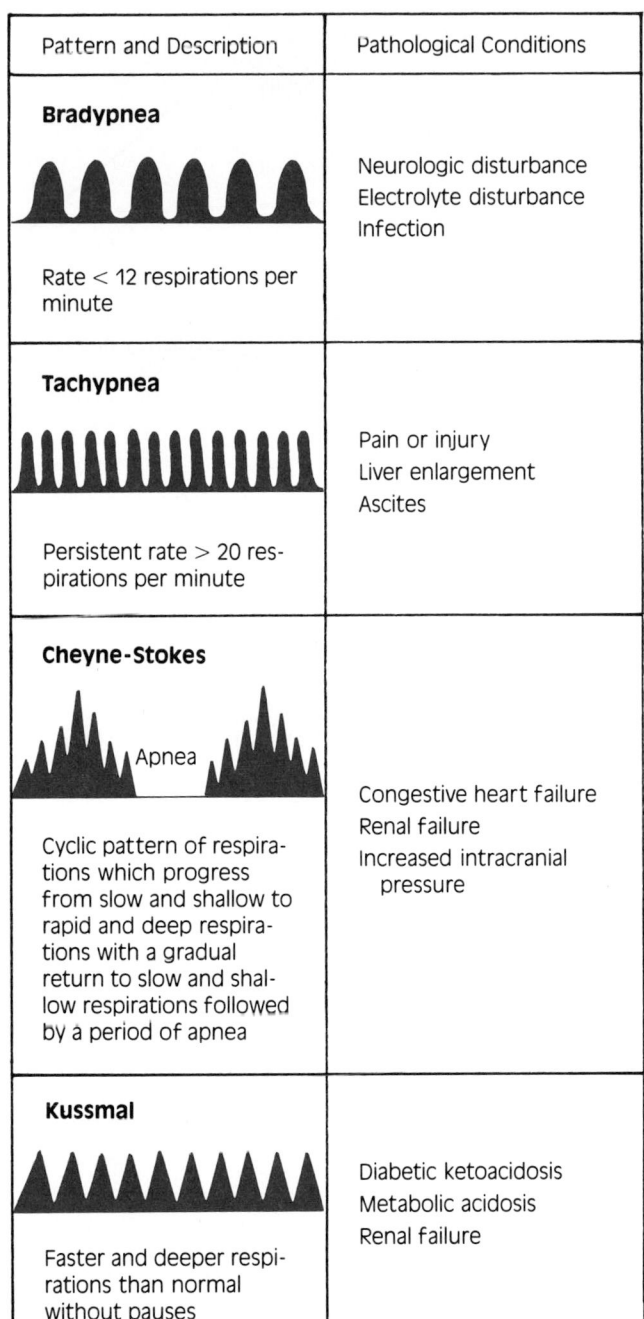

Pattern and Description	Pathological Conditions
Bradypnea Rate < 12 respirations per minute	Neurologic disturbance Electrolyte disturbance Infection
Tachypnea Persistent rate > 20 respirations per minute	Pain or injury Liver enlargement Ascites
Cheyne-Stokes Apnea Cyclic pattern of respirations which progress from slow and shallow to rapid and deep respirations with a gradual return to slow and shallow respirations followed by a period of apnea	Congestive heart failure Renal failure Increased intracranial pressure
Kussmal Faster and deeper respirations than normal without pauses	Diabetic ketoacidosis Metabolic acidosis Renal failure

FIGURE 24-37
Abnormal breathing patterns.

Auscultation. Auscultation is used to detect air flow within the respiratory tract. A stethoscope is used to listen to the sounds of inspiration and expiration over the chest wall in a pattern similar to that used with percussion. Normally, breath sounds result from the free movement of air into and out of all parts of the bronchial tree. The nurse listens for the duration, pitch, and intensity of the sounds; normally these vary over different parts of the lung. The client should be placed in a sitting position and asked to breathe slowly and deeply through the mouth. The warmed diaphragm of the stethoscope is placed over the thoracic landmarks, and breath sounds are auscultated in the same sequential pattern as used for palpation and percussion (Fig. 24-38).

Normally, *bronchial* sounds are heard over the trachea and are high in pitch and intensity, with expiration being longer than inspiration. **Bronchovesicular** sounds are heard over the mainstem bronchus, and are moderate in pitch and intensity, with inspiration equal to expiration. **Vesicular breathing** sounds are soft, low-pitched sounds, heard over the normal lung tissue throughout the lung fields; inspiration is longer than expiration.

Adventitious breath sounds are breath sounds not normally heard in the lungs. One type is called **rales**, which are abnormal breath sounds that originate in small bronchioles, alveolar ducts, or the alveoli. Rales are discrete and noncontinuous sounds produced by moisture in the tracheobronchial tree. The sound is similar to the fizzing sound of a newly opened carbonated beverage or of puffed-rice cereal when milk is added. Rales are best heard on inspiration and are described as fine or coarse. **Rhonchi** are also abnormal breath sounds, characterized by coarse, gurgling sounds in the bronchial tubes and are best heard on expiration. A *wheeze* is a squeaky sound heard best on expiration. Rhonchi are low-pitched sounds, whereas wheezes are higher-pitched sounds; both result from air flow across passages that are narrowed by fluid, tumors, or swelling. A **pleural friction rub** is a grating sound, caused by an inflamed pleura rubbing against the chest wall (see Fig. 24-39). If a productive cough occurs during the examination, the sputum should be assessed for color, consistency, and amount.

Cardiovascular and Peripheral Vascular Systems

The heart is a hollow, muscular, contractile organ that lies in the thoracic cavity behind the sternum to the left of the midline, and is enclosed in a sac known as the *pericardium*. The heart has four chambers: the right and left atria that serve as receiving chambers, and the right and left ventricles that serve as pumping chambers. The four chambers of the heart are connected by two sets of valves, the atrioventricular and semilunar valves. The atrioventricular valves, located between the atria and the ventricles, are the tricuspid and mitral valves. The tricuspid valve leads from the right atrium to the right ventricle; the mitral valve is located between the left atrium and the left ventricle. These valves respond to pressure changes as they open to allow blood flow to enter into their chamber, and are forced to snap closed to prevent any backflow of blood. The aortic and pulmonic valves, which allow blood flow from the ventricles to the lungs and body, are known as *semilunar valves* because of their half-moon shape. The closure of the four valves is responsible for normal heart sounds (Fig. 24-40).

Bronchial or Tubular

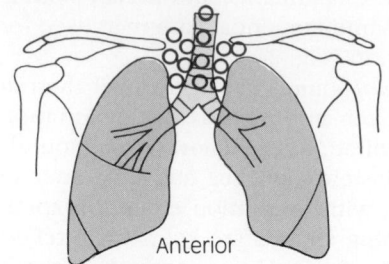

Anterior

Blowing, hollow sounds auscultated over the trachea

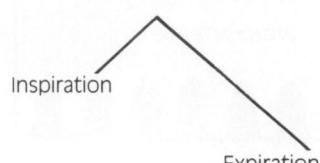

Ratio of inspiration to expiration

Inspiration

Expiration

Inspiration is shorter than expiration
Expiration is longer, lower, and
higher-pitched than inspiration

Bronchovesicular

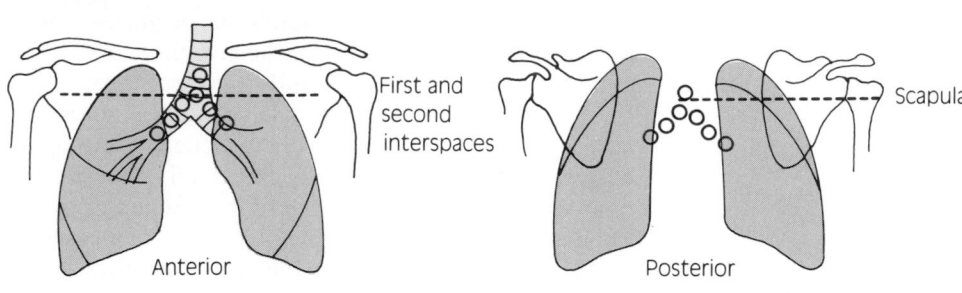

First and
second
interspaces

Anterior

Scapula

Posterior

Medium-pitched, medium intesity, blowing sounds auscultated over the
first and second interspaces anteriorly and the scapula posteriorly

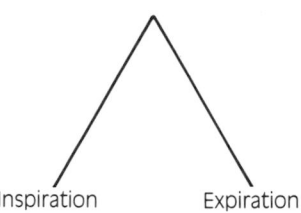

Inspiration   Expiration

Inspiration and expiration have
similar pitch

Vesicular

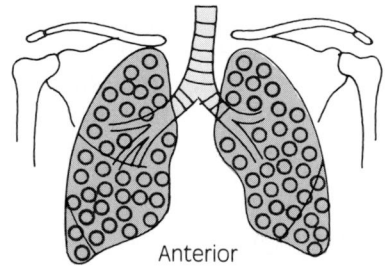

Anterior

Posterior

Soft, low-pitched sounds auscultated over the lung periphery

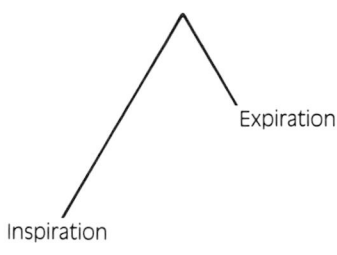

Expiration

Inspiration

Inspiration is longer, louder, and
higher-pitched than expiration

F I G U R E   24-38
Normal breath sounds.

Heart

This examination includes assessment of the **precordium** and heart. Risk factors for consideration during this assessment include nutritional status, cholesterol levels, triglyceride levels, hypertension, congenital disorders, stress, use of tobacco, alcohol consumption, and use of medications.

The techniques used for assessment of the heart include inspection, palpation, and auscultation. (Inspection and palpation, although discussed separately here, are usually combined.) Equipment used in this examination are a stethoscope with a bell and diaphragm and a sphygmomanometer. The client is in a sitting or supine position with the head raised approximately 30 degrees. Adequate lighting is essential for inspection of color and

pulsations. A quiet environment is necessary for accurate auscultation of heart sounds. The nurse is usually positioned at the right side of the client.

Inspection. The neck and precordium are observed for visible pulsations. Generally, there are no visible pulsations, except the apical impulse (or the point of maximal impulse [PMI]), located approximately at the fourth or fifth intercostal space at the left midclavicular line. Inspect the epigastric area at the tip of the sternum for pulsation of the abdominal aorta. Findings of neck vein distention or visible pulsations in precordial areas other than the PMI are considered abnormal.

Palpation. The precordium (aortic, pulmonic, tricuspid, and apical areas, as illustrated in Fig. 24-40) is pal-

Breath Sounds	Characteristics
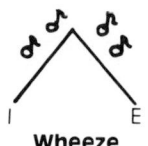 **Wheeze**	Musical or squeaking High-pitched and continuous sounds Auscultated during inspiration or expiration Occurs in small air passages
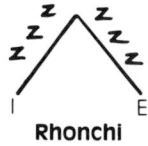 **Rhonchi**	Sonorous or coarse Low-pitched and continuous sounds Auscultated during inspiration or expiration Occurs in large air passages (Coughing may clear the sound)
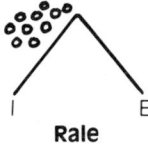 **Rale**	Bubbling, crackling, popping Low to high-pitched; discontinuous sounds Auscultated during inspiration Occurs in small air passages and alveoli
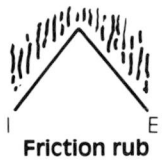 **Friction rub**	Rubbing or grating Loudest over lower lateral anterior surface Auscultated during inspiration and expiration

FIGURE 24-39
Abnormal breath sounds.

pated for the presence of pulsations. The nurse's hands, which should be warm, are used to gently palpate with the four fingers held together. Palpation proceeds in a systematic manner, with assessment of specific cardiac landmarks: the aortic (Fig. 24-41A), the pulmonic (Fig. 24-41B), and the tricuspid and mitral areas (Fig. 24-41C).

Each area is palpated to determine if a pulsation is felt. Identify the PMI and record the apical impulse by interspace and relationship to the midsternal line or midclavicular line. Identify any precordial **thrills**, which are fine, palpable, rushing vibrations over the right or left second intercostal space; and **lifts** or **heaves**, which are risings along the border of the sternum with each heartbeat.

Normal findings include no pulsation palpable over the aortic and pulmonic areas, with a palpable pulsation at the PMI. Abnormal findings include visible pulsations, palpable thrill at the aortic, pulmonic, tricuspid, or mitral area, and lifts or heaves.

Auscultation. Auscultation is used to determine the heart sounds caused by closure of the heart valves. A systematic approach is used as the nurse attentively listens at all cardiac landmarks (Fig. 24-42). Auscultation is done systematically, beginning at the aortic area, then moving to the pulmonic, then to the tricuspid, and last to the apical. The client should breathe normally. The stethoscope diaphragm is first used to listen to high-

pitched sounds, followed by use of the stethoscope bell to listen to low-pitched sounds. The nurse focuses on the overall rate and rhythm of the heart and the normal heart sounds (S_1 and S_2).

During auscultation, the first heart sound heard is the "lub" of "lub-dub." This sound occurs when the mitral and tricuspid valves close and corresponds with the onset of ventricular contraction (Fig. 24-43). The sound, low-pitched and dull, is called S_1, and is heard best at the apical area. The second heart sound, S_2, occurs at the termination of systole and corresponds with the onset of ventricular diastole. It is the "dub" or "lub-dub," and represents the closure of the aortic and pulmonic valves. The sound of S_2 is higher pitched and shorter than S_1. The two sounds occur within 1 second or less, depending on the heart rate.

Normal findings include S_1 to be louder at the tricuspid and apical areas, with S_2 louder at the aortic and pulmonic areas. Abnormal findings include extra heart sounds at any of the cardiac landmarks, and abnormal rate or rhythm.

Extra heart sounds may be S_3, S_4, murmurs, or bruits. S_3, known as the *third heart sound,* often is represented by a "lub-dub-dee" pattern ("dee" being S_3); this sound is best heard with the stethoscope bell at the mitral area, with the client lying on the left side. S_3 is considered normal in children and young adults and abnormal in middle-aged and elderly adults. S_4 is the fourth heart sound, represented by "dee-lub-dub." S_4 is considered normal in elderly clients but abnormal in children and adults. Heart *murmurs* are extra heart sounds caused by some disruption of the flow of blood through the heart. The characteristics of a murmur depend on the adequacy of valve function, rate of blood flow, and the size of the valve opening. Table 24-6 illustrates the grading of heart murmurs. **Bruits** are sounds similar to murmurs and are heard over major blood vessels. The sound is indicative of a partially blocked or overextended artery, causing blood to swirl rather than flow straight. Bruits are most

TABLE 24-6
A Common Grading System for Heart Murmurs

Grade	Description
I	A murmur so faint that it can only be heard with great effort
II	A faint murmur but one that can be easily detected
III	A moderately loud murmur
IV	A very loud murmur that is usually associated with a thrill sound
V	An extremely loud murmur
VI	An exceptionally loud murmur that can be heard while the stethoscope is lifted off the skin

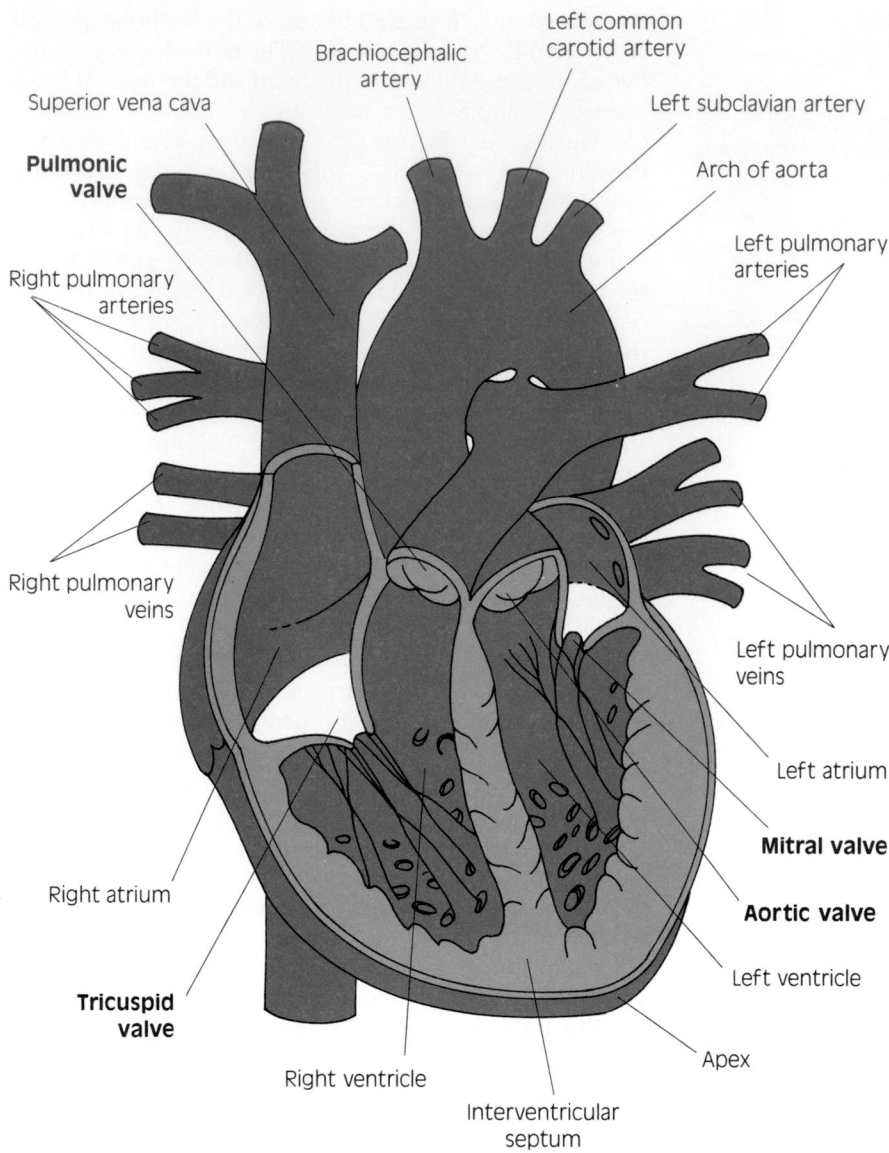

Superior vena cava

Brachiocephalic artery

Left common carotid artery

Left subclavian artery

Arch of aorta

Pulmonic valve

Right pulmonary arteries

Left pulmonary arteries

Right pulmonary veins

Left pulmonary veins

Left atrium

Right atrium

Mitral valve

Aortic valve

Left ventricle

Tricuspid valve

Apex

Right ventricle

Interventricular septum

F I G U R E   24-40
View of the interior of the heart showing the atrioventricular and semilunar valves responsible for normal heart sounds.

commonly heard over the carotid arteries, over the abdominal aorta, and over the femoral arteries.

Peripheral Vascular System

The peripheral vascular assessment includes measuring the blood pressure, assessing peripheral vascular pulses, and assessing peripheral vascular perfusion. Assessments are done by inspection and palpation, with the client in the sitting or supine position. Peripheral vascular assessments may be combined with assessment of other body areas.

Inspection.   The skin of the extremities is inspected for color and temperature (as described previously for assessment of the integument), venous patterns, and

edema. There should be no venous patterns evident (*e.g.,* varicosities, rashes, or ulcers) on the lower extremities. There should also be no edema present.

Palpation.   To palpate peripheral pulses, use the pads of the index and middle fingers and palpate the pulse for rate, rhythm, amplitude, and symmetry. Palpate the *carotid* pulses (one at a time and with caution); the *brachial* pulses, located at the groove between the biceps and triceps muscles; the *radial* pulses, located in the wrist above the thumb in the radial groove; the *femoral* pulses, located in the inguinal area; the *popliteal* pulses, located behind the knee; the *dorsalis pedis* pulse, located on the dorsum of the foot; and the *posterior tibial* pulses, located behind the ankle. Figure 24-44 illustrates the palpation of each of these peripheral pulses.

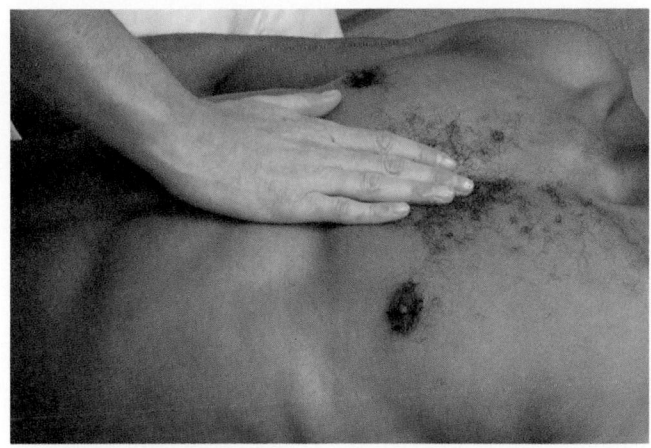

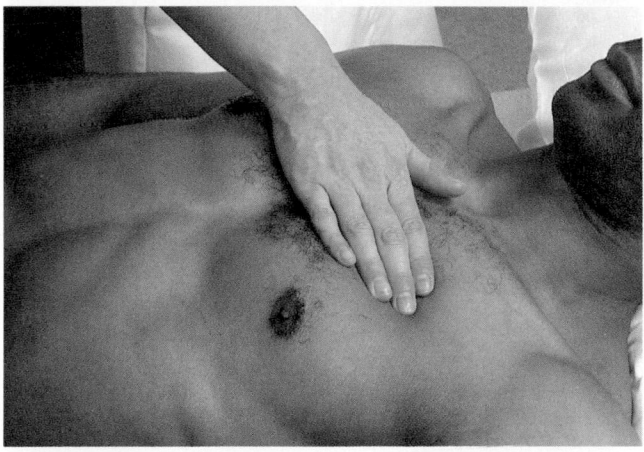

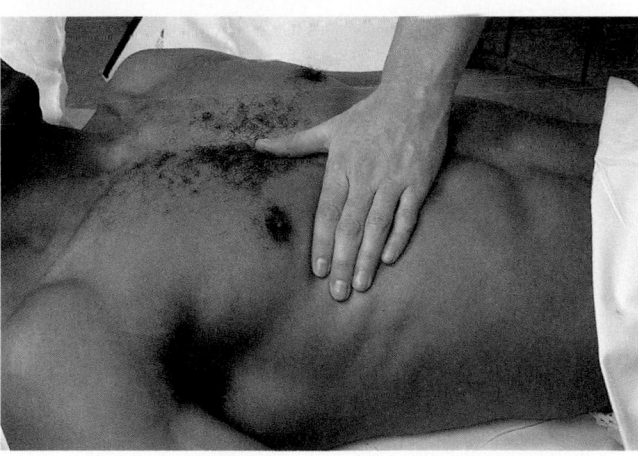

FIGURE 24-41

Palpation of areas of the precordium: (A) aortic area, (B) pulmonic area, and (C) apical and tricuspic area. (Photo © Ken Kasper)

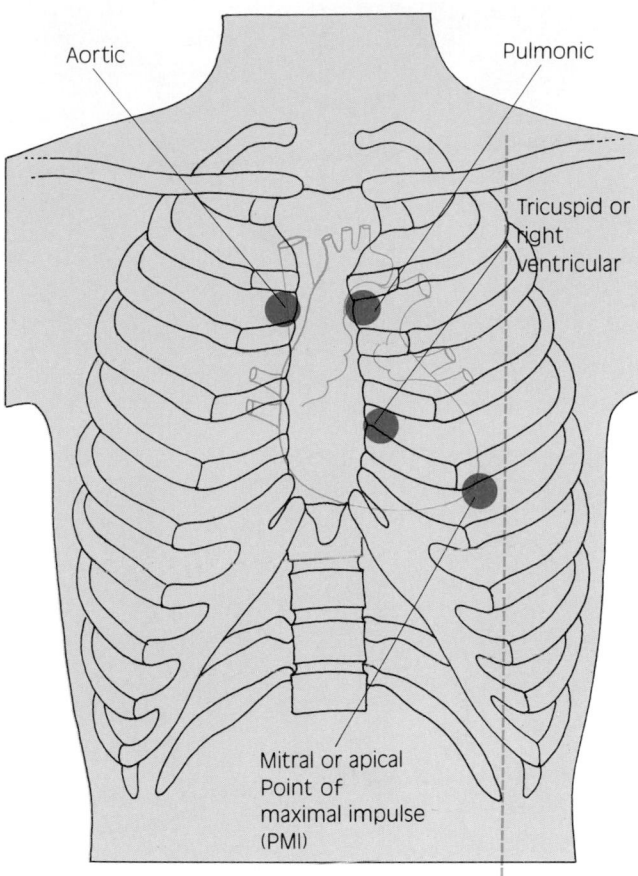

FIGURE 24-42

Cardiac landmarks and sequence of examination using auscultation.

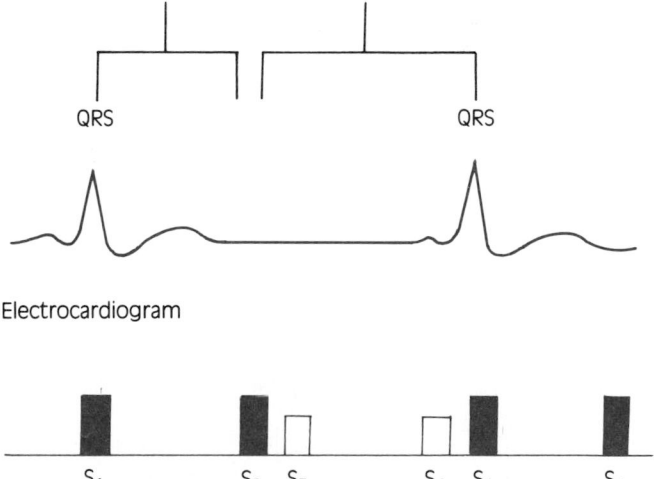

FIGURE 24-43

Heart sounds in relation to the cardiac cycle and an electrocardiogram.

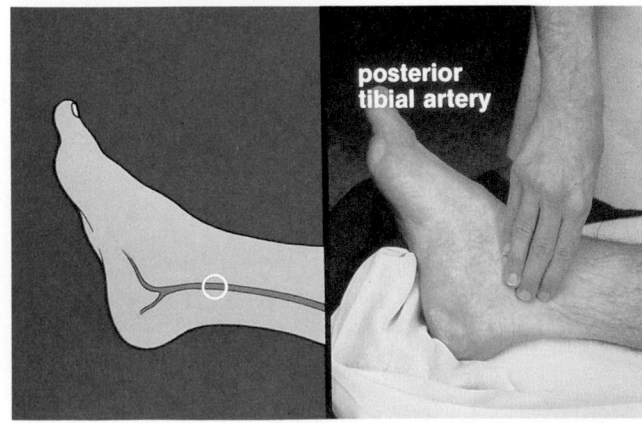

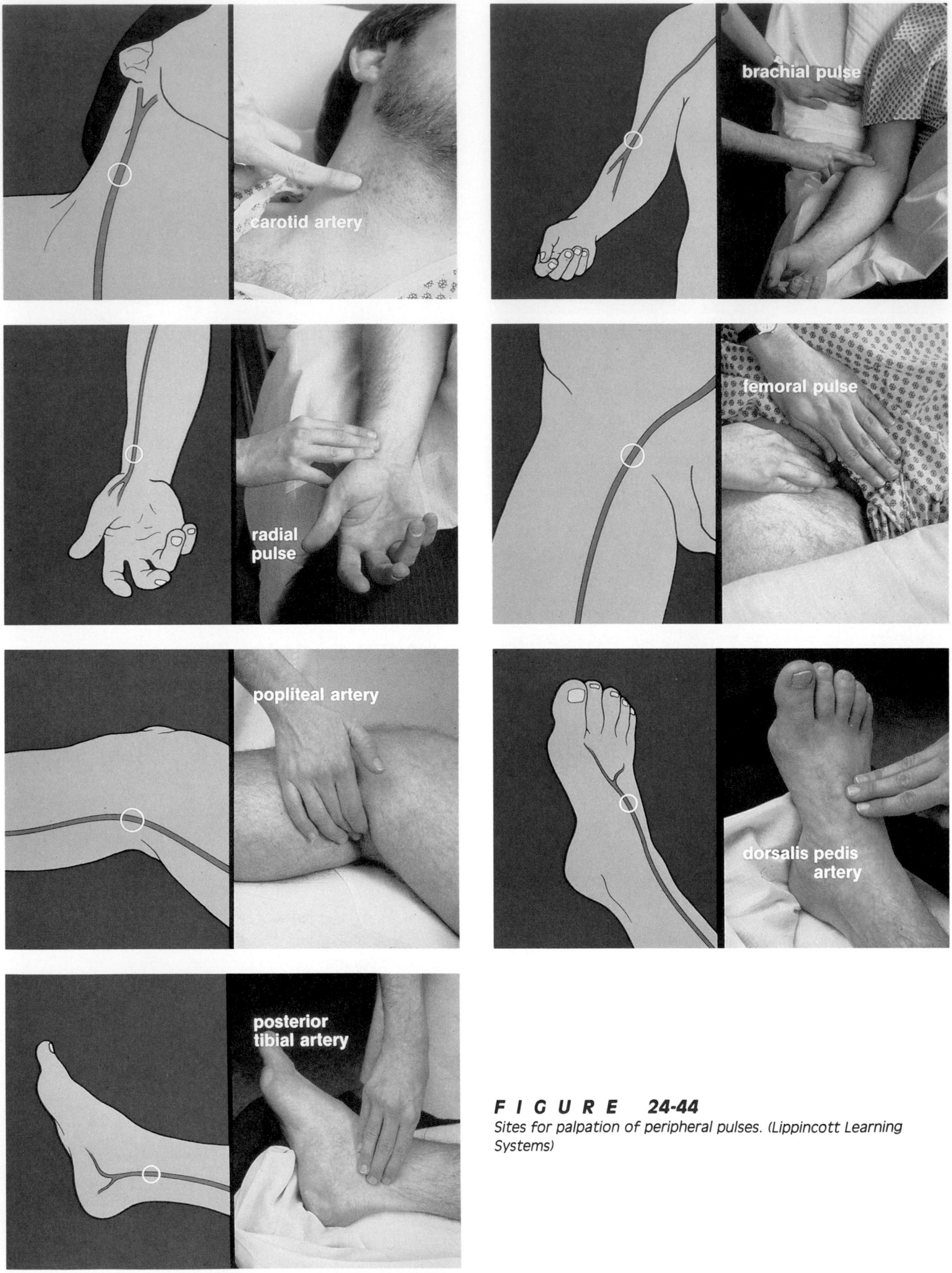

F I G U R E   24-44
*Sites for palpation of peripheral pulses. (Lippincott Learning
Systems)*

The pulse rate should range between 60 and 90 beats per minute, with a regular rhythm and strong and equal pulses bilaterally. It is not necessary to determine rate on all peripheral pulses (*e.g.,* a strong palpable dorsalis pedis pulse is significant of good peripheral circulation). Abnormal findings include an increased or decreased rate, irregular rate, regularity with pauses or skipped beats, weak or thready pulse, forceful or **bounding pulse**, and asymmetry of pulses. Related abnormal assessments include cold, pale, cyanotic skin; edema; and varicosities.

The blood pressure may be taken at this time or during the initial stage of the assessment.

Breasts and Axillae

The breasts are located on the anterior chest wall and extend from the second or third rib to the sixth or seventh rib. The breast is composed of glandular, fibrous, and subcutaneous fatty tissue. The areola, a brown pigmented area, is located centrally on the breast and surrounds the nipple. Each breast is composed of a lymphatic network that drains into the underlying axilla (Fig. 24-45). Although assessments and disorders focus on the female breast, both male and female clients should have breast examinations. Men as well as women may have diseases of the breast.

Risk factors for consideration when assessing the breasts include age, changes in breast tissue, pain, discharge from the nipple, and knowledge and practice of breast self-examination (the latter is discussed in Chap 38). Inspection and palpation are the techniques used in the assessment. The client may be in a sitting or lying position. If sitting, the client should sit erect, arms at sides or abducted overhead. If supine, the client's hands are under the head.

Inspection.   The breasts and axilla are inspected for size, shape, symmetry, color, texture, and skin lesions. The breasts should be relatively symmetrical, although variations are normal. The size varies among individuals. The shape of the breasts is round and smooth, and there should be no skin depressions (*retraction*) or puckering (*dimpling*). The color should be consistent with the rest of the skin, and the texture of the skin should be soft.

The areola and nipples are inspected for size and shape; the nipples are inspected for discharge, crusting, and inversion. The areolar and nipple areas should be equal in size, round or oval, with a smooth surface. Montgomery tubercles are a normal component of the areola. The nipples are normally everted. The skin is intact and without discharge.

Palpation.   The primary purpose of palpation is to detect any abnormal masses or lumps. The breast is divided into four quadrants: the outer upper and lower quadrants, and the inner upper and lower quadrants (Fig. 24-46). Using the pads of the first three fingers, each quadrant of each breast is palpated using a systematic,

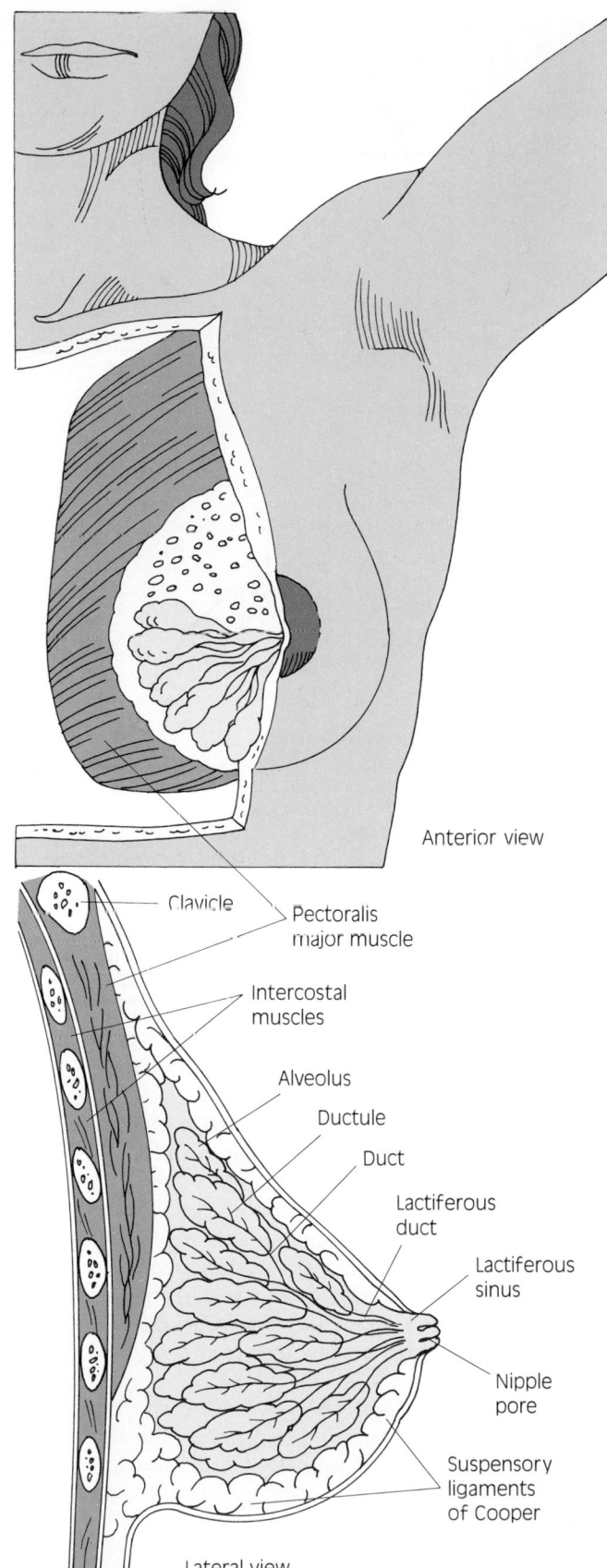

Anterior view

Clavicle
Pectoralis major muscle
Intercostal muscles
Alveolus
Ductule
Duct
Lactiferous duct
Lactiferous sinus
Nipple pore
Suspensory ligaments of Cooper

Lateral view

FIGURE 24-45
Anterior and lateral views of the female breast.

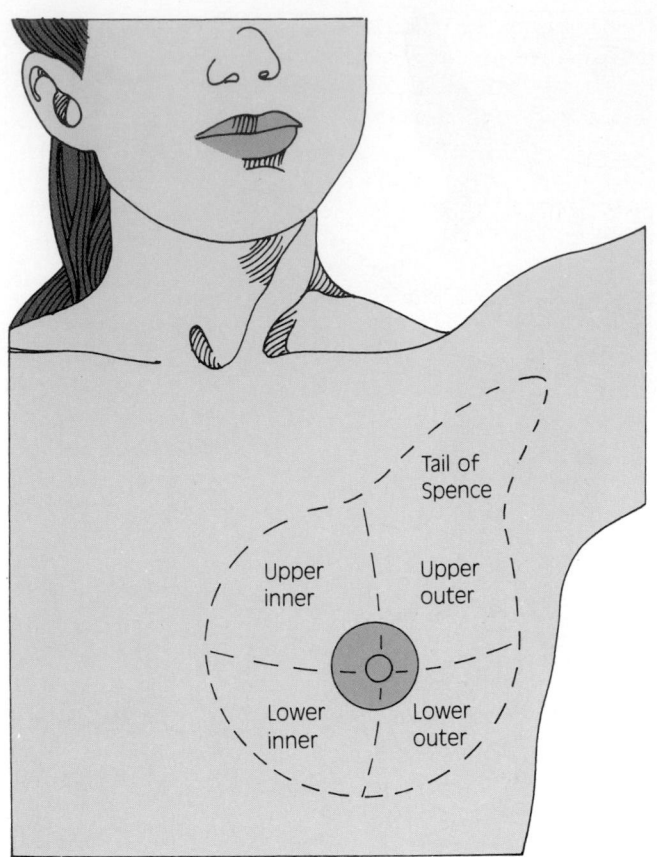

ucts. The liver, located in the right upper quadrant, is responsible for carbohydrate, fat, and protein metabolism. The gallbladder, located on the inferior surface of the liver, concentrates and stores bile. The pancreas lies behind the stomach and functions as an exocrine gland to produce hormones and digestive juices. The spleen is in the left upper quadrant above the kidney and functions as part of the reticuloendothelial system. The kidneys are responsible for filtration, reabsorption, and secretion of water and electrolytes and for eliminating wastes. The urinary bladder, located behind the symphysis pubis, collects and eliminates urine.

Factors to consider during assessment of the abdomen include nutrition, use of alcohol, stress, urine and stool characteristics, bowel habits, infectious diseases, trauma, and medications. A warm stethoscope, adequate lighting, and warm hands with short fingernails are needed for abdominal assessment. The client is placed in the supine position with the head slightly elevated and arms at sides. Small pillows may be placed under the head and knees. The client should have an empty bladder and be warm. These measures, as well as the position, help prevent contraction of the abdominal muscles.

To better locate organs and to make documentation more specific, the abdomen can be divided into four

F I G U R E　24-46
Location of assessment findings of the breast are identified by quadrant.

clockwise direction as the breast tissue is gently compressed against the chest wall (Fig. 24-47). The breast tissue should be smooth and firm with a granular consistency. If a mass is detected, the location, size, shape, consistency, and tenderness should be carefully assessed.

The nipple and aerola are palpated, and the nipple is gently compressed between the thumb and forefinger to assess for discharge.

The axillary areas are palpated for lymph nodes, which normally are not palpable and are nontender. If any nodes are palpable, assess location, size, shape, consistency, tenderness, and mobility. The lymph nodes (Fig. 24-48) are the supraclavicular, subclavian, intermediate, brachial, scapular, mammary, and internal mammary.

Abnormal findings when assessing the breast include presence of a lump, dimpling, nipple discharge, lesions, asymmetry, and palpable lymph nodes.

Abdomen

The abdominal cavity (Fig. 24-49) contains several vital organs. The stomach, the small intestine, and the large intestine ingest and digest food; absorb essential nutrients, electrolytes, and water; and excrete waste prod-

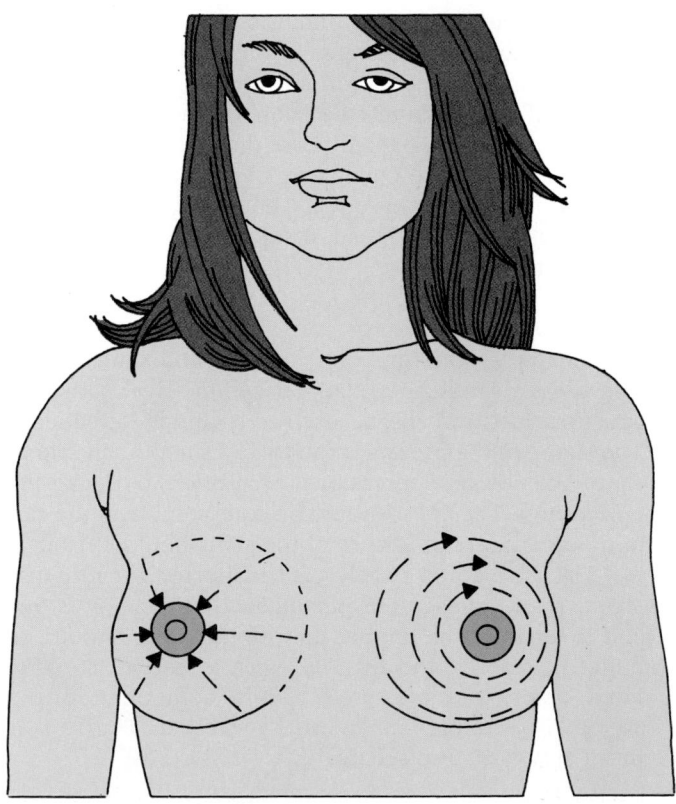

F I G U R E　24-47
Two techniques for palpation of the breast. (Left) Working in a clockwise direction, the examiner palpates the breast from the periphery toward the aureola at "hour" positions. (Right) The breast is palpated from the outer periphery in smaller and smaller circles moving toward the aureola.

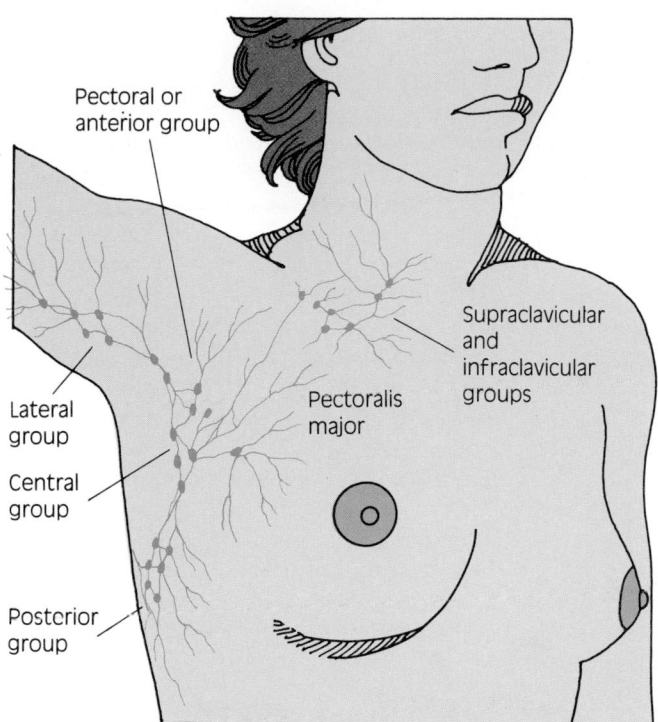

FIGURE 24-48
Location of the cervical, axillary, and mammary lymph nodes.

quadrants: right upper, right lower, left upper, and left lower (Fig. 24-50). Some examiners prefer to further divide the abdomen into nine sections: the right and left hypochondriac, lumbar, and inguinal; and the epigastric, umbilical, and hypogastric.

The sequence of techniques used to assess the abdomen is inspection, auscultation, percussion, and palpation. Percussion and palpation stimulate bowel sounds and so are done after auscultation of the abdomen.

Inspection. The nurse inspects the abdomen while sitting at the right side of the client, allowing a tangential view that enhances shadows and contours. Inspection is made of skin color and surface characteristics, including the umbilicus, contour, symmetry, **peristalsis**, pulsations, and masses. The skin color may be slightly lighter than exposed areas. Fine white or silver lines (**striae**) may be present and are caused by stretching from weight gain or pregnancy. The umbilicus should be centrally located and normally may be flat, rounded, or concave. The abdomen should be evenly rounded or symmetrical, without visible peristalsis. In thin persons, an upper midline pulsation may normally be visible.

Auscultation. Auscultation is used to assess bowel sounds and vascular sounds. Auscultation is performed in a systematic manner, using the four quadrants as a guide. The stethoscope is warmed, and the flat diaphragm is placed lightly on the abdomen in one of the selected quadrants. Listen carefully for bowel sounds, and note their frequency and character; they are heard as

clicks and gurgles and usually occur every 5 to 20 seconds. Move the stethoscope in a clockwise manner, assessing all four quadrants systematically. Using the bell of the stethoscope, auscultate over the aorta, renal arteries, and iliac arteries for bruits. Normal findings include increased, decreased, or absent bowel sounds (established after auscultating each quadrant for 5 minutes) and bruits.

Percussion. All four quadrants are percussed in a systematic, clockwise manner to identify fluid, masses, or air. The nurse should note the distribution of sounds. Normal sounds are tympany over the abdomen, dullness over the liver, and dullness over a full bladder. The predominate percussion note in abdominal assessment is tympany. Abnormal findings include decreased tympany and increased dullness (possibly caused by fluid or a mass).

Palpation. The pads of the fingers are used to palpate with a light, gentle, dipping motion. Watch the client's face for nonverbal signs of pain during palpation. Palpate each quadrant in a systematic manner, noting muscular resistance, tenderness, enlargement of the organs, or masses. The abdomen should normally be soft, relaxed, and free of tenderness. Abnormal findings include involuntary rigidity, spasm, and pain.

Male and Female Genitalia

This section discusses inspection and palpation of the genitalia. Further discussion of male and female anatomy is found in Chapter 38. An outline of an internal pelvic examination is also included here, although individual health agency policies vary on whether this is included as part of the nursing examination. Equipment required includes a vaginal speculum, a good light source, and disposable gloves. The client should have an empty bladder.

Female Genitalia

The external female genitalia consist of the mons pubis, labia majora and minora, clitoris, vestibular glands, vaginal vestibule, vaginal orifice, and urethral opening (Fig. 24-51). Factors in assessing the female genitalia include menstrual history, sexual history, use of contraceptives, and frequency of pelvic examinations. The woman is placed in the lithotomy position on the examination table, legs in stirrups, and draped so that only the genitalia are exposed. She should be told about the procedure and helped to relax as it is carried out. The nurse wears gloves during this assessment.

Initially, the external genitalia are inspected. The pubic area is inspected for color, size, lesions, and discharge. The vulva normally has more pigmentation than other skin areas, and the mucous membranes will be dark pink and moist. The skin and mucosa should be smooth, without lesions or swelling. There may nor-

(Text continues on p. 469.)

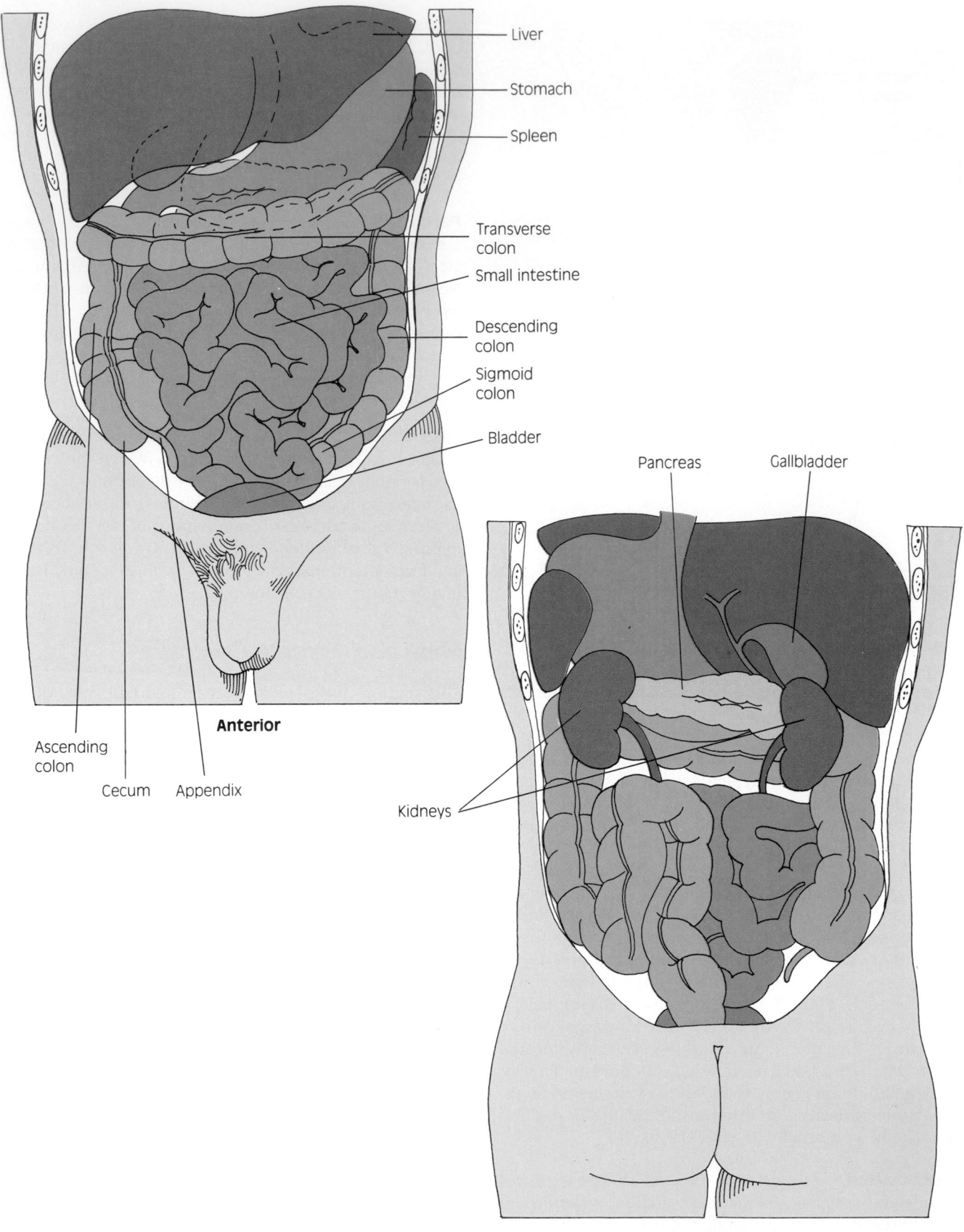

Anterior

Ascending
colon

Cecum   Appendix

Liver

Stomach

Spleen

Transverse
colon

Small intestine

Descending
colon

Sigmoid
colon

Bladder

Pancreas   Gallbladder

Kidneys

Posterior

F I G U R E   24-49
Organs of the abdominal cavity.

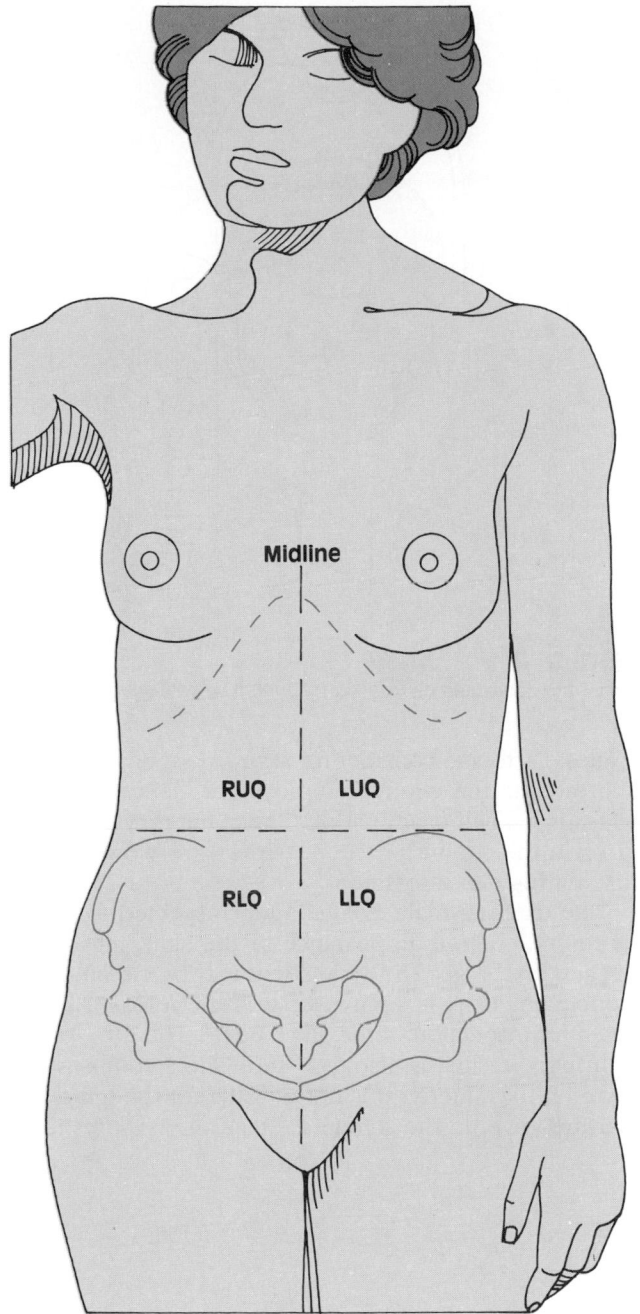

Right Upper Quadrant

Pylorous
Duodenum
Gallbladder
Liver
Right kidney and adrenal
   gland
Hepatic flexure of the
   colon
Head of the pancreas

Left Upper quadrant

Stomach
Spleen
Left kidney and adrenal
   gland
Splenic flexure of the colon
Body of pancreas

Right Lower Quadrant

Cecum
Appendix
Right ovary and fallopian
   tube (female)
Right ureter and lower
   kidney pole
Right Spermatic cord
   (male)

Left Lower Quadrant

Sigmoid colon
Left ovary and fallopian
   tube (female)
Left ureter and lower
   kidney pole
Left spermatic cord (male)

Midline

Urinary bladder
Uretus (female)

F I G U R E   24-50
Diagram of abdominal quadrants and outline of underlying organs.

mally be a small amount of clear or whitish vaginal discharge.

A speculum is used to inspect the cervix and vagina (Fig. 24-52). An outline of the procedure is as follows:
- Explain the procedure to the client.
- Warm the speculum under warm, running water; if cytolic specimens are to be taken, the water will serve as the lubricant; if no specimens are needed, a water-soluble lubricant may be used.
- Using two fingers placed just inside the vagina, press down gently on the posterior vaginal wall.

- Insert the speculum blades into the vagina, posterior in direction at a 45-degree angle. Be sure no pubic hair is caught in the speculum.
- Turn the speculum so that the handle is down and the blades are in a horizontal position.
- Open the blades and close the screw that locks the blades open.
- Inspect the cervix and os for size, color, shape, lesions, and discharge.
- Withdraw the blades slowly, observing the vaginal walls.

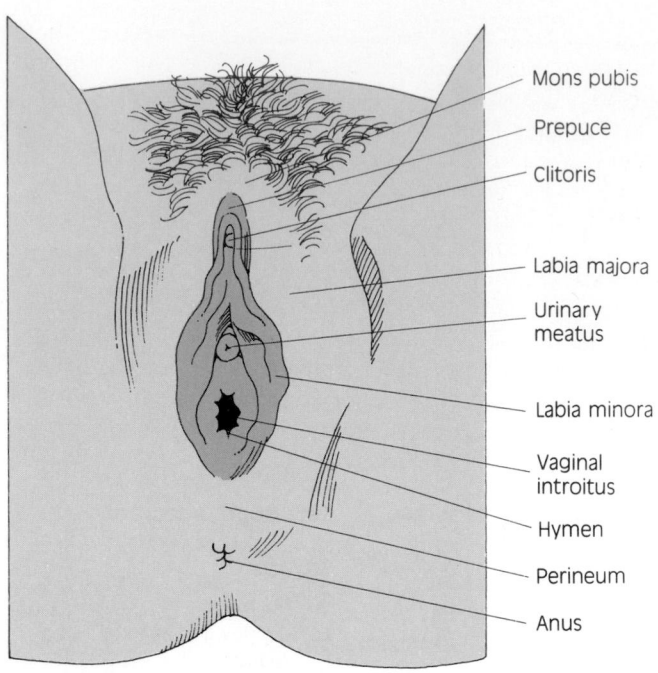

F I G U R E   24-51
External female genitalia.

- When the speculum blades are clear of the cervix, release the screw so that the blades close, and withdraw the speculum from the vagina.

Abnormal findings include redness, swelling of glands, discharge, lesions, and pain. For related assessments, such as the urinary tract and sexually transmitted diseases, see Chapters 33 and 38, respectively.

Male Genitalia

The male genitalia (Fig. 24-53) include the penis, testicles, epididymis, scrotum, prostate gland, and seminal

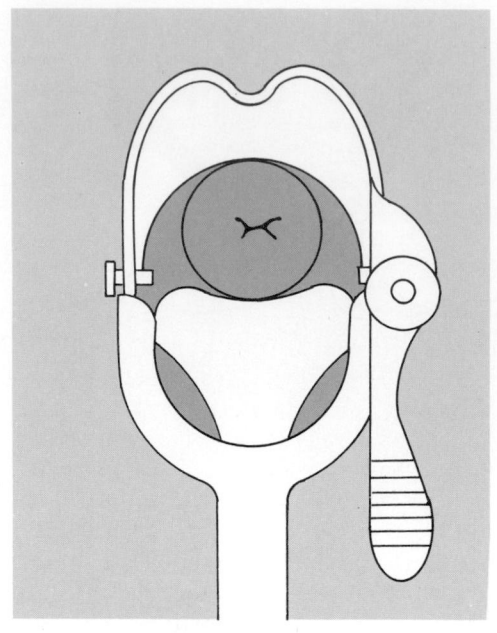

F I G U R E   24-52
View of the cervix and cervical os through a vaginal speculum.

vesicles. Factors to consider for assessment of male genitalia include the client's employment, sexual history, and testicular self-examination. The client may be standing or in the supine position. Gloves are worn by the nurse during this assessment.

The external male genitalia are inspected for size, placement, contour, appearance of the skin, inflammation, and discharge. The male client may be circumcised or uncircumcised; if uncircumcised, the foreskin is retracted for inspection of the glans penis. The location of the urinary meatus is also assessed. The scrotum is inspected for symmetry; it is not unusual for the left testicle to lie lower in the scrotal sac than the right testicle.

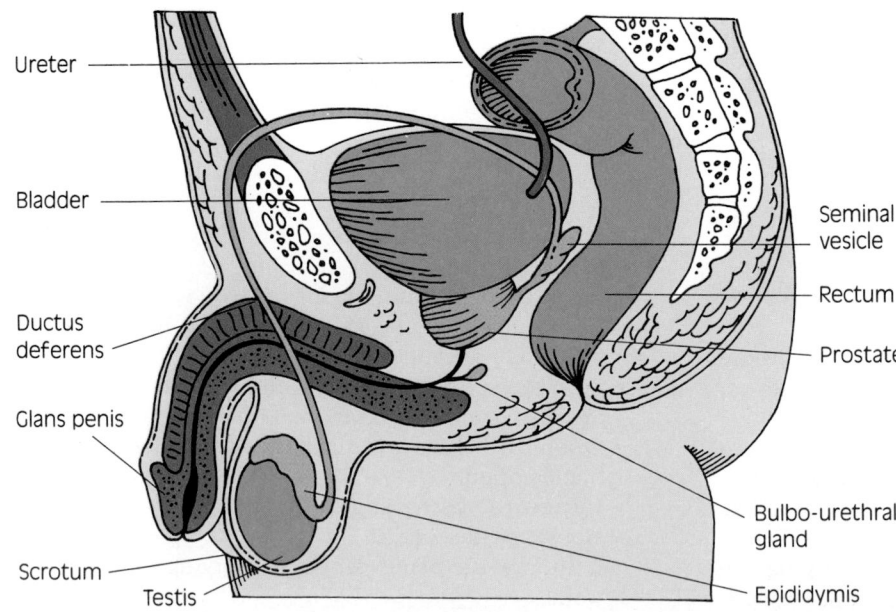

F I G U R E   24-53
Organs of the male urogenital system.

The size, shape, and consistency of the scrotal contents should be similar. Abnormal findings are the presence of lesions, pain, discharge, fluid-filled masses in the scrotum, and displacement of the urinary meatus or difficulties with voiding. (See Chaps 33 and 38 for further discussion of the male urinary tract and sexually transmitted diseases.)

Rectum and Anus

The rectum and anus form the last portion of the gastrointestinal tract. The anal canal is approximately 2 cm to 4 cm in length and opens onto the perineum. Techniques used for examination of the rectum and anus are inspection and palpation. Necessary equipment includes lubricant and good lighting. The nurse wears gloves during this assessment. The client may be in the Sims, knee-chest, or lithotomy position, or may be standing while leaning over the examination table.

Inspection is used to assess the anal area. The area normally has increased pigmentation and some hair growth. Palpation is used to assess the rectum, using a well-lubricated, gloved index finger. Sphincter tone at the anus should be good, and the mucosal lining smooth. (Fecal specimens may be taken at this time if necessary.) The prostate gland in men can be assessed for size, shape, and consistency through the anterior rectal wall; the gland is normally smooth, firm, and approximately 1¾ inches (4 cm) in size. In women, the cervix may be felt as a small, round mass when palpating the anterior rectal wall.

Abnormal findings include relaxed musculature; cracks, nodules, or hemorrhoids at the anal sphincter; bleeding; discharge; and hard or abnormally colored stools.

Musculoskeletal System

The primary structures of the musculoskeletal system are the bones, muscles, cartilage, ligaments, tendons, and joints. The musculoskeletal system provides movement, protection, and support. Assessments are made of muscles, bones, and joints. During the assessment, the client assumes a variety of positions, including standing, sitting, and supine. Assessments of the musculoskeletal system can be integrated into the assessment of other body systems. Factors to consider during this examination include a history of arthritis, trauma, or neurologic disorders; pain; and loss of or altered function.

Muscles

The muscles are examined by inspection and palpation of muscle groups and by testing muscle tone and strength. Muscle groups are observed for bilateral symmetry and palpated for tenderness; normally they are symmetrical and nontender. Muscle *tone* (the normal condition of a muscle at rest) is evaluated by putting each joint and extremity through passive range of mo-

tion. Bilateral equal resistance should be present. Muscle strength is assessed by asking the client to move against resistance. Observe muscle contraction and determine muscle strength exerted. An individual's dominant side is normally stronger than the nondominant side. Techniques for testing muscle strength are illustrated in Figure 24-54A through J. Muscle strength should be bilaterally equal with slight increase on the dominant side.

Muscles are normally firm, with good strength and tone. Abnormal findings include *atrophy,* a decrease in size; *tremors,* involuntary movements; and *flaccidity,* weakness of muscles. Other abnormal findings are loss of strength and tone, decreased range of motion, uncoordinated movements, swelling, and pain.

Bones

Bones are palpated for normal contour and prominences, as well as for bilateral symmetry. Abnormal findings include pain, enlargement, and changes in contour.

Joints

Joints are assessed by inspection and palpation. Normally, each joint will have full range of motion, be nontender, and move smoothly. Each joint is put through full range of motion (ROM), and the degree of ROM is assessed. Joint movements include flexion, extension, hyperextension, abduction, adduction, supination, and pronation. Joints are palpated for the abnormal findings of pain, swelling, nodules, and *crepitation* (a grating sound heard on movement).

Neurologic System

The neurologic system, which is responsible for cognitive, behavioral, and involuntary processes, is the most complex of the body systems and integrates all other body systems. The central nervous system, composed of the brain and spinal cord, is responsible for receiving sensory stimuli from the environment, using adaptive processes to maintain body functions, controlling cognitive and voluntary behavioral processes, and controlling unconscious and involuntary body functions.

The neurologic assessment is conducted by observation of the client to detect normal and abnormal findings for cerebral function, cranial nerve function, cerebellar function, motor and sensory function, and reflexes.

Cerebral function is assessed by observing the client's behavior throughout the interview and assessment, and includes mental status, memory, emotional status, cognitive abilities, and behavior. Fine motor skills, coordination, and balance are evaluated to assess cerebellar function. The sensory system is assessed by having the client identify various sensory stimuli, and the reflexes are evaluated by contraction of specific muscles.

(Text continues on p. 474.)

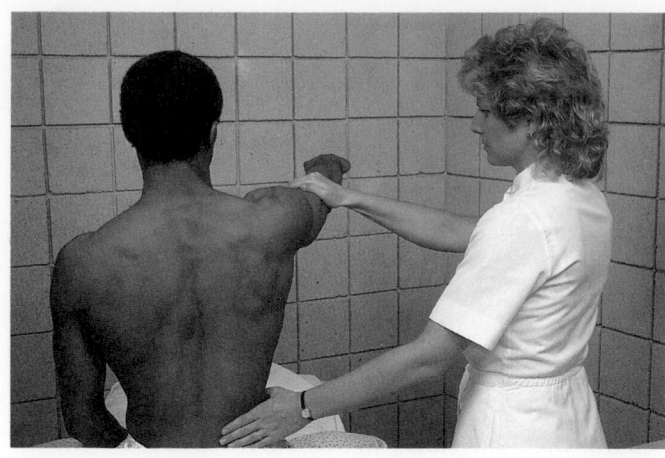

The client flexes shoulder muscle against resistance of examiner's hand.

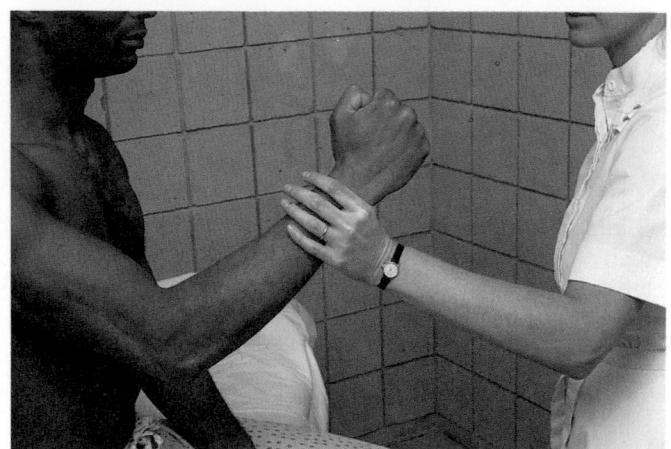
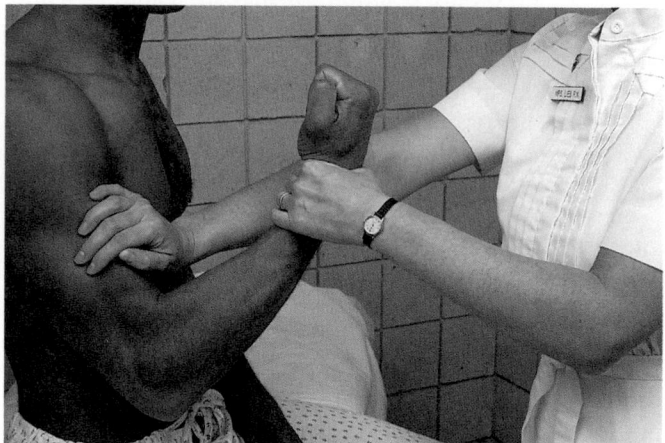

Elbow extension and flexion. The client first extends elbow against resistance by the examiner, then flexes elbow against resistance.

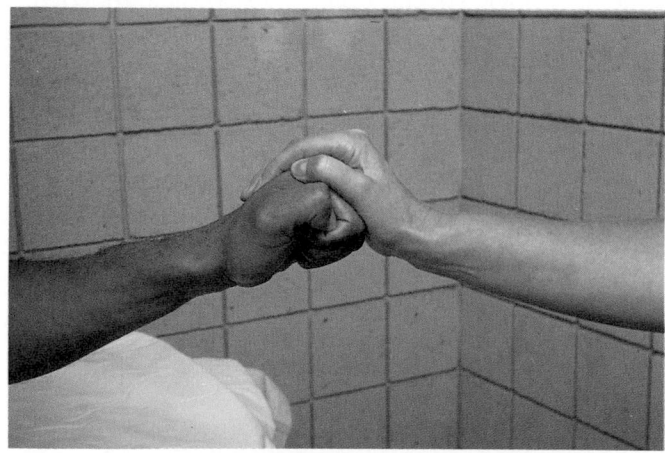
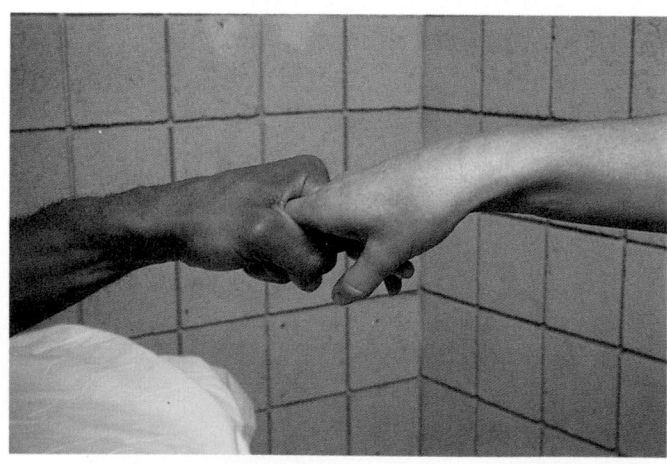

Wrist extension. The client makes a fist and resists the examiner's attempts to pull wrist down.

Testing grip. Client squeezes examiner's index and middle fingers.

F I G U R E   24-54
Techniques for testing muscle strength. (Photos © Ken Kasper)

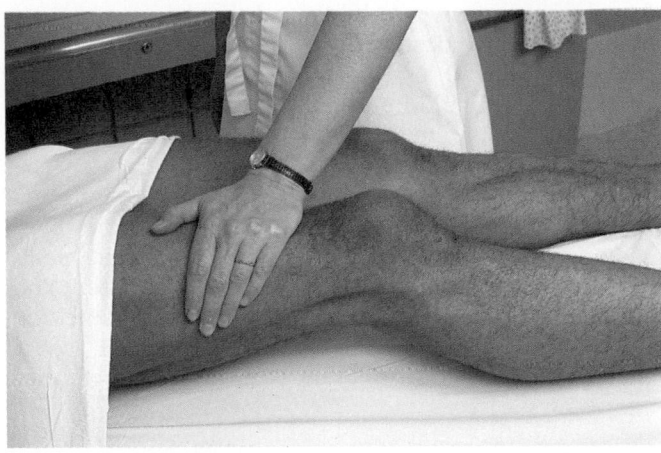

Hip flexion. Client attempts to raise his thigh against examiner's resistance.

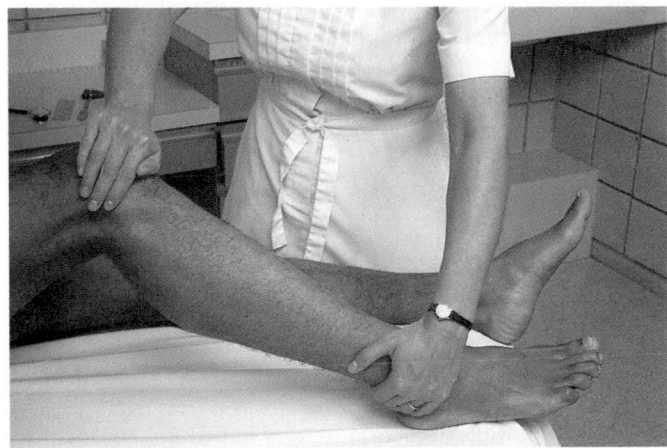

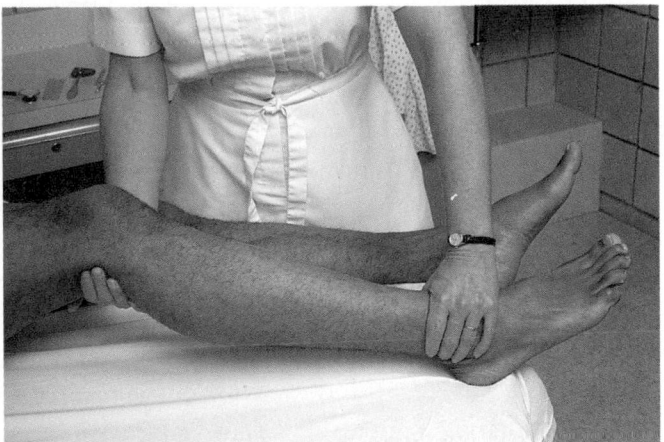

Knee flexion and extension. With the client's knee bent and foot on the examining table, the client attempts to keep foot down while examiner attempts to straighten the client's leg to test flexion. To test extension, the examiner supports client's knee, and the client attempts to straighten his leg against examiner resistance at the ankle.

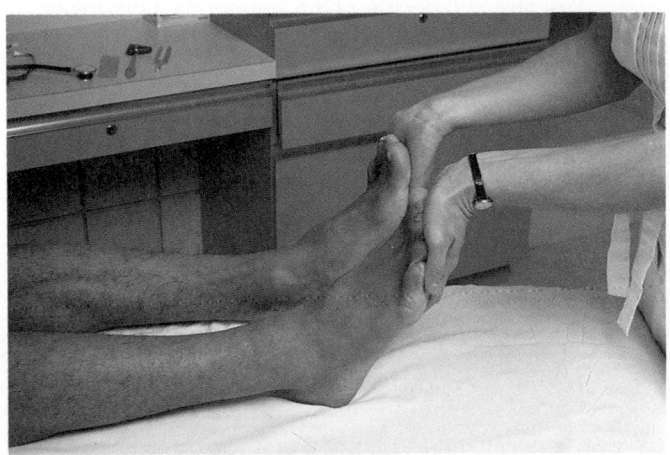

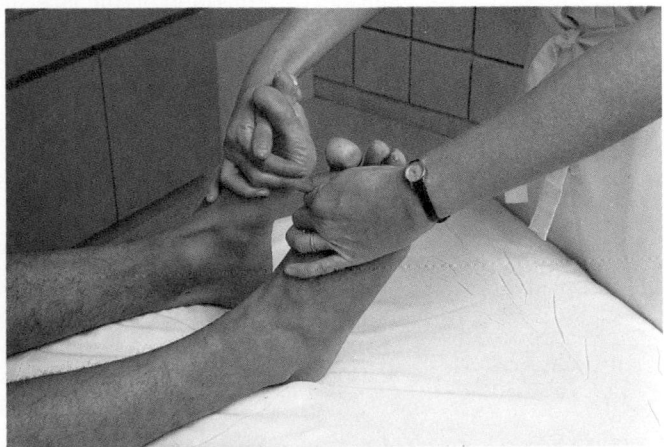

Ankle plantar flexion and dorsiflexion. The client first pushes the balls of the feet against resistance of examiner's hands, then attempts to pull against examiner's resistance.

Factors for consideration in this examination include environmental hazards (exposure to lead, insecticides, chemicals), emotional and intellectual status, use of alcohol or other chemicals, medication, and history of seizures, dizziness, weakness, or numbness.

Equipment for this examination includes vials of aromatic substances (such as peppermint and vanilla), visual acuity devices, a penlight, a sharp object, cotton balls, vials of solution to test taste (*e.g.*, salt, sugar), tuning fork, tongue depressor, reflex hammer, and familiar objects (*e.g.*, a key or coin). The client should be in a sitting position, and the environment should be quiet and nondistracting.

Examination of Mental Status

On initial contact, the nurse begins to evaluate the client's orientation level to person, place, and time, as well as cognitive abilities and affect (*e.g.*, does the client know who he is, where he is, and the day or month or year). The nurse observes the client's appearance, general behavior, and responses to questions. Any variation in responses should be noted. The nurse also assesses the client's ability to speak clearly (refer to the discussion under General Survey, earlier in this chapter). The client should have a clean, neat appearance with erect posture; be oriented to person, place, and time; have memory recall (both short-term and long-term memory); and have the ability to demonstrate coherent and logical thought processes. Abnormal findings include poor hygiene, inappropriate dress, disorientation, absent memory recall, and incoherent or illogical thought processes.

Examination of Cranial Nerve Function

The function of the twelve cranial nerves is assessed primarily during the neurologic examination, although

T A B L E   24-7
Cranial Nerves

Nerve (Number)	Type	Functions	Methods for Examining Nerve
Olfactory (I)	Sensory	Sense of smell	Test each nostril for smell reception and interpretation.
Optic (II)	Sensory	Sense of vision	Test vision for acuity and visual fields.
Oculomotor (III)	Motor	Pupil constriction Raise eyelids	Test pupillary reaction to light and ability to open and close eyelids
Trochlear (IV)	Motor	Downward inward eye movement	Test for downward and inward movement of the eye.
Trigeminal (V)	Motor	Jaw movements—chewing and mastication	Ask client to open and clench jaws while palpating the jaw muscles.
	Sensory	Sensation on the face and neck	Test face and neck for pain sensations, light touch, and temperature.
Abducens (VI)	Motor	Lateral movement of the eyes	Test ocular movement in all directions.
Facial (VII)	Motor	Muscles of the face	Ask the client to raise eyebrows, smile, show teeth, and puff out cheeks.
	Sensory	Sense of taste on the anterior two thirds of the tongue	Test for the taste sensation with various agents.
Acoustic (VIII)	Sensory	Sense of hearing	Test hearing ability.
Glossopharyngeal (IX)	Motor	Pharyngeal movement and swallowing	Ask the client to say "ah," and have client yawn to observe upward movement of the soft palate. Elicit the gag response. Note ability to swallow.
	Sensory	Sense of taste on the posterior one third of the tongue	Test for taste with various agents.
Vagus (X)	Motor	Swallowing and speaking	Ask the client to swallow and speak. Note hoarseness.
Spinal accessory (XI)	Motor	Movement of shoulder muscles	Ask the client to shrug shoulders against your resistance.
Hypoglossal (XII)	Motor	Movement of the tongue Strength of the tongue	Ask the client to protrude tongue. Ask client to push tongue against cheek.

parts of cranial nerve function are assessed with other body systems (*e.g.,* pupillary response). The cranial nerves are outlined in Table 24-7. Each nerve has a specific function and is evaluated individually.

Olfactory (I) Nerve. The olfactory nerve is a sensory nerve and its function is the sense of smell. Two or three vials of liquids with aromatic odors, such as coffee, vanilla, or peppermint, should be available. The client is asked to close the eyes and occlude one nostril (by pressing a finger against the side of the nose). The client is then asked to take a breath as the vial is placed under the open nostril, and to identify the odor; the process is then repeated for the opposite nostril. Normal findings are equal and bilateral sense of smell; abnormal findings are the inability to identify the odor or absence of smell.

Optic (II) Nerve. The optic nerve is a sensory nerve and its function is vision. Vision is tested for acuity and visual fields, as described earlier in this chapter in the discussion on examination of the eye. Abnormal findings include changes in vision, blurring of vision, or inability to identify letters, numbers, or pictures.

Oculomotor (III), Trochlear (IV), and Abducens (VI) Nerves. The oculomotor, trochlear, and abducens nerves are motor nerves that control movement of the eyes through the cardinal fields of gaze; pupil size, shape, response to light, and accommodation; and opening of the upper eyelids. These assessments are discussed in the examination of the eye, earlier in this chapter. Normal responses include round pupils that are equal in size, direct and consensual pupillary response, lid margin flush with the surface of the eyeball, equal and complete bilateral lid closure, and parallel movements of the eyes. Abnormal findings include asymmetrical eye position, a portion of the eye not covered by the eyelid, lesions, edema, abnormal eye movements, and inability for one or both eyes to follow the cardinal fields.

Trigeminal (V) Nerve. The trigeminal nerve is a sensory and motor (sensorimotor) nerve. Motor function is assessed by observing the facial muscles for deviation of the jaw to one side and by instructing the client to clench the jaw and palpating the tone of the muscles. Sensory status of the nerve is assessed by testing for the ability to discriminate between sharp, dull, and light touch. The client is asked to close the eyes, and as the nurse touches each side of the client's face with a needle or paper clip, to report whether the sensation is sharp or dull. The same procedure is used for light touch, using a wisp of cotton and asking the client to tell you when and where on the face the sensation is felt. Normally, the client will correctly identify sharp, dull, and soft sensation of the face and neck bilaterally. Abnormal findings are decreased or absent sensations unilaterally or bilaterally.

Facial (VII) Nerve. The facial nerve is a sensorimotor nerve that innervates the muscles of the face and functions also to provide the taste sensation of the anterior two thirds of the tongue. Motor function is evaluated by observing a series of expressions that you ask the client to make: raise the eyebrows, smile and show the teeth, and puff out the cheeks. Facial expressions should be symmetrical. The taste sensation of the tongue is tested by placing a small amount of various taste solutions (such as sugar, salt, lemon) on the anterior two thirds of the tongue as the client, with eyes closed, protrudes the tongue. Various substances should be normally correctly identified; abnormal findings include incorrect identification of substances or the inability to taste.

Acoustic (VIII) Nerve. The acoustic nerve is a sensory nerve that is tested by assessing hearing ability, as described previously in assessment of the ear. The client should be able to hear bilaterally; abnormal findings are the inability to hear unilaterally or bilaterally.

Glossopharyngeal (IX) Nerve. The glossopharyngeal nerve is a sensorimotor nerve that allows tongue movement and swallowing, as well as taste sensations of the posterior one third of the tongue. The motor function of this nerve is assessed with the vagus (X) nerve, and the taste function is assessed with the facial (VII) nerve. The client should be able to identify various taste substances correctly, have a gag reflex, and be able to move the tongue.

Vagus (X) Nerve. The vagus nerve is a motor nerve that is assessed by asking the client to open the mouth and say "ah" as the upward movement of the soft palate is observed. The uvula should remain midline and rise symmetrically. The swallowing reflex can be assessed by having the client sip and swallow water.

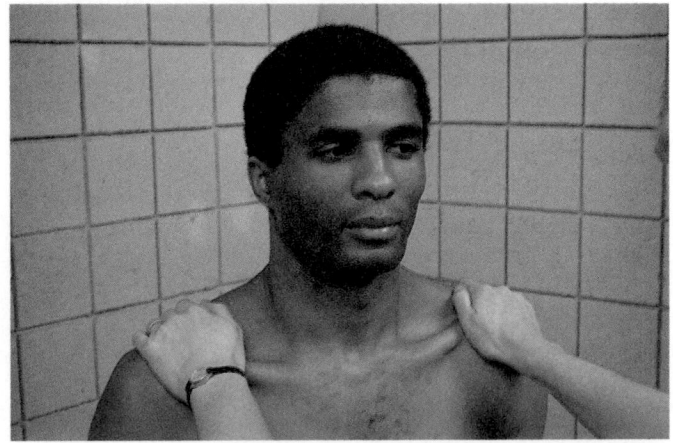

FIGURE 24-55
Test of the spinal accessory nerve. The client shrugs his shoulders against the resistance of the examiner's hands. (Photo © Ken Kasper)

Spinal Accessory (XI) Nerve. The spinal accessory nerve is a motor nerve that controls the movement of the head and houlders. Ask the client to shrug the shoulders upward and turn the head against the resistance of your hands (see Fig 24-55). There should be equal movement and strength of the muscles of the shoulder and head bilaterally.

Hypoglossal (XII) Nerve. The hypoglossal nerve is a motor nerve that affects the movement and strength of the tongue. Ask the client to protrude the tongue forward and to push out the cheek with the tongue. The protrusion should be symmetrical, and the cheek should have a puffed-out appearance. Abnormal findings include asymmetry of tongue movements, drooping, weakness, tremors, and loss of strength.

Assessment of Motor, Sensory, and Reflex Abilities

This part of the neurologic assessment includes the motor, sensory, and reflex abilities of the client. Motor ability is assessed by balance, gait, and coordination; sensory function is assessed by sensory discrimination of pain, light touch, and vibrations; and deep tendon reflexes are evaluated to determine the functioning ability of specific spinal segment levels.

Motor Abilities

Balance and Gait. Balance and gait are evaluated by having the client walk across the room on the toes, on the heels, and heel-to-toe. The nurse observes posture, balance, and arm and leg movements. The posture should be erect, with slight swaying in the standing position, and the gait even with simultaneous arm movements. Abnormal findings include loss of balance, shuffling, wide-based gait, and abnormal patterns of gait.

Motor Function and Coordination. Motor function and coordination are evaluated by having the client rapidly touch each of finger with the thumb, rapidly pat the hand on the thigh, and tap the foot against the floor (or against your hand, if the client is supine). Normally, the movements should be coordinated.

Sensory Abilities.

Sensory perception is tested by evaluating the client's response to pain, light touch, and vibratory sensation. With the client's eyes closed, a sharp object and a soft object are used randomly to touch upper and lower extremities to test sensation. This examination proceeds from distal (hands, arms, feet, legs) to proximal (trunk). The client should be able to distinguish between sharp (pain) and soft or dull touch. The same process is repeated by using the tuning fork to test for vibratory sensation, placing the fork on bony prominences. Abnormal findings include inability to perceive pain or light touch, inability to identify the location of touch, and absence of vibratory sensation.

Reflex Function. The reflexes are tested to evaluate the function of specific spinal segment levels. The reflex hammer is used to elicit muscle contraction and reflexes. The client may be either sitting or supine. The reflexes are illustrated in Table 24-8.

Biceps Reflex. The client's arms should be partially flexed at the elbow, with the palms down. Place your thumb or finger firmly on the client's biceps muscle, and strike with the reflex hammer, aimed directly toward your finger. Observe for flexion at the elbow, and feel for contraction of the biceps muscle.

Triceps Reflex. Flex the client's arm at the elbow, with the client's palm facing the body, and position it across the client's chest. Strike the triceps tendon above the elbow. Observe for contraction of the triceps muscle and extension at the elbow.

Brachioradialis or Supinator Reflex. Rest the client's forearm on the abdomen on in the lap, with the palm facing downward. Strike the client's radius approximately 1 to 2 inches above the wrist. Observe for flexion and supination of the forearm.

Patellar or Knee Reflex. The client is placed in a sitting or supine position while the nurse supports the client's knee in a flexed position. Briskly tap the patellar tendon just below the patella, and observe for contraction of the quadriceps with knee extension.

Grading of Reflexes

Reflexes are usually graded on a 0 to 4+ scale:

- 4+ Very brisk, hyperactive; often indicative of disease; often associated with clonus (rhythmic oscillations between flexion and extension)
- 3+ Brisker than average; possibly but not necessarily indicative of disease
- 2+ Average; normal
- 1+ Somewhat diminished; low normal
- 0   No response

Achilles Tendon Reflex or Ankle Reflex. The client's leg should be slightly flexed at the knee, with dorsiflexion of the foot at the ankle joint. Strike the Achilles tendon, and observe for plantar flexion at the ankle.

Reflexes are graded according to their response, with a +2 considered a normal or active response (see the accompanying box for further grading).

(Text continues on p. 479.)

T A B L E   24-8
Normal Responses of Commonly Tested Reflexes

Reflex	How to Test Reflex	Normal Response
Biceps	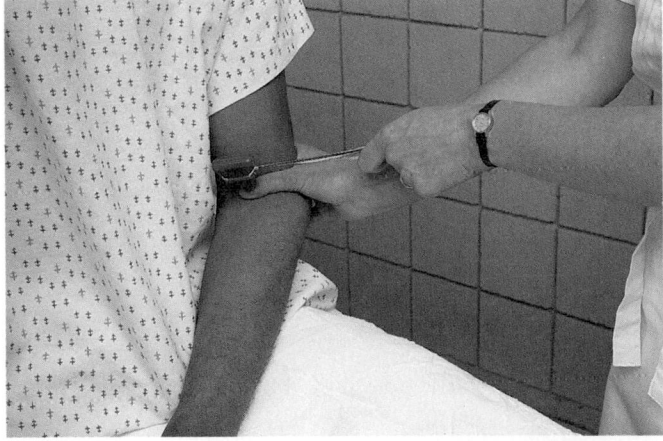	The contraction of the biceps can be seen and felt. To test the biceps reflex, the elbow is slightly bent, and the palm faces downward. The examiner's thumb is placed on the biceps tendon at the bend in the elbow. The percussion hammer strikes the examiner's thumb.
Triceps	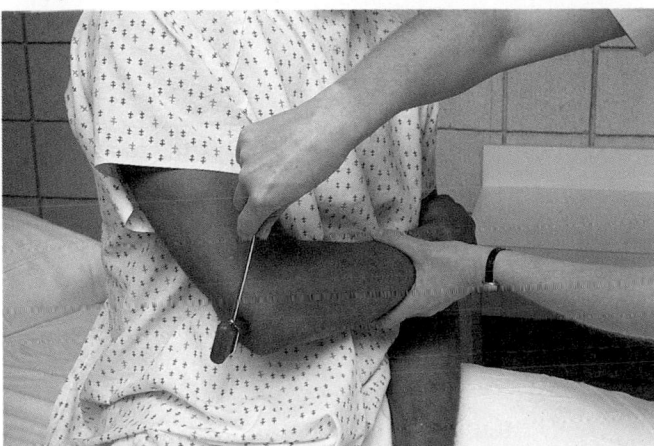	The contraction of the triceps can be seen as the elbow extends. To test the triceps reflex, the client's elbow is sharply bent; the forearm is placed across the chest wall with the palm turned toward the body. The triceps muscle is struck with the percussion hammer just above the elbow.
Knee	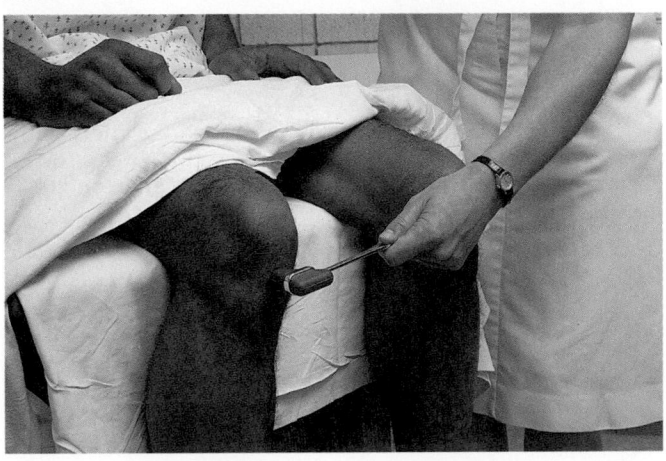	The contraction of the quadriceps causes the knee to extend. To test the knee reflex, the client is in the sitting position. The patellar tendon just below the patella is struck with the percussion hammer. If the client is lying down, the reflex is tested while the examiner's hands are placed under the knees to bend them.

(Continued)

T A B L E   24-8
Normal Responses of Commonly Tested Reflexes   (Continued)

Reflex	How to Test Reflex	Normal Response

Ankle

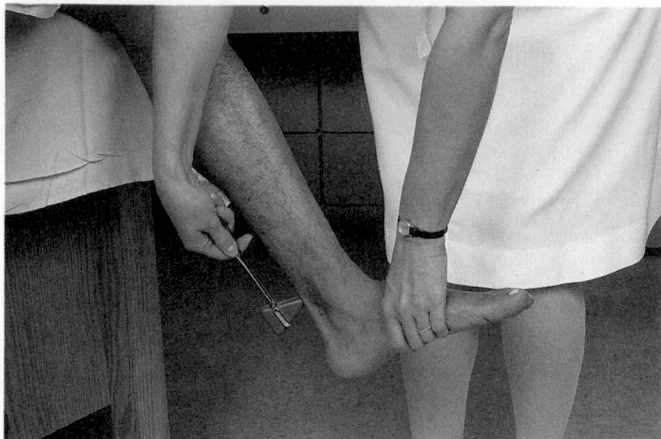

The foot jerks and moves downward.

To test the ankle reflex, the leg is bent at the knee and the foot is supported in a walking position. The Achilles tendon is struck with the percussion hammer.

Plantar

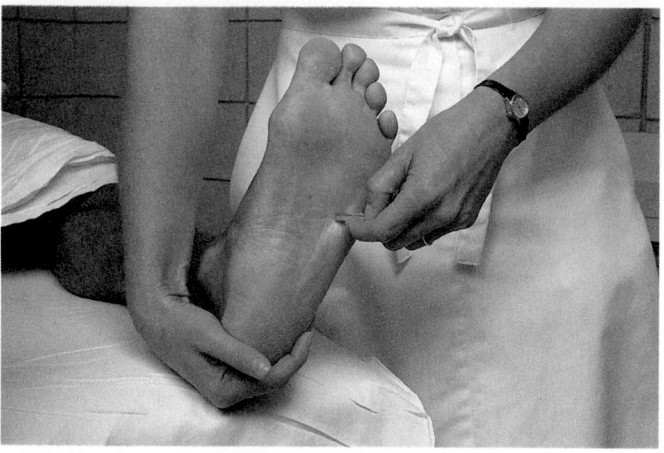

The toes bend or curl.

The lateral aspect of the sole of the foot is stroked with an object, such as a key or a thumbnail, from the heel to the ball of the foot.

Abdominal

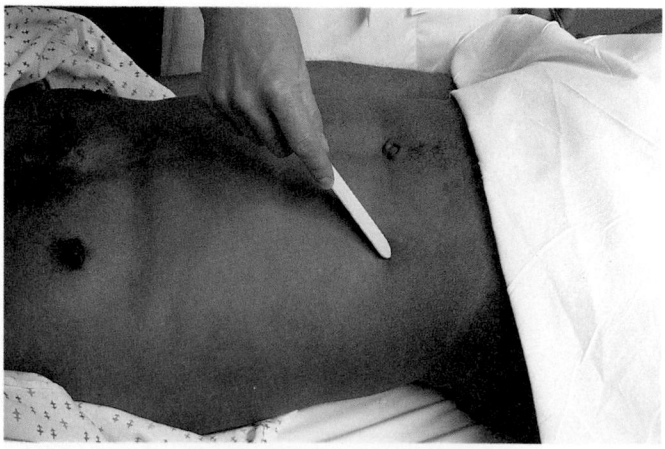

The contraction of abdominal musculature can be seen.

To test the abdominal reflex, with the client lying on the back, each side of the abdomen is stroked from the sides toward the center with a tongue blade or key.

(Photos © Ken Kasper)

DOCUMENTING THE DATA

After completing the nursing history and examination, the nurse organizes all assessment data accurately and completely for the purpose of identifying actual and potential problems, making nursing diagnoses, planning appropriate care, and evaluating the client's responses to treatment. Often a pattern is established that begins during the history and is confirmed during the physical examination.

The data are documented, with each system recorded individually. Documentation of the nursing examination, using a format based on functional health patterns, and integrating the health history and physical assessment, is illustrated in the box entitled Documentation of Health History and Physical Assessment to demonstrate the application of nursing assessment skills in the clinical setting.

Documentation of Health History and Physical Assessment

Holistic Assessment and Diagnosis
Complete History and Physical History

I. Client Profile
L.N. is a 66-year-old white man, who lives in a rural midwestern community. Married and lives with 64-year-old wife. Education level: 8th grade. Catholic religious affiliation. Sources and reliability of information: client alert and oriented.
Medical diagnosis and previous hospitalizations:
1. Hemorrhoidectomy in 1964. History of hemorrhoids from early 1930s. No complications of surgery.
2. Heart attack in 1980. No complications.
3. Prostate surgery in 1980. No complications.
4. Present diagnosis: chest pain, rule out myocardial infarction.
No known allergies for drug, food, environmental.

II. Major Reason for Seeking Health Care
Intermittent chest pain beginning 3 days prior to admission. Pain began without physical exertion while lying in bed. Denies anxiety or emotional incident precipitating the event. Pain substernal radiating to both shoulders and arms. Denies nausea and vomiting, palpitations, dizziness, or diaphoresis. States "I have difficulty breathing with pain." Rates pain as 9 on a scale of 1 to 10. Denies nitroglycerin administration for pain. States "I had some of those pills a long time ago but the wife couldn't find them. I kept thinking it was indigestion or arthritis but when it didn't go away I got worried. My wife wanted me to come in to the hospital to be checked out. So I did and they gave me some nitroglycerin in the emergency room and it helped the pain. I feel okay now. I haven't had any pain since I've been here."

III. Health Perception–Health Management Pattern
A. *Client Rating of Health Scale: 10 = Best, 1 = Worst*
5 years ago—10. Now—5. 5 years from now—5. "I've had a little problem with my heart but other than that I'm not in too bad of shape." Seeks health care only when ill. Last physical exam 1984.
B. *Medication: Prescribed*
   Lanoxin, 0.125 mg = one a day
   Cardizem, 30 mg = three times a day
   Nitroglycerin, 0.4 mg = as needed
Preparation H cream every 2 or 3 months
Ex-Lax, two to three times a week for bowel movements
"I still have a few hemorrhoids and I don't want to cause them to act up." Takes prescribed medications daily. Depends on wife for taking medications on time. Unable to verbalize medication rationale, side-effects, dosages, or administration times.

IV. Developmental Level
Integrity versus despair: Oldest of five children. Lived on a farm with parents until age 18 years. At that time, married and began employment as truck driver. Retired from work in 1987 at age 65. States "I'm not worried about dying, I just don't want to go any sooner than I have to." States "I like being retired. I have got time to do all the things I want to do, like fishing." Client lives with spouse in a two-bedroom home. Talks about selling home and moving into a senior-citizen apartment with wife where they have several friends. Visits with grandchildren 3 to 4 times a week. Expresses affection and pride in children. Denies financial difficulties. States "It's really expensive getting by nowadays but we do

(Continued)

Documentation of Health History and Physical Assessment (Continued)

okay. I have my social security and pension from work and my wife has hers.''

V. Biophysical Assessment

A. Nutritional Metabolic Pattern
Current height: 69 inches (175.26 cm)
Current weight: 175 lb (79.4 kg)
Weight stable at this time. Denies significant loss or gain. States ''The doctor prescribed a low-salt and low-cholesterol diet when I was in the hospital for my heart attack. My wife tries to keep me on it but I don't always follow it.'' Denies dietary instruction with previous hospitalization. States ''It might do me some good if I had a list or something to check with on what I can eat. My wife is the one who really needs to understand the diet stuff.'' Voices no particular likes or dislikes. Client wears full dentures. Last dental exam when teeth were extracted 1976. Denies difficulties with eating, chewing, swallowing, sore throat, tongue, or colds. Denies nausea and vomiting, abdominal pain, or excessive gas. Denies intolerance to heat or cold, voice change, polyuria, polydipsia, and polyphagia. Denies bruising, pruritus. Denies problems with wound healing.

B. Elimination Patterns
Bladder pattern: voids 7 to 8 times daily. Clear yellow urine. Denies dysuria, hematuria, polyuria, incontinence, or nocturia. Bowel habits: hard stool if laxative not taken. States ''I take a laxative 3 or 4 times a week because I don't want my hemorrhoids to act up.'' Has been taking Ex-Lax for five years to avoid cramps and straining. Stools soft, light brown, and moderate in amount. Denies mucus in stool, rectal bleeding, changes in color, consistency, or habits. States ''I have a small hemorrhoid or two that sometimes bother me.'' Uses Preparation H cream for soreness once every 2 or 3 months.

C. Activities/Exercise Pattern
1. Average day: arises at 6:00 AM. Dresses and shaves. Watches news or reads paper. Eats breakfast. Works in garden or yard for an hour or two. Drives to visit with friends or grandchildren. Eats lunch around 12 noon. Takes afternoon nap on occasion for 1 hour. Watches television in evening. Plays cards with friends occasionally. Goes fishing at nearby lake one or two times weekly, weather permitting. Takes shower around 8:00 PM. Denies chest pain, fatigue, wheezing, cramping, stiffness, joint pain, or swelling with activity. Patient happy with activities of daily living (ADLs) and

states he has not had to alter his activities because of chest pain.
2. Hygiene: showers daily. Uses commercial denture cleaners. Shaves daily with electric razor. Washes hair 3 times weekly.
3. Denies use of tobacco or illicit drugs.

D. Sleep–Rest Pattern
Retires at 8:30 PM consistently. Denies difficulties falling asleep or remaining asleep; feels well and rested upon arising at 6:00 AM. Denies using over-the-counter sleep aid. Denies orthopnea, nocturnal dyspnea.

E. Sensory–Perceptual Pattern
1. Eyes: wears glasses to read and drive and for close-up work. Glasses prescribed around age 40. Last eye check-up 1987. Average check-up every other year. Denies diplopia, itching, excessive tearing, discharge, redness, or trauma to eyes.
2. Ears: does not wear hearing aid. Cannot recall last hearing test. Responds appropriately to inquiries without need of repeating. Denies tinnitus, pain, discharge, or trauma to ears.
3. Nose: denies difficulties with smell, pain, postnasal drip, sneezing, or frequent nosebleeds.
4. Head: denies headaches, dizziness, vertigo, or trauma to head.

F. Sexuality
Actively engages in coitus twice weekly average. States sexual activity is satisfying. Denies chest pain or dyspnea with sexual activity. Denies difficulty with erection or orgasm.

VI. Psychologic Assessment

A. Cognitive Pattern
Speaks English clearly with regular pattern. Follows verbal cues. Expresses ideas and feelings clearly. States he has had some memory loss over past 4 years. He has difficulty recalling long-ago dates and times. Demonstrates no difficulty with short-term recall. States no difficulty in learning. New material is mastered by reading and studying several times.

B. Self-Perception/Self-Concept
Describes self as an outgoing person. Speaks with ease about self and life-style. Verbalizes no specific concerns. Smiles frequently. Posture erect and eye contact good. Appears confident, relaxed.

C. Coping–Stress Tolerance Pattern
Makes own decisions. Discusses alternatives of decisions with wife, various friends, and children on occasion. States he and neighbors share daily conversations, problems. Walks to relieve tension. States

(Continued)

Documentation of Health History and Physical Assessment (Continued)

"I really don't get too excited about things any more. Most things will work themselves out."

VII. Social Cultural Assessment

A. Role-Relationship Pattern

Client has been married to spouse for 48 years. Retired truck driver. Describes relationship as very good; socializes with neighbors and friends often.

VIII. Spiritual Assessment

A. Belief in God

Attends Catholic church weekly. Active in church activities (i.e., helps with fish fries, Church picnics). Prayer important to client and participates in weekly prayer group. States "Belief in God gives me hope and strength."

IX. Physical Assessment

A. General

Height: 5' 8" (175.26 cm)
Respiration: 20/min
Weight: 175 lb (79.4 kg)
Blood pressure: right arm—136/84
Radial pulse: 70
Left arm—113/80
Sitting comfortably and smiling

B. Skin

1. Hair: short, gray, straight, clean, fine texture, distributed evenly on head. No scalp lesions or flaking noted.
2. Nails: short, rounded, medium thickness. No clubbing, Beau's lines, or other abnormalities noted. Capillary refill time less than 1 second bilaterally.
3. Skin: tan, warm, and dry to touch with good turgor. Skin fold returns to place in 1 second when lifted over wrist. Multiple brown "age spots" over dorsal hands and forearms bilaterally. Scattered macules noted on facial area, approximately 4 cm each.

C. Mouth and Pharynx

Lips moist, pink, and without cracking, ulcers, or lesions. Dentures removed, gums are pink, moist, no bleeding apparent, no redness or discoloration. Hard and soft palates are smooth in appearance without lesions or masses. Tongue midline and good strength. Cranial nerves are intact. Uvula in midline and rises symmetrically when client says "ah."

D. Eyes—With Glasses: Vision 20/30

Glasses off, client has blurred vision 3 feet away from object, but can identify number of fingers. Eyelids pink without drainage, ptosis, or edema. Sclera white. Conjuctiva slightly reddened without lesions noted. Corneal reflexes present. Iris green bilaterally. EOMs intact bilaterally. Red reflexes present bilaterally. Optic discs round, cream colored, equal with grayish crescents, temporal borders, physiologic cups present and equal. No lesions, hemorrhages, or exudates.

E. Assessment of Ear

Auricles without deformity, lumps, lesions, or tenderness. Preauricular and postauricular nodes nonpalpable. Whisper test: client identifies 3 of 3 words. Weber test: bilateral equal lateralization. Rinnie's test: AC > BC bilaterally.

F. Assessment of Nose and Sinuses

External structure without deformity, asymmetry, or inflammation. Nares patent, and identifies smells without difficulty (cranial nerve #1 intact). Nasal mucosa pale pink, without swelling, exudate, or bleeding. Nasal septum midline without bleeding, perforation, or deviation. Turbinates pink without polyps. Frontal and maxillary sinuses nontender to palpation.

G. Neck

Neck symmetrical without masses, scars, or pulsations. ROM equal in strength to all positions; shrugs shoulders against resistance. Lymph nodes nonpalpable. Trachea in midline. Thyroid nonpalpable. Carotid arteries palpable without bruit.

H. Thorax, Throat, and Lungs

Skin pale pink. No scars, retractions, or lesions noted. Fine gray hair over sternum area. Thorax expands evenly. Slope of ribs 40 degrees. No auxiliary respiratory usage or nasal flaring noted. Anteroposterior diameter = 1:2. Respirations even and unlabored (20/min). No cough noted. No tenderness, crepitus, or masses noted bilaterally. Symmetrical thoracic excursion anteriorly and posteriorly. Tactile fremitus decreases below T6 bilaterally, posteriorly, and 5th intercostal space anteriorly bilaterally. Thoracic lung sounds resonant throughout.

I. Breasts

Breasts symmetrical and nontender. No lumps, masses, lesions, or discharge noted.

J. Heart

No pulsations visible. No heaves, lifts, or thrills in any areas. PMI: 5th ICS, LMCL. Pulmonic area: S_1 and S_2 heard, no S_3 or S_4 noted. Early systolic grade 2 murmur noted. Aortic area: same as pulmonic area. Tricuspid area: S_1 louder than S_2, no S_3 or S_4 auscultated. Mitral area: S_1 and S_2 present, no S_3 or S_4 noted. Apical pulse 74/min regular and strong. Client states "systolic murmur present since childhood."

(Continued)

Documentation of Health History and Physical Assessment (Continued)

K. Peripheral Vascular System

Arms equal in size and symmetry bilaterally. Radial pulses equal in rate and strength. No bruit noted. Brachial pulses strong, equal, and even. Epitrochlear nodes nonpalpable. Legs equal in size and symmetry. Upper and lower extremity skin pale pink, warm, and dry to touch without edema, bruising, lesions, or increased vascularity. Superficial inguinal, horizontal, and vertical lymph nodes nonpalpable. Femoral pulses, popliteal pulses, dorsalis pedis, and posterior tibial pulses strong and equal. Edema to feet = 1+ bilaterally. Toenails thick and yellowed.

L. Abdomen

Umbilicus in midline without herniation, swelling, or discoloration. Abdomen rounded, symmetrical without masses, lesions, pulsations, or peristalsis noted. Bowel sounds low and gurgling at 20/min in all four quads. Aortic, renal, and iliac arteries without bruit. No tenderness or masses noted with light and deep palpation in all four quadrants.

M. Musculoskeletal

Stands erect with shoulders slightly forward. No asymmetry noted. Normal concave curve of cervical and lumbar spine. Convex thoracic spine noted. *No* joint deformities, tenderness, or crepitations. Full active range of motion of all extremities without pain.

N. Neurologic

Mental Status: alert and oriented to person, time, and place. Smooth fine and gross motor movements. Facial expression symmetrical and matches mood. Speech clear and appropriate. Follows through with train of thought. Expresses feelings and ideas clearly. Attentive and able to focus on exam during entire interaction. Short-term memory and long-term memory intact. General information questions answered correctly 100% of the time. Vocabulary suitable to educational level. Abstract reasoning intact. Gives semiabstract answers. Identifies similar-ities 5 seconds after asked. Answers to judgment question in realistic manner.

Cranial nerves:

I–XII intact (integrated throughout exam) Cerebellar Function: Alternates finger to nose with eyes closed. Rapidly opposes fingers to thumb without difficulty. Alternates pronation and supination of hands rapidly without difficulty. Coordinates heel to shin. Gait steady and even. No involuntary movements noted.

Sensory: Identifies superficial and deep touch sensations over trunk, face, and extremities. Identifies position of toes and fingers and location of points. Motor Function: Muscle size and tone equal bilaterally. Muscle strength equal in all extremities. Reflexes intact.

Nursing Diagnoses

1. Alteration in health management related to lack of knowledge of importance of regular check-ups
2. Knowledge deficit: prescribed medication and dietary regimen
3. Knowledge deficit: management and causes of constipation related to lack of prior exposure to information
4. Alteration in bowel elimination related to fear of painful defecation and laxative use
5. Potential for alterations in comfort: acute chest pain
6. Potential for alterations in cardiac output: decreased

Client's Strengths

Positive attitude and outlook

Spouse support and participation in health-care regimen

Interest and motivation regarding acquiring health-care knowledge

Religious belief and supports

Health history and physical assessment documentation provided by Janet R. Weber, RN, MSN, Faculty, Department of Nursing, Southeast Missouri State University, Cape Girardeau, Missouri.

KEY POINTS

■ Data collection during the assessment step of the nursing process includes a nursing history and nursing (physical) assessment. Data from nursing examinations are used to formulate nursing diagnoses.

■ There are four techniques used in performing a nursing assessment: inspection, palpation, percussion, and auscultation.

- The nurse should plan the nursing examination at a time that is appropriate for both the client and the nurse. The nurse should prepare the room, gather instruments and equipment, ensure privacy, and meet the client's physical and psychologic needs.

- There are various positions used during the nursing examination. The client's privacy and comfort should be considered in each position.

- Each body system is assessed for normal and abnormal findings; included are the integument, the head and neck, the thorax and lungs, the breasts and axilla, the abdomen, the male and female genitalia, the rectum and anus, the musculoskeletal system, and the neurologic system. The techniques of assessment are used to assess the health status of the client systematically.

- The nurse carefully documents normal and abnormal findings.

BIBLIOGRAPHY

Assessing Your Patients. *Nursing Photobook Series.* Horsham, PA, Intermed Communications, 1980

Bates B: A Guide to Physical Examination, 4th ed. Philadelphia, JB Lippincott, 1987

Block G, Nolan J: Health Assessment for Professional Nursing, 2nd ed. Norwalk, CT, Appleton-Century Crofts, 1986

Brunner LS, Suddarth DS: Textbook of Medical-Surgical Nursing, 6th ed. Philadelphia, JB Lippincott, 1988

Dennison R: Cardiopulmonary assessment. Nursing '86 16(4): 34–39, April, 1986

Koeckerizt J: How to coax out a frank patient history. RN 56–61, October, 1981

Smith C: With good assessment skills you can construct a solid framework for patient care. Nursing '84 14(12):26–31, December, 1984

25 Safety and Asepsis

OBJECTIVES

After studying this chapter, the learner should be able to

Define key terms used in the chapter.

Identify factors that may be safety hazards in the client's environment.

Describe ways in which the client's safety can be promoted in the home and health-care setting.

Identify clients at risk of falling.

Describe preventive strategies to decrease the incidence of client falls.

Identify nursing diagnoses associated with a client in an unsafe situation.

Describe nursing responsibilities for fire safety.

Explain the infection cycle.

Describe nursing interventions used to break the chain of infection.

List the stages of an infection.

Identify clients at risk of developing an infection.

Identify factors that reduce the incidence of nosocomial infection.

Identify situations in which handwashing is indicated.

Identify nursing diagnoses associated with a client who has an infection or is at risk of developing an infection.

Identify protocols for each isolation category.

Describe recommended techniques for medical and surgical asepsis.

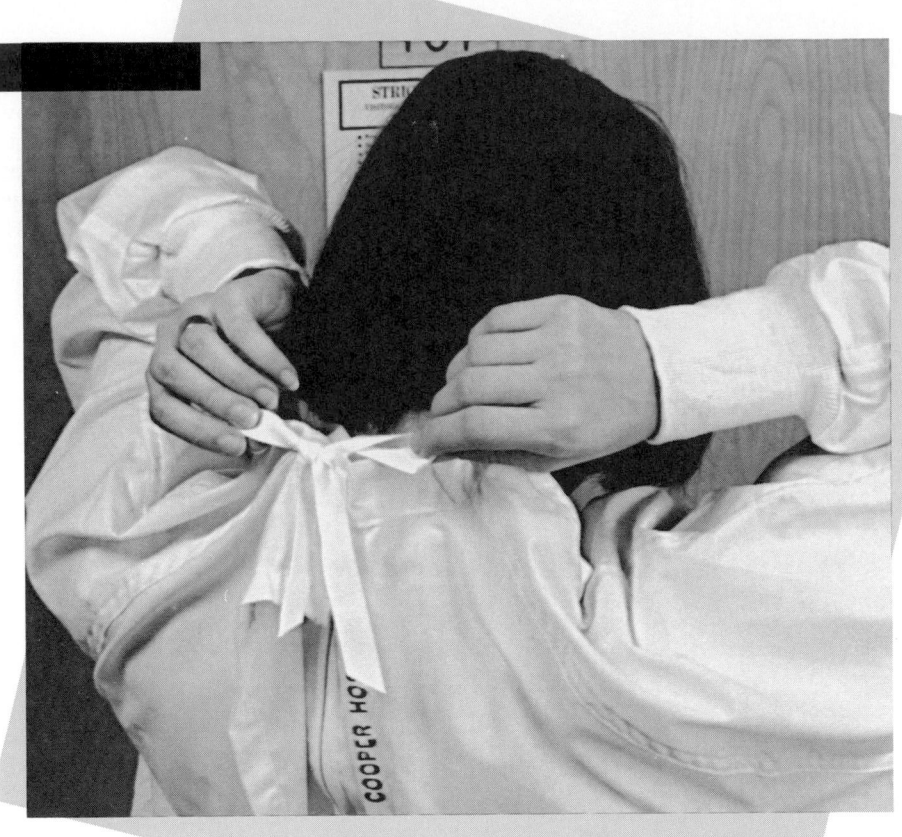

Safety and security are basic human needs. Safety is a paramount concern underlying all nursing care and is a responsibility for all health-care providers in every environment. The focus on safety encompasses the acute and extended care facilities as well as the home, workplace, and community. Each population is at risk. The nursing process further defines the specific hazards confronting each age group and situation. The focus of this chapter is environmental safety in both the home and health-care agency, infection control and prevention, and isolation and communicable diseases.

ENVIRONMENTAL SAFETY

The prevention of accidents affects the wellness of all persons. Table 25-1 lists statistics for accidental deaths.

Factors Affecting Safety

Nursing strategies that identify potential hazards and promote wellness evolve from an awareness of the various factors that affect safety in the environment.

Developmental Considerations

Nurses interact with clients at varying developmental levels. Each age has its own particular risks. Promoting safety and preventing injury is a dual responsibility. The nurse and client or family cooperate and together strive to eliminate or reduce accident risks in the home, community, or any health-care setting. Education to promote awareness of potentially dangerous situations must begin as early as possible and continue throughout the life span.

The infant or young child has a limited awareness of danger. Parents need encouragement to teach children as early as possible what can potentially cause injury. Many childhood accidents are preventable. As motor skills develop, the environment expands and potential hazards multiply. Protecting an infant or young child may involve childproofing activities in the home, simple instruction about potentially dangerous situations such as crossing a street, or careful observation during routine activities.

Adolescents are particularly at risk from accidents in motor vehicles. Conflicts with parental values coupled with peer pressure may lead to experimentation with drugs and alcohol creating more potential accident hazards. Young and middle-aged adults become more accident prone when alcohol is used in response to stressful situations.

Although elderly people have more experience with their environment, illness or some degree of motor or sensory impairment may increase their risk for accidents. They are vulnerable to falls, exposure to unfavorable environmental conditions, and fire hazards. Realistic con-

KEY TERMS

antigen
antibody
asepsis
   medical asepsis
   surgical asepsis
carrier
Centers for Disease Control
colonize
convalescent period
disinfectant
disinfection
endogenous
exit from the reservoir
exogenous
fomite
full stage of illness
ground
host
iatrogenic infection
immune response
incident report
incubation period

infection
inflammatory response
isolation
localized symptoms
macroshock
microshock
normal flora
nosocomial infection
pathogen
portal of entry
prodromal stage
reservoir
resident bacteria or flora
restraint
sterilization
suffocation
susceptibility
systemic symptoms
transient bacteria or flora
vector
vehicle
virulence

T A B L E   25-1
Principal Types of Accidental Deaths in the United States for 1985

Type	Total Number	Death Rates Per 100,000 Population
Motor vehicle	45,600	19.1
Falls	11,300	4.7
Drowning	5,700	2.4
Fires, burns	4,900	2.1
Other poisons	3,800	1.6
Ingestion of food, object	3,200	1.3
Fire-arms	1,600	0.7
Poison by gas	1,200	0.5

(Adapted from National Data Book and Guide to Sources, Statistical Abstract of the United States. US Department of Commerce, Bureau of Statistics, 1987)

cerns exist for elderly clients with slowed reflexes who continue to operate motor vehicles in an overly cautious or inadvertently careless manner. Noncompliance to a medication regimen may be related to failing sight, hearing difficulties, memory lapses, or inadequate communication from the health-care provider.

The majority of hospitalized clients who fall are over age 60. Mortality associated with a fall increases as age progresses. Older women fall more often coinciding perhaps with statistics indicating increasing numbers of females in this age group. More than one-third of falls in the elderly population are associated with the need to urinate. Checklists that can be used to assess the potential for a fall occurring in the home or health-care setting are included in the discussion of nursing implementations later in this chapter.

Life-Style

Certain occupations and environments place individuals in more hazardous situations. A worker who operates heavy industrial machinery, functions in perilous settings, or is involved with chemical agents on a consistent basis is at greater risk of accidental injury. Some people, by their nature, are more inclined to take risks and place themselves at jeopardy. Failure to wear seat belts or abide by safety precautions is common behavior for some clients. Stress may precipitate unhealthful lifestyles involving drug or alcohol abuse. Although much has been done to identify and control environments affected by pollutants, certain areas may statistically prove more hazardous and may expose residents to potentially unhealthy circumstances.

Living in an area where crime is prevalent may pose an additional threat to physical and emotional well-

being. Security measures, such as locks and adequate exterior lighting, provide additional safety reassurances.

Mobility

Any limitation in mobility is potentially unsafe. An elderly client with an unsteady gait is prone to falling, and an unfamiliar setting may further aggravate the situation. Someone with paralysis or a spinal cord injury may require assistance with even the simplest movement. Supportive devices, such as canes, walkers, or wheelchairs, may facilitate movement, but they necessitate careful instruction and preparation for safe use. Recent surgery or a prolonged illness can temporarily affect mobility and necessitate special precautions to prevent accidental falls or injuries. Nurses must assess a client's potential for accidental injury with a view toward maintaining independence and fostering self-esteem while providing a safe, predictable environment.

Sensory Perception

Alterations in sensory perception can have a devastating effect on safety. Any impairment in sight, hearing, smell, taste, or sense of touch can reduce sensitivity to the environment. Visual changes may cause an individual to stumble, lose his balance, and fall. A hearing deficit interferes with normal communication and may result in a client who is insensitive to safety alarms, traffic horns or sirens, as well as unable to clearly understand instructions relating to health care. Reduction in one's ability to distinguish odors may mean failure to detect leaking gas or smoke. Loss of taste bud receptors can foster unsafe eating habits or result in ingestion of tainted food. A client whose tactile sense is impaired may be unable to perceive extremes in temperature as a threat to safety.

Knowledge

An awareness of safety precautions is crucial in promoting and maintaining wellness. A client needs instruction to adhere accurately to his medical regimen or follow safety precautions when oxygen is in use. He requires a certain amount of knowledge to manage new equipment and unfamiliar procedures. Nursing assessment includes identification and recognition of potentially threatening circumstances. Recommendations for specific safety precautions are included throughout this chapter.

Ability to Communicate

Communication between the environment and the senses is basic to safety. The nurse must be sensitive to any factor that influences the client's ability to receive and send messages. Fatigue, stress, medication, aphasia, and language barriers are examples of situations that can affect any personal interchange and interfere with an accurate perception of events. A valid assessment by the nurse not only identifies the client's level of understanding but facilitates a positive communication experience.

Health State

Anything affecting the health state of the client potentially has the ability to impact on the safety of the environment. When an individual is chronically ill or in a weakened health state, the focus of health care includes preventing accidents as well as promoting wellness and restoring the client to a healthy state. The nurse caring for a client recovering from a stroke identifies his neuromuscular impairment and also pays particular attention to health teaching concerning maintaining his sense of balance and carefully assisting with ambulation to prevent falls. Many of the clients who fall have a primary or secondary diagnosis of cardiovascular disease. The nurse strives to maximize the client's potential for return to a healthy state by considering safety factors as nursing care plans are developed.

Psychosocial State

Stressful situations tend to narrow an individual's attention span and make him more prone to accidents. Stress may be sustained over long periods of time, but the effects tend to be more devastating in the later years when there is less adaptive and coping capacity. Depression, when it develops, may result in confusion and disorientation accompanied by reduced awareness or concern about environmental hazards. Lack of social contact or social isolation may be responsible for a reduced level of concentration, errors in judgment, and diminished awareness to external stimuli.

Assessing

Environmental safety hazards result in falls, fires, poisoning, suffocation, and accidents involving motor vehicles, equipment, and procedures.

Identifying clients at risk and unsafe situations requires a knowledge of the various factors mentioned above that influence safety and predispose individuals to accidents. Recognition of these considerations facilitates development of an individualized plan of care and has implications for nursing interventions aimed at protecting the client. Assessment includes risk factors in the home and health-care agency.

Falls

Statistics verify that falls are the major safety problem in hospitals as well as the leading cause of accidental death for the elderly in the home. The nurse needs to be aware of those clients who are most likely to fall as well as situations and settings consistently that have been implicated as hazards.

Assessing for falls includes use of the nursing history and nursing examination. Sample questions to be asked in the nursing history are listed in the box on page 488. The nursing examination includes examining for faulty vision and hearing, mobility problems such as alterations in gait or posture, and postural hypotension.

Falls occur at both ends of the life continuum. Infants and older people are at risk for falls.

A client is considered a high-risk candidate for a fall if

- Age is greater than 60.
- Previous falls are documented.
- Vision or sense of balance is impaired.
- Alterations in gait or posture are present.
- Medication regimen includes diuretics, tranquilizers, sedatives/hypnotics, analgesics.
- Postural hypotension is recorded.
- Reaction time is slowed.
- Confusion or disorientation is apparent.
- Mobility is impaired.

Continuous surveillance of environmental hazards in the health-care facility and of clients who are at risk for falls must be made. A checklist for preventing falls is given in the box on page 489.

History of Accidents

Some persons seem more likely to have accidents. Once an older adult has suffered one fall it is likely he will fall again. It is not uncommon for some children to be involved in multiple mishaps resulting in a fractured bone. Some adolescent drivers have repeated motor vehicle accidents. They appear unable to predict situations that may prove hazardous. Opinion varies as to the probable cause of this accident-prone behavior. Some suggest an emotional link, but the consensus is that a client with a history of accidents is likely to have another one.

Fires

A prominent cause of fires is smoking in bed or watching television and falling asleep while smoking on a sofa or chair. Kitchen stoves, candles, and electric heaters are other causes of home fires. Faulty wiring and unsafe electrical equipment cause fires in homes and health-care facilities. Assessment involves determining risk factors by assessing knowledge of clients and families. Such questions might be

Do you smoke?
At what places in the house?
Do you smoke in bed?
While watching television?
Do you remain in the kitchen when you are cooking?
Do you use grease and fry foods often?
At what time of the day do you cook?

Elements of an Environmental Assessment for Falls in the Home

Home exterior

Are sidewalks uneven? _____

Are steps in good repair? _____

Do steps have handrails? _____

Are handrails securely fastened? _____

Is there adequate lighting? _____

Can client sit down and get up
from outdoor furniture easily? _____

Home interior

Are lights bright enough to compensate for any limited vision? _____

Are stairways adequately lit? _____

Are there enough night lights to improve vision during darkness? _____

Do throw rugs have secure rubber
backings? _____

Are rooms uncluttered to permit
easy mobility? _____

Do chairs and stools provide sufficient support for sitting down
and getting up? _____

Is temperature within a comfortable range (70°–75°F)? _____

Do door thresholds impair
mobility? _____

Stairs

Are stairways well illuminated? _____

Are steps in good repair? _____

Are step edges clearly marked with
colored tape? _____

Are handrails available on both
sides of stairways? _____

Are handrails securely fastened to
walls? _____

Kitchen

Is the gas stove pilot light in good
repair? _____

Are chairs of proper height for ease
in sitting down and getting up? _____

Are storage areas easily reached? _____

Are floors slippery? _____

Is there adequate light? _____

Are mats nonskid? _____

Bathroom

Is there a mat or skidproof strips in
the tub or shower? _____

Does the tub/toilet have grab bars
nearby? _____

Will the client need an elevated
toilet seat to get on and off
easily? _____

Is the medication cabinet well illuminated? _____

Bedroom

Are the bed and chairs of adequate
height to allow for getting on
and off easily? _____

Are rugs/carpets nonskid or well
anchored to the floor? _____

Are night lights available? _____

Are light switches accessible? _____

Is there adequate lighting? _____

(Adapted from Tideiksaar R: Geriatric falls in the home. Home Healthcare Nurse 4(2):21, 1986)

Do you ever cook late at night when other family
members are asleep?

How do you heat your house?

Do you have electricity? gas? oil?

It is also proper to question how a client heats the house
if they have a limited income and you suspect they may
have had electricity or gas turned off.

Smoke detectors save lives.

Does the client have smoke detectors in the house?
Where and how many?

Are the batteries working properly?

It is a law that safety boards be set up in hospitals and
that regular inspection be made of the facilities for possible hazards. Equipment must be checked regularly, and
escape routes must be kept open. Nurses in their daily
care procedures should be aware of equipment and its
proper functioning and should assess when and how
often drills are performed.

Poisoning

Although the incidence of childhood poisoning has
been reduced dramatically in the last 10 years, accidental
poisoning remains a concern in teenage and adult age
groups (Spencer, 1989). Causes of fatalities from poisoning are listed in Table 25-2. However not all poisonings result in death. Table 25-3 lists categories of ingested poisonous substances by age groups.

Checklist for Preventing Falls

Client's Name: _____ Age: _____
Diagnosis: _____
Nursing Unit & Station: _____

	YES	NO	COMMENTS
1. Are restraints needed? If yes, what type?	☐	☐	_____
2. Are side rails up?	☐	☐	_____
3. Is bed in low position?	☐	☐	_____
4. Are bed wheels locked? Wheelchair brakes on?	☐	☐	_____
5. Is call light within the client's reach?	☐	☐	_____
6. Does the client understand how to use the call light?	☐	☐	_____
7. Is the night-light on?	☐	☐	_____
8. Does the room have any physical hazards (*e.g.,* is the floor slippery because of damp mopping)?	☐	☐	_____
9. What type of footwear does the client have on?	☐	☐	_____
10. Are the client's water, tissues, and urinal within reach?	☐	☐	_____
11. If the client is a surgical patient, how many hours or days postop is he?			_____
12. Does the client have any previously identified limitations?	☐	☐	_____
13. Is the client aware of his activity limitations?	☐	☐	_____
14. Is the client showing any physical or mental limitations now?	☐	☐	_____
15. Has the client received any analgesics, hypnotics, sedatives, or relaxants? If yes, what are they?	☐	☐	_____
16. Is he receiving other medications that could cause him to fall? If yes, what are they?	☐	☐	_____

T A B L E 25-2
Poisoning Deaths by Age and Most Common Cause

Age	Agent/Cause
5 years and under	Carbon monoxide resulting most commonly from improperly vented gas space heaters
10–17 years	Carbon monoxide from motor vehicle Drugs Methaqualone Alcohol in combination
18–19 years	Drugs Diazepam Antidepressants Heroin Cocaine Methadone Phencyclidine Alcohol in combination
Adults	Drugs Alcohol in combination, usually with heroin Heroin Codeine Amitriptyline Diazepam Propoxyphene Phenobarbital Cocaine

(Data from Massachusetts Poison Control System: Clinical Epidemiology of Serious Poisonings. Clin Toxicol Rev 5:11, 1983; printed in Spencer RT et al: Clinical Pharmacology and Nursing Management, 3rd ed. Philadelphia, JB Lippincott, 1989)

Younger children are more apt to ingest household chemicals while older children may swallow medicines in a suicide attempt. Experimentation with drugs by adolescents or young adults may result in accidental poisoning and death. An elderly client may inadvertently consume an overdose of a medication due to confusion or forgetfulness. Poor vision is also a factor in accidental poisoning in the elderly population.

These developmental considerations must be taken into account while making assessments. Many poison control centers provide checklists for poison proofing a home and lists of toxic household items. Reviewing these items will help in assessing and teaching the family about poisonous materials.

Suffocation

Suffocation may occur in any age group, but the incidence is greater in children.

Common causes of suffocation include drowning, choking on a foreign substance inhaled into the trachea, or gas or smoke poisoning. An infant may suffocate when a pillow or piece of plastic inadvertently covers his nose and mouth. A young child may be accidentally strangled by the shoulder harness of a seat belt. Old unused refrigerators may be responsible for death by suffocation when a young child crawls into it while playing and becomes entrapped.

Drowning is another form of suffocation. Nearly half of all drowning accidents occur in children under age 5. In younger children the cause is mostly inadequate supervision in the bathtub and in pools, even small wading pools. Older children die more often in swimming or boating accidents.

Educating the public on the various causes of suffocation is the strongest factor in promoting wellness in this category. Assessing the knowledge level of clients, and especially parents, is vitally important.

Diagnosing

Once the nurse has identified a client at risk and an unsafe situation, the nursing diagnosis and care plan should reflect this. The actual or potential statement of the client's health status must be followed by the appropriate contributing or risk factors to individualize the nursing care plan.

Samples of nursing diagnoses pertaining to safety risks include the following:

Potential for injury related to visual/auditory sensory deficits; history of falling; unsteady gait; substance abuse; refusal to use seat belt/child safety seat; effects of medication; age greater than sixty (60); generalized weakness

Impaired home maintenance management related to insufficient finances; substance abuse; physical disability

Knowledge deficit concerning safety related to confusion; language barrier; unfamiliarity with fire prevention guidelines

Planning: Client Goals

Many accidental injuries and deaths are preventable. The nurse considers the varied factors and environment that affect the client's safety and formulates client goals uniquely suited to each situation and circumstance. Nursing interventions focus on meeting these safety needs.

Client goals that promote safety and prevent injury may include the following:

Client will identify unsafe situations present in his environment.

Client will identify potential hazards in the environment.

Client will use safety measures to prevent accidents.

Client will establish safety priorities with family members or significant others.

Client will demonstrate familiarity with his environment.

Client will identify resources for safety information.

T A B L E **25-3**

Summary of General Categories of Poisonous Substances Most Frequently Ingested in 1980

	Age			Total
Agent	Under 5 Yr	Over 5 Yr	Unknown	All Ages
Medicines	29,786	22,472	2,386	54,644
Medicine combination	773	5,454	396	6,623
Medicine, external	8,234	2,744	411	11,389
Medicine, internal	20,779	14,274	1,579	36,632
Medicine, internal—aspirin	2,812	955	114	3,881
Cleaning and polishing agents	11,074	3,648	687	15,409
Plants and plant substances	9,650	1,706	505	11,861
Cosmetics	7,600	794	301	8,695
Pesticides	4,044	2,395	570	7,009
Turpentine, paints	2,913	1,644	276	4,833
Petroleum products	2,045	1,710	187	3,942
Paint	915	358	55	1,328
Gases and vapors	102	1,035	139	1,276
Solvents and thinners	555	578	76	1,209

(National Clearinghouse for Poison Control Centers: Poison Control Case Report Summary, June 14, 1982)

Implementing

Safety measures are an integral part of the nursing care plan. The nurse intervenes to control or modify the environment and promote client safety. These safety recommendations apply to health agency settings, the home, and the community. Nursing implementations are discussed for each developmental level as well as for specific hazards in the environment. Teaching is an important step in accident prevention and health promotion.

Teaching to Prevent Accidents

Many teaching opportunities concerning safety measures arise while the nurse performs regular client care. Careful assessment, diagnosis, and planning will prepare the nurse to use these opportunities wisely.

Assessment data and statistical information often prove helpful to health-care personnel who are developing a safety program for clients at risk. Safety education classes, in addition to situational health teaching, can be worthwhile for the hospitalized client and family. Recent studies have demonstrated that early assessment of vulnerable clients and preventive education programs can decrease the incidence of falls (Gray-Vickrey, 1984; Knight, 1985; Lee and Pash, 1983).

A school nurse has multiple opportunities and a ready audience for health teaching about safety, including screening programs, fire prevention sessions, or classes on a variety of accident prevention techniques. Management of minor accidents that involve children at school provides a forum for additional preventive strategies.

Table 25-4 lists types of injuries and safety topics that should be taught to parents and in the schools for various age groups. The material in the remainder of this section on environmental safety is adaptable to teaching.

Considering Developmental Levels

Infant. The nurse has many opportunities for education about safety and accident prevention for infants and young children. The lack of mobility in early infancy limits opportunities for hazardous activity, but minimal safeguards are vital if accidents are to be prevented.

Safe care of an infant entails never leaving the child unattended, using crib rails, and monitoring objects that may be placed in his mouth and swallowed. As infancy progresses and the child becomes more active, parents and caregivers must be alert to hazards that a curious, mobile infant may encounter. All items within reach must be carefully inspected and, if dangerous, secured in a safe place. Household products, medicines, electric outlets, and sharp instruments may cause injury and death. Because an infant frequently climbs or pulls up on objects, scalding hot liquids must be placed out of reach. Lead-free paint on all furniture and toys ensures that the infant will not be exposed to lead poisoning. Many states mandate the need for safe infant car seats and carriers when transporting a child in a motor vehicle. Additional safety counseling measures which focus on tasks and behavior typical for this developmental level are included in Table 25-4.

(Text continues on p. 493.)

T A B L E   25-4
Developmental Considerations and Safety Topics to be Taught

Developmental Age	Accidents	Safety Topics
Newborn	Falls	Newborn supervision Proper method of caring for newborn Environment—Crib, bath, and changing area Infant car seats Use of vitamins, iron medications Feeding
Infant (first half year)	Falls Injuries from toys Burns	Many of above topics Infant supervision Development—Rolling over and falls Toy safety—Size, construction, lead-free paint Flame-retardant clothes and inflammable toys Smoke alarms Sunburns, bathwater temperature, smoking, hot beverages Kitchen safety Electric cords and outlets Using medications
Infant (second half year)	Falls Injuries from toys Burns Suffocation/drowning Inhalation/ingestion Foreign bodies	Many of above topics Close supervision for active child Development—Crawling, pulling up to stand, and pulling down objects: curiosity Safety on stairs (gates) Teaching siblings about infant safety Plastic bags Tub and pool safety Childproofing entire house and houses infant visits Poisonous plants Child-resistant packaging of medications and all poisonous substances Poison Control Center and instructions for emergencies
Toddler	Falls Cuts from sharp objects Burns Suffocation/drowning Inhalation/ingestion Foreign bodies	Many of above topics Toddler supervision Development—Inquisitive nature Outdoor safety—Cars, driveways, parking lots Safety glass on doors, lock doors and windows, screens Animal safety—Pets and strange animals Child car seats Storage of hazardous substances (indoors and outdoors) Poisonous plants (indoors and outdoors) Car safety (car seats, unattended children, cars parked in sun) Storage of matches, use of "hot" liquids Water safety—Tubs and wading and swimming pools, swimming lessons
Preschooler	Falls Cuts Burns Drowning Inhalation/ingestion Guns and weapons	Many of above topics Safe play areas (equipment and supervision, streets) Tricycles, scissors, other toys Guns or rifles in the house Begin to teach safety measures to child Fire safety—Prevention, emergency measures, fire drills
School-age Child	Burns Drowning Broken bones Inhalation/ingestion Guns and weapons Substance abuse	Many of above topics Safety on way to school (traffic, child abuse) Play equipment—Bicycle, skateboards, roller skates Competitive sports Use of machinery (farm, lawn, cooking) Teaching safety measures (bicycle, use of phone in emergencies, policeman as helper, substance abuse) Parental role modeling

(Continued)

Developmental Age	Accidents	Safety Topics
Adolescent	Drowning Vehicle accidents Guns and weapons Inhalation/ingestion	Many of above topics Responsibilities of new freedoms of being a teenager Driving (driver education, traffic safety, drinking and driving, motorcycles and snowmobiles) Competitive sports (proper equipment, physical examination before beginning sports or going to camp) Safety around water and water sports Emergency procedures, first-aid training Gun safety Substance abuse and role modeling for siblings Stress and coping

Toddler and Preschooler. To prevent accidental injury and death during the toddler and preschool years, the focus of parental responsibility is on childproofing the environment. Play areas must allow for exploration but must provide for safety. Vigilant supervision by parents and guardians should anticipate hazardous elements and protect with precautionary devices such as safety locks, guard rails, and electric outlet covers. Ingestion of poisons or medications is a major threat for the preschooler. Their overconfidence and initiative make them more likely to dart into the street while chasing a ball, climb into an unused refrigerator, or play with matches. Nursing measures that provide for safety of the toddler or preschooler are included in Table 25-4.

School-Age Child. As the child becomes more independent during the school years, accidents continue as a leading cause of death. Though increasingly independent behavior is typical of this age group, children need assistance to evaluate activities that are potentially dangerous. The nurse counseling parents of school age children about safeguarding their child's environment needs to discuss specific interventions that provide for safety at home, at school, and in the neighborhood (Table 25-4 and Fig. 25-1).

Adolescent. Nurses and parents must collaborate to reinforce safety behaviors in the adolescent. Much of the adolescent's time is spent away from home, with his peer group, or in automobiles. Education must focus on safe driving skills including wearing a seat belt, discussions about drug and alcohol use, and formulation of a healthful life-style in response to the stress of daily living. Providing safety information is crucial in helping the adolescent to make mature decisions about the health hazards particular to this age group (Table 25-4).

Adult. Young and middle-aged adults need reminders about the effect of stress on their life-style. Coping with the demands of raising a family and establishing and promoting a career may lead to development of unsafe health practices and reliance on drugs or alcohol. It is possible to modify and change unsafe behaviors, but this requires considerable effort and commitment. The nurse may be directly involved in health education and counseling measures or may suggest resources adult clients can contact for additional support.

The Elderly. Most of the accidents that occur to elderly client are preventable. Falls, fires, and motor vehicle accidents are significant hazards for this age group. Many risk factors for falls (listed earlier in this chapter) apply to the elderly person.

Visual changes and slowed reaction time are realistic concerns affecting the elderly driver. Some become overly cautious, while others are prone to careless responses. Interventions aimed at helping the elderly client drive safely include maintaining the automobile in optimum driving condition, scheduling regular eye examinations, wearing corrective lenses when necessary, and keeping noise from radio and other equipment to a minimum. Some states require additional testing for the elderly client to renew a driving license.

The elderly person is at greater risk of suffering injuries from burns. Confusion, forgetfulness, and diminished visual and olfactory senses are factors. More fires occur in the home, and smoke inhalation is frequently the cause of death. Nursing interventions directed at helping to promote a fire-safe environment for the elderly client at home include admonitions not to smoke in bed, recommendations for installation of a smoke detecting device, and encouragement to wear nonflammable clothing.

Preventing Falls

Major causes of falls in the home include slippery surfaces, poor lighting, clutter, and improperly fitting

3-prong plug adapters with
grounding wire

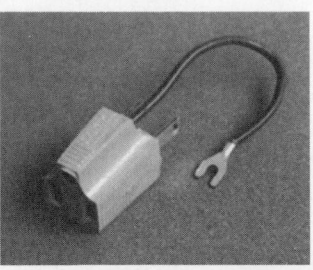

Outlet covers protect curious
tots from electrical shock

All-purpose fire extinguishers
for the home

Smoke detectors for the home

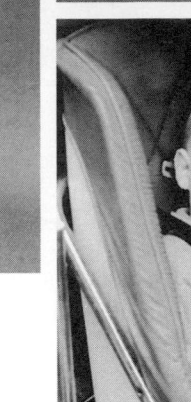

Car seats for infants and
small children

Toddler gates at stairs and
doors

F I G U R E   25-1
*The nurse's responsibility in home safety is primarily that of education and counseling, in-
cluding providing information about home-safety devices and sources for additional information.*

clothing or slippers. The living room, hall, bedroom, and
stairs are the home areas where most falls occur. Measures as simple as hand rails in bathrooms and on stairs,
good lighting, and discarding or repairing broken
equipment about the home will decrease accidents. The
following safety measures are recommended to reduce
the number of falls in acute- and extended-care facilities
(see also Fig. 25-2):

• Thorough orientation to surroundings
• Careful survey of physical surroundings for hazards
• Bed wheels locked and bed in low position
• Call bell and personal articles within client's reach
• Examination of client's footwear
• Use of restraints when necessary.

Side rails, common equipment on agency beds, provide support and aid equilibrium but are especially important for the safety of clients who are likely to be disoriented, restless, confused, or unconscious. When in
doubt about the client's mental status, it is better to err in
the overuse of side rails than to contribute to a situation
that results in a client falling out of bed. A confused
client may attempt to climb over side rails or out the foot
of the bed. The client may fall out of bed or may disturb
tubes, equipment, dressings, or wounds. This may necessitate the use of restraints with raised side rails to
protect the client. An explanation frequently facilitates
cooperation with their use.

Using Restraints.   **Restraints** are devices used to limit
the client's movement in bed. They can be used to restrict the movement of an extremity when an infusion is
running. They are helpful in preventing unconscious or

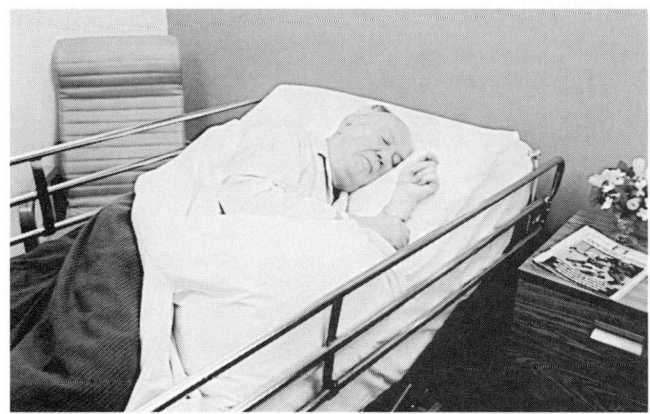

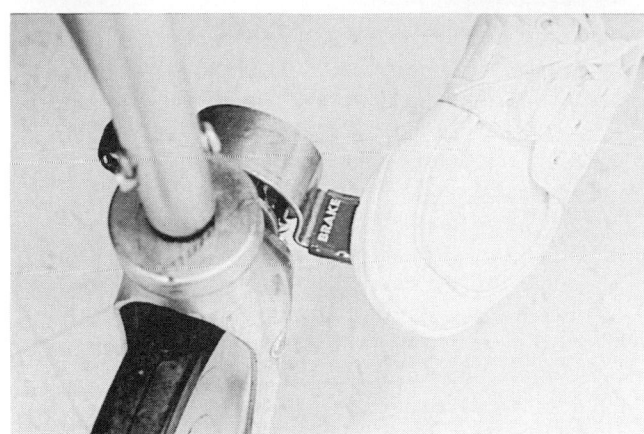

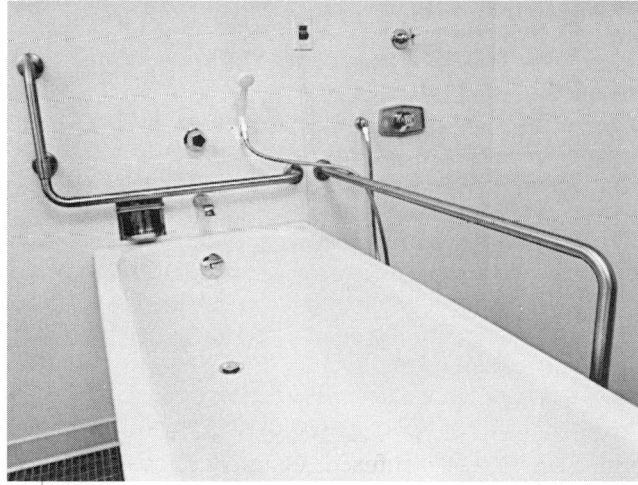

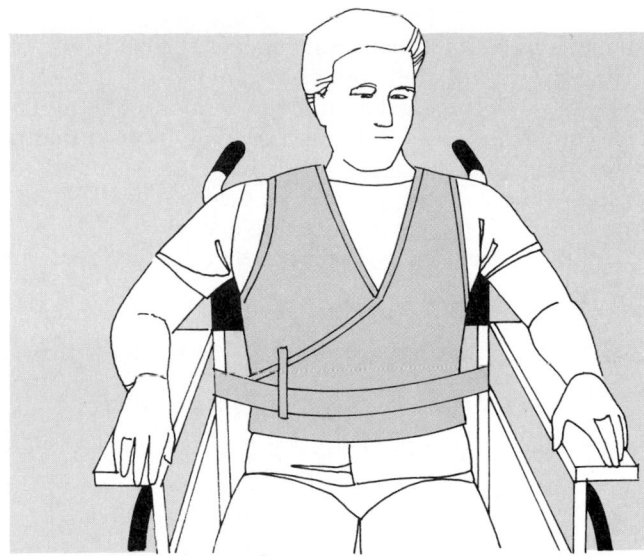

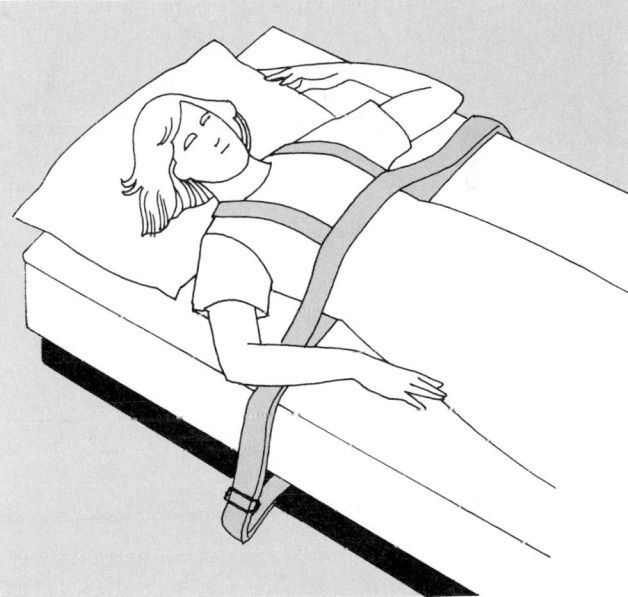

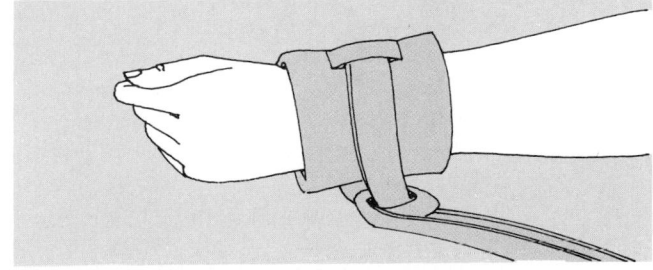

FIGURE 25-2
Side rails on beds, locking devices on wheeled equipment, and hand rails in bath facilities are some of the safety devices used in health-care agencies to prevent falls.

FIGURE 25-3
Restraints that can be adjusted to the specific activity limitation desired are more likely to be accepted by the client and his family. The purpose of restraints is to help prevent the client from being harmed. They should not interfere with physiologic functioning, such as impairing circulation, limiting muscular activity to the point of immobilization, or interfering with respiration.

delerious clients from pulling at wound dressings and tubings leading from the body. They prevent clients who are unsteady and in danger of falling when trying to get out of bed or up from a chair. Figure 25-3 illustrates types of restraints.

It is important to convey to the client and family the reason for the application of restraints by explaining that

it is a protective device and not a punishment measure. Some clients find it helpful to consider the restraint as a reminder to limit their movements. There are some clients who become so fearful and agitated by the use of restraints that the stress induced by their presence is felt to be more detrimental than the movement. The frightened client will often relax and become more comfortable if someone stays and calms him. Quiet talking to even the client who appears to be unaware of surroundings will generally have a soothing effect.

A physician's order is ordinarily required to apply restraints, but some agencies allow nurses to apply them under certain emergency situations. The nurse is advised to consult with appropriate personnel whenever in doubt and to obtain an order at the earliest convenience when using restraints in an emergency. The client should be assessed carefully before applying restraints, and they should be applied with care. See Nursing Guidelines for Applying Restraints.

Nursing Guidelines for Applying Restraints

- Determine if there is need for the restraint. For example, is the client confused and likely to harm himself if not restrained? Is he likely to remove dressings or tubes? Know that nurses can be faulted for applying restraints when there was no need, for applying them incorrectly, and for failing to apply them when needed to ensure the client's safety. Careful documentation should always accompany a decision to restrain a client, to remove restraints, or to use other alternatives to ensure safety.
- Be familiar with the agency policy on the use of restraints. When a physician's order is indicated make sure it is on the client's record.
- Explain to the client and family why restraints are being used. Make every effort to orient the confused client. For example, explain who you are and where he is; provide equipment in his room to help orient him such as a clock and calendar; eliminate unnecessary and monotonous noises as much as possible. Talk quietly and try to calm the frightened and agitated client. Stay with the client as much as possible.
- Apply the restraints with care, according to the manufacturer's directions, so they do not interfere with circulation and respirations:
  1. The restraints should allow the greatest degree of mobility possible without defeating their purpose (*e.g.,* a client may be restrained so he cannot fall out of bed but is still able to turn from side to side).
  2. Pad bony prominences to prevent skin breakdown.
  3. Ensure that the extremity being restrained is in a normal anatomic position.
  4. Use a knot that will not tighten when pulled (*e.g.,* a clove hitch).
  5. Fasten the restraint to a movable part of the bed frame (if the head of the bed is elevated and the restraint is tied to the side rail or to the fixed bed frame, the restraint will pull tightly against the client and may compromise respiration and circulation).

6. Ensure that the restraint can be removed quickly in an emergency.
7. Remove restraints every 2 hours to 4 hours according to agency policy and client need, and assess the skin at this time for signs of decreased circulation (paleness, coolness, decreased sensation, tingling, numbness, pain) or abrasion.
8. When restraints are removed, range-of-motion exercises should be performed to increase circulation in the restrained extremity.
9. Apply restraints as inconspicuously as possible to reduce client and family embarrassment.
10. Take extra time to reassure client and to provide comfort and nursing care. It may be necessary to remove one restraint at a time to provide care.
11. A careful explanation of restraints should be given to the client and the family. Include the purpose of the restraint, how care will be given, and that the use of restraints is usually temporary.
12. Assess for signs of sensory deprivation, such as increased sleeping, day dreaming, anxiety, panic, and hallucinations.

- Documentation should include
  Description of client behavior that led to the decision to use restraints
  Type of restraint used
  Times the restraint was applied and removed
  Frequency of nursing assessment and the type of nursing care given while the restraint was in place
  Client's response to being restrained
- Under no circumstances should the use of restraints be looked on as alleviating the nurse's responsibility to observe the client. These observations are intended to see that the restraints need to be continued, that they are properly placed, and that they are not likely to lead to complications and further health problems.

Preventing Fires and Maintaining Fire Safety

Health-care personnel regard fire as a serious emergency. Careless smoking in bed and faulty electric equipment are most frequently implicated as causes in hospital fires while cigarettes, grease, and electric problems are often responsible for fires in the home.

Home.   The focus of nursing education for home fire safety includes a plan of action similar to one used in a health-care setting. Priorities and practical suggestions include the following:

- Have emergency numbers near the telephone.
- Evacuate family members as soon as smoke or fire is detected.
- Use stairs to exit. Do not use elevator.
- Use a fire extinguisher if one is available and fire is small.
- Close doors to rooms. Open or break window only if necessary to obtain fresh air.
- Remain close to floor because smoke rises.
- Cover nose and mouth with wet washcloth to prevent smoke inhalation.
- Do not run if clothing catches fire. Lie down and roll over to douse flames. Another person may smother flames with an available blanket or coat.
- Have approved smoke detectors installed in recommended locations.
- Rehearse response to fire and fire evacuation routes with family members before an emergency ever occurs.

Health-Care Agency.   Orientations to health-care agencies stress fire prevention information. The nurse is responsible for the client's safety and needs to be familiar with the agency's fire safety plan, exits, location and operation of fire extinguishers, and any special directions to report the fire.

Most hospital procedures emphasize the following priorities:

- Move anyone in immediate danger out of the area first.
- Call for help and activate the fire code system.
- Use the appropriate fire extinguisher on the fire (Fig. 25-4).

Additional activities to safeguard clients include closing all windows and doors, feeling any door for heat before opening, and never using elevators as an escape route during a fire. If a bed-ridden client needs to be moved, try to move the entire bed or carefully transfer him by an evacuation carry. It may be necessary to lower him to a blanket and slide him along the floor toward an exit. Remember that smoke rises so stay near the floor if it is dense. Any oxygen near the vicinity of the fire needs to be discontinued immediately because oxygen supports combustion. A review session after any fire situation may suggest alternate responses to better safeguard clients as well as yourself.

Preventing Poisoning

Concerted efforts by individuals, communities, and state and national governments have reduced the number of accidental deaths by poisoning. Childproof containers are primarily responsible for this reduction.

Nursing intervention involves health education aimed at preventing accidental poisoning in the home. Parents need to be aware of hazardous substances that could result in poisoning if ingested. Plants are frequently implicated as a dangerous poison available in or near the home. Toxic household substances should be removed or stored safely out of a child's reach. Many local poison control centers will provide lists of poisonous substances found in or near the home. Additional suggestions for childproofing homes are listed in the

Household Principles for Prevention of Childhood Poisoning

1. Keep all medications and toxic products in original containers.
2. Keep childproof caps on toxic products if children live in the home or are frequent visitors.
3. Keep all medications, including vitamins, out of the reach of children, in a locked chest.
4. Keep household chemical products out of the reach of children.
5. Do not treat medicines as candy.
6. Do not take or give medicine in the dark.
7. Read labels carefully before using drugs or toxic products.
8. Keep emergency poison control telephone numbers handy.
9. Have emergency drugs in the home—syrup of ipecac and Epsom salts.
10. Use toxic chemical products in a well-ventilated area.
11. Do not mix common household cleaning products.
12. Destroy all old medications.
13. Destroy unused medications by flushing down toilet or washing down sink rather than by throwing in trash.
14. Use childproof containers when available.
15. Identify any poisonous houseplants, and keep seeds, bulbs, leaves, and fruits of such plants away from children.

(Spencer RT et al: Clinical Pharmacology and Nursing Management, 3rd ed. Philadelphia, JB Lippincott, 1989)

Type of Extinguisher \ Type of Fire	Class "A" Fire in wood, paper, rags and extinguished by reducing the heat.	Class "B" Fire in flammable liquids, etc. Best extinguished by blanketing or smothering action. Fast spreading fire.	Class "C" Fire in energized electrical equipment. Smothering with a nonconducting extinguishing agent is of prime importance. Never use water or solutions with water.
Pressurized Water	**YES** Water soaks burning material and prevents rekindling.	**NO** Water will spread fire. Causes grease to splatter.	**NO** Water conducts electricity.
Carbon Dioxide (CO_2)	**NO** Has limited range. For small surface fires only.	**YES** Carbon dioxide smothers flames. Does not affect equipment or food.	**YES** Carbon dioxide is a non-conductor. Does not damage equipment.
Dry Chemical	**NO** Has limited range. For small surface fires only.	**YES** Chemical absorbs heat and smothers the flames.	**YES** Chemical is a non-conductor.
All Purpose	**YES** Coats material with a fire-retardant blanket to prevent reflash.	**YES** Covers fire with fast, flame-choking smothering action.	**YES** Chemical is a non-conductor.

F I G U R E   25-4
Chart detailing appropriate fire extinguisher usage for specific types of fires.

box. The nurse may counsel parents and children to affix warning labels such as "Mr. Yuk" on any potentially poisonous household product (see Fig. 25-5).

It is vital that every household have the telephone number of the nearest poison control center available should a poisoning emergency occur. The nurse should emphasize to parents that calling the poison control center must be the first priority before attempting any home remedy. Parents may be instructed to induce vomiting with syrup of ipecac or instructed to bring the child immediately to an emergency facility for treatment. The focus of emergency treatment of poisoning is to stabilize vital bodily functions, prevent the absorption of the poison, and encourage excretion of the toxic substance.

Preventing Suffocation

Suffocation, or asphyxiation, is the stoppage of breathing or the lack of air reaching the lungs. Unconsciousness results almost immediately, followed by respiratory and cardiac arrest. Emergency measures are necessary immediately and involve removing any obstruction and initiating cardiopulmonary resuscitation (see Procedures 34-6, 34-7, and 34-8).

The educated, aware parent can decrease the risk of suffocation occurring in the home. The nurse may be involved in child care instruction that emphasizes careful supervision of children when they are drinking from a bottle, eating, bathing, or playing near a swimming

chair wheels can result in client injury. Using suction devices with inadequate vacuum and rate regulators or infusion equipment that delivers erratic amounts of solution have also resulted in equipment-related accidents.

Electric equipment can present a particular safety hazard to both clients and health practitioners when safety measures are ignored. Most electric equipment used in hospitals is equipped with three-prong plugs. The third prong, when inserted into a properly wired wall outlet, provides a ground for the piece of equipment. A **ground** is a connection from an electricity source to the earth through which electric current leakage can be harmlessly conducted. Current leakage is not uncommon in electric equipment, but a grounding system renders the equipment safe.

Most persons have experienced a tingling sensation in the extremities and trunk resulting from an electric current passing through a relatively large area of the body. This is known as **macroshock**, and while unpleasant, it is usually not harmful. Macroshock often results from an ungrounded appliance or one in which the electric wiring has been damaged.

Microshock is the transmission of an electric current through a relatively small area of the body, usually directly into the heart. Because of the sensitivity of the myocardium to electric impulses, microshock can cause serious or even fatal heart irregularities. Persons with tubes, wires, or electrodes implanted in the chest or heart are susceptible to microshock dangers because the

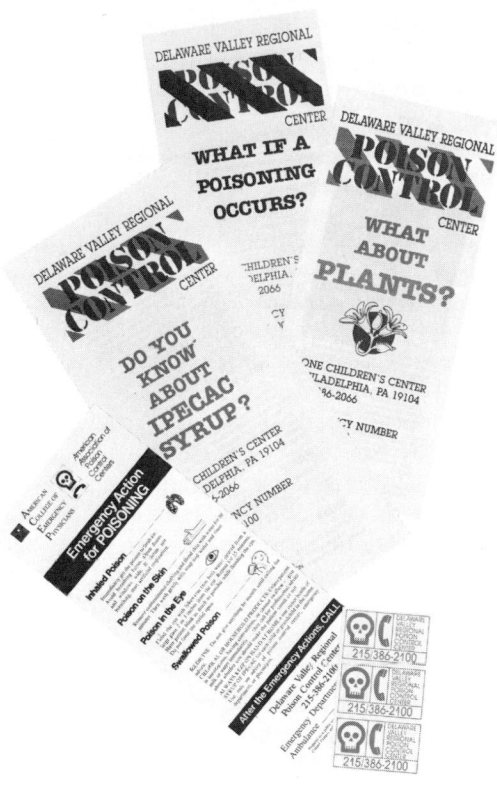

F I G U R E   25-5
Most local poison control centers provide printed information on poison control in and around the home. Educational packets may include emergency action instructions in the event of a poisoning and stickers of the control center phone number to be pasted on or near the phone. The nurse should be aware of such community services and alert clients to their availability and usefulness. (Courtesy of Delaware Valley Regional Poison Control Center)

pool. When traveling in a motor vehicle, a child less than 55 inches tall needs to be restrained in the appropriate car seat rather than using an adult seat belt and shoulder harness which can slip with impact and cause neck injury. Health education is a valuable preventive force.

Preventing Equipment-Related Accidents

With the marked increase of highly sophisticated equipment, it is especially important for health practitioners to learn to use equipment properly and to know how to recognize signs that indicate the equipment is not functioning correctly. For example, failure to use protective belts or side rails on carts and neglecting to lock wheel-

Guidelines To Help Decrease Equipment-Related Accidents

- Use equipment only for the use for which it was intended.
- Do not operate equipment with which you are unfamiliar.
- Handle equipment with care to prevent damaging it.
- Use three-prong electric plugs whenever possible.
- Do not twist or bend electric cords. The wires inside the cord may break.
- Be alert to signs that indicate equipment is faulty, such as breaks in electric cords, sparks, smoke, electric shocks, loose or missing parts, and unusual noises or odors. Report signs of trouble immediately.
- Make certain that electric cords are not in a position to be trapped as beds are raised or lowered. This can strip insulation covering the electric wires.
- Be alert for wet surfaces on areas where electric cords or connections are present.

tubing or wire can conduct leakage electricity directly to the heart muscle. Particularly because of microshock dangers, only equipment with three-prong plugs is recommended for use in health-care agencies. Suspicion of ungrounded current leakage, including even a slight tingling sensation when touching a piece of equipment, or any other malfunction of electric equipment should be reported immediately.

Accidents in the home frequently result from using equipment carelessly or using malfunctioning or poorly maintained equipment. Many injuries and accidental deaths from electric shock can be avoided. Overload of electric circuits, faulty appliances, frayed wires, careless use of electric equipment, and handling of electric devices and cords when shoes and hands are wet often result in injury and death. The box on page 499 lists guidelines to help decrease equipment-related accidents.

Preventing Procedure-Related Accidents

The nurse must always be cautious and alert when caring for clients to prevent a procedure-related accident. The potential for an error exists when the nurse is administering medications or intravenous solutions, transferring a client, changing a dressing, or applying external heat to a client's extremity. It is vital that the nurse follow correct procedures when administering care. Safeguards to prevent errors include careful attention to ensure the client is always identified properly (Fig. 25-6). A system of checking and rechecking further assures safety. The availability and use of resources further corroborate any question about correct procedure and prevent procedure-related accidents.

Filing An Incident Report

An accident in a health-care agency requires the completion of an **incident report**, a confidential document that objectively describes the circumstances of the accident. The report also provides detail concerning the client's response and the examination and treatment of the client after the incident. The nurse completes the incident report immediately following an accident and is also responsible for recording the occurrence of the accident and its effect on the client in the medical record.

All incident reports are reviewed carefully to detect any potentially threatening situation or pattern. The focus of a conference after the incident report has been filed is prevention of a similar occurrence and continuation of efforts to deliver quality nursing care. Chapter 6 discusses incident reports in greater detail.

Transferring the Client

Transferring Within the Agency. Clients may be transferred within an agency. After diagnostic procedures, a client may be transferred from a medical unit to a surgical unit. A client's condition may dictate transfer to a special care unit, such as a coronary care unit. Conversely, the client may be well enough to transfer from a special care unit to a general unit. A client who has been admitted to a semiprivate room may be transferred to a private room. Whatever the reason for moving the client,

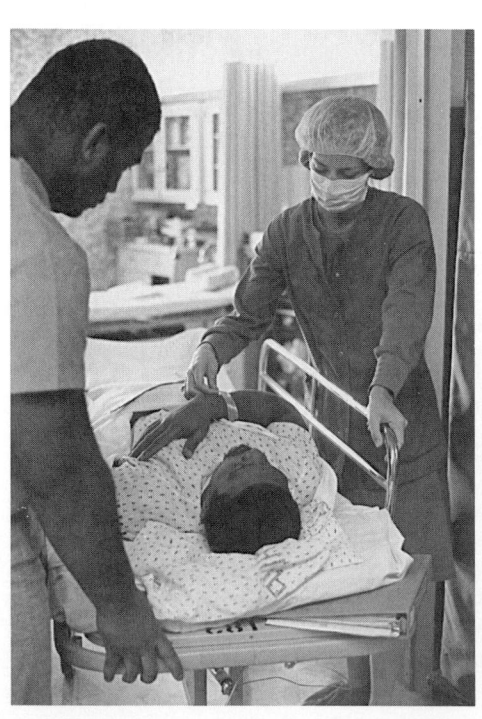
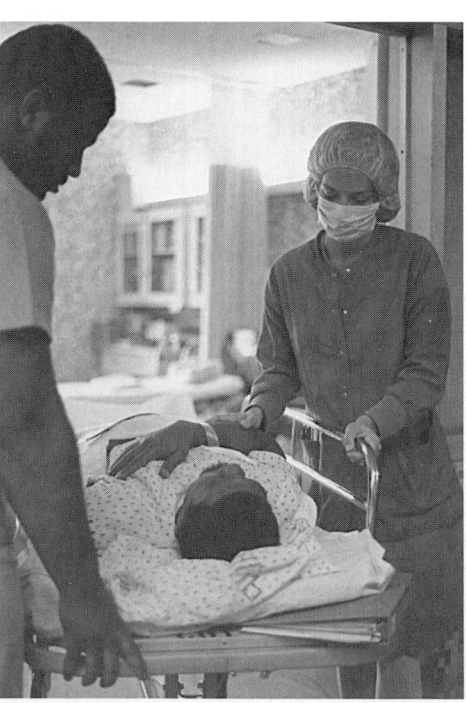

F I G U R E   25-6
Safeguards to prevent procedure-related accidents are based on a system of checking and rechecking. Careful attention should be paid to identifying the patient properly, checking or communicating necessary client records, and preparing the client physically and psychologically for any procedure or transfer. (Photo by Gates Rhodes, courtesy of the School of Nursing, University of Pennsylvania)

the procedures for transferring the client are similar to those for discharge, except that a visit to the business office is not required. (Discharge is discussed in Chap 26.)

The client should be prepared both physically and psychologically for the transfer. If he has not requested the transfer himself, he should be told why he is being moved and where he is going. If at all possible, nursing personnel from the new unit should visit the client prior to the transfer.

Admission of the client to the new unit should include the same basic procedures as for the admission of any new client. (Admission procedures are discussed in Chap 26.) The transfer may be traumatic for some clients. For example, the client who has been accustomed to the security of cardiac monitoring and constant surveillance may feel anxious when the equipment is no longer being used and he is transferred to a less acute care unit. Certain recommended techniques help make the transfer of the client from one unit to another as comfortable as possible:

- Explain about equipment and procedures that may be different in the unit to which the client is being transferred.
- Introduce the client to new nursing personnel and allow him to visit the new surroundings, if possible.
- Orient the client to the new surroundings.
- Make sure family members and friends are notified of the client's transfer.
- To provide continuity, review the client's previous hospital record with nurses taking over responsibility for his care.
- Alert staff on new unit to any special safety precautions that need to be incorporated into the client's plan of care.

Transferring to Another Agency. The nurse should be sure that all arrangements have been made when the client is being transferred to another agency, such as a nursing home. The discharge order is written by the physician, and procedures are the same as when the client is discharged to his home. If the client is leaving the hospital in an ambulance, arrangements should be made concerning the time the client will be ready to leave. Financial arrangements are made in the same manner as for any other discharge.

Evaluating

The nurse must evaluate the effectiveness of interventions to promote environmental safety and prevent injury. If client goals have been met and evaluative criteria have been satisfied, the client will

- Correctly identify real and potential unsafe environmental situations
- Implement safety measures in his environment
- Use available resources for safety information
- Incorporate accident prevention practices into his activities of daily living.

INFECTION: PREVENTION AND CONTROL

In addition to environmental safety, a major concern of health practitioners is the danger of spreading microorganisms from person to person and from place to place. Microorganisms are naturally present in the environment. Some are beneficial and some are not. Some are harmless to most people, and others are harmful to many persons. Still others are harmless except in certain circumstances.

The efforts of many persons are involved in maintaining a microorganism-safe environment. Government agencies at the international, national, state, and local levels; health personnel; citizens from every walk of life; and family members are all involved in making and keeping the environment as free from harmful organisms as possible. Such efforts include mass immunization programs, laws concerning safe sewage disposal, regulations for the control of communicable diseases, hospital infection-surveillance programs, and so on. As medical science continues to grapple with increasingly virulent organisms and immunologically compromised hosts, prevention of infection becomes a major focus for the nurse. As the primary caregiver, the nurse needs to be involved in identifying, preventing, controlling, and teaching the client about infection. Consistent application of the nursing process can prove critical in breaking the chain of infection.

Infection Cycle

An **infection** is a disease state resulting from the presence of pathogens in or on the body. A **pathogen** is a disease-producing microorganism. An infection occurs as a result of a cyclical process as illustrated in Figure 25-7. The six components in the infection cycle are

- Infectious agent
- Reservoir
- Portal of exit
- Vehicle of transmission
- Portal of entry
- Susceptible host

Infectious Agent. Agents capable of causing infection include bacteria, fungi, viruses, and yeast. Bacteria are the most significant and most commonly observed agents causing infections in health-care institutions. An organism's potential to produce disease depends on a variety of factors including

- Number of organisms
- **Virulence** of the organism or its ability to cause disease

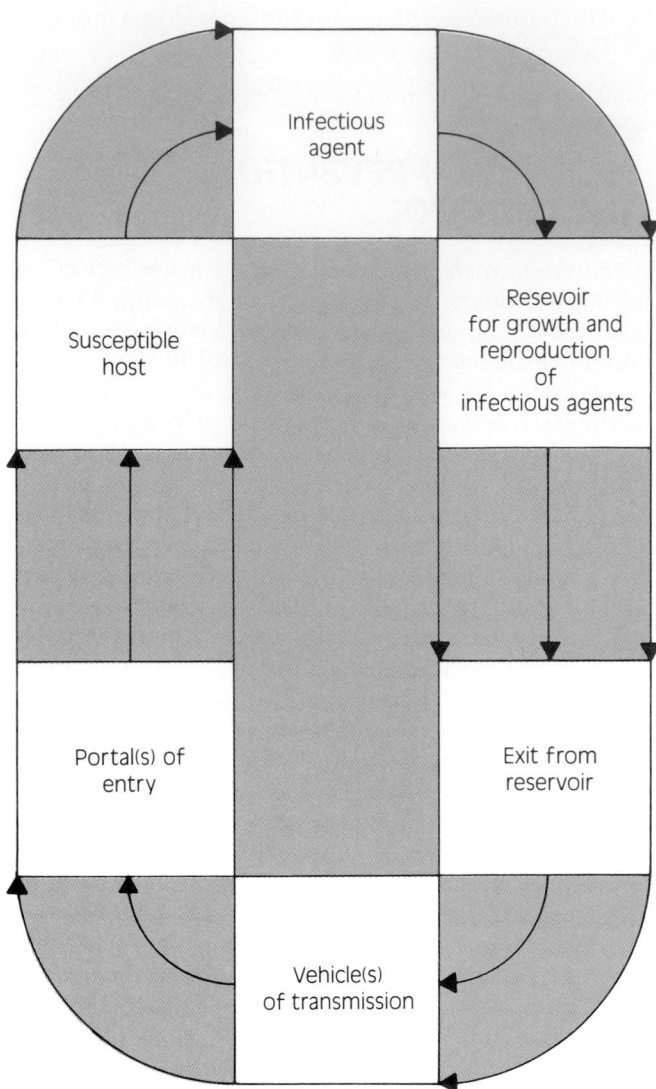

F I G U R E   25-7
Infection process cycle. An infection occurs as a result of interrelated factors. An infection will not develop if the sequence is interrupted. Hence efforts to control infections are directed toward interrupting the sequence.

- Competence of a person's immune system
- Length and intimacy of the contact between an individual and the microorganism.

Under normal conditions an organism may not produce disease. Other factors may intervene and cause this relatively harmless organism, which normally resides in, or **colonizes,** various tissue and organ systems, to become the source of an infection. Microorganisms that normally inhabit various body sites and are part of the body's natural defense system are referred to as **normal flora** (see Table 25-5). For example, *Escherichia coli,* which normally resides in the intestinal tract, may produce infection when it migrates into the urinary tract.

Reservoir.   The **reservoir** for growth and multiplication of microorganisms is the natural habitat of the organism.

Possible reservoirs that support organisms pathogenic to humans include other humans and animals, as well as food, water, milk, and inanimate objects.

Other Humans.   The tubercle bacillus and the spirochete causing syphilis are examples of pathogens whose reservoirs are inhabited by the infectious agent and exhibit symptoms of disease while others are **carriers** of the disease but do not show any symptoms of illness. For example, an individual who has tested positive after an HIV antibody test most likely has been infected with HIV. Even though symptoms of AIDS may not be present, it is believed the virus may be transmitted by intimate sexual contact, sharing a contaminated needle and syringe, transfusion with contaminated blood or blood products, and from an infected mother to child during pregnancy or birth. The individul's own normal flora can serve as a reservoir of pathogens.

Animals.   The rabies virus is an example of a pathogen whose reservoir is various animals, notably dogs, squirrels, and raccoons.

Soil.   Organisms causing gas gangrene and tetanus are examples of pathogens whose reservoir is soil.

Portal of Exit.   The **exit from the reservoir** is the point of escape for the organism. The organism cannot extend its influence unless it moves away from its original source. Most often, there is a primary exit route for each type of microorganism. In humans, common escape routes are the respiratory, gastrointestinal, and genitourinary tracts, as well as breaks in the skin. Blood and tissue can also serve as an exit for pathogens.

Vehicle of Transmission.   Various **vehicles** act as means for transmitting organisms from one place to another. Organisms can enter the body by direct contact such as touching, kissing, or sexual intercourse. Contaminated food, water, or inanimate objects (**fomites**) can be vehicles of transmission. **Vectors,** such as mosquitoes, ticks, and lice can transmit organisms. Microorganisms can also be spread by droplet nuclei via coughing, sneezing, and talking or by becoming attached to dust particles. This is known as the airborne mode of transmission. Table 25-6 presents a summary of the vehicles of transmission and examples of diseases they transmit.

Portal of Entry.   The organism must find a portal of entry on a host. The **portal of entry** is the point at which organisms enter a host. The entry route is often, though not exclusively, the same as the exit route. The urinary, respiratory, and gastrointestinal tracts and the skin are common entry points.

Susceptible Host.   For microorganisms to continue to exist, they must find a source that is acceptable (a **host**)

T A B L E 25-5
System-by-System Guide to Infection Detection

System	Normal Flora	Common Signs and Symptoms	Laboratory Data	Special Considerations
Gastrointestinal tract	Esophagus: anaerobes *Corynebacterium* (except *C. diphtheriae*), *Diplococcus pneumoniae, Hemophilus, Klebsiella, Neisseria, Proteus, Staphylococcus epidermidis, Streptococcus,* yeasts Stomach: sterile Large intestine: anaerobes, *Enterobacteriaceae,* enterococci, *Klebsiella, Lactobacillus, Proteus, Pseudomonas,* yeasts Small intestine: anaerobes, *Lactobacillus, Streptococcus*	Diarrhea, watery or purulent stools Severe abdominal pain Nausea and vomiting	Stool culture showing known pathogen, such as *Staphylococcus aureus,* enteropathogenic *E. coli,* Salmonella, or *Shigella* Polymorphonuclear leukocytes on Gram's stain Stool specimen may show parasites.	Handle bedpans as contaminated.
Upper respiratory tract	Nose: *Corynebacterium* (except *C. diphtheriae*), *D. pneumoniae, Hemophilus, Klebsiella, Neisseria, Proteus, Staphylococcus epidermidis, Streptococcus* Mouth: anaerobes, *Hemophilus, Staphylococcus epidermidis, Streptococcus,* yeasts Throat: *Corynebacterium* (except *C. diphtheriae*), *E. coli, Hemophilus influenzae, Hemophilus parainfluenzae, Mycoplasma pneumoniae, Neisseria*	Sneezing Watery discharge from nose Malaise Sore throat Throat abscesses	Data are difficult to obtain because most organisms are viruses or have uncertain origins.	Wear gloves when handling drainage. Advise patient to cover nose and mouth when sneezing or coughing.
Lower respiratory tract	Trachea: normally sterile Bronchi: normally sterile Lungs: normally sterile	Cough Pleuritic chest pain Fever Rales Dullness Purulence	Chest x-ray showing infiltration Sputum culture showing *D. pneumoniae,* beta-hemolytic streptococci, *E. coli, Proteus, Pseudomonas, Staphylococcus aureus, Enterobacteri, Serratia* Polymorphonuclear leukocytes on Gram's stain	Must rule out congestive heart failure, postoperative atelectasis and pulmonary embolism. Wear gloves on both hands when suctioning. Restrict respiratory equipment for this patient's exclusive use. Mark equipment as contaminated and send it for processing. Deterioration of patient's condition may indicate superinfection.
Urinary tract	Urethra: *Corynebacterium* (except *C. diphtheriae*), enterococci, *E. coli, Lactobacillus, Mycobacterium smegmatis, Mycoplasma, Proteus,* sporophytic yeasts, *Spirochaeta, Staphylococcus, Streptococcus*	Fever Dysuria Frequent urination Tenderness over costovertebral angle Suprapubic tenderness	Colony count greater than 100,000 microorganisms per ml Consistent isolation of 10,000 or more microorganisms per ml in a random clean-catch specimen or specimen from catheter	When handling a Foley catheter bag from a colonized or infected patient, wear gloves or wash your hands scrupulously afterward.

(Continued)

T A B L E   25-5
System-by-System Guide to Infection Detection   (Continued)

System	Normal Flora	Common Signs and Symptoms	Laboratory Data	Special Considerations
Skin	C. albicans, Corynebacterium (except C. diphtheriae), Enterobacteriaceae, enterococci, E. coli, Klebsiella, Proprionibacterium, Proteus, Staphylococcus aureus, Staphylococcus epidermidis, Streptococcus	Purulence Redness Edema Pain Rash	Positive culture Polymorphonuclear leukocytes on Gram's stain	Wear gloves or use instruments to handle dressings. Before inserting an IV line, clean the site scrupulously. Keep the site clean. Rotate the site every 48 hr to 72 hr.

(Jones I: You can drive back infection . . . if you know where to make your stand. Nursing '85 4:50–52, 1985; reprinted with permission)

T A B L E   25-6
Vehicles of Transmission

Route	Means	Disease
Contact	*Direct*—Person to person involving close proximity	Staphylococcal infection Gonorrhea or syphilis Herpes simplex virus
	Indirect—Personal contact with inanimate contaminated object	Measles Hepatitis B
Vehicle	Water (usually fecal contamination)	Cholera, typhoid
	Blood	Hepatitis B and non-A, non-b HIV
	Food (contaminated by improper handling or storing)	Salmonellosis Staphylococcus gastroenteritis
	Medicines, drugs	Pseudomonas
Air	Droplet nuclei—Dried droplets of secretions or excretions suspended in the air and disseminated by air currents	Chickenpox Diphtheria Influenza Tuberculosis
	Dust	Aspergillosis
Vectors	Insects—Mosquitos, fleas, ticks, lice, and mites	Malaria Bubonic plague Rocky Mountain spotted fever
	Animals—Cows, pigs	Brucellosis

(Adapted from Hargiss CO: Nurs Clin North Am 15(4):673, 1980)

and overcome any resistance mounted by the host's defenses. **Susceptibility** is the degree of resistance the potential host has to the pathogen. It is not uncommon for a person admitted to a hospital to be in a weakened state of health due to illness. Many factors influence a host's susceptibility and are discussed later in the chapter.

Stages of Infection

An understanding of the stages in the development of an infection is necessary if the nurse is to intervene and disrupt the infection cycle. An infection progresses through the following phases:

- Incubation period
- Prodromal stage
- Full stage of illness
- Convalescent period

The course and severity of the infection as well as the client's response influence the extent and type of nursing care provided.

Incubation Period. The **incubation period** is the interval between the invasion of the body by the pathogen and the appearance of symptoms of infection. During this stage the organisms are growing and multiplying, and the length of incubation may vary. For example, the common cold develops in 1 to 2 days whereas tetanus has an incubation period ranging from 2 to 21 days.

Prodromal Stage. A person is most infectious during the **prodromal stage.** Early signs and symptoms of disease are present but are vague and nonspecific ranging from fatigue and malaise to a low-grade fever. This period lasts from several hours to several days at the most.

Full Stage of Illness. The presence of specific signs and symptoms indicates the **full stage of illness.** The type of infection determines the length of the illness and the severity of the manifestations. Symptoms that are limited or restricted to a discrete area are referred to as **localized symptoms** while **systemic symptoms** are manifested throughout the entire body.

Convalescent Period. The **convalescent period** represents recovery from the infection. The signs and symptoms disappear, and the person returns to a healthy state. Convalescence may vary according to the severity of the infection and the client's general condition.

Body's Defense Against Infection

In addition to the normal flora that inhabit various body sites (see Table 25-5 and discussion on handwashing later in this chapter), other defense systems help the individual combat infection.

The **inflammatory response** is a protective mechanism that eliminates the invading pathogen and allows for tissue repair to occur. The inflammation process is discussed in detail in Chapter 42.

The **immune response** involves specific reactions in the body as it responds to an invading foreign protein such as bacteria, or even in some cases, the body's own proteins. The complex mechanisms that comprise the immune response occur as the body attempts to protect and defend itself. The foreign material is called an **antigen**, and the body commonly responds to the antigen by producing an **antibody**. This antigen–antibody reaction is one component of the overall immune response and is also known as humoral immunity. The cell-mediated defense, or cellular immunity, involves an increase in the number of lymphocytes (a white blood cell) for the pur-

pose of destroying or reacting specifically with cells the body recognizes as harmful. Although not completely understood, it is known that these complicated chemical and mechanical responses help defend the body specifically against bacterial, viral, and fungal infections as well as malignant cells.

Factors Affecting Risk of Infection

The susceptibility of the host is influenced by a variety of factors including

- Intact skin and mucous membranes protect the body against microbial invasion.
- The normal *p*H levels of gastric secretions and of the genitourinary tract help ward off microbial invasion.
- The body's white blood cells influence resistance to certain pathogens.
- Age, sex, race, and hereditary factors have been shown to influence susceptibility, although reasons are not always entirely clear. Newborns and elderly persons appear to be more vulnerable to infection.
- Immunization, natural or acquired, acts to resist infection.
- Fatigue, climate, nutritional and general health status, the presence of preexisting illnesses, previous or current treatments, and some kinds of medications may play a part in the susceptibility of a potential host.
- Stress may adversely affect the body's normal defense mechanisms.
- The increasing use of invasive or indwelling medical devices is providing more potential sources of disease-producing organisms, particularly in a client whose defenses are already weakened by disease.

Terminology in Infection Control

A knowledge of certain terms, described in Table 25-7, is necessary to understanding basic concepts of infection control.

Asepsis. The nurse uses principles of aseptic technique to halt the spread of microorganisms and minimize the threat of infection. To control the number of organisms, medical and surgical asepsis are vital. The practice of **asepsis** includes any activities that prevent infection or break the chain of infection and is divided into two types: medical asepsis and surgical asepsis. **Medical asepsis,** or clean technique, involves procedures and practices that reduce the number and transfer of pathogens. **Surgical asepsis,** or sterile technique, includes practices used to render and keep objects and areas free from microorganisms.

Several processes are used to destroy microorganisms. **Disinfection** destroys all pathogenic organisms except spores while **sterilization** is the process by which all

T A B L E   25-7
Terms Commonly Used to Describe Medical and Surgical Asepsis, Sterilization, and Disinfection

Term	Description
Asepsis	The absence of disease-producing microorganisms; being free of infection
Pathogen	A disease-producing microorganism
Nonpathogen	A microorganism that does not normally cause disease
Host	An animal or person upon which or within which microorganisms live
Medical asepsis	Practices designed to reduce the number and transfer of pathogens: also called *clean technique*
Surgical asepsis	Practices that render and keep objects and areas free of microorganisms: also called *sterile technique*
Isolation technique	Practices designed to prevent the transmission of microorganisms
Contamination	Process by which something is rendered unclean or unsterile
Disinfection	Process by which pathogens, but not necessarily spores, are destroyed
Disinfectant	Substance, usually intended for use on inanimate objects, that destroys pathogens but generally not spores
Antiseptic	Substance, usually intended for use on persons, that inhibits the growth of pathogens but does not necessarily destroy them
Bactericide	Substance that destroys bacteria but not necessarily spores: also called a *germicide*. A *fungicide* destroys fungi; a *virucide* destroys viruses.
Sterilization	Process by which all microorganisms, including spores, are destroyed

microorganisms, including spores, are destroyed. Disinfection and sterilization of contaminated or infected objects and good handwashing diminish and often eliminate microorganisms as potential sources of infection.

Nosocomial Infections.   For a variety of reasons and sometimes despite best efforts, certain clients in health agencies develop infections that were not noted to be present upon admission. The term **nosocomial** is used to describe a hospital-acquired infection. In its broad meaning, nosocomial means that the infection results while the client is receiving health care, and the source may be either exogenous or endogenous. An **exogenous** infection means the causative organism is acquired from other persons while an **endogenous** infection means the causative organism comes from microbial life the person himself harbors. An infection is referred to as **iatrogenic** when it occurs as a result of a treatment or diagnostic procedure. Not all nosocomial infections have an iatrogenic component.

Most hospital-acquired infections are caused by bacteria. According to 1983 statistics from the Centers for Disease Control, urinary tract infections, surgical wound infections, and pneumonia are the most common nosocomial infections. Streptococci, staphylococci, and multiresistant strains of gram-negative organisms have previously been implicated as common causative organisms. The increasing use of biomedical equipment is responsible for 42% of nosocomial infections since 1975 (Gillis, 1984). The devices most often implicated include urinary catheters, pressure monitoring lines, hemodialysis equipment, and respiratory equipment. Often the hands of the person using the instruments are responsible for the contamination.

Nosocomial infections will continue to be a problem. The increasing technologic emphasis and the population of immunosuppressed patients present many challenges to the medical and nursing professions. Health agencies have found the following measures to be successful in reducing the incidence of nosocomial infections:

- Constant surveillance by infection-control committees and nurse epidemiologists. These committees and nurses are charged with the responsibility of studying nosocomial infections closely so that precise information is obtained concerning the who, what, where, and why of hospital-acquired infections. Their work has been noted to reduce infections significantly when better control measures resulting from their findings are initiated.
- Having written guidelines for health personnel to observe when caring for clients with infections. Typical guidelines are described later in this chapter. When health personnel are well-acquainted with these guidelines and follow them precisely, nosocomial infections have been observed to decrease.
- Using practices to help promote and keep clients in the best possible physical condition. Measures include meeting the client's needs for nutrition, fluids, rest, oxygen, and physical and psychologic comfort and security.
- Following techniques of medical and surgical asepsis with precision. This measure includes the strict observance of isolation techniques required by a client and of practices of asepsis for all clients. Using careful techniques is of special importance when introducing a catheter into the urinary system, maintaining urinary drainage with an indwelling catheter, giving wound care, using intravenous therapy, and introducing and suctioning tubes used to support respiratory functioning.

The cost of nosocomial infections is estimated to be millions of dollars each year (US Department of Health and Human Services, 1983). The Centers for Disease Control (CDC) recently completed a 12-year nationwide study in an effort to produce infection-control guidelines to reduce incidence of infection and produce considerable financial savings for hospitals. The study concluded that a hospital infection-control program should include

- Intensive epidemiologic surveillance with feedback to hospital staff members
- Intensive intervention and control activities to reduce or eliminate identified risk factors
- A full-time infection control nurse per 250 occupied hospital beds
- A physician with special training in infection control to act as a full or part-time infection control advisor to the medical staff

Implementation of these recommendations resulted in a 32% decrease in infections while hospitals not using these strategies averaged an 18% increase (Haley, 1985). Diligence in observing techniques described in this chapter will help reduce infections, as well as much unnecessary suffering imposed on clients.

Assessing

The nurse's critical role in controlling infection begins with early detection and surveillance techniques. The extent of the nursing interventions is determined by the susceptibility of the host and the virulence of the organism as well as the client's signs and symptoms.

To formulate an individualized nursing care plan, the nurse inquires about the client's immunization status and previous or reoccurring infections, observes nonverbal cues, and elicits information regarding the history of the current disease process. (See Chap 42 for a detailed description of signs and symptoms of an infection.) A review of laboratory data provides further insights into the presence of an infectious process. This compilation of assessment data comprises a unique nursing data base which suggests nursing interventions for those at risk of infection or those clients in whom an infection is already present.

Diagnosing

The potential for infection or the actual presence of an infection in a client suggest possible nursing diagnoses. The direction or focus of nursing care depends on a nursing diagnosis that accurately reflects the client's condition.

Examples of nursing diagnoses that relate to an infectious process are the following:

Potential for infection related to presence of chronic disease; altered immune response; effects of medication; altered skin integrity; malnutrition; presence of invasive or indwelling medical device; lack of proper immunization

Social isolation related to presence of communicable disease

Altered oral mucous membranes related to ineffective dental hygiene; trauma

Diversional activity deficit related to lack of visitors; restrictions imposed by isolation precautions

Planning: Client Goals

Effective nursing interventions can control or prevent infection. The nurse reviews the assessment data, considers the cycle of events that result in the development of an infection, and incorporates principles of infection control as client goals are formulated. Planning client goals that prevent infection or interfere with the infection cycle provides an exciting challenge for the nurse and an opportunity to see positive results because of these efforts.

The following client goals are appropriate to prevent infection:

Client will demonstrate effective handwashing.
Client will identify the signs of an infection.
Client will maintain adequate nutritional intake.
Client will demonstrate proper disposal of soiled articles.
Client will use appropriate cleansing and disinfecting techniques.
Client will demonstrate an awareness of the necessity of proper immunizations.
Client will use stress reduction techniques.

Implementing

Using Medical Asepsis

Medical asepsis is used continuously both within and outside health agencies because it is always assumed that pathogens are likely to be present. For example, public drinking cups are unsanitary because pathogens may be present on the cup after being used by someone who is possibly harboring pathogens. In a health-care facility, if a specific pathogen is known to be present, special methods of medical asepsis are used to isolate and pre-vent further spread of the organism. Nearly every nursing activity includes practices of medical asepsis. Breaking the chain of infection is the nurse's responsibility. It involves giving safe client care and protecting the client as well as one's self from microorganisms that have at least the potential to cause disease. See the boxed material for basic practices of medical asepsis nurses should use when giving care to clients.

Teaching Asepsis to Clients. Clients should be taught to use basic principles of asepsis at home and in public facilities. These involve activities of daily living (refer to Chap 27 for discussion of personal hygiene). The following are typical examples of medical asepsis practices recommended in the home:

- Wash hands before preparing food and before eating.
- Prepare foods at temperatures sufficiently high to ensure they are safe to eat, the most common example being the preparation of fresh pork.
- Use care with cutting boards and utensils and wash hands before and after handling raw chicken.
- Keep foods refrigerated, especially those containing mayonnaise.
- Wash raw fruits and vegetables before serving them.

Basic Practices of Medical Asepsis in Client Care

- Wash hands frequently but especially before handling foods, before eating, after using a handkerchief, after going to the toilet, and before and after each client contact.
- Keep soiled items and equipment from touching the clothing. Carry soiled linens or other used articles so that they do not touch the uniform.
- Do not place soiled bed linen or any other items on the floor, which is grossly contaminated. It increases contamination of both surfaces.
- Avoid having clients cough, sneeze, or breathe directly on others. Provide them with disposable tissues, and instruct them, as indicated, to cover their mouth and nose to prevent spread by airborne droplets.
- Move equipment away from you when brushing, dusting, or scrubbing articles. This helps prevent contaminated particles from settling on the hair, face, and uniform.
- Avoid raising dust. Use a specially treated cloth or a dampened cloth. Do not shake linens. Dust and lint particles constitute a vehicle by which organisms may be transported from one area to another.
- Clean the least soiled areas first and then the more soiled ones. This helps prevent having the cleaner areas soiled by the dirtier areas.
- Dispose of soiled or used items directly into appropriate containers. Wrap items that are moist from body discharge or drainage in waterproof containers, such as plastic bags, before discarding into the refuse holder so that handlers will not come in contact with them.
- Pour liquids that are to be discarded, such as bath water, mouth rinse, and the like, directly into the drain so as to avoid splatterings in the sink and onto you.
- Sterilize items that are suspected of containing pathogens. Following sterilization, they can be managed as clean items, if appropriate.
- Use practices of personal grooming that help prevent spreading microorganisms. Examples include shampooing the hair regularly, keeping it short or pinned up to limit the possibility of carrying microorganisms on hair shafts, keeping the fingernails short and free of broken cuticles and ragged nail edges, and avoiding wearing rings with grooves and stones that may harbor microorganisms.
- Follow guidelines conscientiously for isolation technique as prescribed by agency.

- Use pasteurized milk.
- Wash hands after using the bathroom.
- Use individual personal care items, such as washcloths, towels, and toothbrushes.

Observe infection prevention in public facilities by following these guidelines:

- Wash hands after using any public bathroom.
- Use paper towels or hot air dryers in restrooms.
- Use individually wrapped drinking straws.
- Use tongs to lift food from common service trays in cafeterias, food stores, or salad bars.

The community reinforces medical asepsis practices in a variety of ways, including

- Use of sterilized combs and brushes in barber and beauty shops
- Examination of food handlers for evidence of disease
- Enforcement of frequent handwashing by food handlers

Handwashing. *Handwashing is, without a doubt, the single most effective way to help prevent the spread of organisms.* Differences of opinion persist about proper cleaning agents, length of time, and ideal frequency of adequate handwashing, but everyone agrees that handwashing is the most important procedure in the prevention of nosocomial, or hospital-acquired, infections. Attention needs to be refocused on this simple procedure which can interrupt the chain of infection.

Bacterial Flora on Hands. Two types of bacterial flora are normally found on the hands: transient bacteria or flora and resident bacteria or flora. **Transient bacteria,** normally picked up by the hands in the usual activities of daily living, are relatively few on clean and exposed areas of the skin. They are attached loosely to the skin, usually in grease, fats, and dirt, and are found in greater numbers under the fingernails. Transient bacteria, pathogenic as well as nonpathogenic, can be removed with relative ease by washing the hands thoroughly and frequently. **Resident bacteria or flora,** normally found in creases in the skin, are relatively stable in number and type. They cling tenaciously to the skin by adhesion and adsorption, and considerable friction with a brush is required to remove them. Also, they are less susceptible to the action of antiseptics than transient bacteria are. For practical purposes, it is not considered possible to clean the skin of all bacteria.

Transient bacteria may adjust to the environment of the skin if the flora are present in large numbers over a long enough time. They then become resident bacteria. If pathogenic organisms become resident bacteria on the skin, the hands are then carriers of the particular organism. Therefore, it is important that the hands be cleaned promptly after each contact with contaminated materials to help prevent transient bacteria from becoming resident bacteria on the hands.

Cleansing Agents. Various products are available for handwashing. Soaps and detergents are generally considered adequate for routine mechanical cleansing of the hands and removal of most transient microorganisms. They help remove soil because they lower surface tension and act as emulsifying agents. Bar, liquid, or other forms of soap have all proved effective, but the factor that determines selection may prove to be preference of personnel.

Using soaps or detergents containing an antiseptic tends to cause skin dryness and irritations. These irritations defeat the purpose of decreasing the number of surface organisms because irritated skin harbors organisms and is difficult to clean adequately. Therefore, handwashing with only soap or detergent and water under routine circumstances is generally recommended for health personnel. Handwashing with antimicrobial-containing products kills or inhibits microorganisms and is used when a surgical scrub is required.

Recommended Techniques. Recommended handwashing techniques are listed in Procedure 25 1. The techniques are intended for use with medical asepsis. Cleaning the hands prior to performing certain procedures incorporating surgical asepsis, such as for operative procedures and for deliveries, is described in texts dealing with operating and delivery room procedures. A 10-second to 30-second scrub before and after giving client care is recommended when exposure to contamination is minimal. It may take from 1 minute to 4 minutes to wash thoroughly hands that are visibly soiled.

Some authorities recommend that rings be removed prior to handwashing, but a recent study indicated that thorough handwashing reduced the bacterial count in ring wearers to that of non-ring wearers even though the former demonstrated a higher number of bacteria on the hands before the wash (Jacobsen et al: 1985). Removal of all jewelry, except a plain wedding band, is considered the best procedure.

Handwashing is indicated in the following situations:

- Any prolonged contact with a client
- When assisting with or performing invasive procedures
- Caring for particularly susceptible clients such as those who are immunologically suppressed, newborn infants, or the aged adult
- Wherever gloves are used
- Handling of blood and body fluids, secretions or excretions, or any contact with mucous membranes
- Contact with any inanimate object that may be contaminated, such as dressings, urine collection devices
- Whenever there is a question about the necessity of handwashing

Unfortunately, knowledge and awareness of recommendations do not guarantee compliance. Another recent study documented poor compliance with handwashing

(Text continues on p. 512.)

PROCEDURE 25-1
Handwashing

Equipment

Liquid or bar soap   Paper towels   Lotion (optional)
Orangewood stick

Action

1 Stand in front of the sink. Do not allow your uniform to touch the sink during the washing procedure.

2 Remove jewelry.

3 Turn on water and adjust force. Regulate the temperature until the water is warm.

4 Wet the hands and wrist area. Keep hands lower than elbows to allow water to flow toward fingertips.

5 Use about 1 teaspoon liquid soap from dispenser or lather thoroughly with bar soap. Rinse bar and return to soap·dish.

6 With firm rubbing and circular motions, wash the palms and backs of the hands, each finger, the areas between the fingers, the knuckles, wrists, and forearms. Wash up the forearms at least as high as contamination is likely to be present.

Rationale

The sink is considered contaminated. Uniforms may carry organisms from place to place.

Removal of jewelry facilitates proper cleansing. Microorganisms may accumulate in settings of jewelry.

Water splashed from the contaminated sink will contaminate your uniform. Warm water is more comfortable and has less tendency to open pores and remove oils from the skin. Organisms can lodge in roughened and broken areas of chapped skin.

Water should flow from the cleaner area toward the more contaminated area. Hands are more contaminated than forearms.

Rinsing the soap removes the lather that may contain microorganisms.

Friction caused by firm rubbing and circular motions helps to loosen dirt and organisms that can lodge between the fingers, in skin crevices of knuckles, on palms and backs of the hands, as well as the wrists and forearms. Cleaning less contaminated areas (forearms and wrists) after hands are clean prevents spreading organisms from the hands to the forearms and wrists.

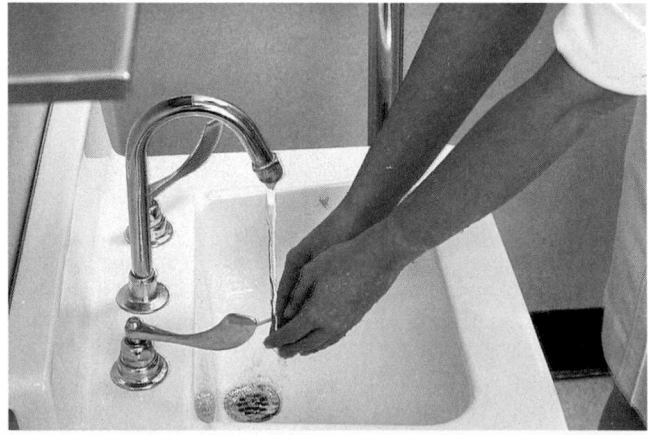

Step 4: Wetting hands and wrists.

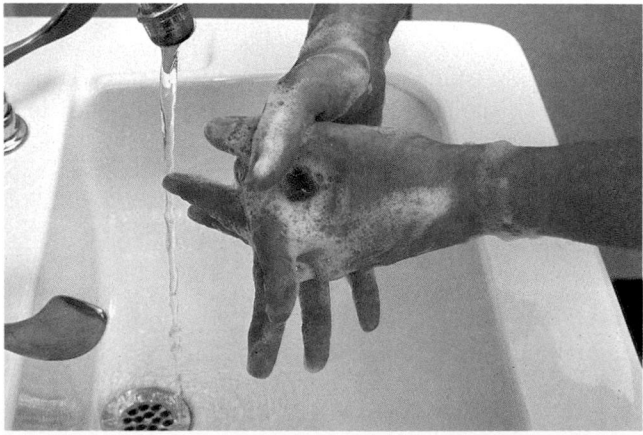

Step 6: Washing hands and forearms with firm rubbing and circular motions.

(Continued)

Action	**Rationale**
7 Continue this friction motion for 10 to 30 seconds.	Length of handwashing is determined by degree of contamination.
8 Use fingernails of the other hand or a clean orange-wood stick to clean under fingernails.	Organisms can lodge and remain under the nails where they can grow and be spread to others.
9 Rinse thoroughly.	Running water rinses organisms and dirt into the sink.
10 Dry hands and wrists with a paper towel. Use paper towel to turn off faucet.	Drying the skin well prevents chapping. Dry hands first because they are the cleanest and least contaminated area. Turning the faucet off with a paper towel protects the clean hands from contact with a soiled surface.

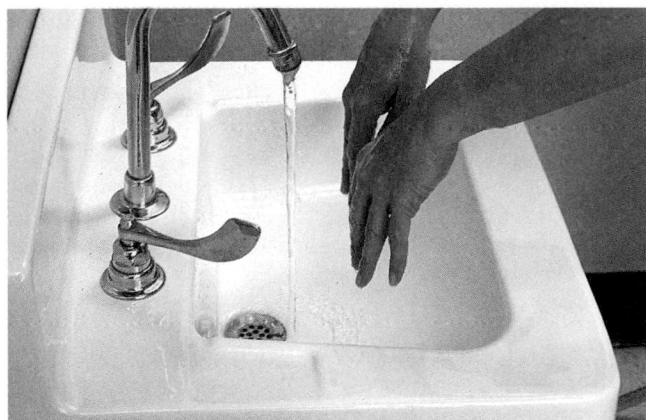

Step 9: Rinsing thoroughly.

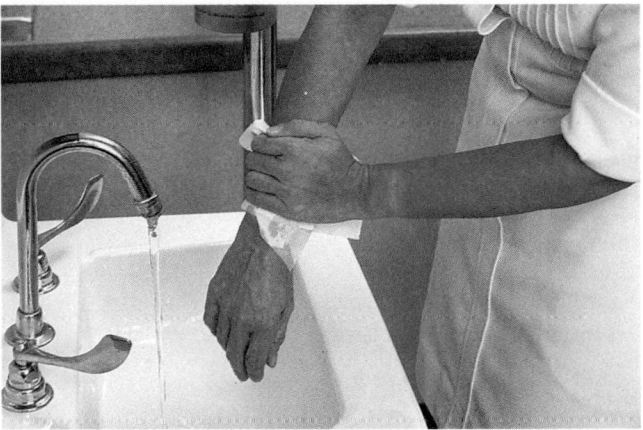

Step 10: Drying with a paper towel.

11 Use lotion on hands if desired.	Lotion helps to keep the skin soft and prevents chapping.

Age Considerations

Instruct children at early age in proper handwashing techniques.

Special Considerations

Special scrubbing techniques can reduce the risk for nurses who do not remove their rings. Research by Jacobsen demonstrated that a 1-minute scrub using liquid soap and a scrub brush, followed by a 1-minute rinse can remove any additional surface bacteria (Jacobsen, 1985).

Sinks with various faucet controls are available. In addition to the more common hand faucets, knee- and foot-operated controls may be used. Sinks with elbow controls are generally used in a surgical setting.

recommendations by physicians and nurses in an ICU setting (Albert and Condie, 1981). The importance of handwashing cannot be overstressed.

Controlling Infectious Agents by Sterilization and Disinfection

Cleansing, disinfection, and sterilization help to break the chain of infection and prevent nosocomial disease. Most health agencies provide items for client care that are sterile when purchased and disposed of after use. Some items, such as pitchers, water glasses, and thermometers, may be used repeatedly but by one client only; they are then discarded or sent home with the client upon discharge.

Health agencies usually maintain a central supply unit where most reusable equipment is cleaned, kept in good working order, and sterilized as indicated. There are times, especially in homes and in some small health agencies, when the nurse is required to make decisions about how to prepare equipment and supplies so that they are safe for client use. Although nurses may not be directly involved in the actual process, they must be aware of the critical role they play in the prevention of infection.

Factors in Selecting Method.   Various factors must be considered when selecting sterilization and disinfection methods.

Nature of Organisms Present.   Some organisms are destroyed easily while others are able to withstand certain commonly used sterilization and disinfection methods. The tubercle bacillus is relatively resistant to most disinfection processes while the meningococcus is fragile and easily destroyed. Spores are particularly resistant to destruction. Although not a great deal is known about transferring viruses by contaminated supplies and equipment, the CDC recommends precautions particularly to minimize nosocomial transmission of HIV and HBV. The disease-causing viruses can be spread by needles and scalpel blades contaminated with blood. A simple prick of the skin with a contaminated needle or scalpel blade may result in illness.

Number of Organisms Present.   The more organisms that are present on an article, the longer it takes to destroy them. If organisms are protected by coagulated proteins or harbor under a layer of grease, it will take longer to sterilize or disinfect the article. Articles cleaned prior to sterilization or disinfection will be made sterile or clean more quickly and with more certainty than an article that has not been cleaned.

Type of Equipment.   Equipment with small lumens, crevices, or joints that are difficult to clean and to expose requires special care. For example, if a reusable tube

(catheter) is placed in a chemical solution, disinfection will be ineffective if the solution does not fill the inside of the tube. Also, certain articles are damaged by various sterilization and disinfection methods, an example being equipment with lens mountings. Such equipment requires special handling to keep it safe for use and in good condition. Some plastic items cannot tolerate heat and may need gas sterilization rather than steam autoclaving.

Intended Use of Equipment.   If equipment is being used when medical asepsis is practiced, it is safe for it to be free of pathogenic organisms. But when surgical asepsis is required, equipment must be sterile. Although in some instances it may be safe to use equipment and supplies that are clean, most health agencies follow a policy of using sterilized articles for patient care whenever feasible.

Available Means for Sterilization and Disinfection. Sterilization and disinfection may be accomplished by physical or chemical means. There is no one ideal way. The choice is made on the basis of the nature and number of organisms, the type and intended use of the equipment, and the availability and practicality of the means.

Time.   Time is a key factor when sterilizing or disinfecting articles. Failing to observe recommended time periods is gross negligence, except in the most dire emergencies when, even then, very careful judgment should prevail.

Cleaning Supplies and Equipment.   Proper cleaning of items used in health care prior to their being sterilized or disinfected is essential to reduce the number of organisms and to dislodge them from crevices and from under layers of contaminating substances. The following techniques are recommended for cleaning equipment:
- Wear waterproof gloves if the articles are contaminated with organic materials such as feces, blood, pus, mucous, and if you have skin abrasions on the hands.
- Rinse the articles first with cold running water to remove organic material. Heat coagulates certain organic material, which makes removal more difficult.
- Wash the articles, after rinsing them, in warm water containing detergent or soap. The combination of warm water and soap facilitates emulsification and removal of dirt and debris.
- Use a brush with stiff bristles as indicated to clean the articles thoroughly. Friction aids in the removal of organisms and debris from difficult to reach areas (see Fig. 25-8).
- Rinse and dry the article thoroughly.

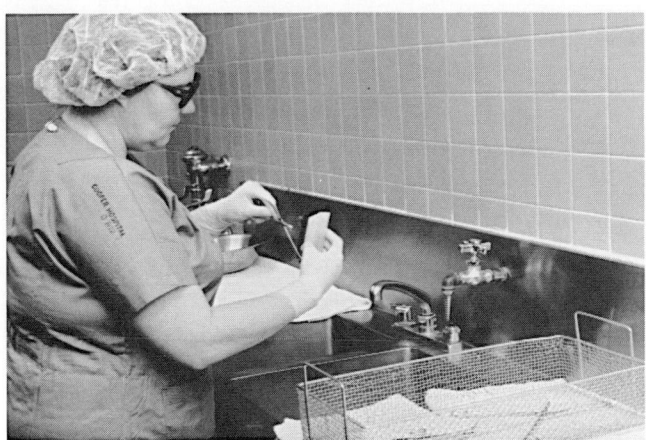

FIGURE 25-8
Proper cleaning of items used in health care prior to sterilization is essential. Items should be rinsed in cold running water, washed in warm water using soap or detergent and a brush, rinsed, and dried in preparation for sterilization or disinfection.

- Prepare the cleaned equipment for sterilization or disinfection.
- Consider the brush, gloves, and the sink or basin in which the articles were cleaned as highly contaminated, and treat or discard them accordingly.

Physical Means of Sterilization and Disinfection.
Physical means of sterilization and disinfection involve using heat or radiation. Dry heat kills organisms by an oxidation process, while moist heat coagulates protein within the cells. Radiation causes the death of microorganisms by altering their essential metabolic processes.

The following are the primary physical means of sterilization and disinfection:

Steam. Steam under pressure or moist heat is the most dependable and practical means for the destruction of all forms of microbial life. Its primary disadvantage is that items that are sensitive to high temperatures, such as most plastics, lensed instruments, drugs, and thermometers, are damaged by steam under pressure. The autoclave is a pressure-steam sterilizer. The home pressure cooker operates on the same principles as an autoclave.

The amount of pressure in an autoclave has nothing to do with the destruction of organisms. It is the higher temperature resulting from higher pressure that destroys organisms, and the higher the temperature, the more quickly organisms will die. It is generally recommended that saturated steam at 121°C to 123°C (250°F to 254°F) under 15 lb to 17 lb of pressure per square inch can achieve sterilization of items in 15 to 45 minutes.

Free-flowing steam, although inexpensive, has limited practical value because it only reaches the boiling point (100°C or 212°F), and this is insufficient for killing all pathogens. Certain bedpan flushers use free-flowing steam. These flushers do not render equipment sterile despite some manufacturers' claims.

Boiling Water. Two advantages of using boiling water are that it is inexpensive and simple. A disadvantage is that spores and some viruses are resistant to boiling. Boiling water is commonly used in homes. Although authorities differ, it is believed boiling an item for a minimum of 15 minutes can achieve disinfection.

Dry Heat. Dry heat is rarely used in health-care agencies. It has the advantage of being harmless to objects that are damaged by moisture, such as the cutting edges of sharp instruments, the ground surfaces of glass, and powders. Its disadvantage is that the penetration ability of dry heat is not believed sufficient to destroy all microorganisms. Dry heat may be used in some home situations to achieve disinfection. An ordinary baking oven can be used for this purpose. Authorities agree that, for most articles, disinfection occurs when a temperature of 160°C (320°F) is maintained for 2 hours.

Radiation. Ionizing radiation is used for pharmaceuticals, foods, plastics, and other heat-sensitive items. The major advantage is that it is believed to be extremely effective for many items that are otherwise difficult to sterilize. The primary disadvantage is that the facilities and equipment for the use of ionizing radiation rays are complex and expensive.

Chemical Means of Sterilization and Disinfection
Ethylene Oxide Gas. Ethylene oxide gas is a chemical sometimes used for sterilization. The gas destroys microorganisms by interfering with metabolic processes in cells, and it has been found to have lethal action on spores as well as vegetative cells. Its penetrating qualities are excellent, and it has the advantage of being useful for sterilizing such heat-sensitive items as oxygen and suction gauges and blood-pressure equipment. The major disadvantage of ethylene oxide is that it is considered to be toxic to humans in high concentrations. It is extremely important that health personnel adhere to recommendations for adequate ventilation of the sterilizer and aeration of the sterilized materials.

Chemical Solutions. Chemical solutions are generally used for instrument and equipment disinfection and for housekeeping disinfection. **Disinfectants** destroy organisms by disturbing their structure or their metabolic processes through coagulation and alterations of the cell membrane and cell protein. The time of exposure, concentration and temperature of the chemical, and the type of organism are key factors in achieving disinfection.

The major classes of chemical solutions used in health agencies are chlorine compounds, iodine, and alcohol. Chlorines are useful for disinfecting water and for housekeeping disinfectants. They should not be used on metals because of their tendency to cause corrosion.

Iodine has an effective bactericidal effect but also an undesirable staining quality. This characteristic is reduced when a detergent is added to the solution. The combination is distributed as iodophors which have a fairly rapid germicidal effect and are relatively nontoxic. Ethyl (grain) and isopropyl (rubbing) alcohols are most commonly used as antiseptics, although they occasionally are used as disinfectants. They act as germicides. Extensive use of alcohol is drying to the skin and can damage plastics.

Using Surgical Asepsis

Surgical asepsis techniques, used regularly in the operating room, labor and delivery areas, and certain diagnostic testing areas, are also used by the nurse at the client's bedside. Procedures involving insertion of a urinary catheter, sterile dressing changes, and preparing an injectable medication are examples of surgical asepsis techniques. An object is considered sterile when all microorganisms, including pathogens and spores, have been destroyed. For example, the needle for an injection is handled so that it is sterile when inserted into a client. A sterile forceps or sterile gloves are used to handle sterile dressings to protect from contamination. Basic principles of surgical asepsis are listed in the accompanying box.

In observing medical asepsis, areas are considered contaminated if they bear, or are suspected of bearing, pathogens. In observing surgical asepsis, areas are considered contaminated if touched by any object that is not also sterile. One of the most important aspects of surgical and medical asepsis is that the effectiveness of both depends on the faithfulness and the conscientiousness of those carrying them out. It is far better to err on the side of safety when using surgical asepsis than to take the slightest chance of possible contamination.

Explanation of the surgical asepsis procedure (Fig. 25-9) facilitates cooperation of the client. An awareness of which objects and areas may not be touched as well as directions to avoid sudden movements are vital for the client to assist the nurse in maintaining the sterility of the procedure.

Handling Sterile Objects. Sterile gloves or sterile forceps are used for handling items when maintaining sterility is necessary.

Putting on Sterile Gloves. Sterile gloves are donned so that only the inside of the glove comes in contact with the hands. Procedure 25-2 illustrates the proper technique for putting on sterile gloves. After the gloves are on, sterile items may be handled with the sterile-gloved hands. Careful removal of the gloves reduces any hand contact with contaminated materials.

Putting on Surgical Cap and Mask. For a sterile surgical procedure the nurse puts on a disposable paper or

Basic Principles of Surgical Asepsis

- Only a sterile object can touch another sterile object. Unsterile touching sterile means contamination has occurred.
- Open sterile packages so that the first edge of the wrapper is directed away from the worker to avoid the possibility of a sterile surface touching unsterile clothing. The outside of the sterile package is considered contaminated. Opening a sterile package is illustrated and described in Figure 25-9.
- Avoid spilling any solution on a cloth or paper used as a field for a sterile setup. The moisture penetrates through the sterile cloth or paper and carries organisms by capillary action to contaminate the field. A wet field is considered contaminated if the surface immediately below it is not sterile.
- Hold sterile objects above the level of the waist. This will help ensure keeping the object within sight and preventing accidental contamination.
- Avoid talking, coughing, sneezing, or reaching over a sterile field or object. This will help to prevent contamination by droplets from the nose and the mouth or by particles dropping from the worker's arm.
- Never walk away from or turn your back on a sterile field. This will prevent possible contamination while the field is out of the worker's view.
- All items brought into contact with broken skin, or used to penetrate the skin in order to inject substances into the body, or to enter normally sterile body cavities, should be sterile. These items include dressings used to cover wounds and incisions, needles for injection, and tubes (catheters) used to drain urine from the bladder.
- Use dry, sterile forceps when necessary. Forceps soaked in disinfectant are not considered sterile.
- Consider the edge (outer 1 inch) of a sterile field to be contaminated.
- Consider an object contaminated if you have any doubt as to its sterility.

clean cloth cap. All hair must be covered. The mask, with the rigid strip on the uppermost edge, is held by the upper two strings and tied securely at the back of the head. The lower two ties are fastened around the neck. In the operating room, once the mask has become moistened it must be covered with a second mask rather

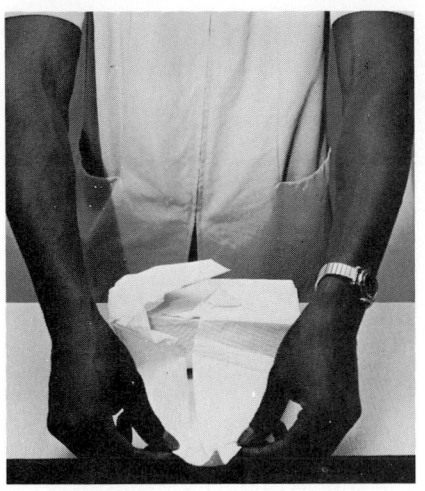
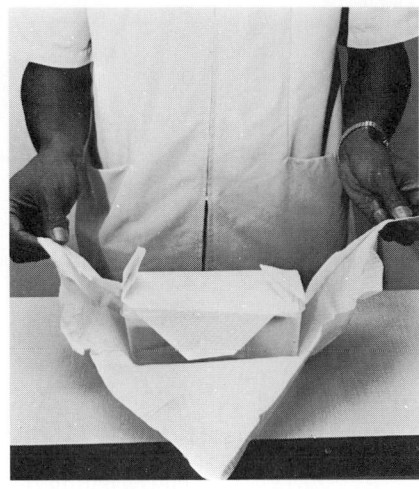
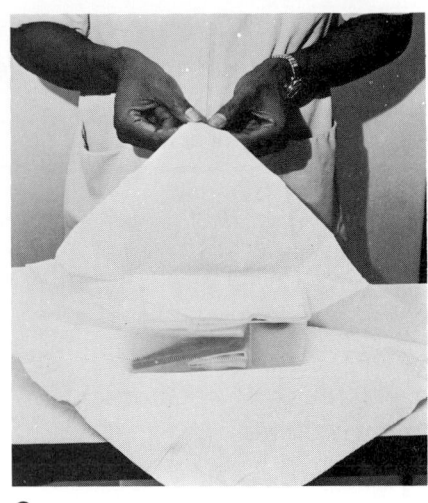

A   B   C

F I G U R E   25-9
(A) The nurse opens a sterile set or tray by folding the top-most part of the covering wrapper away from him. This leaves sterile equipment and supplies well covered so that they cannot be contaminated by the nurse's reaching across the set or tray to open the wrapper. (B) Next, the nurse opens the second layer of the wrapper to the sides of the set or tray. This still leaves sterile equipment and supplies covered with the last layer of the wrapper. (C) As the last step, the nurse opens the final layer of the wrapper toward himself. The wrapper can now become the sterile field immediately surrounding the sterile set or tray. Note that at no time did the nurse reach across an uncovered sterile field or sterile equipment and supplies.

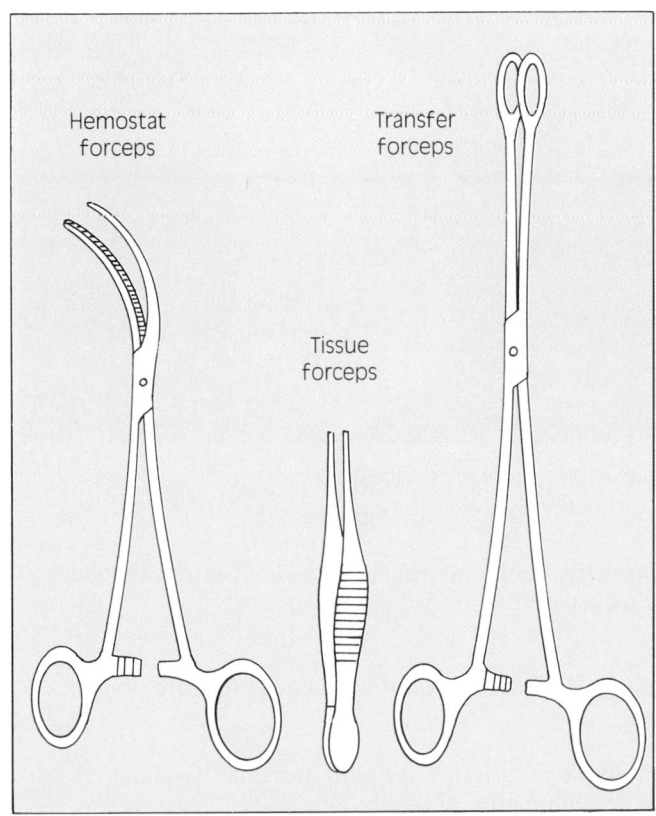

Hemostat forceps

Transfer forceps

Tissue forceps

F I G U R E   25-10
Examples of sterile forceps used for sterile procedures.

than remove the original and contaminate adjacent objects.

Prior to removing the mask and cap the nurse must remove the sterile gloves and wash hands. The mask is then untied and is removed holding it by the strings. Both cap and mask should be discarded in the proper container (see Procedure 25-3).

Using Sterile Forceps. Various forceps are available for use in sterile procedures (see Fig. 25-10). The practice of considering forceps sterile that were stored in a germicidal solution and then reused is outdated and unsafe. As with other sterile objects, forceps should be kept above waist level. If handled with the bare hand, only the tips can be considered sterile. Sterile forceps should not touch the edge of a container or sterile wrapper because this outer area is considered unsterile. The forceps' tips need to be held down, particularly if they become wet, so fluid will not flow from a contaminated area to a sterile one.

Pouring Sterile Solutions. Care is necessary when pouring sterile liquids onto a sterile dressing or into a sterile basin. The outer surface of the bottle and cap are unsterile. Remove the cap carefully and do not allow the inner surface of the lid to touch an unsterile area. Pour a small amount of the solution into a sink or waste container to clean the lip of the bottle. Be sure the label side of the container is uppermost when pouring so that the

(Text continues on p. 519.)

PROCEDURE 25-2
Donning and Removing Sterile Gloves

Equipment

Sterile gloves (Size of gloves is indicated on outer wrapping. Select appropriate size.)

Action	Rationale
To Apply Gloves	
1 Wash and dry hands carefully.	Handwashing deters the spread of microorganisms. Gloves are easier to don when hands are dry.
2 Place sterile glove package on clean, dry surface above your waist.	Moisture could contaminate the sterile gloves. Any sterile object held below the waist is considered contaminated.
3 Open the outside wrapper by carefully peeling the top layer back. Remove inner package, handling only the outside of it.	Maintains sterility of gloves in inner packet
4 Carefully open the inner package and expose the sterile gloves with the cuff end closest to you.	The inner surface of the package is considered sterile.

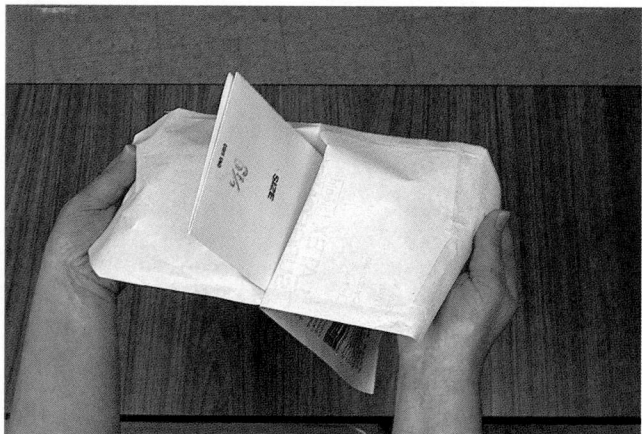

Step 3: Peeling back top layer of outer package.

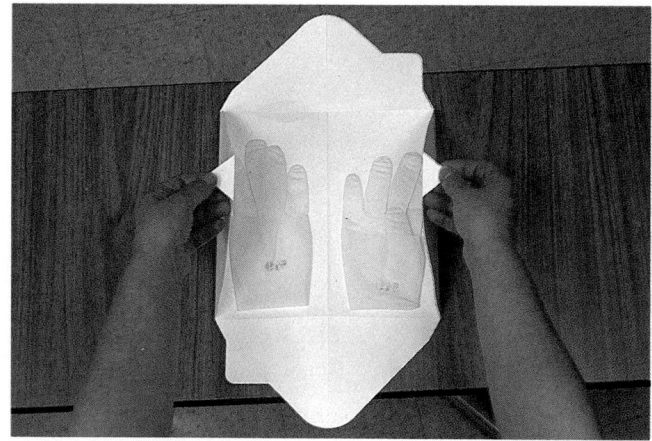

Step 4: Opening inner package.

Action	Rationale
5 With the thumb and forefinger of nondominant hand, grasp the top edge of the folded cuff of the sterile glove for dominant hand.	Unsterile hand only touches inside of glove. Outside remains sterile.
6 Lift and hold glove with fingers down. Be careful it does not touch any unsterile objects.	Glove is contaminated if it touches unsterile object.
7 Carefully insert the dominant hand into glove and pull glove on. Leave cuff folded down until other hand is gloved.	Attempts to turn upward with unsterile hand may result in contamination of sterile glove.

(Continued)

Action	**Rationale**

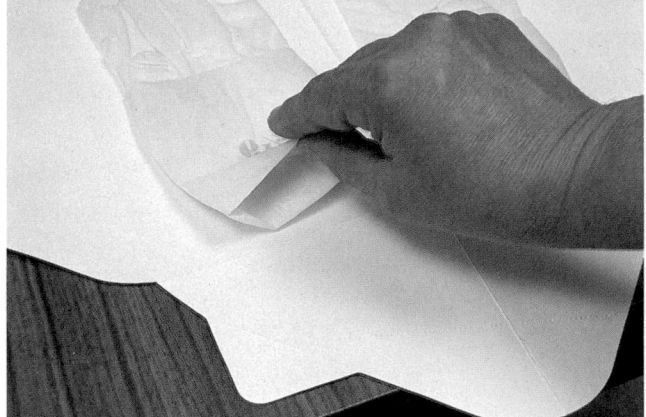

Step 5: Grasping edge of folded cuff.

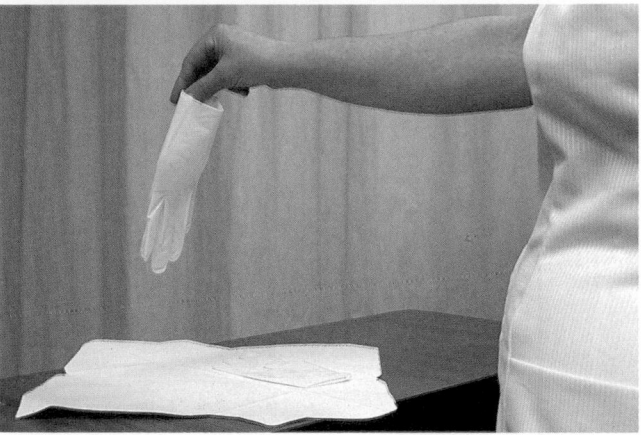

Step 6: Lifting and holding glove with fingers down.

8 Holding thumb outward, slide fingers of gloved hand under cuff of remaining glove and lift glove upward.

Thumb is less likely to become contaminated if held outward.

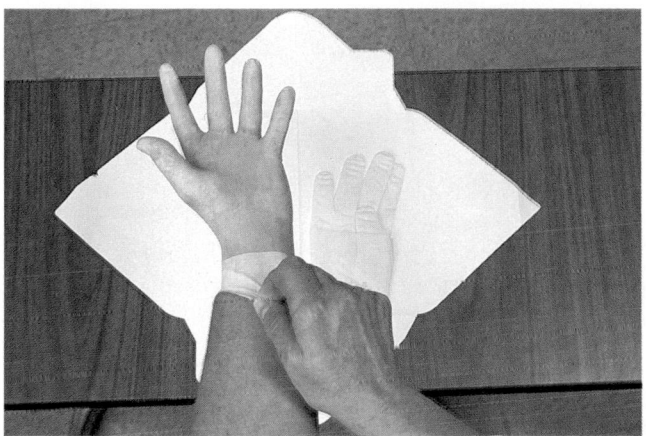

Step 7: Pulling first glove on with cuff folded.

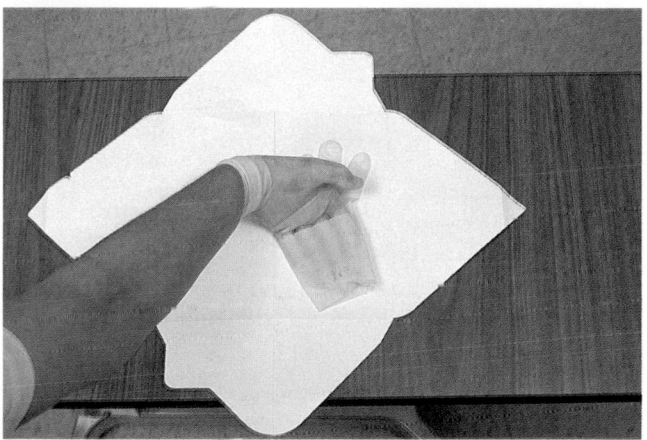

Step 8: Sliding fingers of gloved hand under cuff of second glove.

9 Carefully insert nondominant hand into glove. Adjust gloves on both hands touching only sterile areas.

Sterile surface touching sterile surface prevents contamination.

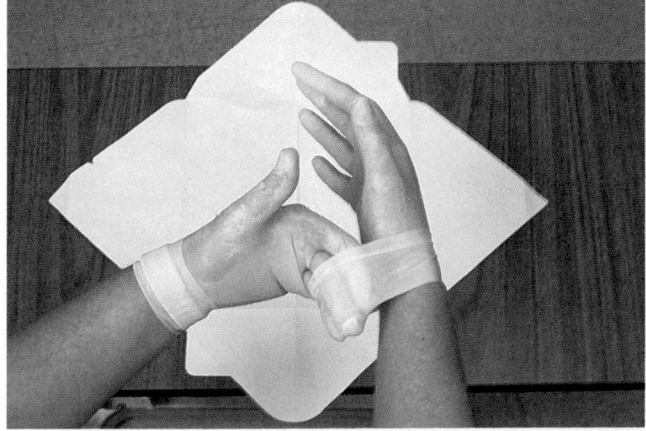

Step 9: Inserting hand with cuff folded.

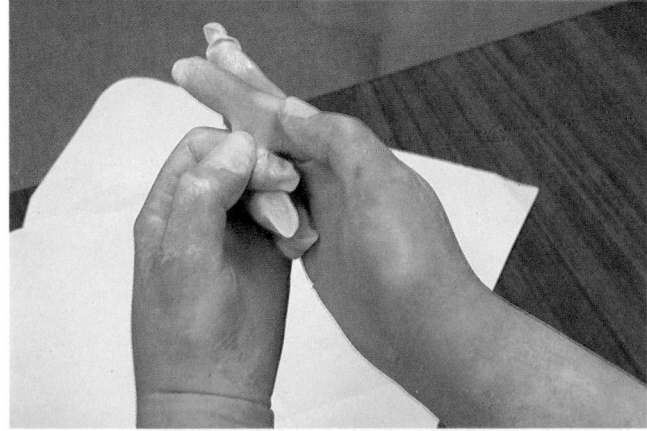

Step 9: Adjusting gloves on both hands.

(Continued)

Action

Rationale

To Remove Gloves

1 Using dominant gloved hand, grasp other glove near cuff end and remove by inverting it, keeping the contaminated area on the inside. Continue to hold onto glove.

Contaminated area will not come in contact with hands or wrists.

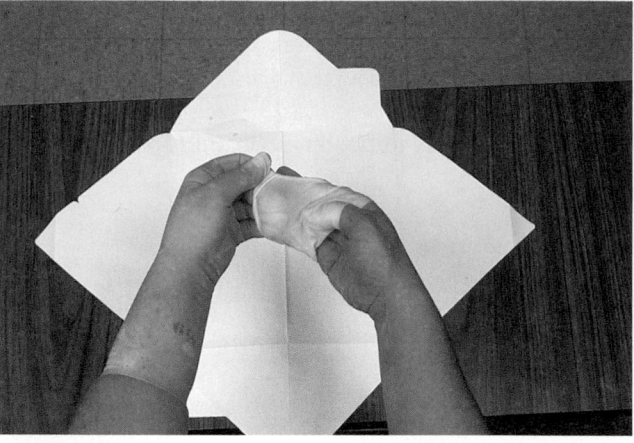

Step 1: Inverting glove as it is removed.

2 Slide fingers of ungloved hand inside the remaining glove. Grasp glove on inside and remove by turning inside out.

Contaminated area does not come in contact with hands or wrists.

3 Discard gloves in appropriate container and wash hands.

Handwashing reduces the spread of microorganisms.

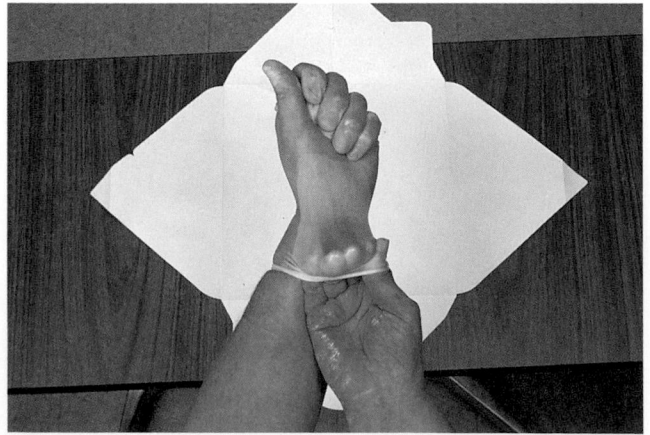

Step 2: Sliding ungloved fingers inside second glove.

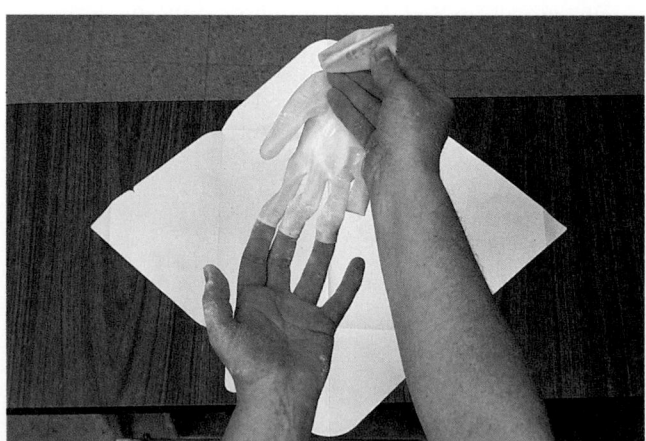

Step 2: Removing second glove inside out.

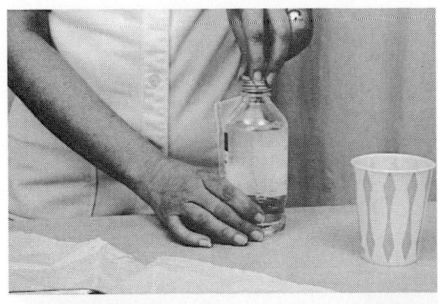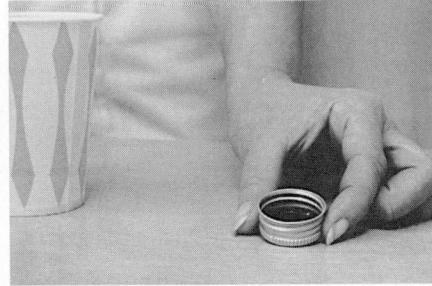
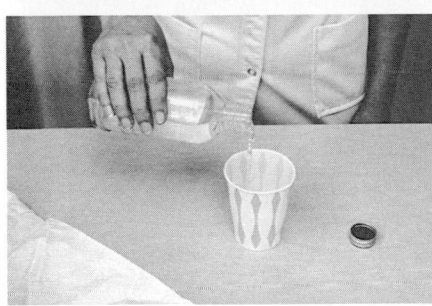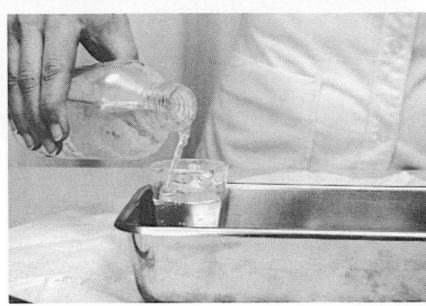

FIGURE 25-11
Pouring sterile liquids. (Top) Working outside the sterile field, the nurse opens the
bottle of sterile liquid, being careful to
touch only the outside of the cap. (Bottom
left) The nurse pours a small amount of
the liquid into a container that will later be
discarded to cleanse the lip of the sterile
liquid bottle. (Bottom right) The nurse
pours the sterile liquid into the graduate,
carefully holding the bottle to the outside
of the sterile tray and field.

label does not become wet and soiled. Hold the bottle
outside the edge of the sterile field and pour carefully so
as not to splash the solution. The tip of the bottle should
never touch the sterile container or dressing. Touch only
the outside of the cap when recapping (see Fig. 25-11).

Adding Sterile Supplies to a Sterile Field. It may be
necessary on occasion to add additional items to the
sterile field. The nurse should open the sterile item and
drop it onto the sterile field from a safe distance being
careful that the outside wrapper does not touch the sterile field. If the item is wrapped in a sterile cloth, the
nondominant hand should be used to secure the loose
ends away from the item and protect them from contaminating the sterile field.

Applying Sterile Drapes. The sterile drape, which ideally is waterproof, may be applied to extend the sterile
working area. Using sterile gloves to apply the drape
allows the nurse to handle the entire surface. For protection when positioning, the upper edges of the drape
should be folded over the sterile-gloved hands (see Fig.
25-12). When sterile gloves are not worn, the nurse is
only allowed to touch the outer 1 inch of the drape.
Caution must be used when shaking the drape open so as
not to touch the uniform or an unsterile object. Holding
the drape by the 1-inch upper edge, the nurse positions
the drape over the desired area. The nurse must not
reach over the drape because this would contaminate a
sterile area.

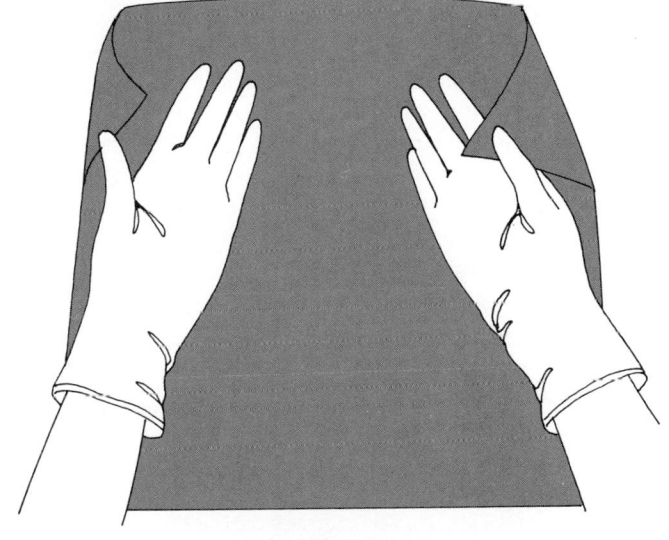

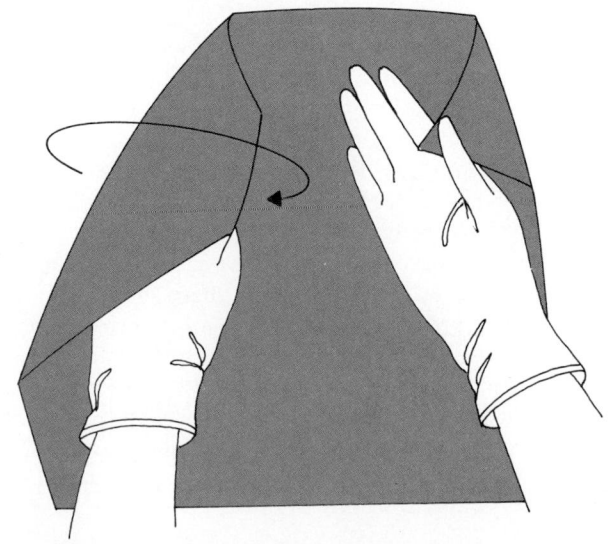

FIGURE 25-12
Techniques of cuffing a sterile drape over gloved hands.

Universal Precautions: Prevention of Transmission of Human Immunodeficiency Virus, Hepatitis B Virus, and Other Bloodborne Pathogens in Health-Care Settings

Under universal precautions, blood and certain body fluids of all patients are considered potentially infectious for human immunodeficiency virus (HIV), hepatitis B virus (HBV), and other blood-borne pathogens. Blood is the single most important source of HIV, HBV, and other bloodborne pathogens in health care settings. Infection control efforts for HIV, HBV, and other bloodborne pathogens must focus on preventing exposures to blood as well as delivery of HBV immunization.

Epidemiologic evidence has implicated only blood, semen, and vaginal secretions, and possibly breast milk in transmissions. Although the risk is unknown, universal precautions also apply to tissues and to the following fluids: cerebrospinal fluid, synovial fluid, pleural fluid, peritoneal fluid, and amniotic fluid. Universal precautions do not apply to feces, nasal secretions, sputum, sweat, tears, urine, and vomitus unless they contain visible blood. The risk of transmission of HIV and HBV from these materials is extremely low or nonexistent.

Health-care workers are at risk for exposure to blood from clients infected with HIV, HBV, and other bloodborne pathogens. Health-care workers must consider *all* clients as potentially infected with bloodborne pathogens and must adhere rigorously to infection-control precautions for *all* clients.

Precautions to Prevent Transmission of HIV

General Precautions

- Consider *all* clients as potentially infected.
- Wear gloves when touching blood, body fluids containing blood, and body fluids to which universal precautions apply and for handling items or surfaces soiled with blood or applicable fluids, and for performing venipuncture, and other vascular access procedures. Change gloves after each contact with a client.
- Use protective barriers, i.e., wear masks, protective eyewear or face shields and gowns or aprons when performing procedures that may produce blood or body fluid droplets or splashes.
- Wash hands and skin surfaces immediately and thoroughly if contaminated with blood or other body fluids to which universal precautions apply.
- Take precautions to prevent injuries from needles, scalpels, and other sharp instruments during procedures, when cleaning instruments, during disposal, or when handling. To prevent needle-stick injuries, needles should not be recapped, purposely bent or broken by hand, removed from disposable syringes, or otherwise manipulated by hand. After they are used, disposable syringes and needles, scalpel blades,

and other sharp items should be placed in puncture-resistant containers for disposal.

Special Considerations

- Health-care workers who have exudative lesions or weeping dermatitis should refrain from all direct patient care and from handling patient-care equipment until the condition resolves.
- Pregnant health-care workers are not known to be at greater risk of contracting HIV infection than health-care workers who are not pregnant; however, if a health-care worker develops HIV infection during pregnancy, the infant is at risk of infection resulting from perinatal transmission. Because of this risk, pregnant health-care workers should be especially familiar with and strictly adhere to precautions to minimize the risk of HIV transmission.

Precautions for Invasive Procedures

(Here an invasive procedure is defined as any surgical entry into tissues, cavities, or organs or repair of major traumatic injuries.) General blood and body fluid precautions listed above, combined with the precautions listed below, should be the *minimum precautions for all such invasive procedures.*

- All health-care workers who participate in invasive procedures must routinely use appropriate barrier procedures to prevent skin and mucous membrane contact with all patients' blood and other body fluids to which universal precautions apply.
- Gloves and surgical masks must be worn for all invasive procedures.
- Protective eyewear or face shields should be worn for all procedures that commonly result in generation of droplets, splashing of blood, body fluids containing blood, and other applicable body fluids.
- Gowns or aprons made of materials providing an effective barrier should be worn during invasive procedures likely to result in the splashing of blood or other pertinent body fluids.
- All health-care workers who perform or assist in vaginal or cesarean delivery should wear gloves and gowns when handling the placenta or the infant until blood and amniotic fluid have been removed from the infant's skin. Gloves should be worn until post-delivery care of the umbilical cord.
- If a glove is torn or a needle-stick or other injury occurs, the glove should be removed and a new glove used as promptly as patient safety permits; the needle or instrument involved in the incident should also be removed from the sterile field.

(Source: Centers for Disease Control: Recommendations for prevention of HIV transmission in health care settings. MMWR 36:Suppl. 25: 1987. Centers for Disease Control: Update: Universal precautions for prevention of transmission of human immunodeficiency virus, hepatitis B virus, and other bloodborne pathogens pathogens in health-care settings. MMWR 37:24, 1988.)

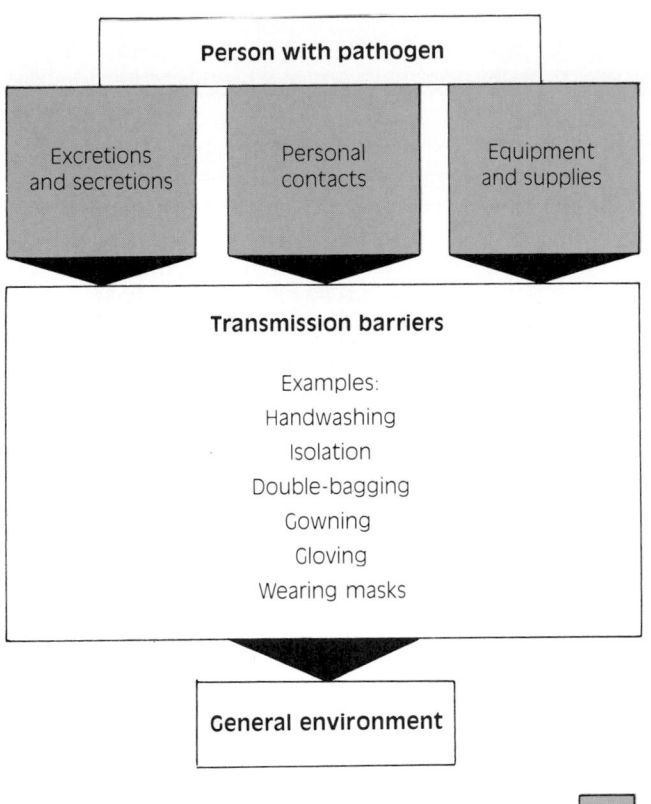

FIGURE 25-13
The transmission barriers are communicable disease or isolation techniques. Note that the transmission barriers prevent common vehicles from transporting pathogens from the infected person to the general environment.

Providing Isolation and Control of Communicable Disease

Isolation is a protective procedure that limits the spread of infectious diseases among hospitalized clients, hospital personnel, and visitors. The transfer of pathogens from person to person can be decreased when dissemination of pathogens is limited. The most practical means of accomplishing this is to develop barriers that prevent common vehicles from transmitting them. Figure 25-13 demonstrates the ability of barriers to break the infection cycle.

Isolation procedures are based on the manner in which the pathogen leaves the person (reservoir) and its ability to survive and be transmitted to another person. Some health-care institutions refer to isolation precautions as protective aseptic techniques or barrier techniques because of an unfavorable connotation associated with isolating a person.

Types of Isolation Practices. In 1983 the Centers for Disease Control revised their isolation guidelines to include disease-specific isolation categories and category-specific isolation systems. The disease-specific format identifies necessary precautions to interrupt transmission of each disease. As the category system implies, precautionary measures have been assigned to each of the major modes of transmitting infectious diseases (see Fig. 25-14). Hospitals may modify these guidelines to meet their specific needs but the CDC protocols are viewed as the minimum protection standards. The types of isolation, purpose, and specifications for each category are described in Table 25-8.

With any type of isolation the client needs to be located in a physical environment in which it is feasible to carry out the intent of whatever precautions are necessary. Handwashing facilities and adjoining bathing and toilet facilities are important. Adequate space separating the person harboring the pathogen from others helps to decrease the possibility of transmission. A separate room with a door that can be kept closed is essential in certain situations. Special ventilation which results in slight negative pressure in the room in relation to adjoining areas is desirable for some infections.

Handwashing before and after the care of a client with a communicable illness is mandatory for all health personnel.

Previous CDC guidelines included a protective or reverse isolation category. Current protocols do not include this category because strict observance of handwashing policy has proved just as effective in protecting most immunosuppressed persons. Guidelines are available for special infection problems related to compromised patients.

Specially constructed rooms or commercial devices can be used to provide an environment as free from organisms as possible. The special space should be under slight positive pressure with respect to adjacent areas so that air flow from the protected room or area moves to the adjoining areas. After thorough handwashing, persons caring for the client wear a sterile "space suit" type of apparel or work through special sealed openings in the plastic walls of the area. All substances coming in

(Text continues on p. 523.)

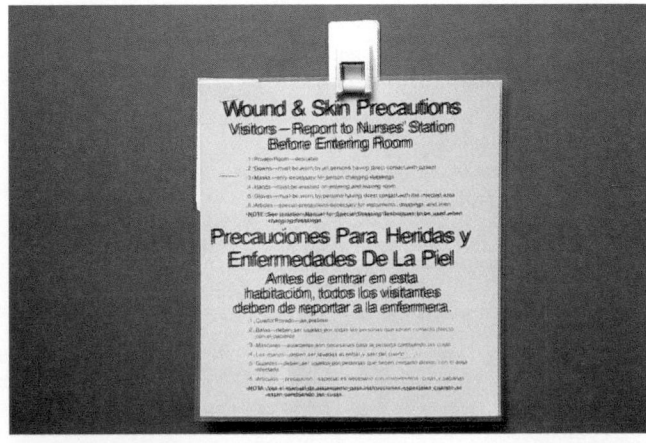

FIGURE 25-14
Example of a category-specific precaution sign.

T A B L E 25-8
Category-Specific Isolation System

Type	Purpose	Specifications*						Diseases Requiring Isolation
		Private Room	Handwashing	Gowns	Masks	Gloves	Articles	
Strict	Prevents transmission of highly contagious or virulent infections spread by air and contact	×	×	×	×	×	Discard or bag and label and send for decontamination and reprocessing	Diphtheria (pharyngeal) Lassa fever Smallpox Varicella
Contact	Prevents transmission of highly transmissible infections that do not require strict isolation	×	×	Wear if soiling is likely	Wear in close contact with client	Wear if touching infective material	Discard or bag and label and send for decontamination and reprocessing	Acute respiratory infections in infants and young children Herpes simplex Impetigo Multiple resistant bacterial infections
Respiratory	Prevents transmission of infectious diseases primarily over short distances by air droplets	×	×	——	Wear in close contact with client	——	Discard or bag and label and send for decontamination and reprocessing	Measles Meningitis Pneumonia, *Hemophilus influenza* in children Mumps
Tuberculosis	For client with pulmonary TB who has a positive sputum or chest x-ray that indicates active disease	×	×	Wear if soiling is likely	Wear if client is coughing and does not consistently cover mouth	——	Rarely involved in transmission of TB. Should still be thoroughly cleaned and disinfected	Tuberculosis
Enteric precautions	To prevent infections that are transmitted by direct or indirect contact with feces	Indicated if client's hygiene is poor and there is risk of contamination with infective materials	×	Wear if soiling is likely	——	Wear if touching infective material	Discard or bag and label and send for decontamination and reprocessing	Hepatitis, viral (type A) Gastroenteritis caused by highly infectious organism Cholera Diarrhea, acute with infectious etiology
Drainage-secretion precautions	To prevent infections that are transmitted by direct or indirect contact with purulent material or drainage from infected site	——	×	Wear if soiling is likely	——	Wear if touching infective material	Discard or bag and label and send for decontamination and reprocessing	Abcess Burn infection Conjunctivitis Decubitus ulcer Skin or wound infection
Blood–body fluid precautions	To prevent infections that are transmitted by direct or indirect contact with blood or body fluid	Only if client's hygiene is poor	×	Wear if soiling with blood or body fluids is likely	——	Wear if touching blood or body fluids	Discard or bag and label and send for decontamination and reprocessing	AIDS Hepatitis, viral (type B) Malaria Syphilis, primary and secondary

* × = necessary; —— = not necessary.

contact with the patient (air, linen, food, medications, equipment, and supplies) may be sterilized.

Isolation Precautions for Personnel. Many healthcare agencies use isolation carts stocked with all the necessary equipment and supplies which can be placed outside the client's room. Care must be taken to see that supplies are replenished as necessary.

There are several common practices to help control the transmission of organisms by personal contact. These include handwashing and wearing a gown, mask, and gloves. (See the Centers for Disease Control Recommendations.)

Gowns. In most instances, gowns are worn to prevent soiling of clothing when caring for clients. They should be stored immediately outside the client's room and should be donned immediately before entering the client's room. Individual gown technique is recommended. This means gowns are worn only once and then discarded. The recommended practices when gowns are in use for a client on isolation precautions are included in Procedure 25-3.

Masks. Masks are intended to prevent the wearer from inhaling large-particle aerosols, which generally travel short distances (about 3 feet), and small-particle droplet nuclei, which can remain suspended in the air and travel longer distances. Masks also discourage the wearer from touching eyes, nose, and mouth thus limiting contact of organisms with mucous membrane.

Various practices are observed in the use of masks. In some instances, all personnel and all of the client's visitors wear masks; in others, the client wears the mask when he is transported outside his room. Recommended practices when wearing a mask are included in Procedure 25-3.

A mask should be worn only once and should *never* be lowered around the neck and then brought back over the mouth and nose for reuse. The length of time to wear one mask while caring for one client is debatable. It should certainly be changed before it becomes damp from the wearer's exhalations.

Gloves. The CDC (1983) recommends that caregivers wear gloves for three reasons.
- They reduce likelihood of contact with infectious microorganisms.
- They limit transmission of one's own endogenous flora to clients.
- They reduce the possibility of becoming transiently colonized with microorganisms which could then be transmitted to other clients.

Because of the danger of AIDS virus transmission in health facilities, the CDC (1988) has updated its advice on wearing gloves (see Centers for Disease Control Recommendations, page 520). Gloves are worn only once and then discarded appropriately, according to agency policy. Gloves should be changed after direct handling of potentially contaminated drainage and before completing the client's care. When gloves are worn, handwashing is recommended to protect against possible perforation of a glove. Disposable gloves are recommended and used in most health agencies.

Isolation Precautions with Equipment and Supplies. A second common vehicle for transmitting organisms is equipment and supplies. The following are commonly recommended practices to help control the transmission of organisms by equipment and supplies:
- Such equipment as a sphygmomanometer, a stethoscope, and other items used for a physical examination should be left in the client's room until the illness has subsided and is no longer infectious. Terminal disinfection of the equipment should be appropriate for the type of equipment used and the causative organism involved.
- Disposable thermometers are preferred. A reusable thermometer should be left at the bedside for the duration of the client's illness. It is recommended that electronic thermometers not be used for clients in isolation because of the difficulty of rendering them safe for the next client.
- Soiled linens should be removed from the client's room using the double-bag technique. This technique is described in Procedure 25-3.
- Contaminated linens may be placed in a hot-water-soluble bag that can be placed directly in the washing machine. As an additional precaution these linen containers need to be double-bagged because the inner bag may dissolve if linen is wet or may tear easily.
- When changing bed linens, vigorous movements should be avoided to prevent air movements, which help spread microorganisms in the environment.
- Gas sterilizers are usually used for personal items that cannot be washed when they become contaminated.
- In general, disposable dishes are preferred, and these are handled according to the agency policy for disposable equipment. Reusable dishes and utensils that have been contaminated with infective material need to be bagged and labeled for return to the food service department. Waterproof gloves should be worn when dishes contaminated with pathogens are handled.
- The client's chart should not be allowed to come into contact with infective microorganisms.

Isolation Precautions with Excretions and Secretions. A third common vehicle for transmitting organisms is through excretions and secretions. The following are common practices to help control the transmission of organisms through excretions and secretions:
- The contents of urinals and bedpans can be dis-

(Text continues on p. 527.)

Caring for Client on Isolation Precautions

Action	Rationale
1 Check physician's order for type of isolation and review precautions in Infection Control Manual.	Mode of transmission of organism determines type and degree of precautions.
2 Plan nursing activities and gather necessary equipment prior to entering client's room. Supplies may include:	Organization facilitates performance of task and adherence to isolation precautions.

Bed linens
Gown and personal hygiene items
Equipment to measure vital signs

Medications
Water pitcher, cups, and water
Specimen collection equipment

Isolation apparel
Isolation disposal supplies

Action	Rationale
3 Provide instruction about isolation precautions to client, family members, and visitors.	An explanation encourages cooperation of client and family and reduces apprehension about isolation procedures.
4 Wash your hands.	Handwashing deters the spread of microorganisms.
5 Put on gown, gloves, and mask if recommended as isolation precaution:	Interrupts chain of infection. Protects client and nurse.
a. Tie gown securely at neck and waist.	Gown should protect entire uniform.
b. Use clean disposable gloves. If worn with gown draw glove cuffs over gown sleeves.	Protect hands and wrists from microorganisms.
c. Mask must be securely tied and fitted to face.	Protects nurse from droplet nuclei and large particle aerosols.

Step 5a: Tying gown at neck and waist.

Action	Rationale
6 Enter client's room with necessary equipment. Place on paper towel if necessary to avoid contamination. Leave chart and flow sheets outside room on isolation cart.	Avoids direct contact with infected material
7 *Measure vital signs* using client's equipment in room (thermometer and sphygmomanometer). Stethoscope and watch should not come into contact with contaminated material. Place them on a clean paper towel. Vital sign recording may also be noted on clean towel placed on top of first paper towel.	Leaving equipment in room prevents spread of microorganisms to other clients. Alcohol may be used to cleanse nurse's equipment prior to being used for another client.

(Continued)

Action

8 *Assist client with care.* Discard his gown and linens in isolation laundry bag and discard paper products in isolation waste container bag.

9 *Administer medications* as ordered by physician. Discard syringes in disposal container kept in room.

10 *Collect specimens* and label appropriately. Place in plastic bag held by assistant outside of room for transport to laboratory.

11 *Dispose of linen bags and waste bags* when necessary and, usually, at the end of each shift:

a. Tie bags securely.

b. Double bag by placing linen in clean disposable bag opened and held by assistant with top edge cuffed over assistant's hands. Use same technique and place waste bag in duplicate container for disposal according to agency policy.

c. Assistant will seal or label outer bag as necessary and transport to appropriate area for safe disposal.

Rationale

Identifies need for special precautions with waste disposal and laundry process

Reduces risk of needle stick with contaminated needle

Outer wrap is not contaminated, and label indicates isolation precautions.

Double bagging ensures safe transporting of contaminated material. Cuffed clean bag protects assistant from soiled items in client's room.

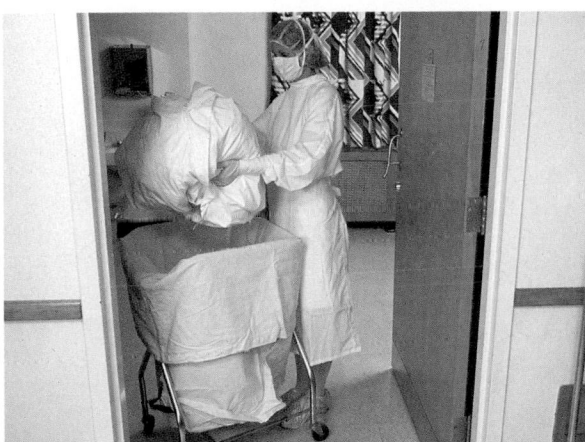

Step 11: Disposing of soiled linens in agency-specified laundry bag.

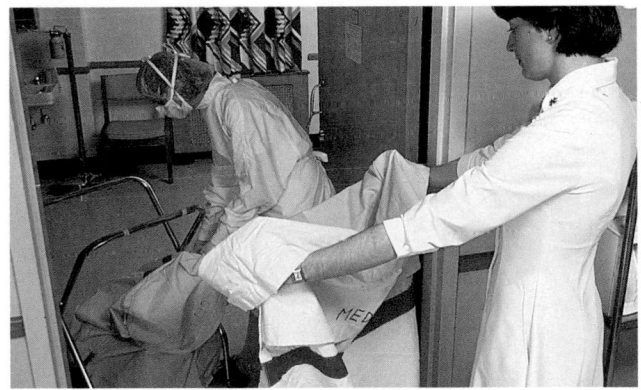

Step 11b: Assistant nurse preparing to double-bag laundry bag.

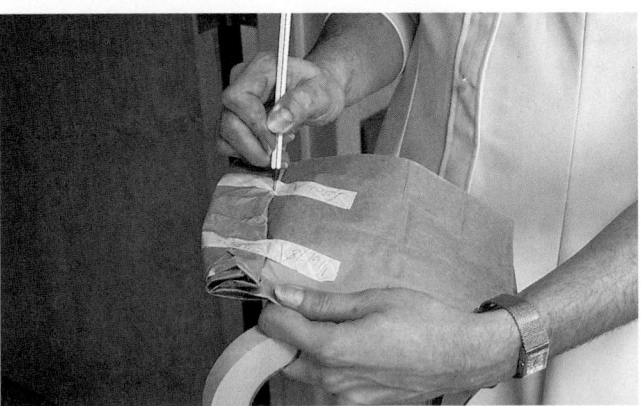

Step 11c: Assistant nurse sealing and labeling outer waste bag.

(Continued)

Action	**Rationale**
d. Have assistant hand you replacement supplies and place them in room.	
12 Remove gloves, gown, and mask before leaving and place in appropriate receptacle.	
a. Untie waist strings of gown first. Grasp outside of one glove and turn inside out to remove. Drop in waste container. Repeat procedure with second glove.	Ungloved hand is clean and should not touch contaminated areas. Waist strings of gown are considered contaminated.
b. Untie mask and drop by strings into waste container.	Center of mask is contaminated. Strings are considered clean.
c. Untie neck strings of gown. Remove gown without touching outside of gown. Neck band may be grasped to pull off gown. Turn gown inside out and drop in laundry bag.	Neck strings are considered clean. Outside of gown is contaminated.

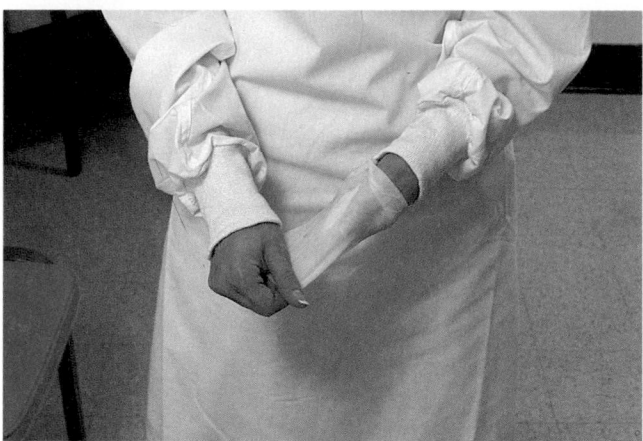

Step 12a: Removing gloves, touching only inside.

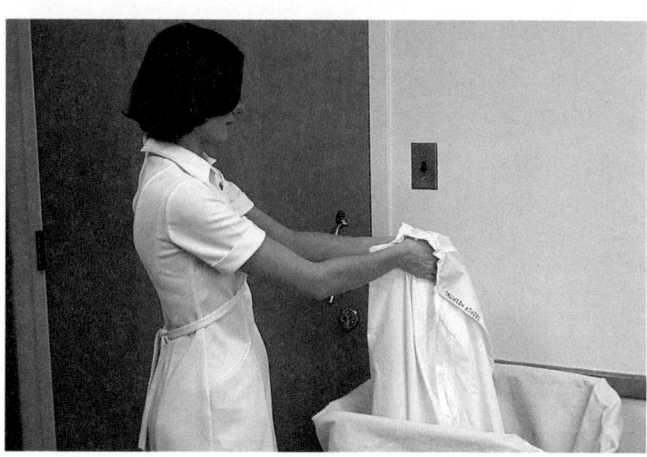

Step 12c: Disposing of gown, touching only inside.

13 Wash hands thoroughtly.	Prevents spread of microorganisms
14 Retrieve stethoscope and watch and check notation of vital signs.	Clean hands may touch clean equipment
15 Close door to room when leaving.	May depend on type of isolation. Check agency policy.
16 Record maintenance of isolation precautions and client's response in chart.	Ensures adequate documentation. Clients may require additional emotional support due to sensory deprivation and feelings associated with being isolated for a disease process.

COMPUTER APPLICATIONS IN NURSING

Computerized Help in Infection Control

The infection control nurse of the future, with the aid of analysis programs, will be able to identify trends in the rate of infection, causative infection agents, degree of treatment success, and means of transmission of infection. With this information, nurse-executives will be able to make recommendations through the Infection Control Committee.

Reference

McHugh M, Schultz S: Computer technology in hospital nursing departments: Future applications and implications. Proceedings of the Sixth Annual Symposium on Computer Applications in Medical Care. Silver Spring, MD, IEEE Computer Society Press, 1982

(Adapted from Walker MB, Schwartz C: What Every Nurse Should Know About Computers. Philadelphia. JB Lippincott, 1984)

carded in a toilet in most communities because the sewage disposal systems are adequate to destroy pathogens.

- Disposable bedpans are preferred when excretory matter is likely to carry pathogens. The safest practice for handling reusable bedpans and urinals is to empty them, rinse them thoroughly with cold water, and wash them with soap or detergent and water. They should be sterilized with steam under pressure before reuse by another client, or before reuse by the same client if the client is discharging organisms with which he could be reinfected.
- Paper tissues and dressings contaminated with wound, oral, nasal, penile, or vaginal drainage should be treated as vehicles for the transmission of organisms. The contaminated tissues and dressings should be placed in a waterproof bag and closed tightly. When the double-bag technique is being used, the bag is removed from the client's room and then discarded according to agency policy for eventual incineration.
- Gloves should be worn when handling any potentially infective material.

Specimens of body secretions and excretions may be needed for laboratory analysis. The collection container should have a lid that fits securely so leakage will not occur during transport. It is important that the outer side of the specimen container not be contaminated with pathogens for the protection of laboratory personnel. The best technique is to place the specimen container into a larger, clean container so that a barrier between the pathogens and persons handling the specimen is provided. A label on the outside of the container should clearly indicate infective material.

Meeting Psychologic Needs of Clients in Isolation.

The psychologic implications of isolation precautions are usually great, whether the client is strictly separated from others or whether he needs to observe relatively simple precautions. The feeling of being undesirable to others is generally intense for clients. They often feel frightened, lonely, unclean, guilty, and rejected. The likelihood of suffering with sensory alteration is also an undesirable accompaniment. Friends and relatives as well as health-care personnel may be inclined to spend less time with the client because of fear of contracting the disease or the inconvenience of coping with isolation procedures.

Nursing measures to help prevent sensory alteration are discussed in Chapter 37.

Teaching and supportive measures are probably the two biggest contributions the nurse can make during this period of a client's illness. The client and his family need to have an accurate understanding of the pertinent epidemiologic facts of the situation and of how to carry out the specific precautions. The idea that it is the pathogenic organism that is unwanted, not the person, must be emphasized. The client who resents and ignores precautions needs help also in being accepted as a person and in constructively expressing his feelings.

Studies have shown that extensive separation of persons from others can be very traumatic. The goal now is to minimize the extent of the precautions and the length of time they must exist as much as can be safely done. The problem of striking a balance between what is best for both the client and others is a delicate one that often requires the nurse's utmost skill and ingenuity.

A well-informed nurse who understands how to protect self and clients and a well-informed client who is cooperating in his care are superior communicable disease precautions.

Educating About Infection Control

Teaching about medical asepsis and infection control is a challenging nursing responsibility. Clients need an awareness of techniques that prevent the spread of infection. Consistent application of the nursing process protects both the client and the nurse.

In the home, medical asepsis techniques are generally appropriate for most procedures with the exception of self-injection technique. The client frequently must make adjustments and improvise with the resources and supplies available for his use. The nurse emphasizes effective handwashing and hygiene practices that interrupt the infection chain.

In the hospital, the infection control nurse is responsible for educating clients and staff about effective infection control techniques and for collecting statistics about infections. Many hospitals rely on this specialized practitioner to survey laboratory reports and review records for clients at risk as well as suggest approaches to potentially dangerous situations. Intensive investigative strategies create a positive environment to significantly reduce the incidence of nosocomial infections in health-care facilities. The infection control nurse is aware of the devastating effects of infection and is intent on promoting health and fostering a systematic approach to infection control.

KEY POINTS

■ Safety is the responsibility of all health-care providers in every environment.

■ Falls are the major safety problem in hospitals as well as the leading cause of accidental death for the elderly.

■ Those clients at high risk of falling include the elderly and those clients who have previously fallen.

■ Careless smoking in bed and faulty electric equipment are frequently implicated as causes in hospital fires.

■ Restraints that are correctly applied limit the client's mobility but do not interfere with his circulation or respirations.

■ Orientation to new surroundings, introduction to staff members, and explanations about equipment and procedures facilitate the client's transfer to a new health-care setting.

■ The infection chain consists of six components and can be interrupted by measures that halt the spread of disease.

■ The stage of an infection as well as the client's response will influence the extent and type of nursing care provided.

■ Sterilization and disinfection may be accomplished by physical or chemical means based on the nature and number of organisms, the type and intended use of equipment, and the availability and practicality of the means.

■ Handwashing is the single most effective way to prevent the spread of infection and decrease the incidence of nosocomial infection.

■ The most common nosocomial infections are urinary tract infections, surgical wound infections, and pneumonia.

■ Medical asepsis, or clean technique, is concerned with reducing the number of pathogens.

■ Surgical asepsis, or sterile technique, includes practices that keep objects and areas free from microorganisms.

■ Isolation procedures develop barriers that prevent common vehicles from transmitting pathogens.

BIBLIOGRAPHY

Adams A: External Barriers to Infection. Nurs Clin North Am 20(1):145–148, March 1985

Albert RK, Condie F: Handwashing patterns in medical intensive units. N Engl J Med 304(14):1465–1466, June 11, 1981

Barbieri EB: Patient falls are not patient accidents. J Gerontol Nurs 9(3):165–173, March 1983

Carpenito L: Nursing Diagnosis: Application to Clinical Practice, 2nd ed. Philadelphia, JB Lippincott, 1987

Carroll M: Infection control in long-term care. Geriatric Nurs 5(2):100–103, March–April 1984

Centers for Disease Control: Guideline for Handwashing and Hospital Environmental Control. Atlanta, US Department of Health, Education, and Welfare, Public Health Service, 1985

Centers for Disease Control: Guidelines for Prevention and Control of Nosocomial Infections. Atlanta, US Department of Health, Education, and Welfare, Public Health Service, 1983

Centers for Disease Control: Recommendations for Prevention of HIV Transmission in Health-Care Settings. Atlanta, US Department of Health, Education, and Welfare. MMWR 36 (Suppl. 28), 1987

Centers for Disease Control: Update: Universal precautions for prevention of transmission of human immunodeficiency virus, hepatitis B virus, and other bloodborne pathogens in health-care settings. Atlanta, US Department of Health, Education, and Welfare. MMWR 37:24, 1988

Cooper S: Common concern: Accidents and older adults. Geriatr Nurs 2(4):287, April 1981

Garner JS et al: CDC guidelines for the prevention and control of nosocomial infections: Guideline for isolation precautions in hospitals. Am J Infect Control 12(2):103–163, April 1984

Gillis A: Hospital acquired infections: Past, present, future. Dimens Health Serv 61(2):40, 42–43, February 1984

Gray-Vickrey M: Education to prevent falls. Geriatr Nurs 5(3):179–183, May–June 1984

Haley R: Infection control strategies save $250,000 annually. Hospitals 59(22):63–65, November 16, 1985

Jacobsen G et al: Handwashing: Ring-wearing and number of microorganisms. Nursing Res 34(3):186–188, May–June 1985

Kasal SE: Infractions in aseptic technique. AORN J 41(3):611, 613, 616–617, March 1985

Knight MR: Our safety net keeps patients from falling. RN 48(12):9–10, December 1985

Larson E: Current handwashing issues. Infect Control 5(1):15–17, January 1984

Lee PS, Pash BJ: Preventing patient falls. Nursing 83 13(2):118–120, February 1983

Morse JM et al: The patient who falls . . . and falls again

. . . defining the aged at risk. J Gerontol Nurs 11(11):15–18, November 1985

National Data Book and Guide to Sources, Statistical Abstract of the United States, 107th ed. US Department of Commerce, Bureau of Statistics, 1987

Parent B: Moral, ethical, and legal aspects of infection control. Am J Infect Control 13(6):278–280, December 1985

Riffle KL: Falls: Kinds, causes and prevention. Geriatr Nurs 3(3):165–169, May–June 1982

Rotter ML: Hygienic hand disinfection. Infect Control 5(1):18–22, January 1984

Spencer RT et al: Clinical Pharmacology and Nursing Management, 3rd ed. Philadelphia, JB Lippincott, 1989

Strumpf NE, Evans LK: Physical restraint of the hospitalized elderly: Perceptions of patients and nurses. Nurs Res 37(3):132–137, 1988

Venglarik JM et al: Which client is high risk? . . . patient safety to prevent falls. J Gerontol Nurs 11(5):28–30, May 1985

Webster M: Hospital-acquired infection: Control measures. Nurs Times 82(6):26–28, February 1986

Williamson KM, Selleck CS, Turner JG et al: Occupational health hazards for nurses: Infection. Image 20(1):48–53, 1988

Wyatt DM: Are you prepared for a hospital fire? Nursing 85 15(2):51, February 1985

26 Admitting, Discharge, and Home Visits

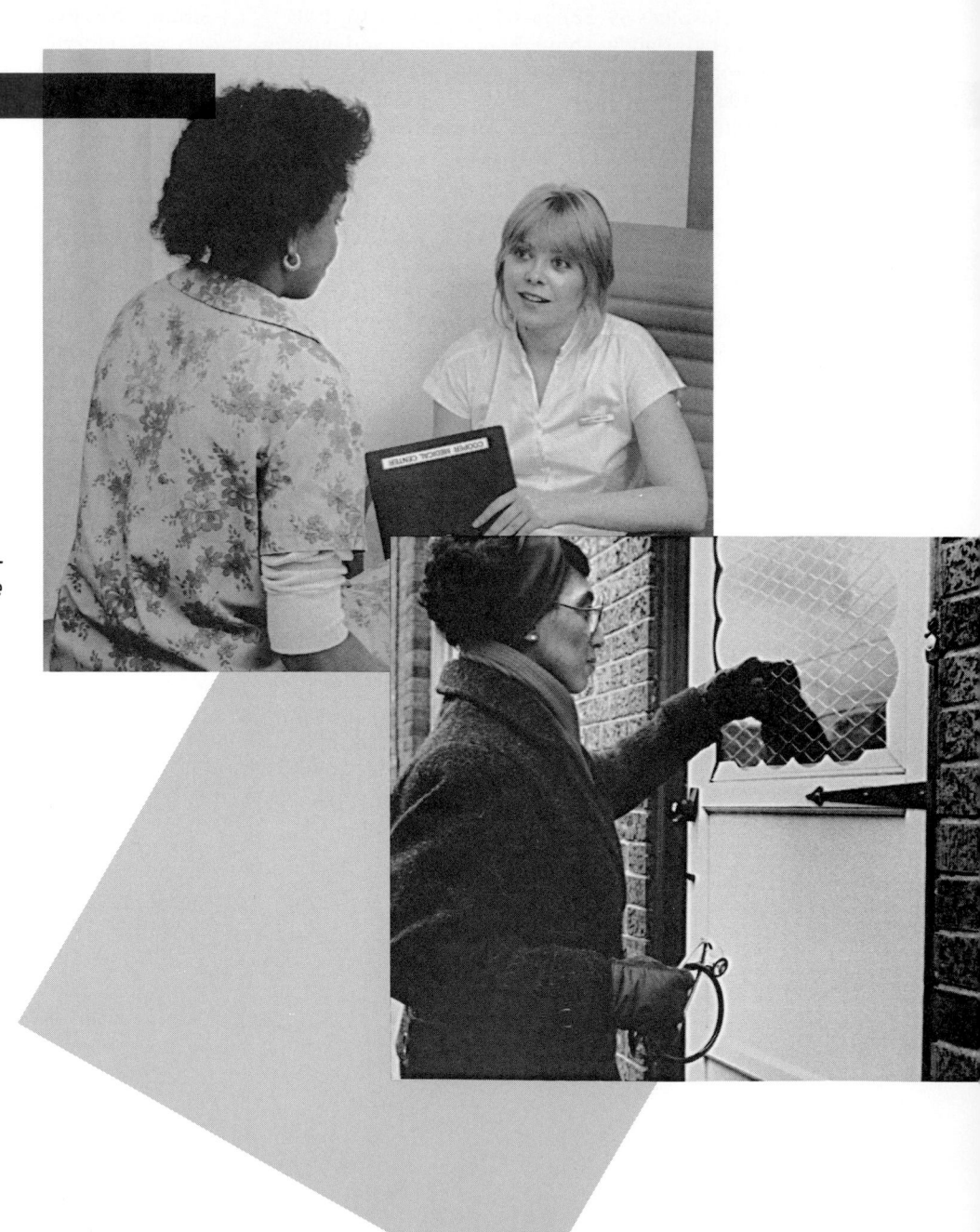

OBJECTIVES

After studying this chapter, the learner should be able to

Define key terms used in the chapter.

Identify differences and similarities between nursing care in the hospital and home.

Develop possible nursing diagnoses for a client in the hospital and develop it for home situation.

Perform a discharge assessment on a hospitalized client and family.

Be aware of constraints relating to reimbursement in the provision of home health care.

Name factors that influence planning at the individual and family level.

KEY TERMS

admission
compliance
discharge planning
home health care
intensive level care
intermediate level care

maintenance level care
noncompliance
psychiatric nurse specialist
rehabilitative level care
respite care

Today's health-care system is a large and complex entity affected by a variety of factors. Because of increasing costs and a reimbursement system that is prospective instead of retrospective, lengths of hospital stays are decreasing. This means people are discharged earlier with more instabilities and needing more care. This chapter deals with some of the ways nurses holistically promote wellness, prevent further illness, restore health, and facilitate coping in the hospital and the home.

Admission to the hospital can be a traumatic experience. Most people are not used to such structure and regimentation. Taking a sick person from the home environment and placing that person in a strange and lonely place with strange people and regulations is traumatic. The person loses identity, independence, and control of daily activities.

Going home after discharge can also be traumatic. Usually the client is sent home weakened and ill and sometimes apprehensive about a new diagnosis.

Although the person is anxious to get home there are some real fears associated with leaving the hospital —How will I manage? Who will take care of me? What about my sick husband? What happens if . . . ? All these are real fears which have an effect on the person's well-being and recuperation. The family is also concerned about its ability to manage the care of the client in the home.

The nurse is one of the most important persons clients meet on their journey through the health system. The establishment and maintenance of continuity in the delivery of care are the responsibility of the nurse. The manner in which the client is admitted to the hospital can help to diminish some of that anxiety and fear. Establishing rapport and a trusting nurse–patient relationship is important. Assisting the family to provide care in the home is done effectively by early planning and teaching. The establishment of a plan of care to be followed and coordinated in the home helps to ensure the continuity of comprehensive health care.

ADMITTING THE CLIENT

Care that was once delivered primarily in hospitals is now provided in many other settings. Ambulatory care settings and short procedure units are examples of the expansion of health-care delivery systems. Regardless of where clients enter the system or how long the stay will be, a variety of unknown factors precipitate client fear and anxiety.

The nurse plays a significant role in assuring that the admission of a client to a health agency meets basic needs. The nurse acts not only as a practitioner during the admission process, but also as a person concerned about the welfare of client and family. The admission period corresponds to the orientation phase of the helping relationship, discussed in Chapter 20.

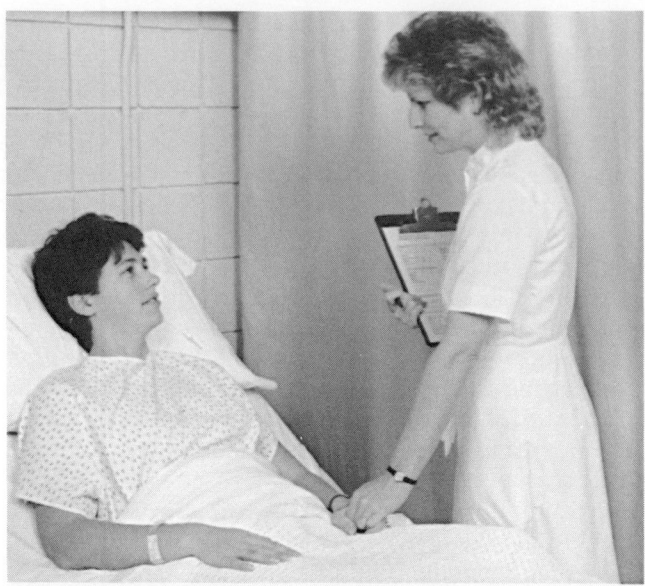

F I G U R E   26-1
Admission to the hospital can be a traumatic experience. The manner in which the client is admitted can help diminish some of the fear and anxiety. Establishing rapport and a trusting nurse–client relationship is important. (Photo © Ken Kasper)

Preliminary Admission Procedures

In most hospitals, except in emergency situations, the **admission** of clients begins in an admitting office, where basic information is obtained, for examples the person's name, address, age, occupation, type of insurance, next of kin, reason for admission, and the admitting physician. The information may be entered into a computer and placed on an admission sheet which accompanies the client to the assigned hospital unit.

The client is assigned a permanent hospital identification number when admitted. The number is used to identify the client's record during hospitalization. An identification bracelet, which contains the identification number, the client's name and room number, the physician's name, and any other information required by the agency, is placed on the client's wrist. The bracelet is important for identifying the client at times such as before administering medications and treatments and before performing surgery. Identification bracelets are especially important for identifying comatose and incoherent clients, as well as infants and children.

After the necessary forms have been completed in the admitting office, clients who are not in acute distress are generally directed to the unit to which they will be assigned. Because of cost-containment measures, lab studies and x-rays are often performed on an outpatient basis before the day of admission.

Preparing the Room for Admission

The admitting office should notify the unit prior to the patient's arrival so the room can be prepared. The fol-

lowing activities should be carried out by the nurse in anticipation of the client's arrival:

- Position the bed. For the ambulatory client, the bed should be in its lowest position. Place the bed in its highest position if the client will arrive on a stretcher. Make sure furniture in the room has been arranged to ensure easy access to the bed.
- Open the bed. Fold back the bedspread, top blanket, and top sheet.
- Assemble necessary equipment and supplies. A hospital admission pack, which contains such items as a bath basin, pitcher, drinking glass, thermometer, tissues, and lotion, is ordered for each client. A hospital gown should be available, although the client may choose to wear personal bed attire. Equipment for obtaining the client's blood pressure should also be available.
- Assemble special equipment and supplies. The client may require oxygen therapy, cardiac monitoring, or suction equipment. The nurse makes sure equipment is functioning properly and is ready for the patient's use upon arrival.

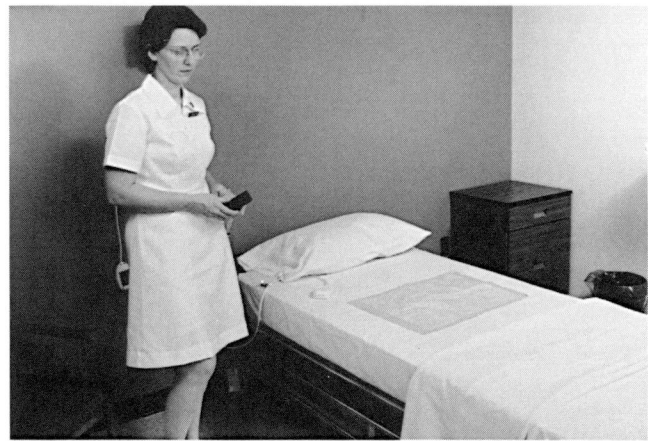

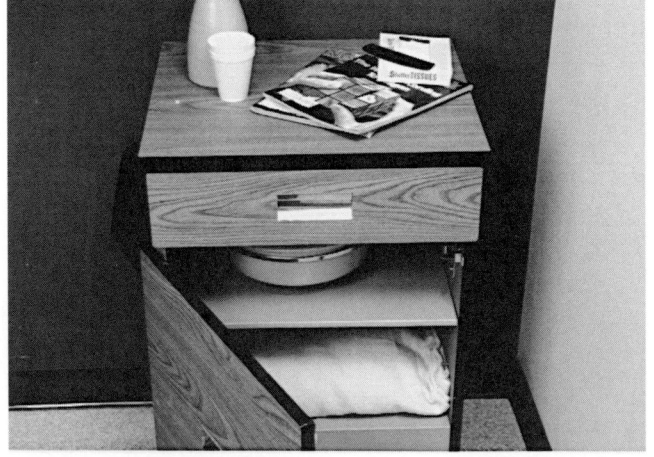

F I G U R E   26-2
In anticipation of the client's arrival, the nurse should open the bed, position the bed, and assemble necessary equipment and supplies.

PROCEDURE 26-1
Admitting a Client to the Unit

Action

1 Check the clients' identification band. Greet the client and relatives. Introduce yourself to the client and the client to his roommate(s).

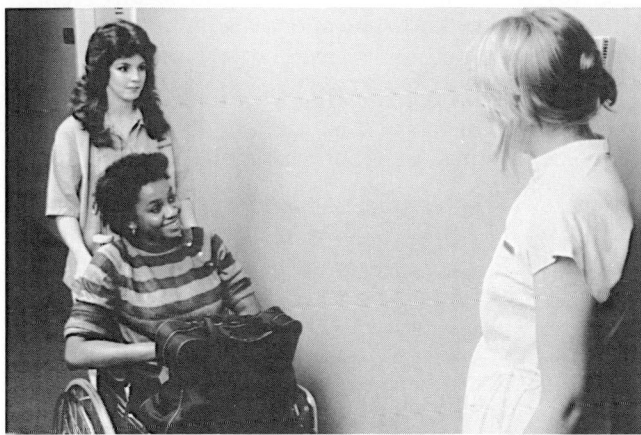

2 Explain use of the bathroom and agency equipment, such as the call system, adjustable bed, television, telephone, and so on. Explain agency routines, such as meal times, visiting hours, and so on.

3 Place the signal device and other equipment so that they will be convenient for the client to use.

4 Obtain the client's temperature, pulse and respiratory rates, and blood pressure. Obtain a urine specimen at a convenient time during the admission procedure.

5 Provide for privacy. Ask relatives to leave unless they will assist with undressing the client.

6 Help the client to undress, if indicated, and assist the client into a comfortable position in bed.

Rationale

Calling the client by name, extending common courtesies, and welcoming the client and relatives often help them to feel at ease and less frightened.

Step 1: Greeting the client.

Explaining agency routines and how to use equipment helps put the client at ease. Knowing how to use equipment helps prevent accidents.

Being unable to call for help is unsafe and can result in accidents. When equipment is handy for clients, accidents, such as falling, are less likely to occur.

Obtaining these signs and specimen is an important part of the clients' admission physical examination and is the nurse's responsibility.

Providing privacy shows respect and interest in the client.

Assisting the client to undress and into bed conserves strength, helps prevent accidents, and prepares the client for care. If he has no functional limitations, it is important to allow the client the opportunity to change alone.

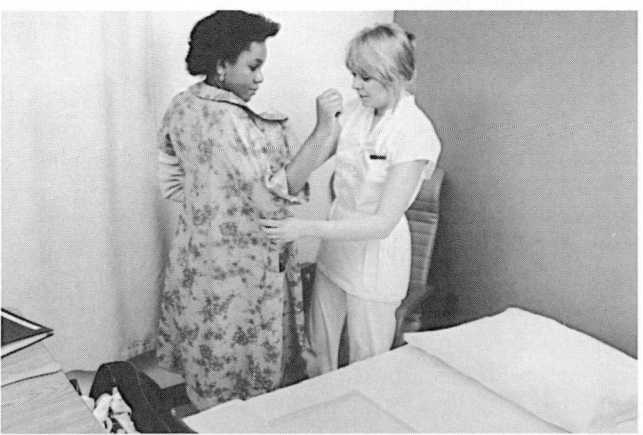

Step 6: Helping the client change into bed clothes.

(Continued)

P R O C E D U R E 26-1
Admitting a Client to the Unit (Continued)

Action

7 Take care of the client's clothing and valuables. Follow agency procedure.

8 Indicate to relatives that they may return to the client's bedside.

9 Take this time to tell the client what will be happening and what to expect.

Rationale

Losing items is upsetting to the client and can result in legal problems.

Relatives have worries and fears too and usually feel better when they know the client is admitted, settled, and comfortable.

It is very stressful not knowing what to expect. This explanation may decrease some anxiety. It will also give you some information about what the client perceives as the problem.

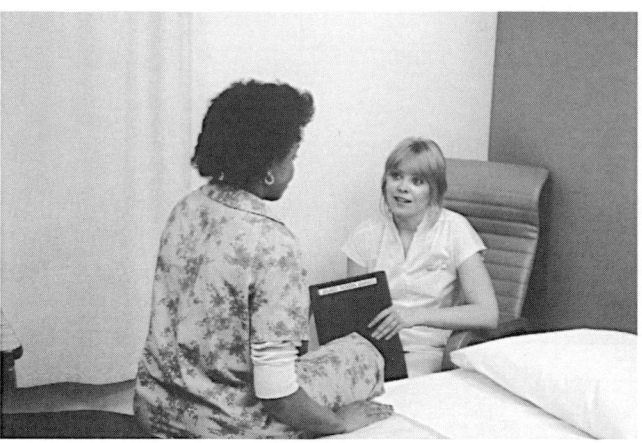

Step 9: Talking to the client about what to expect.

10 Do necessary recording on client's record, following agency policy. Begin the nursing history and assessment—it may or may not be advisable to have the family in the room.

11 After the family has left continue the history and assessment.

The information is an important part of the client's permanent record. Presence of family may inhibit the responses of the client.

The client may divulge important information that he did not want family to know.

• Adjust the physical environment of the room. This may include turning on lights and setting the room temperature.

Arrival of the Client on the Unit

The nurse becomes accountable for the client's comfort and well-being upon arrival. The person who initially meets the client assumes responsibility for making him feel that he will be receiving individualized attention and quality nursing care. The admitting practices carried out by the nurse will be directed primarily by the physio-

logic and psychologic status of the client. Procedure 26-1 presents techniques generally used by the nurse when admitting the client. Documentation must be made of the client's arrival, and all pertinent information must be charted.

The nurse should welcome the client in the same courteous manner used in welcoming guests into one's home. The nurse must assess the role the family plays as a support to the client. It may be necessary for them to be present for client support and to provide information for the nursing history. If the family needs to wait outside the room, direct them to a comfortable area and check

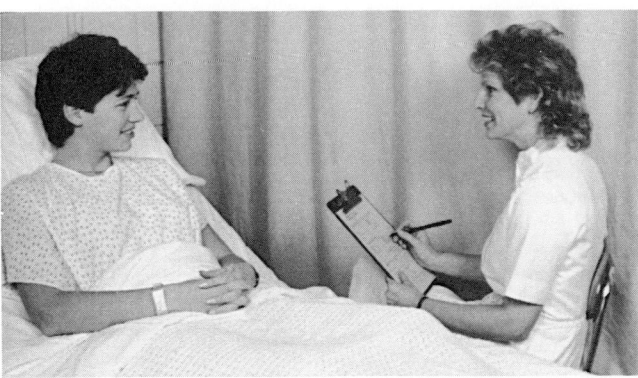

F I G U R E 26-3
The admission data base is used for the present hospitalization and for discharge and home-care planning. (Photo © Ken Kasper)

on them periodically. Both client and family need attention, especially if it is a first encounter with the health-care system.

After the client is made comfortable, the nurse uses a form to gather the admission data base (see sample form based on Gordon's functional health patterns, pp. 536–537). Each facility has its own form. The data base is used for the present hospitalization and also for discharge planning and home care.

DISCHARGE PLANNING

Many hospitalized clients are in an acute state of illness and are sent home earlier than the previous prctice but with many skilled nursing needs.

Clients and their families are expected to adhere to very complicated, highly technical treatment plans. If they are not adequately prepared, the result may be that the client is rehospitalized with an exacerbation of the illness or a more severe complication. This be prevented by providing the client with comprehensive health care to ensure ongoing needs are met. Discharge planning is an integral component of comprehensive health care.

Discharge planning is defined as a systematic process for preparing the client to leave the health-care agency and for continuity of care. The key to successful discharge planning is an exchange of information among the client, the present caregivers, and those responsible for care after release. Coordination of aspects of discharge is generally the nurse's responsibility.

Discharge planning is virtually the same as the nursing process. It is a process by which a multidisciplinary team anticipates and plans for the needs of a client and family after discharge from a health-care facility. The ultimate goal in assisting the client and family is the achievement of an optimal level of wellness. Effective discharge planning will also guarantee continuity of care in the least stressful manner.

For discharge planning to be effective, it must begin at the time of admission. With shorter hospital stays and increased acuity in client status, it is crucial to plan for discharge early. The nurse must anticipate needs and prepare the client and family for a smooth transition.

There are a number of ways in which discharge planning can occur. Each institution has its own organizational structure that should be adhered to. Discharge planning must be

- Coordinated
- Interdisciplinary
- Initiated as early as possible
- Carefully planned
- Involving the client, family or significant others who are caregivers

Initiation of the process involves identifying clients who need discharge planning. All clients need this service, but certain clients are at higher risk for specific needs and services. The nurse who conducts the initial nursing assessment is in the best position to determine these special needs. Burgess (1983) describes characteristics that indicate the need for a formal discharge plan and referral to another agency:

- Lack of knowledge of treatment plan
- Social isolation
- Newly diagnosed chronic disease
- Major surgery
- Radical surgery
- Prolonged recuperation from major surgery or illness
- Emotional or mental instability
- Complex home-care regimen
- Financial difficulties
- Lack of available or approximate referral sources
- Terminal illness

Discharge planning is also indicated when a client is to be placed in a nursing home or other continued care setting. The American Nurses Association has published the following in support of discharge planning.

Continuity of care planning in an organized health care system establishes a process designed to meet the needs of the patient or client during every phase of care. The process involves admission planning, discharge planning, referral and follow up (ANA, 1975).

Assessing

Assessment involves collecting and organizing data about a client. (Assessment and interviewing are covered in detail in Chaps 15 and 20.) When assessing the client for discharge, the family is included as the unit of care. The client and family must be actively involved in the discharge process if the transition from hospital to home is to be effective.

A sample data base form, including information for discharge planning, was printed in the Admitting section of this chapter. It follows Gordon's (1980) organizing
(Text continues on p. 538.)

Doe, Jane   Age 73

1200 West Elm

Jackson, MO

00011000

(Area must be completed by RN or LPN)

PATIENT'S HEALTH HISTORY

What is reason for admission? (Patient's own words)

"I had trouble breathing and a bad cough"

Past Hospitalization and/or illnesses: (Medical, surgical, emotional problems)

1980 Heart Problems
1982 Colon Resection

Saint Francis Medical Center

NURSING ADMISSION DATA BASE
(Entire area can be completed by any patient care staff)

Date: 12-2-89   Time: 0900

ADMISSION

- ☐ Ambulatory ☒ Wheelchair ☐ Stretcher
- ☐ Correct identification band ☐ Allergy band

Admitted From: ☒ Home ☐ Nursing Facility ☐ Emergency Room ☐ Other _____

Information Given By: ☐ Family member ☐ Friend ☒ Patient ☐ Unable to take history, patient unresponsive/ not accompanied by family or friend

Orientation to Room
- ☒ Visiting hours ☒ Call light system (bedside/bath)
- ☒ Smoking policy ☒ Use of phone
- ☒ Bedrails up at H.S. unless ordered otherwise

Valuables: ☐ None ☒ Sent home ☐ To safe

Allergens: (Drugs, food, tapes, dyes, other) ☐ NKA ☒ Allergy Bracelet Applied

Allergen	Symptoms	Treatment
Pollens	stuffy nose	none
Penicillin	rash	avoid drug

(Area must be completed by the RN or LPN)

Medications Prescribed And Non-Prescribed	Dosage	Usual Times Taken	Time Of Last Dose	Patient's Understanding Of Purpose/Problems
Aspirin	3 tabs	8-12-6	12/2: 8AM	for arthritis
Lanoxin	0.125 mg	8 Am	12/2: 8Am	for heart
Diuril	500 mg	8-6	12/2: 8Am	for heart
Milk of Magnesia	1½ oz.	bedtime	11/30/89	as needed for constipation

Medications sent ☒ To Pharmacy ☐ Home With whom? _____

FUNCTIONAL HEALTH PATTERN ASSESSMENT

(All areas of the Functional Health Pattern Assessment MUST be completed by the RN with the exception of #1 of Objective Data. See *)   (√) Box if data is pertinent)

SUBJECTIVE DATA:

1. Health Perceptions/Health Management Pattern

General health __Good__

Use of: ☐ Tobacco How much ∅ How long? ____
☐ Alcohol How much? ∅ How long? ____
Last Drink _____
☒ Other drugs type(s) __see above__

2. Nutritional/Metabolic Patterns

Special diet __Low Salt__

Meals/day __3__   Snacks/day __1__

Weight: ☐ Gain ☒ Loss ☐ How much? __5 pounds__
☐ No problems

3. Respiration/Circulation Patterns

History of: ☒ Shortness of breath ☒ With exercise
☐ Without exercise
☒ Cough ☒ Sputum (phlegm)
☐ No problems Sleeps on __2__ pillows

History of: ☐ Chest pain ☒ Pedal Edema ☐ No problems
☐ Pacemaker ☐ Rate ☐ Arrhythmias

640-009-816/0800053

OBJECTIVE DATA: *(#1 of objective data can be completed by any patient care staff)

1. Clinical Data

Height __64"__   Weight __142__ ⊙ Actual/approx ____
Temperature __99.8°__ Pulse __102__ Respirations __30__
Blood pressure Right arm __120/72__ Left arm __124/76__
☐ Sitting ☒ Lying

2. Nutritional/Metabolic Pattern

Oral Mucosa: ☒ Color __pink__ ☐ Lesions __NO__ Moistness __yes__
Teeth: ☒ Dentures ☒ Upper ☒ Lower
Skin integrity: ☒ Turgor normal ☐ Other ____
☐ Intact ☒ Other __Sl. pedal edema__

3. Respiration/Circulation Pattern

Breath sounds __Rales and Rhonchi, both lower lung bases__
Cough: ☐ Non-Productive ☒ Productive ☒ Sputum Color __Rusty__
Apical Rate __104__ Rhythm: ☒ Regular ☐ Irregular
Pedal edema: ☒ Present ☐ Absent
Right dorsalis pedal pulse: ☒ Strong ☐ Weak ☐ Absent
Left dorsalis pedal pulse: ☒ Strong ☐ Weak ☐ Absent
Homan's sign Positive R ☐ L ☐ Negative R ☒ L ☒

(Used with permission of St. Francis Medical Center, Cape Girardeau, MO)

(continued)

SUBJECTIVE DATA (Cont'd)

4. Elimination Pattern

History of: ☐ Nausea   ☐ Vomiting   ☐ Dysphagia
☒ No Problems

Bowel Habits: Stools/Day __1/q 3 days__ ☐ Soft/Formed
☒ Constipation   ☐ Diarrhea
☐ Incontinence   ☐ Melena   Last BM __12/1/89__

Bladder habits: Urinates/Day __4-5X__ ☒ No problem
☐ Self-Cath   ☐ Urgency   ☐ Frequency
☐ Nocturia   ☐ Dysuria   ☐ Hematuria
☐ Incontinence

5. Activity/Exercise Pattern

Energy level: ☒ Tires easily   ☐ Average
☐ High/Energy

Exercise Program: ☒ None   ☐ Other _____

Able to: ☒ Feed self   ☒ Bathe self   ☐ With assist
☒ Ambulate   ☒ Climb stairs
☒ Can do household chores

Adaptive devices: ☐ Cane   ☐ Walker   ☐ Crutches
☐ Wheelchair   ☐ Other __Ø__

6. Sleep/Rest Pattern

Sleep problems: ☐ Trouble falling asleep
☒ Early AM waking   ☐ Other
☐ No Problems

7. Cognitive/Perceptual Pattern

Communication: Language spoken __English__
Understands __German__
Able to: ☒ Read   ☒ Write   ☐ Lip read
Cognition: ☒ No problems   ☐ Recent memory change
☐ Difficulty learning
Discomfort/pain: ☐ No   ☒ Yes   Where? __L. Thorax__
How do you manage your pain? __use medicines,__
__go to bed, read Bible__

8. Role/Relationship Pattern

Marital Status: ☒ Married   ☐ Single   ☐ Widowed
☐ Divorced
Children (#) __3__
Occupation __Housewife__
Retirement activities: (Hobbies) __Knits, reads__

Family concerns about hospitalization? __Worried about__
__long-term effects of illness__

9. Sexuality/Reproductive Pattern (if appropriate)

Last menstrual period __20 years ago__
Menstrual problems ☐ Yes   ☒ No
Birth control measures __N/A__
Any sexual concerns related to illness (optional)
__NO__

Signature __P. Le Mone R.N.__
Date __12/2/89__

OBJECTIVE DATA (Cont'd)

4. Elimination Pattern

Abdomen: ☒ Soft   ☐ Firm
☒ Non-tender   ☐ Tender
☐ Non-distended   ☐ Distended _____ girth
☒ Bowel sounds   ☐ Bowel sounds absent
☐ Ostomies/tubes   ☐ Type _____

Urinary devices _____

5. Activity/Exercise Pattern

ROM: ☐ Full   ☒ Other __Arthritic changes__
Balance and gait: ☒ Steady   ☐ Unsteady
Hand grasps: ☒ Equal   ☐ Strong
Weakness/paralysis: ☐ Right   ☐ Left
Leg muscles: ☒ Equal   ☐ Strong
☐ Weakness/Paralysis ☐ Right   ☐ Left
☐ Disorientation at night
☐ Prone to falling

7. Cognitive/Perceptual Pattern

Level of consciousness: ☒ Alert   ☒ Responds to pain
☐ No response
Oriented to: ☒ Time   ☒ Place   ☒ Person
Mood: ☒ Calm   ☐ Sad   ☐ Angry   ☐ Withdrawn
☐ Other _____
Pupils: ☒ Equal   ☒ Reactive   ☐ Other _____
Cognition: ☒ Able to follow simple commands
☒ Responds appropriately to questions
☐ Unable to follow commands
☐ Other
Hearing: ☒ Normal   ☐ Impaired   ☐ Left ear
☐ Right ear   ☐ Aid
Vision: ☐ Normal   ☒ Impaired   ☒ Glasses
☐ Contact Lenses
Pain: Location and type __L. lower thorax__

Discharge Planning Evaluation

		A	B
1. Do you live at home alone?		Yes ☐	No ☒
2. Who lives with you? __husband, Carl__			
3. Do you live in a house, apartment, or trailer? __house__			
Do you live in a nursing home or boarding home?		Yes ☐	No ☒
4. Do you have any problems caring for yourself at home?		Yes ☐	No ☒
5. What relatives or friends are willing to help with your care if needed:			
Name: __Son, Joe__			
Phone: __111-2222__			
6. Have you been receiving help from any person or agency while at home?		Yes ☐	No ☒
Name of person: _____			
Name of agency(s): _____			
7. Will you need any help with care to be able to return home?		Yes ☐	No ☒
8. Discharge planning coordinator or social service indicated at admission?		Yes ☐	No ☒
If yes, notify appropriate person.			

Elements of a Discharge Planning Assessment

Health data

Clients' age, sex, height, weight, diagnosis, past medical history, current health problems, surgery, functional limitations such as amputations, wheelchair or walker use, blindness

Personal data

Ascertain how the client feels about discharge (is he anxious? frightened?), expectations for recovery—are they realistic? What are the caregivers' expectations and fears? What has been their coping ability in the past—effective or ineffective? What are their attitudes and beliefs about health and illness, health habits? Values, religious beliefs, and cultural practices that may affect treatments, such as diet, restriction on blood products; Who are the caregivers—age, sex, relationship, any illness or disability, past experience with this treatment or illness? Does caregiver live with client? What is educational level of client and caregiver? Any language barriers?

Environment

Include both home and community. Are there any structural barriers that would inhibit function—narrow stairs for a wheelchair-bound elderly client or caregiver; assistive devices in bathroom; hot water, heat, available space; Rural or urban community; availability of health care in close proximity; transportation availability; known hazards (water, air).

Client/Family Knowledge

Assess the understanding of treatment plan and care regimen—medication, side-effects, diet diagnosis, and prognosis; emergency measures, complications, and symptoms of impending problems.

Financial/Support Services

A financial profile should be completed here. What will be the expenses, including new medication and treatments? All available resources to assist this family (Medicaid, food stamps, Meals on Wheels) If this client is alone and home bound, what support services are available? If the client is not homebound, where can he go to obtain these services?

framework based on functional health patterns (see Chap 15). Important elements of a discharge planning assessment are listed in the box on this page. Whatever assessment tool is used, it must be a holistic assessment that encompasses all aspects of the client/family life. The medical record and physician orders must also be consulted for the exact medication and treatment plan before a nursing care plan can be developed.

Diagnosing

In the development of the nursing diagnosis, the needs of both the client and family must be recognized. The family is the unit of care, and the health status of the client greatly influences the others. Examples of nursing diagnoses for a client being discharged from the hospital are:

> Self-care deficit related to inability to dress self secondary to neuromuscular impairment
> Knowledge deficit related to dietary and insulin management of diabetes mellitus
> Ineffective family coping related to lack of support systems
> Impaired home management related to chronic debilitating disease

It is important to note whether these are actual or potential problems. For example, if the client and family cannot administer insulin on the day of discharge, that is an actual problem in knowledge deficit. But you may not be certain that a client leaving the hospital with an order for daily dressing changes to a leg wound will do well if the caregiver is also elderly and has limited mobility. There is potential here for poor management of the situation. Reassessment of goals and learning needs is necessary.

Planning

Goals must be mutually set to ensure success. **Compliance** is the act of completing what is expected of one; **noncompliance** is a disregard of orders or not completing what is expected of one. Goals that are acceptable to all will encourage compliance. Noncompliance will occur shortly after discharge if goals are not realistic.

METHOD Approach. The METHOD approach to discharge planning (p. 539) focuses on six critical areas of teaching, to be addressed prior to the client's departure from the hospital.

Interdisciplinary Approach. The nurse as coordinator of services initiates all contacts and consults with other disciplines. Their expertise must be used in the provision of comprehensive health care.

In the following example the interdisciplinary approach is described. Mr. Smith is a 55-year-old, married man with a diagnosis of cerebral vascular accident (stroke) with left hemiparesis (weakness). He also has

METHOD Discharge Planning

M: Medication

The client will know
- Drug name
- What dosage to take and when
- Purpose of drug
- Effect(s) the drug should have
- Symptoms of possible adverse effects, and which ones to report. (Repeat for each drug prescribed)

E: Environment

The client will be assured of
- Adequate instruction in necessary homemaking skills
- Investigation and correction of any physical hazards in the home environment
- Adequate emotional support
- Investigation of sources of economic support
- Investigation of transportation means to appointments and/or clients

T: Treatment

The client and family will
- Know the purpose of any treatment to be continued at home
- Be able to demonstrate correct performance of the treatment

H: Health Teaching

The client will
- Describe how his or her disease or condition affects body function
- Describe the means necessary to maintain present level of health, or achieve a higher level of health

O: Outpatient Referral

The client will
- Know when and where to keep clinical appointments
- Know where and whom to call for medical help
- Take home written discharge instructions

D: Diet

The client will be able to
- Describe the purpose of his or her prescribed diet
- Plan several typical menus using the prescribed diet

(Rosemarie A. Cucuzzo: METHOD of Discharge Planning Supervisory Nurse 7:43–45, 1976; reprinted with permission)

difficulty communicating verbally and has a history of hypertension for 10 years. He is to be discharged from the hospital in 3 days if his blood pressure remains stable. He will be going home with four new medications, a Foley catheter, and feeding tube. After reviewing the medical record, the nurse interviews Mr. and Mrs. Smith. The assessment reveals Mr. Smith is limited in his ability to transfer from bed to chair. Both Mr. and Mrs. Smith are fearful of discharge, but Mr. Smith believes he will be able to return to work as an accountant in 3 weeks, and Mrs. Smith thinks he'll never work again. They have never faced a life-threatening illness in the past, but he has had severe hypertension and hasn't been compliant with diet or medication regimen. Mr. Smith believes he will be fine soon and hates the thought of being an invalid at his age. They are both Catholic but have no strong cultural preferences in terms of diet. They have two adult children living out of state with their own families. Mrs. Smith does have a younger sister living nearby. They are both college educated. The Smiths live in a suburban area in a two-story home with narrow stairs leading to two baths and three bedrooms on the second floor. They have adequate plumbing but no as-

sistive devices. Their doctor's office is about a mile away, and shopping is nearby.

Mrs. Smith does not believe she can manage care of the feeding tube and Foley catheter. She also needs instruction in the new medication and diet regimen. She is terrified that she may not be able to handle an emergency in the middle of the night.

Financially, this two-income family has quickly become one and will shortly have no income. Mr. Smith is not 65 and not yet eligible for Medicare.

How would the nurse coordinate this discharge plan? The physician must be consulted for diet, medication, and other treatment orders. Physical therapy has already been initiated at the hospital. Occupational therapy also needs to evaluate Mr. Smith's ability to perform activities of daily living (ADLs) and to fit him with assistive devices. The nutritionist needs to counsel the Smiths on the 1-g sodium diet and on creative ways to prepare low-salt meals. The social worker has been called for financial assessment to determine exactly what services the Smiths can expect to have reimbursed by their insurance carrier, and how they will manage their out-of-pocket expenses. The nurse will begin to formulate a teaching plan for medications and treatment. Mrs. Smith must learn about the Foley catheter and feeding tube before discharge to feel more in control. Hopefully, some of their fears will be dealt with, and new coping strategies will develop. The nurse will also make a referral to the local visiting nurse association to continue physical therapy and nursing care and to evaluate if any more teaching is necessary at home.

Teaching Plan. The teaching plan has been discussed in great detail in Chapter 21. Review of the sample teaching plan in Chapter 21 will aid the student in understanding the steps and strategies of discharge planning. All aspects of teaching may not be completed in the hospital, and referral to a home-care agency may be necessary for follow-up care and teaching.

Implementing

Implementation is the actual carrying out of the teaching plan and referrals. All teaching should be documented in the nurse's notes and the discharge summary (p. 541). Written instructions are given to the client. Return demonstrations must be satisfactory. The client and caregiver must have exposure to and practice with the equipment they will be using at home.

The home-care referral is made before the client is actually discharged. As much information as possible about the client and the hospitalization should be given to the agency. Such information includes the kind of surgery, medication (including need for intravenous

fluids at home), the client's physical and mental status, and significant social factors (*e.g.,* frail caregiver with health problem, no caregiver), and expected needs of the family. Transportation should be arranged at this time.

For a home-care referral to be made and subsequent home visits to be reimbursed, there must be a written order by the physician for all services. Clients must meet certain criteria to have home-care services reimbursed by Medicare and other third-party payors. Reimbursement issues are briefly discussed in the home-visit section. The guidelines for discharge of a client are presented in Procedure 26-2.

Discharging a Client Against Advice. The client who is leaving the hospital *against medical advice* (sometimes abbreviated AMA) must sign a form releasing the hospital and physician from responsibility and any ill effects that may result from such action. The client has the right to terminate health care, but the nurse has an obligation to discuss with the client the possible outcomes of this decision. Each agency has its own form for clients who choose to leave against medical advice. It is required that the client's signature on the form be witnessed and that financial arrangements be completed through the business office.

Evaluating

Evaluation of the discharge plan is crucial in making this process work. Planning and referrals must be scrutinized to ensure quality and appropriateness of services. Evaluation is ongoing, and the need for revision of plans also changes.

Further evaluation of the discharge process is usually conducted a few weeks after the client has been home. It may be carried out by a telephone call, a questionnaire, or a home visit.

Case Study

The following case study illustrates nursing care of a client with and without discharge planning.

Mr. Sam Jones is a 75-year-old retired truck driver. He lives with his wife, who has just recently suffered a heart attack. She is on oxygen and frequently complains of chest pain and shortness of breath. Activity restriction, a low-salt diet and a number of medications have been ordered for her. She is also incontinent of urine. Mr. Jones is the primary caretaker. He has recently complained of increased urination, thirst, and hunger, as well as periods of weakness, headache, and blurred vision. He was admitted to the hospital, and diabetes mellitus was diagnosed. He is to be discharged this morning (day 4) on NPH insulin and a 1500-calorie diabetic diet.

Case Study Without Effective Discharge Planning.

Insulin was not ordered for Mr. Jones until the day before discharge. His primary nurse could not begin teach-

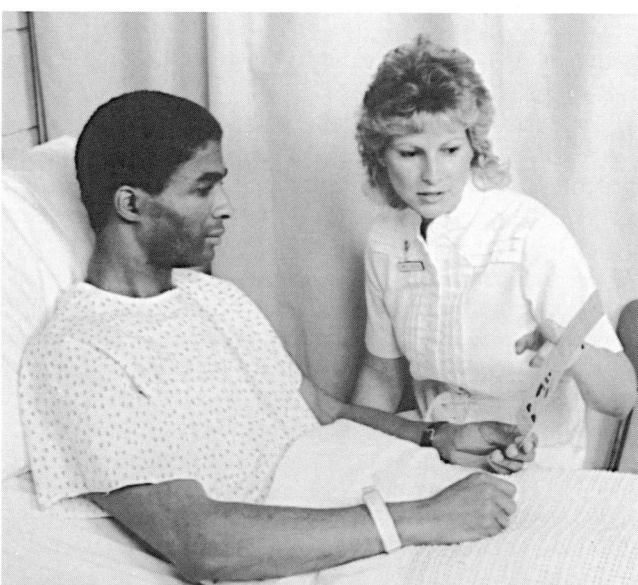

F I G U R E 26-4
Written instructions for continuing self-care at home should be given to the client. The nurse should review the instructions with the client to ensure that they are clearly understood. (Photo © Ken Kasper)

Doe, Jane
1200 West Elm
Jackson, Mo.
000 11 000

Age 73

ST. FRANCIS MEDICAL CENTER
211 ST. FRANCIS DRIVE
CAPE GIRARDEAU, MO. 63701

PATIENT DISCHARGE SUMMARY

I

MEDICATION (NAME/DOSAGE)	6 AM	7 AM	8 AM	9 AM	10 AM	11 AM	12 NOON	1 PM	2 PM	3 PM	4 PM	5 PM	6 PM	7 PM	8 PM	9 PM	10 PM	11 PM	12 PM	1 AM
ASA gr $\overline{XV}$			X				X						X							
Lanoxin 0.125 mg			X																	
Diuril 500 mg			X										X							
Cefaclor 500 mg			X								X								X	

WEEKLY SCHEDULE (For alternating dosage)

NAME / DOSAGE	SUNDAY	MONDAY	TUESDAY	WEDNESDAY	THURSDAY	FRIDAY	SATURDAY

☒ **PRESCRIPTION GIVEN TO PATIENT**   ☐ **HOME MEDICATIONS RETURNED**   ☒ **HANDOUT GIVEN IF APPLICABLE**

MEDICATIONS SHOULD BE TAKEN IN ACCORDANCE WITH YOUR PHYSICIAN'S PRESCRIPTION. THIS FORM IS PROVIDED AS A SERVICE BY ST. FRANCIS MEDICAL CENTER. ANY CHANGE IN AMOUNT OR DOSAGE OF MEDICATION MUST BE APPROVED BY YOUR PHYSICIAN.

II   **SPECIAL DISCHARGE INSTRUCTIONS** (Side Affects to Medications, Activities, Diabetes, Cardiac Rehab., P.T., R.T., Wound or Dressing Care, Irrigation, etc.)

1) Take antibiotic (Cefaclor) with food; report rash or GI upset to MD

2) Use good handwashing to prevent spread of infection and dispose of sputum and tissues in paper bag

3) Rest for one hour each afternoon

4) Drink extra fluids for this week

INSTRUCTED BY P. LeMone R.N.   PATIENT UNDERSTANDS ☒ YES ☐ NO   CARBON COPY GIVEN TO PATIENT ☒

III   M.D. OFFICE VISIT ☐ NO ☒ YES   1 week - appointment made

IV   **METHOD OF DISCHARGE**

☒ RELEASE SIGNED

☐ AMA WITH RELEASE SIGNED BY PATIENT ☐ YES ☐ NO

DR. NOTIFIED   Date _____ Time _____

D/C BY DR. James
D/C DATE 12-2-89   Time 1000
HOW D/C ☒ VOLUNTEER, OTHER and husband
TRANSPORTED BY ☐ STRETCHER ☒ W/C ☐ AMBULATORY

V   **DISCHARGED TO:**

☒ HOME WITH WHOM husband
☐ NURSING HOME _____
☐ TRANSFER TO OTHER FACILITY _____

VI   **GENERAL CONDITION ON DISCHARGE**

☒ ALERT	☐ LETHARGIC	☒ PAIN CONTROLLED	☐ DECUBITUS	☒ SELF
☒ ORIENTED	☐ COMATOSE	☒ AFEBRILE	☐ INCISION HEALING	☐ WITH HELP
☐ CONFUSED	☐ PAIN FREE	☐ RASH	☐ DRAINING WOUND	☐ ROOM ONLY
			☒ AMBULATORY	☐ HALL

Signature P. LeMone R.N.   Date 12-2-89

640-260-812/0800048

(Used with permission of St. Francis Medical Center, Cape Girardeau, MO)

CHART

Discharging a Client from a Health-care Agency

Action	**Rationale**
1 Check to see that the client has a discharge order.	It is the physician's responsibility to discharge a client.
2 Make sure the client or support person has had discharge instructions (*i.e.,* regarding diet, medications).	The client or a support person should be able to continue with necessary care after discharge when properly instructed.
3 Have all necessary equipment and supplies ready for the client.	Having equipment and supplies ready saves time and the annoyance of having to wait for them when the client is ready to leave.
4 Check to see that proper financial arrangements have been made by the client or support person. Obtain valuables. Observe agency policies.	These actions help to avoid legal problems.
5 Assist the client to dress and pack belongings. Make sure the client has all personal belongings.	Assisting the client conserves client strength. Time and trouble are saved when the client leaves with all belongings.
6 If the client needs reimbursement for future home visits, be sure the physician has given a written order for all services.	There must be a physician's order for reimbursement by Medicare and other third-party payers.
7 Transport the client and belongings to a car and assist the client into the car as necessary.	Assisting the client conserves client strength. Such assistance is courteous and helps the client feel that personnel are interested in the client's welfare.
8 Make necessary recordings on the client's records and complete the discharge summary.	It is important legally and for hospital records to complete the client's permanent record.

Special Considerations

If the client is leaving without a physician's consent, check to see that the proper form has been completed. If the client refuses to sign the form, document your explanation to the client and consequent refusal to sign release form; notify the physician. Because a person cannot be held legally in an institution against one's wishes, a properly signed form releases the agency and physician from responsibility should problems arise because the client refused further care.

ing him how to administer insulin until yesterday afternoon. The client is quite anxious to return home to his ailing wife, who is being cared for by neighbors. He quickly demonstrates insulin administration on the morning of discharge and is sent home with a few syringes and an insulin prescription.

The nutritionist has been informed of this client only yesterday and could schedule a consult only on the day of discharge. She sees him for a few minutes and gives him a diet to follow. By this time, Mr. Jones is counting the minutes until departure.

The client is sent home with a neighbor in time for lunch. He is so busy preparing lunch for his wife and excited about being home that he forgets to eat. At dinner, he feels nauseous and weak, and he doesn't feel like eating. At 8 PM, Mrs. Jones calls the ambulance after her husband has lost consciousness. Mr. Jones is readmitted with the diagnosis of insulin shock.

Case Study: Effective Discharge Planning. Mr. Jones first meets the discharge planning nurse on the day of his admission and learns what he should expect during the hospitalization and why he has been admitted. Mr. Jones seems quite anxious; during the intake interview, he states concern about his wife who is homebound and recovering from a recent heart attack. He explains that he is the sole caretaker and has left her alone with only neighbors checking in on her and bringing her meals.

After an initial assessment, the discharge planner confers with the physician, and both agree a home-care referral will be in order for Mrs. Jones and most probably Mr. Jones upon his discharge.

The local home-care agency now becomes involved with the family. A visiting nurse will see Mrs. Jones to monitor her medication regimen and cardiac status. A home health aide will visit to attend to her personal needs. The neighbors will continue to prepare meals and check in. Mr. Jones is much more at ease now that he knows his wife will be taken care of.

The discharge planner is coordinating this client's care. The nutritionist is called in to discuss the new diet he must follow. His food likes and dislikes, life-style, cultural and religious preferences are all taken into account during the preparation of this diet. The primary nurse, physician, and discharge planner are all involved in the care plan for this client. He is taught about his disease and insulin administration during his stay but is still unsure of himself. All agree that a home-care referral is necessary to ensure accurate compliance and support for Mr. Jones.

On the day of discharge, Mr. Jones is sent home with syringes and insulin. He knows that a visiting nurse will visit him this afternoon to obtain a 3 PM blood sugar and make sure all is well. The nurse will continue to visit to teach him the proper technique for insulin administration and the overall treatment plan. The nurse will also make sure he can adequately care for Mrs. Jones.

Can you see the difference in these two case studies? The discharge planner made the difference in the smooth transition from hospital to home and actually prevented a second more costly hospitalization for this client. The key is adequate preparation and involvement initiated as early as possible with an interdisciplinary team approach.

HOME VISITS

Caring for the sick at home is not a new phenomenon. Modern community health nursing practice developed from a history of providing health care to the sick and indigent in their homes. Today it has become a highly

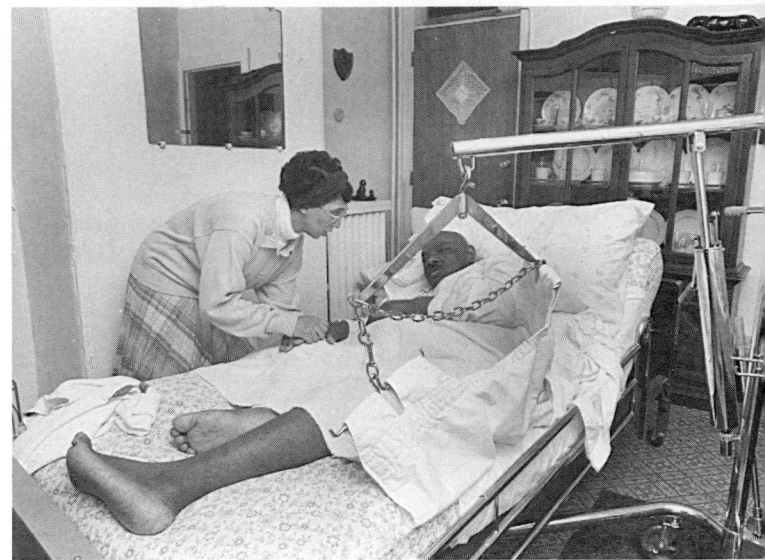

F I G U R E   26-5
Caring for the sick at home is not new but has become a highly specialized area of health care and a major component of a continuum of comprehensive health care. (Photo by Robert Coldwell, courtesy of Community Home Health Services of Philadelphia)

specialized area of health care requiring professionals with great skill and creativity.

Home health care is that component of a continuum of comprehensive health care in which health services are provided to individuals and families in their places of residence for the purpose of promoting, maintaining or restoring health, or of maximizing the level of independence while minimizing the effects of disability and illness, including terminal illness (Warhola, 1980).

Home health services are provided by a variety of agencies with an employed staff or on a contractual basis. Services include skilled care (nursing, physical therapy, speech therapy, occupational therapy), social services (to coordinate financial and long-term placement issues), counseling for family and client, and personal services (home health aide, housekeeping, companion). An agency can be hospital based, free-standing, for-profit, voluntary, not-for-profit, or official. For an agency to receive government reimbursement from the Medicare program it must be Medicare certified and must adhere to the guidelines set forth by the Health Care Financing Administration (HCFA).

Factors Affecting Home Care

The importance of home health care today is evidenced by many factors:

- The prospective payment system of reimbursement (DRG), which encourages early discharge from the hospital, has created a new acutely ill population needing skilled care at home.

- There is a greater percentage of elderly people, living longer with multiple chronic illnesses, who are not institutionalized.
- With more sophisticated technology, a person can be kept alive and relatively comfortable in their own home.
- Health-care consumers demand that services be humane with provisions for a dignified death at home.

Reimbursement.   Cost containment is an important factor in home health care. Services must be carefully coordinated and planned to ensure reimbursement. Reimbursement is affected by three levels of care in home health services: intensive, intermediate, and maintenance.

Intensive level care indicates that a client's condition warrants close observation, monitoring, or treatment, and requires skilled care (*e.g.,* a client who needs sterile

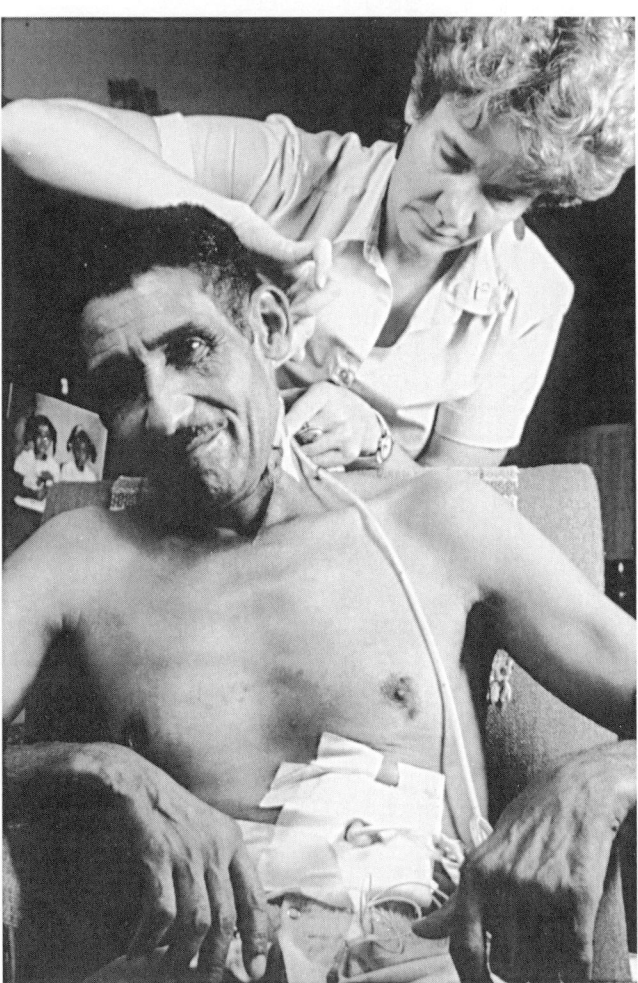

F I G U R E   26-6
Intensive-level home health care requires the services of a highly skilled professional. The client requiring sterile dressing changes, monitoring of indwelling catheters or tubes, and special training for the caregiver needs intensive-level care. (Photo by Robert Coldwell, courtesy of Community Home Health Services of Philadelphia)

dressing changes to a large abdominal wound which is draining copious amounts of purulent discharge). This client's family needs the services of a nurse to assess the wound for healing or infection, to monitor the amount and type of drainage, to perform the dressing changes, and to teach the caregiver the procedure. This family also needs teaching on medications, high-protein diet, and vitamins to promote wound healing, fluid balance, and complications of immobility. The client may also be receiving intravenous antibiotics.

Intermediate or **rehabilitative level care** indicates the client with an expected change or improvement in function, warranting skilled services (*e.g.,* client with a stroke who no longer needs nursing services but may still need physical or speech therapy). This level is reimbursed by insurance.

Maintenance level care indicates a client for whom there is no expected change in condition. This client's family needs assistance with personal care and homemaker services. Such care is not reimbursed by Medicare and most other insurance carriers. These services are usually paid out of pocket by the family or by state grants through Area Agencies on Aging (AAA).

The major criteria to be met in order to have skilled services reimbursed by Medicare are the following:
- The client must be homebound.
- The care must be intermittent.
- There must be a responsible physician ordering the care.

Home Environment.   Nursing care in the home is quite different from nursing care in the hospital. The family, not the individual client, is the unit of care. In the hospital the nurse may never meet the caregiver, but in the home it is essential to do so.

In the hospital the client is forced to comply. Dressing changes, tube feedings, turning in bed, and medications are all given on a schedule. If the client doesn't want to perform a treatment or the caregiver doesn't give a medication in the home, it is their choice. No one will be there to make sure treatments are carried out every 2 hours. The client is on "home turf," and the nurse must respect that. But the nurse must make every effort to promote care and give support and instruction whenever possible.

Preparing for Visiting

The key to an effective home visit is preparation and organization. Although home health nursing is only a small part of community health nursing, the four basic assumptions described by Tinkham and Voorhees (1977) are relevant to understanding the role of home health nursing.
- The family has the right and responsibility to make its own decisions.
- The Community Health Nurse (CHN) assists the family in determining its health needs and problems, in developing the plan of action and evaluat-

ing the outcomes (sometimes referred to as either implicit or explicit contracting).

- The family is involved early in the decision-making process.
- To be effective in their nursing practice with families, CHNs must trust in the ability of families to solve their own health problems with the support and guidance of the nurse.

All available information must be reviewed in preparation for the visit. There will be some type of brief intake history from the discharge planner at the hospital. These data should identify health problems and family needs. A thorough understanding of the physician's plan of treatment is essential. It is necessary to have the physician's phone number on the chart in case a call must be made from the home to report significant findings, clarify an order, or request other services and equipment which may be needed.

Cultural Sensitivity. Home-care nurses must be sensitive to the cultural values of their clients and aware of their own biases and beliefs. If they are not, the care of those clients may be compromised. The nurse should be aware of cultural background before visiting a client. Because a person belongs to a particular ethnic group, however, does not mean the person adheres to cultural practices of that group. Each client is an individual. Refer to Chapter 8 for a discussion on culture and ethnicity.

Planning. Once all available data have been reviewed, objectives for the visit should be developed. The nurse needs to set realistic and specific objectives and determine what baseline information is needed and what treatments need to be completed. Anticipating teaching needs prior to the visit is helpful, but it is unlikely that an extensive teaching plan can be carried out on the first visit.

Arranging the Visit. Preparation includes finding directions to the home and checking all supplies before leaving the office. If the family has a telephone, call and arrange for a convenient time to visit. If no telephone is available in the home, hopefully the number of a friend or relative in the vicinity has been given. This pre-visit contact is important in preparing the family psychologically as well as physically for the visit. Identify yourself and the agency you represent, the purpose of the visit, and determine if any special supplies are needed.

The Visit

A skillful home-care nurse can get much accomplished in one visit. The first visit will give the nurse and the client information about each other. It is the first step in establishing a trusting and therapeutic nurse–client relationship.

Entering the home may be the first test for the nurse. Roles are now reversed. The nurse must show respect for the people in the home. Introduce yourself and the

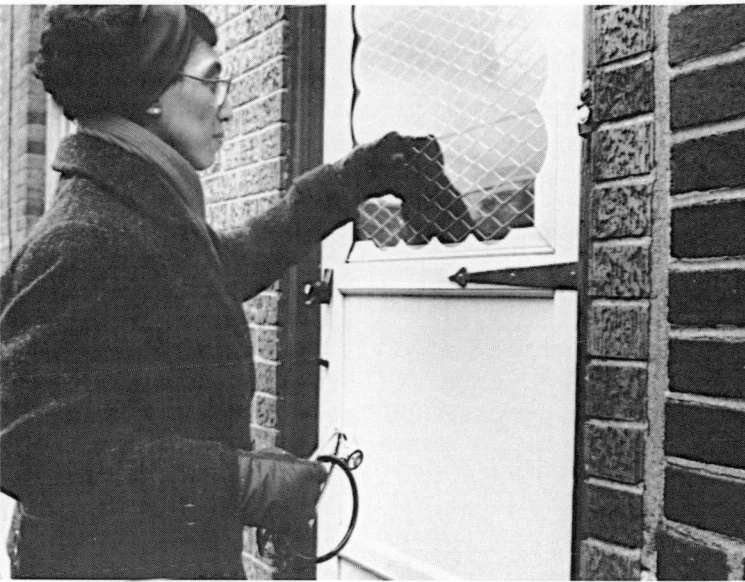

FIGURE 26-7

The home health-care nurse must demonstrate utmost respect for clients in their personal surroundings, arrive fully prepared and equipped, and have a plan with realistic and specific objectives for the visit. (Photo by Robert Coldwell, courtesy of Community Home Health Services of Philadelphia)

agency you are from. If the caregiver will not let you in, do not force the issue. After explaining who you are and the importance of the visit, give them the option of setting up another visit. In most cases, the family will be eagerly awaiting your arrival and greet you warmly.

Obviously personal safety is an important factor to consider when making a home visit. Both the nurse and client have concerns in this area. The nurse should wear a uniform and identification to display to the client who may be wary of strangers. Most home-care nurses are assigned a certain district or community. They are generally well known to neighbors and are familiar with the area. When visiting in certain areas of the city or very rural areas it would be wise to discuss problems with your supervisor and consider precautions to take. Generally, common sense is the best precaution.

The visit should be organized around the nursing process to facilitate prioritizing care. Before the end of the first visit, the nurse should explain the findings with the client and family. They should be aware of the short-term goals, indicated services, and a schedule of future visits. Any information that is unclear should be discussed.

Assessing

Many clients requiring care in their home are coping with chronic illness. They may have been hospitalized for an acute exacerbation of that illness and are now home with additional therapy requirements. To facilitate coping, promote a higher level of wellness, prevent further illness or complications, and avoid undue depen-

Elements of a Home Visit Assessment

Progress

Has the client made progress since the last contact with health-care personnel? Have goals been reached? Why not?

Current Problem

Is it the same for which the client was hospitalized? Is there a new problem? Or has one in the background come to the forefront?

Functional capacity

Is the client able to function in normal activities of daily living? Why not? What changes need to be made to improve functional capacity?

Family

Names, ages, and sex of other family members. What is their relationship, occupation, education, and language? Are there family members not living at this address who help provide care? What are their addresses and phone numbers? Is the family adapting to the medical diagnosis, prognosis, and care? How will this illness affect their normal patterns of living? Have the roles of family members changed?

Psychosocial needs

How have the client and family adjusted to this illness and the change in their routine? Is the client motivated to self-care? Is the family supportive and willing to help with the treatment plan? What is their ability to meet the needs of this client? Does the client and family know the diagnosis and prognosis? What are the emotional resources? What are the strengths and limitations? Does this family have any outside support systems, neighbors, relatives?

Primary Caregiver (Support Person)

Is this a member of family? Friend? Neighbor? Does this person have health problems? Is this person able to perform the care? Does this person have any respite time? What other responsibilities does this person have? What are this person's psychosocial and physical needs?

Environment

Are the living arrangements and space sufficient for this family? Does the client share a bedroom or bathroom? Is there enough privacy for the client and family members? What are the barriers? Are there steps or small doorways where a wheelchair could not maneuver through? Is there a bath or shower? Are there safety devices for bathing? Does the plumbing work? Is electricity, heat, and hot water available? Are there any electric hazards? Where are the smoke alarms, if any? Can the client leave the house quickly in case of an emergency? Is there an emergency plan for escape? Is there infection control? How are supplies handled? Are they kept away from pets? Are there any rodents or insects? Is the house dirty? Are there soiled linens on the bed or in the bath?

Medications

What type? How frequently? What is the system for administering and timing medications? What is the expiration date? What are they? How are they ordered to be taken? What is the expiration date on the bottle? Does the client have prescriptions? How do they get them—does their pharmacy deliver? What is their system for administering them? Is timing and frequency correct? Side-effects?

Nutrition

Who prepares meals? Is a special diet required? What is the meal planner's knowledge of the diet? Who buys the food? Has there been a recent weight gain or loss? Weight now? Was this planned or unplanned? What is the client's appetite like? Have there been any changes? What foods does the client like or dislike? Are there any religious instructions? Much of this information will be obtained during the health history and surgical exam.

(continued)

Elements of a Home Visit Assessment (continued)

Involvement with Other Health-Care Personnel

What other health-care providers are delivering service to this family? Is there more than one physician involved? Does the client have a cardiologist, rheumatologist, and surgeon? Is the medical plan being coordinated?

Financial Status (or Financial Concerns)

What is the financial state of this family? Are finances adequate for their needs (food, rent, utilities)? How much more is needed for added medication and supply costs? Do they have insurance? What carrier do they have, and how much is reimbursed? Is the family in need of assistance? Are they eligible for food stamps, rent and energy rebate, medication subsidy?

---

dency, nursing service should fill the gaps that clients and their families have in meeting care requirements (Eliopoulos, 1981). Skillful assessments are essential in determining how well basic and illness-imposed needs are being met.

The effectiveness of the discharge plan should be evaluated. Many factors affecting the client in the home should be assessed. Sample factors to be considered are listed in the box. Whatever format is being used, it is important to be complete.

Depending on circumstances, the nursing examination is usually an important part of the home nursing assessment. The review of systems and nursing examination indicate changes since hospitalization and indicate data needed to proceed with or revise a nursing care plan.

Expert assessment skills are important because the nurse identifies any needs for medical intervention. It is crucial for the nurse to be able to note changes in the client's physical status and report them to the physician. The physician will then either change the treatment and have the nurse continue to monitor the response to the new treatment, continue with the same treatment or medication, or request rehospitalization.

Why a need is not being fulfilled must be identified as part of the assessment (Eliopoulos, 1981). The nursing diagnosis is based on those needs, and specific services may be ordered based on those needs.

Diagnosing

When assessment is completed, nursing diagnoses are developed. Diagnoses may remain the same as at discharge or may need to be revised. Determining and prioritizing the problem list (discussed in Chap 16) must be family centered because the basic unit of care is the family and compliance is more realistic when the family is involved.

Planning

Planning home care is a multifaceted process. The nurse, client, and family must agree on both short- and long-

term goals. Long-term goals for clients with chronic conditions provide a projected outcome of care and include preventive health maintenance, restorative care, or support (Eliopoulos, 1981). Short-term goals serve as a guide to care and can be changed with each nursing visit. An example of a long-term goal is the client's independent management of diabetic care including insulin administration. The short-term goal would be that the client correctly prepares the insulin after three skilled nursing visits.

Another aspect of planning care is the coordination of services. The nurse will request the services of the physical, occupational, or speech therapists as well as a social worker or home health aide. During the visit the nurse obtains data indicating what other services are required and if the client and family are agreeable to this, the nurse proceeds with plans. The physician must be contacted for orders regarding the initiation of services.

Implementing

Home-care nurses possess a wide range of skills to provide the nursing actions required in the care of the homebound. Table 26-1 illustrates care categories in which home-care nurses work (Hewner, 1986).

Monitoring Health Status. The nurse makes assessments, performs nursing examinations, and observes the client's physical and mental status on each visit. The nurse will also perform laboratory tests such as glucose levels, blood counts, and any other blood tests ordered by the physician.

Teaching to Restore Health. Instructing the client and caregiver on the disease and treatment plan is crucial to the family's success and to avoiding rehospitalization. The nurse teaches about the disease process, medications, safety, emergency measures, and basic nursing care such as turning, lifting, bathings, skin care, mouth care, and comfort measures. Clients and families must learn to care for themselves because nursing services will be provided for only a relatively short period of

TABLE 26-1
Home Health Care Nursing Interventions by Care Category

Care Categories	Nursing Intervention
Monitoring health status	Physical exam as appropriate: vital signs, functional assessment, mental status exam, laboratory tests
Teaching to restore health	Education on disease, safety, emergency measures, basic nursing care, preventive measures, instruction on all treatments, medications, diet. Basic nursing care includes skin care, turning and positioning bed-bound clients, lifting, feeding, mouth care, comfort measures.
Supporting caregivers	Evaluate for caregiver burnout. Offer respite. Suggest caregiver support group. Provide support in home. Assess health status.
Monitoring medications	Teach medication administration. Monitor use of medications.
Managing bowel and bladder	Prevent constipation/dehydration. Instruct in toileting regimen. Provide toileting aids. Instruct in skin care and decubitus prevention.
Evaluating the environment	Evaluate home. Recommend adaptive equipment and home modification. Arrange for occupational therapy evaluation. Teach home safety, check for smoke alarms, fire and electric hazards.
Providing skilled nursing treatments	Complicated dressings. Monitor wound healing. Change gastric tubes and urethral catheters. Insert nasogastric tubes. Intramuscular injections.
Meeting psychosocial needs	Instruct caregiver on managing behavioral problems. Reality orientation. Allow ventilation of feelings. Provide structured environment in home.
Providing hygiene needs	Monitor ability to bathe self. Cut nails. Instruct in footcare. Arrange podiatry follow-up.
Referring clients	Coordinate all services and providers such as physical therapy, occupational therapy, speech therapy, home health aide social work. Communicate with physician.

(Hewner SJ: Bringing home the health care: Nurses make a difference. J Gerontol Nurs 12[2]:33, 1986)

time. For example, Foley catheter care, insulin administration, diet planning, feeding, and medication administration, must be mastered by the family. Treatments such as complicated wound care, dressing changes, and IV/central line maintenance must be learned by the client and family. The nurse is not available 24 hours a day, unless part of a hospice program, and families must be able to troubleshoot and act accordingly.

Nutrition instruction is also important. A thorough nutritional assessment elicits problem areas. If the client is in a debilitated state or has poor wound healing, the importance of an adequate diet rich in protein cannot be overly stressed. Clients on special diets such as 1-g salt, 1500-calorie diabetic, or low-protein diets must have in-

struction on how to manage these diets at home. They may not be able to cook or shop and may have financial limitations. (See Chap 31 for nursing care involving nutrition.)

A specific plan with outlined time intervals for teaching is drawn up. The client and caregiver must be approached at their level at that particular time. An elderly caregiver with rheumatoid arthritis may need more time to become proficient with a dressing change than a young person with no physical limitations. The plan must be specific and always reviewed and reinforced. Information must be timed, and the teaching goal must be realistic. (For more information, see Chap 21 on teaching plans.)

Supporting Caregivers. The caregiver has a 24-hour-a-day job that is physically and emotionally exhausting. Sometimes this person is elderly and has a chronic condition which is being treated. The caregiver has an increased chance of burnout, and care must be taken to avoid this. The nurse can assist by involving other services and trying to mobilize other family members or neighbors to help. If a home health aid can come to the home two to three times a week for bathing, linen change, and other personal care, the caregiver can find some free time to shop, run errands, or simply take a nap.

Monitoring Medications. Many medications have severe adverse effects and can interact with each other. The family and client must be aware of the wide range of possibilities and when to call the nurse and the doctor.

The nurse must monitor the effects of the medication on each visit and report any adverse findings to the physician. The efficiency of the treatment plan depends on this communication.

It is not uncommon to find people taking expired medications. It is important to teach clients to take current medications and follow the prescription as ordered. Lack of finances is a definite deterrent to medication compliance. This must be assessed, and a plan of action must be formulated. A social service consult for the possibility of medication assistance should be ordered. Many states have programs that subsidize the cost of medications to those who qualify.

Some homebound people have elaborate ways of remembering how and when to take their pills. Some people use charts with samples of pills taped or drawn on them. Others use tape on the caps with numbers of times to take the medication. Others, especially those who have poor vision may mark each bottle with rubber bands using a different number for each drug. Those with caregivers may have all their drugs prepared in the morning or even prepared for the week. Such methods may seem complicated to an outsider but, if the method is accurate, safe, and helps with compliance, it should not be changed. Changing it will cause confusion and perhaps noncompliance.

Managing Bowel and Bladder. Bowel and bladder management often goes unnoticed when a client is hospitalized for a short stay. However bowel and bladder function should be assessed. Bowel function can affect all other areas of care. Constipation can cause pain and discomfort, nausea, and anorexia, which may also speed the process of skin breakdown. If there is a problem, the first intervention when possible should be dietary; increase fluids and high-fiber fruits and vegetables if this is not medically contraindicated. If diet is not effective, obtain an order for laxatives or other aids from the physician. A bowel and bladder program should be initiated as appropriate (see Chaps 32 and 33).

Bladder and urinary tract infections are a source of discomfort to many elderly clients. Thorough genitourinary assessment is the key to avoiding serious discom-

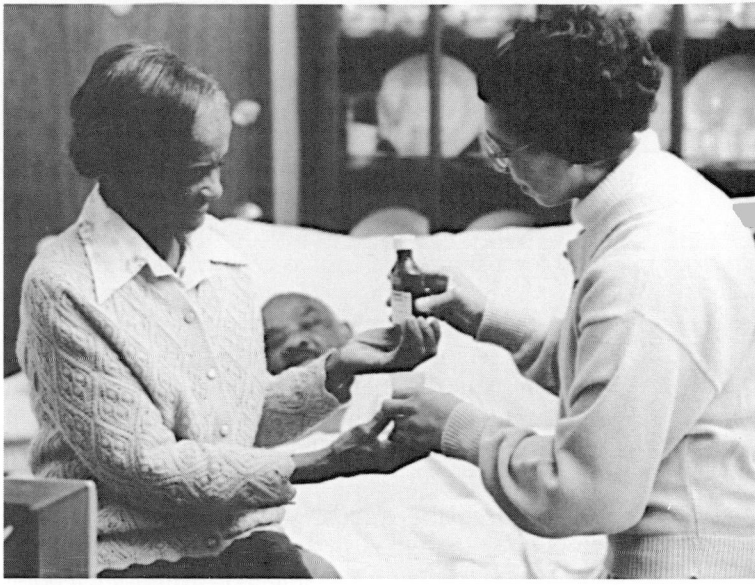

FIGURE 26-8
The client or caregiver must be taught special skills such as medication administration, diet planning, or feeding so that they can care for themselves when nursing services are no longer provided. (Photo by Robert Coldwell, courtesy of Community Home Health Services of Philadelphia)

fort. This includes asking about fluid intake, urine output, dysuria, and hematuria. If the client is catheterized, assessment must be made of urine, including color, odor, sediment, leakage. (See Chap 33 on Foley catheter care.) Good skin care is crucial for incontinent clients. Skin breakdown and decubitus ulcers can be the cause of serious septic infections and prolonged treatment. Any client who is immobilized or has decreased ambulation is at risk for skin breakdown. Preventive skin care must be taught to client and caregivers.

Evaluating the Environment. Assessment of the environment was discussed earlier. If the nurse finds the environment lacking the actions to be taken vary. An occupational therapist may be needed to help a client reorganize the kitchen with adaptive devices for cooking. A physical therapist may be contacted for obtaining certain bathroom equipment or teaching the client to use a walker, crutches, or cane.

Electric safety should be taught, and smoke alarms may be purchased.

Providing Nursing Interventions. Many skilled treatments are performed in the home (*e.g.,* dressing and catheter changes—IV, central, or Foley—and nasogastric and other feeding tubes. Certain IV medications can only be given by an RN or physician. Certain large, very complicated dressings on wounds that are difficult to reach can only be performed by the RN. Most of the treatments a nurse performs in the hospital can be done at home, with only some slight modifications.

Meeting Psychosocial Needs. Assessment and intervention of psychosocial factors should be ongoing. Preventive measures such as counseling and offering emotional and physical support should be implemented. Before the client and caregiver become exhausted and despondent, the nurse should have intervened. **Respite care**—someone coming into the home for a few hours or a day to relieve the caregiver, or sending the client to a facility for a short time (not as readily available)—is an option for many families. Respite care allows both the caregiver and the client to have a break in the routine.

If the client is clinically depressed with a deteriorating health status, the help of a **psychiatric nurse specialist**, a community health nurse with a speciality in psychiatric nursing, is indicated. Therapy is given in the home.

Providing Hygiene Needs. The nurse must monitor the ability of the client or the caregiver to administer personal care. If they are unable to provide care a home health aide may be warranted.

Referring Clients. Numerous organizations provide services, many of them free of charge (*e.g.,* American Cancer Society and Arthritis Association). There are also support groups: the Zipper Club for people who have undergone open heart surgery; Reach for Recovery for women with breast cancer; Alzheimers groups for families of persons with Alzheimers disease. A quick resource for the nurse is the blue section in the back of the local phone directory.

A social worker may be called in to arrange for the family to receive certain benefits for which they are eligible (*e.g.,* food stamps, WIC, energy and fuel rebates, prescription discounts, Meals on Wheels).

Supervising Other Personnel. The nurse must be able to supervise other personnel. If a client requires the services of a home health aide to assist with personal care and ADLs, the nurse must direct and supervise the care. The aide reports to the nurse and must be directly supervised in the home at least once every 2 weeks. The nurse will review the plan of care and evaluate the aide's performance. The nurse will also decide the frequency of the aide's visits.

Managing Finances. Financial concerns can be a problem during an illness. If a family is on a fixed income,

medical bills can be devastating. It is important to complete a financial assessment on the family.

When planning for care, the nurse must be aware of what services are reimbursed. Medicare guidelines are specific. The nurse must fill the role of financial manager. The nurse must be able to plan for appropriate quality care and basically stay within the "reimbursement budget" as well as the family budget. Skill and creativity are important in finding a less expensive and equally effective method of carrying out treatments. The nurse develops conservation skills and learns not to waste any supplies. The nurse must reuses when it's appropriate and improve when there is no other alternative. Families are also adept in developing less expensive ways of carrying out procedures. Some people have been caring for their families for such a long time, and their methods may be routine and work well for them. As long as they are safe, effective, and follow the treatment plan, allow them to continue.

Documenting Care. Communication is an important skill in effective management of a homebound client. To coordinate the plan of care the nurse needs to communicate with many health-care professionals who may be providing other services to the home. One way to ensure effective communication is through accurate documentation. Documentation takes a large part of the nurse's time after the home visit. When the nurse returns to the agency there are numerous telephone calls to be made to follow up on the visit, and many forms to be completed. After the charting is done, the care plan must be updated. A verbal order form must be mailed to the physician to sign if any treatment changes have been made. Referrals for other services must be made if appropriate. This must be carried out each day for the nurse's caseload (a typical day may be as many as seven or eight visits for one nurse).

Evaluating

Evaluation of the effectiveness of the plan of care is ongoing. The plan changes as goals change. The nurse and client evaluate the progress made and together reformulate priorities and goals. Frequency of visits may decrease or increase, other services may be added or discharged, medications and treatments may be changed. All of these are depend on the skilled planning involved in the client's care and the evaluation of that care.

K E Y   P O I N T S

■ The establishment and maintenance of continuity of care is the nurse's responsibility. Developing a plan of care to be followed and coordinated from admission to discharge to the home helps ensure the continuity of comprehensive health care.

■ Basic information obtained in the admitting office includes the person's name, address, age, occupation, type of insurance, next of kin, reason for admission, and the admitting physician. The client is assigned a permanent hospital identification number. An identification bracelet, containing the client's identification number, name, and room number and the physician's name, is placed on the client's wrist.

■ The unit nurse prepares the room for admission upon notification from the office and greets the client upon arrival on the floor. The client's arrival is documented, and all pertinent information is charted.

■ Discharge planning is a process by which a multi-disciplinary team anticipates and plans for the needs of the client and family after discharge from a health-care facility. Optimally, discharge planning begins at admission.

■ Discharge planning must be coordinated and inter-disciplinary. It is initiated as early as possible, is carefully planned, and must involve the client and family or significant-other caregiver.

■ Implementation of the discharge plan is the actual carrying out of the teaching plan and referral.

■ In order for a home care referral to be made and fees for subsequent home visits reimbursed, there must be a written order by the physician for all services.

■ Cost containment is an important factor in home health care, and services must be carefully coordinated and planned to ensure reimbursement.

■ There are three levels of care in reimbursement of home health services: intensive, intermediate, and maintenance.

■ Expert assessment skills are necessary skills for home health-care nurses. It is the nurse who identifies any changes in needs for medical intervention.

■ To obtain compliance, the nurse, client, and family must agree on both short- and long-term goals. Short-term goals can be changed with each nursing visit.

■ The home health-care nurse is the coordinator of services, requesting the services of physical, occupational, and speech therapists, social workers, and the home health aide. The physician must be contacted for orders regarding the initiation of such services.

■ The nurse communicates with other health-care professionals who may be providing services. Accurate documentation is an important aspect of effective communication.

BIBLIOGRAPHY

American Nurses Association: Continuity of care and discharge planning programs in institutions and community agencies. A statement of the American Nurses Association Division on Medical Surgical Nursing practices and the Division on Community Health Nursing Practice. Kansas City, MO, American Nurses Association, 1975

Bulechek GM, McClosky JC: Nursing Interventions: Treatments for Nursing Diagnosis. Philadelphia, WB Saunders, 1985

Burgess W, Ragland EC: Community Health Nursing: Philosophy, Process, Practice. Norwalk, Appleton-Century-Crofts, 1983

Carpenito LJ: Nursing Diagnosis Application to Clinical Practice. Philadelphia, JB Lippincott, 1987

Christopher MA: Home care for the elderly—in three part harmony . . . assessment of the patient's health, home, and community. Nursing 86 16(7):50–55, 1986

Clemen-Stone S, Eigsti DG, McGuire SL: Comprehensive Family and Community Health Nursing. New York, McGraw-Hill, 1987

Eggland ET: Nurse's guide to home health care. Nursing 17(10):75–81, 1987

Eliopoulos C: Chronic Care and the Elderly: Impact on the Client, the Family and the Nurse. Aspen, 1981

Friedemann ML: Manual for Effective Community Health Nursing Practice. Monterey, CA, Wadsworth, 1983

Gordon M: Historical perspective: The national group for classification of nursing diagnoses. In Kim MJ, Moritz DA (eds): Classification of Nursing Diagnoses, p 3. New York, McGraw-Hill, 1982

Hewner SJ: Bringing home the health care: Nurses make a difference. Journal of Gerontological Nursing, 12(2): 1986

Mezzanotte ET: A checklist for better discharge planning. Nursing 17(10):55, 1987

Tinkham C, Voorhees E: Community Health Nursing: Evolution and Process, 2nd ed. New York, Appleton-Century-Crofts, 1977

Warhola C: Planning for Home Health Services: A Resource Handbook. Pub. #HRA (80-14017). Washington DC: Publication of Department of Health and Human Services, August 1980

Promoting Healthy Physiologic Responses

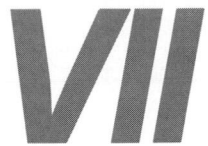

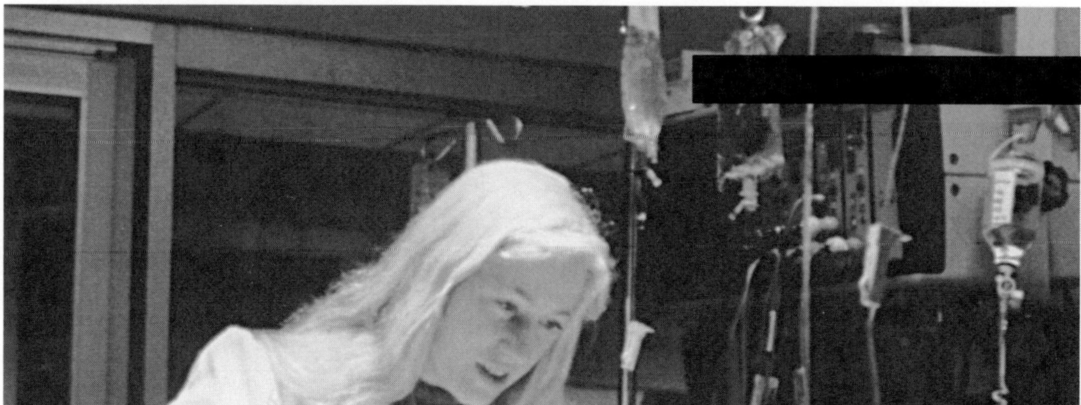

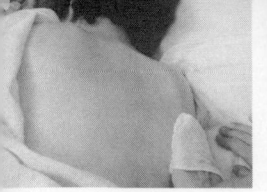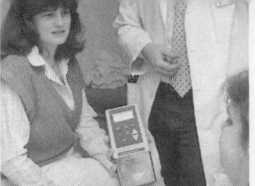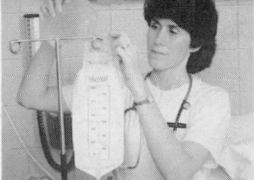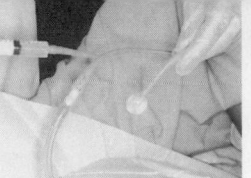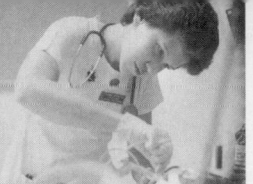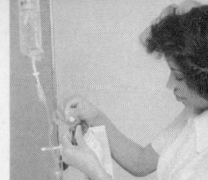

The art and science of caring are blended when nurses implement actions to meet basic human needs and promote healthy physiologic responses. The chapters in Unit VII focus on information and guidelines essential to nursing practice in a wide variety of clinical settings and involving both healthy and ill clients of all ages. Included are nursing interventions to promote safety and comfort and to meet basic physiologic needs—hygiene, activity and rest, nutrition, elimination, oxygenation, and fluid/electrolyte balance.

Each basic physiologic need is discussed by first reviewing concepts pertinent to the specific area of human function and response and then presenting factors that affect need satisfaction. The steps of the nursing process are utilized to provide guidelines and information necessary for making accurate assessments; establishing goals; and planning, implementing, and evaluating specific nursing interventions to meet needs and promote wellness. A section entitled Nursing Process in Clinical Practice at the end of each chapter provides application of knowledge by providing a case study, selected nursig diagnoses, and a care plan, illustrating how skilled nursing interventions and caring are combined to resolve problems and meet needs.

The content of Unit VII allows utilization of the nursing process in the clinical setting, integrating knowledge and skills to provide holistic care while meeting basic human needs and promoting healthy physiologic responses.

Hygiene

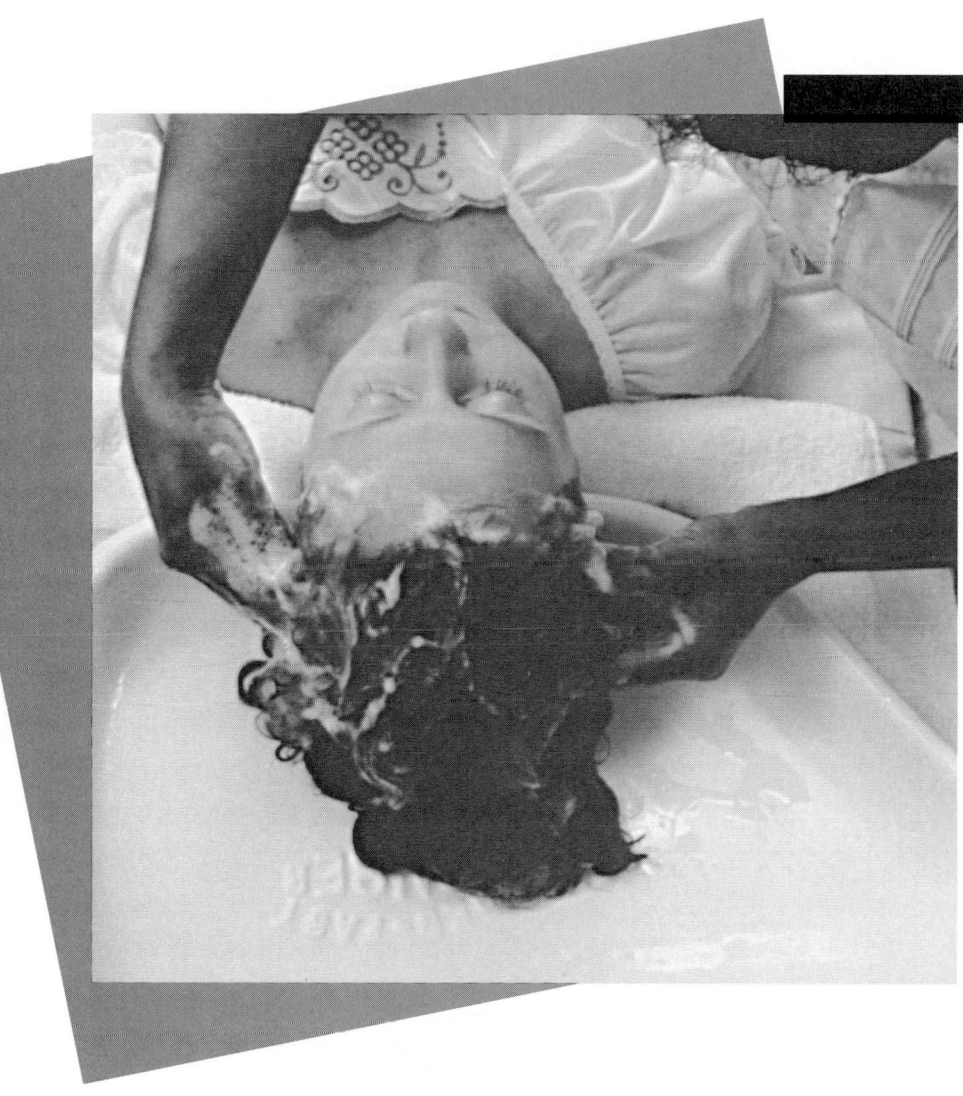

After studying this chapter, the learner should be able to

List five functions of the skin, three factors influencing the skin's condition, and four basic principles that guide practices of skin care.

Identify factors affecting skin condition and personal hygiene.

Assess the integumentary system and the adequacy of hygiene self-care behaviors using appropriate interview and physical assessment skills.

Develop nursing diagnoses related to deficient hygiene measures.

Describe the priorities of scheduled hygienic care, early morning care, morning care, afternoon care, and evening care.

Demonstrate the back massage, identifying at least four reasons for including the back massage in daily nursing care.

Demonstrate techniques used when assisting clients with hygiene measures, including those used when administering various types of baths and those used in cleaning each part of the body.

Describe agents commonly used on the skin and scalp and precautions to observe in their use.

Plan, implement, and evaluate nursing care for common problems of the skin and mucous membranes.

Describe the prevention and treatment of pressure ulcers.

Ordinarily, the well person is responsible for self-hygiene. Through teaching, the nurse may assist the well person to develop personal hygiene habits when these are found to be wanting.

Illness, hospitalization, and institutionalization may demand modifications in hygiene practices. In these situations, the nurse helps the client to continue sound hygienic practices and has an opportunity to teach the client and family members regarding hygiene.

The nurse who assists a client with basic hygiene respects individual client preferences and administers only that amount of care the client cannot or should not provide for self.

PERSONAL HYGIENE

Measures for personal cleanliness and grooming that promote physical and psychologic well-being are called **personal hygiene**. Personal hygiene practices vary widely from one person to another. The time of day for bathing or the frequency of shampooing the hair and changing the bed linens and sleeping garments is relatively unimportant. What is important is that personal care be carried out conveniently and often enough to promote personal hygiene.

This chapter provides the nurse with knowledge of the multiple factors that affect personal hygiene and of nursing measures that promote personal hygiene. A practical guide for assessing the adequacy of personal hygiene behaviors is presented. Since the data the nurse collects when assisting with hygiene may lead to the identification of multiple nursing diagnoses and collaborative problems, samples of these are provided. Client goals are presented, as are descriptions of specific nursing strategies used when performing care of the skin; mouth; eyes, ears, and nose; and feet; and perineal and vaginal areas.

In the section Nursing Process in Clinical Practice, focused assessment, diagnosis, planning, implementation, and evaluation guides are offered for caring for clients with pressure ulcers. These guides and the concluding case study (feminine hygiene) illustrate how the nurse's knowledge of personal hygiene practices and the integumentary system is combined with specific nursing interventions to successfully resolve nursing diagnoses and promote the client's general sense of well-being.

Physiology of the Skin

The term **integument** refers to the skin. The **integumentary system** consists of the skin and its appendages, that is, the hair, glands in the skin, and the nails. The skin is one of the body's vital organs and is essential for maintaining life.

The skin consists of three layers. The superficial portion is called the **epidermis** and is made up of layers of stratified epithelial cells. These cells are fused to form a protective, water-proof layer of keratin material. Epithelial cells have no blood vessels of their own and depend on underlying tissues for nourishment and waste removal. When well nourished, epithelium regenerates relatively easily and quickly.

The next layer of skin is called the **dermis** and consists of smooth, muscular tissue; nerves; hair follicles; certain glands and their ducts; arteries; veins and capillaries; and fibrous, elastic tissue. Each hair consists of the shaft, which projects through the dermis beyond the surface of the skin, and the hair follicle, which lies in the dermis. The *hypodermis* consists of a subcutaneous fatty tissue layer that anchors the other skin layers and serves as a heat insulator for the body. This fatty tissue layer contains blood and lymph vessels, nerves, and fat cells.

The skin covers the entire body and is continuous with the mucous membrane at normal body orifices. A cross-section of normal skin is illustrated in Figure 27-1. Glands in the skin include the sebaceous glands, the sweat glands, and the ceruminal glands. The **sebaceous glands** secrete an oily substance called **sebum**, which lubricates the skin and hair and keeps the skin and scalp pliant. The sweat glands secrete perspiration. The **cerumen** in the external ear canals, consisting of a heavy oil and brown pigment, is secreted by **ceruminal glands**.

Functions of Skin and Mucous Membranes

The skin serves six major functions:
- Protects the body
- Regulates body temperature
- Senses stimuli from the environment and transmits these sensations (pain, temperature, touch, pressure)
- Excretes waste products
- Helps maintain water and electrolyte balance
- Produces and absorbs vitamin D

These functions are described further in Table 27-1.

Mucous membranes line body cavities that open to the outside of the body and can also be found in the digestive tract, the respiratory passages, and the urinary and reproductive tracts. Epithelium covers the mucous membrane surfaces and contains cells that secrete mucus. Connective tissue lies beneath the epithelium. Mucous membranes have receptors that offer the body

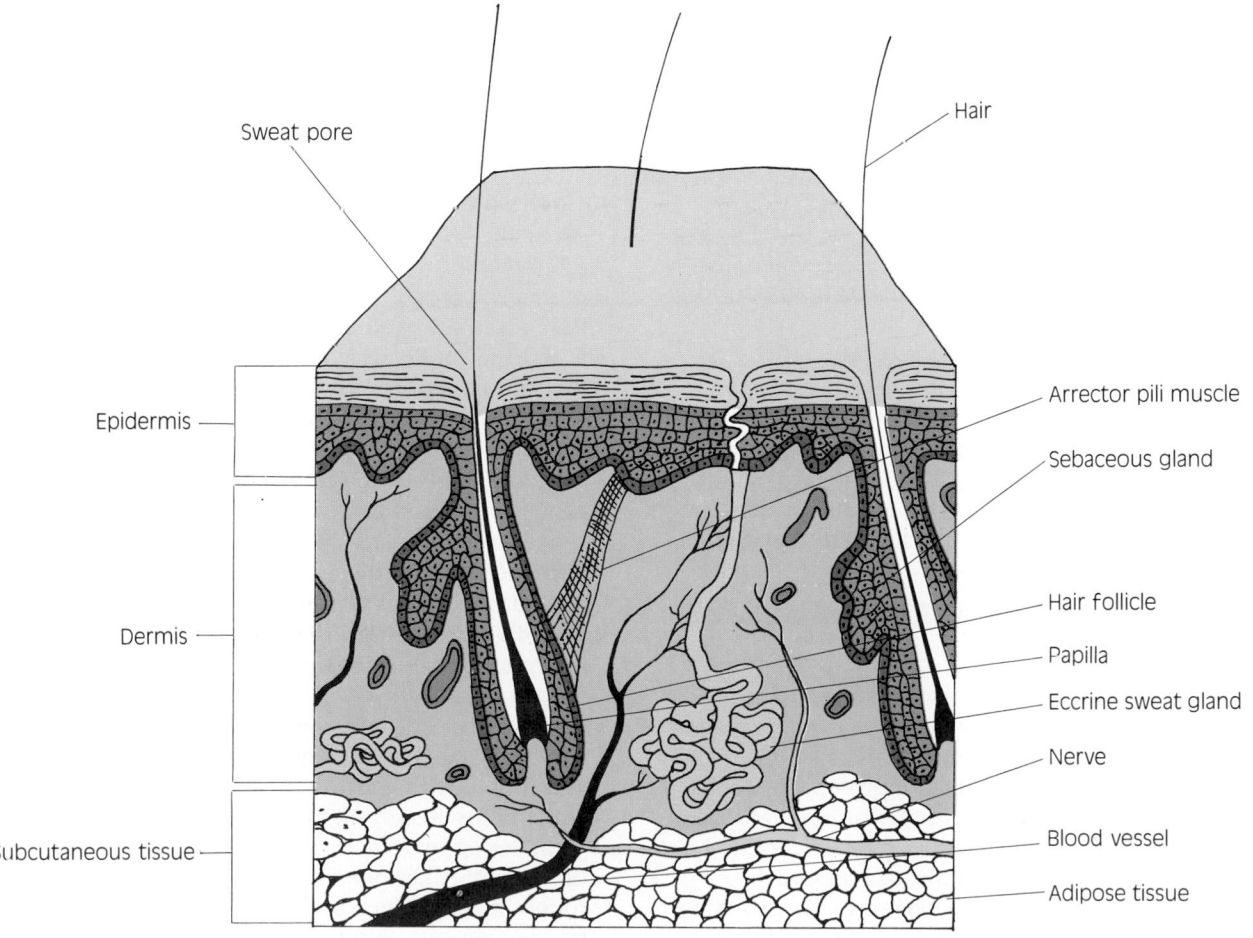

Sweat pore

Hair

Epidermis

Dermis

Subcutaneous tissue

Arrector pili muscle

Sebaceous gland

Hair follicle

Papilla

Eccrine sweat gland

Nerve

Blood vessel

Adipose tissue

FIGURE 27-1
A cross section of normal skin.

T A B L E   27-1
Functions of the Skin

Function	Mechanisms
The skin protects the body.	Invasion of the body by bacteria is prevented by intact skin. Injury to underlying tissues and organs is decreased by intact skin.
The skin helps regulate body temperature.	The production of perspiration and its loss by evaporation help cool the body. Much heat is lost from the body by radiation and by conduction when the blood supply to the skin is increased by vasodilatation. Lack of perspiration and vasoconstriction help the body retain heat. The phenomenon of producing gooseflesh, which is caused by contraction of pilomotor muscles in the skin, helps conserve body heat because the hair standing on end forms a layer of air on the body for insulation.
The skin is a sense organ.	There are receptors for pain, touch, pressure, and temperature in the skin that help the body receive stimuli from the environment.
The skin is an excretory organ.	Water, salts, and nitrogenous wastes are lost from the skin, although in much smaller quantities than are lost from the kidneys.
The skin helps maintain water and electrolyte balance.	The escape of excess water and electrolytes from the body is prevented by the skin.
The skin produces and absorbs vitamin D.	A precursor for vitamin D is present in the skin, which in conjunction with ultraviolet rays from the sun produces vitamin D.

protection; for example, an irritating substance in the upper respiratory tract will cause a person to sneeze, and food caught in the larynx or trachea will cause a person to cough. Sneezing and coughing are protective mechanisms that help rid the body of foreign materials. Mucous membranes are insensitive to temperature, except in the mouth and rectum, but are sensitive to pressure.

Mucous membranes also function to absorb substances from their surface; for example, digested food is absorbed through the mucous membrane in the small intestine.

Principles of Skin Care

A knowledge of the functions of the skin and mucous membranes and of factors affecting them point up certain basic principles that become important in their care:

Unbroken and healthy skin and mucous membranes serve as the first lines of defense against harmful agents.

Resistance to injury of the skin and mucous membranes varies among people. Factors influencing resistance include a person's age, the amount of underlying tissues, and illness conditions.

Adequately nourished and hydrated body cells are resistant to injury. The better nourished the cell, the better its ability to resist injury and disease.

Adequate circulation is necessary to maintain cell life. The cells are inadequately nourished and wastes are poorly removed when circulation is impaired for any reason.

Factors Affecting Skin Condition and Personal Hygiene

Skin Condition

A person's developmental stage and health condition influence the skin in various ways.

Developmental Considerations

- An infant's skin and mucous membranes are easily injured and subject to infection. Careful handling of infants is required to prevent injury and infection of the skin and mucous membranes.
- A child's skin becomes increasingly resistant to injury and infection. However, the skin requires special care because of the toilet and play habits of children.
- An adolescent's skin ordinarily has enlarged sebaceous glands and increased glandular secretions, caused by hormonal changes in the body. These characteristics predispose to acne, which is discussed later in this chapter.
- Secretions from the skin glands are at their maximum during adolescence and up to approximately 50 years of age.
- Changes that occur in the skin with aging are irreversible. The skin becomes thinner and less elastic and supple with aging. Subcutaneous fat that normally helps absorb injury to the skin decreases. Wrinkles appear, most of which are deep in the dermis. The skin becomes dry, often scaly, and rough in appearance because less oil is secreted from sebaceous glands. Brown spots, called *liver spots,* often appear. They may begin appearing as early as age 35 and tend to become more numer-

ous and larger with aging. These spots result from exposure to the wind and sun and are not caused by liver disease.

Illness

- Very thin and very obese people tend to be more susceptible to skin irritation and injury.
- Fluid loss through fever, vomiting, or diarrhea reduces the fluid volume of the body and is called *dehydration*. Dehydration makes the skin appear loose and flabby.
- Excessive perspiration, often associated with being ill, predisposes to skin breakdown, especially in areas where the skin folds.
- Jaundice, a condition caused by excessive bile pigments in the skin, results in a yellowish skin color. The skin is often itchy and dry in the presence of jaundice.
- Diseases of the skin are usually characterized by various lesions that require special care to promote personal hygiene and to carry out therapeutic regimens.

Personal Hygiene

The nurse caring for clients from diverse backgrounds quickly learns that hygiene practices vary widely among individuals. All of the factors described below may influence personal hygiene behaviors.

Culture. Many people in North America place a high value on personal cleanliness and feel unclean unless they shower or bathe at least once daily. They consider bathing incomplete without the use of multiple products to reduce or mask normal body odors. People from other cultures often find a weekly bath sufficient and feel no need to mask normal body odors. Culture may also dictate whether bathing is a private or communal activity.

Socioeconomic Class. Financial resources often define the hygiene options available to individuals. A single person renting one room in a boarding house may have limited or no access to tubs or showers and limited finances for the purchase of soap, shampoo, shaving cream, and deodorants. Homeless persons, who often carry all their belongings in a car or shopping cart, may welcome the warm running water and soap available in a roadside or other public restroom. Other persons may refrain from using public restrooms because they are perceived as being dirty.

Religion. Religion may dictate ceremonial washings and purifications, which may be a prelude to prayer or eating. For example, in the orthodox Jewish tradition, ritual baths are required for women after childbirth and menstruation. Contact with a deceased person or a deceased rodent may make a person "unclean."

Developmental Level/Knowledge Level. Children learn different hygiene practices while growing up. Family practices may dictate morning or evening baths, the frequency of shampooing, feelings about nudity, frequency of clothing changes, and so on. A teenager may experience the need to change hygiene measures practiced throughout childhood and begin to take long, frequent hot showers. The elderly often experience the need to decrease bathing times and the use of deodorant soaps because these may excessively dry the skin.

Health State. Disease or injury may adversely affect an individual's ability to perform hygiene measures or motivation to follow usual hygiene habits. Weakness, dizziness, and fear of falling may prevent an individual from entering a tub or shower or from bending to wash the lower extremities. Illness may also create a demand for new or modified hygiene measures.

Personal Preferences. Different people have different personal preferences with regard to hygiene practices. Showers versus tub baths, bar soap versus liquid soap, washing to wake oneself or to relax before sleep are personal preferences. One's self-concept and sexuality are also personal influences on hygiene.

Nurse as Role Model

Nurses consistently serve as role models for clients in regard to personal hygiene. Before attempting to teach clients healthy hygiene practices, it is important that nurses evaluate their own practices. If unable to meet the following goals, you may wish to take the time now to examine your own hygiene practices.

- The nurse's physical appearance and body scents give evidence of adequate hygiene practices:
    - Hair is clean and neatly styled.
    - Skin is clean.
    - Mouth evidences satisfactory oral hygiene.
    - Nails are neatly manicured.
    - Body is free of unpleasant odors.
- The nurse's diet and exercise habits contribute to clean and intact skin.
- The nurse brushes teeth after each meal, flosses daily, and goes to the dentist for a check-up at least once a year.
- The nurse's care of clients demonstrates an appreciation for the relationship between hygiene and overall well-being.
- The nurse consistently uses appropriate aseptic safeguards (handwashing, use of gloves) to prevent the transmission of microorganisms.

Assessing

A comprehensive assessment of the skin and mucous membranes includes

- Collection of data about usual hygiene practices
    Showering or bathing practices
    Skin, hair, and scalp care
    Eye, ear, nose, and mouth care
    Nail and foot care
    Perineal care
- Assessment of any sensory, cognitive, endurance, mobility, or motivation deficit that interferes with the individual's hygiene practices
- Identification of any existing problems of the skin or mucous membranes, as well as associated care and its effectiveness
- Nursing examination of the skin and mucous membranes

Skin and basic hygiene assessment guidelines follow. Focused assessment criteria for select body parts appear later in the chapter.

Nursing History

While assessing hygiene practices, it is important to remember that different individuals and families possess different ideas regarding personal cleanliness. Bathing practices and cleansing habits and rituals vary widely. Before a nurse decides that an individual's hygiene practices are "inadequate," a clear threat to health must exist.

The following questions are helpful in eliciting data from a client about health practices:

"Tell me about your daily and weekly bathing habits . . ."
"Has anything happened recently to cause a change in these habits?"
"Does anything interfere with your ability to be as clean as you would like to be?"
"Are you allergic to any cleansing or cosmetic products?"
"Is there any special way nursing can help you with regard to hygiene?"

At times it may be appropriate to ask the client direct questions about specialized aspects of hygiene:

"I notice that your gums look inflamed. How do you clean your teeth and gums? Have you seen a dentist about this problem?"
"Do you follow any special hygiene practices during menstruation? What type of feminine hygiene products (pads, tampons, douches) do you use?"

The nurse assessing the adequacy of hygiene practices evaluates whether or not the individual possesses the knowledge, attitude, skills, and resources to care for the skin and mucous membranes. See the box entitled Elements of a Hygiene History.

The nursing history also includes data about problems of the integumentary system. The client should be questioned about any past or present problems such as rashes, lumps, itching, dryness, lesions, ecchymoses, masses, or specific changes in the hair or nails. When skin problems are present, the client should be asked

Elements of a Hygiene History

Usual hygiene practices (showering or bathing practices; skin, hair, and scalp care; eye, ear, nose, and mouth care; nail and foot care; perineal care)
    "Tell me about your daily and weekly bathing habits . . ."
    "Are there special bathing or hygiene products you routinely use or can't use?"
    "How can nurses best help you to meet your hygiene needs?"
Factors interfering with the individual's hygiene practices (sensory, cognitive, endurance, mobility, or motivational deficits)
    "What recently or in the past has interfered with your hygiene practices?"
    "Tell me about anything that keeps you from being as clean as you would like . . ."
History of skin or mucous membrane problems (nature, onset of problem and frequency, causes, severity, symptoms, interventions attempted and results)
    "Describe any skin problems with rashes, lumps, itching, dryness, lesions, ecchymosis, or masses . . ."

"How long have you had this problem?"
"Does it itch or bother you?"
"How does it bother you?"
"Have you found any care helpful in relieving these symptoms?"

Sample entries in a nursing history follow:

Hygiene: "Showers twice daily, once in the A.M. and after working out in the evening. Skin tends to be very dry, and moisturizing creams are used daily. Oilated Aveeno baths prn. Allergic to deodorant soaps."

Integument: "History of athlete's foot since high school days with outbreaks every 2–3 months. Knowledgeable about appropriate foot care. Uses Tinactin ointment and Mexsana powder."

Nursing Examination

The inspection and palpation skills utilized to assess the integumentary system are described in detail in Chapter 24. The nurse who assists a client with basic hygiene measures has an excellent opportunity to examine the client's skin carefully. Many individuals are unaware of skin lesions such as precancerous moles, which if untreated could prove fatal. Early detection and treatment of skin problems are important nursing functions.

In examining the skin, the nurse pays careful attention to cleanliness, color, texture, temperature, turgor, moisture, sensation, vascularity, and the presence of lesions. If a lesion is detected, the nurse documents the type, color, size, distrbution and grouping, location, and consistency. Terminology helpful in describing these findings is presented in Chapter 24. General guidelines for assessing the skin are the following:

- Proceed systematically in head-to-toe fashion.
- Utilize a good source of light, preferably daylight.
- Compare bilateral parts for symmetry.
- Utilize standard terminology to report and record findings.
- Allow data obtained in the nursing history to direct the skin assessment.
- Identify any variables known to cause skin problems: deficient self-care abilities, immobility, malnutrition, decreased hydration, decreased sensation, vascular problems (altered tissue perfusion or venous return), presence of irritants (body secretions or excretions on the skin, other chemicals, mechanical devices).

Since life-style factors, changes in health state, illness, and certain diagnostic and therapeutic measures may adversely affect the skin, the nurse needs to identify high-risk populations and perform the appropriate skin assessment. Knowing *when* to perform the skin assessment and incorporating this into the client's plan of care is as important as knowing *how* to do this well. Table 27-2 identifies sample factors that place an individual at high risk for skin alterations.

Sample entries under integumentary system in the nursing examination follow:

"Skin is pink, warm, dry, and elastic; no petechiae, lesions, or excoriation; multiple moles of small size and regular border and surface."

"Red, macular rash generalized over trunk and thighs; semi-confluent lesions measure 1 mm to 2 mm; abrupt onset."

Diagnosing

A careful assessment of the skin and mucous membranes may lead to the identification of numerous client problems that can be classified as nursing diagnoses. Problems concerning deficient hygiene are categorized as self-care deficits. These may be general, such as Self-care deficit: personal hygiene, or very specific, such as Self-care deficit: care of artificial eye. It is important to identify the etiology of these problems correctly. If hygiene is deficient because of insufficient knowledge, health education can quickly remedy the problem. If, however, the individual attaches low priority to hygiene, or lacks the physical ability to perform hygiene measures, these problems must be addressed before health education can be effective.

Sample nursing diagnoses related to hygiene and skin problems follow:

Self-care deficit: personal hygiene *related to* sensory, cognitive, endurance, mobility, or motivation deficits

Altered comfort *related to* skin or mucous membrane alterations

Ineffective individual coping *related to* chronic skin problems

Altered health maintenance (dental caries, peridontal disease, halitosis) *related to* deficient oral hygiene practices

Knowledge deficit *related to* new therapeutic regimen to manage skin or mucous membrane alteration

Impaired physical mobility *related to* painful foot condition (calluses, corns, plantar warts)

Altered oral mucous membrane *related to* inadequate oral hygiene, stomatitis, malnutrition/dehydration

Potential for infection *related to* broken skin or traumatized tissue

Self-concept, disturbance in body image, *related to* visible integumentary problems, body odors

Altered sexual patterns *related to* fear of transmitting or acquiring sexually transmitted disease, painful genital lesions

Impaired skin integrity *related to* altered circulation, nutritional and fluid deficit or excess, impaired mobility, irritants (chemical, thermal, mechanical, radiation)

Impaired social interaction *related to* negative body image (*e.g.,* acne, alopecia)

Impaired swallowing *related to* reddened, irritated oropharyngeal cavity

Impaired tissue integrity (cornea, mucous membrane, integumentary, or subcutaneous) *related to* altered circulation, nutritional and/or fluid deficit/excess, impaired mobility, irritants (chemical, thermal, mechanical, radiation)

Additional diagnoses are discussed in this chapter under specific body parts.

Date collected during the nursing assessment may also lead to the identification of a collaborative problem. A nurse caring for a client receiving intravenous chemotherapy should carefully check the infusion site every shift, realizing that phlebitis commonly occurs with certain chemotherapeutic agents. Careful preparation and administration of the drug according to the manufacturer's instructions, adherence to nursing protocols for the maintenance of intravenous infusions, and ongoing nursing assessment may decrease the likelihood of phlebitis. If redness, warmth, tenderness, or swelling is noted with any intravenous infusion, immediate collaborative intervention is indicated.

Similarly, a nurse may notice a 1.5-cm mole with an irregular border on a client's back during the bath. Prompt reporting of this finding to the physician may lead to the detection and early, successful treatment of the medical diagnosis—malignant melanoma.

T A B L E   27-2

Factors Placing an Individual at High Risk for Skin Alterations

Factor	Nursing Implications
Life-Style Variables	
Homosexual male, with a history of multiple sexual partners; drug users; hemophiliacs; bisexual male; partners of the above	• High-risk profile for acquired immunodeficiency syndrome (AIDS) • Assessment needs to include careful examination of the skin for purple blotches that may be indicative of Kaposi's sarcoma.
Occupation that gives a fair thin-skinned individual prolonged exposure to the sun	• Places individual at high risk for developing skin cancer, which has an excellent prognosis if detected and treated in its early stages but which may be fatal if treatment is delayed • Assessment needs to include careful examination for a sore that does not heal or a change in size or color of a wart or mole.
Changes in Health State	
Dehydration/malnutrition	• If fluid, protein, and vitamin C intake is deficient, skin loses elasticity and becomes prone to breakdown. • Nursing care is directed toward preventing skin breakdown: frequent changes of client's position with skin assessment at each change, special mattresses and protection of bony prominences; use of lotions; attention to fluid and nutritional status.
Reduced sensation (paralysis, local nerve damage, circulatory insufficiency)	• Client's inability to sense temperature extremes, pressure, friction, and other such factors can easily result in injury. • Nursing care incorporates special attention to safety.
Illness	
Diabetes mellitus	• Numerous factors combine to cause skin problems in diabetics: cuts and sores that do not heal; lesions on the lower extremities that ulcerate and become necrotic; recurrent bacterial and fungal infections. • The diabetic must be taught special hygiene measures to prevent trauma to the skin and learn to assess the skin carefully to detect any alteration.
Diagnostic Measures	
Gastrointestinal (GI) series	• The GI cleansing preparations administered to clients having GI studies done may result in diarrhea, which irritates the sensitive skin in the perianal area—especially if the client had bouts of diarrhea prior to the studies. Anticipating the problem, noting redness/inflammation, and beginning warm baths/ointments are welcome nursing measures that clients may be too embarrassed to seek.
Therapeutic Measures	
Bedrest	• Bedrest predisposes clients to skin breakdown; the harsh detergents used on hospital laundry compound this problem. • Pressure points need to be examined frequently and protected.
Casts	• Casts easily irritate the skin; careful assessment, covering the rough edges of the cast, and skin care are indicated.
K-thermia unit	• Moist wet heat has therapeutic benefit but if applied to the skin too long may macerate the skin; follow protocol in length of application, examine skin carefully between treatments, and allow to dry.
Medications	• Medications may cause allergic skin reactions, such as rashes. • When evaluating the client's response to a new drug, examine the skin for redness and itching.

Planning

Each plan of nursing care identifies nursing measures to assist the client develop or maintain hygiene practices that contribute to a sense of well-being. Appropriate client goals include the following:

- The client will verbalize feeling comfortable and clean.
- The client will participate fully in necessary hygiene measures according to cognitive, sensory, mobility, and endurance abilities.
- The client will maintain intact skin and mucous membranes.
- The client will demonstrate correct skin care measures (when indicated).
- The client will demonstrate signs of healing in existing lesions.

Client goals related to specific body parts are presented later in the chapter.

Implementing

The nurse, in performing general personal hygiene skills, respects the client's personal preferences in hygiene measures, allows and encourages as much self-care as the client can perform, meets the client's needs for privacy, and promotes physiologic and psychologic wellness. In the following sections general hygiene measures are discussed, including providing scheduled care, helping with bathing, massaging, bedmaking, and providing environmental care. Nursing care for specific body parts is discussed later in this chapter.

Providing Scheduled Hygienic Care

When clients require nursing assistance with personal hygiene, it is important to schedule this care at regular intervals. In most hospitals and long-term care settings, the following types of hygienic care are provided. These are individualized to clients according to their personal and cultural preferences.

Early Morning Care. Shortly after awakening, the client is assisted with toileting if necessary and then provided comfort measures designed to refresh the client and in preparation for breakfast (or diagnostic tests). Nursing measures include washing the face and hands

R E S E A R C H   I N   N U R S I N G   *Making a Difference*

Personal Hygiene

An integral component of self-esteem and comfort in clients who are unable to carry out self-care activities is nursing intervention aimed at maintaining skin integrity to prevent breakdown and facilitating healing when breakdown has occurred. Nursing research has been carried out to examine this problem from various perspectives.

Related Research

Diekmann J: Use of a dental irrigating device in the treatment of decubitus ulcers. Nurs Res 33:303–305, 1984

Diekmann conducted this study to determine if the dental irrigating device could be successfully used to treat decubitus ulcers. Although the results did not support this hypothesis, the device was useful for debridement and stimulation of circulation.

Wells P, Geden E: Paraplegic body-support pressure on convoluted foam, waterbed, and standard mattresses. Research in Nursing and Health 7:127–133, 1984

This study examined the pressure over selected bony prominences in contact with a foam mattress, a waterbed, and a standard mattress. Results indicated that prevention of decubitus ulcers depends on reducing the intensity and duration of pressure, accomplished by changing the client's position every 1 to 2 hours and by selecting a mattress, such as a waterbed, that distributes the body weight over a larger surface area.

Whitney J, Fellows B, Larson E: Do mattresses make a difference? Journal of Gerontological Nursing 10(9):20–25, 1984

This study focused on the prevention of bedsores by examining different types of mattresses. No significant difference was found in skin condition between clients using an alternating-pressure mattress and clients using a foam mattress. Until further research is done, the authors recommend mattress use be based on cost, client preference, and ease of maintenance.

Nursing care is often implemented to maintain skin integrity in clients on bedrest so as to promote comfort and self-esteem. The use of research findings can help provide effective nursing care; further research can identify risk factors and improve nursing management when alterations in skin integrity are present.

and mouth care. Agency policy dictates whether the nurses on night shift or day shift are responsible for early morning care. This is an excellent time to note if the supplies needed for morning care are available and to order any that are lacking.

Morning Care (AM Care).

After breakfast the nurse completes morning care. Depending on the client's self-care abilities, the nurse offers assistance with toileting, oral care, bathing, back massage, special skin care measures (*e.g.,* decubitus care), hair care (includes shaving if indicated), cosmetics (if desired), dressing, and positioning for comfort. Agency policies are followed in refreshing or changing bed linens, and the client's bedside area is tidied. When morning care is completed, the client should feel refreshed and be in a comfortable and safe environment. For some clients this may mean positioning the call light within reach and using protective devices such as bed rails or restraints.

Morning care is often characterized as self-care, partial care, or complete care. *Self-care* clients are capable of managing their personal hygiene independently once oriented to the bathroom. These clients should still be offered a back massage and receive quality nursing time directed to assessing their day-to-day needs. *Partial care* clients most often receive morning hygiene care at the bedside or seated near the sink in the bathroom. Because of weakness, these clients may be able to wash only the parts of their bodies that are within easy reach. The nurse washes the back and legs and sometimes the axillae and perineum since these body parts have the most secretions and are difficult to reach. *Complete care* clients require nursing assistance with all aspects of personal hygiene. A complete bed bath is done or the client is taken to the shower or tub.

Afternoon Care.

Since hospitalized clients frequently receive visitors in the afternoon or evening, or use this time to rest when not scheduled for tests, the nurse should ensure the client's comfort after lunch and offer assistance to nonambulatory clients with toileting, handwashing, and oral care. Straightening bed linens and helping clients with mobility problems to reposition themselves comfortably are other welcome nursing measures.

Hour of Sleep Care (hs Care).

Shortly before the client retires the nurse again offers assistance with toileting, washing of face and hands, and oral care. Many clients find that a back massage helps them to relax and fall asleep and this should be offered routinely. Soiled bed linens or clothing should be changed and the client positioned comfortably. If protective devices are indicated for night hours (side rails, restraints) these are applied at this time. The call light and any other objects the client desires (urinal, radio, water glass) should be within easy reach.

As Needed Care (prn Care).

In addition to the scheduled care described above, the nurse offers individual hygiene measures as needed. Some clients require oral care every two hours. Clients who are diaphoretic (sweating profusely) may need their clothing and bed linens changed several times a shift. At other times a nurse may decide to forego hygienic measures because the client's need for undisturbed rest may take precedence.

Helping With Bathing

Purposes of Bathing.

Bathing serves a variety of purposes, including the following:
- It cleanses the skin.
- It acts as a skin conditioner.
- It helps relax a restless person.
- It promotes circulation by stimulating the skin's peripheral nerve endings and underlying tissues.
- It serves as a musculoskeletal exercise through activity involved with bathing and thus improves joint mobility and muscle tonus.
- It stimulates the rate and depth of respirations.
- It promotes comfort through muscle relaxation and skin stimulation.
- It provides the person with sensory input.
- It helps improve self-image.
- It gives the nurse an excellent opportunity to strengthen the nurse–client relationship, to observe the client's physiologic and emotional status closely, to teach the client as indicated, and to demonstrate that the nurse cares for the client and is interested in the client's general welfare.

Shower and Tub Baths.

Using a shower or a tub is the preferred method of bathing for hospitalized persons who are ambulatory. Even though clients can, for the most part, do this on their own, the nurse still has responsibilities:
- Check to see that the bathroom is available, clean, and safe. Showers and tubs should have mats or nonskid strips to prevent the client from slipping and falling.
- See to it that necessary articles, such as soap, a washcloth, a towel, and a gown, are available for the client.
- Provide for a place for a weak or physically handicapped client to sit in a shower. Most health agencies have a stool or chair that can be used in a shower and hand-held shower heads may facilitate the process. Some nurses have reported that a commode chair with the pan removed serves effectively as a shower chair, and it offers the client more support than a stool or chair.
- Assist the client to the shower or bathroom, as indicated. Clients who are beginning ambulation need assistance to help prevent falling and fainting.

- Check to see that the water temperature is safe and comfortable, 43° C to 46° C (110° F to 115° F).
- Help the client get in and out of a bathtub, as indicated. Have the client grasp handrails at the side of the tub. Or, place a chair at the side of the tub. The client sits on the chair and eases to the edge of the tub. After putting both feet into the tub, it is then relatively easy for the client to reach the opposite side and ease down into the tub. The client may kneel first in the tub and then sit in it and can leave the tub in the same manner. Use a hydraulic lift, when available, to lower and lift a helpless and heavy client in and out of a tub.
- Ensure privacy for the client who is safe to shower or bathe independently. See to it that a call device is handy so that the client can obtain help if necessary.
- Keep the bathroom door unlocked. Health personnel should be able to enter with ease if the client needs help. A sign hung on the door ensures privacy. Children should never be left alone in bathrooms.
- Help wash and dry areas of the body that the client cannot reach, such as the back.

Figure 27-2 illustrates several features that add to the safety of a client who takes a shower or tub bath.

Bed Baths.   Some clients must remain in bed as a part of their therapeutic regimen, but they are able to bathe themselves. The nurse helps the client who takes a bath in bed in several ways:

- Provide the client with articles for bathing. Provide a basin of water that is of a comfortable and safe temperature. Place these items conveniently for the client on a bedside stand or overbed table.
- Provide privacy for the client. See to it that the call device is within reach.
- Remove top linens on the client's bed while replacing them with a bath blanket.
- Place make-up items in a convenient place for the

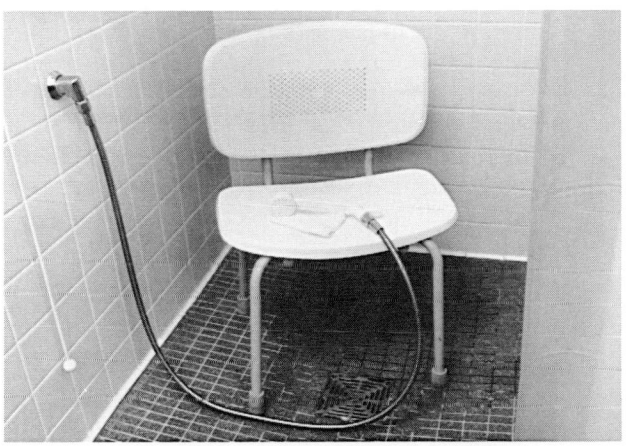

A chair placed in the shower with a hand-held shower head.

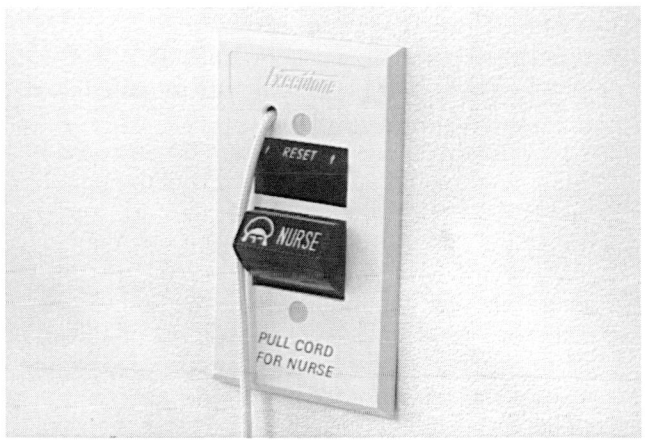

A call bell equiped with a pull cord.

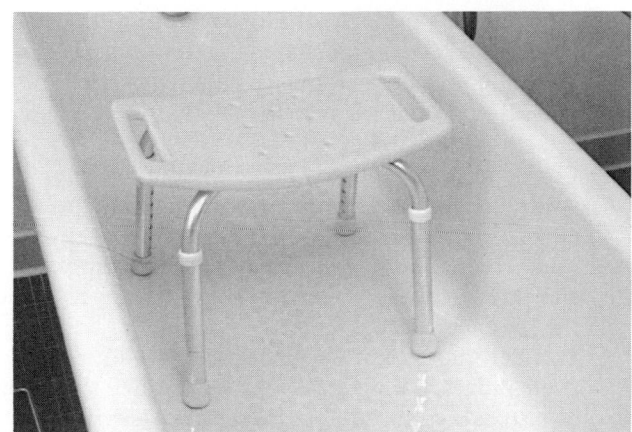

A stool in the bath tub to facilitate getting in and out of the tub and nonslip strips adhered to the bottom of the tub.

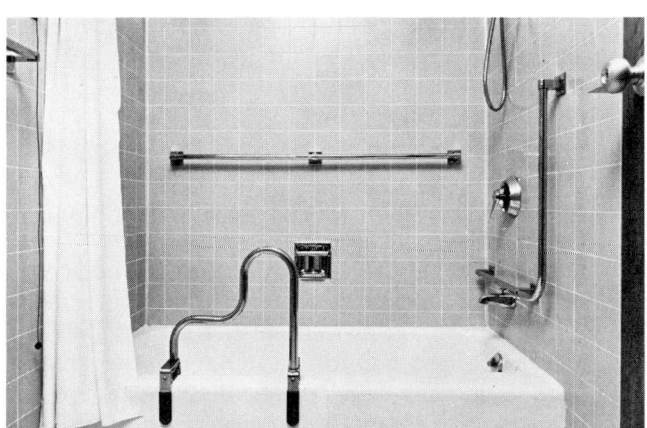

A bath equipped with safety hand rails.

F I G U R E   27-2
Examples of features that add to the safety of a client in the bath.

client's use. Provide a mirror, a good light, and hot water for the male client who wishes to razor shave.

- Assist clients who cannot bathe themselves completely. For example, some clients will be able to wash only the upper parts of the body. The remainder of the bath is then completed by nursing personnel.

Bathing procedures for the client who requires total nursing assistance vary among health agencies. The one described in Procedure 27-1 is offered as a guide. It assumes that the client is able to be raised or lowered in bed and that, although there may be limitation of movement, it is possible for the nurse to manage the client alone.

Towel Baths.

The in-bed towel bath, or lotion bath as it is sometimes called, uses a quick-drying solution containing a cleaning agent, a disinfectant, and a softening agent mixed with water that is 43.3° C to 48.9° C (110° F to 120° F). A commonly used solution developed cooperatively by a nurse and Vestal Laboratories is called Septi-Soft. A recommended procedure for giving the towel bath follows:

1. Place a terry cloth towel, approximately 3 feet wide by 7 feet long, in a plastic bag, and saturate it with the warmed cleaning solution.
2. Wring out the towel well and unroll it over the client while simultaneously removing the upper bed linens.
3. Fold an extra amount of the towel under the client's chin for later use.
4. Use a massaging motion to clean the body, beginning with the client's feet and working up the body.
5. Fold the towel upward as the bath proceeds while a clean sheet is unfolded over the client.
6. Cleanse the client's face, neck, and ears with the part of the towel that is folded under the chin.
7. Fold the towel into quarters, soiled side turned in, and turn the client to the side. The folded towel is used to wash the back and buttocks.
8. Remove the towel after finishing the bath. The back may then be rubbed.
9. Place clean linen on the bed, and dress and position the client.
10. The client need not be dried since the cleaning solution dries in a matter of seconds.

According to reports, the towel bath can be accomplished with little fatigue to the client; the towel remains warm during the short procedure; clients state they feel clean and refreshed; and the oil in the bathing solution eliminates dry, itchy skin. The bathing procedure and linen change take about 10 minutes. The brevity of the bath may be its greatest disadvantage. The nurse has less time with her clients than when giving the traditional bath in bed, which is especially important for developing a helping relationship.

Assisting with Antiembolism Stockings

Antiembolism stockings are often used for clients with limited activity to help prevent phlebitis and thrombi formation (these conditions are described in Chap 28). They are made of elastic material and are manufactured by several companies. Antiembolism stockings help force blood in superficial veins of the legs to deeper veins and prevent stagnation of blood in the veins of the legs.

Antiembolism stockings should always be removed during morning care, the legs inspected, and the stockings reapplied before the client is out of bed. General nursing guidelines for assisting with antiembolism stockings follow:

- Measure the client's leg to ensure that a proper size stocking is used. The manufacturer whose stockings are being used gives directions for measuring. Some stockings fit either leg; others are designated right or left. An improperly fitting stocking is uncomfortable and will do little good and may even harm the client.
- Be prepared to apply the stockings in the morning before the client is out of bed and while the client is lying down. If the client is sitting or has been up and about, have the client lie down with legs and feet well elevated for at least 15 minutes before applying the stockings. After the leg vessels are congested with blood, the effectiveness of using the stockings will have been defeated.
- Do not massage the legs. If a clot is present, it may break away from the vessel wall and circulate in the bloodstream. Put on the stockings as the manufacturer directs; the stocking is rolled down from the top to the inset of the foot, the foot is placed correctly into the foot of the stocking, and the stocking is then pulled up over the legs; or as shown in Procedure 27-2.
- Be sure the client's heel is well positioned in the stocking. The purpose of the stocking is likely to be defeated if the stocking is applied improperly.
- Pull the toes of the stockings slightly to relieve pressure on the toes after the stockings are in place if they have no toe openings.
- Check the legs regularly for redness, blistering, swelling, and pain. Some persons recommend checking the legs at least once every 8 hours; others recommend twice a day. The stockings should be removed completely once a day to bathe the legs and feet.
- Launder the stockings as necessary but at least every 3 days. Soiled stockings will irritate the skin. The stockings should be dried on a flat surface to prevent them from stretching.

Several manufacturers produce men's and women's hose that are capable of applying pressure to the legs from the foot to the mid thigh or higher. Some apply

(Text continues on p. 575.)

PROCEDURE 27-1
Giving the Bed Bath

Equipment

Wash basin
Soap and dish
Washcloths
Bath blanket

Gown or pajamas
Bed linen
Towels (2)
Disposable gloves
    (for anal and
    perineal care)

Personal hygiene
    supplies—de-
    odorant, lotion,
    and others
Bedpan or urinal
Laundry bag or cart

Action

1 Discuss procedure with the client and assess the client's ability to assist in the bathing process as well as personal hygiene preferences. Review the client's chart for any limitations in physical activity.

2 Bring necessary equipment to the bedside stand or overbed table.

3 Close the curtains around the bed and close the door to the room if possible.

4 Offer the client the bedpan or urinal.

5 Wash your hands.

6 Raise the client's bed to the high position.

7 Lower the side rail nearer to you and assist the client to the side of the bed where you will work. Have the client lie on his back.

8 Loosen top covers and remove all except the top sheet. Place bath blanket over the client and then remove the top sheet while the client holds the bath blanket in place. If linen is to be reused, fold it over a chair. Place soiled linen in the laundry bag.

9 Assist the client with oral hygiene, as necessary, and as described in Procedure 27-5.

10 Remove the client's gown and keep the bath blanket in place. If client has an intravenous line, remove the gown from the other arm first. Lower the intravenous container and pass the gown over the tubing and the container. Rehang the container and check the drip rate.

Rationale

This discussion promotes reassurance and provides knowledge about the procedure. Dialogue also encourages client participation and allows for individualized nursing care.

Bringing everything to the bedside conserves time and energy. Arranging items nearby is convenient, saves time, and helps prevent unnecessary stretching and twisting of muscles on the part of the nurse.

This ensures the client's privacy and lessens the possibility of loss of body heat during the bath.

Voiding or defecating before the bath lessens the likelihood that the bath will be interrupted, since warm bath water may stimulate the urge to void.

Handwashing deters the spread of microorganisms.

Having the bed in a high position prevents strain on the nurse's back.

Having the client positioned near the nurse and lowering the side rail help prevent unnecessary stretching and twisting of muscles on the part of the nurse.

The client is not exposed unnecessarily and warmth is maintained. If a bath blanket is not available, the top sheet may be used in place of the bath blanket.

This helps maintain teeth and gums in good condition, alleviates unpleasant odor and taste, and may improve appetite. Some clients may prefer oral care after the bath is completed.

This provides uncluttered access during the bath and maintains warmth of the client. Intravenous fluids must be maintained at the prescribed rate.

(Continued)

Action

11 Raise the side rail. Fill the basin with a sufficient amount of comfortably warm water (between 43° C and 46° C [110° F to 115° F]). Change as necessary throughout the bath. Lower the side rail closer to you when you return to the bedside to begin the bath.

12 Fold the washcloth like a mitt on your hand so there are no loose ends, as illustrated.

Rationale

Warm water is comfortable and relaxing for the client. It also stimulates circulation and provides for more effective cleansing. Side rails maintain client safety.

Having loose ends of cloth drag across the client's skin is uncomfortable. Loose ends cool quickly and will feel cold to the client.

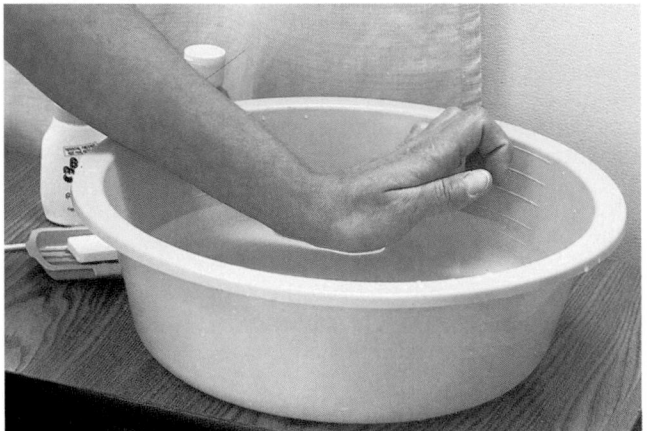

Step 11: Testing water temperature.

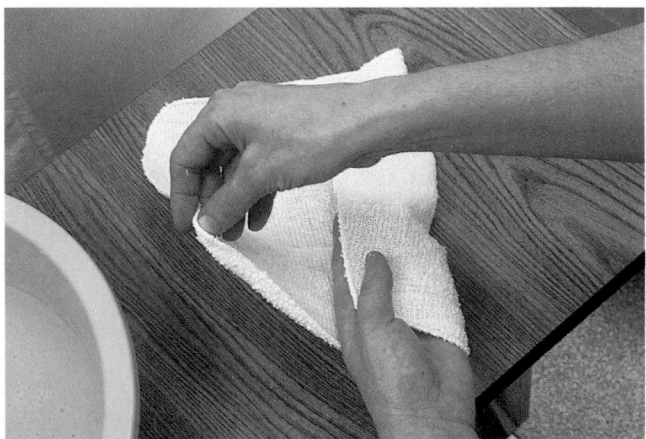

Step 12: Folding washcloth in thirds around hand to make a bath mitt.

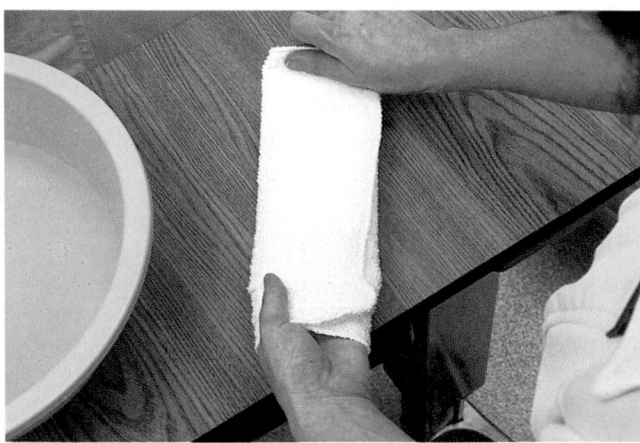

Step 12: Straightening washcloth prior to folding into mitt.

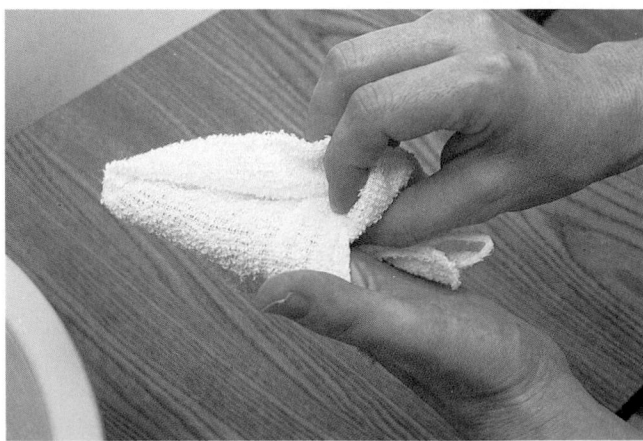

Step 12: Folding ends over and tucking ends under folded washcloth over palm.

(Continued)

13 Lay a towel across the client's chest and on top of the bath blanket.

This prevents chilling and keeps the bath blanket dry.

14 With no soap on the washcloth, wipe one eye from the inner part of the eye, near the nose, to the outer part. Rinse or turn the cloth before washing the other eye.

Rinsing or turning the washcloth prevents spreading organisms from one eye to the other. Soap is irritating to the eyes. Moving from the inner to the outer aspect of the eye prevents carrying debris toward the nasolacrimal duct.

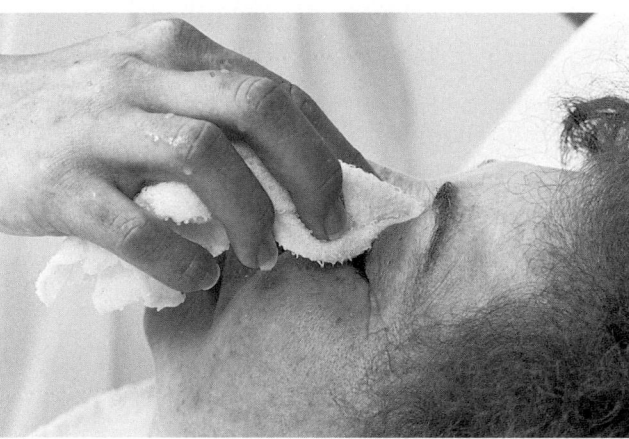

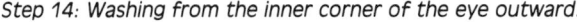
Step 14: Washing from the inner corner of the eye outward.

15 Bathe the client's face, neck, and ears, avoiding soap on the face if the client prefers.

Soap can be drying and may be avoided as a matter of personal preference.

16 Expose the far arm of the client and place the towel lengthwise under it. Using firm strokes, wash the arm and axilla, rinse, and dry.

The towel helps to keep the bed dry. Washing the far side first eliminates contaminating a clean area once it is washed. Gentle friction stimulates circulation and muscles and helps remove dirt, oil, and organisms. Long, firm strokes are relaxing and more comfortable than short, uneven strokes.

17 Place a folded towel on the bed next to the client's hand and put the basin on it. Soak the client's hand in the basin. Wash, rinse, and dry the hand.

Placing the hands in the basin of water is comfortable and relaxing for the client, allows for a thorough washing of the hands and between the fingers, and facilitates removal of debris from under the nails.

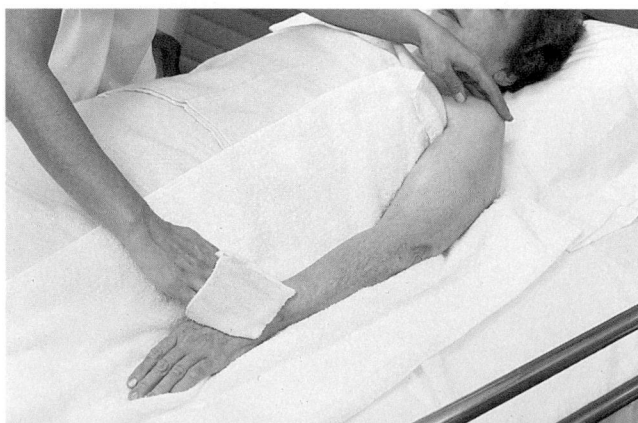
Step 16: Exposing the far arm and washing.

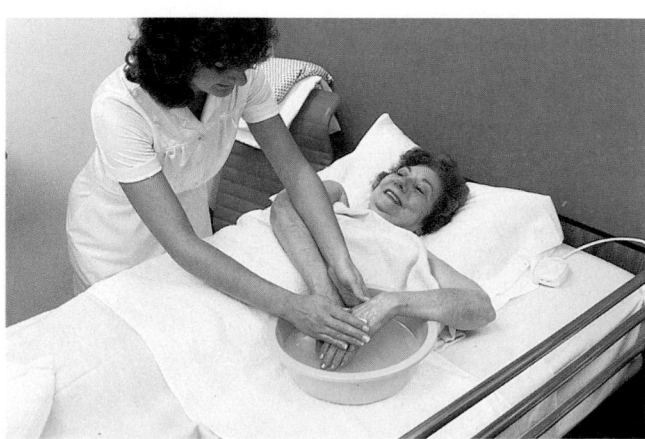
Step 17: Soaking hand in basin.

(Continued)

Action

18 Repeat Steps 16 and 17 for the arm nearer to you.

19 Spread a towel across the client's chest. Lower the bath blanket to the client's umbilicus area. Wash, rinse, and dry the client's chest. Keep the client's chest covered with the towel between the wash and rinse. Pay special attention to skin folds under the breasts of female clients.

20 Lower the bath blanket to the client's perineal area. Place a towel over the client's chest.

21 Wash, rinse, and dry the client's abdomen. Carefully inspect and cleanse the umbilical area and any abdominal folds or creases.

Rationale

Exposing, washing, rinsing, and drying one part of the body at a time avoids unnecessary exposure and chilling. Skin fold areas may be sources of odor and skin breakdown if not cleansed and dried properly.

Keeping the bath blanket and towel in place avoids exposure and chilling.

Skin-fold areas may be sources of odor and skin breakdown if not cleansed and dried properly.

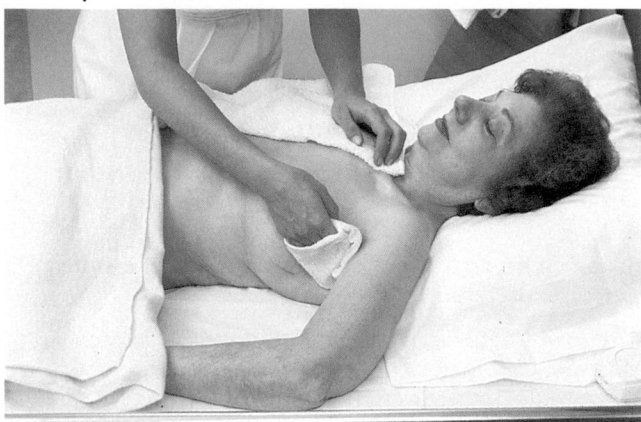

Step 19: Washing the chest area, including the axilla.

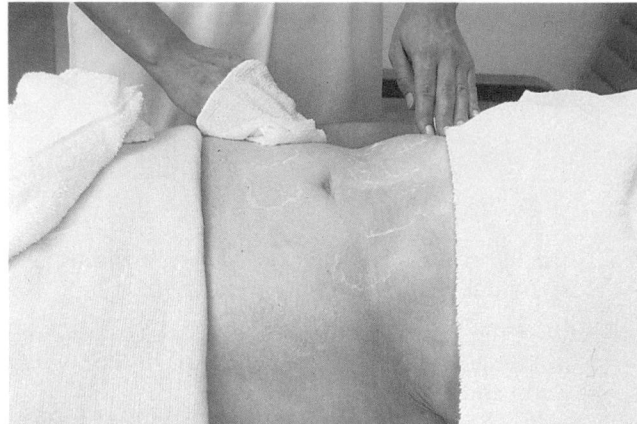

Step 21: Washing the abdomen, with perineal and chest areas covered.

22 Return the bath blanket to its original position and expose the far leg of the client. Place the towel under the far leg. Using firm strokes, wash, rinse, and dry the client's leg from ankle to knee and knee to groin.

The towel protects linens and prevents the client from feeling uncomfortable from a damp or wet bed. Washing from ankle to groin with firm strokes promotes venous return.

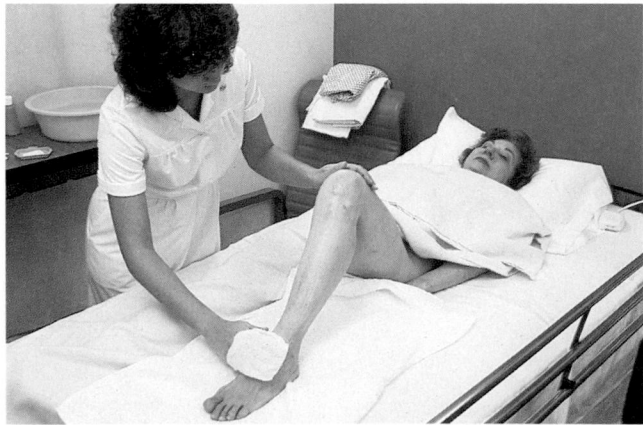

Step 22: Washing and drying far leg, keeping other leg covered.

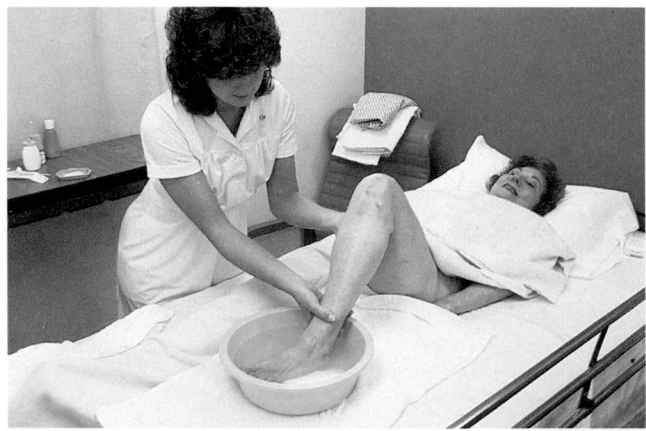

Step 23: Soaking the foot in basin.

(Continued)

23 Fold a towel near the client's foot area and place the basin on it. Place the client's foot in the basin while supporting the client's ankle and heel in your hand and the leg on your arm. Wash, rinse, and dry, paying particular attention to the area between the toes.

Supporting the client's foot and leg helps reduce strain and discomfort for the client. Placing the feet in a basin of water is comfortable and relaxing and allows for a thorough cleaning of the feet and the areas between the toes and under the nails.

24 Repeat Steps 22 and 23 for the other leg and foot.

25 Make sure the client is covered with the bath blanket. Change water at this point or earlier if necessary. Assist the client onto his or her side.

The bath blanket maintains warmth and privacy. Clean, warm water prevents chilling and maintains the client's comfort.

26 Assist the client to a prone or side-lying position. Position the bath blanket and towel so as to expose only the back and buttocks.

Positioning of the towel and bath blanket protects the client's privacy and provides warmth.

27 Wash, rinse, and dry the client's back and buttocks area. Pay particular attention to cleansing between gluteal folds and observe for any indication of redness or skin breakdown in the sacral area.

Fecal material near the anus may be a source of micro-organisms. Prolonged pressure on the sacral area or other bony prominences may compromise circulation and lead to development of decubitus ulcer.

28 If not contraindicated, give the client a back rub, as described in Procedure 30-1. Back massage may be given also after perineal care.

A back rub improves circulation to the tissues and is an aid to relaxation. A back rub may be contraindicated in clients with cardiovascular disease or musculoskeletal injuries.

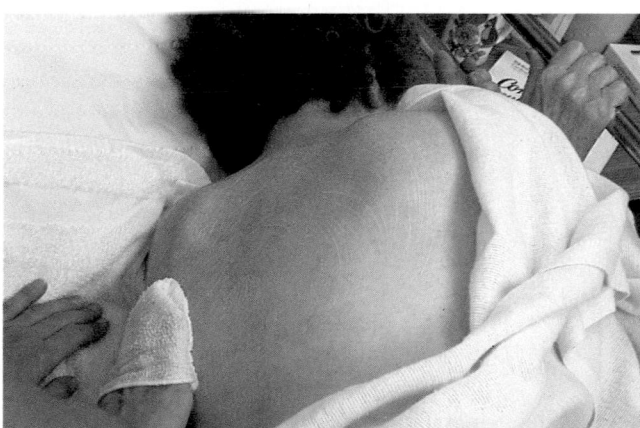

Step 27: Washing the upper back.

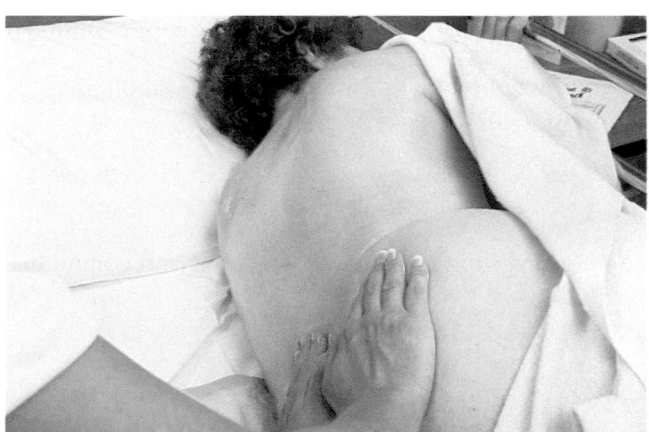

Step 28: Giving a backrub, after washing lower back.

29 Refill basin with clean water. Discard washcloth and towel.

The washcloth, towel, and water are contaminated after washing the client's gluteal area. Changing to clean supplies decreases the spread of organisms from the anal area to the genitals.

(Continued)

Action	**Rationale**
30 Clean the client's perineal area or set up the client so he or she can complete perineal self-care.	Providing perineal self-care may decrease embarrassment for the client. Effective perineal care reduces odor and decreases the chance of infection through contamination.

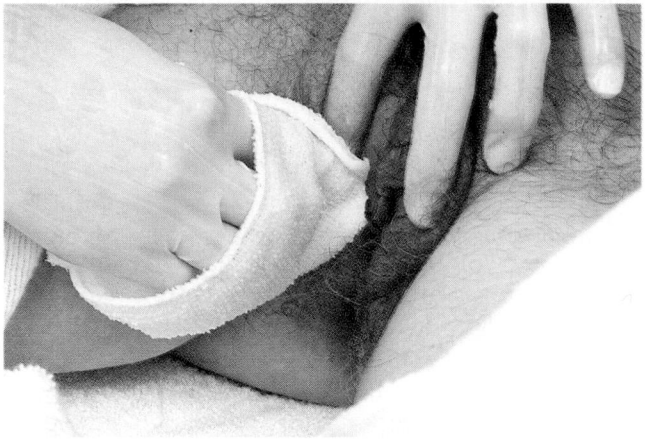

Step 30: Cleansing the perineal area.

31 Help the client put on a clean gown and attend to personal hygiene needs.	This provides for the client's warmth and comfort.
32 Protect the pillow with a towel, and groom the client's hair, as described in the text.	
33 Change bed linens, as described in Procedures 27-3 and 27-4.	
34 Record any significant observations and communication on the client's chart.	A careful record is important for planning and individualizing the client's care.

Age Considerations

When bathing an infant or young child, have all supplies within easy reach and support or hold the child securely at all times to ensure safety. Never leave the child alone.

Check temperature of water, particularly before bathing an older client because sensitivity to temperature may be impaired.

(Continued)

Removal of gown if client has an intravenous line necessitates taking the gown off, uninvolved arm first, and then threading the intravenous tubing and bottle or bag through the arm of the gown after the affected arm has been removed from the gown. To replace the gown, reverse the procedure. Place the clean gown on the unaffected arm first and thread intravenous tubing and bottle or bag from inside the arm of the gown on the involved side. *Never* disconnect intravenous tubing to change a gown because this causes a break in a sterile system and is a potential for infection.

Certain clients may not be able to tolerate lying flat in bed during the bed bath. Position may have to be modified to accommodate needs of such clients.

Change water as often as necessary to maintain at a comfortable temperature. Always change the water after performing perineal care or when the water is soiled.

PROCEDURE 27-2
Applying Elastic Stockings

Equipment

Elastic stockings (in correct size)

For knee-high stockings
- Measure from heel to popliteal space.
- Measure circumference of calf at widest point.

For thigh-high stockings
- Measure from heel to gluteal fold.
- Measure circumference of calf and thigh at widest point.

Measuring tape
Talcum powder (optional)

Action	Rationale
1 Explain the rationale for use of elastic stockings to the client.	Explanation encourages the client's cooperation.
2 Wash your hands.	Handwashing deters the spread of microorganisms.
3 Assist the client to the supine position.	Dependent position of legs encourages blood to pool in the veins.
4 Provide privacy. Expose legs, one at a time, and powder lightly unless client has dry skin. If the skin is dry, a lotion may be used.	Powder and lotion reduce friction and make application of stockings easier.

(Continued)

Applying Elastic Stockings   (Continued)

Action	Rationale
5 Using both hands, gather and bunch stocking down to the heel.	This facilitates the application of the stocking.
6 Ease the foot of the stocking over the client's toes, foot, and heel. Check that the stocking is straight and smooth.	Wrinkles or improper fit interferes with circulation.

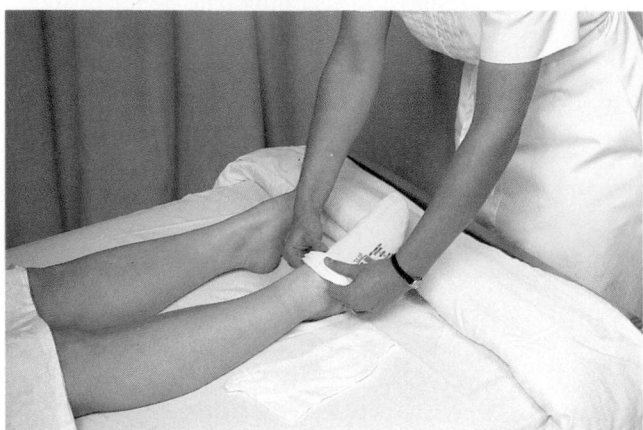

Step 6: Easing stockings over toes and foot.

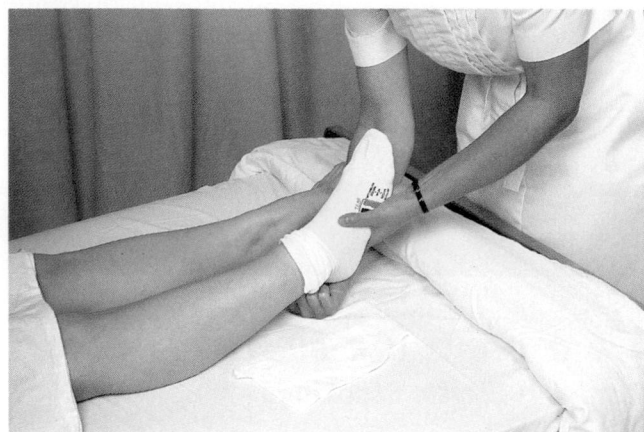

Step 6: Lifting leg slightly to ease stocking over heel.

7 Using your fingers and thumbs, grasp the gathered stocking and ease up smoothly to full height. Check that the stocking is straight and smooth. Readjust as necessary. Repeat for the other leg. Caution the client not to roll stockings partially down.	Easing the stocking carefully into position ensures proper fit of the stocking to the contour of the leg. Rolling stockings may have a constricting effect on veins.
8 Wash your hands.	Handwashing deters the spread of microorganisms.
9 To remove stocking, grasp the top of the stocking with your thumb and fingers and smoothly pull the stocking off inside out to heel. Support the client's foot and ease the stocking over it.	This preserves elasticity and contour of the stocking.

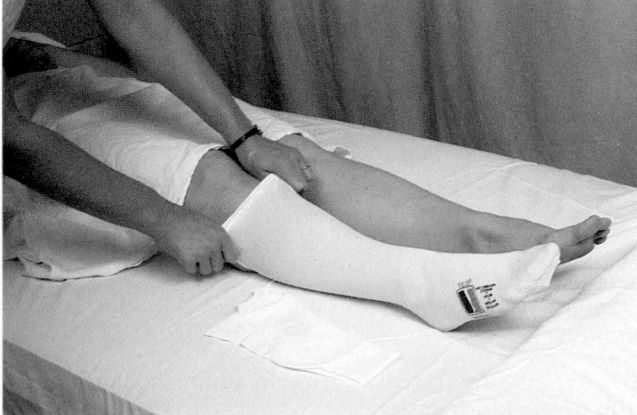

Step 7: Easing stocking up smoothly to full height.

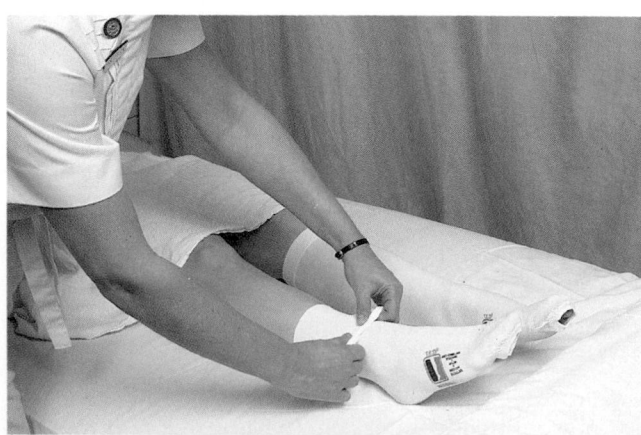

Step 9: Removing stockings by pulling them off inside out.

(Continued)

10 Remove stockings once every shift for 20 to 30 minutes. Wash and air dry as necessary (according to manufacturer's directions).

This allows observation of the client's circulatory status and condition of the skin on the lower extremities.

11 Record the application of elastic stockings as well as assessment of the client's circulatory status and skin condition.

This provides accurate documentation of the procedure.

mild pressure while others are capable of applying pressure equivalent to an elastic bandage. They are available in a variety of colors so that another stocking is not required over them for the ambulatory person. Many persons who are on their feet or remain in one position a great deal, such as homemakers, nurses, salespersons, and business persons, find them very useful. The stockings should be fitted correctly to the person's measurements. Also, they should be applied immediately on awakening, before getting out of bed and before the legs are in a dependent position.

Massaging the Back

A back rub generally follows the client's bath. This acts as a general body conditioner. It can be used as a stimulant or a relaxant, or both. Giving a back rub provides an opportunity for the nurse to observe the skin for signs of breakdown. It improves circulation and provides a means of communication with the client through the use of touch.

Because some clients may consider the back rub a "luxury" and be reluctant to accept it, the nurse should simply say to the client "Now it is time for your back massage." An effective back rub should take 4 to 6 minutes to complete. A lotion for massaging the back is usually used, although alcohol is sometimes recommended when the skin is oily. For the comfort of the client, the lotion or alcohol should be warmed before applying it to the back. The nurse should be aware of the client's diagnosis when a back rub is being considered. A back rub is contraindicated, for example, when the client has had back surgery or has fractured ribs. Position the client on the abdomen or, if this is contraindicated, on the side for a back rub. Recommended techniques for administering a back rub are outlined in Procedure 30-1.

Bedmaking

It is usual procedure to change bed linens after the bath. The bed is made for the client who is up and about in the manner described in Procedure 27-3. If the client is bedridden, the occupied bed is made according to Procedure 27-4.

There are minor variations in the procedure for making the occupied bed. However, these small differences have no real effect on the client's comfort. In some instances, it is necessary for nurses to devise unique ways to change the linens on a client's bed because of the nature of the client's condition, orthopedic appliances on the bed, or treatments that may be in progress.

Providing Environmental Care

Bedside Unit. Since the client's environment contributes positively or negatively to the sense of well-being, it is important for the nurse to ensure that the bedside unit is clean, safe, and pleasant. The term *bedside unit* generally refers to the furnishings and equipment in the space surrounding the client's bed. Basic furniture includes the bed, overbed table, bedside stand, and chairs. Standard equipment in the hospital environment includes the call light, oxygen, suction, and electrical outlets; light fixtures; bath basin; emesis basin; bedpan/urinal; water pitcher/glass; and bed linens. A nursing responsibility is ensuring that necessary equipment and items are in their proper place and functioning properly.

Since the client's personal items are generally stored in the bedside stand, the nurse should request permission of the alert client before opening the stand to obtain the bath basin, lotion, or other items. When assisting with hygiene, respecting the client's right to privacy and ownership of personal goods will decrease the client's sense of powerlessness.

Before leaving the bedside unit, it is good nursing practice to say to the client "Is there anything else I can do to make you more comfortable?" Checking with the client compensates for any oversight on the nurse's part and communicates genuine caring. Limits may need to be set for manipulative clients as to what comfort and hygiene measures the nurse is able to perform.

Elements of a safe bedside unit include the following:

- Client call light functioning and always within reach

(Text continues on p. 584.)

PROCEDURE 27-3
Making an Unoccupied Bed

Equipment

Two large sheets (or one large sheet and one fitted sheet)
Drawsheet
Blankets

Bedspread
Pillowcases
Linen hamper or bag

Bedside chair
Waterproof sheet or protective pad (optional)

Action

1 Assemble equipment and arrange on a bedside chair in the order in which items will be used.

2 Wash your hands.

3 Adjust the client's bed to the high position, and drop the bed side rails.

4 Check bed linens for the client's personal items and disconnect call bell or any tubes from bed linens.

5 Loosen all linen as you move around the bed from the head of the bed on the far side to the head of the bed on the near side.

6 Fold reusable linens, such as blankets or spread, in place on the bed in fourths and hang them over a clean chair.

7 Snugly roll all of the soiled linen inside of the bottom sheet and place directly into the laundry hamper. Do not place them on the floor or on furniture. Do not hold soiled linens against your uniform.

Rationale

Organization facilitates performance of task.

Handwashing deters the spread of microorganisms.

Having the bed in the high position and the side rails down reduces strain on the nurse while working.

It is costly and inconvenient when personal belongings are lost.

Loosening linen helps prevent tugging and tearing on linen. Loosening the linen and moving around the bed systematically reduce strain caused by reaching across the bed.

Folding saves time and energy when reusable linen is replaced on the bed. Folding linens while they are on the bed reduces strain on the nurse's arms.

Rolling soiled linens snugly and placing them directly into the hamper helps prevent the spread of organisms. The floor is heavily contaminated; soiled linen will further contaminate furniture. Soiled linen contaminates the nurse's uniform and this may spread organisms to another client.

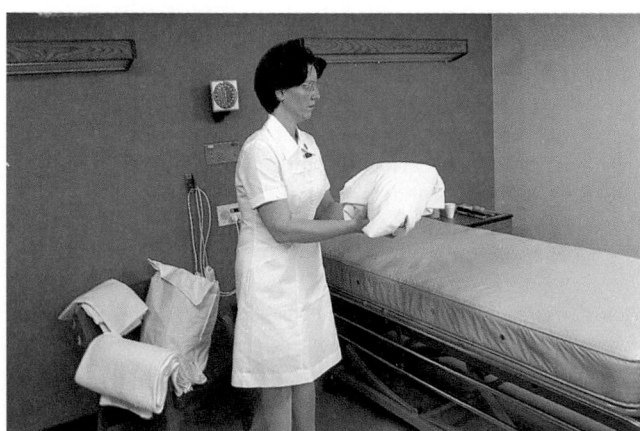

Step 7: Bundling soiled linens in bottom sheet and holding away from body.

8 Grasp mattress securely and shift up to the head of the bed.

This allows more foot room for the client and moves the mattress against the head of the bed.

(Continued)

Action

9 Place the bottom sheet with its center fold in the center of the bed and high enough to have a sufficient amount of the sheet to tuck under the head of the mattress.

10 If a waterproof sheet or protective pad is used, place it over the bottom sheet so that it will be under the client's chest to knee area. Place the cotton drawsheet in the same manner over the waterproof covering. Not all agencies use drawsheets routinely. The nurse may decide to use one.

Rationale

Opening linens on the bed reduces strain on the nurse's arms and diminishes the spread of organisms.

When a client soils the bed, drawsheets can be changed without the bottom and top linens on the bed. Having all bottom linens in place before tucking them under the mattress avoids unnecessary moving about the bed. A drawsheet also is an aid when moving the client in bed.

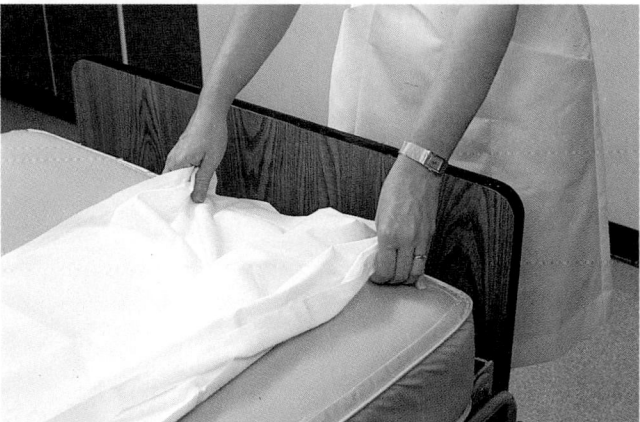

Step 9: Placing clean linens to begin bed making.

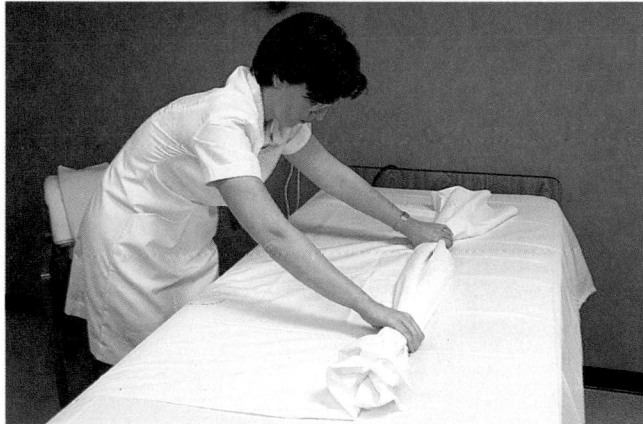

Step 10: Placing the drawsheet on the bed.

11 Tuck the bottom sheet securely under the head of the mattress on one side of the bed, making a corner according to agency policy. A mitered corner is shown in the illustrations. Using a fitted bottom sheet eliminates the need to miter corners. Tuck the remaining bottom sheet and drawsheet securely under the mattress. (At this point, before moving to the other side of bed, top linens may be placed on the bed, unfolded, and secured, allowing the entire side of the bed to be completed at one time as shown in the illustrations.)

Making the bed on one side and then completing the bed on the other side saves time. Having bottom linens free of wrinkles reduces discomfort to the bedridden client.

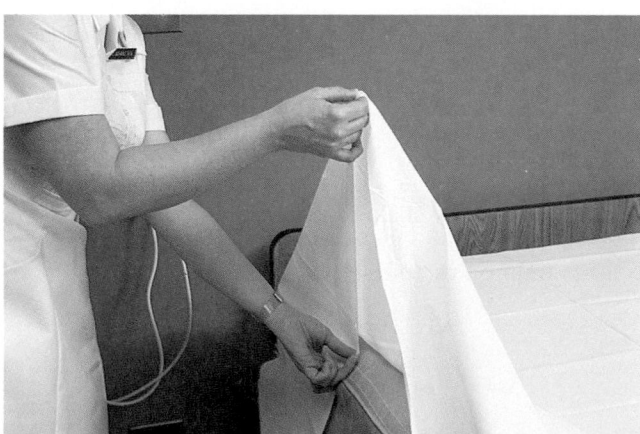

Step 11: Beginning to make mitered corner by creating a triangular fold.

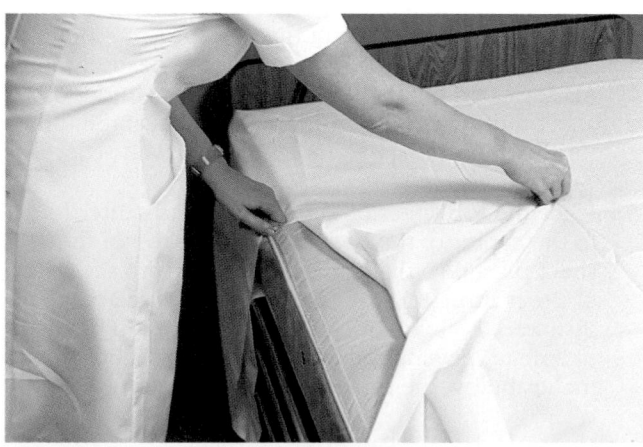

Step 11: Laying triangular fold on top of bed.

(Continued)

Action

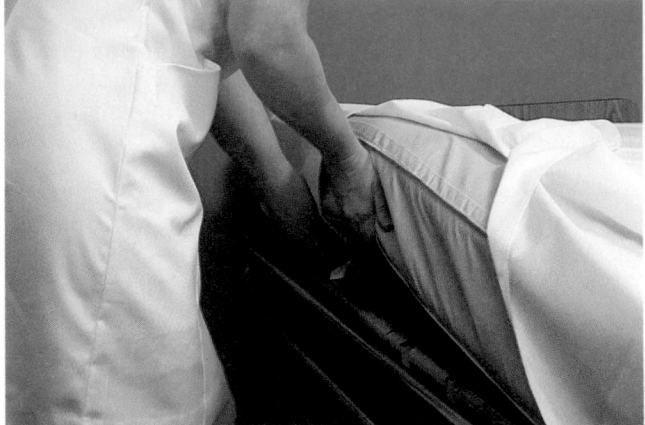

Step 11 (cont.): Tucking end of sheet under mattress.

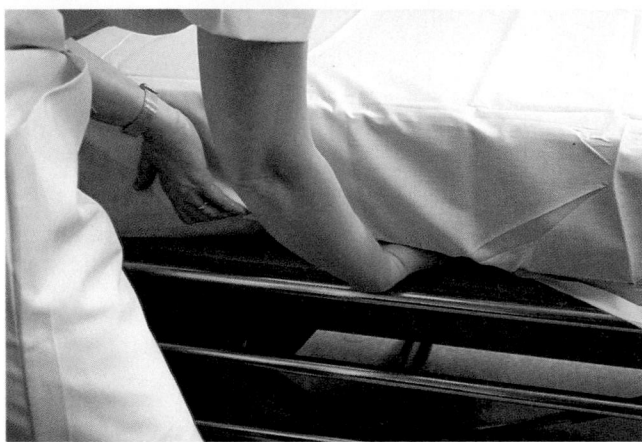

Tucking end of triangular linen fold under mattress to complete mitered corner.

Rationale

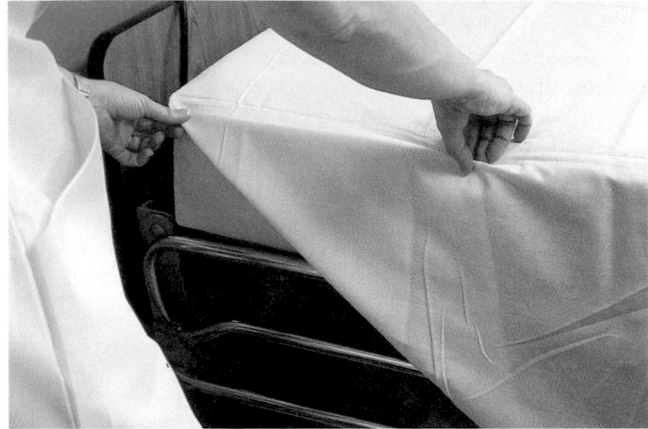

Folding triangular linen fold down over side of mattress.

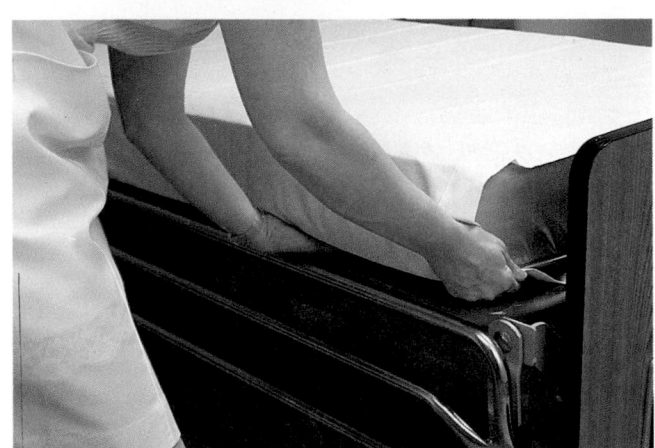

Tucking sheet snugly under foot of mattress.

12 Move to the other side of the bed to secure bottom linens. Secure top of sheet under the head of the mattress and miter the corner. Pull remainder of sheet tightly and tuck under mattress. Do the same for the drawsheet.

This rids bottom linens of any wrinkles that can cause discomfort for the client.

13 Place the top sheet on the bed with its center fold in the center of the bed and with the top of the sheet placed so that the hem is even with the head of the mattress. Unfold the top sheet in place, as illustrated. Follow same procedure with top blanket or spread, placing the upper edge approximately 6 inches below the top of the sheet.

Opening linens by shaking them spreads organisms into the air. Holding linens overhead to open them causes strain on the nurse's arms.

(Continued)

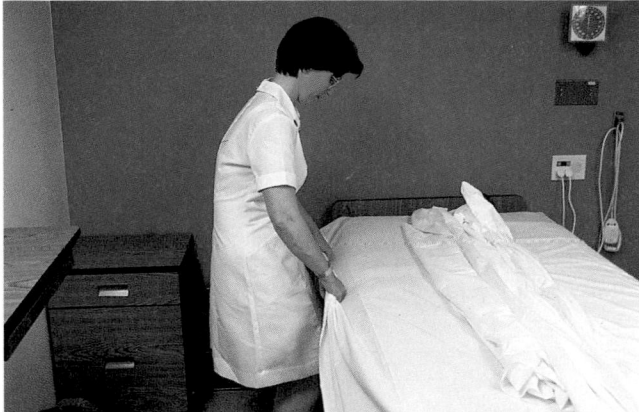

Step 12: Pulling bottom sheet tightly on opposite side of bed.

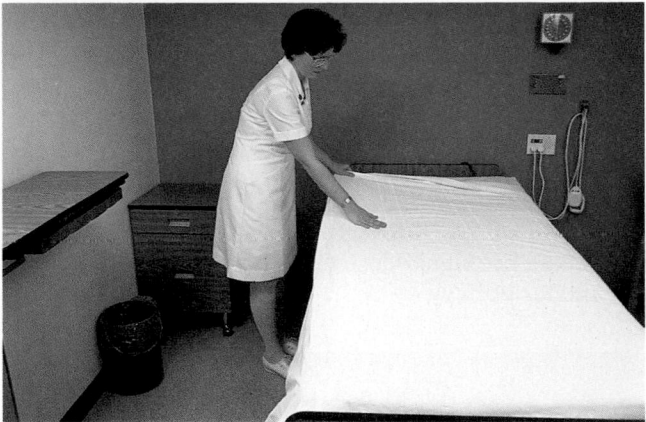

Step 13: Smoothing linens.

14 Tuck the top sheet and blanket under the foot of the bed on the near side. Miter the corners.

This saves time and energy and keeps the top linen in place.

15 Fold the upper 6 inches of the top sheet down over the spread and make a cuff.

This makes it easier for the client to get into bed and pull the covers up.

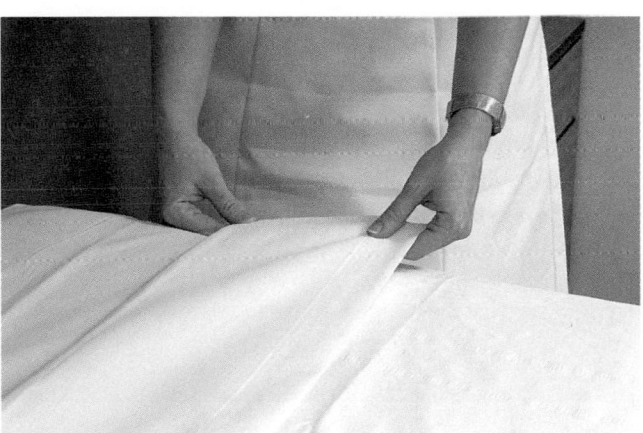

Step 15: Cuffing top linens.

16 Move to the other side of the bed and follow the same procedure for securing top sheets under the foot of the bed and making a cuff.

Working on one side of the bed at a time saves energy and is more efficient.

17 Place the pillows on the bed. Open each pillowcase in the same manner as opening other linens. Gather the pillowcase over one hand toward the closed end. Grasp the pillow with the hand inside the pillowcase. Keeping a firm hold on the top of the pillow, pull the cover onto the pillow.

Opening linens by shaking them causes organisms to be carried about on air currents. Covering the pillow while it rests on the bed reduces strain on the nurse's arms and back.

(Continued)

Action

18 Place the pillow at the head of the bed with the open end facing toward the window.

19 Fan-fold or pie-fold the top linens.

20 Secure the signal device on the bed according to agency policy.

Rationale

This provides for a neater appearance.

Having linens opened makes it more convenient for the client to get into bed.

Having the signal device handy for the client makes it possible for the client to call for assistance as necessary.

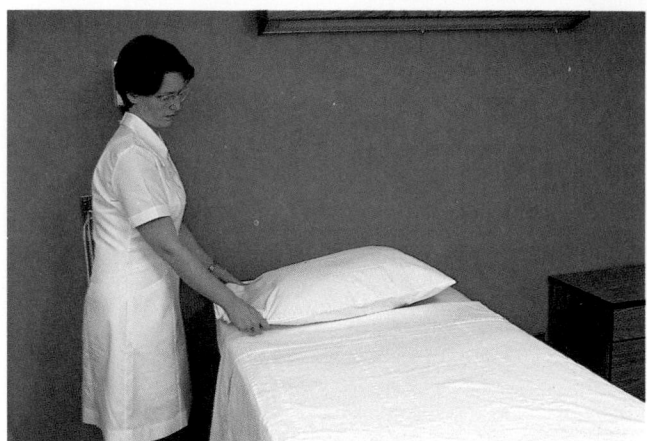

Step 18: Placing pillow with fresh pillowcase.

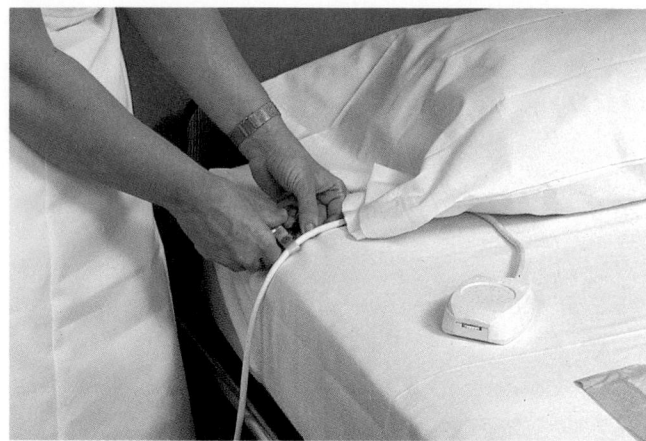

Step 20: Securing the signal device on bed.

21 Adjust the bed to the low position.

22 Dispose of soiled linen according to agency policy. Wash your hands.

Having the bed in the low position makes it easier and safer for the client to get into bed.

This deters the spread of microorganisms.

P R O C E D U R E   27-4
Making an Occupied Bed

Equipment

Two large sheets (or one large sheet and one fitted sheet)
Drawsheet
Blanket (optional)

Bedspread
Pillowcases
Linen hamper or bag (optional)

Bedside chair
Waterproof sheet or protective pad (optional)
Bath blanket (optional)

(Continued)

Action	Rationale
1 Explain the procedure to the client. Check the client's chart for limitations on the client's physical activity.	This facilitates client cooperation and determines level of activity.
2 Wash your hands.	Handwashing deters the spread of microorganisms.
3 Assemble equipment and arrange on the bedside chair in the order the items will be used.	Organization facilitates performance of task.
4 Close door or curtain.	This provides for privacy.
5 Adjust the client's bed to the high position. Lower the side rail nearest you, leaving the opposite side rail up. Place the bed in the flat position if the client can tolerate it.	Having the bed in the high position reduces strain on the nurse while working. Having the mattress flat facilitates making a wrinkle-free bed.
6 Check bed linens for client's personal items and disconnect the call bell or any tubes from bed linens.	It is costly and inconvenient when personal items are lost. Disconnecting tubes from linens prevents discomfort and accidental dislodging of the tubes.
7 Place a bath blanket, if available, over the client. Have the client hold onto the bath blanket while you reach under it and remove top linens. Leave the top sheet in place if a bath blanket is not used. Fold linen that is to be reused over the back of a chair. Discard soiled linen in a laundry bag or hamper.	This provides warmth and privacy.

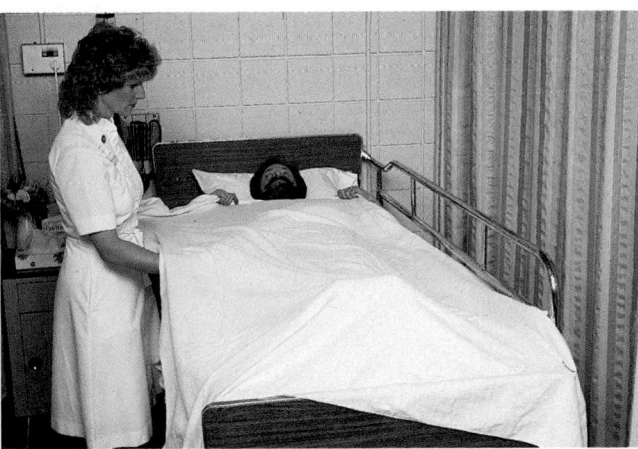

Step 7: Removing top linens from under bath blanket.

Action	Rationale
8 Grasp mattress securely and shift it up to the head of the bed (you may require the assistance of another person).	This allows more foot room for the client and positions the mattress against the head of the bed.
9 Assist the client to turn toward the opposite side of the bed and reposition the pillow under the client's head.	This allows the bed to be made on the vacant side.

(Continued)

Action

10 Loosen all bottom linens from the head and sides of the bed.

11 Fan-fold soiled linens as close to the client as possible.

12 Use clean linen and make near side of bed following Steps 9, 10, and 11 of Procedure 27-3. Fan-fold the clean linen as close to the client as possible.

Rationale

This facilitates removal of linens.

This facilitates removal of linens when the client turns to the other side.

This positions clean linen to make the side of the bed.

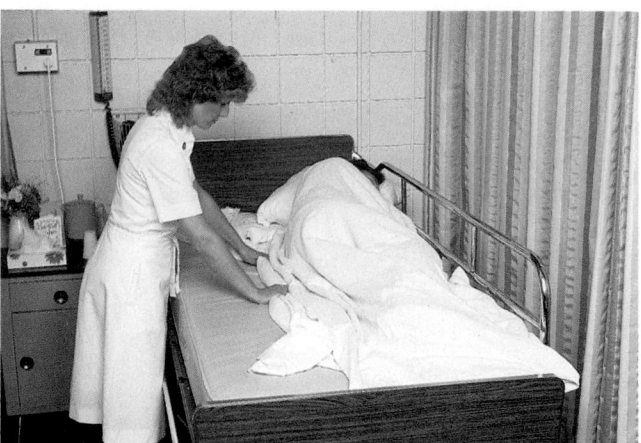

Step 11: Fanfolding soiled linen close to client.

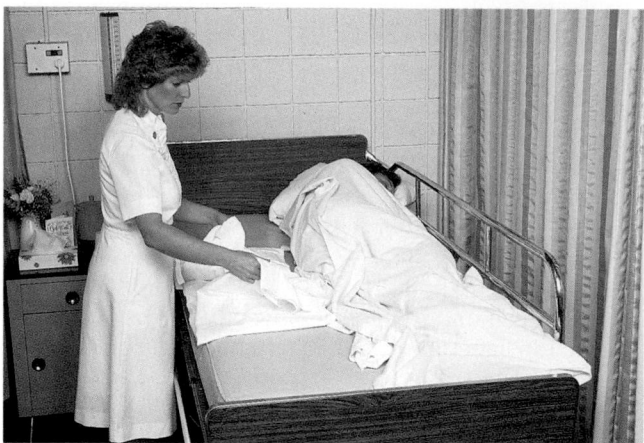

Step 12: Unfolding clean linens.

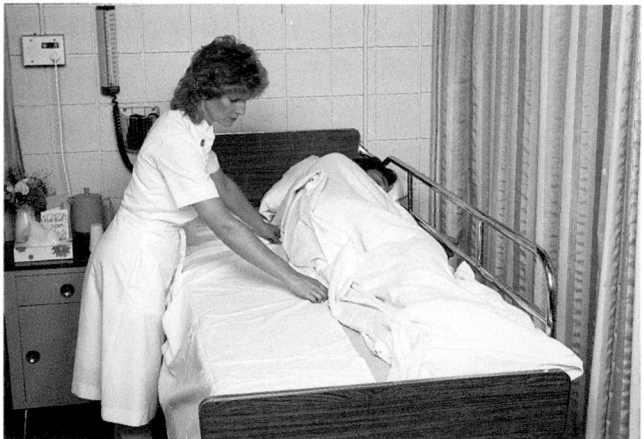

Step 12: Aligning clean bottom sheet on half of bed.

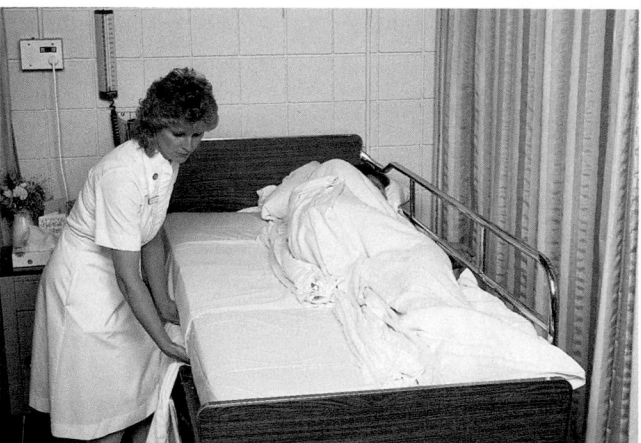

Step 12: Tucking bottom sheet and draw sheet tightly.

13 Raise the side rail. Move to the other side of the bed and lower the side rail. Assist the client to roll over the folded linen in the middle of the bed and toward the other side. Reposition the pillow and bath blanket or top sheet.

This ensures client safety. The movement allows the bed to be made on the other side. The bath blanket provides warmth and privacy.

(Continued)

Action	**Rationale**

14 Loosen and remove all bottom linen. Place these in a linen bag or hamper. Hold soiled linen away from your uniform.

Proper disposal of soiled linen prevents spread of microorganisms.

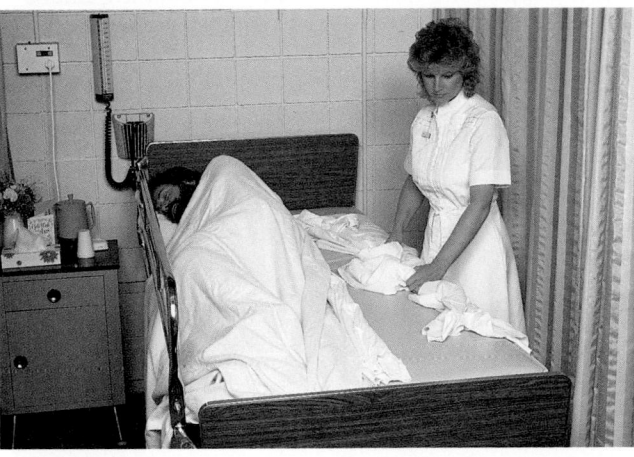

Step 14: Removing soiled bottom linens from other side of bed.

15 Ease the clean linen from under the client. Pull taut and secure the bottom sheet under the head of the mattress. Miter corners. Pull the side of the sheet taut and tuck under the side of the mattress. Repeat this with the drawsheet.

This removes wrinkles and creases in the linens, which are uncomfortable to lie on.

16 Assist the client to return to the center of the bed. Remove the pillow and change the pillowcase before replacing, with open end facing toward the window.

This provides for a neater appearance.

17 Apply top linen so that it is centered and top hems are even with the head of the mattress. Have the client hold onto the top linen so the bath blanket can be removed.

This allows bottom hems to be tucked securely under the mattress and provides for privacy.

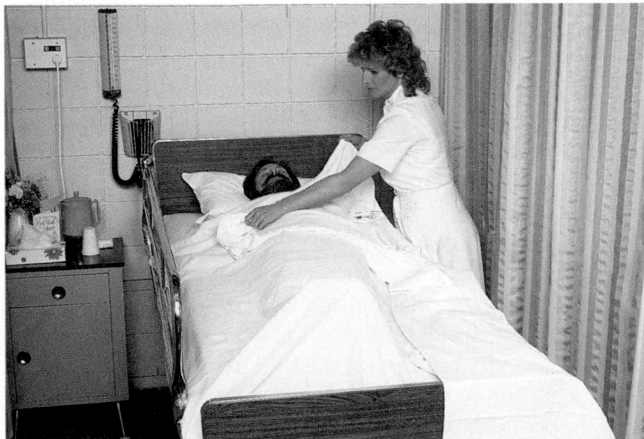

Step 17: Applying top linen over bath blanket.

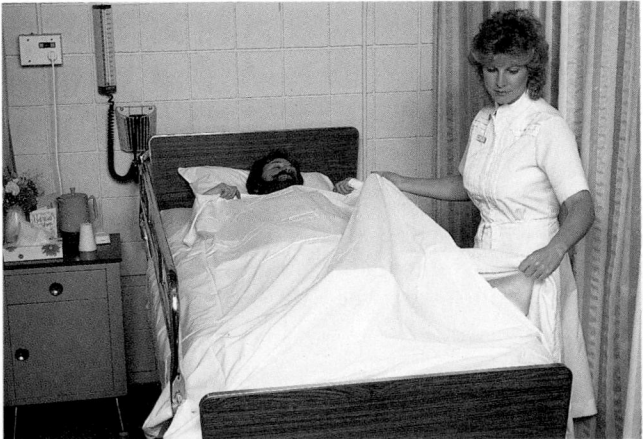

Step 17: Removing the bath blanket from under the top linens.
(Photos © Ken Kasper)

(Continued)

Action	**Rationale**
18 Secure top linens under the foot of the mattress and miter corners. Loosen top linens over the client's feet by grasping them in the area of the feet and pulling gently toward the foot of the bed.	This provides for a neat appearance. Loosening linens over the client's feet gives more room for movement.
19 Raise the side rail. Lower bed height and adjust the head of the bed to a comfortable position. Reattach call bell and drainage tubes.	This provides for the client's safety.
20 Dispose of soiled linens according to agency policy. Wash your hands.	This prevents spread of microorganisms.

- Bed positioned properly and at the appropriate height
- Side rails and restraints safely used when indicated
- Principles of medical asepsis followed
- Electrical equipment safely grounded
- Uncluttered walk space

Elements of providing a comfortable bedside unit include attention to ventilation, odors, room temperature, lighting, and noise.

Ventilation and Odors. Because of all the pathogens in hospitals and unpleasant odors associated with body secretions and excretions (urine, stool, vomitus, draining wounds, body odors), good ventilation in client rooms is imperative. Since many clients are sensitive to drafts, it is often wise to "air" the room during times when clients are out of their rooms for diagnostic or therapeutic procedures. Odors may be decreased by promptly emptying bedpans, urinals, and emesis basins, and by being careful not to dispose of soiled dressings or anything with a strong odor in the waste receptacle in the client's room. Deodorizers may need to be employed.

Room Temperature. Whenever possible client preferences (which may vary widely) should be followed regarding room temperature. In general, the room temperature should fall between 20° C and 23° C (68° F and 74° F).

Lighting and Noise. Since many clients find it difficult to sleep in the hospital and may need to be disturbed frequently for assessment or treatment purposes, the nurse should be careful to reduce harsh lighting and noises whenever possible. However, adequate lighting should be provided for all nursing procedures. Clients

may enjoy sunlight or find it disturbing, and drapes may be arranged accordingly. Whenever possible, conversations should not be carried on immediately outside the client's room. Many clients find this stressful both because the noise disturbs them and because they believe whatever is being said involves them.

Beds. Since many persons who are ill spend a large portion of the day—if not the entire day—in bed, the bed is an important part of the client's environment. Nursing responsibilities include ensuring both a safe and comfortable bed.

Bed Safety. The typical hospital bed has a motorized metal frame in three sections, which allows the height of the bed to be raised or lowered as well as the head and foot of the bed to be adjusted. It is important that the nurse know how to operate the bed and explain this to the client. Bed positions are described in Chapter 28. Since certain positions may actually be harmful to some clients, the client and family should be instructed about advisable bed positions and use of the bed controls. Hospital beds are generally 66 cm (26 inches) from the floor. This is higher than most beds at home and enables the nurse to reach the client without undue musculoskeletal strain. Whenever the client's condition indicates the need for upper or lower side rails, these should be used to prevent dangerous falls. The wheels (or casters) on the hospital bed should be locked whenever the bed is stationary to prevent the bed from "slipping away" from a client who is transferring from the bed to an upright position or to a stretcher. The headboard of most hospital beds is removable to allow close client contact in an emergency situation.

In summary, before leaving the client's bedside, ensure that

- The bed is in its lowest position
- The bed position is safe for the client
- The bed controls are functioning (bed is electrically safe)
- Side rails (upper and lower) are raised if indicated
- The wheels or casters are locked

Bed Comfort.   The hospital mattress is firm and generally covered with a water-repellent material that can be easily wiped down with a bactericidal solution between clients. Since many clients find it uncomfortable to rest with just a sheet between them and the rubberized mattress, the nurse may need to find creative solutions—especially for clients at high risk for skin impairment. The egg crate mattress (Fig 27-3, top) is often an acceptable solution. Clients with arthritis and vascular problems often find the rubberized mattress cold; the use of sheep skins (Fig 27-3, bottom) or a soft bath blanket or flannelette blanket used under or as a substitute for the bottom sheet may solve this problem. Pillows covered with water-repellent material can be especially uncom-

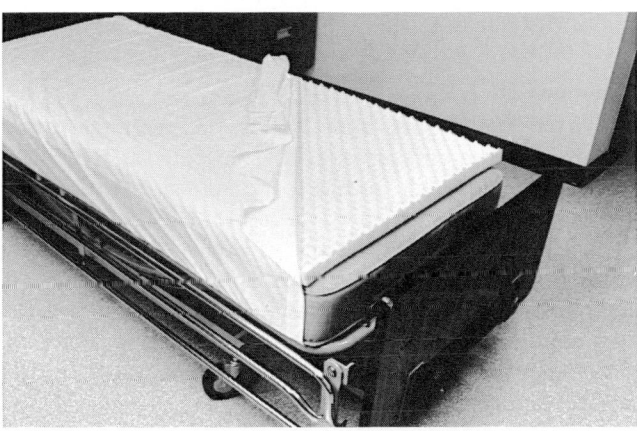

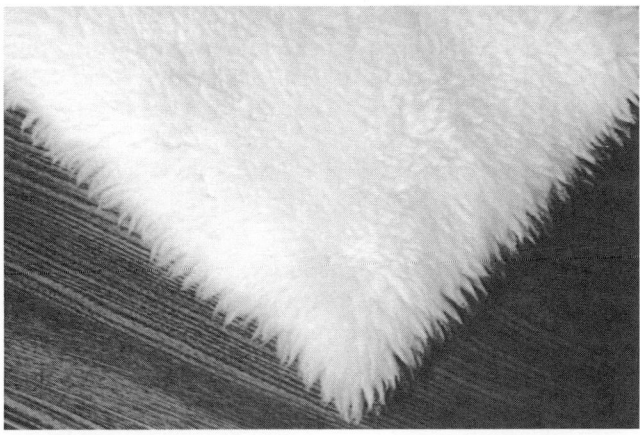

F I G U R E 27-3
The eggcrate mattress (top) adds to comfort and helps distribute body weight evenly to reduce the risk of pressure sores. Sheepskin (bottom) laid over the bottom sheet is softer and warmer than just a bottom sheet over the rubberized mattress.

fortable to clients. Clients spending many days in bed may find that having a pillow from home greatly aids their rest.

Agency policies usually dictate the availability and use of bed linens. Bed linens include mattress covers, sheets, drawsheets, incontinent pads, pillow cases, blankets, bedspreads, and bath blankets. Towels, washcloths, and patient gowns are often included in linen packs. Devices to support and protect the client confined to bed are described in Chapter 28. In some settings, making the bed is not nursing's responsibility. However, ensuring client comfort is always a priority in nursing, and this often involves creating a comfortable bed environment.

Before leaving a client, the nurse should ensure that
- Linens are clean and wrinkle-free
- The client feels comfortably warm
- Pressure points on the client at high risk for skin impairment are protected from rough sheets, hem edges, and water-repellent materials

Teaching Clients About Skin Problems and Skin Care

The nurse can share information with the client during assessment and care procedures. Occasionally clients will ask for specific information. The following concerns skin problems and skin care.

Skin Problems

Dry Skin.   Dry skin is characteristically flaky and is easily susceptible to injury and irritation. Suggestions for persons whose skin is dry and injured easily are the following:
- Bathe less frequently, especially when the outdoor temperature and humidity are low.
- Rinse off soaps or detergents well when they are used for cleansing the skin. Residue left on the skin predisposes to skin irritation and breakdown.
- Avoid defatting agents, such as alcohol, on dry and easily injured skin.
- Avoid wearing garments made of woolen fabrics since wool tends to irritate dry skin.
- Wash garments made of wrinkle-resistant fabrics once or twice before wearing them. The chemical impregnated in the fabric tends to irritate dry skin.
- Add moisture to the air through a humidifier when the skin is dry.
- Increase fluid intake when the skin is dry.
- Try using a bath oil when the skin is dry. These oils make bathtubs slippery, and care should be used to prevent falls. Bubble-bath preparations, which often contain oil, should be mixed well in the bath water before the person sits in the tub. Urinary tract infections have been correlated with the use of bubble bath preparations.
- Use an **emollient**, which is an agent used to soften, soothe, and protect dry skin after it is cleansed. Emollient or moisturizing creams do not add mois-

ture to the skin. Rather, the film they leave on the skin retards normal moisture evaporation and helps to hold down the scaly skin surfaces. Cocoa butter, petroleum jelly, and lanolin are effective emollients and are used in many emollient creams.
- Use creams to clean skin that is very dry or allergic to soaps and detergents.

Acne.   Oily skin is especially bothersome during adolescence, when hormones cause enlargement of the sebaceous glands and increased glandular secretions. Blackheads and pustules appear when these secretions become dammed up in the sebaceous ducts, and inflammation with infection occurs. The condition is referred to as **acne** and most often appears on the face, neck, shoulders, and back. From a health standpoint, acne is not a serious condition, although it can lead to permanent scarring and psychologic problems for the person suffering from it. There are various recommended ways to help control acne and minimize scarring:
- The infected areas should not be squeezed or picked. This tends to cause a spread of the infection and scarring of the skin.
- The person with acne should wash the skin and shampoo hair with soap or detergent and hot water frequently to remove oil and debris.
- Oily cosmetics, cleansing creams, and emollients should be avoided. They tend to make the condition worse.
- Cosmetics should be used sparingly to avoid further blocking of sebaceous gland ducts.
- Sunshine or exposure to an ultraviolet lamp helps keep acne under control in many instances. However, caution should be exercised to prevent burning the skin.
- Foods that are found to aggravate the condition should be eliminated from the diet. Chocolate, nuts, cola beverages, and foods containing iodine tend to make acne worse for some people.

In severe cases, the services of a physician are recommended. Treatment modalities vary.

Skin Rashes.   Rashes are eruptions or inflammations of the skin that may be found anywhere on the body. Rashes may be precipitated by the skin's contact with an allergen (*e.g.,* chemicals in cleansers and soaps) or by overexposure to the sun or to moisture. They may also result from systemic causes such as the body's response to medications or to certain diseases. Rashes may be described as flat or raised, pruritic or nonpruritic, localized or systemic, dry or wet. Scratching a rash may result in inflammation and infection.

Interventions include the following:
- Wash the area thoroughly with a mild cleansing agent and rinse well.
- Use a moisturizing lotion on a dry rash to prvent itching and to promote healing.
- Use a drying agent on a wet rash.

- Tepid baths or soaks may relieve inflammation and itching.
- Antiseptic sprays or lotions may be useful in lessening itching, promoting healing, and preventing skin breakdown.
- A number of over-the-counter products such as caladryl lotion and hydrocortisone creams may be useful, depending on the nature of the rash. Read the manufacturer's recommendations and cautions before testing a new product.
- If the causative agent is known; avoid exposure to it.
- Refer to a physician if symptoms do not respond to treatment.

Pressure Ulcers.   Pressure ulcers are areas of cellular necrosis caused by the lack of blood circulation to the involved area. At best they are extremely painful and debilitating to clients and at worst they may be life-threatening. They offer a persistent challenge to even the most experienced nurse. Preventing pressure ulcers whenever possible and identifying and treating them at the earliest stage possible are critical nursing responsibilities, and this topic will be explored in detail at the end of this chapter.

Skin Care

Soaps, Detergents, and Creams.   A great variety of soaps and detergents are available. Expensive cleansing agents have not been found to be superior to the less expensive ones. For most persons, the best way to cleanse the skin is with soap or detergent and water. Soaps are made from vegetable and animal fats. Most detergents are made from petroleum derivatives and are especially satisfactory when the water is hard, cold, or salty. Persons who are sensitive to soap often find they can use detergents without difficulty.

Cold creams consist of an oil or wax, water, and perfume. The cream feels cold because the water evaporates, producing a feeling of coolness. The oil and wax liquify on the skin and loosen and suspend dirt, oily secretions, perspiration, bacteria, cosmetics, dead cells, and other foreign material. They are then removed with a tissue or a soft cloth.

Cleansing creams are similar to cold creams except they contain little or no water.

Deodorants and Antiperspirants.   Perspiration is essentially odorless, although it contains some waste products, such as uric acid and ammonia. The odor of perspiration occurs when bacteria, normally present on everyone's skin, act on the skin's normal secretions.

Keeping the body and clothing clean is the prime requisite for preventing body odors. Deodorants and antiperspirants may be used *after* the skin is clean. Antiperspirants are intended to reduce the amount of perspiration. They act as astringents and tend to close the exits of the sweat glands. Antiperspirants and deodorants should be used with care and according to directions to prevent irritation of the skin.

Cosmetics. Cosmetics frequently enhance the appearance of clean and healthy skin, although certain cultural and religious groups would not agree with this opinion. Make-up used judiciously helps disguise blemishes, improve skin coloring, and make wrinkles appear less obvious. Creams and lotions made by reputable concerns are safe to use.

From time to time, cosmetics containing harmful ingredients, such as various dyes used to color cosmetics, have appeared on the market. The nurse should be alert to such agents and help consumers avoid their use. The Food and Drug Administration of the United States Department of Health and Human Services enforces federal laws on the purity of foods, drugs, and cosmetics and on the advertising claims of their manufacturers. The agency is a good source of information about these products. Similar agencies exist in Canada.

It has been found that cosmetics often become contaminated with bacteria and fungus. It is best to discard cosmetics after they are approximately four months old, especially those applied near the eyes. Make-up applicators and puffs should be kept immaculately clean.

Evaluating

Daily contacts with the client while hygiene measures are being performed enable the nurse to frequently evaluate whether the client is meeting hygiene goals. Evaluative criteria include

- Level of client's participation in hygiene program
- Elimination, reduction in or compensation for factors interfering with the client's independent execution of hygiene measures (*e.g.,* weakness, decreased motivation, lack of knowledge)
- Client's achievement of goals related to specific skin problems is evaluated by giving attention to (1) the healing of skin lesions, (2) the elimination or reduction of causative factors, and (3) the client's ability to manage the prescribed treatment program independently.

ORAL CARE

The mouth is the first part of the alimentary canal and is an adjunct of the respiratory system. The ducts of the salivary glands open into the vestibule of the mouth. The teeth and the tongue are accessory organs in the mouth and play an important role in beginning digestion by breaking up food particles and mixing them with saliva. Saliva is also important as a mechanical cleaner of the mouth.

General good health is as essential as cleanliness for maintaining a healthy mouth and teeth. The relationship, for example, between good teeth and a diet sufficient in calcium and phosphorus along with vitamin D, which is necessary for the body to utilize these minerals, is well established.

There are several benefits for maintaining good oral hygiene and dental care. There is aesthetic value in having a clean and healthy mouth. Having one's own teeth contributes to an intact body image. The beginning of the digestive process and gustatory pleasure are enhanced when the mouth and teeth are in good condition.

Assessing

Nursing History. Identify the client's normal oral hygiene practices: brushing, flossing, use of rinses, presence and care of dentures or other orthodontic devices, frequency of dental examinations, and variables influencing these. Note the history of any oral problems and related treatments.

Nursing Examination. Examine the lips for color, moisture, lumps, ulcers, lesions, and edema. Examine the buccal mucosa for color, moisture, lesions, nodules, and bleeding. Examine the color of the gums and surface of the gums for lesions, bleeding, edema, and exudate. Examine for loose, missing, or carious (decayed) teeth. Note the presence of dentures or other orthodontic devices. Examine the tongue for color, symmetry, movement, texture, and lesions. Examine the hard and soft palates for intactness, color, patches, lesions, and petechiae. Examine the oropharynx: movement of the uvula, condition of tonsils if present. Note unusual mouth odors. Assess adequacy of mastication and swallowing.

High-Risk Variables. Identify any variables known to cause oral problems: deficient self-care abilities, poor nutrition and excessive intake of refined sugars, family history of periodontal disease, ingestion of chemotherapeutic agents that produce oral lesions, and other such factors. Clients at high risk for oral problems include those who are seriously ill, comatose, dehydrated, confused, depressed, or paralyzed. Clients who are mouth breathers, who can have no oral intake of nutrition or fluids (NPO), who have nasogastric tubes or oral airways in place, and who have had oral surgery are also at increased risk.

Common Oral Problems

When inspecting the oral cavity, the nurse frequently observes oral problems that at best are benign and only mildly annoying to clients but that may also be life threatening. It is imperative to identify the problem and its cause and to initiate the appropriate treatment. This may require consultation with a dentist or physician.

Dental Caries. The decay of teeth with the formation of cavities is called **caries.** Caries result from the failure to remove **plaque**, an invisible, destructive, bacterial film that builds up on everyone's teeth and eventually leads to the destruction of tooth enamel. A successful plaque-fighting program includes (1) elimination of sweet snacks between meals, such as soft drinks, candy, gum, jams, and jellies; (2) thorough cleansing; and (3) regular dental check-ups. The use of antiplaque, fluoride tooth pastes and mouth rinses helps prevent dental caries.

Periodontal Disease.   The major cause of tooth loss in adults over 35 years of age is gum disease. **Gingivitis** is an inflammation of the **gingiva**, the tissue that surrounds the teeth.

Periodontitis is a more marked inflammation of the gums and also involves the alveolar tissues; it is commonly called **pyorrhea** or *periodontal disease.* Symptoms include bleeding gums; swollen, red, painful gum tissues; receding gum lines with the formation of pockets between the teeth and gums; pus that appears when gums are pressed; and loose teeth. If unchecked, plaque builds up and, along with dead bacteria, forms hard deposits called **tartar** at the gum lines. The tartar attacks the fibers that fasten teeth to the gums and eventually attacks bone tissue also. The teeth then loosen and fall out. A strong mouth odor (**halitosis**) or persistent bad taste in the mouth may be the first indication of periodontal disease. Regular dental treatment by a dentist is imperative.

Other Oral Problems.   Other oral problems that the nurse may observe when inspecting the oral cavity include the following:

Stomatitis is an inflammation of the oral mucosa with numerous causes, such as bacteria, virus, mechanical trauma, irritants, nutritional deficiencies, and systemic infection. Symptoms may include heat, pain, increased flow of saliva, and halitosis. Manifestations include such diverse problems as aphthous ulcers, herpetic ulcers (fever blisters), fungal ulcers (*Candida albicans*–induced thrush), and chemotherapy-induced stomatitis.

Glossitis is an inflammation of the tongue.

Cheilosis is an ulceration of the lips (reddened fissures at the angles of the mouth) most often caused by vitamin B complex deficiencies (especially riboflavin).

Dry oral mucosa may simply be related to dehydration or may be caused by mouth breathing, an alteration in salivary functioning, or by certain medications (*e.g.,* the anticholinergics).

Oral malignancies appear as lumps or ulcers; it is critical that these be distinguished from benign mouth problems since early detection may be the difference between cure and radical dissecting surgery and death. Teach clients if they notice white or red patches, persistent sores, swelling, bleeding, numbness, or pain in the mouth to see their dentist right away.

Diagnosing

Make a judgment about the adequacy of the client's oral hygiene practices, identifying any factors contributing to deficiencies. An example is

Self-care deficit: oral hygiene related to low value attached to regular brushing, flossing, and dental examinations

Identify actual or potential oral problems that nurses can treat, noting contributing factors. Identify "unhealthy" client responses to oral problems. Examples are

Altered comfort: oral pain *related to* chemotherapy-induced oral ulceration

Potential for infection *related to* breaks in oral mucosa and inadequate secondary defenses

Altered nutrition: less than body requirements, *related to* painful oral lesions (ill-fitting dentures, gingivitis)

Altered oral mucous membrane *related to* dehydration (ineffective oral hygiene, medication)

Impaired swallowing related to neuromuscular impairment

Body image disturbance *related to* loss of teeth, halitosis, or dental caries

Planning

Identify nursing measures that will assist the client to develop or maintain oral hygiene practices to promote oral health and general well-being and resolve identified nursing diagnoses. Plan to achieve the following client goals:

• Client's lips, oral mucosa, gums, and tongue are intact, moist, and free of inflammation and lesions.
• Client's teeth (or dentures) are clean.
• The client demonstrates the ability to masticate and swallow food.
• Oral lesions demonstrate signs of healing.
• Client demonstrates correct oral hygiene measures: brushing and flossing.
• Client verbalizes importance of fluoride use and regular dental examinations.

Pertinent nursing measures to include in the plan of care are the following:

• Teaching proper brushing and flossing techniques; instructing clients about fluoride use and the importance of regular dental examinations
• Teaching correct denture care or providing this when necessary
• Performing mouth care for the unconscious client (cleaning the mouth with swabs dipped in dilute mouth rinse or in a solution of 1 part hydrogen peroxide to 3 parts water; suctioning as necessary to prevent aspiration; applying petroleum jelly to the lips)
• Performing mouth care for clients with oral lesions (cleansing to prevent infection and numbing if indicated to encourage eating)

In the plan of care, identify any supplies needed to carry out the specified oral care and the timing and frequency of oral hygiene measures.

Implementing

While carrying out the plan of care the nurse utilizes each nurse–client interaction for ongoing assessment of the client's oral cavity and evaluation of the adequacy of the plan of care. Described in this section are techniques for administering and teaching oral care. See the accompanying box for sample documentation of oral hygiene care.

Administering Oral Hygiene

The mouth must be cared for even during illness. However, there are times when care must be modified to meet the specific needs of a client. If the client is able to assist with mouth care while bedridden, the nurse provides necessary materials (see Procedure 27-5). If the client is helpless, the nurse will need to make certain that attention is given to the patient's mouth as often as necessary to keep it clean and moist, as often as every hour or two if necessary. This is especially true for patients who are unable or are not permitted fluids by mouth. Procedure 27-6 gives techniques for administering oral hygiene to the dependent client. Moisten the mouth with water, if allowed, and lubricate the lips sufficiently frequently to keep the membranes well moistened.

Studies suggest that the procedure of cleaning the mouth thoroughly is more important than the agent used. This finding supports the personal experience of many people that no mouthwash, breath freshener, ointment, or paste replaces a thorough mechanical cleaning of the oral cavity.

Denture Care. Keeping dentures out for long periods permits the gum line to change, thus affecting their fit. If the client has been instructed to remove dentures while sleeping, a disposable denture cup is convenient and easy to use. Dentures should not be wrapped in toilet tissue or disposable wipes because these are likely to be thrown away. It is recommended that dentures be stored in water to prevent drying and warping of plastic materials (Fig 27-4). A deodorant solution of water and a few drops of ammonia or white vinegar can be used. A few drops of essence of peppermint may be added also. Dentures made of vulcanite, which is a porous material, are especially prone to develop unpleasant odors.

The person with dentures is more likely to keep them in the mouth when dentures are kept clean. When the client is unable to care for them, th nurse is responsible for seeing to it that they are clean.

Care should be exercised when handling a client's dentures. They represent a considerable financial investment, and damage or loss becomes expensive. When cleaning dentures, the nurse should hold them over a basin of water or over a soft towel so that if they slip from the nurse's grasp, they will not fall onto a hard surface and break. Warm water should be used to cleanse them. Hot water may warp the plastic material from which most dentures are made. The use of a brush and a nonabrasive powder or paste is also recommended. There are also preparations in which to soak dentures to help remove stain and hardened particles. The dentures are rinsed well in warm water after cleaning.

Teaching Oral Hygiene

Toothbrushing and Flossing. A toothbrush should be small enough to reach all teeth. The bristles should be sufficiently firm to clean but not so firm that they are likely to injure tooth enamel and gum tissue. Brushes should be cleaned and dried between uses. There is a difference of opinion as to the best way to brush teeth. When assisting and teaching a client, the nurse should follow the preference of the client's dentist. One recommended brushing regimen is illustrated in Figure 27-5.

(Text continues on p. 594.)

Sample Documentation of Oral Hygiene

10/20/88 Client generally breathes with mouth open. Sordes present on palate, teeth, gums, and oral mucosa. Toothettes dipped in 1 part hydrogen peroxide/3 parts water solution used for cleansing q 4 hours. Petrolatum jelly to lips.

C. Moser, RN

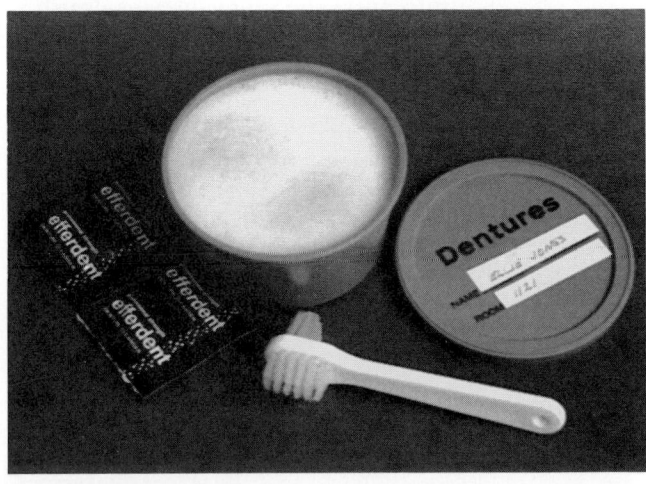

FIGURE 27-4
Dentures should be stored in water to prevent warping. Many health-care agencies provide denture cups for storage and cleaning. Soaking dentures in special cleaning preparations helps remove stains and hardened particles.

PROCEDURE 27-5
Assisting the Client With Oral Care

Equipment

Toothbrush	Towel	Denture-cleansing
Toothpaste	Mouthwash	equipment (if
Emesis basin	(optional)	necessary)
Glass with cool water	Dental floss	Denture cup
	(optional)	Denture cleaner
		Gauze 4 × 4
		Washcloth or
		paper towel
		Petroleum jelly (op-
		tional)

Action

1 Explain the procedure to the client.

2 Assemble equipment on an overbed table within the client's reach.

3 Wash your hands.

4 Provide privacy for the client.

5 Lower side rail and assist client to sitting position if permitted, or turn the client onto the side. Place the towel across the client's chest. Raise the bed to a comfortable working position.

6 Encourage the client to brush own teeth or assist if necessary:

    a. Moisten the toothbrush and apply toothpaste to bristles.

    b. Place brush at a 45-degree angle to gum line and brush from gum line to crown of each tooth. Brush outer and inner surfaces. Brush back and forth across biting surface of each tooth.

Rationale

Explanation facilitates cooperation.

Organization facilitates performance of task.

Handwashing deters the spread of microorganisms.

Client may be embarrassed if cleansing involves removal of dentures.

The sitting or side-lying position prevents aspiration of fluids into the lungs. The towel protects the client from dampness.

Water softens the bristles.

This facilitates removal of plaque and tartar. The 45-degree angle of brushing permits cleansing of all surface areas of the tooth.

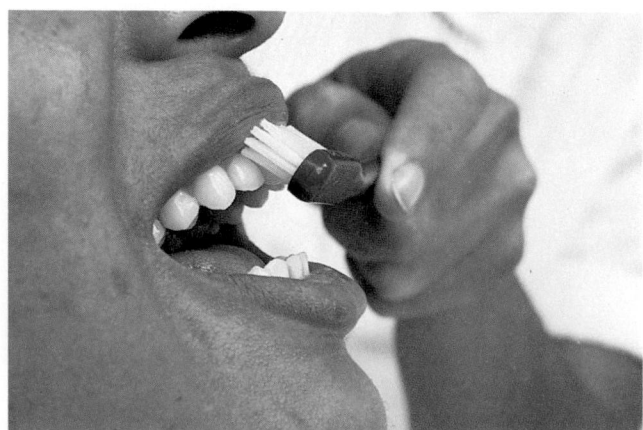

Placing brush at a 45° angle to the gum line.

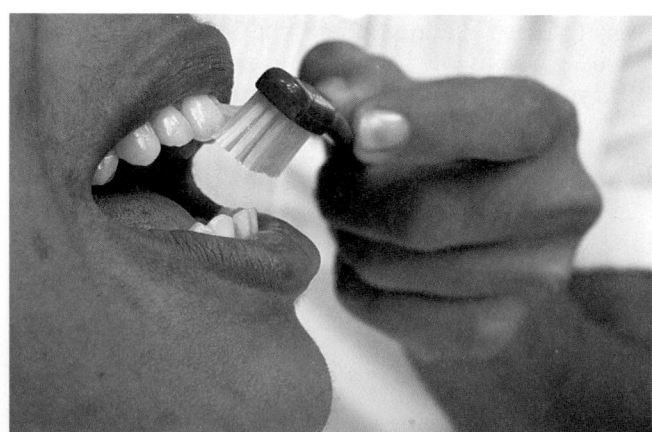

Brushing from the gum line to the crown of each tooth.

(Continued)

c. Brush tongue gently with toothbrush.

This removes coating on the tongue. Gentle motion does not stimulate gag reflex.

d. Have the client rinse vigorously with water and spit into emesis basin. Repeat until clear.

The vigorous swishing motion helps to remove debris.

e. Assist the client to floss teeth if necessary.

Flossing aids in removal of plaque and promotes healthy gum tissue.

f. Offer mouthwash if the client prefers.

Mouthwash leaves a pleasant taste in the mouth.

7 Assist the client with removal and cleansing of dentures if necessary:

a. Apply gentle pressure with 4 × 4 gauze to grasp upper denture plate and remove. Place it immediately in the denture cup. Lift the lower denture using slight rocking motion, remove, and place in the denture cup.

Rocking motion breaks suction between the denture and gum. Using 4 × 4 gauze prevents slippage and discourages spread of microorganisms.

b. If the client prefers, add denture cleanser to the cup with water and follow directions on preparation or brush all areas thoroughly with toothbrush and paste. Place paper towels or washcloth in sink while brushing.

Dentures collect food and microorganisms and require daily cleansing. Paper towels or washcloth in the sink protects against breakage.

c. Rinse thoroughly with water and return dentures to the client.

Water aids in removal of debris and acts as a cleansing agent.

d. Offer mouthwash if the client prefers.

Mouthwash leaves a pleasant taste in the mouth.

e. Apply petroleum jelly to lips if needed.

Petroleum jelly prevents cracking and drying of lips.

8 Remove equipment and assist the client to a position of comfort. Record any unusual bleeding or inflammation. Raise side rail and lower the bed.

This promotes oral hygiene and provides for oral assessment. Elevated side rails and lowered bed position maintain safety for bedridden clients.

9 Wash your hands.

This deters spread of microorganisms.

PROCEDURE 27-6
Providing Oral Care for the Dependent Client

Equipment

Toothbrush	Mouthwash	Sponge toothette or
Toothpaste	Denture-cleansing	tongue blades
Emesis basin	equipment (if	padded with 4 ×
	necessary)	4 gauze sponges

(Continued)

PROCEDURE 27-6
Providing Oral Care for the Dependent Client (Continued)

Equipment

Disposable gloves
   (optional)
Cup with cool water
Towel

Denture cup
Washcloth or
   paper towel

Irrigating syringe
   with rubber tip
   (optional)
Cleansing agent (hy-
   drogen peroxide
   at half strength)
Lubricating jelly
Suction catheter
   with suction
   apparatus
   (optional)

Action

1 Explain the procedure to the client.

2 Assemble equipment on overbed table within reach.

3 Wash your hands and, if preferred, don disposable gloves.

4 Provide privacy for the client. Adjust the height of the bed to a comfortable position. Lower one side rail and position the client on the side with head turned toward you and tilted toward the mattress. Place the towel across the client's chest and emesis basin in position under the chin.

5 Open the client's mouth and gently insert a padded tongue blade between the back molars if necessary.

Rationale

Explanation facilitates cooperation.

Organization facilitates performance of task.

Handwashing and disposable gloves deter the spread of microorganisms.

The side-lying position with head turned down prevents aspiration of fluid into lungs. Towel and emesis basin protect client from dampness.

Padded tongue blade keeps mouth open for easier cleaning and prevents the client from biting the nurse's fingers.

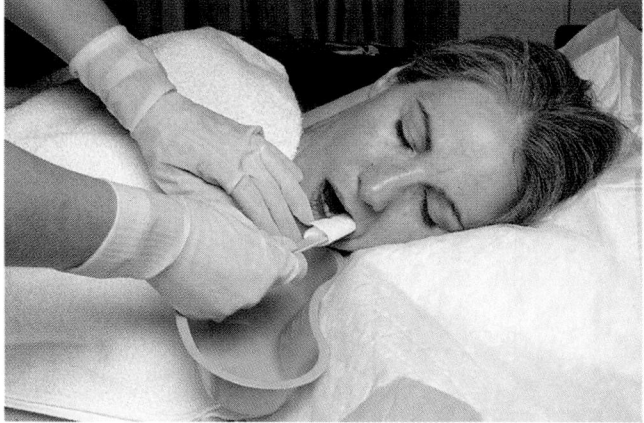

Step 5: Gently inserting padded tongue blade between back molars.

6 If teeth are present, brush carefully with toothbrush and paste. Remove dentures if present and clean before replacing (see Step 7 of Procedure 27-5). Use toothette or gauze-padded tongue blade moistened with hydrogen peroxide gently to cleanse gums, mucous membranes, and tongue.

Toothbrush or padded tongue blade provides friction necessary to clean areas where plaque and tartar accumulate. Hydrogen peroxide solution effectively cleans and removes encrustations from the oral cavity.

(Continued)

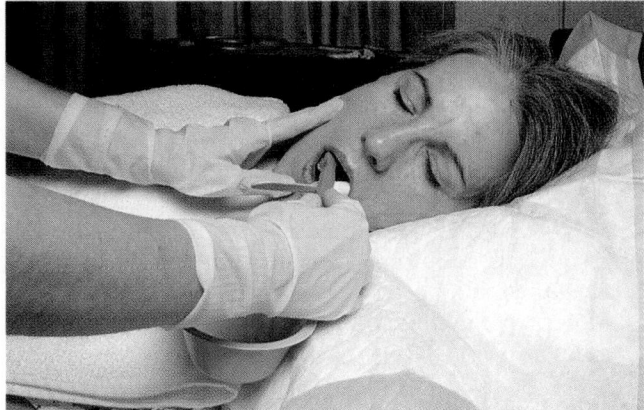

Step 6: Carefully brushing client's teeth.

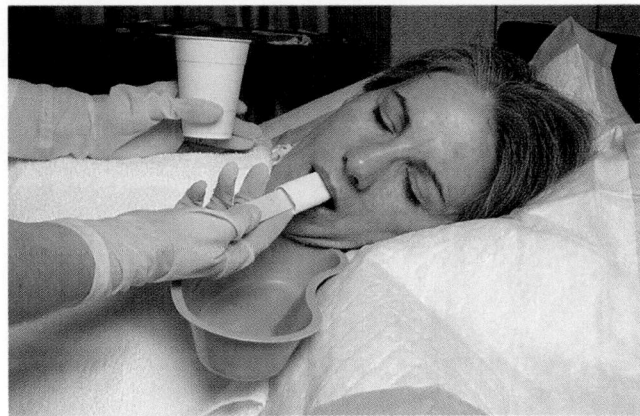

Step 6: Using moistened padded tongue blade to cleanse gums, mucous membranes, and tongue.

7 Use gauze-padded tongue blade dipped in mouthwash solution to rinse the oral cavity. If desired, insert the rubber tip of the irrigating syringe into the client's mouth and rinse gently with a small amount of water. Position the client's head to allow for return of water or use suction apparatus to remove the water from oral cavity.

Rinsing helps to cleanse debris from the mouth. Solution that is forcefully irrigated may cause aspiration.

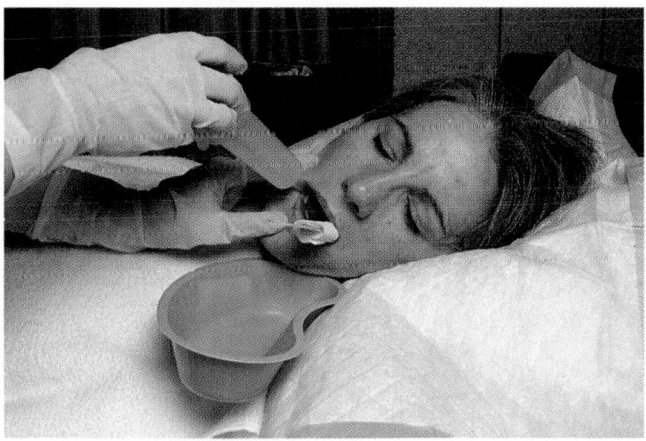

Step 7: Using irrigating syringe and a small amount of water to rinse mouth.

8 Apply lubricating jelly to the client's lips.

This prevents drying and cracking of lips.

9 Remove equipment and return the client to a position of comfort. Raise the side rail and lower the bed. Record any unusual bleeding or inflammation.

This promotes oral hygiene and provides for oral assessment. Raised side rail and lowered bed maintain client safety.

10 Wash your hands.

Handwashing deters spread of microorganisms.

Special Considerations

A client receiving chemotherapy medication may have bleeding gums and extremely sensitive mucous membranes. Use a soft sponge toothette for cleaning or substitute a salt water rinse (½ tsp salt in 1 cup of warm water) for brushing of teeth.

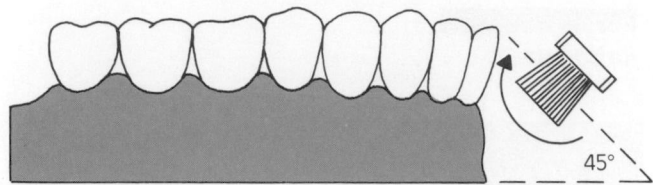

To clean gum line, surfaces, and between teeth, hold the tooth-brush with the bristles at a 45° angle to the gum line and brush from the gum line to the crown of each tooth with a short, semi-circular wrist action.

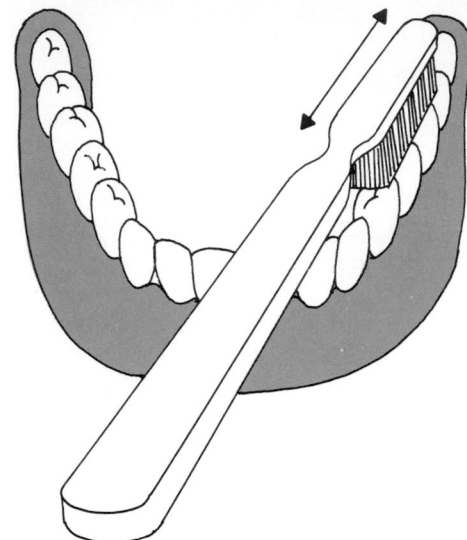

To clean biting and chewing surfaces of the teeth, hold the top of the bristles parallel to the tooth surface and brush back and forth.

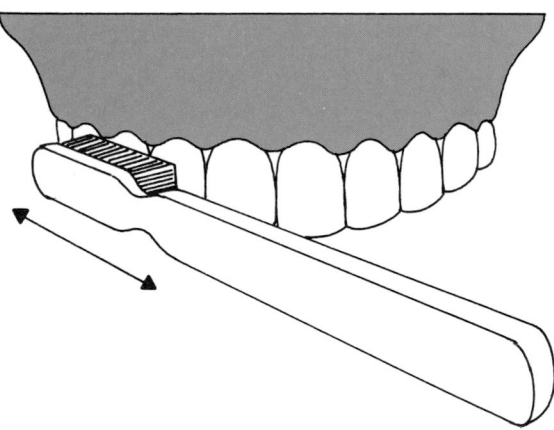

To polish the sides of the teeth, hold the brush bristles parallel to the surface of the teeth and gently brush back and forth.

F I G U R E   27-5
Techniques for brushing teeth.

Most damage is done by bacteria directly after eating. Therefore, it is ideal practice to brush the teeth immediately after eating or drinking. The tongue also should be cleaned with the brush.

Automatic toothbrushes, electric or battery-oper-ated, have been found to be simple to use and as good as hand brushes in removing debris and plaque. Water-spray units are available to assist with oral hygiene. However, if an undue amount of water pressure is used, particles of debris may be forced into tissue pockets and damage may occur to gum tissue. Therefore, it is recommended that their use be discussed with a dentist.

The toothbrush cannot effectively reach areas between the teeth where food lodges; hence, flossing once a day is recommended. The practice not only removes what the brush cannot, but helps to break up colonies of bacteria. Figure 27-6 illustrates a flossing technique. The following are additional recommended techniques for flossing the teeth:

- Keep about 1 inch of floss held taut between the fingers.

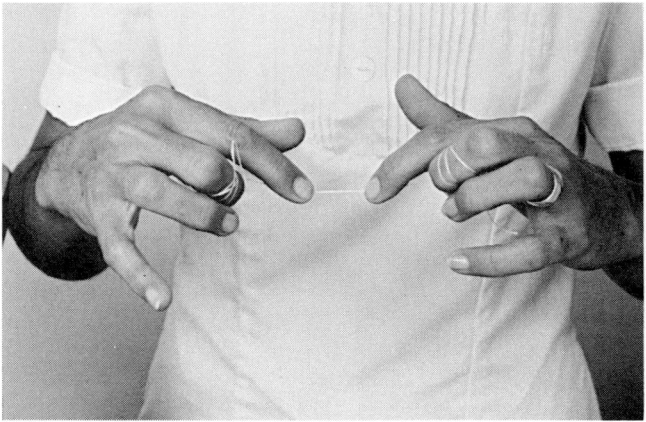

Floss may be wrapped around the middle fingers of each hand or simply grasped in each hand in such a way that it can be stretched and held taut between the controlling fingers.

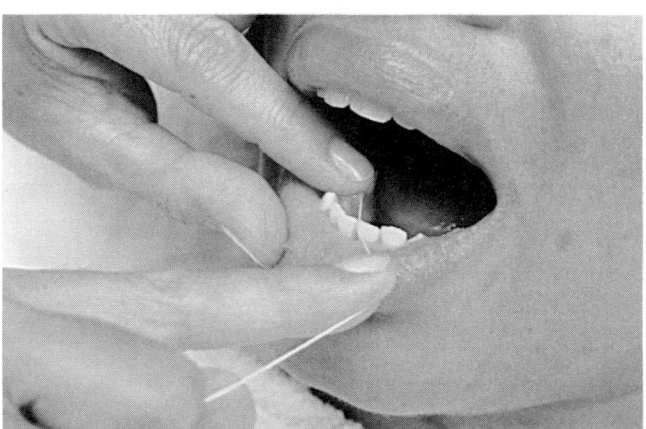

Gently insert the floss between the teeth and move it with a saw-ing motion up from the gum line along the side of each tooth.

F I G U R E   27-6
Dental flossing is necessary for removal of plaque and tartar between teeth. Flossing helps prevent gum disease as well as tooth decay by removing debris just below the gum line.

- Keep the fingers controlling the floss no more than 1.3 cm (½ inch) apart.
- Do not force the floss between the teeth, but insert it gently by moving it back and forth where teeth touch each other.
- Move the floss up and down while using *both* fingers, first on the side of one tooth and then on the side of the other tooth, until the surfaces are squeaky clean.
- Go to the gum tissue with the floss but not into the gum, since this may result in discomfort, soreness, or bleeding.
- Advance the floss from one hand to the other to bring up a fresh section of floss when it has become frayed or soiled.
- Rinse the mouth *well* with water after flossing to remove food particles and plaque that have been loosened. Also, rinse after eating when flossing or brushing is not possible.

Toothpastes and powders aid the brushing process, usually have a pleasant taste, and often encourage brushing, especially among children. Most dentrifrices are safe to use, but those containing harsh abrasives may scratch the enamel of the teeth and therefore are not recommended. Salt, sodium bicarbonate, or precipitated chalk are just as effective for cleaning the mouth and the teeth and are far less expensive than proprietary products on the market. Dentrifrices containing stannous fluoride and antiplaque rinses have proven to be effective in helping to decrease dental caries and hence are recommended by many dentists.

Mouthwashes. An offensive breath or **halitosis** is often systemic in nature. For example, the odor of onions and garlic on the breath comes from the lungs, where the oils are being removed from the bloodstream and eliminated with respiration. A mouthwash cannot remove halitosis when odors are being eliminated by respiration.

If the cause of halitosis is poor oral hygiene, cleaning will reduce the odor. Commercial mouthwashes may be helpful and many persons enjoy their fresh aftertaste. If concentrated mouthwashes are used frequently for debilitated clients they may injure oral tissue, and infection and additional odor may result.

Evaluating

At designated intervals, evaluate whether or not the client has met the goals established during planning and revise the plan of care if indicated.

Example. 10/26/88 Goal partially met. Client's oral mucosa is intact, but thick, dry secretions continue to build on oral mucosa and gums despite q 4 hour care.

Revision. Increase frequency of oral hygiene to q 2 hours. Instruct family.

CARE OF THE EYES, EARS, AND NOSE

Assessing

Nursing History. Identify any special eye, ear, or nose care the client performs. Include the use and care of visual aids or prostheses (glasses, contact lenses, artificial eye) and hearing aids. Note any history of eye, ear, and nose problems and related treatments.

Nursing Examination. In the eye examination, note the position, alignment, and general appearance of the eye. Check that eyelashes are equally distributed and curl outward. Note the presence of lesions, nodules, redness, swelling, crusting, flaking, excessive tearing, or discharge of eyelids. Check the color of the conjunctivae, presence of blink reflex, and visual acuity (ability to read newsprint).

In the ear examination, note the position, alignment, and general appearance of the ear. Pay particular attention to a build-up of wax in the canal, dryness, crusting, or the presence of any discharge or foreign body. Check hearing acuity.

During examination of the nose, note its position and general appearance, patency of nostrils, and presence of tenderness, dryness, edema, bleeding, discharge, or secretions.

Diagnosing

Make a judgment about the adequacy of the client's self-care practices related to eye, ear, and nose care, identifying any factors that contribute to deficiencies. For example

Self-care deficit: care of artificial eye, *related to* knowledge deficit

Identify actual or potential eye, ear, and nose problems that nurses can treat, noting contributing factors. Identify "unhealthy" client responses to eye, ear, and nose problems, for example

Sensory–perceptual alteration (visual, auditory, or olfactory) *related to* psychologic stress

Health maintenance deficit *related to* perceptual impairment (visual or auditory)

Impaired social interaction *related to* visual or auditory impairment

Fear *related to* sudden loss of vision or hearing

Anticipatory grieving *related to* increasing visual or auditory impairment

Potential for injury *related to* visual impairment

Planning

Identify nursing measures that will assist the client develop or maintain eye, ear, and nose care measures that will contribute to healthy eye, ear, and nose functioning and to the client's general sense of well-being. Plan to achieve the following client goals:

- Client demonstrates healthy functioning of eyes, ears, and nose.
- The client's eyes, ears, and nose appear clean.
- Sensory impairment (visual, auditory, olfactory) shows signs of healing (if realistic—specify these signs), *or* client seeks aids appropriate to impairment.
- Client demonstrates correct eye, ear, and nose care measures, including the proper use and care of visual or auditory aids.

Pertinent nursing measures to include in the plan of care are as follows:

Eye

- Clean the eye from the **inner canthus** to the **outer canthus**, using a wet, warm washcloth, cotton ball, or compress to soften crusted secretions. Carefully avoid cross-contamination.
- When the blink (corneal) reflex is decreased or absent (*e.g.,* in the comatose client), use artificial tear solution or normal saline at least every 4 hours to keep the eyes moist and protected from drying; a protective shield may be necessary to keep the lids closed.
- Offer correct eyeglass, contact lens, or artificial eye teaching and care.

Ear

- Clean the external ear with a washcloth-covered finger, instructing the client never to insert objects into the ear for cleaning purposes.
- Assist with the softening and removal of excessive wax deposits.
- Offer hearing aid teaching and care.

Nose

- Clean the nose by instructing the client to blow the nose while both nares are patent (nasal suctioning with a bulb syringe may be indicated) unless contraindicated (*e.g.,* following brain surgery or head trauma).
- Remove crusted secretions around the nose and keep this tissue intact by applying a non–water-soluble ointment (*e.g.,* petroleum jelly).

In the plan of care, identify any supplies needed to carry out the specified eye, ear, and nose care and the timing of these measures.

Implementing

Carry out the plan of care, remembering to use each nurse–client interaction for ongoing assessment of the client's eyes, ears, and nose and for evaluation of the adequacy of the plan of care. The following sections describe select nursing measures related to eye, ear, and nose care. See accompanying box for sample documentation of eye care.

Cleaning the Eyes

Normally, the eyes are clear and kept clean with lacrimal secretions. During illness, the eyes may produce more secretions than they normally do and appear glasslike. The following techniques are recommended when secretions adhere to the eyelashes and become dry and crusty, or when there is discharge present:

- Use water or normal saline and cotton balls or a clean washcloth or compress to clean the eyes. Boric acid solution, once popular for cleaning the eyes, is no longer recommended because of its toxicity when absorbed from mucous membrane. The eyes are never cleaned with soap because of its irritating effects on eye tissues.
- Position the client on the same side as the eye to be cleaned so that solution and debris will not run across the bridge of the nose and contaminate the other eye.
- Dampen a cotton ball with the solution of choice and wipe *once* while moving the cotton ball from the inner canthus to the outer canthus of the eye. This technique minimizes forcing debris into the area drained by the nasolacrimal duct. Discard the used cotton ball.
- Continue this technique, using one cotton ball for each stroke, until the eye is clean.
- Turn the client to the opposite side and clean the other eye in the same manner.

Sample Documentation of Eye Care

10/20/88 #4
Self-care deficit: care of artificial eye related to knowledge deficit, fear, and nonacceptance
S: "I can't believe they expect me to take care of this eye. I don't even want to touch it."
O: One week postenucleation; to date has not participated in care
A: Fear, nonacceptance of loss of eye, and lack of knowledge are all limiting client's ability to develop new eye care skills.
P: Encourage client to verbalize feelings about the artificial eye.
Begin to implement the prepared teaching plan for care of an artificial eye.
Demonstrate artificial eye care q AM and encourage a return demonstration until client performs this independently.

N. Glynn, RN

- Wipe the lashes dry with a paper tissue or a *clean* washcloth, exposing a clean area of the tissue or cloth with each stroke.

Caring for the Unconscious Client's Eyes

Clients with diminished or absent blink (corneal) reflexes and clients whose eyelids remain open require frequent eye care (at least every 4 hours). If the eye is not kept moist, corneal ulceration may result from excessive drying of the eye. Nursing measures include using saline or artificial tears to lubricate the eye and a protective eye shield to keep the eye closed.

Providing Eyeglass Care

Eyeglasses are essential for many persons and represent a considerable financial investment. The nurse should take precautions to prevent their breakage or loss. Clients needing glasses should be encouraged to wear them to avoid eye strain.

Plastic lenses are popular because they are considerably lighter in weight than glass lenses and as accurate in correction as glass. The one decided disadvantage of plastic is that the material scratches very easily.

Eyeglasses should be cleaned over a terry towel so that if they slip they will not become scratched or broken. Glasses are cleaned with warm water and soap. Hot water may warp plastic lenses and frames. Or, a special cleansing preparation may be used for cleaning them. The glasses should be rinsed well when cleansed with soap and water. They should be dried with a clean, soft cloth, such as a cotton handkerchief or napkin. Paper products are made of wood pulp and are likely to scratch the lenses. Eyeglasses should not be cleaned with a dry paper tissue or cloth.

Providing Care of Contact Lenses

A contact lens is a small disc worn directly on the eyeball. It stays in place by surface tension of the eye's tears. Hard lenses are made of a nonpliable and nonabsorbent material. Soft lenses are of a plastic material that absorbs water to become soft and pliable. They are brittle when dehydrated and absorb water when placed in solution, usually normal saline, or when in contact with tears.

Persons wearing contact lenses need to take special precautions to keep them free of microorganisms that may lead to eye infections and to use them in a manner that will not injure or scratch the surface of the eye. Hands must always be washed before touching eye surfaces and lenses. Lenses are to be removed before showering, swimming, or sunbathing and when the person is in the presence of irritating vapors or smoke. The lenses should not be in contact with cosmetics, soaps, or hair sprays because eye irritation may result. It is recommended that any adverse reaction to their use be reported to the prescribing physician immediately.

The cornea, which consists of dense connective tissue, does not have its own blood supply. It is nourished primarily by oxygen from the atmosphere and from tears. When wearing contact lenses, the cornea requires more than its normal supply of oxygen because its metabolic rate increases. To allow the cornea to receive a maximal supply of oxygen, hard lenses should be removed before sleeping and should not be worn more than 12 to 16 hours. Extended-wear soft lenses can be left in place for as long as 14 to 30 days. Excessive tearing, pain, and redness signal the need to remove lenses.

There may be times when the nurse may be required to remove lenses if a patient cannot do so. To leave them in place for long periods of time could result in permanent eye damage. This may occur, for example, when the nurse is attending an unconscious patient. Figure 27-7 illustrates and describes how to remove hard contact lenses when the person is unable to do so independently.

Soft lenses are removed by gently grasping the lens near the lower edge, between the forefinger and thumb. Each lens "folds up" with this technique and is then lifted from the eye. Soft lenses are cleaned, rinsed, and placed in a container of solution for storage. The lenses should be identified as being for the right or left eye since the two lenses are not necessarily identical. The nurse should not try to remove lenses, however, if an eye injury is present, because of the danger of additional injury.

Providing Care of an Artificial Eye

Most clients who wear an artificial eye prefer to take care of it themselves, and they should be encouraged to do so when possible. The necessary equipment includes a small basin, soap and water for washing, and solution for rinsing the prosthesis. Normal saline or tap water can be used for rinsing. Most persons have their own method for cleaning the eye socket and the area around it. The nurse should ask the client how he or she does this and make it possible for the client to continue with the usual practice. The client should be lying down so that the eye does not accidentally fall to the floor. The socket is ordinarily flushed with normal saline before replacing the eye.

Providing Ear Care

Other than cleaning the outer ears, little more is needed for routine hygiene of the ear. After the ears are washed, they should be dried carefully with a soft towel so that water and cerumen (wax) are removed by capillary action. Forcing the towel into the ear for drying may aid in the formation of wax plugs.

If a wax plug is present in the auditory canal, it is removed by gentle irrigation of the ear. The stream of water should be directed toward the side of the canal to prevent injury to the drum (see Chap 40 for the proce-

(Text continues on p. 599.)

Removing hard contact lenses

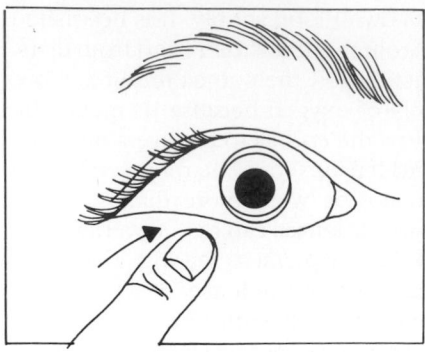

If the lens is not centered over the cornea, apply gentle pressure on the lower eyelid to center the lens.

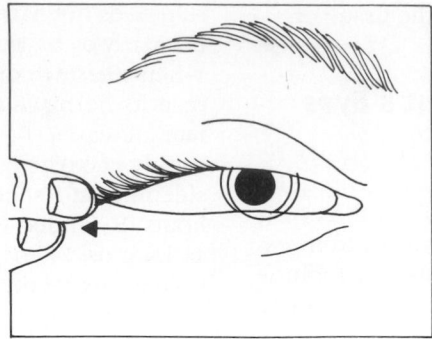

Gently pull the outer corner of the eye toward the ear.

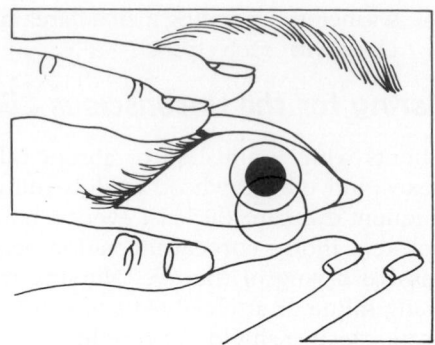

Position the other hand below the lens to receive it and ask the client to blink.

or

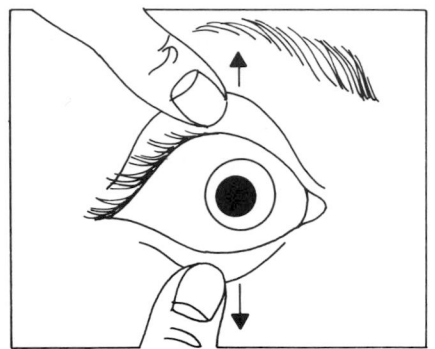

Gently spread the eyelids beyond the top and bottom edges of the lens.

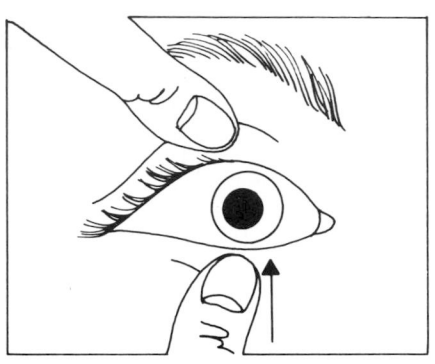

Gently press the lower eyelid up against the bottom of the lends.

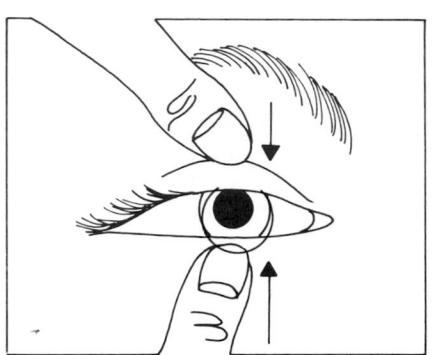

After the lens is tipped slightly, move the eyelids toward one another to cause the lens to slide out between the eyelids.

Removing soft contact lenses

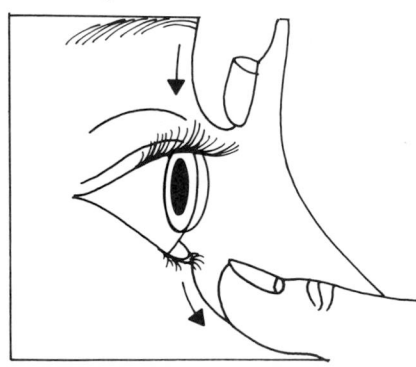

Have the client look forward. Retract the lower lid with one hand. Using the pad of the index finger of the other hand, move the lens down to the sclera.

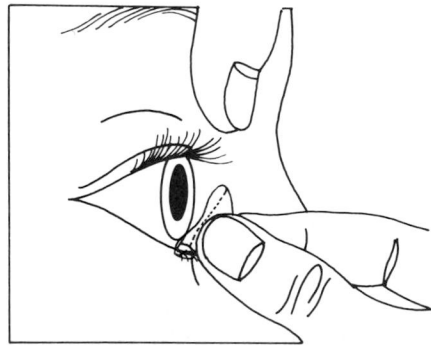

Using the pads of the thumb and index fingers grasp the lens with a gentle pinching motion and remove.

Storing lenses

Because lenses may be different for each eye, storage cases are marked L and R designating left and right lenses. It is important to place the first lens in its designated cup in the storage case before removing the second lens to avoid mixing them up.

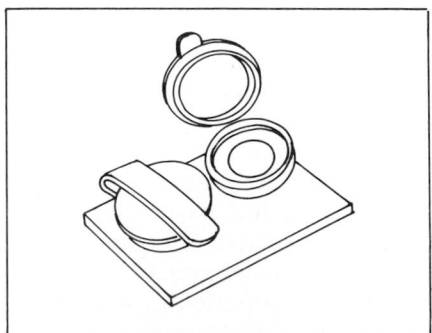

F I G U R E **27-7**
Removing contact lenses.

dure for ear irrigations). Using bobby pins, hairpins, paperclips, or fingernails to remove wax from the ear is extremely dangerous because these may injure or puncture the eardrum. Use of cotton-tipped applicators is also discouraged because they may impact cerumen.

Hearing Aids. If the client uses a hearing aid, batteries should be checked routinely and the earpieces cleaned daily with mild soap and water.

Providing Nose Care

The best way to clean the nose is to blow it gently. Both nostrils should be open while doing this. Closing one nostril adds to the danger of forcing debris into the eustachian tubes. Irrigations are usually contraindicated because of the possible danger of forcing material into the sinuses.

If the external nares are crusted, applying mineral or cotton seed oil helps to soften and remove the crusts. Disposable paper tissues are recommended for nasal secretions. A cotton applicator may be used to clean the nares but with great care to avoid injury. The applicator should never be introduced into the nares.

Evaluating

At designated intervals evaluate whether or not the client has achieved the goals established during planning. Revise the plan of care if indicated.

Example. 10/24/88 Goal met. Client demonstrated correct care (cleaning) of artificial eye for the last two mornings. States "I guess I should be happy to be alive and still able to see."

N. Glynn, RN

HAIR CARE

Hair is an accessory structure of the skin. Good general health is essential for attractive hair and skin, and cleanliness helps in keeping these attractive. Illness affects the hair, especially when endocrine abnormalities, increased body temperature, poor nutrition, or anxiety and worry are present. Changes in the color or condition of the hair shaft are related to changes in hormonal activity or to changes in the blood supply to hair follicles.

Assessing

Nursing History. Identify the client's usual hair and scalp care practices, including styling preferences. Note any history of hair or scalp problems, possible etiologies for changes in the distribution, texture, or amount of hair, and related treatments.

Nursing Examination. Assess the condition of the hair (texture, cleanliness, oiliness) and scalp (scaling, lesions, inflammation, infection).

Risk Factors. Identify any factors known to cause hair or scalp problems or that require special care: deficient self-care abilities, immobility, malnutrition, treatments known to result in hair loss (*e.g.,* irradiation of the head, certain chemotherapeutic agents).

Common Scalp and Hair Problems

Dandruff. Dandruff is a condition characterized by itching and flaking of the scalp that may be further complicated by the embarrassment it causes. Persistent severe cases usually require medical attention. Daily brushing and shampooing with a medicated shampoo may be all that is needed to keep the scalp free of dandruff.

Hair Loss. Hair growth and hair loss are ongoing, daily processes. Hair loss from plaiting, excessive back combing and "teasing," or the use of hair rollers is usually temporary, and hair returns when the tension on the hair shaft is halted. Some people experience hair loss owing to illness with high fever, certain medications, x-ray therapy of the head, childbirth, and general anesthesia. There appears to be no evidence that hair loss occurs as a result of wearing wigs or excessive shampooing. It is believed by some that an excessive intake of vitamin A may play a role in hair loss. Some permanent thinning of hair normally accompanies aging.

Baldness is called **alopecia**. It is common in men but rare in women, and it is believed to be hereditary. There is no known cure for baldness; although some external medications are being developed, their long-term efficacy is not known. Hairpieces, frequently worn by persons who are bald, require the same care as normal hair, but less frequent washing.

A surgical procedure for baldness is the hair transplant. Hair is taken from donor sites, usually from the back or sides of the scalp, and transplanted to areas with no hair. The procedure is long and expensive but reportedly has decided benefits for persons who find baldness psychologically unpleasant. Complications include serious scalp infections.

Pediculosis. Infestation with lice is called **pediculosis**. There are three common types of lice: *Pediculus humanus* var *capitis,* which infests hair and scalp; *Pediculus humanus* var *corporis,* which infests the body; and *Phthirus pubis,* which infests the shorter hairs on the body, usually the pubic hair and the axillary hair. Lice lay eggs, called **nits**, on the hair shafts. Nits are white or light gray and look like dandruff, but they cannot be brushed or shaken off the hair. Frequent scratching and scratch marks on the body and the scalp suggest the presence of pediculosis. Although anyone may become infested with lice, the continued presence of pediculosis is usually a result of uncleanliness. Pediculosis can be spread directly by contact with infested areas or indirectly through clothing, bed linen, brushes, and combs. Teaching clients, especially children, not to share personal items is a good way to prevent transmission. The linen and personal-care items of a patient with pediculosis require separate and careful handling to prevent spreading from person to person.

There are any number of preparations, called **pediculicides**, for the treatment of pediculosis, some of which will destroy the nits as well as the lice. Several treatments are usually necessary before all the nits are destroyed. The procedures and the medications used for the treatment of pediculosis vary among health agencies. Shaving off the infested hair may be done, especially when pubic hair and axillary hair are infested. Sexual partners must be notified if the lice were sexually transmitted.

Ticks.   Ticks are small, gray–brown, blood-sucking parasites important because of their ability to transmit serious diseases such as Rocky Mountain spotted fever and tularemia. Ticks should never be forcibly pulled out of the skin. Since oil suffocates the tick, covering the tick with oil or petroleum jelly facilitates its removal.

Diagnosing

Make a judgment about the adequacy of the client's self-care practices. Identify factors contributing to deficiencies, for example

> Self-care deficit: hair care *related to* continuous bed rest

Identify actual or potential hair or scalp problems that nurses can treat, noting contributing factors. Identify "unhealthy" client responses to these problems, for example

> Altered comfort *related to* pediculosis
> Potential for scalp infection *related to* hair transplant
> Disturbance in body image *related to* baldness
> Impaired skin integrity *related to* scalp laceration (head bandages)

Planning

Identify nursing measures that will assist the client develop or maintain needed hair and scalp care practices or that otherwise resolve nursing diagnoses. Specify any special products needed for hair care. Plan to achieve the following client goals:

- Hair is clean and neatly styled.
- Scalp lesions (or infestation) are decreased or absent.
- Client verbalizes satisfaction with appearance.
- Client participates in hair and scalp care as able.

Implementing

Carry out the plan of care remembering to utilize scheduled hygienic care interactions for ongoing assessment of the client's hair and scalp and for evaluating the adequacy of the plan of care. The following discussions give suggestions for grooming hair, shampooing hair, caring for beards and mustaches, and assisting with unwanted hair removal.

Daily brushing of the hair helps to keep it clean and distributes oil along the shaft of each hair. Brushing also stimulates the circulation of blood in the scalp.

Grooming the Hair

There are many cultural overtones associated with hair; however, styles also change within a culture from decade to decade. The nurse shows consideration when hair is groomed in the style preferred by the client. Hair that becomes entangled is difficult to comb. Combing of tiny sections of hair at a time may be necessary if a client's hair has not been combed for even one day. The best way to protect long hair from matting and tangling is to ask the client for permission to braid it. Clients usually will consent to the procedure if it provides them with more comfort. Parting the hair in the middle on the back of the head and making two braids, one on either side, prevents the discomfort of lying on one heavy braid on the back of the head.

Occasionally, a client's hair is almost hopelessly matted, and cutting the hair may be necessary. Before a client's hair is cut, it is usual procedure to have the client sign a written consent. It is also recommended that the nurse discuss the necessity for cutting the hair with an immediate member of the client's family.

The care of the black person's hair usually requires special attention. The hair is normally dry, very curly, and becomes easily matted and tangled. The comb used for arranging the hair should have widely spaced teeth. Oil should be used, and white petrolatum or mineral oil is often recommended. However, a skin lotion has been used effectively also. Braiding the hair of a black person is usually the best way to prevent matting and tangling.

Shampooing the Hair

The hair is exposed to the same dirt and oil as the skin. It should be washed as often as necessary to keep it clean. The comb and the brush should be washed each time the hair is washed and as frequently as necessary between shampoos. Many health agencies have beauticians and barbers to assist with the care of the client's hair, including shampooing it. However, the convenience does not relieve the nurse of responsibility.

Before shampooing the hair, it is recommended that the nurse, or the client if able, brush and comb the hair well to stimulate the scalp and undo tangled hair. The patient may then shampoo the hair while showering, if able. In some hospitals a physician's order is required for shampooing a client's hair.

The following techniques are recommended for shampooing the hair of a client on bed rest (Fig 27-8):

- Prepare several pitchers of water of a suitably warm temperature for a thorough washing and rinsing,

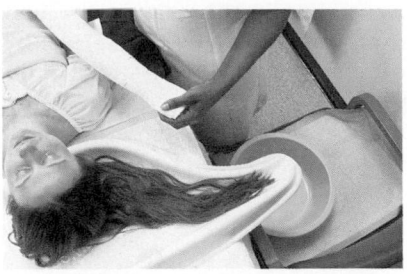

Place a waterproof pad under the client's shoulders, neck, and head. Position the shampooing trough under the client's head with the drainage spout extending over the edge of the bed. Place a recepticle below the spout to catch the water. Place a rolled towel under the client's neck at the edge of the trough.

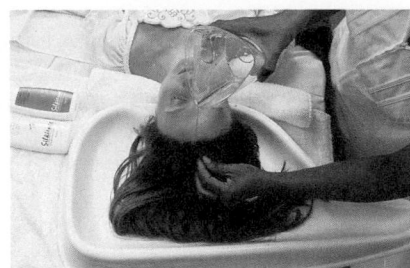

Using a pitcher of comfortably warm water, wet the client's hair completely.

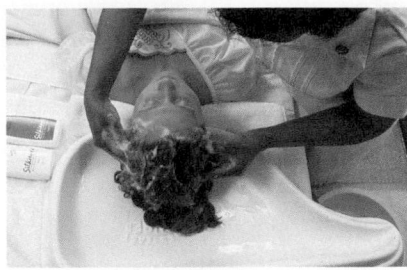

Apply shampoo and lather using both hands and working from the front to the back of the head.

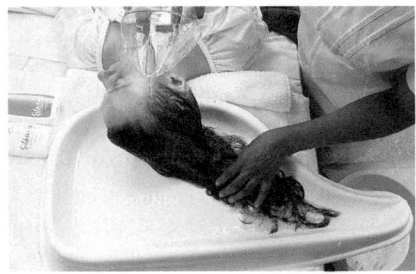

Rinse hair completely. Repeat shampooing and rinsing if necessary. Apply conditioner if requested and rinse again.

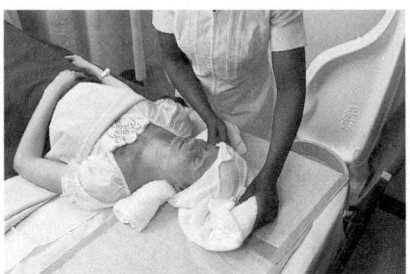

Wrap the client's head in towels to remove as much moisture as possible from the scalp and hair. Dry the client's face and neck.

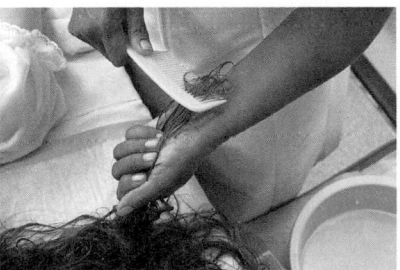

Comb gently to remove tangles. Complete drying of the hair using a dryer or towel according to agency policy.

FIGURE 27-8
Technique for shampooing a client's hair in bed.

shampoo soap, one or two towels for drying, and a receptacle to receive wash and rinse water.

- Place a protective pad under the head.
- Place the client in a position over the pad so that there will be constant drainage of water directed into the receptacle.
- Wet the hair, apply soap, and massage the scalp well while washing the hair.
- Rinse the hair and apply soap for a second washing, if indicated.
- Rinse the hair *thoroughly* after washing it with soap and water.
- Apply conditioner if requested.
- Dry the hair as quickly as possible to prevent the client from becoming chilled, and arrange the hair according to the client's preference.

Dry Shampoo. Dry shampoos cannot replace the cleaning benefits of regular shampoos, but they are helpful in removing at least some of the dirt, oils, and odors from the hair of clients too ill or incapacitated to have a wet shampoo. Dry shampoos or powders are not recommended for black persons because of their normally dry hair and scalp.

The dry shampoo or powder is applied and then combed or brushed from the hair. The teeth of a comb can be pulled through gauze, which will help remove and capture the powder.

Caring for Beards and Mustaches

Most male clients with beards or mustaches are able to groom these independently. Dependent clients will require nursing assistance to keep the beard and mustache clean, especially after eating. For no reason should a nurse trim or shave off a client's beard or mustache without the client's consent.

Shaving

Individual preferences for shaving methods are based on such factors as the type of skin, the quality of the beard, the frequency with which one shaves, the presence of skin problems, and convenience. Blade razors tend to give a closer shave than electric razors, but many men find electric razors convenient and practical. They are especially convenient for the ill and bedridden client.

F I G U R E   27-9
To shave a client's face with a razor, first apply shaving cream or warm soap lather to soften the beard. Shave the face by gently pulling the skin taut and using short, firm strokes in the direction of hair growth. After shaving, wash off any residual lather and dry the client's face. After-shave lotion may be applied if requested.

The technique for shaving a client who is unable to shave himself is described here and illustrated in Figure 27-9.
- Shaving cream or a warm soap lather is first applied to the skin to soften the facial hair and prevent pulling.
- The skin of the face is pulled taut.
- Short, firm strokes in the direction of hair growth are used. The client often can give suggestions on how he shaves.
- Wash the client's face of residual lather and dry.
- Aftershave lotion may be applied. Aftershave preparations tend to make the face feel good and have a cosmetic rather than a therapeutic effect.

Evaluating

At designated intervals, evaluate whether or not the client has achieved the goals established during planning and revise the plan of care if indicated.

Example.   10/27/86 Goal partially met. Client reports that she is not comfortable wearing a wig yet but feels better since its purchase

Revision.   Since client still has many questions about effects of chemotherapy, continue teaching and utilize opportunities to build self-esteem.

C. Moser, RN

NAIL AND FOOT CARE

The nails are an accessory structure of the skin and are composed of epithelial tissue. The body of the nail is the exposed portion; the root lies in the skin in the nail groove where the nail grows and is nourished. Healthy nails have a pink color and are convex and evenly curved. With certain pathologic conditions, and to some extent with aging also, the nails become ridged and areas become concave.

Assessing

Nursing History.   Identify the client's normal nail and foot care practices, the type of footwear worn, and any history of nail or foot problems and their related treatments.

Nursing Examination.   Examine nails for intactness and cleanliness; note capillary refill and the contour of the nailbed; observe the nail base for redness, swelling, bleeding, discharge, and tenderness. Examine the feet for cleanliness and intactness of skin, and note the presence of swelling, inflammation, lesions, tenderness, or orthopedic problems. Examine carefully the skin between the toes.

High-Risk Factors.   Identify any variables known to cause nail and foot problems: deficient self-care abilities; vascular disease; arthritis; diabetes mellitus; history of biting nails or trimming them improperly; frequent or prolonged exposure to chemicals or water; trauma; ill-fitting shoes; obesity.

Diagnosing

Make a judgment about the adequacy of the client's self-care practices related to nail and foot care, identifying any factors that contribute to deficiencies. An example is
   Self-care deficit: diabetic foot care related to
      knowledge deficit and weakened physical state
   Identify actual or potential nail or foot problems that nurses can treat, noting contributing factors. Identify "unhealthy" client responses to these problems. For example
      Altered comfort: foot pain related to corns (calluses, plantar warts, ingrown nails)
      Impaired physical mobility related to painful foot condition (specify)
      Potential for infection related to traumatized nail base or deficient nail or foot care
      Impaired skin integrity (feet) related to altered circulation

Planning

Identify nursing measures that will assist the client develop or maintain healthy nail and foot care practices. Plan to achieve the following client goals:
- Nails are intact, clean, and manicured.
- Foot skin is intact, clean, and free of lesions.
- Nail and foot problems (specify: calluses, corns,

plantar warts, ingrown nails, athlete's foot) are reduced or absent.

- Client demonstrates correct nail and foot care measures.
- Client verbalizes nails and feet contribute to general sense of comfort and well-being.

Pertinent nursing measures to include in the plan of care are

- Soaking nails and feet and assisting with cleaning of nails and trimming nails (if not contraindicated)
- Massaging the feet to promote relaxation and comfort
- Teaching correct nail and foot care

In the plan of care, identify any supplies needed to carry out the specified nail and foot care and the timing of these measures.

Implementing

Carry out the plan of care remembering to utilize bath times to continually assess the status of the client's nails and feet and to evaluate the adequacy of the plan of care. Described in this section are techniques for providing fingernail and foot care. See the accompanying box for sample documentation of foot care.

Providing Care of Fingernails

The following are recommended techniques for the care of fingernails:

- File the nails to form an oval at the ends. Do not trim so far down on the sides that injury to the skin and cuticles occurs.
- Remove hangnails, which are broken pieces of cuticle, by cutting them off. Take special care to avoid injury to tissue with the cuticle scissors.

Sample Documentation of Foot Care

10/20/88 #7
Impairment of skin integrity: right toe related to altered circulation
S: "I guess I cut that nail too short . . . that toe's been hurting for two months now." History of adult-onset diabetes since 1975
O: Great toe on right foot is swollen, red, and painful; skin at base of nail is white. Limps when walking
A: Healing of traumatized tissue right toe delayed because of altered circulation (diabetes mellitus)
P: Soak feet after each bath and dry carefully afterward. Consult with physician.

C. Moier, RN

- *Gently* push cuticles back off the nail after they are soft and pliable following a soaking in warm water.
- Push back cuticles with a blunt instrument or a terry cloth.
- Apply an emollient to the cuticle to help prevent hangnails.
- Clean under the nails with a blunt instrument or the large end of a toothpick, being careful to prevent injuring the area where the nail is attached to the underlying tissue.

Splitting and peeling of the nails are usually caused by dryness. It is helpful to avoid contact with soap and water as much as possible, use a good hand cream frequently, and avoid the use of nail polish and polish remover, both of which have a tendency to dry the nails.

Providing Foot Care

Proper foot care is important at any age. It becomes even more so with aging and when such conditions as circulatory disturbances or diabetes mellitus are present. Techniques for foot care follow:

- Bathe the feet thoroughly in a basin of soap or detergent and water solution. Be sure to clean the interdigital areas.
- Rinse the feet to remove soap or detergent residue, which irritates the skin if not properly removed.
- Continue to soak the feet in a basin of warm water if the toenails are brittle, thick, and striated before attempting to trim them. Or, wrap the feet in damp cloths and place them in plastic bags to soften the nails, if this is more convenient.
- Trim the nails straight across and not so short that tender areas of skin are exposed to the normal friction from shoes and stockings when the client is walking. In many institutions, a physician's order is necessary for cutting nails.
- When trimming the nails, avoid digging into or cutting the toenails at the lateral corners. These practices predispose to ingrown nails. Clients with ingrown toenails, especially older people and clients with circulatory disorders or diabetes mellitus, may require the services of a physician or podiatrist.
- Clean under the nails with a blunt instrument or the large end of a toothpick, being careful to prevent injury to the area where the nail is attached to the underlying tissue.
- Apply powder to the feet and interdigital areas. If the skin is dry, use a lanolin cream instead.
- Bathe the feet at least daily but more often if they tend to perspire freely. Using a foot powder containing a nonirritating deodorant is helpful when foot odor is due to excessive perspiration. Foot powders are more absorbent than regular bath powders and often contain menthol, which makes the skin feel cool.

Improperly fitting and extremely worn or soiled hosiery contributes to foot problems. For some persons with allergies or skin infections, nylon hosiery is contraindicated.

The nurse should be alert to any signs of foot problems, including infection, inflammation, ingrown nails, breaks in the skin in the interdigital areas, corns, calluses, bunions, and pressure areas, that may result in ulcerations. This is especially important for the client with diabetes.

Providing Foot Care for the Diabetic

A diabetic client is especially prone to foot problems owing to skin irritation, infection, and ulcers, which, without proper precautions, can result in gangrene. There are certain additional precautions that should be observed and taught to the client with diabetes:

- File the toenails. Scissors are too likely to slip and injure tissues.
- Do not cut off corns or calluses. Also, do not use commercial removers because they contain ingredients that often lead to irritation, infection, and ulcers. A physician or podiatrist should be consulted when corns and calluses are present.
- Do not use nonprescription preparations to treat athlete's foot and ingrown toenails because they may contain ingredients that lead to infection and ulcers. A physician or **podiatrist** should be consulted when athlete's foot or ingrown nails are present. The causative fungi of athlete's foot are species of *Trichophyton* or *Epidermophyton floccosum* and are capable of attacking the hair and nails as well as the skin.
- Avoid using heating pads and hot-water bottles applied to the feet because of the danger of blistering and burning the feet.
- Teach the client to avoid wearing round garters and stockings with elastic tops and not to sit with the knees crossed to prevent obstruction of circulation to the lower extremities and feet.
- Prop the feet up above the level of the hips a few minutes several times a day if the feet swell.
- Explain the dangers of going barefoot. The client may injure the skin of the feet or acquire athlete's foot in such places as public showers.
- Keep the feet dry and warm in shoes and stockings that provide plenty of room.
- Break in new shoes gradually; begin with a half hour of wear the first day and increase the time by about an hour a day. Improperly fitting shoes are a major cause of foot problems and can lead to corns, calluses, bunions, and blisters. The back of the shoe, or the counter, should fit snugly but not tightly. A heel offering safe support is recommended. When standing, there should be about ¾ inch of space in the shoe beyond the great toe and also at the widest part of the shoe. In a shoe that fits well, the arch of the foot will lie comfortably over the arch in the shoes. The soles should be flexible and nonslippery. Shoes with rough ridges,

wrinkles, or tears in the linings should be discarded or repaired.

Evaluating

At designated intervals, evaluate whether or not the client has achieved the goals established during planning and revise the plan of care if indicated.

Example. 10/24/88 Goal met. Client correctly verbalized rationale for diabetic foot care program and expressed interest in attending the diabetic classes.

C. Moser, RN

PERINEAL AND VAGINAL CARE

The perineal area is dark, warm, and often moist, which favors bacterial growth. The client unable to clean the perineal area will need the nurse's assistance for this important part of personal hygiene. To neglect cleaning the perineal area of the client unable to provide self-care often results in physical and psychologic discomfort for the client, a breakdown in the skin, and offensive odors.

Assessing

Nursing History. Identify any special perineal and vaginal hygiene practices the client performs, products used, and variables influencing these practices. Note any history of perineal or vaginal problems and related treatments.

Nursing Examination. Examine the male genitalia (penis, scrotum, and perineum) for lesions, swelling, inflammation, excoriation, tenderness, and discharge (amount, color, odor, and source); examine the female genitalia (pubic area, labia, clitoris, urinary meatus, and perineum) for color, size, lesions, masses, swelling, inflammation, excoriation, tenderness, and discharge (amount, color, odor, and source). Examine the anal area for cracks, nodules, distended veins, masses, or polyps; note strong perineal odors.

Risk Factors. Identify any variables known to cause perineal or vaginal problems or to create a need for special care: urinary or fecal incontinence, indwelling Foley catheters, childbirth, rectal or genital surgery, diseases such as urinary tract infection, diabetes mellitus, and certain sexually transmitted diseases (*e.g.,* herpes).

Diagnosing

Make a judgment about the adequacy of the client's perineal (vaginal) self-care practices, identifying any factors that contribute to deficiencies. An example is

Self-care deficit: perineal care *related to* cognitive impairment

Next, identify actual or potential perineal and vaginal problems that nurses can treat, noting contributing factors, and identify "unhealthy" client responses to these problems. Examples of these are

Altered comfort: perineal pain *related to* excoriated perineal area

Potential for infection *related to* client's deficient perineal hygiene

Knowledge deficit: advisability of using deodorized feminine hygiene products *related to* inexperience and a desire to "be clean"

Disturbance in body image *related to* genital lesions

Altered sexuality patterns *related to* painful genital lesions

Potential impairment of perineal skin integrity *related to* urinary and fecal incontinence

Planning

Identify nursing measures that will assist the client to develop or maintain healthy perineal (vaginal) care practices that will contribute to the client's general sense of well-being. Plan to achieve the following client goals:

- Client's perineal area is clean with skin intact.
- Perineal lesions, excoriations show sign of healing (discharge is decreased or absent).
- Client demonstrates correct perineal/vaginal hygiene measures.

Pertinent nursing measures to include in the plan of care include:

- Cleaning the male genitalia (penis, scrotum, perineum, and rectal area) or the female genitalia (pubic area, labia, clitoris, urinary meatus, perineum, and rectal area)
- Instructing the client on perineal hygiene practices

Implementing

Carry out the plan of care, remembering to utilize bath time, when appropriate, for ongoing assessment of the client's perineum and for evaluation of the adequacy of the plan of care. Described in this section are procedures for perineal and vaginal care. See the accompanying box for sample documentation of teaching care of genitalia.

Providing Perineal Care

It is not always possible for male nurses to attend to male patients and female nurses to attend to female patients. When the perineal cleaning is carried out in a matter-of-fact and dignified manner, patients generally do not find care by a person of the opposite sex to be offensive or embarrassing.

Some nurses use a sitz tub to clean the client's perineal and anal areas. The portable type is especially handy when it is cumbersome to move a client to a stationary sitz tub. The procedure may be carried out while the client remains in bed. The following techniques are recommended to administer perineal care to clients (Fig 27-10):

- Assemble supplies and provide for privacy.
- Explain the procedure to the client and don disposable gloves.

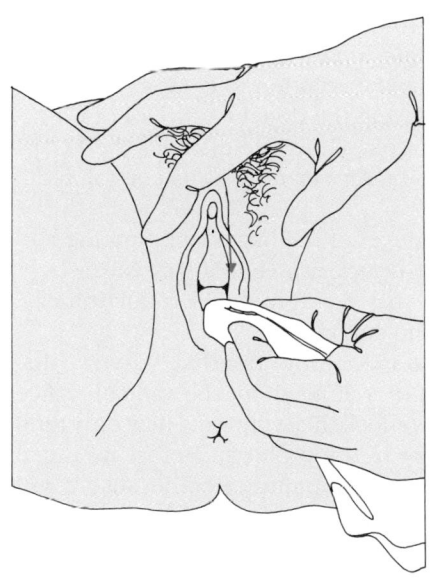 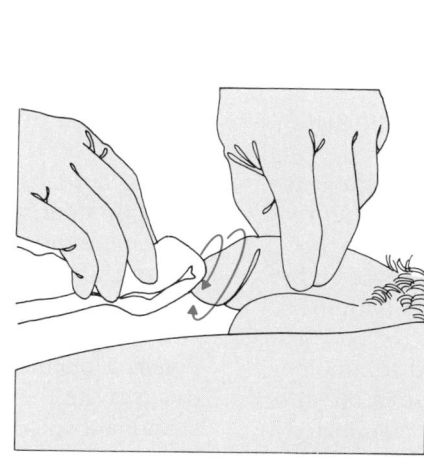 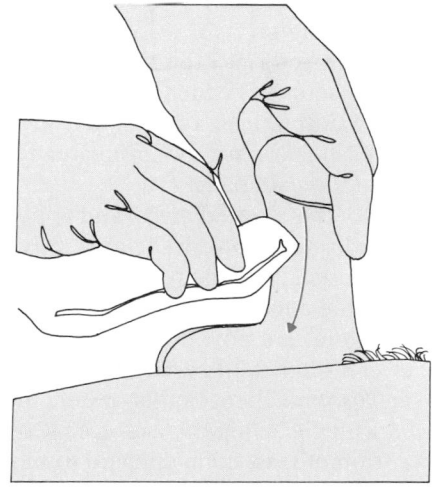

Female

Spread the labia to expose the urethral meatus and the vaginal orifice. Using a washcloth, cleanse from the pubic area toward the anus in one stroke. Repeat, using a clean portion of the cloth for each stroke, cleansing around the labia minora, clitoris, and vaginal orifice.

Male

Cleanse the tip of the penis from the urethral meatus outward in a circular motion. Clean the shaft of the penis from the tip toward the scrotum.

FIGURE 27-10
Performing normal perineal care.

Sample Documentation of Teaching Care of Genitalia

10/20/88 Child presented with large amount of smegma under the foreskin and painful urination. Mother and child were instructed in the need for and correct technique for cleansing the uncircumcised penis. Child correctly returned the demonstration.

C. Maier, RM

- Wash and rinse the groin area for both the male and female client.
- Always proceed from the least contaminated area to the most contaminated area. For a female client, spread the labia and move the washcloth from the pubic area toward the anal area to prevent carrying organisms from the anal area back over the genital area. Use a clean portion of the washcloth for each stroke. For a male client, move the washcloth in a spiral motion from the tip of the penis down its length toward the pubic area.
- In an uncircumcised male client, retract the foreskin (prepuce) while washing the penis. Rinse well with plain water.
- Rinse the washed areas well with plain water.
- Pull the uncircumcised male client's foreskin back into place over the glans penis to prevent constriction of the penis, which may result in edema and tissue injury.
- Wash and rinse the male client's scrotum. Handle the scrotum, which houses the testicles, with care because the area is very sensitive.
- Wash and rinse the groin area for both the male and female patient.
- Dry the cleaned areas, and apply an emollient as indicated. Powder the area only if the patient requests it. For the female client, powder may become a medium for the growth of bacteria, and studies are now linking use of powder with increased risk of cervical cancer.
- Turn the client on his or her side and continue with cleansing the anal area. Continue in the direction of least contaminated to most contaminated area. In the female, cleanse from the vagina toward the anus. In both female and male clients, change the washcloth with each stroke until the area is clean. Rinse and dry the area.

Providing Vaginal Care

In normal, healthy women, regular daily internal douching is believed to be both unnecessary and unwise. The practice tends to remove normal bacterial flora from the vagina, and if the solution is high in acid content, it may irritate or injure normal cells. Many women use douches for personal hygiene reasons after intercourse. The practice is satisfactory when the solution is nonirritating. There are many products on the market that can be used safely in douching solutions. Many gynecologists apparently feel that a mild white-vinegar solution, using a tablespoon or two in a quart of warm water, or normal saline, is just as satisfactory. Douching more often than twice a week is not recommended for normal personal hygiene purposes.

The following are recommended techniques for administering a vaginal douche for therapeutic reasons:

- Fill a douche bag with a quart or two of the warmed solution of choice, and allow the tubing and tip to fill with solution. Bulb syringes are available for douching but are less frequently recommended because of the danger of injecting solution with too much force and forcing it into the cervix.
- Place the client on a bedpan. The woman may lie in a bathtub if she is able to administer the douche herself. Standing up in the tub is not recommended because it requires too much force to carry solution to the vagina for thorough cleaning.
- Hold the bag or hang it on a standard so that it is about 24 to 36 inches (60 cm to 90 cm) above the level of the hips.
- Separate the labia with gloved fingers, and insert the douche tip by directing it downward and backward to follow the normal contour of the vagina. Allow the solution to begin flowing.
- Hold the vulva snugly to close the vaginal orifice or ask the client to contract her muscles around the orifice to allow solution to collect and distend the vagina; then allow the solution to escape. Repeat this procedure during the douche until all of the solution is used. This technique distends the vagina and permits better cleaning of its convoluted walls.
- Do not raise the level of the bag containing the solution during the douche since this may cause undue force that may result in the introduction of organisms into the cervix.

Medical attention is recommended when a discharge or irritation and itching about the vaginal orifice persist. Douching to relieve the symptoms may only tend to aggravate the cause of the problem. Before a vaginal examination, a douche is contraindicated because it will remove secretions and discharge needed for specimens necessary for diagnostic procedures. Most authorities recommend not having a vaginal douche for 24 to 48 hours before a vaginal examination.

Deodorants to control odor around the vaginal orifice may be applied directly to the area or placed on sanitary napkins. Although these deodorants do not contain aluminum salts, which are irritating to the mucous membrane, they are intended for external use only. They should not be used on tampons. Some have been reported as possibly harmful when sprayed into the vagina.

Repeated use is not generally recommended because of reported irritation and rashes, nor should they be used on broken skin areas. No therapeutic benefit from their use has been proven to date. These special deodorants cannot replace cleanliness of the area.

Evaluating

At designated intervals, evaluate whether or not the client has achieved the goals established during planning, and revise the plan of care if indicated.

Example. 11/20/88 Goal partially met. Child returned to clinic with clean perineal area and relief of painful urination. Mother reports child spends half time with her and half with father (parents separated) and that father is uncommitted to hygiene practices.

Revision. Stress again to child importance of retracting foreskin during perineal care.

C Maier, RN

NURSING PROCESS in Clinical Practice

Approximately 75,000 of the 1 million clients hospitalized each year in the United States develop pressure ulcers (Shannon, 1984), and the statistics in Canada are similar. The threat these ulcers pose to the client's physical and mental well-being and the amount of nursing energy they consume make them one of nursing's persistent top-priority challenges. For this reason, the nursing diagnosis Impairment of skin integrity related to pressure ulcer will now be explored.

Impaired Skin Integrity Related to Pressure Ulcer

Description

A **pressure ulcer** is an area of cellular necrosis that is caused by the lack of blood circulation to the involved area. **Necrosis** means that there is death of cells. The terms **pressure ulcer**, **decubitus ulcer**, and **bedsore** are used synonymously.

The term *decubitus* derives from a Latin word meaning lying down. However, lying down does not cause a decubitus ulcer, and a client need not be bedridden to develop one. Therefore, some persons prefer the term *pressure ulcer* because pressure is the most prominent underlying cause of a decubitus ulcer.

Pathologic changes at the site of a decubitus ulcer are caused by the collapse of blood vessels in the area of the ulcer, especially the arterioles and capillaries. The damage to vessels is a result of pressure, usually from body weight. When the blood supply is occluded owing to the pressure on vessels, cells are not adequately nourished, and cell wastes accumulate. Death of cells eventually occurs, leading to the characteristic ulcer of a pressure sore. The steps of this process are as follows: pressure → compression of small nutrient vessels of skin and underlying tissue → tissue anoxia and ischemia → necrosis of tissue cells → sloughing and ulceration → invasion by microorganisms → infection → sepsis → involvement of underlying fascia, muscle, and bone → rapidly irreversible condition (Brunner and Suddarth, 1988, p 222).

The first sign that a pressure sore may be developing is a blanching of the skin over the area under pressure. Instead of a healthy, pink color, the skin becomes pale and white. In the non-Caucasian, this blanching is more difficult to see. However, insufficient blood circulation in the capillaries makes the skin appear pale when compared with areas where circulation is good. Local anemia owing to poor circulation in the area is called **ischemia**, which means containing little blood.

When pressure is relieved, ischemia is rapidly followed by hyperemia. The area appears red and feels warm. In the non-Caucasian, hyperemia may best be detected by touch. The skin will feel warm. Hyperemia is a compensatory mechanism. The body literally floods the area with blood in order to nourish and remove wastes from the cells. This phenomenon is called **reactive hyperemia**. If pressure is not relieved, the area remains red, but circulation cannot occur to the extent necessary for cell survival, and the tissue cells eventually will die. The skin breaks, and a shallow crater or ulcer develops. The pressure sore then is often called superficial and with proper care ordinarily will heal with relative ease.

A decubitus ulcer is usually described as deep when a superficial pressure sore extends and involves underlying tissues. Shearing forces are often responsible for deep decubitus ulcers. A **shearing force** results when layers of tissue move on each other. Small blood vessels and capillaries are stretched and may even tear, thus resulting in poor circulation to tissue cells under the skin. The area of skin over an area damaged by a shearing force usually appears bluish in color, and sometimes a lump can be felt under the skin. A small break in the skin, which leads to necrotic tissue in the underlying area, eventually appears. Figure 27-11 illustrates how shearing forces occur.

The skin can tolerate considerable pressure without cell death but for short periods only. Duration is more

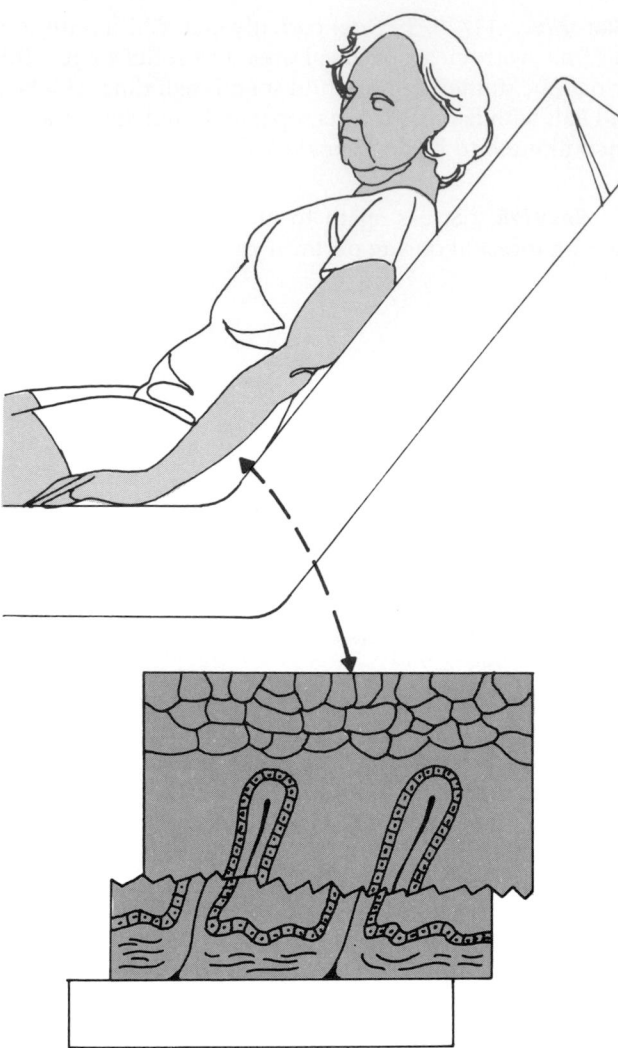

F I G U R E   27-11

Shearing force can occur when a client is moved carelessly or slides down in bed. Friction causes resistance on the surface layers of the skin, while underlying tissue moves in the direction of the body movement. Capillaries in underlying tissue are stretched and torn in pressure areas by the opposing forces of movement.

important than the amount of pressure in the formation of a decubitus ulcer.

Common Sites for Pressure Ulcers

Decubitus ulcers usually occur over bony prominences where body weight is distributed over a small area that does not have many subcutaneous tissues to cushion damage to the skin. Common sites for decubitus ulcers are illustrated in Figure 27-12. Of the susceptible areas, most pressure sores occur over the sacrum and coccyx.

Risk Factors

There are numerous factors that predispose to pressure sores. Usually a combination of factors cause their development.

Pressure

The most formidable predisposing factor for a decubitus ulcer is pressure over an area, which results in occluded blood capillaries and poor blood circulation to tissues. This lack of sufficient circulation causes cell death and ulcer formation.

Immobility

The person who sits or lies most of the time is a candidate for a pressure sore because immobility predisposes to prolonged pressure on body areas. The up-and-about person does not develop decubitus ulcers since no part of the body suffers from prolonged pressure. During sleep, the well person tends to move about in bed freely. Unconscious and paralyzed clients are subject to pressure sores if allowed to remain in one position in bed. So also are emotionally depressed persons who do not ordinarily tend to move about very much.

Shearing Forces

Clients who are moved in bed or from beds to stretchers or chairs carelessly will suffer from shearing forces as skin and underlying tissues are pulled over each other. A client who is partially sitting up in bed is susceptible when skin sticks to the sheet and underlying tissues move downward with the body. This may occur also in the client who sits in a chair but slides down while skin sticks to clothing and the back of the chair.

Friction

The client who lies on wrinkled sheets is likely to suffer tissue damage owing to friction. The skin over the elbows and heels often suffers when clients lift and help move themselves in bed with the use of their arms and feet. Friction burns also occur on the back when clients are pulled or slid over sheets in bed or on a stretcher.

Edema

Water imbalances and the accumulation of excessive fluid in tissues interfere with proper cell nourishment.

Moisture

Prolonged moisture on the skin reduces its resistance to trauma. Warmth increases the cells demands for oxygen. Hence, moisture and warmth will eventually lead to cell destruction, especially when pressure is present. If personal hygiene is poor, the skin will contain many organisms that thrive in the warm, moist environment. This adds to the danger of developing a decubitus ulcer that will become infected.

Malnutrition

Malnutrition predisposes to pressure sore formation because poorly nourished cells are easily damaged. For example, vitamin C deficiency causes capillaries to become fragile, and poor circulation to the area results when they break. Negative nitrogen balance and electrolyte imbalances also predispose to pressure sore formation.

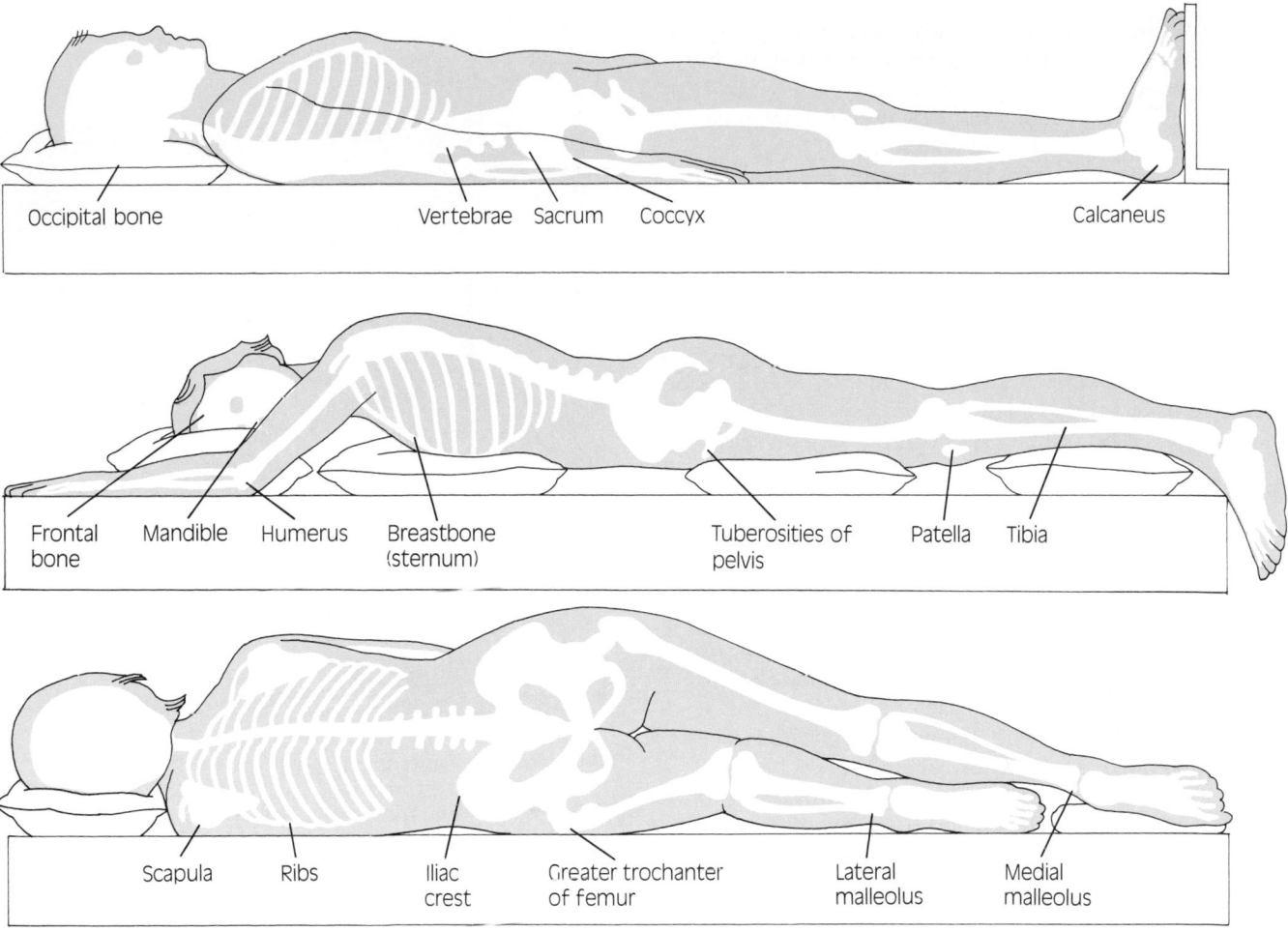

F I G U R E   27-12
Common sites for development of decubitus ulcers.

Incontinence

Urinary or fecal incontinence increases the risk of an individual developing a decubitus ulcer that will become infected.

Mental Status

The more alert an individual is the more likely he or she is to protect skin integrity by relieving pressure periodically and managing adequate skin hygiene. Apathy, confusion, or a comatose state can diminish these self-care abilities and increase the likelihood of skin breakdown.

Miscellaneous Factors

There are additional factors that predispose to decubitus ulcers:

- Older persons whose skin is wrinkled and forms folds because of loss of subcutaneous fat are good candidates for developing pressure sores because the skin is very susceptible to injury.
- Persons with debilitating diseases are likely candidates for developing decubitus ulcers since skin nourishment ordinarily becomes poor.
- Destruction of tissues leading to pressure sores becomes relatively easy when illness causes an ele-

vated temperature and normal functioning of body cells is altered in any way.
- Clients whose skin is very dry and those whose skin has been irritated with adhesive tape are candidates for decubitus ulcers.
- Various kinds of debris in bed or on a chair, such as crumbs, hairpins, buttons, pencils and pens, and pieces of silverware, irritate and damage the skin so that a decubitus ulcer is likely to develop.

Nursing Management
Assessment

Identify those at risk and note predisposing factors: pressure, immobility, shearing forces, friction, edema, moisture, incontinence, health management deficits, malnutrition, debilitating disease. When a pressure ulcer is noted

- Describe the pressure ulcer as to site, size, edema, warmth, color, odor, eschar, slough, drainage, and surrounding skin. Description of the ulcer must be ongoing. Many agencies utilize a special pressure ulcer assessment form.
- Describe the skin in general: turgor, dryness or moisture, sensation in pressure areas, and warmth.

- Describe contractures or any predisposing environmental factors (*e.g.,* casts, wrinkled linen, rubber drawsheet).
- Describe the client's self-care abilities: hygiene, mobility, nutrition, and continence.
- Describe the current nursing care: special skin care, pressure-relief measures, nutritional support, and incontinence management or devices.

Diagnosis

Unless the institution specifies a different classification system, diagnose the pressure ulcer according to the four-stage classification system commonly used by rehabilitation specialists (Cassell, 1986) (see Fig 27-13).

Stage 1: The primary sign is redness. The skin doesn't return to a normal color when the pressure is relieved, but there is no induration; the skin and underlying tissues remain soft.

Stage 2: Redness persists, usually accompanied by edema and induration. The epidermis may blister or erode.

Stage 3: There is an open lesion and a crater, exposing subcutaneous tissue. You may be able to see fascia at the base of the ulcer.

Stage 4: Necrosis will extend through the fascia and may even involve the bone. Eschar is a common finding. Bone destruction can lead to periostitis, osteitis, and osteomyelitis.

Sample nursing diagnoses read

Impaired skin integrity: stage 2 sacral pressure ulcer related to incontinence and malnutrition as manifested by persistent redness and edema in sacral area

Impaired skin integrity: stage 4 heel pressure ulcer related to immobility as manifested by 3-cm black necrotic area on the left heel involving fascia

Goals

- Pressure ulcer demonstrates signs of healing.
- Predisposing factors are eliminated or their effects are reduced.
- Client (if able) demonstrates appropriate self-care behaviors:
  - Demonstrates satisfactory hygiene
  - Shifts weight and changes position every 1 to 2 hours
  - Eats nutritious diet (high in protein, iron, vitamin C; zinc supplements; sufficient fluids)
  - States rationale for treatment measures
- Client develops no new areas of skin breakdown.

Nursing Interventions

There are a variety of nursing measures to help prevent pressure sores:

FIGURE 27-13
Stages of development of decubitus ulcers.

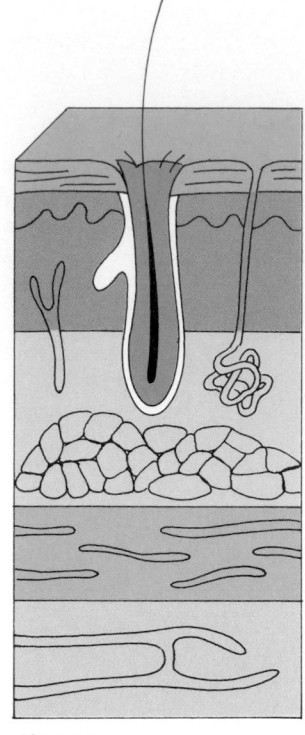

Stage 1
The primary sign is redness. The skin doesn't return to a normal color when the pressure is relieved, but there is no induration—the skin and underlying tissues remain soft.

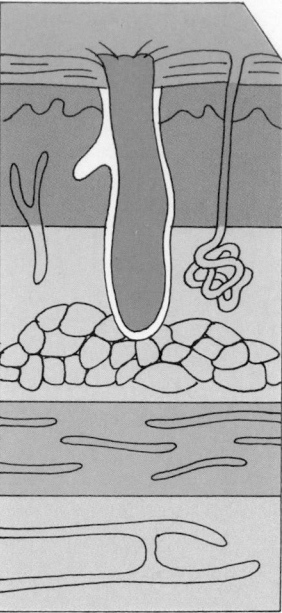

Stage 2
Redness persists, usually accompanied by edema and induration. The epidermis may blister or erode.

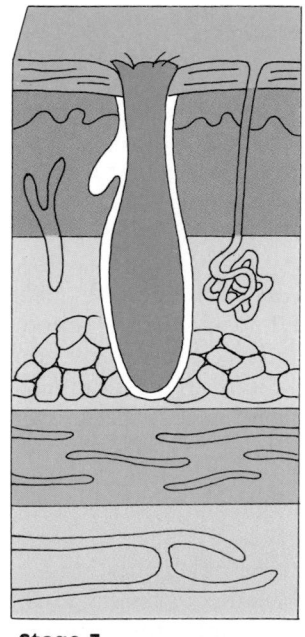

Stage 3
There is an open lesion and a crater exposing subcutaneous tissue. You may be able to see fascia at the base of the ulcer.

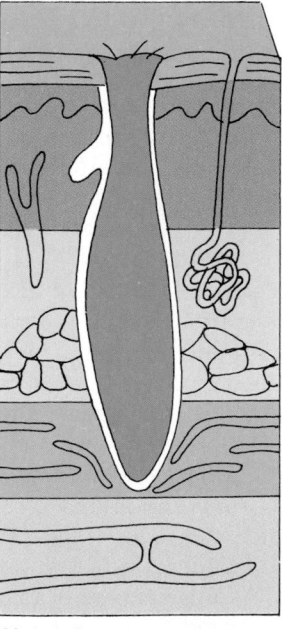

Stage 4
Necrosis will extend through the fascia and may even involve the bone. Eschar is a common finding. Bone destruction can lead to periosteitis, osteitis, and osteomyelitis.

- Change the client's position *frequently* to relieve pressure, which, if unrelieved, is the most important cause of a decubitus ulcer. This should be done every 1 to 2 hours for clients who are candidates for developing a decubitus ulcer. The back-lying position should be used as infrequently as possible because it causes the greatest amount of pressure to many vulnerable areas of the body. The right and left side-lying positions and lying on the abdomen are preferred.

- Do everything possible to keep the client in the best possible physical condition. This includes seeing to it that the client eats nutritious meals, takes plenty of fluids, has sufficient rest, and receives active and passive activity, including ambulation. Healthy, well-nourished cells are less likely to deteriorate.

- Keep the skin dry and clean. Dampness and uncleanliness predispose to skin breakdown and infection.

- Use a mild soap or detergent and water when cleaning the skin, and rinse soap or detergent from the skin. Soap and detergent residues are very irritating and predispose to skin breakdown. Blot tender skin dry to prevent friction. Some agencies use a special skin care program for high-risk clients that includes a water-repellent ointment for the perineal area.

- Avoid using waterproof material on the client's bed. It tends to cause the client to perspire and prevents evaporation of moisture. Pads made of synthetic fibers or closely cropped wool may be placed under pressure-prone areas. The spaces between the tufts allow air circulation and help keep the area dry.

- Massage areas carefully and frequently where there is pressure on the body except when redness is already present. This stimulates circulation to the area. Alcohol for massaging is drying but tends to toughen the skin. A lotion or cream adds moisture, but if it is not allowed to dry well, it may soften the skin and predispose to breaks in the skin.

- Protect areas especially prone to pressure, such as the coccyx, heels, and elbows. There are various devices on the market to protect such areas as the heel and elbow. Also, consider using packs filled with gelatinous material under parts of the body where pressure is present. They are available in various sizes and shapes to fit different parts of the body.

- Prevent friction on the skin when moving the client. Avoid sliding the client on bed linens or on a chair. Friction burns predispose to pressure-sore formation.

- Support clients in bed and in a chair securely so that they do not slip down and cause a shearing force to occur. It is recommended that an ulcer-prone patient not have the head of the bed elevated more than 30 degrees to prevent sliding down in bed.

- Avoid using air-inflated rings, or use them only with the greatest care. They may relieve pressure over an area, but they restrict circulation where the body part rests on the ring. This pressure may cause more problems than the ring may prevent

- Keep bed linens free of wrinkles, and dry and clean them to prevent friction and irritation to the skin.

- Avoid applying top linens on the client's bed so that they restrict freedom of movement. Also, avoid pressure and irritation from casts, adhesive, tubing, arm boards, and the like.

- Protect areas of the skin especially susceptible to pressure sores. A silicone and zinc oxide mixture dispensed in aerosol has been used effectively. So also has tincture of benzoin.

- Use pressure-relieving devices such as sheepskin, air mattresses, egg crate mattresses, air–fluid support systems, and low air-loss bed systems:

    The *Clinitron bed* minimizes pressure and eliminates shear, friction, and maceration by means of the fluidization principle. The client floats on a dry fluid created by forcing a gentle flow of temperature-controlled air upward through a mass of fine ceramic microspheres. The client's body fluids pass downward through a specially designed filter shell. This elimination of moisture and the desiccating effect on the warm, dry air flow provide a clean immediate environment hostile to bacterial growth. Maceration is virtually eliminated so there is reduced need for dressings, topicals, and antibiotics.

- A low air-loss system is provided by a variety of beds consisting of the bed and an air-supply system. The frame provides ease in position changes, allowing the client's head and trunk to be elevated, the feet and thighs to be raised, and the knees flexed. Other systems allow for side-to-side rotation. The client lies directly on vapor-permeable air sacs, controlled by preset dials determined by client size and comfort. The sacs are machine washable, and drawsheets may be used for the incontinent client.

- Many topical agents have been used for the treatment of pressure ulcers. The following agents have been reported in the literature within the last few years: skin barriers (*e.g.,* karaya powder, Stomahesive); antiseptic plastic sprays; aerosol sprays containing a corticosteroid and an antibiotic; absorbable gelatin sponges (Gelfoam); enzymatic debriding agents; transparent, elastic, self-adhesive film (Op-Site), dextranomer (Debrisan); and absorption dressing (Bard Absorption Dressing). Also used are tannic acid, oxygen under pressure, sugar and sugar paste, gold leaf, whipped egg whites, and antacids. According to reports, success with certain persons is reported with each agent. However, as can be seen by the number of agents being tried, an effective treatment appears more illusive than real.

Because of the lack of consensus on pressure ulcer management, it is generally recommended that the nurse follow agency guidelines for the treatment of pressure ulcers in each of their four stages. If these do not exist, detailed nursing management and wound care guidelines (supportive measures, physical measures, mechanical devices, specifics of wound care) have been developed by the skin care task force of Beth Israel Hospital in Boston, Massachusetts, for each stage of pressure ulcers (American Journal of Nursing, August, 1984). Debridement guidelines (stage 3 and 4 ulcers), cleansing and rinsing solutions, and dressing treatment should be specified. Wound irrigations are described in Chapter 42.

Evaluative Criteria
Client meets the above goals.

CASE STUDY

Glenda Davis is a nurse practitioner who works in a campus health clinic at a state university. She is frequently approached by women who ask questions about feminine hygiene. Realizing that each woman who presents with a question probably represents many other women with similar unvoiced questions, she decides to develop an insert entitled *Self-Care: Feminine Hygiene* for the campus newspaper.

Assessment Findings
- Heterogeneous female population of various ages, cultures, religions, and family/life-style backgrounds
- Knowledge about feminine hygiene varies widely from almost no knowledge to students who are well read or members of women's health professions.
- Students who present with questions are mostly concerned about dangers of certain products (*e.g.,* tampons and toxic shock syndrome) or have questions related to intercourse (*e.g.,* advisability of douching, how to avoid getting a sexually transmitted disease, and so forth).
- Numerous students report to the clinic with vaginal infections and urinary tract infections.
- Interest is high; ability to comprehend written material is high.

Nursing Diagnosis
Self-care deficit: feminine hygiene related to knowledge deficit

Planning
Ms Davis talks with other nurses at the campus health clinic and together they decide to make education about feminine hygiene a priority for the year. Ms Davis volunteers to develop a standardized care plan as well as a feminine hygiene health education hand-out for publication in the campus newspaper and distribution at the clinic. After discussion, the staff agrees on the following goals:

Long-Term Goals
Female students consistently demonstrate positive ownership of their bodies and practice good personal hygiene.

Short-Term Goals
Students will express positive body image valuing their uniqueness.
Students will correctly describe feminine hygiene self-care behaviors that they are willing to incorporate into their daily life-styles.
Campus health clinic records will demonstrate a reduction in both new and recurrent genitourinary infections.

The short-term goals may be evaluated at each client visit or at periodic time intervals, for example, 6 months after development and use of hand-out on feminine hygiene.

Implementation
To develop better feminine hygiene self-care abilities successfully, the nurse needs the following specialized abilities:
- Strong interpersonal skills: the ability to communicate to women of many different backgrounds concern for their health questions and fears and the commitment to work with women to develop healthier self-care behaviors
- Attentive listening and other interviewing skills to assess the health-care needs of this population correctly
- Knowledge of feminine hygiene and advantages and disadvantages of various women's health-care practices and products
- The ability to communicate to women acceptance and understanding of the female body: body parts (appearance, odor) and cycles
- Teaching and counseling skills to work one-on-one with women who come to the campus health clinic
- Written communication skills to develop a self-care feature on feminine hygiene for campus publication
- Accountability; self-direction

Documentation

Sample documentation of a nursing intervention. Recorded is a SOAPIE note written after a teaching session with a client who presented at the campus clinic.

6/15/86 #1 Self-care deficit: feminine hygiene related to knowledge deficit 3 PM

S: Became sexually active this year; sexual intercourse once or twice weekly

"Many of my friends use douches . . . are there any douche products you particularly recommend?"

Expresses concern about contracting sexually transmitted disease from partners

O: —

A: Lacks knowledge about feminine hygiene practices related to intercourse

P: *Diagnostic:* Assess accuracy of what she has learned about feminine hygiene in general and specifically related to intercourse; explore her knowledge and feelings about her body.

Educative: Using the *Self-Care: Feminine Hygiene* hand-out, instruct regarding self-care practices. Clarify misconception regarding the advisability of douching. Counsel about her right to talk with a sexual partner about sexually transmitted diseases and previous contacts with infected individuals; advise refraining from contact or to use condom when she has any doubts about partner.

I: Above carried out

E: Client reports feeling more "in charge" of body and better able to care for it.

Evaluation

Goal achievement is ongoing, once the nursing staff in the campus health clinic is committed to improving the self-care feminine hygiene behaviors of students and identifies this as a priority. Using the standardized care plan, short-term goal achievement may be evaluated at the conclusion of each client visit or at designated time intervals (*e.g.,* 6-month evaluation). See the care plan for related evaluative statements.

NURSING CARE PLAN for Female University Students

Nursing Diagnosis:	Self-care deficit: feminine hygiene related to knowledge deficit
	Signs and symptoms: female students present to the campus clinic with questions about feminine hygiene; high incidence of vaginal and urinary tract infections; negative attitudes about feminine body frequently expressed
Long-Term Goal:	Female students consistently demonstrate positive ownership of their bodies, practicing good personal hygiene

Goals	Nursing Actions	Rationale	Evaluative Statement
Students will express positive body image, valuing their uniqueness.	With each student who presents at the clinic for help with a gynecologic concern or problem take the time to *assess* her knowledge of the female body, and her acceptance of *her body* and comfort with it. Counsel appropriately.	The women's health movement has encouraged women to feel ownership of their bodies, to appreciate their uniqueness as women, and to increase their awareness of their physical bodies and the feelings associated with them. Many women still feel that the genital area and cyclic phenomena such as the menstrual cycle and the female sexual response cycle are "dirty" and symptoms in this area may evoke fear, guilt, anxiety, and shame. It is important for nurses to provide women with information about their bodies.	*Six-month evaluation:* 6/30 Goal partially met: students are beginning to discuss gynecologic concerns more freely yet great hesitancy persists. *Revision:* Continue to help women to know, understand, and accept their bodies and to talk about their bodies. Make this a priority of the nursing staff at the clinic. *G. Davis, RN*

N U R S I N G   C A R E   P L A N   (Continued)

Goals	Nursing Actions	Rationale	Evaluative Statement
Students will correctly describe feminine hygiene self-care behaviors they are willing to incorporate into their daily life-styles.	Assess with each client her knowledge of feminine hygiene practices (correct any misconceptions) and motivation to utilize them consistently. Address specific concerns related to menstruation, intercourse, other maturational events. Distribute the *Self-Care: Feminine Hygiene* hand-out and discuss this with the client. Teach the importance of using preventive hygiene measures to reduce the likelihood of acquiring a urinary tract or vaginal infection.	Many women have never been instructed about feminine hygiene and harmful practices may be "picked up" from the media and other sources (*e.g.*, the use of frequent douching and deodorants to eliminate normal body odors). Maturational events, such as menstruation, becoming sexually active, and pregnancy, may result in a need for new or modified hygiene practices. It is better to *prevent* a genitourinary infection than to *treat* it.	6/30 Goal met. Following publication of the *Self-Care: Feminine Hygiene* feature and one-on-one counseling using this printed hand-out, clients are knowledgeable about preventive hygiene measures. *G. Davis, RN*
Campus health clinic records will demonstrate a reduction in both new and recurrent genitourinary infections.	Educate women to distinguish normal from abnormal findings (vaginal discharge, pain, bleeding, problems with urination) and to seek help when appropriate. Educate women regarding preventive hygiene measures (refer to the hand-out). Document new and recurrent genitourinary infections; identify predisposing factors.	Early treatment of genitourinary infections reduces the likelihood of residual problems. Nursing measures include teaching preventive measures, instructing in recognition of symptoms, and assisting with self-care activities to prevent and treat infections, including the securing of medical assistance when indicated.	6/30 Goal met. Six months following publication and use of the *Self-Care: Feminine Hygiene* hand-out, the incidence of genitourinary infections is reduced 10%. Will continue to keep education in this regard a priority. *G. Davis, RN*

SELF-CARE: Feminine Hygiene

Many women have concerns about feminine hygiene. Personal health-care practices are influenced by past experiences, cultural knowledge, and societal expectations. It is important for women to feel comfortable with their bodies and to be knowledgeable about self-care practices that promote health and well-being and prevent infection and disease. If this is a concern for you, take a few minutes to respond to the questions below and read the accompanying information.

ASSESSMENT GUIDE
(Check the phrase that best describes you.)   *SELF-CARE KNOWLEDGE—ATTITUDE—SKILLS**

——— I feel comfortable with my body. I accept its uniqueness.

A woman's health and sense of self can be uniquely influenced by her sexuality and its expression and by several changes in her physiology:

ASSESSMENT GUIDE
(Check the phrase that best describes you.)

SELF-CARE KNOWLEDGE—ATTITUDE—SKILLS*

_____ My body often makes me feel uncomfortable (fearful, anxious, guilty).

the onset of menstruation, pregnancy, interruption of pregnancy, childbirth, postpartum, nursing, and menopause.

By virtue of ownership, women have the right to control their own bodies. This includes *knowing* their bodies, accepting their uniqueness, and caring for their bodies appropriately.

Distorted ideas that the genital area is somehow "dirty" and needs special deodorizing and scenting or that it is "shameful" to discuss problems in this area or to talk about related concerns need to be replaced by healthier attitudes. Often these ideas are deep-seated and reinforced by culture, religion, and society (advertising world).

_____ I am knowledgeable about feminine hygiene practices and products. I value preventive measures that promote health and reduce the likelihood of infection.

_____ I have never thought much about feminine hygiene nor discussed this with anyone.

Each woman can be an expert in the care of her own body. Feminine hygiene practices that promote health and prevent infection include the following:

- Wash the perineal area at least once daily to remove perspiration and smegma accumulations; pat rather than rub the area dry; towels and washcloths should be clean and never shared.
- Always wipe from front to back after voiding and defecation to avoid introducing bacteria into the vagina or urethra.
- Sprays, soaps, powders, deodorants, and tampons and pads that are perfumed or irritating in any way should not be used; any chemicals that irritate the skin or vaginal mucosa or alter the vaginal environment should be avoided.
- Avoid clothing that is too tight, does not allow free air flow to the perineum, or traps moisture; underpants and pantyhose should always have a cotton crotch.
- Douching should be avoided or kept to a minimum; douching can strip the vagina of its normal flora, introduce bacteria, and aggravate inflammation.
- If tampons are used during menstruation, choose the smallest absorbency needed to absorb flow; change regularly (every 3 to 4 hours), and use good handwashing techniques prior to insertion; women who have had toxic shock syndrome should not use tampons until *Staphylococcus aureus* is no longer present in the vaginal flora.
- Sexual partners should be clean: it is "ok" to discuss this with partners prior to intercourse; advise use of condoms; if any doubts exist about partner, refrain from contact; void before and after intercourse; if lubricant is needed during intercourse, a sterile, water-soluble type should be used. A final cautionary note: "Don't put anything in your vagina you wouldn't put in your mouth."

_____ I understand that changes in vaginal discharge, pain, and bleeding may indicate pathology or disease or may be a normal variation of the menstrual cycle.

_____ I know when to seek help.

_____ Changes in my body make me feel uncomfortable. I would probably delay seeking help with discomforting symptoms because of my anxieties.

Throughout her life, the average woman will experience bleeding, pain, or discharge associated with her reproductive organs or functions. These may cause discomfort, interference with life style, and distress, both physical and emotional. At times professional assistance may be required to distinguish the normal from the abnormal, to identify pathology, and to explore the meaning of the symptom or illness.

Symptoms frequently experienced that may require the assistance of a health-care professional include abnormal vaginal discharge and itching of the vulva and vagina, gynecologic pain, differences in cyclic bleeding patterns or bleeding that is perceived as abnormal, and problems with urinary elimination.

Every woman should have a health-care professional she trusts with whom she can discuss gynecologic problems. The nurses at the campus health clinic are committed to helping women with gynecologic problems.

* Adapted from Fogel CI, Woods NF: Health Care of Women: A Nursing Perspective, pp 220–255. St Louis, CV Mosby, 1981

KEY POINTS

■ Personal hygiene refers to measures of personal cleanliness and grooming that promote physical and psychologic well-being.

■ People differ in personal hygiene practices, which may be affected by culture, socioeconomic class, religion, developmental level, knowledge level, health state, and personal preferences.

■ A comprehensive assessment of the skin and mucous membranes includes the collection of data about usual hygiene practices (showering or bathing practices; skin, hair, and scalp care; eye, ear, nose, and mouth care; nail and foot care; and perineal care); an assessment of any sensory, cognitive, endurance, mobility, or motivational deficit that interferes with the individual's hygiene practices; the identification of any existing problems of the skin or mucous membranes and associated care and its effectiveness; and a physical examination of the skin and mucous membranes.

■ Since life-style factors, changes in health state, illness, and certain diagnostic and therapeutic measures may adversely affect the skin, the nurse needs to identify high-risk populations and perform the appropriate skin assessment, teach the client how to examine and care for the skin, and institute preventive skin care measures.

■ Nursing diagnoses may be written that specifically address problems of deficient hygiene (self-care deficit: personal hygiene) or that identify the effects problems of the skin, hair, scalp, eye, ear, nose, mouth, nail, feet, or perineum have on other areas of human functioning (comfort, mobility, nutrition).

■ The individual with cognitive, sensory, endurance, mobility, or motivational deficits may require nursing assistance with any or all aspects of personal hygiene. The nurse promotes independence in these measures consistently. Whenever possible the nurse offers assistance compatible with the individual's preferences and usual routines. When indicated, the client and family are taught necessary hygiene measures.

■ Hospitalized clients receive scheduled hygienic care. This care includes careful attention to ensuring the safety and comfort of the client's bedside unit. Because of the long hours many ill clients spend in bed, the condition of bed linens is checked periodically throughout the day.

■ Pressure ulcers continue to be a priority nursing problem. Identifying high-risk clients and immediately initiating a plan of preventive care are nursing's first concerns. When a pressure ulcer develops, ongoing assessment, diagnosis (staging), planning, treatment, and evaluation are imperative. The numerous treatment strategies available and absence of any one clearly successful modality underscore the need for preventive care.

BIBLIOGRAPHY

Barnhill SE, Chenoweth EE: Cleansing the perineum. Am J Nurs 66(3):566, 1966

Beaver MJ: Mediscus low air-loss beds and the prevention of decubitus ulcers. Critical Care Nurse 6(5):32–39, 1986

Bergstrom N, Braden BJ, Laguzza A, Holman V: The Braden scale for predicting pressure sore risk. Nurs Res 36(4):205–210, 1987

Blaney GM: Mouth care—Basic and essential. Geriatric Nursing 7(5):242–243, 1986

Braden B: A conceptual schema for the study of the etiology of pressure sores. Rehabilitation Nursing 12(1):8–12, 1987

Bristow JV, Goldfarb EH, Green M: Clinitron therapy: Is it effective? Geriatric Nursing 8(3):120–124, 1987

Brunner LS, Suddarth D: Textbook of Medical–Surgical Nursing, 6th ed. Philadelphia, JB Lippincott, 1988

Byrne N, Feld M: Preventing and treating decubitus ulcers. Nursing '84 14(4):55–57, 1984

Cardin RG: The ins and outs of contact lenses. RN (2):48–50, 1985

Cuzzell JZ, Willey T: Wound care forum: Pressure relief perennials. Am J Nurs 87(9):1157, 1987

Davis E: Give a bath? Am J Nurs 70(11):2366–2367, 1970

Davis M: Getting to the root of the problem: Hair grooming for blacks. Nursing '77 7(4):60–65, 1977

Dyer ED, Monson M, Cope M: Dental health in adults. Am J Nurs 76(7):1156–1159, 1976

Fakouri C et al: Relaxation Rx: Slow stroke back rub. Journal of Gerontological Nursing 13(2):32–35, 1987

Gannon EP, Kadezabek E: Giving your patients meticulous mouth care. Nursing '80 10(3):70–75, 1980

Goldstone LA, Goldstone J: The Norton scale: An early warning of pressure sores? J Adv Nurs 7(5):419–426, 1982

Hauk L: Enabling clients to manage dentures. Geriatric Nursing 7(5):254–255, 1986

Holder L: Hearing aids: Handle with care. Nursing '82 12(4):64–67, 1982

Holmes R, Macchiano R, Jhangiani S et al: Combating pressure sores—nutritionally. Am J Nurs 87(10):1301–1303, 1987

Jackson G: Step-by-step massage techniques. Canadian Nurse 79(4):32–35, 1983

Jones PL, Millman A: A three-part system to combat pressure sores. Geriatric Nursing 7(2):78–82, 1986

Judd CO: Selected topical agents in the treatment of pressure sores. Canadian Nurse 77(7):32–33, 1981

Kamenir S, Fothergill R: Hands-on skills for dealing with hearing aids. Canadian Nurse 78(11):44–45, 1982

Kerr JC, Stinson SM, Shannon ML: Pressure sores: Distinguishing fact from fiction. Canadian Nurse 77(7):23–28, 1981

King PA: Foot problems and assessment. Geriatric Nursing 1(5):182–186, 1980

Lincoln R et al: Use of the Norton pressure scale risk assessment scoring system with elderly patients in acute care. Journal of Enterostomal Therapy 13(4):132–138, 1986

MacMillan K: New goals for oral hygiene. Canadian Nurse 77(3):40–43, 1981

Meissner JE: A simple guide for assessing oral health. Nursing '80 10(4):84–85, 1980

Michelson D: Giving a great back rub. Am J Nurs 78(7):1197–1199, 1978

Mondoux LCA (ed): Pressure ulcers. Nurs Clin North Am 22(2):357–494, 1987

Morley M: Sixteen steps to better decubitus ulcer care. Canadian Nurse 77(7):29–31, 1981

Pajik M et al: Investigating the problem of pressure sores. Journal of Gerontological Nursing 12(7):11–16, 1986

Shannon ML: Five famous fallacies about pressure sores. Nursing '84 14(10):34–41, 1984

Smiler I: Foot problems of elderly diabetics. Geriatric Nursing 3(3):177–181, 1982

Phipps M et al: Staging care for pressure sores. Am J Nurs 84(8):999–1003, 1984

Preston K: Dermal ulcers: Simplifying a complex problem. Rehabilitation Nursing 12(1):17–21, 1987

Wagnild G, Manning R: Convey respect during bathing procedures. Journal of Gerontological Nursing 11(12):6–10, 1985

Wells R, Trostle K: Creative hairwashing techniques for immobilized patients. Nursing '84 14(1):47–51, 1984

Wisser SH: When the walls listened. Am J Nurs 78(6):1016–1017, 1978

Zuchnick MM: Care of an artificial eye. Am J Nurs 75(5):835, 1975

28 Activity

OBJECTIVES

After studying this chapter, the learner should be able to

Define key terms used in this chapter.

Describe the role of the skeletal, muscular, and nervous systems in the physiology of movement.

Identify seven variables that influence body alignment and mobility.

Differentiate isotonic, isometric, and isokinetic exercise.

Describe the effects of exercise and immobility on major body systems.

Assess body alignment, mobility, and activity tolerance, utilizing appropriate interview questions and physical assessment skills.

Develop nursing diagnoses that correctly identify mobility problems amenable to nursing therapy.

Utilize proper body mechanics when positioning, moving, lifting, and ambulating clients.

Design exercise programs.

Plan, implement, and evaluate nursing care related to select nursing diagnoses involving mobility problems.

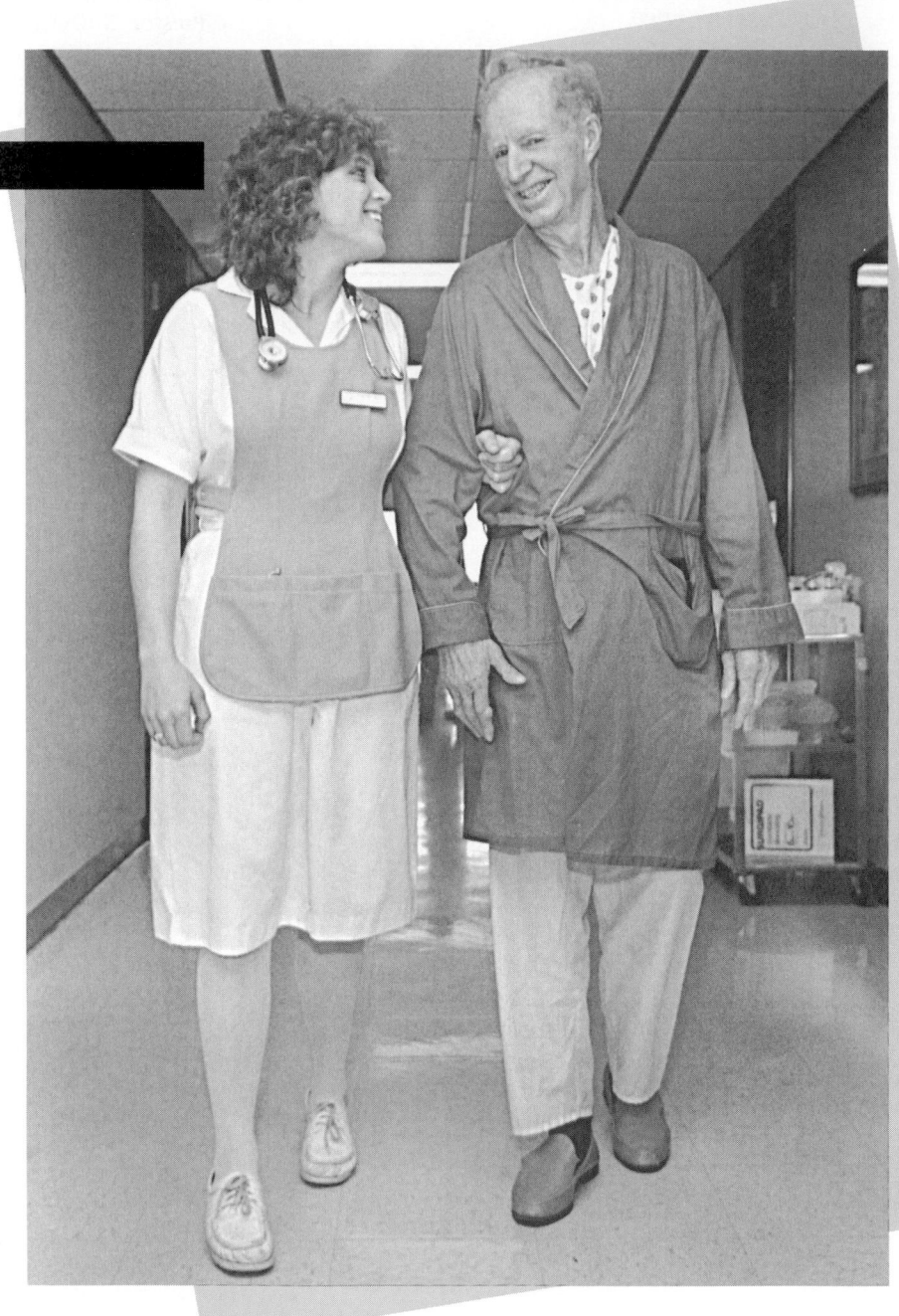

For the majority of healthy individuals, the ability for movement is taken for granted. We simply expect our amazingly complex skeletal, skeletal muscle, and nervous systems to work together smoothly and on command to enable us to stand upright, to walk, and to reach for and to grasp what we want. Often little thought is given to the need to care for the systems that promote and coordinate healthy movement until disuse, trauma, or illness cripples some aspect of movement. Although exercise and fitness are valued by some, many persons live over-whelmingly inactive life-styles that limit their ability to experience and enjoy life to its fullest and that openly invite degenerative and chronic diseases such as hypertension, ischemic heart disease, diabetes, and others.

The ability to move is closely related to the fulfillment of other basic human needs. Although breathing continues during rest, movement facilitates pulmonary functioning and increases peripheral blood flow. Since regular exercise contributes to the healthy functioning of each body system and, conversely, immobility negatively affects each body system, nurses actively promote exercise to promote wellness, prevent illness, and restore health. It is now generally accepted that there are more serious health consequences related to a sedentary life-style than there are risks related to exercise.

Study of this chapter provides the student with knowledge of the physiology of movement, the principles of body mechanics, and factors affecting body alignment and mobility. A comprehensive section on exercise differentiates types of exercise, explores the role of exercise in disease prevention and health promotion, notes risks related to exercise, and allows the design of individualized exercise programs. The effects of immobility on body systems are presented with a full discussion of related nursing interventions. A practical guide to assessing body alignment and mobility states is offered with pertinent interview questions and physical assessment techniques. Analysis of mobility data may lead to the nursing diagnoses of impaired physical mobility or activity intolerance or to diagnoses identifying the effect of mobility problems on other areas of human functioning. Examples of nursing diagnoses are included. Client goals are identified and specific nursing strategies are presented. In the section entitled Nursing Process in Clinical Practice, focused assessment, planning, implementation, and evaluation guides are offered for select nursing diagnoses of common mobility problems: Activity intolerance; Impaired physical mobility; Potential for injury: complications of immobility; and Alteration in health maintenance: lack of exercise program. These guides and the concluding case study illustrate how the nurse's knowledge of body mechanics and mobility is combined with specific nursing interventions and caring to successfully promote fitness and to resolve mobility problems.

KEY TERMS

abduction
active exercise
active-assistive exercise
adduction
aerobic exercise
ankylosis
atelectasis
atrophy
base of support
body mechanics
center of gravity
contractures
dangling
disuse osteoporosis
dorsiflexion
endurance
eversion
extension
external rotation
fitness
flaccidity
flexibility
flexion
footdrop
Fowler's position
hemiplegia
hyperextension

internal rotation
inversion
isokinetic exercise
isometric exercise
isotonic exercise
line of gravity
movement/daily life
  activities
orthopedics
osteoporosis
paraplegia
passive exercise
plantar flexion
pronation
prone position
range of motion
rotation
semi-Fowler's position
spasticity
strength
strength and endurance
  exercises
stretching exercises
supination
supine position
Sims' position
synovial joints
tonus
target heart range

PHYSIOLOGY OF MOVEMENT

Purposeful coordinated movement of the body requires the integrated functioning of the skeletal, skeletal muscle, and nervous systems of the body. A review of the physiology of movement is given here.

Skeletal System

The framework of bones and cartilages that protects our organs and allows us to move is called the *skeletal system*. Functions of this system include the following:

- It *supports* the soft tissues of the body (maintains body form and posture).

- It *protects* the delicate structures of the body (brain, lung, heart, spinal cord).
- It *furnishes surfaces for the attachments of muscles, tendons, and ligaments,* which in turn pull on the individual bones and produce *movement.*
- It serves as *storage areas* for mineral salts and fat.
- It produces blood cells (hematopoiesis).

The 206 bones in the human body are classified on the basis of their shape. *Long bones* are found in the upper and lower extremities; they contribute to height and length. *Short bones* are located in the wrist and ankle and they contribute to movement. *Flat bones* are relatively thin (*e.g.,* ribs and several of the skull bones) and contribute to shape (structural contour). And *irregular bones* are all those bones not included in the above classifications (*e.g.,* bones of the spinal column and jaw).

T A B L E 28-1
Terms Commonly Used to Describe Body Positions and Movements

Term	Definition and Example
Abduction	Lateral movement of a body part away from the midline of the body. Example: A person's arm is abducted when it is moved away from the body.
Adduction	Lateral movement of a body part toward the midline of the body. Example: A person's arm is adducted when it is moved from an outstretched position to a position alongside the body.
Flexion	The state of being bent. Example: A person's cervical spine is flexed when the head is bent forward chin to chest.
Extension	The state of being in a straight line. Example: A person's cervical spine is extended when the head is held straight on the spinal column.
Hyperextension	The state of exaggerated extension. It often results in an angle greater than 180 degrees. Example: A person's cervical spine is hyperextended when looking overhead, toward the ceiling.
Dorsiflexion	Backward bending of the hand or foot. Example: A person's foot is in dorsiflexion when the toes are brought up as though to point them at the knee.
Plantar flexion	Flexion of the foot. Example: A person's foot is in plantar flexion in the footdrop position.
Rotation	Turning on an axis; the turning of a body part on the axis provided by its joint. Example: A thumb is rotated when it is moved to make a circle.
Internal rotation	A body part turning on its axis to ward the midline of the body. Example: A leg is rotated internally when it turns inward at the hip and the toes point toward the midline of the body.
External rotation	A body part turning on its axis away from the midline of the body. Example: A leg is rotated externally when it turns outward at the hip and the toes point away from the midline of the body.
Special Movements	
Pronation	The assumption of the prone position. Examples: A person is in the prone position when lying on the abdomen: a person's palm is prone when the forearm is turned so that the palm faces downward.
Supination	The assumption of the supine position. Examples: A person is in the supine position when lying on the back; a person's palm is supine when the forearm is turned so that the palm faces upward.
Inversion	Movement of the sole of the foot inward (occurs at the ankle)
Eversion	Movement of the sole of the foot outward (occurs at the ankle)

Since bones are too rigid to bend without damage, all movements that change the positions of the bony parts of the body occur at joints. The terms *articulation* and *joint* refer to the area where bones come into close contact with one another. Joints are classified according to the amount of movement they permit. Of concern here are the freely movable joints called *diarthroses* or **synovial joints**, in which there is a space between the articulating bones. Movements possible at diarthrotic joints include abduction, adduction, flexion, extension, and rotation. Special movements of the forearm, ankle, and clavicle include supination, pronation, inversion, and eversion. These are defined in Table 28-1 and illustrated in Figure 28-11. Types of freely movable joints include

- *Ball-and-socket joint:* Rounded head of one bone fits into a cup-like cavity in the other; flexion–extension, abduction–adduction, and rotation are permitted (*e.g.,* shoulder and hip joints).
- *Condyloid joint:* Oval head of one bone fits into a shallow cavity of another bone; flexion–extension and abduction–adduction are permitted (*e.g.,* wrist joint).
- *Gliding joint:* Articular surfaces are flat; flexion-extension and abduction–adduction are permitted (*e.g.,* carpal bones of wrist and tarsal bones of feet).
- *Hinge joint:* Spool-like surface fits into a concave surface; only flexion–extension is permitted (*e.g.,* elbow, knee, and ankle joints).
- *Pivot joint:* Ring-like structure that turns on a pivot; movement is limited to rotation, for example, turning a doorknob (*e.g.,* joints between the atlas and axis and between the proximal ends of the radius and the ulna).
- *Saddle joint:* Bone surfaces are convex on one side and concave on the other; movements are side to side and back and forth (*e.g.,* joint between the trapezium and metacarpal of the thumb).

The strength and flexibility of the skeletal system also depend on ligaments, tendons, and cartilage. Ligaments are tough, fibrous bands that bind joints together and connect bones and cartilages. Tendons are strong, flexible, inelastic fibrous bands that attach muscle to bone. Cartilage is nonvascular connective tissue found in the joints as well as in the nose, ear, thorax, trachea, and larynx.

Muscular System

Bones and joints provide form to the body and serve as the levers and fulcrums that make body movement possible. It is the contraction and relaxation of skeletal muscles, however, that actually produce movement by pulling on bones. The excitability, contractility, extensibility, and elasticity of muscles enable them to perform three important functions for the body through contraction:

- Motion
- Maintenance of posture (Skeletal muscle contractions hold the body in stationary positions.)
- Heat production (Skeletal muscle contractions produce heat and help maintain body temperature.)

There are actually three types of muscles: skeletal, cardiac, and smooth or visceral. The skeletal muscle system includes the skeletal muscle tissue and connective tissues that make up individual muscle organs, such as the biceps. Movement is the result of a skeletal muscle contracting and exerting force on a tendon; which in turn pulls on a bone. Muscles have two differing points of attachment: attachment of a muscle to the more stationary bone is called the *point of origin* and attachment to the more movable bone is the *point of insertion*. Between these two points is the fleshy "belly" of the muscle. Figure 28-1 illustrates the relationship of skeletal muscles to bones and the use of bones as levers and joints as fulcrums to produce body movement.

Nervous System

The skeletal and muscular systems cannot produce purposeful movement without a functioning nervous system. It is a nerve impulse that stimulates muscles to contract. More specifically

- The afferent nervous system conveys information from receptors in the periphery of the body to the central nervous system (*e.g.,* light pressure on nose).
- Nerve cells called *neurons* are responsible for conducting impulses from one part of the body to another.
- This information is processed by the central nervous system (CNS) and a response is decided on (*e.g.,* "There is a fly on my nose I want to brush it off").
- The efferent system conveys the desired response from the CNS to skeletal muscles by way of the somatic nervous system (*e.g.,* muscles in the arm, wrist, and hand contract and the fingers brush the fly from the face).

Body Mechanics

Body mechanics is the efficient use of the body as a machine and as a means of locomotion. Body mechanics is directly related to the effective functioning of the body. The correct use of body mechanics should be evident in every activity and even during periods of rest.

Because correct use of the body is another phase of prevention of illness and the promotion of health, the nurse has a major responsibility to teach, both directly and indirectly by example. To be able to evaluate the client's musculoskeletal needs, the nurse must understand and utilize correct body mechanics. Every activity

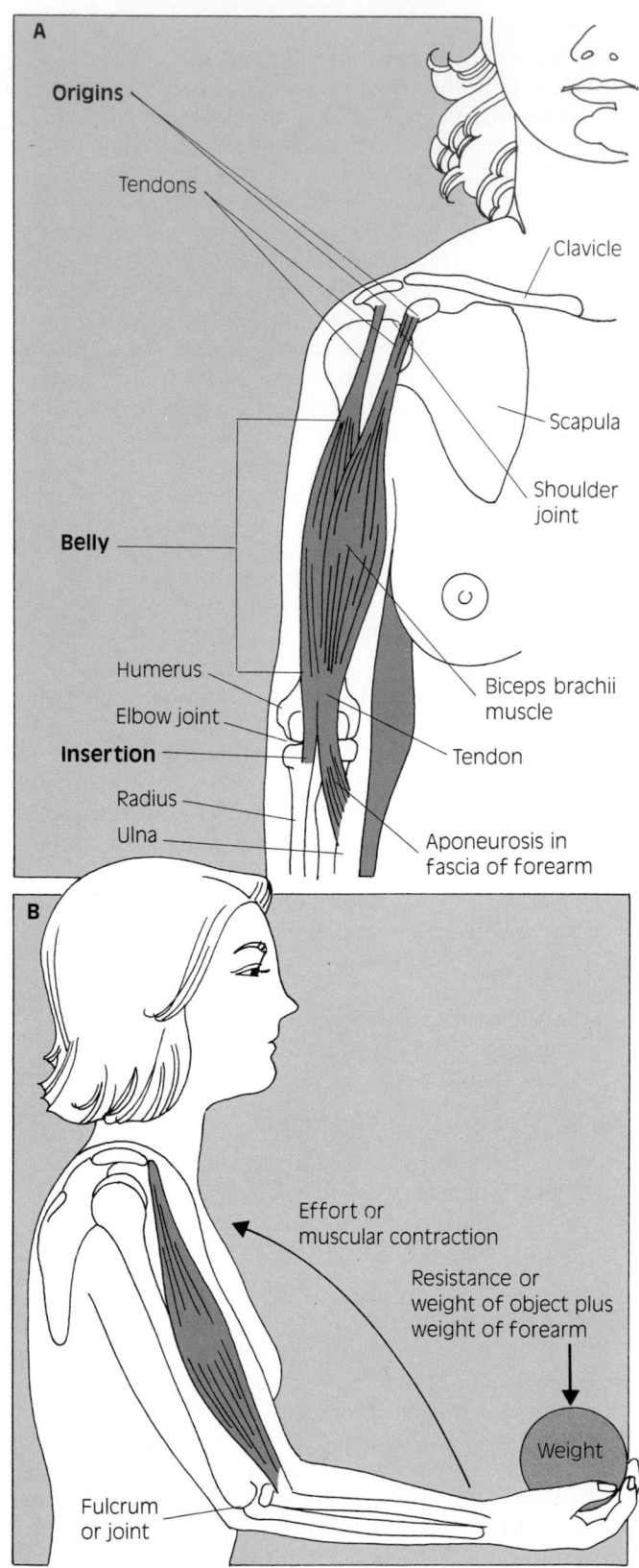

F I G U R E 28-1

Relationship of skeletal muscles to bones. (Top) Skeletal muscles produce movements by pulling on bones. (Bottom) Bones serve as levers, and joints act as fulcrums for the levers. The lever–fulcrum principle is illustrated by the movement of the forearm lifting a weight.

in which the nurse engages will require understanding and use of these principles, from as simple an activity as moving a chair to lifting a client out of bed.

Orthopedics means the correction or the prevention of disorders of the body's structures for locomotion. Nurses have long recognized that basic orthopedic principles are applicable to all areas of nursing, not just to the client who has a bone fracture or some other pathologic skeletal change. For example, the person who has a sedentary occupation and engages in little physical activity may have poorly developed muscles. The client who is on complete bed rest is in danger of losing muscle tonus. **Tonus** is the term used to describe the state of slight contraction in which we normally find skeletal muscles. Should the bed rest be prolonged, there is danger of developing contractures if the client does not have exercise and joint motion and if provision is not made for maintaining good posture. Functioning of various internal body processes is also influenced by position and movement or by their absence.

Concepts of Body Mechanics

Concepts most helpful to the understanding of body mechanics are body alignment, balance, and coordinated movement.

Body Alignment or Posture. Good posture or good body alignment is that alignment of body parts that permits optimal musculoskeletal balance and operation and promotes healthy physiologic functioning. A person in correct alignment is experiencing no undue strain on the joints, muscles, tendons, or ligaments while balance is maintained. Criteria for correct alignment in the standing, sitting, and reclining positions are presented in the assessment section later in this chapter.

Balance. A body in correct alignment is balanced. An object is balanced when (1) its center of gravity is close to its base of support, (2) the line of gravity goes through the base of support, and (3) the object has a wide base of support. The **center of gravity** of an object is the point at which its mass is centered. In humans, the center of gravity when standing is located in the center of the pelvis approximately midway between the umbilicus and the symphysis pubis. The **line of gravity** is a vertical line that passes through the center of gravity. The **base of support** is the foundation that provides for an object's stability. The wider the base of support and the lower the center of gravity, the greater the stability of the object. Figure 28-2 illustrates body balance.

Nurses can increase body balance when working by spreading their feet farther apart (broadening the base of support) and by flexing their hips and knees (lowering the center of gravity). These two simple maneuvers are important principles in body mechanics by which nurses can decrease musculoskeletal strain.

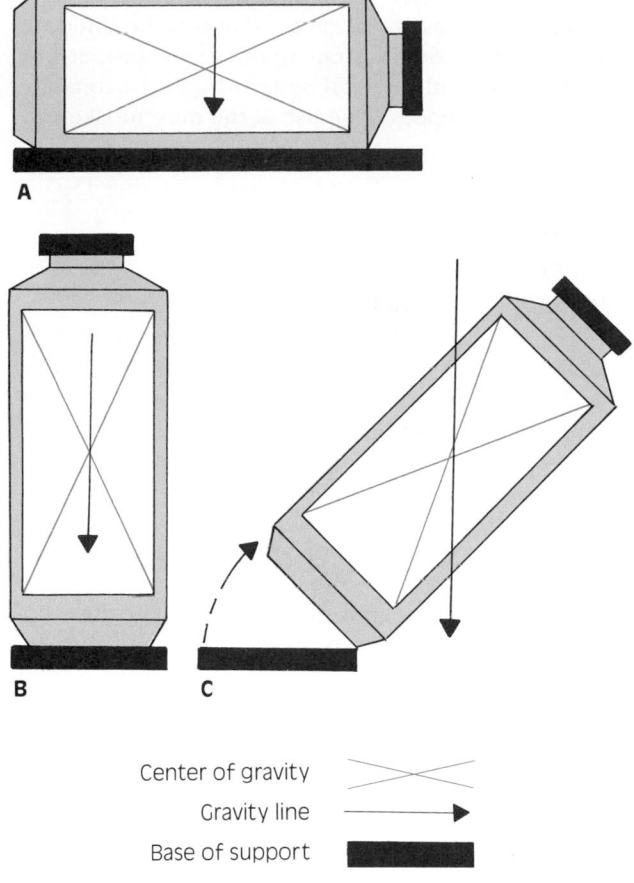

Center of gravity ⊠
Gravity line →
Base of support ▮

FIGURE 28-2
The effect of the base of support and gravity on balance is shown. (A) The line of gravity passes through the wide base of support. This object is the most stable of the three. (B) The line of gravity also passes through the base of support, although the base is narrower. This object is less stable than the one on the left. (C) The line of gravity does not pass through the base of support. This object is unstable.

Coordinated Body Movement. Since the nurse providing direct client care must frequently use the body to assist in positioning, turning, and lifting both clients and equipment, it is important to do this knowledgeably to avoid musculoskeletal strain and injury. This work is facilitated when the nurse uses major muscle groups rather than weaker ones and takes advantage of the body's natural levers and fulcrums. For example, rather than attempt to push a client to the opposite side of the bed, the nuse flexes the knees, positions the forearms above and below the client's buttocks (preferably under a pull sheet), and rocks backward sliding the client toward self. This one coordinated movement illustrates the following principles:

- The nurse is using major muscle groups—flexors, extensors, and abductors of the thighs; flexors and extensors of the knees; flexors and extensors of the upper and lower arms—rather than weaker ones.
- Use of the arm bones as levers and the elbows as

fulcrums facilitates lifting a weight against resistance (force of gravity)—lever–fulcrum principle.
- Using a pull sheet and smooth, dry, firm bed foundation decreases the effects of friction, which increases the amount of effort required to move an object. Rough, wet, or soiled surfaces contribute to friction's effect.
- By positioning the arms under the client's center of gravity (hips) and sliding it back toward self, the nurse is working close to the object to be moved and decreasing the effort involved.

Postural Reflexes

Integrated functioning of the musculoskeletal and nervous systems is essential for body alignment and balance. Postural tonus, the sustained contraction of select skeletal muscles that keeps the human body in an upright position against the force of gravity, depends on the functioning of several postural reflexes:

Labyrinthine Sense: This is provided by the sensory organs in the inner ear, which are stimulated by body movement (changes in head position) and transmit these impulses to the cerebellum.

Proprioceptor or Kinesthetic Sense: This informs the brain of the location of a limb or body part as a result of joint movements stimulating special nerve endings in muscles, tendons, and fascia.

Visual or Optic Reflexes: Visual impressions contribute to posture by alerting the person to spatial relationships with the environment (nearness of ceilings, walls, furniture, condition of floor, and so on).

Extensor or Stretch Reflexes: Conceivably the force of gravity could exert enough force to flex the body at the hip and knees; when extensor muscles are stretched beyond a certain point (*e.g.,* when knees buckle under) their stimulation causes a reflex contraction that reestablishes erect posture.

Body Mechanics Used for Work

The following guidelines are offered for the use of body mechanics when the person is at work:

- Develop a habit of erect posture (correct alignment) and whenever necessary begin activities by broadening the base of support and lowering the center of gravity.
- Use the longest and the strongest muscles of the arms and the legs to help provide the power needed in strenuous activities. The muscles of the back are less strong and are easily injured when used improperly.
- Use the internal girdle and a long midriff to stabilize the pelvis and to protect the abdominal viscera when stooping, reaching, lifting, or pulling. The in-

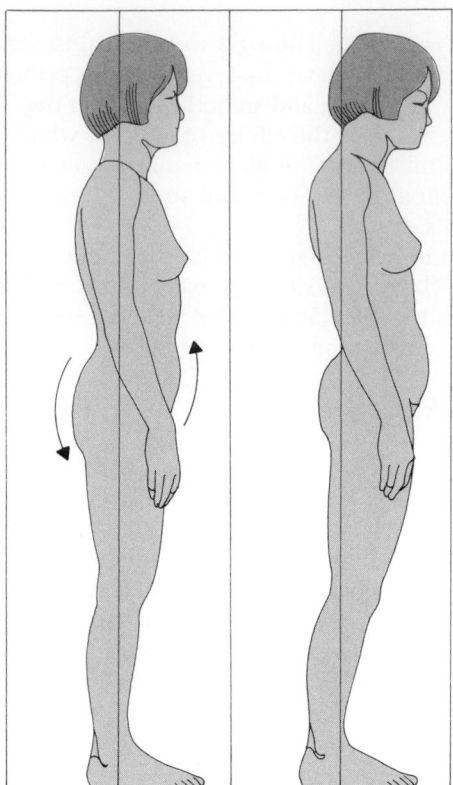

F I G U R E   28-3
(Left) *Internal girdle "on." Abdominal muscles contracted, giving a feeling of upward pull, and gluteal muscles contracted, giving a downward pull.* (Right) *Slouch position, showing abdominal muscles relaxed and body out of good alignment.*

ternal girdle is made by contracting the gluteal muscles in the buttocks downward and the abdominal muscles upward. It is helped further by making a long midriff. This is done by stretching the muscles in the waist. Figure 28-3 illustrates the internal girdle.

• Work as close as possible to an object that is to be lifted or moved. This brings the body's center of gravity close to that of the object being moved, thereby permitting most of the burden to be borne by the leg and arm muscles. Figure 28-4 illustrates a proper and an improper way to pick up an object.

• Use the weight of the body as a force for pulling or pushing, by rocking on the feet or leaning forward or backward. This reduces the amount of strain placed on the arms and the back.

• Slide, roll, push, or pull an object rather than lift it to reduce the energy needed to lift the weight against the pull of gravity.

• Use the weight of the body to push an object by falling or rocking forward, and to pull an object by falling or rocking backward. Sliding a client in bed while rocking backward is illustrated in Figure 28-5.

• Place the feet apart to provide a wider base of support when increased stability of the body is necessary.

• Flex the knees, put on the internal girdle, and come down close to an object that is to be lifted.

The nurse can demonstrate to others the proper way of using the musculoskeletal system if good habits are consciously developed in the use of the musculoskeletal system.

FACTORS AFFECTING BODY ALIGNMENT AND MOBILITY

Numerous factors, including growth and development, physical health, mental health, life-style variables, attitude and values, fatigue/stress, and external factors such as weather, influence an individual's posture, movement, and daily activity level.

Developmental Considerations

A person's age and degree of neuromuscular development markedly influence body proportions, posture,

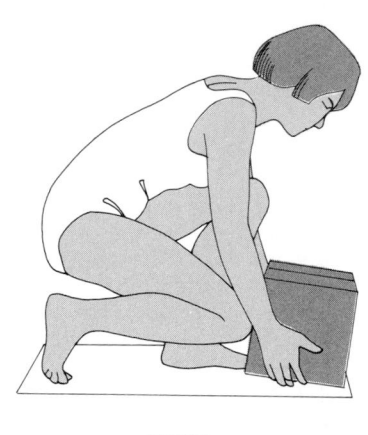

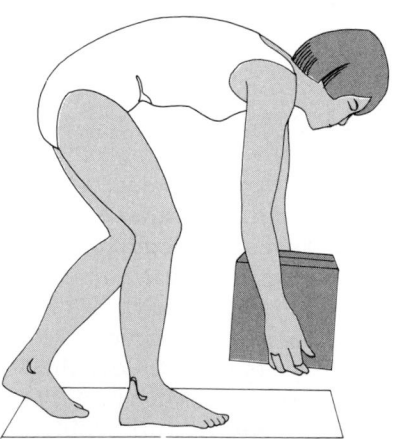

F I G U R E   28-4
(Top) *A good position for lifting is illustrated. This person is using the long and strong muscles of the arms and legs and holding the object so that the line of gravity falls within the base of support.* (Bottom) *This is a poor position for lifting because pull is exerted on the back muscles and leaning causes the line of gravity to fall outside the base.*

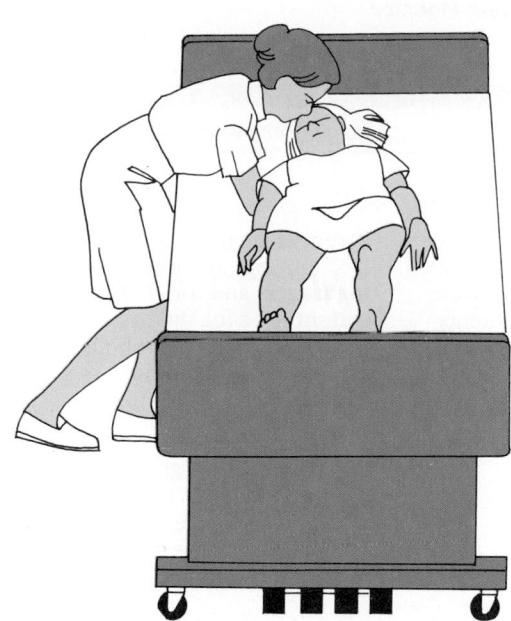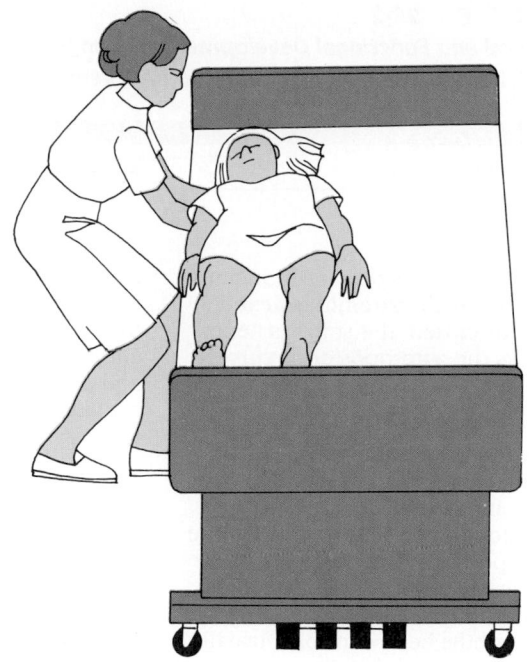

FIGURE   28-5
Before sliding a client to the edge of the bed, establish a wide base of support with one knee near the edge of the bed and both knees flexed. Place arms under the client as far as possible while close to and leaning over the client. Rock backward, using your own body weight to assist in moving the client toward you.

body mass, movements, and reflexes. To promote neuromuscular development in clients of all ages and to facilitate each client's use of the body to perform self-care actions, the nurse needs to be familiar with developmental variations in body proportions and neuromuscular development. These are presented in Table 28-2 with related nursing assessment priorities and nursing interventions.

Physical Health

Problems in the musculoskeletal or nervous systems can have a negative influence on body alignment and movement. Similarly, illness or trauma involving other body systems may also interfere with movement either because of the underlying pathology or the treatment regimen. Examples of these follow. Nurses need to develop sensitivity to how both acute and chronic health problems affect a client's general appearance (posture, body proportions, and movements) and ability to move purposefully to perform the activities of daily living. When assessing a client's response to a mobility deficit, the nurse

- Reinforces behaviors that promote healthy functioning (*e.g.,* congratulates a client who manages transfers well despite left-sided weakness or paralysis)
- Corrects behaviors that over time will compound the mobility deficit (*e.g.,* client with arthritis who

severely restricts movement because of joint stiffness and tenderness learns successful adaptive strategies that can be shared with other clients and families; or energy conservation measures used by clients with emphysema who have greatly decreased activity tolerance)

Musculoskeletal Problems

Congenital or Acquired Postural Abnormalities.
The newborn with congenital hip dysplasia or a clubfoot, the teenager with scoliosis (lateral curvature of the spine), and the elderly person with kyphosis (increased convexity in the curvature of the thoracic spine) are all experiencing postural abnormalities that affect appearance and mobility. Nursing responsibilities may include the following:

- Early detection and referral of these problems
- Client education, counseling, and support as treatment options are explored and selected
- Careful attention to positioning, transfers, and exercise
- Education of the client and family regarding safe self-care activities

Problems with Bone Formation or Muscle Development.   Problems with bone formation may be
- *Congenital,* such as achondroplasia, in which premature bone ossification leads to dwarfism, or os-

(Text continues on p. 628.)

T A B L E   28-2
Structural and Functional Developmental Changes in Body Alignment and Mobility With Related Nursing Assessment and Intervention Priorities

Developmental Changes	Assessment Priorities	Nursing Interventions

Infant

Structure: The newborn term infant usually lies with extremities flexed and hands closed; the spine is flexed and lacks the anteroposterior curves of the adult.

Function: The infant's spontaneous activity varies greatly. Periods of activity and alertness alternate with quiet periods and sleep.
• By 3 months of age the infant in the prone position is generally able to raise the chest and head from the floor.
• By 5 months head control is usually achieved in both the sitting position and when being held erect.

Newborn assessments should include attention to structure of spine and extremities (deformities), muscle tone and strength (abnormal movements and tremors), reflex responses, and activity level/alertness (jitteriness, lethargy, paresis).

3- to 6-month assessment
• Head control
• Ability to sit

6- to 9-month assessment
Gross motor
Ability to
• Sit steadily
• Roll over adeptly
• Creep on all fours
• Pull to a standing position

Fine motor
• Improved hand–eye coordination

9- to 12-month assessment
Gross motor
• Progress toward unassisted walking

Fine motor
• Skill in using hands—ability to pick up even tiny objects

Parents may need the nurse's help in "examining" their baby (*e.g.,* counting fingers and toes). This is an excellent time for the nurse to respond to any concerns parents have about minor variations in their newborn's appearance or behavior.

Nurses may need to explain to parents that there is great individual variation in total activity patterns and neuromuscular development among infants and children.

Toddler

Structure: The young toddler's long trunk, short legs, and undeveloped abdominal musculature (potbelly) give the toddler a top-heavy, sway-backed appearance. Growth during this period is rapid and faster in the legs than in the trunk. The young toddler walks on a broad base with flat feet that tend to toe in or out. Balance is achieved slowly.

Function: Both gross and fine motor development continue rapidly. By 15 months most toddlers can walk unassisted, they are running at 18 months of age and jumping by 2 years. By 3 years of age most toddlers can stack blocks, string large beads, work simple puzzles, and dress themselves.

Assess progress in walking, running, and jumping.

Assess small muscle coordination as evidenced in everyday skills: ability to dress themselves, wash hands, brush teeth.

Distinguish slow developers who fall within normal ranges from those whose developmental lags may indicate deprivation of environmental stimulation or retardation.

Since individual differences in motor activity, balance, and grace become very evident during this period, help parents to learn and accept their child's uniqueness.

Teach parents (1) the importance of providing a safe environment in which the toddler is free to explore, to satisfy curiosity, and to develop skill in motor control; (2) that reinforcement, enthusiasm, and praise for progress will stimulate the toddler's mastery of new skills; and (3) that limits need to be set so the toddler does not overextend himself in his newfound drive for mastery.

(Continued)

Developmental Changes	Assessment Priorities	Nursing Interventions

Toddler (continued)

The sense of mastery achieved through safe exploration and the practice of motor skills lays the foundation for all later physical, social, and intellectual pursuits.

Child

Structure: Between ages 3 and 6 the child's arms and legs continue to grow rapidly relative to the trunk and the child develops better balance. By age 6 the child has replaced "baby fat" with muscle, developed increased tone in abdominal muscles (loss of potbelly), and developed a more prominent chest.

Function: Muscles, bones, and the nervous system are developing a harmony that allows greater gross and fine motor control.
- By 4 years of age most children can negotiate stairs without using a hand rail, walk backwards, and hop on one foot.
- By 5 years most children have learned to skip, to play in running games, to jump rope, and to jump off heights of several steps.
- Progress in fine motor development is reflected in the child's manipulation of writing materials.
- By the time children enter school they have acquired all the basic mechanisms for physical locomotion they will use later in life.

Utilize developmental charts to assess gross and fine motor development.

Since important attitudes about the body and exercise are developed during childhood, parents should be questioned about these during the nursing history. Teach or counsel as appropriate.

Adolescent

Structure: There is considerable increase and change of the musculoskeletal system, resulting in increased size as well as the appearance of secondary sex characteristics. The adolescent growth spurt gives the adolescent an awkward, gangling appearance, and there is an increase in muscle mass and a decrease in fat, especially in boys.

Function: For the physically fit adolescent this can be a time of boundless energy and great athletic performance. Life-style factors (inactivity, poor nutrition) may begin a lifelong unhealthy pattern of immobility and disuse.

Interview the client to determine present activity level and type of regular exercise. Evaluate safety of recreational choices. Note history of any musculoskeletal or neurologic problems.

During the physical assessment note posture and alignment. Screening for scoliosis (lateral curvature of the spine) should be made prior to the adolescent's peak growth velocity and a referral made when there is more than a 15-degree curvature of the spine.

Examine muscle mass, tone, and strength and joint mobility.

Adolescents have many questions about their changing bodies and will often value nursing input although they seldom seek "professional" advice.

Life-style counseling regarding the importance of exercise and fitness is critical. Adolescents may need (1) encouragement to exercise regularly or (2) help in gauging their physical limits and a caution not to "push too hard."

(Continued)

T A B L E   28-2
**Structural and Functional Developmental Changes in Body Alignment and Mobility
With Related Nursing Assessment and Intervention Priorities   (Continued)**

Developmental Changes	Assessment Priorities	Nursing Interventions
Adult		
Structure: The healthy adult stands and sits erect and is capable of balanced and coordinated purposeful movement. During pregnancy the developing fetus shifts the mother's center of gravity forward and the mother compensates by leaning backward and walking with a broader base of support.	Assess the balance between activity and rest in the client's life-style and note any life-style factors or illnesses that interfere with the client's mobility or ability to carry out activities of daily living.	For most adults the most important nursing intervention is fitness counseling, which includes clarifying misconceptions about exercise and designing and monitoring safe exercise programs.
Function: Activity levels vary greatly among adults and are influenced by numerous factors explained in this chapter.		Clients with mobility alterations require special care.
Older Adult		
Structure: There is increased convexity in the thoracic spine (kyphosis) from disc shrinkage and decreased height, flexed posture, loss of muscle tone, and increased prominence of bony structure because of subcutaneous fat loss. Arthritic joint changes are often present.	Assess general ease of movement and gait; alignment; joint structure and function; and muscle mass, tone, and strength.	Teach/counsel clients about • Importance of regular exercise • Need to maintain appropriate weight to reduce stress on joints • Need for high-protein, calcium and Vitamin D–enriched diet • To pace activities to compensate for decreased strength • To use assistive devices safely when needed • To safety-proof homes to reduce likelihood of falls
Function: General slowness of movement with progressive decrease in activity tolerance.		

teogenesis imperfecta, which is characterized by excessively brittle bones and multiple fractures both at birth and later in life
• *Dietary related,* for example, vitamin D deficiency, which results in deformities of the growing skeleton (rickets)
• *Disease related,* such as in Paget's disease where excessive bone destruction and abnormal regeneration result in skeletal pain, deformities, and pathologic fractures
• *Age related,* such as osteoporosis, in which bone destruction exceeds bone formation; the resultant thin, porous bones fracture easily.

The muscular dystrophies are a group of genetically transmitted disorders that have in common progressive degeneration and weakness of skeletal muscles. They vary in terms of the muscle groups involved and their clinical course. Myasthenia gravis is a weakness of the skeletal muscles caused by an abnormality at the neuromuscular junction that prevents muscle fibers from contracting.

Nursing responsibilities with problems of bone formation and muscle development and functioning include
• Careful collaboration with the physician and health-care team to determine the motor capacities of the individual
• Client and family education aimed at developing optional mobility
The nurse must be knowledgeable about the underlying disease process and be able to position, lift, transfer, and exercise the client safely, with attention to client comfort.

Problems Affecting Joint Mobility.   Inflammation, degeneration, and trauma can all interfere with joint mobility. The term *arthritis* describes more than twenty diseases, all characterized by inflammation in one or more joints and possibly pain and stiffness in adjacent body parts. *Degenerative joint disease,* also termed *osteoarthritis,* is a noninflammatory, progressive disorder of movable joints, particularly weight-bearing joints, characterized by the deterioration of articular cartilage and pain with motion. Spurs form, which restrict joint movement. Trauma to a joint may result in either (1) a *sprain,* in which the wrenching or twisting of a joint results in a partial tear or rupture to its attachments, or (2) a *dislocation,* that is, the displacement of a bone from a joint with tearing of ligaments, tendons, and capsules. Any condition restricting joint mobility has potentially crippling effects.

The nurse caring for clients with joint problems works collaboratively with the physician and physical therapist to maintain joint mobility. Client education is directed to the client's mastery of an exercise and care program, which fosters tissue repair and maximal independence in activities of daily living.

Problems Affecting the Central Nervous System

A problem in any of the principal parts of the brain or spinal cord concerned with skeletal muscle control can affect mobility:

- *Cerebral motor cortex:* Assumes the major role of controlling precise, discrete movements. A cerebrovascular accident (stroke) or head trauma may damage the motor cortex and produce temporary or permanent voluntary motor impairment.
- *Basal ganglia:* Integrate semivoluntary movements such as walking, swimming, and laughing. In Parkinson's disease there is progressive degeneration of the basal ganglia of the cerebrum. Unnecessary skeletal movements result in tremors and muscle rigidity, which interfere with voluntary movement.
- *Cerebellum:* Assists the motor cortex and basal ganglia by making body movements smooth and coordinated. In multiple sclerosis, the myelin sheaths of neurons in the CNS deteriorate to hardened scars or plaques. Plaque formation in the cerebellum may produce lack of coordination of one hand.
- *Pyramidal pathways:* Voluntary motor impulses are conveyed from the brain through the spinal cord by way of two major pathways: the pyramidal and extrapyramidal pathways. With trauma to the spinal cord, transection of these motor pathways results in complete bilateral loss of voluntary movement below the level of the trauma.

The overwhelming complaint of clients with injury to the CNS is that no one talks with them (or with their families) about how the disease will progress and affect their functioning. Nurses caring for these clients need knowledge about the pathology and clinical course of these diseases so that appropriate client education and counseling can take place.

Trauma to the Musculoskeletal System

Injury to the musculoskeletal system can result in fractures and soft tissue injuries. A fracture is a break in the continuity of the structure of bone or cartilage. It may result from a traumatic injury or occur as a result of some underlying disease process. Healing requires realignment of the bone fragment, immobilization, and restoration of the bone's function. Soft tissue injuries include sprains, strains, and dislocations. Dislocations and sprains are discussed above, under Problems Affecting Joint Mobility. A strain, the least serious of these injuries, is a stretching of a muscle. Nurses need to be knowledgeable in first-aid measures for musculoskeletal trauma as well as in acute and rehabilitative care.

Problems Involving Other Body Systems

The pathology of numerous other acute and chronic illnesses may also affect mobility. Chronic obstructive lung disease and conditions such as ascites may alter posture. Any illnesses that interfere with oxygenation at the cellular level decrease the amount of oxygen available to the muscles for work and thus decrease activity tolerance. These illnesses include anemia, angina, cardiac arrhythmias, congestive heart failure, and chronic obstructive pulmonary disease. Diseases characterized by negative nitrogen balance (*e.g.,* anorexia nervosa and certain cancers) result in muscle wasting and decreased physical energy for movement and work. Symptoms accompanying many illnesses such as fatigue, muscle aches, and pain may also immobilize clients. Finally, bed rest is an important component of the treatment regimen for many diseases or trauma states such as myocardial infarction, surgery, and fractures. Although rest is integral to the healing process, immobility may cause its own problems (see Table 28-8). Nurses need to be vigilant in determining the impact any injury or illness will have on mobility and in providing care that facilitates optimal mobility.

Mental Health

Just as an individual's physical health influences body appearance and movement, so also does mental health. Bodily processes tend to slow down in depression and there is a lack of visible energy and enthusiasm. The depressed person often sits with the head bowed and shoulders slumped and may lack the energy to feed or even toilet self. Even facial movement may be decreased to the point where the individual's face registers no emotion (termed a *flat affect*). On the other hand, "high-energy" individuals have erect posture and animated facial features.

Life-Style Variables

Whether an individual opts for an active or sedentary life-style is influenced by many factors. Among the most important are an individual's occupation, leisure activity preferences, and cultural influences. Since the majority of professional occupations as well as many blue-collar jobs are sedentary in nature, individuals wishing to exercise regularly need to plan leisure activities that give the body a workout. Cultural influences may encourage or discourage exercise. For example, currently in North America it is popular for both male and female professionals to engage in some form of aerobic exercise. In the not so distant past it was considered "unladylike" for women to be involved in most sports activities. Other life-style variables that influence mobility include a person's diet and smoking history.

Attitude and Values

In some families, such as those that hike together, swim together, and play ball together, children learn early to value regular exercise. As these children mature they often continue to value exercise and find new ways to incorporate regular exercise into their daily routine. Similarly, children may be raised in sedentary families where watching sports is the closest anyone comes to exercise. This attitude may also be internalized for a lifetime. Many individual values also explain the exercise options persons make. Individuals who place a high value on physical attractiveness may be highly committed to regular exercise because it produces the body they want. Another individual may exercise because of the desire for physical strength, relating strength with power. Someone more disposed to intellectual pursuits may perceive body development as simply wasting time that could be better utilized to develop the mind.

Fatigue/Stress

Chronic stress may deplete body energy to the point that fatigue makes even the thought of exercise overwhelming. Ironically, regular exercise is energizing and can better equip a person to deal with daily stresses. At the same time, excessive exercise may stress the body in a harmful way and lead to injury as well as to fatigue.

External Factors

Many external factors can influence mobility. Among these, weather probably exerts the greatest influence. A brisk, clear day is invigorating and invites increased activity. High humidity and high temperatures, on the other hand, discourage any extra movement. Sufficient financial resources for exercise memberships and equipment, safe outdoor parks and sports areas, support persons, and occupational or insurance rewards for exercise can all encourage regular exercise. Detractors include insufficient funds, air pollution, unsafe neighborhoods, and lack of support and reinforcement.

EXERCISE

Active exertion of muscles involving the contraction and relaxation of muscle groups is termed *exercise.* There are many different types of exercise and each type has the potential to produce different physiologic and psychologic benefits.

Types of Exercise

Muscle Contraction. Exercise may be categorized according to the type of muscle contraction involved as being isotonic, isometric, or isokinetic (Fig 28-6).

Isotonic exercise involves muscle shortening and active movement. Examples include carrying out activities of daily living, independently performing range-of-motion exercises, and swimming, walking, jogging, and bicycling. Potential benefits include increased muscle mass, tone, and strength; improved joint mobility; increased cardiac and respiratory function; increased circulation; and increased osteoblastic activity. When the nurse or family member performs passive range-of-motion exercises for a client, the client's muscles do not exert effort and potential benefits are reduced to improved joint mobility and increased circulation.

Isometric exercise involves muscle contraction without shortening (*i.e.,* there is no movement or a minimum shortening of muscle fibers). Examples include contractions of the quadriceps and gluteal muscles. Potential benefits are increased muscle mass, tone, and strength; increased circulation to the exercised body part; and increased osteoblastic activity. Nurses encourage both isotonic and isometric exercises for hospitalized clients with limited mobility.

Isokinetic exercise involves muscle contractions with resistance, varying at a constant rate produced by a device with a capacity for variable resistance. Examples include rehabilitative exercises for knee and elbow injuries. Using the isokinetic device the muscles and joint are taken through a complete range of motion without stopping with resistance at every point.

Body Movement. Exercise activities may also be categorized according to the type of body movement involved and the health benefits they produce. Hill and Smith (1985) offer the following breakdown.

- **Aerobic exercise:** Sustained (often rhythmical) muscle movements that increase blood flow, heart rate, and metabolic demand for oxygen over a period of time promote cardiovascular conditioning. Activities that *may* be aerobic are swimming, jogging, cross-country skiing, aerobic dance, bicycling, jumping rope, and racquetball. (Aerobic exercise may be further distinguished as having high versus low impact. The number of injuries, such as

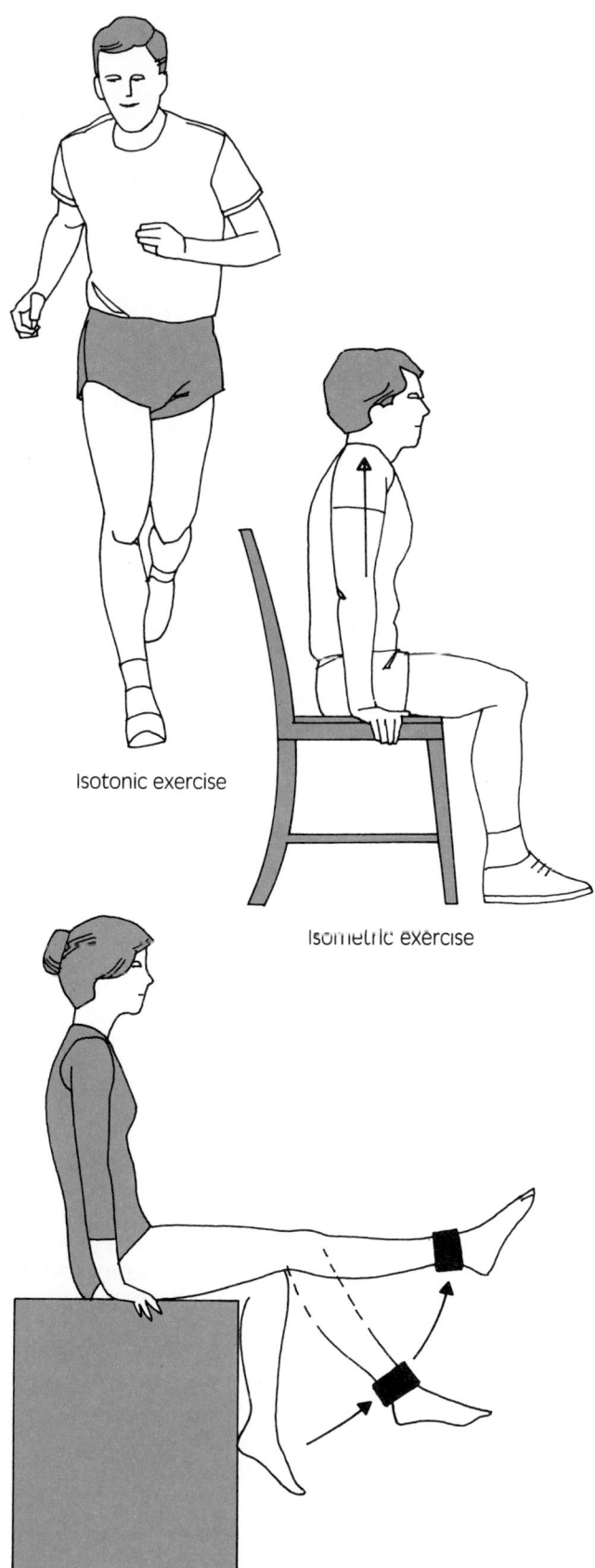

Isotonic exercise

Isometric exercise

Isokinetic exercise

shin splints, related to high-impact aerobic workouts led to the development of low-impact workouts that place less stress on the musculoskeletal system.)

- **Stretching exercises**: Movements that allow muscles and joints to be stretched gently through their full range of motion increase flexibility. Specific warm-up and cool-down exercises, hatha yoga, 'tai 'chi,' and some forms of dance are examples. Benefits include increased range of joint movements, improved circulation and posture, and relaxation.
- **Strength and endurance exercises**: A variety of muscle-building programs fall into this category. Weight training, calisthenics, and specific isometric exercises can build both strength and endurance, increasing the power of the musculoskeletal system and generally improving the whole body. They may or may not have aerobic benefit.
- **Movement/daily life activities**: House cleaning, running after playful toddlers, climbing stairs instead of riding in elevators, all have an impact on health. Increased fitness does not require a gym.

Effects of Exercise and Immobility on Major Body Systems

The human body was designed for motion, and regular exercise is necessary for its healthy functioning. Individuals who choose inactive life-styles or who are forced to inactivity by illness or injury place themselves at high risk for serious health problems. The effects of both regular exercise and immobility on major body systems are explored in this section. Just as individuals differ in the benefits they receive from exercise, so, too, complications resulting from immobility differ in their occurrence and severity according to the client's age and overall health state.

Cardiovascular System

Effects of Exercise.   In order to meet the demand for oxygen created by the rhythmic contraction and relaxation of skeletal muscle groups, the supply of oxygenated blood to skeletal muscle needs to be increased. The cardiovascular system meets this challenge by increasing the heart rate, increasing the contractile strength of the myocardium, and increasing stroke volume (volume of blood ejected), thus increasing cardiac output. Arterial (systolic) blood pressure is increased and blood is

---

F I G U R E   28-6
Three types of exercise: isotonic, involving muscle shortening and active movement; isometric, involving muscle contraction without shortening; and isokinetic, involving muscle contraction with resistance.

R E S E A R C H I N N U R S I N G *Making a Difference*

Exercise

Exercise is an essential component in improving circulation and maintaining muscle strength and joint mobility. Nursing interventions have traditionally been carried out to prevent the complications associated with immobility, but nursing research has expanded the scope of nursing in this area by analyzing exercise as a therapy in maximizing the health status of clients at all levels of wellness.

Related Research

Byers P: Effect of exercise on morning stiffness and mobility in patients with rheumatoid arthritis. Research in Nursing and Health 8(3):275–281, 1985

Byers carried out this research to test the hypothesis that exercise before evening bedtime would reduce morning stiffness and improve joint mobility in clients with rheumatoid arthritis. Findings from the study supported this hypothesis; effects of exercise were significant in decreasing stiffness and improving joint mobility. Byers suggests that nurses who prescribe exercises for the arthritic client should evaluate both subjective and objective data when determining effectiveness.

Estok P, Rudy E: Marathon running: Comparison of physical and psychosocial risks for men and women. Research in Nursing and Health 10:79–85, 1987

The purpose of this study was to compare physical, psychologic, and addictive behavioral effects reported by male and female runners. There was no difference found in incidence or kind of self-esteem or negative addiction to running. Physical injuries significantly related to running were torn ligaments and hematuria. The researchers noted a relationship between running and positive life-style changes despite the musculoskeletal injuries.

Summary

Nursing research in the area of exercise and physical fitness has important implications for promoting wellness and preventing illness. Life-style changes to behaviors that promote normal physiologic functioning have lifelong effects, and exercises to improve alterations in tissue function are beneficial in improving self-care and independence.

---

shunted from the nonexercising tissues to the heart and muscles. Exercise also improves venous return as the contracting muscles compress superficial veins and push blood back to the heart against gravity. Over time, with cardiovascular conditioning, regular exercise produces the following benefits:

- Increased efficiency of the heart
- Decreased heart rate and blood pressure
- Increased blood flow to all body parts
- Increased circulating fibrinolysin (substance that breaks up small clots)

Effects of Immobility. The primary and serious effects of immobility on the cardiovascular system include increased cardiac workload, orthostatic hypotension, and venous thrombosis.

Immobility results in an increased workload for the heart. It has been demonstrated that the heart works more when the person is resting; probably because there is less resistance offered by the blood vessels and because there is a change in the distribution of blood in the immobile person. As a result, the heart rate, cardiac output, and stroke volume increase.

Immobility predisposes to thrombi formation owing to venous stasis, especially in the legs, where normal muscular activity helps move blood toward the central circulatory system. Thrombus formation is also caused by an increased rate in the coagulation of blood, one reason being that during periods of immobility, calcium leaves bones and enters the blood, where it has an influence on blood coagulation.

The immobile person is more susceptible to developing orthostatic hypotension. The person tends to feel weak and faint when the condition occurs. The phenomenon is probably due to a decrease in the neurovascular reflexes, which normally cause vasoconstriction, and to a loss of muscle tone. The result is that blood pools and does not squeeze from veins in the lower part of the body to the central circulatory system.

Pertinent nursing diagnoses and collaborative problems related to immobility include

Increased cardiac workload related to prolonged bed rest

Potential for injury: deep vein thrombosis related to venous stasis, hypercoagulability, and decreased muscle activity

Potential for injury: falls related to orthostatic hypotension

Respiratory System

Effects of Exercise.   The respiratory and cardiovascular systems work together to make increased oxygen available to the muscles. During exercise, the depth of respiration, respiratory rate, gas exchange at the alveolar level, and rate of carbon dioxide excretion are increased. Over time, regular exercise leads to improved pulmonary functioning.

Effects of Immobility.   Immobility's effects on the respiratory system are related to decreased ventilatory effort and increased respiratory secretions. Immobility causes a decrease in the depth and rate of respirations owing at least partially to a reduced need for oxygen by body cells. When areas of lung tissues are not used over a period of time, atelectasis may occur. **Atelectasis** is an incomplete expansion or collapse of lung tissue.

Immobility results in a poor exchange of carbon dioxide and oxygen, upsets their balance in the body, and results eventually in an acid–base imbalance.

When a person is immobile, the movement of secretions in the respiratory tract is decreased, resulting in the pooling of secretions and in respiratory tract congestion. These conditions predispose to respiratory tract infections. *Hypostatic pneumonia* is a type of pneumonia that results from inactivity and immobility. The situation worsens when the person is dehydrated or using pharmaceutical agents that increase the tenacity of secretions, depress the coughing mechanism, and depress respirations.

Decreased movement in the thoracic cage during respirations also results from immobility. This decrease may be due to loss of tonus in muscles involved with respirations, to pressure on the chest wall owing to the client's position in bed, and to depression of the respiratory apparatus by various pharmaceutical agents.

Pertinent nursing diagnoses related to immobility include

Ineffective breathing patterns related to limited chest expansion

Ineffective airway clearance related to decreased position changes, ineffective coughing, and stasis of secretions

Impaired gas exchange related to decreased respiratory movement (loss of muscle tonus)

Musculoskeletal System

Effects of Exercise.   The rhythmic contraction and relaxation of muscle groups during exercise result in increased muscle mass, tone, and strength and increased joint mobility. The more a person exercises, the more strength he or she has to exercise or work in the future. Regular exercise produces the following benefits:

• Increased muscle efficiency (strength) and flexibility

• Increased coordination
• Increased efficiency of nerve impulse transmission

Regular exercise is also believed to slow the effects of aging (*i.e.,* it helps prevent osteoporosis associated with aging).

Effects of Immobility.   Effects of immobility on the musculoskeletal system are rapidly seen in clients confined to bed. Persons attempting to walk after several days of bed rest are often surprised to find how weak their legs have become. Immobility (musculoskeletal disuse) leads to decreased muscle size (**atrophy**), tone, and strength; decreased joint mobility and flexibility; bone demineralization; and limited endurance, resulting in problems with activities of daily living.

Immobility is often the cause of **contractures**, which are permanent contraction states of muscle (muscle shortening), and **ankylosis**, which is a consolidation and immobilization of a joint. Contractures result from atrophy of muscles with resulting incompetence, and from a decrease in the muscle's strength, coordination, and endurance. A joint can be permanently fixed when ankylosed.

The process of bone demineralization (**osteoporosis**) is also increased in the immobile client. Normally the stress and strain of weight-bearing activity stimulate bone formation and balance destruction. With immobility, however, bone formation slows while breakdown increases, with a net loss of bone calcium, phosphorus, and matrix. This condition is termed **disuse osteoporosis** and is characterized by bones that may be either spongy or brittle. Bone demineralization may result in (1) pathologic fractures related to the bone's brittleness; (2) bone deformities related to the bone's sponginess; (3) arthropathy (joint disease) related to calcium depletion in the joints; and (4) renal calculi (stones) related to the excessive excretion of calcium through the kidneys and urinary tract.

Pertinent nursing diagnoses and collaborative problems related to immobility include

Activity intolerance related to decreased muscle mass, tone, and strength

Impaired physical mobility related to muscle atrophy (contractures) and limited joint mobility (ankylosis)

Potential injury: pathologic fracture related to excessive bone demineralization (disuse osteoporosis)

Self-care deficits related to decreased muscle strength and decreased flexibility

Metabolic System

Effects of Exercise.   The metabolic rate increases during exercise so that sufficient glucose and fatty acids can be converted to provide the energy needed for increased muscle function. During strenuous exercise the metabolic rate can increase to up to 20 times normal. Increased body heat and waste products are also produced. With regular exercise the body develops

- Increased efficiency of metabolic system
- Increased efficiency of body temperature regulation

Effects of Immobility.   Since the resting body requires less energy, the cellular demand for oxygen is decreased and this is reflected by a decreased metabolic rate. In many immobilized clients, however, factors such as fever, trauma, chronic illness, or poor nutrition can actually increase the body's metabolic demands and increase catabolism (the breakdown of the body's protein stores to provide energy to meet the body's energy requirements). If unchecked, this process results in muscle wasting. When more protein is being broken down than manufactured, the body excretes more nitrogen than it takes in and *negative nitrogen balance* occurs. Anorexia, or decreased appetite, often accompanies and compounds this problem. Negative nitrogen balance and poor nutrition thus worsen the muscle atrophy and weakness already resulting from immobility. Numerous fluid and electrolyte imbalances, alterations in the exchange of nutrients and gases at the cellular level, and gastrointestinal problems can all result from the above metabolic disturbances.

Pertinent nursing diagnoses related to immobility include

Altered nutrition: less than body requirements related to negative nitrogen balance and anorexia

Altered nutrition: more than body requirements related to imbalance between calories ingested and burned off

Fluid volume excess: dependent edema related to fluid shifts (intravascular to interstitial compartments) secondary to negative nitrogen balance

Figure 28-7 summarizes the effects of exercise and immobility by body system.

Gastrointestinal System

Effects of Exercise.   During exercise blood is shunted away from the stomach and intestines to the exercising muscles—hence the advice never to exercise on a full stomach. With regular exercise

- Appetite is increased.
- Intestinal tone is increased, which improves digestion and elimination.

Effects of Immobility.   Immobility leads to disturbances in appetite, decreased food intake, altered protein metabolism, and poor digestion and utilization of food. If individuals increase food intake while decreasing energy expenditure, weight gain will result.

Normal muscular activity in the gastrointestinal tract also slows down in the immobile person, which often

results in constipation, poor defecation reflexes, and an inability to expel feces and gas adequately.

Pertinent nursing diagnoses related to immobility include

Altered bowel elimination: constipation related to decreased gastric motility and muscle tone

Altered nutrition: more than body requirements related to imbalance between food intake and activity (decreased energy expenditure)

Urinary System

Effects of Exercise.   Regular exercise increases blood circulation, including improved blood flow to the kidneys. This allows the kidneys more efficiently to maintain the body's fluid balance and acid–base balance and excrete body wastes.

Effects of Immobility.   In the nonerect client, the kidneys and ureters are level and urine stays longer in the renal pelvis before being expressed against gravity into the ureters and bladder. Urinary stasis favors the growth of bacteria, which when present in sufficient quantities may cause urinary tract infections. Poor perineal hygiene, incontinence, decreased fluid intake, or an indwelling Foley catheter can increase the risk of urinary tract infection for an immobile client.

Immobility also predisposes to renal calculi, or "stones," which are a consequence of high levels of urinary calcium; urinary retention and incontinence resulting from decreased bladder muscle tone; the formation of alkaline urine, which facilitates growth of urinary bacteria; and decreased urinary volume.

Pertinent nursing diagnoses related to immobility include

Alterations in comfort: acute pain related to inability to pass renal calculi

Urinary retention related to prolonged immobility

Potential for urinary tract infection related to urinary stasis and increased urine alkalinity

Skin

Effects of Exercise.   Increased circulation resulting from regular exercises nourishes the skin and promotes its general health.

Effects of Immobility.   In elderly or debilitated immobile clients, the impaired circulation that accompanies immobility may result in serious skin breakdown. Prolonged pressure over bony prominences produces areas of breakdown, or pressure ulcers, which can progress from stage I, redness, to stage IV, destruction of subcutaneous tissue and muscle. Pressure ulcers are described in detail in Chapter 27.

(Text continues on p. 636.)

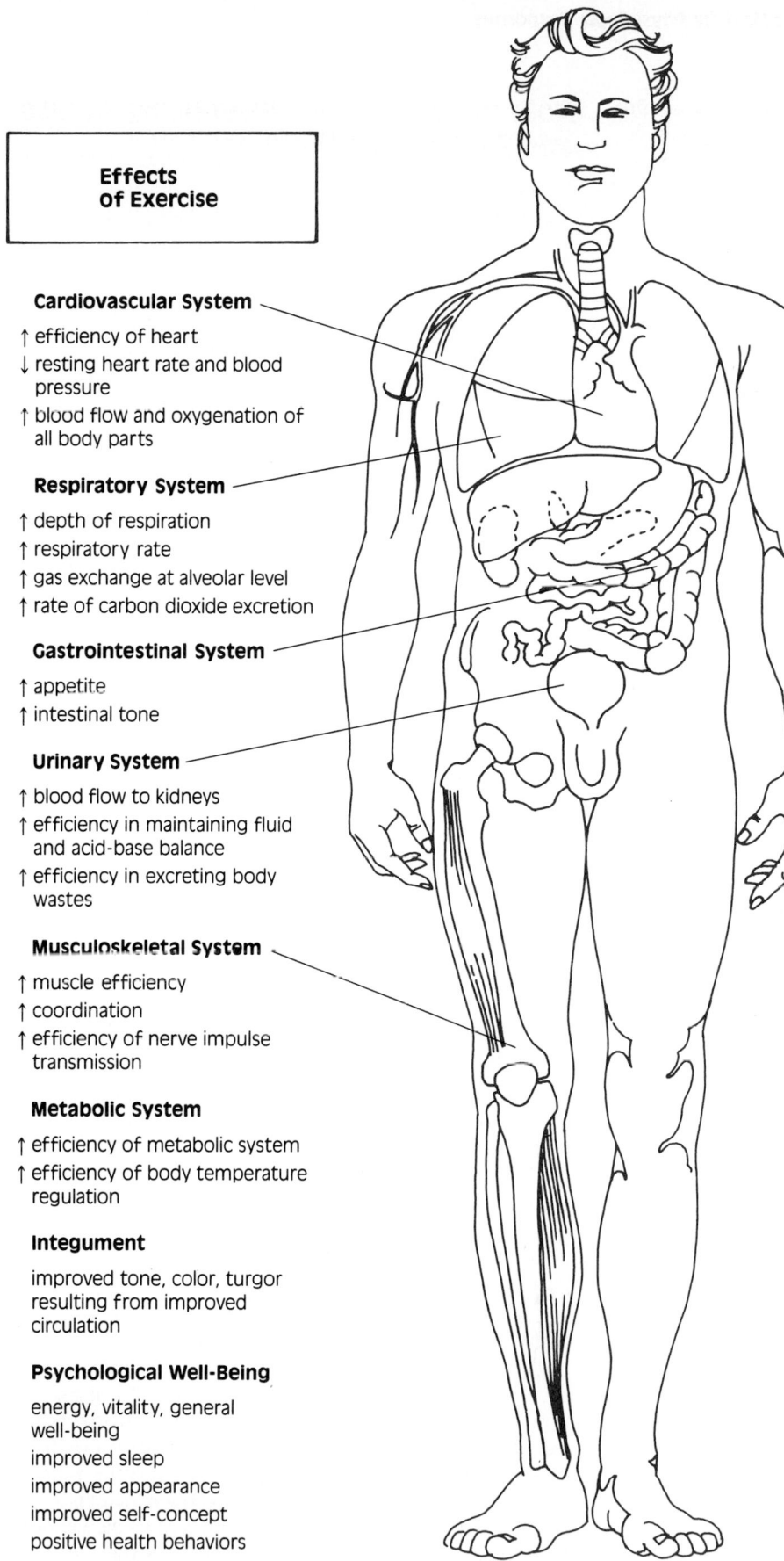

Effects of Exercise

Cardiovascular System

↑ efficiency of heart
↓ resting heart rate and blood pressure
↑ blood flow and oxygenation of all body parts

Respiratory System

↑ depth of respiration
↑ respiratory rate
↑ gas exchange at alveolar level
↑ rate of carbon dioxide excretion

Gastrointestinal System

↑ appetite
↑ intestinal tone

Urinary System

↑ blood flow to kidneys
↑ efficiency in maintaining fluid and acid-base balance
↑ efficiency in excreting body wastes

Musculoskeletal System

↑ muscle efficiency
↑ coordination
↑ efficiency of nerve impulse transmission

Metabolic System

↑ efficiency of metabolic system
↑ efficiency of body temperature regulation

Integument

improved tone, color, turgor resulting from improved circulation

Psychological Well-Being

energy, vitality, general well-being
improved sleep
improved appearance
improved self-concept
positive health behaviors

Effects of Immobility

Cardiovascular System

↑ cardiac workload
↑ risk of orthostatic hypotension
↑ risk of venous thrombosis

Respiratory System

↓ depth of respiration
↓ rate of respiration
pooling of secretions
impaired gas exchange

Gastrointestinal System

disturbance in appetite
altered protein metabolism
altered digestion and utilization of nutrients

Urinary System

↑ urinary stasis
↑ risk of renal calculi
↓ bladder muscle tone

Musculoskeletal System

↓ muscle size, tone and strength
↓ joint mobility, flexibility
bone demineralization
↓ endurance, stability
↑ risk of contracture formation

Metabolic System

↑ risk of electrolyte imbalance
altered exchange of nutrients and gases

Integument

↑ risk of skin breakdown and formation of decubitus ulcers

Psychological Well-Being

↑ sense of powerlessness
↓ self-concept
↓ social interaction
↓ sensory stimulation
altered sleep-wake pattern
↑ risk of depression

FIGURE 28-7
A summary and comparison of the effects of exercise and immobility by body system.

Pertinent nursing diagnoses related to immobility include

Impairment of skin integrity (specify stage of pressure ulcer) related to decreased circulation and pressure on skin overlying bony prominences

Psychologic/Social

Effects of Exercise.   Some of the most important benefits of regular exercise are psychologic. These include

• Increased energy, vitality, and general well-being
• Improved sleep
• Improved appearance (body image)
• Improved self-concept
• Increased positive health behaviors

Effects of Immobility.   When a person can no longer move the body purposefully and needs to depend on someone else for assistance with simple self-care activities, the sense of self is often threatened. Skeletal deformities can influence body image; an inability to meet role expectations can decrease self-concept; and a prolonged period of lying dependent in bed can lead to feelings of worthlessness and diminished self-esteem.

Immobility can produce exaggerated emotional responses to the stresses of everyday living. Persons who become apathetic, possibly because of decreased sensory stimulation, often exhibit altered thought processes. Lack of mobility can also diminish an individual's opportunities to interact socially and deprive that person of normal support systems. Coping difficulties are common in both the immobilized client and the client's family.

Finally, the amount of time the immobilized client spends resting often disrupts usual sleep–wake patterns and may interfere with both the quantity and quality of sleep.

Pertinent nursing diagnoses related to immobility include

Disturbance in self-concept (body image, self-esteem, personal identity) related to immobility and need to depend on others (and other variables)

Powerlessness related to increasing dependency in basic self-care activities

Impaired social interaction related to immobility

Altered thought processes: disorientation related to decreased stimulation to maintain orientation

Knowledge deficit related to decreased motivation to learn

Ineffective individual coping related to prolonged bed rest and increasing activity intolerance

Altered sleep–wake pattern related to increased bedtime/napping and decreased physical exercise

Role of Exercise in Preventing Illness and Promoting Wellness

Haskell and Superko (1984) reviewed the literature on the health benefits of exercise and identified three categories of benefits:

• Health benefits with the most substantial scientific basis: (1) maintenance of optimal body weight; (2) prevention of coronary heart disease; (3) normalization of fat and carbohydrate metabolism
• Probable benefits—less persuasive supporting data: (1) prevention of hypertension; (2) maintenance of bone density with aging; (3) prevention of low back pain syndrome; (4) improved psychologic status
• Probable benefits—if individuals with certain diseases exercise they tend to show clinical improvement although there is no evidence that exercise prevents these disorders: (1) insulin-dependent diabetes mellitus; (2) chronic obstructive pulmonary disease; (3) renal failure; (4) type II hyperlipidemia; (5) arthritis

Risks Related to Exercise

Among the reasons many persons offer for not exercising is fear of causing some personal harm. Nurses need to respond to these fears with realistic knowledge of the risks associated with exercise and specific prevention strategies.

Avoiding Exercise.   The greatest risk associated with exercise is viewing it as too much of a chore and avoiding it.

Precipitating a Cardiac Event.   Although the risk of exercise precipitating a major cardiac event in a healthy individual is minimal, the risk is much higher for individuals with known or documentable cardiovascular disease. Thus, a pre-exercise medical examination, medical supervision during exercise, and an individually designed exercise plan are recommended for sedentary persons over 35 years of age and for any person with a past or current cardiovascular condition.

Orthopedic Discomfort and Disability.   The most common injuries associated with exercise are orthopedic in nature and are caused by irritation of bones, tendons, ligaments, and sometimes muscles. This irritation may result from added weight-bearing stress or from collision with the ground, an object, or another person. Teach clients when injured to rely on the acronym RICE: rest, ice, compression, and elevation. A physician should be contacted immediately for diagnosis of the extent of the injury. Exercise should not be continued until the injury is healed, or further damage may be done.

Other Health Problems. Many other types of health problems may be associated with different types of exercise, depending to a large extent on external factors (temperature on a given day, humidity, pollution index, safety of the neighborhood) as well as internal factors (age, history of previous injury, overuse, obesity, health history).

NURSE AS ROLE MODEL

Nurses who wish to role model healthy mobility behaviors to clients will demonstrate a commitment to using the principles of body mechanics in both their leisure and work activities and to exercising regularly to promote fitness. Since nurses who work closely with clients providing physical care are at high risk for developing musculoskeletal problems if they do not use their bodies properly, they also have a personal reason for being attentive to the use of good body mechanics. Similarly, the work of nursing places heavy demands on a nurse's psychic and physical energy and the nurse who is physically fit is better able to respond to these challenges. Nurses who are effective role models easily meet the following goals. The nurse will:

- Consistently utilize sound principles of body mechanics in both leisure and work activities
- Incorporate regular periods of physical exercise into life-style (minimum of three 20-minute aerobic exercise activities weekly)
- Demonstrate a preference for an active versus a sedentary life-style (*e.g.,* uses stairs in preference to elevators, walks rather than drives short distances, balances active leisure alternatives with sedentary options)
- Appear physically fit to clients and colleagues (appropriate weight for height; adequate muscle mass, tone, and strength; performs work activities without becoming short of breath or excessively fatigued)

PROMOTING WELLNESS

Exercise

Use the following assessment checklist to determine how well you are meeting your need for exercise. Then develop a prescription for self-care by choosing appropriate behaviors from the list of suggestions.

Assessment Checklist

almost always / some times / almost never

☐ ☐ ☐ 1. My life-style demonstrates that I place a high value on exercise as a component of wellness (*e.g.,* I walk stairs instead of using elevators).

☐ ☐ ☐ 2. I exercise for 30 to 45 minutes three to four times/ week.

☐ ☐ ☐ 3. I have sufficient energy for each day's tasks.

☐ ☐ ☐ 4. I maintain my target weight.

Self-Care Behaviors

1. Decide to make the most of everyday opportunities for exercise: use stairs instead of elevators, walk instead of ride, park your car farther from your destination than usual and walk the distance briskly, etc.
2. Choose exercise activities you enjoy and plan three to four, 30- to 45-minute exercise sessions weekly.
3. Obtain medical clearance for exercise if you fall in a high-risk group. Learn and observe the appropriate exercise safeguards (*e.g.,* wear running shoes with the proper support).
4. Alternate types of exercise to avoid boredom.
5. Use part of your lunchtime for brisk walking or other exercise.
6. Invite a friend to exercise with you so you have the added support of a buddy.
7. Join a spa, health club, or exercise group.
8. Build up exercise sessions gradually to avoid overexertion and injury to muscles.
9. Evaluate your life-style to see what prevents you from exercising regularly and address these factors (low value attached to health or exercise, low motivation, lack of time, lack of rest, faulty nutrition, etc.).

Elements of a Mobility/Exercise History

1. Daily activity level
   "Describe the activities you normally carry out during a routine day."
   "What type of physical exercise is a part of your daily life-style?"
   - Activities of daily living
   - Type, frequency, duration of physical exercise
   - Past history of activity/exercise; recent changes
2. Endurance
   "Describe how much and what type of activity makes you tired."
   - History of dizziness, dyspnea, frequent pauses in activity to rest, or marked increase in respiratory rate after moderate activity
3. Exercise/fitness goals
   "What exercise or fitness goals are you currently working on?"
   - Attitudes about exercise and physical fitness
   - Knowledge of the benefits of exercise
   - Motivation to exercise
   - Current exercise/fitness goals
4. Mobility problems
   "Do you experience any problems with movement or with more vigorous activity or exercise?" If yes, "Describe these please."
   - Nature of the problem
   - Onset of disturbance and frequency
   - Known cause(s)
   - Severity
   - Symptoms
   - Effect of problem on everyday functioning
   - Interventions attempted and results
5. Physical or mental health alterations
   "Are there any physical or mental health problems that may be affecting your mobility?" "Tell me about them."
   - Decrease of strength or endurance (*e.g.,* myocardial infarction, congestive heart failure, cardiomyopathy, chronic obstructive pulmonary disease, cancer, gastrointestinal disorders)
   - Neuromuscular impairment (multiple sclerosis, Parkinson's disease, spinal injuries)
   - Musculoskeletal impairment (arthritis, fractures, muscular dystrophy)
   - Perceptual/cognitive impairment (cerebrovascular accident, brain tumor or trauma, vision disorders)
   - Pain/discomfort (burns, rheumatoid arthritis, chronic pain syndrome, post-operative pain)
   - Depression/severe anxiety (neurosis, schizophrenia)
6. External factors affecting mobility
   "Is there anything else you can think of that limits or affects your ability to get around?"
   - Environmental factors (stairs, lack of railings or other assistive devices, unsafe neighborhood)
   - Financial resources

ASSESSING

The nurse performing a comprehensive nursing assessment uses both interview and physical assessment skills to elicit data about the client's mobility status. When alterations in a client's physical or mental health state result in impaired mobility, more detailed assessment skills are needed.

Nursing History

During the nursing history the nurse interviews the client regarding daily activity level, endurance, exercise/fitness goals, mobility problems, physical or mental health alterations that affect mobility, and external factors affecting mobility.

It is important to question clients about their fitness goals. This interviewing strategy communicates to clients that you expect them to be exercising and is itself a powerful teaching tool.

The history of a client's mobility status is brief if initial questioning reveals no problems. The accompanying box illustrates elements common to a mobility status history. When a problem exists (*e.g.,* loss of joint mobility or decreased tolerance for physical activity), the nurse assesses (1) the nature of the problem, (2) onset and frequency, (3) known causes, (4) severity, (5) symptoms, (6) effect of problem on everyday functioning, and (7) interventions attempted by the client and results obtained.

Nursing Examination

Physical assessment of mobility status includes an assessment of general ease of movement and gait; alignment, joint structure, and function; muscle mass, tone, and strength; and endurance. See Table 28-3 for normal findings and significant alterations. The nurse performing this assessment directs attention to both structure and function. The client's ability to stand, walk, sit up, and grasp are important because these enable the client to wash, dress, feed self, and perform other basic activities of daily living.

General Ease of Movement and Gait

The nurse begins the examination of the ambulatory client the moment the client walks into the room. Voluntarily controlled, fluid, and coordinated body movements are keys to the integrated functioning of the skeletal, skeletal muscle, and nervous systems. Significant

T A B L E   28-3
An Overview of the Physical Assessment of Mobility Status

Component	Normal Finding	Significant Alterations
General ease of movement	Body movements are • Voluntarily controlled (purposeful) • Fluid • Coordinated	Involuntary movements • Tremors • Tics • Chorea • Athetosis • Dystonia • Fasciculations • Myoclonus • Oral–facial dyskinesias
Gait	• Head erect, vertebrae are straight • Knees and feet point forward • Arms at side with elbows flexed • Arms swing freely in alternation with leg swings • While one leg is in the stance phase the other is in the swing phase	Abnormalities of gait and posture • Spastic hemiparesis • Scissors gait • Steppage gait • Sensory ataxia • Cerebellar ataxia • Parkinsonian gait • Gait of old age • Use of assistive devices for ambulation
Alignment	Independent maintenance of correct alignment: In the standing and sitting position a straight line can be drawn from the ear through the shoulder and hip; in bed, the head, shoulders, and hips are aligned.	• Abnormal spinal curvatures • Inability to maintain correct alignment independently
Joint structure and function	Absence of joint deformities Full range of motion	• Limitation in the normal range of motion • Increased joint mobility • Swelling or tenderness in or around the joint • Heat or redness • Crepitation • Deformities • Muscle atrophy, nodules, skin changes • Asymmetry of involvement
Muscle mass, tone, and strength	Adequate muscle mass, tone, and strength to accomplish movement/work	• Atrophy, hypertrophy • Hypotonicity (flaccidity), spasticity • Paresis or paralysis
Endurance	Ability to turn in bed, maintain correct alignment when sitting and standing, ambulate, and perform self-care activities	Physiologic or psychologic inability to tolerate an increase in activity • Significantly increased pulse, respirations, blood pressure after rest • Shortness of breath, dyspnea • Weakness • Pallor • Confusion • Vertigo

findings include the presence of any of the following involuntary movements:

- *Tremors:* Relatively rhythmic oscillatory movements
  Resting tremors: Most prominent at rest and may decrease or disappear with voluntary movement
  Intention tremors: Appear with activity and may increase in severity as the target is neared
  Postural tremors: Appear when the affected part is maintaining a posture; may be aggravated by anxiety or fatigue
- *Tics:* Brief, repetitive, stereotyped, coordinated movements occurring at regular intervals (*e.g.,* repetitive winking, grimacing)
- *Chorea:* Brief, rapid, jerky, irregular, and upredictable movements that occur at rest or interrupt normal, coordinated movements; seldom repeat themselves
- *Athetosis:* Movements that are slower, more twisting and writhing than chorea movements and have a larger amplitude; commonly involve the face and distal extremities
- *Dystonia:* Movements similar to athetosis but that involve larger portions of the body, including the trunk; may result in grotesque, twisted postures
- *Fasciculations:* Fine, rapid, flickering, or twitching movements originating in relatively small groups of muscle fibers; vary irregularly in frequency and extent, but rarely move a joint
- *Myoclonus:* Sudden, brief, rapid, unpredictable jerks, usually involving the limbs or trunk; may be single or repetitive
- *Oral–facial dyskinesias:* Repetitive, bizarre movements that chiefly involve the face, mouth, jaw, and tongue
  (Bates, 1987, pp 518–520)

The nurse also notes if the body movements are quick and sure or slow and deliberate. These observations communicate both a sense of the person's emotional status and self-care abilities.

The gait of the ambulatory client is also noted. The client's movements while walking should be coordinated and the posture well balanced. The arms should swing freely in alternation with leg swings. Figure 28-8 illustrates stance and swing, the two phases of the normal gait. The heel of the right foot strikes the ground (stance) while the toe of the left foot pushes off and leaves the ground, moving the leg from behind to in front of the body (swing). While one leg is in the stance phase the other is in the swing phase.

Gait abnormalities should be noted because they may place the individual at risk for injury and also because they may be indicative of intoxication or a neuromuscular disorder. Common abnormalities of gait and posture are illustrated in Figure 28-9.

If a client uses a brace, cane, walker, or crutches to

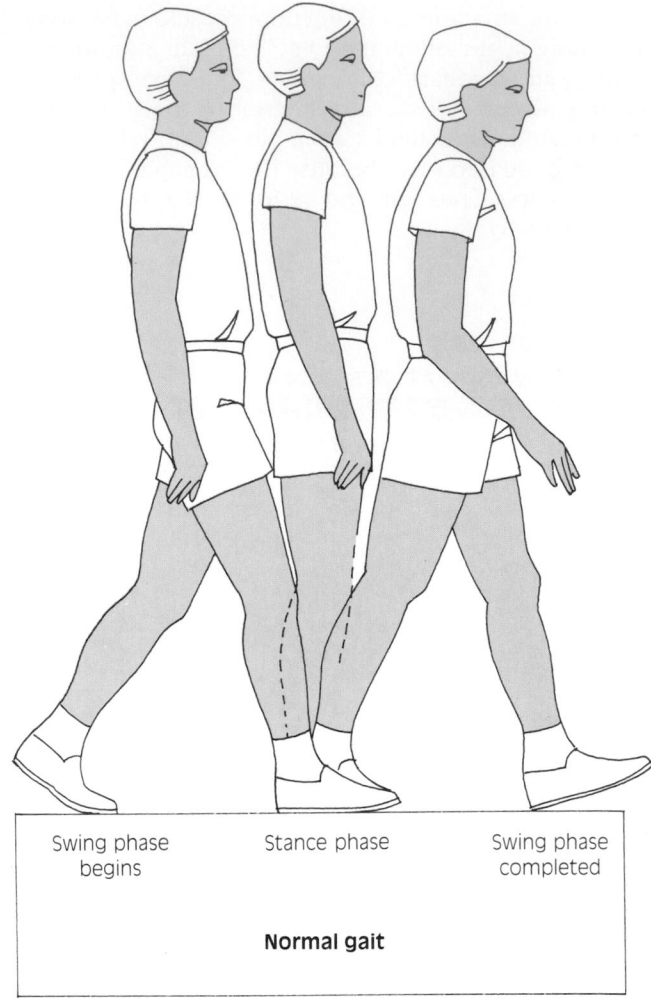

| Swing phase begins | Stance phase | Swing phase completed |

Normal gait

F I G U R E   28-8
The stance and swing phases of normal gait.

assist with ambulation, this should be noted. The nurse also determines if this aid is meeting the client's needs and is being used safely. The use of a wheelchair is also noted.

Alignment

Correct body alignment permits optimal musculoskeletal balance and operation and promotes good physiologic functioning. Deviations in body alignment may result from chronic poor posture, trauma, muscle damage, or nerve dysfunction. Fatigue and a person's mental and emotional status may also influence alignment. Alignment may be observed when a client is standing, sitting, or lying (Fig. 28-10). The nurse notes whether the client is able to maintain correct alignment independently.

Correct body alignment when standing is as follows:
- The head is held erect.
- The face is in the forward position, in the same direction as the feet.

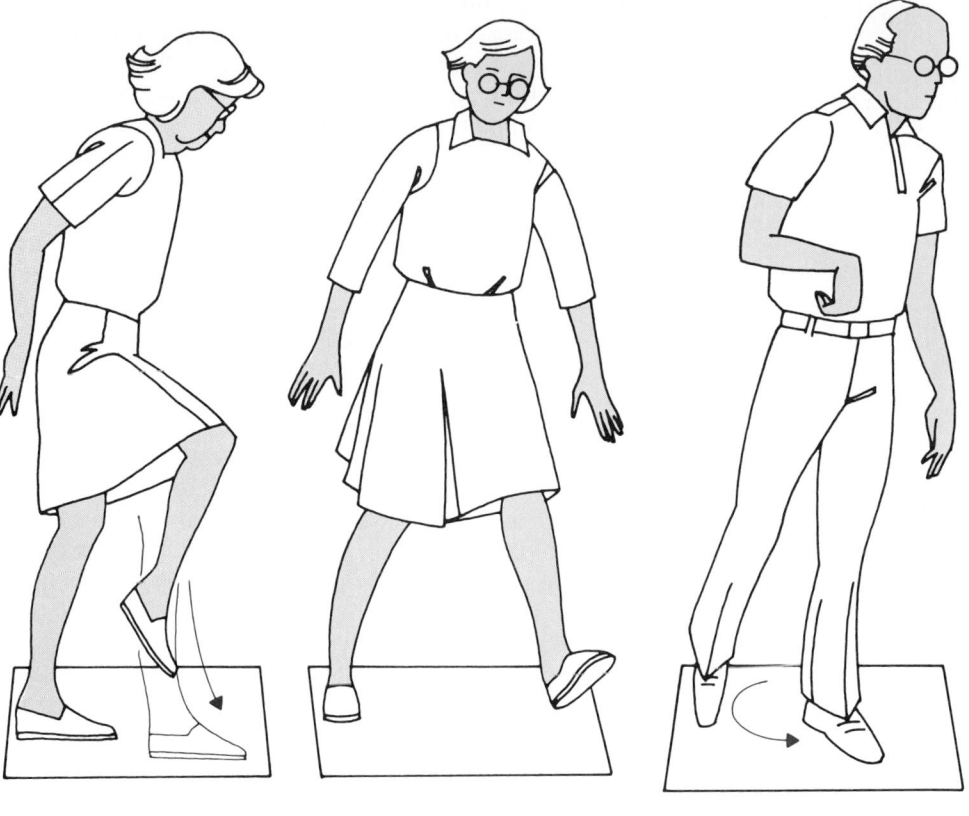

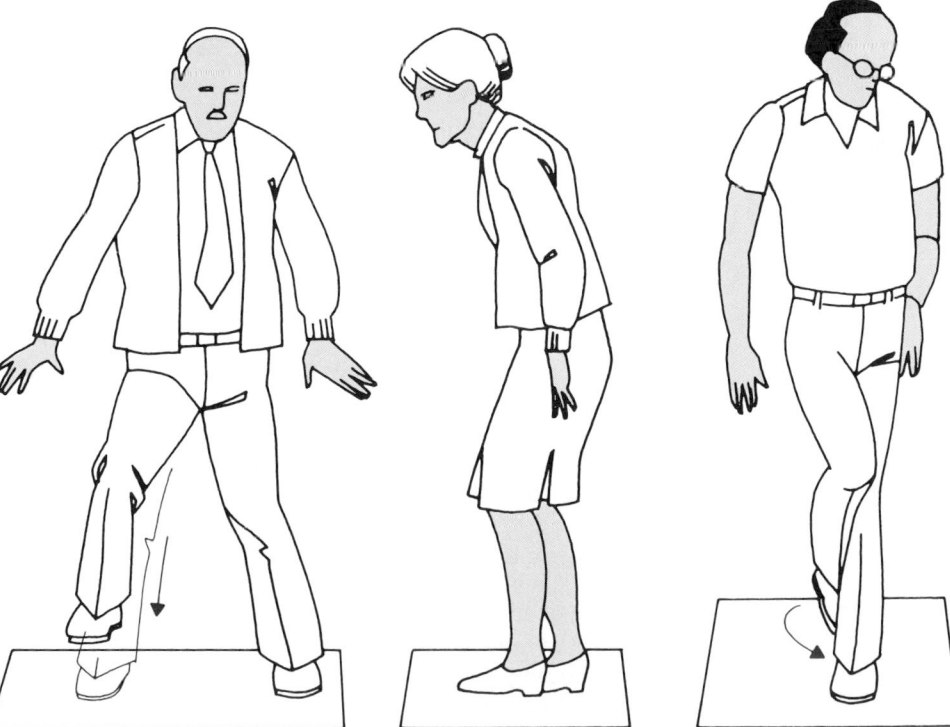

FIGURE 28-9
Gait abnormalities. (Adapted from Bates B: A Guide to Physical Examination. Philadelphia, JB Lippincott, 1980)

(Top left) Steppage gait is associated with footdrop usually secondary to lower motor neuron disease. The feet are lifted high, with knees flexed, and then brought down with a slap on the floor. The patient looks as if he were walking up stairs.

(Top middle) Cerebellar ataxia is associated with disease of the cerebellum or associated tracts. The gait is staggering, unsteady, and wide-based, with exaggerated difficulty on the turns. The patient cannot stand steadily with feet together, whether eyes are open or closed.

(Top right) Spastic hemiparesis is associated with unilateral upper motor neuron disease. One arm is flexed, close to the side, and immobile; the leg is circled stiffly outward and forward (circumducted), often with dragging of the toe.

(Bottom left) Sensory ataxia is associated with loss of position sense in the legs. The gait is unsteady and wide-based (the feet are far apart). The feet are lifted high and brought down with a slap. The patient watches the ground to guide his steps. He cannot stand steadily with feet together when his eyes are closed (positive Romberg test).

(Bottom middle) Parkinsonian gait is associated with the basal ganglia defects of Parkinson's disease. The posture is stooped, the hips and knees slightly flexed. Steps are short and often shuffling. Arm swings are decreased and the patient turns around stiffly—"all in one piece."

(Bottom right) Scissors gait is associated with bilateral spastic paresis of the legs. Each leg is advanced slowly and the thighs tend to cross forward on each other at each step. The steps are short. The patient looks as if he were walking through water.

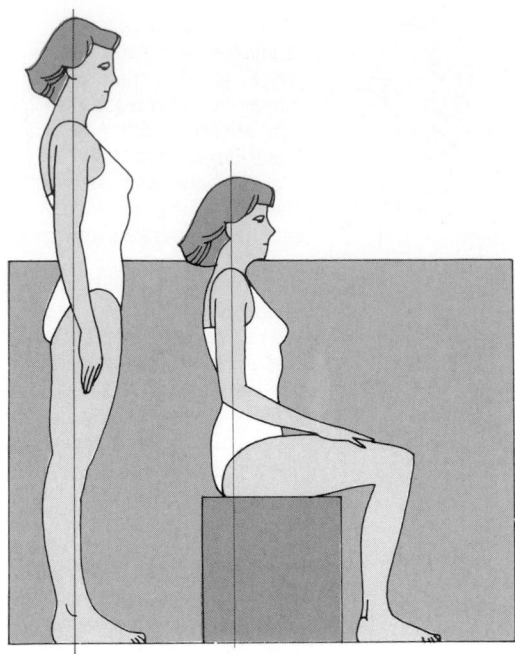

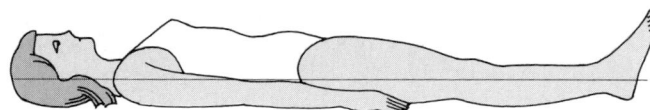

F I G U R E   28-10
Adequate posture. Note that in sitting and standing positions a straight line can be drawn from the ear through the shoulder and hip. In bed, the head, shoulders, and hips are aligned.

- The chest is held upward and forward.
- The spinal column is elongated, and the curves of the spine are within normal limits.
- The abdominal muscles are held upward and the buttocks downward.
- The knees are extended—not bent or hyperextended in the knee-locked position.
- The feet are at right angles to the lower legs.
- The line of gravity goes through the center of the knees and in front of the ankle joints.
- The base of support is on the soles of the feet and weight is distributed through the soles and heels.

Correct body alignment when sitting is similar to correct alignment when standing except the hips are flexed, the knees are flexed and not crossed, and the base of support is on the buttocks and upper thighs. The popliteal area should be free of the edge of the chair to prevent circulatory stasis and possible nerve injury.

Joint Structure and Function

The nurse uses inspection and palpation to examine joints, their range of motion, and the surrounding tissue.

Range of motion is the complete extent of movement of which a joint is normally capable. Figure 28-11 illustrates the range of motion of selected joints. When assessing joint mobility, Bates (1987) recommends notation of

- Any limitation in the normal range of motion or any unusual increase in the mobility of a joint (instability). Range of motion varies among individuals and decreases with aging.
- Any swelling in or around the joint. Swelling may involve the synovial membrane, which then feels boggy, or doughy, to your fingers, or may be produced by excessive synovial fluid within the joint space. Swelling sometimes originates not in the joint itself but in tissues around it, such as bones, tendons, tendon sheaths, bursae, and fat.
- Tenderness in or around the joint. Try to define the specific anatomic structure that is tender.
- Increased heat. Use the backs of your fingers to compare the joint with the symmetrical joint on the opposite side or, if both joints are involved, with the tissues near them.
- Redness of the overlying skin
- Crepitation, a palpable or even audible crunching or grating sensation produced by motion of the joint
- Deformities, such as bony enlargement, subluxation (partial dislocation), or contracture
- Condition of the surrounding tissues, including muscle atrophy, subcutaneous nodules, and skin changes
- Muscular strength
- Symmetry of involvement. Note whether arthritic changes involve several joints symmetrically on both sides of the body or affect only one or perhaps two joints.
  (Bates, 1987, pp 442–443)

Muscle Mass, Tone, and Strength

Adequate skeletal muscle mass, tone, and strength are prerequisites to body movement and work performance. Mass refers to muscle size. The term **atrophy** is used to describe muscle mass that is decreased through disuse or neurologic impairment. *Hypertrophy* refers to increased muscle mass resulting from exercise or training. The examiner assesses muscle mass throughout the body and may also compare one muscle group to another using tape measurements. Clients experiencing muscle wasting as a result of a chronic disease process such as cancer may report visible changes in muscle mass.

The slight residual tension that remains in a resting normal muscle with an intact nerve supply is termed *muscle tone*. Muscle tone may be assessed by flexing and extending the elbow or knee and noting the degree of resistance to these movements. Decreased tone, hypotonicity, or **flaccidity** results from disuse or neurologic impairments. **Spasticity**, increased tone that interferes with movement, is also caused by neurologic impairments.

(Text continues on p. 645.)

Neck

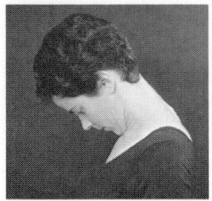
Flexion

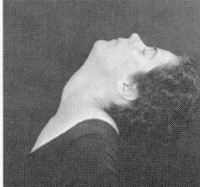
Hyperextension

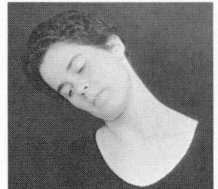
Lateral flexion

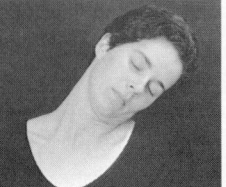

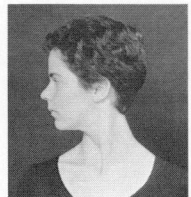
Rotation

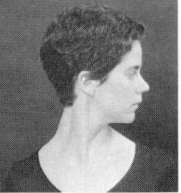

Shoulder

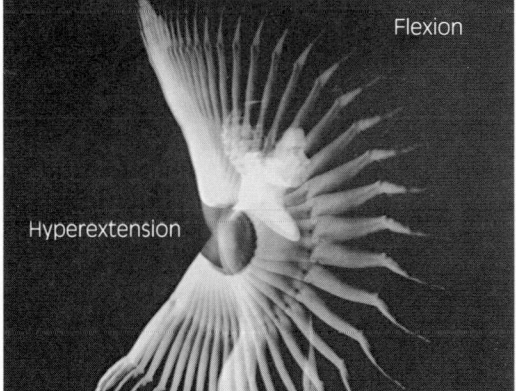
Flexion
Hyperextension
Extension

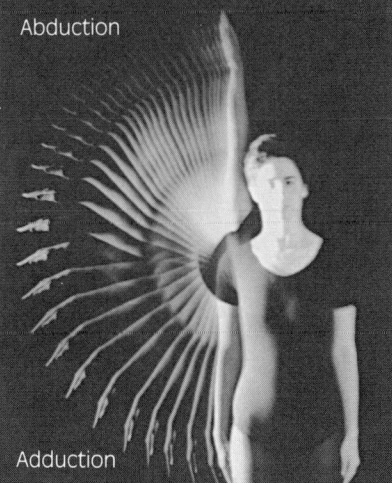
Abduction
Adduction

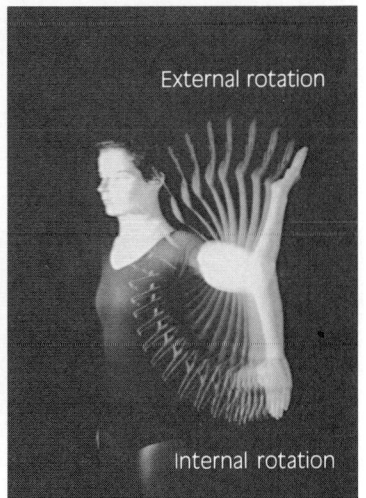
External rotation
Internal rotation

Elbow

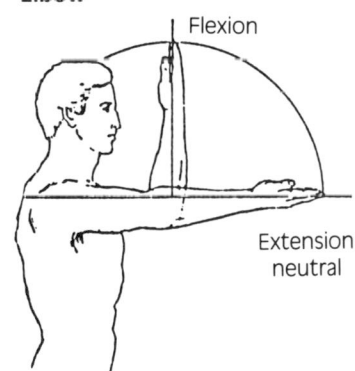
Flexion
Extension neutral

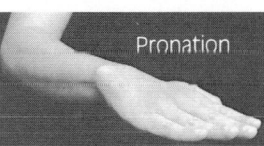
Pronation

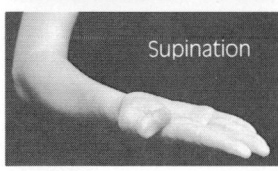
Supination

Wrist

Hyperextension
Extension neutral
Flexion

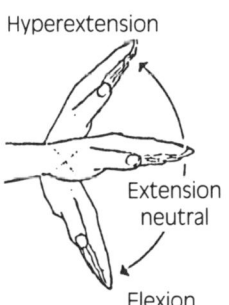
Radial deviation

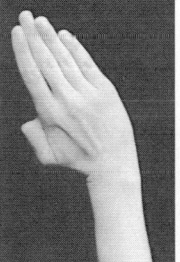
Ulnar deviation

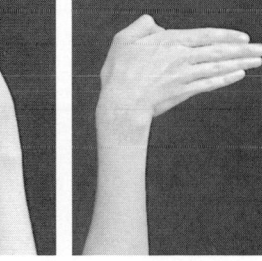

Fingers

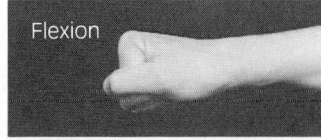
Flexion

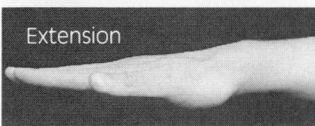
Extension

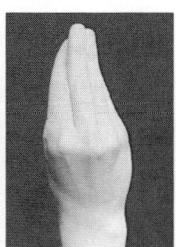
Abduction

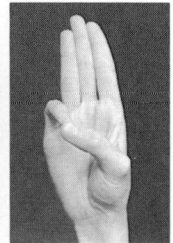
Adduction

Apposition of thumb to finger

F I G U R E   28-11
Normal range of motion of selected joints.

Hip

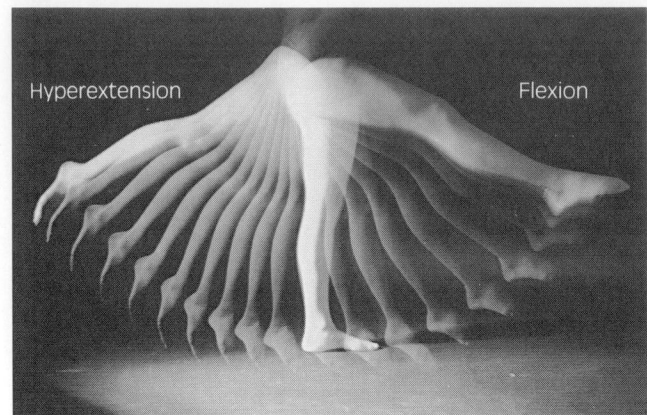

Hyperextension

Flexion

Extension

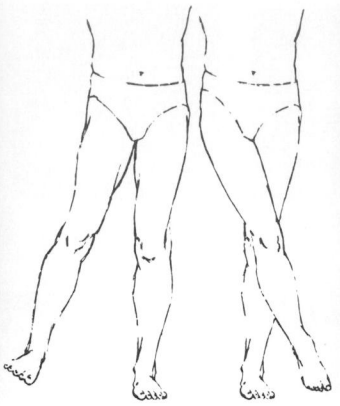

Abduction Adduction

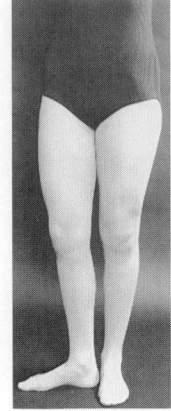

External rotation

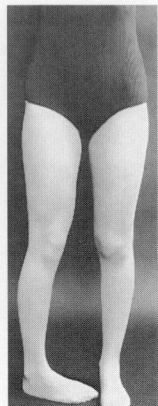

Internal rotation

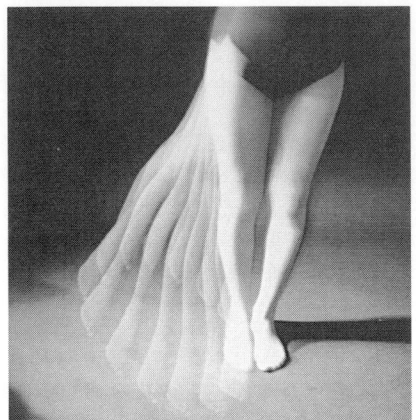

Rotation

Knee

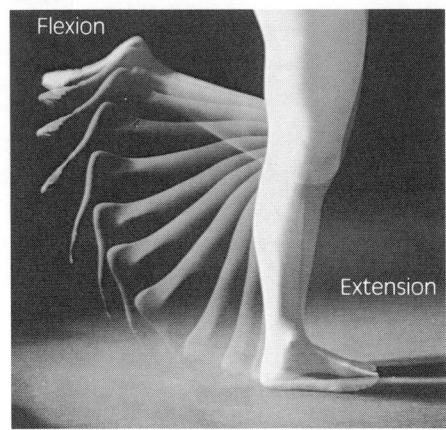

Flexion

Extension

Ankle

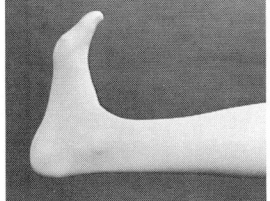

Dorsiflexion

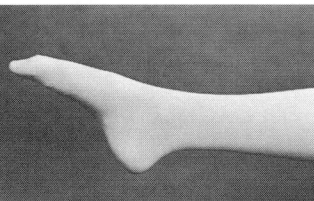

Plantar flexion

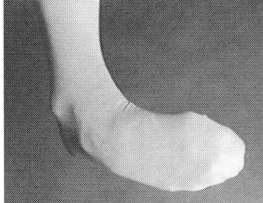

Inversion

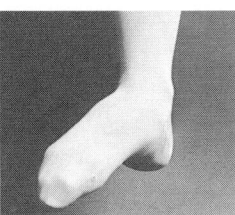

Eversion

Toes

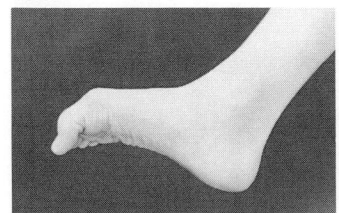

Flexion

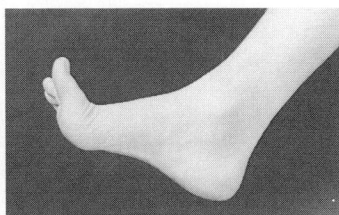

Extension

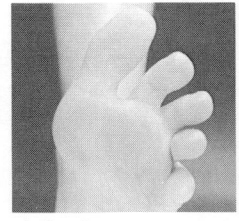

Abduction

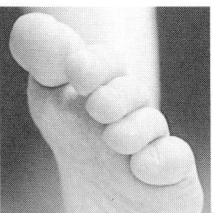

Adduction

F I G U R E   28-11   (Continued)

Muscle **strength** varies greatly from one individual to another and within the same individual, and is affected by muscle use. Muscle strength is tested by asking the client to move actively against resistance. For example, the client may be instructed to push the examiner's palms apart or to push the foot against the examiner's palm. When comparing muscle groups it is important to remember that a person's dominant side tends to be stronger.

Impaired muscle strength or weakness is termed *paresis*. Absence of strength secondary to nervous impairment is *paralysis*. *Hemiparesis* refers to weakness of one half of the body, and **hemiplegia** to paralysis of one half of the body. **Paraplegia** is paralysis of the legs, and *quadriplegia* is paralysis of all four limbs.

Nursing's concern is that the client's muscle strength is adequate for the performance of tasks the client deems necessary. For example, a client whose primary means of ambulation is a wheelchair requires upper body strength.

Endurance

When assessing **endurance**, the nurse evaluates the client's ability to (1) turn in bed, (2) maintain correct alignment when sitting or standing, (3) ambulate, and (4) perform self-care abilities. When a physical or psychologic factor is believed to be affecting endurance, the nurse

- Takes the vital signs while the client is at rest
- Instructs the client to perform the activity (*e.g.,* ambulation)

- Observes the client's response during and after the activity
- Takes the vital signs immediately after the activity
- Reassesses the vital signs after the client has rested for 3 minutes

Significant findings include significantly increased pulse, respirations, and blood pressure; shortness of breath; dyspnea; weakness; pallor; confusion; and vertigo.

DIAGNOSING

The nurse must recognize cues that indicate both potential and actual problems when analyzing data about a client's mobility status. Since the problems accompanying immobility can seriously undermine well-being and often require complex and costly treatment, nursing energies are directed to preventing these problems whenever possible. The plan of care for the client with an alteration in mobility should contain nursing diagnoses that identify the complications of immobility for which the client is at greatest risk.

Nursing diagnoses specifically addressing problems of mobility include activity intolerance and impaired physical mobility. Examples of pertinent etiologies and defining characteristics may be found in Table 28-4.

Examples of nursing diagnoses that describe the effect of mobility alterations on other areas of human functioning follow. This list is by no means exhaustive.

T A B L E 28-4
Nursing Diagnoses for Mobility Problems

Problem/Title	Etiologic or Contributing Factors	Sample Defining Characteristics
Activity intolerance	Any condition that interferes with the transport of oxygenated blood to tissue (*e.g.,* cardiac problems such as congestive heart failure and arrhythmias; respiratory problems, especially chronic obstructive pulmonary disease; circulatory problems; diabetes mellitus)	Decreased ability to perform basic self-care activities: turning in bed, changing position, ambulating, washing, dressing, eating, and so on.
	Any condition that causes fatigue (depression, pain, sleep disturbances, prolonged bed rest, sedentary life-style)	Altered response to activity • Dyspnea, shortness of breath, excessive increase in respiratory rate • Week pulse, excessive increase in pulse rate, change in rhythm • Blood pressure that fails to increase with activity or that decreases • Weakness, pallor, confusion, vertigo
Impaired physical mobility	• Neuromuscular impairment (arthritis, stroke, Parkinson's disease) • Musculoskeletal impairment • Decreased strength and endurance • Pain/discomfort • Depression	• Physical inability to move purposefully or a reluctance to move • Limited range of motion • Decreased muscle mass, tone, or strength • Therapy-related restrictions on movement (*e.g.,* an order for bed rest, traction, cast, or splints)

There are multiple etiologies possible for many of these problem statements.

Ineffective airway clearance related to prolonged bed rest, decreased position changes, ineffective coughing related to weakness

Altered bowel elimination: constipation related to inactivity, decreased muscle tone

Ineffective breathing pattern related to limited chest expansion (prolonged bed rest, muscle disuse, atrophy, loss of muscle coordination)

Altered comfort related to inability to change body position independently

Altered comfort: painful movement of joints related to limited range of motion and muscle atrophy

Ineffective individual or family coping related to loss of ability to move purposefully in environment, spouse's need for assistance with all self-care activities

Altered fluid volume: excess related to prolonged bed rest

Impaired gas exchange related to decreased respiratory movement

Altered health maintenance related to lack of mobility to procure needed services—no support persons

Impaired home maintenance management related to immobility

Potential for urinary tract infection related to urinary retention secondary to immobility

Potential for injury: falls related to orthostatic hypotension secondary to immobility

Potential for injury: venous thrombosis related to immobility

Potential for injury: Musculoskeletal problems related to infrequent, excessive exercise

Knowledge deficit: exercise program related to having no previous experience with regular exercise

Noncompliance with exercise prescription related to decreased endurance, decreased motivation

Powerlessness related to inability to move self

Self-care deficit related to physical weakness (decreased muscle mass and strength), altered mobility (upper and/or lower extremities)

Altered self-concept (body image, self-esteem, personal identity) related to postural deviation, inability to perform self-care activities, inability to meet role expectations

Sexual dysfunction related to neuromuscular impairment

Impaired skin integrity related to inability to change positions independently, prolonged bed rest

Sleep pattern disturbance related to lack of exercise (sedentary life-style)

Impaired social interaction related to decreased activity tolerance

Urinary retention related to prolonged bed rest

Increased work of heart related to prolonged supine position and greater volume of circulating blood

PLANNING: CLIENT GOALS

If the client is not experiencing any mobility problems, client goals are directed toward the promotion of physical fitness. For example

- Client will follow a program of regular physical exercise that improves cardiovascular function, endurance, flexibility, and strength.

In order to achieve this long-term goal, numerous short-term goals may be needed. Examples of these follow:

By the next visit, 2/20, the client will
1. Identify four personal benefits of regular exercise
2. Describe an exercise program (activities, frequency, duration) client is willing to follow
3. Identify the target heart range
4. Obtain medical clearance for the exercise program if at high risk for complications
5. List support systems that will reinforce exercise efforts

Clients at high risk for developing specific mobility problems require different goals:

- Client will demonstrate correct body alignment whenever observed (alignment).
- Client will adhere to an every-two-hour positioning schedule (alignment).
- Client will demonstrate full range of joint motion (joint mobility).
- Client will demonstrate adequate muscle mass, tone, and strength to perform functional activities of daily living (muscle mass, tone, and strength).

Specific goals for the client at risk of developing complications related to immobility may be found in Table 28-8. Goals for more specific problems, for example, for the client learning to walk with crutches or needing to master transfer techniques with only upper body mobility, need to be individualized to the client.

IMPLEMENTING

Nursing strategies designed to promote correct body alignment, mobility, and fitness are described in this section. Techniques for positioning clients; performing range-of-motion exercises; moving, lifting, and ambulating clients; and designing exercise programs are highlighted.

Positioning Clients

Positioning that maintains correct body alignment and facilitates physiologic functioning contributes to the client's psychologic and physical well-being. The force of gravity pulls parts of the body out of alignment unless adequate support is provided. Various positions are therefore protective in nature only when the client is positioned properly.

Common Devices to Promote Correct Alignment

There are many devices to help maintain good body alignment and muscle tonus while the client is in bed and to alleviate discomfort or pressure on various parts of the body.

Pillows. Pillows are used primarily to provide support or to provide elevation of a part. Pillows of different sizes are useful for different parts of the body. Those intended for the head are usually full- or large-sized pillows. Small pillows are ideal for support or elevation of the extremities, shoulders, or incisional wounds. Specially designed heavy pillows are useful to elevate the upper part of the body when an adjustable bed is not available, such as in a home situation.

Mattresses. For a mattress to be comfortable and supportive, it must be firm but have sufficient "give" to permit good body alignment. A client who must remain in a bed with a nonsupportive mattress might very well complain of backache and other discomforts.

A well-made and well-supported foam-rubber mattress retains a uniform firmness. This mattress is made of natural or synthetic rubber, or both in combination. A large volume of air is incorporated. The foam-rubber mattress conforms to the contours of the body and supplies support at all points. Its greatest advantage is that it does not form slopes and valleys as the inner-spring mattresses are likely to do. Nor does the foam-rubber mattress create as much pressure against bony prominences, such as the ankles, the elbows, the scapulae, and the coccyx.

Special mattresses and pads used to help prevent decubitus ulcers are discussed in Chapter 27.

Bed Board. If the mattress does not provide sufficient support, a bed board may help to keep the client in better alignment. Bed boards usually are made of plywood or some other firm composition. The size varies with the needs of the situation. For home use, full bed boards are available commercially or can easily be made at home from available materials.

Adjustable Bed. The head of an adjustable bed can be elevated to the desired degree. This positioning is discussed later in this chapter. The foot of an adjustable bed can also be elevated to the desired degree. Some adjustable beds allow the bed to be "broken," or gatched, so that the client can rest the knees over an elevated portion of the mattress. This position is rarely

recommended or is used only for brief periods because it may cause nerve injury and decreased circulation.

The adjustable bed can also be changed so that the distance of the bed to the floor can be altered. The client can get in and out of bed easier when the bed is in the lowest position. The higher positions are used by health-care workers so they do not strain their backs while giving bed care.

Rocking Bed. The rocking bed, although used primarily in the care of clients with vascular or respiratory diseases, is also of great value in the care of immobile clients. This bed is mounted on a frame that can be made to rock rhythmically up and down. The bed is adjusted to rock at the frequency of the client's respirations. The rocking aids respiration by shifting the abdominal viscera, which in turn helps move the diaphragm up and down, helping air to be forced out and into the lungs. The constant changing of position also helps the flow of blood.

Chair Bed. Another type of bed used in the care of clients requiring bed rest is one that can be placed into a chair position. These beds were designed primarily for clients with heart ailments. They permit the client to be in a semisitting position, which may aid the client's cardiac output.

Circular Bed. The electric circular bed is a 6-foot or 7-foot metal frame with a diameter support for the client. The direction of the support can be changed so the client can be placed in a variety of positions. This bed is especially useful for the client who will be completely helpless for an extended period.

Stryker Frame. The Stryker frame is a narrow support that can be turned 360 degrees. The client can be alternated between the supine and prone positions without changing alignment. This bed is particularly useful for the totally immobilized client, such as one who is paralyzed.

Footboards. The greatest danger to the feet occurs when they are not supported in the dorsal flexion position. The toes drop downward, and the feet are in plantar flexion. Because of the pull of gravity, this position of the feet occurs naturally when the body is at rest. If maintained for extended periods of time, plantar flexion can cause an alteration in the length of muscles, and the client may develop a complication called **footdrop**. In this position, the foot is unable to maintain itself in the perpendicular position, heel–toe gait is impossible, and the patient will experience extreme difficulty in walking. The use of a foot support, such as the footboard, helps avoid this complication. The footboard also provides a firm surface against which the feet of the bedfast client can be placed for proprioceptor stimulation.

Commercial footboards, such as the one pictured in

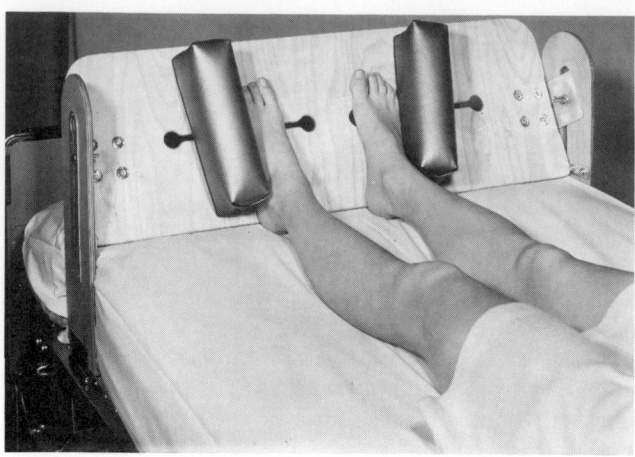

F I G U R E   28-12
Adjustable footboard, used to keep the client's feet in dorsal flexion. (JT Posey Company, Arcadia, California)

Figure 28-12, are available. They are generally adjustable for clients of different heights. The footboard must come far enough up from the foot of the bed so that the client's feet rest firmly against it without the client sliding down in bed. Also, the footboard should not be so far from the foot of the bed that the client's knees are flexed when the feet are against it.

If the client is in a sitting position while in bed, the footboard must be placed at an angle. This prevents hyperextension of the knees, which would result if the feet were kept in dorsiflexion while the trunk was flexed forward. Some clients at risk for developing footdrop are also being advised to wear canvas sneakers while on bed rest in conjunction with the footboard.

Cradle.   If top bedding must be kept off the client's lower extremities, a device called a *cradle* is used. A cradle is usually a metal frame that supports the bed linens away from the client while providing privacy and warmth. Some cradles are equipped with lightbulbs, which provide extra heat. There are any number of sizes and shapes of cradles. If used, the cradle should be fastened securely to the bed so that it does not slide or fall on the client.

Sandbags.   Sandbags immobilize an exremity and support body alignment. Their value is enhanced if they are available in various sizes. When properly filled, they are not hard or firmly packed. They should be pliable enough to be shaped to body contours and to give support. They should be placed so they do not create pressure on a bony prominence.

Trochanter Rolls.   Trochanter rolls are used to support the hips and legs so that the femurs do not rotate outward. Figure 28-13 illustrates and describes how to use trochanter rolls. Properly placed pillows can also be

used to help prevent the thighs from turning outward, but they tend to slip out of place and require frequent adjusting to be effective.

Hand–Wrist Splints.   If a client is paralyzed or unconscious it may be necessary to provide a means for keeping the thumb in the correct position, that is, slightly adducted and in apposition to the fingers. A commercial plastic or aluminum splint may be used to hold the thumb in place no matter what position the hand is in. Clients who are not moving their fingers should be encouraged to do finger exercises with special attention to having the thumb touch the tip of each finger.

Bed Side Rails.   One of nursing personnel's greatest safety concerns is to prevent clients from falling out of bed. Many hospitals today require that side rails be present on all beds and used except when the client is receiving care or is ambulating. The use of side rails requires explanation to clients and their families. Clients should be helped to understand how the side rails offer protection if they are weak or receiving certain drugs and cannot prevent themselves from falling should they roll to the edge of the bed. They also help to remind clients that they are not in their usual environment, should they awaken during the night and wish to get out of bed.

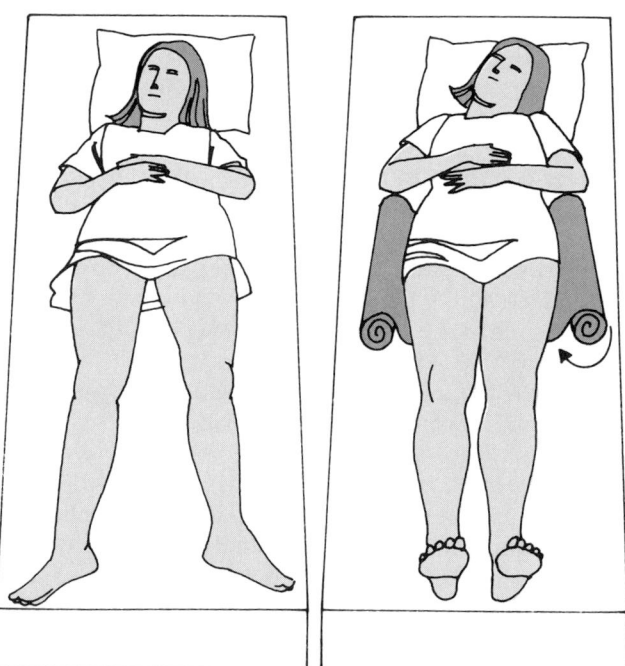

F I G U R E   28-13
Trochanter rolls prevent the external rotation of the hips of a bedridden client. The client is placed on a folded sheet so that the top edge is at the hips and the lower edge is about one third of the way down the thighs. Towels or a bath blanket is rolled under each side until the roll is snugly against the client's hips and thighs. The support cannot unroll, and the weight of the client keeps it secure.

Side rails make it possible for a client to roll from one side to the other or to sit up without calling for assistance. This in itself is a very good activity: it helps the client retain or regain muscle efficiency.

Bed side rails may not deter some clients from getting out of bed. Many a client has crawled over the foot of the bed. It is now recommended that side rails extend only for three fourths of the length of the mattress. Then, if clients do attempt to get out of bed, they do not have to climb over the side rail or the foot of the bed and further increase the danger of falling. When a client sleeps restlessly or has frequent involuntary movements of the extremities and is in danger of harming self against the side rails, protective padding may be ordered.

Trapeze Bar. A *trapeze bar* is a handgrip suspended from a frame near the head of the bed. The client can grasp the bar with one or both hands and then raise the trunk from the bed. The trapeze makes moving and turning considerably easier for many clients and facilitates transfers into and out of bed. It can also be used to perform exercises that strengthen some muscles of the upper extremities.

Protective Positioning

Clients accustomed to an active life-style who generally only use a bed for sleep are often unaware of the importance of correct body alignment and regular position changes when on prescribed bed rest. Whenever possible, nurses should teach both the client and family
- Correct positioning techniques
- The need to change positions frequently, at least every 2 hours
- The importance of using the time allotted to position changes to exercise the extremities and to assess and massage pressure area (*Note:* Reddened areas should not be massaged.)

When the client is unable to change position independently, a turn schedule should be posted at the bedside so that nurses assist with and document the rotation of positions. Table 28-5 describes nursing measures to prevent complications associated with common bed positions.

Fowler's Position. The semisitting position is called **Fowler's position** and calls for the head of the bed to be elevated from 45 degrees to 60 degrees. This position is often used to promote cardiac and respiratory functioning because abdominal organs drop in this position and thereby provide maximal space in the thoracic cavity. This is also the position of choice for eating, conversation, vision, and urinary and intestinal elimination.

Variations of Fowler's position include high Fowler's and low Fowler's or **semi-Fowler's position.** In the high Fowler's position the head of the bed is elevated 90 degrees. When a bedside table with a pillow on top of it is placed in front of the client in high Fowler's

position, the client can lean forward and rest the arms on the pillow, assuming a posture that allows for maximal lung expansion. In the low or semi-Fowler's position the head of the bed is elevated 30 degrees.

In Fowler's position, the buttocks bear the main weight of the body. Other skin areas that require assessment and massage include the heels, the sacrum, and the scapulae.

The arms and feet need particular attention when the client is in a semisitting position. Unless properly supported, the arms fall to the bed and pull on the shoulders, and the feet fall into a footdrop position. Supportive devices may be necessary, including pillows supporting (1) the upper back and head, (2) the elbows and wrist joints, (3) the lower back, (4) the thighs, and (5) the ankles; trochanter rolls; and a foot board. The correct positioning and nursing actions to prevent complications associated with the Fowler's position are presented in Table 28-5.

Supine or Dorsal Recumbent Position. In this position the client lies flat on the back with the head and shoulders slightly elevated with a pillow unless contraindicated. The pillow under the head and upper shoulders may not be allowed following a spinal anesthetic or surgery on the spinal vertebrae.

The body areas in need of attention when in the supine position are the feet and neck. Pillows are almost always used to support the head to tilt it forward so that the person's vision is improved. This causes flexion of the cervical spine. The feet will fall into a plantar flexion position unless support is provided. Table 28-5 describes nursing actions to prevent complications associated with this position and illustrates correct alignment in the supine position.

Side-Lying or Lateral Position. In the side-lying position the client lies on the side and the main weight of the body is borne by the lateral aspect of the lower scapula and the lateral aspect of the lower ilium. Since many people routinely fall asleep in the side-lying position, this is a comfortable alternate to the supine position for the client on bed rest. Although it relieves pressure on the scapulae, sacrum, and heels and allows the legs and feet to be comfortably flexed, support pillows are needed for correct positioning. Areas of the body in need of particular attention when in the side-lying position are the arm and leg on the side opposite the one on which the person is lying. Unless properly supported, the arm will interfere with proper breathing and will be adducted, and the leg adducts and rotates internally. Table 28-5 describes and illustrates the protective side-lying position.

A variation of the lateral position is the **Sims' position.** In this position the client again lies on the side but the lower arm is behind the client and the upper arm is flexed at both the shoulder and the elbow. Since in this position the main body weight is borne by the anterior

(Text continues on p. 652.)

T A B L E   28-5
Common Bed Positions and Protective Nursing Actions

	Complication to Be Prevented	Suggested Preventive Actions
Fowler's Position		
	Flexion contracture of the neck	Allow the head to rest against the mattress or be supported by a small pillow only.
	Exaggerated curvature of the spine	Use a firm support for the back. Position the client so the angle of elevation starts at the hips.
	Dislocation of the shoulder	Support the forearms on pillows to elevate them sufficiently so that no pull is exerted on the shoulders.
	Flexion contracture of the wrist	Support the hand on pillows so it is in natural alignment with the forearm.
	Edema of the hand	Support the hand so it is slightly elevated in relation to the elbow.
	Flexion contractures of the fingers and abduction of the thumbs	Provide hand–wrist splints if necessary.
	Impaired lower extremity circulation and knee contracture, pressure on heels	Elevate the knees for only brief periods of time. Place one or two pillows under the lower legs from below the knees to the ankles. Avoid pressure on the popliteal vessels. Avoid using the knee gatch.
	External rotation of the hips	Use trochanter roll.
	Footdrop	Support the feet in dorsal flexion. Use footboard.
Protective Supine Position		
	Exaggerated curvature of the spine and flexion of the hips	Provide a firm supportive mattress. Use a bed board if necessary.
	Flexion contracture of the neck	Place pillow(s) under the upper shoulders, the neck, and the head so that the head and the neck are held in the correct position.
	Internal rotation of the shoulders and extension of the elbows (hunch shoulders)	Place pillows or arm supports under the forearms so that the upper arms are alongside the body and the forearms are pronated slightly.
	Flexion of the lumbar curvature	Place rolled towel or small pillow under lumbar curvature if needed.
	Extension of the fingers and abduction of the thumbs (clawhand deformities)	Use hand–wrist splints if appropriate
	External rotation of the femurs	Place sandbags or a trochanter roll alongside the hips and the upper half of the thighs.

(Continued)

	Complication to Be Prevented	Suggested Preventive Actions
	Hyperextension of the knees	Place a pillow under the lower legs from below the knees to the ankles.
	Footdrop	Use a footboard or make an improvised firm foot support to hold the feet in dorsal flexion.

Protective Side-Lying or Lateral Position

	Complication to Be Prevented	Suggested Preventive Actions
	Lateral flexion on the neck	Place a pillow under the head and the neck.
	Inward rotation of the arm and interference with respiration	Place a pillow under the upper arm. Lower arm should be flexed and positioned comfortably.
	Extension of the finger and abduction of the thumbs	Provide hand–wrist splint if necessary.
	Internal rotation and adduction of the femur	Use one or two pillows as needed to support the leg from the groin to the foot.
	Twisting of the spine	Make sure that the two shoulders are aligned with the two hips.

Protective Sims' Position

	Complication to Be Prevented	Suggested Preventive Actions
	Lateral flexion of the neck	Place a small pillow under the head unless the drainage of oral secretions is desired.
	Damage to nerves and blood vessels in the axillae of the lower arm	Carefully position lower arm behind and away from client's back.
	Internal shoulder rotation and adduction	Abduct the upper shoulder slightly so that shoulder and elbow are flexed. Place a pillow between the chest and upper arm.
	Internal rotation and adduction of the hip; lumbar lordosis	Place a pillow under the upper flexed leg from the groin to the foot.
	Twisting of the spine	Make sure that the two shoulders are aligned with the two hips.
	Footdrop	Support the lower foot in dorsal flexion with a sandbag.

Protective Prone Position

	Complication to Be Prevented	Suggested Preventive Actions
	Flexion on the cervical spine	Place a small pillow under the head.
	Hyperextension of the spine; impaired respirations	Place some suitable support under the client between the end of the rib cage and the upper abdomen if this facilitates breathing and if there is space there.
	Footdrop	Move the client down in bed so that the feet are over the mattress, or support the lower legs on a pillow just high enough to keep the toes from touching the bed.

aspects of the humerus, clavicle, and ilium, the major pressure points differ from those in the lateral and other bed-lying positions (see Table 28-5).

Prone Position. In the **prone position**, the person lies on the abdomen with the head turned to the side. The body is "straightened out" in the prone position since the shoulders, head, and neck are in an erect position, the arms are easily placed in correct alignment with the shoulder girdle, the hips are extended, and the knees can be prevented from flexing or hyperextending. When clients on bed rest use this position periodically it helps to prevent flexion contractures of the hips and knees. However, the pull of gravity on the trunk when the client lies prone produces a marked lordosis. The position is thus contraindicated for persons with spinal problems. The pull of gravity on the feet may result in plantar flexion unless the legs and feet are positioned carefully. Table 28-5 illustrates correct alignment in the prone position and describes nursing activities to prevent complications.

Turning the Client in Bed

Frequently, the client is unable to turn in bed without assistance. Nurses need to use correct body mechanics and knowledge of correct alignment to turn the client from the back onto the side, from the back onto the abdomen, and from the abdomen onto the back. These techniques are described and illustrated in Procedure 28-1. Mastering these turning techniques will help the nurse to adhere to an every-two-hours turn schedule for an immobile client.

Assisting with Range-of-Motion Exercises

Range of motion is the complete extent of movement of which a joint is normally capable. Engaging in routine tasks, such as bathing, eating, dressing, and writing, helps utilize muscle groups that keep many joints in effective range of motion. When all or some of normal activities of daily living are impossible, attention should be given to the joints not being used at all or to those that are limited in their use.

Unless contraindicated, active, active-assistive, or passive range-of-motion exercises should be encouraged regularly and included in the client's plan of care. In **active exercise**, the client independently moves joints through their full range of motion (isotonic exercise). In **active-assistive exercise**, the nurse may provide minimal support, whereas in **passive exercise** the client is unable to move independently and the nurse moves each joint through its range of motion. Both active and passive exercises improve joint mobility and increase circulation to the affected part, but only active exercise increases muscle mass, tone, and strength and improves cardiac and respiratory functioning. Thus, exercises should be as ac-

tive as the client's physical condition permits. It is also helpful to teach isometric exercises to clients to increase muscle mass, tone, and strength.

In the following section specific guidelines are offered for providing range-of-motion exercises for clients. In some institutions nurses work closely with physiotherapists in designing and implementing exercise programs.

Directives should be included in the nursing care plan for range-of-motion exercises. The nursing orders should explain what, how, and when, so that all who care for the client observe the same routine. The following are basic guidelines for the nurse when helping to put the client's joints through range of motion:

- Teach the client what exercising is being undertaken, why, and how it will be done. Using a show-and-tell technique is often helpful.
- Avoid overexertion and using exercises to the point that the client develops fatigue. The exercises are not to exhaust or tax the client. Certain exercises may need to be delayed until the client's condition allows.
- Start gradually and work slowly. All movements should be smooth and rhythmic. Irregular and jerky movements are uncomfortable for the client.
- Move each joint until there is resistance but not pain. Uncomfortable reactions should be reported and exercises halted until further instructions are obtained.
- While exercising joints the nurse uses a variety of support measures to prevent muscle strain or injury to the client.
    Cupping: Placing a cupped hand under the joint to support it (*e.g.,* under the ankle)
    Cradling: Supporting the joint with one hand while "cradling" the distal portion of the extremity with the remaining arm (*e.g.,* the calf or forearm might be cradled while the knee or elbow is supported)
    Supporting the joint by holding the adjacent distal and proximal muscular areas (indicated when a joint is painful): Grasping muscle groups or major tendons is likely to cause injury to the tissues.
- Return the joint to a neutral position, that is, its normal position of alignment, when finishing each exercise.
- Keep friction at a minimum when moving extremities to avoid injuring the skin.
- Use range-of-motion exercises twice a day, and do the exercises regularly to build up muscle and joint capabilities. Each exercise is carried out two to five times. Many of the exercises can be carried out when the client is being bathed and become part of that procedure. Routine tasks, such as eating, dressing, self-bathing, and writing, also help to put certain joints through range of motion and should be encouraged.

PROCEDURE 28-1
Turning a Client in Bed

Action

1 Explain the procedure to the client.

2 Wash your hands.

3 Raise the bed to your waist level. Adjust to flat position or as low as the client can tolerate. Lower side rail nearest you and raise the opposite side.

4 Position the client closer to the far side of the bed in the supine position.

5 Place the client's arms across the chest and cross the client's far leg over the near one.

6 Stand opposite the client's center with your feet spread and one foot ahead of the other. Tighten your gluteal and abdominal muscles and flex your knees.

Rationale

This facilitates the cooperation of the client.

Handwashing deters the spread of microorganisms.

This position facilitates the turning maneuver and minimizes strain on the nurse yet keeps the client safe.

The client will be in the center of the bed after turning is accomplished.

This facilitates the turning motion and protects the client's arms during the turn.

This positions the turner opposite the center of the body mass. It places the nurse in a stable position with good body alignment and prepared to use large muscle masses to turn the client.

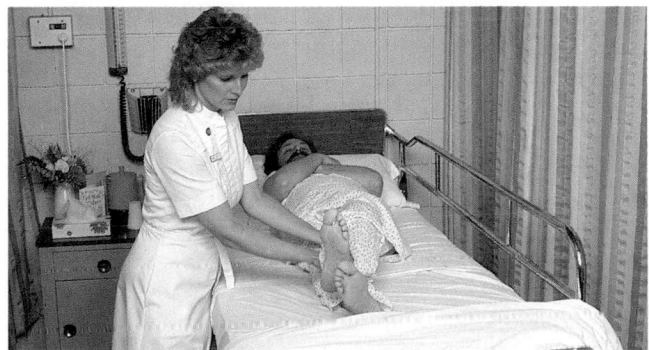

Step 5: Positioning client's arms and legs.

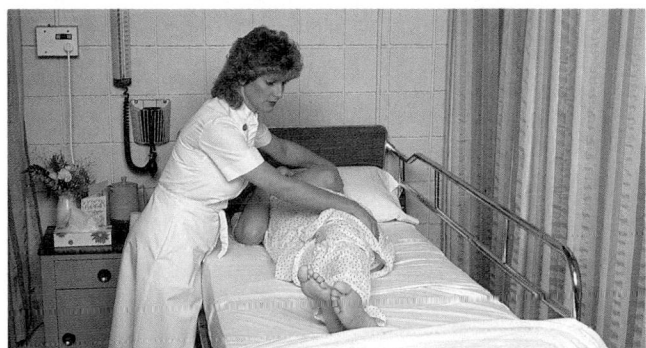

Step 6: Preparing to turn client.

7 Position your hands on the client's far shoulder and hip and roll the client toward you.

8 Make the client comfortable and position in proper alignment.

This maneuver supports the client's body and makes use of the nurse's weight to assist with turning.

This ensures that the client will be able to maintain desired position.

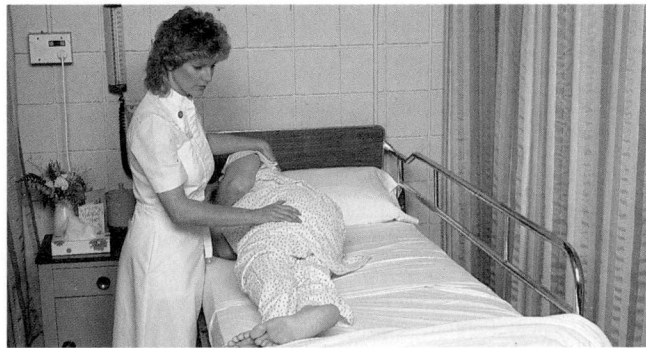

Step 7: Turning client.

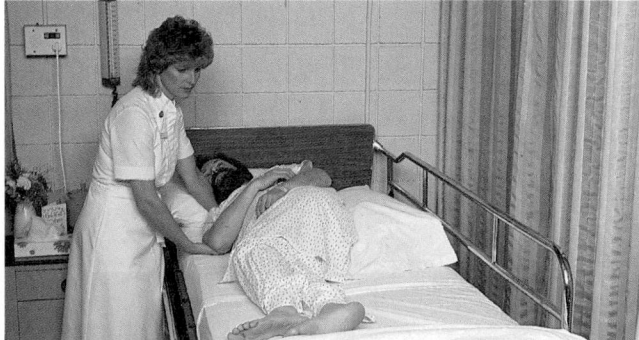

Step 8: Making client comfortable.

9 Readjust the bed height and position and raise side rail if appropriate.

10 Wash your hands.

This ensures the client's safety.

Handwashing deters the spread of microorganisms.

- Expect the client's respiratory and heart rate to increase during exercising, which is good. These rates should return to normal within a few minutes. If they do not, the exercises are probably too strenuous for the client.
- Use passive exercises as necessary, but encourage active exercises of the same kind when the client is able to do so independently. Exercises should continue at home after a period of hospitalization, as necessary.

The goal of range-of-motion exercises is to keep the client in the best possible physical state while bed rest is necessary. When range-of-motion exercises are not considered as routine measures, the client's physician should be consulted. Figure 28-14 illustrates a series of passive range-of-motion exercises.

Moving and Lifting the Client

Frequently it is necessary to move a helpless client. The client must be kept in good alignment and protected from injury while being moved. There are certain recommended guidelines the nurse should follow when moving and lifting clients:

- Know the client's diagnosis, capabilities, and any movement not allowed. Place braces or any device the client wears before helping from bed.
- Plan carefully what you will do before moving or lifting a client. Assess mobility of attached equipment. You may injure the client or yourself if you have not planned well. If necessary, enlist the support of another nurse. This reduces the strain on all involved.
- Explain to the client what you plan to do. Then, use what abilities the client has to assist you. This technique often decreases work and possible injury to yourself.
- If the client is in pain, administer the prescribed analgesic sufficiently in advance of the transfer to allow the client to participate in the move comfortably.
- Remove obstacles that may make moving and lifting inconvenient.
- Elevate the bed as necessary so that you are working at a height that is comfortable and safe for you.
- Lock the wheels of the bed, wheelchair, or stretcher so that they do not slide about while you are moving the client.
- Observe principles of body mechanics while you work to prevent injuring yourself.
- Be sure the client is in good body alignment while being moved and lifted to protect the client from strain and muscle injury.
- Support the client's body well. Avoid grabbing and holding an extremity by its muscles.
- Avoid causing friction on the client's skin during moving. Friction can be reduced by sprinkling powder or cornstarch on bed linens and on the client's skin.
- Move your body and the client in a smooth, rhythmic motion. Jerky movements tend to put extra strain on muscles and joints and are uncomfortable for the client.
- Use mechanical devices such as a Hoyer lift or turning board when they are available for moving clients. Be sure that you understand how the device operates and that the client is properly secured and informed of what will occur. Clients who do not understand or are afraid may not be able to cooperate and may suffer injury as a result.
- Be realistic about how much you can safely do without injury. Two small persons cannot lift or move an obese client without risking muscle strain and injury.

Moving the Client Up in Bed

Children and lightweight adults are relatively easy to slide toward the head of the bed without the assistance of a second person. A technique used to move a client up in bed when the client is able to assist is described and illustrated in Procedure 28-2. The procedure also describes and illustrates how two nurses can move the client up in bed.

Using a Sheet to Move the Client Up in Bed. Although the methods just described may be convenient, the amount of effort expended by the nurse can be reduced when moving a client up in bed. A drawsheet or a large sheet may be placed under the client so that it extends from the client's head to below the buttocks, and can be used to lift the client. When using the sheet lift, the friction that must be overcome is between the lift sheet and the bed linen. Therefore, the client's skin is spared the effects of abrasion and friction.

Moving the Client from Bed to Stretcher

Considerable care must be taken when moving a client from a bed to a stretcher, or *vice versa,* to prevent injury to the client. If the client is unconscious or helpless, additional nurses are needed to support the extremities and the head. The skills are explained in Procedure 28-3. For clients who are obese, use of a transfer board or roller board will facilitate the move from stretcher to bed and ensure that the client's body is properly aligned during the transfer. When returning the client to the bed from the stretcher, the same techniques are observed. However, the carriers should first move the client from the stretcher onto the edge of the bed. Then, one member of the team supports the client on the edge of the bed to prevent falling off while the other two team members go around to the opposite side of the bed and place their arms underneath the client. After the two persons on the opposite side of the bed have a good grip

(Text continues on p. 664.)

FIGURE 28-14

In this example of a passive range-of-motion exercise regimen, the nurse begins with the neck and works down to the toes on one side of the client's body then up the opposite side. The nurse then turns the client over and works head to toe down one side and toe to head up the other side. All exercises should be done slowly, evenly, smoothly, and gently. Joints should be moved to the point where resistance is felt, but never to the point of pain. Each exercise should be repeated the prescribed number of times. When supporting a body part, the nurse grasps firmly above and below the joint with fingers together. After each movement, the body part is returned to its normal anatomical position.

Neck

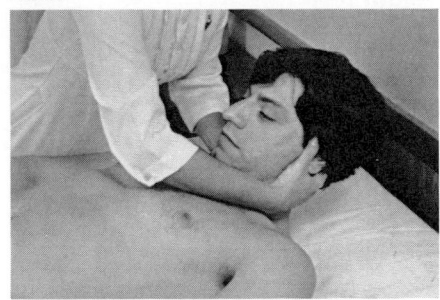

Flexion
Flex the head forward trying to place the chin to the chest.

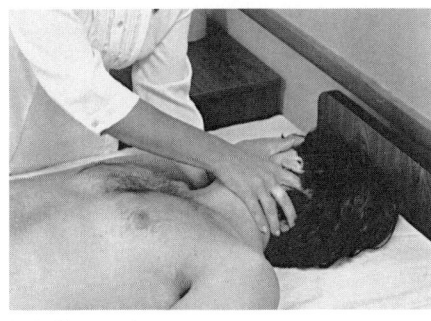

Rotation
Rotate the head to each side trying to place the chin on the shoulder.

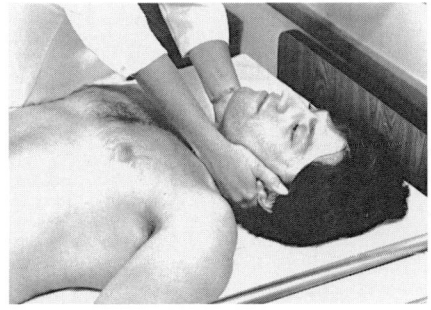

Lateral flexion
Tilt the head to each side trying to place the ear on the shoulder.

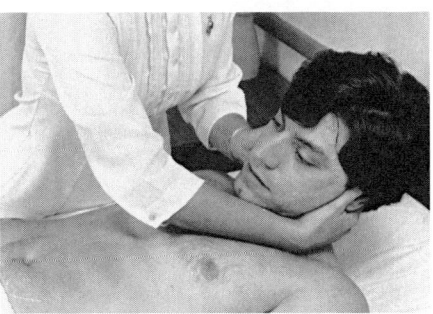

Rotation
Flex the neck and circumduct the head from side to side in as wide a semi-circle as possible.

Shoulder

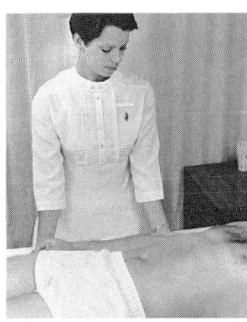
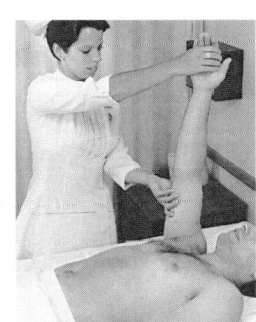
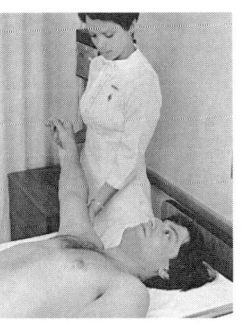

Flexion
Support the arm above the elbow with one hand. With the other hand grasp the client's hand. Extend the arm upward above the head.

Abduction, Adduction
Abduct the shoulder by moving arm away from body to the side. Adduct the shoulder by returning the arm to the neutral position.

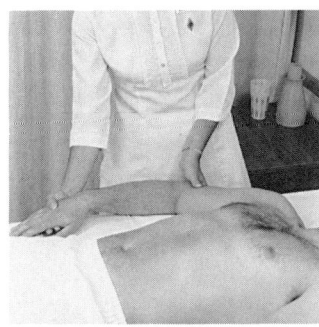
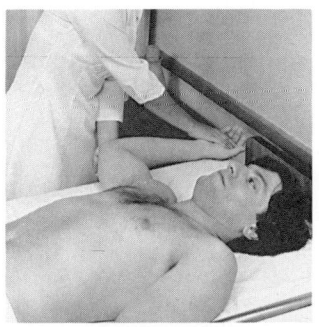

External/Internal rotation
Position the arm with the upper arm perpendicular to the body and the lower arm parallel to the body. Rotate the shoulder

through a 180 degree arc and return to neutral position. With the elbow extended and the arm supported above the elbow, circumduct the shoulder in as wide a semi-circle as possible.

Elbow

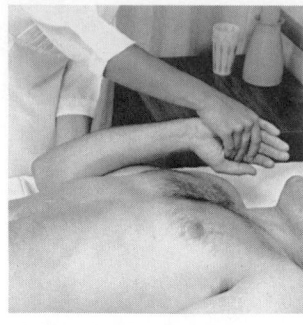
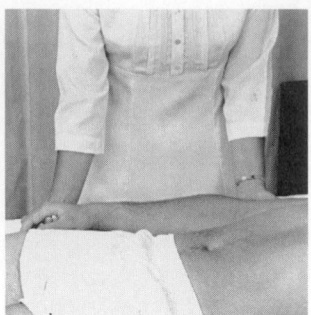

Flexion and Extension
With the client's upper arm at his side, flex and extend the elbow.

Wrist

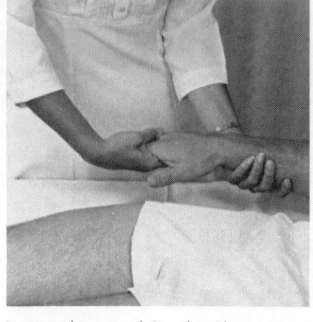

Pronation and Supination
Support the forearm with one hand. With the other, grasp the client's hand. Pronate the hand, then supinate it.

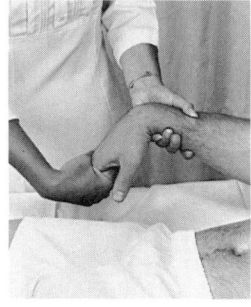
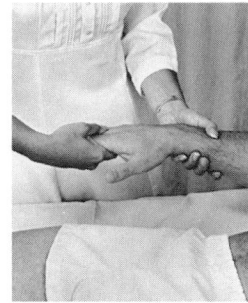
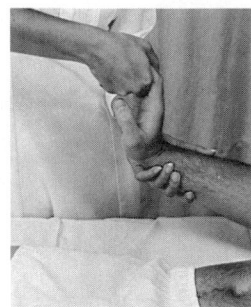

Flexion and Extension
Flex the wrist, extend the wrist and hyperextend the wrist.

Radial and Ulnar deviation
With the palm down, perform a radial deviation of the wrist and an ulnar deviation of the wrist.

Fingers and Thumb

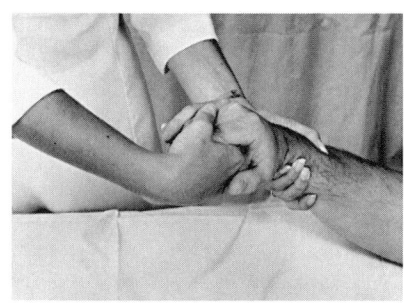
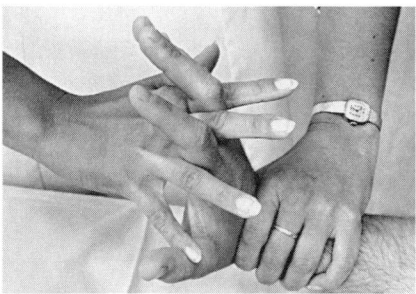

Rotation
Slowly and gently move the wrist in as wide a circle as possible, first in one direction and then the other.

Abduction/Adduction
Abduct the fingers by interlacing your fingers with the client's. Then adduct them moving the thumb across the palm as far as possible.

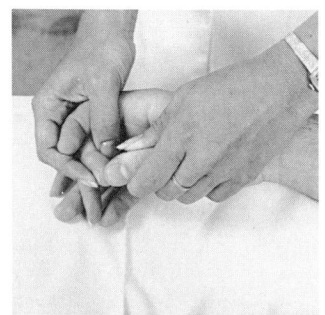
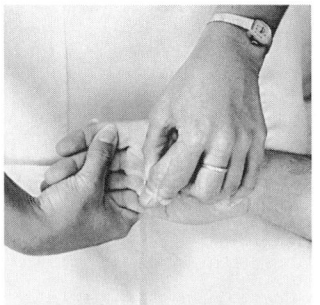
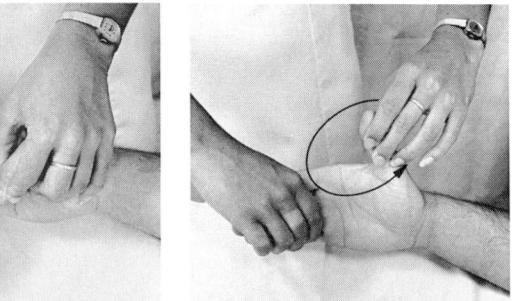

Flexion/Extension and Opposition
Flex fingers individually by touching each fingertip with the tip

of the thumb. Circumduct the thumb in a wide circle in one direction and then the other.

Trunk

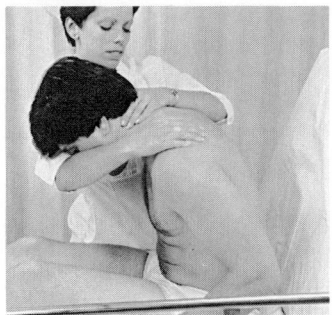 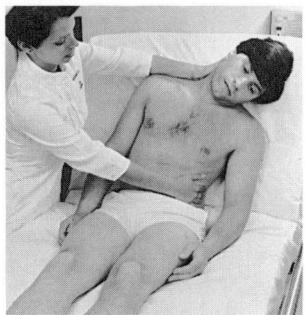 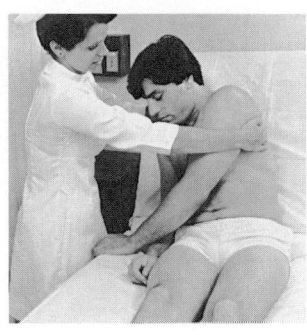 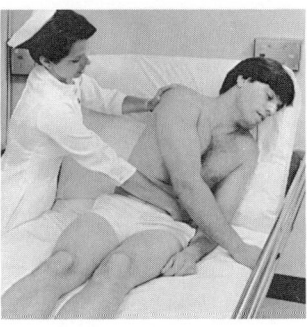

Flexion
With the head of the bed raised and the client in a sitting position, flex the trunk by bending the client forward. Lateral flexion occurs as you pull the client's waist toward you while pushing his neck and shoulders away from you.

Rotation
Rotate the trunk by placing the client's forearm across waist, grasping the upper body just below the shoulders and rocking backward, pulling the client toward you.

Hip and Knee

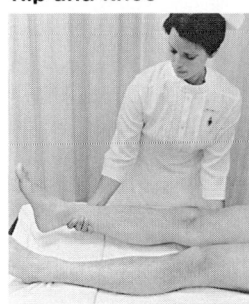 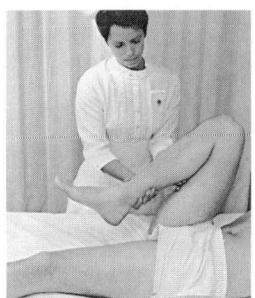 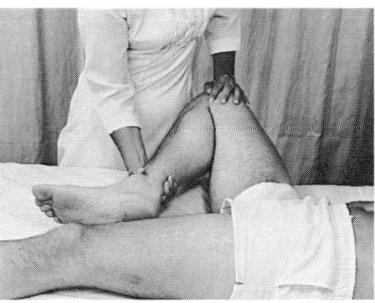 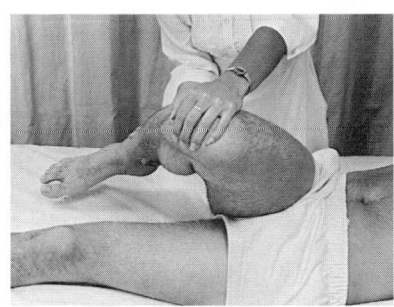

Flexion/Extension
With the client in a supine position and bed flat, combine flexion of hip and knee. Supporting the upper leg and the heel, lift the leg as far as possible while flexing the knee. Extend the leg.

Internal/External Rotation
Flex the knee and place the client's foot on the bed next to the other knee. Lift the foot just off the sheet and swing the knee toward you maintaining flexed postion. This motion produces external rotation of the hip. Internal rotation is effected by moving the foot away from the midline while moving knee across the midline and down.

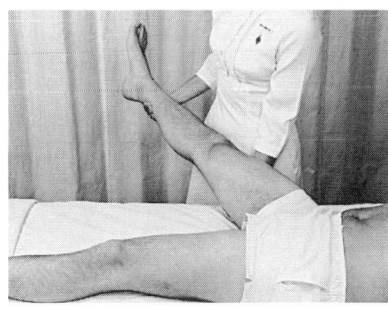 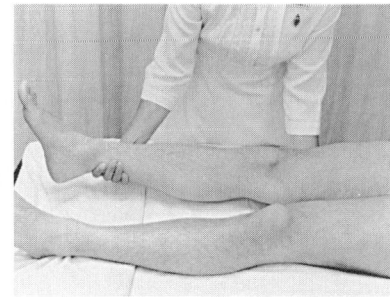 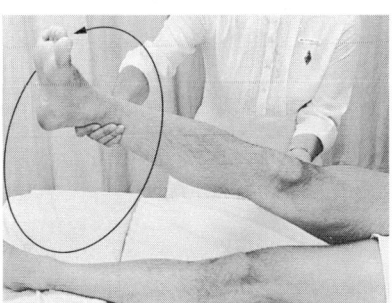

Abduction/Adduction
Abduct and adduct the hip as for the shoulder.

Rotation
Rotate the hip in as large a semi-circle as possible.

Ankle

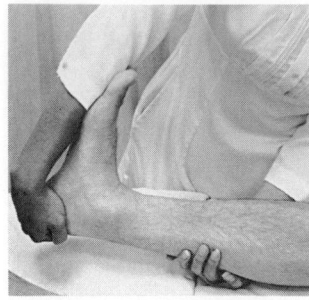 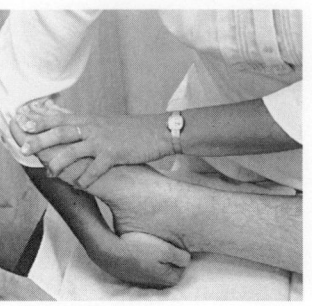 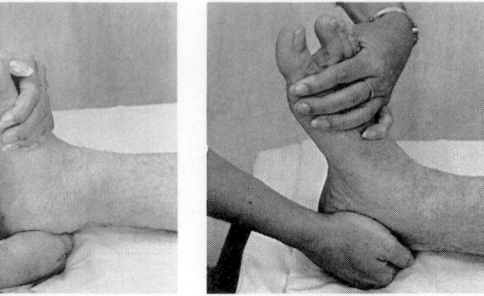

Dorsiflexion/Plantarflexion
Cupping the heel and resting the sole of the foot on your forearm, produce dorsiflexion by pressing against the ball of the foot with your forearm.

Inversion/Eversion
Cupping the heel and grasping the distal portion of the foot, turn the foot to point the sole toward the midline, then away form the midline to effect inversion and eversion of the ankle.

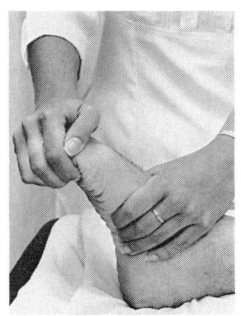 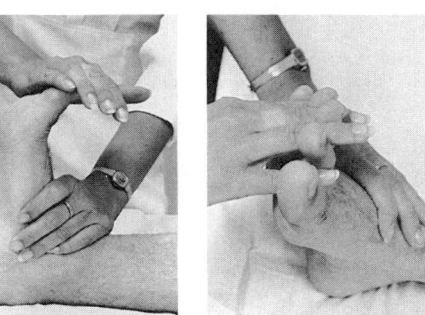

Rotation
Rotate the ankle in as wide a circle as possible, first in one direction and then the other.

Flexion/Hyperextension
Manually flex and hyperextend the toes as shown.

Abduction/Adduction
Abduct and adduct the toes as for the fingers.

Having completed exercises on both sides of the client in the supine position, turn the client over.

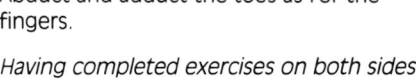

Neck　　　　　　　　　　　　　　　　　　**Shoulder**

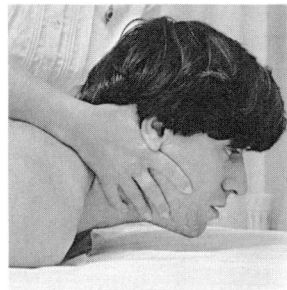 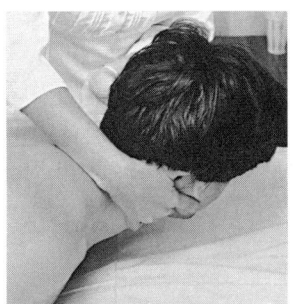 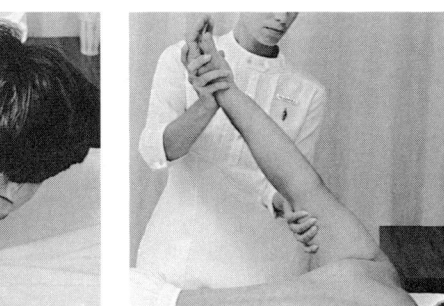 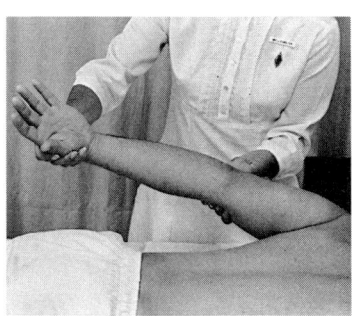

Hyperextension
Hyperextend the neck gently.

Rotation
Rotate the neck in as large a semi-circle as possible.

Hyperextension
Hyperextend the shoulder.

Rotation
Rotate the shoulder in as large a semi-circle as possible.

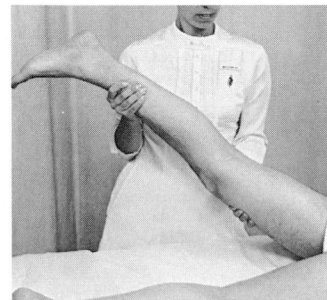 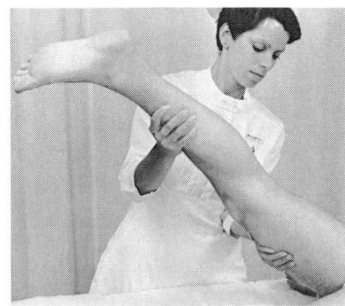

Hip

Hyperextension
Hyperextend the hip by lifting the leg with the knee extended.

Rotation
Rotate the hip in as large a semi-circle as possible.

PROCEDURE 28-2
Moving a Client Up in Bed

One Nurse

Action	**Rationale**
1 Explain the procedure to the client.	This facilitates cooperation of the client.
2 Wash your hands.	Handwashing deters spread of microorganisms.
3 Raise the bed to a comfortable position for you. Adjust the bed to flat position if the client can tolerate it. Lower the side rail nearest you.	This position facilitates moving the client upward and minimizes strain on the nurse.
4 Remove the pillow and place it at the head of the bed.	This reduces friction and protects the client's head from striking the top of the bed.
5 If able to assist, have the client flex the knees with the feet flat on the bed.	The client is prepared to push upward by using a major muscle group.
6 Assist the client to grasp the overhead trapeze bar or, if unable to assist, fold the client's arms across the chest.	This provides assistance and reduces friction.
7 Instruct the client to flex the neck with the chin on the chest.	This prevents hyperextension of the neck.
8 Stand opposite the client's center with your feet spread and turned toward the head of the bed. Position one foot slightly forward.	This positions the mover opposite the center of the body mass. It places the nurse in a stable position, with good alignment.

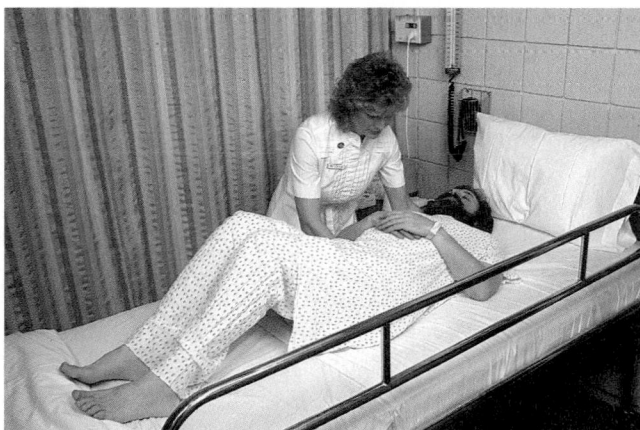

Step 5: Preparing client for move.

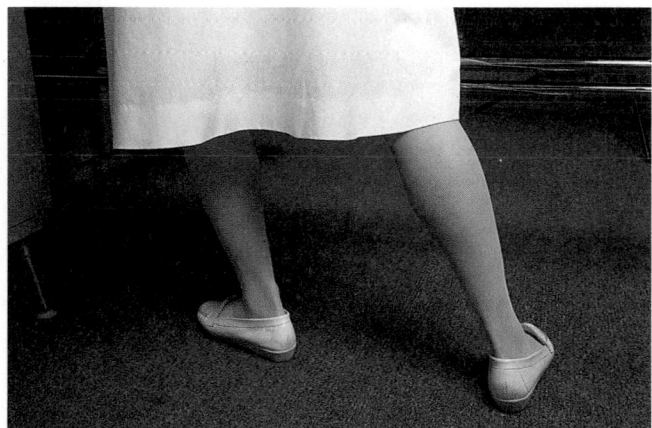

Step 8: Placing legs and feet for stable position.

9 Flex your knees and hips. Place one arm under the client's neck and shoulders, grasping the far shoulder with your hand. Place your other arm under the client's upper thighs. Pull the client closer to your side of the bad. Move the client's head and legs into alignment.	This prepares the nurse to use a large muscle mass to aid in lifting. The placement of the arms supports and evenly distributes the weight of the client.
10 Review the plan of movement with the client. Tighten your abdominal and gluteal muscles. Assume the position to move the client (see Step 9).	These muscles stabilize the pelvis prior to the lifting maneuver.

(Continued)

One Nurse

Action

11 Shift your weight back and forth from back leg to front leg, and on count of three, move the client upward in bed. If possible, the client should push with the legs and assist movement upward by grasping the trapeze. Repeat if necessary.

Rationale

The rocking motion uses your weight to counteract the client's weight when moving the client up in bed. If the client assists, less effort is required by the nurse.

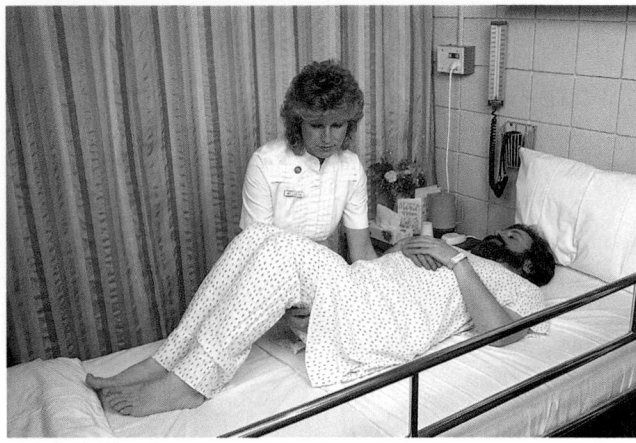

Step 11: Moving client.

12 Assist the client to a comfortable position in the center of the bed. Reposition the pillow. Raise the side rail and adjust the bed position, if necessary.

This ensures the client's safety.

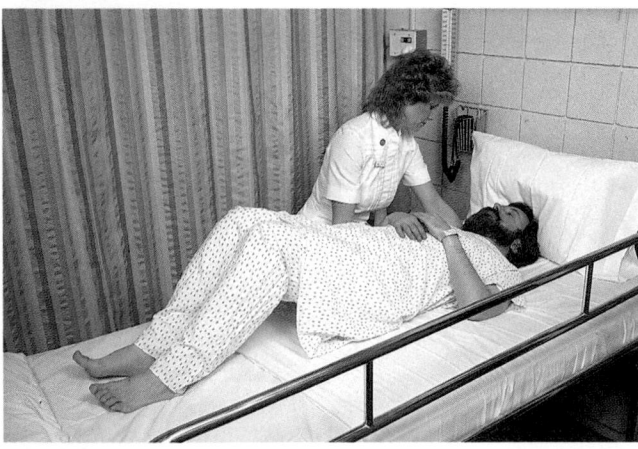

Step 12: Assisting client in new position.

13 Wash your hands.

Handwashing deters the spread of microorganisms.

Special Considerations

1 Two nurses on opposite sides of the bed may move a client up in bed by interlocking their arms under the client's shoulders and thighs and lifting as described above.

2 Two nurses on opposite sides of the bed may move a client up in bed by using a drawsheet placed under the client from shoulder to thigh area. Fold or bunch the drawsheet close to the client and lift as described above.

PROCEDURE 28-3
Transferring a Client from Bed to Stretcher

Action	**Rationale**
1 Explain the procedure to the client.	This facilitates the cooperation of the client.
2 Wash your hands.	Handwashing deters the spread of microorganisms.
3 Move the bed and equipment in the room to make room for the stretcher. Make sure that assistants are available. Close the door or curtain.	This facilitates transfer movement and provides for privacy.
4 Raise the bed to the same height as the stretcher and adjust the head of the bed to the flat position if the client can tolerate it. Lower side rails.	Pushing and pulling require less effort than lifting. This position facilitates moving the client.
5 Place a drawsheet under the client if one is not already there. Use the drawsheet to move the client to the side of the bed where the stretcher will be placed.	This facilitates movement of the client to the stretcher.
6 Position stretcher next to the bed and parallel to it. Lock wheels on the stretcher and bed. Remove the pillow from the bed and place it on the stretcher.	Positioning of the stretcher and locking the wheels facilitate safe transfer of client.
7 To move the client:	
a. The first nurse should kneel on far side of the bed away from the stretcher. Position the knee at the upper torso closer to the client than the other knee. Grasp the drawsheet securely.	The nurse uses a major muscle group to assist in movement. The nurse's flexed hips help avoid back injury.
b. The second nurse should reach across the stretcher and grasp the drawsheet at the head and chest areas of the client.	This promotes safe transfer by supporting the client's head and upper body.
c. The third nurse should reach across the stretcher and grasp the drawsheet at the client's waist and thigh area. Ask the client to fold arms across the chest.	This supports the lower part of the client's body for safe transfer.
d. At a signal given by the first nurse, the second and third nurses pull while the first nurse lifts the client from the bed to the stretcher.	Working in unison distributes the work of moving the client and facilitates the transfer.

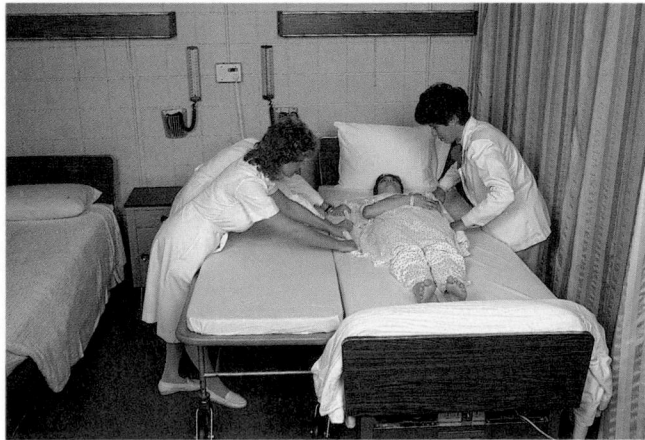

Step 5: Using drawsheet to move client to side of bed.

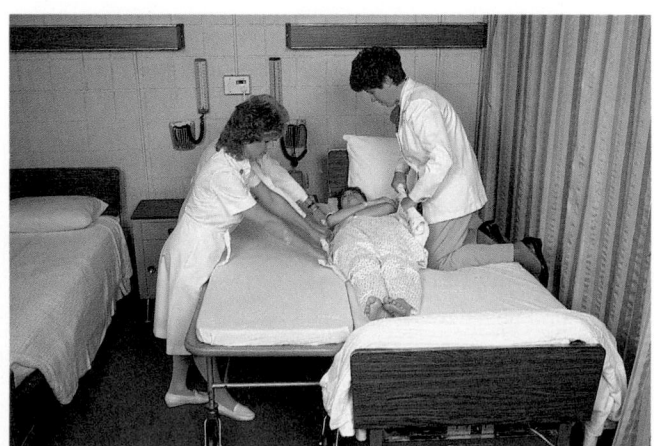

Step 7: Moving client to stretcher.

(Continued)

PROCEDURE 28-3
Transferring a Client from Bed to Stretcher (Continued)

Action	Rationale
8 Secure the client on the stretcher until side rails are raised. Assist the client to a comfortable position with the covering in place. Leave the draw-sheet in place for transfer back to bed.	This ensures client safety and comfort.
9 Wash your hands.	Handwashing deters the spread of microorganisms.

PROCEDURE 28-4
Transferring a Client from Bed to Stretcher (Three-Carrier Lift)

Action	Rationale
1 Explain the procedure to the client.	This facilitates the cooperation of the client.
2 Wash your hands.	Handwashing deters the spread of microorganisms.
3 Place the stretcher at a right angle to the foot of the bed. Lock the wheels of the bed and the wheels of the stretcher. Raise the bed to the height of the stretcher.	The stretcher will be in position for the carriers after they pivot away from the bed.

4 Decide on responsibility for the lift. Each person must support one section of the body:
 	
   a. Head, shoulders, and chest
   b. Hips
   c. Thighs and legs
	Opinions differ about how to determine who lifts which area. The recommendations are that the strongest helper should support the heaviest body area or that the tallest person with the longest reach should support the client's head and shoulders.

5 In preparation for the lift, flex your knees and separate your feet, with the foot closest to the stretcher slightly forward.	Broad-based stance improves balance and lowers the lifter's center of gravity.

(Continued)

Action	**Rationale**
6 Slide your arms under the client as far as possible and, on signal, all helpers should simultaneously roll the client toward their chests.	"Logrolling" the client onto the carriers brings the centers of gravity of all objects closer, thereby increasing the stability of the group and reducing strain on the carriers.
7 On signal, the helpers should stand up and steady the client securely against their chests.	Flexed knees and body position allow workers to lift with strong leg muscles.

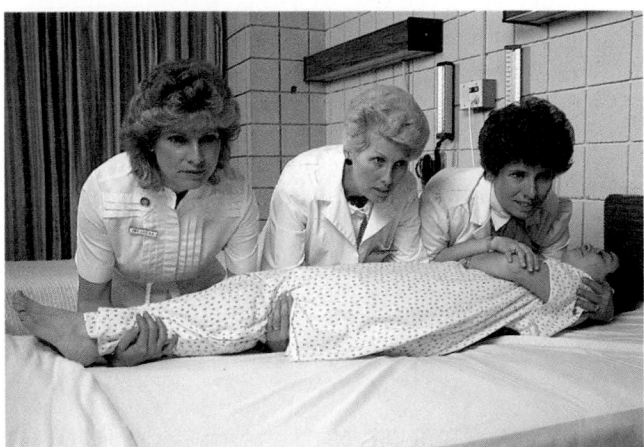

Step 6: Positioning client close to lifters.

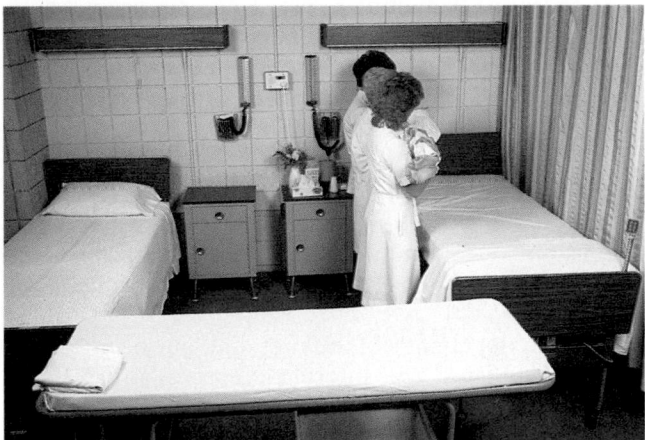

Step 7: Standing with client held to chest.

8 Helpers should step back together, pivot around to the stretcher, and, on signal, lower the client onto the stretcher.	This lets the large leg and arm muscles do the work of lowering the client.

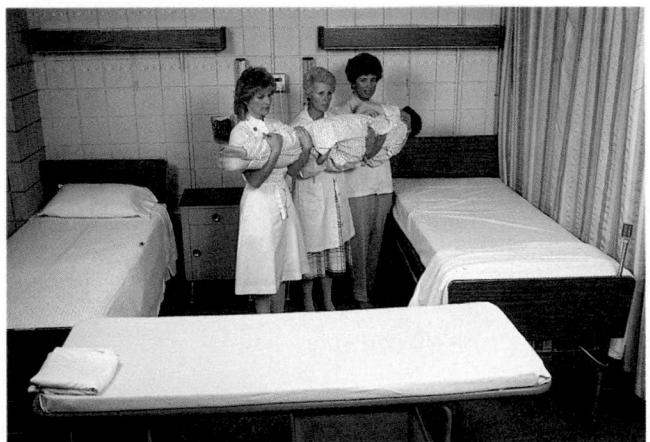

Step 8: Pivoting to stretcher.

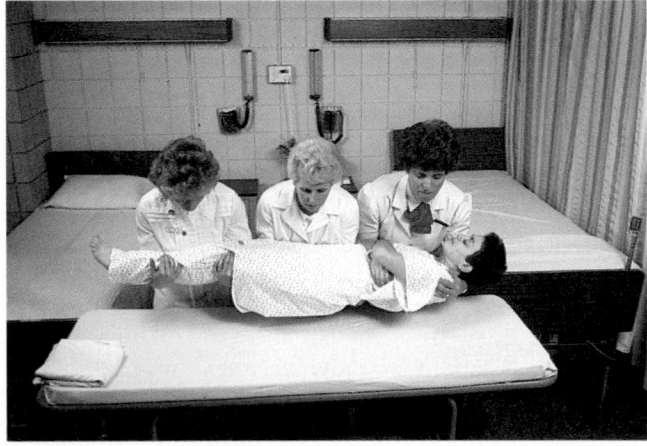

Step 8: Lowering client to stretcher.

9 The client should be covered with a sheet or blanket and positioned as necessary. Stretcher side rails should be raised.	This ensures comfort and safety of the client.
10 Wash your hands.	Handwashing deters the spread of microorganisms.

on the client, the third person is able to join them and assist in sliding the client to the center of the bed.

There are instances when clients must be lifted and carried. This can be done by means of a three-carrier lift. If done properly, the client will feel secure, and those lifting will not suffer strain. The three-carrier lift is described and illustrated in Procedure 28-4.

The three-carrier lift is used in various other situations, such as lifting a client who has fallen to the floor and is unable to get up independently, or lifting a client out of a chair into the bed.

For clients who present special problems because of their excessive weight or a cast, it may be necessary to have an additional person to support the heaviest or most cumbersome part of the client. The persons distribute their arms while carrying so that the heaviest part is well supported.

Assisting the Client Out of Bed

The patient's safety and comfort are enhanced when certain precautions are taken prior to assisting the client out of bed:

- Obtain the client's blood pressure, pulse, and respiratory rates. This information serves as baseline data before the client is out of bed.
- Have a walker, cane, or crutches available if the client needs a device to assist with walking.
- Place a chair or wheelchair parallel to the head of the bed if the client is to move from the bed to a chair without walking. If the client has weakness or paralysis in the lower extremities and the plan is to pivot the client from the bed to the chair, place the chair on the client's unaffected side. Be sure the wheels of a wheelchair are locked and the foot pedals are in the up position so that they are not in the way of the client.
- Place the client's bed in its lowest position so that feet touch the floor easily.
- Help the client to the dangling position on the side of the bed.
- Help the client to dress. Clothing should be sufficient to prevent embarrassment, but should not be too warm. Clothing should not impede the client's movements. Supportive shoes with nonskid soles should be worn by the client.

When the client is ready, the nurse next assists the client to move from the bed.

- Face the client, give yourself a wide base of support, put one foot forward between the client's feet, and flex your knees to give yourself stability.
- Have the client place the hands on your shoulders, around your waist or rib cage (never around your neck), and then grasp the client at the side of the upper chest, never in the axillary areas. Grasping the client on the chest wall is uncomfortable and restricts breathing.
- Ask the client to lift self as you help lift the upper part of the body.

- Allow the client to stand a few seconds to be sure he or she is not feeling faint. If feelings of faintness occur, allow the client to rest on the bed before proceeding.
- If the client is standing comfortably, instruct the client to take several deep breaths since the standing posture facilitates lung expansion.
- Pivot yourself and the client while maintaining a wide base of support if the client is without feelings of faintness.
- Lower the client into the chair or wheelchair by bending your knees and keeping your back straight. Have the client assist by holding onto the armrests on a chair or wheelchair while being lowered into it.
- Check the client's vital signs to determine how they have been affected by the activity. The pulse rate can be expected to increase temporarily. However, no prolonged significant change in blood pressure should be expected. If the client's pulse rate or blood pressure is significantly affected, stay with the client until it returns to normal.

Moving the Client from Bed to Chair and from Chair to Bed

It is possible for only one person to get a helpless client from a bed to a chair, although two people simplify matters. The one-person technique is valuable for nurses to know for the home care of invalids and for emergency use. More than one person should be available if the bed and chair seat are not the same height. The technique by which one person moves a client from a bed to a chair and vice versa are described in Procedure 28-5. The technique for transferring a client by two nurses is described in Procedure 28-6.

Helping Clients Ambulate

Fortunately for most clients, prolonged periods of bed rest are no longer considered necessary during most illnesses. Activity, even as mild as a stroll around the room, down the hall, from the bedroom to the living room, or out into the yard, is a protective measure for the body.

Physical Conditioning

Clients who are not confined to bed for long periods, who sleep well, and who experience possibly short periods of rest during the day may not require special considerations for increased physical activity in preparation for ambulation. However, there are others who will have to be prepared for the day when ambulation is resumed. Certain exercises that strengthen the overall efficiency of the musculoskeletal system can be done in bed.

Quadriceps Drills (Sets). Quadriceps drills are an **isometric exercise**, which is defined as an exercise in which muscle tension occurs without a significant change in

(Text continues on p. 668.)

PROCEDURE 28-5
Assisting a Client to Transfer from Bed to Chair

Action	**Rationale**
1 Explain the procedure to the client. Offer bedpan.	This facilitates cooperation of the client. Empty bladder will increase client comfort.
2 Wash your hands.	Handwashing deters the spread of microorganisms.
3 Assess the client's ability to assist with transfer. Move equipment as necessary to make room for the chair. Close the door or curtain.	This ensures client safety and facilitates the transfer. Closing the door or curtain provides for privacy.
4 Place the bed in the low position.	This facilitates transfer to chair.
5 Assist the client to put on a robe and slippers.	These provide warmth. Slippers provide protection and stability.
6 Position the chair at the bedside:	
a. *For a client with unimpaired mobility:* Bring chair close to the bedside facing the foot of the bed and, if possible, brace the back of the chair against a bedside table.	This increases stability and ensures client safety during the transfer.
b. *For a client with impaired mobility:* Position the chair facing the head or foot of the bed. When sitting on the side of the bed; the client should be able to steady self by using the hand on the unaffected side to grasp the arm of the chair.	This uses the strong side to provide balance and improve stability during the transfer.
7 Lock the wheels on the chair and bed if appropriate.	This ensures client safety.
8 Raise the head of the bed to the highest position.	Moving from the sitting to the standing position requires less energy.
9 Assist the client to sit on the side of the bed by supporting the client's head and neck while moving the client's legs off the bed to dangle. Steady the client in that position for a few minutes.	The sitting position facilitates transfer to the chair and allows the circulatory system to adjust to a change in position.

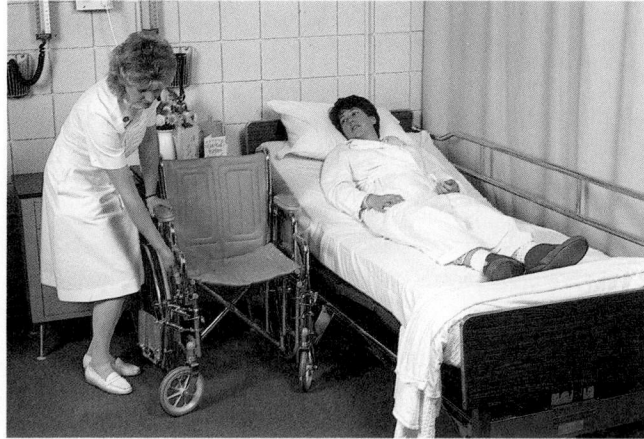

Step 6: Placing chair at bedside.

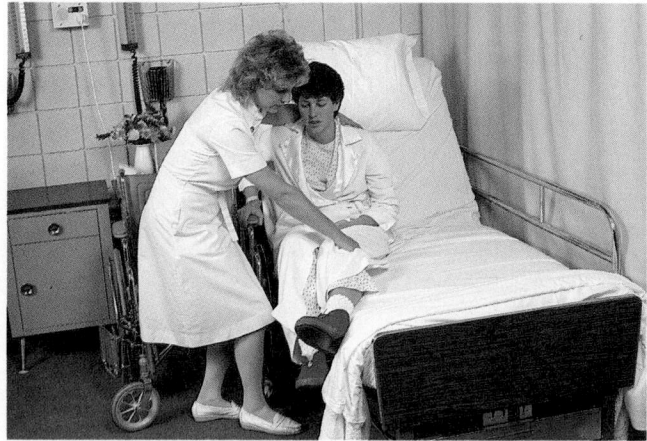

Step 9: Supporting client while moving legs off bed.

(Continued)

Action

10 Assist the client to the standing position:

a. *For a client with unimpaired mobility:* Face the client and brace your feet and knees against the client. Place your hands around the client's waist while the client places arms around your shoulders. Raise the client to the standing position.

b. *For a client with impaired mobility:* Face the client and brace your feet and knees against the client, especially against the affected extremity. Place your hands around the client's waist. The client may place the unaffected arm around your shoulder or use the unaffected arm to reach for the arm of the chair and to push up while raising to the standing position.

11 Pivot the client (on the unaffected limb if applicable) into position in front of the chair with legs positioned against the chair.

12 The client may use one arm (the unaffected limb if applicable) to place on the arm of the chair and steady self while slowly lowering to the sitting position. Continue to brace the client's knees with your knees and flex your own hips and knees when seating the client.

Rationale

This provides for stability and for use of major muscle groups to facilitate movement.

This provides for stability and makes use of the unaffected extremities to facilitate movement.

This provides security and proper position prior to sitting.

The client uses own arm for support and stability. The nurse flexes the knees and hips to use a major muscle group to aid in movement and reduce strain on the back.

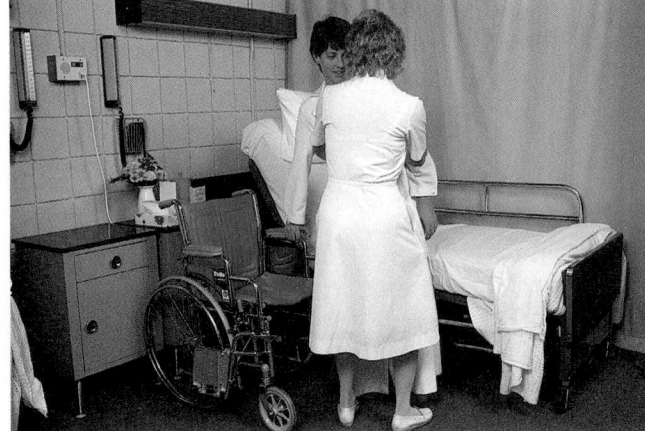

Step 10B: Assisting client to stand.

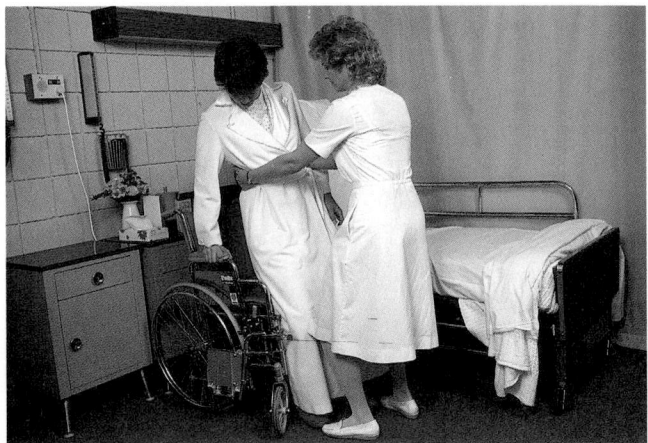

Step 12: Bracing client's knees while lowering client to chair.

13 Adjust the client's position using pillows where necessary. Cover the client and use restraint if necessary. Position the call bell so it is available for use.

14 Wash your hands.

15 Document the client's tolerance of the procedure and length of time in the chair.

This maintains proper body alignment and provides for comfort and safety.

Handwashing, deters the spread of microorganisms.

This provides accurate documentation and ensures continuity of care.

PROCEDURE 28-6
Transferring a Dependent Client from Bed to Chair (Two Nurses)

Action	Rationale
1 Explain the procedure to the client.	This facilitates cooperation of the client.
2 Wash your hands.	Handwashing deters the spread of microorganisms.
3 Move equipment as necessary to make room for the chair. Close the door or curtain. Assist the client to put on a robe and slippers.	This ensures client safety and facilitates transfer. It provides for privacy and warmth.
4 Move the client to the near side of the bed and cross the client's arms across the chest if possible. Lock the wheels of the bed.	This requires less effort to move the client. Locked wheels will prevent the bed from moving if the client leans against it.
5 Position the chair next to the bed near the upper end and with the back of the chair parallel to the head of the bed. (If wheelchair, remove the armrest closer to the bed if possible). Lock the wheels if appropriate.	Positioning the chair next to the bed facilitates easier movement into the chair.
6 Adjust the bed to a comfortable level for nurses or at the level of the armrest if one is present on the chair.	This facilitates transfer with minimal muscle strain on the nurses.
7 Prepare to lift the client from the bed to the chair:	Two people lifting the client distributes weight and decreases the effort needed for transfer.
a. The first nurse should stand behind the chair. Slip the arms under the client's axillae and grasp the client's wrists securely.	
b. The second nurse should face the wheelchair and support the client's knees by placing the arms under them.	
c. On a predetermined signal, both nurses flex their hips and knees and simultaneously lift the client gently to the chair.	

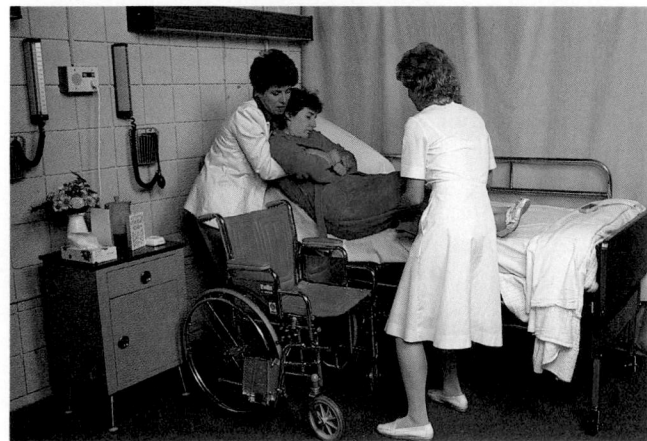

Steps 7A&B: First nurse slipping arms under client's axillae and grasping wrists; second nurse supporting client's knees.

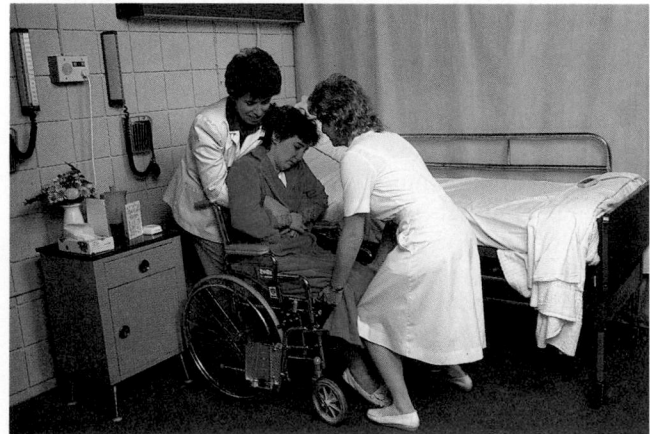

Step 7C: Lowering client into chair.

(Continued)

Transferring a Dependent Client from Bed to Chair (Two Nurses)   (Continued)

Action	Rationale
8 Adjust the client's position using pillows where necessary. Cover the client and use restraint if necessary. Position the call bell so it is available for use.	This maintains proper body alignment and provides for comfort and safety.
9 Wash your hands.	Handwashing deters the spread of microorganisms.
10 Document the client's tolerance of the procedure and length of time in the chair.	This provides accurate documentation and ensures continuity of care.

the length of the muscle. One of the most important muscle groups used in walking is the quadriceps femoris. This muscle group helps extend the leg and flexes the thigh. To help reduce weakness and make first attempts at walking easier, bedridden clients should be encouraged to contract this muscle group frequently. The following are techniques for quadriceps drills:

- Have the client contract the muscles on the front of the thighs by pulling the kneecaps toward the hips. The client has the feeling of pushing the knees downward into the mattress and pulling the feet upward.
- Have the client hold the position just described while counting slowly to four, and then relax the muscles for an equal amount of time. Emphasize that relaxation is important to prevent muscle fatigue.
- Caution the client not to hold the breath during these exercises as this places strain on the heart.
- Teach the client to do quadriceps drills two or three times each hour, four to six times a day.
- Instruct the client to stop the exercise short of muscle fatigue.

The muscles in the buttocks can be exercised in the same way by pinching the buttocks together and then relaxing them. This is called *gluteal settings*. Tightening and holding the abdominal muscles for 6 seconds and then relaxing them also strengthens this muscle group and facilitates walking.

Push-Ups.   The muscle strength of the arms and shoulders also may need to be improved before the client is ready to be out of bed. Exercises should improve the strength needed to hold onto or get into a chair and to move about better. They are part of the preparation for clients who must learn to walk on crutches.

A trapeze attached to the bed of a client who has limited use of the lower part of the body helps the client to move about in bed and strengthens muscles in the upper part of the body. However, this does not strengthen the triceps, which is the muscle group necessary for crutch walking or for moving from a bed to a chair. More suitable exercises are push-ups, which are done as follows:

- Sitting up in bed without support is one type of push-up exercise. Instruct the client to lift the hips off the bed by pushing down with the hands on the mattress. If the mattress is too soft, a block of books can be placed on the bed under the client's hands.
- Push-ups may also be done with the client lying in bed on the abdomen. Instruct the client to place the hands near the outstretched body at approximately shoulder level, with palms down on the mattress and elbows bent sharply. Then have the client straighten the elbows while lifting the head and shoulders off the bed.
- Push-ups may also be done when the client sits in an armchair or wheelchair. The client places the hands on the arms of the chair and then raises the body out of the seat.

Push-ups are usually done three or four times a day, with the number increased as upper body strength is increased.

Dangling.   Dangling refers to the position in which the person sits on the edge of the bed with legs and feet over the side of the bed. This exercise helps prepare the client for being out of bed also. It is carried out as follows:

- Place the client in the sitting position in bed for a few minutes. This will accustom the client to this position and help prevent feelings of faintness.

- Place the bed in the low position or have a footstool handy on which the client can rest the feet while dangling.
- Move the client toward the side of the bed near you so that you do not stretch and strain while turning the client.
- Pivot the client a quarter of a turn by supporting the shoulders and legs. Swing the client's legs over the side of the bed. The client may place the hands on your shoulders.
- Rest the client's feet on the floor or on a footstool. This gives a sense of security, and the client is less likely to slide from the bed.
- Have the client pick up and put down the feet alternately in a marching motion. This promotes circulation in the legs.
- Remain with the client, and be ready to put the client in a lying position if feeling faint so that the client does not fall out of bed.

Daily Activities for Purposeful Exercise. Many activities in addition to those just described can be carried out with benefit to the client. These include placing the bedside stand so that the client must use shoulder and arm muscles to reach what is needed instead of placing it so as to require little effort to take things from it; placing the signal cord so that the client must engage in either arm or shoulder action in order to reach it; encouraging the client to sit up and reach for the overbed table, to pull it close, and then to push it back in place; encouraging a client to try to wash the back; and having the client put on socks while still in bed. There are innumerable ways in which clients can be helped to exercise, and when they understand the purpose, they very often adopt other exercises for themselves.

Assisting the Client to Walk

Many clients who have been confined to bed for a long time find that they must almost learn to walk all over again. Often, it is the nurse who plays a major role in the client's recovery and mental outlook, hope and faith, especially when a rigid and often difficult schedule of reeducating muscle groups must be adhered to. It has been noted that a client able to raise the leg only 2.5 cm (1 inch) from the bed possesses sufficient power to permit walking.

When the major problem of muscle reeducation presents itself, the client will need the assistance of experts in physical medicine. However, nurses assist clients out of bed and help them to walk when a physical therapist is not present. The nurse should also plan to walk with a client who is using this activity for the first few times after a period of bed rest.

Before getting the client out of bed, the nurse

- Assesses the client's ability to walk and need for assistance (one nurse, two nurses, walker, cane, walking belt, or crutches)
- Explains to the client exactly what is to be done: transfer technique from bed to erect position, projected distance to be ambulated, assistance available and the correct manner of using it; the client is instructed to alert the nurse immediately if feeling dizzy or weak.
- Ensures that the client has a clear path for ambulation

The nurse then slowly assists the client to an erect position and ambulation, pausing after the client is seated at the edge of the bed and again after the client first stands to ensure that the client feels steady. The nurse reminds the client to take deep breaths to promote good aeration of the lungs while walking. Clients who are fearful of walking often tend to look at their feet and may need to be reminded to stand erect and to hold the head high to achieve the full benefits of walking. Since it is not unusual for clients who are walking for the first time after prolonged bed rest to feel faint or weak, a short distance should be planned. As this distance is increased, it is helpful to have chairs readily available should the client need to rest. Should a client faint or begin to fall while walking, the nurse stands with feet apart to create a wide base of support and rocks the pelvis out on the side facing the client. With arms under the client's axillae and encircling the client, the nurse slides the client down the nurse's own body to the floor, carefully protecting the client's head. This maneuver should be practiced before it is needed in an emergency situation.

One-Nurse Assist. The client who requires minimal nursing assistance may ambulate well with the nurse walking alongside and keeping the arm that is near the client under the client's arm in an arm-to-arm position. Should the client fall in this position, however, the nurse will find it difficult to lower the client to the floor by supporting the client's weight against the nurse's body, and the client's shoulder joint may be dislocated if the nurse holds onto it tightly.

The nurse better supports the client by standing at the client's side and placing both hands at the client's waist. Use of a walking belt (Fig. 28-15) with handgrasps for the nurse at the sides and back facilitates this type of support. By supporting the client at the waist the nurse helps the client maintain an erect posture and is prevented from pulling the client unintentionally to one side.

When a client has weakness or paralysis on one side, the nurse has two options:

- For the moderately weak client, the nurse walks at the client's affected side, with the near arm under the client's near arm and the near hand grasping the inferior aspect of the client's near upper arm. The nurse's far hand then grasps the client's near lower arm or hand (Fig. 28-15).
- For the very weak client, the nurse walks on the client's unaffected side and places the near arm around the client's waist. The near arm of the

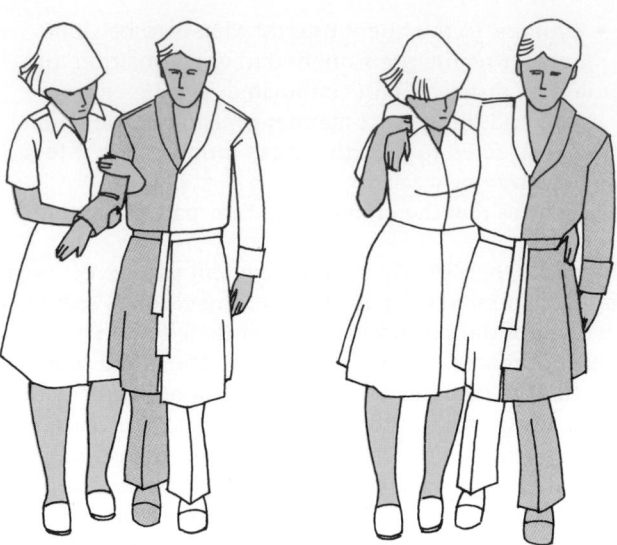

F I G U R E 28-15
Two techniques to assist a client to walk. The shaded area indicates the affected side of the client with hemiparesis or hemiplegia.

client is placed around the nurse's shoulders and the nurse grasps this hand with the far hand. In this position both the nurse and client step forward on their inside feet. When the client advances the outer leg, which is the weaker, the nurse's outer leg is also put forward, providing a wide base of support. A transfer belt should always be used with clients who are unstable.

Two-Nurse Assist.   There are two methods of ambulation that two nurses can safely use to support a client. In the first, the nurses stand at the client's sides with their near hands grasping the inferior aspect of the client's near upper arm and their far hands holding the client's lower arm or hand. The second position provides more support to the client but requires the three persons involved to be of similar heights. The nurses again position themselves at the client's sides, slipping their near arms under the client's arms and around the client's back, grasping one another's wrists. The client stretches the arms around the nurses' shoulders and the nurses grasp the client's hands with their far hands. In both these positions the nurses and the client step in unison. See Figure 28-16.

Utilizing Mechanical Aids for Walking

Various devices can assist a client with walking. The most common are walkers, canes, braces, and crutches. Most often a client is fitted for these devices and instructed in their use in a department of physical medicine or physical therapy. In this instance, nursing's concern is chiefly to reinforce the teaching the client has received and to make sure the client continues to use the device properly to assist in safe ambulation. However, in some work settings nurses may be responsible for fitting

clients for these devices. Whenever a nurse assesses a client who has been using a walker, cane, brace, or crutches over a period of time, it is important to determine if the device is still needed, if it continues to meet the client's needs, and if the client continues to use it properly.

General guidelines for helping clients who need the assistance of a walker, cane, brace, or crutches are the following:

- Whenever possible, instruct the client and family members in the correct use of the device before it is needed (*e.g.,* prior to surgery). If family members are knowledgeable, they can reinforce the teaching as needed.
- When ready to begin ambulation with the new device, make sure the client is wearing rubber-soled,

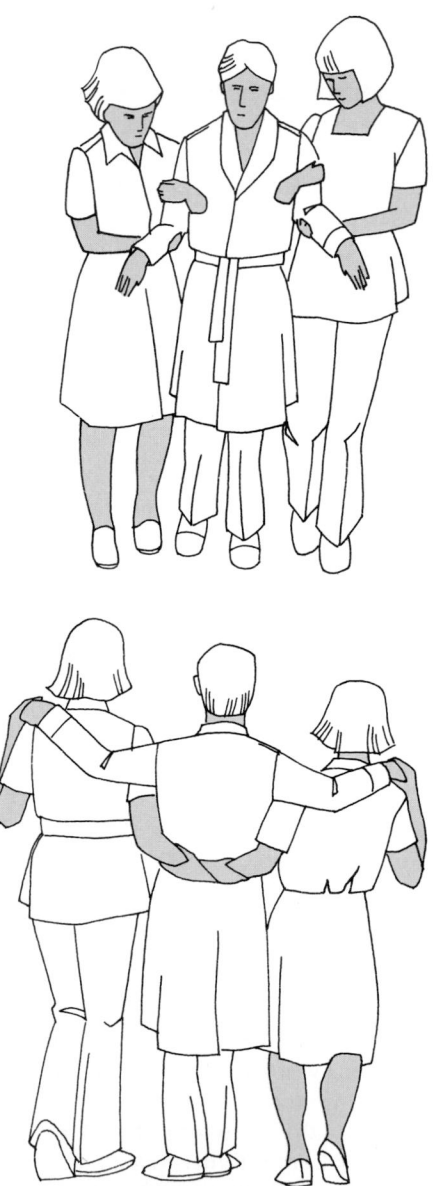

F I G U R E 28-16
Two techniques for two nurses to safely assist a client to ambulate.

well-fitting shoes and that there is a clear path for ambulation (clean, flat, dry, and well lighted). If the client is at high risk for falls, use a walking belt for added support.

- Before moving, make sure the client is steady on the feet when standing; instruct the client to stand erect, looking straight ahead, and walk behind and slightly to one side of the client (in cases of hemiparesis or hemiparalysis, walk on the client's affected side). Should the client lose balance, be prepared to grasp the client's shoulder and the transfer belt to steady the client.

Walker. A walker is a lightweight metal frame (usually aluminum) with four legs (Fig. 28-17). The walker provides a sense of security and support. There are several variations of walkers, and they are specified according to the arm strength and balance of the client.

When the client stands between the back legs of the walker, the walker should extend from the floor to the client's hip joint; the client's elbows should be flexed about 30 degrees. Rubber tips should be intact to prevent slipping. Generally the client lifts the walker ahead of self and steps into it. However, the gaits may be specified. The elderly frequently develop dangerous walking patterns with a walker and may require close observation.

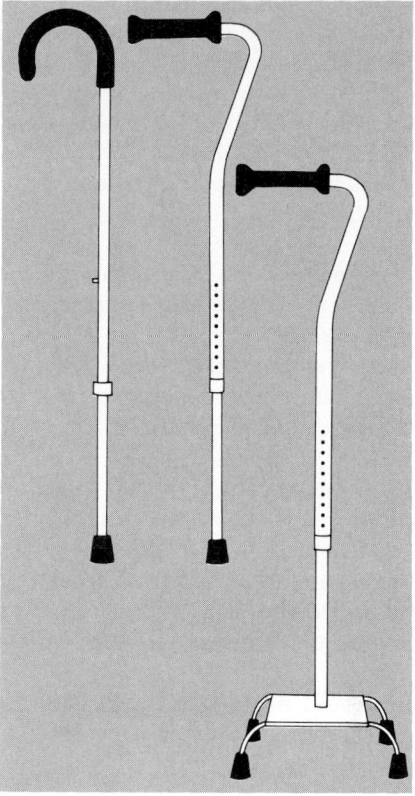

FIGURE 28-18

Three types of canes. Single-ended canes with half-circle handles are recommended for clients requiring minimal support. Single-ended canes with straight handles are recommended for clients with hand weakness. Three or four prong canes are recommended for clients with poor balance.

Canes. Canes come in basically three variations (Fig. 28-18):

- *Single-ended canes with a half-circle handle* are recommended for clients requiring minimal support and if the client will be using stairs frequently.
- *Single-ended canes with straight handles* are recommended for clients with hand weakness because their handgrips are easier to hold; they are not recommended for clients with poor balance.
- *Canes with three or four prongs or legs to provide a wide base of support* (tripod or quad cane) are recommended for clients with poor balance. Instruct the client to use a cane with as small a base as possible, and eventually to progress to a single-ended cane if possible. The smaller the base, the less the client relies on the cane for support.

Many canes are adjustable and should be fitted so that when the client stands with the cane's tip 4 inches (10 cm) to the side of the foot, the cane extends from the floor to the client's hip joint. The elbow should be flexed at a 30-degree angle when holding the cane. Rubber tips on the cane prevent slipping and accidents. They should be inspected regularly for this reason. Clients should be taught to stand erect when walking with a cane and not to lean out over the cane.

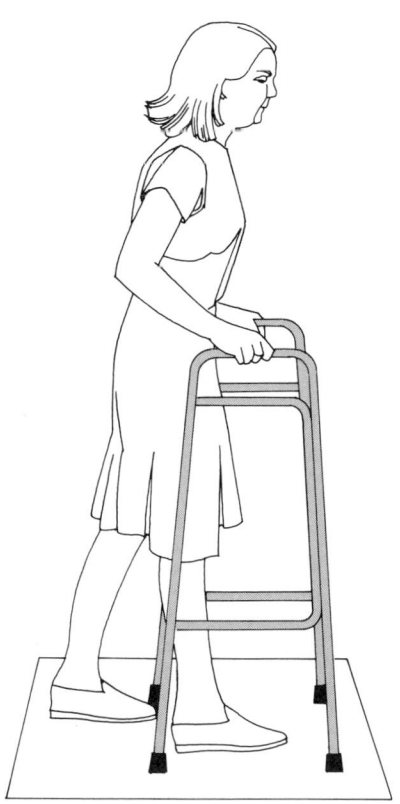

FIGURE 28-17

A walker is a light-weight metal frame with a broad, four-point base of support. The walker should be adjusted to the height of the client's hip joint so that the client's elbows are flexed about 30 degrees.

When walking with a cane, clients are generally instructed to hold the cane on the unaffected side to provide additional support for the weaker leg. Ambulation proceeds in the following fashion:

1. The client stands with weight evenly distributed between the feet and the cane.
2. The cane is held on the client's stronger side and is advanced 4 inches to 12 inches (10.2 cm to 30 cm).
3. Supporting weight on the stronger leg and the cane, the client advances the weaker foot forward, parallel with the cane.
4. Supporting weight on the weaker leg and the cane, the client next advances the stronger leg forward ahead of the cane (heel slightly beyond the tip of the cane).
5. Finally, the weaker leg is moved forward until even with the stronger leg and the cane is once again advanced as in Step 2.

When less support is required from the cane the client can advance the cane and stronger leg forward while the cane and weaker leg support the client's weight.

Clients should be taught to position their canes within easy reach when they sit down so that they can rise easily.

Braces.   Braces that support weakened leg muscles are available in many variations. Nursing responsibilities include (1) learning with the client when the brace is to be worn and the correct technique for applying the brace; (2) monitoring the client's correct use of the brace; and (3) observing for any untoward problems the brace might be causing (*e.g.,* skin irritation). Muscle changes such as those occurring with growth and development or brought about by illness (atrophy) may result in the brace needing to be refitted to maintain its effectiveness.

Crutches.   Sometimes, it is necessary for clients to use crutches for a time to avoid using one leg or to help strengthen one or both legs. This procedure is taught best by a physical therapist; however, there are numerous instances when the nurse is called on to measure clients for crutches and to teach them to use them. Even if a client is being taught to crutch walk by a physical therapist, it is necessary for the nurse to understand the client's progress and the gait being taught. The nurse must often guide the client at home or in the hospital after the initial teaching is completed. The two types of crutches most commonly used are the underarm or axillary crutches and the forearm support crutches (Fig. 28-19).

Measuring for Axillary Crutches.   The following techniques are used to measure the client for axillary crutches:

- Have the client lie flat in bed on the back while wearing shoes to be used when walking.

- Measure the distance from the anterior fold of the axilla straight down to the heel, and then add 5 cm (2 inches). Or measure the distance from the anterior fold of the axilla diagonally out to a point 15 cm (6 inches) away from the heel.
- After proper crutches are obtained, have the client stand to adjust the handgrips. Secure the handgrips

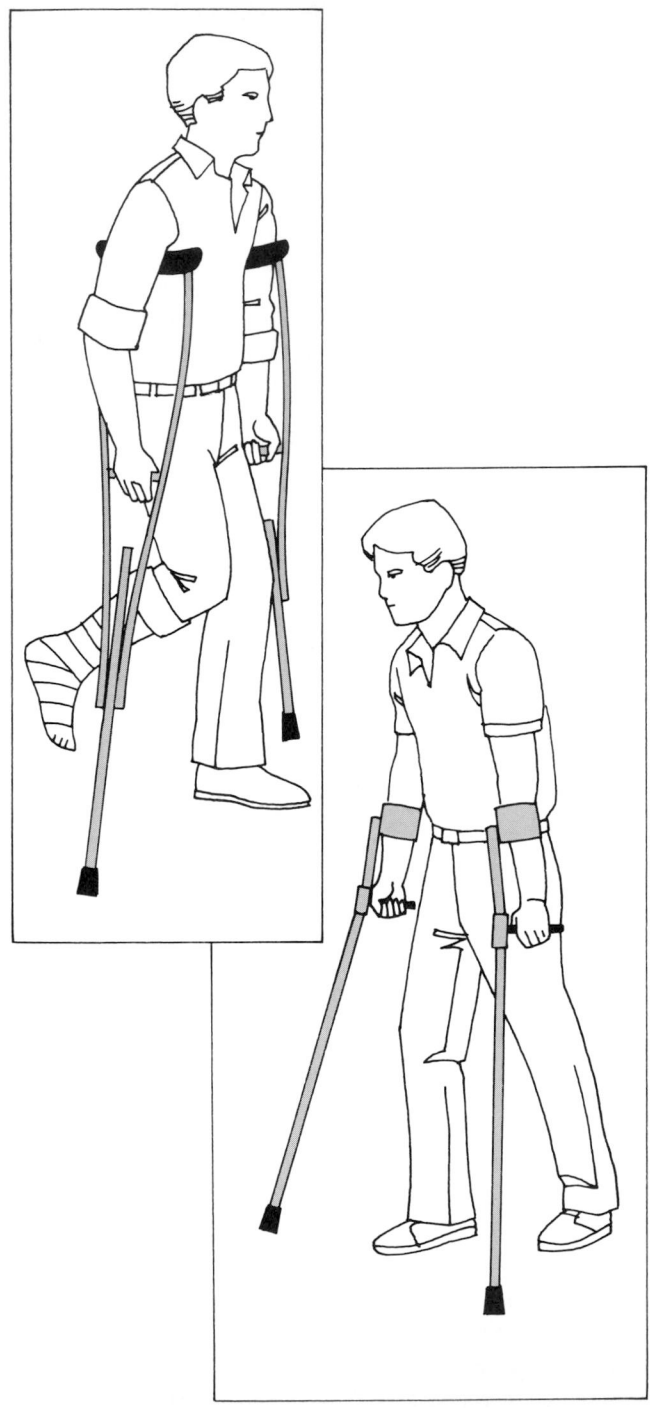

F I G U R E   28-19
Axillary and forearm support crutches.

while the client grasps them in the hands with elbows slightly bent and wrists bent backwards.

- Teach the client that the support of body weight should come primarily on the hands and arms while using the crutches, *not* in the axillary areas, where pressure may damage nerves and cut off circulation. Also, the crutches should not be forced into the axillae each time the body moves forward.

It is important that axillary crutches are properly fitted and used correctly to prevent damage to nerves and circulation in the axillae from being cut off, and to provide well-balanced support.

There are crutches available that have no axillary support. A supportive frame extends beyond the handgrip for the lower arm to help guide the crutch. These crutches are more likely to be used by clients who have permanent limitations and will always need crutch assistance for ambulation.

Exercises to Prepare for Crutch Walking. Before being asked to use the crutches, several exercises will help the client to be more confident and skillful. The client begins by strengthening the arm and the shoulder muscles. The push-up exercise described earlier is most helpful. The muscles of the hand must also be strengthened. Squeezing a rubber ball 50 times a day by flexing and extending the fingers helps to do this.

The client should be assisted into a chair that is close to the wall and then helped to stand against the wall and the crutches placed in the client's hands. Next, standing slightly away from the wall, the client should sway on the crutches from side to side. This accustoms the hands and the arms to weight-bearing.

After this, the client should be asked to lean against the wall and pick one crutch up about 15 cm (6 inches) from the floor and then place it down. This should be repeated with the other crutch, and the whole exercise should be done six to eight times. Then, still leaning against the wall, the client should be asked to pick up both crutches from the floor and place them down. This too should be repeated several times.

After these exercises, it will be possible to judge the client's ability to hold and manage the crutches without the added concern for movement. If judged capable, the client proceeds to the practice of a gait. If possible, it is recommended that the client begin with the four-point gait.

Crutch Gaits. There are four crutch gaits: four-point, three-point, two-point, and swing-through. These gaits are described in Table 28-6.

The swing-through gait is used by some clients when they become accustomed to the use of crutches and wish to get about quickly. The gait is also used by clients who have had a leg amputated. A disadvantage of this gait is that it does not simulate normal walking. Its extended use will lead to atrophy of the muscles in the lower extremity that is not being used, or in both legs if they both swing through.

TABLE 28-6
Crutch-Walking Gaits

Gait	Walking Pattern
Four-point gait	Weight-bearing is permitted on both legs. Pattern: Right crutch forward, left foot forward, left crutch forward, right foot forward.
Two-point gait	Weight-bearing is permitted on both feet. The pattern is a speed-up of the four-point gait. Pattern: Right crutch and left foot forward at the same time, left crutch and right foot forward at the same time.
Three-point gait	Weight-bearing is permitted on only one foot. The other foot cannot support, but acts as a balance. Pattern: Both crutches and the nonsupportive leg go forward, then the weight-bearing leg comes through; the crutches are brought forward immediately, and the pattern is repeated.
Swing-through gait	Weight-bearing is permitted only on one foot. Pattern: Unaffected foot bears weight while both crutches are brought forward; then both legs swing through between the crutches, and weight-bearing returns to the unaffected leg. Swing-through gait can also be used by the paraplegic client with weight-bearing on both feet.

Designing Exercise Programs

The benefits of exercise on each of the major body systems are so important that designing individualized exercise programs for clients is an important nursing responsibility. These programs incorporate activities of daily living and planned exercise sessions. Depending on the physical condition of the client, exercise is designed to promote optimal **fitness**.

An individual's commitment to a program of regular exercise rests on the following:

- Knowledge of the benefits of exercise and problems related to immobility
- Appreciation of the fact that in today's society sedentary life-styles are common and most people must consciously choose to exercise
- Belief that each person is responsible for self-health and that exercise is essential to well-being

Nurses can foster a commitment to regular exercise by teaching and counseling clients about exercise. To do this the nurse needs knowledge of the types and benefits of exercise as well as of the risks associated with exercise (presented earlier in this chapter).

The nurse working with a client to develop an indi-

Characteristics of a Successful Exercise Program

- The program is individually designed (takes into account the individual's fitness goals, interests, skills, exercise opportunities, and exercise capacity).
- The program specifies warm-up and cool-down activities and a variety of major exercise activities—variety is preferable to a single exercise activity.
- The program specifies frequency, intensity, and duration of exercise.

- The program is convenient to perform, compatible with the individual's life-style, and *fun!*
- The individual in such a program should understand the program and feel confident that exercise will result in definite health benefits.

Prevention Strategies to Avoid Risks Associated With Exercise

Persons beginning exercise programs should be familiar with the following guidelines:

- Obtain a pre-exercise medical examination and medical supervision during exercise if over age 35 and sedentary or if there is any past or current cardiovascular condition.
- Begin a new exercise program slowly and allow your body's support structure time to accommodate to the new stress.
- Know your body and respect its limitations. Never force a joint beyond its natural range of motion.

- Respect fatigue. Whenever you feel tingling, pain, or burning in a muscle stop and rest the muscle for 15 minutes before continuing to exercise.
- Follow the safety guidelines for specific exercises; for example, joggers are recommended (1) to run on soft surfaces as opposed to cement or asphalt, (2) to wear well-constructed shoes with thick soles and arch supports, and (3) to run in a safe environment with a low pollution index.

vidualized exercise prescription completes the following process.

- Explore the client's fitness goals, interests, skills, exercise opportunities, and exercise capacity.
- Assist the client in obtaining medical clearance for exercise.
- Explore feasible exercise activities with the client, considering health benefits sought, time involved, cost, need for special equipment, precautions, and risk.
- Develop an exercise program that specifies warm-up and cool-down activities (walking, stretching) and three or four major exercise activities from which the client can choose. Specify the frequency, duration, and intensity of the exercise activity. Recommended *frequency* is at least three times a week (but may work up to five or six times a week). For recommended *duration* and *intensity*, a person should be able to converse normally without getting out of breath or should maintain a **target heart rate** (60 to 90% of maximal heart rate [220 minus age]).
- Encourage the client to complement the exercise program with everyday activities that require exercise.
- Try to identify with the client potential threats to the exercise program's successful implementation. Plan support strategies.

- Utilize ongoing evaluation to determine if the exercise prescription is meeting the client's needs and if the client is adhering to the prescription.

The accompanying box identifies characteristics of a successful exercise program and prevention strategies to avoid risks associated with exercise.

EVALUATING

When evaluating the effectiveness of a plan of care designed to help clients enhance, maintain, or regain mobility and fitness goals, the nurse uses each nurse–client interaction to evaluate the client's

- General ease of movement and gait
- Alignment
- Joint structure and function
- Muscle mass, tone, and strength
- Endurance

An excellent time to assess these essential ingredients of well-being is when the client is performing simple everyday tasks such as ambulation, hygiene measures, dressing, and eating. Since illness and enforced inactivity can affect all of the above negatively, ongoing evaluation is necessary if serious problems are to be avoided. Specific criteria for evaluating individualized plans of care follow.

N U R S I N G   P R O C E S S   *in Clinical Practice*

Once a mobility problem is detected, the nurse implements each phase of the nursing process to ensure correct identification and treatment of the problem. The nurse who wishes to identify and manage the mobility problem correctly and to prevent complications related to immobility must possess the knowledge and clinical skills described earlier in this chapter. The following discussion outlines the assessment priorities, client goals, nursing interventions, and evaluative criteria for the following nursing diagnoses:

> *Activity intolerance*
> *Impaired physical mobility*
> *Potential for injury*: complications of immobility
> *Altered health maintenance*: lack of exercise program

In the case study that follows, a plan of care is developed to address the mobility needs of a client with left-sided hemiplegia following a cerebrovascular accident (stroke).

Activity Intolerance

Nurses working with clients with chronic illnesses that affect oxygen transport or with immobilized clients will frequently observe in these clients a reduced ability to perform the activities of daily living. Activity intolerance is the diagnostic label describing the physical or psychologic inability to tolerate an increase in activity. For one client this may translate into an inability to climb the four sets of stairs leading to an apartment, whereas for another client it may mean the inability to walk the few steps from the bed to the bathroom without becoming winded.

Any factor causing fatigue or interfering with the amount of oxygen being delivered to the muscles for the work of contraction and relaxation can produce activity intolerance. Common etiologies include

- Developmental factors (decreased strength in an older person
- Pathophysiologic factors (illnesses altering oxygen transport: *cardiac*—congestive heart failure, arrhythmias, angina, myocardial infarction; *respiratory*—chronic obstructive pulmonary disease; *circulatory*—anemia, peripheral arterial disease; other chronic diseases; malnourishment)
- Situational (prolonged bed rest or inactivity, depression, decreased motivation, pain, anything causing fatigue)

Assessment

- Note complaints of fatigue, weakness, or an inability to perform usual tasks without dizziness, dyspnea, or frequent pauses to rest.
- Identify any contributing factors that increase fatigue or compromise oxygen transport.

- Assess the client's response to activity:
  Take resting vital signs and note the client's mental status and skin characteristics.
  Have the client perform an activity (*e.g.,* ambulation) and take the vital signs immediately after the activity and after the client rests for 3 to 5 minutes.

While it is customary for the pulse, blood pressure, and respiratory rate to rise with exercise, they should return to the baseline rate after rest. Weakness, pallor, diaphoresis, confusion, and vertigo may all signal activity intolerance.

Client Goals

The client will

- Identify factors contributing to activity intolerance
- Reduce or eliminate these factors to the extent possible
- Increase endurance to the point of being able to perform key activities of daily living (specify)
- Demonstrate energy conservation measures
- Demonstrate decreased signs of anoxia (sustained increases in pulse rate, blood pressure, respiratory rate, dyspnea, pallor)

Interventions

- Set daily realistic activity goals with the client and offer immediate reinforcement if the goal is met. Explore the client's motivation to increase the activity level.
- Assist the client to reduce or eliminate factors contributing to the decreased tolerance (*e.g.,* improve quantity and quality of sleep, offer pain medication prior to the client's activity, inspire client with a sincere "can do" mentality).
- Pace the activities according to the client's strength and intersperse activities with periods of rest.
- Teach the client and family how to progress activities gradually and how to conserve energy for priority activities.

Evaluative Criteria

Client meets above goals.

Impaired Physical Mobility

Since impaired physical mobility may interfere with an individual's ability to meet other human needs (*e.g.,* obtain, prepare, and eat food; bathe and dress self; toilet self) as well as with self-concept, it is important that problems affecting physical mobility be correctly identified and worked up in the plan of care. Mobility impairments may affect the upper or lower limbs, or both. Possible etiologies include

- Developmental factors (muscle weakness or painful movement of joints in the elderly)

- Pathophysiologic factors (neuromuscular or musculo-skeletal impairment)
- Situational factors (need for bed rest; devices such as casts, splints, and braces; pain; nonfunctioning or missing limbs; effects of medications)

Assessment

- Observe the client to determine the precise nature of the mobility impairment:

    Inability to maintain body alignment

    Inability to execute coordinated, purposeful movements (includes bed mobility, transfers, ambulation—gait)

    Decreased muscle strength or control (motor function in all four extremities—strong, weak, absent, spastic; weight-bearing potential)

Limited joint mobility

Impaired perception of position or presence of body parts

- Identify all etiologic factors. Carefully assess the client's motivation to be mobile and the effect of any secondary gains being derived from the immobility.
- When illness or trauma is causing the mobility problems, consult with the physician to determine both the immediate and future effects of the mobility deficit on human functioning so that realistic client counseling can be planned.

Client Goals

Depending on the nature of the mobility impairment, the following goals will need to be individualized. The client will

---

T A B L E   28-7

Problems of Immobility With Related Etiologies, Assessment Priorities, Client Goals, and Nursing Interventions

Problems Related to Immobility	Etiologies	Assessment Priorities	Client Goals	Nursing Interventions
Cardiovascular				

Increased cardiac workload	Supine position contributes to greater volume of circulating blood, which must be pumped by the heart; decreased vascular resistance	• Assess apical and peripheral pulses.
		• Note increased heart rate; presence of third heart sound; weakened peripheral pulses.
		• Note the presence of edema (check sacrum, legs, feet).
			Client will maintain baseline vital signs.	• When possible encourage the client to sit in the Fowler's position; avoid lying supine for prolonged intervals.
				• Avoid any activities that increase intrathoracic pressure:
				    Discourage straining while moving or defecating (Valsalva maneuver).
				    Exhale through mouth while exercising.

Thrombus formation	Venous stasis secondary to a lack of muscular contraction in the legs Calcium leaving bones and entering blood increases its coagulability External pressure on the veins (*e.g.,* that exerted by the knee gatch of the hospital bed) (note: poor positioning can result in partial or total occlusion of the blood vessels.)	• Assess for complaints of pain, especially calf pain; signs of warmth, redness, swelling, tenderness—compare one extremity to the other. • Daily calf or thigh circumference measurements may be indicated (mark spot to be measured).	Client will show signs of adequate venous return (absence of dependent edema, thrombi, emboli).	• Encourage active exercise of legs (range of motion and quadriceps settings) three to four times daily. • Elevate legs periodically. • Position clients carefully, following agency guidelines; avoid prolonged knee and hip flexion. • Apply antiembolism stockings if ordered. • Assess for signs of thrombosis. *Never* rub or massage the legs—especially if the client complains of pain.
Orthostatic hypotension	Skeletal muscle weakness and decreased vessel tone (failure of arteriole vasoconstriction on assuming an erect position) Hypovolemia	• Assess for complaints of light-headedness, dizziness, seeing spots, or fainting. • Compare blood pressure prior to position change with that taken immediately afterwards.	Client will change from a lying to a sitting or standing position safely without injury.	• If not contraindicated, have client sleep sitting up or in an elevated position. • Encourage client to change position very gradually and with support if needed: supine to Fowler's to sitting at edge of bed to standing (each change may require 15 to 20 minutes stabiliza-

(Continued)

- Maintain (or increase) muscle strength and control in the upper/lower/right/left extremities
- Demonstrate correct execution of isometric/isotonic exercise program
- Independently (or with the correct use of adaptive devices) demonstrate correct alignment, transfers, and ambulation
- Demonstrate correct use of safety measures to prevent injury
- Perform activities of daily living with greatest degree of independence possible

Interventions

- Whenever possible, reduce or eliminate factors contributing to immobility (fear of falling, apathy, effects of nonessential medications).
- If pain is contributing to immobility, administer the prescribed analgesic prior to the client's activity.
- Ensure that the client is positioned in correct alignment and changes position every 2 hours.
- Develop an exercise program that includes complete range-of-motion exercises, isometric "setting" exercises, and ambulation (as possible).
- Encourage maximal participation in activities of daily living.
- Provide the appropriate nursing care for casts, traction devices, slings, braces, and prosthetic devices.
- Teach the client how to transfer and ambulate safely using a cane, walker, crutches, or wheelchair.
- Be vigilant for the development of any of the complications of immobility. Identify high-risk clients and include preventive care in the plan of care. See Table 28-7.

(Text continues on p. 680.)

Problems Related to Immobility	Etiologies	Assessment Priorities	Client Goals	Nursing Interventions
				tion time); instruct client never to "jump to feet" and begin walking. • Use waist-high antiembolism stockings. • Encourage leg exercises. • Encourage client to increase time out of bed as condition allows; gradually increase the frequency and duration of ambulation.
Respiratory				
Ineffective breathing patterns	Limited chest expansion: Prolonged sitting or lying position Muscle disuse—atrophy Loss of muscle coordination Depressant pharmacologic agents: analgesics, sedatives, anesthetics	• Assess rate, rhythm, and quality of respirations; note a decrease in the depth and rate of respirations. • Assess the symmetry of chest wall movements.	Client will maintain baseline respiratory rate and depth. Client coughs and deep breathes every 1 to 2 hours.	• Adhere to an every-2-hour position change schedule. • If the client is allowed out of bed, encourage deep breathing when the client stands/ambulates. • Teach the client to cough and deep breathe every 1 to 2 hours. • If abdominal binders or rib supports are in place, remove them every 2 hours and encourage deep breathing.
Ineffective airway clearance	Altered function of mucous membranes and cilia Decreased position changes Ineffective coughing secondary to weakness, incisional pain, depressant pharmacologic action Dehydration Stasis of secretions	• Auscultate the entire lung region and note regions of diminished breath sounds, rales, rhonchi, or wheezes. • Percuss the chest and note any dull area. • Assess sputum (color, texture, odor); culture and sensitivity test may be ordered.	Client's lungs will be clear to auscultation. Client will remain free of signs of respiratory tract infection (fever, productive cough, chest pain)	• See above. • Keep client well hydrated. • Initiate chest physiotherapy. • Suction as needed.

(Continued)

T A B L E   28-7
Problems of Immobility With Related Etiologies, Assessment Priorities, Client Goals, and Nursing Interventions (Continued)

Problems Related to Immobility	Etiologies	Assessment Priorities	Client Goals	Nursing Interventions
Impaired gas exchange (O_2/CO_2 ratio)	Decreased respiratory movement Pooling of secretions	• Note any changes in the client's behavior, mental status. • Compare clinical picture with changes in arterial blood gas values or pulmonary function test values.	Client will maintain an adequate O_2/CO_2 ratio	• See above.
Musculoskeletal				
Activity intolerance (self-care deficits) Impaired physical mobility	Decreased muscle mass, tone, and strength (atrophy) Contractures Stiffness and pain in the joints Limited range of motion Joint degeneration (ankylosis) Decreased stability Bone demineralization (disuse osteoporosis) Decreased endurance	• Assess for weakness, fatigue, complaints of muscle pain or joint pain or tenderness. • Assess for decreased muscle mass (anthropometric measurements, tape measurements), decreased muscle tone and strength. Test joint flexibility. Note any contractures or ankyloses.	Client will maintain adequate muscle strength and joint mobility to perform basic self-care activities.	Incorporate range-of-motion exercises (as client's condition permits) and isometric "setting" exercises into client's daily routine (at least three to four times daily).
Potential for injury: pathologic fractures	Excessive bone demineralization (disuse osteoporosis)	• Bone demineralization is not detectable via physical assessment. • Relate clinical picture to blood chemistries (note elevated serum calcium and phosphorus levels).	Client will remain free of contractures, ankyloses, pathologic fractures.	Increase client's activity tolerance gradually: • Participates in positioning in bed • Transfers from bed to chair • Ambulates • Gradually increases frequency and duration of sitting out of bed and frequency and distance of walks • Progresses to independence in all self-care activities
Metabolic				
Nutritional alterations: less than body requirements Nutritional alterations: more than body requirements Fluid volume excess: dependent edema	Negative nitrogen balance Anorexia Imbalance between calories ingested and "burned off" Fluid shifts secondary to negative nitrogen balance	• Assess diet history and note problems with anorexia, digestion, or elimination. • Monitor intake and output and correlate client's clinical picture with laboratory studies that evaluate fluid and electrolyte status. • Evaluate muscle atrophy via anthropometric measurements (height, weight, mid-upper arm circumference, and triceps skin-fold measurements). • Assess skin turgor and wound healing.	Client will maintain appropriate weight for height. Client's fluid output will approximately equal intake. Client's electrolyte values and serum protein will fall within normal range. Client's skin will demonstrate adquate turgor.	• Provide client with high-protein, high-calorie diet. Explore parenteral and enteral (nasogastric, gastrostomy, or jejunostomy tubes) alternatives if the client is unable to eat. • Serve small, frequent feedings in a pleasant environment. • Monitor intake and output.

(Continued)

Problems Related to Immobility	Etiologies	Assessment Priorities	Client Goals	Nursing Interventions
Gastrointestinal				
Alteration in bowel elimination: constipation	Decreased gastric motility and muscle tone Decreased fluid intake	• Assess frequency and consistency of bowel movements (use of elimination aids). • Examine for bowel sounds, abdominal tone, and anal sphincter tone.	Client will have a formed, semisolid stool every 1 to 3 days. Client will be free of signs of fecal impaction (distended abdomen, no bowel movement for several days or liquid bowel movement, lethargy)	• Respect client's usual elimination schedule. • Offer assistance with the bedpan or commode if needed and provide privacy. • Increase fluid intake and roughage. • Caution about Valsalva maneuver (straining with mouth closed).
Urinary				
Alterations in patterns of urinary elimination Urinary retention Potential for urinary tract infection	Renal calculi Urinary stasis	• Assess voiding patterns —time and amount (note history of small, frequent voidings); question about urgency, dysuria, pain. • Monitor fluid output. • Examine for bladder distention. • Examine urine for cloudiness or odor (culture urine if indicated).	Client will maintain usual voiding pattern (frequency and amount). Client will be free of renal calculi. Client will be free of signs of urinary tract infection (urgency, burning, flank pain, fever).	• Keep the client well hydrated (aim is for client to void large amounts of dilute urine). • Maintain usual voiding pattern. • If needed, provide assistance with bedpan or urinal—respect client's privacy.
Skin				
Impairment of skin integrity (pressure ulcer)	Decreased local blood circulation to the tissues Prolonged pressure on the skin	• Examine skin, especially pressure points, for beginning signs of breakdown with each position change (at least every 2 hours). • Assess for factors that place client at high risk for breakdown (malnutrition, incontinence, and so on).	Client's skin will show no sign of breakdown.	• Reposition client in correct alignment at least every 1 to 2 hours and ensure protection of pressure points where possible (*e.g.,* heel and elbow protectors). • Decrease effects of shearing forces. • Massage pressure points and keep skin clean and dry. • Keep bed linens dry and free of wrinkles.
Psychologic/Social				
Disturbance in self-concept (body image, self-esteem, personal identity) Powerlessness Impaired social interaction Alteration in thought processes Knowledge deficit	Inability to move body voluntarily Dependency on others Inability to fulfill role expectations Pain experience Skeletal deformities Exaggerated emotional and behavioral responses Loss of mobility to contact friends Decreased stimuli to maintain orientation Immobility-induced depression	• Assess client for changes in behavior, emotional status, and mental abilities. • Explore with the client and family possible reasons for these changes. • Assess the adequacy of the client's and family's coping strategies. • Assess sleep–wake patterns.	Client will identify personal strengths. Client will verbalize positive body image. Client will describe successful coping strategies. Client will demonstrate ability to problem solve.	• Utilize care contacts with client to explore immobility's effects on the client's mental status and behavior. • Explore means to meet client's needs for socialization. • Increase stimuli to maintain client's orientation. • Encourage client to be as independent as possible and to structure daily activities and schedule as closely as possible to pre-immobilization. Encourage wearing of personal clothes, use of makeup, and so on.

(Continued)

T A B L E   28-7
Problems of Immobility With Related Etiologies, Assessment Priorities, Client Goals, and Nursing Interventions (Continued)

Problems Related to Immobility	Etiologies	Assessment Priorities	Client Goals	Nursing Interventions
Psychologic/Social (continued)				
	Decreased motivation to learn			• Challenge client intellectually. Communicate that you expect the client to reason, to problem solve.
	Decreased ability to learn and decreased retention			• Explore impact of client's illness on family and counsel appropriately.
	Decreased motivation to solve problems			
Ineffective individual and family coping	Increased need for assistance with self-care abilities			
	Exaggerated emotional responses			
Altered sleep–wake patterns	Decreased physical exercise			
	Increased bedtime/napping			

Evaluative Criteria
Client meets above goals.

Potential for Injury: Complications of Immobility

The effects of immobility on major body systems as well as on an individual's psychosocial functioning are presented earlier in this chapter. Nursing's challenge is to identify clients at high risk for developing problems related to immobility and to institute nursing measures immediately to prevent these problems. Because the problems are multiple, they are presented in table format according to body system with specific etiologies, assessment priorities, client goals, and related nursing interventions (Table 28-7). Nursing care plans for immobilized clients should reflect nursing's concern to prevent immobility problems.

Altered Health Maintenance: Lack of Exercise Program

Although in recent years a "fitness craze" has prompted many individuals to develop more active life-styles, many persons still live overwhelmingly sedentary lives. Reasons for the lack of regular physical exercise are many.

- Science and technology have developed complex machines and services to aid in the performance of the activities of daily living, which formerly required an expenditure of physical energy. In the past, persons who wished to survive had no choice but to be active. Today an individual must consciously choose to be active.
- Convenience (reduced energy expenditure) has come to be valued over activities requiring more effort.
- Children are quickly socialized into valuing sedentary activities such as watching television or listening to the radio.
- Our society's fetish for cleanliness leads some persons to abhor any activities that produce "sweat."
- There is still lack of knowledge and much confusion about the benefits of regular exercise.
- Some individuals become discouraged from being more active following unsuccessful attempts.
- Physical injury or discomfort resulting from a poorly designed exercise program may cause a person to discontinue the activity.
- Some persons believe that exercise is simply "too much bother."
- Some persons are unable to find the time for regular exercise.
- Embarrassment may be related to an individual's appearance, ability, or physical condition.
- Some persons erroneously believe that the need for exercise decreases with age and eventually disappears.
- Some persons overrate the benefits of light, sporadic exercise.
- Some persons underrate their own abilities and exercise capacity.

Assessment
- Interview the client to determine (1) past and present history of exercise, (2) knowledge about the benefits of exercise, (3) motivation to adhere to a regular program of exercise, (4) exercise preferences, (5) feasibility of these preferences (time involved, cost, need for special equipment, pres-

ence of support systems, safety concerns), (6) any contraindications for beginning to exercise without medical supervision (*e.g.,* history of chest pain or pressure with activity, past or current cardiovascular or respiratory problems, degenerative joint diseases or other orthopedic problems), and (7) ability to design and follow safe exercise program.

- Identify factors likely to sabotage the client's efforts to exercise (decreased motivation, multiple demands on time, lack of funds for child care, and so on).
- Perform a physical examination to rule out any physical contraindications (*e.g.,* obesity, high blood pressure, musculoskeletal problems) to exercising without medical clearance. (Note: Stress testing is mandatory for sedentary persons over age 35 and for anyone with a past or current cardiovascular condition.)

Client Goals

Long-Term
Client will adhere to a regular program of exercise, which promotes cardiovascular function, endurance, flexibility, and strength.

Short-Term
Client will
- Identify four personal benefits of exercise
- Identify personal factors that tend to prevent regular exercise
- Develop a feasible and safe exercise program, including specifics for
  Warm-up activities
  A variety of exercise activities including aerobic and stretch exercises (type, frequency, duration)
  Cool-down activities
- Identify the risks inherent in this program and the precautions that will be taken

- Obtain medical clearance for exercise program if needed
- Describe three means to reinforce exercise goals (reward system, exercise partner, utilization of other supports)

Interventions
- Teach the client
  Four components of fitness (cardiovascular function, endurance, **flexibility**, strength)
  Benefits of regular exercise
  Types of exercise
- Assist the client to determine exercise preferences by comparing and contrasting different types of exercise: (1) time required, (2) place, (3) equipment needed, (4) cost, (5) aerobic versus anaerobic value, (6) advantages, (7) disadvantages, and (8) precautions and risks.
- Assist the client to develop an individualized exercise program:
  Choose warm-up, major, and cool-down activities.
  Set objectives for duration, intensity, and frequency.
  Teach the client how to take a radial pulse and how to determine his target heart rate if necessary.
  Consider the best setting for the activity and the equipment and money needed to perform the exercise safely.
  Identify risks and safety factors.
  Explore with the client potential threats to the exercise program and existing supports.
- Help the client to develop a strategy to evaluate the attainment of the exercise goals. A self-contract with or without additional nursing intervention may be sufficient.

Evaluative Criteria
Client meets above goals.

CASE STUDY

Mr. Adams is an alert 57-year-old married man who was admitted to the hospital with a diagnosis of right cerebrovascular accident secondary to thrombosis. He has a history of hypertension. This is his fifth hospital day and the attending physicians have termed the stroke a *completed stroke,* that is, Mr. Adams' neurologic deficits have been unchanged for two days and he is now believed to be ready for more aggressive rehabilitative treatment.

Assessment Findings
On hospital day 5 an assessment of Mr. Adams' mobility status and ability to participate in activities of daily living revealed the following data:

- *Mental status:* Client is basically alert and able to follow simple commands; expresses his needs verbally when encouraged but speech is slow; seems forgetful of usual routine for basic self-care activities.
- *Neuromuscular status:* Hemiplegia; severe motor and sensory deficits of the left side of the face and the left arm and leg
  Muscle mass, tone, and strength: Well-developed muscles in all extremities; history of a life-time of sports, most recently played tennis two to four times weekly; decreased muscle tone (hypotonicity, flaccidity) in

left arm and leg; motor function is absent in left arm and very weak in left leg; strong motor function on right extremities. Incapable of weight-bearing on left side. Incapable of independent turning, sitting, standing, transferring, or ambulation.

Joint Mobility: Decreased on left side; otherwise full range of motion; no contractures

Endurance: Fatigues quickly (*e.g.*, during complete bath)

Some deficit in spatial–perceptual orientation (*e.g.*, ignores objects on his left side) but difficult to assess this completely yet

Nursing Diagnoses

Impaired physical mobility (turning in bed, sitting, standing, transferring, and ambulating) related to left hemiplegia and weakness

Self-care deficit related to decreased alertness and left-sided motor and sensory deficits

Planning

Since it is not known to what extent Mr. Adams is able to comprehend his illness, the nurse operates on the assumption that he is able to understand a simple explanation of how the stroke is affecting his motor function and how he can best work together with his family and the nurse to regain motor function. After assessing both his past and present motor abilities the nurse shares with Mr. Adams and his wife and son the following short-term goals:

- Whenever observed the client will be in correct body alignment with (1) each joint on the left side higher than the joint proximal to it and (2) supportive devices appropriately in place (bed board, footboard, trochanter roll, hand–wrist splint, shoulder sling, pillows).
- By hospital day 10, the client will

  Replace the passive range-of-motion exercises the nurse is now performing four times daily to all joints with (1) active exercise of his left arm and leg and (2) active range of motion of all other joints

  Perform quadriceps settings, gluteal settings, and abdominal settings five times daily

  Participate in the every-two-hour positioning schedule by assisting with turning to the degree he is able

  Utilize a sling on the left arm when upright so long as the arm muscles are hypotonic

  Keep the left arm and hand elevated with a pillow to prevent dependent edema

  Demonstrate a safe pivot transfer from bed to chair and chair to bed

  Demonstrate standing balance

  Show beginning ability to resume self-care activities despite motor and sensory deficits on left side

- On discharge from the acute-care hospital to the rehabilitation center, the client will

  Be free of contractures

  Show signs of physical and mental readiness to acquire increasing independence in self-care

Both the client and family express great willingness to work to achieve these goals. Later the wife confides to the nurse "It's been so awful just sitting here not knowing what was going to happen. At least now I feel like we have something to work for!"

See the Nursing Care Plan for Mr. Adams for details of the nursing strategies utilized to achieve these goals.

Implementation

In implementing the plan of care the nurse needs the following specialized abilities:

- The belief that nursing can make a difference in the quality of this family's present and future life and the commitment of nursing energies to help Mr. Adams reach his full rehabilitative potential
- Strong assessment skills (interviewing and primarily physical assessment) to determine how the neurologic dysfunction is influencing the client's mobility and coordination
- Knowledge of how the skeletal, muscular, and nervous systems function to produce purposeful and coordinated movement
- Interpersonal skills to communicate to Mr. Adams and his family empathy for their situation and to mobilize their energies for the long process of rehabilitation
- Excellent use of body mechanics when positioning Mr. Adams and assisting him with transfers (and when teaching these techniques to the family)
- Vigilant caregiver skills directed to preventing complications and maintaining muscle strength and joint mobility to facilitate an optimal return of function.
- Teaching and counseling skills to enable Mr. Adams to regain independence in self-care activities
- Interpersonal and leadership skills to motivate the entire nursing staff to value Mr. Adams' rehabilitation
- Ability to work collaboratively with many other members of the health-care team while coordinating all their efforts into a comprehensive care plan
- Accountability and patience

Documentation

Sample documentations of nursing interventions follow. The first is a typical entry on the client record using the traditional note format; the second is a sample of a SOAP note.

Nursing 1/25/88 3 PM Dr. Steel examined the client at 1:00 PM and noted he is now in "completed stroke stage and ready for more aggressive rehabilitative treatment." This was explained to client, his wife, and his son. The

(Text continues on p. 687.)

NURSING CARE PLAN *for Mr. Adams*

Nursing Diagnosis: Impaired physical mobility (turning in bed, sitting, standing, transferring, and ambulating) related to left hemiplegia and weakness

Signs and Symptoms: Motor function is absent in left arm and very weak in left leg; muscles are well developed but hypotonic; decreased joint mobility in left extremities; fatigues quickly

Long-Term Goal: Client will regain independence in turning, sitting, standing, transferring, and ambulating.

Goals	Nursing Actions	Rationale	Evaluative Statement
1/25 Whenever observed the client will be in correct body alignment with (1) each joint on the left side higher than the joint proximal to it and (2) supportive devices in place (bed board, footboard, trochanter roll, hand–wrist splint, shoulder sling, pillows).	1. At each position change (as dictated by every-2-hour turn schedule posted at the bedside) make sure that the client is in correct alignment. Follow agency positioning guidelines for the supine, side-lying (lies on unaffected side) and prone positions. 2. Utilize the following supportive devices: firm mattress with bed board; footboard, trochanter roll, shoulder sling when client is in upright position, volar resting splint, and pillows. 3. Teach both the client and family the importance of correct positioning. Allow the family to participate in helping the client to get comfortable in the different positions.	Correct positioning prevents contractures, relieves pressures, and maintains alignment. 1. Firm mattress and bed board provide skeletal support. 2. Footboard during flaccid period prevents footdrop, heel cord shortening, and plantar flexion. 3. Trochanter roll prevents external rotation of hip when client is in dorsal position. 4. Shoulder sling during flaccid period prevents shoulder subluxation and shoulder-hand syndrome. 5. Volar resting splint supports the wrist and hand in a functional position. 6. A pillow in the axilla of the left side prevents adduction of the affected side. 7. Positioning each joint higher than the preceding one prevents edema and its resulting fibrosis. 8. Placing the client in the prone position for 30 minutes two to three times daily helps prevent knee and hip flexion contractures.	1/27 Goal being met. Every-2-hour positioning schedule being followed with client in correct body alignment to prevent contractures. *S. Beecher, RN*

N U R S I N G C A R E P L A N (Continued)

Goals	Nursing Actions	Rationale	Evaluative Statement
By hospital day 10 (1/30) the client will Replace the passive range-of-motion exercises the nurse is now performing four times daily to all joints with (1) his active exercise of the left arm and left leg and (2) his active range-of-motion exercises for all other joints	1. Assess the client's knowledge of the importance of exercise and ability and motivation to exercise. 2. Teach the client how to exercise his left arm and leg by using his unaffected (right) extremities. 3. Demonstrate a complete set of range-of-motion exercises to the client and family and have the client return the demonstrations.	Unless the client understands the reason for exercise and is physically, mentally, and attitudinally capable of exercise, he will not follow through. Active exercise maintains joint mobility, prevents contracture development in the paralyzed extremity, prevents further deterioration of the neuromuscular system, helps to regain motor control and increases circulation. Involving the family helps ensure the success of the exercise program because it requires a big time and effort commitment.	1/30 Goal partially met. Client has successfully demonstrated complete set of range-of-motion exercises (to both left and right sides); however, he tires during the exercises and stops unless verbally encouraged. *Revision:* Monitor client's exercise four times daily; continue to enlist family's support. *S. Beecher, RN*
Perform quadriceps, gluteal, and abdominal settings five times daily	Teach the client and family how to tighten these muscles and hold them for 6 seconds (slow count to 4) before relaxing. A 2-minute rest should be allowed between contractions and the client cautioned not to hold his breath during these exercises because this places strain on the heart. The exercises should be stopped short of muscle fatigue.	These exercises will maintain muscle mass, tone, and strength (while the client is on bed rest) and prevent atrophy. They also increase circulation to the exercised body parts.	1/30 Goal partially met. Client has demonstrated exercises correctly; however, he needs to be reminded to perform them. Family is very effective in this regard. *Revision:* Compliment family on excellent job they are doing and reinforce importance of exercise to maximize rehabilitative potential. *S. Beecher, RN*
Participate in the every-2-hour positioning schedule by assisting with turning to the degree he is able	Teach the client how he can help to reposition himself by grabbing onto the side rail with his right hand and also by placing his unaffected leg under the left one in order to move himself.	The more the client can do independently, the more in control he will feel. These activities will pave the way to increasing independence in self-care activities.	1/27 Goal met. Client consistently assists in repositioning. Seems pleased to be able to help the nurses in this way. *S. Beecher, RN*
Demonstrate a safe pivot transfer from bed to chair and chair to bed	Assess the stage of recovery of muscle function.	Most clients will begin to show signs of spasticity with exaggerated reflexes within 48 hours—this denotes progress. If muscles are still flaccid after several weeks, prognosis for regaining function is poor.	1/30 Goal met. Client can safely transfer from bed to chair and chair to bed but requires nursing assistance. *S. Beecher, RN*

(Continued)

NURSING CARE PLAN (Continued)

Goals	Nursing Actions	Rationale	Evaluative Statement
Demonstrate standing balance	1. Assess activity tolerance. 2. Take vital signs before attempting balance training and transfers. 3. Precede transfers with balance training. Assist the client to a sitting position at the edge of the bed and observe for steadiness and the ability to maintain an erect posture. 4. Place the chair by the bed on the client's unaffected side and assist the client to dress. Initially the nurse helps the client to stand by placing his or her right knee against the client's strong knee, grasping the client around the waist with both arms, and pulling the client forward while rocking back on the left leg (nurse's knees are slightly flexed). 5. Once the client is standing, assess standing balance and observe for signs of activity intolerance (pallor, shortness of breath, excessive increase in pulse rate, perspiration). Direct the client to (1) grab the far arm of the chair with his strong arm, (2) turn on his strong foot, and (3) sit down. The nurse's right leg and the client's strong leg are used as a pivot. 6. Pivot client out of bed to chair tid (may pivot out of bed to bedside	Vital signs and the client's physical condition should be assessed prior to a new activity, during the activity, and shortly afterwards to assess activity tolerance. The client needs sitting and standing balance before progressing to harder tasks. Dizziness or syncope may signal vasomotor instability. This prevents the client's knees from buckling and the pressure of the nurse's knee forces the client to straighten the strong knee and bear weight on it. In this position the client's feet cannot slip forward. In this position the nurse is using good principles of body mechanics.	1/30 Goal not met. Client has not demonstrated standing balance; falls to left side without nursing support. *Revision:* allow more time for goal achievement. *S. Beecher, RN*

N U R S I N G   C A R E   P L A N (Continued)

Goals	Nursing Actions	Rationale	Evaluative Statement
	commode). Gradually increase time in chair based on client's tolerance. Correctly align client in chair using supportive devices as necessary.		
Upon discharge to rehabilitation center client will be free of contractures.	Implement above nursing actions.		1/31 Goal met. Client has no contractures. *S. Beecher, RN*

Nursing Diagnosis: Self-care deficit (all basic self-care activities) related to decreased alertness and left-sided motor and sensory deficits

Signs and Symptoms: Unable to use left arm for any activities; client's right side is dominant; incapable of ambulation at present; basically alert but seems forgetful of usual routine for self-care activities; tires quickly

Long-Term Goal: Client demonstrates increasing independence in self-care abilities.

Goals	Nursing Actions	Rationale	Evaluative Statement

By hospital day 10 (1/30) the client will demonstrate beginning ability to resume self-care activities despite motor and sensory deficits of left side; uses right arm to
    Assist in AM hygiene
    Feed himself (finger foods, beverages)
    Exercise
	1. Continue to assess extent of client's motor and sensory deficits and ability to perform self-care activities.
	2. Set realistic short-term goals for each session with client and reward progress: "This morning we'll see how much of your bath you are able to manage yourself!" "It must feel good to be able to do this for yourself again . . ."
	3. Approach client from his unaffected side and place call light, bedside table, phone, and so on, on this side.
	4. Teach client how to transfer all self-care activities to the unaffected side and how to use one-handed techniques and adaptive equipment.
		Adding *realistic* new tasks for each day gives the client a goal to work toward; a pattern of *noticed* success encourages continued efforts.
		
		This helps the client to compensate for alterations in sensory perception.
		
		There is never only one way to do anything.
			1/29 Goal met. For the last two days client has washed his left arm, abdomen, and legs; combed his hair; fed himself; and performed range-of-motion exercises.
			
			S. Beecher, RN

NURSING CARE PLAN (Continued)

Short-Term Goals	Nursing Actions	Rationale	Evaluative Statement
	5. Encourage client to brush his teeth, comb his hair, bathe and feed himself, and to assist in toileting. Explain to the family why it is critical to allow him to do these things himself, even if movements are tiring, clumsy, and initially frustrating. 6. Continually reevaluate the client's need for TLC vs firm, directive encouragement. Involve the family in this process.	Emotional lability is common following stroke. Clients will fluctuate between heroic efforts toward independent self-care and whining demands to be totally cared for. The appropriate nursing response varies from moment to moment and runs the range of TLC to unrelenting firm direction. All nursing responses need to communicate the nurse's sincere care for the client and commitment to developing his *best* potential.	
Upon discharge to rehabilitation center the client will show signs of physical and mental readiness to acquire increasing independence in self-care.	Implement above nursing actions.		1/31 Goal met. Client's muscle strength and joint mobility maintained during hospitalization. Client is now participating in self-care activities and is eager to learn skills to become more independent. *S. Beecher, RN*

client smiled and seemed to understand that he is out of immediate danger. Initial instructions given to the client as to how he can assist with position changes and actively exercise his left arm and leg. Correctly demonstrated these maneuvers with verbal cueing. Motor function still absent in left arm and weak in left leg. Care plan revised to incorporate new exercise goals.

Susan Beecher, RN

1/27/88 #2 Self-care deficit related to decreased alertness and left-sided motor and sensory deficits

S: "Get out of here."

O: Client threw washcloth at nurse during bath and refused to assist with bathing; later observed crying

A: Temporary setback influenced by frustration with absent motor function in left arm and emotional lability

P: *Educative:* Explain to client that most persons in his position get frustrated and that his behavior is normal. Reinforce the importance of his continued efforts to regain independence in self-care activities.

Therapeutic: Make determined effort to compliment his progress to date (assistance with turning, range-of-motion exercises, feeding). Communicate warm acceptance of client and understanding of his anger and frustration.

KEY POINTS

■ The fulfillment of most human needs depends, at least partially, on the body's ability to move. Purposeful, coordinated movement of the body requires the integrated functioning of the skeletal, muscular, and nervous systems of the body.

■ Bones and joints provide form for the body and serve as the levers and fulcrums that make body movement possible. It is the contraction and relaxation of skeletal muscles, however, that actually produce movement by pulling on bones, and it is nerve impulses that stimulate the muscles to contract.

■ Good body mechanics is the efficient use of the body as a machine and as means of locomotion. In order to role model healthy body mechanics, the nurse pays special attention to body alignment, balance, and coordinated body movement during work and leisure activities.

■ Factors that influence body alignment and mobility include developmental considerations, physical health, mental health, life-style variables, attitudes and values, fatigue/stress level, and external factors.

■ The active exertion of muscles involving the contraction and relaxation of muscle groups is termed *exercise.* Isotonic exercise involves muscle shortening and active movement, and its potential benefits include increased muscle mass, tone, and strength; improved joint mobility; increased cardiac and respiratory function; increased circulation; and increased osteoblastic activity. Isometric exercise involves contraction without movement, and potential benefits are increased muscle mass, tone, and strength; increased circulation to the exercised body part; and increased osteoblastic activity.

■ Individuals who chose to live inactive life-styles place themselves at high risk for serious health problems. Problems of immobility include increased cardiac workload, thrombus formation, orthostatic hypotension, ineffective breathing patterns, ineffective airway clearance, impaired gas exchange, activity intolerance, potential for injury: pathologic fractures, nutritional alterations, fluid volume excesses, alterations in bowel and urinary elimination, potential for urinary tract infection, impairment of skin integrity, disturbances in self-concept, powerlessness, impaired social interaction, altered thought processes, ineffective coping, and altered sleep–wake patterns.

■ Persons beginning exercise programs should be familiar with the following guidelines: begin program slowly and allow the body time to adjust to the new stress, know your body and respect its limitations, and follow the safety guidelines for specific exercises.

■ When assessing mobility status, interview the client regarding daily activity level, endurance, exercise/fitness goals, mobility problems, physical or mental problems that affect mobility, and external factors that affect mobility. The physical assessment of mobility status includes an assessment of general ease of movement and gait; alignment; joint structure and function; muscle mass, tone, and strength; and endurance.

■ Nursing diagnoses for mobility problems include activity intolerance and impaired physical mobility. Both problem statements have multiple etiologies. Since mobility influences so many other areas of human functioning, many nursing diagnoses have as their etiology a problem with mobility.

■ The aim of nursing care for both well and ill clients is that the client follow a program of regular physical exercise that improves cardiovascular function, endurance, flexibility, and strength.

■ Nursing strategies that promote mobility for clients on bed rest include (1) careful attention to positioning that maintains correct alignment and facilitates physiologic functioning; (2) safe transfer of client from bed to chair or stretcher; (3) and the early and safe ambulation of clients. The nurse may also play a key role in teaching clients to use mechanical aids for walking.

■ Clients require specialized nursing care if they have the following mobility diagnoses: Activity intolerance, Impaired physical mobility, Potential for injury: complications for immobility, and Alteration in health maintenance: lack of exercise program.

B I B L I O G R A P H Y

Bates B: A Guide to Physical Examination, 4th ed. Philadelphia, JB Lippincott, 1987
Bennett-Canclini S: The kinetic treatment table: A new approach to bedrest. Orthopedic Nursing 4(2):61–70, 1985
Booth CL et al: Infant massage and exercise: Worth the effort? Matern-Child Nurs J 10(3):184–189, 1985
Brower P, Hicks D: Maintaining muscle function in patients on bedrest. Am J Nurs 72(7):1250–1253, 1972

Brown BS: Fitting fitness into your life. Nursing Economics 1(2):93–96, 1983
Casperson CJ et al: Physical activity, exercise, and physical fitness: Definitions and distinctions for health-related research. Public Health Rep 100(2):126–131, 1985
Ciuca R, Bradish J, Trombly S: Active range-of-motion exercises. Nursing '78 8(8):45–49, 1978
Cohen S, Viellion G: Teaching a patient how to use crutches. 79(6):1111–1126, 1979

Cozen LN: Walking aids: Select the right one, teach its use, and avoid damage elsewhere. Consultant 24(1):268–273, 276, 1984

Dehn MM: The effects of exercise. Am J Nurs 80(3):435–440, 1980

Dionne KE: The no-strain approach to back-breaking work. RN 48(1):45–47, 1985

The Fit Body: Building Endurance. Alexandria, VA, Time-Life Books, 1987

Ford JR, Duckworth B: Moving a dependent patient safely, comfortably. Nursing '76 part 1, 6(1):27–36; part 2, 6(2):25–32, 1976

Foss G: Use your head and save your back: Body mechanics. Nursing '73 3(5):25–32, 1973

Goldberg L, Elliot D (eds): Symposium on medical aspects of exercise. Med Clin North Am 65(1), 1985

Gordon JE: CircOlectric beds: Circumventing the trauma of positioning. Nursing '77 7(2):42–47, 1977

Gordon M: Assessing activity tolerance. Am J Nurs 76(1):72–75, 1976

Haskell WL, Superko R: Designing an exercise plan for optimal health. Family and Community Health 7(1):72–88, 1984

Hill L, Smith N: Self-care Nursing. Englewood Cliffs, NJ, Prentice-Hall, 1985

Hirschberg GG, Lewis L, Vaugh P: Promoting patient mobility and preventing secondary disabilities. Nursing '77 7(5):42–47, 1977

Howden L: Basic back care: It doesn't have to hurt. Canadian Nurse 77(7):46–50, 1981

Jacobs B, Young M: Transferring patients safely and efficiently. Nursing '81 11(8):64–67, 1981

Johnson S: Jump to it. Women's Sports and Fitness 9(8):34–38, 1987

Johnson-Pawlson J: Exercise is for everyone. Geriatric Nursing 6(6):322–325, 1985

Jordan-Marsh M: Development of a tool for diagnosing changes in concern about exercise: A means of enhancing compliance. Nursing Res 34(2):103–107, 1985

Kelly MM: Exercises for bedfast patients. Am J Nurs 66(10):2209–2213, 1966

Koplan JP et al: The risks of exercise: A public health view of injuries and hazards. Public Health Rep 100(2):189–195, 1985

Leinweber E: Belts to make moves smoother. Am J Nurs 78(12):2080–2081, 1978

Maier P: Take the work out of range-of-motion exercises . . . continuous passive motion machine. RN 49(9):46–49, 1986

Mandzak-McCarron K et al: Ambulation aids. Rehabilitation Nursing 12(3):139–141, 1987

Marchette L et al: Back injury: A preventable occupational hazard. Orthopedic Nursing 4(6):25–29, 1985

Public health aspects of physical activity and exercise—Special section. Public Health Rep 100(2):113–224, 1985

Rodts MF: An orthopedics assessment you can do in 15 minutes. Nursing 13(5):65–73, 1983

Roy S: Injuries of exercise. Med Clin North Am 69(1):197–209, 1985

Sivarajan ES, Halpenny CJ: Exercise testing. Am J Nurs 79(12):2162–2170, 1979

Snyder M, Baum R: Assessing station and gait. Am J Nurs 74(7):1256–1257, 1974

Thomas DF: An ambulation assessment system you can count on. Nursing '86 16(11):58–59, 1986

Tyler ML: (1984). The respiratory effects of body positioning and immobilization. Respiratory Care 29(5):472–483, 1984

Winslow EH, Weber TM: Progressive exercises to combat the hazards of bedrest. Am J Nurs 80(3):440–445, 1980

29 Rest and Sleep

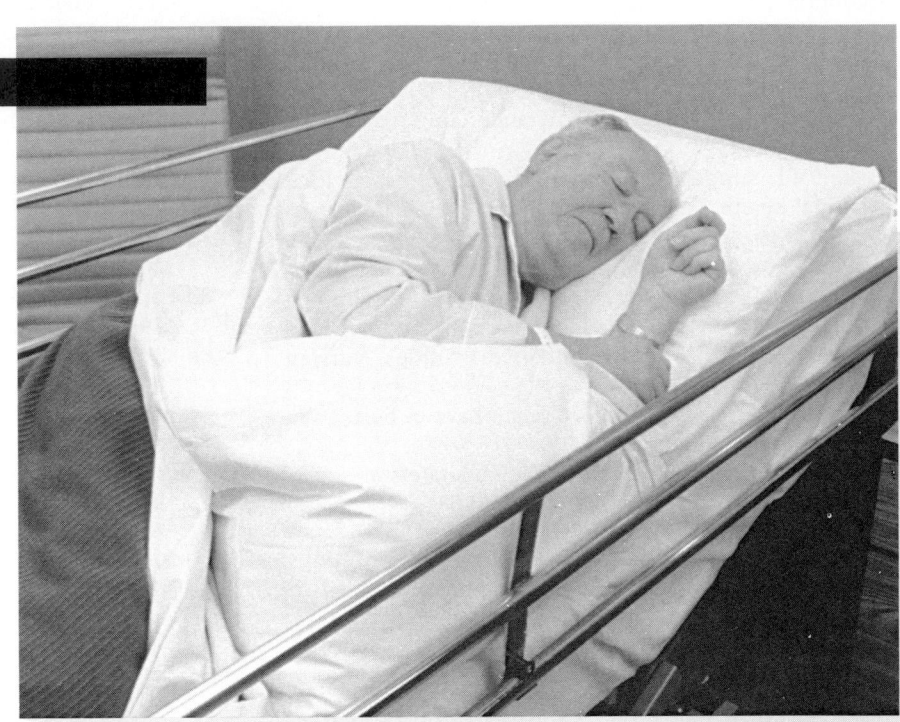

OBJECTIVES

After studying this chapter, the learner should be able to

Define key terms used in this chapter.

Describe the functions and physiology of sleep.

Identify 11 variables that influence rest and sleep.

Describe nursing implications for age-related differences in the sleep–wakefulness cycle.

Perform a comprehensive sleep assessment using appropriate interview questions, a sleep diary when indicated, and physical assessment skills.

Describe common sleep disorders noting key assessment criteria.

Develop nursing diagnoses that correctly identify sleep problems that may be treated by independent nursing intervention.

Describe nine nursing strategies to promote rest and sleep, and identify their rationale.

Plan, implement, and evaluate nursing care related to select nursing diagnoses involving sleep problems.

On the average, people spend a third of their lives asleep. While the exact purpose of sleep is not clear, sleep's functions are usually characterized as being protective and restorative. The advice "everything will look better after a good night's sleep" is based on the belief that sleep

- Restores physical well-being
- Relieves stress and anxiety
- Restores the ability to cope and to concentrate on activities of daily living

In this chapter **rest** is used to connote a condition in which the body is in a decreased state of activity with the consequent feeling of being refreshed, and **sleep** is used to mean a state of altered consciousness throughout which varying degrees of stimuli produce wakefulness. Sleep is an active and complex rhythmic state involving a progression of repeated cycles, each representing different phases of body and brain activity.

Most persons can fall asleep easily and remain asleep until the desired waking time; on the other hand, some individuals rarely fall asleep without a struggle and, even then, their sleep is fragmented. Many persons' sleep disturbances go undetected for years, progressively undermining energy and destroying sense of self. The discomfort produced by physical and mental illness and the need for hospitalization and treatment may interfere dramatically with a client's ability to sleep. Consequently, nurses need to be vigilant in both detecting and treating sleep disturbances.

Study of this chapter provides the nurse with knowledge of (1) the functions and physiology of sleep, (2) dreams and dream theories, and (3) factors affecting sleep. Practical suggestions for performing a comprehensive sleep assessment are given. Sample interview questions for both a general and focused sleep history are presented along with information on sleep diaries and pertinent physical assessment data. The importance of analyzing these data is noted and numerous examples of nursing diagnoses are offered. Client goals and specific nursing strategies for promoting rest and sleep are described. In the section entitled "Nursing Process in Clinical Practice" focused assessment, diagnosis, planning, implementation, and evaluation guides are offered for select nursing diagnoses related to the sleep disturbances: insomnia and sleep deprivation. These guides and the concluding case study illustrate how the nurse's knowledge of rest and sleep, combined with skilled nursing interventions and caring, can successfully resolve sleep problems.

KEY TERMS

circadian rhythm
circadian synchronization
delta sleep
electroencephalograph (EEG)
electromyogram (EMG)
electrooculogram (EOG)
enuresis
hypersomnia
insomnia
narcolepsy
nocturnal myoclonus
nonrapid eye movement (NREM)
parasomnias
rapid eye movement (REM)
rest
sleep
sleep apnea
sleep cycle
sleep deprivation
somnambulism

PHYSIOLOGY OF SLEEP

Two systems in the brainstem, the reticular activating system and the bulbar synchronizing region are believed to work together to control the cyclic nature of sleep.

The reticular formation (Fig. 29-1) is found in the brain stem. It extends upward through the medulla, the pons, the midbrain, and then into the hypothalamus. It is composed of many nerve cells and fibers. The fibers have connections that relay impulses into the cerebral cortex and into the spinal cord. The reticular formation facilitates reflex and voluntary movements, as well as cortical activities related to a state of alertness. During sleep, the reticular system experiences few stimuli from the cerebral cortex and the periphery of the body. Wakefulness occurs when the reticular system is activated with stimuli from the cerebral cortex and from periphery sensory organs and cells. For example, an alarm clock wakens us from sleep to a state of consciousness when we realize that we must prepare for work. Sensations such as pain, pressure, and noise will produce wakefulness by means of periphery organs and cells. Wakefulness is activated by the cerebral cortex and body sensations. During sleep, stimuli from the cortex are minimal.

The hypothalamus has control centers for several involuntary activities of the body, one of which is concerned with sleeping and waking. Injury to the hypothalamus may cause a person to sleep for abnormally long periods.

It has been shown that some compounds play a role as neurotransmitters and are involved with the sleeping process. Norepinephrine and acetylcholine, followed by dopamine, serotonin, and histamine, are involved with

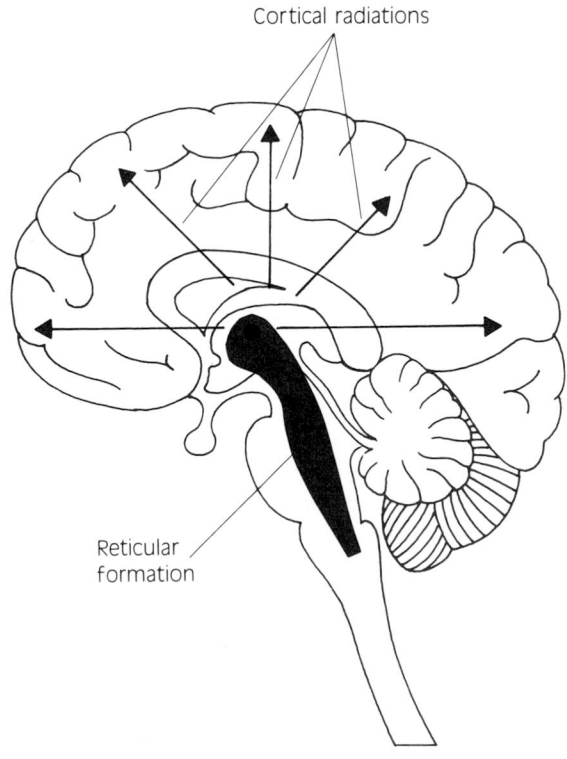

F I G U R E   29-1

Reticular formation in brain stem and diencephalon with radiations to the cerebral cortex.

excitation. Gamma-aminobutyric acid (GABA) appears to be necessary for inhibition. However, research has yet to prove exactly how biochemical changes and hormones function in sleep.

Circadian Rhythms

Rhythmic biologic clocks are now known to exist in plants, animals, and humans. Influenced by both internal and external factors, they regulate select biologic and behavioral functions in humans. Some cycles are monthly, such as a woman's menstrual cycle. Circadian rhythms complete a full cycle every 24 hours. Fluctuations in heart rate, blood pressure, body temperature, hormone secretions, metabolism, and in an individual's performance and mood depend in part on **cir-cadian rhythm**.

Sleep is one of the body's most complex biologic rhythms. **Circadian synchronization** exists when an individual's sleep–wake patterns follow the inner biologic clock. That is, when physiologic and psychologic rhythms are high or most active, the person is awake, and when these rhythms are low, the person sleeps. Although light and dark appear to be powerful regulators of the sleep–wake circadian rhythm, they do not exert primary control. The regulating mechanism is an individualized biologic clock subject to occupational demands, social pressures, and so forth. The nurse who works the night shift may routinely sleep from 2 PM to 8 PM and peak physiologic activity may occur between 10 PM and 6 AM during work. Problems of desynchronization occur when sleep–wake patterns are frequently altered and an individual attempts to sleep during high activity rhythms and to work when the body is physiologically prepared to rest.

Stages of Sleep

Research illustrates that there are two major stages of sleep: **nonrapid eye movement (NREM)** and **rapid eye movement (REM)**. These stages have been studied and analyzed with the help of the **electroenciphalograph (EEG)**, which receives and records electrical currents from the brain; the **electrooculogram (EOG)**, which records eye movements; and the **electromyogram (EMG)**, which records muscle tone.

NREM Sleep. NREM sleep consists of four stages. Stages I and II, consuming about 5% to 50%, respectively, of a person's sleep, are light sleep, and the person can be aroused with relative ease. Stages III and IV, each comprising about 10% of total sleep time, are deep-sleep states termed **delta sleep**, or slow-wave sleep (SWS). The arousal threshold (intensity of stimulus required to awaken) is usually greatest in stage IV NREM. Throughout the stages of NREM sleep the parasympathetic branch of the autonomic nervous system dominates, and decreases in pulse, respiratory rate, blood pressure, metabolic rate, and body temperature are observed. Characteristics of the four stages of NREM sleep are summarized in Table 29-1.

REM Sleep. It is more difficult to arouse a person during REM sleep than during NREM sleep. In normal adults, the REM state consumes 20% to 25% of a person's nightly sleep. If persons are awakened during the REM state, they almost always report that they have been dreaming. Many researchers state that everyone dreams; those persons who say they do not simply are unable to recall their dreams.

During REM sleep the pulse, respiratory rate, blood pressure, metabolic rate, and body temperature increase while general skeletal muscle tone and deep tendon reflexes are depressed. REM sleep is believed to be essential to mental emotional equilibrium and to play a role in learning, memory, and adaptation.

When a person is deprived of REM sleep for several nights he will generally spend more time in REM sleep 'on successive nights. This phenomenon is termed REM rebound and allows the total amount of REM sleep to remain fairly constant over time. Characteristics of REM sleep are summarized in Table 29-2.

TABLE 29-1
Characteristics of NREM (Nonrapid Eye Movement) Sleep

Stage	Characteristics
Stage I	Transitional stage between wakefulness and sleep The person is in a relaxed state but still somewhat aware of his surroundings. Involuntary muscle jerking may occur and waken the person. The stage normally lasts only for minutes. The person can be aroused very easily. Comprises only about 5% of our total sleep.
Stage II	The person falls into a stage of sleep. The person can be aroused with relative ease. Comprises 50%–55% of our sleep.
Stage III	The depth of sleep increases and arousal becomes increasingly difficult. Comprises about 10% of our sleep.
Stage IV	The person reaches the greatest depth of sleep, which is called *delta sleep.* Arousal from sleep is difficult. Physiologic changes in the body include the following: Slow brain waves are recorded on an electroencephalogram. Pulse and respiratory rates decrease. Blood pressure decreases. Muscles are very relaxed. Metabolism slows and the body temperature is low. Comprises about 10% of our sleep

TABLE 29-2
Characteristics of REM (Rapid Eye Movement) Sleep

Item	Characteristics
Eyes	Dart back and forth quickly
Muscles	Small-muscle twitching, such as on the face Large-muscle immobility, resembling paralysis
Respirations	Irregular; sometimes interspersed with apnea
Pulse	Rapid and/or irregular
Blood pressure	Increases or fluctuates
Gastric secretions	Increase
Metabolism	Increases; body temperature increases
Brain waves	Encephalogram tracings active
Sleep cycle	REM sleep enters from stage II of NREM sleep and reenters NREM sleep at stage II: arousal from sleep difficult

Sleep Cycle

During a **sleep cycle** a person normally passes consecutively through the four stages of NREM sleep. Then, the person reverses this pattern and returns from stage IV to stage III to stage II. Instead of reentering stage I and awakening, the person enters into the stage of REM sleep, after which he reenters NREM sleep at stage II and returns to stages III and IV. If a person is awakened from sleep at any time, he returns to sleep again by starting at stage I of NREM sleep.

It is typical to go through four or five cycles of sleep each night. On the average, each cycle lasts about 90 to 100 minutes. The cycles tend to become longer as morning approaches. Ordinarily, more sleep occurs in the delta stage in the first half of the night, especially if one is tired or has lost sleep.

Figure 29-2 illustrates the normal sleep pattern of young adults. Variations in the sleep cycle are observed according to age, as Figure 29-3 illustrates.

Sleep Requirements and Patterns

For no known reason, 8 hours of sleep every night has been the accepted standard, despite obvious variances shown in the general population. There is no rigid formula for normal periodicity and duration of sleep. It is important, however, that each person follow a pattern of rest that maintains well-being.

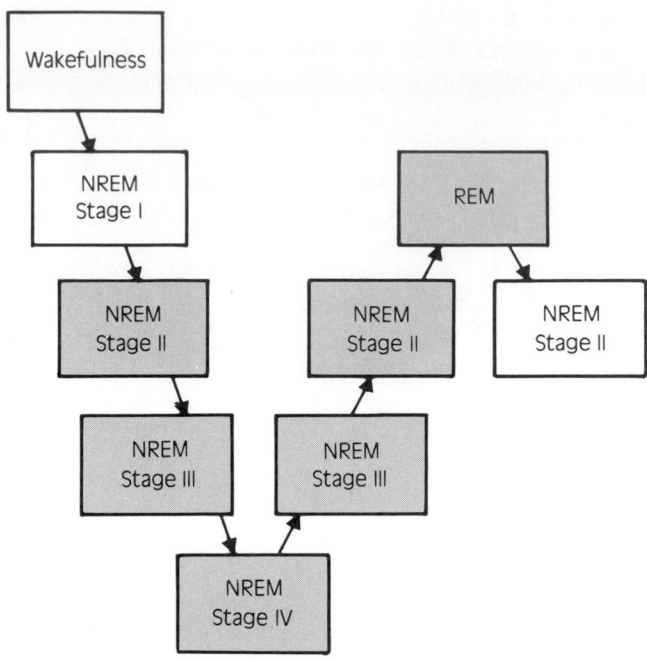

F I G U R E   29-2
A single normal sleep cycle. In the normal nocturnal pattern, the shaded cycle is repeated four or five times. Periods of REM sleep generally increase in duration, and periods of deep sleep (stage IV) progressively decrease as morning approaches.

Despite variations, some generalities can be stated. On the average, infants sleep from 14 to 20 hours each day. Growing children require from 10 to 14 hours of sleep. Adults average 7 to 9 hours, although a 4-hour

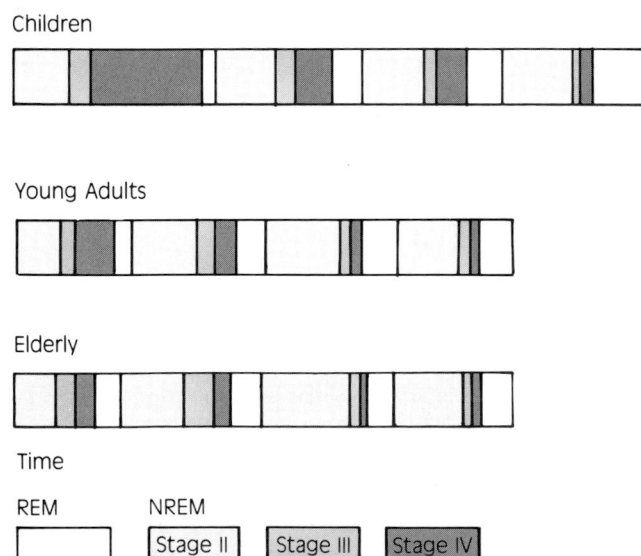

F I G U R E   29-3
A comparison of developmental differences in NREM-REM cycles during nocturnal sleep. Age affects the duration of sleep-cycle stages without affecting the number of cycles. (Adapted from Kales A [ed]: Sleep: Physiology and Pathology, p 45. Philadelphia, JB Lippincott, 1969)

range has been observed in many normal adults. Those who are able to relax and rest easily, even while awake, often find that less sleep is needed, while others may find that more sleep is required to overcome fatigue. Fatigue can be considered a normal, protective body mechanism and nature's warning that sleep is necessary. Chronic fatigue is abnormal and is often a symptom of illness.

Sleep patterns of the elderly vary. However, the elderly are characterized by requiring a longer time to go to sleep, waking earlier, and being less able to cope with changes in their usual sleep patterns than younger persons. Elderly persons tend to nap during the day, which often results in sleeping fewer hours at night.

Patterns of sleep periodicity appear to be learned. For example, most people learn to sleep at night and to be awake and work during the day. However, many night workers learn to sleep equally well during the day.

FACTORS AFFECTING SLEEP

A variety of factors influence both the quality and quantity of sleep.

Developmental Considerations. Age variations also exist in sleep–wakefulness cycles. These are presented with related nursing interventions in Table 29-3.

Physical Activity. Activity and exercise influence sleep by increasing fatigue and, in many instances, by promoting relaxation that is followed by sleep. It appears that physical activity increases both REM and NREM sleep.

Psychologic Stress. Illness and situations in daily living that cause psychologic stress tend to disturb sleep. Generally, psychologic stress affects sleep in two ways: the person experiencing stress tends to find it difficult to obtain the amount of sleep he needs, and REM sleep decreases in amount, which tends to add to anxiety and stress.

Motivation. A desire to be wakeful and alert helps overcome sleepiness and sleep. For example, a tired person may be wakeful and alert when at a party or when attending an interesting play or concert. The opposite is also true—when there is minimal motivation to be awake, sleep generally follows.

Diet. It is believed that the amino acid L-tryptophan acts to promote sleep. It is a precursor of serotonin, a neurotransmitter. A diet containing adequate protein enhances normal sleep while a diet lacking in essential protein may well interfere with it. It has been theorized that elderly people who have difficulty falling asleep and remaining asleep may have diets lacking in sufficient protein or may be absorbing protein poorly.

(Text continues on p. 698.)

TABLE 29-3
Developmental Variation In The Sleep–Wakefulness Cycle

Age Group	Sleep–Wakefulness Cycle	Nursing Implications
Infants	The infant exhibits six states or levels of arousal 1. Regular sleep—Muscle tonus is low, eyelids are closed and still, respirations are about 36 breaths per minute, even, and of regular rhythm. 2. Irregular sleep—Muscle tonus is greater, movements follow no sequence, grimaces are frequent, there is intermittent gross mouthing (*i.e.,* chomping, chewing, and licking), respirations are irregular, and the mean rate is greater than during regular sleep. 3. Periodic sleep (intermediate between regular and irregular sleep)—Respiratory rates are periodic (*i.e.,* bursts of rapid shallow breathing alternate with bursts of deep, slow respirations similar to Cheyne-Stokes respiration). 4. Drowsiness—Less activity than in irregular or periodic sleep but more activity than in regular sleep, the eyes have a dull glazed appearance, open and close intermittently, and just before closing may roll upward, generally regular respirations may become tachypneic, there may be a high-pitched squeal. 5. Alert inactivity—The eyes are open and bright and make conjugate movements in the vertical and horizontal plane, the face is relaxed, respirations are more variable and faster than in regular sleep, not seen before 3½ weeks of age 6. Crying—Vocalization accompanied by gross motor activity, open or closed eyes, tears can been seen as early as 24 hr after birth; characteristic patterns of crying identifiable as early as the first 5 days of life In older infants, a state of active wakefulness is seen, during which they explore their world. This becomes increasingly evident as they mature. Each infant has a unique sleep pattern. Generally, by 8 to 16 weeks the infant's biologic rhythms coincide with daytime and nighttime hours, and he or she will sleep through the night. The younger infant may sleep 17 to 20 hr a day. The 12- to 16-week-old infant will sleep 14 to 18 hr, and by the end of the first year the infant may sleep from 12 to 16 hr a day. Young infants spend much time in irregular or rapid eye movement (REM) sleep. This is believed to furnish great quantities of functional excitement to the higher brain centers.	Nurses may need to help parents understand the infant's sleep and wakefulness patterns. The eye movements, groaning, moving, grimacing, and irregular breathing and gasping are normal and require no attention. Most infants are content to sleep on their abdomens, and this position prevents the aspiration of mucous or regurgitated milk. During waking hours infants enjoy stimulation and play. The nurse should determine if the parents provide visual, auditory, and tactile stimulation for the infant when the child is awake. The parent's perception of the amount of sleep and activity the infant needs and the type of schedule provided should also be assessed. Guide and counsel as needed.
Toddlers	The toddler averages from 10 to 15 hr of sleep in a 24-hr period. Two naps per day are more common in the early toddler period; the number and length of naps generally decline as the child approaches the preschool years. Awakening two or three times during the night occurs with most toddlers. This may be due to sepa-	Establishing a regular bedtime routine with the toddler will facilitate sleep. Routines can include a parent reciting or reading a story, singing a lullaby, rocking the child, or giving the child a bottle of water to suck on. Such activities provide the toddler with love and security and a time to settle down after a busy day.

(Continued)

Age Group	Sleep–Wakefulness Cycle	Nursing Implications
	ration anxiety, loneliness, teething pains, illness, nightmares, or a stressful family situation. Often the toddler is able to fall back to sleep, but some may need attention and comfort from a parent. A circadian sleep–wakefulness rhythm can be identified by the age of 3 months, and a gradual maturation of this cycle occurs between the ages of 2 and 10 years in children. Thus, the toddler should manifest an individual pattern of night sleep, naps, and awake time in a 24-hr period.	To avoid behavioral or emotional disruptions caused by alterations in the toddler's cycle, it is important that parents learn to allow the child to follow a routine sleep pattern, with only occasional interruptions in the pattern.
Preschoolers	Most authorities agree that by the age of 2 to 3, the child's sleep–wakefulness cycle, physiologic rhythms, and hormonal cycles are established. The sleep–wakefulness cycle is fully developed by age 2. The REM pattern (rapid eye movement) of sleep is like an adult pattern by the preschool era. In children, naps represent approximately 12% of sleep for toddlers, 5% for 4-year-olds, and 0% for 5-year-olds. It is estimated that children from age 2 to 5 need about 9 to 16 hr of sleep per day, which decreases as the child gets older.	When assessing the sleep–wakefulness cycle it is essential that the nurse explore the parents' perception of the amount of sleep the child needs and elicit information regarding the schedule the parents use for the child's sleep and rest times. Also, the sleeping patterns of the family should be determined so that congruency or conflict with the preschooler's pattern can be identified. If the child's primary caregiver is unable to obtain sufficient rest the nurse needs to explore alternative ways to help her or him to get more rest so that health and caretaking responsibilities are not jeopardized. The nurse should determine if there are any external factors that might interfere with the child's sleep. Some significant factors include noise, heat, light, and disturbance from siblings. The nurse should offer the parents suggestions on how to change or eliminate any problematic environmental conditions.
School-aged children	Normally children require an average of 8 to 10 hr of sleep, but this will vary with each individual. During periods of increased physical growth, the need for sleep may increase.	Parents may need reassurance that it is not uncommon for interruptions in sleep/rest patterns to occur at this age. Frequently, sleep disturbances are the result of increasing awareness of the concept of death. This knowledge, usually gained through television and books, can be frightening to the child, who views himself or herself as powerless in face of the perceived danger. Preparing the child for sleep in a relaxed manner (*e.g.,* through quiet talking or reading sessions) and establishing bedtime routines (*e.g.,* prayers) may help diminish anxiety. Adults, through their presence and support, can increase the child's own coping resources and help alleviate fears.
Adolescents	Adolescent clients may have an unusual sleep–wakefulness cycle, especially if they live outside the family. Older adolescents tend to prefer sleeping late in the morning and going to bed late at night whenever possible. The sleep needs of different teenagers vary widely.	It is important to assess the amount of sleep the teenager needs and is able to obtain during each 24-hr period. Because adolescents are sensitive about their personal habits, the nurse should always be careful to ask questions about these subjects in a nonjudgmental manner. Questions such as, "Do you feel rested when

(Continued)

Age Group	Sleep–Wakefulness Cycle	Nursing Implications
		you wake after sleeping?" or "Do you feel you get enough sleep?" or "How would you describe the way you sleep?" allow the client to describe personal perceptions (questions about dreams and waking during the sleep period should be included). A teenager may often have complaints about fatigue or inability to do well in school because of poor sleeping patterns.
Young adults	Of all the rhythmic patterns, the most important for the young adult is the sleep–wakefulness cycle. Many factors influence the need for rest and sleep, including physical health, type of occupation, and amount of daily exercise. The young adult is generally full of energy and participates in many activities —attending school, participating in family responsibilities, and working. All of these activities present new and exciting frontiers to explore as an adult, with minimal or no parental influence.	If there is a problem in sleep habits, the nurse needs to explore the client's current life-style to see if adequate time is being allocated for sleep. If stress is hindering sleep, means other than medication should be established for handling and decreasing the problem. The client might be encouraged to take a brief rest period during the day or to participate in stress-reduction exercises. Such activities may prevent sleepless nights. Brief periods of watching television, reading, or sewing may be just enough to bring easy rest at the end of the day.
	The young adult often maintains an active life-style, interrupting sleep patterns along the way. Traditionally, it has been thought that the young adult requires 7 to 8 hr of sleep per night, but some members of this age group seem to do well with less.	Whatever the prescription, the young adult needs to know the impact that a sustained, frantic, exhausting schedule will have over time. Good sleep habits established during the young adult years will not only have a significant impact on sustaining current health but on maintaining long-term wellness as the client ages.
	The percentage of time spent in each stage of sleep decreases with age; however, interestingly enough, the percentage of time spent in stage I REM (rapid eye movement) sleep does not change through life, consistently comprising 20% to 25% of total sleep time. This particular biologic rhythm is thought to be very important for maintaining a stable psychologic balance in each individual, no matter what age.	
	Frequently, the young adult will take medication to alter sleep patterns. Because of significant stress (*e.g.,* trying to achieve, to maintain a family, to establish meaningful relationships, to participate in extracurricular activities), the young adult may have difficulty falling asleep. He or she becomes overtired and increasingly worried about the inability to sleep. Medications may seem a logical way to get some rest quickly. All too often the potential hazards of sleep medications are overlooked, and the young adult may become a prime target for some specific health problems.	
	Sleep medications significantly decrease REM sleep. If these medications are taken consistently, there is a gradual return to the normal amount of REM sleep. However, when the medication is stopped, the individual may undergo withdrawal symptoms, including insomnia, nightmares, fatigue, and increased sensitivity to pain. These symptoms may last up to 5 weeks.	

(Continued)

T A B L E   29-3
Developmental Variation in The Sleep–Wakefulness Cycle   (Continued)

Age Group	Sleep–Wakefulness Cycle	Nursing Implications
Middle adults	For the middle adult, gradual changes in the sleep patterns develop in earlier life and continue through middle adulthood. Specifically, total sleep time decreases, with a particular decrease in the amount of stage IV sleep. The number of sleep arousals increases, and the percentage of time in bed spent awake begins to increase. This will be exaggerated in people who follow previously established sleep patterns after their sleep requirements have decreased.	Because of the multiple changes and stresses in middle age, sleep disturbances are common. However, any sleep aberration should be investigated to exclude the possibility of underlying anxiety or depression which can be reflected by difficulty in falling asleep, early-morning awakening, or alternatively, hypersomnia. Sleeping pills or other aids may be used by middle adults, and such use should be determined during the health history.
Older adults	Sleep–wakefulness patterns are altered in the aged. Old people know they no longer sleep deeply. Luce (1973) discusses the influence of circadian rhythms in elderly clients. "The proportion of rapid eye-movement REM sleep in the cycle remains the same throughout life unless a person has suffered brain damage from cardiovascular or other diseases. Some changes in sleep rhythms are an indication of illness within the maturing and aging brain, but others may only mean that the restrictions of society have loosened their hold on the individual who no longer needs to meet daily schedules of job and family. Hoch and Reynolds (1986) describe the following sleep alterations for the elderly. The proportion of REM and NREM sleep time changes with age. There is an increased quantity of stage I sleep and a 25% increase in light sleep (stage II). However, slow-wave sleep (stages III and IV) decreases by 50% or more. Some elderly people have no stage IV sleep. REM sleep occurs as often in younger adults but the length of each episode shortens. These changes are reflected in the common sleep related complaints of older adults: • Spending more time in bed • Taking longer to fall asleep • Awakening more often • Being sleepy in the daytime • Needing longer to adjust to changes in the usual sleep–wake schedule.	Sleep disturbances in the elderly, while common, are not trivial. Age-related changes in sleep–wake patterns, concurrent medical or psychiatric disorders, and environmental changes may produce an array of sleep-related complaints. Comprehensive assessment and individualized intervention can be effective in the long-term care of these individuals.

(Data from Jones DA, Lepley MK, Baker BA: Health Assessment Across the Lifespan. New York, McGraw-Hill, 1984)

Alcoholic Intake.   Alcoholic beverages, when used in moderation, seem to help induce sleep in some people. However, large quantities have been found to limit REM and delta sleep. This effect may partially explain the phenomenon of hangover after excessive alcohol consumption.

Caffeine-Containing Beverages.   Caffeine is a central nervous system stimulant. For many people, beverages containing caffeine interfere with the ability to fall asleep. Examples of beverages containing caffeine include coffee, tea, most cola drinks, and chocolate.

Environmental Factors.   Most people sleep best in their usual home environments. Sleeping in a strange or new environment tends to influence both REM and NREM sleep for most.

Life-style.   Various life-styles affect the ability to sleep well. Persons working a shift other than the day shift must reorganize their priorities. Developing a sleep pattern is especially difficult if the shift changes periodically. The type of television watched in the evening, involvement in emotionally stirring outside activities, and the amount of activity or exercise in which one participates can all affect sleep. Moderate exercise is a healthy way to promote sleep, but excessive exercise can defeat sleep. One's ability to relax from work-related pressures or to regard or disregard conflict in the home are important factors in the ability to fall asleep.

Illness. Illness acts as a physiologic and psychologic stressor and, as a result, influences sleep. Certain illnesses are more closely related to sleep disturbances than others. Several examples follow.

Gastric secretions increase during REM sleep. Many persons with peptic ulcers awaken at night with pain. They find that eating a snack to help neutralize stomach acidity is often helpful to relieve discomfort and promote sleep.

The pain associated with diseases of the coronary arteries and the occurrence of myocardial infarctions is often associated with REM sleep. Seizure attacks owing to epilepsy are most likely to occur during NREM sleep and appear to be depressed by REM sleep. Liver failure and encephalitis tend to cause a reversal in day–night sleeping habits. Hypothyroidism tends to decrease the amount of NREM sleep, especially stages II and IV.

Some research, especially when children were studied, has demonstrated that asthma attacks appear to occur less frequently during stage IV sleep, and efforts to increase this stage of sleep are recommended. One method is to increase exercise to assist in promoting

extended periods of deep sleep; the type of exercise should be one the patient can tolerate.

Most persons suffering from infectious diseases require more than normal amounts of sleep to overcome fatigue. Infectious hepatitis requires marked increases in the quantity of sleep. The fatigue associated with this disease extends well into the convalescing period.

Medications. Sleep quality is also influenced by certain drugs. Some examples of drugs that decrease REM sleep are barbiturates, amphetamines, and antidepressants. Chloral hydrate and flurazepam (Dalmane) appear to influence the quality of sleep least and promote normal sleep.

NURSE AS ROLE MODEL

It is difficult for clients to work collaboratively with a nurse to achieve sleep and rest goals, when the nurse's appearance and behavior demonstrate inadequate rest and sleep. Because professional, personal, and family demands can all outrank sleep on a nurse's list of priorities, nurses often find themselves showing up for work with inadequate rest and energy. Nurses who value their own well-being and who wish to be role models of

PROMOTING WELLNESS

Rest and Sleep

Use the assessment checklist to determine how well you are meeting needs for rest and sleep. Then develop a prescription for self-care by choosing appropriate behaviors from the list of suggestions.

Assessment Checklist

almost always / some times / almost never

☐ ☐ ☐ 1. I feel rested and refreshed when I get up in the morning.

☐ ☐ ☐ 2. I have energy to carry out normal activities of daily living.

☐ ☐ ☐ 3. I understand the normal changes in sleep and rest requirements and patterns that occur with aging.

☐ ☐ ☐ 4. I set aside time for quiet recreation and restful activities each day.

Self-Care Behaviors

1. Follow a regular routine for bedtime and morning awakening.
2. Accept individual differences in need for sleep.
3. Use relaxation exercises to relax before bedtime, especially if feeling stressed.
4. Avoid caffeine and alcohol before bedtime.
5. Adjust bedcoverings, room temperature, and lighting to your preferences.
6. Drink a glass of milk before going to bed.
7. Be aware of the potential dangers of sleeping pills.
8. Use some part of each day for quiet, enjoyable activities, such as crafts, hobbies, reading, watching television, listening to music, visiting with friends.

healthy sleep self-care behaviors must develop life-styles supportive of the following nurse goals:

The nurse will
- Routinely obtain the amount of sleep necessary to provide energy for the next day's work (specify number of hours)
- Incorporate three to four periods of regular exercise into each week
- Perform some relaxing activity 1 hour prior to retiring
- Evaluate the use of nicotine, caffeine, alcohol, and any pharmacologic sleep aids
- Limit as far as possible shift rotations and working two shifts back-to-back to prevent disrupting usual circadian rhythm

ASSESSING REST AND SLEEP

Sleep History

Because rest and sleep are important components of general health, a sleep history should be included in each comprehensive nursing history. Interview questions are used to identify the client's sleep–wakefulness patterns, the effect of these patterns on everyday functioning, sleep aids, and the presence of sleep disturbances and contributing factors. The sleep history may be brief (four questions) if the client's sleep is adequate and posing no problems, or it may be detailed (see accompanying box).

If the client is being admitted to a care facility it is important to assess the client's usual times for retiring and waking, bedtime rituals, and client preferences regarding sleep environment so that these can be incorporated into the plan of care if possible. Sensitivity to small matters can make the difference between a good night's sleep and no sleep.

When a sleep disturbance is noted the history should determine
1. The nature of the problem
2. Its cause
3. The related signs and symptoms
4. When it first began and how often it occurs
5. How it affects everyday living
6. The severity of the problem and whether it can be treated independently by nursing or needs to be referred to another professional
7. How the client is coping with the problem and the success of any treatments attempted.
Sample questions follow:

Sleep–Wakefulness Pattern
How have you been sleeping?
How many hours of sleep do you usually get in a day?
How much sleep do you think you need to feel rested?

Elements of a Sleep History

1. Usual sleep–wakefulness pattern; recent changes
   "Tell me about your sleep."
   - Usual sleeping and waking times
   - Number of hours of undisturbed sleep
   - Quality of sleep
   - Number and duration of naps
2. Effect of sleep pattern on everyday functioning
   "In what ways does the sleep you get each day affect your everyday living?"
   - Energy level (ability to perform activities of daily living)
3. Sleep aids
   "What do you do to help yourself fall asleep? Do you take any sleep medications?"
   - Means of relaxing prior to bedtime
   - Bedtime rituals
   - Sleep environment
   - Pharmacologic aids
4. Sleep disturbances/contributing factors
   "Is your sleep causing any problems now?"
   - Nature of the sleep disturbance
   - Onset of disturbance and frequency
   - Causes (physical, psychosocial, medicine related)
   - Severity
   - Symptoms
   - Interventions attempted and results

Do you have any difficulty falling asleep?
Do you wake up frequently during the night?
Do you wake up earlier in the morning than you would like and find it difficult to fall back asleep?
Do you take naps throughout the day?
Have there been any recent changes in your usual sleep–wake patterns? If yes, describe them and tell me if they are causing any problems for you.
Do you usually go to bed and wake up at about the same time each day?
Do you dream at night?
Are your dreams frightening?
When the client's response to any of the above questions indicates a potential problem, open-ended questions may be used to gather more data.

General
Why do you think you are only getting 4 hours of sleep a night?
When you wake up during the night what do you do?

Effect of These Patterns on Everyday Functioning

Do you feel rested and ready to start the day when you wake up?

Are there times during the day or during certain activities when you feel especially tired?

What happens when you don't get enough sleep?

Sleep Aids

What do you do to relax before you get ready for bed?

Describe what you usually do to help yourself fall asleep.

Do you take any medications to help you sleep? Are you taking any medicine at all?

Tell me how you like your room (lights, noises, ventilation, position of door, temperature), and bed (mattress, pillows, blankets) when you are sleeping.

Sleep Disturbances/Contributing Factors

Tell me about your sleep problem.

When did this problem begin?

How often does it occur?

Are you doing anything differently now that might be causing the problem?

Can you tell me about any worries or anxieties that might be affecting your sleep?

Are there any illnesses or medications that might be affecting your sleep?

How does this problem affect your everyday life?

What have you been doing to deal with the problem?

Interview questions may be directed to the client, to his bed partner, or to a caregiver. The client record may also contain pertinent information (*e.g.,* a history of illnesses that influence sleep or a history of drug dependency or withdrawal).

Sample recordings of a sleep history in a comprehensive nursing assessment:

> Reports needs 8 to 9 hours of sleep to feel his best and usually gets this without problem. Generally retired at 11:30 PM and rises at 7:30 AM. No special sleep rituals.

> Mother reports toddler has erratic sleep patterns. May nap at anytime in the afternoon or evening and sleep from 1 to 3 hours. Depending on nap, goes to bed anywhere from 7 PM to 11 PM and sleeps about 11 to 13 hours. Resists falling asleep and wants "water, story, snack, kisses, etc." Parents life-style is constantly changing—little consistency for the child regarding sleep expectations.

Common Sleep Disorders

The nurse interviewing a client to obtain a sleep history needs to be knowledgeable about common sleep disturbances in order to recognize significant data. A brief description of these disturbances follows. Specific interview questions may be found in Table 29-4.

Primary Sleep Disorders. Primary sleep disorders are those in which the sleep disturbance is the main symptom or sign of the problem. Examples include insomnia, hypersomnia, narcolepsy, and sleep apnea.

Insomnia is characterized by difficulty in falling asleep, intermittent sleep, or early awakening from sleep. Usually, persons complaining of insomnia have been observed to fall asleep more quickly and sleep more than they report they do. But the condition can lead to such distress that further wakefulness results. It is the most common of all sleep disorders.

Hypersomnia is a condition characterized by excessive sleep, particularly sleep during the daytime. Although this condition may result from medical conditions, it is frequently used as a coping mechanism when someone has no desire or energy to face a new day.

Narcolepsy is a condition characterized by an uncontrollable desire to sleep. The person with narcolepsy can literally fall asleep standing up, while driving a car, in the middle of a conversation, or while swimming. It is considered to be a neurologic disorder. The condition usually begins in susceptible persons during adolescence or early adulthood and continues through life. Agrypnotic drugs that cause wakefulness are used to control narcolepsy. Persons using such drugs should take them faithfully because if they are discontinued, the uncontrollable desire to sleep returns.

Sleep apnea refers to periods of no breathing between snoring intervals. The person may not breathe for periods of 15 seconds to as long as 2 minutes. During long periods of apnea, there is a drop in the oxygen level of the blood, the pulse usually becomes irregular, and the blood pressure often increases. Although most commonly seen in middle-aged men, women and persons of other ages may also experience it. Fortunately, sleep apnea is not particularly common. Some investigators have theorized that sleep apnea possibly may explain certain cases of death that occur during sleep.

Parasomnias. Parasomnias refers to patterns of waking behavior that appear during sleep. Common examples include **somnambalism** (sleepwalking), sleeptalking, nocturnal erections, bruxism (grinding of teeth during sleep), and **enuresis** (bedwetting during sleep).

Sleep Deprivation. Sleep deprivation may result from decreased REM sleep, NREM sleep, or from total sleep deprivation. Causes are multiple, and manifestations progress from irritableness and impaired mental abilities to a total disintegration of personality. The strange environment of the hospital, physical discomfort and pain, the effects of medications, and the need for 24-hour nursing care may all contribute to sleep deprivation in the hospitalized client.

Sleep Diary

A sleep diary or log will provide more specific data of the client's sleep–wakefulness patterns over a prolonged pe-

(Text continues on p. 704.)

T A B L E   29-4
Common Sleep Problems: Description and Pertinent Interview Questions

Sleep Problem	Description	Sample Interview Questions
Primary Sleep Disorders (sleep alteration is the only symptom or sign of a problem)		
Insomnia	Shortened sleep period; may be characterized by difficulty in falling asleep (initial insomnia), frequent or prolonged awakening (maintenance or intermittent insomnia), or early morning awakening (terminal insomnia). In imaginary or subjective insomnia the client has actually slept but claims he has not.	*Initial insomnia* Are you able to fall asleep easily? How long does it ordinarily take you to fall asleep? What are you doing, thinking about, feeling, before you fall asleep? *Maintenance insomnia* Do you find yourself waking up in the night after you have fallen asleep? Tell me how often this happens on a usual night? What do you do once you are awake? *Terminal insomnia* What time do you normally wake up? What might be causing you to wake up so early? How often does this happen? How does this affect the rest of your day?
Hypersomnia	Excessive sleep—in particular, sleep during the day. May occur from medical conditions (diabetic acidosis, increased intracranial pressure, hypothyroidism), but is more often a coping mechanism used when the individual has no desire or ability to face the day (depression, hysteria).	Tell me again how many hours you sleep per day? Is this all at one time or does it include naps? What are you thinking when you first wake up in the morning? Do you get out of bed as soon as you wake up? If no, what do you do? Do you know of any medical conditions that might be causing you to sleep more?
Narcolepsy	A condition characterized by an uncontrolled and abrupt onset of "sleep attacks"—during normally alert activities (*e.g.,* while eating, driving a car, talking. Undiagnosed, the narcoleptic is potentially dangerous to himself and others. Clients with narcolepsy tend to (1) fall asleep quickly, (2) find it difficult to wake up, (3) sleep fewer hours than others, and (4) sleep restlessly. Common symptoms include sleep attacks, cataplexy (abrupt weakness or paralysis of voluntary muscles), hypnagogic hallucinations (frightening "dream attack" that occurs while the person is falling asleep), and sleep paralysis (skeletal muscle paralysis while falling asleep or waking up).	Do you ever fall asleep suddenly during the day? If yes, tell me more about that? Has anyone ever teased you about falling asleep on them, right in the middle of your work, a conversation, or a meal? Have you ever had an attack of muscle weakness or paralysis? Wanted to move and couldn't? If yes, what were you doing when this occurred? How often does it happen? Do you ever experience dreams right as you are falling asleep? What are they like? Does sleep pose any particular problems for you?
Sleep apnea	Period of no breathing during sleep—may last for periods of 15 seconds to as long as 2 minutes. During periods of apnea, there is a drop in the oxygen level of the blood, the pulse may become irregular, and the blood pressure may increase. Many persons experience sleep apnea without symptoms. At high risk for complications are middle-aged men in whom repeated episodes may cause anginal attacks, cardiac arrhythmias, and pulmonary hypertension. It is now postulated that sleep apneas are related to mortality which occurs during sleep. *Obstructive apnea*—Caused by pharyngeal obstruction in the upper airway	Has anyone ever told you that there are times during sleep when you stop breathing for awhile and then start back up again? If yes, tell me what this means to you. Do you have any concerns about this habit? Do you snore? Is there someone who can describe your snoring? Any recent problems with headache and nausea? (related to low oxygen levels) Do you have a history of any heart or lung problems? Chest pain? Are you aware of any changes in your mental abilities or any emotional changes?

(Continued)

Sleep Problem	Description	Sample Interview Questions
	Central apnea—Stoppage of all attempts to breathe; may be related to defects in the respiratory center in the brain Mixed apnea—Combination of central sleep apnea followed by an obstructive apnea Hypopnea—Reduction in the amplitude of ventilation Hypersomnia-sleep apnea—Obesity and airway deformities place both men and women at risk for this syndrome in which sleep is restless and interrupted by snoring and periods of apnea; daytime sleepiness is common. Sleep deprivation affects the mental and emotional functioning of these individuals in whom anxiety, depression, and jealousy are common.	Inspect body build Observe for airway deformities (short neck, thick tongue, deviated nasal septum) In the hospitalized client, compare vital signs during apnea with baseline signs. A report from a bed partner or a tape recording of the client's sleep may be helpful in establishing a diagnosis.

Secondary Sleep Disorders (sleep alterations which caused by another clinical disorder)

	Numerous clinical problems can cause sleep alterations. Among the most common are • Hypothyroidism—Decreased stages III and IV sleep time • Hyperthyroidism—Increased stages III and IV sleep time • Chronic renal insufficiency—Sleep disturbances just before dialysis • Depression—Difficulty falling asleep, more rapid transition from stage to stage, more frequent awakening, less slow-wave sleep, less total sleep time, and more REM activity. • Schizophrenia—Reduction in REM sleep, reduced stages III and IV • Alcoholism REM deprivation • Anorexia nervosa—Reduction of deeper sleep, stages III and IV, as well as of REM sleep; increased stage I sleep but reduction of total sleep time.	Are there any medical or psychiatric illnesses that might be affecting your sleep? (These may be unknown to the client but present on the client record) Have you noticed any changes in your sleep since this disease began? Or since you started treatment for this illness? If yes, please describe these for me.

Parasomnias (patterns of waking behavior that appear during sleep)

	Somnambulism (sleep walking)—Occurs during stages III and IV of NREM sleep; danger is that somnambulist may hurt himself; protective environment is required. Sleep talking—Occurs prior to REM sleep, rarely presents a problem unless annoying to others Nocturnal erections—Occur during REM sleep Bruxism (grinding of teeth during sleep)—Usually occurs during stage II sleep Enuresis—Bedwetting during sleep (see Chap 33)	These questions may be directed to the client: Has anyone ever told you that you walk in your sleep, talk in your sleep, and so forth? Or the questions may be directed to a child's parent: Have you ever noticed your child walking in his sleep? talking while asleep? and so forth With yes to any of these questions: Are you aware of any stressful event or emotional conflict prior to these sleep events? Describe a typical day and what you might have been feeling before one of these events. Does this sleep activity pose any problems for you? Tell me how you are dealing with it.

(Continued)

T A B L E 29-4
Common Sleep Problems: Description and Pertinent Interview Questions (Continued)

Sleep Problem	Description	Sample Interview Questions
Sleep Deprivation	There are basically three types of sleep deprivation: • REM deprivation (absence of dreaming) characterized by irritableness, insecurity, impaired concentration, and anxiousness. Increased sensitivity to pain and increased appetite may result. • NREM deprivation (slow-wave sleep deprivation) characterized by fatigue, lethargy, depression, and difficulty in executing repetitive tasks of everyday living • Total sleep deprivation—Rarely occurs except in laboratory setting; characterized by weariness progressing to total disintegration of personality	In what way is your sleep shortened? What might be causing this? How do you feel when you get up? In what ways do you think your lack of sleep is affecting you?

(Data from Malasonas L et al: Health Assessment, 2nd ed, pp 120–124. St Louis, CV Mosby, 1981)

riod of time. Generally the diary is kept for 14 days and includes

1. A graph of the total number of hours of sleep per day. Depending on the nature of the problem, graphs may be made of the number of undisturbed hours of sleep, number of awakenings, and so forth.
2. A daily record of
   • Time client decided to retire
   • Time client actually tries to fall asleep
   • Approximate time client falls asleep
   • Time of any awakenings during the night and when sleep was resumed
   • Time of awakening in the morning
   • Presence of any stressors client believes are affecting his sleep
   • A record of any food, drink, or medication client believes has positively or negatively influenced his sleep (include time of ingestion)
   • Record of physical activities—type, duration, and time
   • Record of mental activities—type, duration, and time
   • Record of activities performed 2 to 3 hours before bedtime, bedtime rituals, changes in sleep environment
   • Presence of any worries or anxieties client believes are affecting his sleep

It is helpful if the client has a bed partner who can assist with the diary. It should be stressed to the client that the diary is simply a diagnostic tool. If keeping the diary causes too much stress for the client and further interferes with his ability to sleep restfully, it should be discontinued.

Nursing Examination

Physical findings during the nursing examination should either confirm that the client is getting sufficient rest to provide energy for the day's activities or validate the existence of a sleep disturbance which is decreasing the quantity or quality of sleep. Key findings include energy level (presence of physical weakness, fatigue, lethargy); facial characteristics (narrowing or glazing of eyes, swelling of eyelids, decreased animation); behavioral characteristics (yawning, rubbing eyes, slow speech, slumped posture). Data suggestive of potential sleep problems (*e.g.,* obesity, enlarged neck, deviated nasal septum) may also be noted.

If the nurse or a bed partner is able to observe the client sleeping, other sleep characteristics to assess include restlessness, sleep postures, and sleep activities such as snoring or leg jerking (nocturnal myoclonus).

Snoring. Snoring is caused by an obstruction to the air flow through the nose and mouth. Other than disturbing persons sharing the same bedroom, snoring is ordinarily not considered to be a sleeping disorder. However, snoring accompanied by apnea can present a problem. When snoring changes from the characteristic "sawing wood" sound to a more irregular silence followed by a snorting this is indicative of obstructive apnea.

Nocturnal Myoclonus. Observed in 10% to 20% of chronic insomniacs, **nocturnal myoclonus** involves marked muscle contraction which results in the jerking of one or both legs during sleep. The jerking lasts about

28 seconds and may arouse the sleeper. *Restless leg syndrome* is a different condition in which the awake individual is unable to lie with his body and especially his legs still long enough to fall asleep. Both conditions may contribute to insomnia.

DIAGNOSING

When assessment data point to a sleep problem which is amenable to nursing therapy it receives the label "sleep pattern disturbance" and may then be further specified as

Insomnia: difficulty falling asleep
Insomnia: difficulty remaining asleep
Insomnia: premature awakening
Hypersomnia: excessive daytime sleeping
Sleep deprivation
Altered sleep–wake patterns

Common etiologies for sleep pattern disturbances include

Physical discomfort or pain
Emotional discomfort or pain caused by anxiety and stress
Changes in bedtime rituals or sleep environments
Disruption of circadian rhythm
Exercise just before sleep
Caffeine or alcohol after dinner
Drug dependency and withdrawal
Symptoms of physical illness

Sample nursing diagnoses in which the sleep disturbance is the primary problem are presented in Table 29-5.

Sleep pattern disturbances may affect many other areas of human functioning. In the nursing diagnoses which follow the sleep pattern disturbance is the etiology of another problem.

Anxiety related to inability to fall asleep, inability to control behavior while asleep, sleep apnea —threat of death
Altered comfort related to sleep deprivation
Ineffective individual coping related to insomnia: insufficient quantity and quality of sleep
Fear related to narcoleptic's potential to harm himself or others
Impaired gas exchange related to sleep apnea (oxygen saturation of the blood)
Potential for injury related to somnambulism, narcolepsy, sleep apnea
Knowledge deficit (specify: *e.g.,* nonpharmacologic remedies for insomnia) related to misinformation, lack of interest in learning, cognitive limitation
Disturbance in self-concept related to effects of

sleep deprivation hypersomnia–sleep apnea syndrome
Decreased self-esteem related to nocturnal enuresis
Impaired social interaction related to excessive daytime sleeping, sleep deprivation
Altered thought processes related to chronic insomnia, sleep deprivation

Because the *problem statement* of the nursing diagnosis identifies what is wrong with the client and suggests the client goals, and the *etiology* of the problem directs nursing interventions, it is important for the nurse analyzing the assessment data to decide if the sleep data (1) are indicative of the problem, (2) are contributing to a different problem, or (3) are signs or symptoms of the problem. For some reason sleep data seem to fit well in all three categories. For example, when altered sleep–wake patterns are noted in the graduate nurse who is getting adjusted to a new full-time job, shift work, and increased independence, three different diagnoses might be written.

Sleep pattern disturbance: altered sleep–wake pattern (insomnia) related to shift work and stress of new job as manifested by complaints of always feeling tired and never getting enough sleep anymore.

Altered sleep–wake patterns are the problem statement; priority nursing energies will be directed to changing these patterns and to helping the client achieve both the necessary quantity and quality of sleep.

Ineffective individual coping related to multiple stresses of new job and altered sleep–wake patterns (→ sleep deprivation) as manifested by statements like "I don't know how much longer I can do this." "I'm always tired anymore and all I want to do is sleep." "I'm so grouchy—people must hate me!"

Here, the altered sleep–wake patterns are *one* of the factors contributing to the client's problem of ineffective coping; priority nursing energies will be directed toward improving the client's coping skills; one of the means used will be teaching the client how to increase the quantity and quality of sleep.

Ineffective individual coping related to multiple stressors and lack of destressing rituals as manifested by inability to fall asleep (altered sleep–wake patterns), excessive fatigue, and feelings that personality is changing.

In this instance, altered sleep–wake patterns are merely a symptom of the client's actual problem; ineffective coping; it is expected that when the coping problem is resolved, the symptom will disappear.

No one of the above diagnoses is more correct than the others. With each client the nurse must make a decision with each cluster of significant data and pull out the key problem, contributing factors, and related signs and symptoms. How the diagnosis is developed will direct the nursing interventions.

(Text continues on p. 707.)

T A B L E   **29-5**
Nursing Diagnoses for Common Sleep Problems

Title	Etiologic or Contributing Factors	Sample Defining Characteristics
Sleep pattern disturbance: difficulty falling asleep	Worries about family and lack of destressing rituals	• "At least four of five nights a week I lay in bed awake for 3 or 4 hours before I finally fall asleep. Sometimes it is two or three in the morning and I'm still awake worrying about the kids. I've tried getting up and reading or paying my bills, but even that doesn't make me sleepy." • Reports problem falling asleep for last 6 months; is widowed and very concerned about two teenage sons. Never sleeps until both sons are home. States she does nothing special to relax. Feels her worries are "her business"—no support person with whom she shares these.
Sleep pattern disturbance: difficulty remaining asleep	Noise of hospital environment and need for periodic treatments	• Admitted to hospital 3/6; cholecystectomy 3/7 • "I don't think I've had one decent night's sleep since my surgery. I've been falling asleep about 9 PM and then someone wakes me up for my medicine. I just about get back to sleep and someone's putting the light on to poke at my dressing or to check this tube. I know I'm getting grouchy." • Orders include every 4 hour vital signs; nursing assessment of the incision, nasogastric tube, IV; and medication for pain and for sleep.
Sleep pattern disturbance: premature awakening	Barbiturate dependency and lack of knowledge of nonpharmacologic aids for insomnia	• Client has history of mild to moderate depression, related to loss of job and perceived role inadequacy, for the last 3 years; has been taking secobarbital (Seconal), a barbiturate hypnotic, 100 mg PO nightly for the last year and a half. • "I seem to be waking up earlier and earlier, can't fall back asleep, and I start each day feeling like I have a hangover." • "I'd like to get off these drugs, but I'm terrified that without them I won't sleep at all."
Sleep pattern disturbance: excessive daytime sleeping	Altered sleep cycle and inability to cope with multiple stresses	• Only child, first-year college student who is living away from home for the first time. Shares a dormitory room with a roommate. Sleep patterns are erratic and depend on school and social demands. Has recently broken up with high school boyfriend. Fears she is failing three courses. Has no desire to do anything but sleep. "When I get up my only thought is: when can I go back to bed? I often sleep through class."
Sleep pattern disturbance: excessive daytime sleeping	Effects of biologic aging (moderate increase in stage I and II sleep; slow-wave sleep, stages III and IV, decreases by 50% or more)	• Male client, age 74, complains during his annual physical that he seems to be napping more during the day, yet when he tries to fall asleep at night he often can't. • "I'm spending more time in bed, but I'm less rested. Worst of all is not knowing whether or not I'll be awake enough to drive my car or enjoy a good card game."
Sleep pattern disturbance: altered sleep–wake patterns	Frequent rotations of shift and overtime	• 24-year-old graduate nurse who has been working on a busy medical floor for 6 months; rotates 11–7 and 7–3 shifts; recently, a problem with staffing has necessitated frequent rotations. Client often volunteers (two or three times a week) for overtime. • "I don't know what is wrong with me. I'm so tired anymore and don't feel at all like myself. All I want to do when I'm off is to sleep—but often I can't fall asleep when I lay down. Please help!"

PLANNING

Rest and sleep are essential components of well-being. Planning for client care, especially in the hospital involves planning with the client suitable measures to promote rest and sleep.

Client Goals

Whenever nurses care for a client, nursing measures are supportive of the following client goals:

The client will
- Maintain a sleep–wake pattern that provides sufficient energy for the day's tasks
- Demonstrate self-care behaviors that provide a healthy balance between rest and activity

When the client's physical, psychosocial, or spiritual condition contributes to sleep disturbances individualized client goals are developed. For example,

By 1/10, the client will identify two destressing rituals that enable him to fall asleep more easily. The client will demonstrate decreased signs of sleep deprivation by 3/8:
- Attentive to conversation
- Ability to concentrate on complex task (*e.g.,* learning about new medication)
- Verbalizes feeling less fatigued and more "in control" of situation

IMPLEMENTING

Because sleep problems are often not the primary reason for a client's interaction with the health-care system, the key to their detection is often the attitude the nurse communicates to the client. Clients who believe the nurse is generally concerned about their well-being will not be reluctant to discuss insomnia or voice concern about a child who is a bedwetter. Fundamental to the success of any nursing measure to correct a sleep problem is the client's belief that the nurse cares and is readily available for extra help to promote rest and sleep.

Preparing a Restful Environment

Having a comfortable bed helps promote rest and sleep. The bottom linen should be tight and clean. The upper linen, while secure, should allow freedom of movement and should not exert pressure, especially over the legs and feet. Having the body in good alignment is conducive to relaxation. For clients who must assume unusual positions because of their illness, ingenuity and skill are necessary in order to keep muscle strain and discomfort at a minimum. For example, the client who must remain in the orthopneic position to aid breathing should be well supported in a manner that relieves muscle strain.

A quiet and darkened room, with privacy, is relaxing for nearly everyone. In a strange environment, unfamiliar noises, such as people walking or entering and leaving the room, and the closing of elevator doors, bring complaints from most hospitalized clients. Although some of these sources are difficult for the nurse to control, every effort should be made toward reducing disturbances to promote relaxation and sleep.

The temperature of the room, the amount of ventilation, and the quantity of bed covering are matters of individual choice, and the client's wishes should be met whenever it is at all possible.

Promoting Bedtime Rituals

Most people have bedtime rituals to help relaxation and promote sleep. Reading, listening to the radio, watching television, talking to a family member, and praying are common before-sleep activities. Similarly children may search out a favorite doll, stuffed toy, or blanket before going to bed; insist on a bedtime story; kiss everyone goodnight; and say night-time prayers before bed. Readiness for sleep is preceded by a personal hygiene routine for many persons, such as brushing teeth, washing hands and face, voiding, or taking a bath or shower. Snacks are important elements in the bedtime rituals of many children and adults. Whereas, it is true that eating the wrong foods may produce a bad night's sleep, going to bed hungry may also interfere with sleep.

The nurse should be alert to the clients bedtime rituals and make every effort to observe them as far as possible to aid in promoting relaxation and sleep. These rituals should appear in the client's plan of care so that all health personnel can observe them.

Offering Appropriate Bedtime Snacks and Beverages

Because the amino acid L-tryptophan helps promote sleep, there now appears to be justification for offering a high-protein beverage, such as milk, or high-protein snacks, such as cheese or nuts, prior to bedtime when this is allowed in the client's regimen. An alcoholic beverage helps to promote sleep for some people, but, generally, alcohol after dinner should be avoided. For most, beverages containing caffeine should be avoided for at least 4 to 5 hours before bedtime. It is best that the client take fluids during the daytime and avoid excessive fluid intake prior to bedtime to help prevent the necessity of using the bathroom during sleeping hours.

Promoting Relaxation

One can relax without sleeping, but sleep rarely occurs until one is relaxed. Stress and anxiety-producing situations tend to interfere with a person's ability to relax, rest, and sleep. Effective means for dealing with worries include (1) dealing with problems as they arise; (2)

R E S E A R C H   I N   N U R S I N G   *Making a Difference*

Sleep

The human body uses sleep for rest, recuperation, and adaptation to physical and emotional stress. Although sleep disturbances may occur at any age, it has been documented that the older adult often experiences difficulty in achieving restful sleep. Sleep disturbances in this age group have been the topic of nursing research, with the goal of developing nursing interventions to promote rest and sleep.

Related Research

Bahr Sr R, Gress L: The 24-hour cycle: rhythms of healthy sleep. Journal of Gerontological Nursing 11(4):14–17, 1985

Bahr and Gress studied the sleep–wakefulness patterns of elderly institutionalized adults and found individual variability among subjects. This study provides useful baseline data for further studies.

Johnson J: Drug treatment for sleep disturbance. Journal of Gerontological Nursing 11(8):9–12, 1985

This study examined the effects of drug therapy on nocturnal sleep patterns and daytime behavior of older adults. Subjects who took benzodiazepine at night reported more frequent patterns of sleep disruption, were less refreshed on awakening, and were less satisfied with their sleep. Subjects who took no medication or took acetaminophen at bedtime skipped fewer daytime activities and had fewer problems with physical activity than those who took benzodiazepine. These research findings suggest that drugs should not be given routinely for sleep, unless ordered by the physician or requested by the client, because of disruptive effects on sleep patterns and daytime activities.

Steffes R, Thralow J: Do uniform colors keep patients awake? Journal of Gerontological Nursing 11(7):6–9, 1985

This study determined that there was an increase in somnolence in visually impaired elderly clients when the staff wore colored uniforms, and a corresponding higher level of wakefulness on nights when white uniforms were worn. No significant relationship was found between uniform color and restfulness of sleep in nonvisually impaired subjects. In meeting the special needs of the physiologic changes associated with aging, these results present a valid argument for use of other than the traditional white uniform.

Summary

Implications from nursing research about sleep in the elderly include teaching the older adult about normal age-related changes in sleep patterns, using nonpharmacological sleep interventions, such as back rubs, relaxing music, and temperature control to encourage sleep, and assessing the desirability of traditional uniform color.

---

conditioning oneself to worry only during preset times; (3) teaching oneself that worrying never solves problems and is counterproductive; and (4) giving the worries over to another (a trusted family member or friend, caregiver, or God). The distraction and relaxation techniques described in Chapters 9 and 30 may be beneficial when counseling a client whose worries are contributing to a sleep disturbance. Back rubs, warm baths, and face washing if the client is bedridden are typical nursing measures to help the client relax. The technique for back massage is given in Procedure 30-1.

Promoting Comfort

One of the greatest deterrents to rest and sleep is pain; it is often a realistic experience when illness is present. Depending on the cause and severity of the discomfort or pain, appropriate nursing measures include remaining with a lonely and frightened child or adult, using the simple strategy of caring presence and touch, offering a back massage, obtaining an extra blanket, or administering an analgesic. These and other nursing techniques to promote comfort are described in Chapter 30. However, the nurse must be sensitive to the client's discomfort before he or she can relieve it.

Respecting Normal Sleep–Wake Patterns

Every effort should be made to observe the client's normal periods of sleep. In many instances, it is hardly necessary to insist that all client's retire and awaken at specific times. For example, is there a good reason to waken a client at 7 AM when he ordinarily sleeps until 9 AM? It is also recommended that a client's normal napping habits be followed when possible. It has been observed that REM sleep is common during morning naps while NREM sleep is common during naps later in the day. With this knowledge, the nurse can help the client plan napping periods that best fit individual needs and that interfere least with nighttime sleeping.

Scheduling Nursing Care to Avoid Unnecessary Disturbance

Common client complaints are that they are awakened to take sleeping pills and are aroused at early morning hours to prepare for breakfast long before it is served. These common observations should be taken into account when planning care that will help most to promote rest and sleep.

Every effort should be made to time care during periods when the client is normally awake. When this cannot be done, it is preferable to avoid awakening the client during REM sleep, when the rapid eye movements can be observed. Since a client's need for sleep is important, priorities should be examined. For example, the nurse should ask if checking a vital sign or carrying out a particular nursing measure is more important than the client's sleep.

Using Medications to Produce Sleep

Medications for sleep are often ordered for clients. Sedative-hypnotics induce sleep; antianxiety drugs reduce anxiety and tension. The sleep produced by hypnotic-sedatives is an unnatural sleep. All these drugs disturb either REM or NREM sleep to some degree. While most hypnotic-sedatives provide several nights of excellent sleep, the medication often loses its effect after a week or two. At this point many people increase the dosage of the medication or complement the drug with alcohol. Vigorous nursing intervention is needed to prevent a client from developing a pattern of drug dependency and alcohol abuse.

Nurses also need to be alert to the dangers of withdrawal symptoms that can accompany the abrupt cessation of barbiturate sedative-hypnotics. Progressive withdrawal symptoms include weakness, tremulousness, restlessness, insomnia, increased pulse and heart rates, anxiety, convulsions, psychosis, continued seizures, and death.

Flurazepam (Dalmane), a popular nonbarbiturate sedative hypnotic, disturbs NREM slow-wave sleep which results in daytime drowsiness and the morning "hang over" effect. Some persons counteract this side-effect by taking amphetamines or "uppers." The antianxiety medications, once hoped to be the answer to the sleeping pill dilemma, are increasingly implicated in physical and psychologic dependence.

Many times these medications are ordered on a PRN or as needed basis. The nurse should administer these medications only when indicated and always with full knowledge of their limitations. Thorough client teaching should accompany their use. Nurses should aid clients in developing other self-care strategies including developing healthy sleep and life-style behaviors.

Teaching the Client About Rest and Sleep

A well-informed person is better able to cope with distressing situations. Helping clients and their families understand the nature of rest and sleep and their importance to well-being through teaching is an important nursing function. Teaching should include aspects of normal variations in sleep patterns and common measures to promote relaxation and sleep. Also, the care plan should be discussed with the client for acceptability. When sleep disorders become a problem and common nursing measures are inadequate, the nurse can assist and teach by recommending the services of health practitioners especially prepared to deal with them.

NURSING PROCESS *in Clinical Practice*

When identifying and treating sleep disturbances categorized as nursing diagnoses the nurse uses each phase of the nursing process. Quality care is dependent on the nurse's possession of the knowledge and clinical skills described earlier in this chapter. What follows in outline format are the assessment priorities, client goals, nursing interventions, and evaluative criteria for two common types of sleep problems treated by nurses: insomnia and sleep deprivation.

> **Sleep pattern disturbance: insomnia (difficulty falling asleep, difficulty remaining asleep, or premature awakening)**
> **Sleep pattern disturbance: sleep deprivation**

Sleep Pattern Disturbance: Insomnia

An inability to obtain the quantity or quality of sleep that is essential for an individual's healthy functioning is termed insomnia. The knowledge base for insomnia was discussed in Table 29-4. Insomnias may also be classified as situationally related or as a persistent problem (Lareau and Bonnet, 1985). Situational insomnia is defined as a difficulty in falling asleep or staying asleep which has existed for 3 weeks or less and is associated with significant life change. Nursing intervention is directed to helping the client understand the relationship between his sleep problem and the stressor. Persistent insomnias last for longer than 3 weeks and are the most common complaint reported by clients seen in sleep disorder centers. Lareau and Bonnet identify the following conditions as well-established causes of persistent insomnia:

- Biologic rhythm disturbances related to irregular sleep–wake habits (*e.g.,* jet lag, shift work, or sleep pattern irregularities)
- Drug dependence or withdrawal of medication
- Psychophysiologic abnormalities due to a combination of chronic tension/anxiety or inappropriate reinforcement for sleeping
- Psychiatric disturbance (insomnia is a symptom of the psychiatric disturbance and not the disorder itself)
- Sleep apnea syndrome
- Nocturnal myoclonus

Insomnia may also be reported by clients suffering from pain with chronic medical illness, by shortsleepers, or by the elderly.

Assessment

- Use interview questions directed to the client and his bed partner, and direct observation when possible, to determine if the insomnia is caused by difficulty falling asleep, periodic awakenings, or early morning awakenings. Determine if the client's perception of his sleep–wakefulness pattern corresponds to reality.
- Explore the client's life-style and physical and mental health for contributing factors. Because problems in sexual adjustment or functioning may contribute to insomnia, a sexual history may be indicated.
- Instruct the client to keep a sleep diary which may or may not include a graph of undisturbed hours of sleep per night. Use the diary to relate factors causing or correcting the insomnia to sleep–wakefulness patterns.
- Assess for signs of sleep deprivation.
- Assess the actual and perceived degree of control the client has over his insomnia.
- Assess the safety and effectiveness of aids client has used to deal with insomnia.

Client Goals

The client will

- Report that his regular pattern is reestablished or that a new pattern characterized by ease in falling asleep and diminished or absent nightime and early morning awakenings is established.
- Identify the reversible causes of his insomnia.
- Institute life-style changes to eliminate factors contributing to insomnia (*e.g.,* decrease caffeine intake).
- Incorporate appropriate destressing rituals into prebedtime activities (*e.g.,* listening to soothing music, progressive relaxation, prayer).

Interventions

Interventions for insomnia vary according to its cause and severity. Life-style counseling includes the recommendation, when appropriate, for

- Eating high-protein food before bedtime, such as cheese or milk. It is thought that tryptophan from digested protein helps to induce sleep.
- Eliminating caffeine and alcohol in the evening because both are known to disrupt the normal sleep cycle.
- Decreasing or stopping smoking because nicotine withdrawal can occur 3 hours after the last cigarette and cause sleep restlessness, altered sleep cycle, and early awakening to obtain a new cigarette.
- Incorporating a period of regular exercise into each day—but not before bedtime. Avoiding any stimulating activity before attempting to fall asleep.
- Setting aside time for some destressing rituals (relaxation exercises, music, conversation, prayer) immediately before retiring. Having someone with whom one can share fears, worries, and anxieties is often helpful.
- Trying to sleep only when sleepy and not when wakeful.
- Observing a regular bedtime hour and awakening hour because biologic clocks are affected by staying up later or rising later in the day.
- Avoiding naps during the day and evening because for some persons the ability to fall asleep is related to the time interval since the last sleep period.
- Leaving the bed and bedroom when awake. Even if this occurs during the night, the client should take up a quiet, nonstimulating activity (reading, television, music) in another room—so that the bed remains firmly associated with sleep.

Independent nursing measures for insomnia may include all those described earlier in the chapter. The nurse may also need to collaborate with the physician in determining the best course of action if the client's insomnia is drug-related. Clients who have used hypnotic medications for a long period of time will most likely benefit most from a gradual program of withdrawal and will value nursing support throughout this process. On the other hand, a short course of treatment with a sedative-hypnotic or antianxiety agent may be indicated, in which case the nurse works collaboratively with the prescribing physician and teaches the client the action of the drug, the reason it is being used, safe administration particulars, side-effects to watch for and to report, and potential dangers of overreliance on medication.

For severe problems of insomnia referral for psychiatric evaluation and treatment may be necessary. Clients may also be referred to a sleep disorder clinic (for listings write: The Association of Sleep Disorders Centers, P.O. Box 2604, Del Mar CA 92014, 619-755-6566).

Evaluative Criteria

Client meets above goals.

Sleep Pattern Disturbance: Sleep Deprivation

Shortchanging one's sleep occasionally rarely results in any serious problems but a prolonged pattern of sleep deprivation will produce symptoms progressing from irritableness and fatigue to generalized personality disintegration. There are basically three types of sleep deprivation:

1. REM deprivation (absence of dreaming)—Causes: certain drugs (especially alcohol and barbiturates), general sleep disturbances (shift work, travel, hospitalization—especially in intensive care setting). When persons are denied dreaming during normal REM sleep, they become irritable, insecure, and anxious. Also, their sensitivity to pain increases, they are unable to concentrate, and they exercise poor judgment. Relationships with other people suffer. Depression is a common mental symptom, and in extreme cases, a person's ethical standards have been known to deteriorate. Symptoms of psychoses have appeared in rational people after prolonged REM sleep deprivation. These same subjects, when allowed to sleep uninterrupted, experience more frequent REM periods, as if the body were trying to make up for losses. It has been observed that when persons are denied REM sleep for whatever reason, REM sleep with dreaming, often including nightmares, increases. Similarly, when stage IV NREM sleep is denied, the person will try to catch up on lost NREM sleep. If both REM and NREM sleep are insufficient, stage IV NREM sleep increases.

2. NREM deprivation (delta sleep or slow-wave sleep deprivation)—Causes: may be same as above; also, continual interruption of the sleep cycle (*e.g.,* with frequent treatments); certain medications: (*e.g.,* diazepam (Valium), flurozepam (Dalmane), and morphine); and conditions such as sleep apnea, hypothyroidism, and diseases causing respiratory distress. The elderly frequently experience lack of NREM sleep. Symptoms include fatigue, lethargy, depression, and difficulty in executing the repetitive tasks of everyday living.

3. Total sleep deprivation—Rarely occurs except in controlled laboratory situations. Symptoms of total sleep loss occur in a relatively slow but predictable pattern, mounting as time goes on. As weariness begins, normal performance fades off with lapses in attention and concentration. Unpleasant sensations, such as blurred vision, glazed and itching eyes, nausea, and headache are common symptoms of fatigue. Hallucinations and illusions eventually become vivid, and mental confusion and inability to determine reality occur. There may be a lack of memory, a decrease in intellectual effort, and an attitude of not caring what happens.

Exactly why sleeplessness leads to ill effects is not known. It is not known whether irreversible damage to body tissue results from prolonged or chronic sleep deprivation. However, the fact that sleep deprivation produces changes in physical and mental functioning supports observations that sleep is essential for well-being.

Assessment

- Use interview questions directed to the client and family and observation skills to determine (1) the type of sleep deprivation, (2) its probable causes, (3) its effect on everyday functioning, and (4) the severity of the problem.
- Instruct the client to keep a sleep diary and note increases or decreases in quality sleep and the factors that contribute to or detract from quality sleep.
- Assess the actual and perceived amount of control the client has over his sleep–wakefulness patterns.

Client Goals

The client will

- Keep a sleep diary (if feasible) until factors causing sleep deprivation and factors that facilitate sleep are identified
- *If indicated:* Change or eliminate life-style behavior contributing to sleep deprivation
- Increase REM and NREM sleep until usual sleep cycle is reestablished (specify)
- Increase REM and NREM sleep until behaviors indicating sleep deprivation (specify) are no longer present

Interventions

As soon as the cause of the sleep deprivation has been identified, nursing measures are instituted to eliminate the cause or to modify either it or the client's response.

- If insomnia is the cause, the nurse institutes the interventions for insomnia described earlier.
- If hospitalization is the cause, appropriate nursing measures include
  1. Familiarizing the client with the hospital environment
  2. Recreating the client's usual sleep environment as much as possible: favorite pillow, dim light or darkness, ventilation, door open or closed, child's favorite toy.
  3. Respecting the client's presleep habits and rituals when these are sleep-producing: evening snack of milk, watching the 11 PM news, listening to music, taking a warm shower or bath, using relaxation exercises, prayer.
  4. Using good nursing care measures to ensure the client's comfort prior to falling asleep: body is repositioned and in good alignment, supported if necessary; bed linens are clean and straightened; client is free of pain; tubes are patent and draining; equipment is functioning optimally (if frequent checks are needed throughout the night [*e.g.,* with an I.V.] keep-

ing a soft night light on continuously may be less distressing than having each nurse fumble for a light); finally, if pharmacologic aids are to be used to promote sleep, a determination should first be made that they are not negatively interfering with REM or NREM sleep.

5. Carefully evaluating the need for nursing interventions throughout the night which are likely to awaken the client and to schedule nursing care to allow the client the longest periods of undisturbed rest.

- If medications are contributing to sleep deprivation, the nurse needs to consult with the physician regarding the advisability of their use and possible substitutes.
- When alcohol is contributing to sleep deprivation, the nurse needs to teach the client about alcohol's effects in the body and counsel the client about decreasing or eliminating alcohol intake.
- When sleep deprivation results from shift work, travel, and so forth, the nurse must explore with the client the need for this activity and suggest means to compensate if the activity is necessary.

Evaluative Criteria

Client meets the above goals.

C A S E   S T U D Y

Mr. Bitner is an 86-year-old alert, black, widowed male who was admitted to a nursing home 2 months ago. He is ambulatory and performs most of his self-care. Admitting medical diagnoses included diabetes mellitus and hypertension. He adds to this list "a touch of arthritis." His daughter complains to the charge nurse that her dad seems to be spending more and more time during the day napping and that he says he doesn't sleep well at night.

Assessment Findings

A comprehensive sleep assessment of Mr. Bitner following his daughter's expression of concern revealed the following data:

Sleep-Wakefulness Pattern

Client goes to bed between 8 PM and 9 PM and gets out of bed between 7 AM and 8 AM because the staff are getting his roommate out of bed at this time. He states he never falls asleep before midnight because he always watched the late news at home. He usually wakens twice during the night to void and often cannot fall back asleep. During the day he is frequently observed dozing in his chair. If not discouraged he returns to his room midmorning and afternoon for a 1-hour nap.

Effect of Sleep Pattern on Everyday Living

"I'm always tired. I don't seem to have much energy anymore." Client has not socialized yet with other residents and without strong encouragement does not participate in group activities. From his point of view, life holds little for him to be awake for. "I worked for the railroad for almost 50 years and I never overslept once."

Sleep Aids

Denies ever using medication to fall asleep. States he often relaxed at home in the evening with a couple of beers. Likes a dim light on during the night so he can find the bathroom easily and likes his bedroom door ajar. Sleeps with two blankets and is often still cold.

Sleep Disturbances and Contributing Factors

"Ever since my wife died I'm just not getting enough sleep and since I came here its worse. I don't know why I don't fall asleep when I go to bed or why I wake up so much. It sure makes the nights long." He has no regular periods of exercise and drinks black coffee with every meal and one or two diet colas in the evening.

Nursing Diagnosis

Sleep pattern disturbance: Difficulty falling asleep and remaining asleep related to new sleep environment and schedule, evening caffeine intake, and insufficient meaningful daytime activity.

Planning

Mr. Bitner is eager to do anything that will help him to get a better night's sleep, and his daughter is supportive. During the planning process it is important to communicate to Mr. Bitner and his daughter that some of his sleep disturbance may be an unavoidable result of aging. It is not that less sleep is needed, but that the ability to sleep well seems to diminish with age. Planning will be directed toward strengthening the sleep–wake cycle rhythm and combating the age-related tendency to develop several brief sleep episodes in a 24-hour period (see Nursing Care Plan). During a family conference attended by Mr. Bitner, his daughter, the primary nurse, and the unit's social worker, and the activity director, Mr. Bitner endorsed the following goals:

Short-term goals

By the next monthly assessment, 1/20, the client will

1. Retire after viewing the 11 o'clock news in the TV room with Mr. Sparter
2. Report that he falls asleep within 1 hour of getting into bed
3. Decrease nightime awakenings to one, after which he returns to a sound sleep
4. Attend the center's exercise sessions Monday–Friday at 10 AM
5. Substitute noncaffeine beverages for coffee and cola at supper and evening snack
6. Report obtaining a minimum of 6 hours of quality sleep nightly

To assist in the above Mr. Bitner's daughter will bring her father noncaffeine cola and include a walk in her visits to her father.

Long-term goals

Mr. Bitner establishes a new sleep–wakefulness pattern which provides sufficient energy for daytime activities:

• 6 to 7 hours of quality sleep nightly
• Daytime napping decreased to one nap anytime before evening meal

Implementation

In implementing the care plan the nurse needs the following specialized abilities:

• Strong assessment skills and knowledge of how aging affects sleep–wakefulness patterns. The following common sleep complaints of older adults are related to changes in the proportion of REM and NREM sleep and to alterations in the quality of sleep which are consistent signs of biologic aging: spending more time in bed, taking longer to fall asleep, awakening more often, being sleepy in the daytime, and needing longer to adjust to changes in the usual sleep–wake schedule (Hoch and Reynolds, 1986).
• Knowledge of the multiple factors that contribute to insomnia and its severity; knowledge of which insomnias can be independently treated by nursing.
• Interpersonal skills to communicate to both Mr. Bitner and his daughter that something can be done to improve the duration and quality of his sleep and that nursing is committed to helping.
• Teaching and counseling skills to help Mr. Bitner understand the relationship between life-style factors (decreased exercise, caffeine, lack of meaningful activity) and his sleep difficulty and to initiate the necessary changes.
• Interpersonal and leadership skills to motivate the nursing staff to value Mr. Bitner's goals and to work collaboratively with the social worker and activities director.

Documentation

Sample documentation of the family conference follows in the traditional note format:

12/20/88   Family conference to discuss Mr. Bitner's sleep disturbance—initiated by daughter's concern. Present were Mr. Bitner and his daughter (A. Jelner), K. Behner (social worker), W. Quing (activity director), and M. LeBon (primary nurse). Primary nurse presented findings from comprehensive sleep assessment; Nursing diagnosis: difficulty falling asleep and remaining asleep related to new sleep environment and schedule, evening caffeine intake, and insufficient meaningful daytime activity. Discussion centered on strategies to (1) help Mr. Bitner develop interests in the center including possibilities for increased physical exercise, (2) decrease his evening caffeine intake (daughter to bring noncaffeine colas), and (3) reestablish usual retiring and waking times. See care plan. Client's progress will be evaluated at next monthly assessment, 1/20/89.

M. LeBon, RN

SOAP documentation

12/20/88   #3 Difficulty falling asleep and remaining asleep 2 PM

S: "Ever since my wife died I'm just not getting enough sleep and since I came here it's worse."
   Reports less than 5 hours sleep nightly with frequent awakenings.
   Reports drinking coffee at every meal and cola in the evening.
O: Frequently observed to be awake at night; often found asleep in chair during the day; rarely observed at center's activities
A: Above sleep pattern disturbance is related to new sleep environment and schedule, evening caffeine intake, and insufficient meaningful daytime activity (exercise).
P: 1. Attempt to reestablish his usual retiring and waking times
   2. Decrease caffeine intake—especially in the evening
   3. Increase his participation in center activities—especially exercise program

Reevaluate sleep status at next monthly assessment, 1/20/89.

M. LeBon, RN

Evaluation

Short term goal achievement is evaluated at next monthly assessment. See the care plan for related evaluative statements and revisions of the plan of care. Long-term goal achievement is an ongoing evaluation.

N U R S I N G   C A R E   P L A N   *for Mr. Bitner*

Nursing Diagnosis: Sleep pattern disturbance: Difficulty falling asleep and remaining asleep related to new sleep environment and schedule, evening caffeine intake, and insufficient meaningful daytime activity.

Long-Term Goal: Client establishes a new sleep–wakefulness pattern which provides sufficient energy for daytime activities: (1) 6 to 7 hours of quality sleep nightly, (2) daytime napping decreased to one consistent nap time anytime before evening meals.

Goals	Nursing Actions	Rationale	Evaluative Statement
By the next monthly assessment, 1/20, the client will: 1. Retire after viewing the 11 o'clock news in the TV room with Mr. Sparter	Assess advisability of reestablishing Mr. Bitner's usual retiring pattern of going to bed after the 11 o'clock news. Assess how client spends the time from the evening meal to 11 PM—explore relaxing alternatives with him. Investigate possibility that he and Mr. Sparter might become social partners.	Strengthens the natural rhythm of his sleep–wake cycle. Elimination of evening naps will facilitate his falling asleep more easily.	1/18 Goal met. Client does not go to bed until after the news and has been observed talking with Mr. Sparter. *Recommendation:* Continue to develop evening activities with him—he finds that the time after supper "drags." *M. LeBon, RN*
2. Report that he falls asleep within 1 hr of getting into bed	Continue to assess how long it takes client to fall asleep after getting into bed. Explore with client means to relax prior to falling asleep: deep breathing, imagery, prayer. Teach the importance of using the bed only as a place to sleep. Advise client when he cannot sleep to get out of bed and to go to another room where he can perform some monotonous activity (watching television, listening to radio).	Activities that calm and relax the person prepare the body for sleep. This maintains the bed as a powerful stimulus for sleep and helps to prevent "conditioned" insomnia ("Well, here I am in bed now and I know sleep won't come.")	1/18 Goal partially met. Three to four nights a week he falls asleep within 30 min of going to bed. States he really misses comfort of his wife. *Revision:* Investigate his sense of loss and need for touch. May be a good candidate for pet therapy program. *M. LeBon, RN*
3. Decrease nighttime awakenings to one after which he returns to a sound sleep	Assess and manipulate factors that contribute to nighttime awakenings: • Need to void (time of day diuretic is taken, amounts of fluid intake in the evening) • Roommate's wakefulness, snoring, or need for care • Uncomfortableness in strange environment • Comfort (*e.g.,* temperature)	Individualizing the client's bedtime environment and meeting comfort needs (warmth, soft light, and so forth) promote sleep onset and maintenance.	1/18 Goal partially met. Nighttime awakenings vary from none to three nightly. See above revision. *M. LeBon, RN*

(Continued)

N U R S I N G   C A R E   P L A N   (Continued)

Goals	Nursing Actions	Rationale	Evaluative Statement
	Teach client upon awakening how to concentrate on breathing until he falls back to sleep.	Uses power of positive thinking to facilitate return to sleep	
4. Attend the center's exercise sessions Monday–Friday at 10 AM	Assess if client understands the relationship between daily exercise and his ability to sleep. Determine how his exercise needs can best be met (*i.e.,* through a group program or an individualized program of walking, or other program) Use positive verbal reinforcement to communicate to client that someone cares that he is using positive means to remedy his sleep disturbance and increase his well-being. Encourage client's daughter to go for walks with him when she visits and to question him about his exercise program.	Regular exercise throughout the day is known to increase physical fatigue and to promote sleep. Exercise or stimulating activities immediately prior to retiring interfere with sleep's onset.	1/20 Goal met. Client has become an enthusiastic participant in exercise sessions—attends daily. *L. Fox, RN*
5. Substitute noncaffeine beverages for coffee and cola at supper and evening snack	Assess client's willingness to substitute decaffeinated beverages for coffee and cola. Consult with dietary department and his daughter about options. Experiment with options until his preferences are determined. Gradually reduce his caffeine intake, especially from evening meal onwards. Offer a high-protein evening snack.	To avoid stimulating effects of caffeine	1/20 Goal met. Client now drinks Sanka with meals and milk in the evening. Dislikes noncaffeine sodas. *M. LeBon, RN*
6. Report obtaining a minimum of 6 hours of quality sleep nightly	Assess Mr. Bitner's progress weekly. Continue to identify factors that contribute to better sleep or interfere with his sleep.	Because multiple factors influence sleep–wakefulness cycles in the elderly, ongoing assessment is needed.	1/20 Goal partially met. Mr. Bitner is pleased he is sleeping better but still reports "two or three bad nights" a week. Continue to implement plan and reassess 2/20. *M. LeBon, RN*

KEY POINTS

- Most persons spend approximately one third of their lives asleep; sleep of some quality and duration is an essential component of well-being.

- Sleep is a state of altered consciousness throughout which varying degrees of stimuli produce wakefulness. It is an active and complex rhythmic state, a progression of repeated cycles.

- The cyclical nature of sleep is controlled by the reticular activating system and bulbar synchronizing region in the brain stem. Biochemical changes and hormones also influence the sleep process.

- Circadian synchronization occurs when an individual's sleep–wake patterns follow the inner biologic clock. Shift work, traveling across time zones, and irregular sleep–wake patterns can easily lead to desynchronization and poor quality sleep and decreased work performance.

- There is both nonrapid eye movement (NREM) sleep and rapid eye movement (REM) sleep. During a sleep cycle a person passes through the four stages of NREM sleep and through REM sleep. The average person has four to five complete sleep cycles each night.

- Factors affecting sleep include age, physical activity, psychologic stress, motivation, diet, alcoholic intake, caffeine intake, environment, life-style, illness, and medications. Most persons with sleep disturbances can initiate life-style changes that will improve sleep.

- Nurses should explore parents' perceptions about the amount of sleep their infant or child needs and the schedule the parent uses for sleep and rest times. Developmental variations and the need for consistent sleep–wake patterns and bedtime rituals may need to be taught.

- For the young adult, the sleep–wakefulness cycle is the most important of all the rhythmic patterns and the one most likely to be abused. Multiple stressors can interfere with the young adult obtaining sufficient rest and sleep and can encourage the use of alcohol or sleep medications. Teaching needs to include the importance of developing good sleep habits to promote long-term wellness.

- The nurse who wishes to be an effective role model in promoting rest and sleep uses appearance and energy level to communicate to clients the value of proper rest and sleep self-care behaviors.

- A comprehensive sleep history includes data on sleep–wakefulness pattern, the affect of the sleep pattern on everyday functioning, sleep aids, and sleep disturbance/contributing factors.

- When a sleep disturbance exists, the assessment attempts to identify the nature of the problem, its cause, related signs and symptoms, onset and frequency, effect on everyday living, severity, if the problem can be treated independently by nursing, and the coping means the client has used and their success. A sleep diary and information from a bed partner may be needed to establish a diagnosis.

- Common sleep problems include insomnia, hypersomnia, narcolepsy, sleep apnea, parasomnias (sleep walking, sleep talking, enuresis), and sleep deprivation.

- Nursing diagnoses may be written to specifically address sleep pattern disturbances (insomnia: difficulty falling asleep, difficulty remaining asleep, or premature awakening; hypersomnia) or to identify the effect sleep pattern disturbances have on other areas of human functioning (*e.g.,* anxiety, comfort, coping, alteration in thought process).

- Nursing interventions to promote rest and sleep include establishing a trusting relationship, preparing a restful sleep environment, attending to bedtime rituals, offering appropriate bedtime snacks, promoting relaxation and comfort, respecting normal sleep–wake patterns, scheduling nursing care to avoid disturbances, using medications to promote sleep, and teaching the client about rest and sleep.

BIBLIOGRAPHY

Bahr RT: Sleep–wake patterns in the aged. Journal of Gerontological Nursing 9(10):534–537, 540–541, 1983

Block AJ: Respiratory disorders during sleep. Part 1. Heart Lung 9(6):1011–1024, 1980

Bower B: Recurrent dreams: Clues to conflict. Science News 129:197, March 29, 1986

Burgener S: Circadian rhythms: Implications for evaluation of the critically ill patient. Critical Care Nurse 5(5):43–48, 1985

Deters GE: Circadian rhythm phenomenon. MCN 5(4):249–251, 1980

Edgil AE, Wood KR, Smith DP: Sleep problems of older

infants and preschool children. Pediatric Nursing 11(2):87–89, 1985

Fabijan L, Gosselin MD: How to recognize sleep deprivation in your ICU patient and what to do about it. The Canadian Nurse 78(4):20–23, 1982

Hayter J: The rhythm of sleep. Am J Nurs 80(3):457–461, 1980

Hayter J: Sleep behaviors of older persons. Nurs Res 32(4):242–246, 1983

Hayter J: To nap or not to nap? Geriatr Nurs 6(2):104–106, 1985

Hoch C, Reynolds C: Sleep disturbances and what to do about them. Geriatr Nurs 7(1):24–27, 1986

Lareau SC, Bonnet H: Sleep disorders: Insomnias. Nurs Pract 10(8):13, 16–17, 20, 23–24, 1985

Luce CG: Body time. New York, Bantam Books, 1973

Lukasiewicz-Ferland P: When your ICU patient can't sleep. Nursing 17(11):51–53, 1987

Malasanos L, Barkauskas V, Moss M, Stoltenberg-Allen K: Health Assessment, 3rd ed. St Louis, CV Mosby, 1986

Milne B: Sleep–wake disorders and what we can do about them. The Canadian Nurse 78(4):24–27, 1982

Ross MM, Hare K, McPherson M: When sleep won't come: Helping our elderly clients. The Canadian Nurse 82(9):14–18, 1985

Schirmer M: When sleep won't come. Journal of Gerontological Nursing 9(1):16–21, 1983

Walseben J: Sleep disorders. Am J Nurs 82(6):936–940, 1982

Weaver T, Millman RP: Broken sleep. Am J Nurs 86(2):146–150, 1986

30 Comfort

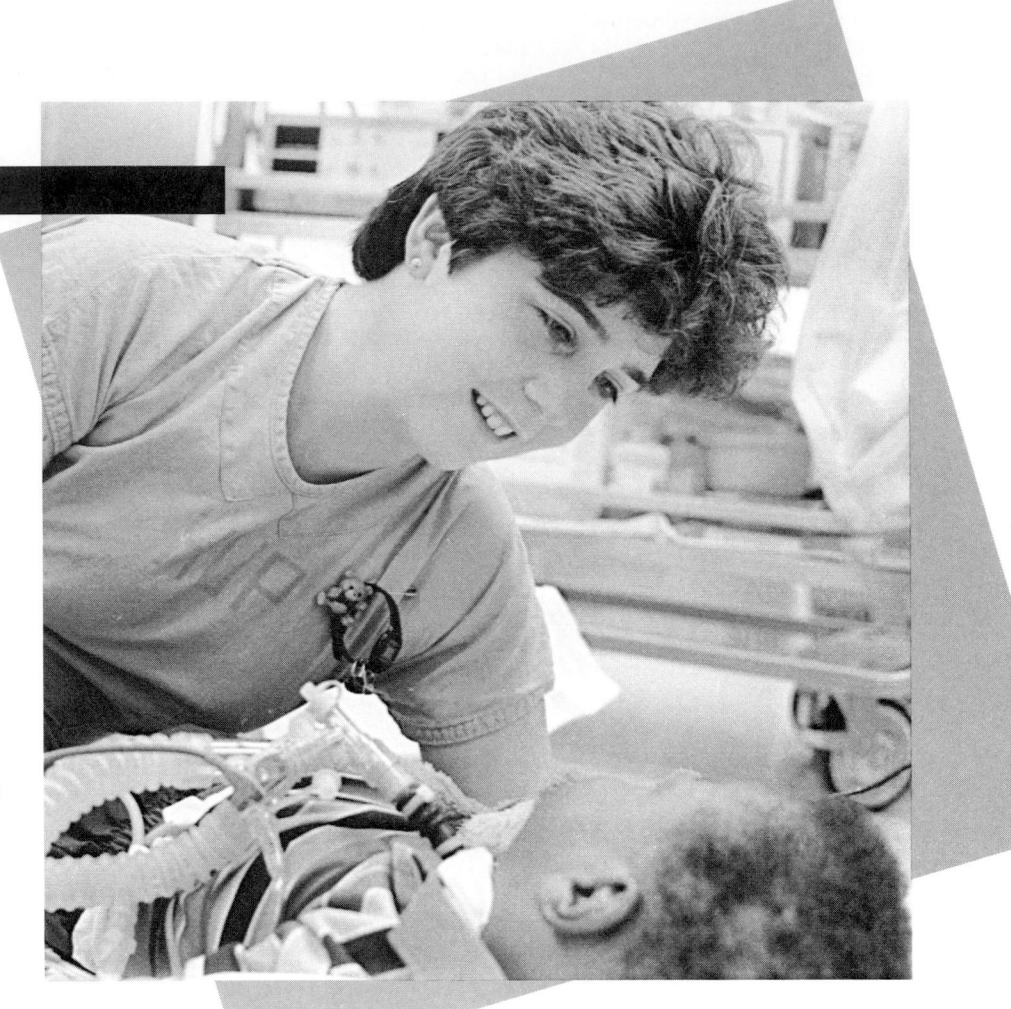

OBJECTIVES

After studying this chapter, the learner should be able to

Define the list of key terms used in the chapter.

Describe specific elements in the pain experience.

Compare and contrast acute and chronic pain.

Identify factors that may affect an individual's pain experience.

Obtain a complete pain assessment utilizing appropriate interviewing and physical assessment skills.

Develop nursing diagnoses that correctly identify pain problems and demonstrate the relationship between pain and other areas of human functioning.

Demonstrate the correct use of noninvasive pain-relief measures: distraction, relaxation, cutaneous stimulation.

Administer analgesic agents safely to produce the desired level of analgesia without causing undersirable side-effects.

Collaborate with the members of other health disciplines employing different treatment modalities to promote pain relief.

Plan, implement, and evaluate nursing care related to select nursing diagnoses for pain problems.

Utilize teaching and counseling skills to empower clients to direct their own pain management programs.

The person in pain often experiences pain as an all-consuming reality and wants only one nursing intervention: pain relief. If pain relief were as simple as rubbing a back or administering a prescribed analgesic, nursing's task would be easy. However, no two persons experience pain exactly the same way. Differences in individual pain perception and response to pain as well as the multiple and diverse etiologies of pain require highly specialized abilities of the nurse seeking to promote comfort and relieve pain. The most essential of these are the nurse's (1) belief that the client's pain is real, (2) willingness to become involved in the client's pain experience, and (3) competence in developing effective pain management regimens. Nursing studies repeatedly indicate that although pain is often an all-consuming priority for clients, it is frequently a low priority for nurses because it is an intangible commodity. Unfortunately, it is easier to ignore a client's poorly communicated pain than it is to ignore a dressing that needs to be changed, a client who requires assistance with ambulation, or a prescribed medication. Nurses who somehow manage to practice nursing while remaining insensitive to the comfort needs of their clients do a grave disservice to these clients and to the nursing profession itself.

Nurses are not alone in undervaluing the need for pain management. Although pain is the single most common reason for seeing a physician and the number one reason why people take medication, medical science is still ill equipped to deal with pain. A special *Time* magazine report (June 11, 1984) contained the following:

> A 1983 survey by Bonica of 17 standard textbooks on surgery, medicine, and cancer found that only 54 pages out of a total of 22,000 provided information about pain.
> The National Cancer Institute . . . spends little more than one-fifth of 1% of its $1.08 billion budget on pain research, even though the dread of terminal cancer pain has become a national phobia.

Study of this chapter will provide the student with knowledge of the pain experience and factors that influence it. A detailed guide to assessing alterations in comfort is presented, including specific questions and approaches to use when assessing various pain factors. Numerous examples of nursing diagnoses are offered that either identify specific alterations in comfort or the effects of these alterations on other areas of human functioning. Specific nursing strategies for promoting comfort and assisting clients to achieve pain management goals are detailed. These include establishing a trusting nurse–client relationship, teaching the client about pain, manipulating factors that affect the pain experience, initiating noninvasive pain-relief measures (distraction, relaxation, cutaneous stimulation), assisting with the pain therapies of other disciplines (analgesic administration, hypnosis, acupuncture, biofeedback, local anesthesia, neurosurgery, and electrical nerve stimulation), and evaluating the effects of the plan of care.

KEY TERMS

acupressure	intermittent pain
acupuncture	mild pain
acute pain	moderate pain
analgesic drug	pain
brief pain	pain threshold
cutaneous stimulation	pain tolerance
continuous pain	phantom limb pain
contralateral stimulation	placebo
chronic pain	psychogenic pain
diffuse pain	referred pain
dull pain	relax
endorphins	severe pain
excruciating pain	sharp pain
gate control theory	shifting pain
hypnosis	slight pain
imagery	somatic pain
	transient pain
	visceral pain

In the section Nursing Process in Clinical Practice, focused assessment, planning, implementation, and evaluation guides are offered for nursing diagnoses of acute and chronic pain problems. These guides and the concluding case study illustrate how the nurse's knowledge of and sensitivity to the client's pain experience may be combined with specific nursing interventions to resolve pain problems successfully.

THE PAIN EXPERIENCE

Definition

Pain is an elusive and complex phenomenon, and despite its universality its exact nature remains a mystery. It is one of the human body's defense mechanisms that indicates the person is experiencing a problem. Aristotle defined pain as well as anyone when he wrote that it is the antithesis of pleasure, the epitome of unpleasantness. Richard Sternback, a psychologist, is credited with the classic definition of pain, which expresses both its sensory and reactive components: "Pain is an abstract concept which refers to (1) a personal, private sensation of hurt; (2) a harmful stimulus which signals current or impending tissue damage; (3) a pattern of responses which operate to protect the organism from harm" (1968, p 12). The definition of pain that is probably of greatest benefit to nurses and their clients is that offered by Margo McCaffery: "Pain is whatever the experiencing person says it is, existing whenever he (or she) says it does" (1979, p 11). This definition rests on the belief that the only one who can be a real authority on whether or not an individual is experiencing pain is that individual.

In summary, pain is present whenever a person says it is, even when no specific cause of the pain can be found. Health practioners must rely on the client's description of the pain because it is a subjective symptom, which only the client can identify and describe.

Origins of Pain

Pain is somatic or visceral in origin. **Somatic pain** pertains to the body wall, and **visceral pain** refers to internal organs in the thorax, cranium, and abdomen. Superficial or cutaneous somatic pain involves a localized area of disturbance. Deep somatic pain is diffuse and originates in tendons, ligaments, bones, blood vessels, and nerves. Visceral pain is also poorly localized and originates in body organs.

Pain may originate from physical causes, that is, a physical cause for the pain can be identified. Pain may also have a psychogenic origin (**psychogenic pain**), that is, a physical cause for the pain cannot be identified. However, it has been observed that a *pure* origin is probably rare, and pain usually has both physical and psychogenic concomitants. Furthermore, pain that results from

a mental event can be just as intense as pain that results from a physical event.

When the threshold of perception for pain has been reached and when there is injured tissue, it is believed that the injured tissue releases chemicals that excite nerve endings. A damaged cell releases histamine, which excites nerve endings. Lactic acid accumulates in tissues injured by lack of blood supply and is believed to excite nerve endings and cause pain or to lower the threshold of nerve endings to other stimuli (*e.g.,* heat or pressure).

New research has shown that bradykinin, a powerful vasodilator that increases capillary permeability and constricts smooth muscle, plays an important role in the chemistry of pain at the site of injury even before the pain message gets to the brain.

- Bradykinin binds to receptors on the pain nerve, firing it and amplifying the pain impulse; it may also make the nerve more sensitive to gentle heat or light touch.
- Bradykinin triggers the release of histamine, which widens the junctions between cells in the capillary wall, causing more fluid and the infection-fighting white blood cells to leak out; this leads to swelling, redness, and tenderness.
- Nerve centers in the brain or spinal cord order the nerve ending to release substance P, which also boosts histamine production.
- Bradykinin binds to many nearby cells, setting in motion a chain reaction that produces prostaglandins, which bind to the nerve, making it fire and itensifying the pain. Prostaglandins also promote swelling.
- In summary, bradykinin initiates the pain impulse and prostaglandins initiate additional pain impulses. The area stays swollen, red, and tender until infection is suppressed and healing starts. (McKean, 1986, pp 86–89)

Receptors in the skin and superficial organs, although incapable of responding selectively, are stimulated by mechanical, thermal, chemical, and electrical agents. Friction from bed linens and pressure from a cast are mechanical stimulants. Sunburn and cold water on a tooth with caries are thermal stimulants. An acid burn is the result of a chemical stimulant. The jolt of a static charge is an electrical stimulant.

Stretching of the hollow viscera, pulling on the omentum, and muscle spasms result in pain. Some investigators believe that at least some of the deep-lying organs have their own individual pain receptors, the uterus being an example. Some organs, such as the lungs, are insensitive to pain.

It has been observed that pain may be present without injury and may not be present with injury. Therefore, tissue injury does not necessarily accompany pain in all instances. For example, tissue injury is present when the client experiences pain owing to a first- or second-degree burn. On the other hand, although physiologic changes do occur, tissue injury or destruction is not necessarily present when the client has a headache owing to psychologic tension. In addition, intensity of pain may not accurately relate to the seriousness of a particular condition giving rise to the pain. Thus, the client may not experience pain until the ravages of a malignancy are beyond control, whereas the severe pain that usually accompanies a bunion is not in keeping with the degree of pathology involved.

Pain Syndromes. While the causes of pain are many, certain major pathologic pain syndromes have been identified to describe the conditions most frequently associated with producing severe or prolonged pain. Common pain syndromes highlighted in Table 30-1 include peripheral pain syndromes (causalgia, postherpetic neuralgia, and phantom limb pain), central pain syndromes (thalamic syndrome, trigeminal neuralgia), and pain with underlying pathology syndromes (musculoskeletal pain syndromes, headache, cancer pain syndrome). Since appropriate treatment of these syndromes is often delayed because of misdiagnosis, nursing can play an important role in their early detection.

Transmission of Pain Stimuli

Pain sensations are conducted along pathways that have been rather clearly defined in certain areas but are still somewhat questionable in other areas. There are no specific pain organs or cells in the body. Rather, an interlacing network of undifferentiated free nerve endings receive painful stimuli. Free nerve ending pain receptors include (1) A delta-fibers, for fast-conducting, acute, well-localized pain, and (2) C fibers, for slow-conducting, diffuse, chronic pain. It is estimated that there are several million of these nerve endings in the body. They are numerous in the layers of the skin and in some internal tissues, such as the joint surfaces. In the deeper tissues of the body, the pain receptors are diffusely but unevenly spread.

Somatic sensation is carried to the dorsal gray horn cells of the spinal cord, then to the spinothalamic tract, and eventually to the cerebral cortex. Although the autonomic nervous system is an efferent system—that is, it carries impulses *from* the central nervous system—pain sensations from the viscera apparently course along the autonomic system. Through that system, these sensations from deep-lying structures reach the spinal cord by way of the dorsal roots and then continue along the same pathways as sensations from the skin and superficial body structures. Pain impulses are also carried by the cranial nerve to the central nervous system. There is integration of the sensory impulses of pain along its entire central nervous system route, but the highest level of integration occurs in the cortex.

Figure 30-1 illustrates the transmission of the pain sensation and the initiation of response.

Referred pain is pain in an area removed from that in which stimulation has its origins. The phenomenon has been well described, as follows:

(Text continues on p. 723.)

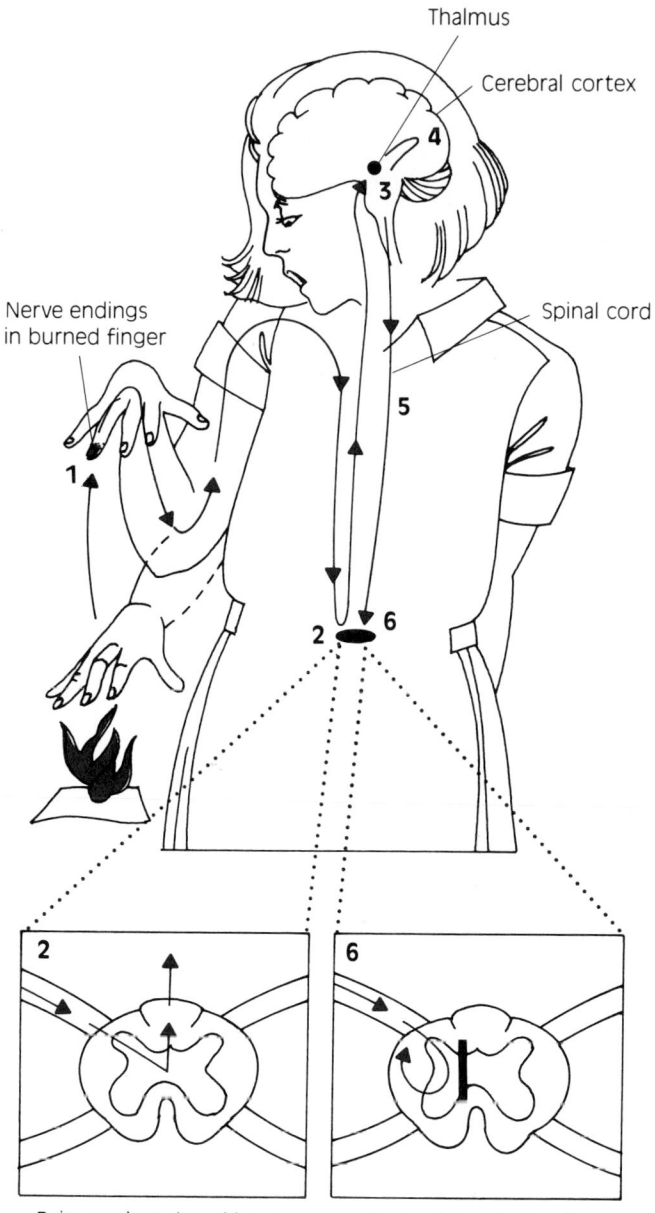

F I G U R E 30-1

Pain sensation and relief. (1) Pain's path begins as a message is received by nerve endings in a burned finger. Potent chemicals (substance P, bradykinin, prostaglandins) are released, sensitizing the nerve endings, helping to transmit the pain message from the injured finger toward the brain, and setting the stage for healing (inflammatory response). (2) The pain signal from the burnt finger travels as an electrochemical impulse along the length of the nerve to the dorsal horn on the spinal cord (a region that runs the length of the spine and receives signals from all over the body). (3) The message is relayed to the thalamus, a sensory center in the brain where sensations like heat, cold, pain, and touch first become conscious. (4) It then travels on to the cortex, where the intensity and location of pain are perceived. Little is known about factors that influence the individual's perception of pain at this point, the meaning attributed to the pain, and the voluntary responses elicited. (5) Pain relief begins as a signal from the brain descends via the spinal cord. (6) In the dorsal horn, chemicals like endorphin S are released to diminish the pain message from the injured finger. (Adapted from Unlocking pain's secrets. Time, pp 58–66, June 11, 1984)

T A B L E   30-1
Common Pain Syndromes

Pain Syndrome	Description
Peripheral Pain Syndromes	
Causalgia	Pain occurs in the area of a partially injured peripheral nerve (the most common lesions are of the brachial plexus or median or sciatic nerve). The pain is described as burning, severe, diffuse, and persistent and occurs most commonly on the palms of the hands, soles of the feet, and in the digits. Hyperalgesia (excessive sensitivity to pain) and hyperesthesia (excessive sensitivity to stimuli) are often so severe that any stimuli (*e.g.,* contact with clothing) can trigger the dreaded pain.
Postherpetic neuralgia	Pain syndrome that follows an acute central nervous system infection primarily of the dorsal root ganglia by the varicella-zoster (herpes) virus. The *herpes syndrome* is characterized by a vesicular eruption and neuralgic pain, which is usually unilateral and encircles the body in band-like clusters. The severity of the pain may be mild to severe and the quality may be burning, sharp, or dull. In the postherpetic syndrome, severe, intractable pain persists for months and years, with episodes of lightning-like pain in the area of the original eruption.
Phantom limb pain	May occur in any person who has had a body part amputated either surgically or traumatically. Pain varies and may be a severe, burning, firey sensation, crushing; cramping; a sense that the limb is edematous; or a sensation that the limb is being twisted and distorted. It may be triggered by many things including touching the stump, the occurrence of another illness, fatigue, atmospheric changes, and emotional stress.
Central Pain Syndromes	
Thalamic syndrome	Syndrome characterized by severe, spontaneous, and often continuous pain and hyperesthesia on the contralateral side of the lesion in the thalamus. This pain syndrome is often accompanied by a myriad of symptoms resulting from a disturbance in the major relay function of the thalamus.
Trigeminal neuralgia	Paroxysms of lightning-like stabs of intense pain in the distribution of one or more divisions of the trigeminal nerve, the fifth cranial nerve. Pain is usually experienced in the mouth, gums, lips, nose, cheek, chin, and surface of the head and may be triggered by everyday activities like talking, eating, shaving, or brushing one's teeth. Serious consequences of this syndrome are dehydration, wasting, and exhaustion because clients will refrain from anything that triggers the pain.
Pain With Underlying Pathology Syndromes	
Musculoskeletal pain syndromes	Many conditions are capable of causing severe pain in the musculoskeletal structures —the bones, joints, cartilage, synovial membranes, fibrous sheath, muscles, and tendons. Clients may present with pain that is acute or chronic and local or referred, and that varies in intensity.
Myofascial pain syndrome	Pain in the muscles and fascia; these syndromes are among the most frequent causes of severe disabling pain; characterized by the presence of trigger points in muscles or connective tissue together with a specific syndrome of pain: muscle spasm, tenderness, stiffness, limitation of motion, weakness, and occasionally autonomic dysfunction. Pain is described as dull and aching and its intensity varies from mild to severe and disabling.
Intervertebral disc syndrome	Pain syndrome caused by ruptured, herniated, or prolapsed intervertebral discs; most often occurs in the lower back or cervical area. Pain and limitation are the most frequent symptoms.
Arthritis	Chronic, systemic, often very painful disease of connective tissue; one of the major disabling chronic diseases in North America. Rheumatoid arthritis (joint and muscle involvement) is characterized by pain, inflammation, swelling, tenderness, and stiffness in the involved joints. In contrast, osteoarthritis occurs primarily in weight-bearing joints and is benign and slowly progressive.

(Continued)

Pain Syndrome	Description
Headache	The most common type of deep, somatic pain; experienced by about 90% of the population in some form or another. Headaches have multiple intracranial and extra-cranial causes. A careful analysis of the quality of the pain (dull, deep aching; sharp, throbbing; pressure, tightness); its location; its onset, duration, frequency, and time course; and prodromal signs and symptoms is important in accurately diagnosing the headache.
Cancer pain syndrome	Pain syndromes in cancer patients may develop due to the progression of the disease, as a result of the therapy directed at the control or cure of the disease, or unrelated to the disease.

All of these pain syndromes are capable of causing severe pain.

(Adapted from Meinhart NT, McCaffery M: Pain: A Nursing Approach to Assessment and Analysis, pp 213–237. Norwalk, CT, Appleton-Century-Crofts, 1983).

The afferent neurons that conduct such (pain) impulses from receptors in the viscera to the spinal cord come in contact with central neurons in the spinal cord whose axons form the lateral spinothalamic tracts. Some of these impulses, such as those from serous membranes, have a private pathway to the brain, somewhat like a private telephone line. Other impulses are not so fortunate; being on a party telephone line, they must share the central neurons with impulses from cutaneous areas. Thus, the axons of the central neurons do double duty by conducting impulses from visceral pain receptors and from cutaneous pain receptors to the same areas in the thalamus and the cerebral cortex. This arrangement is called convergence, and sometimes it can lead to confusion as you will see.

In the first case, in which there is a private wire to the cerebral cortex, the pain can be localized accurately as it is projected to the point of stimulation with ease. As an example of this, the patient with pleurisy can point to a certain spot where he experiences a sensation of pain on the chest, and the physician will hear a friction rub over this area, which means that the pleural membrane is inflamed in this particular spot.

In the second case, in which there is a party line, the sensation of pain is aroused in the brain as usual. However, it is projected to the cutaneous area from which impulses come to the same area in the brain. This happens since cutaneous pain is of more frequent occurrence than visceral pain, and the brain projects over the well-trod path (Chaffee, 1980, p 265).

Figure 30-2 illustrates cutaneous areas to which pain from various organs is usually referred.

Stimulation of sensory receptors and intactness of their nerve supply are neither necessary nor sufficient conditions for pain. It would seem that a receptor for pain and a nerve route that eventually carries the impulse to the brain are necessary when pain is present. Yet it is well-known that this is not always necessary. The pain that is often referred to an amputated leg where receptors and nerves are clearly absent is a very real experience for the client. This type of pain is called **phantom limb pain** and is without demonstrated physiologic or pathologic substance.

Gate Control Theory of Pain.   The **gate control theory** of pain is related to the transmission of painful stimuli. The theory states that certain nerve fibers, those of small diameter, conduct excitatory pain stimuli toward the brain, but nerve fibers of a large diameter appear to inhibit the transmission of pain impulses from the spinal cord to the brain. There is a gating mechanism that is believed by some to be located in substantia gelatinosa cells in the dorsal horn of the spinal cord. The exciting and inhibiting signals at the gate in the spinal cord determine the impulses that eventually reach the brain. Thus, only a limited amount of sensory information can be processed by the nervous system at any given moment. When too much information is sent through, certain cells in the spinal column interrupt the signal as if closing a gate. The brain also appears to influence the gating mechanism. Past experiences and learned behaviors, which are interpreted by the brain, have the effect of regulating or adjusting the eventual behavioral responses to pain. This helps explain why similar painful stimuli are interpreted differently by different people. While not everyone accepts the gate control theory, it has been widely discussed in nursing, and certain nursing measures to relieve pain (*e.g.*, massage, guided imagery) are believed to be effective because of the gating mechanism. Table 30-2 further describes the gate control theory of pain.

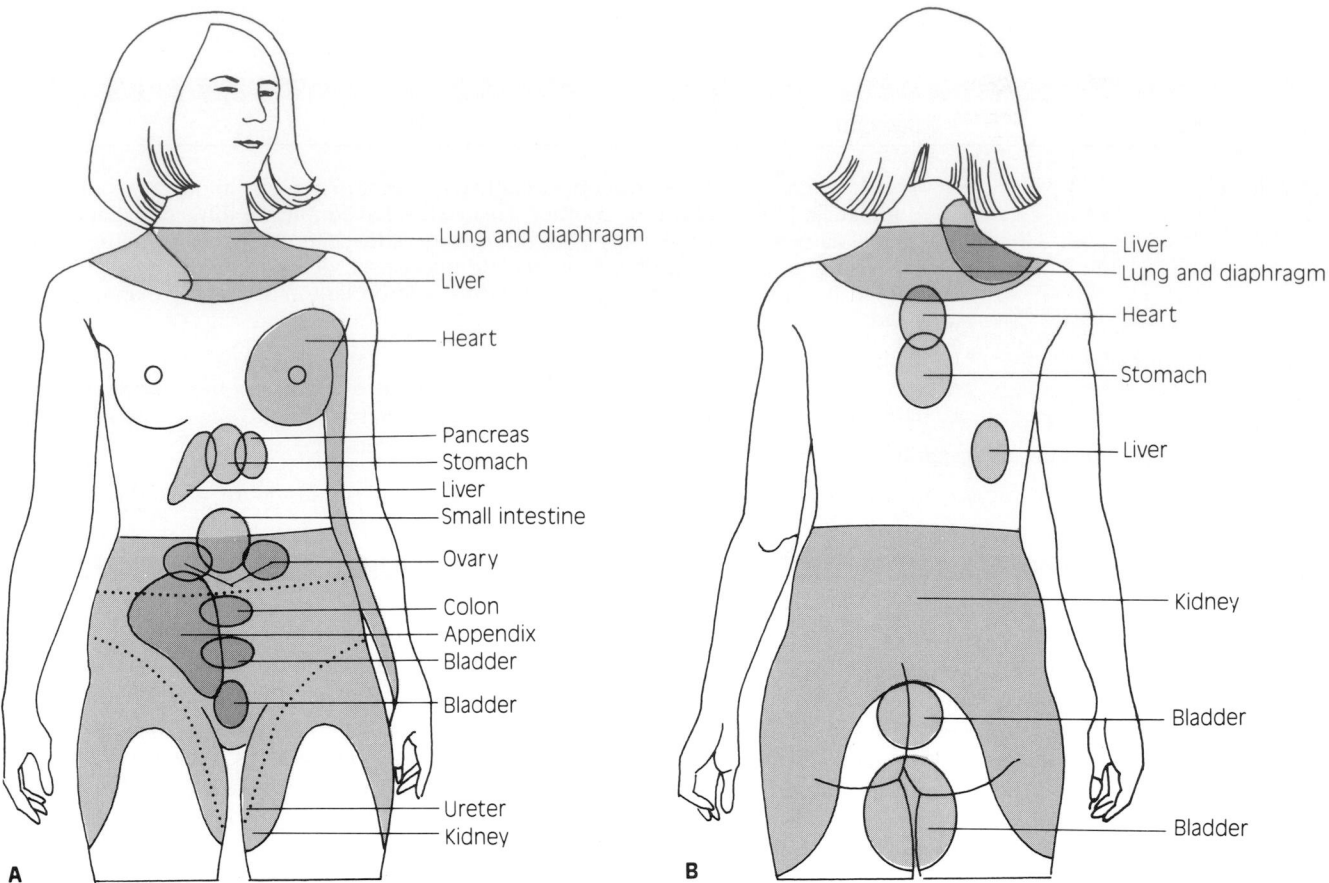

F I G U R E   30-2
These drawings representing the anterior (A) and posterior (B) views of the body illustrate areas to which various organs refer pain. (Redrawn from Chaffee EE, Lytle IM: Basic Physiology and Anatomy, 4th ed, pp 265–266. Philadelphia, JB Lippincott, 1980)

T A B L E   30-2
Nature of the Gate Control Theory of Pain
The transmission of potentially painful impulses to the level of conscious awareness may be affected by a gating mechanism, possibly located at the spinal cord level of the central nervous system.

Structures Involved	No Pain or Decreased Intensity of Pain	Pain
Spinal cord (?)	Results from closing the gate by	Results from opening the gate by
Nerve fibers	1. Activity in the *large-diameter nerve fibers* (*e.g.,* caused by skin stimulation)	1. Activity in the *small diameter nerve fibers* (*e.g.,* caused by tissue damage)
Brain stem	2. Inhibitory impulses from the *brain stem* (*e.g.,* caused by sufficient or maximum sensory input arriving through distraction or guided imagery)	2. Facilitory impulses from the *brain stem* (*e.g.,* caused by insufficient input from a monotonous environment)
Cerebral cortex and thalamus	3. Inhibitory impulses from the *cerebral cortex* and *thalamus* (*e.g.,* caused by anxiety reduction based on learning when the pain will end and how to relieve it).	3. Facilitory impulses from the *cerebral cortex* and thalamus (*e.g.,* caused by fear that the intensity of pain will escalate and will be associated with death)

(Adapted from McCaffery M: Nursing Management of the Patient With Pain, 2nd ed., p 26. Philadelphia, JB Lippincott, 1979)

Perception of Pain

The perception of pain involves the sensory process when a stimulus for pain is present. It includes the person's interpretation of the pain. The threshold of perception is the lowest intensity of a stimulus that causes the subject to recognize pain. This threshold is remarkably similar for everyone. Still, it is theorized by at least some authorities that a phenomenon of adaptation does occur; that is, the **pain threshold** can be changed within certain ranges. This phenomenon has been studied, for example, when prisoners of war reported that the pain of repeated torture was not as acute as it would have been under different circumstances. Many factors might well have played a role, but at least some adaptation appears likely.

Adaptation may also be present when a person's hand is immersed in warm water. A sensation of pain eventually occurs as the water is heated. However, the person can tolerate a higher temperature as water is gradually heated to the pain level than if the hand had been plunged into hot water without any preparation.

Endorphins. Although many questions remain, research has produced some evidence that the body produces substances called **endorphins**, which are morphine-like compounds. These powerful pain-blocking chemicals, which occur naturally in the brain and spinal cord, appear to alter the perception of pain. It is suggested that endorphins may be released when certain measures are used to relieve pain, such as skin stimulation and relaxation techniques, and when certain pain-relieving drugs are used. Many questions remain about endorphins. Current findings have revealed several types of natural opiates and nonopiates produced in the body that can alter the pain message. Some of these chemicals are called *neurotransmitters* and are also involved in emotional responses such as depression.

Pain is a highly personal experience. A person learns to know what causes unpleasantness and what to interpret as pain. Each person's interpretation is influenced by background, such as how he or she has experienced and dealt with pain in the past and what cultural factors have taught about pain. Through past experiences, each person also learns to differentiate among the various types of pain and to associate pain with certain descriptive words.

Duration, Severity, Quality, and Periodicity of Pain

Pain is a mixed sensation and occurs in varying degrees. It is also associated with other sensations, such as the sensations of stretching, pulling, pressure, squeezing, heat, or cold. Terms commonly used to describe the duration, severity, quality, and periodicity of pain are listed in Table 30-3. Usually, the more intense the stimulation, the more likely it will produce pain and the more

TABLE 30-3
Terms Used to Describe the Duration, Severity, Quality, and Periodicity of Pain

Duration

Acute	An episode that lasts for seconds to less than about 6 months
Chronic	An episode of pain that lasts for 6 months or longer. The pain may be intermittent or continuous.

Quality

Sharp	Pain that is sticking in nature and is intense
Dull	Pain that is not as intense or acute as sharp pain, possibly more annoying than painful. It is usually more diffuse than sharp pain.
Diffuse	Pain that covers a large area. Usually the client is unable to point to a specific area without moving the hand over a large surface, such as the entire abdomen.
Shifting	Pain that moves from one area to another, such as from the lower abdomen to the area over the stomach.

Other terms used to describe the quality of pain include *sore, stinging, pinching, cramping, gnawing, cutting, throbbing, shooting, vise-like pressure.*

Severity

Severe or **excruciating** **Moderate** **Slight** or **mild**	These terms depend on the client's interpretation of pain. Behavioral and physiologic signs help assess the severity of pain. On a scale of 1 to 10, slight pain could be described as being between about 1 and 3; moderate pain, between about 4 and 7; and severe pain, between about 8 and 10.

Periodicity

Continuous	Pain that does not stop
Intermittent	Pain that stops and starts again
Brief or **transient**	Pain that passes quickly

likely the pain will be severe. For example, there normally is pressure from a cast on the body part to which it has been applied but the sensation of the pressure is not painful. However, if there is abnormal swelling of the body part within the cast, the pressure may exceed the pain threshold and be perceived as pain. Pain perception will be sharply increased if tissue injury results from unrelieved cast pressure.

Responses to Pain

There are three types of responses to pain: physiologic, behavioral, and affective. These responses are summarized in Table 30-4.

The severity of pain and its duration affect responses to pain. **Mild pain** experienced briefly may produce little or no behavioral responses while intense pain experienced briefly usually brings forth reflex action to escape the cause. Pain that continues for a relatively short time, such as for a few days or a week, is very often accepted by the client without its being all-consuming. The client expects relief and believes the cause is self-limiting. However, anxiety is ordinarily present. On the other

T A B L E 30-4
Common Responses to Pain

Response	Comments
Behavioral (Voluntary) Responses	
Moving away from painful stimuli	The person moves self or a part of the body away from the source of pain. It is one of the body's protective mechanisms.
Grimacing, moaning, and crying	These responses are normal in many cultures when they are in keeping with the amount of pain the client experiences.
Restlessness	Restlessness keeps the person alert and probably also serves as a distraction from pain. Pacing the floor is an example.
Protecting the painful area and refusing to move	The person assumes a posture to protect the painful area, such as holding a painful hand or drawing the knees up when abdominal pain is present. The client may assume a posture and then refuse to move.
Physiologic (Involuntary) Responses	
Typical Sympathetic Responses When Pain Is Moderate and Superficial Increased blood pressure Increased pulse and respiratory rates Pupil dilation Muscle tension and rigidity Pallor (peripheral vasoconstriction) Increased adrenalin output Increased blood glucose	These signs are the body's responses to promote homeostasis. The body is preparing for emergency action, or the fight-or-flight phenomenon, as described in Chapter 9.
Typical Parasympathetic Responses When Pain Is Severe and Deep Nausea and vomiting Fainting/unconsciousness Decreased blood pressure Decreased pulse rate Prostration Rapid and irregular breathing	The body shows signs of being unable to cope with the stressor of pain.
Affective (Psychologic) Responses	
Exaggerated weeping and restlessness Withdrawal Stoicism Anxiety Depression Fear Anger Anorexia Fatigue Hopelessness Powerlessness	A person's previous experience with pain and sociocultural background play an important role in the emotional responses to pain. Emotional responses differ according to whether pain is acute or chronic. Anxiety is most often associated with acute pain and is very frequently present when pain is anticipated. Depression is most often associated with chronic pain. Emotional responses tend to intensify the reactions to pain, causing a vicious cycle that may be difficult to break. Emotional responses help explain why some persons experience pain that seems to be without physiologic cause or why some tend to complain of pain more than others when circumstances are similar. Pain is real as reported by the person, but for some, pain may help relieve feelings of guilt or serve as a way to gain attention and relieve loneliness.

hand, chronic pain tends to consume the entire person. It demands total attention so that the client has limited resources to take care of other matters in daily living. It is physically and emotionally exhausting and tends to result in depression and irritability. Chronic fatigue usually accompanies chronic pain.

Lack of an obvious response to pain does not mean the client is without pain. Careful assessment is especially important to understand what the client is experiencing.

Acute versus Chronic Pain

Pain is classified in many ways. Perhaps the most common distinction is between acute and chronic pain.

Acute pain is generally rapid in onset, varies in intensity from mild to severe, and may last from a very brief period up to any period less than 6 months. Acute pain is protective in nature, that is, it warns the individual of tissue damage or organic disease. Once its underlying cause is resolved, acute pain disappears. Causes of acute pain include a pricked finger, sore throat, or surgery.

Chronic pain is pain that may be limited, intermittent, or persistent, but that lasts for 6 months or longer. Pain associated with cancer or other progressive disorders is termed *chronic malignant pain* and pain in persons whose tissue injury is nonprogressive or healed is termed *chronic nonmalignant pain.*

Nearly one third of the North American population have persistent or recurrent chronic pain, according to Seattle anesthesiologist John Bonica, founder of the International Association for the Study of Pain. According to Bonica, chronic pain disables more people than cancer or heart disease and costs the public $70 billion a year in medical costs, lost working days, and compensation (*Time,* June 11, 1984, p 59). Unlike acute pain, chronic pain is often perceived as meaningless and may lead its host to withdrawal, depression, anger, frustration, and dependency.

Comparing clients with chronic cancer pain to those with noncancer chronic pain, Bonica (1980) noted these differences:

- The physiologic and psychologic impact of cancer pain on the person is greater than that of non-cancer chronic pain.
- Persons with cancer have greater physical deterioration due to loss of appetite, nausea, vomiting, and sleep disturbances.
- Persons with cancer develop greater emotional reactions of anxiety, depression, hypochondriasis, somatic focusing, and neuroticism than noncancer chronic pain sufferers.
- The effects of uncontrolled cancer pain (interpersonal problems, family stress, loss of employment, client feelings of dependency and uselessness) are more serious.

As any nurse who has experienced chronic pain or struggled through the experience with a loved one knows, chronic pain can be the most debilitating and destructive force in a person's life, one that totally drains energies and narrows perspective on living. Mary Schmitt (1977, pp 627, 629) a nurse who had lived with chronic pain for over 20 years, described her pain's positive dimensions:

> Pain is one of the greatest teachers we have, for it holds our attention as very few teachers can. The body does not want pain—it uses it only as a means to tell us that all is not well, that something needs attending to. . . . Nothing cares more or has more knowledge or more capacity to give direction, fulfillment, and happiness than one's own being. It speaks on many levels, in many symbolic languages, and at the oddest moments. . . . If the body is speaking to us in the language of pain, it is telling us extremely important truths. . . . The body will continue to do its utmost to heal itself. All that any of us can do, whether sufferer or helper, is to try to remove the impediments and give the body our love, which is all the energy it needs for assistance.

FACTORS AFFECTING THE PAIN EXPERIENCE

Many factors influence the comfort status of a person at any given moment. When an individual experiences pain, almost anything can influence how the painful stimulus is transmitted to the brain, how it is perceived, and the response that is made to it.

Culture

Since cultural norms dictate much of our daily behavior, attitudes, and values, it is natural to assume that culture will influence the individual's response to pain. It is important for nurses to understand that there are ways other than their own of responding to pain. A form of pain expression that is frowned upon in one culture may be desirable in another cultural group. The nurse studies cultural variations not to stereotype clients of different cultural backgrounds but to develop an understanding of cultural influences on

- Appropriate, acceptable, and effective behavioral responses to pain
- When, how, and by whom pain should be treated
- The meaning or significance of the pain (Meinhart and McCaffery, 1983)

Ethnic Variables. Much research has now been done on cultural influences on pain. The classic study on behavioral responses to pain present in groups of people of similar ethnic origin was done by Zborowski (1969). He studied males in four cultural groups: Old American (American-born, white, Protestant, and without identification with any foreign group), Jewish, Italian, and Irish. A summary of his findings follows.

Old American. A man of this background describes his pain efficiently to health-care practitioners, minimizes his pain when with family and friends, carefully controls his expression of pain, and tends to withdraw when his pain is severe—he wants to be alone. The Old American finds little value in pain and expects to have it relieved.

Jewish. A man of Jewish background tends to be more vocal about his pain and uses pain to elicit sympathy and support from others. Like the Old American he is future-oriented and concerned with the significance of his pain but he is less confident that modern medicine will cure the cause of the pain. He often seeks the advice of several physicians, including specialists.

Italian. He finds it natural to respond to pain with cries, moans, complaints, gestures, and body movements. Unlike the Old American and Jew, the Italian is present-oriented and is concerned with the sensation of pain itself rather than with its significance. The Italian wants quick pain relief and willingly accepts pain-relief measures.

Irishman. Like the Old American, the Irishman is calm and unemotional about pain, feeling that complaining serves no purpose; he wants to be alone with his pain. He takes pride in his ability to handle pain, generally using two strategies: relaxing and fighting. The Irishman may struggle with his pain for a long time before consulting a physician.

Other. The nurse working with other ethnic groups will find pertinent studies in the literature.

Family, Sex, and Age Variables.

Variables related to culture are family, sex, and age. Children growing up in different families may quickly learn to ignore pain, to exploit pain as a means to secure the attention and services of family members, or to value pain as a means the body uses to teach important truths. Similarly, children may learn that there are gender differences in pain expression; whereas it may be acceptable for a little girl to run home crying with a scraped knee, a little boy may be told that he should be brave and not cry. Adult men and women may hold onto gender expectations regarding pain communication and incorrectly interpret the presence or absence of pain expressions in others. Finally, there are different beliefs and norms for different age groups regarding pain sensation and response. At one time the infant's inability to communicate pain led health-care practitioners to the erroneous assumption that pain sensation was diminished or absent. It is now generally believed that infants and small children are sensitive to pain.

Among the elderly, pain has often been viewed as a natural component of the aging process and is often ignored when present as an indicator of a treatable condition. On the other hand, conditions normally painful in young adults (*e.g.* myocardial infarction) may present minimal pain complaints in the elderly. These variables, which influence pain sensation, perception, and response, make pain assessment a complex task for the nurse.

Religion

Religious beliefs may powerfully influence the individual's experience of pain. In some religions individuals view pain and suffering not as good in themselves, but as means of purification or as a means of "making up" for individual and community sin. This meaning helps the individual to cope with pain and becomes a source of strength. Clients with this belief may refuse analgesics and other pain-relief measures, feeling that this lessens their offering. On the other hand, illness and pain may also be viewed as punishment from a vengeful God. Individuals may find their faith shaken and question the existence of a loving God. How can belief in a loving God be compatible with their present experience of pain? Anger, resentment, and depression may then compound the pain experience. Clients may find it helpful to confer with a spiritual advisor about their pain experience.

Meaning of Pain/Coping Strategy

The meaning an individual attaches to illness, pain, and suffering significantly influences the coping strategies employed. Lipowski (1970) and Archer Copp (1974) worked with the following categories of meaning: challenge, enemy, punishment, weakness, relief, strategy, loss, or value. Often the degree to which an individual feels control over pain determines both the type of coping strategy effected and its success. Specific coping strategies may be chosen to consciously minimize pain or to focus it vigilantly. It is important for the nurse to assess the adequacy of each client's pain meaning and coping strategies since what works for one person may prove detrimental to another. Misconceptions about pains (*e.g.,* equating pain with death when the pain's underlying cause is highly treatable), need to be corrected as these can powerfully influence an individual's unhealthy response to pain. Table 30-5 illustrates a coping model that identifies five common views of pain and related views of persons with pain and their situation (Copp, 1985).

Environment/Support Persons

An individual's environment and the presence or absence of caring support persons may also influence the

T A B L E   30-5
Coping Model

Pain/Self-Image	Language	Self-Situation	Coping
Type One			
Pain: powerful	Merciless	Fragile	Skepticism
Coper: passive victim	Cosmic	Helpless	Fate
	Overwhelming	Dread-filled	Ritual
	Continuous	Abandoned	Magic
	Irrevocable	Alone	
	Irreparable	Suffering	
	Irrational		
Type Two			
Pain: invading	Episodic	Fighter	Counterpain
Coper: combatant	Strong	Coper	Muscle language
	Sharp	Survivor	Delegates
	Dominating	Soldier	Assigns tasks
	Testing	Confronter	Armamentarium
Type Three			
Pain: reality	Testing	Confronter	Meditating
Coper: responsive	Demanding	Endurer	Focusing
	Mysterious	Suffering	Searching for
	Hidden	Analyzing	meaning
	Cosmic	Strategizing	
Type Four			
Pain: cunning	Hidden	Watcher	Anticipating
Coper: reactive	Faceless	Waiter	Rehearsal
	Sneaky	Monitor	Review
	Sly	Vigilant	Early warning
	Invading	Ready	Not risking
	Degrading		Avoidance
Type Five			
Pain: demanding	Intense	Cooperator	Contractual
Coper: interactive	Persistent	Collaborator	Arrangement
	Sharp	Communicator	Permission
	Probing	Contractor	Compliant
	Treacherous	Dependent	Bonding
	Ill-tempered	Reporter	Rule keeper
	Strong	Consumer	Sets limits

(Copp LA: Pain coping. In Copp L (ed): Perspectives of Pain. Recent Advances in Nursing Series. Edinburgh, Churchill-Livingstone, 1985)

experience of pain. Many people find that the strangeness of the hospital environment, and especially the lights, noise, and constant activity of a critical care unit, compound the experience of pain. The sense of powerlessness that accompanies admission to an institution may decrease the individual's ability to cope with pain. Depersonalization, separation from a favorite pillow, pet, or source of music, may further decrease the person's sense of comfort. For some, the presence of a loved family member or friend is essential to their sense of well-being. Others prefer to be alone when in pain and may become agitated in the presence of a family member.

Some clients may "use their pain" to acquire secondary gains, such as special attention and services from their families. Since this tendency, if unchecked, usually leads to resentment and anger in family members and their eventual avoidance of the client, the nurse should intervene and attempt an honest discussion of this problem when noting its occurrence.

Anxiety/Other Stressors

Anxiety, which is almost always present when pain is anticipated or being experienced, tends to increase the perceived intensity of pain. The threat of the unknown is ordinarily more devastating and anxiety producing than a threat for which one has been prepared. Studies have indicated that clients who were taught preoperatively about what to expect postoperatively did not require as much medication for pain as those who had similar operative procedures but were not taught preoperatively.

Pain is ordinarily aggravated when anxiety, muscular tension, and fatigue are present. A vicious cycle can easily develop when pain interferes with rest and relaxation, and tension and fatigue will almost always aggravate the discomfort. The rested and relaxed person can often cope with great discomfort.

The individual who is greatly fatigued and who has no competing demands requiring attention may experience pain acutely. For example, many persons have discovered that the pain of a footache or ingrown toenail that was only mildly annoying during the day's work became unbearable at night when there was nothing else to distract the mind from the pain. Similarly, athletes can be so determined to win a game that they are oblivious to the pain of a serious sports injury. Following the game and particularly if the game was lost and the effort seemingly useless, the pain becomes overpowering.

Past Pain Experience

Whether or not an individual has experienced pain in the past and the qualities of that experience profoundly affect new pain experiences.

- Some clients have never known severe pain and have no fear of pain, not realizing how intense the sensation can be.
- Some clients have experienced severe acute or chronic pain in the past but received immediate and adequate pain relief. These clients are generally unafraid of pain and initiate appropriate requests for assistance.
- Some clients have known severe pain in the past and were unable to secure relief. Even the suggestion of new pain can throw these clients into a frenzy of fear and feelings of despair and hopelessness.
- The individual whose past pain experience led to correction of unhealthy behavior and produced a greater sense of health and well-being may respect and value pain and study the meaning and significance of a new pain carefully.
- In general, persons who have experienced more pain than usual in their lifetimes tend to anticipate more pain and to exhibit increased sensitivity to pain.
- Some pain memories are virtually unerasable and new contact with conditions similar to those that caused the earlier pain can provoke a violent response.

NURSE AS ROLE MODEL

The nurse who wishes to role model healthy pain management behaviors to clients

- Balances work and leisure activities to promote optimal personal well-being (consistently communicates to self "I care about you!")
- Respects pain as the body's means of signaling that all is not well
- Treats what is producing pain as opposed to simply trying to eradicate pain
- Utilizes an effective coping model (pain view and view of self) when responding to personal pain
- Routinely incorporates comfort measures into nursing care
- Practices nursing sensitive to the pain needs of clients and is committed to pain relief
    - Communicates to clients the belief that their pain experience is real and that help is available
    - Assigns high nursing priority to assisting clients (and family members) to develop effective pain management strategies compatible with their belief systems
    - Designs varied pain management programs that incorporate noninvasive and invasive interventions; works collaboratively with other health professionals
    - Supports pain management programs with attention to the client's overall nutrition, hydration, elimination, rest, activity, and stimulation
- Continuously updates knowledge of pain theories, assessment strategies, and treatment modalities

ASSESSING THE PAIN EXPERIENCE

Because the pain experience is unique to each individual, the nurse who wants to understand a client's pain so as to help the client achieve pain control needs sophisticated pain assessment skills. It is recommended that nurses assume that all clients are experiencing some type of discomfort or pain (Jacox and Stewart, 1973, p 152) and take the initiative in pain assessment.

Misconceptions. Many client misconceptions interfere with the client's ability to communicate pain. Among these are the following:

- The nurse will know when I am in pain and do something to relieve it if this is possible.

- The doctor has ordered pain-relieving medication for me, which I will be given routinely.
- If I ask for something for my pain I may become addicted to the medication.
- I should somehow be able to control my pain. It is immature to talk about pain.
- It is better to wait until the pain gets "real bad" before asking for help.

Misconceptions and prejudices about pain and pain relief that hamper the *nurse's* assessment of the client with pain have been summarized by McCaffery (1979) and are presented in Table 30-6. In a later work, Meinhart and McCaffery (1983) added to this list the misconceptions that infants and young children do not perceive as much pain as adults and that when they do perceive pain it is not remembered. On the contrary, research has shown that the younger the child, the lower the pain-perception threshold and that the memory of pain may occur as early as 6 months of age.

Components of Pain Assessment

Various forms used to help guide the assessment of pain have been described in nursing literature. The primary purposes of using a guide to assess pain are to eliminate guesswork and biases when dealing with the client's pain, to understand what the person is experiencing, and to analyze findings that will help prepare an appropriate nursing care plan for the client. For the most part, these guides contain common elements. Donovan and Girton (1984) include the following as aspects of a comprehensive pain assessment:

- Determination of whether or not pain exists
- Descriptive characteristics of the pain
- Physiologic responses, which may or may not be present, depending on the chronicity of the pain
- Behavioral responses, if any are present
- Affective responses
- How the pain is affected by interaction with others
- The degree to which the pain is interfering with the client's life
- How the client perceives the pain and what meaning, if any, it has for the client
- Adaptive mechanisms used to cope with the pain

Characteristics of pain generally assessed include the pain's location, duration, quantity, quality, chronology, aggravating factors, and phenomena associated with pain. A guide for assessing pain that suggests questions

T A B L E   30-6
Misconceptions that Hamper Assessment of the Patient With Pain

Misconception	Correction
1. Health team members are the authorities on the existence and nature of the client's pain.	The client is the authority on the pain. Pain is whatever the experiencing person says it is, existing whenever that person says it does. The client is believed.
2. The client who uses pain to obtain benefits or preferential treatment does not hurt as much as he or she says and may not hurt at all.	The client who uses pain to personal advantage may nevertheless be experiencing the pain.
3. The client's pain can always be verified by the presence of certain behavioral and/or physiologic expressions of pain.	Physiologic and behavioral adaptations occur, leading to periods of little or no signs of pain. Lack of pain expression does not mean lack of pain.
4. All "real" pain has an identifiable physical cause.	Not all physical causes of pain can be identified. All pain is real, regardless of its cause. Calling pain imaginary does not make it go away.
5. Psychogenic pain does not really hurt and is almost the same as malingering.	A localized sensation does exist in psychogenic pain.
6. The severity and duration of pain can be predicted accurately on the basis of the stimuli for pain.	There is no direct and invariant relationship between any stimulus and the perception of pain.
7. All clients can and should be encouraged to have a high tolerance for pain.	Pain tolerance is the individual's unique response, varying among clients and in the same client from one situation to another.
8. Health team members tend to make accurate inferences about the severity and existence of the client's pain.	Health team members tend to infer less pain than the client experiences.

(McCaffery M: Nursing Management of the Patient With Pain, 2nd ed, p 21. Philadelphia. JB Lippincott, 1979)

McGill - Melzack Pain Questionnaire

Patient's Name _____ Date _____ Time _____ am/pm
Analgesic(s) _____ Dosage _____ Time Given _____ am/pm
_____ Dosage _____ Time Given _____ am/pm

Analgesic Time Difference (hours):   +4   +1   +2   +3

PRI: S _____ A _____ E _____ M(S) _____ M(AE) _____ M(T) _____ PRT(T) _____
      (1-10)   (11-15)   (16)   (17-19)   (20)   (17-20)   (1-20)

PPI _____   COMMENTS:

1 FLICKERING	11 TIRING
QUIVERING	EXHAUSTING
PULSING	12 SICKENING
THROBBING	SUFFOCATING
BEATING	13 FEARFUL
POUNDING	FRIGHTFUL
2 JUMPING	TERRIFYING
FLASHING	14 PUNISHING
SHOOTING	GRUELLING
3 PRICKING	CRUEL
BORING	VICIOUS
DRILLING	KILLING
STABBING	15 WRETCHED
LANCINATING	BLINDING
4 SHARP	16 ANNOYING
CUTTING	TROUBLESOME
LACERATING	MISERABLE
5 PINCHING	INTENSE
PRESSING	UNBEARABLE
GNAWING	17 SPREADING
CRAMPING	RADIATING
CRUSHING	PENETRATING
6 TUGGING	PIERCING
PULLING	18 TIGHT
WRENCHING	NUMB
7 HOT	DRAWING
BURNING	SQUEEZING
SCALDING	TEARING
SEARING	19 COOL
8 TINGLING	COLD
ITCHY	FREEZING
SMARTING	20 NAGGING
STINGING	NAUSEATING
9 DULL	AGONIZING
SORE	DREADFUL
HURTING	TORTURING
ACHING	PPI
HEAVY	0 No pain
10 TENDER	1 MILD
TAUT	2 DISCOMFORTING
RASPING	3 DISTRESSING
SPLITTING	4 HORRIBLE
	5 EXCRUCIATING

CONSTANT
PERIODIC
BRIEF

ACCOMPANYING SYMPTOMS:
NAUSEA
HEADACHE
DIZZINESS
DROWSINESS
CONSTIPATION
DIARRHEA
COMMENTS:

SLEEP:
GOOD
FITFUL
CAN'T SLEEP
COMMENTS:

FOOD INTAKE:
GOOD
SOME
LITTLE
NONE
COMMENTS:

ACTIVITY:
GOOD
SOME
LITTLE
NONE

COMMENTS:

Key:
PPI = present pain intensity
PRI = pain rating index
  S = sensory components of pain
  A = affective, or emotional, components of pain
  E = evaluative terms
  M = miscellaneous terms

Combinations of words can be identified: M(S) and M(AE) and the entire number totaled: PRI(T). (Copyright 1970. Ronald Melzack)

or approaches helpful in assessing the various pain factors is illustrated in Assessment of the Pain Experience.

Some pain centers ask clients to complete a self-questionnaire. The McGill-Melzack Pain Questionnaire (above) is an example of such a questionnaire. Using this questionnaire, an individual checks words that fit the description of the pain experience. Marks can be made on the figure to show pain location. Comparison of changes on subsequent questionnaires aids in determining an individual's improvement or regression. When a client presents with severe pain, the pain requires quick assessment and relief. The comprehensive pain assessment should be performed when the client is more comfortable and better able to respond to questions. There is a McGill Comprehensive Pain Questionnaire that can be used in such instances.

Assessment in the Cognitively Impaired.

Assessment of pain in children and in persons who are cognitively impaired presents special challenges to nurses. It is now generally recognized that children and cognitively impaired adults are frequently undertreated. Needed are special efforts to identify accurate means of assessing pain in individuals in early or altered stages of cognitive development who are unable to express concepts such as pain magnitude. While these tools are being devel-

Assessment of the Pain Experience

Factors to Assess	Questions/Approaches
Characteristics of the pain	
Location	Where is your pain? Is it external or internal? (Asking the client with acute pain to point to the painful area with one finger may help to localize the pain. Clients with chronic pain may have difficulty trying to localize their pain, however.)
Duration	How long have you been experiencing pain? How long does a pain episode last? How often does a pain episode occur?
Quantity	Ask the client to indicate the degree (amount) of pain currently experienced on the scale below:

0	1	2	3	4	5	6	7	8	9	10
No pain		Mild		Moderate			Severe			Pain as bad as it can be

It is also helpful to ask how much pain the client has (on the same scale) when the pain is at its least and at its worst:
Least ____ Worst ____

Factors to Assess	Questions/Approaches
Quality	What words would you use to describe your pain? (Useful in research, this characteristic is least useful in day-to-day clinical practice).
Chronology	How does the pain develop and progress? (If pattern can be identified, interventions early in a pain sequence will often be far more effective than those employed after the pain is well-established.) Has the pain changed since it first began? If so, how?
Aggravating factors	What makes the pain occur or increase in intensity?
Alleviating factors	What makes the pain go away or lessen? What methods of relief have you tried in the past? How long were they used? How effective were they? (Methods of relief currently in effect for hospitalized clients should be apparent from the chart. It is important to verify the use of current orders and their effectiveness with the client. Outpatients may need to be asked to record a medication profile, a thorough and accurate account of all medications they are taking.)
Associated phenomena	Are there any other factors that seem to relate consistently to your pain? Any other symptoms that occur just before, during, or after your pain?
Physiologic responses	
Vital signs (blood pressure [BP], pulse [P], respirations)	Signs of sympathetic stimulation commonly occur with acute pain. Signs of parasympathetic stimula-

(Continued)

Assessment of the Pain Experience (Continued)

Factors to Assess	*Questions/Approaches*
Skin color Perspiration Pupil size Nausea	tion ($\downarrow$ BP, $\downarrow$% P, pupil constriction, nausea and vomiting, and warm, dry skin) may be present, especially in prolonged, severe pain, visceral, or deep pain.
Muscle tension	Observe. Ask the client if he is aware of any tight, tense muscles.
Anxiety	Are signs of anxiety evident? (May include decreased attention span or ability to follow directions, frequent asking of questions, shifting of topics of conversation, avoidance of discussion of feelings, acting out, somatizing.)
Behavioral responses Posture, gross motor activities	Does client rub or support a particular area? Make frequent position changes? Walk, pace, kneel, or assume a rolled-up position? Does client rest a particular body part? Protect an area from stimulation? Lie quietly? (In acute pain, postural and gross motor activities are often altered; in chronic pain, the only signs of change may be postures characteristic of withdrawal.)
Facial features	Does the client have a pinched look? Are there facial grimaces? Knotted brow? Overall taut, anxious appearance? (A look of fatigue is more characteristic of chronic pain.)
Verbal expressions	Does the client sigh, moan, scream, cry, repetitively use the same words?
Affective responses Anxiety	Do you feel anxious? Are you afraid? If so, how bad are these feelings?
Depression	Do you feel depressed, "down," or low? If so, how bad are these feelings? Are your feelings about yourself mostly good or bad? Do you have feelings of failure? Do you see yourself or your illness as a burden to those you care about?
Interactions with others	How does the client act when he is in pain in the presence of others? How does the client respond to others when he is not in pain? How do significant others and caregivers respond to the client when he is in pain? When he is not in pain?
Degree to which pain interferes with client's life (use past performance as baseline)	Does the pain interfere with sleep? If so, to what extent? Is fatigue a major factor in the pain experience? Is the conduct of intimate or peer relationships affected by the pain? Is work function affected? Participation in recreational–diversional activities? (An activity diary is often very helpful, sometimes crucial. One to several weeks of hourly

(Continued)

Assessment of the Pain Experience (Continued)

Factors to Assess	Questions/Approaches
	activity recorded by the client may be necessary. Levels of pain, intake of food, and sleep–rest periods are noted along with activities performed. Separate diaries for inpatient and outpatient episodes may be necessary, as hospitalization markedly affects the nature and type of activities performed.)
Perception of pain and meaning to client	Are you worried about your illness? Do you see any connection between your pain and the nature or course of illness? If so, how do you see them as related? Do you find any meaning in your pain? If so, is this beneficial or detrimental to you? Are you struggling to find some meaning for your pain?
Adaptive mechanisms used to cope with pain	What do you usually do to relieve stress? How well do these things work? What techniques do you use at home to help cope with the pain? How well have they worked? Do you use these in the hospital? If not, why not?
Goals	What would you like to be doing right now, this week, this month, if the pain was better controlled? How much would the pain have to decrease (on the 0–10 scale) for you to begin to accomplish these goals?

(Adapted with permission from Donovan MI, Girton SE: Cancer Care Nursing, 2nd ed. Norwalk, CT, Appleton-Century-Crofts, 1984)

oped, nurses must rely on careful assessments and their empathic qualities as a guide to pain management.

DIAGNOSING

Pain is such a complex phenomenon that its analysis often requires the collaboration of different members of the health team. While nursing has much to offer individuals experiencing both acute and chronic pain, the data collected by the nurse during the comprehensive pain assessment will most benefit the client when shared with physicians and other members of the health-care team.

Initially, pain must be viewed as a symptom and its physical etiology pursued. Interventions for pain done prior to an accurate assessment may mask the true cause of the patient's pain, thus causing further suffering and possibly even death by allowing the progression of signs, symptoms, and the disease process. A thorough assessment provides the opportunity of ascribing the accurate meaning to a given set of behaviors and variables such as a pain pattern.

Only after all physiological causes which are treatable by traditional medical and surgical techniques are ruled out does one treat pain as a disease entity. Even when pain becomes a treatable disease, vigilance must be maintained for *any changes and new symptoms*. Additional information may provide a more accurate diagnosis, therefore, possibly, a different treatment plan will be devised (Meinhart and McCaffery, 1983, pp 27–28).

The nurse who notes a pattern of headaches in a client and relates this to the client's description of recent stress (divorce, relocation, new job) may erroneously assume that the headaches are merely stress related and devise and implement a plan of relaxation exercises. A more careful analysis of client data, however, may reveal that the headaches are of vascular origin, migraine in nature, and medical intervention is indicated. The headaches may also be symptomatic of intracranial disease such as a brain tumor and delay in diagnosis may decrease the possibility of treatment and cure.

When a nursing diagnosis of acute or chronic pain is developed the diagnostic statement and plan of care should identify
- Type of pain
- Etiologic factors, to the extent that they are known and understood
- The client's behavioral, physiologic, and affective responses

• Other factors affecting pain stimulus, transmission, perception, and response

Examples of nursing diagnoses developed to describe common pain problems are given below. Many diagnoses could be developed for pain problems. The importance of the nurse identifying these problems and including them as priorities in the plan of care cannot be overstated. In general, it is not recommended that the medical diagnosis be used as the etiology of the problem statement in the nursing diagnosis. However, when stating nursing problems of comfort alteration it may at times be difficult to avoid this without sacrificing the specificity desired. Remember that the purpose of the etiology is to direct the nursing interventions.

Altered comfort: acute postoperative pain related to fear of taking prescribed analgesics

Altered comfort: left leg pain related to fractured femur and multiple lacerations and unsuccessful attempts to determine effective analgesic

Altered comfort related to prolonged labor (dystocia) and commitment to natural childbirth

Altered comfort: heightened pain anticipation related to child's history of undergoing frequent painful procedures

Altered comfort: chest pain related to decreased blood supply to myocardium (angina)

Altered comfort: chronic headaches related to inadequate pain management secondary to belief that client somehow "deserves this pain"

Altered comfort: chronic malignant pain related to inadequate pain management of metastic cancer involving bone

Altered comfort: chronic pain related to rheumatoid arthritis

Table 30-7 offers sample defining characteristics for these problems.

Since the experience of pain affects so many other aspects of human functioning, pain may be the etiology of numerous other nursing diagnosis statements. Examples of these follow:

Ineffective airway clearance related to postoperative incisional pain

Severe anxiety related to pain anticipation and inadequate pain management in the past

Altered bowel elimination: constipation related to chronic use of narcotic analgesics

Ineffective family coping related to father's inability to allow family to share his pain experience

Ineffective individual coping related to failure of chronic pain management strategies to date

Altered health maintenance related to loss of will to live secondary to prolonged chronic pain

Hopelessness related to belief that present pain means imminent death

Potential for injury related to decreased pain sensation

Knowledge deficit: angina pain management related to belief that nothing will help the pain

Impaired physical mobility related to arthritic pain

Altered nutrition. less than body requirements related to gastrointestinal distress

Self-care deficit related to painful movement of joints

Altered sexuality patterns related to painful intercourse

Sleep pattern disturbance: inability to fall asleep related to pain's worsening at night

Spiritual distress related to belief that God is unfairly causing this pain as some sort of undeserved punishment

Altered thought processes related to effects of chronic pain and overmedication

Potential for self-directed violence related to loss of will to live with unrelieved chronic pain

PLANNING: CLIENT GOALS

Once the diagnosis of a pain problem is made, it is critical for nurses to develop a plan of care that, when implemented, demonstrates nursing's commitment to assist the client to develop effective pain management strategies. Table 30-8 illustrates possible outcomes of two very different nursing responses to a client with low back pain.

Nursing measures are directed toward the achievement of the following client goals for the client whose pain is acute in nature (*i.e.*, it is expected that with healing the pain will subside and eventually disappear):

Long-Term Goals
• Client will verbalize that pain is eliminated (if client is nonverbal, the absence of the signs that indicated the presence of pain is sought).

Short-Term Goals
• Client will describe a gradual reduction of pain using a scale of 0 (no pain) to 10 (pain as bad as it can be).
• Client will demonstrate competent execution of successful pain management program (specify).

For the client whose pain is chronic in nature, the long-term goals differ somewhat:

Long-Term Goals
• Client will verbalize (demonstrate) the ability to control pain to the point of being able to manage/enjoy key elements of everyday living.
• Family/significant others will relate feeling better able to share and to cope with the pain experience of the client.

An important short-term goal for the client with chronic pain may be contacting a hospice or a pain clinic.

T A B L E   30-7
Nursing Diagnoses for Common Pain Problems

Diagnosis	Etiologic or Contributing Factors	Sample Defining Characteristics
Altered comfort: acute postoperative pain	Fear of taking prescribed analgesics	Recent cholecystectomy Face is pale and drawn: vital signs elevated from baseline States "I don't like to ask for anything for pain because I know people often get addicted."
Altered comfort: left leg pain	Fractured femur and multiple lacerations; unsuccessful attempts to determine effective analgesic	Recent motor vehicle accident Grimaces whenever left leg is moved Directs abusive language to anyone who touches left leg Refused to have dressing changed on left leg Reports analgesic "only takes the edge off" the pain
Altered comfort	Prolonged labor (dystocia) and commitment to natural childbirth	Admitted to labor unit 18 hours ago with moderate contractions 2 minutes apart Strength of contractions weakening; progress of dilatation and effacement slow; failure to progress "I'll feel like a failure if I take anything for pain. I want to 'go natural.' I know I can do it. Besides, the drugs would only hurt my baby."
Altered comfort: heightened pain anticipation	Child's history of undergoing frequent painful procedures	Child diagnosed at age 3 with acute nonlymphoid leukemia History of bone marrow aspirations, spinal taps, platelet transfusions, chemotherapy, and other such procedures Child "freezes" when unfamiliar health-care worker enters room
Altered comfort: chest pain	Decreased blood supply to myocardium (angina) and fear	"I never know when it will grab me next. I get this crushing pain in my chest and can't do anything. Usually one or two of those nitro tablets bring me relief. I'm always scared, though, that the pain won't go away."
Altered comfort: chronic headaches	Inadequate pain management secondary to belief that somehow client "deserves this pain"	Reports history of migraine headaches for last 5 years Never sought treatment "My mother told me that we all get the pain in life that we deserve—and goodness, I've been no saint." "I can't help feeling, though, that no one is meant to live like this."
Altered comfort: chronic pain	Inadequate pain management of metastatic cancer involving bone	Diagnosed with cancer of bladder 2 years ago; presently metastic spread to spine Rates pain 10 on a scale of 1 (minimal) to 10 (greatest) "I haven't been taking as much of this pain medicine as the doctor said I could because if I get used to it now nothing will work when the pain gets even worse later." "When I told the nurse in the hospital about my pain she said I'd have to get used to it." "I don't want to burden my wife and kids with my pain."
Altered comfort: chronic pain	Rheumatoid arthritis and inappropriate activity during exacerbations	Stiffness of joints, limitation of motion, heat, swelling, and tenderness States pain is often intense after activity "I can't accept not being able to do all I want to do for my husband and children."

T A B L E   30-8
Different Outcomes for A Client With Low Back Pain

Client

A 32-year-old married man, father of two, presents to the hospital with complaints of dull and aching low back pain, weakness, and stiffness. Pelvic traction, heat treatments, and anti-inflammatory medication are ordered.

Situation A	Situation B

Nursing Priorities During Client's Hospitalizations

Situation A	Situation B
• Administer medications. • Set up pelvic traction and instruct client in its use. • Inquire how heat treatments "are going." No detailed pain assessment performed	• Nursing and medicine collaborate in detailed pain assessment. • Once a diagnosis of degenerative disc disease is made the nurses teach the client about the disease and related self-care measures (these include alternate methods of pain control, including use of heat, activity, massage, and progressive relaxation). • Intensive inhospital care includes use of pelvic traction, administration of medications, and heat treatments.

Typical Nursing Comments

Situation A	Situation B
"Did you injure your back to get a couple of days off? I've often thought of doing that myself." (Some nurses are upset about shortstaffing and angry with two nurses claiming work-related back injuries.)	"Gee, it must be awfully hard for someone as healthy as you've been to suddenly find yourself in bed with all this pain. How's it going?" "How do you think your back problem will affect you once you get home?"

Client's Discharge/Evaluation of Care

Situation A	Situation B
• Client withdrawn during hospitalization; discharged after 5 days of treatment reporting relief of symptoms • Tells family: "No one in there believed I had pain—or if they did, they sure didn't care. I wish someone would have wanted to help me. I won't go that route again!"	While hospitalized, client experiences an increased sense of self-respect and worth as well as hope that relief from his pain will be found. Many years later when the disc herniates he returns to the hospital confident in the health-care team's ability and willingness to help him.

Aftermath of Hospitalization

Situation A	Situation B
• Client tries to ignore pain when it recurs. • Irreversible musculoskeletal damage occurs from prolonged muscle spasm. • Weakness, endocrine imbalance (loss of weight), and sleep disturbance • Irritability, depression, feelings of worthlessness, powerlessness, personality changes, decreased motivation, suicidal ideation • Inability to meet role expectations: spouse, father, friend, employee→divorce, unemployment, destruction of the quality of his life and that of his family	Early treatment and life-long care of back complemented by general health behaviors (*e.g.,* good nutrition, regular exercise, stress management), prevent the development of symptoms related to the gradual build-up of paravertebral spasms. Health status and quality of life are actually improved following client's hospitalization.

IMPLEMENTING

Once the plan of care is developed the nurse implements the nursing strategies that are most likely to assist the client to achieve pain-relief goals. Nursing interventions described in this chapter include establishing a trusting nurse–client relationship, teaching the client about pain, manipulating factors that affect the pain experience, initiating the appropriate noninvasive pain-relief measures (distraction, relaxation, cutaneous stimulation), and assisting with the pain therapies of other disciplines.

Establishing a Trusting Nurse–Client Relationship

Most clients with pain feel better, suffer less, and experience less anxiety when they believe that a competent nurse cares about their experience of pain and is available for help and support. Without the confidence developed in a good nurse–client relationship, nothing seems to work. With it, often amazing results have been obtained by using measures that ordinarily are only modestly effective. Measures that help strengthen the nurse–client relationship and promote pain relief include discussing pain with the client, allowing the client to help decide on a method of pain relief, and visiting and remaining with the client in pain. These measures promote a collaborative relationship in which the client's pain is treated with respect.

Teaching the Client About Pain

The well-informed person can often cope better with the distress of pain and tends to experience less anxiety about pain. In many situations, teaching about pain should include family members so that they understand and may help the person in pain.

The following are examples of information to share with the client and family when pain is present:
- Function of pain
- Cause of pain
- When pain can be anticipated and when it need not be anticipated
- Quality and duration of pain to expect
- Assurance that it is acceptable to express feelings about pain
- What pain-control measures can and will be used
- Assurance that the client's complaints about pain are believed
- Knowledge that it is easier to control pain before it is allowed to become severe

Play may often be used very effectively to discover a child's experience of pain and to teach the child how to

---

RESEARCH IN NURSING *Making a Difference*

Comfort

The relief of pain has long been a subject for study. Pain is a physical response to malfunction of an organism but can also occur in the absence of an organic cause. Despite the cause, the person still responds with alterations in comfort (pain). Increased anxiety also interferes with the benefits of rest and so prevents comfort. Nursing research in these areas continues to explore appropriate interventions.

Related Research

Randolph G: Therapeutic and physical touch: Physiological response to stressful stimuli. Nursing Res 33(1):33–36, 1984
Randolph conducted this study to determine the physiologic difference between groups reacting to stressful stimuli when treated by either therapeutic touch or personal touch. Although the benefits of therapeutic touch are increasingly discussed in the literature, this study found no significant difference in response when it was used.

Taylor A, Skelton J, Butcher J: Duration of pain condition and physical pathology as determinants of nurses' assessments of patients in pain. Nursing Res 33(1):48, 1984

This study explored the client responses to pain that best accounted for differential assessments and interventions by nurses. Results indicated that (1) the amount of active intervention received by a client is significantly influenced by the presence or absence of depression and the type of complaint, (2) clients with objective signs of pathology were viewed more positively as having pain, and (3) chronic pain was believed to be less intense than acute pain.

There are many implications for nursing from these studies. It is the responsibility of the nurse to promote maximum well-being for all clients, and to accept that pain is a unique and individual response deserving appropriate therapeutic interventions.

cope with pain. Children are usually receptive to using dolls to act out pain experiences.

Manipulating Factors Affecting the Pain Experience

Removing or Altering the Cause of Pain.
Removing or altering the cause of the pain is ideal and sometimes possible. Ways of doing this include removing or loosening a tight binder, if permissible; seeing to it that a distended bladder is emptied; taking steps to relieve constipation and flatus; changing body positions and ensuring correct body alignment; and changing soiled linens and dressings that may be irritating the skin. The hungry or thirsty client may need a snack or a drink to feel more comfortable.

Certain drugs are useful for removing or altering the intensity of painful stimuli. For example, drugs that decrease smooth muscle spasms in the gastrointestinal tract and those that decrease contractions of skeletal muscles reduce discomfort.

Altering Factors that Decrease Pain Tolerance.
The nurse's pain assessment and the establishment of a trusting relationship should result in the identification of factors that decrease **pain tolerance** and increase the pain experience. These should also be alleviated whenever possible. For example, a client whose family has never acknowledged his pain and who has repeatedly been told that his pain is all in his head may experience a greater ability to deal with his pain when someone finally takes his pain seriously. Nursing measures include communication to the client that responses to pain are acceptable as well as education of the client's family.

Fatigue tends to increase pain, and promoting rest is then helpful. The client in pain usually feels more comfortable when the environment is quiet and restful. Although sensory restrictions such as eliminating unnecessary noise, bright lights, and so on are usually indicated, it is rarely helpful to leave the client alone in an environment with little sensory input. The client will then be more likely to focus on self and the discomfort.

Lack of knowledge, finding no meaning in the pain, being pessimistic about its relief, and fear may also interfere with the client's ability to deal with pain. Common fears include a fear of losing control and embarrassing oneself by not being able to deal with the pain maturely, and the fear of taking pain-relief medication because this may be viewed as a sign of weakness, may become addictive, or will lose its effectiveness later.

Initiating Noninvasive Relief Measures

Distraction

Conscious attention often appears to be necessary to experience pain, whereas preoccupation with other things has been observed to distract the client from pain. Dis-

traction requires the client to focus attention on something other than the pain. It is not entirely clear whether distraction raises the threshold of pain or increases pain tolerance. Many clients whose pain is relieved by distraction report being able to place pain in the periphery of awareness. This is compatible with the theory that if the reticular formation in the brain stem receives sufficient sensory input it can ignore or block out select sensations such as pain. The Lamaze method of childbirth illustrates one common use of distraction.

Distraction is best used before pain begins or very soon thereafter. Persons in mild to severe pain can successfully utilize distraction, but distraction cannot generally be practiced for long periods of time and may result in an increased sense of pain and fatigue at its completion. In general, clients who are experiencing chronic pain need a greater variety of distractions than clients with pain of short duration.

Distraction may be successfully used with children. In order for distraction to be effective, the individual must be aware of activities or situations that are the most exciting, interesting, or absorbing. Distractions may be visual, auditory, tactile kinesthetic, or "project" (see the accompanying box entitled Techniques That Distract Attention).

Imagery

The client who uses **imagery**, an example of mind–body interaction, to decrease pain sensation imagines some-

---

Techniques that Distract Attention

Visual Distractions
- Staring at an object or spot and describing it in detail
- Counting objects
- Reading or watching television

Auditory Distractions
- Listening to music

Tactile Kinesthetic Distractions
- Holding or stroking a loved person, pet, or toy
- Rocking
- Slow, rhythmic breathing

"Project" Distractions
- Playing a challenging game (puzzles, card game, computer game)
- Performing meaningful play/work (hobby, vocational work, creative work: writing a journal, taping memoirs, and other such projects)

thing that involves one or all of the senses, concentrates on that "image," and gradually becomes less aware of the pain. Imagery may be as simple as a child thinking of "happy things" (a beloved pet, lollipops, Christmas morning, grandmom's lap) or as involved as an adult recreating a favorite place and then experiencing the healing presence or touch of a loved person or the healing energies of nature in that setting. Imagery has also been used to create an image in which the cause of the pain is visualized and then overcome, counteracted, by some more powerful image.

Imagery has been found to be more effective for the client with chronic pain than for the client with acute, severe pain. The nurse can teach a client to use imagery by performing "guided imagery." The nurse sits close to the client but not touching the client and in a gentle voice invites the client to use all five senses to recreate a favorite restful scene. This scene would have been previously described to the nurse by the client. If the client becomes restless or upset, the imagery experience is terminated and attempted later when the client seems better disposed. Guided imagery is discussed in Chapter 9.

Relaxation

To **relax** means to become less rigid, to slacken effort, and to decrease tension and anxiety. The positive effects of relaxation on an individual's mental and physical health include

- Relief of fatigue
- Increased ability to cope with anxiety
- Relief of the kind of stress that contributes to cardiac and circulatory disease
- Conservation of the body's energy
- Reduction of the tendency to smoke, drink, or use drugs
- Facilitation of sounder sleep
- Increased alertness and ability to sleep
  Relaxation affects pain specifically by
- Reducing pain caused by muscle tension
- Reducing anxiety-related pain
- Giving the relaxer something to do before, during, and after a pain experience
  (Witt, 1984)

Most relaxation techniques can be learned with little practice and with relative ease. Some require the help and guidance of a person experienced in the technique, such as zen or yoga. Practices producing relaxation generally have four elements in common:

- Assuming a comfortable position with the body in good alignment
- Being in quiet surroundings

- Repeating a certain word, sound, phrase, or prayer
- Adopting a passive attitude when distracting thoughts enter the individual's consciousness

Relaxation is most effective as a pain alleviator when combined with slow, deep, easy breathing from the abdomen or diaphragm while the eyelids are closed or with the individual focusing on a real or imagined fixed spot. Relaxation techniques are discussed in Chapter 9. Many tapes are now available to direct this process. (A free catalogue of tapes on relaxation and imagery may be obtained from Psychology Today Cassettes, PO Box 278, Pratt Station, Brooklyn NY 11205.) Other techniques that promote relaxation include listening to restful music or nature sounds while concentrating on relaxing; thinking about something that is relaxing, such as lying on a beach while listening to the roar of the waves; meditation; yoga; zen; biofeedback; systematic desenzitization; and operant conditioning.

Cutaneous Stimulation

The success of techniques that stimulate the skin's surface in relieving pain is often explained on the basis of the gate control theory. The gate control theory of pain postulates that cutaneous nerve fibers are large-diameter fibers carrying impulses to the central nervous system. When the skin is stimulated, pain is believed to be controlled by closing the gating mechanism in the spinal cord. This decreases the number of pain impulses that reach the brain for perception.

Cutaneous stimulation techniques include

- Massage (with or without stimulants such as liniments or menthol ointments; see Procedure 30-1
- Application of heat or cold, or both intermittently
- Vibration
- Pressure

One example of pressure is myotherapy, which is a modern-day Western descendant of acupuncture. The therapist using this technique applies pressure for 4 to 7 seconds on select trigger points, starving the area of needed oxygen and thus relieving the pain. Trigger points are highly irritable, painful muscle spots at which the pain from various body pathologies is registered.

Contralateral stimulation is a technique that involves stimulating an area opposite the painful area. For example, if the left arm is painful, skin stimulation is used on the right arm. The reason contralateral stimulation works is not understood.

Cutaneous stimulation is limited in that (1) unless the pain can be localized it is most likely too diffuse to benefit from these techniques and (2) most individuals cannot tolerate stimulation of the painful area but may be

(Text continues on p. 743.)

PROCEDURE 30-1
Giving a Back Massage

Equipment

Massage lubricant or lotion   Bath blanket   Towel

Powder

Action	**Rationale**
1 Explain the procedure and offer back massage to the client.	Back massage can facilitate circulation and promote relaxation.
2 Wash your hands.	Handwashing deters the spread of microorganisms.
3 Close the curtain and/or door.	Privacy increases relaxation.
4 Assist the client to the prone position or side-lying position with the back exposed from the shoulders to the sacral area. Use the bath blanket to drape the client. Raise the bed to the high position and lower the side rail closest to you.	This position exposes an adequate area for massage with privacy and warmth maintained. Having the bed in the high position reduces back strain for the nurse.
5 Warm the lubricant or lotion in the palm of your hand or place the container in warm water.	Cold lotion causes chilling and uncomfortable sensation.
6 Using light strokes (effleurage), apply lotion to client's shoulders, back, and sacral area.	Effleurage relaxes the client and lessens tension.
7 Place your hands beside each other at the base of the client's spine and stroke upward to the shoulders and back downward to the buttocks in slow, continuous strokes. Continue for 3 to 5 minutes.	Continuous contact is soothing and stimulates circulation and muscle relaxation.
8 Massage the client's shoulders, entire back, areas over iliac crests, and sacrum with circular stroking motion. Keep your hands in contact with the client's skin. Continue for 3 to 5 minutes, applying additional lotion as necessary.	A firmer stroke with continuous contact promotes relaxation.
9 Knead the client's skin by gently alternating grasping and compression motions (pétrissage).	Kneading increases blood circulation to areas.
10 Complete the massage with additional long stroking movements.	Long stroking motion is soothing and promotes relaxation.
11 During massage, observe the client's skin for reddened or open areas. Pay particular attention to the skin over bony prominences.	Pressure may interfere with circulation and lead to development of decubitus ulcers. Back rub stimulates circulation to these areas.
12 Use the towel to pat the client dry and to remove excess lotion. Apply powder if the client requests it.	This provides additional comfort for the client.
13 Wash your hands.	Handwashing deters the spread of microorganisms.
14 Assess the client's response and record your observations on the client's chart.	This provides accurate documentation of the procedure and condition of the client's skin.

helped by stimulation of the surrounding or contralateral area.

Assisting With Pain Therapies of Other Disciplines

A team of health-care professionals is often involved in the client's care and nurses work collaboratively with other team members to secure pain relief for the client. One of nursing's important functions is to assist the client to explore pain-relief alternatives by providing or securing information about different treatment modalities. These modalities may range from simple folk remedies to complex surgical treatments. The nurse's role is not to make decisions for the client but to provide the support and knowledge that enable the person in pain to secure helpful assistance. Depending on the nature of the person's pain, this assistance may be provided by a family member, a member of the clergy, a folk healer, a clinical psychologist, a nurse, or a physician. Nursing interventions may include referral assistance as well as support and protection during the treatment.

Analgesic Administration

An **analgesic drug** is a pharmaceutical agent that relieves pain. Analgesics function to reduce the person's perception of pain and to alter the person's responses to discomfort. There are three general classes of drugs used as analgesics:

- Non-narcotic analgesics (*e.g.,* aspirin, acetaminophen, nonsteroidal anti-inflammatory agents)
- Narcotic analgesics (all controlled substances; (*e.g.,* morphine, codeine, meperidine, methadone)
- Narcotic antagonists (nalorphine, levallorphan, pentazocine)

These classes are compared in Table 30-9.

The nurse administering analgesics needs to combine a healthy respect for the drug being administered with thorough knowledge of its mechanism of action, side-effects, and administration guidelines. This respect for the drug should result in analgesics being utilized wisely to produce their desired effect. McCaffery (1987b) offers an equianalgesic drug chart illustrating how different drugs relate to the traditional analgesic standard (10 mg of subcutaneous morphine). Compara-

T A B L E   30-9
Comparison of Narcotic and Non-narcotic Analgesic Agents

Agents	Development of Tolerance and Physical Dependency	Analgesic Efficacy	Site and Mechanisms of Analgesic Effect	Common Side-Effects
Narcotic analgesics (morphine-like)	Yes; discontinuance of narcotic administration or administration of a narcotic antagonist (*i.e.,* precipitated withdrawal after prolonged use) causes withdrawal syndrome	Greater efficacy: can relieve pain of a more severe nature In sufficient dosage are considered capable of relieving pain of virtually every nature	Produce analgesia by central nervous system (*i.e.,* brain and spinal cord) mechanisms	Nausea, vomiting, dizziness, mental clouding, sedation, constipation, respiratory depression
Non-narcotic analgesics (aspirin-like, anti-inflammatory)	No	Less efficacy: limited to relief of mild to moderate pain (*e.g.,* headache, muscle and joint pain) regardless of the dose administered	Chiefly produce analgesia by peripheral mechanisms ouside of the central nervous system (*e.g.,* via interference with the biosynthesis of prostaglandins)	Nausea, vomiting, dyspepsia, gastric ulceration, decreased blood clotting
Narcotic antagonist (pentazocine-like)	When administered in the presence of an opioid, precipitates a withdrawal syndrome almost instantly Physical dependence can result from chronic use of these drugs for analgesia.	Most are not generally employed as analgesics *per se* but do possess analgesic efficacy; pentazocine is widely employed as an analgesic for mild to moderate pain.	Similar to narcotic analgesics	Nausea, vomiting, sweating, lightheadedness, sedation, psychomimetic effects (anxiety, nightmares, hallucinations, distorted body image, depersonalization)

tive knowledge of common analgesics enables the nurse to tailor the client's regimen and communicate professionally with physicians about a client who is being undermedicated or who needs a different drug or route of administration.

At no time should analgesics be used as a substitute for good nursing care that includes other measures to relieve discomfort. If the administration of "pain-killers" is the only treatment strategy a nurse consistently employs to deal with pain, then care is grossly deficient. On the other hand, nurses should not refrain from using analgesics or reduce their doses because of an unrealistic fear of their potency and side-effects.

Repeated studies have demonstrated that pain is usually undertreated in hospitalized individuals. Physician, nurse, and client variables all contribute to this outcome. Physicians often prescribe insufficient analgesic doses because of a tendency to (1) overestimate the efficacy and duration of analgesics; (2) underestimate the pain experience; and (3) worry excessively about the possibility of respiratory problems and addiction. Nurses who ideally spend the most time with the client and who

---

Flow Sheet—Pain—Example

Patient _____   Date _____

Rx _____

Purpose: *To evaluate the safety and effectiveness of the analgesic(s).*

Analgesic order _____

Pain Rating Scale used _____

I. Time	II.* Pain rating	III. Analgesic	IV. R	V. P	VI. BP	VII. Level of arousal	VIII.** Other	IX. Plan & comments

***Pain rating:** A number of different scales may be used. Indicate which scale is used and use the same one each time. Two common examples:
• 0 to 10 with 0 being no pain and 10 being as bad as it can be.
• Melzack's scale: 0 = no pain; 1 = mild; 2 = discomforting; 3 = distressing;
  4 = horrible; 5 = excruciating.

****Possibilities for other columns:** respiratory depression, nausea and vomiting, bowel function, other pain relief measures, etc. Identify the side effects of greatest concern to patient, family, physician, nurses, etc.

F I G U R E   30-3

Pain flow sheet. Possibilities for other columns are respiratory depression, nausea and vomiting, bowel function, other pain relief measures, etc. Identify the side-effects of greatest concern to client family, physician, and nurses. (Reproduced with permission from Meinhart NT, McCaffery M: Pain: A Nursing Approach to Assessment and Analysis. Norwalk, CT, Appleton-Century-Crofts, 1983)

are supposed experts in human responses, for example, such as the response to pain, often compound this problem by further reducing the insufficient analgesic dose or by not administering the medication at all. Nurse variables include the low priority nurses give to pain management; arbitrary pain assessments and erroneous judgments about a client's pain and need for analgesia; and fear of being the person who administers the drug that causes respiratory depression or another serious side-effect. The inability of many clients to discuss their pain and to request pain assistance perpetuates this problem.

General Principles for Administering Analgesics

Goals for Pain Relief. When using medications for pain relief the nurse must first understand the client's and family's goals for pain relief. Donovan and Girton (1984) recommend consideration of

- The nature of the process causing the pain (whether it is temporary or chronic)
- The life expectancy of the client
- The functions the client desires or is required to perform
- Client preference regarding the desired degree of control over pain (in light of the risks and side-effects associated with the method of control)
- The client's financial status (cost of various drugs and medication regimens)
- The character of the pain (whether it is intermittent, continuous, intense, mild)
- The risk, nature of, and client's willingness to tolerate side-effects of drug regimens

Ongoing Assessment. Just as the pain experience of each client is unique, so is the response of each client to a prescribed analgesic. The nurse needs continually to (1) evaluate whether or not the medication is producing the desired analgesic effect; (2) identify changes in the client's condition (correction or worsening of pathology, increased drug tolerance) that necessitate changes in the analgesic agent, dose, or route of administration; and (3) identify the development of side-effects of the analgesic that may warrant its discontinuance. As long as the client's pain exists, the need for ongoing assessment is imperative. The flow chart in Figure 30-3 facilitates this assessment. Basic to this assessment is the knowledge of the basic action, doses, routes of administration, side-effects, and administration guidelines of the analgesic being administered.

Timing. Timing is an important consideration when administering analgesics. Their effect is usually greatest when administered before pain occurs or becomes severe. To time analgesics appropriately the nurse needs to know the average duration of action for the drug and time administration so that the peak analgesic effect occurs when the pain is expected to be most intense. For example, an analgesic would be offered before ambulating a client postoperatively.

A prn (as needed) drug regimen may meet the needs of many persons experiencing acute pain. However, with a prn protocol the client usually has to request the pain medication and has no guarantee that the nurse will administer it promptly. Often there is a long delay between the client's request for pain medication and the nurse's administration of the drug, which is a source of frustration for both clients and nurses.

The prn protocol is totally inadequate for clients experiencing chronic pain. Regular administration of analgesics has been shown to offer superior pain management for chronic pain. Figure 30-4 illustrates the deficiencies in chronic pain treatment of the regular use of a short-acting drug such as meperidine (Demerol), the use of a prn medication, and the use of a medication whose dosage is insufficient. Comparing Figure 30-4 with Figure 30-5 will quickly demonstrate the superiority of a regularly administered effective analgesic.

Patient-Controlled Analgesia

Patient-controlled analgesia (PCA) is an innovative technique developed to provide effective individualized, client-controlled analgesia and comfort. The PCA unit is an infusion pump that holds a vial of an intravenous analgesic that allows the client to regulate the intravenous infusion of small amounts of a narcotic at short intervals (Fitzgerald, 1987). Advantages of this approach to pain management include the following:

- Consistent analgesia is maintained rather than the inconsistent analgesia obtained with periodic intramuscular injections, which result in sharp rises and falls of serum narcotic levels.

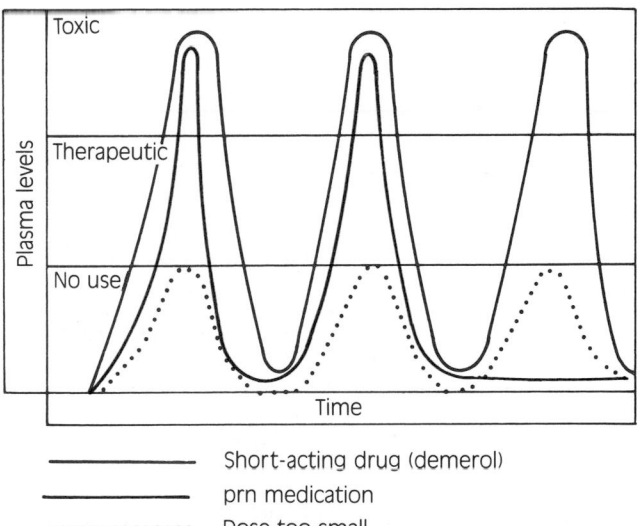

FIGURE 30-4
Inadequacy of a short-acting drug, prn medication, and insufficient dosage to relieve continuous pain. (From Dr. Tom West, St. Christopher's Hospice, London; National Conference on Pain, Discomfort, and Humanitarian Care, NIH, Bethesda, MD, 1979)

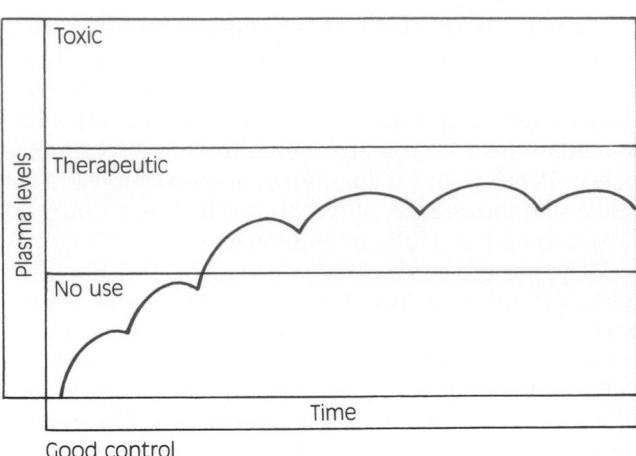

FIGURE 30-5

Regularly administered effective analgesic. (From Dr. Tom West, St. Christopher's Hospice, London; National Conference on Pain, Discomfort, and Humanitarian Care, NIH, Bethesda, MD, 1979)

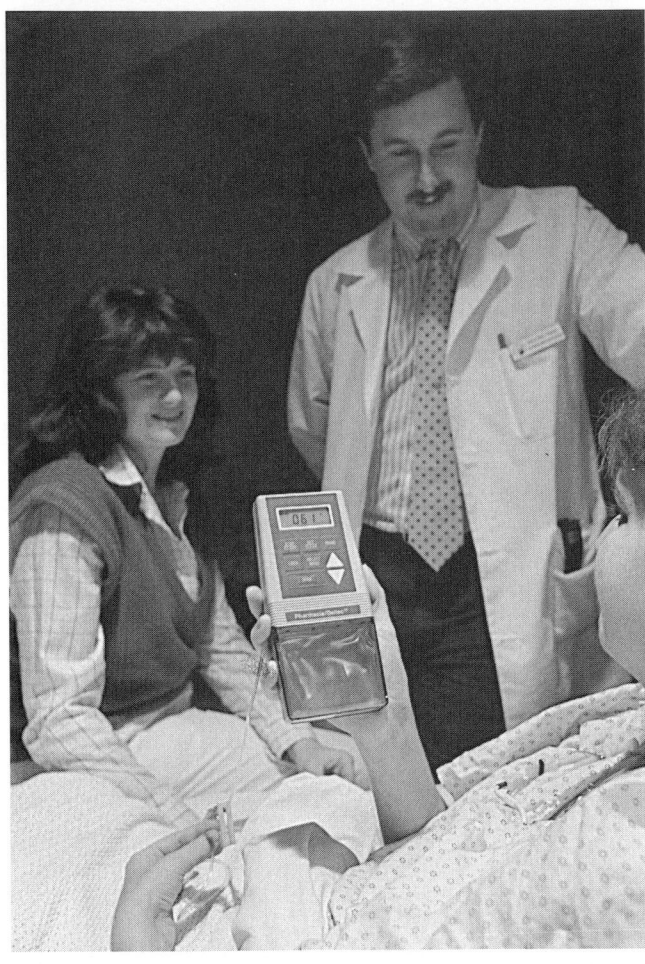

FIGURE 30-6

A self-controlled analgesia unit (PCA) allows the client to regulate the intravenous infusion of small amounts of analgesic as needed. (Photo by Don Walker, courtesy of Thomas Jefferson University)

- The narcotic is delivered intravenously so that absorption is faster and more predictable than with the intramuscular route.
- The client is in charge of the pain management program.

The PCA unit has two settings (appropriate dose and lock-out interval), which, once set, limit the amount of narcotic the client can receive. Built-in safety features help to prevent narcotic theft and overdose. Nursing responsibilities include

- Identifying clients who are good candidates for PCA (alert and capable of controlling the unit; no prior history of drug or alcohol abuse)
- Setting up the PCA unit and ensuring that it is functioning properly
- Educating clients in the use of PCA
- Evaluating the effectiveness of this type of pain management control for the client

A broader definition of PCA is advocated by McCaffery (1987a), for whom PCA encompasses any drug-administration method (oral, PCA pump, intravenous, subcutaneous, or spinal route) that allows the client to exercise control. She recommends that all analgesics be given on the basis of this concept, provided the client is able and willing to participate and safe limits are set.

The Placebo Controversy

The term **placebo** is a Latin word meaning "I shall please." It consists of an inactive substance often given to satisfy a person's demand for a drug. The person, unaware of the placebo's properties, may find it to be effective for the relief of pain because of the perception that it will provide comfort and because of belief in the person administering it. It is an injustice to judge a person experiencing relief from pain after the use of a placebo as a malingerer or as mentally ill. If the pain is relieved, the placebo has served its purpose. Many believe that the placebo has its place in health care to help prevent addiction to certain drugs, to offer relief when an analgesic is contraindicated, and to substitute an innocuous agent when a person seems dependent on drug therapies that are deemed unnecessary.

The use of placebos, however, raises serious ethical questions. Can the good done by the placebo justify lying to a client? The nurse who administers a placebo must be willing to risk the possible consequence of the client becoming aware of the duplicity and then refusing to trust the nurse or any other health-care professional ever again. Clients who feel themselves to be in pain are vulnerable. If such a client discovers a seeming "plot" to "trick him" into feeling better, it is not likely that the client will respect or appreciate the good intentions of the physicians and nurses involved. The long-term effects of this practice would seem to outweigh its benefits. It is recommended that nurses decide their stand on placebos before encountering a situation in practice where they are expected to administer one. The nurse has firm legal and ethical grounds for refusing to administer a placebo but must also communicate the basis for refusal to the appropriate authorities.

Hypnosis

Hypnosis, a technique that produces a subconscious condition accomplished by suggestions made by a hypnotist, has been used successfully in many instances to control pain. The person's state of consciousness is altered by suggestions so that pain is not perceived as it normally would be. According to many hypnotists, it also alters the physical signs of pain. Many persons can be taught autohypnosis, that is, self-induced hypnosis, for the control of pain. It is generally believed that a successful response to hypnosis is related to the individual's openness to suggestion, belief that hypnosis will work, and emotional readiness.

Acupuncture

Acupuncture is a technique that utilizes needles of various lengths to prick specific parts of the body to produce insensitivity to pain. After the needles are inserted into the body, they are twirled or used to conduct a mild electrical current. The technique was developed in China and has been used for centuries in many Oriental countries. It is beginning to gain acceptance in the Western world and is being investigated as a possible tool to help control discomfort. The relief of pain by acupuncture is generally explained on the basis of the gate control theory. The needles are believed to stimulate large diameter nerve fibers and thereby the gating mechanism is closed and pain impulses do not reach the brain for perception. Self-hypnosis may also account for some of acupuncture's success. Repeated treatments are often needed.

Acupressure is the application of pressure or massage, or both, to usual acupuncture sites. It is usually applied with the thumb, a finger, the palm of the hand, or a fingernail. Its effectiveness may be explained on the basis of the gate control theory.

Biofeedback

Biofeedback is a technique that utilizes a teaching machine with a feedback signal to help a client learn by trial and error to control the supposedly involuntary body mechanisms (e.g., poor circulation, muscle spasms) that may cause pain. The technique decreases the individual's pain (1) by reducing the anxiety associated with lack of control over bodily functions, (2) by distracting the person's attention from the pain to concentration on the person's inner state and the feedback signal, and (3) by reducing the cause of the pain. Limitations for this method include the high degree of motivation needed and difficulty of maintaining control at the end of the training program.

Local Anesthesia

Anesthetic agents may be applied topically to the skin or mucous membranes or injected into the body to produce a temporary loss of sensation and motor and autonomic function in a localized area. The agents work by chemically blocking the nerve pathways involved in pain sensation and response and are sometimes called *nerve blocks*. Many persons have experienced nerve blocks during dental work.

Nursing measures include (1) noting any allergic responses the client has had in the past to anesthetic agents, (2) alerting the client to the pain the initial injection of the anesthetic may cause if the physician does not numb the area first, (3) offering emotional support to the client during the procedure and observing for any untoward effects, and (4) protecting the client from injury until sensory and motor functions return.

Neurosurgery

Transmission of pain may be interrupted permanently by surgical (or thermocoagulation) neural destruction. Because the destruction is permanent it is usually used only as a last resort for intractable pain. In persons for whom psychologic elements contribute heavily to the pain experience, the pain may persist following nerve transection. These procedures require highly skilled neurosurgeons and anesthesiologists and their execution varies from medical center to medical center. Common procedures include the following.

Neurectomy. This is a partial or total excision of a peripheral or cranial nerve to relieve localized pain. It may result in total loss of sensation and some paralysis of the affected area.

Rhizotomy. This is an interruption (by surgical resection) of the posterior root just outside the posterior horn cells of the spinal cord. This procedure offers the benefit of relief of both localized acute pain and deep visceral pain (interrupts sensory function) while preserving motor function. A surgical rhizotomy is indicated for localized pain in the neck, chest, back, and perineum if the client is in good physical condition.

Cordotomy. This is a surgical resection of the spinal and cerebral tracts carrying painful impulses and is used for advanced disease and intractable pain. Ideally, pain and temperature sensation below the level severed are obliterated while the senses of touch and position are retained. This procedure carries a heavy risk of complications, and permanent paralysis may result from accidental resection of the motor nerves. This open surgical procedure has been largely replaced by percutaneous thermoregulation.

Sympathectomy. This is a severing of the sympathetic afferent nerve pathways that is used primarily for causalgias, phantom pain, and pain due to vascular disorders.

Electrical Nerve Stimulation

Selective electrical stimulation of large-diameter fibers has now been successfully used to inhibit transmission of painful impulses carried over small-diameter fibers. All the electroanalgesia methods use electrodes attached to or implanted in the area to be stimulated. The gate control theory is used to explain the success of these methods as is the theory that the analgesia is produced through the release of endorphins both in the spinal cord and centrally.

Types of nerve fiber stimulation include
- Transcutaneous nerve stimulation (TNS) or transcutaneous electrical nerve stimulation (TENS)
- Dorsal column stimulation (DCS)
- Percutaneously implanted spinal cord epidural stimulation (PISCES)
- Central gray stimulation

Specific indications, application and care procedures, and cautions exist for each of the above types.

EVALUATING

As soon as a pain problem is identified and a treatment plan developed and implemented, evaluation becomes ongoing. Evaluation is directed toward the changing nature of the pain experience, the treatment modalities (pain management program), and the client and family's response to the plan of care. Obviously all three overlap.

The Pain Experience. The pain the client is experiencing may change in many ways and the nurse must be careful not to make a judgment about this too quickly. For example, if the pain lessens in intensity or disappears, it may mean that the underlying cause of the pain is diminished or absent and that treatment should be stopped, or it may mean that the pain management program is effective and should be continued. When pain intensity is increased, it may simply indicate the need for more aggressive therapy, or it may be a warning that the underlying pathology has changed or worsened and that new medical intervention is required. Often a new problem very amenable to treatment is masked by "old pain" and its detection may be delayed to the point that treatment is useless.

Treatment Modalities. The use of both noninvasive and invasive therapies must be continually evaluated to determine if they are the best possible means the client could use to obtain pain relief and if they are effective with only minimal risk to the client. Too often a client "stays with" the first analgesic prescribed without questioning if it is the most effective drug for the particular pain, if the dosage and timing guidelines are correct for the client, and if the analgesic is perhaps producing annoying or even harmful side-effects that another drug would not produce. Similarly, one client may "take to" progressive relaxation exercises and find them very helpful whereas another may obtain similar benefits from a daily walking program. Nursing time spent evaluating the effectiveness of each pain-relief therapy is well spent and results in a pain management program that is truly individualized to the client.

Client and Family Response. Ultimately, the plan of care is not successful unless the client and family are satisfied with the results it is producing. A successful plan of care results in the achievement of specified client goals that the client values. Whenever possible, nursing care should terminate when the client and family can independently direct the pain management program with the assistance of appropriate resources.

N U R S I N G   P R O C E S S   *in Clinical Practice*

Once a pain problem is suspected the nurse implements each phase of the nursing process to ensure its correct identification and treatment. The knowledge and clinical skills described in this chapter will enable the nurse to manage these problems successfully. The following outlines specific assessment priorities, client goals, nursing interventions, and evaluative criteria for nursing diagnoses representative of the two major classifications of pain—acute and chronic:

Altered comfort: acute postoperative pain
Altered comfort: chronic malignant pain

The case study following the discussion of these diagnoses presents a woman suffering from the discomforts of premenstrual syndrome. Although her symptoms considered individually hardly constitute a "pain problem," together they afford the client sufficient discomfort to interfere with her everyday functioning. This case illustrates the close relationship between an individual's comfort level and functional abilities.

Altered Comfort: Acute Postoperative Pain

Once the anesthesia administered during surgery begins to wear off, the surgical client generally experiences pain. Etiologies for the above diagnoses vary. The nature and degree of surgical trauma, the physical and mental health of the client, and the presence of other discomforting conditions (*e.g.,* nausea and vomiting, flatulence, drains and dressings, multiple tubes and equipment) contribute to the client's pain experience. The client's lack of knowledge of pain-relief measures and self-imposed restrictions on pain expression or use of relief measures, as well as deficient pain management skills of health-care professionals, may compound the client's pain.

Assessment

Initiate this assessment preoperatively and continue postoperatively.

- Conduct a thorough assessment of the client's pain experience (see Assessment of the Pain Experience). Note in particular the accuracy of the client's knowledge about pain (*i.e.,* its protective function) and assess the client's ability to manage pain appropriately by using both invasive (drug) and noninvasive treatment modalities.
- Never rely on the client to communicate the need for pain medication or assistance with pain relief. Anticipate the client's need for help and initiate a pain assessment during times when pain is probable. Communicate that the client's pain responses are "OK."

Client Goals

The client will

- Identify pain as the body's means to protect itself
- Request prescribed analgesic or initiate appropriate noninvasive relief modalities (1) before pain becomes severe and (2) prior to beginning a painful activity
- Report a gradual reduction in pain and its eventual elimination

Interventions

- Teach the client preoperatively about the purpose of pain and its value in alerting us to certain body conditions. Inform the client that pain-relieving medications will be available (on request if prn protocol is in place) and that they are most effective when taken before the pain becomes severe. Correct any misconceptions the client has and counsel regarding fears.
- During the immediate postoperative period, carefully assess the lessening of anesthetic effect and the need for pharmacologic analgesia. Initial doses of narcotics may need to be reduced if the client is hypotensive; however, the pain may also be causing the hypotension.
- Utilize good nursing care to keep the client as comfortable as possible. This includes assistance with turning, positioning, and ambulation (as ordered); assistance with coughing and deep breathing; assistance with hydration and nutrition (mouth

care for the patient who is allowed no oral intake of nutrition or fluids); wound care; massage; help with bathing; and attention to bed linens and elimination needs. Family members may be shown how to comfort clients through massage, repositioning, feeding, and other comfort measures.
- Administer analgesic medications as needed, carefully assessing whether they are producing the desired analgesia without producing undesired side-effects. Collaborate with physicians in noting when dosages need to be increased or decreased or when a different medication is needed. Use the power of suggestion to enhance the analgesic effect: "Here is your Demerol. You should be feeling good relief shortly . . . let me know."
- Assist the client to develop a good repertoire of noninvasive pain-relief modalities (distraction, relaxation, cutaneous stimulation) that he can utilize both while hospitalized and at home.

Evaluative Criteria

The client meets above goals.

Altered Comfort: Chronic Malignant Pain

Pain associated with cancer or other progressive disorders, which lasts for more than 6 months, is termed *chronic malignant pain.* As compared with acute pain, which is often described as meaningful, protective, purposeful, and reversible, clients frequently describe chronic malignant pain as hopeless, cyclical, all-consuming, meaningless, and as leading to fear, anxiety, depression, and helplessness. Yasko (1983) identifies common etiologies of chronic malignant pain:

- Infiltration of nerves, blood vessels, or lymphatic channels by tumor cells
- Compression of nerves by tumor
- Disruption of the nerve pathways due to pathologic fractures
- Tumor infiltration or distention of tissues that are pain-sensitive, such as fascia or periosteum
- Obstruction of a hollow viscus such as intestine or ureter
- Occlusion of blood vessels by infiltrating tumor, causing venous engorgement or arterial ischemia
- Inflammation, infection, or necrosis of tissue affected by neoplastic growth

Other factors contributing to the presence and severity of chronic pain include

- Discomfort associated with diagnostic procedures and cancer treatment
- Decreased mobility
- Anxiety and fear associated with the diagnosis of cancer, physical disfigurement, financial concerns, role changes, and disruption of personal relationship

In addition to these etiologies, problems of pain may be compounded by the client's inability to communicate pain or the need for assistance with pain relief as well as by the possibly deficient pain management skills of health-care professionals.

The seven aims of therapy in cancer pain are the following:

- Identify the cause.
- Prevent the pain.
- Erase the pain memory.
- Maintain an unclouded sensorium.
- Maintain a normal affect.
- Provide ease of therapy delivery (high touch, low tech).
- Prevent physical side-effects. (Levy, 1982).

Achieving these aims most often involves the energies of a multidiscipline health-care team and the active involvement of the client and family. Many nursing interventions are collaborative in nature.

Assessment

- Conduct a thorough assessment of the client's pain experience and update this as necessary. Note any difficulty the client has in communicating/expressing pain or the need for pain relief.
- Assess

    Characteristics of the pain (location, duration, quantity, quality, chronology, aggravating and alleviating factors, associated phenomena)

    Physiologic responses

    Behavioral responses

    Affective responses

    Interactions with others

    Degree to which pain interferes with the client's life

    Perception of pain and its meaning to the client

    Adequacy of adaptive mechanisms used to cope with pain

- Collaborate with the medical team to identify the physiologic reasons for the client's pain.
- Continually assess the client's response to treatment modalities and note any changes in the client necessitating a change in the plan of care; be especially sensitive to the development of discomforting or harmful side-effects.
- Assess the impact of the client's pain on the family and note the family's coping strategies.

Client Goals

The client will

- Relate ability to draw strength (sense of control) from the conviction that the pain will be treated
- Identify persons and resources that can be utilized to secure assistance with pain relief
- Describe a gradual reduction of the pain using a scale of 0 (no pain) to 10 (pain as bad as it can be)
- Demonstrate competent execution of pain management program

Analgesics (produce desired pain relief with minimal side-effects: sedation, respiratory depression, gastrointestinal problems)

Noninvasive pain-relief measures

- Demonstrate the ability to control pain by managing/enjoying key elements of everyday living

The family will report feeling better able to deal with the client's pain.

Interventions

- Establish a trusting nurse–client–family relationship within which the client can freely express pain, fears, and concerns. Be alert to misconceptions about pain and specific fears (fear of losing control, of being abandoned, of addiction; the family's fear that the client will use pain for secondary gains). Whenever possible, assure the client that he need never (or never again) feel overwhelmed by pain and then work to make this promise *real.*
- Work closely with the physician to develop effective pain control with narcotic analgesics. Realize that addiction is generally not a problem with this type of pain. Continual experimentation with drug dosage is usually necessary to keep the dose in the zone between oversedation and recurrence of pain; use of the pain flow sheet (see Fig 30-3) is helpful. The client in severe pain needs relief with narcotic analgesics before noninvasive treatment modalities will be helpful. When in severe pain the client does not have sufficient psychic energy for hypnosis, imagery, or progressive relaxation.

    Analgesic options are varied. For rapid and flexible control initially, intramuscular or subcutaneous morphine has been unsurpassed. Since the goal for maintenance management is an oral drug, opiate cocktail mixtures were used for years. More recently a sustained-release oral morphine has been used quite successfully. Severe, intractable cancer pain has also been treated with morphine administered by continuous intravenous drip. With the continuous drip route more uniform pain control is achieved with lower doses of the drug. Safe administration is facilitated with use of an infusion pump and requires close monitoring of vital signs. A narcotic antagonist, for example, naloxone (Norcan), should be readily available to reverse respiratory depression if needed. Depending on the client, other narcotic and non-narcotic analgesics may become the drug of choice. Nursing responsibilities with all drug therapy include client education, safe administration, and the reduction or elimination of drug side-effects.

- Identify other factors that compound the client's pain experience and work with the health-care team to resolve these problems. Common disturbances include

    Anxiety and depression: Interventions include simple psychologic support; attention to social, financial, and legal problems; and administration of low doses of tricyclic antidepressants or anxiolytic agents.

Gastrointestinal symptoms: Common problems include anorexia and dysphagia, mouth problems, nausea and vomiting, intestinal obstruction, constipation and diarrhea, and ascites. Because each of these problems can cause discomfort to the client, nursing needs to identify them quickly and initiate measures for their management and control.

Skin problems: Decubitus ulcers, other open lesions, pruritus

Fever

Weakness

Respiratory symptoms

- Collaborate with the client and family in initiating appropriate noninvasive pain-relief measures: distraction, relaxation, cutaneous stimulation; remember that these may have little effect on severe, intractable pain.
- Work with the client and family to improve the self-care abilities that promote the life-style they desire.
- Assist the family to respond optimally to the client's pain experience.

- If necessary, refer the client and family to a hospice or a pain clinic for assistance.

Resources

American Pain Society
340 Kingsland Street
Nutley, NJ 07110
(201) 235-0587

National Hospice Organization
1311 Dolly Madison Boulevard
McLean, VA 22101
(703) 356-6770

Palliative Care Foundation
288 Bloor Street West
Toronto, Ontario
M5S/V8

For directions on pain clinics

Committee on Pain Therapy
American Society of Anesthesiologists
515 Busse Highway
Park Ridge, IL 60068

CASE STUDY *

Patti Potter is a 26-year-old white woman. She is unmarried and has no children. Presently, she is employed at a large company as a computer programmer. Over the past 7 months, Patti has been experiencing periodic fatigue, anxiety, irritability, depression, and mood swings. Her general health is excellent. The nurse practitioner at the gynecologist's office believes Ms. Potter may be suffering from premenstrual syndrome (PMS).

Assessment Findings

The nurse practitioner who interviewed Ms. Potter noted the following data:

Generalized discomfort: fatigue, anxiety, irritability, depression, and mood swings, approximately 1 week prior to her menses; subside after onset of menses

Discomforts are believed to be heightened by stress at work but are not dependent on this. Client denies any new or unusual stress in life at present but feels symptoms are affecting her job performance and relationships.

Relates history of "bad cramps" ever since periods started. Client lacks knowledge of appropriate dietary and stress management techniques.

* Case Study and accompanying plan contributed by Ruth E. Gordon, RNC, MSN, Assistant Professor, Holy Family College, OB/GYN Nurse Practitioner.

Relates she has occasionally taken some of her friend's "tranquilizers" to ease her through a bad day—but she prefers not to take medication.

Nursing Diagnosis

Ineffective individual coping related to irritability, anxiety, depression, and mood swings

Planning

The nurse practitioner collaborates with Ms. Potter in establishing a two-step plan of care. First, the client needs to establish a daily record of her symptoms to identify if they are directly related to her menstrual cycle. If so, Ms. Potter and the nurse practitioner will outline a plan of care to relieve the symptoms of PMS.

Ms. Potter has provided positive feedback and acceptance of the following client goals:

By the completion of one menstrual cycle the client will

1. List all symptoms that cause her the most difficulty
2. Complete a daily record of all symptoms from her list as they occur
3. Return for office visit with her daily record at the completion of one menstrual cycle

Documentation

Traditional Note: 8/13/86 Consultation with client regarding apparent symptoms of PMS. She states she experiences fatigue, anxiety, irritability, depression, and mood swing approximately 1 week prior to her menses. She states these symptoms interfere with her job performance and relationships. She also states that these symptoms seem to subside after onset of her menses. Client admits to use of "tranquilizers" but prefers not to use medication. Advised client to keep daily record of symptoms for one complete menstrual cycle. Client indicated understanding of all instructions. She will return to office after completion of daily record for its analysis and to begin treatment, if indicated.

R. Gordon, RNC

SOAP Note: 8/13/86—Ineffective individual coping related to irritability, anxiety, depression, and mood swings

S: "I'm really flakey before I get my period and its starting to affect my job."

O: 26-year-old white female, no history of pregnancy

A: General health excellent, eager to collaborate on plan of care

P: Keep daily record of all symptoms for one menstrual cycle and return to office for analysis and treatment if indicated.

R. Gordon, RNC

Ms. Potter returned to the office with her daily record of symptoms complete after one menstrual cycle. Her record revealed that her symptoms were occurring largely from 10 days prior to her menses to the day her menses began. She experienced one full week of no symptoms following her menses. This information validates that she is suffering from PMS.

Revised Nursing Diagnosis

Ineffective individual coping related to discomforts of premenstrual symptoms

Planning

The nurse practitioner outlined a treatment plan for Ms. Potter to alleviate her premenstrual symptoms. The plan includes the general areas of relaxation, diet, exercise, and vitamin supplements.

Long-Term Goal

Client will verbalize symptom-free menses that will enable her to work at optimal effectiveness.

Short-Term Goals

See the care plan.

Implementation

The nurse needs to possess the following specialized abilities to implement the plan of care:

- Assessment skills: interviewing and physical assessment skills
- Knowledge of women's health and of current modes of treatment of PMS
- Interpersonal skills to collaborate with client for a plan of care that will work for her
- Teaching skills to provide client with the knowledge she needs to control discomforts of PMS
- Counseling skills to listen and empathize with client regarding her symptoms and how they are affecting her job performance and relationships

Evaluation

Short-term goals will be evaluated monthly. Long-term goal will be evaluated at 6 months.

N U R S I N G   C A R E   P L A N   *for Ms. Potter*

Nursing Diagnosis: Ineffective individual coping related to discomforts of premenstrual symptoms

Signs and Symptoms: Client complains of fatigue, anxiety, irritability, depression, and mood swings.

Long-Term Goal: Client will verbalize symptom-free menses that will enable her to work at optimal effectiveness.

Goals	Nursing Actions	Rationale	Evaluative Statement
By the next monthly assessment client will: 1. Utilize relaxation techniques during periods of anxiety	• Assess client's knowledge of relaxation techniques and motivation to use them. • Instruct client regarding the use of progressive relaxation exercises and controlled breathing during periods of anxiety. For example	Relaxation and controlled breathing are utilized to decrease anxiety and increase coping mechanisms.	10/30 Goal partially met, client utilized relaxation techniques during two periods of anxiety. Was driving on expressway during another period of anxiety which made relaxation difficult. *R. Gordon, RNC*

(Continued)

NURSING CARE PLAN (Continued)

Goals	Nursing Actions	Rationale	Evaluative Statement
	"Find a quiet, comfortable place and sit down. Consciously contract and relax the muscles of the whole body starting at the head and neck and working down to the feet until completely relaxed. At the same time, take slow, rhythmic breaths. Continue until anxiety passes."		
2. Utilize meal plan that includes three balanced meals per day and excludes caffeine, sugar, and sodium	• Assess client's nutritional intake. • Teach client rationale for decreasing intake of caffeine, sugar, and sodium. • Have client identify current food preferences high in the above and discuss substitutes. • Instruct client in developing meal plan that includes three balanced meals per day.	Refined sugar and caffeine contribute to feelings of tension and irritability. Sodium contributes to water retention in the body.	10/30 Goal met. Client utilized meal plan for 3 balanced meals per day and alleviated all sugar, caffeine, and sodium from diet. *R. Gordon, RNC*
3. Incorporate exercise into routine	• Assess value client attaches to physical fitness and regular periods of aerobic exercise; explore preferences. • Instruct client in use of regular daily exercise; design exercise prescription.	Exercise can alleviate symptoms of depression, tension, anxiety, fatigue, and irritability. Exercise also serves as a distraction from discomforts. The fitness produced by regular exercise contributes to self-esteem.	10/30 Goal met. Client includes daily brisk walk around her neighborhood in her routine. *R. Gordon, RNC*
4. Supplement her diet with 50 mg of vitamin B_6 daily	Instruct client on daily use of vitamin B_6.	Vitamin B_6 may be effective in relieving symptoms of irritability, fatigue, and depression.	10/30 Goal met. Client supplements her diet daily with 50 mg of vitamin B_6. *R. Gordon, RNC*
5. Continue use of daily record of PMS symptoms	Instruct client to continue use of daily record of PMS symptoms throughout the menstrual cycle.	To evaluate effectiveness of plan of care	10/30 Goal met. Client continued daily record, which illustrated drastic reduction in occurrence of PMS symptoms. Client expressed delight in greater feeling of control she now has over how she feels. "I never realized that so many things affect my comfort level and health." *R. Gordon, RNC*

KEY POINTS

■ Pain is a universal human experience, yet no two individuals experience and respond to pain exactly the same way. The most important services nurses offer a client experiencing pain are (1) belief that the client's pain is real, (2) willingness to become involved in the client's pain experience, and (3) competence in developing effective pain management regimens.

■ Pain may originate from physical (somatic or visceral) causes or mental/emotional (psychogenic) causes. Most often pain is a blend of both. There is no direct and constant relationship between a stimulus for pain and its perception. Little is understood about what causes individuals to perceive pain differently.

■ The transmission of pain stimuli is a complex process involving (1) the release of potent chemicals that sensitize the nerve endings, help transmit the pain message, and set the stage for healing; (2) transmission of the pain signal as an electrochemical impulse along the length of the nerve to the dorsal horn of the spinal cord; and (3) relay of the pain signal to the thalamus and eventually to the cortex.

■ The gate control theory of pain transmission postulates that only a limited amount of sensory information can be processed by the nervous system at any given moment. The effectiveness of many nursing measures to relieve pain (cutaneous stimulation, imagery) may result from their "overstimulation" of nerve fibers and the "closing of the gate" to pain stimuli.

■ Pain is a mixed sensation and occurs in varying degrees. Pain characteristics include duration, severity, quality, and periodicity. Pain responses may be physiologic, behavioral, or affective.

■ Many factors influence the pain experience. Among these are culture, religion, meaning and coping strategy, environment, support persons, anxiety and other stressors, and past experience with pain.

■ Numerous misconceptions about pain by both clients and health-care professionals interfere with the client's communication of pain and relief needs and with pain assessment and management.

■ It is helpful for nurses to assume that all clients are experiencing some degree of discomfort or pain and to initiate a pain assessment rather than waiting for the client to indicate experiencing pain.

■ Pain flow sheets clearly demonstrate the effectiveness of treatment modalities and the development of undesirable side-effects.

■ Multiple nursing diagnoses may be written that specifically address pain problems or identify the effect of pain problems on other areas of human functioning. Nursing diagnoses developed for pain problems should identify (1) type of pain; (2) etiologic factors; (3) client responses; and (4) other factors affecting pain stimulus/transmission, perception, and response.

■ Client goals regarding pain are directed toward the reduction and elimination of discomfort and pain and, whenever possible, to the client's management of a pain-relief program that makes possible the client's desired life-style patterns.

■ Nurses are often reluctant to become involved in pain management because of a natural tendency to avoid pain and because pain in the past has evoked in them feelings of fear, frustration, inadequacy, uselessness, and incompetence.

■ The unique relationship that can be developed among a client, the family, and the nurse makes the nurse a critical member of the pain management team. Nursing skills are ideal for developing in the client and family the needed self-care behavior to direct an effective pain management program.

■ Nursing interventions for pain relief include education, empowerment, manipulating factors that affect the pain experience, initiation of noninvasive treatment modalities (distraction, relaxation, cutaneous stimulation), safe and effective administration of analgesics, and participation in the treatment modalities of other health-care professionals.

■ Cancer pain requires specialized nursing skills. The chief objective with severe cancer pain is to prevent rather than treat the pain and this most often involves regular doses of narcotic analgesics. Until the client with cancer pain trusts that the pain can be effectively managed, he or she has little psychic energy for other life activities. The nurse's vigilant control of newly developing symptoms can contribute greatly to the client's comfort.

■ Evaluation of the plan of care necessitates the nurse's ongoing attention to the client's pain experience and the continual modification of pain therapies as needed. Integral to evaluation is feedback from the client and family regarding their feelings about themselves and their present ability to deal with pain.

BIBLIOGRAPHY

Ahles TA: Psychological approaches to the management of cancer-related pain. Seminars in Oncology Nursing 1(2):141–146, 1985

Bonica JJ: Pain research and therapy: Past and current status and future needs. In Ng LK, Bonica JJ (eds): Pain, Discomfort, and Humanitarian care. Proceedings of the National Conference, NIH, Bethesda, MD, February 15–16, 1979. New York, Elsevier/North Holland, 1980

Broome ME: The child in pain: A model for assessment and intervention. Critical Care Journal 8(1):47–55, 1985

Burden LL: Assessing chest pain and intervening efficiently. Nursing Life 6(2):33–40, 1986

Catalano RB: Pharmacology of analgesic agents used to treat cancer pain. Seminars in Oncology Nursing 1(2):126–140, 1985

Chaffee EE, Lyttle IM: Physiology and Anatomy, 4th ed. Philadelphia, JB Lippincott, 1980

Copp LA: Pain coping model and typology. Image 17(3):69–71, 1985

Copp LA: Perspectives of pain. Recent Advances in Nursing Series. Edinburgh, Churchill-Livingstone, 1985

Copp L: The spectrum of suffering. Am J Nurs 74(3):491–495, 1974

Donovan MI: Nursing assessment of cancer pain. Seminars in Oncology Nursing 1(2):109–115, 1985

Donovan MI: Relaxation with guided imagery: A useful technique. Cancer Nursing 3(1):27–32, 1980

Donovan MI, Girton SE: Cancer Care Nursing, 2nd ed. Norwalk, CT, Appleton-Century Crofts, 1984

DeCrosta T: Relieving pain: Four noninvasive ways you should know more about. Nursing Life 4(2):28–33, 1984

Escobar PL: Management of chronic pain. Nurse Pract 10(1):24–25, 29–30, 32, 1985

Fitzgerald JJ: Let your patient control his analgesia. Nursing '87 17(7):48–51, 1987

Forshee T: Track down the what, where, when, and how of chest pain. Nursing '86 16(5):34–42, 1986

Gaston-Johansson F: A baseline study for the development of an instrument for the assessment of pain. J Adv Nurs 10(6):539–546, 1985

Geach B: Pain and coping. Image 19(1):12–15, 1987

Hurley A, Whelan EG: Cognitive development and children's perception of pain. Pediatr Nurs 14(1):21–24, 1988

Jacox A: Pain: A Source Book for Nurses and Other Health Professionals. Boston, Little, Brown & Co, 1977

Jacox A, Stewart M: Psychosocial Contingencies of the Pain Experience. Iowa City, University of Iowa, College of Nursing, 1973

Larkin DM, Zahourek RP (eds): Stress, coping, and pain. Holistic Nurs Practice 2(3):entire issue, 1988

Leib RA: Epidural and intrathecal narcotics for pain management. Heart Lung 14(2):164–174, 1985

Levy M: Symptom control manual. In Cassileth BR, Cassileth PA (eds): Clinical Care of the Terminal Cancer Patient, pp 214–262. Philadelphia, Lea & Febiger, 1982

Lipowski ZJ: Physical illness, the individual, and the coping process. Psychiatric Medicine 1:91–101, 1970

McCaffery M: Patient-controlled analgesia: More than a machine. Nursing '87 17(11):62–64, 1987a

McCaffery M: A practical, "postable" chart of equianalgesic doses. Nursing '87 17(8):56–57, 1987b

McCaffery M: Would you administer placebos for pain? These facts can help you decide. Nursing '82 12(2):22–27, 1982

McCaffery M: Nursing Management of the Patient With Pain, 2nd ed. Philadelphia, JB Lippincott, 1979

McGuire L: Continuous narcotic infusion: It's not just for cancer patients. Nursing '84 14(12):50–56, 1984

McGuire L: Seven myths about pain relief. RN 46(12):30–31, 1983

McKean K: Pain. Discover 7(10):82–92, 1986

Meinhart NT, McCaffery M: Pain: A Nursing Approach to Assessment and Analysis. Norwalk, CT, Appleton-Century-Crofts, 1983

Schmitt M: The nature of pain, with some personal notes. Nurs Clin North Am 12(4):621–629, 1977

Steeves RH, Kahn DL: Experience of meaning in suffering. Image 19(3):114–116, 1987

Sternback RA: Pain: A Psychophysiological Analysis. New York, Academic Press, 1968

Tartaglia MJ: Managing chronic cancer pain effectively. Nursing Life 7(5):49–56, 1987

Weaver MT: Acupressure: An overview of theory and application. Nurse Pract 10(8):38–39, 42, 1985

West BA: Understanding endorphins: Our natural pain relief system. Nursing '81 11(2):50–53, 1981

Whipple B: Methods of pain control: Review of research and literature. Image 19(3):142–146, 1987

Witt JR: Relieving chronic pain. Nurse Pract 9(1):36–38, 78, 1984

Wong DL, Baker CM: Pain in children: Comparison of assessment scales. Pediatr Nurs 14(1):9–17, 1988

Yasko J: Guidelines for Cancer Care: Symptom Management. Reston, VA, Prentice-Hall, 1983

Zborowski M: People in Pain. San Francisco, Jossey-Bass, 1969

31 Nutrition

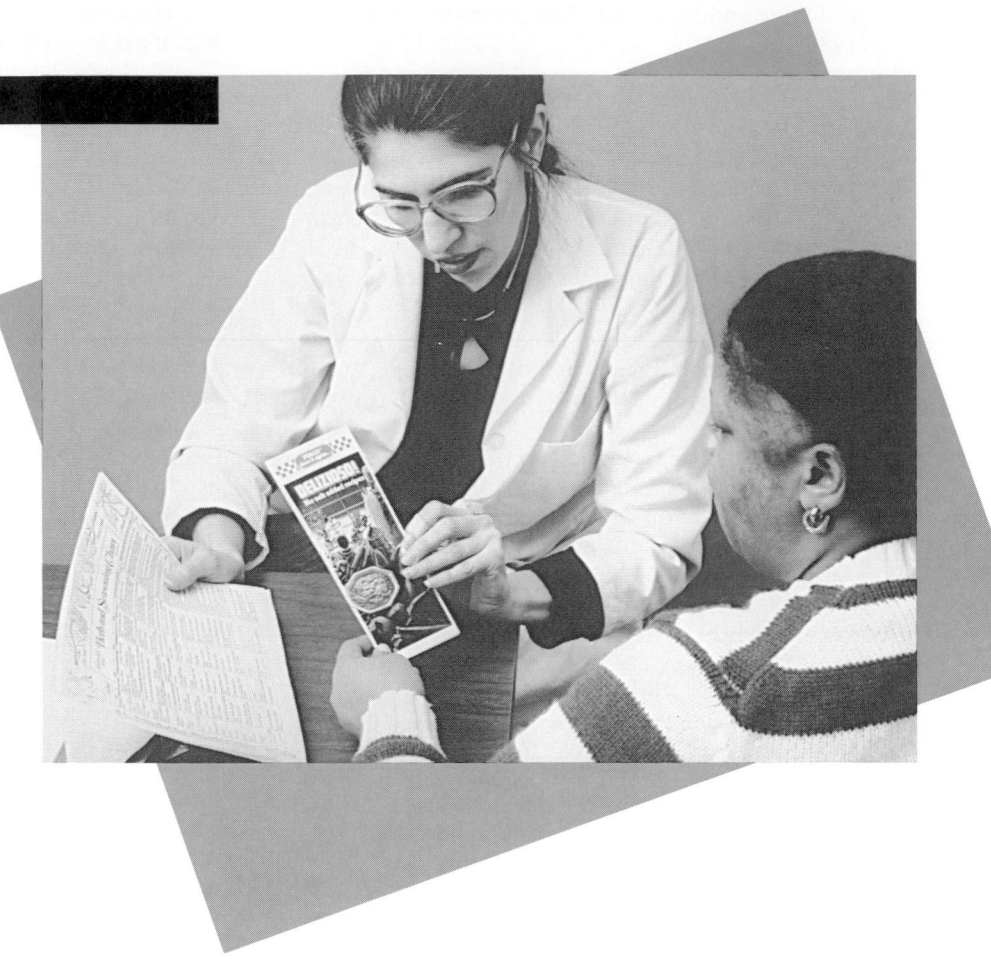

OBJECTIVES

After studying this chapter, the learner should be able to

Define key terms used in the chapter

List the six classes of nutrients and explain the significance of each, including variables affecting nutrient requirements.

Evaluate a diet using the food group approach.

Identify dietary, medical-socioeconomic, anthropometric, clinical, and biochemical risk factors for poor nutritional status.

Describe nutritional implications of growth and development throughout the life cycle.

Perform a nutritional assessment using appropriate interview questions, a 24-hour food recall when indicated, and a nursing examination.

Describe common nutritional problems noting key assessment criteria.

Develop nursing diagnoses that correctly identify nutritional problems which may be treated by independent nursing intervention.

Describe nursing interventions to help clients achieve their nutritional goals.

Plan, implement, and evaluate nursing care related to selected nursing diagnoses involving nutritional problems.

KEY TERMS

amino acid	minerals
anorexia	monosaccharides
anorexia nervosa	nitrogen balance
anthropometric	nutrition
basal metabolism	obesity
bulimia	overweight
calorie	polysaccharides
cholesterol	recommended dietary allowances
complete proteins	
disaccharides	specific dynamic action
fatty acid	trace elements
incomplete proteins	triglycerides
lipid	vitamins

Nutrition is a basic human need that changes throughout the life cycle and along the wellness–illness continuum. Food provides nutrition for the body and the mind. Eating has evolved from being simply a necessity; it may be a source of pleasure, a pasttime, a social happening, a political statement, a religious symbol, a cultural emblem, or an integral component of medical treatment. As such, food, eating, and nutrition take on different meanings to different individuals, and changing a person's eating behaviors may be a difficult and slow process. However, because nutrition is vital for life and health and because poor nutrition can seriously decrease one's level of wellness, nutrition is a vital component of nursing.

This chapter provides a knowledge base of basic nutrition theory, focusing on the six classes of nutrients, energy balance, choosing an adequate diet, food patterns and habits, and factors affecting nutrition. Components of simple screening and in-depth nutritional assessments are outlined. Two sets of nursing diagnoses are provided, and client goals for healthy nutrition are discussed. In the section entitled "Nursing Process in Clinical Practice," focused assessment, diagnosis, planning, implementation, and evaluation guides are offered for select nursing diagnoses related to nutritional alterations: more than body requirement, less than body requirement, and knowledge deficit related to a new medical diet. These guides and the concluding case study illustrate the significance of nutrition in nursing care.

PRINCIPLES OF NUTRITION

The science of **nutrition** encompasses the study of nutrients and how they are handled by the body as well as the impact of human behavior and environment on the process of nourishment. As such, this discipline includes physiology, psychology, and socioeconomics.

Nutrients are specific biochemical substances used by the body for growth, development, activity, reproduction, lactation, health maintenance, and recovery from illness or injury. Because the metabolic processes involved in these functions are complex, most nutrients tend to work better together than they do alone. Also, nutrient needs change throughout the life cycle in response to changes in body size, activity, growth, development, and state of health.

Some nutrients are considered essential because they are either not synthesized in the body or they are made in insufficient amounts; essential nutrients must be provided in the diet or through supplements. Nonessential nutrients do not have to be supplied through exogenous sources because either they are not required for body functioning or the body synthesizes them in adequate amounts. Some nutrients can be converted to others in the body. For instance, the body converts excess carbohydrates and protein into fat and stores them as triglycerides.

Of the six classes of nutrients, three supply energy (carbohydrates, protein, and lipids) and three regulate body processes (vitamins, minerals, and water).

Energy Balance

Energy in the diet is measured in the form of kilocalories, commonly abbreviated as **calories** or cal (kilojoule—KJ—in Canada). Only carbohydrates, protein, and fat (and alcohol) provide energy; vitamins and minerals are needed for the metabolism of energy but do not provide calories. Total energy intake for a meal, a day, or longer, can be calculated by using food composition tables: the values given for total calories for each food eaten can simply be added or the grams of carbohydrate, protein, and fat for each food eaten can be added and multiplied by the appropriate calorie level (4, 4, and 9 calories, respectively).

Energy in the body is used to carry on any kind of activity, whether voluntary or involuntary. A person's total daily energy expenditure is the sum of all the calories used to

Perform Physical Activity.

The amount of energy a person expends on physical activity depends on the intensity and duration of the activity and also on the person's weight. Obviously, heavier people expend more energy than lighter people doing the same activity because more energy is required to move their bodies. Mechanization and an increase in leisure time (that we tend to use observing activity rather than participating in it) have led to a general decrease in peoples' energy expenditure.

Maintain Basal Metabolism.

Basal metabolism is the amount of energy required to carry on the involuntary activities of the body at rest, such as maintaining body temperature and muscle tone, producing and releasing secretions, propelling food through the GI tract, inflating the lungs, and beating the heart. As the amount of energy used on physical activity declines, the proportion of calories used for basal metabolism increases; it accounts for more than half of most people's total energy requirements. Because of their larger muscle mass males have a higher basal metabolic rate (BMR) than females. Other factors that increase BMR include growth, infections, fever, emotional tension, extreme environmental temperatures, and elevated levels of certain hormones, especially epinephrine and thyroid hormones. Aging, prolonged fasting, and sleep all decrease BMR. Generally, BMR is about 1 cal/kg of body weight/hr for men and 0.9 cal/kg/hr for women.

Digest, Absorb, and Metabolize Food, Otherwise Known as Specific Dynamic Action (SDA).

Because the metabolism of protein requires a lot of energy, high-protein meals may increase BMR by as much as 15% to 30%. However, the SDA of a normal, mixed diet is about 6% to 10% of the total calorie intake. For instance, a person

eating a 2,000-calorie diet uses about 120 to 200 calories to process food.

A person's state of energy balance can be determined by comparing energy intake to energy output. A person is in a neutral energy balance (*i.e.*, maintaining their weight) when energy intake equals output. A positive balance occurs (*i.e.*, weight gain) when calorie input exceeds output. A negative energy balance and weight loss result when calorie input is less than calorie output.

Ideal body weight (IBW) is an estimate of optimal weight for optimal health. Although numerous tables and approaches have been devised for determining ideal

T A B L E   31-1

1983 Metropolitan Life Insurance Co. Height and Weight Tables

Height	Small Frame	Medium Frame	Large Frame
		lb	
Men*			
5' 2"	128–134	131–141	138–150
5' 3"	130–136	133–143	140–153
5' 4"	132–138	135–145	142–156
5' 5"	134–140	137–148	144–160
5' 6"	136–142	139–151	146–164
5' 7"	138–145	142–154	149–168
5' 8"	140–148	145–157	152–172
5' 9"	142–151	148–160	155–176
5' 10"	144–154	151–163	158–180
5' 11"	146–157	154–166	161–184
6' 0"	149–160	157–170	164–188
6' 1"	152–164	160–174	168–192
6' 2"	155–168	164–178	172–197
6' 3"	158–172	167–182	176–202
6' 4"	162–176	171–187	181–207
Women†			
4' 10"	102–111	109–121	118–131
4' 11"	103–113	111–123	120–134
5' 0"	104–115	113–126	122–137
5' 1"	106–118	115–129	125–140
5' 2"	108–121	118–132	128–143
5' 3"	111–124	121–135	131–147
5' 4"	114–127	124–138	134–151
5' 5"	117–130	127–141	137–155
5' 6"	120–133	130–144	140–159
5' 7"	123–136	133–147	143–163
5' 8"	126–139	136–150	146–167
5' 9"	129–142	139–153	149–170
5' 10"	132–145	142–156	152–173
5' 11"	135–148	145–159	155–176
6' 0"	138–151	148–162	158–179

* Weights at ages 25 to 59 based on lowest mortality. Weight in pounds according to frame (in indoor clothing weighing 5 lb, shoes with 1-inch heels).

† Weights at ages 25 to 59 based on lowest mortality. Weight in pounds according to frame (in indoor clothing weighing 3 lb, shoes with 1-inch heels). (Courtesy of Statistical Bulletin, Metropolitan Life Insurance Company)

weight (see Table 31-1), opinion varies as to what method is most accurate. A general guideline for adult women is to allow 100 lb for the first 5 feet of height and add 5 lb for each additional inch. A range spanning 10% below and above is considered normal depending on body frame size. For men, the guidelines suggest 106 lb for the first 5 feet of height, with an additional 6 lb for each additional inch of height. Again, this weight can be adjusted up or down by 10%, depending on body frame. (Height and weight tables are generally used for infants and children.) Usually, a person is considered **overweight** if he weighs 10% to 20% more than ideal and obese if he weighs more than 20% above ideal weight for height.

Just like ideal body weight can be determined in a variety of ways, so can a person's calorie requirements (Table 31-2*). The National Academy of Sciences has also published recommended energy intake ranges based on age and sex (Table 31-3). The Bureau of Nutritional Sciences of the Department of National Health and Welfare (Canada) has developed a similar energy requirement table (Appendix D-1).† After calorie requirements have been determined, adjustments can be made for weight gain or loss as needed. For instance, 1 lb of body fat equals about 3,500 cal. Therefore, to gain or lose 1 lb in a week, daily calorie intake should be increased or decreased, respectively, by 500 cal (3,500 cal divided by 7 days = 500 cal/day). Similarly, a weight gain or loss of 2 lb per week would require an adjustment of 1,000 cal/day. Because it becomes increasingly difficult to plan an adequate diet as the calorie level drops, diets resulting in more than a 2 lb weight loss per week are not recommended.

* Tables 31-2, 31-4 to 31-6, 31-8, 31-9, and 31-11 to 31-13 from Dudek SG: Nutrition Handbook for Nursing Practice; Philadelphia, JB Lippincott, 1987.

† All tables referring to nutrition for Canada have been placed together in Appendix D.

TABLE 31-2
Three Methods of Calculating Calorie Requirements

Method I

Adults

Multiply ideal body weight (IBW) by 10 to determine basal body requirements. Depending on activity level, multiply IBW by the appropriate number indicated below and add to the basal body requirement.

Activity	Calories
Sedentary	Basal calorie needs × 3
Moderate	Basal calorie needs × 5
Heavy	Basal calorie needs × 10

Children (under 12 years old)

Generally allow 1000 calories plus 100 calories/year of age. For example, a 4-year-old child needs approximately 1000 + (100 calories × 4) = 1400 calories.

Method II

Depending on activity level, multiply IBW in pounds by the appropriate number of calories.

Activity	Cal/lb of IBW
Sedentary	11–12
Light	13–14
Moderate	15–16
Heavy	18–19

Method III: USDA Guidelines for Calculating Calorie Requirements

Based upon activity level, multiply IBW in pounds by the appropriate number of calories/pound according to sex.

Activity	Cal/lb of IBW	
	Males	Females
Sedentary	16	14
Moderate	21	18
Heavy	28	22

T A B L E   31-3
Mean Heights and Weights and Recommended Energy Intake*

Age	Weight		Height		Energy Needs (with range)	
(Years)	(kg)	(lb)	(cm)	(in)	(kcal)	(MJ)
Infants						
0.0–0.5	6	13	60	24	kg × 115 kg × (95–145)	kg × .48
0.5–1.0	9	20	71	28	kg × 105 kg × (80–135)	kg × .44
Children						
1–3	13	29	90	35	1300 (900–1800)	5.5
4–6	20	44	112	44	1700 (1300–2300)	7.1
7–10	28	62	132	52	2400 (1650–3300)	10.1
Males						
11–14	45	99	157	62	2700 (2000–3700)	11.3
15–18	66	145	176	69	2800 (2100–3900)	11.8
19–22	70	154	177	70	2900 (2500–3300)	12.2
23–50	70	154	178	70	2700 (2300–3100)	11.3
51–75	70	154	178	70	2400 (2000–2800)	10.1
76+	70	154	178	70	2050 (1650–2450)	8.6
Females						
11–14	46	101	157	62	2200 (1500–3000)	9.2
15–18	55	120	163	64	2100 (1200–3000)	8.8
19–22	55	120	163	64	2100 (1700–2500)	8.8
23–50	55	120	163	64	2000 (1600–2400)	8.4
51–75	55	120	163	64	1800 (1400–2200)	7.6
76+	55	120	163	64	1600 (1200–2000)	6.7
Pregnant					+300	
Lactating					+500	

* The data in this table have been assembled from the observed median heights and weights of children together with desirable weights for adults for the mean heights of men (70 inches) and women (64 inches) between the ages of 18 and 34 years as surveyed in the United States population (HEW/NCHS data).

The energy allowances for the young adults are for men and women doing light work. The allowances for the two older groups represent mean energy needs over these age spans, allowing for a 2% decrease in basal (resting) metabolic rate per decade and a reduction in activity of 200 kcal/day for men and women between 51 and 75 years, 500 kcal for men over 75 years and 400 kcal for women over 75. The customary range of daily energy output is shown in parentheses for adults and is based on a variation in energy needs of ±400 kcal at any one age, emphasizing the wide range of energy intakes appropriate for any group of people.

Energy allowances for children through age 18 are based on median energy intakes of children of these ages followed in longitudinal growth studies. The values in parentheses are 10th and 90th percentiles of energy intake, to indicate the range of energy consumption among children of these ages.

(National Academy of Sciences: Recommended Dietary Allowances, 9th rev. ed. Washington, DC, 1980)

Energy Nutrients

Carbohydrates

Significance. Carbohydrates, commonly known as sugars and starches, are organic compounds composed of carbon, hydrogen, and oxygen. Generally, carbohydrates serve as the structural framework of plants; the only animal source of carbohydrate in the diet is lactose, or "milk sugar."

The significance of carbohydrates cannot be overstated. Because they are relatively easy to produce and store, carbohydrates are the most abundant and least expensive source of calories in the diet worldwide. In fact, carbohydrate intake is correlated to income: as income increases, carbohydrate intake decreases and protein intake, a more expensive form of energy, increases. In countries where grains are the dietary staple, carbohydrates may contribute as much as 90% of total calories. In the United States, the average person consumes about 45% of total calories from carbohydrates, an amount many health professionals believe should be higher. In Canada the amount is 40% (Recommended Nutrient Intakes for Canadians, 1983).

Classification. Depending on the number of molecules within the structure, carbohydrates are classified as either simple sugars (monosaccharides and disaccharides) or complex (polysaccharides). **Monosaccharides** are composed of only one sugar molecule; as the simplest sugar, they are absorbed without undergoing digestion. Monosaccharides with nutritional significance include glucose (dextrose), fructose, and galactose.

Disaccharides are double sugars composed of glucose and one other monosaccharide. Disaccharides (*i.e.,* sucrose, lactose, and maltose) must be broken down by enzymes within the intestinal tract before they can be absorbed.

Polysaccharides, like starch, glycogen, cellulose, and other types of fiber, are complex molecules composed of hundreds to thousands of glucose units. They are not sweet and vary in their degree of digestability. Table 31-4 summarizes the sources, functions, and significance of dietary carbohydrates.

Metabolism. Carbohydrates are more easily and quickly digested than protein and fat. Generally, 90% of carbohydrate intake is digested, although the percentage decreases as fiber intake increases.

Although a small amount of cooked starch may begin to be digested in the mouth, the primary site of chemical digestion is the small intestine. Polysaccharides and disaccharides are broken down into monosaccharides through the action of pancreatic and intestinal enzymes, which are complex protein molecules that facilitate chemical reactions without undergoing change themselves. Monosaccharides are absorbed through the intestinal mucosa and transported to the liver through the portal blood circulation. Cellulose and other undigestible fibers cannot be digested by human enzymes and are therefore excreted in the feces unchanged.

In the liver, monosaccharides are converted to glucose, which may then be released into the bloodstream to keep serum glucose levels within a normal range (Fig. 31-1). Under normal conditions, certain tissues, particularly the central nervous system, rely on glucose as their sole source of fuel; therefore a constant supply of glucose is necessary. Hormones, especially insulin and glucagon, are responsible for keeping serum glucose levels fairly constant during both feasting and fasting.

Through a series of steps, cells oxidize (burn) glucose to provide energy, carbon dioxide, and water. Depending on a person's state of energy balance, the period between carbohydrate consumption and when it is used

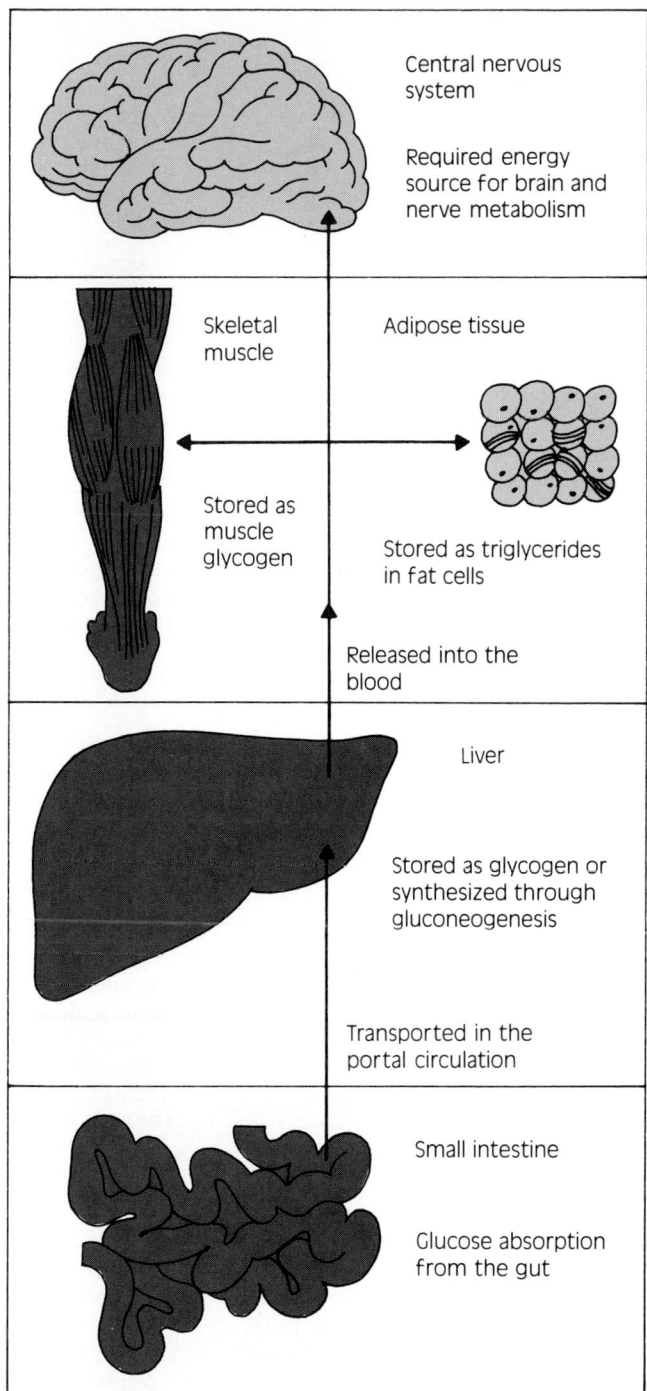

FIGURE 31-1

Glucose is an efficient fuel on which certain tissues, particularly the central nervous system, relies almost exclusively as an energy source. Glucose ingested in the diet is transported from the gastrointestinal tract, through the portal vein, to the liver. The liver stores glucose and regulates its entry into the blood. (Adapted from Porth CM: Pathophysiology: Concepts of Altered Health States, 2nd ed, p 604. Philadelphia, JB Lippincott, 1986)

T A B L E   31-4
Sources, Functions, and Significance of Carbohydrates, Protein, and Fat

Nutrient	Sources	Functions	Significance
Carbohydrates			
Simple sugars and starch	Fruits Vegetables Grains: rice, pasta, breads, cereals Dried peas and beans Milk (lactose) Sugars: white and brown sugar, honey, molasses, syrup	Provide energy Spare protein so it can be used for other functions Prevent ketosis from inefficient fat metabolism	Provide about 46% of the calories in the typical American diet (40% in Canadian); many believe carbohydrate intake should be increased to 50%–60% of total calories Low carbohydrate intake can cause ketosis; high simple sugar intake increases the risk of dental caries.
Cellulose and other water-insoluble fibers	Whole wheat flour and wheat bran Vegetables: cabbage, peas, green beans, wax beans, broccoli, brussel sprouts, cucumber skins, peppers, carrots Apples	Absorbs water to increase fecal bulk Decreases intestinal transit time	Is nondigestable, therefore it is excreted Helps relieve constipation North Americans are urged to eat more of all types of fiber. Excess intake can cause gas, distention, and diarrhea.
Water-soluble fibers	Oat bran and oatmeal Dried peas and beans Vegetables Prunes, pears, apples, bananas, oranges	Slow gastric emptying Lower serum cholesterol Delay glucose absorption	Help improve glucose tolerance in diabetics
Protein			
	Milk and milk products Meat, poultry, fish Eggs Dried peas and beans Nuts	Tissue growth and repair Component of body framework: bones, muscles, tendons, blood vessels, skin, hair, nails Component of body fluids: hormones, enzymes, plasma proteins, neurotransmitters, mucus Help regulate fluid balance through oncotic pressure Help regulate acid–base balance Detoxify harmful substances Form antibodies Transport fat and other substances through the blood Provide energy when carbohydrate intake is not adequate	Most North Americans consume twice the RDA (RNI) for protein. Experts recommend we eat less animal protein and more vegetable protein. Protein deficiency is characterized by edema, retarded growth and maturation, muscular wasting, changes in the hair and skin, permanent damage to physical and mental development (in children), diarrhea, malabsorption, numerous secondary nutrient deficiencies, fatty infiltration of the liver, increased risk of infections, and high mortality. Except for the elderly, fad dieters, hospitalized clients, and people of low income, protein deficiency is rare in the US and Canada.
Fat			
	Butter, oils, margarine, lard, salt pork, salad dressings, mayonnaise, bacon Whole milk and whole milk products High fat meats Nuts	Provides energy Provides structure Insulates the body Cushions internal organs Necessary for the absorption of the fat-soluble vitamins	Fat supplies about 42% of total calories in the typical North American diet; experts suggest a reduction to 30%–35% or less. High-fat diets increase the risk of heart disease and obesity, and are correlated with an increased risk of colon and breast cancers.

for energy may vary from minutes to months or longer. Unlike protein and fat, glucose is burned efficiently and completely and does not leave a toxic product for the kidneys to excrete.

When the supply of glucose exceeds what is needed for energy and to maintain serum levels, it is stored. If muscle or liver glycogen stores are deficient, glucose is converted to glycogen and stored (glycogenesis). Conversely, glycogen is broken down in time of need to supply a ready source of glucose (glycogenolysis). When glycogen stores are adequate, the body converts excess glucose to fat and stores it as triglycerides in adipose tissue.

Functions and Recommended Dietary Allowance (RDA). The primary function of carbohydrates is to supply energy. Except for undigestable fiber, all carbohydrates provide 4 cal/g regardless of the source. Carbohydrates also function to spare protein (*i.e.,* using carbohydrates for energy "spares" protein so it can be used to carry on functions specific for protein, like building and repairing tissue). Carbohydrates are also needed to efficiently burn fat for energy and thereby prevent ketosis. Although an exact requirement for carbohydrates has not been established, at least 50 g to 100 g are needed daily to prevent ketosis. In terms of an optimum diet, most health experts recommend that carbohydrates provide 50% to 60% of the diet's total calories, mostly in the form of complex carbohydrates.

Protein

Significance. Protein is a vital component of every living cell. Within the human body, more than a thousand different proteins are made by combining various amounts and proportions of the 22 basic building blocks known as **amino acids.** Although amino acids contain carbon hydrogen, and oxygen like carbohydrates, they differ in that amino acids also contain nitrogen. Nine amino acids are classified as essential because they cannot be synthesized in the body; the remaining amino acids are no less important, but because the body can make them if a supply of nitrogen is available, they are termed nonessential.

Classification. Dietary proteins may be labeled complete (high quality) or incomplete (low quality) based on their amino acid composition. **Complete proteins** contain sufficient amounts and proportions of all the essential amino acids to support growth, whereas **incomplete proteins** are deficient in one or more essential amino acids. Generally, animal proteins (eggs, dairy products, and meats) are complete and plant proteins (grains, legumes, and vegetables) are incomplete. However, because different sources of plant proteins lack different amino acids, plant proteins can be "complemented," and its quality made high, by combining them with a different plant protein or by adding a small amount of an animal protein. Examples of complementary vegetable proteins include corn tortilla and refried beans and lentil rice soup (Fig. 31-2). Complementary proteins using a small amount of animal protein are cereal with milk, rice pudding, and cheese sandwiches.

Metabolism. Chemical digestion of protein begins in the acid medium of the stomach; however, most pro-

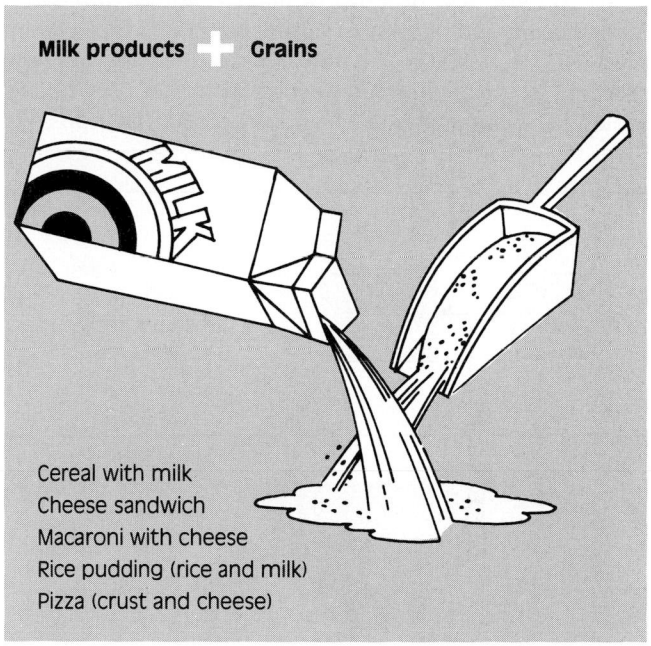

Milk products + Grains

Cereal with milk
Cheese sandwich
Macaroni with cheese
Rice pudding (rice and milk)
Pizza (crust and cheese)

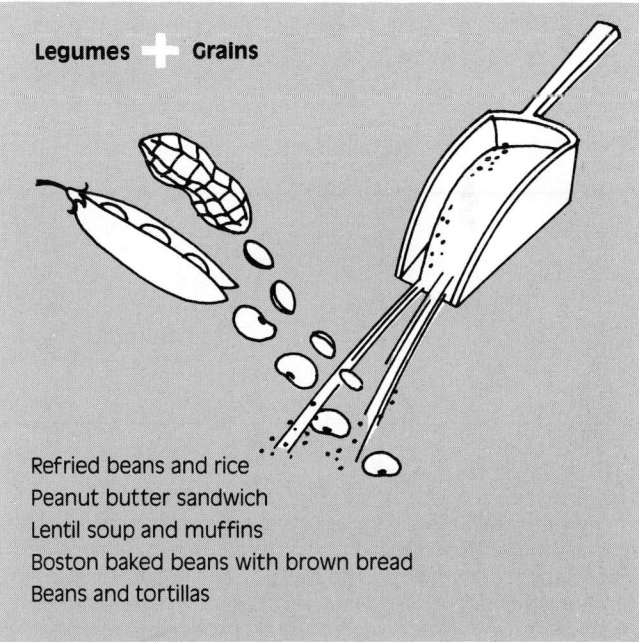

Legumes + Grains

Refried beans and rice
Peanut butter sandwich
Lentil soup and muffins
Boston baked beans with brown bread
Beans and tortillas

FIGURE   31-2
Combinations of legumes and grains, and milk products and grains in appropriate quantities at the same meal provide high-quality proteins in complement.

tein digestion occurs in the small intestine through the action of pancreatic and intestinal proteases. Amino acids are absorbed through the intestinal mucosa into the portal blood circulation for transportation to the liver. Newborns are uniquely able to absorb whole proteins, namely antibodies from breast milk, which affords them a certain degree of immunity from infections. Normally only a small amount of ingested protein remains undigested and is excreted in the feces.

Once in the liver, amino acids can then be recombined to form new proteins or may be released into the bloodstream and carried to tissues and cells for protein synthesis (Fig. 31-3). The body's protein tissues are in a constant state of flux: tissues are continuously being broken down (catabolism) and replaced (anabolism).

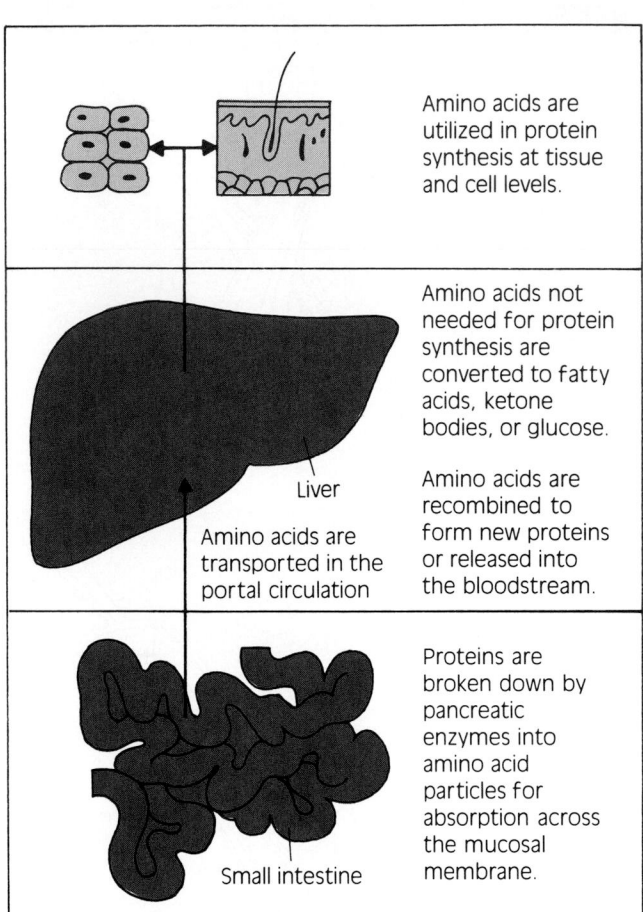

Amino acids are utilized in protein synthesis at tissue and cell levels.

Amino acids not needed for protein synthesis are converted to fatty acids, ketone bodies, or glucose.

Liver

Amino acids are recombined to form new proteins or released into the bloodstream.

Amino acids are transported in the portal circulation

Proteins are broken down by pancreatic enzymes into amino acid particles for absorption across the mucosal membrane.

Small intestine

F I G U R E   31-3

Dietary protein is broken down into amino acid particles by pancreatic enzymes in the small intestine and absorbed through the intestinal mucosa for transportation to the liver. In the liver, amino acids are recombined into new proteins or are released into the bloodstream for use in protein synthesis by tissues and cells. Excess amino acids are converted to fatty acids, ketone bodies, or glucose, and stored or used as metabolic fuel. Proteins are essential for the formation of all body structures, including genes, enzymes, muscle, bone matrix, and hemoglobin. Amino acids are the building blocks of protein.

Nitrogen balance, a comparison between catabolism and anabolism, can be measured by comparing nitrogen intake (protein intake) and nitrogen excretion (nitrogen lost in urine, urea, feces, hair, nails, and skin). When catabolism and anabolism are occurring at the same rate, like in healthy adults, the body is in a state of neutral nitrogen balance (*i.e.,* nitrogen intake equals nitrogen excretion). A positive nitrogen balance occurs when nitrogen intake is greater than excretion, like during periods of growth, pregnancy, lactation, and recovery from illness. A negative nitrogen balance, an undesirable state such as starvation and the catabolism that immediately follows surgery, illness, trauma, and stress, indicates that more nitrogen is being excreted than consumed.

Functions. The major function of protein is to maintain body tissues that break down from normal "wear and tear" and to support the growth of new tissue. Protein is also a component of the body's framework (bones, muscles, tendons, blood vessels, skin, nails, hair), many essential secretions and fluids (hormones, enzymes, neurotransmitters, breast milk, mucus, sperm, bile acids), and body compounds like the blood clotting factor thrombin. Protein plays a role in fluid balance and acid–base balance, helps to detoxify harmful foreign substances, and forms antibodies to help the body resist infection and certain diseases. It helps move fat, fat-soluble vitamins, minerals, and other substances through the blood. Lastly, protein can be oxidized to provide 4 cal/g. However, using protein for energy is not only more financially expensive than using carbohydrates, but is physiologically costly as well: the nitrogen remaining after protein is metabolized burdens the kidneys and requires energy in order to be excreted. Like carbohydrates, protein consumed in excess need can be converted to and stored as fat.

RDA. The recommended daily dietary allowance for protein for adults is 0.8 g/kg, or about 44 g for the average woman and 56 g for the average man (National Research Council, 1980). In Canada the figures are 0.74 g/kg for adult females and 0.82 g/kg for adult males (Recommended Nutrient Intakes for Canadians, 1983). Most Americans consume twice as much protein as this, mostly in the form of animal proteins. Many experts agree that protein intake should be modified to include more plant proteins and less animal proteins, which tend to be high in saturated fat and cholesterol. Table 31-4 summarizes the sources, functions, and significance of protein.

With the exception of elderly persons, hospitalized clients, fad dieters, some pregnant women, and people of low socioeconomic status, protein deficiency is rare in North America. However, in developing countries, protein deficiency alone (kwashiorkor) or combined with calorie undernutrition (marasmus), is a leading cause of infant death. Signs and symptoms of protein deficiency include edema, retarded growth and maturation, mental apathy, muscular wasting, and changes in the hair and skin.

Lipids

Significance. Lipids, commonly known as fats, are insoluble in water and therefore insoluble in blood. Like carbohydrates, they are composed of carbon, hydrogen, and oxygen. Ninety-five percent of the lipids in the diet are in the form of fats and oils, otherwise known as simple lipids. Compound lipids (like phospholipids, where a lipid is combined with another substance) and derived lipids (like cholesterol) constitute the remainder of the lipid intake.

Triglycerides are the predominant form of fat in food and also the major storage form of fat in the body. Triglycerides are composed of a glycerol molecule and three fatty acids, which vary in length and degree of saturation. Most food fats are composed of long chain fatty acids (*i.e.*, they contain more than 12 carbon atoms).

Classification. Saturated fatty acids are not able to hold any more hydrogen atoms; their carbon bonds are all saturated. Unsaturated fatty acids have one (monounsaturated) or more (polyunsaturated) double bonds between carbon atoms; therefore they have the potential to hold more hydrogen atoms if the double bonds are broken. Food fats contain mixtures of both saturated and unsaturated fatty acids. Generally, animal fats are considered saturated because they contain proportionately more saturated fatty acids then unsaturated fatty acids. Conversely, most vegetable fats are considered unsaturated because they contain more unsaturated than saturated. Commercially, the addition of hydrogen atoms to unsaturated fats (hydrogenation) makes a fat more saturated and thereby increases its shelf life and stability. However, saturated fats tend to raise serum cholesterol levels whereas unsaturated fats lower serum cholesterol.

Cholesterol is a fatlike substance found only in animal products. It is not essential that cholesterol be provided in the diet because the body synthesizes about twice as much cholesterol as most people in North America eat. Cholesterol is an important component of cell membranes and is especially abundant in brain and nerve cells. Cholesterol is also used to synthesize bile acids and is a precursor of the steroid hormones and vitamin D. Although cholesterol serves many important functions in the body, high serum levels are clearly associated with an increased risk of atherosclerosis. To help lower serum cholesterol levels, researchers recommend limiting cholesterol intake, eating less total fat, especially saturated fat, eating more unsaturated fat, and increasing fiber intake, which increases fecal excretion of cholesterol.

Linoleic acid is the only fatty acid the body cannot synthesize; therefore it is labeled essential. Linoleic acid is important for capillary strength and cell membrane structure, is a precursor of prostaglandins, and helps decrease serum cholesterol levels. Because the requirement for linoleic acid is so small (about 2% to 3% of total calories), a deficiency is rare. The best sources of linoleic acid are polyunsaturated vegetable oils like sunflower, soybean, and corn.

Metabolism. Fat digestion occurs largely in the small intestine. Bile, secreted by the gallbladder, emulsifies fat to increase the surface area so that pancreatic lipase can break down fat more effectively. Through a complex series of events, most fats are absorbed into the lymphatic circulation with the help of a protein carrier and are transported to the liver (Fig. 31-4). Of 100 g eaten, only about 3 g are excreted in the feces.

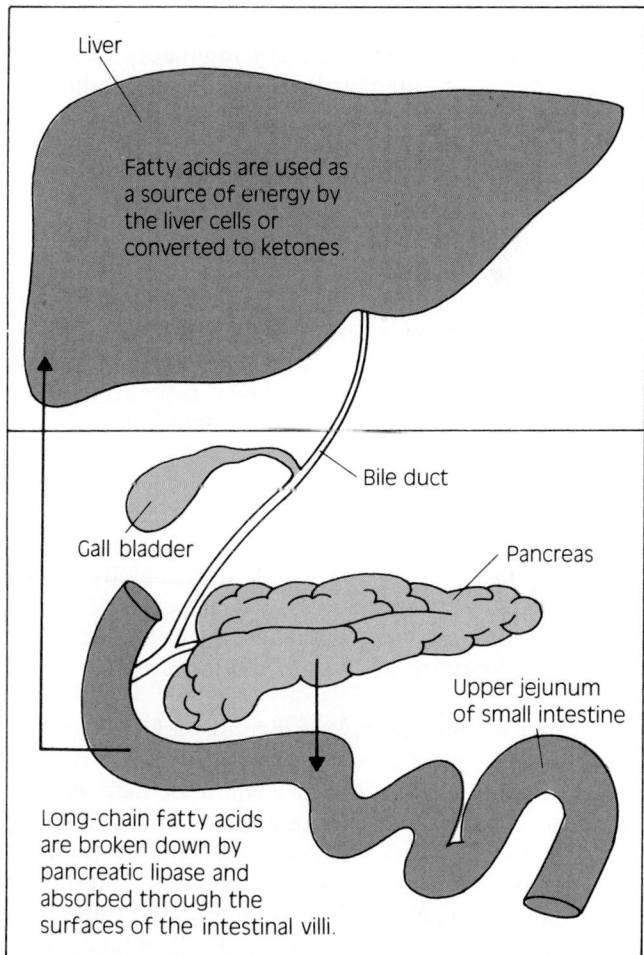

Liver

Fatty acids are used as a source of energy by the liver cells or converted to ketones.

Bile duct

Gall bladder

Pancreas

Upper jejunum of small intestine

Long-chain fatty acids are broken down by pancreatic lipase and absorbed through the surfaces of the intestinal villi.

FIGURE 31-4

The average adult consumes 60 to 100 grams of fat daily, mostly as triglycerides. These triglycerides are broken down by pancreatic lipase and are absorbed primarily in the upper jejunum. Fatty acids transported to the liver are used by the liver cells as a source of energy or are converted to ketones.

Functions. Fats are the most concentrated source of energy in the diet, providing 9 calories for every gram. Fat increases the palatability of the diet (*e.g.,* to most people, filet mignon tastes better than flank steak) and has a high satiety value because it delays gastric emptying time. In the body, fat aids in the absorption of the fat-soluble vitamins and provides insulation, structure, and temperature control. Table 31-4 summarizes the source, functions, and significance of fat.

RDA. Because fat can be synthesized in the body from carbohydrates and protein, a recommended daily dietary allowance for fat has not been established. Currently, Americans and Canadians consume about 42% of their total calorie intake in the form of fat. Most experts agree that fat should not contribute more than 30% to 35% of the day's calorie intake.

Regulatory Nutrients

Vitamins, minerals, and water are regulatory nutrients because they are needed by the body for the metabolism of energy nutrients.

Vitamins

Vitamins are organic compounds needed by the body in small amounts. Most vitamins are active in the form of a coenzyme, which together with enzymes, facilitate thousands of chemical reactions in the body. Although vitamins do not provide energy (calories), they are needed for the metabolism of carbohydrates, protein, and fat. Because most vitamins are not synthesized in the body, or are made in insufficient quantities, vitamins are essential in the diet.

Vitamins are present in foods in only small amounts. Because vitamins may be destroyed by light, heat, air, and during preparation, fresh foods are generally higher in vitamins than processed foods. The exception is in the case of fortification, where vitamins that don't occur naturally in a food are added (*e.g.,* Vitamin D fortified milk).

In North America severe vitamin deficiencies are rare. However, mild or subclinical deficiencies of vitamin A, vitamin C, folate, and vitamin B_6 may affect a significant proportion of the population, especially those who (1) are members of certain age groups (infants, adolescents, pregnant and lactating women, and the elderly), (2) smoke, abuse alcohol, or use medications on a long-term basis, (3) are chronically ill, either physically or psychologically, and (4) are poor or finicky eaters, like chronic dieters, strict vegetarians, and food faddists.

Vitamins are classified as either water-soluble or fat-soluble. The water-soluble vitamins are vitamin C and the B-complex vitamins. Water-soluble vitamins are absorbed through the intestinal wall directly into the bloodstream. Although some tissues are able to hold limited amounts of water-soluble vitamins, they are generally not stored in the body. Deficiency symptoms are apt to develop quickly when intake is inadequate; therefore a daily intake is recommended. Because water-soluble vitamins are not stored, amounts consumed in excess of need are excreted in the urine. Toxicities are not likely, although megadoses of certain water-soluble vitamins can be harmful.

Vitamins A, D, E, and K, the fat-soluble vitamins, are absorbed with fat into the lymphatic circulation; like fat, they must be attached to a protein in order to be transported through the blood. Secondary deficiencies of the fat-soluble vitamins can occur any time fat digestion or absorption is altered, like during malabsorption syndromes and pancreatic and biliary diseases. The body stores excesses of the fat-soluble vitamins mostly in the liver and adipose tissue. Because they are stored, a daily intake is not imperative, and deficiency symptoms may take weeks to months to years to develop. Excessive intakes, particularly of vitamins A and D, are toxic.

Table 31-5 summarizes water- and fat-soluble vitamins. (Canadian Recommended Nutrient Intakes [RNIs] are listed in Appendix D-2.)

Minerals

Minerals are inorganic elements found in all body fluids and tissues in the forms of salts (*e.g.,* sodium chloride) or combined with organic compounds (*e.g.,* iron in hemoglobin). Some minerals function to provide structure within the body, whereas others help regulate body processes. Because they are elements, they are not broken down or rearranged in the body, but are contained in the ash that remains after digestion. Although excessive soaking and cooking in water can cause loss of minerals from food, they are generally not destroyed by food processing. Calcium, phosphorus, and magnesium are considered macrominerals because they are found in the body in amounts greater than 5 g and are needed by the body in amounts greater than 100 mg/day. Microminerals, also known as **trace elements**, are found in the body in amounts less than 5 g and are needed in only very small amounts (18 mg or less). Trace elements with an established RDA and RNI (Canada) include iron, iodine, and zinc. Ranges of estimated safe and adequate daily intakes have been suggested for copper, manganese, fluorine, chromium, selenium, molybdenum; no recommendations have been made for cobalt, nickel, vanadium, arsenic, and silicon. Macro- and microminerals are summarized in Table 31-6. (Canadian RNIs are listed in Appendix D.)

Water

As the major body constituent present in every body cell, water accounts for between 50% and 60% of the adult's total weight; infants have proportionately more water.

(Text continues on p. 771.)

TABLE 31-5
Summary of Water- and Fat-Soluble Vitamins*

Nutrient and Adult RDA	Sources	Functions	Signs and Symptoms of Deficiency	Signs and Symptoms of Excess	Pharmacologic Uses
Water-Soluble Vitamins					
Vitamin C (ascorbic acid) 60 mg	Citrus fruits and juices, guava, broccoli, brussel sprouts, green pepper, strawberries, "greens," tomatoes, cabbage	Collagen formation, protects other nutrients from oxidation, enhances iron absorption, converts folic acid to its active form, involved in the metabolism of certain amino acids	Scurvy, characterized by bleeding gums; hemorrhaging; muscle degeneration; delayed wound healing; softening of the bones; soft, loose teeth; anemia; increased susceptibility to infection, hysteria and depression	Kidney stones, scurvy upon withdrawal, nausea, abdominal cramps, diarrhea, false-positive test for urinary glucose	Only proven effective use is to treat scurvy; there is no evidence that it cures or prevents colds, cures cancer, or improves breathing in asthmatics
Vitamin B complex B₁ (thiamine) 1.0 mg– 1.4 mg	Pork, liver, organ meats, whole grain and enriched grains, nuts, dried peas and beans, eggs	Energy metabolism, especially the metabolism of carbohydrates, normal nervous system functioning	Beriberi, mental confusion, fatigue, peripheral paralysis, muscle weakness, painful calf muscles, anorexia, edema, enlarged heart, heart failure	None known	Used only to treat thiamine deficiency
B₂ Riboflavin 1.2 mg– 1.7 mg	Milk and dairy products, organ meats, eggs, enriched grains, green leafy vegetables	Carbohydrate, protein, and fat metabolism; other metabolic functions	Ariboflavinosis, dermatitis, cheilosis, glossitis, photophobia, reddening of the cornea	None known	Used only to treat riboflavin deficiency
Niacin 13 mg–19 mg	Kidney, liver, poultry, lean meat, fish, yeast, peanut butter, enriched and whole grains, dried peas and beans, nuts	Carbohydrate, protein, and fat metabolism	Pellagra, dermatitis, diarrhea, dementia, death	Flushing and itching, nausea, vomiting, diarrhea, hypotension, tachycardia, hypoglycemia, and liver damage	To treat niacin deficiency and pellagra; megadoses of nicotinic acid used to lower serum cholesterol in people who do not respond adequately to diet and weight loss
B₆ 2.0 mg– 2.2 mg	Yeast, wheat germ, pork, organ meats, egg yolk, whole grain cereals, potatoes	Amino acid metabolism, blood formation, maintenance of nervous tissue, conversion of tryptophan to niacin	Dermatitis, cheilosis, glossitis, abnormal brain wave pattern, convulsions, anemia	Difficulty walking, numbness of the feet and hands, sensations of shock	Used to treat vitamin B₆ deficiency; used experimentally to relieve malaise and depression in women using oral contraceptives; used with some success to relieve nausea and vomiting during pregnancy and following radiation therapy
Folic acid (folacin)	Green leafy vegetables, as-	RNA and DNA synthesis, for-	Macrocytic anemia: fatigue, weakness,	None known	Used to treat folic acid deficiency; used

* See Appendix D for Canadian RNIs.

(Continued)

T A B L E   31-5

Summary of Water- and Fat-Soluble Vitamins*   (Continued)

Nutrient and Adult RDA	Sources	Functions	Signs and Symptoms of Deficiency	Signs and Symptoms of Excess	Pharmacologic Uses
400 µg	paragus, broccoli, liver, organ meats, milk, eggs, yeast, wheat germ	mation and maturation of RBC, amino acid metabolism	pallor, diarrhea, weight loss, glossitis		prophylactically to prevent anemia during pregnancy
B_{12} (cobalamin) 3.0 µg	Only foods of animal origin: meat, fish, seafood, poultry, eggs, milk, dairy products	RNA and DNA synthesis, myelin formation: carbohydrate, protein, and fat metabolism; folic acid metabolism	Pernicious anemia (B_{12} deficiency related to impaired absorption related to the lack of intrinsic factor): macrocytic anemia, pallor, dyspnea, weakness, fatigue, palpitations, glossitis, anorexia, indigestion, recurring diarrhea or constipation, weight loss, paresthesia of the hands and feet, poor muscle coordination, poor memory, irritability, depression, paranoia, delirium, hallucinations	None known	Used only to treat B_{12} deficiency; no evidence exists to support claims that B_{12} relieves infectious hepatitis, multiple sclerosis, poor appetite, poor growth, aging, or fatigue
Pantothenic acid 4 mg–7 mg	Liver, kidney, salmon, egg yolk, fresh vegetables, yeast, whole grain cereals	Carbohydrate, protein, and fat metabolism	None known	None known	Has been credited with improving the burning-food syndrome
Biotin 100 µg–200 µg	Liver, organ meats, peanuts, mushrooms, egg yolk, milk, yeast	Carbohydrate, protein, and fat metabolism; conversion of tryptophan to niacin	Produced by adding large amounts of raw egg white to a biotin-deficient diet. Raw egg white contains avidin, which prevents biotin absorption. Symptoms include dry, scaly dermatitis, anorexia, nausea, vomiting, glossitis, and depression	None known	None known

Fat-Soluble Vitamins

Vitamin A (retinol, retinal, retinoic acid) 800 RE–1000 RE	Liver; egg yolk; fortified milk, dairy products, margarine, breakfast ce-	Visual acuity in dim light, formation and maintenance of skin and	Night blindness; dry, rough skin; dry mucous membranes; dry eyes (xerosis); decreased saliva se-	Anorexia, nausea, vomiting, abdominal pain, diarrhea, weight loss, irritability, fatigue,	To treat vitamin A deficiency; to treat severe, resistant forms of acne (Accutane); used experimentally

(Continued)

Nutrient and Adult RDA	Sources	Functions	Signs and Symptoms of Deficiency	Signs and Symptoms of Excess	Pharmacologic Uses
	reals; dark green and yellow vegetables, such as sweet potatoes, winter squash, carrots, broccoli, spinach, "greens"; peaches; apricots; cantaloupe	mucous membranes, normal growth and development of bones and teeth	cretion leading to difficulty chewing and swallowing, impaired digestion and absorption, diarrhea; increased susceptibility to respiratory, urinary tract, and vaginal infections; impaired bone and teeth development	ascites and portal hypertension, loss of hair, dry skin, bone pain and fragility, spleen enlargement, extensive liver damage, hydrocephalus (in infants and children)	to block the conversion of precancerous cells into cancerous cells
Vitamin D (cholecalciferol, ergosterol) 5 µg–10 µg	Sunlight; fortified milk, margarine, and breakfast cereals; butter; egg yolk; liver; fish liver oils	Calcium and phosphorus metabolism, stimulates calcium absorption, mobilizes calcium and phosphorus from the bone, stimulates reabsorption of calcium and phosphorus by the kidney	Rickets in infants and children: retarded bone growth, bone malformation, enlargement of ends of long bones, malformed teeth, tooth decay; osteomalacia in adults: bone deformities, pain, easy fracture, involuntary muscle twitching and spasms	Excessive calcification of the bones, kidney stones, nausea, vomiting, headache, weakness, weight loss, constipation, polyuria, polydipsia. Mental and physical growth retardation and failure to thrive in children. Drowsiness and coma in severe cases	Used to treat hypocalcemia diseases: rickets, renal osteodystrophy, postoperative tetany, idiopathic tetany, hypoparathyroidism
Vitamin E (tocopherol) 8 mg–10 mg	Vegetable oils, wheat germ, whole grain products	Protects vitamin A and polyunsaturated fatty acids from oxidation, helps maintain cell membrane integrity, heme synthesis	Increased RBC hemolysis and macrocytic anemia in premature infants	Relatively nontoxic, although large doses can cause depression, fatigue, diarrhea, cramps, blurred vision, and headaches; also interferes with normal blood clotting and vitamin A metabolism	Only to treat vitamin E deficiency. Claims that vitamin E treats coronary heart diseases, infertility, cancer, diabetes, ulcers, skin disorders, burns, shortness of breath, and muscular dystrophy are unfounded, as are claims that it increases physical performance and sexual potency and slows the aging process.
Vitamin K 70 µg–140 µg	Dark green leafy vegetables, vegetables of the cabbage family; synthesized in the intestines from gut bacteria	Synthesis of certain proteins necessary for blood clotting	Hemorrhagic disease of the newborn, delayed blood clotting	Hemolytic anemia and liver damage with synthetic vitamin K	Used to treat coagulation disorders related to impaired vitamin K synthesis or absorption; used prophylactically to treat hemorrhagic disease of the newborn; used to treat oral anticoagulant-induced prothrombin deficiency

T A B L E 31-6
Summary of Macro- and Microminerals*

Nutrient and Adult RDA	Sources	Functions	Signs and Symptoms of Deficiency	Signs and Symptoms of Excess
Macrominerals				
Calcium 800 mg	Milk and dairy products, canned fish with bones, green leafy vegetables	Bone and tooth formation, blood clotting, nerve transmission, muscle contraction, cell membrane permeability, activation of certain enzymes	Osteomalacia; osteoporosis; hypocalcemia leads to tetany: intermittent, tonic contractions of the extremities, muscular cramps, uncontrolled seizures, possible convulsions	Hypercalcemia can cause nausea, vomiting, anorexia, abdominal pain, constipation, polyuria, polydipsia, calcium kidney stones, excessive calcification of the bones and soft tissues. Coma and death result if not treated.
Phosphorus 800 mg	Milk and milk products, meat, poultry, fish, eggs, dried peas and beans, nuts, soft drinks, processed foods	Bone and tooth formation, acid–base balance, energy metabolism, cell membrane structure, component of nucleic acids, regulates activity of hormones and coenzymes, fat absorption and transportation, glucose absorption	Hypophosphatemia: anorexia, weakness, circumoral paresthesia, hyperventilation	Hyperphosphatemia: symptoms of hypocalcemia tetany
Magnesium	Green leafy vegetables, nuts, dried peas and beans, grains, seafood, cocoa, chocolate	Bone and tooth formation, smooth muscle relaxation, protein synthesis, carbohydrate metabolism, cell reproduction and growth, hormonal activity	Hypomagnesemia: increased neuromuscular and CNS irritability, loss of muscular control, tremors, disorientation, tetany, convulsions	Hypermagnesemia: CNS depression, coma, hypotension
Sulfur	Meat, fish, poultry, eggs, milk, dried peas and beans, nuts	Store and release energy; structural component of nucleic acids, some vitamins, some amino acids, insulin, and heparin; promotes certain enzyme reactions; detoxification	None known	None known
Sodium 1100 mg–3300 mg†	Salt, sodium-containing preservatives and additives, processed foods, canned meats and vegetables, condiments, pickled foods, soft water, ham, foods prepared in brine solutions, milk, meat, carrots, celery, beets, spinach	Fluid balance, acid–base balance, muscular irritability, cell permeability, nerve impulse transmission	Hyponatremia: cold, clammy skin, decreased skin turgor, apprehension, confusion, irritability, anxiety, hypotension, tachycardia, headache, tremors, convulsions, abdominal cramps, nausea, vomiting, diarrhea	Edema, weight gain; hot, flushed, dry skin; dry red tongue; intense thirst; restless agitation; oliguria or anuria
Potassium 1875 mg–5625 mg†	Whole grains, legumes, fruits, leafy vegetables, broccoli, sweet potatoes, potatoes, meat, tomatoes	Fluid balance, acid–base balance, nerve impulse transmission, striated skeletal and cardiac muscle activity, carbohydrate metabolism, protein synthesis, catalyst for many metabolic reactions	Hypokalemia: muscular cramps and weakness, including cardiac muscle weakness, anorexia, nausea, vomiting, mental depression, confusion, drowsiness, abdominal distention, increased urine output, shallow respiration, irregular pulse	Hyperkalemia: irritability, anxiety, listlessness, mental confusion, nausea, diarrhea, poor respirations, GI hyperactivity, muscular weakness, numbness of the extremities, hypotension cardiac arrhythmia, heart block, cardiac arrest
Chlorine 1700 mg–5100 mg†	Salt	Component of HCl in the stomach, fluid balance, acid–base balance	Hypochloremia: muscle spasms, alkalosis, depressed respiration, possible coma	Hyperchloremia: acidosis

* See Appendix D for Canadian RNIs.

(Continued)

Nutrient and Adult RDA	Sources	Functions	Signs and Symptoms of Deficiency	Signs and Symptoms of Excess
Microminerals				
Iron 10 mg–18 mg	Liver, lean meats, enriched and whole grain breads and cereals	Oxygen transport via hemoglobin and myoglobin, constituent of enzyme systems	Microcytic anemia, pallor, decreased work capacity, fatigue, weakness, spoon-shaped fingernails	Hemosiderosis, acute iron poisoning from accidental overdose leads to GI cramping, nausea, vomiting, possible shock, convulsions, coma
Iodine 150 mg	Iodized salt, seafood, food additives, dough conditioners, dairy disinfectants	Component of thyroid hormones	Goiter	Acne-like skin lesions, "iodine goiter"
Zinc 15 mg	Oysters, liver, meats, poultry, dried peas and beans, nuts	Tissue growth, development, and healing; sexual maturation and reproduction; enzyme formation; immune response	Impaired growth, sexual maturation, and immune system functioning; skin lesions; decreased sense of taste and smell	Anorexia, nausea, vomiting, diarrhea, muscle pain, lethargy, drowsiness, bleeding gastric ulcers, decreased serum levels of high-density lipoproteins (HDL)
Copper 2.0 mg–3.0 mg†	Liver, kidney, shellfish, grains, dried peas and beans, dried fruit, fresh fruit	Bone and blood formation, formation and activity of some enzymes, integrity of heart and large arteries	Anemia, altered bone formation, hypercholesterolemia	Nausea, vomiting, headache, dizziness, heartburn, weakness, diarrhea
Manganese	Whole grain, nuts, dried peas and beans, fruit	Needed for bone formation, reproduction, and blood clotting; protein and energy metabolism	Poor reproductive performance, growth retardation, abnormal bone and cartilage formation, impaired glucose tolerance	None known
Fluorine 1.5 mg–4.0 mg†	Fluoridated water, fish, tea	Tooth formation and integrity, bone formation and integrity	Tooth decay, may increase the risk of osteoporosis	Mottling and discoloration of tooth enamel
Chromium 0.05 mg–0.2 mg†	Whole grains, meat	Cofactor for insulin, proper glucose metabolism	Impaired glucose tolerance, insulin resistance	None known
Selenium 0.05 mg–0.2 mg	Wheat (if grown in high selenium soil), organ meats, other meat, seafood	Antioxidant	None known	Loss of hair, brittle fingernails, fatigue
Molybdenum 0.15 mg–0.5 mg†	Liver, whole grains, dried peas and beans, organ meats	Oxidizes sulfur and products of sulfur and nucleic acid metabolism	None known	Interferes with copper metabolism
Cobalt	Organ meats	Essential component of vitamin B_{12}	None known	None known

† Estimated safe and adequate intake.

About two-thirds of the body's water is contained within the cells (intracellular fluid or ICF); the remainder is called extracellular fluid (ECF) and includes all other body fluids like plasma and interstitial fluid. Total body water and ECF decreases with age; ICF increases with an increase in body mass.

Water is more vital to life than food because it provides the fluid medium necessary for all chemical reactions, it participates in many reactions, and is not "stored" in the body. Water acts as a solvent that dissolves many solutes, thereby aiding the processes of digestion, absorption, circulation, and excretion. Through evaporation from the skin, water helps regulate body temperature. As a lubricant, water is needed for mucous secretions and between moving joints.

Sources of water in the diet include not only beverages, but also solid foods, which range from 10% to 98% water. Water is also produced through the metabolism of carbohydrates, protein, and fat. Water leaves the body through urine, feces, expired air, and perspiration. Generally, water intake (average of 1500 ml–3000 ml/day) equals water output. However, water balance may be seriously affected when either intake (*i.e.,* in comotose states) or output (*i.e.,* altered renal function, profuse perspiration, diarrhea, vomiting, fistulas, drainage tubes, hemorrhage, severe burns) is altered.

CHOOSING AN ADEQUATE DIET

An adequate diet obviously provides a balanced intake of all essential nutrients in amounts appropriate for the individual: what constitutes an adequate diet is less obvious. Although a major problem in developing countries, malnutrition related to poor dietary intake is not common in North America. Rather, nutritional concerns tend to focus more on problems of overnutrition. Tools for planning or evaluating a diet for adequacy include food groups, the Recommended Dietary Allowances (RDA), Recommended Nutrient Intakes (RNI) in Canada, dietary recommendations and guidelines issued from health and U.S. government agencies, Nutrition Recommendations for Canadians, and Canada's Food Guide.

Food Groups.   The food group approach to diet planning suggests how many servings of food, not the quantity of particular nutrients, a person should consume daily from each of four or more food groups (Fig. 31-5). Generally, food groupings are made on the basis of vitamin and mineral content: the calorie, fat, sodium, and fiber content of foods are not usually addressed. Portion sizes are suggested, and the recommend number of servings per day varies according to age. The plan provides only about 1,200 calories (4,000 KJ to 6,000 KJ) for adults, therefore additional servings may be added depending on the person's calorie requirements and appetite. A variety of foods is encouraged.

Recommended Dietary Allowances and Recommended Nutrient Intakes.   Recommended dietary allowances or RDA, prepared by the Committee on Dietary Allowances of the Food and Nutrition Board, and the RNI, prepared by the Health Promotion Directorate, National Health and Welfare in Canada, are recommendations for average daily amounts of nutrients considered to be adequate to meet the known nutritional needs of practically all healthy persons (Table 31-7). (A summary of Canadian RNIs is in Appendix D-3.) Unlike a requirement, which is the amount of a nutrient needed to prevent a deficiency, an allowance has a safety factor built in to account for individual variations. However, because the RDA and RNI are intended for populations and not individuals, some people may not be able to meet their individual requirements despite consuming the RDA or RNI. Likewise, it is possible for some people to eat less than the RDA or RNI and still avoid deficiencies. Although RDAs and RNIs are defined for age and sex and are revised about every 5 years as new information becomes available, they have not been established for all

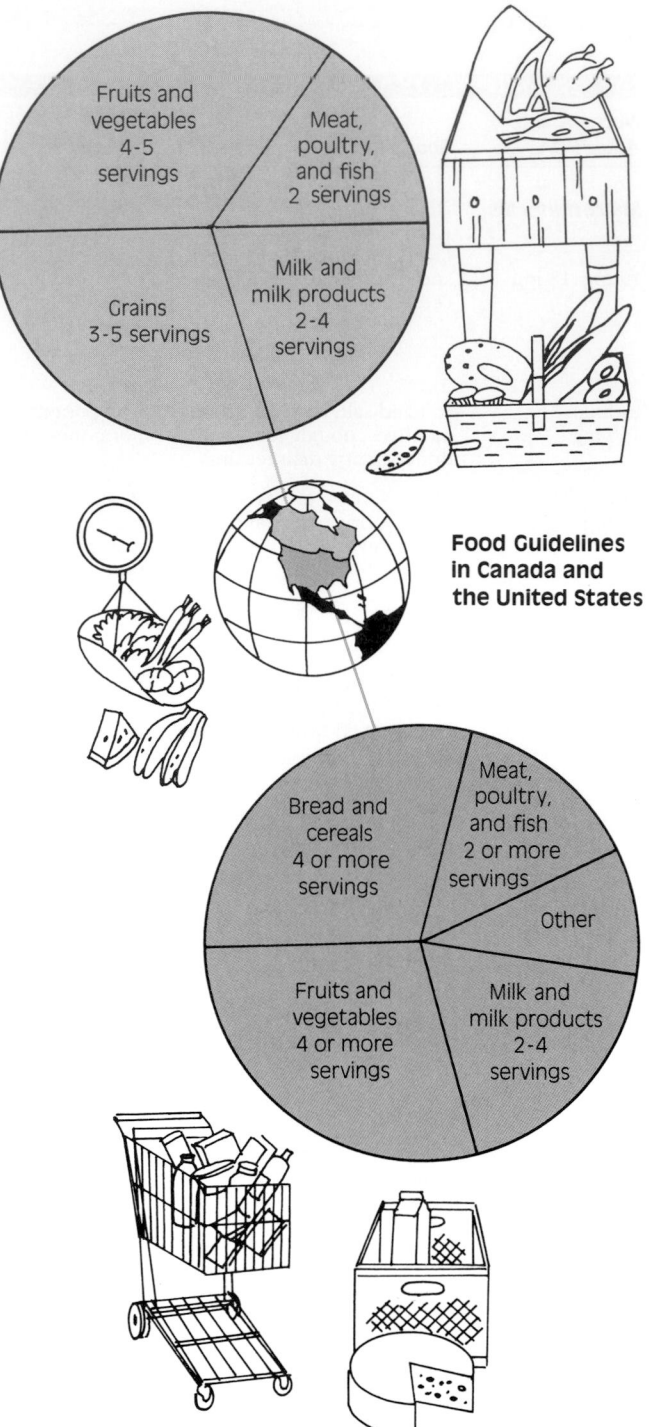

Food Guidelines in Canada and the United States

F I G U R E   31-5
United States and Canadian recommendations for daily dietary intake by food groups.

nutrients. Like the food group approach, variety is recommended.

USRDA and Nutrition Labeling Regulations.   The USRDA are standards for food labeling derived from the 1968 RDA tables. Nutritional labeling regulations in

COMPUTER APPLICATIONS IN NURSING

Computer-Generated Nutritional Analysis

Computer software is now available to allow the user to key daily food intake into the computer and to receive as output a complete nutritional analysis. Anyone who has manually computed nutritional values and who remembers the extensive mathematical calculations and tedium involved will enjoy these programs. Output generally includes two charts showing the client's *recommended dietary* *amounts* based on the client's age, sex, height and weight, and his or her *actual nutrition intake.* Also included are tables showing the amount of dietary fiber in each item, as well as the amounts of thiamine, riboflavin, niacin, folacin, pyridoxine, cobalamin, folacin, calcium, iron, magnesium, phosphorus, potassium, sodium, and zinc. These data are very useful for counseling clients on special diets.

Canada derive from the 1983 RNI. They represent the highest regular RDA and RNI for each nutrient. For instance, the USRDA for iron is 18 mg (the RDA for adult women), even though the RDA for men is 10 mg. (Canadian nutrition labeling regulations state 14 mg for adult women and 8 mg for men.) Thus, a serving of food that provides 100% USRDA for iron actually provides 18 mg of iron (14 mg in Canadian nutrition labeling regulations).

Dietary Recommendations. Unlike the food group approach to diet planning and the RDAs and RNIs, current diet recommendations and guidelines proposed by numerous government and health agencies focus not on getting enough, but on avoiding nutritional excesses. Although these diet recommendations do not guarantee to prevent diseases in individuals, many experts believe Americans and Canadians in general can reduce their risk of chronic diet-related diseases like type II diabetes, certain types of cancer, and heart disease by modifying the typical diet. Specific recommendations vary somewhat among sources, however, most experts agree that persons should

- Eat a variety of foods
- Eat more starch and fiber
- Consume less sugar, salt, cholesterol, total fat, and saturated fat
- Use alcohol only in moderation
- Maintain ideal weight

Food Patterns and Habits. Although nutritional adequacy is an important consideration in planning a diet, an individual's food patterns and habits may have a greater impact on a person's overall food intake. Food habits are a product of many evolving variables, such as physical factors (like geographic location, food technology, and income), physiologic factors (like health, hunger, and stage of development), and psychosocial factors (like culture, religion, tradition, education, politics, social status, food ideology, and learned aversions). Although not static, conservative traditional influences like culture, geographic region, and religion tend to have a stabilizing effect on food habits.

FACTORS AFFECTING NUTRITION

A variety of factors are known to influence nutrition, either by affecting nutritional requirements or by altering nutrient intake.

Factors Influencing Nutrient Requirements

Developmental Considerations. Throughout the life cycle, nutrient needs change in relation to growth, development, activity, and age-related changes in metabolism and body composition. Periods of intense growth and development, such as during infancy, adolescence, pregnancy, and lactation, cause an increase in nutrient needs. Nutrient needs tend to stabilize during adulthood, although elderly persons may need more or less of some nutrients.

Age influences not only nutrient requirements, but also food intake. The consistency of food, eating patterns, and the significance of food change with physical and psychosocial development. Nutrient needs and developmental landmarks are summarized in Table 31-8.

Sex. Men have somewhat different nutrient requirements than women related to differences in body composition and reproductive function. Males' larger muscle mass translates into higher calorie and protein requirements (and therefore slightly higher needs for B vitamins that metabolize calories and protein) because it is more metabolically active than adipose tissue, of which females proportionally have more. Women of childbearing age have higher iron requirements related to menstruation.

State of Health. The alteration in nutrient requirements that results from illness and trauma varies with the intensity and duration of the stress. For instance, fevers

T A B L E *31-7*
Recommended Daily Dietary Allowances,* Revised 1980†

Age (years)	Weight (kg)	(lb)	Height (cm)	(in)	Protein (g)	Fat-Soluble Vitamins		
						Vitamin A (μg)†	Vitamin D (μg)§	Vitamin E (mg α)‖
Infants								
0.0–0.5	6	13	60	24	kg × 2.2	420	10	3
0.5–1.0	9	20	71	28	kg × 2.0	400	10	4
Children								
1–3	13	29	90	35	23	400	10	5
4–6	20	44	112	44	30	500	10	6
7–10	28	62	132	52	34	700	10	7
Males								
11–14	45	99	157	62	45	1000	10	8
15–18	66	145	176	69	56	1000	10	10
19–22	70	154	177	70	56	1000	7.5	10
23–50	70	154	178	70	56	1000	5	10
51+	70	154	178	70	56	1000	5	10
Females								
11–14	46	101	157	62	46	800	10	8
15–18	55	120	163	64	46	800	10	8
19–22	55	120	163	64	44	800	7.5	8
23–50	55	120	163	64	44	800	5	8
51+	55	120	163	64	44	800	5	8
Pregnant								
					+30	+200	+5	+2
Lactating								
					+20	+400	+5	+3

* The allowances are intended to provide for individual variations among most normal persons as they live in the United States under usual environmental stresses. Diets should be based on a variety of common foods to provide other nutrients for which human requirements have been less well defined.

† See Appendix D-4 for Canadian RNIs.

‡ Retinol equivalents. 1 Retinol equivalent = 1 μg retinol or 6 μg β carotene.

§ As cholecalciferol. 10 μg cholecalciferol = 400 IU vitamin D.

‖ α-tocopherol equivalents. 1 mg d-α-tocopherol = 1 α TE.

do increase the need for calories and water; however unlike fevers related to septicemia, fevers caused by a mild case of the flu require few dietary adjustments.

Trauma, like major surgery, burns, and crush injuries, is followed by hormonal changes that profoundly affect the body's use of nutrients. To preserve or replenish body nutrient stores and promote healing and recovery, nutrient requirements increase dramatically in the adaptive phase following stress. In some cases of severe trauma, like major burns, the rehabilitative phase of recovery characterized by the gradual normalization of nutrient needs, may last for years.

Chronic disorders, like diabetes mellitus, renal disease, hypertension, heart disease, GI disorders, and cancer, can alter nutrient requirements by influencing nutrient intake, digestion, absorption, metabolism, utilization, or excretion.

Alcohol Abuse. Alcohol can alter the body's use of nutrients, and therefore its nutrient requirements, by numerous mechanisms. The toxic effect of alcohol on the intestinal mucosa interferes with normal nutrient absorption: thus requirements increase as the efficiency of absorption decreases. Need for B vitamins increases be-

Water-Soluble Vitamins							Minerals					
Vitamin C (mg)	Thiamine (mg)	Riboflavin (mg)	Niacin (mg NE)#	Vitamin B$_6$ (mg)	Folacin** (μg)	Vitamin B$_{12}$ (μg)	Calcium (mg)	Phosphorus (mg)	Magnesium (mg)	Iron (mg)	Zinc (mg)	Iodine (mg)
35	0.3	0.4	6	0.3	30	0.5††	360	240	50	10	3	40
35	0.5	0.6	8	0.6	45	1.5	540	360	70	15	5	50
45	0.7	0.8	9	0.9	100	2.0	800	800	150	15	10	70
45	0.9	1.0	11	1.3	200	2.5	800	800	200	10	10	90
45	1.2	1.4	16	1.6	300	3.0	800	800	250	10	10	120
50	1.4	1.6	18	1.8	400	3.0	1200	1200	350	18	15	150
60	1.4	1.7	18	2.0	400	3.0	1200	1200	400	18	15	150
60	1.5	1.7	19	2.2	400	3.0	800	800	350	10	15	150
60	1.4	1.6	18	2.2	400	3.0	800	800	350	10	15	150
60	1.2	1.4	16	2.2	400	3.0	800	800	350	10	15	150
50	1.1	1.3	15	1.8	400	3.0	1200	1200	300	18	15	150
60	1.1	1.3	14	2.0	400	3.0	1200	1200	300	18	15	150
60	1.1	1.3	14	2.0	400	3.0	800	800	300	18	15	150
60	1.0	1.2	13	2.0	400	3.0	800	800	300	10	15	150
60	1.0	1.2	13	2.0	400	3.0	800	800	300	10	15	150
+20	+0.4	+0.3	+2	+0.6	+400	+1.0	+400	+400	+150	‡‡	+5	+25
+40	+0.5	+0.5	+5	+0.5	+100	+1.0	+400	+400	+150	‡‡	+10	+50

1 NE (niacin equivalent) is equal to 1 mg of niacin or 60 mg of dietary tryptophan.

** The folacin allowances refer to dietary sources as determined by *Lactobacillus casei* assay after treatment with enzymes (conjugases) to make polyglutamyl forms of the vitamin available to the test organism.

†† The RDA for Vitamin B$_{12}$ in infants is based on average concentration of the vitamin in human milk. The allowances after weaning are based on energy intake (as recommended by the American Academy of Pediatrics) and consideration of other factors such as intestinal absorption.

‡‡ The increased requirement during pregnancy cannot be met by the iron content of habitual American diets nor by the existing iron stores of many women; therefore, the use of 30 mg to 60 mg of supplemental iron is recommended. Iron needs during lactation are not substantially different from those of nonpregnant women, but continued supplementation of the mother for 2 to 3 months after parturition is advisable to replenish stores depleted by pregnancy.

(National Academy of Sciences: Recommended Dietary Allowances, 9th rev. ed. Washington, DC, 1980)

cause they are used to metabolize alcohol. Alcohol can also influence nutrient metabolism by impairing nutrient storage, increasing nutrient catabolism, and increasing nutrient excretion. Alcohol abuse resulting in liver damage has profound effects on the body's nutrient metabolism and requirements.

Medication. Many drugs have the potential to influence nutrient requirements. *Nutrient absorption* may be altered by drugs that (1) change the *p*H of the GI tract, (2) increase GI motility, (3) damage the intestinal mucosa, or (4) bind with nutrients, rendering them unavail-

able to the body. *Nutrient metabolism* can be altered by drugs that (1) act as nutrient antagonists, (2) alter the enzyme systems that metabolize nutrients, or (3) alter nutrient degradation. Some drugs alter the renal reabsorption of nutrients, and therefore may increase or decrease *nutrient excretion*.

Megadoses of Nutrient Supplements. Because some nutrients compete against each other for absorption, an excess of one nutrient can lead to a deficiency (or increase the requirement) of another, especially if one is absorbed preferentially. For instance, a delicate balance

(Text continues on p. 779.)

T A B L E   31-8

Nutritional Implications of Characteristic Developmental Landmarks Throughout the Life Cycle

Age	Characteristic Development	Nutritional Implications
Infants (birth to 1 year)	Most rapid period of growth after birth; birth weight doubles in 4 to 6 months and triples by age 1; length increases 50% in first year	Nutritional needs per unit of body weight are greater than at any other time in the life cycle.
	Inborn reflexes, such as rooting, sucking, swallowing, and gagging, disappear between 4 and 6 months.	Milk feedings are most appropriate for the first 4 to 6 months.
		Breastfeeding is recommended as the major source of nutrition for the first 6 months; supplements of vitamin C, vitamin D, fluoride, and iron may be prescribed.*
		A variety of routine and special infant formulas are available if mothers choose not to breastfeed or if breastfeeding is contraindicated because of medical problems in the infant or mother.
	Muscular control of the head, neck, jaw, and tongue develops, as does hand–eye coordination and the ability to sit and self-feed.	Spoon feeding becomes possible. Solids may be introduced between 4 and 6 months of age. Common progression is iron-fortified infant cereals followed by strained vegetables, noncitrus fruits, noncitrus fruit juices.
		Texture increases gradually to table food at 1 year.
		Finger foods and drinking from a cup may begin around 6 months.
	Stomach capacity is limited at birth, peristalsis is rapid.	Initially, small frequent feedings are necessary.
	Pancreatic amylase (starch-digesting enzyme) is limited at birth until 3 months of age.	Starch digestion (*i.e.,* cooked cereal) does not develop until 3 months of age.
	Iron stores present at birth start to become depleted between 3 and 4 months.	Exogenous iron is necessary. Cow's milk given too early (*i.e.,* before the infant is eating the equivalent of 1 1/2 jars of baby food a day) contributes to iron deficiency anemia.
	Immune system matures between 4 and 6 months.	Solid foods given too early may trigger allergic reactions.
		New foods should be introduced one at a time for 5 to 7 days so that allergic reactions can be noted.
		Egg whites should not be given until age 1.
Toddlers and preschoolers	Dramatic decrease in growth rate	Dramatic decrease in appetite; appetite becomes erratic; calorie needs per unit of body weight decline.
	Maturation of biting, chewing, and swallowing continues.	Able to eat a variety of textures
	Develop greater mobility, autonomy, and coordination	Completely self-feed by the age of 2 Can seek food independently May use food to manipulate parents; food jags begin around 15 months.
	Muscle mass and bone density increase.	Need adequate amounts of protein, calcium, and phosphorus
	Language skills increase.	Can associate food with its name; verbalize food likes and dislikes

* In Canada, vitamin B_{12} may be prescribed if mothers are strict vegetarians.

(Continued)

Age	Characteristic Development	Nutritional Implications
	Food attitudes develop between ages 3 and 5.	Inappropriate use of food (*i.e.,* to punish, reward, bribe, or convey love) may lead to inappropriate food attitudes.
School-aged children (6 to 12 year olds)	Erratic, uneven growth pattern; wide variations in growth rate among individuals	Appetite improves but may still be irregular; calorie needs per unit of body weight gradually decline.
	Digestive system matures.	Can eat larger meals and eat less frequently
	Permanent teeth erupt.	Fluoride, vitamin A, vitamin D, calcium, and phosphorus are important for dental health.
	Socialization and independence increase.	Parents' role as primary gate keepers of what their children eat diminishes; advertising impacts on food choices; variety of food eaten increases.
	Reserves are laid down for upcoming adolescent growth spurt.	Nutrient needs increase toward the end of school-aged period in preparation for growth spurt.
Adolescents	Period of rapid physical emotional, social, and sexual maturation	Nutrient needs, especially for calories, protein, calcium, and iron, increase to support growth.
	Growth spurt begins at different ages among individuals, begins earlier for girls than boys.	Physiologic age is a more valid indicator of need than chronologic age.
	Boys experience an increase in muscle mass, lean body tissue, and bones.	Iron needs increase; boys have higher calorie needs than girls to maintain larger muscle mass.
	Girls begin menstruation and experience fat deposition.	Iron needs increase; body fat requires fewer calories to be maintained, therefore girls need fewer calories than boys.
		Weight consciousness becomes compulsive in 1 out of 100 teenaged girls and results in **anorexia nervosa,** an eating disorder characterized by extreme weight loss, muscle wasting, arrested sexual development, refusal to eat, and bizarre eating habits.
		An estimated 1 in 5 teenage girls suffer from **bulimia,** an eating disorder characterized by gorging followed by purging with self-induced vomiting, diuretics, and/or laxatives.
		Teenage pregnancy occurring within 3 to 4 years after menstruation begins places mother and fetus at increased nutritional risk.
	Period of intense psychosocial growth, family conflict, social and peer pressure	Nutritional needs may be hard to meet because fewer meals are eaten at home, peer influence, busy schedules, and because independence may be expressed through diet.
Adults	Growth ceases.	Nutrient needs level off.
	Basal metabolic rate (BMR) declines each decade.	Fewer calories are required for BMR; weight gain occurs if adjustments in intake are not made.
	Physical activity may decline.	Also contributes to weight gain if caloric intake does not decrease
Pregnant women	Dramatic growth of fetus, maternal tissues, and placenta	Nutrient needs increase to support growth and maintain maternal homeostasis.

(Continued)

T A B L E   31-8

Nutritional Implications of Characteristic Developmental Landmarks Throughout the Life Cycle   (Continued)

Age	Characteristic Development	Nutritional Implications
		Key nutrients include protein, calories, iron, folic acid, calcium, and iodine. Iron and folic acid supplements are necessary to meet needs.
		Actual nutrient needs increase little during the first trimester in a well-nourished mother but increase steadily throughout the remainder of pregnancy.
	Weight gain occurs.	Recommended pattern: 2 lb–4 lb (1 kg–3 kg) during the first trimester; 0.8 lb–0.9 lb (0.45 kg) per week during second and third trimesters; underweight women may need more, overweight women less.
		Pattern of weight gain is more significant than total amount.
	GI changes occur that may cause nausea, vomiting, heartburn, or constipation.	Dietary changes may help relieve unpleasant symptoms.
Lactating Women	The quantity of milk produced is dependent on an adequate supply of nutrients.	Calorie needs are higher for lactation than pregnancy, as are the requirements for vitamin A, niacin, riboflavin, iodine, zinc, and fluid. Calcium and protein are also important.
		Calories may come from diet or fat mobilized from adipose tissue.
	The quality of milk is generally not affected by maternal diet, with the exception of vitamin C, riboflavin, thiamine, and fat.	The nutritional quality of breast milk is generally maintained at the expense of maternal nutrition if the diet is inadequate.
Elderly Persons	Energy expenditure decreases related to a decrease in BMR, decrease in physical activity, and loss of lean body mass.	Calorie needs decrease.
	Loss of teeth, periodontal disease, and jaw bone disease may result in difficulty chewing.	Food intake may be limited to soft, easy-to-chew foods; meat is the food most commonly eliminated.
	Constipation is a common problem related to decreased activity, decreased peristalsis due to a loss of abdominal muscle tone, inadequate fluid and fiber intake, or secondary to drug therapy.	Increasing fiber and fluid may help relieve constipation.
	Digestive disorders may occur related to normal changes in GI function.	Diet modifications may be necessary to relieve discomfort.
	Loss of taste begins between 55 and 59 years of age; people lose tastes of sweet and salt; bitter and sour remain.	Taste threshold increases, which may lead to an increase in sugar and salt intake or anorexia.
	Sensation of thirst decreases	The elderly are prone to dehydration.
	Physical disabilities may develop related to arthritis or strokes.	Food preparation may be difficult or impossible.
	Income becomes "fixed."	Most sacrificed items on a limited food budget are milk and meats.
	Degenerative diseases and the use of medications are more common with aging.	Nutrient intake, digestion, absorption, metabolism, or excretion may be altered.
	Social isolation, poor self-esteem, or being institutionalized may affect intake.	Lack of interest in eating is common.

exists between zinc and copper. People who take therapeutic levels of zinc run the risk of developing a copper deficiency, which is otherwise quite rare, unless they also increase their intake of copper.

Factors Influencing Nutrient Intake

Food intake may decrease for a variety of reasons. **Anorexia**, or the lack of appetite, may be related to systemic and local diseases; numerous psychosocial causes like fear, anxiety, and depression; pain; impaired ability to smell and taste; or may occur secondary to drug therapy or medical treatments. People who have difficulty chewing and swallowing correspondingly eat less, and those on inadequate food budgets may have no choice but to limit their intake.

Ironically, problems like fear, anxiety, and depression, which cause anorexia in some people, can stimulate others to overeat. Also, some drugs like antihistamines, psychotropic drugs, tricyclic antidepressants, and steroids increase the appetite.

NURSE AS ROLE MODEL

A nurse's credibility as a health practitioner may be severely questioned if he or she appears badly nourished, or displays poor eating habits, weight problems, or other clinical signs of nutritional deficiencies. As a role model for health behaviors, the nurse should adopt the following goals:

- Attain and maintain ideal body weight.
- Use recommended dietary guidelines for adequate nutrient intake.
- Maintain appropriate balance between food intake and exercise.
- Limit intake of alcohol, fats, sugar, salt, and red meats.
- Eat foods high in fiber.

ASSESSING NUTRITIONAL STATUS

Nutritional status has a significant impact on both health and disease. For well clients, good nutritional status can help maintain health, promote normal growth and development, and help protect against disease. During illness, good nutritional status can reduce the risk of complications and speed recovery time. Conversely, poor nutritional status can increase the risk of illness or death (Salmond, 1980).

The nature of the nurse–client relationship affords nurses the opportunity to incorporate nutritional assessment in the nursing process. Like other aspects of nurs-

---

PROMOTING WELLNESS

Nutrition

Use the assessment checklist to determine how well you are meeting your nutritional needs. Then develop a prescription for self-care by choosing appropriate behaviors from the list of suggestions.

Assessment Checklist

almost always	some times	almost never	
☐	☐	☐	1. I know and use the recommended dietary guidelines and servings.
☐	☐	☐	2. My weight is within 10% of the ideal for my height and body frame.
☐	☐	☐	3. I maintain an appropriate balance between exercise and food intake.
☐	☐	☐	4. I limit my fat, sugar, salt, and red meat intake.

Self-Care Behaviors

1. Maintain desirable weight, eating a variety of foods in adequate amounts from each of the four food groups.
2. Eat slowly, take smaller portions, and avoid second helpings if trying to control overeating.
3. Eat a variety of foods low in calories and high in nutrients to lose weight.
4. Obtain medical clearance before starting a weight-loss program.
5. Avoid too many foods high in cholesterol (milk, egg yolk, organ meats, fats, oils); instead choose lean meat, fish, poultry, and beans.
6. Eat foods high in fiber: whole-grain breads and cereals, fruits, vegetables, dry beans.
7. Avoid excess use of salt and sugar.
8. Begin an exercise program, and maintain it.
9. Learn healthy eating habits; read labels, become familiar with healthy fast-food and restaurant menus, drink alcohol moderately (if at all).
10. Substitute healthy rewards for yourself that do not include high-calorie, low-nutrition snacks and beverages.

Elements of a Nutritional Assessment

Dietary Data

Screen
24-hour food recall
Food frequency record

In-depth: add
Food diary
Diet history

Medical–Socioeconomic Data

Screen
Brief personal and family history

In-depth
Sequential history, including present and past health status, social history, and family history

Anthropometric Data

Screen
Height
Weight
Ideal body weight (IBW)
Usual body weight (UBW)

In-depth: add
Triceps skinfold (TSF)
Mid-arm circumference (MAC)
Mid-arm muscle circumference (MAMC)
Body mass index (BMI)

Clinical Data

Screen and in-depth
Observe for signs and symptoms of malnutrition

Biochemical Data

Screen
Serum hemoglobin, hematocrit, and albumin
Total lymphocyte count (TLC)

In-depth: add
Serum transferrin
Antigen skin testing
24-hour urinary creatinine excretion
Urinary urea nitrogen (UUN)

---

ing care, nutritional assessment is a systematic approach used to identify the client's actual or potential needs, formulate a plan to meet those needs, initiate the plan or assign others to implement it, and evaluate the effectiveness of the plan. As such, nutritional assessment is appropriate for all clients, although the level of assessment may range from simple screening to a comprehensive in-depth assessment depending on individual circumstances (see box). Nurses can collect assessment data through history taking (dietary and medical-socioeconomic data), physical assessments (anthropometric and clinical data), and laboratory data.

Dietary Data

Dietary data may be collected from the client or his family and can be evaluated according to the food group approach, dietary guidelines, or the RDA (RNI in Canada), depending on the purpose of the assessment.

The most simple and easy way to collect dietary data is to obtain a 24-hour recall of all food and beverages the client normally consumes throughout the course of an average day. It includes the client's usual portion sizes, meal and snack patterns, meal timing, and the place where food is eaten. Unfortunately, because this method relies on memory and accurate interpretation of portion sizes, information may not be very reliable. Food frequency questionnaires or food diaries may provide a better overall picture of nutrient intake because the client records all food and beverages consumed in a specified period of time, usually 3 days to 7 days.

A more comprehensive approach to diet assessment is the diet history. In addition to a 24-hour food recall and food frequency record, interview questions are geared to provide information on past and present food intake and habits. Sample questions follow:

Does your present intake differ from your usual intake? If so, is the reason due to a loss of appetite, changes in smell or taste, difficulty chewing and swallowing, hospitalization, a modified diet?

Do you have any food allergies or intolerances?

Who does the food shopping? Who prepares the meals?

How is the food normally prepared? For instance, is food usually fried, baked, or broiled?

Do you have adequate food storage space and preparation equipment?

Do you now, or have you in the past, followed a modified diet prescribed by a doctor?

Do you now, or have you in the past, used a fad diet, health foods, or self-prescribed supplements?

These findings are considered dietary risk factors for poor nutritional status:

- Inadequate food intake, fad dieting, numerous food intolerances or allergies
- Use of inadequate modified diet (*i.e.,* clear liquid) for more than 3 days without adequate supplementation
- NPO with simple IV therapy for longer than 3 days
- Inadequate tube feedings
- Difficulty chewing or swallowing
- Changes in taste, smell, or appetite

Medical-Socioeconomic Data

Medical, social, and economic factors, as well as cultural and psychologic influences, should be evaluated for their impact on nutritional requirements and food choices. Table 31-9 outlines medical-socioeconomic data for assessment.

The following findings are considered medical-socioeconomic risk factors for poor nutritional status:

- Medical conditions that alter intake or nutrient requirements: cancer, malabsorption, diarrhea, hyperthyroidism, severe infection, recent surgery, hemorrhage, physical or mental disabilities, multiple wounds or fractures, extensive burns
- Persistent fever above 37°C for more than 2 days
- Chronic use of drugs that affect nutritional status
- Alcohol abuse
- Inadequate food budget

Anthropometric Data

Anthropometric measurements measure body dimensions. In children, anthropometric measurements are used to assess growth rate; in adults, they can give indirect measurements of body protein and fat stores. In order for the data to be accurate and reliable, standardized equipment and procedures must be used and the data must be compared to the appropriate reference standards for the client's age and sex.

Height and weight, the most common anthropometric measurements, should be made when the client is admitted to the hospital and periodically thereafter. A client should be weighed on the same scale each time, and at the same time of day, preferably before breakfast. Weight should be compared to ideal body weight and usual body weight. Because actual weight may be inflated if the client has edema, hydration status should be considered. Although self-reported weight may be recorded when actual weight is unobtainable, it is highly inaccurate and should be duly noted.

In-depth anthropometric measurements include triceps skinfold measurements (TSF), a measure of subcu-

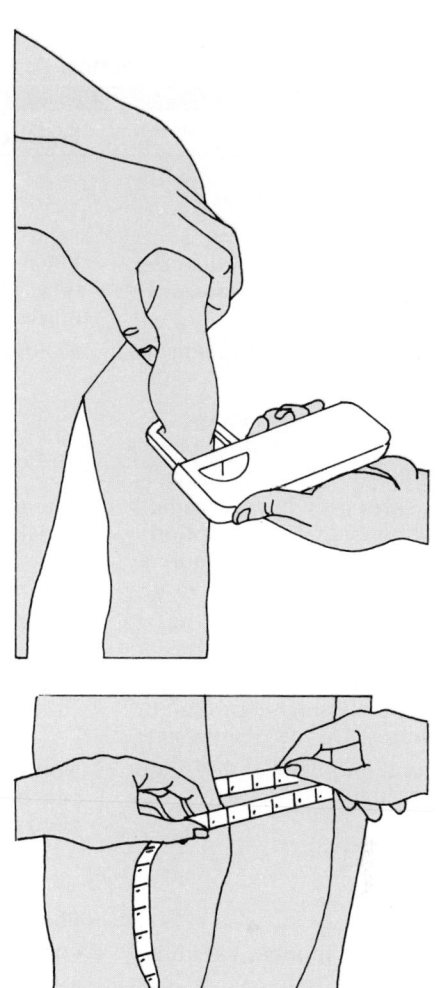

F I G U R E   31-6
Two anthropometric measurements to assess nutritional status. (A) triceps skin-fold measurement and (B) midarm muscle circumference.

taneous fat stores (see Fig. 31-6); mid-arm circumference (MAC), a measure of skeletal muscle mass; and mid-arm muscle circumference (MAMC), a measure of both skeletal muscle mass and fat stores.* Reference standards have been determined for men and women for all three measures, as have figures representing 90%, 80%, 70%, and 60% of standard.

---

* In Canada, the Quetelet or Body Mass Index:

$$BMI = \frac{weight\ (kg)}{height\ m^2}$$

T A B L E   31-9
Medical-Socioeconomic Data for Nutritional Assessment

Collect	Evaluate
Medical Data	
Past medical history: type of disorder, treatment (including diet and drug)	Effect on intake, digestion, absorption, metabolism, and excretion of nutrients
Current illness or chief complaint	Need for diet modifications
Family medical history	
Past surgical history: type, date, length of hospitalization, development of complications	
Past and present drug history: name of prescription and nonprescription drugs used on a regular basis, purpose, dosage, duration of use	Potential or actual effects on nutritional status; need for diet modification
History of drug dependence; drug abuse	
Ability to chew and swallow (Does the client have missing teeth? Full or partial dentures? Do the dentures fit?)	Impact on food intake
Appetite, food intolerances and allergies, bowel habits	Normal pattern, recent changes, impact on intake and nutritional status, need for diet modification
Social Data	
Age, sex	Effect on nutritional requirements
Position in family; number in family; life-style	Outside support systems; social aspects of eating
Occupation; frequency and intensity of physical exercise; usual number of hours of sleep/day	Effect on calorie requirements and meal timing
Religious affiliation, cultural and ethnic background	Effect on food choices and aversions
Educational background	Ability to comprehend diet instruction; appropriate teaching materials and methods
Use of alcohol and tobacco	Effect on food intake, food budget, and nutrient requirements
Economic Data	
Source of income	Reliability and adequacy; eligibility for social assistance
Food budget	Adequacy

The following findings are considered anthropometric risk factors for poor nutritional status:

- Weight 20% greater than ideal or 10% less than ideal
- Recent unintentional weight loss greater than 10% of weight
- Arm muscle circumference or triceps skinfold less than 85% of standard
- Inconsistent growth rates in children or abnormal weight for height

Clinical Data

Although signs and symptoms of malnutrition may be observed during a physical assessment (Table 31-10), they usually do not appear until malnutrition is advanced. In addition, further investigation is necessary to determine whether abnormal findings are actually caused by a nutritional deficiency, possibly related to a nutritional deficiency, or unrelated to nutritional status.

TABLE 31-10
Clinical Observations for Nutritional Assessment

Body Area	Signs of Good Nutritional Status	Signs of Poor Nutritional Status
General appearance	Alert, responsive	Listless, apathetic, and cachexic
General vitality	Endurance, energetic, sleeps well, vigorous	Easily fatigued, no energy, falls asleep easily, looks tired, apathetic
Weight	Normal for height, age, body build	Overweight or underweight
Hair	Shiny, lustrous, firm, not easily plucked, healthy scalp	Dull and dry, brittle, loss of color, easily plucked, thin and sparse
Face	Uniform skin color; healthy appearance, not swollen	Dark skin over cheeks and under eyes, flaky skin, facial edema (moon face), pale skin color
Eyes	Bright, clear, moist, no sores at corners of eyelids, membranes moist and healthy pink color, no prominent blood vessels	Pale eye membranes, dry eyes (xerophthalmia); Bitot's spots, increased vascularity, cornea soft (keratomalacia), small yellowish lumps around eyes (xanthelasma), dull or scarred cornea
Lips	Good pink color, smooth, moist, not chapped or swollen	Swollen and puffy (cheilosis), angular lesion at corners of mouth or fissures or scars (stomatitis)
Tongue	Deep red, surface papillae present	Smooth appearance, beefy red or magenta colored, swollen, papillae, hypertrophy or atrophy
Teeth	Straight, no crowding, no cavities, no pain, bright, no discoloration, well-shaped jaw	Cavities, mottled appearance (fluorosis), malpositioned, missing teeth
Gums	Firm, good pink color, no swelling or bleeding	Spongy, bleed easily, marginal redness, recessed, swollen and inflamed
Glands	No enlargement of the thyroid, face not swollen	Enlargement of the thyroid (goiter), enlargement of the parotid (swollen cheeks)
Skin	Smooth, good color, slightly moist, no signs of rashes, swelling, or color irregularities	Rough, dry, flaky, swollen, pale, pigmented, lack of fat under the skin, fat deposits around the joints (xanthomas), bruises, petechiae
Nails	Firm, pink	Spoon shaped (koilonychia), brittle, pale, ridged
Skeleton	Good posture, no malformations	Poor posture, beading of the ribs, bowed legs or knock-knees, prominent scapulas, chest deformity at diaphragm
Muscles	Well developed, firm, good tone, some fat under the skin	Flaccid, poor tone, wasted, underdeveloped, difficulty walking
Extremities	No tenderness	Weak and tender, presence of edema
Abdomen	Flat	Swollen
Nervous system	Normal reflexes, psychologic stability	Decrease in or loss of ankle and knee reflexes, psychomotor changes, mental confusion, depression, sensory loss, motor weakness, loss of sense of position, loss of vibration, burning and tingling of the hands and feet (paresthesia)
Cardiovascular system	Normal heart rate and rhythm, no murmurs, normal blood pressure for age	Cardiac enlargement, tachycardia, elevated blood pressure
GI system	No palpable organs or masses (liver edge may be palpable in children)	Hepatosplenomegaly

(Adapted from Christakis G [ed]: Nutritional Assessment in Health Programs. Washington, DC, American Public Health Association, 1973 and Williams SR: Nutrition and Diet Therapy, 5th ed. St Louis, Times Mirror/Mosby, 1985)

Biochemical Data

Laboratory tests, which measure blood and urine levels of nutrients or biochemical functions that are dependent on an adequate supply of nutrients, can objectively detect nutritional problems in their early stages. Most routine biochemical tests measure protein status; measures of body vitamin, mineral, and trace element status are also available.

Hemoglobin, the oxygen-carrying protein of the red blood cells, and hematocrit, the volume of red blood cells packed by centrifugation in a given volume of blood, are measures of plasma protein also used to assess iron status. Protein status can also be measured by serum albumin, transferrin, and total lymphocyte count. Twenty-four hour urine tests used to measure protein metabolism are urinary creatinine excretion and urinary urea nitrogen.

The following findings are considered biochemical risk factors for poor nutritional status:

- Low hemoglobin and hematocrit
- Decrease in lymphocyte count
- Serum albumin less than 3.5 g/dl
- Elevated or decreased cholesterol level

DIAGNOSING

Assessment data may reveal actual or potential nutritional problems such as

Nutrition, altered: less than body requirements related to NPO, inadequate tube feeding, prolonged use of a clear liquid diet, numerous food intolerances or allergies, excessive dieting, anorexia, chewing/swallowing difficulties, nausea and vomiting, chronic diarrhea; malabsorption, psychologic eating disorders (anorexia nervosa, bulimia), alcoholism, metabolic and endocrine disorders, inappropriate use of supplements

Nutrition, altered: more than body requirements related to overeating, inactivity, metabolic and endocrine disorders, inappropriate use of supplements

Nutrition, altered: potential for more than body requirements related to inappropriate eating, closely spaced pregnancies, metabolic and endocrine disorders, inappropriate use of supplements

Samples of three of these diagnoses are given in Table 31-11.

Nutritional problems may affect other areas of human functioning. In the following nursing diagnoses, the nutritional problem is the cause of another problem.

Activity intolerance related to inadequate calorie intake, obesity, iron deficiency anemia

Anxiety related to obesity

Bowel elimination, altered: constipation related to inadequate fluid and/or fiber intake

Bowel elimination, altered: diarrhea related to

T A B L E   31-11

Nursing Diagnoses for Common Nutritional Problems

Nursing Diagnosis	Etiologic or Contributing Factors	Sample Characteristics
Nutrition, altered: less than body requirements	Malabsorption	- "I seem to eat all day long and yet I keep losing weight." - Reports losing 15 lb within the last 3 weeks. Has 8 to 10 bowel movements daily of frothy, odorous stools that float. Fecal fat excretion test indicates steatorrhea. Client appears fatigued and undernourished; muscle wasting is evident. Laboratory data reveal low serum albumin (protein deficiency) and iron deficiency anemia.
Nutrition, altered: more than body requirements	Decreased thyroid function leading to a decrease in metabolism	- I don't eat enough to keep a bird alive, but I just keep getting fatter and fatter. I don't know what else to do unless I stop eating altogether." - Client reports a 10-lb weight gain within the last month despite following a 1200-calorie diet. Other symptoms noted include fatigue, amenorrhea, and dry skin. Laboratory data indicate low serum thyroxine (T_4), elevated thyroid-stimulating hormone, low protein-bound iodine, and increased serum cholesterol. Radioactive iodine (RAI) uptake was low.
Nutrition, altered: potential for more than body requirements	Inappropriate use of supplements	- "I sent a sample of my hair away for a nutritional analysis, and the report came back saying that I should take supplements of zinc, iron, potassium, and magnesium." - For the last week, client has been taking supplements of 500% the USRDA for zinc and magnesium. She takes twice as much iron as recommended, and large doses of potassium ad lib.

overeating, excessive fiber intake, excessive sorbitol intake (sugar alcohol)

Fluid volume, deficit, related to inadequate fluid intake

Infection, potential for, related to inadequate calorie intake, inadequate protein intake

Knowledge deficit related to new medical diet, nutrition misinformation, lack of interest in nutrition, intellectual deficit

Noncompliance (to a particular diet order) related to lack of motivation, misinformation

Self-concept, disturbance in related to obesity

Skin integrity, impaired, related to protein malnutrition, vitamin A deficiency

Sleep pattern disturbance related to excessive caffeine intake

Social isolation related to obesity

PLANNING: CLIENT GOALS

Client goals evolve from the actual or potential nutritional problems diagnosed. The following are general client goals:

- Client will attain and maintain ideal body weight.
- Client will eat a diet adequate but not excessive in all nutrients.
- Client will eat a variety of food in each of three or more meals.
- Client will follow the appropriate modified diet, when necessary, to restore health, avoid disease recurrences, and prevent or delay potential complications.

IMPLEMENTING

Providing proper and adequate nourishment to the hospitalized client is a team effort: diet orders are written by the physician, confirmed by the dietitian, and usually delivered by the nurse. The nurse may also be responsible for observing intake and appetite, evaluating the client's tolerance, assisting the client with eating, administering tube and parenteral feedings, consulting with the dietitian and physician when dietary problems arise, obtaining more food or snacks for the client when appropriate, monitoring food brought by visitors, and conducting or reinforcing diet instructions.

Stimulating Appetite

To the hospitalized client, food and eating may take on much greater meaning. Loss of control over food choices, the way food is prepared, when and how food is served, and eating alone may do little to encourage normal eating. In addition, pain, illness, anxiety, and medications can contribute to anorexia and poor intake. Every effort must be made to ensure that not only is the proper food served, but that it is also eaten. The following measures may help stimulate appetite:

- Serve small frequent meals to avoid overwhelming the client with large amounts of food.
- Solicit food preferences and encourage food from home, if possible.
- Provide encouragement and a pleasant eating environment.
- Be sure the client's tray looks attractive.
- Schedule procedures and medications at a time when they are least likely to interfere with appetite.
- Control pain, nausea, or depression with medications.
- Offer alternatives for items the client cannot or will not eat.
- Encourage or provide good oral hygiene.

Providing Special Diets

A variety of "normal" and modified diets are available in the hospital setting. "Normal" or "house" diets are designed to maintain a client's good nutritional status by providing adequate amounts of all nutrients. The diet's actual composition varies with the quantity and type of foods selected: the average calorie content ranges from 1400 to 2500 calories.

Liquid diets are used most often as transitional diets when eating resumes after acute illness, surgery, or parenteral nutrition. *Clear liquid diets* contain only foods that are clear liquids at room or body temperature: gelatin, fat-free broth, bouillon, popsicles, clear juices, carbonated beverages, regular and decaffeinated coffee, and tea. Because clear liquid diets are inadequate in calories, protein, and most nutrients, they should be progressed as soon as possible.

Full liquid diets contain milk, plain frozen desserts, pasteurized eggs, cereal gruels, and milk and egg substitutes in addition to clear liquids. High-calorie, high-protein supplements are recommended if the diet is used for more than 2 or 3 days.

Soft diets are usually regular diets that have been modified to eliminate hard to digest and hard to chew foods, including items high in fiber, high in fat, and highly seasoned. Soft diets are adequate in calories and nutrients and may be used on a long-term basis.

Other modified diets are listed in Table 31-12.

Assisting With Eating

The loss of independence that comes with the inability to self feed can be a severe blow to a client's self-esteem. The following nursing measures may help a client maintain dignity while being fed:

- Involve the client as much as possible. Solicit his preferences with regard to the order of items eaten and the eating pace.
- Engage the client in pleasant conversation to ease tension.
- Place a "napkin," not a "bib," over the client's clothes for protection.

T A B L E 31-12
Normal and Modified Diets

"Normal" ("Regular" or "House") Diets for

Adults
Infants, children, and adolescents
Pregnancy and lactation
Vegetarians

Diets Modified in Consistency and Texture

Clear liquid diet
Full liquid diet
Soft diet
Mechanical soft diet
Tube feedings
Low-residue diet
High-fiber diet
Bland diet

Calorie-Modified Diets

High-calorie diet
Low-calorie diet
Calorie-controlled diet (*i.e.,* diabetic diets)

Modified Nutrient Diets

High-carbohydrate diet
Restricted carbohydrate diet
High-protein diet
Low-protein diet
Low-fat diet
Modified fat diet
Low-cholesterol diet
Low-potassium diet
Low-sodium diet
Fluid-restricted diet
Force fluids

Modified Diets Restricting or Eliminating Certain Foods

Gluten-free diet
Low-lactose or lactose-free diet
Purine-restricted diet
Elimination diets for allergies
Tyramine-restricted diet
Phenylalanine-restricted diet

Withholding Food

Hospitalized clients may be ordered NPO (nothing by mouth) for several reasons. Food is prohibited before surgery to prevent aspiration related to anesthesia, and after surgery until bowel sounds return. NPO may also be necessary for clients undergoing certain medical tests and for clients experiencing severe nausea and vomiting, an inability to chew or swallow, coma, various acute or chronic GI abnormalities, and labor and delivery.

Well-nourished clients can easily withstand the stress of NPO for a short period of time. Clients with increased nutritional requirements or who will be NPO for more than 1 day to 2 days may require nutritional support from tube feedings and/or parenteral nutrition.

The following measures may provide comfort to clients who are NPO:
- Encourage or provide good oral hygiene.
- Provide the client with ice chips, sips of water, hard candies, or gum as allowed.
- Let the client chew his favorite foods without swallowing.
- Urge the client to avoid watching others eat. Suggest alternate activities at mealtime.

Feeding by Tube

Whenever possible, clients are given oral diets. However, if the client's GI tract is functional but the client is unable or unwilling to consume an adequate oral intake, a tube feeding may be used to deliver total or supplemental nutrition. One choice is *gastric gavage,* the introduction of nourishment into the stomach by mechanical means. A gavage is usually indicated when no stomach or duodenal pathology is present to interfere with normal digestive processes.

Inserting Tubes. Tubes may be inserted nonsurgically through the nose into the stomach (nasogastric, NG), the duodenum (nasoduodenal, ND), or the jejunum (nasojejunal, NJ) or may be surgically implanted into the esophagus, stomach, or jejunum. The nasal method of insertion is used most often. It requires a smaller tube and skill in insertion, but resistance to insertion is lower in this method. Insertion of the nasogastric tube is discussed in Procedure 31-1.

Irrigating the Tube. Irrigate the client's gastric tube at regular intervals to determine and maintain patency. Irrigation of the nasogastric tube is done upon the physician's orders. The actions and rationale for irrigation are discussed in Procedure 31-2. NG feedings have the advantage of using the stomach as a reservoir: formula that is held and released at a controlled rate from the stomach does not cause "dumping syndrome," a reaction that occurs when food or liquids are quickly "dumped" into the small intestine in high concentrations. Immediate reactions include gas, bloating, pain, and diarrhea which may be followed by hypoglycemia. Unfortunately, NG feedings have a high risk of aspiration and are contraindicated if the client has uncontrolled vomiting, upper GI bleeding, or a complete intestinal obstruction (Cataldo, 1980).

Types of Tubes. Short tubes, used for placement in the stomach, are usually about 127 cm (approximately 4

(Text continues on p. 792.)

PROCEDURE 31-1
Inserting a Nasogastric (NG) Tube

Equipment

Nasogastric tube of appropriate size (12–18 French)

Small basin filled with ice (optional)

Water-soluble lubricant

Tongue blade

Flashlight

Stethoscope

Normal saline (for irrigation only)

Asepto bulb syringe or Toomey syringe (20 ml–50 ml)

Tape (1 inch wide)

Tissues

Glass of water with straw

Suction apparatus

Bath towel or disposable pad

Safety pin and rubber band

Clamp

Emesis basin

Disposable gloves (optional)

Action	**Rationale**
1 Check physician's order for insertion of nasogastric tube.	Clarifies procedure and type of equipment required
2 Explain procedure to client.	Explanation facilitates client cooperation.
3 Gather equipment.	Provides for organized approach to task
4 If nasogastric tube is rubber, place it in basin with ice for 5 min–10 min (optional).	Cold will stiffen the rubber tube making it easier to insert. Plastic tube is usually firm enough.
5 Assess client's abdomen.	Determines presence of bowel sounds and amount of abdominal distention
6 Wash your hands.	Handwashing deters the spread of microorganisms.
7 Assist the client to high Fowler's position, and drape his chest with bath towel or disposable pad. Have emesis basin and tissues handy.	An upright position is more natural for swallowing and protects against aspiration, should the client vomit. Passage of tube may stimulate gagging and tearing of eyes.
8 Check the nares for patency by asking the client to occlude one nostril and breathe normally through the other. Select the nostril through which air passes more easily.	Tube will pass more easily through the nostril with the largest opening.
9 Measure the distance to insert the tube by placing tip of tube at client's nostril and extending to tip of earlobe and then to tip of xiphoid process. Mark tube with a piece of tape.	The measurement ensures that the tube will be long enough to enter the client's stomach.
10 Lubricate the first 10 cm–20 cm (4 inches–8 inches) of the tube with a water-soluble jelly.	Lubrication reduces friction and facilitates passage of the tube into the stomach. Water-soluble lubricant will not cause pneumonia if tube accidentally enters the lungs.
11 Ask the client to lift his head, and insert the tube into the nostril while directing the tube downward and backward. The client may gag when the tube reaches the pharynx.	Following the normal contour of the nasal passage while inserting the tube reduces irritation and the likelihood of mucosal injury. The gag reflex is readily stimulated by the tube.

(Continued)

Inserting a Nasogastric (NG) Tube   (Continued)

Action

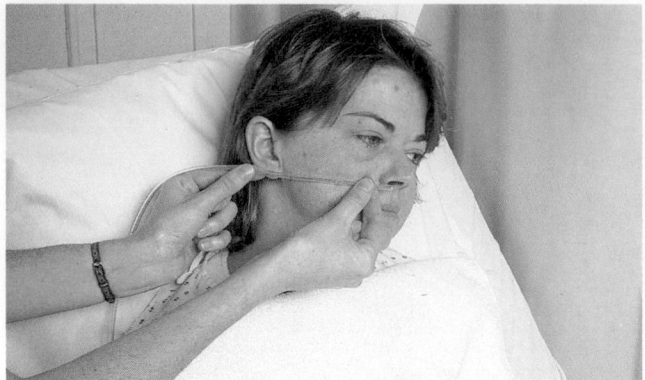

Step 9A: Measuring distance from nostril to tip of earlobe.

Rationale

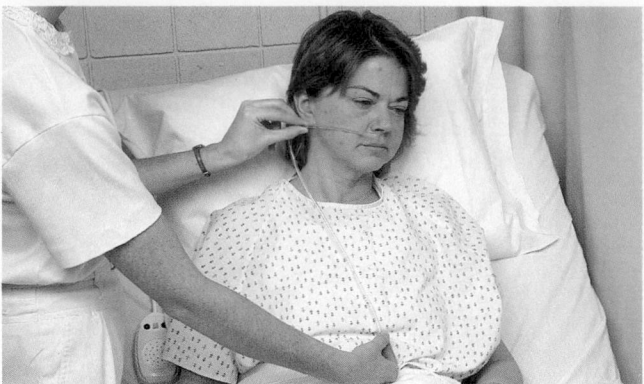

Step 9B: Measuring distance from earlobe to tip of xiphoid process.

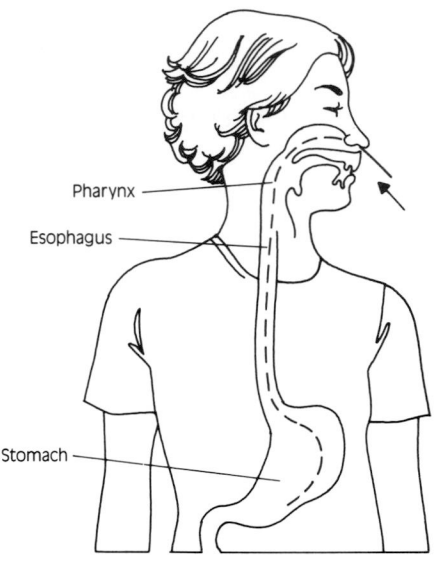

Pharynx

Esophagus

Stomach

Path of the tube.

12 Instruct the client to bring his head forward. Advance the tube in a downward and backward direction. Swallowing or sipping water through a straw may be helpful. If gagging and coughing persist, check placement of tube with a tongue blade and flashlight. Keep advancing the tube until the tape marking is reached. Do not use force. Rotate the tube if it meets resistance.

Bringing the head forward helps close the trachea and open the esophagus. Swallowing helps advance the tube and causes the epiglottis to cover the opening of the trachea. Excessive coughing and gagging may occur if the tube has curled in the back of throat. Forcing the tube may injure mucous membranes.

13 Discontinue the procedure and remove the tube if there are signs of distress, such as gasping, coughing, cyanosis, and the inability to speak or hum.

The tube is not in the esophagus if the client shows signs of distress and is unable to speak or hum.

14 Determine that the tube is in the client's stomach:

a. Attach the syringe to the end of the tube and aspirate 10 ml–20 ml of stomach contents.

The tube is in the stomach if its contents can be aspirated.

b. Place 10 ml–20 ml of air in syringe and inject air into the tube. Simultaneously auscultate over the epigastric area with a stethoscope.

A whooshing sound can be heard when the air enters the stomach through the tube.

(Continued)

Action

15 Secure the tube with tape to the client's face. Be careful not to pull the tube too tightly against the nose:

   a. Cut a 4-inch piece of tape and split bottom 2 inches.

   b. Place unsplit end over bridge of client's nose.

   c. Wrap split ends under the tubing and up and over onto the nose.

16 Attach tube to suction or clamp the tube with a screw-type clamp according to the physician's orders.

17 Secure tube to the client's gown by using a rubber band or tape and a safety pin.

18 Wash hands. Remove all equipment and make client comfortable.

19 Record the insertion procedure, type and size of tube, description of gastric contents, and client's response.

Rationale

Constant pressure of the tube against the skin and mucous membranes causes tissue injury.

Suction will provide for decompression of stomach and drainage of gastric contents.

This prevents tension and tugging on the tube.

Handwashing deters the spread of microorganisms.

Facilitates documentation and provides for comprehensive care

---

PROCEDURE 31-2
Irrigating a Nasogastric (NG) Tube

Equipment

Nasogastric tube connected to continuous or intermittent suction

Irrigation set (Asepto or Toomey syringe and container for irrigating solution)

Normal saline for irrigation

Stethoscope

Disposable pad or bath towel

Clamp

Disposable gloves (optional)

Action

1 Check physician's order for irrigation. Explain procedure to client.

2 Gather necessary equipment. Check expiration dates on irrigating saline and irrigation set.

Rationale

Clarifies schedule and irrigating solution. An explanation encourages client cooperation and reduces apprehension.

Provides for organized approach to task. Agency policy dictates safe interval for reuse of equipment.

(Continued)

Irrigating a Nasogastric (NG) Tube   (Continued)

Action

Rationale

3 Wash your hands.

Handwashing deters the spread of microorganisms.

4 Assist client to semi-Fowler's position unless this is contraindicated.

Minimizes risk of aspiration.

5 Check placement of NG tube:

a. Attach Asepto or Toomey syringe to the end of tube and aspirate gastric contents.

The tube is in the stomach if its contents can be aspirated.

b. Place 10 ml–20 ml of air in syringe and inject into the tube. Simultaneously auscultate over the epigastric area with a stethoscope.

A whooshing sound can be heard when the air enters the stomach through the tube.

c. Ask client to speak.

If tube is misplaced in trachea, client will not be able to speak.

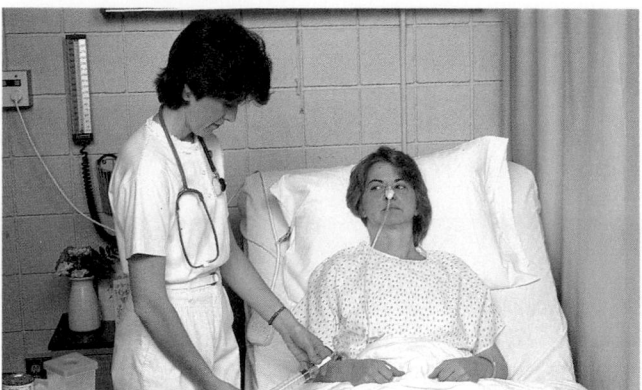

Step 5a: Aspirating gastric contents.

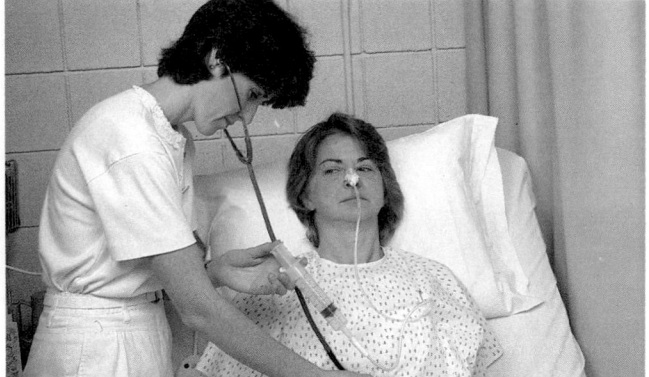

Step 5b: Listening for sound of air entering stomach.

6 Clamp suction tubing near connection site. Disconnect NG tube from suction apparatus and lay on disposable pad or towel.

Protects client from leakage of NG drainage.

7 Pour irrigating solution into container. Draw up 30 ml of saline (or amount ordered by physician) into syringe.

Delivers measured amount of irrigant through NG tube. Saline compensates for electrolytes lost through NG drainage.

8 Place tip of syringe in NG tube. Hold syringe upright and gently insert the irrigant (or allow solution to flow in by gravity if agency or physician indicates). Do not force solution into NG tube.

Position of syringe prevents entry of air into stomach. Gentle insertion of saline (or gravity insertion) is less traumatic to gastric mucosa.

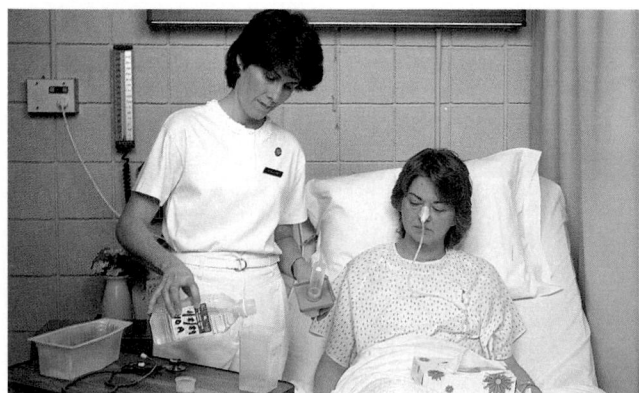

Step 7: Preparing irrigant.

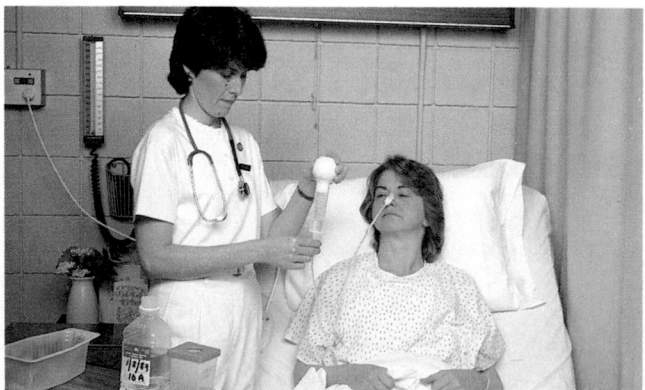

Step 8: Introducing irrigant into tube.

Action	**Rationale**
9 If unable to irrigate tube, reposition client and attempt irrigation again. Check with physician if repeated attempts to irrigate tube fail.	Tube may be positioned against gastric mucosa making it difficult to irrigate.
10 Withdraw or aspirate fluid into syringe. If no return, inject 20 ml of air and aspirate again.	Injection of air may reposition the end of tube.
11 Reconnect NG tube to suction. Observe movement of solution or drainage.	Determines patency of NG tube and correct operation of suction apparatus
12 Measure and record amount and description of irrigant and returned solution.	Irrigant placed in NG tube is considered intake; solution returned is recorded as output.
13 Rinse equipment if it will be reused.	Promotes cleanliness and prepares equipment for next irrigation
14 Wash your hands.	Handwashing deters the spread of microorganisms.
15 Record irrigation procedure, description of drainage, and client's response.	Facilitates documentation of procedure and provides for comprehensive care

R E S E A R C H   I N   N U R S I N G   *Making a Difference*

Nutrition

Current interest in nutrition and fitness has created a focus on the dietary behavior of our society. Negative nutrition has been indicated as a risk factor in illness and health maintenance. Achieving and maintaining an optimal level of nutrition for clients should be the concern of all nurses.

Related Research

Dixon J: Effect of nursing intervention on nutritional and performance status in cancer patients. Nurs Res 33(6):330–335, 1984

Dixon based this study on the need for preventing undernutrition in clients with cancer. Various elements found to be positive in improving nutrition (dietary management, client education, oral supplements, behavior techniques) were integrated into nursing interventions. This particular study found that the use of relaxation techniques was very effective in maintaining or improving nutrition in clients with cancer.

Marrale J, Shipman J, Rhodes M: What some college students eat. Nutrition Today Jan/Feb: 16–21, 1986

This study explored dietary patterns of undergraduate college students at a large metropolitan university. Of the subjects surveyed, three-fourths were rated as fair or poor in adequate nutrition, and more than half were dieting. The results suggest that sound childhood nutritional habits may not persist into adulthood, and that nutritional counseling and weight control programs are needed on college campuses.

Martyn P, Hansen B, Jen K: The effects of parenteral nutrition on food intake and gastric motility. Nurs Res 33(6):336–342, 1984

This study investigated the effects of parenteral nutrition on food intake and gastric motility in healthy subjects. It was found that high-calorie parenteral infusions suppressed appetite and oral intake. These results suggest that hunger in clients receiving venous feedings may be due to factors other than a need for calories.

Nursing research about nutrition is applicable in promoting good nutrition through counseling clients with altered responses to health, in teaching dietary guidelines to the community, and in providing individualized interventions to meet specific needs of hospitalized clients with altered nutrition.

ft) long. Single-lumen tubes (the lumen is the inner open space) without air vents come in several sizes. Levin tubes are an example of single-lumen tubes. Single-lumen tubes lack a venting system; therefore, mucosal damage may result if they are suctioned for decompression. Double-lumen sump tubes are a tube-within-a-tube. One lumen empties the stomach while the second lumen provides for a continuous flow of air. The air-flow lumen controls suction by preventing the drainage lumen from pulling stomach mucosa into the tube's eyes and irritating the stomach lining. Suction can be continuous rather than intermittent, as is required when a single-lumen tube is used. Salem and Ventrol sump tubes are examples. There are some new, smaller tubes available that are softer and more pliable. Usually placement of these tubes is confirmed by x-ray procedure before the feeding is started.

Feedings. The nutritional composition of tube feedings depends on the feeding route, the client's ability to digest and absorb nutrients, and his nutrient and fluid requirements. Other considerations include the availability and cost of the formula, medical conditions requiring diet modifications, food intolerances and allergies, and "taste." Even though the client cannot truly taste a tube feeding, its appearance and aroma influence palatability and acceptance.

Nourishment can be given by gastric gavage on a continuous basis by the gravity drip method. An infusion pump is used in some agencies and has the advantage of maintaining accuracy in the administration of the feeding. The basic method for gastric gavage feeding is outlined in Procedure 31-3.

Implementing Care. Agency protocols may differ and should be followed, but nursing actions that may contribute to successful tube feedings usually include the following measures (Cataldo, 1980):

- Check the placement of an NG tube before beginning a new or intermittent feeding. After ensuring proper placement, instill a small amount of water to make sure the tube is patent and to prevent the formula from sticking to it.
- Before feedings, check the amount of residual; if it is more than 150 ml, investigate reasons for delayed emptying.
- Initially, dilute the formula to half strength and administer slowly to give the client time to adapt to the tube feeding. The small intestine can tolerate changes in volume better than changes in concentration; therefore, the volume should be increased gradually to the optimal level before the concentration is increased to full strength.
- Avoid giving fluids by mouth. Fluids flush important electrolytes from the stomach. Occasionally, ice chips or very limited quantities of fluid may be

allowed to help relieve thirst and moisten mucous membranes. This fluid should be recorded as intake.
- Administer oral hygiene frequently to prevent drying of tissues and to relieve thirst. Lubricate the lips generously.
- Keep the nares clean, especially around the tube, where secretions tend to accumulate. Using a lubricant after cleaning the nares is recommended.
- Help control local irritation from the tube in the throat. The following measures are recommended: use analgesic throat lozenges, spray the area with a local anesthetic, or apply lidocaine viscous to the area.
- Clean feeding equipment as needed.
- Allow the client to verbalize feelings.

The nurse has the responsibility of assessing a client receiving nourishment by gastric gavage for indications of complications:

- *Dehydration, diarrhea, and intestinal cramping.* These symptoms are often present when the nourishment being used is highly concentrated and high in carbohydrate content. They can usually be controlled by reducing the strength of the formula and by introducing it more slowly.
- *Spilling of glucose in the urine (glycosuria) and frequent urination.* These signs are due to a high carbohydrate load from the nourishment. They can usually be relieved by reducing the strength of the formula and by introducing it more slowly. Insulin may need to be used in some instances.
- *Nausea.* Nausea is usually the result of delayed emptying of the stomach. The feedings should be stopped and the patient examined for gastric residual. Slowing the rate of the administration of the nourishment is ordinarily indicated.
- *Aspiration of nourishment.* This complication is serious! It can usually be prevented by keeping the client in a semisitting position so that the nourishment is less likely to enter the esophagus and be aspirated.
- *Vomiting.* Vomiting tends to occur when the nourishment does not leave the stomach. The gastric residue should be checked and the amount of feedings reassessed.

The placement of the tube is checked upon insertion and before each intermittent gavage feeding. Procedure 31-4 gives additional nursing actions in monitoring the client with a nasogastric tube in place.

Removing the Tube. The tube must be removed as carefully as it is inserted to provide as much comfort as possible to the client. Oral hygiene follows removal of the tube. This is especially important to remove disagreeable tastes and odors and should be done thoroughly when the tube has been in the intestinal tract and in contact with intestinal contents. Directions for removing the nasogastric tube are given in Procedure 31-5.

(Text continues on p. 797.)

PROCEDURE 31-3
Feeding by Gastric Gavage

Equipment

Tube feeding at room temperature

Stethoscope

Asepto or Toomey syringe, feeding bag, or prefilled tube feeding set

Clamp (Hoffman or butterfly)

Disposable pad or towel

Water

Sterile gauze

Rubber band

Enteral feeding pump (if ordered)

IV pole

Action	Rationale
1 Explain procedure to client.	Facilitates cooperation and provides reassurance for client
2 Assemble equipment. Check amount, concentration, type, and frequency of tube feeding on client's chart.	Provides for organized approach to task. Ensures the correct feeding will be administered.
3 Wash your hands.	Handwashing deters the spread of microorganisms.
4 Position client with head of bed elevated at least 30 degrees or as near normal position for eating as possible.	Minimizes possibility of aspiration into trachea
5 Unpin tube from client's gown and check to see that the gastric tube is properly located in the stomach, as described in Procedure 31-1, Step 14.	Even when initially positioned correctly, a gastric tube left in place can become dislodged between feedings. The instillation of water or nourishment could lead to serious respiratory problems if a gastric tube is in the trachea or a bronchus, rather than in the stomach.
6 Aspirate all gastric contents with a syringe and measure. Return immediately through tube and proceed with feeding if amount of residual does not exceed policy of agency or physician's guideline. Disconnect syringe from tubing.	This indicates gastric emptying time. A residual more than 50% of the previous hour's intake is significant and must be reported to physician. Fluid should be returned to stomach so as not to cause any fluid or electrolyte losses.
7 When using Asepto or Toomey syringe:	
a. Remove plunger or bulb from syringe and attach syringe to nasogastric tube which has been pinched with finger and introduce the prescribed amount slowly.	The syringe acts to receive the nourishment. Introducing the nourishment slowly gives the stomach time to accommodate the fluid and decreases gastrointestinal distress.
b. Hold the syringe approximately 12 inches above the stomach. Allow solution to run in by gravity. Raise the syringe to increase the rate of flow, and lower the syringe to decrease the rate of flow.	Nourishment enters the stomach by gravity when gastric gavage is used.
c. Do not let the syringe empty while introducing the nourishment.	This technique prevents air from being forced into the stomach when the syringe is refilled.

(Continued)

Action

d. Introduce 30 ml–60 ml (1 oz–2 oz) of water into the tube after the nourishment is introduced.

e. Clamp the gastric tube immediately after the nourishment and water are instilled. Disconnect the syringe and cover end of tubing with gauze secured with rubber band.

8 When using a feeding bag:

a. Hang bag on IV pole and adjust to about 12 inches above the stomach. Clamp tubing and pour formula into the bag. Release clamp enough to allow formula to run through tubing. Close clamp.

b. Attach tubing to nasogastric tube, open clamp, and regulate drip according to physician's order.

c. Add 30 ml–60 ml (1 oz–2 oz) of water to feeding bag when feeding is almost completed and allow it to run through tube.

d. Clamp the tubing immediately after water has been instilled. Disconnect from nasogastric tube. Clamp nasogastric tube and cover end with gauze secured with a rubber band.

Rationale

Washing the gastric tube with water forces remaining nourishment in the tube into the stomach and prevents nourishment from adhering to the tube and souring.

Clamping the tube prevents nourishment from draining back into the tube and air from entering the stomach. Cover on end of tube deters entry of microorganisms and protects client and linens from any fluid leakage from tube.

Formula displaces air in the tubing.

Introducing the formula at a slow, regular rate allows the stomach to accommodate to the feeding and decreases gastrointestinal distress.

Water rinses the feeding from the tube and helps to keep it patent.

Clamping the tube prevents air from entering the stomach. Cover on end of nasogastric tube deters entry of microorganisms and protects client and linens from any fluid leakage from tube.

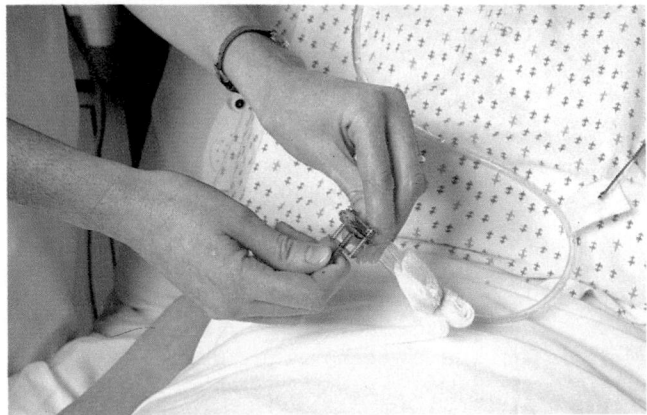

Step 7A: Introducing nourishment slowly.

Step 7E: Clamping the tube after feeding.

(Continued)

Action

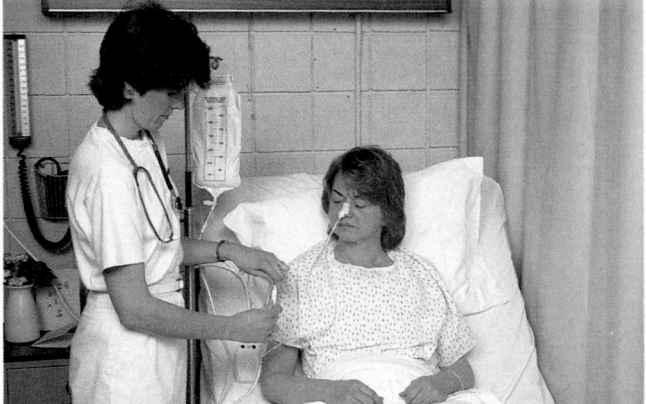

Step 8B: Attaching feeding-bag tubing to NG tube.

Rationale

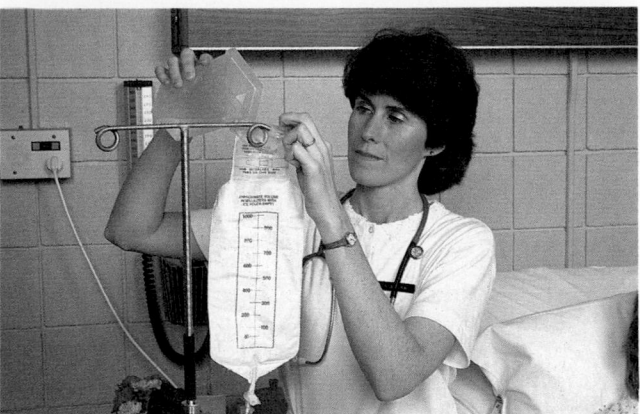

Step 8C: Adding water to rinse feeding tube.

9 When using pre-filled tube feeding set-up:

a. Remove screw-on cap and attach administration set-up with drip chamber and tubing. Hang set on IV pole and adjust to about 12 inches above the stomach. Clamp tubing and squeeze drip chamber to fill one-third to one-half of capacity. Release clamp and run formula through tubing. Close clamp.

Formula displaces air in tubing.

b. Follow steps 8b, 8c, and 8d. Feeding pump may be used with tube feeding set-up to regulate drip.

10 Observe client's response during and after tube feeding.

Pain may indicate stomach distention which may lead to vomiting.

11 Have client remain in upright position for at least 30 min after feeding.

This position minimizes risk of backflow and discourages aspiration should any vomiting occur.

12 Wash and clean equipment or replace according to agency policy. Wash your hands.

Prevents contamination and deters spread of microorganisms

13 Record type and amount of feeding and client's response. Monitor urine or blood glucose if ordered by physician.

Provides accurate documentation of procedure. Many feedings contain high loads of carbohydrate.

P R O C E D U R E   31-4
Monitoring a Nasogastric (NG) Tube

Action

1 Confirm physician's order for NG tube, type of suction, and directions for irrigation.

Rationale

Ensures correct implementation of physician's order

(Continued)

Action	**Rationale**
2 Observe drainage from NG tube. Check amount, color, consistency, and odor. Hematest drainage to confirm presence of blood in drainage.	Normal color of gastric drainage is light yellow to green in color due to the presence of bile. Bloody drainage may be expected after gastric surgery but must be monitored closely. Presence of coffee-ground type drainage may indicate bleeding.
3 Inspect suction apparatus. Check that setting is correct for type of suction (continuous or intermittent), range of suction (low, medium, high), and that movement of drainage through tubing is present.	Ensures correct implementation of physician's order. Ensures that suction is present and correctly adjusted. Loose connections or a kink or blockage in tube may interfere with suction.
4 Assess placement of NG tube. See Procedure 31-2. Irrigating a Nasogastric Tube, step 5.	NG tube may be displaced into trachea through movement or manipulation.
5 Assess comfort of client. Check for presence of nausea and vomiting, feeling of fullness, or pain.	May indicate incorrect operation of NG suction or blockage in tube.
6 Assess client's abdomen for distention and auscultate for presence of bowel sounds.	Abdominal distention may be related to the accumulation of gas or internal bleeding. Presence of bowel sounds indicates the return of peristalsis.
7 Assess mobility of client and respiratory status.	Turning from side to side in bed and ambulation when permitted encourage the return of peristalsis and facilitate drainage. Presence of NG tube may discourage client from coughing and deep breathing necessary for adequate respiratory exchange.
8 Observe condition of client's nostrils and oral cavity.	Nostrils need cleansing and lubrication with water-soluble lubricant and tape must be changed when necessary to minimize irritation from NG tube. Frequent mouth care (at 2-hr intervals) improves comfort and maintains moisture in oral mucosa.
9 Monitor overall safety of client with NG tube.	NG tube that is secured to client's nose with tape and pinned to gown allows easier movement. Call bell within reach allows client ready access to nursing assistance. Any kinks or obstruction interferes with patency of NG tube. A semi-Fowler's position facilitates drainage and minimizes any risk of aspiration.
10 Monitor NG tube and suction apparatus at least every 2 hr. Irrigate at interval ordered by physician. See Procedure 31-4.	Promotes safe operation of system. Any change in client's condition or type of drainage necessitates more frequent observation and notification of physician.
11 Record and measure NG irrigations and drainage on intake/output chart according to schedule and agency protocol. Document description of drainage and client's response on chart.	Irrigations are recorded as intake. Drainage from NG tube is measured as output every 8 hr. If drainage is copious, more frequent emptying of collection container will be necessary. Documentation provides accurate record of client's response to NG drainage.
12 Replenish supplies and maintain equipment according to agency policy and manufacturer's recommendations.	Ensures availability of necessary supplies. Provides for safe operation of equipment and efficient drainage of client's gastric contents.

PROCEDURE 31-5
Removing a Nasogastric Tube

Equipment

Tissues
Bath towel or dis-
    posable pad

Plastic disposal bag

Clean disposable
    glove

Action	**Rationale**
1 Check physician's order for removal of nasogastric tube.	Ensures correct implementation of physician's order
2 Explain procedure to client.	Explanation facilitates client cooperation.
3 Gather equipment.	Provides for organized approach to task
4 Wash your hands. Don clean disposable glove on hand that will remove tube.	Handwashing deters the spread of microorganisms. Glove protects hand from contact with abdominal secretions.
5 Discontinue suction and separate tube from suction. Unpin tube from client's gown and carefully remove adhesive tape from bridge of nose.	Allows for unrestricted removal of nasogastric tube.
6 Place towel or disposable pad across client's chest. Hand tissues to client.	Protects client from contact with gastric secretions. Tissues are necessary if client wishes to blow his nose when tube is removed.
7 Instruct client to take a deep breath and hold it.	Prevents accidental aspiration of any gastric secretions in tube
8 Clamp tube with fingers. Quickly and carefully remove tube while client holds his breath.	Minimizes trauma and discomfort for client. Clamping prevents any drainage of gastric contents in tube.
9 Place tube in disposable plastic bag. Remove glove and place in bag.	Prevents contamination with any microorganisms
10 Offer mouth care to client and make client comfortable.	Provides for comfort
11 Measure nasogastric drainage. Remove all equipment and dispose according to agency policy. Wash your hands.	Measuring nasogastric drainage provides for accurate recording of output. Proper disposal deters spread of microorganisms.
12 Record removal of nasogastric tube, client's response, and measurement of drainage.	Facilitates documentation and provides for comprehensive care.

Feeding by Vein

Clients with nonfunctional GI tracts, who are comatose, or who cannot consume a nutritionally adequate diet enterally (*e.g.,* clients undergoing aggressive cancer therapy, or recovering from extensive burns, sepsis, multiple fractures) may require parenteral nutrition. Sterile infusions of nutrients normally found in the blood may be delivered peripherally (isotonic solutions) or through the central vein if nutrient needs are great (hypertonic solutions). Although all the client's nutritional needs can be met through **total parenteral nutrition** (TPN), it is expensive, requires constant monitoring, and has potential infectious, metabolic, and mechanical complications (Table 31-13). TPN should be used only when an enteral intake is inadequate or contraindicated, and should be gradually discontinued as soon as possible.

T A B L E   31-13
Potential Complications of Total Parenteral Nutrition

Infection and Sepsis Related to

Catheter contamination during insertion
Long-term in-dwelling catheter
Catheter seeding from blood-borne or distant infection
Contaminated solution

Metabolic Complications

Dehydration
Hyperglycemia
Rebound hypoglycemia
Hyperosmolar, hyperglycemic nonketotic coma
Azotemia
Electrolyte disturbances
    Hypocalcemia
    Hypophosphatemia, hyperphosphatemia
    Hypokalemia
    Hypomagnesemia
High serum ammonia levels
Deficiencies of
    Essential fatty acid
    Trace elements
Altered acid–base balance
Elevated liver enzymes

Mechanical Complications Related to Catheterization

Catheter misplacement
Hemothorax (blood in the chest)
Pneumothorax (air or gas in the chest)
Hydrothorax (fluid in the chest)
Hemomediastinum (blood in the mediastinal spaces)
Subcutaneous emphysema
Hematoma
Arterial puncture
Myocardial perforation
Catheter embolism
Air embolism
Endocarditis
Nerve damage at the insertion site
Laceration of lymphatic duct
Chylothorax
Lymphatic fistula
Thrombosis

Teaching Nutritional Information

For the greatest chance of success, diet instructions should be individually tailored to the client's life-style, intellectual ability, and level of motivation. While strict guidelines and printed handouts may be viewed as the ideal, in practice, simplicity and compromise are often the keys to client compliance. Although specific instructions vary according to the diet order, the following guidelines are applicable for all types of diets:

- Provide simple verbal instructions. When appropriate, include family members and provide written teaching aids (Fig. 31-7).
- Advise the client to eliminate any foods not tolerated.
- Advise the client to alert the physician if the diet conflicts with religious beliefs, if adverse side-effects develop, or if special foods required are too costly or difficult to locate.
- Offer support and encouragement.
- If possible, spread diet instructions out over a period of days or weeks, so as not to overwhelm the client with too much information at one time and to allow the client time to internalize the information and form questions.
- Evaluate the client's level of understanding; assess the need for reinforcement or elaboration.

EVALUATING

The effectiveness of the plan of care is evaluated as the last step in the nursing care process. On an ongoing basis, the nurse should:

- Evaluate the client's progress toward meeting his nutritional goals.
- Evaluate the client's tolerance and adherence to the diet, when appropriate.
- Assess the client's level of understanding of the diet and his need for further diet instruction or reinforcement.
- Communicate findings to other members of the health-care team.
- Revise the plan of care, as needed, or terminate nursing care.

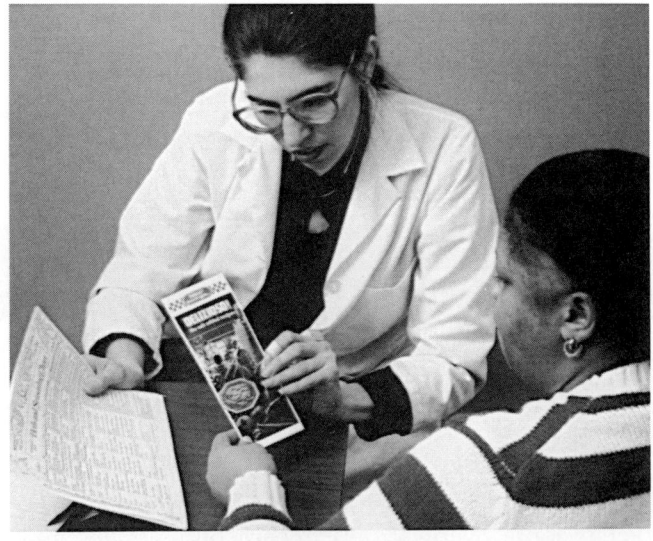

F I G U R E   31-7
Diet instructions should be individually tailored to the client's lifestyle, abilities, and level of maturation. Printed information is ideal.

NURSING PROCESS   in Clinical Practice

Nursing diagnoses related to the client's nutritional status can be made after assessment data have been collected and analyzed. Nursing diagnoses may cite actual or potential nutritional problems, may deal with how nutritional problems affect other areas of human functioning, or may be related to nutritional knowledge deficits. The following three examples of nutritional diagnoses include assessment priorities, client goals, nursing interventions, and evaluative criteria.

Altered Nutrition, More Than Body Requirement: Obesity

Obesity is defined as body weight 20% or more above ideal weight (Brownell, 1984). A positive calorie balance, resulting from an excess calorie intake and/or a decrease in energy expenditure, leads to the gradual accumulation of weight. Although society tends to assume obese people gorge themselves with food, studies have shown that obese people actually tend to eat less than their thin counterparts. The cascading effect of increased weight gain leading to a decrease in activity and social isolation perpetuates the problem of obesity.

It is estimated that approximately 88 million Americans (and 26% to 39% of Canadian adults) are overweight; 40 million of those are obese (Brownell, 1984). Obesity strikes all segments of society, although an increase in socioeconomic status is related to an increase in the risk of obesity for men and decreases the risk of obesity in women. Obesity can occur at any age and affects approximately 25% of all American children (5% to 25% of Canadian children).

Obesity is probably multifactorial in origin, with different factors contributing to its development in different people. Numerous theories have been proposed, such as the following genetic theories:

- Faulty ATP production causes obese people to use less energy performing metabolic functions.
- Familial traits: The weight of natural children is highly correlated to that of their natural parents, whereas there is only a slight correlation between the weight of adopted children and their adopted parents.

Physiologic theories regarding the development of obesity include:

- Fat cell theory: Obese people have more fat cells in their body, which have the propensity to store fat.
- "Set point" theory: The hypothalamus determines the body's ideal biologic weight (set point) and struggles to maintain that weight, even when calorie intake is restricted, by lowering metabolic rate. As metabolic rate decreases, it becomes increasingly difficult to lose weight, without further reducing calories, which causes a further reduction in metabolic rate.

- Brown fat: Obese people have less brown fat, and thus use less energy producing heat through nonshivering or diet-induced thermogenesis.
- Insulin response: Obese people respond more readily to external cues (the sight, sound, or smell of food) which stimulate the release of insulin and lead to a decrease in serum glucose and the sensation of hunger accompanied by an increase in fat formation.
- Hormonal imbalances: An undersecretion of thyroid hormones causes a decrease in metabolic rate and therefore a decrease in energy expenditure.

The following environmental theories have also been proposed:

- Food environment: Some people may be lured into overeating because of the abundance of food.
- Family environment: Obesity tends to run in families. For instance, a child with no obese parents has a 10% chance of becoming obese, the risk increases to 40% if one parent is obese, and children who have two obese parents have an 80% chance of becoming obese.
- Work environment: Since the turn of the century, mechanization, shorter work days, and shorter work weeks have led to a decrease in energy expenditure.

Psychologic theories suggest that obese people overeat

- Because they suffer from a compulsive behavioral disorder similar to alcoholics and drug abusers
- As an emotional crutch
- To compensate for lack of affection, love, and companionship
- To relieve boredom, tension, anxiety, frustration, and feelings of inadequacy

Obesity presents a serious health problem physically, socially, and emotionally. Obesity increases the risk of numerous medical problems, such as hypertension, hyperlipidemia, cardiovascular diseases, diabetes mellitus, respiratory disorders, and osteoarthritis; increases the risks associated with surgery; increases the risk of complications during pregnancy, labor, and delivery; and increases morbidity and mortality. Socially, obese people are often discriminated against in social, educational, and employment settings. And in a society that values thinness, obesity can cause feelings of failure, desperation, frustration, and rejection.

Obesity is resistant to treatment, and weight loss is usually temporary at best. According to Brownell, obesity is harder to "cure" than many forms of cancer, if cure is defined as attaining and maintaining ideal body weight for 5 years (Brownell, 1984).

The following assessment criteria, client goals, nursing interventions, and evaluative criteria are for a client diagnosed with obesity related to overeating.

Assessment

A thorough assessment to determine not only the degree of obesity, but also whether the client is likely to succeed in a weight loss program must be performed before a plan of care can be devised. Although all obese clients have the potential to benefit from weight loss, not all clients are motivated enough to lose weight and to keep it off. In addition, static obesity may be less harmful than frequent weight loss and regain. Thrusting weight loss diets on unmotivated clients may also cause "negative contagion," which may spread to others in a group setting; failure, which can have devastating consequences that preclude later attempts at dieting when the client may have had a better chance of success; and loss of morale among the health-care professionals (Brownell, 1984).

To determine the severity of the obesity and the client's level of motivation

- Use interview questions to assess pertinent dietary factors, such as the pattern and frequency of eating; the social environment surrounding eating; the client's actual and perceived reasons for eating; the client's previous use of weight loss diets; cultural, familial, religious, and ethnic influences on eating habits and their relative importance to the client; and nutritional knowledge.
- Explore the client's life-style and physical and mental health for factors contributing to obesity.
- Instruct the client to keep a food diary for a period of 3 days to 7 days to determine his level of motivation as well as to gain knowledge about his eating habits.
- Assess the client's present weight and ideal body weight and determine the percentage of excess body weight.
- Obtain body measurements, such as bust/chest, waist, hips, and thighs, for use in ongoing evaluation. Skinfold measurements may also be helpful in determining body fatness and measuring weight loss progress.
- Assess for the presence of complications: hypertension, diabetes, heart disease, osteoarthritis.
- Assess the duration of obesity: age of onset, family history.
- Assess activity patterns and how activity is affected by obesity.
- Assess the actual and perceived degree of control the client has over food.
- Assess the client's feelings about obesity and weight loss diets, his sense of body image and self-esteem.
- Determine if outside support systems are present.
- Assess the safety and effectiveness of weight loss aids the client has used in the past.

Client Goals

The client who undertakes a weight control program will
- Identify eating attitudes and behaviors that contribute to obesity

- Practice behavior modification techniques to control factors contributing to overeating
- Incorporate some type of physical activity into his daily routine, gradually increasing the intensity and duration of activity
- Enlist the support of family and friends, and attend group weight loss sessions, if possible

Interventions

Interventions for obesity vary according to its cause and severity. Weight loss programs should combine dietary changes, social support, exercise, and behavior modification.

Dietary Interventions

- Decrease calories for a gradual, weekly weight loss of 1 lb to 2 lb (0.5 kg to 1.0 kg/week).

  Low calorie intakes can be achieved by several methods, depending on the amount of weight the client has to lose and his level of motivation. For clients who don't have a lot of weight to lose, simply eliminating second helpings and snacks may be adequate. Counting total calories consumed throughout the day may work, but unfortunately it does not ensure nutritional adequacy. A more effective and realistic approach uses exchange lists that state the size and number of servings allowed daily from each of six or more food group lists.

  Traditional low-calorie diets may produce too gradual a weight loss for clients who are moderately to morbidly obese (*i.e.,* greater than 40% and 100% above ideal weight, respectively). In such cases, a medically supervised very low calorie diet (VLCD), otherwise known as a protein-sparing modified fast, may be indicated. VLCD provide 1.5 g of high biologic value protein/kg of body weight, either in the form of meat, fish, poultry, or powdered protein supplement. Supplemental vitamins and minerals are given, based on the client's laboratory data, and the client is closely monitored for tolerance, weight loss, and complications. Although the average weight loss in a 12-week period is about 45 lb, weight loss tends to be poorly maintained after the diet is discontinued.

Social Support

- Enlist the support of family and friends.
- Encourage the client to enroll in a group weight loss program, which tend to be more successful than individual programs.

Exercise

- Incorporate a period of exercise into each day, gradually increasing its intensity and duration.

Behavior Modification Techniques

(which suggest "how to" and "how not to," as opposed to stipulating "do's" and "don'ts")
- Think thin, by making a list of reasons why the client wants to lose weight, setting long-term

weight loss goals, rewarding successes periodically with nonfood items, and by avoiding talk about food.

- Plan strategies: Keep food only in the kitchen and avoid the kitchen except for meal time, cook only as much food as is needed for each meal, avoid tasting food while cooking, position low-calorie food in the front of the refrigerator and higher calorie items in the back, keep tempting items out of sight, preferably out of the house; limit the list of forbidden foods.
- Change eating habits: Wait 10 minutes after feeling the urge to eat, eat slowly, never skip meals, eat only in one designated place and don't do anything else while eating, eat low-calorie foods first, use a small plate, chew food thoroughly and eat slowly, leave some food on your plate.
- Modify shopping habits: Never shop while hungry, always shop from a list, buy only as much food as needed, don't buy items that you know are your "weakness."
- Incorporate life-style changes: Keep busy with projects and hobbies; accept changes in eating as a way of life, not a short-term hurdle to overcome; trim recipes of extra fat and sugar; don't weigh yourself too frequently; accept set backs or infrequent cheating without giving up on the plan—they are inevitable.

Although numerous prescription and over-the-counter drugs are promoted as diet aids, they are inappropriate and ineffective when used alone. At best, some drugs may be useful on a short-term basis when combined with other weight loss measures. If drugs are prescribed, the nurse instructs the client about the action of the drug, the reason for its use, side-effects to be aware of and to report, and the potential dangers of the drug.

Surgical intervention, such as gastric stapling, may be used as a last resort in a client who (1) cannot lose weight by nonsurgical methods, (2) is at increased risk of illness because of obesity, and (3) whose obesity poses a greater risk than the risk of surgery. A row of staples across the stomach forms a small pouch which initially holds 1 oz to 2 oz of food. Because the pouch can eventually expand to hold more food, and because the staples can burst under too much pressure, it is also imperative that a low-calorie diet of small frequent meals be used.

Clients suffering from compulsive overeating may benefit from Overeaters Anonymous, a self-help program designed to identify and cope with feelings that lead to overeating. Other options include referral for psychiatric evaluation.

Evaluative Criteria

Client meets above goals.

Altered Nutrition, Less Than Body Requirement: Iron Deficiency Anemia

One of iron's major functions in the body is to form heme, the pigment that combines with the protein globin in the blood to form hemoglobin. Hemoglobin is responsible for carrying oxygen from the lungs to the tissues, and therefore it is needed by all body cells for the release of energy.

Iron deficiency anemia, characterized by small (microcytic), pale (hypochromic) red blood cells (RBC), is a common nutritional deficiency disorder worldwide. Without sufficient iron, the body cannot produce enough hemoglobin, which hinders oxygen transport and leads to fatigue, weakness, and pallor.

Iron deficiency anemia has a 10% to 50% (10% to 60% in Canada) incidence rate among high-risk population groups who simply do not consume enough dietary iron to meet their requirements: infants and children under age 2, menstruating women, the elderly, people in low-income groups, and vegetarians. Iron deficiency anemia is commonly related to an inadequate intake for two reasons. First, iron is not widespread in the diet and there are few excellent sources: liver, other organ meats, muscle meats, clams, liver sausage, oysters, pork loin, sardines, shrimp, dark poultry meat. These animal sources are known as "heme" iron. "Nonheme" sources of iron include enriched and fortified grains and cereals, dried fruit, dried peas and beans, nuts, and "greens." Secondly, on the average, only 10% of dietary iron is absorbed, with a 15% to 35% absorption rate for heme iron, and a 3% to 8% absorption rate for nonheme iron. Unlike heme iron, nonheme iron absorption is greatly influenced by other dietary factors. For instance, vitamin C, heme iron, and certain animal proteins enhance nonheme iron absorption while tea, coffee, bran, phosphates, oxalates, phytates, and antacids inhibit its absorption.

Iron deficiency anemia may also occur secondary to an increase in iron requirement related to

- Chronic blood loss. Bleeding ulcers, gastritis, malignancy, parasites, closely spaced pregnancies
- Inadequate absorption: Chronic diarrhea, malabsorption syndrome, partial or total gastrectomy, pica, poor iron bioavailability of foods consumed
- Accelerated growth: Pregnancy, infancy, and puberty

The following assessment criteria, client goals, nursing interventions, and evaluative criteria are for a toddler diagnosed with iron deficiency anemia related to inadequate intake.

Assessment

Observe for signs and symptoms of iron deficiency anemia, which vary with severity and chronicity: fatigue and weakness, pallor, sensitivity to cold, anorexia, dizziness and headaches, thin, spoon-shaped fingernails, sore tongue, sore mouth, pica (ingestion of nonfood substances, such as dirt, clay, laundry starch).

Interview the client or primary caregiver to determine the amount and sources of iron normally consumed. Be aware that toddlers consuming more than a quart of milk daily are at risk of iron deficiency anemia because milk displaces the intake of foods rich in iron.

Assess intake for the influence of nonheme iron inhibitors and enhancers.

Assess medical-socioeconomic data to determine whether the child's inadequate intake is related to low socioeconomic status or compounded by another medical problem.

Interview the client or primary caregiver to determine whether the person has ever or is currently taking iron supplements: symptoms of iron overload may mimic iron deficiency anemia.

Client Goals

The client will

- Increase iron intake, especially heme iron.
- Eat a source of heme iron at every meal.
- Include a rich source of vitamin C at each meal (*i.e.,* citrus fruits and juices, broccoli, tomatoes, strawberries, cantaloupe, green pepper, brussels sprouts).
- Avoid tea, coffee, and antacids immediately before and after eating because of their inhibitory effect on nonheme iron absorption.

Interventions

Instruct the client or family on ways to increase the iron content of the diet.

- Encourage the use of iron-fortified infant cereals until the child is 18 months old, if possible, because its iron is absorbed more readily than the iron in other cereals.
- Eat organ meats, muscle meats, and dark meat of poultry more often.
- Eat meat at every meal, if possible.
- Limit milk intake to less than 1 quart a day to avoid displacing other iron-rich foods.
- Add dried fruits to cereals and cookies; use as a snack or dessert.
- Use crushed iron-fortified cereals as a breading for meat, fish, poultry, and vegetables; mixed with butter for a casserole topping; as a meat extender in meatloaf, meatballs, and burgers; sprinkled on ice cream, fruit salad, yogurt, pudding.
- Substitute whole grains for refined products.
- Cook in iron pots whenever possible, especially acidic foods (tomatoes, foods with vinegar or lemon).

Instruct the family on ways to increase iron absorption

- Eat meat at every meal, if possible.
- Include a rich source of vitamin C at every meal.
- Do not give a child tea or coffee, which interfere with iron absorption.

Instruct the client and family that if the person is anorexic or a finicky eater, small frequent meals may be better tolerated.

Advise the client and family to avoid acidic and salty foods, strong spices, coarse breads, raw vegetables, and hot foods and beverages if the oral mucosa is inflamed.

If inadequate food budget is contributing to poor iron intake, refer the client to the appropriate social service.

If iron supplements are prescribed, teach when they should be taken, the possible side-effects to anticipate, and the dangers of overuse.

Evaluative Criteria

Client meets the above goals.

Knowledge Deficit Related to a New Medical Diet

The following assessment criteria, client goals, nursing interventions, and evaluative criteria may be used for a client who is being discharged from the hospital on a high-fiber diet (for diverticulum) which he has been receiving for 3 days.

Assessment

Through interview questions, obtain a diet history to determine

- Quantity and sources of fiber in the client's usual diet
- Client's tolerance of a high-fiber diet while in the hospital. Potential adverse side-effects of initiating a high-fiber diet too quickly include flatus, distention, cramping, and diarrhea.
- Client's willingness to make the appropriate dietary changes
- Who shops and prepares the client's meals

Client Goals

The client will

- Eat a variety of high-fiber foods daily
- Substitute high-fiber foods for foods of lower fiber content
- Add bran to the diet slowly to decrease the likelihood of developing flatus and distention
- Drink at least six to eight glasses of water daily
- Recognize the signs and symptoms of eating too much fiber

Interventions

Instruct the client and family that a high-fiber diet will increase stool bulk, stimulate peristalsis, and reduce pressure within the bowel to avoid aggravating his diverticulum.

Instruct the client and family that many different types of fiber exist in the diet; some are effective as laxatives, others tend to lower serum cholesterol levels and influence glucose levels in diabetics.

Advise the client and family that the following dietary changes should be incorporated gradually:

- Eat more raw vegetables and fresh fruit, preferably with the skin on
- Substitute whole grain breads and cereals for refined grains

- Add up to 3 tablespoons of coarse bran to the diet. The fiber in bran is the type most effective as a laxative. Bran can be sprinkled over cereal, applesauce, or eggs; added to muffins, quick breads, casseroles, and meatloaves before baking; mixed with fruit juice or milk.
- Drink at least six to eight glasses of water daily; fiber absorbs water in the gut to increase fecal bulk.

Inform the client about the potential adverse side-effects of eating too much fiber too quickly: flatus, distention, diarrhea. Advise the client to reduce fiber intake if symptoms appear.

Evaluative Criteria
Client meets above goals.

CASE STUDY

Mrs. Oakland is a 21-year-old woman who was seen at the prenatal clinic for her first pregnancy at 5 weeks gestation. On her next visit 4 weeks later, Mrs. Oakland complained of nausea and vomiting and had lost 3 lb.

Assessment Findings
A comprehensive nutritional assessment revealed the following data:

Anthropometric Data
Usual body weight: 112 lb
Weight at 9 weeks gestation: 109 lb
Height: 5'5"
Ideal body weight: 125 lb (range of 113–137)
Expected weight gain for 9 weeks gestation: 1 lb to 2 lb

Biochemical Data
Laboratory data revealed low hemoglobin and hematocrit.

Medical–Socioeconomic Data
Client complains of nausea and vomiting, which begins in the morning and continues until midafternoon. Appetite is poor. Also states "I'm always tired."

Client and her husband are first semester graduate students; their source of income is graduate assistantships so their food budget is limited.

Client states that she did not intend to become pregnant, but both she and her husband are excited about becoming parents. Client plans to take a leave of absence from school for one semester when the baby is born; wants to breastfeed.

Clinical Data
Client appears pale. No other abnormal physical findings were noted.

Dietary Data
Client's 24-hour recall revealed an inadequate intake from the milk group and a marginal intake from the grain and meat groups. Client avoids breakfast because of a hurried schedule, which is now complicated by nausea; lunch consists of soup, salad, and fruit; dinner is usually chicken, cooked vegetables, pasta, rice, or potatoes, and fruit. Client dislikes red meat and eats it only once or twice a month. Also dislikes milk—she substitutes sugar-free soft drinks and water. Before becoming pregnant she drank five to six cups of black coffee a day, but now she avoids it. Snacks usually consist of fresh fruit and vegetables.

Client is very weight conscious; periodically "crash" diets to maintain her weight at 112.

Client does not take vitamins, medications, or drugs; drinks socially.

Nutritional problems and contributing factors are the following:

Inadequate intake of milk and calories in general contributed to by nausea and vomiting, dislike of milk, limited food budget, weight consciousness

Poor iron intake contributed to by lack of good sources of iron in her diet, no supplemental iron intake

Meal skipping contributed to by nausea and vomiting, hurried schedule

Underweight or losing weight contributed to by weight consciousness, nausea and vomiting

Nursing Diagnosis
Nutritional alteration, less than body requirement related to increased requirements imposed by pregnancy; nausea and vomiting; weight consciousness; hurried schedule; and food dislikes.

Planning
Mrs. Oakland is very concerned about her pregnancy and willing to make dietary changes for the sake of the baby. Her husband is also very supportive. Planning will focus on maintaining good dietary habits, improving overall intake and meal patterns to meet the demands of pregnancy and subsequent lactation, initiating dietary

changes aimed at avoiding nausea and vomiting, and increasing iron intake.

Short-term goals agreed upon by the client include
By the next monthly assessment, the client will
1. Report that she eats three or more small meals a day
2. Eat dry crackers, bread sticks, or dry cereal 30 minutes before getting up in the morning to help avoid nausea
3. Drink water between meals instead of with meals
4. Avoid diet soft drinks
5. Eat the recommended number of servings from each of the food groups suggested by the daily food guide for pregnancy
6. Gain 1 lb to 2 lb; realize weight gained during pregnancy is necessary and that excess weight can be lost during lactation after the baby is born
7. Take prenatal vitamins as prescribed

Long-term goals:

Mrs. Oakland establishes new dietary habits and patterns that provide adequate nourishment for herself, the baby, and subsequent lactation, such as
1. An adequate intake from each of the food groups according to the daily food guide for pregnancy
2. Gradually gains 22 lb to 27 lb
3. Avoids hunger by eating three meals and two to three snacks daily
4. Drinks six to eight glasses of fluid daily
5. Takes supplements as prescribed by the physician
6. Avoids the use of sugar substitutes, alcohol, and caffeine

Implementation

Instruct the client and husband
- On the importance of nutrition for maternal and infant health
- On the optimum amount and rate of weight gain
- How to modify her diet to avoid nausea and vomiting: eat dry crackers, bread sticks, or cereal before rising; don't drink fluid with meals; eat small frequent meals to avoid hunger; avoid high fat foods and foods the client does not tolerate. Assure the client that nausea and vomiting usually subside by the end of the third month of pregnancy.
- How to modify her diet to meet the increase in nutritional requirements: eat more whole grain breads and cereals; use yogurt, cheese, and puddings as substitutes for milk; eat at least three meals a day
- To take supplements as prescribed by the physician
- To avoid alcohol during pregnancy
- To avoid all drugs and medications unless approved by the physician

Investigate the client's eligibility for WIC, a federal nutrition program for women, infants, and children. In Canada it is called Nutrition and Financial Support Systems for a Pregnant Woman.

Conduct ongoing assessment and evaluation at each visit. Provide dietary instructions as needed to reinforce previous instructions or to meet the client's changing needs.

Documentation

Sample documentation of the prenatal visit follows in the traditional note format:

Mrs. Oakland was seen for routine prenatal checkup at 9 weeks gestation. Assessment findings reveal the client is underweight, has lost 3 lb in the last 4 weeks, is experiencing nausea and vomiting, has a deficient hemoglobin and hematocrit, and is fatigued. Nursing diagnosis: nutritional alteration, less than body requirement related to increased requirements imposed by pregnancy; nausea and vomiting; weight consciousness, hurried schedule, food dislikes. Discussion centered on maintaining good dietary habits, improving overall intake and meal patterns to meet the demands of pregnancy and subsequent lactation, initiating dietary changes aimed at avoiding nausea and vomiting, and increasing iron intake. See care plan. Client's progress will be evaluated at the next monthly visit.

L. Swift, RN

SOAP documentation:
Nutritional alteration, less than body requirement
S: "Who can eat with nausea and vomiting? And anyway, I'm often too tired to cook and eat nowadays."
"I don't really like red meat. Besides, its too expensive when you're on a limited food budget like we are. I don't care for milk either."
"I've always tried to stay slim, but with the baby coming, I guess that will have to change."
O: Underweight; 3-lb weight loss within 4 weeks, deficient hemoglobin and hematocrit
A: Above nutritional alteration is related to the increase in nutritional requirements imposed by pregnancy, nausea and vomiting, weight consciousness, hurried schedule, and food dislikes.
P: 1. Increase overall intake to meet the daily food guide recommendations for pregnancy.
2. Modify meal patterns and intake to avoid nausea and vomiting.
3. Recognize the importance of adequate weight gain during pregnancy.
4. Alter schedule to allow for regular meals and snacks.
5. Substitute acceptable alternatives to red meat (for iron) and milk (for calcium) in the diet.
6. Reevaluate nutritional status at the next monthly checkup.

L. Swift, RN

Evaluation

Short-term goal achievement is evaluated at next monthly assessment. See the nursing care plan for related evaluative statements and revisions of the care plan. Long-term goal achievement is an ongoing evaluation.

N U R S I N G   C A R E   P L A N   *for Mrs. Oakland*

Nursing Diagnosis: Nutritional alteration: Less than body requirement related to increased requirements imposed by pregnancy; nausea and vomiting; weight consciousness; hurried schedule; food dislikes.

Long-Term Goals: Client meets the increased nutritional requirements imposed by pregnancy by: (1) adequate intake from each of the food groups as recommended by the daily food guide for pregnancy, (2) gradually gaining 22 lb to 27 lb, (3) eating three meals a day with two to three small snacks, (4) drinking six to eight glasses of fluid daily, (5) taking prenatal supplements as prescribed by the physician, (6) avoiding sugar substitutes, alcohol, and caffeine.

Goals	Nursing Actions	Rationale	Evaluative Statement
By the next monthly assessment, the client will: 1. Eat three or more small meals a day	Determine how the client's schedule may be altered to allow time for meals. Encourage the client to have easy-to-eat foods available for quick snacks, like cartons of yogurt, cheese and crackers, muffins, and fresh fruit. Advise the client that nausea may be lessened by avoiding periods of hunger, and that later in the pregnancy, avoiding hunger will help ensure a steady supply of nutrients to the fetus.	Client complained that her current schedule prevents regular meals. Easy-to-eat foods may be more acceptable than, and can be nutritionally comparable to, traditional meals. Low blood glucose may contribute to nausea early in pregnancy; later in pregnancy, low blood glucose and resultant ketosis may be harmful to the fetus.	Goal met. Client eats three meals daily. Tries snacking on easy-to-eat foods when possible. *Recommendation:* Encourage more snacking to increase overall food intake. *L. Swift, RN*
2. Eat dry crackers, bread sticks, or dry cereal 30 minutes before rising	Advise the client to eat a source of dry carbohydrates before getting up in the morning.	Eating dry carbohydrates 30 minutes before rising helps avoid nausea.	Goal met. Client eats dry crackers every morning 30 minutes before getting out of bed. Reports that it prevents morning nausea. *L. Swift, RN*
3. Drink water between meals	Advise the client to avoid fluid with meals. Recommend fluids be consumed 1 hr before or 2 hr after eating.	Fluid with meals may contribute to nausea.	Goal met. Client avoids liquids with meals. Nausea is occurring less frequently throughout the day. *L. Swift, RN*
4. Avoid diet soft drinks	Advise client to avoid diet soft drinks. Recommend acceptable nutritional alternatives to the client.	The effects of saccharin and aspartame on the fetus have not been proven safe.	Goal partially met. Client reports that she drinks two or three cans of diet soft drinks a week at school to relieve thirst because nothing else is available. *Recommendation:* Recommend the client bring something to drink

(Continued)

N U R S I N G   C A R E   P L A N (Continued)

Goals	Nursing Actions	Rationale	Evaluative Statement
			during the day from home, such as frozen drink boxes of 100% fruit juice which will thaw at room temperature or a thermos of ice water or milk flavored with vanilla (dislikes plain milk). *L. Swift, RN*
5. Eat the recommended number of servings from each food group as suggested by the daily food guide for pregnancy	Provide the client with a daily food guide for pregnancy and explain the rationale for the increased recommendations. Investigate acceptable alternatives for red meat and milk, which the client normally does not consume.	Because this is the client's first pregnancy, she is not aware of the recommendations for eating during pregnancy. Although no one particular food is essential during pregnancy, red meat is essential during pregnancy and an excellent source of iron and milk is an excellent source of calcium, two minerals important for the developing fetus. If the client is not provided with nutritionally equivalent alternatives, her diet may not be optimal, even if she consumes the recommended number of servings from the meat and milk groups (*i.e.,* client may not be getting as much iron as she can from her diet if she relies on fish, cheese, and white-meat poultry to satisfy the meat group recommendations).	Goal partially met. Client's intake is improved: intake from the grain and meat groups is adequate instead of marginal. However, the client still has difficulty consuming enough items from the milk group. *Recommendation:* Continue encouraging the client to consume more items from the milk group, such as cheese, yogurt, and pudding. Will advise the client to add skim milk powder whenever possible to fortify home-cooked and home-baked products. Will recommend the client increase her intake of nondairy sources of calcium, such as broccoli, spinach, and "greens." *L. Swift, RN*
6. Gain 1 lb to 2 lb	Advise the client on the recommended rate and amount of weight gain. Stress the importance of quality weight gain.	Client needs to understand that a 22-lb to 27-lb gradual weight gain is considered optimal for fetal development, and results in little gain in maternal fat tissue. However, because the fetus and maternal tissues require nutrients along with calories, it is essential that the weight gain comes from eating nutrient-dense calories instead of empty calories.	Goal met. Noting a relief from nausea and an increase in the number of daily meals, the client gained 2 lb.

(Continued)

NURSING CARE PLAN (Continued)

Goals	Nursing Actions	Rationale	Evaluative Statement
7. Take prenatal vitamins as prescribed by the physician	Advise the client to take the supplement as prescribed and that the supplements are not a substitute for an adequate diet. Advise the client that the iron content in the supplements may cause constipation and the stools to become black.	Supplements are intended to be used in conjunction with an optimal diet, not in place of one, because they do not provide optimal amounts of all required nutrients. Because the requirements for folic acid and iron during pregnancy are usually not met through diet alone, supplements of these two nutrients in particular are necessary. Common side-effects of large iron doses are constipation and black stools.	Goal met. Client reports taking supplement as prescribed. No side-effects noted. *Recommendation:* Will continue to monitor client's tolerance of supplement. Will continue to implement plan and reassess at next monthly appointment. *L. Swift, RN*

KEY POINTS

- A person's state of energy balance can be determined by comparing calorie intake with calorie expenditure, which is the sum of calories used during physical activity, for basal metabolism, and for specific dynamic action.

- The six classes of nutrients needed by the body are carbohydrates, protein, lipids, vitamins, minerals, and water.

- Carbohydrates provide the majority of calories in the diet. Glucose, the only carbohydrate present in systemic circulation, may be burned for energy, stored as glycogen, or converted to fat and stored as adipose.

- Protein is broken down by the body into amino acids, which are then recombined to form proteins. Eight to nine amino acids are considered essential because they cannot be made in the body and must be supplied in the diet. Protein is used in the body for tissue growth and repair, as well as the production of enzymes, hormones, antibodies, blood and other substances, and secretions; it may also be oxidized for energy. Excess protein is converted to fat and stored as adipose.

- Lipids provide more than twice the calories per unit than either carbohydrates and protein. Essential fatty acids cannot be made by the body and therefore must be supplied through the diet. Dietary fat not used for immediate energy is stored as adipose.

- Vitamins and minerals do not provide calories but are needed for the metabolism of energy.

- Water provides the medium for all chemical reactions within the body; it is more vital to life than food.

- Tools used to evaluate a diet for adequacy include food groups and recommended dietary allowances (RDA) and recommended nutrient intake (RNI). Dietary guidelines issued from health and government agencies tend to focus on avoiding excesses, rather than on obtaining sufficient quantities of nutrients. Most experts recommend that Americans and Canadians eat a variety of food, maintain their ideal weight, reduce their intake of fat, saturated fat, cholesterol, and salt and eat more complex carbohydrates and fiber.

- A person's food habits are a product of many variables, such as physical factors (geographical location, food technology, income), physiologic factors (state of health, hunger, stage of development), and psychosocial factors (culture, religion, tradition, education, politics, social status, food ideology).

- Factors that influence nutrient requirements include age, sex, state of health, alcohol abuse, the use of medications, and megadoses of nutrient supplements. Nutrient intake can be affected by numerous physiologic and psychologic factors.

■ A systematic approach is used to identify the client's actual or potential needs, formulate a plan to meet those needs, initiate the plan or assign others to implement it, and evaluate the effectiveness of the plan.

■ Nutritional assessment data can be collected through history taking (dietary data and medical-socioeconomic data), nursing examination (anthropometric data and clinical data), and laboratory data.

■ Nursing diagnoses may be written to specifically address nutrition problems (nutrition, alteration in: less than body requirement, more than body requirement, potential for more than body requirement) or to identify the effect nutritional problems have on other areas of human functioning (e.g., activity intolerance, anxiety, alterations in bowel elimination).

■ Implementing a plan of care may involve nursing actions concerned with stimulating appetite, providing special diets, assisting with eating, withholding food, feeding by tube, feeding by vein, and conducting diet instructions.

BIBLIOGRAPHY

American Dietetic Association: Cultural Food Patterns in the USA. Chicago, American Dietetic Association, 1976

Brownell KD: The psychology and physiology of obesity: Implications for screening and treatment. J Am Diet Assoc 84:406, 1984

Canada's Food Guide Handbook (revised). Ottawa, Canada, Department of National Health and Welfare, 1982

Cataldo CB, Smith L: Tube Feedings: Clinical Applications. Columbus, OH, Ross Laboratories, 1980

Christakis G (ed): Nutritional Assessment in Health Programs. Washington, DC, American Public Health Association, 1979

Dudek SG: Nutrition Handbook for Nursing Practice. Philadelphia, JB Lippincott, 1987

Fisher MC, Lachance PA: Nutrition evaluation of published weight-reducing diets. J Am Diet Assoc 85:450, 1985

Five-Year Federal-Provincial Plan on Nutrition in Health Promotion for Pregnant Women. Ottawa, Canada, Federal-Provincial Advisory Committee on Health Promotion, 1983

Fry ST: New ANA guidelines on withdrawing or withholding food and fluid from patients. Nurs Outlook 36(3):122–123, 148–150, 1988

Henneman A, Houfek JF, Morin P, Weise R: Teaching nutritional assessment to nursing students. J Am Diet Assoc 78:498, 1981

Hertzler AA, Owen C: Culture, families, and the change process—A systems approach. J Am Diet Assoc 84:535, 1984

Information Letter—Nutrition Labelling. Ottawa, Canada, Department of National Health and Welfare, 1986

Lecos C: Diet and the elderly. FDA Consumer, Nov 1984

Mertz W: The essential elements: Nutritional aspects. Nutr Today 19:22, 1984

Mertz W: Our most unique nutrients. Nutr Today 18:6, 1983

Mertz W: The essential trace elements. Science 213:1332, 1981

National Research Council: Recommended Dietary Allowances, 9th ed. Washington, DC, National Academy of Sciences, 1980

Nutrition: Canada National Survey. Ottawa, Canada, Department of National Health and Welfare, 1973

Nutrition in Pregnancy—National Guidelines. Ottawa, Canada, The Federal-Provincial Subcommittee on Nutrition, Department of National Health and Welfare, 1986

Pipes PL: Nutrition in Infancy and Childhood, 2nd ed. St. Louis, CV Mosby, 1981

Recommended Nutrient Intakes for Canadians. Ottawa, Canada, Bureau of Nutritional Sciences, Department of National Health and Welfare, 1983

Rivlin RS: Nutrition and the health of the elderly. Arch Intern Med 143:1200, 1983

Rivlin RS: Nutrition and aging: Some unanswered questions. Am J Med 71:337, 1981

Rosenberg IH, Solomons NW: Biological availability of minerals and trace elements: A nutritional overview. Am J Clin Nutr 35:781, 1982

Roe DA: Nutrition and the elderly. Professional Perspectives, June 1982

Salmond SW: How to assess the nutritional status of acutely ill patients. Am J Nurs 80:922, 1980

Scherer JC: Lippincott's Nurses' Drug Manual. Philadelphia, JB Lippincott, 1985

Starkey JF, Jefferson PA, Kirby DF: Taking care of a percutaneous endoscopic gastrostomy. Am J Nurs 88(1):42–45, 1988

Stern JS: Obesity treatment. J Am Diet Assoc 84:405, 1984

Suter CB, Ott DB: Maternal and infant nutrition recommendations: A review. J Am Diet Assoc 84:572, 1984

United States Department of Agriculture, United States Department of Health and Human Services: Dietary Guidelines for Americans, 1985

Waitzkin B: The fat child. Parents 58:111, 1983

Wharton R, Crocker RW: Adolescent obesity. Children Today 13:12, 1984

Whitney EN, Cataldo CB: Understanding Normal and Clinical Nutrition. St. Paul, West Publishing Company, 1983

Williams SR: Nutrition and Diet Therapy, 5th ed. St Louis, Times Mirror/Mosby, 1985

Young EA: Nutrition, aging, and the aged. Med Clin North Am 67:295, 1983

Bowel Elimination

32

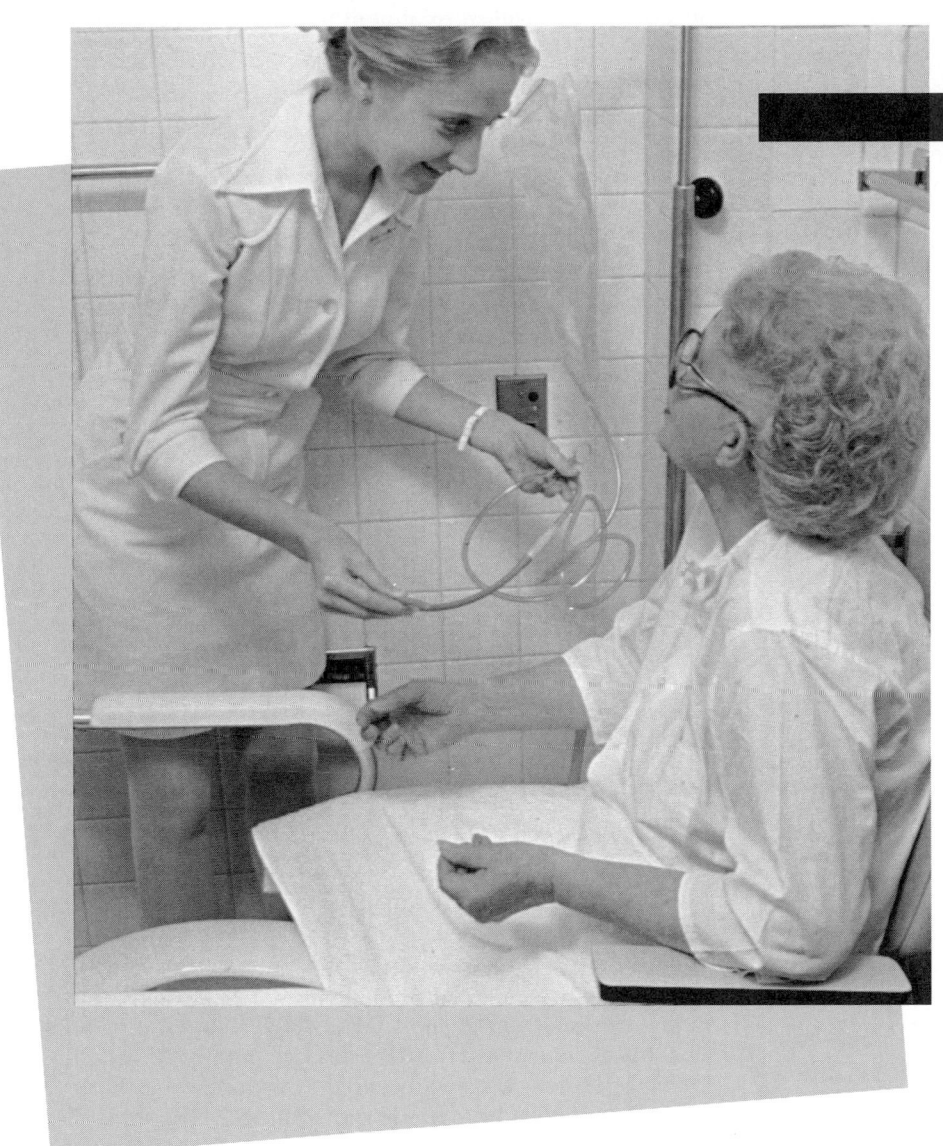

Define key terms used in the chapter.

Describe the physiology of bowel elimination.

Identify ten variables that influence bowel elimination.

Assess bowel elimination using appropriate interview questions and physical assessment skills.

Assist with the following diagnostic measures: stool collection for laboratory analysis and direct and indirect visualization studies of the gastrointestinal tract.

Develop nursing diagnoses that correctly identify bowel elimination problems amenable to nursing therapy.

Demonstrate how to (1) promote regular bowel habits (timing, positioning, privacy, nutrition, exercise); (2) use cathartics, laxatives, and antidiarrheals; (3) empty the colon of feces (enemas, rectal suppositories, rectal catheters, digital removal of stool); (4) design and implement bowel training programs; and (5) use comfort measures to ease defecation.

Plan, implement, and evaluate nursing care related to select nursing diagnoses involving bowel problems.

KEY TERMS

bowel movement	hemorrhoids
bowel training program	impaction (fecal)
cathartic	incontinence (fecal)
chyme	laxative
colon	occult blood
constipation	ostomy
diarrhea	peristalsis
endoscopy	stoma
enema	stool
feces	suppository
flatulence	Valsalva maneuver
flatus	

Elimination of the waste products of digestion is a natural process critical to human functioning. Clients differ widely in their expectations regarding bowel elimination, their usual pattern of defecation, and in the ease with which they can and do speak of bowel problems. Although most persons have experienced minor acute bouts of diarrhea or constipation some clients experience severe or chronic bowel elimination alterations which affect fluid and electrolyte balance, hydration, nutritional status, skin integrity, comfort, and very importantly, self-concept. Because many of the clients nurses encounter are experiencing illnesses that affect bowel elimination or undergoing diagnostic testing and pharmacologic or surgical treatment that affects functioning, nurses need to be knowledgeable in both preventing and treating bowel problems.

Study of this chapter will provide the student with knowledge of the physiology of bowel elimination and the multiple factors that influence this process. A practical guide to assess bowel elimination is presented which includes a description of nursing responsibilities related to diagnostic studies of the gastrointestinal tract. Numerous examples of nursing diagnoses are offered.

Goals are suggested for both the nurse and client, and nursing strategies are described in detail. In the section entitled "Nursing Process in Clinical Practice," focused assessment, planning, implementation, and evaluation guides are offered for select nursing diagnoses of common bowel elimination problems: constipation, fecal impaction, diarrhea, fecal incontinence, and flatulence/abdominal distention. These guides and the concluding case study illustrate how the nurse's knowledge of bowel elimination may be combined with specific nursing interventions and caring to successfully resolve bowel elimination problems.

PHYSIOLOGY

Large Intestine

The large intestine, the primary organ of bowel elimination, is the lower or distal part of the alimentary tract. It extends from the ileocecal valve to the anus. Waste products of digestion, termed **chyme**, are received by the large intestine from the small intestine. The gastrointestinal tract processes about 10 L of chyme daily, of which 100 g to 300 g are eventually expelled as feces. Functions of the large intestine include the completion of absorption, the manufacture of certain vitamins, the formation of feces, and the expulsion of feces from the body.

The length of the large intestine in adults is approximately 1.5 m (50 inches to 60 inches), but variations have been observed in normal persons. The width of the colon varies. At the narrowest point, the colon is approximately 2.5 cm (1 inch) wide; at the widest point, it is about 7.5 cm (3 inches). Its diameter decreases from the cecum to the anus.

The barrier between the large intestine and the ileum of the small intestine is the ileocecal or ileocolic valve. This valve normally prevents contents from entering the large intestine prematurely and prevents waste products from returning to the small intestine.

The waste contents pass through the ileocecal valve and enter the cecum, which is the first part of the large intestine. It is situated on the right side of the body, and to it is attached the vermiform process or appendix. When waste products enter the large intestine, the contents are liquid or watery in nature. While they pass through the large intestine, water is absorbed. Approximately 800 ml to 1000 ml of liquid are absorbed daily by the intestinal tract. This absorption of water accounts for the formed, semisolid consistency of the normal stool. When absorption does not occur properly, as when the waste products pass through the large intestine at a very rapid rate, the stool is soft and watery. If the stool remains in the colon too long or if too much water is absorbed, the stool becomes dry and hardened.

From the cecum, the contents enter the colon, which is divided into several parts. The ascending colon extends from the cecum up toward the liver, where it turns to cross the abdomen. This turn is the hepatic flexure. The transverse colon crosses the abdomen from right to left. The turn from the transverse colon to form the descending colon is the splenic flexure. The descending colon passes down the left side of the body, from the splenic flexure to the sigmoid or pelvic colon. When the waste products reach the distal end of the colon, they are called **feces**, and when excreted, feces are called the **stool**.

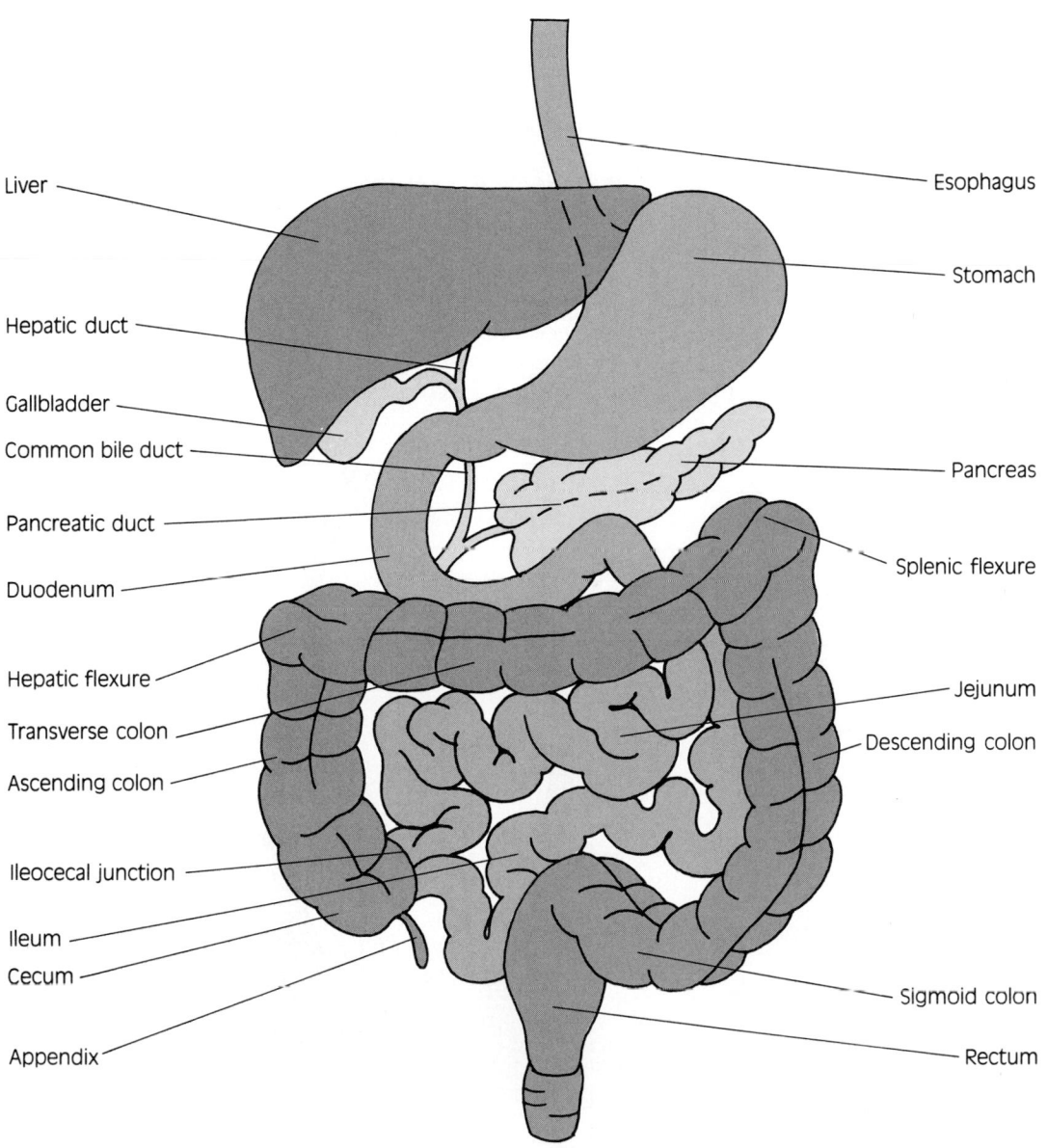

Liver
Hepatic duct
Gallbladder
Common bile duct
Pancreatic duct
Duodenum
Hepatic flexure
Transverse colon
Ascending colon
Ileocecal junction
Ileum
Cecum
Appendix

Esophagus
Stomach
Pancreas
Splenic flexure
Jejunum
Descending colon
Sigmoid colon
Rectum

FIGURE 32-1
Organs of the gastrointestinal system.

The sigmoid colon contains feces ready for excretion and empties into the rectum, which is the last part of the large intestine. The rectum is approximately 12 cm (5 inches) long, 2.5 cm (1 inch) being the anal canal. Normally, three transverse folds of tissue are present in the rectum. These folds may help to hold the fecal material in the rectum temporarily. In addition, there are vertical folds, each of which contains an artery and a vein. Abnormally distended veins are called **hemorrhoids**.

The rectum is usually empty except during and immediately prior to defecation. Feces are excreted from the rectum through the anal canal and the anus, which is about 2.5 cm to 3.8 cm (1 inch to 1½ inches) long.

The anatomy of the gastrointestinal tract is shown in Figure 32-1.

The muscles of the colon are innervated by the autonomic nervous system. The parasympathetic system stimulates movement, and the sympathetic system inhibits movement. Contractions of the circular and longitudinal muscles of the intestine (**peristalsis**) occur every 3 minutes to 12 minutes and continually move waste products along the length of the intestine (Fig. 32-2). Mass peristaltic sweeps occur one to four times each 24-hour period in most persons, propelling the fecal mass forward. This movement is unlike the frequent peristaltic rushes that occur in the small intestine. Mass peristalsis often occurs after food has been ingested. This accounts for the urge to defecate that frequently is observed following meals. Timing nursing interventions to evacuate bowel contents with this natural urge to defecate is helpful. One third to one half of ingested food waste products is normally excreted in the stool within 24 hours and the remainder within the next 24 to 48 hours.

Anal Canal and Anus

The internal sphincter in the anal canal and the external sphincter at the anus control the discharge of feces and intestinal gas, or **flatus**. The internal sphincter consists of smooth muscle tissue and is involuntary. The innervation of the internal sphincter occurs through the autonomic nervous system. Motor impulses are carried by the sympathetic system (thoracolumbar) and inhibitory impulses by the parasympathetic system (craniosacral). These two divisions of the autonomic nervous system function antagonistically to each other in a dynamic equilibrium.

The external sphincter at the anus has striated muscle tissue and is therefore under voluntary control. The levator ani muscle reinforces the action of the external sphincter and is controlled voluntarily. Interference with the normal functioning of elimination from the intestines can occur in health as it can during illness. It can be affected by the amount and quality of fluid or food intake, the degree of activity, and emotional states.

Figure 32-3 illustrates these structures.

Act of Defecation

Defecation is the emptying of the intestines and is often called a **bowel movement**. There are two centers governing the reflex to defecate. One is situated in the medulla, and a subsidiary one is in the spinal cord. When parasympathetic stimulation occurs, the internal anal sphincter relaxes, and the colon contracts. The defecation reflex is

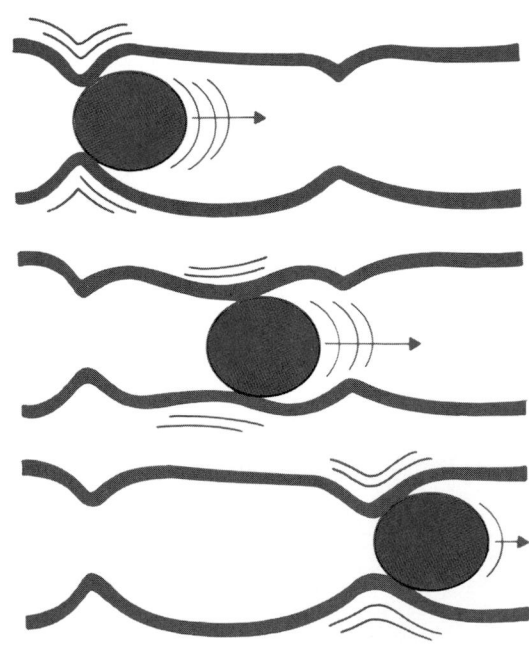

FIGURE 32-2
Peristaltic movements in the intestine.

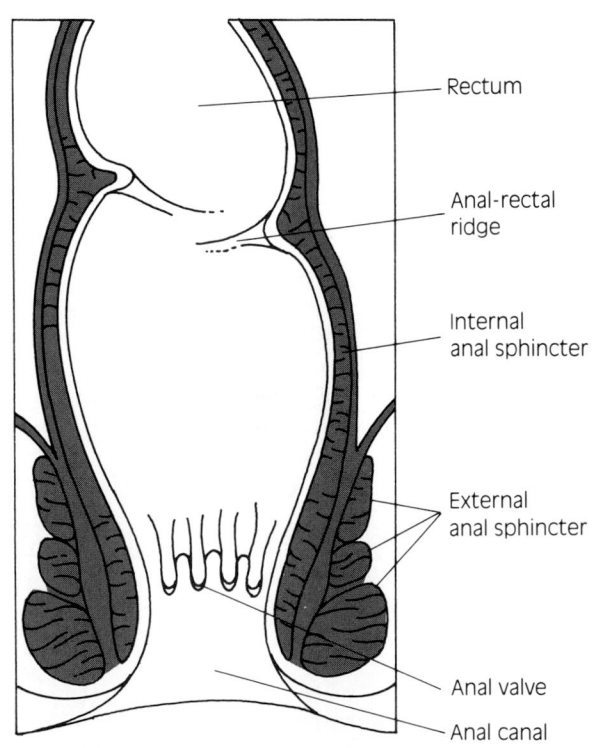

FIGURE 32-3
Interior view of the rectum and the anal canal.

stimulated chiefly by the fecal mass in the rectum. When the rectum is distended, the intrarectal pressure rises, the defecation reflex is stimulated by the muscle stretch, and the desire to eliminate results. The external anal sphincter, controlled voluntarily, is constricted or relaxed at will. If the desire to defecate is ignored, defecation can often be delayed voluntarily.

During the act of defecation, several additional muscles aid the process. Voluntary contraction of the muscles of the abdominal wall, fixing of the diaphragm, and closing of the glottis aid in increasing intra-abdominal pressure up to four or five times the normal pressure that aids in expelling feces. This technique, termed the **Valsalva maneuver,** may be contraindicated in persons with cardiovascular problems and other illnesses. Simultaneously, the muscles on the pelvic floor contract and aid in drawing the anus over the fecal mass.

Ease in defecation is aided by (1) flexing the thigh muscles which increases abdominal pressure and (2) assuming a sitting position which increases downward pressure on the rectum.

Normal Defecation

Normally, the act of defecation is painless. Normality is associated with the regularity and type of stool. If the bowels move at regular intervals and the stools are formed and soft, functional problems of frequency of elimination occur infrequently. However, nurses find that many persons show concern if they do not have a daily bowel movement. The normal frequency of bowel movements cannot be stated arbitrarily. Although many adults pass one stool each day, healthy persons have been observed to have more frequent or less frequent bowel movements. Some persons have a bowel movement two or three times a week; others as often as two or three times a day.

FACTORS AFFECTING BOWEL ELIMINATION

Developmental Considerations

Age affects in part what a person eats and the body's ability to digest nutrients and eliminate wastes. There is a marked difference between the stools of an infant and an older person. Because clients are often reluctant to discuss bowel habits and stool characteristics, nurses need to be familiar with bowel concerns pertinent to each developmental group. These are highlighted in Table 32-1 with related nursing interventions.

Daily Patterns

Most people have regular patterns of bowel elimination which include frequency, timing considerations, position, and place. Changes in any of these may upset a person's routine and actually lead to constipation. For example, many persons defecate after breakfast when the gastrocolic and duodenocolic reflexes cause mass propulsive movements in the large intestine. If this urge to defecate is ignored because the individual finds the time inconvenient, the feces remains in the rectum until the defecation reflex is again initiated. Meanwhile water continues to be absorbed from the unexpelled feces which makes it dry, hard, and painful to pass.

The position most persons assume for defecation is squatting or sitting slightly forward with the thighs flexed. In this position increased pressure is placed on the abdomen as well as downward pressure on the rectum; both facilitate defecation. It is difficult to obtain the same results when seated on a bedpan and embarrassment may further inhibit defecation.

Lastly, for many people defecation is a "private affair" which can only be done easily in the comfort of one's own bathroom. Defecation in a shared hospital room with only a curtain separating one from a roommate or other persons may be extremely difficult.

Food and Fluid

Both the type and amount of foods eaten and the amount of fluids ingested affect elimination. Healthy elimination is facilitated by a high-fiber diet and a daily fluid intake of 2000 ml to 3000 ml. High-fiber foods increase the bulk in fecal material. As the bulk of feces expands, it places pressure on the intestinal wall which serves as a stimulus for peristalsis. When fecal material moves quickly through the intestine, there is less time for water to be reabsorbed and the resultant stool is soft and easily passed. There is also less time for toxins to be absorbed from feces by the colon. Many believe that these toxins play an important role in colon cancer.

People digest and tolerate food very differently. In part this is determined by one's culture. Traveling to a different country and eating the native foods may result in severe indigestion and elimination problems. Differences in water may also affect elimination when traveling. Lactose intolerance is common. Persons who lack the enzyme lactase, which helps break down the simple sugar lactose, found in milk and milk products, cannot digest milk. Food intolerances may result in diarrhea, gaseous distention, and cramping.

In addition to high-fiber, bulk-producing foods, other general food classifications that influence bowel elimination include the following:

Constipating foods: Processed cheese, lean meat, eggs, and pasta

Foods with laxative effect: Certain fruits and vegetables (*e.g.,* prunes), bran, chocolate, spicy foods, alcohol, and coffee

Gas-producing foods: Onions, cabbage, beans, cauliflower

Activity and Muscle Tone

Regular exercise improves gastrointestinal motility and muscle tone while inactivity decreases both. Adequate

R E S E A R C H   I N   N U R S I N G   *Making a Difference*

Bowel Elimination

Normal bowel elimination in clients is an ongoing goal for nurses. Alterations must be identified through assessments, and a plan of care must be developed for the problem. Changes in bowel elimination are distressing to clients; when the nurse helps alleviate this stress, the emotional as well as the physical well-being of the client is maintained.

Related Research

McShane R, McLane A: Constipation. Consensual and empirical validation. Nurs Clin North Am 20:801–807, 1985
McShane and McLane carried out this study to define the characteristics of constipation and validate the diagnosis from the nurse's perspective. As a result, 22 defining characteristics were identified. Implications of the study include: (1) use of these diagnostic indicators in clinical assessment of normal and altered bowel elimination patterns, (2) use of the categories when teaching bowel elimination in nursing programs, and (3) the need for further research to refine and validate the nursing diagnosis

of constipation.

Miller J: Helping the aged manage bowel function. Journal of Gerontological Nursing 11(2):37–41, 1985
This study examined bowel function problems in the elderly, hoping to show that individuals would respond to bulk agents (bran and fluids) and would not need a suppository to stimulate the defecation reflex. Inconclusive results were believed to be due to the short duration of the study. It was noted that in elderly who did well, it was attributed to maintaining an adequate fluid intake, attention to the environment, and sustained and attentive nursing care.

Nursing research of bowel elimination is limited. Studies by other health-care professionals do not provide enough information to help in making nursing decisions. Problems in bowel elimination are commonly identified and treated by nurses, supporting the need for further research on normal and altered patterns of bowel elimination.

---

tone in the abdominal muscles, the diaphragm, and the perineal muscles is essential to ease in defecation. Clients who are on prolonged bedrest are prime candidates for constipation.

Life-style

Many individual, family, and sociocultural variables influence a person's usual elimination habits. The long-term effects of bowel training may result in a person's (1) accepting bowel elimination as a normal life process, (2) preoccupation with bowel elimination, or (3) feeling that bowel elimination is a "dirty" process. Rituals associated with bowel elimination, cleanliness considerations, the language used to talk about bowel elimination or reluctance to discuss it at all, individual responses to involuntary passage of flatus (gas), and so forth, vary widely among individuals. A person's daily schedule, occupation, and leisure activities may contribute to a habit of defecating at regular times or to an irregular pattern.

Psychologic Variables

Emotional stress affects the body in many ways. In certain persons anxiety seems to have a direct effect on

gastrointestinal motility, and diarrhea can be expected during any periods of high anxiety. During the fight or flight response when the body mobilizes itself for intense action, blood is shunted away from the stomach, and intestines and gastrointestinal motility generally slow. Chronic worriers and certain personality types who tend to "hold on" to problems and feelings may experience frequent constipation.

Pathologic Conditions

Numerous pathologic processes may result in changes in a person's usual bowel elimination. When a client reports that his stool is now narrower or ribbonlike in appearance, it is important for the nurse to consider the possibility of a tumor in the colon forming an obstruction to normal stool passage and to report this finding to the physician. Similarly, if a parent reports that a child's stools are frequent, bulky, greasy, and foul smelling, one possible explanation is cystic fibrosis; this would need to be ruled out if other clinical manifestations are present. Changes in stool characteristics or frequency may, therefore, be one of the first clinical manifestations of a disease, and their evaluation may lead to the diagnosis of the disease.

T A B L E 32-1

Developmental Variations in Bowel Elimination with Related Nursing Interventions

	Developmental Variations	Related Nursing Interventions
Infant	Stool characteristics depend on whether the infant is being fed breast milk or cow's milk. Breastfed babies have frequent yellow-to-golden stools of salvelike consistency. With cow's milk feedings, the stools vary from yellow to brown, are firmer, and have a stronger fecal odor because of the decomposition of protein. Both stools may have curds and mucus. Infants have no voluntary control over bowel elimination.	Parents should be advised that the number of stools an infant passes can vary greatly. In the first 4 months breastfed infants average two to four stools daily and bottle-fed infants one to two stools daily. By the time the infant is 1 year old he may only have one stool daily. Parents may mistake the infant's liquid stool for diarrhea. Loose stools may be related to overfeeding or too much corn syrup in the formula. Real diarrhea requires evaluation. The initial treatment for constipation is dietary manipulation; consistent use of suppositories and laxatives is to be discouraged. Infants with persistent constipation should be evaluated for structural defects.
Toddler	Between the ages of 18 and 24 months of age, the nerve fibers innervating the anal sphincter become fully developed and voluntary control of defecation becomes possible. Voluntary defecation requires intact muscular, sensory, and nervous structures. Successful bowel training includes 1. Toddler demonstrates awareness of the need to defecate and communicates this (grunting, tugging at diaper, special word). 2. Toddler wishes to avoid the discomfort of involuntary defecation and wishes to please the significant person managing bowel training. 3. Significant person has clearly and consistently communicated expectations, praises and reinforces successful behavior, does not punish "accidents." Daytime bowel control is normally attained by 30 months.	The parents' approach to toilet training and understanding of the need for physiologic maturity should be assessed. Guidance may be offered to ensure that the process of toilet training strengthens the parent–child relationship. It is critical for parents to understand that a child should never be punished or shamed for elimination accidents or for a lack of readiness to become toilet trained. Toddlers who are toilet trained may regress when hospitalized until they become comfortable in their new environment. Children who feel hostile to parents or staff may retaliate by soiling. Scolding or disgust will only reinforce this behavior and the only constructive approach is to seek out the underlying cause which is most often some form of emotional turmoil.
Child Adolescent Adult	Defecation patterns vary in quantity, frequency, and rhythmicity.	Each comprehensive nursing assessment should include questions about the client's bowel habits. Many persons may not understand the significance of changes in bowel habits or may worry needlessly about normal stool characteristics or bowel habits. The use of over-the-counter laxatives and enemas should be evaluated.
Older adult	Decreased physical activity, decreased gastrointestinal motility, and changes in nutritional habits make constipation a chronic problem for many elderly persons. Abuse of laxatives and enemas may cause rebound diarrhea and may negatively affect other body systems.	Strenuous teaching of the importance of nonpharmacologic remedies for constipation is needed. These include: regular exercise, increased fiber in the diet, decreased animal fat and refined sugar, and increased fluid intake.

Pathologic conditions that may result in diarrhea include diverticulitis, infection, malabsorption syndromes, neoplasms, diabetic neuropathy, hyperthyroidism, and uremia. Conditions predisposing to constipation include diseases within the colon or rectum, injury or degeneration of the spinal cord, and megacolon. Conditions that traumatize the stomach or intestines or that interfere with normal digestion may change the color, contents, odor, and appearance of the stool making stool assessment an important diagnostic task for nursing.

Medications

Medications are available to either promote peristalsis (cathartics and laxatives) or inhibit peristalsis (antidiarrheal medications). These will be discussed later in this chapter.

Other types of medications, however, may affect bowel elimination and stool characteristics. Narcotic analgesics, opiates, and anticholinergic medications all have the potential to cause constipation by decreasing gastrointestinal mobility. Many medications have diarrhea as an undesirable side-effect. The diarrhea may be severe enough to warrant the cessation of the drug. And finally, medications may influence the appearance of the stool for a variety of reasons. Any drug with the potential to cause GI bleeding, (*e.g.,* anticoagulants, aspirin products) may result in the stool appearing pink to red to black; iron salts result in a black stool from the oxidation of iron; antacids may cause a whitish discoloration or speckling in the stool; and antibiotics may cause a green-gray color because of impaired digestion.

Diagnostic Tests

Clients may need to fast for diagnostic studies. Additionally, the stress of hospitalization and waiting for the results of the study combined with changes in food intake can severely alter usual elimination patterns. Bowel cleansing by use of cathartics or enemas is a prerequisite for certain diagnostic studies of the gastrointestinal tract.

Surgery and Anesthesia

Direct manipulation of the bowel during abdominal surgery inhibits peristalsis, causing a condition termed para-lytic ileus. This temporary stoppage of peristalsis normally lasts 24 hours to 48 hours, and during this time food and fluids are withheld. If it persists it may cause distention and symptoms of acute obstruction and may require surgical intervention. General anesthetic agents that are inhaled also inhibit peristalsis by blocking the parasympathetic impulses to the intestinal musculature. Local and regional anesthesia has little effect on peristalsis.

NURSE AS ROLE MODEL

Before intervening to help clients develop healthy bowel elimination patterns it is important for nurses to assess the adequacy of their own bowel elimination habits and patterns. If you are unable to meet the following goals you may wish to take the time now to revise your own health practices so that you will be an effective role model for clients.

The nurse

- Has a soft, formed bowel movement every 1 day to 3 days without discomfort
- Responds to the normal urge to defecate
- Includes in each day's nutritional intake sufficient high-fiber foods and fluid to promote peristalsis and reduce stool retention
- Identifies many different ways to increase fiber and fluid in different types of diets

PROMOTING WELLNESS

Bowel Elimination

Use the assessment checklist to determine how well you are meeting your need for bowel elimination. Then develop a prescription for self-care by choosing appropriate behaviors from the list of suggestions.

Assessment Checklist

almost always	some times	almost never	
☐	☐	☐	1. I have a regular bowel elimination pattern, satisfactory to support comfort and activities of daily living.
☐	☐	☐	2. I eat a diet high in fiber.
☐	☐	☐	3. I exercise regularly.
☐	☐	☐	4. I have an adequate intake of fluids.

Self-Care Behaviors

1. Accept individual patterns of defecation as normal.
2. Eat a balanced diet, including high-fiber foods, such as fruits, vegetables, and nuts.
3. Follow a regular exercise program with 30 minutes to 45 minutes of activity three to four times a week.
4. Do not ignore the urge to defecate.
5. Establish a routine, if needed (1 hour after meals is usually best).
6. Avoid prolonged use of over-the-counter medications or enemas to treat constipation.

- Exercises vigorously for 15 minutes to 30 minutes three to four times/week
- Responds to changes in stool characteristics (or frequency) by seeking their etiology and getting medical assistance when necessary

ASSESSING BOWEL ELIMINATION

Nursing History

Because many clients are reluctant to initiate a discussion of their bowel status, nurses should include pertinent bowel elimination questions in each comprehensive nursing history (see accompanying box). Interview questions are used to identify

- Client's usual patterns of bowel elimination (frequency, time of day, description of usual stool characteristics: amount, consistency, shape, color, odor)
- Recent changes in bowel elimination
- Aids to elimination (liquids, food, laxatives, enemas)
- Problems with bowel elimination (nature of disturbance, onset, frequency, causes, severity, symptoms, interventions attempted and results)
- Presence of artificial orifices (normal routine, history of problems)

If the client is experiencing any disturbance in bowel elimination, a more detailed assessment is conducted with attention directed to each of the factors that may influence bowel elimination (described earlier).

Clients who are critically ill or who have impaired cognition may be incapable of reporting their bowel status accurately. In this instance, nurses need to record the client's daily bowel status in order to be alert to impending problems. While making daily rounds the nurse simply asks the client who is a reliable historian "Did you move your bowels yesterday or today?" and charts the response. If the client cannot offer this information, the nurse assisting with bowel elimination records daily stools.

Nursing Examination

Assessment of bowel elimination includes physical assessment of the abdomen, anus, and rectum. (These are discussed in Chap 24.) Described below are examination techniques helpful when assessing the functioning of the gastrointestinal tract.

Abdomen

The sequence for abdominal assessment proceeds from inspection–auscultation–percussion to palpation. Auscultation is done before palpation because palpation may disturb normal peristalsis. The client is comfortably

---

Elements of a Bowel Elimination History

Usual patterns of bowel elimination
"How often do you move your bowels?"
"Any special time of day?"
"What does your stool look like?"
- Frequency
- Time of day
- Description of usual stool characteristics (amount consistency, shape, color, odor)

Recent changes in bowel elimination
"Have you noticed any changes in your stool recently?"

Aids to elimination
"Do you use anything to help you move your bowels?"
- Natural aids (liquids, food)
- Pharmacologic aids (laxatives)
- Enemas

Problems with bowel elimination
"Are your bowels causing you any problems now?"
- Nature of disturbance
- Onset and frequency
- Causes (*physical:* food and fluid intake, exercise status, history of surgery or illnesses influencing GI tract; *psychosocial; medicine related*)
- Severity
- Symptoms
- Interventions attempted and results

Presence of artificial orifices
"Tell me about your usual routine with your colostomy/ileostomy."
- Normal routine
- History of problems

---

positioned in the supine position with the abdomen exposed and chest and pubic area draped. The bladder should be emptied.

Inspection. The nurse first observes the contour of the abdomen noting any masses or areas of distention. Peristalsis is generally not visible except in very thin clients and when observed (visible waves) may indicate an intestinal obstruction.

Auscultation. The nurse uses a warmed stethoscope to listen for bowel sounds in a systematic clockwise manner in all four abdominal quadrants. The frequency and character of bowel sounds are noted. Bowel sounds are audible "clicks and gurgles" produced by the movement of air and flatus in the gastrointestinal tract. They are usually high pitched, gurgling, and soft. Their frequency may range from 5 to 34 bowel sounds per minute depending on the rate of peristalsis. Of significance are absent or infrequent bowel sounds indicating hypoperistalsis or paralytic ileus (no decision should be made until the nurse has listened for 5 minutes) or abnormally intense and frequent bowel sounds (borborygmus) indicating hyperperistalsis. Bowel sounds are usually described as being audible, hyperactive, hypoactive, or inaudible.

Percussion. The nurse next percusses all four quadrants of the abdomen in a systematic clockwise manner to identify any masses, fluid, or air in the abdomen. A resonate sound or tympany is expected over the abdomen and stomach because these are hollow organs. With practice the nurse can distinguish normal resonance from the hyperresonance which occurs when excess flatus is trapped in the intestines. An intestinal obstruction will percuss dull. Areas of increased dullness may be caused by fluid, a mass, or tumor.

Palpation. Both light and deep palpation in each quadrant are next performed by the skilled nurse, noting muscular resistance, tenderness, enlargement of organs, and masses. The beginning nurse will quickly learn the "feel" of a distended abdomen.

Anus and Rectum

The skill of the nurse examiner will determine the extent of the rectal examination. A superficial examination is performed each time a nurse washes a client's anal area or assists with bowel evacuation. The client is most often positioned in left Sim's position.

Inspection and Palpation. The nurse first examines the anal area for cracks, nodules, distended veins (hemorrhoids), masses, or polyps. A fecal mass may be observed distending the anus. A gloved and lubricated finger is next inserted through the anus into the rectum to examine sphincter tone, smoothness of mucosal lining, and to note the presence of masses, polyps, hardened stool, bleeding, or abnormal discharge. The perineal area is also inspected for areas of skin irritation or breakdown secondary to diarrhea or fecal incontinence.

Stool Characteristics

Nurses are responsible for observing and recording information about the client's stool. Table 32-2 describes characteristics of a normal stool and presents special considerations to take into account when observing a stool. Anything unusual should be reported and re-

corded. Passing little or no gas or unusual amounts should also be recorded and reported.

The frequency with which the client has bowel movements is noted and recorded. Frequency is recorded as I, II, III, or i, ii, iii, and so on. Any unusual observations are described in the nurses' notes on the client's permanent record. Noting and recording the frequency of the client's bowel movements are important parts of nursing care. When auxiliary personnel or the client assumes this responsibility, the nurse should check at regular intervals to see that it is being done correctly.

Focused Assessment

When a client is experiencing constipation, impaction, diarrhea, incontinence, or flatulence/abdominal distention, the nurse conducts a focused assessment to collect more detailed data. Ideally high-risk populations will be identified, and these problems will be prevented or minimized through vigilant nursing care. To perform these assessments accurately, the nurse needs a thorough knowledge of the factors that contribute to these problems and of pertinent assessment priorities. These may be found in the section entitled "Nursing Process in Clinical Practice" later in this chapter.

Assisting with Diagnostic Studies

The nurse is often responsible for caring for clients with elimination problems who are undergoing diagnostic testing. General nursing responsibilities for diagnostic studies are discussed in Chapter 41. In the following section specific guidelines are offered for nursing's role with stool collection, and direct and indirect visualization studies.

Stool Collection. The nurse is responsible for obtaining the specimen according to agency procedure, labeling the specimen, and ensuring that the specimen is transported to the laboratory on time. The institution's policy and procedure manual or laboratory manual must be checked to determine specifics regarding (1) amount of stool needed and time frame during which stool is to be collected, (2) type of specimen container to use, and (3) any special handling precautions.

Medical aseptic techniques are used, and care is taken not to contaminate hands and specimen containers with stool. This admonition also applies when handling the client's bedpan and when disposing of its contents. Organisms in the stool can be spread among health-care personnel and clients when proper precautions are not taken. For clients on isolation precautions utilize correct isolation technique for obtaining, labeling, and bagging the specimen. The client voids first because the labora-

T A B L E 32-2

The Stool: Normal Characteristics and Special Considerations for Observation

Characteristic	Normal Finding	Special Considerations for Observation
Volume	Variable	The volume of the stool depends on the amount the person eats and the nature of the diet. For example, a diet high in roughage produces more feces than a soft, bland diet.
		Consistently large diarrheal stools suggest a disorder in the small bowel or proximal colon; small, frequent stools with urgency to pass them suggest a disorder of the left colon or rectum.
Color	Infant: Yellow Adult: Brown	The brown color of the stool is due to stercobilin, a bile pigment derivative. The rapid rate of peristalsis in the infant causes the stool to be yellow.
		The color of the stool is influenced by diet. For example, the stool will be almost black if the person eats red meat and dark-green vegetables, such as spinach. The stool will be light brown if the diet is high in milk and milk products and is low in meat.
		The absence of bile may cause the stool to appear white or clay-colored.
		Certain drugs influence the color of the stool. For example, iron salts cause the stool to be black. Antacids cause it to be whitish.
		Bleeding high in the intestinal tract causes a stool to be black owing to the digestion of the blood. Bleeding low in the intestinal tract will result in fresh blood in the stool.
		The stool darkens in color with standing.
Odor	Aromatic; may be affected by foods ingested	The characteristic odor of the stool is due to indole and skatole, caused by putrefaction and fermentation in the lower intestinal tract.
		The odor of the stool is influenced by its pH value, which is normally neutral or slightly alkaline.
		Excessive putrefaction causes a strong odor.
		The presence of blood in the stool causes a unique odor.
Consistency	Soft, semisolid, and formed	The consistency of the stool is influenced by fluid and food intake and gastric motility. The less time stool spends in the intestine (or the shorter the intestine) the more liquid the stool. Many pathologic conditions influence consistency.
Shape	Formed stool is usually about 1 inch (2.5 cm) in diameter and has the tubular shape of the colon, but may be larger or smaller depending on the condition of the colon.	A gastrointestinal obstruction may result in a narrow, pencil-shaped stool. Rapid peristalsis thins the stool. Increased time spent in the large intestine may result in a hard, marblelike fecal mass.
Constituents	Waste residues of digestion: bile, intestinal secretions, shedded epithelial cells, bacteria, and inorganic material (chiefly calcium and phosphates); seeds, meat fibers, and fat may be present in small amounts.	Internal bleeding, infection, inflammation, and other pathologic conditions may result in abnormal constituents. These include blood, pus, excessive fat, parasites, ova, and mucus.
		Foreign bodies may also be found in the stool.

tory study may be inaccurate if the stool contains urine. The specimen should also be free of barium and enema solution. Ask the patient to defecate in a clean bedpan, or a sterile bedpan if required. Do not collect a specimen from a toilet bowl because the laboratory study may be hindered by the water. Do not place toilet tissue in the bedpan after the client defecates. Contents in the paper may influence laboratory results.

A portion of the stool is lifted with two clean tongue blades and placed directly into an appropriately labeled specimen container. Usually 1 inch of formed stool and 15 ml to 30 ml of liquid stool are sufficient. If portions of the stool include visible blood, mucus, or pus, include these with the specimen sent.

The specimen is sent to the laboratory immediately because a fresh specimen produces the most accurate results. If this is not possible, the specimen should be refrigerated unless contraindicated. Use commercial tapes, dip sticks, and solution according to manufacturer's directions if testing the stool for blood or *p*H. Clients at high risk for intestinal bleeding should have their stools tested for occult blood (guaiac test). **Occult blood** is blood that is "hidden"; in other words it cannot be seen on gross examination.

Timed Specimens.   Consider the first stool passed by the client as the start of the collection period. Collect a specimen of *every* stool passed within the designated time period (the test may require saving the entire stool passed or only a sample). Follow instructions for sending stools to the laboratory.

Pinworms.   Use clear cellophane tape for collecting a specimen for pinworms. Frosted tape makes examination difficult. The tape is placed directly over the client's anal area, removed immediately, and then placed on a slide. Collect this specimen in the morning, immediately after the client awakens and before the client has a bowel movement or bath. Pinworms tend to come to the anal area during the night and retreat into the anal canal during the day.

Direct Visualization Studies.   **Endoscopy** is the direct visualization of the lining of a hollow body organ using a fiberoptic endoscope (*i.e.,* a long flexible tube filled with glass fibers which transmits light into the organ and returns an image to the scope's optical head). Pincers may also be inserted through the tube for the biopsy of tissues. An endoscope enables the physician to view the integrity of the mucosa, blood vessels, and specific organ parts and is helpful in the diagnosis of inflammatory, ulcerative, and infectious diseases; benign and malignant neoplasms; and other lesions of the esophageal, gastric, and intestinal mucosa. Studies include

- Esophagogastroduodenoscopy: Visual examination of the lining of the esophagus, the stomach, and

the upper duodenum with a flexible, fiberoptic endoscope
- Colonoscopy: Visual examination of the lining of the large intestine with a flexible, fiberoptic endoscope
- Proctosigmoidoscopy: Visual examination of the lining of the distal sigmoid colon, the rectum, and the anal canal using two rigid instruments (tubes): a protoscope and a sigmoidoscope. These tubes also have an attached light source and are equipped to allow biopsy. Being rigid, they may produce greater client discomfort, especially in the client who is not relaxed.

These studies are discussed in Chapter 41. Nursing responsibilities for these studies are highlighted in Table 32-3.

Indirect Visualization Studies.   Indirect visualization of the gastrointestinal (GI) tract is commonly achieved by radiography. The passage of x-radiation through the client creates a radiograph or film depicting body structures. This technique is useful in detecting obstruction, strictures, inflammatory disease, tumors, ulcers, and other lesions, and in diagnosing hiatal hernia and other structural changes in the GI tract. Use of a radiopaque contrast medium such as barium sulfate accentuates the body structures being visualized. In the *upper gastrointestinal examination* (UGI) and *small bowel series,* the client drinks the barium sulfate like a milkshake and the esophagus, stomach, and small intestine are coated and visualized. In the *barium enema or lower gastrointestinal examination,* barium sulfate is instilled into the large intestine by means of a rectal tube inserted through the anus. Fluoroscopy projects the x-ray films onto a screen and permits continuous observation of the flow of the barium.

Nursing responsibilities include
- Preparing the client for the test by describing what will be experienced before, during, and after the test
- Assisting the client to complete a safe dietary and bowel preparation program which will ensure optimal x-rays (institutions vary in the dietary modifications, laxatives, cathartics, and enemas they recommend; individual clients may need special bowel-cleansing strategies because of their bowel status)
- Ensuring that the client eliminates the barium used during the test within 1 day to 3 days after the test to avoid impaction and obstruction
- Encouraging increased fluid intake to maintain hydration and promoting rest following the test

Specific nursing care measures are detailed in Table 32-3.

Scheduling Diagnostic Studies.   Because nurses are commonly involved in the scheduling of diagnostic studies when multiple orders are written, it is helpful to

(Text continues on p. 824.)

TABLE 32-3
Diagnostic Studies of the Gastrointestinal Tract

Test	Purpose	Client Preparation	Nursing Care During Test	Client Aftercare
Esophagogastroduo-denoscopy	• Allows visual examination of the esophagus, stomach, and upper duodenum • Indicated for clients with hematemesis, melena, or substernal or epigastric pain and in post-op clients with recurrent or new symptoms • Assists in the diagnosis of inflammatory, ulcerative, and infectious diseases; tumors; and structural abnormalities • Allows biopsy, removal of foreign objects, and coagulation of bleeding	1. Explain to the client • Nature and purpose of the test • Directions for fasting (6–12 hr before the test; check guidelines) • That the test requires about 30 min and involves the passage of a flexible tube through the mouth (client may experience gagging or sense of fullness; cannot speak during this time) • Dentures need to be removed; mouth guard often used to protect natural teeth • Client will be awake although a sedative (and sometimes an anticholinergic drug to decrease GI secretions) is administered • A bitter tasting local anesthetic is sprayed into the mouth and throat to decrease sensation (tongue will feel swollen temporarily—difficulty swallowing) 2. Ensure that informed consent is signed. 3. Assist client into hospital gown and complete agency protocol for testing (empty bladder, remove jewelry, and so forth) 4. Administer prescribed sedative, anticholinergic, and if ordered, an analgesic.	• Position client in left-lateral or left Sim's position. • Provide emotional support. • Obtain baseline vital signs. • IV in place/administer prescribed medications • Place any tissue or cell specimens in properly labeled containers with preservatives and send to laboratory. • Observe for untoward responses; have emergency resuscitative equipment available.	• Check vital signs according to agency protocol. • Withhold food and fluids until the gag reflex returns. • Observe for signs of perforation: pain, persistent difficulty swallowing, vomiting blood, or black stools. • Explain to the client that it is normal to sense throat soreness and hoarseness for several days; warm, saline gargles, lozenges may help.
Colonoscopy	• Allows visual examination of the large intestine • Indicated for clients with histories of constipation and diarrhea, persistent rectal bleeding, or lower abdominal pain when results of proctosigmoidoscopy and the barium enema are negative or inconclusive • Assists in the diagnosis of inflammatory and ulcerative bowel disease, colonic stricture, and tumors • Allows biopsy, removal of polyps by electrocautery	1. Explain to the client: • Nature and purpose of the test • Directions for dietary and bowel preparation (clear liquid diet for 48 hr prior to test; laxative evening before test; and tap water or sodium biphosphate enema 3–4 hr before test) • Test involves passage of a well-lubricated flexible tube through the anus; air is used to distend the intestine during the procedure; urge to defecate and to pass gas are to be expected • Relaxation is important; breathe deeply and exhale through mouth • Sedative may be administered 2. Ensure that informed consent is signed. 3. If client is unable to complete bowel preparation, administer the prescribed laxative and enema.	• Position client on left side with knees flexed; drape to avoid embarrassment. • Provide emotional support. • Assist in positioning client (client may need to assume supine position to aid scope's advance). • Place any tissue or cell specimens in properly labeled containers with preservatives and send to laboratory. • Watch closely for untoward responses; have emergency resuscitative equipment available.	• Check vital signs according to agency protocol. • Resume usual diet after client recovers from sedation. • Observe for signs of bowel perforation: rectal bleeding, abdominal pain and distention, fever, malaise. • If polyp was removed, inform client it is normal to see some blood in stool. • Inform client it is helpful and usual to expel large amounts of flatus—urge not to withhold.

(Continued)

T A B L E   32-3
Diagnostic Studies of the Gastrointestinal Tract   (Continued)

Test	Purpose	Client Preparation	Nursing Care During Test	Client Aftercare
		4. Assist client into hospital gown and complete agency protocol for testing (empty bladder, remove jewelry, and so forth) 5. Administer sedative if prescribed.		
Proctosigmoidoscopy	• Allows visual examination of the lining of the distal sigmoid colon, the rectum, and the anal canal • Indicated for clients with recent changes in bowel habits, lower abdominal and perineal pain, prolapse on defecation, and passage of mucus, blood, or pus in stool • Assists in the diagnosis of inflammatory, infectious, and ulcerative bowel disease and tumors; and in detection of hemorrhoids, polyps, fissures, fistulas, and abscesses within the rectum and canal	1. Explain to the client • Nature and purpose of the test • That the test involves three steps: a. digital examination b. sigmoidoscopy: a 10-inch to 12-inch (25 cm–30 cm) rigid scope is inserted into the anus to visualize the distal sigmoid colon and rectum c. proctoscopy: a 2 3/4-inch (7 cm) rigid scope is inserted into the anus to examine the lower rectum and anal canal • Directions for dietary and bowel preparation (these vary; check agency protocol; most involve clear liquid diet and possibly fasting and may include an enema before the test) • Both the examiner's finger and the scopes are well lubricated; they may feel cool and stimulate urge to defecate; air is used to distend the intestine and client may feel urge to pass gas • Relaxation is important and eases discomfort; breathe deeply and exhale through mouth 2. Ensure the informed consent is signed. 3. If the client is unable to complete the bowel preparation, administer any prescribed laxatives or enemas. 4. Administer local anesthetic if prescribed to minimize discomfort of rectal inflammation.	• Position client in knee–chest or left-lateral position and drape to avoid embarrassment. • Provide emotional support. • Instruct client to bear down as scope is passed through the anal sphincters. • Place any tissue or all specimens in properly labeled container with preservatives and send to laboratory.	See client aftercare for colonoscopy.
Upper gastrointestinal (UGI) and small bowel series	• Fluoroscopic examination of the esophagus, stomach, and small intestine after ingestion of barium sulfate, a contrast agent • Indicated for clients with upper GI symptoms (difficulty swallowing, regurgitation, burning, or epigastric pain), signs of small	1. Explain to the client • Nature and purpose of the test • Need to maintain a low-residue diet for 2 days to 3 days before the test and to fast and avoid smoking after midnight the day of the test • That the UGI with the small bowel series can take up to 6 hr to complete • That he will be on a rotating x-ray table and will need to assume different positions	A technician in the radiology department cares for the client during the test.	• Before allowing the client to resume food and fluids, check to be sure that additional x-rays have not been ordered. • Encourage fluids to prevent dehydration. • Administer the post-test cathartic prescribed by

(Continued)

Test	Purpose	Client Preparation	Nursing Care During Test	Client Aftercare
	bowel disease (diarrhea, weight loss), and signs of GI bleeding (hematemesis, melena) • Assists in the diagnosis of strictures, ulcers, tumors, regional enteritis, and malabsorption syndrome, and in the detection of hiatal hernia, diverticula, varices, and motility disorders	• That a chalky-tasting barium contrast mixture (16 oz–20 oz) will be given to drink before the test 2. Ensure that an informed consent is signed. 3. Assist client to get into hospital gown and to remove jewelry or any objects that would interfere with the x-ray.		agency policy; if there is any question about its advisability for a particular client check with the physician. • Explain to the client the necessity of his eliminating the barium and that it will lighten the color of his stool the next few days. • If the cathartic and increased fluid intake do not result in the elimination of the barium within 2 days to 3 days, notify the physician. • Encourage extra rest because this test is fatiguing.
Barium enema	• Radiographic examination of the large intestine after rectal instillation of barium sulfate (single-contrast technique) or barium sulfate and air (double-contrast technique) • Indicated for clients with altered bowel habits, lower abdominal pain, or the passage of blood, mucus, or pus in the stool • Assists in the diagnosis of colorectal cancer and inflammatory disease and in the detection of polyps, diverticula, and structural changes in the larger intestine	1. *Nursing Alert:* Review the client's history for any evidence of ulcerative colitis or active GI bleeding which would prohibit the use of the standard bowel preparation procedure of laxatives and enemas. Consult with the physician to determine a safe bowel preparation program. 2. Explain to the client • Nature and purpose of the test (test takes 30 min–45 min) • Importance of following the prescribed dietary and bowel preparation because residual fecal material interferes with accurate test results a. Dietary modifications may include a low-residue diet for 1 day to 3 days before the test, clear liquids the evening before the test, and increased water and clear liquid intake for 12 hr to 24 hr before the test. b. A cathartic is usually administered the afternoon or evening before the test and cleansing enemas (tap water) until clear (not to exceed three) the evening before the test or that morning. • That he will be on a tilting x-ray table and will need to assume different positions	A technician in the radiology department cares for the client during the test.	• Before allowing the client to resume food and fluids, check to be sure that additional x-rays have not been ordered. • Encourage fluids to prevent dehydration. • Encourage rest because this test and the preceding bowel preparation exhaust most clients. • Administer the prescribed cathartic or cleansing enema to promote elimination of the barium and to prevent fecal impaction and bowel obstruction; instruct the client that barium will lighten the color of his stool. • If the barium is not eliminated within 2 days to 3 days, notify the physician.

(Continued)

T A B L E 32-3
Diagnostic Studies of the Gastrointestinal Tract (Continued)

Test	Purpose	Client Preparation	Nursing Care During Test	Client Aftercare
		• That he may experience cramping pains or the urge to defecate as the barium (500 ml–1500 ml) is instilled in his rectum; relaxation and deep breathing may ease this discomfort • That it is important to retain the entire barium enema to get good visualization (keeping the anal sphincter tightly contracted against the rectal tube helps) 3. Ensure that an informed consent is signed. 4. Assist the client into a hospital gown and prepare for transport to radiology following agency protocol.		

(Adapted from Paulfrey ME: Gastrointestinal system. In The Nurse's Reference Library: Diagnostics, pp 831–847. Springhouse, PA, Intermed, 1981)

remember the following guidelines for scheduling studies of the gastrointestinal tract.

1. The following is a logical sequence when more than one test is required for accurate diagnosis of the GI tract:
   - *Fecal occult blood test* to detect GI bleeding
   - *Barium studies* to visualize GI structures and possibly reveal inflammation or ulcers, tumors, strictures, or other lesions
   - *Endoscopics* to directly visualize an abnormality, locate a source of bleeding, and if necessary, to provide a channel for biopsy
2. The barium enema and routine radiography should always precede the upper gastrointestinal series because retained barium from the latter may take several days to pass through the gastrointestinal tract and may cloud anatomic detail on the barium enema studies.
3. Noninvasive procedures generally take precedence over invasive procedures such as endoscopic studies, when sufficient diagnostic data can be obtained. (In some instances endoscopic studies may be done before barium studies to ensure visualization.)

DIAGNOSING

When analysis of assessment data points to a bowel elimination problem which can be prevented or resolved by independent nursing intervention a nursing diagnosis is developed. Common alterations in bowel elimination for which a nursing diagnosis may be identified include:

- Constipation
- Fecal impaction
- Diarrhea
- Incontinence
- Flatulence/intestinal distention

Whenever alterations in bowel elimination require new self-care behaviors (*e.g.*, colostomy management), knowledge deficit may be an appropriate nursing diagnosis. Examples of specific etiologies and defining characteristics for these problems may be found in Table 32-4.

Problems of bowel elimination may also affect other areas of human functioning. In the nursing diagnoses that follow problems of bowel elimination are the etiology for other problems:

Anxiety related to lack of voluntary control of fecal elimination, significant others' response to ostomy

Altered comfort related to intestinal distention, prolonged constipation-impaction, fecal incontinence, hemorrhoids

Ineffective individual coping related to inability to accept permanent ostomy

Fluid volume deficit related to prolonged diarrhea

Altered growth and development related to parents' misconceptions about bowel and bladder training

TABLE 32-4
Nursing Diagnoses for Common Bowel Elimination Problems

Title	Etiologic or Contributing Factors	Sample Defining Characteristics
1. Altered bowel elimination: a. Constipation	• Decreased fiber in diet • Decreased fluid intake • Inactivity • Delaying defecation when urge is present • Abuse of laxatives • Use of constipating medications (antacids, narcotic analgesics, anticholinergics) • Change in routine	• "I feel bloated and know I have to move my bowels but I can't." • "Whenever I'm constipated I feel lethargic and lose my appetite." • Reports straining during defecation with little result • Passes small "marbles" of dry hard stool • Decreased frequency • Decreased frequency of bowel sounds or changes in abdominal growling • Straining often results in small amount of bleeding from swollen external hemorrhoids • Reports feeling rectal fullness or pressure in rectum • Headache
b. Fecal impaction	• Unrelieved constipation • High-risk candidates: clients who are debilitated, confused, or unconscious	• No bowel movement for more than 3 days despite repeated urge to defecate • History of constipation with sudden development of oozing diarrheal stool • Palpable rectal mass of hardened feces • Feelings of lassitude, rectal fullness, back pain, decreased appetite
c. Diarrhea	• Food intolerance (coarse, greasy, or spicy foods) • Food or drug allergies • Abuse of laxatives • Alteration in normal bacterial flora of the intestine (antibiotic therapy) • Emotional stress • Intestinal infection • Colon disease and other diseases • Surgical alterations	• Loose liquid stools, increased frequency • Urgency with soiling • Reports of abdominal pain and cramping • Increased frequency of bowel sounds
d. Incontinence	• Gross constipation with impaction and subsequent overflow • Organic changes in neural innervation of the rectum • Local causes (inflammation, cancer of rectum, prolapsed anus, semifluid stool) • Extreme debilitation	• Involuntary passage of stool (stool characteristics vary) • "I'm sorry, I couldn't get into the bathroom (or onto the bedpan) quickly enough." • "It came so fast I couldn't hold it back."
e. Flatulence/intestinal distention	• Irritating foods (cabbage, beans, onions) • Carbonated beverages • Swallowing large amounts of air • Decreased GI motility (opiates, general anesthetics, abdominal surgery, immobilization)	• Reports of abdominal fullness, pain, and cramping • Changes in abdominal size • Shortness of breath • Decreased ability to pass intestinal gas through the mouth (belching) or the anus
2. Knowledge deficit: Ostomy management	• Surgical procedure resulting in bowel diversion • Difficulty accepting altered body image and function • Desire to remain dependent • Lack of confidence in ability to learn new self-care skills • Limited cognitive ability	• "I don't think I'll ever be able to take care of it." • "How can you touch it?" • Refuses to look at ostomy • Despite encouragement to participate in ostomy care, refuses to cleanse stoma, change the bag, and so forth • "Will they send nurses to me at home to care for this thing?"

Knowledge deficit: bowel training related to no previous experience

Self-care deficit: toileting related to mobility deficit, weakness, confusion

Altered nutrition: less than body requirements related to loss of appetite from flatulence or impaction

Disturbance in body image related to ostomy, need to wear disposable adult briefs

Decreased self-esteem related to need for assistance with toileting, fecal incontinence

Impaired skin integrity related to prolonged diarrhea, fecal incontinence

PLANNING: CLIENT GOALS

Nursing measures for clients without specific bowel elimination problems are directed toward the client's achievement of the following goals:

The client will have a soft, formed bowel movement every 1 day to 3 days without discomfort.

The client will explain the relationship between bowel elimination and dietary fiber, fluid intake, and exercise.

The client will relate the importance of seeking medical evaluation if changes in stool color or consistency persist.

Specific client goals for common bowel elimination problems are presented later in this chapter.

IMPLEMENTING

Promoting Regular Bowel Habits

Regular bowel habits can be promoted in both well and ill clients by attention to timing, positioning, privacy, nutrition, and exercise.

Timing. Once the nurse knows when a client usually experiences the urge to defecate (this occurs most often about an hour after meals when mass colonic peristalsis occurs), the nurse offers whatever assistance is needed to help the client to the bathroom, commode, or bedpan at this time. It is important not to schedule nursing care or treatments during this time. Many clients feel uncomfortable about requesting time for elimination. It is helpful for the nurse to communicate to all clients the importance to heed this natural urge and that postponing it only results in constipation and other problems.

Positioning. The squatting position best facilitates defecation, but most clients routinely use a sitting position while leaning a bit forward. Clients able to use the bedside commode or bathroom toilet generally have lit-

tle difficulty assuming this posture although they may need support. An elevated toilet seat may be ordered for clients with orthopedic problems who cannot lower themselves to a toilet seat.

Clients needing to use the bedpan in bed will benefit from having the head of the bed elevated 30 degrees unless this is contraindicated. This eliminates the hyperextension of the back which occurs when a client who is lying flat attempts to lift his hips onto the pan. Once the head of the bed is elevated the client raises his hips by bending his knees, digging in his heels, and lifting the hips upwards. An overhead trapeze may be helpful to clients with weak lower extremities. The head of the bed should not be raised more than 45 degrees because this makes it harder to lift the hips straight up. Positioning a client with a bedpan is described in Procedure 32-1. Many clients on bedrest appreciate having moistened hand-wipes at the bedside to substitute for handwashing after toiletry. Bedpans should be emptied, cleaned, and returned to the client's bedside stand promptly.

Privacy. Because elimination is considered a private act by most persons, nurses must respect the client's need to be alone while defecating—unless the client's weakness makes this impossible. Bedside drapes should be pulled around the client using a bedside commode or bedpan. Well clients who cannot defecate in a public restroom or strange environment may need assistance in developing a workable schedule of defecation that makes use of private toilet facilities.

Nutrition. Clients with elimination problems may need a dietary analysis to determine which foods and fluids are contributing to their problem and which may help in its treatment. General dietary recommendations to promote regular defecation include a fluid intake of 2000 ml to 3000 ml and a high-fiber intake. Specific recommendations follow:

Constipation. Increase high-fiber foods (fruits, vegetables, whole-grain cereals and bread) and fluid intake (fruit juices, especially prune, and hot liquids).

Diarrhea. Prepare and store food properly. Avoid highly spiced foods or "laxative" type foods such as raw fruits and vegetables. Encourage foods with low fiber content. Replace lost fluids and electrolytes (weak tea, water, bouillon, clear soup, gelatin); if diarrhea is severe intravenous therapy may be needed.

Flatulence. Avoid gas-producing foods such as cabbage, onions, beans, cauliflower, and beer. This may also be helpful for persons with ostomies who are concerned about odor.

Ostomies. Clients with ostomies need to experiment with their diets to see which foods will result in the regular evacuation of a moderate amount of stool. Gen-

PROCEDURE 32-1
Offering and Removing a Bedpan or Urinal

Equipment

Bedpan or urinal
Toilet tissue

Handwashing supplies
Disposable gloves (optional)

Cover for bedpan or urinal (use Chux or disposable cover if others not available)

Action	**Rationale**
1 Bring the bedpan or urinal and equipment to bedside.	Having equipment on hand saves time by avoiding unnecessary trips to the storage area.
2 Warm the bedpan, if it is made of metal, by rinsing it with warm water.	A cold bedpan feels uncomfortable and may make it difficult for the client to void. Plastic bedpans do not require warming.
3 Place an adjustable bed in the high position.	Having the bed in the high position reduces strain on the nurse's back while assisting the client onto the bedpan.
4 Place the bedpan or urinal on the chair next to the bed or on the foot of the bed. Fold the top linen back just enough to allow for placement of bedpan or urinal.	Folding back the linen in this manner prevents unnecessary exposure while still allowing the nurse to place the bedpan or urinal.
5 If the client needs assistance to move onto the bedpan, have him bend his knees and rest some of his weight on his heels. Lift the client by placing one hand under his lower back, and slip the bedpan into place with the other hand.	The client uses less energy as the nurse assists by lifting him onto the bedpan. The nurse uses less energy when the client can assist by placing some of his weight on his heels.
6 If the client is entirely helpless, two people may be required to lift him onto the bedpan. Or, the client may be placed on his side, the bedpan is placed against his buttocks, and the client is rolled back onto the bedpan, as illustrated.	Having two people lift a helpless client causes less strain on the nurse's back. Rolling the client takes less energy than lifting the client onto a bedpan.

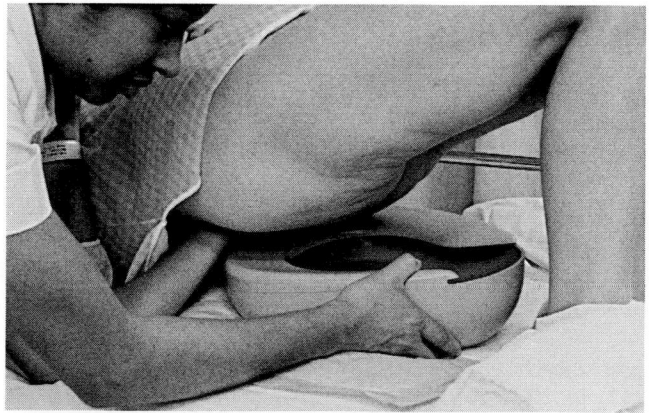

Step 5: Placing bedpan under buttocks while lifting lower back

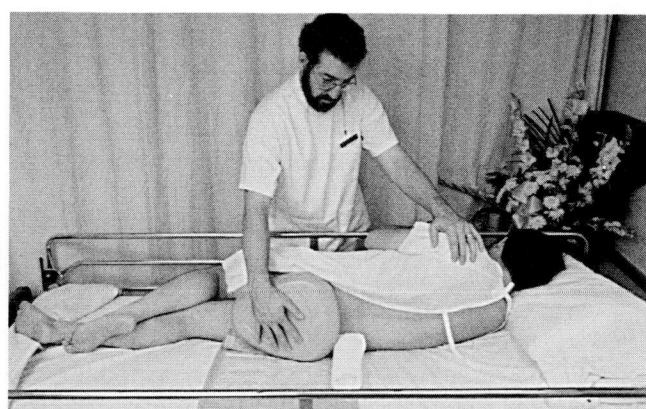

Step 6: Placing bedpan against buttocks while client is on his side.

(Continued)

Action

7 When the bedpan is in the proper place, the client's buttocks rest on the rounded shelf of the bedpan, as illustrated. The urinal is properly placed between slightly spread legs with the penis positioned in it and with the urinal resting on the bed.

8 If permitted, raise the head of the bed as near to the sitting position as tolerated.

9 Place call device and toilet tissue within easy reach. Leave the client if it is safe to do so. Use side rails appropriately.

10 Remove the bedpan in the same manner in which it was offered, being careful to hold it steady. If necessary to assist the client, don disposable gloves, wrap tissue around the hand several times, and wipe the client clean, using one stroke from the pubic area toward the anal area. Discard tissue, and use more until the client is clean. Place the client on his side, and spread the buttocks to clean the anal area. Cover bedpan.

11 Do not place toilet tissue in the bedpan if a specimen is required or if measurement of elimination is required. Have a receptacle handy for discarding the tissue.

12 Offer the client supplies to wash and dry his hands, assisting him as necessary.

13 Empty and clean the bedpan and urinal. Wash your hands. Record according to agency procedure.

Rationale

Having the bedpan or urinal in the proper place prevents spilling contents onto the bed and prevents injury to the skin from a misplaced bedpan.

This position generally makes it easier for the client to void or defecate, avoids strain on the client's back, and allows gravity to aid in elimination.

Falls can be prevented when the client does not have to reach for items he needs. Side rails are an additional safety precaution. Leaving client alone, if possible, promotes self-esteem and respects privacy.

Holding the pan steady prevents spilling its contents. Cleaning an area from front to back minimizes fecal contamination of the vagina and urinary meatus. Cleaning the client after he has used the bedpan prevents offensive odors and irritation to the skin.

Toilet tissue mixed with a specimen makes laboratory examination more difficult and also interferes with accurate output measurement.

Washing hands after using the bedpan or urinal helps prevent the spread of organisms.

Provides adequate documentation. Washing hands helps prevent the spread of organisms.

Modifications

1 A fracture bedpan may be substituted when it is difficult or uncomfortable to use a regular bedpan.

2 If it is difficult to slide client onto the bedpan, powder may be used on the resting surfaces of the pan to eliminate friction. Powder should not be used if a specimen is required because contamination could result.

erally a low-fiber diet is recommended. High-fiber foods, which could block the passage to the stoma, should be avoided; these include foods with skins, seeds, and shells (*e.g.,* raw fruits, popcorns, sunflower seeds, and nuts).

Exercise. Regular exercise improves gastrointestinal motility and aids in defecation. Well clients should be encouraged to incorporate three to five periods of regular exercise into each week's schedule. Ill clients should be ambulated as soon as possible and should be instructed about the relationship between inactivity and constipation/distention/impaction. Bedside exercises may be helpful for the immobilized client.

Clients with weak abdominal and perineal muscles who are using a bedpan may be helped by the following exercises:

Abdominal Settings. Instruct the client who is lying in a supine position to tighten and hold the abdominal muscles for 6 seconds and then to relax them. This should be repeated several times each waking hour.

Thigh Strengthening. Flex and contract the thigh muscles by slowly bringing the knees up to the chest— one at a time—and then lowering them to the bed. This should also be performed several times for each knee each waking hour.

Teaching about Cathartics, Laxatives, and Antidiarrheals

Constipation and fecal impaction are further discussed at the end of the chapter in "Nursing Process in Clinical Practice."

Cathartics and Laxatives

Cathartics and **laxatives** are drugs that induce emptying of the intestinal tract. Sometimes used interchangeably, cathartics exert a stronger effect on the intestines than laxatives. Some of these drugs act chemically by stimulating peristalsis, such as castor oil, cascara, senna, phenolphthalein, and bisacodyl (Dulcolax). Others act by increasing the intestinal bulk, which promotes additional mechanical stimulation on the intestine, such as magnesium sulfate and psyllium hydrophilic mucilloid (Metamucil). Still others act on the fecal material itself by softening it, such as mineral oil and dioctyl sodium sulfosuccinate (Colace). Another frequently used laxative is milk of magnesia. It has antacid properties in small dosages and laxative properties when taken in larger doses (see box entitled Classification of Laxatives).

Laxatives have their rightful place in health care. Laxatives are necessary at times for persons whose activity is limited or whose food intake is poor. They are also used for emptying the intestinal tract in preparation for surgical or diagnostic exploration. Their occasional use is generally not harmful for most persons, but all efforts should be taken to prevent the person from becoming dependent on this means of stimulating defecation. Because many laxatives are available as over-the-counter drugs and because modern advertising promotes their use, many persons take them frequently on their own initiative, whether they need them or not.

Most persons are aware that, because laxatives have a chemical action, they should not be taken when there is abdominal pain because of the danger of intestinal pa-

Classification of Laxatives

Bulk Forming (*e.g.,* methylcellulose, psyllium) Cellulose derivatives that swell in intestinal fluid, stimulating peristalsis by retaining water in the stool; considered the safest and most physiologic type of laxative; each dose should be taken with sufficient water to minimize risk of intestinal or esophageal obstruction; onset of action is usually 12 hr to 24 hr

Emollient/Fecal Softeners (*e.g.,* dioctyl sodium sulfosuccinate) Anionic surfactants, which increase the wetting efficiency of intestinal water, thus softening the fecal mass by facilitating mixture of aqueous and fatty substances; most useful in conditions in which straining is hazardous (*e.g.,* heart disease, perianal disease, hypertension, hernia, rectal surgery); may require several days before an effect is seen

Lubricant (*e.g.,* mineral oil) Softens fecal matter by lubricating the intestinal mucosa, facilitating passage of the stool; may prevent absorption of fat-soluble vitamins and nutrients and delay gastric emptying; do not administer with meals; effects usually occur within 6 hr to 8 hr

Saline/Osmotic (*e.g.,* magnesium citrate, sodium phosphate, lactulose) Nonabsorbable cations (magnesium), anions (phosphate), or sugars (lactulose) that retain water in the intestinal lumen, thus mechanically stimulating peristalsis and altering stool consistency; action is rapid (0.5 hr–2 hr) and should be used only for acute bowel evacuation, except for lactulose which may be administered in chronic constipation

Stimulants (*e.g.,* bisacodyl, castor oil, phenolphthalein) Increase intestinal propulsion by either a direct irritant effect on the mucosa or an activation of sensory nerve endings in intestinal smooth muscle; may produce excessive catharsis, leading to fluid and electrolyte disturbances; prolonged use can result in habituation and laxative dependency; onset of action is generally 6 hr to 8 hr orally

(Malseed RT: Pharmacology: Drug Therapy and Nursing Considerations, 2nd ed, p. 481. Philadelphia, JB Lippincott, 1985)

thology and subsequent harm from increased peristalsis. While many persons take laxatives because they believe they are constipated, most are unaware that habitual use of laxatives is the most common cause of chronic constipation.

Nurses are often in a position to help clients who abuse laxatives. Breaking the laxative habit, from both a physical and psychologic viewpoint, is not easy for a person who has come to depend on laxatives. It often requires a great deal of patience, support, and teaching by the nurse. The person also frequently needs to be helped with diet, fluid intake, activity, and regularity of habits.

Abrams (1987, pp 569–570) offers helpful guidelines for the selection and administration of specific laxatives.

Choice of a laxative or cathartic depends on the reason for use and the client's condition.

1. For long-term use of laxatives or cathartics in clients who are elderly, unable or unwilling to eat an adequate diet, or debilitated, bulk-forming laxatives (*e.g.,* Metamucil, Effersyllium) are usually preferred. However, these agents should not be given to clients with dysphagia, adhesions, or strictures in the gastrointestinal tract because obstruction may occur.
2. For clients in whom straining at stool is potentially harmful or painful, stool softeners (*e.g.,* docusate sodium [Colace]) are agents of choice.
3. For occasional use to cleanse the bowel for endoscopic or radiologic examinations, saline or stimulant cathartics are acceptable (*e.g.,* magnesium citrate, polyethylene glycol-electrolyte solution, castor oil, bisacodyl [Dulcolax]). These drugs should not be used more often than once per week. Frequent use is likely to produce laxative abuse.
4. Oral use of mineral oil may cause potentially serious adverse effects (decreased absorption of fat-soluble vitamins and some drugs, lipid pneumonia if aspirated into the lungs). Thus, mineral oil is not an oral laxative of choice in any condition, although occasional use in the alert client is probably not harmful. Mineral oil is probably most useful as a retention enema to soften hard, dry feces and aid their expulsion. Mineral oil should not be used regularly.
5. In fecal impaction, a rectal suppository (*e.g.,* bisacodyl [Dulcolax]) or an enema (*e.g.,* oil retention or Fleet's enema) is preferred. Oral laxatives are contraindicated when a fecal impaction is present but may be given after the rectal mass is removed. Once the impaction is relieved, measures should be taken to prevent recurrence. If dietary and other nonpharmacologic measures are ineffective or contraindicated, use of a bulk-forming agent daily or another laxative once or twice weekly may be necessary.
6. Saline cathartics containing magnesium, phosphate or potassium salts are contraindicated in clients with renal failure because hypermagnesemia, hyperphosphatemia, or hyperkalemia may occur.
7. Saline cathartics containing sodium salts are contraindicated in clients with edema or congestive heart failure because enough sodium may be absorbed to cause further fluid retention and edema. They also should not be used in clients with impaired renal function or those following a sodium-restricted diet for hypertension. Polyethylene glycol-electrolyte solution (GoLYTELY) causes less sodium absorption than other saline cathartics because it uses sodium sulfate as the major sodium source. In addition, the electrolyte concentrations in this preparation cause virtually no net absorption or secretion of ions. Thus, large volumes may be given without significant changes in water or electrolyte balance.
8. Irritant or stimulant laxatives should usually be avoided in children because of potency and likelihood of promoting laxative abuse.
9. During pregnancy, castor oil should not be used because its irritant effect may induce premature labor. During lactation, danthron or cascara sagrada should not be used because they are excreted in breast milk and may cause diarrhea in the nursing infant.

Antidiarrheals

Antidiarrheal medications are used to relieve the symptom of diarrhea (nonspecific therapy) or the underlying cause of the symptom (specific therapy). (Diarrhea is discussed in the section entitled "Nursing Process in Clinical Practice" at the end of the chapter.) Whatever the type of diarrhea, every effort should be made to identify and eliminate its underlying cause. The most effective antidiarrheal medications are the opiates (*e.g.,* paregoric) and related opiate derivatives (*e.g.,* loperamide) which act systemically to reduce intestinal hypermotility and slow peristalsis. Abrams (1987, p 575) notes that the choice of the antidiarrheal agent depends largely on the cause, severity, and duration of diarrhea.

1. For symptomatic treatment of diarrhea, diphenoxylate with atropine (Lomotil) or loperamide (Imodium) is probably the drug of choice for most people.
2. In bacterial gastroenteritis or diarrhea, choice of antibacterial drug depends on the causative microorganism and susceptibility tests.
3. In ulcerative colitis, sulfonamides and adrenal corticosteroids are the drugs of choice.

4. In diarrhea caused by enzyme deficiency, pancreatic enzymes are given rather than antidiarrheal drugs.
5. In "bile salt" diarrhea, cholestyramine (Questran) is the drug of choice. Colestipol (Colestid), a similar drug, is probably effective also.
6. Although morphine and codeine are contraindicated in chronic diarrhea, they may occasionally be used in the treatment of acute, severe diarrhea. Dosages required for antidiarrheal effects are smaller than those required for analgesia. The following oral drugs and dosages are approximately equivalent in antidiarrheal effectiveness: morphine 4 mg, codeine 30 mg, paregoric 10 ml, diphenoxylate 5 mg, loperamide 2 mg.

Emptying the Colon of Feces

Several methods are used to help promote elimination of feces: enemas, suppositories, rectal catheters, and digital removal of stool.

Enemas

An **enema** is an introduction of a solution into the large intestine, generally for the purpose of removing feces. The instilled solution distends the intestine, may irritate intestinal mucosa, and thus increases peristalsis.

Types of Enemas. Enemas are generally classified as cleansing, retention, or return flow enemas.

Cleansing Enemas. Cleansing enemas are given to remove feces from the colon and are used for four common purposes:
- To relieve constipation or fecal impaction
- To prevent involuntary escape of fecal material during surgical procedures
- To promote visualization of the intestinal tract by x-ray film or instrument examination
- To help establish regular bowel function during a bowel training program

The most frequent types of solutions used for cleansing enemas are tap water, normal saline, soap solution, and hypertonic solution. These are described in Table 32-5. Hypotonic (tap water) and isotonic (normal saline) enemas are large volume enemas which result in rapid colonic emptying. The large volumes of solution (adults, 500 ml to 1000 ml; infants 150 ml to 250 ml) may present a danger to persons with weakened intestinal walls. These solutions often require special preparation and equipment. Hypertonic solutions come commercially prepared and are administered in smaller volumes (adult, 70 ml to 130 ml). These solutions draw water into the colon which stimulates the defecation reflex. They may be contraindicated for clients for whom sodium retention is a problem.

Retention Enemas. Retention enemas are retained in the bowel for a prolonged period for different reasons. They include
- *Oil retention enemas* lubricate the stool and intestinal mucosa making defecation easier. About 150 ml to 200 ml of solution are administered to adults.

TABLE 32-5
Commonly Used Enema Solutions

Solution	Amount	Action	Time to Take Effect	Adverse Side-Effects
Tap water (hypotonic)	500 ml–1000 ml	Distends intestine, increases peristalsis, softens stool	15 min	Fluid and electrolyte imbalance, water intoxication
Normal saline (isotonic)	500 ml–1000 ml	Distends intestine, increases peristalsis, softens stool	15 min	Fluid and electrolyte imbalance, sodium retention
Soap solution	500 ml–1000 ml (concentrate at 3 ml–5 ml/1000 ml)	Distends intestine, irritates intestinal mucosa, softens stool	10–15 min	Rectal mucosa irritation or damage
Hypertonic solutions	70 ml–130 ml	Distends intestine, irritates intestinal mucosa	5–10 min	Sodium retention
Oil solutions (mineral, olive, or cottonseed oil)	150 ml–200 ml	Lubricates stool and intestinal mucosa	30 min	

- *Carminative enemas* help expel flatus from the rectum and provide relief from gaseous distention. Common solutions include the milk and molasses enema (equal parts) and the MGW enema (30 ml magnesium sulfate, 60 ml glycerine, and 90 ml warm water).
- *Medicated enemas* are used to administer medications that are absorbed through the rectal mucosa.
- *Antihelmintic enemas* are administered to destroy intestinal parasites.
- *Nutritive enemas* administer fluids and nutrition rectally.

Return Flow Enemas. *Return flow or Harris flush enemas* are used to expel flatus. For an adult 100 ml to 200 ml of a solution are instilled into the rectum and sigmoid colon and then the solution container is lowered so that the solution flows back into the container. This process is repeated five or six times, and the alternating flow of solution stimulates peristalsis and aids in the expelling of flatus. The procedure is terminated when abdominal distention is relieved. If the return solution becomes thick with feces it is replaced by fresh solution.

Equipment. Commercially prepared enema kits include a flexible bottle containing hypertonic solution with an attached prelubricated firm tip of approximately 5 cm to 7.5 cm (2 inches to 3 inches) in length. Its ease of use makes it particularly convenient for home situations. Clients can readily administer their own enema in many instances.

For the tap-water, saline, or soap solutions, a container for the solution, rubber or plastic tubing with side openings near its distal end, tubing clamp, lubricant, and the solution are necessary. Pitchers with a funnel attached to the tubing for introducing the solution may be used occasionally as solution containers. While the commercially prepared equipment is sterile, and any reusable equipment is sterilized between clients in a health agency, the procedure for administering an enema requires clean or medical-asepsis techniques, not sterile techniques.

Client Preparation. Because the enema is a common procedure, many clients understand its use and how it is administered. Other clients who have not experienced an enema before will need an explanation of its purpose, what they can expect, and how they can participate. The procedure offers an excellent opportunity for health teaching, because many persons are not familiar with the functioning of the intestinal tract. Failure to observe one or more of these principles may be responsible for their considering the procedure a disagreeable one.

Most clients believe that solutions are to be expelled as soon as possible. When a solution is to be retained, care should be taken to have the client understand this.

Administering an Enema Using a Large Volume of Solution. The procedure for administering a cleansing enema using either a large volume of solution or a commercially prepared solution is described in Procedure 32-2.

Administering an Enema Using a Hypertonic Solution. Administering a cleansing enema using a hypertonic solution differs somewhat from the procedure described in Procedure 32-2.

- The equipment is included in the commercially prepared sets. The only additional equipment needed is the bedpan for the bedridden client and a disposable waterproof pad to protect bed linens.
- It is unnecessary to warm the hypertonic solution. Administer it at room temperature, and warm it only if it is very cold.
- The side-lying position is usually used. The knee–chest position helps distribute the solution throughout the lower intestinal tract and is recommended if the client is able to assume the position. It is generally recommended to lubricate rectal tips even though they are prelubricated.
- The solution is forced into the rectum by applying gentle pressure on the collapsible solution container. It should take a minute or two to administer the enema.

Administering an Oil-Retention Enema. The procedure for giving an oil enema differs from that of giving a cleansing enema in certain respects:

- A small rectal tube is used. The small size helps reduce intestinal contractions so that the client can retain the oil more easily. Oil enemas are available in commercial kits similar to the kits for the hypertonic-solution enema. The kits contain a small rectal tube.
- Oil is given at body temperature to minimize muscular contractions caused by a warmer or cooler solution.
- The client should be instructed to retain the oil for at least 30 minutes for best cleansing results.

Rectal Suppositories

A **suppository** is a conical or oval solid substance shaped for easy insertion into a body cavity and designed to melt at body temperature. A variety of rectal suppositories are available. Some act as fecal softeners, others have direct action on the nerve endings in the rectal mucosa, and some liberate carbon dioxide when moistened. Fecal softeners are useful when the stool is very hard, while substances that stimulate the rectal nerves are helpful for persons with weak muscle tone or poor innervation. The carbon-dioxide suppositories liberate about 200 ml of gas, which causes distention, thus producing stimulation and elimination impulses.

PROCEDURE 32-2
Administering a Cleansing Enema

Equipment

Disposable enema set

Water-soluble lubricant

Solution as ordered by physician:

Temperature: For adult—105°F–110°F (40°C–43°C) For children—100°F (37.7°C)

Amount: Will vary depending on type of solution, age of the person, and the client's ability to retain the solution. Average cleansing enema for an adult may range from 750 ml to 1000 ml.

Necessary additives (soap, salt, and so forth)

Bath thermometer

Waterproof pad

Bath blanket

Bedpan and toilet tissue

IV pole

Disposable gloves

Paper towel

Wash cloth, soap, towel or handi-wipes

Action	Rationale
1 Assemble the necessary equipment. Warm solution in amount ordered, and check temperature with a bath thermometer. If tap water is used, adjust temperature as it flows from faucet.	Organization facilitates performance of task. If bath thermometer is not available, warm to room temperature or slightly higher, and test on inner wrist.
2 Explain the procedure to the client and plan with him where he will defecate. Have a bedpan, commode, or nearby bathroom ready for his use.	The client is better able to relax and cooperate if he is familiar with the procedure and knows everything is in readiness when he feels the urge to defecate. Defecation usually occurs within 5 minutes to 15 minutes.
3 Wash your hands.	Handwashing deters the spread of microorganisms.
4 Add enema solution to container. Release the clamp and allow fluid to progress through tube before reclamping.	This causes any air to be expelled from the tubing. Although allowing air to enter the intestine is not harmful, it may further distend the intestine.
5 Position waterproof pad under client.	This protects bed linen.
6 Provide for client's privacy. Position and drape the client on his left side (Sim's position) with anus exposed or on his back, as dictated by his comfort and condition.	The client's comfort and warmth help him relax. The exact position of the reclining person has not been found to alter results of an enema significantly.
7 Put on disposable gloves.	This protects the nurse from microorganisms in the feces.
8 Elevate the solution so that it is 45 cm (18 inches) above the level of the client's anus. Plan to give the solution slowly over a period of 5 minutes to 10	Gravity forces the solution to enter the intestine. The amount of pressure will determine the rate of flow and pressure exerted on the intestinal wall. Giving the solu-

(Continued)

Action

Rationale

minutes. The container may be hung on an IV pole or held in the nurse's hands at the proper height.

tion too quickly causes rapid distention and pressure in the intestine, resulting in too rapid expulsion of the solution, poor defecation, or damage to the mucous membrane.

9 Generously lubricate the end of the rectal tube for 5 cm to 7 cm (2 inches to 3 inches). A disposable enema set may have a prelubricated rectal tube.

This facilitates passage of the rectal tube through the anal sphincter and prevents injury to the mucosa.

10 Lift the buttock to expose the anus. Slowly and gently insert the rectal tube 7 cm to 10 cm (3 inches to 4 inches). Direct it at an angle pointing toward the umbilicus.

Good visualization of the anus helps prevent injury to tissues. The anal canal is approximately 2.5 cm to 5 cm (1 inch to 2 inches) in length. The tube should be inserted past the internal sphincter. Further insertion may damage intestinal mucous membrane. The suggested angle follows the normal intestinal contour. Slow insertion of the tube minimizes spasms of the intestinal wall and sphincters.

11 If the tube meets resistance while inserting it, permit a small amount of solution to enter, withdraw the tube slightly, then continue to insert it. Do not force entry of the tube. Ask the client to take several deep breaths.

Resistance may be due to spasms of the intestine or failure of the internal sphincter to open. The solution may help to reduce spasms and relax the sphincter, thus making continued insertion of the tube safe. Forcing a tube may cause injury to the intestinal wall. Taking deep breaths helps relax the anal sphincter.

12 Introduce the solution slowly over a period of 5 minutes to 10 minutes. Hold tubing all the time that solution is being instilled. Commercial preparations may be administered by compressing container with hands according to package directions.

Introducing the solution slowly helps prevent rapid distention of the intestine and a desire to defecate.

13 Clamp the tubing or lower the container if the client has the desire to defecate or cramping occurs. Client may also be instructed to take small, fast breaths or to pant.

These techniques help relax muscles and prevent the expulsion of the solution prematurely.

14 After solution has been given, clamp the tubing and remove the tube. Have paper towel ready to receive tube as it is withdrawn. Have the client retain the solution until the urge to defecate becomes strong, usually in about 5 minutes to 15 minutes.

This amount of time usually allows muscular contractions to become sufficient to produce good results.

15 Remove disposable gloves from inside out and discard.

This protects the nurse from contact with any microorganism.

16 When the client has a strong urge to defecate, place him in a sitting position on a bedpan or assist him to a commode or to the bathroom.

The sitting position is most natural and facilitates the act of defecation.

17 Record the character of the stool and the client's reaction to the enema. Remind the client not to flush commode before nurse inspects results of enema.

The nurse needs to observe and record the results. Additional enemas may be necessary if physician has ordered enemas "until clear."

18 Assist client if necessary with cleansing of anal area. Offer washcloth, soap, and water to wash his hands.

Deters spread of microorganisms.

(Continued)

19 Leave the client clean and comfortable. Care for the equipment properly.

There is abundant growth of bacteria in the intestine, which can be spread to others when equipment is not properly cared for.

20 Wash your hands.

Handwashing deters the spread of microorganisms.

Age Considerations

For elderly clients, encourage alternative measures to stimulate bowel elimination (prune juice, increased activity level, additional fiber and fluids in diet, regular time).

For elderly clients, discourage regular use of laxatives.

Modify amount of solution according to client's ability to tolerate procedure and size of client.

Home-Care Considerations

Give enema in area that is as close to bathroom as possible. If using bedpan or commode, have them readily accessible.

Inform client about availability of commercially prepared solutions and equipment.

Special Considerations

If client is incontinent or has difficulty retaining enema solution, a baby bottle nipple with the tip cut off may be placed on tubing. This acts as a sphincter and helps to prevent backward leakage of solution and feces.

Reinsert enema tube if there has not been any return of solution within 1 hour. Assist client onto right side and position container lower than his body to allow solution to return by gravity flow.

The following are recommended techniques for inserting a rectal suppository:

- Use a finger cot or a glove to protect the fingers while inserting the suppository.
- Have the client lie on either side, and pie-fold top linens over him.
- Lubricate the suppository and finger tips to reduce irritation on intestinal mucosa while inserting the suppository.
- Separate the buttocks, and then have the client relax by breathing through the mouth while the suppository is inserted.
- Introduce the suppository well beyond the internal sphincter so that the suppository is in the rectum, where its effect is desired.
- Avoid embedding the suppository in the fecal mass. Correct placement when there is stool in the rectum is between the stool and rectal mucosa.
- Be sure the client understands that he is to retain the suppository until he has an urge to defecate,

usually 30 minutes to 45 minutes after insertion. Encourage the client to walk about if he is ambulatory; this often helps promote peristalsis.

Rectal Foley Catheters

Foley catheters are now being used in some institutions for clients with uncontrollable diarrhea following chemotherapy, antibiotics, or tube feedings. Birdsall (1986) reports that they successfully maintain skin integrity and allow liquid stool to be accurately measured. Their chief advantage over a straight rectal tube is that the Foley balloon helps to seal the sphincter and prevents the continuous oozing of stool. They are also used with comatose clients who need retention enemas like polystyrene sulfonate (Kayexalate) and neomycin but who are unable to retain the enema solution.

The procedure includes

- Inserting a 28- or 30-F catheter (for an adult) about 2 inches to 3 inches into the rectum (the catheter should not be introduced into the sigmoid colon). This is a clean, not a sterile procedure.
- Inflating the balloon with saline or air and gently pulling back on the catheter so the balloon sits at the internal sphincter
- Attaching the Foley catheter to a drainage bag
- Deflating the balloon for a few minutes *every hour* to relieve pressure (failure to do this may result in rectal necrosis)
- Changing the rectal Foley catheter and drainage bag every day or more frequently if it becomes messy. (*Recommendation:* Have two catheters for each client, clean each one after use and store in a sterile towel until needed to reduce the risk of nosocomial infections.) The catheter should not be flushed while in place as this may worsen the diarrhea.

Because this is a relatively new procedure there is little research supporting its safety. Some nurses claim that the rectal Foley stimulates sensory nerve fibers in the rectum and then increases peristalsis and worsens diarrhea. Others are concerned about the danger of rectal perforation. A physician's order is needed for this procedure, and the client needs to be carefully monitored.

Digital Removal of Stool

If a client with a fecal impaction is unable to expel the fecal mass voluntarily and oil and cleansing enemas fail to break up the mass, it is necessary to break up the impaction manually. This procedure may cause great discomfort to the client and cause irritation of the rectal mucosa, bleeding, and slowed heart rate by vagal stimulation. A physician's order is necessary for this procedure. The following techniques are recommended:

- Have a second person assist with the procedure. The second person can assure and comfort the client while the first person works to break up the mass.
- Place the client in a side-lying position for the convenience of the nurses.
- Place a bedpan in the bed so that pieces of removed feces can be deposited into it.
- Drape the client by pie-folding top linens back.
- Use clean gloves for the procedure; the intestinal tract is not sterile.
- Lubricate the forefinger generously to reduce irritating the rectum, and insert the finger *gently* into the anal canal. The presence of the finger added to the mass tends to cause discomfort for the client when work is not done slowly and gently.
- Work the finger around and into the hardened mass to break it up, and then remove pieces of it.
- Remove the impaction at intervals if a severe one is present. This helps avoid discomfort as well as irritation, which can injure intestinal mucosa.
- Use an oil-retention enema as necessary. This may be given before attempts are made to break up and remove an impaction digitally. Or, it may be ordered after digital attempts fail. A cleansing enema is often ordered after an oil-retention enema.

Many clients find that a sitz bath or tub bath following this procedure soothes the irritated perineal area.

Designing and Implementing Bowel Training Programs

Clients with a history of chronic constipation and impaction and clients who are incontinent of stool may benefit from a **bowel training program**. The purpose of this program is to manipulate factors within the individual's control (food and fluid intake, exercise, time for defecation) to produce the elimination of a soft, formed stool at regular intervals without laxative support. Steps in a bowel training program include

- Explaining the program and its aim to the client in an effort to enlist the client's full participation
- Assessing the client's bowel elimination patterns and identifying factors promoting and hindering defecation
- Designing a plan to modify contributing life-style variables: (1) increase fluid intake to 2500 ml to 3000 ml—include hot drinks or fruit juices known to promote peristalsis for the client; (2) increase the fiber in the diet; (3) increase exercise if possible
- Starting the program with a clean bowel (rectal examination for impaction—remove if present)
- Maintaining a daily training routine for 14 days to 21 days until a regular pattern of defecation without laxatives is established:
  1. Thirty minutes before the client's usual defecation time (note this in plan) administer a cathartic suppository (*e.g.,* Dulcolax) to stimulate peristalsis.

2. Note the time it usually takes for the suppository to "work" and when the client has an urge to evacuate (usually 15 minutes to an hour). Assist the client to the bathroom or commode or onto a bedpan.

3. Allow the client privacy and ample time for evacuation; avoid both rushing the client and "abandoning" the client on the bedpan or commode for prolonged periods.

4. Share the client's success and offer positive verbal reinforcement and encouragement; refrain from criticizing the client who is unsuccessful.

- Communicating that patience may be necessary before regular elimination patterns resume—project a "can do" mentality

When the client has established a pattern of regular defecation, continue to offer assistance with toileting at the successful time but discontinue use of the laxative.

Meeting Needs of Clients with Bowel Diversions

Surgical procedures are sometimes required to create an opening into the abdominal wall for fecal elimination. The intestinal mucosa is brought out to the abdominal wall, and a **stoma** is formed by suturing the mucosa to the skin. The word **ostomy** is a general term for an opening into the body; it is usually used to refer to an opening created for the excretion of body wastes. An **ileostomy** allows fecal content from the ileum to be eliminated through the stoma. A **colostomy** permits feces from the colon to exit through the stoma. Figure 32-4 presents schematic drawings to illustrate the location of an ileostomy and variously placed colostomies.

An ileostomy or a colostomy may be either temporary or permanent. Temporary ostomies are usually done to allow the intestine to repair itself following inflammatory disease, after some types of intestinal surgery, or following injury. Permanent ostomies are usually done as the result of debilitating intestinal diseases or cancer of the colon or rectum. Clinical texts further discuss pathophysiologic conditions for which ostomies are required.

Colostomy and Ileostomy Care. The person with an ostomy needs physical and psychologic support both preoperatively and postoperatively. This support can come from persons close to the client as well as from members of the health team and from persons who have had similar experiences. The ostomy requires specific physical care for which the nurse is initially responsible. The following are guidelines for helping to promote physical and psychologic comfort for the ostomy client:

- Keep the client as free of odors as possible. The application of a temporary appliance after surgery or during the time of the first dressing change postoperatively can eliminate much of the fecal odor

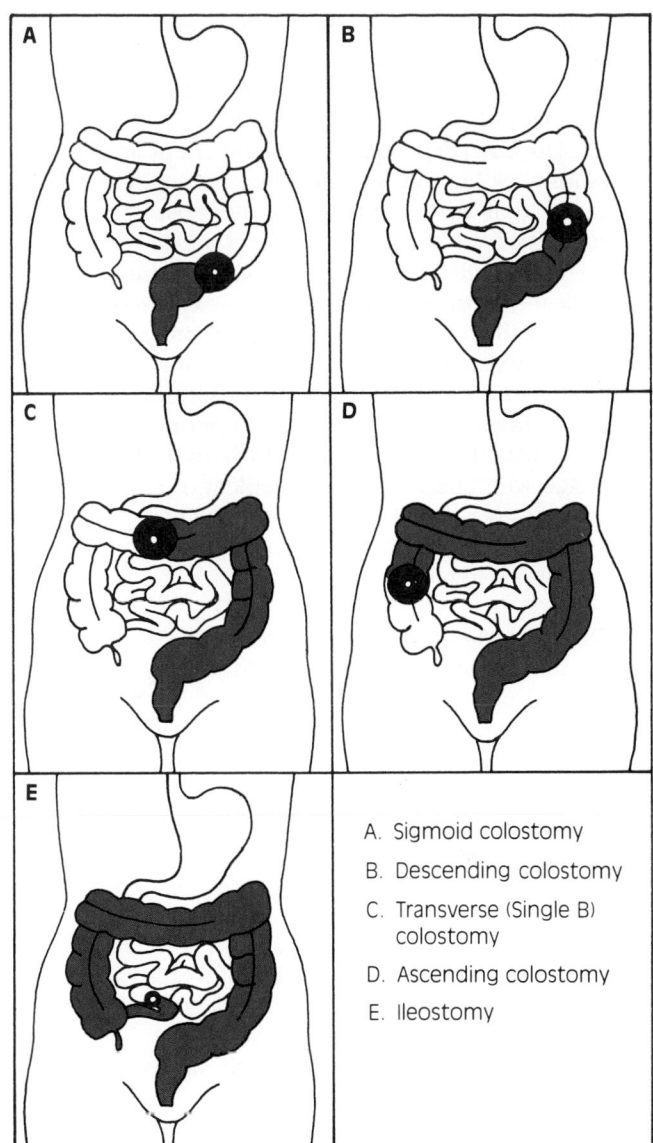

F I G U R E   32-4
Location of various colostomies and the location of an ileostomy.

A. Sigmoid colostomy
B. Descending colostomy
C. Transverse (Single B) colostomy
D. Ascending colostomy
E. Ileostomy

from a bulky dressing. The ostomy appliance should be emptied frequently.

- Check the client's stoma regularly. The color should be dark pink to red. Bleeding around the stoma and its stem should be minimal. Report any abnormal color, bleeding, or excessive edema promptly. If an abdominal dressing is in place, it should also be checked frequently for drainage and bleeding.

- Keep the skin around the stoma site (peristomal area) clean and dry. If care is not taken to protect the skin around the stoma, irritation or infection may occur.

- Measure the client's fluid intake and output. Check the ostomy appliance for the quality as well as the quantity of discharge. Generally, intake and output should be recorded every 4 hours for the first 3 days following surgery. If the client's output decreases while the intake remains stable, the condition should be reported promptly.

- Explain each aspect of care to the client and explain what his role will be when he begins his own care. Client teaching is one of the most important aspects of colostomy care.
- Encourage the client to participate in care and to look at the ostomy. It is generally expected that the client will experience emotional depression during the early postoperative period. The nurse can generally help the client to cope by listening, explaining, being available, and being supportive. The client usually begins to accept his altered body image when he is willing to look at the stoma, makes neutral or positive statements concerning the ostomy, and shows an expression of interest in learning self-care.

Changing the Ostomy Appliance. The ostomy appliance should protect the skin, collect the fecal discharge, and control odor. For the first few days following surgery, most clients wear an open-ended appliance that allows for drainage of fecal material without removing the appliance. The drainage bag is cleansed by injecting warm water into the bag and allowing it to drain, as necessary. When the appliance needs to be changed, the following techniques are recommended:

- Remove the appliance carefully to avoid pulling off the outer layer of skin.
- Use warm water or a mild solvent to facilitate removal of the appliance. If a solvent is used, wash it from the skin with warm water.
- Cleanse the peristomal skin gently with warm

water and a *mild* soap. Avoid hard rubbing and harsh cleansing agents. Some authorities recommend not using any soap because of its irritating effects on the skin.

- Rinse the skin well, gently pat it dry, and apply a protective skin barrier. Use the skin-protecting agent required by agency policy. Karaya Gum Powder is a common agent. Allow the skin barrier to dry thoroughly.
- Measure the stomal size with a measuring guide if a new appliance is to be used.
- Select a bag with the appropriate sized stomal opening, or cut a circle on the adhesive backing of the stomal appliance $\frac{1}{16}$ inch to $\frac{1}{8}$ inch larger than the stoma. Peel back the paper covering the adhesive backing of the stomal appliance. Figure 32-5 illustrates.
- Position the hole of the appliance over the stoma, and place the appliance in position by pressing it gently but firmly on the area immediately around the stoma. Figure 32-6 illustrates the nurse placing the appliance over a colostomy stoma.
- If a belt is to be used, attach it to the stomal appliance. The belt provides extra support for keeping the appliance in place, especially when the client is ambulatory.
- Close the bottom of the appliance with the closure clip if an open-ended one is used. Empty the bag as often as is required.
- Remove the bag every 2 days to 3 days. Make sure the peristomal area is free of irritation or excoriation. *Excoriation* is a breakdown of the epidermis. Protect the skin appropriately.

Colostomy Irrigation. Ileostomies are not irrigated because the fecal content of the ileum is liquid, which cannot be controlled. Irrigations may be used to help in regulating some colostomies. Various factors, such as the site of the colostomy in the colon, and the client's and

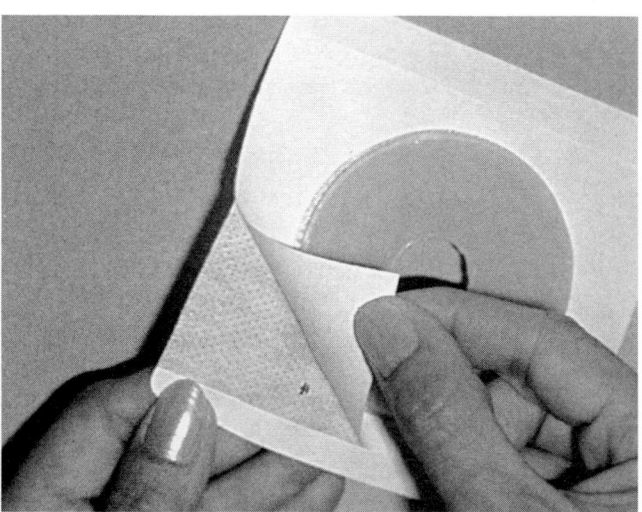

F I G U R E 32-5
The paper is peeled from the adhesive backing of the colostomy appliance before it is placed over the stoma. Note the karaya ring around the opening, which will fit over the stoma. (Courtesy of Convatec, A Squibb Company)

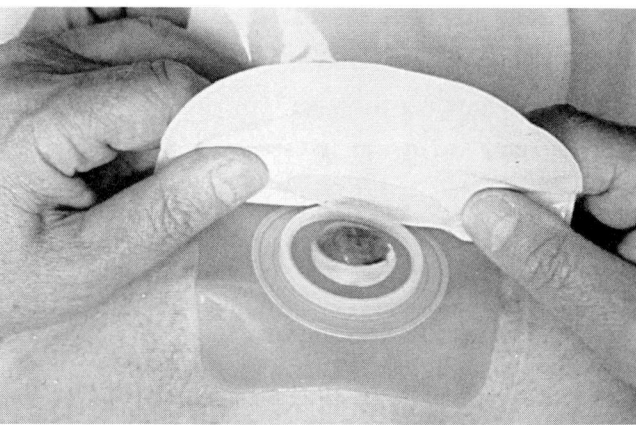

F I G U R E 32-6
The colostomy appliance is pressed into place. The stomal opening should be about ⅛ inch larger than the diameter of the stoma. (Courtesy of Convatec, A Squibb Company)

physician's preferences, determine whether or not a colostomy is irrigated.

If an irrigation is to be done, the nurse should familiarize the client with the technique to be used. The nurse should explain the procedure; demonstrate the equipment; and explain how the return fluid can be directed into a bedpan, commode, or toilet bowl. It is also often helpful to have a family member learn the irrigation techniques in case there are times when the client cannot do the irrigation himself. The procedure for irrigating a colostomy is similar to an enema except that the irrigating catheter is inserted into an abdominal stoma instead of into the anus. A commercially obtained irrigation set usually has all the equipment needed and comes with explicit directions.

In many health agencies, ostomy care, colostomy irrigations, and client teaching are done by specially trained enterostomal therapists.

Long-Term Ostomy Care.   The client can live an active and useful life with an ostomy. He should be aware of community resources to assist him, such as home-visiting nurses, special clinics, and ostomy clubs. The client should be encouraged to seek medical follow-up care on a regular basis.

Ostomy clients are usually encouraged to avoid foods high in fiber content initially, as well as any other foods that cause them to have diarrhea or excessive amounts of flatus. By gradually adding new foods, the ostomy client can generally build up to a normal diet. He may choose to avoid some foods he finds bothersome.

Clients with ostomies should be taught various methods of odor control. The chlorophyll content in dark-green vegetables helps to deodorize the feces when these vegetables are included in the diet. Bismuth subgallots, which can be purchased at drug stores and which can be taken with meals, help to lessen fecal odor.

Some clients can achieve control over fecal elimination from a colostomy by regular irrigations and by habitual emptying of the colon at a certain time each day. Very few clients with an ileostomy gain any degree of control

of the excretion of wastes and rarely may dispense with the use of an appliance, except for short periods of time.

Normal activity, including work, can be resumed. Direct physical contact sports and heavy lifting should be avoided. However, the client can go swimming and needs to wear only gauze or a large Band-Aid over the stoma.

Providing Comfort Measures

Comfort measures related to defecation include working with the client to develop a bowel elimination routine which results in the easy passage of a soft, formed stool, being attentive to perineal hygiene and the maintenance of skin integrity, and using warm moist heat (sitz bath or tub bath) to soothe the perineal area. Clients with hemorrhoids may require special comfort measures such as the application of topical medications to reduce inflammation and the administration of stool softeners.

EVALUATING

The nurse evaluates the effectiveness of a plan of care to promote regular bowel elimination by checking to see if the client has met the individualized client goals specified in the plan. In general, nursing care is considered effective if the client expresses satisfaction with his regular pattern of defecation and ability to comfortably pass a soft, formed stool without the use of medications or laxatives. The plan of care is most successful when the client is able to

- Verbalize the relationship between bowel elimination and nutrition, fluid intake, exercise, and stress management
- Develop a plan to modify any factors that contribute to present bowel problems or which might adversely affect bowel functioning in the future
- Correct unhealthy bowel habits such as ignoring the urge to defecate or abusing laxatives and enemas

NURSING PROCESS   *in Clinical Practice*

Once a bowel elimination problem is detected the nurse implements each phase of the nursing process to ensure its correct identification and treatment. The nurse who wishes to correctly identify and manage the bowel elimination problem must possess the knowledge and clinical skills described earlier in this chapter. What follows in outline format are focused assessment priorities, client goals, nursing interventions, and evaluative criteria for the nursing diagnoses:

> *Altered bowel elimination:* constipation, fecal impaction, diarrhea, fecal incontinence, flatulence/abdominal distention

In the case study that follows, a plan of care will be developed to address the elimination needs of a pediatric client with severe diarrhea.

Altered Bowel Elimination: Constipation

Constipation is the passage of dry, hard stools. Decreased gastric motility slows the passage of feces through the large intestine resulting in increased fluid absorption from the fecal mass and the dry, hard stool. Straining often accompanies defecation. Some persons may be constipated and yet have a daily bowel movement, while others who regularly defecate no more than three times a week are not constipated. The habits of elimination vary greatly among healthy persons.

Assessment

- Assess bowel elimination patterns noting (1) decrease in the usual number of bowel movements, (2) dry, hard stools, (3) straining and difficult evacuation, (4) abdominal distention, (5) swollen hemorrhoids, (6) complaints of headache, lassitude, anorexia, low back pain, or irritability.
- Identify contributing factors: insufficient fluid intake, low-fiber diet, lack of exercise, environmental changes, delaying defecation when urge is present, abuse of enemas or laxatives, use of constipating drugs, mental stress or depression, neurologic degeneration.
- Identify high-risk populations: (1) persons on bed rest who take constipating medications (narcotic analgesics, anticholinergics), (2) persons who reduce fluids or bulk in their diet, (3) depressed persons, and (4) persons with central nervous system disease or local lesions causing pain.

Client Goals

The client will

- Have a soft, formed bowel movement every 1 day to 3 days without straining or discomfort
- Modify life-style variables contributing to constipation (specify, *e.g.,* increase fluid intake to 2000 ml to 2800 ml; increase fiber in diet; incorporate three to five periods of regular exercise into week's routine

Interventions

- Encourage the client to respond to the urge to defecate and to set up a routine for having a bowel movement when the urge is most likely to be present. Ignoring the urge is a common cause of constipation. Most persons experience an urge following a meal, especially breakfast.
- Provide privacy, and allow sufficient time to defecate when stress is at a minimum. Lack of privacy, being under stress, and rushing will usually eliminate quickly the urge to defecate. Emotions tend to cause spasticity, causing *hypertonic* or *spastic constipation.*
- See to it that the client's food and fluid intake are conducive to having a bowel movement. Balanced food content and varied bulk are important to produce fecal matter and to its movement in the intestinal tract. Fresh fruits, vegetables, and bran cereals increase intestinal bulk while such foods as lean meats, rice, and eggs leave little residue. Having sufficient fluids is important to help prevent a dry, hard stool. Many people find taking such fluids as hot water or prune juice upon awakening helps promote elimination. Good-sized, hot meals rather than small, cold meals stimulate peristalsis.
- Teach the client the importance of exercise and ac-

tivity. Studies have shown clearly that lack of activity leads to poor muscle tone, a poor appetite, and sluggish intestinal activity.

- Position the client so that defecation is promoted. The squatting position, which allows maximum use of abdominal muscles, is best, but it is a position few people find comfortable. The sitting position, or semisitting position for bedridden clients, is most often used.
- Encourage the client to seek medical attention when minor rectal or anal problems, such as hemorrhoids or small linear ulcers called *anal fissures,* affect elimination. They generally cause discomfort, which causes the person to ignore the urge to defecate as long as possible.
- Teach the client to minimize the use of over-the-counter constipating drugs and to consult with the physician about limiting the use of constipating drugs when possible.
- Use laxatives, enemas, and suppositories (described earlier in this chapter) as a last resort or temporary treatment. Various measures to stimulate defecation are presented earlier in this chapter.

Evaluative Criteria

Client meets above goals.

Altered Bowel Elimination: Fecal Impaction

A **fecal impaction** is prolonged retention or an accumulation of fecal material, which forms a hardened mass in the rectum. It may be of sufficient size to prevent the passage of normal stools.

It is common for a fecal impaction to prevent the passage of normal stools. Small amounts of fluid may go around the impacted mass. As a matter of fact, liquid fecal seepage and no passage of normal feces are symptomatic of the existence of an impaction.

Assessment

- Assess bowel elimination patterns noting constipation, uncontrolled liquid fecal seepage, frequent urge to defecate but inability to do so, and complaints of rectal pain.
- Introduce a well-lubricated gloved finger into the rectum and palpate for a hard, compacted mass of fecal material.
- Identify contributing factors: anything that predisposes to constipation (see above) also predisposes to the development of a fecal impaction when dry, hard stool becomes lodged in the folds of the rectum. Retained barium following examinations of the large intestine is a frequent cause.
- Identify high-risk populations: clients who are debilitated, confused, or unconscious.

Client Goals

The client will

- Eliminate the fecal impaction with the assistance of the nurse manually removing the stool with or without prior oil enemas

- Resume usual pattern of bowel elimination (evacuate soft, formed stool)
- Avoid recurrence of fecal impaction by program of preventive management (specify, *e.g.,* participate in bowel training program, increase fluid intake to 2000 ml, and so forth)

Interventions

- The nurse follows agency guidelines for removal of fecal impaction. Because vagal stimulation can slow a client's heart rate a physician's order may be necessary for administering oil and cleansing enemas and for manual removal of the stool.
- Oil retention enemas to soften the impaction may be administered before attempts to break up and remove the impaction digitally or after digital attempts fail. A cleansing enema is usually given after an oil retention enema. These procedures are described earlier in this chapter.
- If manual removal of the stool causes perineal discomfort a sitz bath is often greatly appreciated by the client. The warm water reduces discomfort and refreshes the client.
- For 3 days after the removal of the fecal impaction it is appropriate to administer a combination of a stool softener and bowel stimulant.
- A program of preventive management, which modifies the factors contributing to the impaction, needs to be developed to avoid or minimize recurrence of the impaction.

Evaluative Criteria

Client meets above goals.

Altered Bowel Elimination: Diarrhea

Diarrhea is the passage of excessively liquid and unformed stools. Frequent bowel movements do not necessarily mean that diarrhea is present, although clients with diarrhea usually will pass stools at frequent intervals. Diarrhea often is associated with intestinal cramps. Nausea and vomiting may be present, as may blood in the stools. Diarrhea is protective in nature when its cause is the presence of irritants in the intestinal tract.

Diarrhea may have a functional basis. The client may have allergies to ingested food or drugs. The abuse of cathartics, and also certain dietary indiscretions, may cause diarrhea. Diseases in parts of the body other than the intestinal tract may be at the root of the trouble. Examples include uremia and certain cardiac and neurologic disorders.

Diarrhea may be caused by certain intrinsic conditions existing in the intestine itself. These include viral, bacteriologic, fungal, protozoan, or metazoan invasions; alterations in the normal bacterial flora of the intestine; antimicrobial therapy; fistulas; inflammatory conditions, such as ulcerative colitis; and tumors in the intestinal tract.

If the cause of the diarrhea is psychologic in nature, the nurse may be able to play an important part in assisting the client to understand the cause. Situations in daily living may be disturbing to him. However, diarrhea may be associated with deep-seated emotional problems that require the help of psychologic counseling.

Large amounts of fluids and electrolytes may be lost relatively quickly in the presence of diarrhea. This is especially true with infants and young children; if neglected, such loss may easily place a youngster's life in jeopardy. Giving fluids other than by mouth may be necessary when diarrhea is present. If oral intake is possible, cold fluids and rich foods, especially sweets, should be avoided.

Assessment

- Assess bowel elimination patterns noting (1) increased frequency or intensity of bowel movements; (2) increased fluid content in stool, greenish color, mucus, or blood; (3) increased bowel sounds; (4) whether diarrhea is acute, chronic, or recurrent; (5) fecal soiling; (6) being awakened at night to defecate; (7) complaints of abdominal pain and cramping, generalized weakness and fatigue, nausea and vomiting, fever.
- Assess anal and perineal area for excoriation.
- Identify contributing factors: recent travel, food intolerance, food or drug allergies (new medication), emotional stress, abuse of laxatives, alteration in the normal bacterial flora of the intestine (following antibiotic therapy), colon disease and other diseases, intestinal infection, surgical alterations.
- For clients with chronic diarrhea assess effect of person's self-image and physiologic and social functioning. Note problems with hydration, nutritional status, skin integrity, sleep, performance of usual self-care activities, and social interactions. Note abnormal laboratory values (electrolytes and hematocrit).

Client Goals

The client will

- Reestablish usual defecation patterns (soft, formed stool) or experience less diarrhea
- Modify contributing factors when possible (specify, *e.g.,* eliminate certain foods from diet, practice stress management techniques, and so forth)
- Maintain skin integrity in anal and perineal area
- Demonstrate signs of adequate hydration and nutritional status

Interventions

- Recognize that diarrhea is often an embarrassing problem. The client is in need of emotional support and needs to know that the nurse is there to help.
- Answer the client's call signal promptly. The client with diarrhea often cannot control the urge to defecate. It may be necessary to place a bedpan within easy reach but out of sight to prevent embarrassment.
- Whenever possible, remove the cause of diarrhea. Discontinuation of medications causing diarrhea

usually results in a return to normal defecation within 1 day to 3 days.

- If there is any indication of a possible impaction, a rectal examination should be performed before using any antidiarrheal medications.
- Maintain the client's fluid and electrolyte balance. A nonirritating diet is important until symptoms subside. Cold fluids and rich foods tend to aggravate the problem.
- Give special care to the region around the anus, where skin irritation is common. Keep the area clean and dry. Use skin creams, ointments, or powders as necessary. Avoid toilet tissue when it irritates, and use something softer, such as cotton balls, to cleanse and dry the area.
- Foley catheters are now being used in some instances for clients with uncontrollable diarrhea following chemotherapy, antibiotics, or tube feedings. The procedure is described earlier in this chapter.
- Once diarrhea stops it is important to promote a return to normal bowel flora. Fermented dairy products such as buttermilk or yogurt aid this process.
- When diarrhea is a regular or intermittent phenomenon that interferes with daily living, clients need additional counseling regarding judicious use of medications, individualized dietary modifications, fluid balance, skin protection, special clothing, and strategies to permit social interactions (*e.g.,* preplanning seating on a plane or in a theater or restaurant to be near a bathroom).

Evaluative Criteria
Client meets above goals.

Altered Bowel Elimination: Fecal Incontinence

Fecal incontinence is the inability of the anal sphincter to control the discharge of fecal and gaseous material. Usually, the cause of incontinence is an organic disease, resulting either in a mechanical condition that hinders the proper functioning of the anal sphincter or in an impairment in the nerve supply to the anal sphincter. Mental illnesses may also be responsible for the client's indifference to the passage of stool. While fecal incontinence is rarely a threat to life, incontinent clients suffer embarrassment and may become disturbed emotionally.

Assessment
- Assess bowel elimination pattern noting onset of fecal incontinence and regularity and number of incontinent episodes. Note stool characteristics. Rule out impaction by rectal examination.
- Identify contributing factors: gross constipation with impaction and subsequent overflow, organic changes in neural innervation of the rectum, local causes (cancer of rectum, prolapsed anus, semifluid stool), mental illnesses resulting in indifference to passage of stool, extreme debilitation.

- Assess effects of incontinence on self-concept.
- Examine perineal area for skin breakdown.

Client Goals
The client will
- Eliminate incontinent episodes (or reduce their number) if this is realistic
- Demonstrate appropriate self-care measures (or receive related nursing measures): perineal hygiene, use of absorbent pads or waterproof briefs, and so forth
- Demonstrate no signs of perineal excoriation
- Participate in bowel training program to time defecation and reduce the risk of accidents

Interventions
- Take into account that the client suffers embarrassment. The client requires emotional support and understanding.
- Note when incontinence is most likely to occur, and place the client on a bedpan at those times. If there is no pattern, offer a bedpan at regular intervals, such as every few hours.
- Keep the skin clean and dry by using proper hygienic measures. Decubitus ulcers may develop when such measures are overlooked.
- Change bed linens and clothing as necessary to avoid odor, skin irritation, and embarrassment. Disposable bed pads and moisture-proof undergarments are often used. Form-fitting briefs and absorbent pads may be worn by the client.
- Confer with the physician about the use of a suppository or a daily cleansing enema. These measures empty the lower colon regularly and often help decrease incontinence. Bowel training programs may be helpful.

The nurse should keep in mind that emotional problems of clients with diarrhea and fecal incontinence are often as important for the nurse to manage as are the physical problems.

Evaluative Criteria
Client meets above goals.

Altered Bowel Elimination: Flatulence/ Intestinal Distention

Excessive formation of gases in the stomach or intestines is known as **flatulence**. When the gas is not expelled and accumulates in the intestinal tract, the condition is referred to as *intestinal distention* or *tympanites*.

Any disturbance in the ability of the small intestine to absorb gases or in its ability to propel gas along the intestinal tract usually will result in distention. Irritating foods, such as beans and cabbage, often predispose to flatulence and distention. Constipation is a frequent cause of distention. Certain drugs, morphine sulfate for example, tend to decrease peristaltic action, which allows gas accumulation and thus causes distention.

Swallowing large amounts of air while eating and drinking can cause distention. Persons who are tense often can be observed to be swallowing large amounts of air, especially when taking fluids. This habit can be overcome by purposely training oneself to eat and drink without swallowing air. Usually, air swallowers will eructate a great deal, and much air escapes in this manner before it reaches the intestines.

Assessment

- Assess gastrointestinal motility by noting (1) decreased bowel sounds, (2) hyperresonance when percussing the abdomen, (3) increased abdominal girth, (4) taut skin over abdomen, and (5) complaints of abdominal fullness, pain, and cramping, increased or decreased belching, increased or decreased passing of flatus by the anus, and shortness of breath.
- Assess for contributing factors: ingestion of gas-producing foods (cabbage, beans, onions) or carbonated beverages, swallowing large amounts of air, anything that decreases gastrointestinal motility: opiates, general anesthetics, abdominal surgery, immobilization.

Client Goals

The client will
- Expel excess flatus by belching or passing flatus by the anus
- Prevent the recurrence of flatulence and distention by modifying contributing factors

Interventions

- Act on the cause of distention when possible. For example, have the client avoid foods and beverages known to cause distention. Reducing the fat content of meals often helps.
- Have the client move about in bed and walk to help promote peristalsis and the escape of flatus. Reclining after meals should be avoided.
- Use a rectal tube to help gas to escape. The introduction of the tube helps stimulate peristalsis and provides a passageway for the escape of flatus. Sizes 22 Fr. to 34 Fr. are used for adults; smaller sizes are used for children.
- Position the client on his side, and drape the client properly when preparing to insert a rectal tube.
- Lubricate the rectal tube to reduce irritation to mucous membranes when inserting it.
- Separate the buttocks well so that the anus is in plain view, and introduce the rectal tube beyond the anal canal into the rectum for about 10 cm (4 inches). It may be inserted a bit further if it is noted that no flatus is being removed.
- Attach the rectal tube to a piece of tubing of sufficient length to reach a small collection container, which can be attached to the bed frame. Or, place the end of the tube in a specimen container or urinal placed between the client's legs. These techniques will allow any discharge that empties through the rectal tube to be caught.
- Leave the rectal tube in place for a short period of time, no longer than about 20 minutes. The tube no longer acts as a stimulant for peristalsis if left in place longer. If distention is not relieved, use the rectal tube intermittently every 2 hours to 3 hours as necessary.
- Have the client assume various positions to help move flatus along the intestinal tract toward the anus. Gas is lighter than fluids or solids and will rise. Positions that help gas rise include lying on the abdomen, assuming the knee–chest position, and positioning the upper part of the body over the edge of the bed while the lower part rests across the bed. Do not use these positions if they are contraindicated or unsafe for the client.
- Confer with the physician if the above measures bring no relief. An enema (the return flow enema described earlier may be prescribed), a suppository, or a medication may be prescribed to help bring relief.

Evaluative Criteria

Client meets above goals.

CASE STUDY

Jeremy Green, a 4-year-old child, height 45 inches (115 cm), weight 36 lb (16.3 kg), was placed in daycare when his mother returned to work 6 months ago. He presents at the hospital with a diagnosis of viral gastroenteritis.

Assessment Findings

The admitting nurse questions Jeremy's mother about the duration, frequency, and amount of his diarrhea and the appearance and consistency of the stools. Treatment since the onset of diarrhea is noted including any food or fluids the child has taken. Physical assessment is directed to signs of dehydration and the abdominal examination. The nurse records the following assessment note:

5/6   Four-year-old white male child admitted with complaints of diarrhea beginning 3 days ago. Seen by pediatrician today who recommended admission and work-up to rule out causes other than viral. Mother reports liquid stools (no observable pus, blood, or mucus) six to seven times daily beginning 5/4 (amount "one to two cups"). Urgency results in soiling of pants. Child has sipped boiled skim milk and Coke and ate a small amount of broth and a few pretzels but has no appetite; complains of nausea; vomiting ×2 on 5/4. Child is pale, and eyes are sunken. Skin is warm and dry with decreased turgor; mucous membranes are dry. Hyperactive bowel sounds. Ht 45 in, Wt 36 lb, T—99.8 r P—88 R—18. Mother reported several other children in same daycare center are out sick with diarrhea.

D. Levitsky, RN

Nursing Diagnosis

The admitting nurse develops a plan of care for Jeremy which includes several nursing diagnoses. The one that will be developed in this case study is:

Alteration in bowel elimination: diarrhea related to unknown cause (possibly viral, rule out malabsorption of lactose and other causes)

Planning

The nurse works collaboratively with Jeremy and his parents explaining that a plan of care is being developed to maintain Jeremy's well-being until the diarrhea is brought under control. The nurse recognizes Jeremy's distress both at losing control over defecation and at needing to be hospitalized. The family supports the following client goals:

At the time of discharge the client will

1. Voluntarily pass a formed stool of usual consistency (experience less or no diarrhea)
2. Exhibit decreased bowel sounds
3. Demonstrate signs of fluid and electrolyte balance:
   a. Improved skin turgor
   b. Moist mucous membranes
   c. Normal eyeball
4. Demonstrate signs of improved nutritional status
   a. Eat low-fiber diet without abdominal cramping, nausea, or vomiting
   b. Maintain admission weight (or gain weight)
5. Show no signs of skin breakdown in the perianal area

See the nursing care plan which details the nursing strategies used to achieve these goals.

Implementation

In implementing the plan of care the nurse needs the following specialized abilities:

- Strong interpersonal skills to work effectively with children and their families
- Thorough knowledge of child development, normal bowel elimination, causes and manifestations of diarrhea and related problems, and successful treatment strategies
- Strong assessment skills (interviewing and physical assessment) to carefully identify and label the child's problems and their etiology
- Ability to create a secure, comfortable, and developmentally stimulating environment for the child
- Ability to provide safe physical care to the child aimed at promoting optimal functioning of all body systems
- Teaching and counseling skills to meet the child and parents' needs
- Interpersonal and leadership skills to work with the nursing staff and health-care team to implement the plan of care
- Personal accountability

Documentation

Sample documentation of a nursing intervention follows using the SOAP format.

5/7/87 #1. Alteration in bowel elimination: diarrhea related to unknown cause (possible viral, rule out malabsorption of lactose and other causes)

S: "My tummy doesn't hurt so much any more."

O: Liquid stools decreased to two in last 24 hours; negative report on stool culture

A: Diarrhea is resolving—etiology may have been temporary lactose intolerance following acute viral diarrhea (mother had been giving child boiled skim milk)

P: Continue plan of care. Add rice cereal and bananas to diet. Reintroduce milk and milk products last—alert parents to monitor child for lactose intolerance.

D. Levitsky, RN

Evaluation

Short-term goal achievement is evaluated prior to discharge. See the care plan for related evaluative statements and revisions of the plan of care.

N U R S I N G   C A R E   P L A N   *for Jeremy Green*

Nursing Diagnosis: Alteration in bowel elimination: Diarrhea related to unknown cause (possibly viral, rule-out malabsorption of lactose and other causes) as manifested by passage of liquid stools (1–2 cups) × 3 days; urgency with fecal soiling; anorexia, nausea, vomiting × 2 on day 1; signs of dehydration: decreased skin turgor, dry mucous membranes, sunken eyeballs.

Long-Term Goal: Client reestablishes usual pattern of bowel elimination.

(Continued)

![black banner]

N U R S I N G   C A R E   P L A N (Continued)

Goals	Nursing Actions	Rationale	Evaluative Statement
At the time of discharge the client will: 1. Voluntarily pass a formed stool of usual consistency (experience less or no diarrhea)	Assess and chart frequency and amount of diarrhea, stool characteristics, precipitating factors, and accompanying manifestations (GI symptoms, hyperactive bowel sounds).	Assist in identifying the cause of the diarrhea.	5/8 Goal partially met: No recurrence of liquid stools for 24 hr. *Revision:* Continue to monitor. *D. Levitky, RN*
2. Exhibit decreased bowel sounds	Work collaboratively with the physician to identify the etiology of the diarrhea. Obtain stool specimens and send to laboratory.	Correct treatment is dependent on identification of the cause of the diarrhea. Viral diarrhea is usually self-limiting and lasts 24 hr to 72 hr. Prolonged diarrhea after acute viral illness may be from temporary malabsorption of lactose or other simple sugars.	5/8 Goal met: Normal bowel sounds. *D. Levitky, RN*
	Instruct Jeremy and his parents (if they wish to participate in care) on correct enteric precautions for handling stool.	To prevent transmissions of infectious diarrhea to others	
	Increase frequency and length of rest periods and discourage any strenuous activity. Administer prescribed antidiarrheal medication and observe for any side effects.	Exercise and activity stimulate peristalsis.	
3. Demonstrate signs of fluid and electrolyte balance: a. Improved skin turgor b. Moist mucous membranes c. Normal eyeball	Continue to assess hydration status and be alert to signs of electrolyte imbalance.	Reestablishing normal fluid and electrolyte balance by replacing ongoing fluid losses and providing maintenance fluids is a priority for the child with severe and prolonged diarrhea. Diarrhea stools contain large amounts of water and are often relatively low in sodium and high in potassium.	5/8 Goal partially met: Skin turgor improved, eyeballs normal, mucous membranes still dry. *Revision:* Continue to encourage P.O. fluids. Enjoys clear chicken broth and half-strength gelatin products. *D. Levitky, RN*
	Administer prescribed intravenous therapy and clear liquids—note client response as new fluids and foods are added to the diet.	There is no ideal oral replacement fluid. Some may cause diarrhea or provide inappropriate amounts of electrolytes.	
	Chart daily weight.	Daily weights are the most accurate indicator of fluid balance.	

(Continued)

N U R S I N G   C A R E   P L A N (Continued)

Goals	Nursing Actions	Rationale	Evaluative Statement
	Monitor intake and output. Note concentration of urine.	Urine becomes more concentrated when a person is dehydrated.	
4. Demonstrate signs of improved nutritional status: a. Eats low-fiber diet without abdominal cramping, nausea, or vomiting. b. Maintain or increase admission weight.	Discontinue milk products and solid foods. Until the diarrhea resolves, offer a combination of clear liquids (half-strength apple juice or gelatin products; commercial products: Lytren, Pedialyte, 5% glucose water): 30 ml each hour for first 8 hr, then 60 ml–90 ml every 1 hr–2 hr if number of stools lessens. As GI symptoms subside, advance to other liquids and solids (bananas, apple sauce, and rice cereal tend to solidify stool) —milk should be the last liquid added.	If one fluid is used exclusively, inappropriate amounts of electrolytes may be provided. Commercial preparations tend to be expensive. Objective is to provide the necessary water, electrolytes, and minimal calories in a milk-free and solid-free diet—until the diarrhea resolves. Adding new fluids and foods slowly enables intolerances to be quickly detected.	5/8 Goal met. Tolerating rice cereal and bananas. Gained 1 lb since admission. *D. Lovitky, RN*
5. Show no signs of skin breakdown in the perianal area	Assess the perianal area after each passage of stool and note any irritation. Wash and dry the area carefully after each episode of diarrhea and apply protective ointment (as ordered or per agency protocol).	Perianal irritation is a common problem with severe diarrhea. The goal of treatment is prevention. Keeping the skin clean and dry and protected with a waterproof ointment or skin barrier may prevent breakdown.	5/8 Goal partially met. Small area of excoriation around anus. Continue plan. *D. Lovitky, RN*

K E Y   P O I N T S

- Bowel elimination, a natural process in which the body excretes the waste products of digestion, is an essential component of healthy body functioning.

- Problems with bowel elimination may affect fluid and electrolyte balance, nutritional status, skin integrity, and self-concept.

- Healthy bowel elimination presupposes a well-functioning gastrointestinal tract. The large intestine is the primary organ of bowel elimination.

- *Defecation* and *bowel movement* are the terms used to describe the emptying of the intestines. Persons vary in the frequency of their bowel move-

ments. The aim is to have the bowels move regularly and for the stools to be formed, soft, and passed without discomfort.

- Factors affecting bowel elimination include: growth and development, daily patterns, food and fluid intake, activity and muscle tone, life-style variables, psychologic variables, pathologic conditions, medications, diagnostic tests, surgery, and anesthesia.

- A comprehensive assessment of bowel elimination includes the collection of data about usual patterns of elimination; recent changes in these patterns;

aids to elimination; elimination problems; physical assessment of the abdomen, anus, and rectum; and stool characteristics. These findings may need to be correlated with the results of diagnostic studies of the stool and gastrointestinal tract.

■ When caring for a debilitated, confused, or unconscious client, the nurse needs to monitor bowel status daily to identify and treat bowel elimination problems early. Nursing care is directed to the prevention of bowel problems.

■ Endoscopic exams using a lighted tube allow the direct visualization of the gastrointestinal tract and are helpful in the diagnosis of inflammatory, ulcerative, and infectious diseases; neoplasms; and other lesions of the esophageal, gastric, and intestinal mucosa.

■ Indirect visualization of the gastrointestinal tract is achieved through radiography. Important nursing responsibilities are assisting the client to complete a safe and effective dietary and bowel preparation program and ensuring that the client eliminates the contrast medium (barium sulfate) used in the study. Standard bowel preparation agents may be contraindicated for some clients.

■ Nursing diagnoses may be written to specifically address problems in bowel elimination (constipation, impaction, diarrhea, incontinence, flatulence/abdominal distention) and to identify the effect bowel elimination problems have on other areas of human functioning (anxiety, comfort, self-concept, skin integrity).

■ Regular bowel elimination may be promoted in both well and ill clients by attention to timing, positioning, privacy, nutrition, and exercise. Clients need to understand the importance of heeding the urge to defecate and the relationship between bowel elimination and nutrition and exercise.

■ Specific nursing strategies for bowel elimination include use of cathartics, laxatives, and antidiarrheals; techniques for emptying the colon of feces: enemas, rectal suppositories, rectal Foley catheters, and digital removal of stool; bowel training programs; and comfort measures.

■ Although laxatives have valid uses, they are frequently abused. Many persons who take laxatives for what they believe is constipation do not realize that the habitual use of laxatives is the most common cause of chronic constipation.

■ A physician's order may be needed before the nurse digitally removes a fecal impaction because this may result in irritation of the rectal mucosa and bleeding and because vagal stimulation can decrease the heart rate.

■ The purpose of a bowel training program is to manipulate factors within the individual's control (food and fluid intake, exercise, time of defecation) to produce the elimination of a soft, formed stool at regular intervals without laxative support.

■ The client with a bowel diversion will need physical and psychologic support both preoperatively and postoperatively. The nurse works collaboratively with the physician and enterostomal therapist to ensure that the client and family can manage the care of the bowel diversion after discharge.

■ Clients with acute or chronic constipation, impaction, diarrhea, incontinence, or flatulence, require special nursing care. These problems, if uncorrected, may seriously affect the client's comfort, self-concept, and other areas of physical functioning.

BIBLIOGRAPHY

Abrams AC: Clinical Drug Therapy: Rationales for Nursing Practice, 2nd edition. Philadelphia, JB Lippincott, 1987

Alterescu KB: The ostomy: What aboutspecial procedures? Part 2 (2). Am J Nurs 85(12):1363–1367, 1985

Alterescu V: Theoretical foundations for an approach to fecal incontinence. Journal of Enterostomal Therapy 13(2):44–48, 1986

Alterescu V: The ostomy: What do you teach the patient? Part 1 (3). Am J Nurs 85(11):1250–1253, 1985

Becker LB, Stevens SA: Performing in-depth abdominal assessment. Nursing 18(6):59–63, 1988

Behm RM: A special recipe to banish constipation. Geriatr Nurs 6(4):216–217, 1985

Birdsall C: Would you put a Foley in the rectum? Am J Nurs 86(9):1050, 1986

Blackwell AK, Blackwell W: Relieving gas pains. Am J Nurs 75(1):66–67, 1975

Boarini J: The ostomy: What can go wrong? Part 2 (1). Am J Nurs 85(12):1358–1362, 1985

Crowley AA: A comprehensive strategy for managing encopresis. MCN 9(6):395–400, 1984

Davis A et al: Bowel management: A quality assurance approach to upgrading programs. Journal of Gerontological Nursing 12(5):13–17, 1986

Didich JM: Gauging abdominal girth accurately. Nursing 11(7):32–33, 1981

Fry RD: Anorectal disorders. Clin Symp 37(6):2–32, 1985

Johns C: Encopresis. Am J Nurs 85(2):153–156, 1985

Lewis B: Streamlining the process of elimination. Am J Nurs 85(7):774, 1985

Horner MM, McClellan MA: Toilet training: Ready or not? Pediatric Nursing 7(1):15–18, 1981

Mager,-O'Connor E: How to identify and remove fecal impactions. Geriatr Nurs 5(3):158–161, 1984

Maresca JG et al: Assessment and management of acute diarrheal illness in adults. Nurs Pract 11(11):15–16, 18, 21, 1986

McShane RE, McLane AM: Constipation: Consensual and empirical validation. Nurs Clin North Am 20(4):801–808, 1985

Petillo MH (ed): Enterostomal therapy. Nurs Clin North Am 22(2):253–356, 1987

Resnick B: Constipation: Common but preventable. Geriatr Nurs 6(4):213–215, 1985

Smith DB: The ostomy: How is it managed? Part 1 (2). Am J Nurs 85(11):1246–1249, 1985

Sullivan-Bolyai S: Practical aspects of toilet training the child with a physical disability. Issues in Comprehensive Pediatric Nursing 9(2):79–96, 1986

Watt RC: The ostomy: Why is it created? Part 1 (1). Am J Nurs 85(11):1241–1245, 1985

Weight BA et al: The geriatric implications of fecal impaction. Nurs Pract 11(10):53–54, 56, 58, 1986

Urinary Elimination

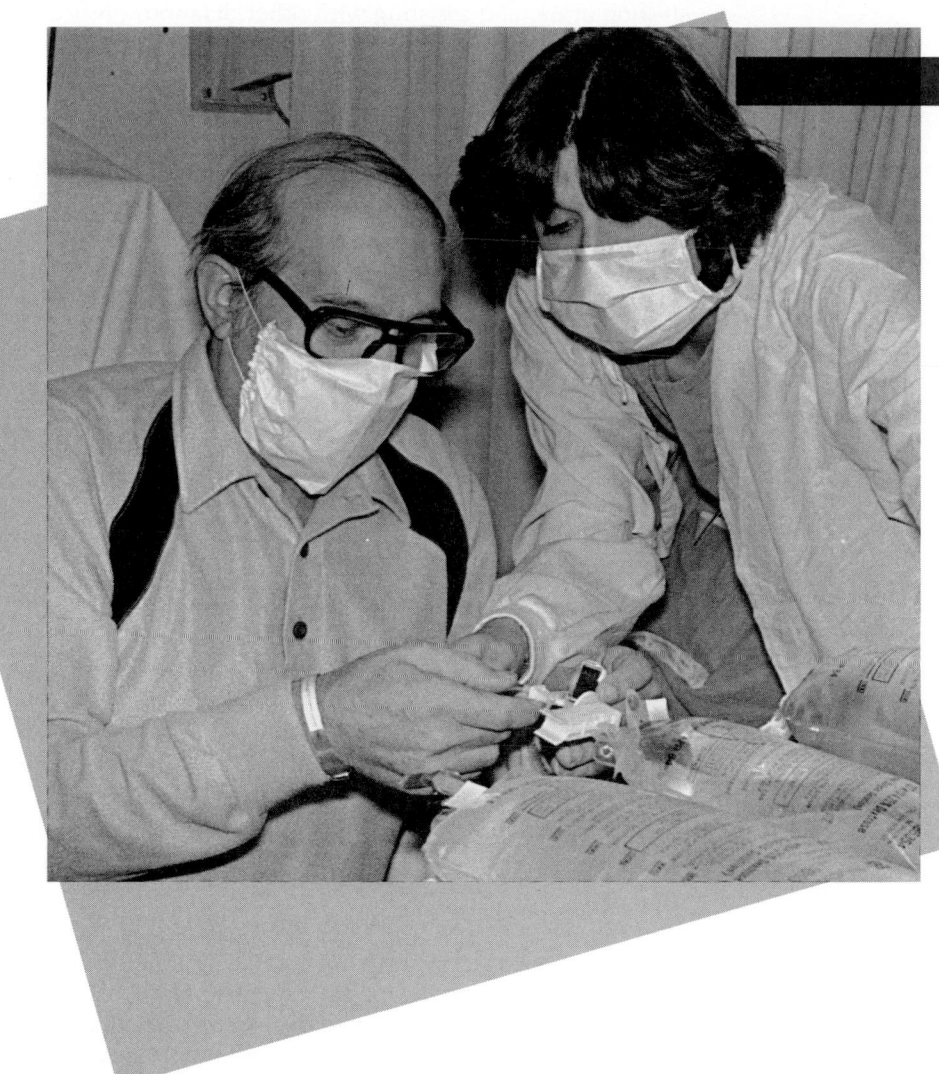

O B J E C T I V E S

After studying this chapter, the learner should be able to

Define key terms used in the chapter.

Describe the physiology of the urinary system.

Identify seven variables that influence urination.

Assess urinary elimination, using appropriate interview questions and physical assessment skills.

Execute the following assessment measures: measure urine output, collect urine specimens, determine the presence of select abnormal urine constituents, determine urine specific gravity, and assist with diagnostic tests and procedures.

Develop nursing diagnoses that correctly identify urinary problems amenable to nursing therapy.

Demonstrate how to promote normal urination; facilitate use of the toilet, bedpan, urinal, and commode; perform catheterizations; and assist with urinary diversions.

Plan, implement, and evaluate nursing care related to select nursing diagnoses involving urinary problems.

KEY TERMS

anuria	oliguria
catheter	orthostatic albuminuria
condom catheter	pneumaturia
cystoscopy	polyuria
dysuria	proteinuria
enuresis	pyuria
Foley catheters	reflex incontinence
frequency	residual urine
functional incontinence	retention
glycosuria	retrograde pyelogram
hematuria	stoma
hesitancy	stress incontinence
hydrometer	suprapubic catheter
ileal conduit	suppression
incontinence	total incontinence
indwelling urethral catheter	urination
intravenous pyelogram	urge incontinence
irrigation	urgency
micturition	urinometer
nocturia	voiding

Elimination from the urinary tract helps rid the body of waste products and materials that exceed bodily needs. The proper functioning of the urinary system is essential to the body's physical well-being, to life itself, and to the individual's general sense of well-being. The nurse assisting a client with urination or intervening to resolve health problems related to urination needs many specialized abilities.

This chapter provides the student with knowledge of the physiology of the urinary system and the multiple factors affecting urination. A practical guide to assessing urinary elimination is presented, including detailed information on specific assessment measures such as monitoring fluid intake, collecting urine specimens, testing urine, and assisting with other diagnostic procedures. Analysis of urinary data may lead to the identification of multiple nursing diagnoses or, when reported to the physician, to the early detection of a medical problem. Numerous examples of nursing diagnoses are offered. Client goals are established in planning care, and specific nursing strategies are presented. The section Nursing Process in Clinical Practice offers focused assessment, diagnosis, planning, implementation, and evaluation guides for select nursing diagnoses of common urinary problems (Alteration in elimination pattern related to dysuria; Alteration in elimination pattern related to maturational enuresis; Urinary incontinence; Urinary retention; Potential for nosocomial infection related to indwelling Foley catheter). These guides and the concluding case study illustrate how the nurse's knowledge of the urinary system and urinary pathology is combined with specific nursing interventions to resolve urinary problems successfully.

PHYSIOLOGY

Kidneys and Ureters

The kidneys are located on either side of the vertebral column behind the peritoneum and in the posterior portion of the abdominal cavity. One of the more significant functions of the kidneys is to maintain the composition and volume of body fluids. They perform this function in a selective manner by filtering and excreting blood constituents that are not needed and retaining those that are. It is estimated that the total blood volume passes through the kidneys for waste removal approximately every half hour. Despite varying kinds and amounts of food and fluids ingested, body fluids remain relatively stable if there is proper kidney functioning. The waste product that the kidneys excrete contains organic, inorganic, and liquid wastes and is called *urine*.

The nephron is the basic unit of kidney structure. There are approximately one million nephrons in each kidney. Urine from the nephrons empties into the pelvis of each kidney. From each kidney, urine is transported by rhythmic peristalsis through the ureters to the urinary bladder. The ureters enter the bladder obliquely, and a fold of membrane in the bladder closes the entrance to the ureters so that urine is not forced up the ureters to the kidneys when pressure exists in the bladder. Figure 33-1 shows views of the male and female urinary systems and shows the position of the kidneys and ureters in the abdominal cavity.

Bladder

The urinary bladder is a smooth muscle sac that serves as a reservoir for urine. There are three layers of muscular tissue in the bladder: the inner longitudinal layer, the middle circular layer, and the outer longitudinal layer. These three layers are called the *detrusor muscle*. At the base of the bladder, the middle circular layer of muscle tissue forms the internal or involuntary sphincter, which guards the opening between the urinary bladder and the urethra. The urethra conveys urine from the bladder to the exterior of the body.

Urinary bladder muscle is innervated by the autonomic nervous system. The sympathetic system carries inhibitory impulses to the bladder and motor impulses to the internal sphincter. These impulses cause the detrusor muscle to relax and the internal sphincter to constrict. This, in turn, causes urine to be retained in the bladder. The parasympathetic system carries motor impulses to the bladder and inhibitory impulses to the internal sphincter. These impulses cause the detrusor muscle to contract and the sphincter to relax. The male and female urinary bladders are illustrated in Figure 33-1.

The bladder normally contains urine under very little pressure, and, as volume of urine increases, the pressure increases only slightly. This adaptability of the bladder wall to pressure is believed to be due to the characteristics of muscle tissue in the bladder and makes it possible for urine to continue to enter the bladder from the ureters against low pressure. When the pressure becomes sufficient to stimulate stretch receptors located in the bladder wall, the desire to empty the bladder becomes apparent.

Urethra

The urethra differs in males and females. The male urethra is common to both the excretory system and the reproductive system. It is approximately 13.7 cm to 16.2 cm (5½ to 6¼ inches) in length and consists of three parts: the prostatic, the membranous, and the cavernous portions. The external urethral sphincter consists of striated muscle and is located just beyond the prostatic portion of the urethra. The external sphincter is under voluntary control.

The female urethra is 3.7 cm to 6.2 cm (1½ to 2½ inches) in length. Its function is to convey urine from the bladder to the exterior. The external or voluntary sphincter is located approximately midurethra. No por-

tion of the female urethra is external to the body as is true in the male. Most literature refers to muscle at the meatus in the female as the external sphincter.

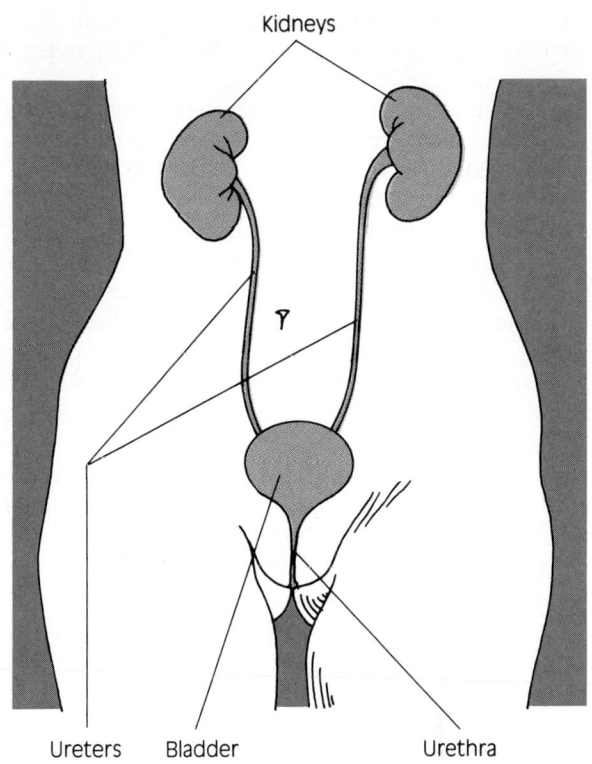

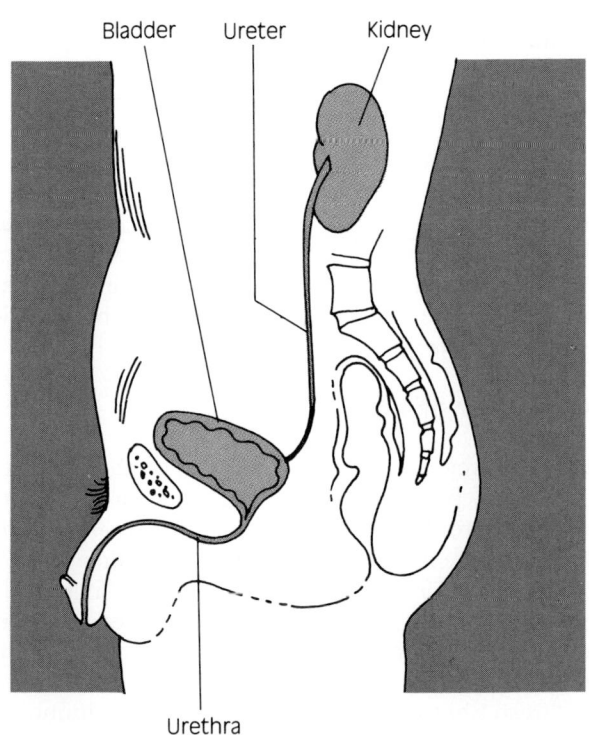

F I G U R E **33-1**
Frontal view of the female urinary tract and lateral view of the male urinary tract.

Act of Micturition

The process of emptying the bladder is known as **micturition**; it is also called **voiding** or **urination**. Nerve centers for micturition are situated in the brain and the spinal cord. Voiding is largely an involuntary reflex act, but its control can be learned.

Following stimulation of the stretch receptors in the bladder as the urine collects, the desire to void is experienced. Usually this occurs when about 100 ml to 200 ml for the child and 200 ml to 300 ml for the adult has collected. If the process of micturition is initiated, the detrusor muscle contracts, the internal sphincter relaxes, and urine enters the posterior urethra. The muscles of the perineum and the external sphincter relax, and micturition occurs. The act consists of relaxation of the internal sphincter, contraction of the detrusor muscle, slight contraction of the muscle of the abdominal wall, and lowering of the diaphragm. The act of micturition is normally painless. During micturition, the pressure within the bladder is many times greater than it is during the time the bladder is filling. The voluntary control of voiding is limited to initiating, restraining, and interrupting the act.

Restraint of voiding is believed to be subconscious when the volume of urine in the bladder is small. But when voiding is delayed, the bladder continues to fill. Discomfort may then be felt when undue distention occurs, and the urgency to void becomes paramount.

Increased abdominal pressure, as occurs with coughing and sneezing, sometimes forces the escape of urine involuntarily, especially in the female, since the urethra is shorter. Strong psychic factors, such as marked fear, may also result in involuntary urination. Under certain conditions, it may be difficult to relax the restraining muscles sufficiently to void, such as when a urine specimen is requested from a shy or embarrassed person.

When the higher nerve centers develop after infancy, the voluntary control of micturition develops also. Until that time, voiding is purely reflex. Persons whose bladders are isolated from control of the brain because of injury or disease also void by reflex only. This is called *autonomic bladder*.

Frequency of Micturition

The frequency of micturition depends on the amount of urine being produced. The more urine produced, the more often voiding is necessary, and *vice versa*. Unless the fluid intake is very large, most healthy persons do not void during normal sleeping hours. The first voided urine of the day is usually more concentrated than urine excreted during the remainder of the day. The nurse should remember that since the first voiding of the day is not "fresh" but rather an accumulation of a number of hours of kidney output, this urine may or may not be used as a specimen for certain tests.

Some persons normally void small amounts at frequent intervals because they habitually respond to the first early urge to void. This habit is insignificant and is not necessarily an indication of disease. Conversely, if this pattern is not a habit but a change in urination routine, it can be an indication of illness.

Other persons have habits that result in infrequent voiding. For example, some people go from 8 to 12 waking hours or longer without urinating. Factors such as a habitual low-fluid intake owing to environmental conditions or age may be the reason. The inaccessibility of toilet facilities owing to travel, work circumstances, or illness, and limitations of mobility can also be the cause of infrequent urination. Persons who habitually urinate infrequently have been found to develop more urinary tract infections and kidney disorders than those who urinate at least every 3 to 4 hours. The reason is believed to be stagnation of urine in the bladder, which serves as a good medium for bacterial growth. Infrequent voiding that is a change in one's urination pattern can also be indicative of a decreased production of urine owing to kidney or circulatory disorders.

FACTORS AFFECTING MICTURITION

Numerous factors affect the amount and quality of urine produced by the body and the manner in which it is excreted.

Developmental Considerations

Infants are born without voluntary control of micturition and with little ability to concentrate urine. Most children develop urinary control between the ages of 2 and 5 years. Daytime control precedes nighttime control and girls often develop control earlier than boys. Older children and adults generally control urination voluntarily and seldom wake to void at night because their kidneys are able to concentrate urine and produce less urine at night because of decreased renal blood flow.

Toilet-Training.   Most children are able to begin to control urination voluntarily at the age of 18 to 24 months. Toilet-training should not begin until the child is able to (1) hold urine for 1 to 2 hours; (2) recognize bladder fullness; and (3) communicate the need to void and control urination until seated on the toilet. The child's desire to gain control is also important. Wanting to be like a parent or older sibling often provides adequate motivation. Lifelong attitudes toward urination, the body, and cleanliness may develop during the time of toilet-training. (Enuresis is discussed in the section Nursing Process in Clinical Practice at the end of this chapter.)

Aging.   Physiologic changes that accompany normal aging may affect urination in the elderly:

- Diminished ability of the kidneys to concentrate urine may result in nocturia.
- Decreased bladder muscle tone may reduce the capacity of the bladder to hold urine and increase frequency.
- Decreased bladder contractility may lead to urine retention and stasis, which increase the likelihood of urinary tract infection.
- Neuromuscular problems, degenerative joint problems, alterations in thought processes, and weakness may interfere with voluntary control and the ability to reach a toilet in time.

Elderly who view themselves as "old, powerless, and neglected" may cease to value voluntary control over urination and simply find toileting "too much bother." Incontinence is often the result.

Food and Fluid

When the body is functioning well, the kidneys preserve a careful balance of fluid intake and output, which generally should be approximately equal. When the body is dehydrated, the kidneys will reabsorb fluid and the urine produced will be more concentrated and decreased in amount. Conversely, with fluid overload, the kidneys will excrete a large quantity of dilute urine.

Caffeine-containing beverages (cola, coffee, tea) have a diuretic effect and increase urine production. Alcohol produces the same effect by inhibiting the release of the antidiuretic hormone. Foods high in water content may increase urine production. Foods and beverages with high sodium content cause sodium and water reabsorption and retention, thereby decreasing urine formation. Also, certain foods may affect the odor of the urine (asparagus, onions) or its color (beets).

Life-style

Many individual, family, and sociocultural variables influence a person's normal voiding habits. For some individuals voiding is a very personal and private act, something one does not talk about. Needing assistance with a bedpan or urinal thus provokes great embarrassment and anxiety, which can be compounded when the bedpan is offered by a nurse of the opposite sex. For others, voiding is a natural act, and these individuals excuse themselves readily to void whenever the urge presents.

Psychologic Variables

Individuals experiencing stress often find themselves needing to void smaller amounts of urine at more frequent intervals. Stress can also interfere with the ability to relax perineal muscles and the external urethral sphincter. When this happens, the urge to void is present but emptying the bladder completely becomes difficult or impossible.

Activity and Muscle Tone

Among the many benefits of regular exercise are increased metabolism and optimal urine production and elimination. With prolonged periods of immobility, decreased bladder and sphincter tone can result in poor urinary control and urinary stasis. Persons with indwelling Foley catheters lose bladder tone because the bladder muscle is not being stretched as the bladder fills with urine. Other causes of decreased muscle tone include childbearing, menopausal muscle or atrophy, and damage to muscles from trauma.

Pathologic Conditions

Certain renal or urologic problems can affect both the quantity and quality of urine produced. Diseases known to be associated with renal problems include congenital urinary tract abnormalities, polycystic renal disease, urinary tract infection, urinary calculi (stones), hypertension, diabetes mellitus, gout, and certain connective tissue disorders.

Diseases that reduce physical activity or lead to generalized weakness such as arthritis, Parkinson's disease, and degenerative joint disease may interfere with toileting. Cognitive deficits and certain psychiatric problems can interfere with an individual's ability or desire to control urination voluntarily. Fever and diaphoresis (profuse perspiration) result in the kidney's conservation of body fluids. Urine production is decreased, and the urine is highly concentrated. Other pathologic conditions such as those present in congestive heart failure may lead to fluid retention and decreased urinary output.

Medications

Medications have numerous effects on urine production and elimination. Of gravest concern are the many prescription and nonprescription drugs known to be nephrotoxic (able to cause kidney damage). Abuse of analgesics such as aspirin has resulted in nephrotoxicity; some antibiotics, such as kanamycin, can be nephrotoxic.

Diuretics ("water pills"), which are commonly used in the treatment of hypertension and other disorders, prevent the reabsorption of water and certain electrolytes in the tubules. Depending on their strength, they cause moderate to severe increases in production and excretion of dilute urine. *Cholinergic* medications stimulate contraction of the detrusor muscle and produce urination. Some *analgesics* and *tranquilizers* that suppress the central nervous system interfere with urination by diminishing the effectiveness of the neural reflex.

Certain drugs cause urine to change color (*e.g.,* phenazopyridine [Pyridium] turns urine orange to red). Anticoagulants may cause hematuria (blood in the urine). Certain antibiotics can interfere with the testing of urine for glucose and yield false-negative results when Clinitest tablets are used.

NURSE AS ROLE MODEL

Before intervening to help clients develop healthy urinary elimination patterns, it is important for nurses to assess the adequacy of their own urinary elimination habits and patterns. If you are unable to meet the following goals, you may wish to take the time now to revise your own health practices so that you will be an effective role model for clients.

The nurse
- Empties the bladder completely at regular intervals
- Responds to the urge to void (*i.e.*, does not routinely postpone voiding because of being "too busy")
- Drinks 8 to 10 glasses of water daily
- Responds to changes in urinary characteristics (or frequency) by seeking their etiology and getting medical assistance when necessary

ASSESSING

A comprehensive nursing assessment of the functioning of the urinary system includes
- The collection of data about voiding patterns, habits, and difficulties and a history of present or past urinary problems
- A physical examination of the kidneys, bladder, and urethral meatus; assessment of skin integrity and hydration; and examination of the urine
- Correlation of these findings with the results of diagnostic tests and procedures for examining urine and the urinary tract

Nursing History

In the initial nursing history the nurse questions the client (or family member providing care/caregiver) about usual voiding habits and the present or past occurrence of voiding difficulties. Terminology should be used that the client understands. Elements of a urinary elimination history are suggested in the accompanying box.

With infants and young children, it is important to assess whether the child has achieved bladder control and if a toileting schedule is established. The nursing history and plan should also note the words the child uses to indicate the need to void.

With older adults, decreased bladder tone may be a problem and the nursing history should note any problems, how the person normally handles these problems,

---

Elements of a Urinary Elimination History

- Usual patterns of urinary elimination
  "Tell me how often you urinate (pass your water) during the day."
  "Do you awaken at night to empty your bladder?"
  "How would you describe your urine?"
- Recent changes in urinary elimination
  "Have you noticed any changes recently in your usual voiding patterns (frequency, amount, force of stream, difficulty, comfort)?"
- Aids to elimination
  "Is there anything you do that helps you to urinate?"
- Present or past occurrence of voiding difficulties (nature of problem, onset, frequency, causes, severity, symptoms, intervention attempted and results)
  "Tell me about any problems you are having now when you urinate (urgency, pain or burning, difficulty starting or stopping stream, dribbling, incontinence)."
  If there is a problem
  "Describe what you feel like before you urinate and while you are urinating."
  "Have you had any urinary problems in the past (any history of urinary tract infections, kidney or bladder disease or problems)?
- Presence of artificial orifices (normal routine, history of problems)
  "Tell me about your usual routine with your ureterostomy."

---

and nursing judgments about the adequacy of the solution.

Persons without bladder control or with limited bladder control as well as persons with urinary diversions usually have well-established routines for emptying the bladder. The procedures and equipment used should be assessed to make sure they follow accepted guidelines and are not predisposing the person to infection or other risk. Any special routine, equipment, or supplies utilized for urinary elimination should be noted in both the history and nursing care plan.

When a problem with voiding is reported, its duration, severity, and precipitating factors should be explored. See the box entitled Common Urinary Problems

Common Urinary Problems

Anuria: Technically, no urine voided; 24-hour urine output is less than 100 ml; synonyms are complete *kidney shutdown* or *renal failure.*

Dysuria: Difficulty in voiding; may or may not be associated with pain; a feeling of warm local irritation occurring during voiding is called *burning.*

Enuresis: Most often used to refer to the child who involuntarily urinates during the night

Frequency: Increased incidence of voiding

Glycosuria: Presence of sugar in the urine; if due to an unusually large intake of sugar or to marked emotional disturbances and is temporary, there is little cause for alarm.

Hematuria: Blood in the urine; if present in large enough quantities, urine may be bright red or reddish brown in color.

Hesitancy: Delay or difficulty in initiating voiding

Incontinence: Inability voluntarily to control the discharge of urine

Nocturia: Frequency of urination during the night

Oliguria: Scanty or greatly diminished amount of urine voided in a given time; 24-hour urine output is 100 ml to 400 ml.

Orthostatic albuminuria: Presence of albumin in urine that is voided after periods of standing, walking, or running; phenomenon of the circulatory system and not necessarily a symptom of kidney disorders

Pneumaturia: Passage of urine containing gas

Polyuria: Excessive output of urine (diuresis)

Proteinuria: Albumin in the urine; indication of kidney disease

Pyuria: Pus in the urine; urine appears cloudy.

Retention: Inability to void although urine is produced by the kidneys and enters the bladder; excessive storage of urine in the bladder

Suppression: Stoppage of urine production; normally the adult kidneys produce urine continuously at the rate of 60 ml to 120 ml/hour.

Urgency: Strong desire to void

---

for definitions of terms used to describe such problems. It is also important to note the client's perception of the problem and the adequacy of the client's self-care behaviors.

Nursing Examination

Physical assessment of urinary functioning includes an examination of the kidneys, urinary bladder, urethral meatus, skin, and urine.

Kidneys

In the normal adult the kidneys are well protected by a considerable amount of fat and connective tissue and are difficult to palpate. The right kidney is at the level of the twelfth rib and is lower than the left kidney. The right kidney may at times be palpated by the nurse if pushed down by the diaphragm when the client inhales. The nurse stands to the right of the supine client and places the left hand under the client's flank while the right hand palpates the abdominal wall. This technique requires deep palpation and should be practiced under supervision. The left kidney is palpated similarly. The contour and size of the kidneys are noted, as is any tenderness or lumps.

An examination of the kidneys includes checking for costovertebral tenderness. The costovertebral angle is formed by the twelfth rib and the spine. When the kidneys are inflamed the client experiences pain when this angle is percussed or struck. The nurse places one palm flat over the costovertebral angle and strikes the back of this hand with the other fist.

Bladder

The bladder is normally positioned below the symphysis pubis and cannot be assessed by the nurse when it is empty. Once the bladder becomes distended, however, it rises above the symphysis pubis and may reach to just below the umbilicus. At this point the nurse observes the lower abdominal wall noting any swelling and palpates this area for tenderness also noting the smoothness and roundness of the bladder. The height of the edge of the bladder above the symphysis pubis may be measured and the bladder may also be percussed. A full bladder produces a dull sound.

Urethral Orifice

The urethral orifice is inspected for any signs of inflammation or discharge. In the female the urethral meatus is a pink slit-like opening below the clitoris and above the vaginal orifice. The female needs to be in the dorsal recumbent position with the inner labia retracted for good visualization of the meatus. In the male the meatus is at the tip of the penis. If the male is uncircumcised, the foreskin may need to be retracted for visualization of the meatus. Foul odors should be noted.

Skin Integrity and Hydration

Because problems with urinary functioning may result in disturbances in hydration and excretion of body wastes, the skin should be carefully assessed for color, texture, turgor, and the excretion of any wastes. The integrity of the skin in the perineal area should also be assessed.

Problems with continence may result in severe excoriation.

Urine

Each time a client's urine is handled it should be assessed for color, odor, clarity, and the presence of any sediment. Abnormalities should be noted. In select clients the pH and specific gravity of the urine will be monitored as well as the presence of abnormal constituents such as protein, blood, glucose, ketone bodies, bac-

T A B L E　33-1
Characteristics of Urine

Characteristic	Normal Findings	Special Considerations
Color	A freshly voided specimen is generally pale yellow, straw-colored, or amber, depending on its concentration.	Urine is darker than normal when it is scanty and concentrated. Urine is lighter than normal when it is excessive and diluted. Certain drugs, such as cascara, L-dopa, and sulfonamides, alter the color of urine.
Odor	Normal urine smell is aromatic. As urine stands it often develops an ammonia odor because of bacterial action.	Some foods cause urine to have a characteristic odor; for example, asparagus causes urine to have a strong, musty odor. Urine high in glucose content has a sweet odor. Urine that is heavily infected has a fetid odor.
Turbidity	Fresh urine should be clear or translucent; as urine stands and cools it becomes cloudy.	Cloudiness observed in freshly voided urine is abnormal and may be due to the presence of red blood cells, white blood cells, bacteria, vaginal discharge, sperm, or prostatic fluid.
pH	The normal pH is approximately 6.0, with a range of 4.6 to 8. (Urine alkalinity or acidity may be promoted through diet to inhibit bacterial growth or urinary stone development or to facilitate the therapeutic activity of certain medications.) Urine becomes alkaline on standing when carbon dioxide diffuses into the air.	A high-protein diet causes urine to become excessively acid. Certain foods tend to produce alkaline urine, such as citrus fruits, dairy products, and vegetables, especially legumes. Certain foods tend to produce acidic urine, for example, meat and cranberry juice. Certain drugs influence the acidity/alkalinity of urine; for example, ammonium chloride tends to produce acidic urine, and potassium citrate and sodium bicarbonate tend to produce alkaline urine.
Specific gravity	This is a measure of the concentration of dissolved solids in the urine. The normal range is 1.010 to 1.025.	Concentrated urine will have a higher than normal specific gravity and diluted urine will have a lower than normal specific gravity. In the absence of kidney disease, a high specific gravity usually indicates dehydration and a low specific gravity indicates overhydration.
Constituents	*Organic* constituents of urine include urea, uric acid, creatinine, hippuric acid, indican, urene pigments, and undetermined nitrogen. *Inorganic* constituents are ammonia, sodium, chloride, traces of iron, phosphorus, sulfur, potassium, and calcium.	*Abnormal constituents* of urine include blood, pus, albumin, glucose, ketone bodies, casts, gross bacteria, and bile.

teria, and so on. Normal characteristics of urine and special considerations for observation are detailed in Table 33-1.

Assessment Measures

In addition to interviewing the client and performing the physical examination, the nurse gathers data about urinary elimination by carrying out the following assessment measures: measuring urine output, collecting urine specimens, determining the presence of abnormal constituents in the urine, and assisting with diagnostic procedures. Discussions of the nursing responsibilities related to each of these measures follow.

Measuring Urinary Output.
Measuring the client's intake and output is an important nursing responsibility. Accuracy of the total fluid intake and output from all sources is essential for the planning of the client's nursing and medical care. The measurement of intake and output is described further in Chapter 35.

The procedure for measuring the urinary output for the client who is voiding is as follows:

- Have the client void into a bedpan or urinal, either in bed or in the bathroom. Urinary devices used to collect or measure urine are illustrated in Figure 33-2.
- Pour urine voided into a bedpan or urinal into the appropriate measuring device provided by the agency. The devices are calibrated in milliliters.
- Place the calibrated container on a flat surface, such as on a shelf, for an accurate reading. Note the amount of urine voided, read at eye level, and record it on the appropriate form. Figure 33-3 illustrates a commonly used form for recording urinary output. The form is kept at the client's bedside or may be taped to the bathroom door. The total amount voided during each shift and 24-hour period is recorded on the patient's permanent record.
- Do *not* discard the urine if a specimen is required. Otherwise, the urine is discarded in the toilet.
- Instruct clients who are ambulatory when their urinary output is to be measured and recorded so that they do not use the bathroom without measuring output. Clients who are willing and able can be taught to measure and record their own output.

When a client has an indwelling Foley catheter in place, the procedure for measuring urinary output is as follows:

- Bring a calibrated measuring device to the bedside and place it beneath the collection bag.
- Place the drainage spout from the collection bag above, but not touching, the calibrated measuring device and open the clamp.
- Allow the urine to flow from the collection bag into the measuring device. Then proceed as described above.

For catheterized clients who are acutely ill, urine may need to be measured hourly. This is facilitated by using a special collection bag with a built-in calibrated measuring chamber, called a urinometer. After the nurse assesses and records the amount of urine produced hourly, the measuring chamber is tilted and this urine empties into the general collection bag. The measuring chamber is now ready to collect the next hour's urine.

Collecting Urine Specimens.
General nursing responsibilities for diagnostic tests are discussed in Chapter 41. Details are explained here.

Routine Urinalysis.
The collection of urine specimens for urinalysis is a nursing responsibility. A sterile urine specimen is not required for a routine urinalysis. The urine is collected by having the client void into a clean bedpan, urinal, or receptacle in the toilet bowl. Care must be taken to avoid contamination with feces. If a woman is menstruating when a urine sample is obtained, this must be noted on the laboratory slip because red blood cells may appear in the urine. The urine is poured into an appropriate container, labeled with the client's name, date, and time of collection, and sent to the laboratory for examination. Urine should not be left standing at room temperature for a long period before being sent to the laboratory because this may alter both the appearance and chemistry of the urine.

Specimens from Infants and Children.
Plastic disposable collection bags are available for infants and small children who have not yet achieved voluntary bladder control (Fig. 33-4). The manufacturer's instructions should be followed and care taken in application and removal not to irritate the sensitive perineal skin.

Clean-Catch or Midstream Specimen.
A clean-catch specimen of urine is required in some situations. Most health agencies specify that a clean-catch specimen be collected during midstream. This means that the client voids a little urine, which is discarded; the specimen is then collected during midstream; and the last urine in the bladder is also discarded. The first voided urine helps flush away organisms that may be near the meatus. The urinalysis findings may be inaccurate if these organisms enter the specimen. Also, it is generally thought that urine voided at midstream is most characteristic of urine the body is producing. A clean-catch midstream specimen from a male is sterile. The female may be catheterized if a sterile specimen is required. Catheterization is discussed later in this chapter.

The client who can carry out proper techniques may collect his or her own clean-catch midstream urine specimen and often prefers to do so. The nurse should provide the appropriate equipment and instructions to carry out the procedure.

(Text continues on p. 859.)

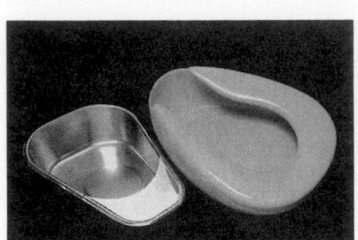

Bedpan and fracture pan
Containers used to collect urine
from nonambulatory clients

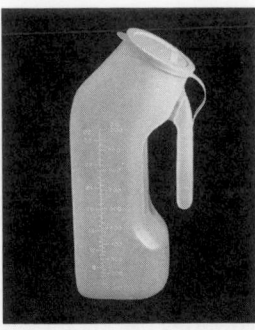

Urinal
Container used to collect
urine from nonambulatory
male clients

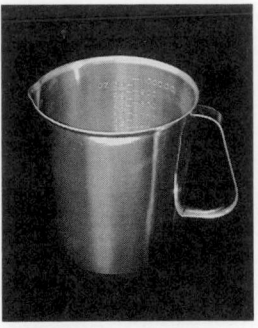

Calibrated measuring
device
Device which makes possi-
ble the recording of an
accurate urine output

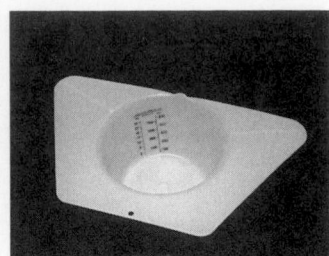

Specimen hat
Container which when placed
anteriorly in the toilet, underneath the seat, collects urine for
measurement or study

Straight catheter and specimen
container
Single lumen catheter which
drains urine from the bladder—
here into a sterile urine specimen
container

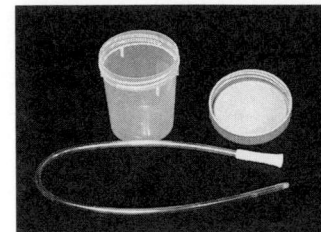

Small urine collection bag well-
suited to ambulatory clients; may
be easily emptied in the toilet;
easily concealed in pants or a
skirt

2-way Foley catheter

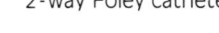
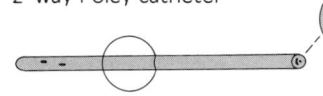
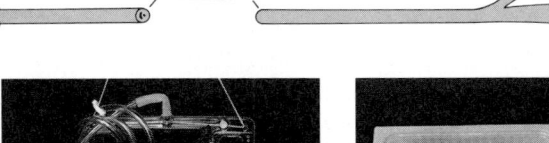

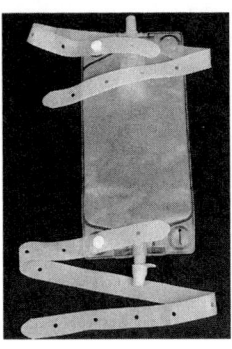

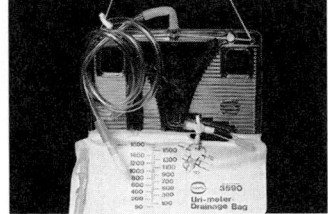

Large urine collection bag—
generally emptied once each
eight-hour shift; provides an
approximate measure of urine

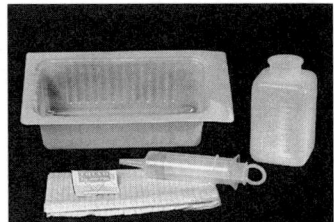

Large urine collection bag with
accurately callibrated small chamber for determining precise
hourly urine outputs

Irrigation tray containing a sterile
piston syringe, a sterile container
for holding the irrigation fluid,
and a sterile tray for collecting
the solution which returns from
the catheter

3000 cc bag of irrigation fluid for
continuous bladder irrigation

3-way Foley catheter
(for continuous bladder
irrigation)

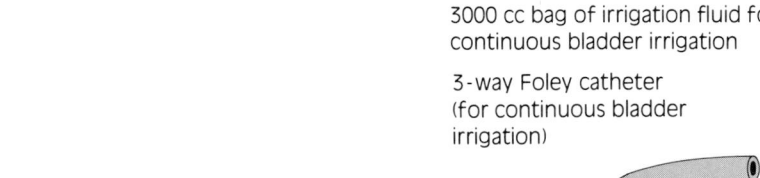
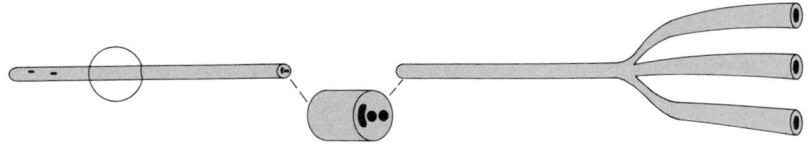

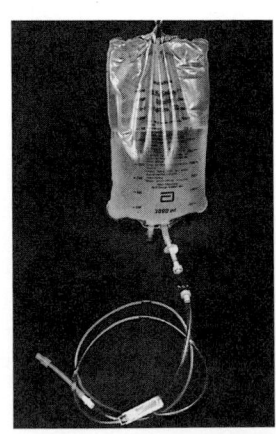

F I G U R E   **33-2**
Devices for collecting and measuring urine.

Intake and Output Chart

7:00 AM _11-18_ to 7:00 AM _11-19_

	Oral	I.V.		Blood	Other	Comments	Urine	Stool	Gastric tube	Drainage tubes		Vomitus	Other	Comments
			Intake							Output				
7-8	250					Force fluids to 1100cc/shift	300							
8-9														
9-10	120													
10-11	60													
11-12	100						250							
12-1	300													
1-2	240													
2-3	100						200							
8 hr Tot	1170						750							voiding 5 discomfort
3-4														
4-5														
5-6														
6-7														
7-8														
8-9														
9-10														
10-11														
8 hr Tot														
11-12														
12-1														
1-2														
2-3														
3-4														
4-5														
5-6														
6-7														
8 hr Tot														
24 hr Tot														

Total intake | | **Total output**

F I G U R E 33-3
An example of a form commonly used for recording intake and output.

Guidelines for obtaining a clean-catch midstream urine specimen from a female client and from a male client are as follows:

Female Client
- Wear sterile gloves.
- Spread the labia well, and keep them apart until the specimen is obtained.
- Clean the area at the external meatus with sterile gauze or cotton balls and antiseptic soap and water. Move the gauze or cotton balls from the meatus toward the anus, and use one piece of gauze or one cotton ball for each stroke.
- Have the client void about 30 ml and discard this urine.

- Position the sterile specimen container near but not touching the meatus and ask the client to void forcibly if she is lying down. This prevents collecting a specimen that has dribbled down and across the perineal area.
- Stop collecting urine before the client empties her bladder. Release the labia. Allow the client to continue emptying her bladder and discard the urine not needed for the specimen.
- Use a sterilized bedpan to collect the midstream specimen if the client has difficulty voiding into the container, and then transfer the urine into the sterile specimen container.
- Label the specimen container appropriately and send the specimen to the laboratory.

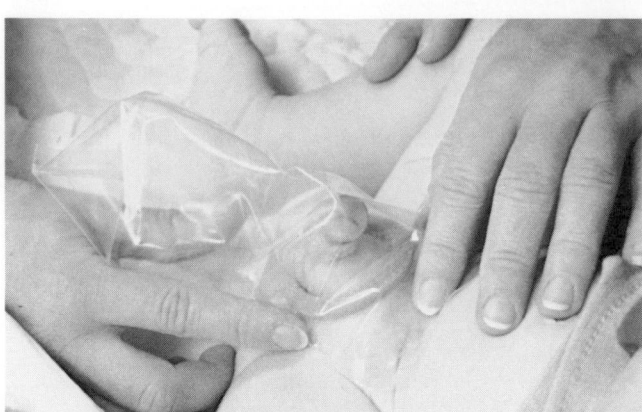

F I G U R E   33-4
Disposable urine-collection devices are available for infants and small children who have not yet achieved voluntary bladder control.

Male Client
- Wear sterile gloves.
- Retract the foreskin to expose the glans penis in the uncircumsized male client.
- Clean the area of the external meatus with sterile gauze or cotton balls and antiseptic soap and water. Move gauze or cotton balls in a circular manner at the meatus, and move down the shaft of the penis a few inches.
- Have the client void about 30 ml and discard this urine.
- Have the client void directly into the sterile container.
- Stop collecting urine before the client empties his bladder. Allow the client to empty his bladder and discard this urine. Return the foreskin to its normal position to prevent swelling and irritation of the glans penis.
- Use a sterilized urinal to collect the midstream specimen if the client has difficulty voiding into the container, and then transfer the urine into the sterile specimen container.
- Label the specimen container appropriately and send the specimen to the laboratory.

Sterile Specimen from an Indwelling Catheter. Sterile urine specimens may be attained using the clean-catch technique, by catheterizing the client (see Procedures 33-1 and 33-2 later in this chapter), or by obtaining the specimen from an indwelling catheter already in place.

When it is necessary to collect a urine specimen from a patient with an indwelling catheter, it should be done from the catheter itself. A specimen from the collecting receptacle (drainage bag) may not be fresh urine, and its use could result in an inaccurate analysis. Sterile technique must be observed.

A sterile 21-gauge needle, a 10-ml or 50-ml syringe,

and an antiseptic swab are needed to collect the specimen. Most catheters have a self-sealing area that tolerates a needle puncture. After locating the area, clean it carefully with the antiseptic swab. Carefully insert the sterile needle into the catheter, and aspirate urine into the syringe. Some manufacturers of indwelling catheters now supply devices for obtaining a sterile urine specimen from a special collection port in the catheter tubing. The device pierces the tubing and aspirates and collects the urine. In this instance the manufacturer's directions should be followed. The specimen is handled according to agency policy.

Care must be taken not to aspirate urine above the Y-junction of the catheter. It is possible for the needle of the syringe to lodge in the lumen of the tube leading to the balloon. In this case, the water inflating the balloon holding the catheter in place will be aspirated instead of urine.

Figure 33-5 illustrates removing urine from an indwelling catheter.

For large samples of urine, the catheter may be clamped for approximately 10 minutes to allow urine to collect in the bladder. Agency policy should be followed for clamping the catheter.

Collecting 24-Hour Urine Specimens. For some types of laboratory studies, 24-hour specimens are required. It is critical that the client and the entire nursing team understand the importance of collecting *all* the urine voided in a 24-hour period. A sign posted on the client's bathroom door is a helpful reminder not to discard urine. The collection is initiated at a specific time (which is recorded) by having the patient empty his bladder. This urine is discarded. All urine excreted for the next 24 hours is collected.

Depending on the type of examination used, the urine from each voiding may be kept in a separately marked container and the time of each voiding recorded. Or, all voidings may be collected in a common receptacle. The laboratory should be contacted to determine whether or not a preservative is needed to retard decomposition and if the specimens are to be refrigerated or kept on ice.

Double-Voided Specimen. When determining the presence of glucose and ketones in the urine, a "freshly" voided specimen is needed. The client is instructed to empty the bladder and discard the urine approximately 30 minutes before the time the test specimen is required. This ensures elimination of urine that has collected in the bladder since the last voiding. The client is instructed to drink a glass of fluid and a fresh specimen is collected in 30 minutes for testing.

Determining Abnormal Constituents in the Urine.
In some situations, the nurse may perform tests on urine specimens, especially when specimens are being tested repeatedly for known abnormalities, when screening

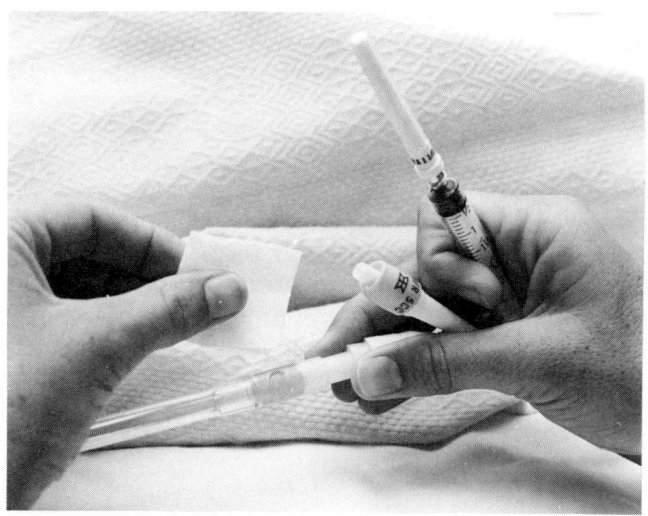

A

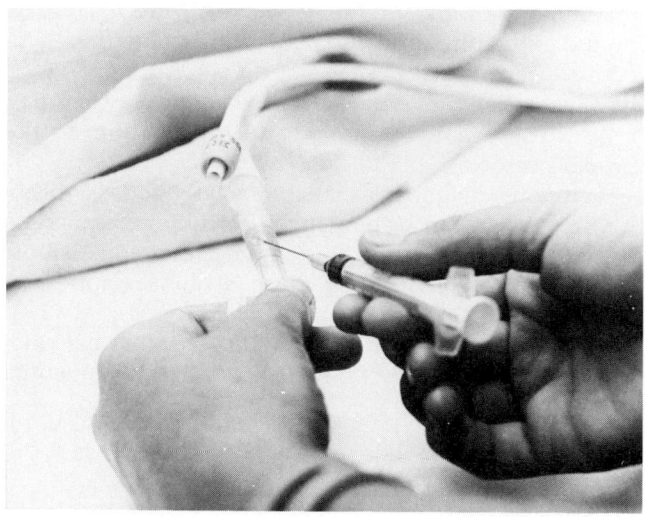

B

F I G U R E   33-5

The nurse is obtaining a urine specimen from a patient using an indwelling catheter. (A) She first cleans the area where she will introduce a sterile needle with a swab moistened with an antiseptic. (B) She then inserts the needle and withdraws a specimen of urine.

tests are being used, or when laboratory facilities are not readily available. For example, a nurse may test urine for the presence of glucose, protein, bilirubin, and blood. The results of the test are recorded on the client's record. Many types of commercially prepared diagnostic kits are available for determining the presence of abnormal substances in the urine. Although the performance of these tests is economical and fast, laboratory analysis is generally recommended when more precise results are needed.

The diagnostic kits generally contain needed equipment and the appropriate reagent, a substance used in a chemical reaction to detect another substance. Reagents are prepared in the form of tablets, fluids, impregnated paper, and plastic strips with a special coating. When the reagent is brought in contact with urine, a chemical reaction occurs, which causes a color change. The reaction is then compared with an accompanying chart that describes the significance of the color.

The precise directions for the amount of the specimen, the time allowance for the chemical reaction, and the significance of the colors vary with the manufacturer. Therefore, it is important to read the directions accompanying the diagnostic kit carefully and to follow them exactly.

Determining Specific Gravity.   Determining the specific gravity of urine requires an instrument called a **urinometer** or a **hydrometer**. The urinometer has a calibrated scale for the measurement of specific gravity. Urine is placed in a cylindrical container, and the urinometer is inserted in a circular motion without touching the bottom or side of the container. The reading on a urinometer should be made at eye level at the bottom of the meniscus formed by the urine. The density of the urine supports the urinometer. If the urine is concentrated, the urinometer will be buoyed up high in the urine container and will register high on the measurement scale. If the urine is diluted, the urinometer will be supported low in the urine, and a low specific gravity reading will result.

Assisting with Diagnostic Procedures.   Various diagnostic procedures, ordinarily performed in an operating room, are used to study the urinary system. The nurse is responsible for preparing the client and giving appropriate aftercare. Anxieties the client may have tend to be reduced when the nurse explains the procedure. Three common diagnostic procedures used to study the urinary system include cystoscopies, intravenous pyelograms, and retrograde pyelograms. A **cystoscopy** provides a direct visualization of the bladder, the ureteral orifices, and the urethra. The instrument used is a cystoscope. An **intravenous pyelogram** involves the injection of a contrast material intravenously, followed by x-ray examination of the kidney and urethra. In a **retrograde pyelogram**, x-ray films are taken of the kidney and urethra after a contrast material is injected into the renal pelvis through the ureter. Descriptions of the preparation and aftercare of the client for each of these procedures are presented in Table 33-2.

DIAGNOSING

The data the nurse collects about the client's urinary functioning may lead to the development of one or sev-

eral nursing diagnoses. Some data are appropriately reported to the physician and may contribute to the physician's identification of a medical diagnosis. It is
important that nurses detect significant urinary findings,
record these appropriately, and report them to the
proper persons.

Nursing diagnoses that specifically address problems in urinary functioning include problems of incontinence, pattern alteration, and urinary retention. Sample
defining characteristics for these diagnoses appear in
Table 33-3.

Difficulty with urination or changes in normal voiding problems may affect other areas of human function-

ing. Examples of nursing diagnoses that may be related
to urinary problems include

Anxiety related to incontinence, diagnostic procedures
Comfort, altered, related to bladder spasms, dysuria, urinary retention, cancer of the bladder,
diagnostic procedures
Infection, potential for nosocomial infection, related to indwelling Foley catheter
Knowledge deficit related to any existing or new
urinary disease or disorder
Self-care deficit: toileting related to parent's lack of
knowledge or motivation to toilet-train child,

T A B L E   33-2
Common Diagnostic Procedures Used to Study the Urinary Tract

Preparation	Aftercare
Cystoscopy	The direct visual examination of the bladder, ureteral orifices, and urethra with a cystoscope
The client is allowed liquids on the morning of the examination.	Tissue swelling, dysuria, and hematuria may occur owing to trauma from the procedure.
Sedation and analgesics are usually prescribed before the procedure.	Encourage a generous fluid intake, and observe and measure urinary output for at least 24 hours.
A signed consent form is required for the procedure.	Observe the client for urinary retention and for signs of infection; nosocomial infection after a cystoscopy is common.
The procedure is ordinarily painless.	
Intravenous Pyelogram	The x-ray examination of the kidney and ureter after a contrast material is injected intravenously
No fluids or food are given for at least 12 hours before the examination so that contrast material will concentrate in the urinary system. Elderly, debilitated, or young clients may not tolerate this dehydration and compromises may need to be made.	Fluids and food may be given immediately after the examination.
	Observe the client for signs of a reaction to the contrast material, such as a skin rash, nausea, and hives.
A laxative the evening before the examination and an enema the morning of the examination are given so that stool and gas do not interfere with visualization.	
The client should void before the examination.	
Retrograde Pyelogram	The x-ray examination of the kidney and ureters after a contrast material is injected into the renal pelvis through the ureter
No fluids and food are given after midnight before the examination.	Foods and fluids may be given, but if anesthesia has been used, this is delayed for several hours.
A laxative the evening before the examination and an enema the morning of the examination are given so that stool and gas do not interfere with visualization.	Check the vital signs regularly if anesthesia has been used.
The client should void before the examination.	Observe the client for signs of a reaction to the contrast material, such as a skin rash, nausea, and hives.
A signed consent form is recommended for the procedure.	Ureteral catheters may be in place and should be connected to drainage receptacles so that the amount and character of drainage from each catheter can be noted.

TABLE 33-3
Nursing Diagnoses for Common Urinary Problems

Title	Etiologic or Contributing Factors	Sample Defining Characteristics
Incontinence, functional	Altered environment Sensory, cognitive, or mobility deficits	"I don't know why Johnny started wetting since he's been hospitalized. He has been toilet-trained for 6 months now." "When I remember to take mother to the toilet she urinates fine. But if I don't remember, I find her wet."
Incontinence, reflex	Neurologic impairment	Individual with spinal cord lesion reports no awareness of bladder filling, no urge to void or feelings of bladder fullness, involuntary loss of urine at somewhat regular intervals.
Incontinence, stress	Age-related degenerative changes High intra-abdominal pressure Incompetent bladder outlet Overdistention between voidings Weak pelvic muscles and structural supports	Obese mother of four reports involuntary dribbling of urine with coughs, sneezes, hearty laughter. Individual "too busy to void" during day reports involuntary leakage of urine with sudden movement, cough, and so on.
Incontinence, total	Neurologic impairment Trauma or disease affecting spinal cord nerves	Constant flow of urine at unpredictable times without distention or uninhibited bladder contractions Nocturia
Incontinence, urge	Decreased bladder capacity Bladder spasms Increased intake of caffeine or alcohol Increased urine concentration Overdistention of bladder	"I can never make it to the bathroom in time." Urgency, frequency, nocturia, bladder contracture/spasm
Urinary elimination, altered patterns	Enuresis (maturational) Dysuria	Parents report 6-year-old son wets bed three to four times/week. Small bladder capacity, less than 300 ml "It hurts when I pass my water." Urinalysis reveals hematuria and proteinuria.
Urinary retention	High urethral pressure caused by weak detrusor Inhibition of reflex arc Strong sphincter Blockage	Elderly male diagnosed with benign prostatic hypertrophy complains of inability to urinate despite feeling bladder is full. Woman 6 hours after delivery has had no urine output since labor; 800 ml IV fluids infused; fundus of uterus is displaced to the right by a full bladder.

neuromuscular impairment or musculoskeletal disorders, immobility, trauma or surgical procedures, confusion, disorientation
Self-concept, disturbance in, related to urinary incontinence, urinary diversion
Sexual dysfunction related to urinary incontinence, urinary diversion
Skin integrity, impaired (actual, potential) related to incontinence
Sleep pattern disturbance related to nocturia

The nurse's challenge is to identify correctly human responses to alterations in urinary elimination that pose specific health problems for the client and family.

PLANNING: CLIENT GOALS

When the client is ambulatory and not experiencing difficulties with the urinary system, the promotion of normal voiding generally is not a problem. Trauma or illness, however, may result in the client's need for nursing assistance with voiding. Nursing interventions (which follow) should be supportive of planned client goals.

- The client will produce urinary output approximately equal to fluid intake.
- The client will maintain fluid and electrolyte balance.
- The client will empty the bladder completely at regular intervals.
- The client will report ease of voiding.
- The client will maintain skin integrity.

Client goals for specific urinary problems follow later in this chapter.

IMPLEMENTING

Promoting Normal Urination

Maintaining Normal Voiding Habits

If the client's voiding habits are adequate, the nurse takes care to maintain these habits to ensure comfort and satisfactory urinary output. Attention to the following variables is helpful:

- *Schedule:* Some clients will report voiding "on demand" in no apparent pattern. Others have inflexible patterns developed over the years and become anxious if these are interrupted. Some clients need assistance voiding and may experience urgency. Adhering to the client's normal voiding patterns as much as possible is recommended.
- *Privacy:* Many adults and children cannot void in the presence of another person. Unless the extreme weakness of the client demands the nurse's assistance, privacy should be offered to the client.
- *Position:* Assisting clients to assume *normal* voiding positions may be all that is necessary to resolve an inability to void. Some males cannot use a urinal lying down or sitting; the nurse should then assist them to void while standing at the bedside unless this is contraindicated. Similarly, some females cannot void easily on a bedpan and respond favorably to the use of a bedside commode.
- *Hygiene:* Individuals confined to bed will find it difficult to perform their usual genital hygiene. Careful cleansing of the perineal and genital area is needed to promote client comfort and to prevent infection. This is easily accomplished for clients on bed rest by placing them on a bedpan and then pouring warm soapy water over the perineal area followed by clear water. Families providing care for ill members at home may also be taught this technique.

Since many individuals customarily wash their hands after toileting, clients confined to bed should be offered a moistened towelette or soap and water to wipe their hands after the nurse removes the bedpan.

Promoting Fluid Intake

Many persons routinely drink less fluid than is optimal to promote healthy urinary functioning. The adult who has no disease-related fluid restrictions should drink 2000 ml to 2400 ml (8 to 10 8-ounce glasses) of fluid daily. A common misperception is that drinking this much fluid causes "water retention" and contributes to weight gain. This is false. If a good proportion of the daily fluid intake is water, the kidneys and urinary structures will be well flushed and waste products will be removed, including potentially harmful bacteria. Fluid intake should be monitored for potentially harmful excesses of caffeine-containing beverages, high-sodium beverages such as diet sodas, and high-sugar beverages.

Fluids of preference, fresh water and juices, should be made available to clients confined to bed. Also, children and confused clients may need to be reminded to drink. With certain diseases, fluid restrictions may be ordered by the physician. In others, forced fluids (above-average intake of fluids) are prescribed. This needs to be incorporated in the plan of care.

Strengthening Muscle Tone

Strengthening muscle tone in the perineal and abdominal muscles can facilitate voluntary control of urination. Clients should be instructed to exercise perineal muscles by voluntarily starting and stopping the stream of urine (Kegel exercises) and by tightening the muscles around the anus. Once the client is familiar with these sensations, these muscles should be contracted and relaxed several times each waking hour for a period of 2 to 3 months. The exercises can be done anywhere and clients should be assisted to incorporate them into their daily activities.

Stimulating Urination

Urinary retention, the inability to void even though the bladder is full, is discussed later in this chapter. Many persons, however, experience hesitancy, a delay, or difficulty in initiating voiding. This may often be resolved by resorting to simple nursing measures.

- Assist the client to void when the urge to void is first experienced. Routine delaying of urination may result in difficulty initiating a stream.
- Make use of the factors noted above to provide a natural environment for voiding: relaxed, private setting and normal position. Squatting or leaning

RESEARCH IN NURSING *Making a Difference*

Urinary Elimination

Urinary incontinence is not a disease but rather a symptom of other underlying medical, psychologic, or environmental problems. It is an embarrassing, potentially disabling, and costly health problem. Until the past decade, incontinence was seen as an inevitable outcome of the aging process. In recent years, nursing research has helped dispel this myth by examining urinary incontinence from three general perspectives: defining or describing types of incontinence, management techniques, and treatment methods.

Related Research

Haeker S: Disposable vs. reusable incontinence products. Geriatric Nursing 6(6):345–347, 1985

Haeker compared the use of disposable undergarments to the use of reusable incontinence products, evaluating the effects of using disposable products on an established toileting program, client's skin condition, and cost-effectiveness. Results showed decreased incontinence and increased toiletings, skin problems, and probable cost with disposable products. Conclusions were that the disadvantages of disposable products outweighed their advantages over washable incontinence garments.

Long M: Incontinence: Defining the nursing role. Journal of Gerontological Nursing 11(1):30–35, 41, 1985

This study was conducted to determine the incidence of urinary incontinence and document the results of nursing assessment and retraining interventions. Nursing interventions focusing on individualized fluid intake, toileting methods, toileting schedules, and incontinence records were evaluated and found to be effective in identifying and resolving urinary incontinence.

Rottkamp B: A holistic approach to identifying factors associated with an altered pattern of urinary elimination in stroke patients. Journal of Neurosurgical Nursing 17(1):37–44, 1985

Rottkamp conducted this study to identify factors affecting urine control in stroke clients. Findings support other studies attempting to isolate factors predictive of urinary dysfunction, illustrating interrelationships between categories of factors (e.g., urologic, psychologic, environmental). It is recommended that nursing management be specific to contributing factors and that continued research be done in this area.

Incontinence research presents implications for changing current methods of nursing practice. For example, analysis of urinary patterns, in addition to traditional intake and output records, would provide significant information about the strength of perineal musculature, an important factor when trying to regain urinary control. Current nursing interventions for incontinence need further study to identify the most successful and clinically realistic methods of care for the incontinent client.

---

forward may assist by putting pressure on the suprapubic area.

- Run tap water within the client's hearing.
- Use a warm bedpan.
- Pour warm water over the perineal area. Measure the amount of water if the voided specimen needs to be measured.
- Pour warm water over the client's fingers.
- Stroke the client's leg or thigh.
- Exert gentle downward pressure over the bladder to facilitate bladder emptying. This technique differs from Credé's maneuver in which manual bladder compression is utilized to stimulate urination by creating a sensation of bladder fullness and relaxing the urethral sphincter. The nurse places one hand on top of the other over the client's bladder (between the umbilicus and symphysis pubis, fingers pointing downward) and exerts downward pressure to compress the bladder walls and forcefully expel urine. This maneuver should only be performed when bladder flaccidity exists and the client is not expected to regain voluntary control. It normally requires a physician's order.

- If urination is being stimulated for the purposes of obtaining a urine specimen and the client is cooperative, having the client forcefully cough will sometimes create sufficient intra-abdominal pressure to stimulate the micturition reflex.

• Ask the client to blow bubbles through a straw in a glass of water

Assisting With Toileting

Toilet. Despite the client's ability to use the bathroom toilet, the nurse is responsible for noting any abnormalities of elimination. In some instances, clients may need to be taught to report abnormalities to the nurse and instructed not to flush the toilet until the nurse checks the urine. In other instances when the urine volume is to be calculated, the client may need to urinate in a bedpan or some other receptable placed on the toilet so the urine can be measured before it is discarded. Although many clients can easily be taught to measure their urinary output, the nurse should observe the urine at least once during a work shift and more frequently if warranted.

A weak client should be assisted to the bathroom. Someone should remain in attendance if there is any danger of the client's falling. Bathrooms should not be locked, and, especially in hospitals, a signal bell should be within easy reach of the client so that help can be summoned easily if the client feels weak and in need of assistance. A hand rail near the toilet is helpful.

Commode. Commodes can be used for clients able to be out of bed but unable to use the bathroom toilet. Commodes are chairs, straight-back chairs, or wheelchairs, with open seats under which there is a shelf or a holder on which a bedpan is placed. The commode can be placed adjacent to the bed, and the client can be assisted to it with minimal exertion.

Bedpan and Urinal. Male clients confined to bed usually use the urinal for voiding and the bedpan for defecation; female clients use the bedpan for both. When a female client is unable to sit up in bed—for example, when she is in a body cast—a female urinal may be used. The bedpan and the urinal are difficult to use and embarrassing to many clients. Privacy is important to almost all clients when they use a bedpan or urinal.

A special bedpan, also called a "fracture" bedpan, is frequently used by persons with fractures of the femur or lower spine. It is smaller and flatter than the ordinary bedpan but is useful for clients who cannot raise themselves easily to use the regular-sized bedpan.

Procedure 32-1 describes and illustrates how to help a client use a bedpan or urinal.

Safety Considerations. Many dangerous situations have been created in the absence of a signal bell or bedpan. Clients confined to bed have gotten up to go to the bathroom to void, sometimes climbing over or around bed side rails or removing oxygen masks or infusion tubings. Offering a bedpan or urinal frequently can save clients from a fractured hip, a dislodged IV infusion, or the embarrassment of soiled linen. A very ill or sedated client may not think to ask in time. As a precaution, family members of clients at home may need to be made aware of this. The nurse is responsible for the client's safety.

Teaching Feminine Hygiene. Female clients often need to be taught the proper technique for perineal care after urination. Drying or washing of the perineal area should be from the front to the back, or from the urethra toward the rectum. A reverse cleaning motion can result in fecal organisms being introduced into the urethra or vagina. This type of contamination is a common cause of urinary tract and vaginal infections.

Catheterizing the Client's Bladder

Urinary catheterization is the introduction of a catheter through the urethra into the bladder for the purpose of withdrawing urine. A **catheter** is a tube for injecting or removing fluids. Catheterization is considered the most prominent cause of nosocomial infections, that is, an infection acquired in a hospital. Whenever possible, it is recommended that catheterization be avoided. When deemed necessary, it should be performed with careful technique. (See Nursing Process in Clinical Practice, later in this chapter.)

Types of Catheters. If a catheter is to remain in place for continuous drainage, an **indwelling urethral catheter** is used. Indwelling catheters are also called **retention** and **Foley catheters**. The indwelling urethral catheter is designed so that it does not slip out of the bladder. These catheters are used for the gradual decompression of an overdistended bladder, for intermittent bladder drainage and irrigation, and for continuous bladder drainage.

Intermittent catheters are used to drain the bladder for shorter periods of time (5 to 10 minutes). Clients can be taught to insert and remove intermittent catheters themselves. Intermittent catheters are discussed later in this section.

Occasionally, a **suprapubic catheter** is used for continuous drainage. This type of catheter is inserted through a small incision above the pubic area. Care of the patient with a suprapubic catheter is more appropriately discussed in clinical texts.

Facts About the Lower Urinary Tract System. Several basic facts about the lower urinary tract system should be borne in mind when considering catheterization:

• The bladder is normally a sterile cavity.
• The external opening to the urethra can never be sterilized.

(Text continues on p. 871.)

PROCEDURE 33-1
Catheterizing the Female Urinary Bladder (Straight and Indwelling)

Equipment

Sterile catheterization kit that contains
  Sterile gloves
  Sterile drapes (one of which is fenestrated)
  Antiseptic solution
  Lubricant
  Cotton balls or gauze squares
  Forceps
  Straight or indwelling catheter (size must be appropriate for client)
  Prefilled syringe
  Basin (base of kit usually serves as this)
  Specimen container

Flashlight or lamp
Urine collection bag and drainage tubing (may be connected to sterile indwelling catheter if a closed drainage system is used)
Velcro leg strap or tape

Disposal bag
Waterproof pad or Chux

Action	Rationale
1 Assemble equipment. Wash your hands. Explain the procedure and its purpose to the client.	Organization facilitates performance of the task. Handwashing deters spread of microorganisms. An explanation encourages client cooperation and reduces apprehension.
2 Provide for good light. Artificial light is recommended (use of a flashlight requires an assistant to hold and position it).	Good lighting is necessary to see the meatus clearly.
3 Provide for privacy by closing the curtains or door.	The procedure may be embarrassing for the client.
4 Assist the client to the dorsal recumbent position with the knees flexed and the feet about 2 feet apart and drape the client. Or, if preferable, the client can be placed in the side-lying position as illustrated in Figure 33-7. Slide the waterproof drape under the client.	Good visualization of the meatus is important. Embarrassment, chilliness, and feeling tense can interfere with introducing the catheter. The client's comfort will promote relaxation. The drape will protect bed linens from moisture.
5 Cleanse the genital and perineal area with warm soap and water. Rinse and dry. Wash your hands again.	Clean technique decreases the possibility of introducing organisms into the bladder.
6 Prepare urine drainage set-up if indwelling catheter is to be inserted and separate urine collection system is used. Secure to bed frame according to manufacturer's directions.	This facilitates connection of the catheter to the drainage system and provides for easy access.
7 Open the sterile catheterization tray on overbed table using sterile technique.	Placement of equipment near the work site increases efficiency. Sterile technique protects the client and prevents the spread of microorganisms.

(Continued)

Action

8 Put on sterile gloves. Grasp the upper corners of the drape and unfold the drape without touching unsterile areas. Fold back a cuff over gloved hands. Ask the client to lift her buttocks and slide the sterile drape under her with gloves protected by cuff.

9 A fenestrated sterile drape may be placed over the perineal area exposing the labia.

10 Place the sterile tray on the drape between the client's thighs.

11 Open all supplies:

   a. *If the catheter is to be indwelling,* test the catheter balloon. Remove the protective cap on the tip of the syringe and attach the syringe prefilled with sterile water to injection port. Inject appropriate amount of fluid. If the balloon inflates properly, withdraw fluid and leave the syringe attached to the port.

   b. Pour antiseptic solution over cotton balls or gauze. Open the specimen container if specimen is to be obtained.

   c. Lubricate 1 to 2 inches of the catheter tip.

Rationale

The drape provides a sterile field close to the meatus. Covering the gloved hands will help keep the gloves sterile while placing the drape.

The drape expands the sterile field and protects against contamination. Use of a fenestrated drape may limit visualization and is considered optional by some practitioners.

This provides easy access to supplies.

A balloon that does not inflate or that leaks needs to be replaced prior to insertion in the client.

It is necessary to open all supplies and prepare for the procedure while both hands are sterile.

Lubrication facilitates the insertion of the catheter and reduces trauma to the tissues.

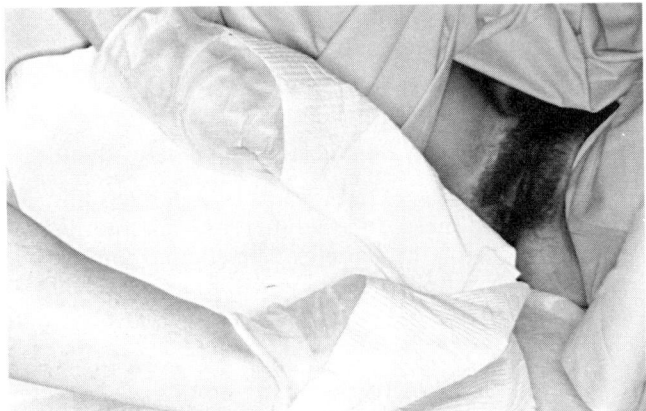

Step 8: Without touching unsterile areas, fold back a cuff over gloved hands.

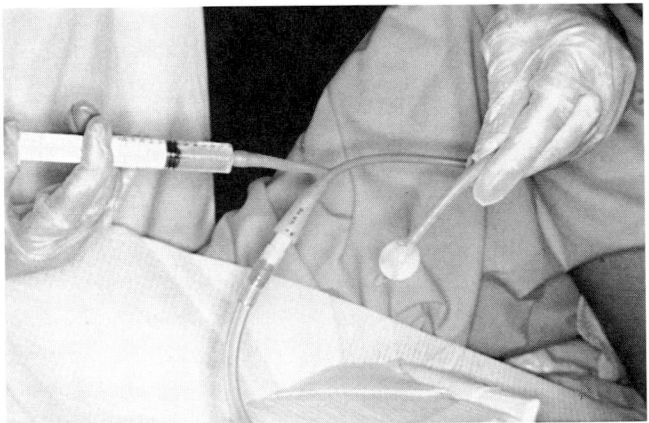

Step 11a: Test the balloon.

12 With the thumb and one finger of your nondominant hand, spread the labia and identify the meatus, as shown in figure. Be prepared to maintain separation of the labia with one hand until urine is flowing well and continuously.

Smoothing the area immediately surrounding the meatus helps to make it visible. Allowing the labia to drop back into position may contaminate the area around the meatus, as well as the catheter. Your nondominant hand is now contaminated.

(Continued)

Action

13 Using cotton balls held with forceps, cleanse both labial folds and then directly over the meatus. Move the cotton ball from above the meatus down toward the rectum. Discard each cotton ball after one downward stroke.

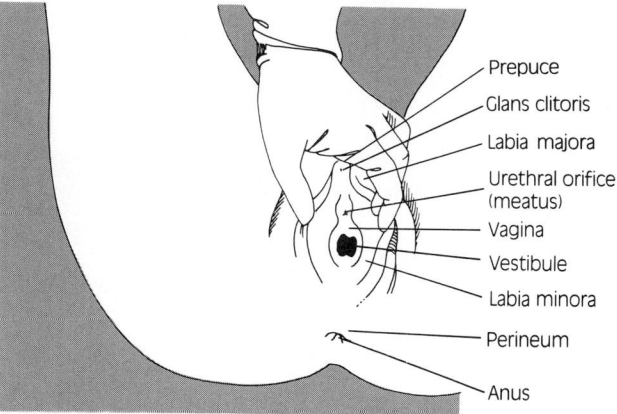

Step 12: With nondominant hand, spread the labia and identify the meatus.

14 With the uncontaminated gloved hand, place the drainage end of the catheter in the receptacle. *For insertion of an indwelling catheter* that is preattached to sterile tubing and drainage container (closed drainage system), position the catheter and set-up within easy reach on the sterile field.

15 Insert the catheter tip into the meatus 5 cm to 7.5 cm (2 to 3 inches) or until urine flows. Do not use force to push the catheter through the urethra into the bladder. Ask the client to breathe deeply, and rotate the catheter gently if slight resistance is met as the catheter reaches the external sphincter. *For an indwelling catheter,* once urine drains, advance the catheter another ½ to 1 inch.

16 Hold the catheter securely with the nondominant hand while the bladder empties. Collect a specimen if required. Continue drainage according to agency policy.

17 Remove the catheter smoothly and slowly if a straight catheterization was ordered.

18 *If the catheter is to be indwelling*

    a. Inflate the balloon according to the manufacturer's recommendations.

    b. Tug gently on the catheter after the balloon is inflated to feel resistance.

    c. Attach the catheter to the drainage system if necessary.

Rationale

Moving from an area where there is likely to be less contamination to an area where there is more contamination helps prevent the spread of organisms. Cleansing the meatus last helps reduce the possibility of introducing organisms into the bladder.

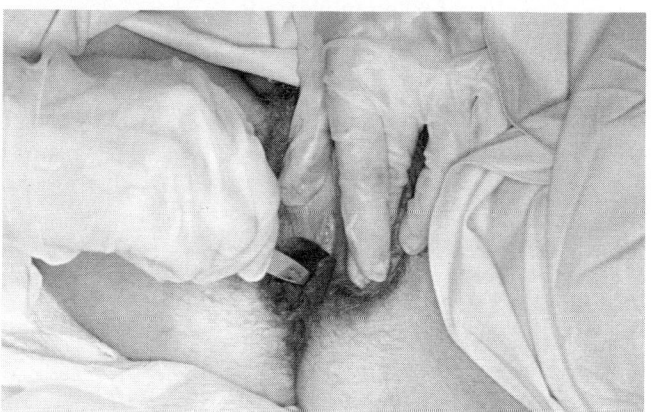

Step 13: Cleanse both labial folds and then directly over the meatus.

This facilitates drainage of urine and minimizes risk of contaminating sterile equipment.

The female urethra is about 3.7 cm to 6.2 cm (1½ to 2½ inches) long. Applying force on the catheter is likely to injure mucous membranes. The sphincter relaxes and the catheter can enter the bladder easily when the client relaxes. Advancing an indwelling catheter an additional ½ to 1 inch ensures placement in the bladder and facilitates inflation of the balloon without damaging the urethra.

Withdrawing and reinserting the catheter increase the chances of cotaminating it. In general, no more than 750 ml of urine should be removed at one time. Pelvic floor blood vessels may become engorged from the sudden release of pressure leading to possible hypotensive episode.

This causes less discomfort to the client.

The balloon anchors the catheter in place in the bladder. Sterile water is used to inflate the balloon as a precaution in case the balloon ruptured.

Improper inflation can cause client discomfort and malpositioning of catheter.

Closed drainage system minimizes the risk of organisms being introduced into the bladder.

(Continued)

Action

d. Secure to the upper thigh with a Velcro leg strap or tape. Leave some slack in the catheter to allow for leg movement.

e. Check that the drainage tubing is not kinked and that movement of side rails does not interfere with catheter or drainage bag.

Rationale

Proper attachment prevents trauma to the urethra and meatus from tension on the tubing.

This facilitates drainage of urine and prevents the backflow of urine.

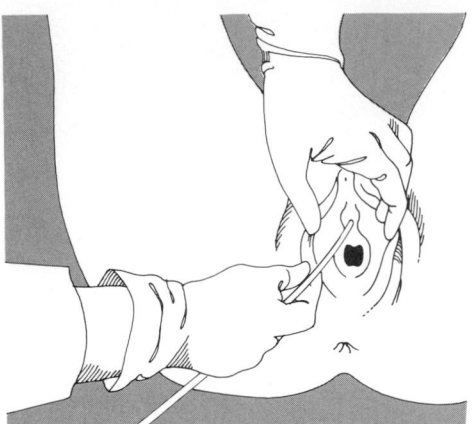

Step 15: With the uncontaminated gloved hand, insert the tip of the catheter into the meatus.

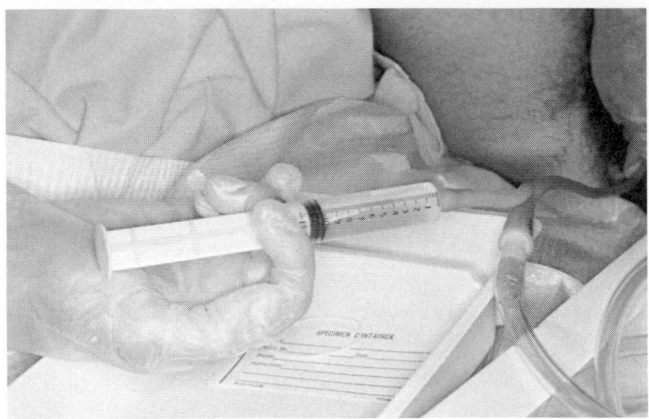

Step 18a: Injecting sterile water to inflate balloon.

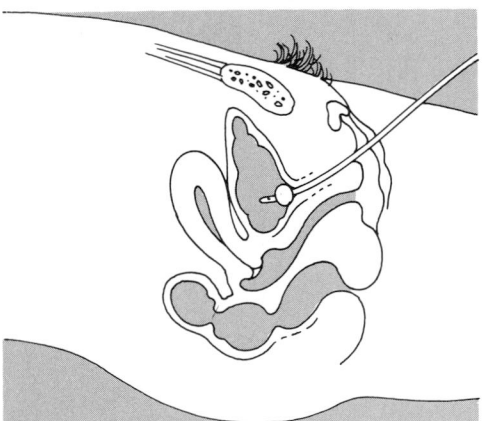

Step 18b: Tug gently on catheter after balloon is in place to feel resistance.

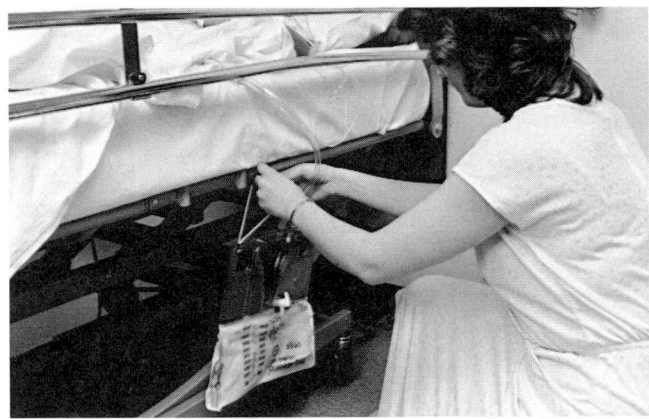

Step 18c: Attach drainage set to bed frame, checking that movement of the side rails will not interfere with catheter and drainage bag.

19 Remove the equipment and make the client comfortable in bed. Cleanse and dry the perineal area, if necessary. Care for the equipment according to agency policy. Send the urine specimen to the laboratory promptly or refrigerate it.

Urine kept at room temperature may cause organisms, if present, to grow and distort laboratory findings.

20 Wash your hands.

Handwashing deters the spread of microorganisms.

21 Record the time of the catheterization, the amount of the urine removed, a description of the urine, the client's reaction to the procedure, and your name.

A careful record is important for planning the client's care.

(Continued)

If the client is a child, the size of the catheter must be adapted accordingly.

Home Care Considerations

If self-catheterization must be performed in the home, clean technique is appropriate. The bladder's natural resistance to microorganisms normally found in the home makes sterile technique unnecessary. Rubber catheters must be washed thoroughly before boiling for 20 minutes. Dry and store properly for next usage.

- The bladder has defense mechanisms. It empties itself of urine regularly and maintains an acidic environment, which has antibacterial advantages. These help to maintain a sterile bladder under normal circumstances and also help in clearing an infection if it occurs.
- Pathogens introduced into the bladder can ascend the ureters and lead to bladder and kidney infection.
- A normal bladder is not as susceptible to infection as an injured one. A client's lowered resistance, present in many diseases and stressful situations, predisposes to urinary infection.

Reasons for Catheterization. The following are common reasons for performing a urinary catheterization:

- Relieve urinary retention
- Obtain a sterile urine specimen from a woman
- Measure the amount of residual urine in the bladder: The client is first asked to void and is then catheterized to determine how much urine stays in the bladder after normal voiding. An amount over 50 ml is considered abnormal.
- Obtain a urine specimen when a specimen cannot be secured satisfactorily by other means: Examples include collecting an uncontaminated specimen from a woman who is menstruating and from an incontinent client.
- Empty the bladder before, during, and after surgery and before certain diagnostic examinations.

Hazards of Catheterization. The hazards of introducing an instrument or a catheter into the bladder are sepsis and trauma. The male urethra is especially vulnerable to injury because of its length. An object forced through a stricture or an irregular opening from the wrong angle can cause serious damage to the urethra. While the urethra in the female is shorter than that in the male, it is also susceptible to damage if a catheter is forced through it. The mucous membrane lining the urethra is delicate and is easily damaged by the friction resulting from the insertion of a catheter. Bacteria can enter the bladder when the catheter is inserted. When the catheter is left in place, the organisms may also move up the catheter lumen or the space between the catheter and the urethral wall.

Equipment. The equipment used during a catheterization is generally prepackaged in a sterile, disposable tray. Most kits already contain a standard-size catheter. The trays used for catheterizing male and female clients are the same. Catheters are graded on the French scale according to the size of the lumen. For the female adult, No. 14 and No. 16 French catheters usually are used. Smaller catheters are generally not necessary, and the size of the lumen is so small that it increases the length of time necessary for emptying the bladder. Larger catheters distend the urethra and tend to increase the discomfort of the procedure. For the male adult, No. 18 and No. 20 French catheters usually are used, but if this appears to be too large, a smaller catheter should be used. No. 8 and No. 10 French catheters are commonly used for children.

An indwelling catheter has a balloon, which is inflated after the catheter is inserted into the bladder. There are several types of indwelling catheters available, but the principles on which they operate are similar.

The indwelling catheter has more than one lumen. In a double-lumen catheter, one lumen is connected directly with the balloon, which is distended with solution, and the other is the lumen through which the urine drains. The triple-lumen catheter provides an additional lumen for the instillation of irrigating solution. Figure 33-6 illustrates double-lumen, triple-lumen, and straight catheters.

Client Preparation. Prior to the catheterization, the client should be given an adequate explanation of the procedure and the reason for it. A catheter being inserted produces a sensation of pressure and some discomfort,

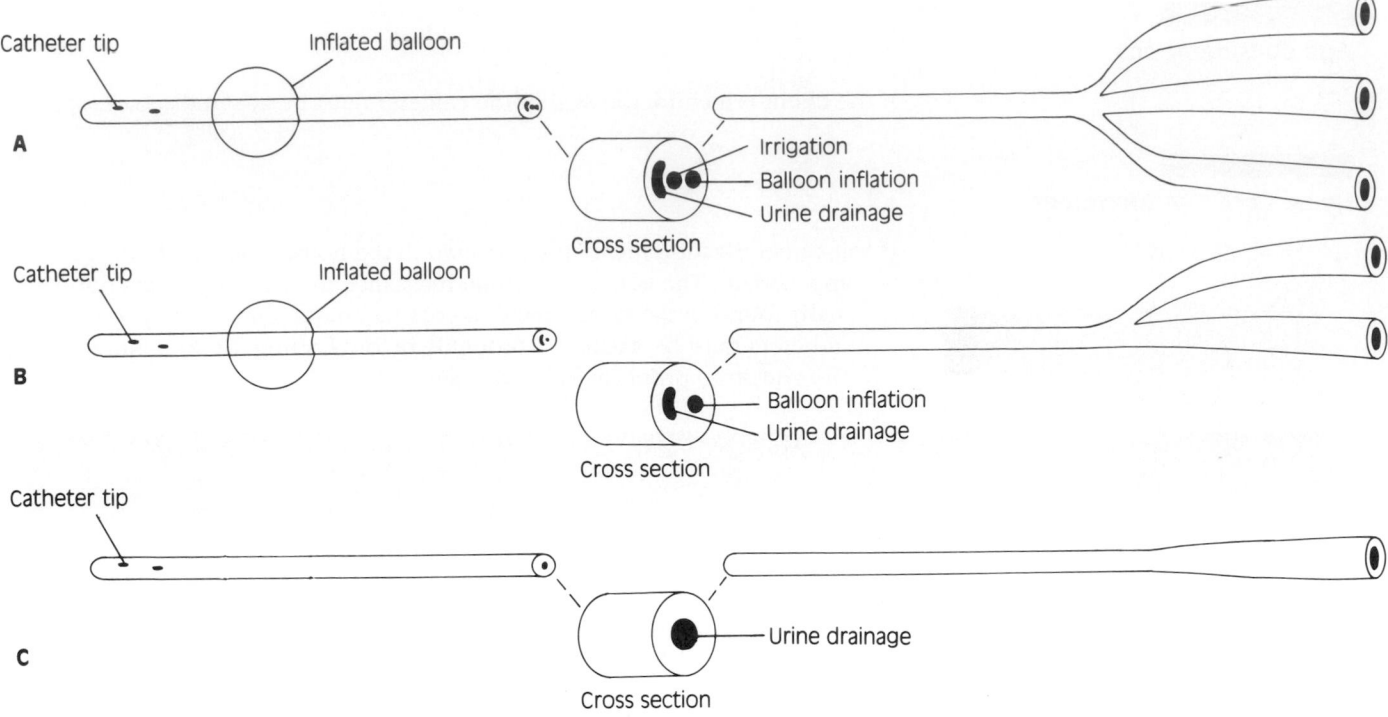

F I G U R E 33-6
(A) Triple-lumen indwelling catheter. (B) Double-lumen indwelling catheter. (C) Straight catheter.

and this should be explained to the client. In addition, the client should be assured that every measure to avoid exposure and embarrassment will be taken. The more relaxed the client can be, the easier it will be to insert the catheter.

The most frequent position for the client is the dorsal recumbent position, preferably on a solid surface, such as a firm mattress or a treatment table. Catheterizing a client in a bed with a soft mattress, especially for the female client, is not as satisfactory because the client's pelvic surfaces are not supported firmly, and visualization of the meatus is difficult. Also, the client may sink into the bed, causing the bladder to be lower than the outlet of the catheter. If the client is in bed; supporting the buttocks on a firm cushion is helpful.

The Sims or lateral position can be an alternate position for the female client. This position may allow for better visualization and make the client more comfortable, especially if hip and knee movements are difficult. A reduced area of exposure also can result in less psychic discomfort for the client. The client may lie on either side, depending on which position is easiest for the nurse and best in terms of the client's comfort. The client's buttocks are placed near the edge of the bed with her shoulders at the opposite edge and her knees drawn toward her chest. The nurse lifts the upper buttock and labia to expose the urinary meatus. This positioning is illustrated in Figure 33-7.

Procedure.   Catheterization of the urinary bladder for female and male clients is described in Procedures 33-1 and 33-2. Techniques of surgical asepsis are of ex-

traordinary importance when catheterizing a client to help prevent urinary tract infection.

Indwelling Catheters

Inserting and Connecting to the Drainage System. The procedure for inserting an indwelling catheter is the same as for inserting a straight, single-lumen catheter with the following differences:

- Inflate the balloon with the prefilled syringe before inserting the catheter to check for balloon patency. Aspirate the fluid back into the syringe when it is determined that the balloon is patent.
- Hold the catheter with one hand, and inflate the balloon, according to the manufacturer's instructions, as soon as the catheter is in the bladder and urine has begun to drain from the bladder. Usually 4 ml to 5 ml *more* sterile water than the size of the balloon is used. This additional water remains in the tube leading to the balloon.
- If the client complains of pain after the balloon is inflated, allow it to empty and replace the catheter with another one. The balloon is probably located in the urethra and is causing discomfort owing to distention of the urethra.

Technique to Complete Closed Urinary Drainage System.   The following techniques are used to complete the closed urinary drainage system:

- Check to see that the drainage tubing is not kinked. Do not place it under a part of the leg, where it may be compressed. Also, do not place it

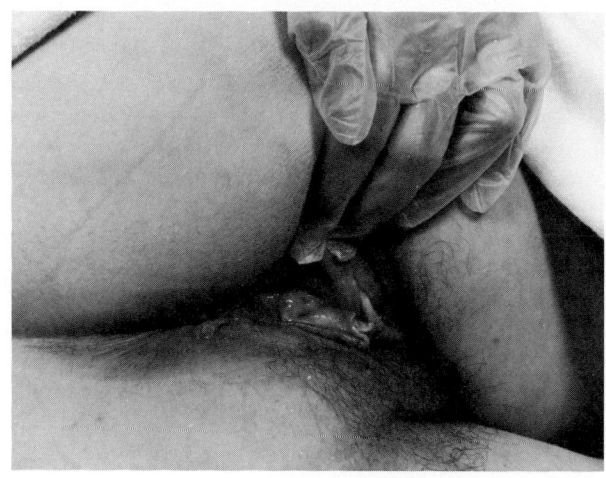

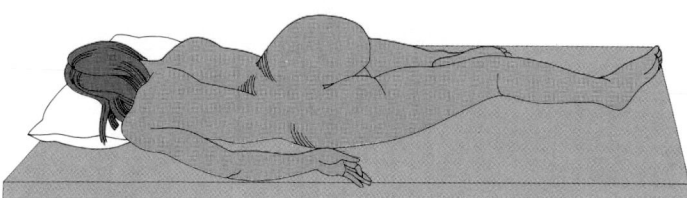

FIGURE 33-7
The side-lying position and how to expose the urinary meatus when catheterizing a female patient.

in a manner so that it moves above the level of the bladder. This may cause the client's bladder to drain by suction rather than by gravity, risking injury to the bladder mucosa.

- Pin the drainage tubing to the bottom bed linen to help hold the drainage tube in the proper place while the client is in bed. This helps prevent pooling of urine in the drainage tubing.
- Keep the drainage bag off the floor at all times to reduce the risk of infection. The floor is grossly contaminated!

Irrigating the Indwelling Catheter. The flushing of a tube, canal, or area with solution is called **irrigation**. The purpose of a catheter irrigation is to restore or maintain its patency. Procedures 33-3 and 33-4 describe how to irrigate an indwelling catheter.

Occasionally, continuous or frequent irrigations are ordered when blood clots or other debris threaten to block the catheter. In the past, the procedure was done

routinely for almost all indwelling catheters, but because this is another means of introducing pathogens, it is now recommended that an irrigation should be done only when there is a demonstrated need. "Natural" irrigation of the catheter through an increased fluid intake by the client is the preferred technique.

Preferably, the client who needs frequent irrigation in order that the catheter and tubing remain patent will have a triple-lumen catheter with continuous irrigation (Procedure 33-5).

Caring for the Client. The following are nursing measures used when caring for a client with an indwelling catheter:

- Be sure to wash hands before and after caring for a client with an indwelling catheter.
- Clean the perineal area thoroughly, especially around the meatus, twice a day and after each bowel movement.
- Use soap or detergent and water to clean the perineal area, and rinse the area well. Do not use powders and lotions after cleaning. Some authorities recommend cleaning the area around the meatus with an antiseptic, for example, povidone-iodine (Betadine).
- Apply a topical antibiotic ointment at the meatus, as ordered.
- Make sure that the client maintains a generous fluid intake. This helps prevent infection and irrigates the catheter naturally by increasing urinary output.
- Encourage the client to be up and about, as ordered.
- Note the volume and character of urine, and record observations carefully. The urine can be observed through the drainage tubing and in the collecting container. The usual procedure is to note and record the amount of urine every 8 hours on the client's intake-and-output record. The collecting container is calibrated. However, the volume markings are usually only approximations. The urine should be emptied into a graduated container that is accurately calibrated for correct determination of output.
- Do not open the drainage system to obtain urine specimens or to measure urine. If the tubing becomes disconnected, wipe the ends of both tubes with antiseptic solution before reconnecting. When emptying the drainage bag, make sure the drainage spout does not touch a contaminated surface.
- Teach the client the importance of personal hygiene, especially the importance of careful cleaning after having a bowel movement and thorough washing of hands frequently.
- Report any signs of infection promptly. These include a burning sensation and irritation at the meatus, cloudy urine, a strong odor to the urine, an elevated temperature, and chills.
- Help keep the urine acid in character since acidity retards bacterial growth. Plain water in increased

(Text continues on p. 882.)

PROCEDURE 33-2
Catheterizing the Male Urinary Bladder (Straight and Indwelling)

Equipment

Sterile catheterization kit that contains
Sterile gloves
Sterile drapes (one of which is fenestrated)
Antiseptic solution
Lubricant
Cotton balls or gauze squares
Forceps
Straight or indwelling catheter
Prefilled syringe
Basin (base of kit usually serves as this)
Specimen container

Flashlight or lamp
Urine collection bag and drainage tubing (may be connected to sterile indwelling catheter if a closed drainage system is used)
Velcro leg strap or tape

Disposal bag
Waterproof pad or Chux

Action

1 Assemble the equipment and follow Steps 1 through 3 for female catheterization in Procedure 33-1.

2 Position the client on his back with the thighs slightly apart. Drape the client so that only the area around the penis is exposed.

3 Follow Steps 5 to 7 for female catheterization in Procedure 33-1.

Rationale

This prevents unnecessary exposure.

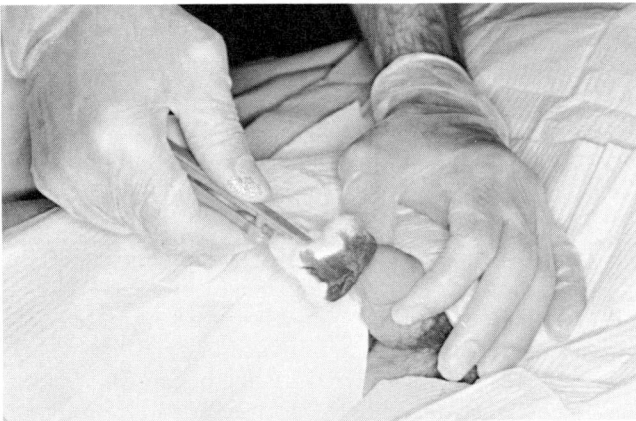

Step 3: Cleanse the area of the meatus.

4 Put on sterile gloves. Open the sterile drape and place on the client's thighs. Place the fenestrated drape with the opening over the penis.

This maintains a sterile working area.

(Continued)

Action	**Rationale**

5 Place the catheter set on or next to the client's legs on the sterile drape.

The sterile set-up should be arranged so that the nurse's back is not turned to it, nor should it be out of the nurse's range of vision.

6 Open all supplies:

a. *If the catheter is to be indwelling,* test the catheter balloon. Remove the protective cap on the tip of the syringe and attach the syringe prefilled with sterile water to the injection port. Inject appropriate amount of fluid. If balloon inflates properly, withdraw fluid and leave syringe attached to port.

A balloon that does not inflate or that leaks must be replaced prior to insertion in the client.

b. Pour antiseptic solution over cotton balls or gauze. Open the specimen container if specimen is to be obtained.

It is necessary to open all supplies and prepare for the procedure while both hands are sterile.

7 *Generously* lubricate the catheter for about 15 cm to 18 cm (6 to 7 inches).

Generous lubrication is especially important because of the length and tortuousness of the male urethra. The lubricant decreases friction.

8 Lift the penis with your nondominant hand, which is then considered contaminated. Retract the foreskin in the uncircumcised male client. Cleanse the area at the meatus with a cotton ball held with a forceps. Use a circular motion, moving from the meatus toward the base of the penis for three cleansings.

The hand touching the penis becomes contaminated. Cleansing the area around the meatus and under the foreskin in the uncircumcised male client helps prevent infection. Moving from the meatus toward the base of the penis prevents bringing organisms to the meatus.

9 Hold the penis with slight upward tension and perpendicular to the client's body. Ask the client to bear down as if voiding. With your dominant hand, place the drainage end of the catheter in the receptacle. *For insertion of an indwelling catheter* that is preattached to sterile tubing and drainage container (closed drainage system), position the catheter and set-up within easy reach on the sterile field.

Holding the penis up with slight traction helps straighten the urethra.

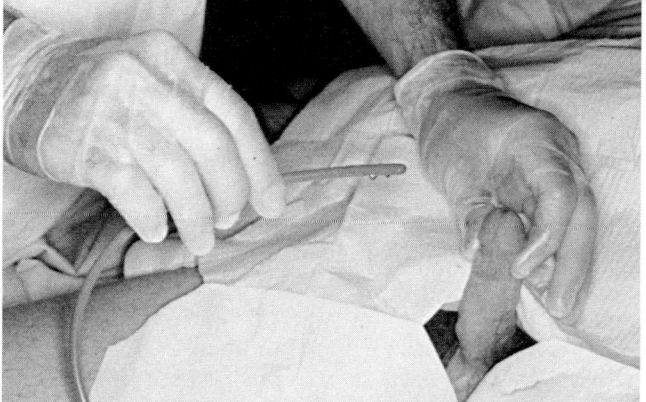

Step 9: Preparing to insert the catheter.

(Continued)

Action

10 Insert the tip into the meatus. Advance the catheter 15 cm to 20 cm (6 to 8 inches) or until urine flows. Do not use force to introduce the catheter. If the catheter resists entry, ask the client to breathe deeply and rotate the catheter slightly. *For an indwelling catheter,* once urine drains, advance the catheter another ½ to 1 inch. Lower the penis.

11 Follow Steps 16 through 21 for female catheterization in Procedure 33-1 except that the catheter may be secured to the upper thigh or lower abdomen with the penis directed toward the client's chest. Slack should be left in the catheter to prevent tension.

Rationale

The male urethra is about 20 cm long. Deep breaths or slight twisting of the catheter may ease the catheter past resistance at the sphincters. Advancing an indwelling catheter an additional ½ to 1 inch ensures its placement in the bladder and facilitates inflation of the balloon without damaging the urethra.

This is done to prevent irritation at the angle of the penis and scrotum.

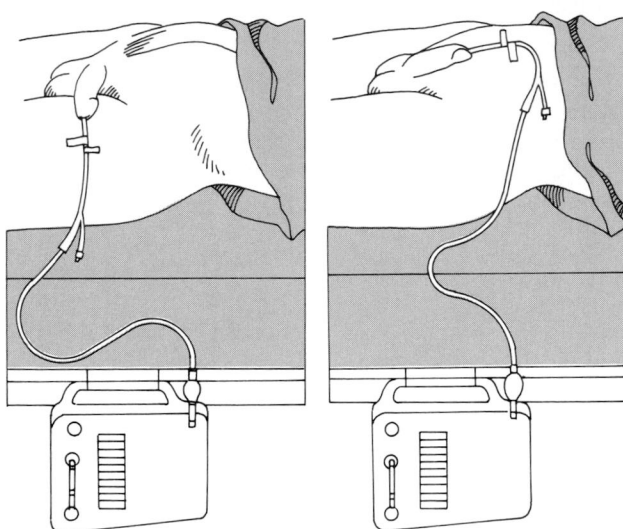

Step 11: Secure the catheter to the upper thigh or lower abdomen, allowing slack to prevent tension.

Age Considerations

If the client is a child, the size of the catheter must be adapted accordingly.

Home Care Considerations

If self-catheterization must be performed in the home, clean technique is appropriate. The bladder's natural resistance to microorganisms normally found in the home makes sterile technique unnecessary. Rubber catheters must be washed thoroughly before boiling for 20 minutes. Dry and store properly for next usage.

PROCEDURE 33-3
Irrigating the Catheter Using the Closed System

Equipment

Sterile basin or container

Gauze squares or cotton balls with disinfectant or alcohol swabs

Waterproof drape

30-ml to 50-ml syringe with 18-gauge or 19-gauge needle

Sterile irrigating solution (at room temperature or warmed to body temperature)

Bath blanket

Action

1 Assemble equipment. Wash your hands. Explain the procedure and its purpose to the client.

2 Provide for privacy by closing the curtains or door and draping the client with the bath blanket.

3 Assist the client to a comfortable position and expose the aspiration port on the catheter set-up. Place the waterproof drape under the catheter and aspiration port.

4 Open the sterile supplies. Pour sterile solution into the sterile basin. Aspirate irrigant (30 ml to 50 ml) into the sterile syringe and attach the capped sterile needle.

5 Disinfect the aspiration port with alcohol swabs or gauze square with antiseptic solution.

6 Clamp or fold the catheter tubing distal to the aspiration port.

7 Remove the cap and insert the needle into the port. Gently instill solution into the catheter.

8 Remove the needle from the port. Unclamp the tubing and allow irrigant and urine to drain. Repeat the procedure as necessary.

9 Assess the client's response to the procedure and the quality and amount of drainage. Document on the client's chart.

10 Record the amount of irrigant used on the intake and output record. Subtract this from the urinary output when totaled.

11 Remove equipment and discard uncapped needle and syringe in appropriate receptacle. Wash your hands. Make client comfortable.

Rationale

Organization facilitates performance of task. Handwashing deters spread of microorganisms. An explanation encourages client cooperation and reduces apprehension.

The procedure may be embarrassing for the client.

This provides for adequate visualization. The drape protects the client and the bed from leakage.

This prevents the spread of microorganisms.

This prevents the spread of microorganisms.

This directs the irrigating solution into the bladder.

Gentle irrigation prevents damage to the lining of the bladder.

Gravity aids drainage of urine and irrigant from the bladder.

This provides accurate documentation of the procedure.

Subtracting irrigant total from drainage in urine collection bag provides accurate recording of urine output.

Handwashing deters the spread of microorganisms. Proper disposal of needle prevents the nurse accidentally puncturing self.

PROCEDURE 33-4
Irrigating the Catheter Using the Open System

Equipment

Sterile irrigation tray
with
  Sterile container
    and basin
  Sterile Asepto or
    Toomey syringe
Disposable gloves
  (optional)

Gauze squares or
  cotton balls with
  disinfectant or
  alcohol swabs
Sterile irrigating so-
  lution (at room
  temperature or
  warmed to body
  temperature)

Bath blanket
Sterile cover for tip
  of drainage tub-
  ing

Action	**Rationale**
1 Follow steps as 1 and 2 in Procedure 33-3.	
2 Assist the client to a comfortable position and expose the connection between the catheter and the drainage tubing. Position a waterproof drape under the catheter.	This provides for adequate visualization. The drape protects the client and the bed from leakage.
3 Open the sterile supplies. Pour sterile solution into the sterile container. Remove the tip from the Asepto syringe and aspirate irrigant (30 ml) into the syringe.	This prevents the spread of microorganisms.
4 Cleanse the catheter junction with a gauze pad and disinfectant or alcohol swab.	This prevents the spread of microorganisms into bladder tissue.

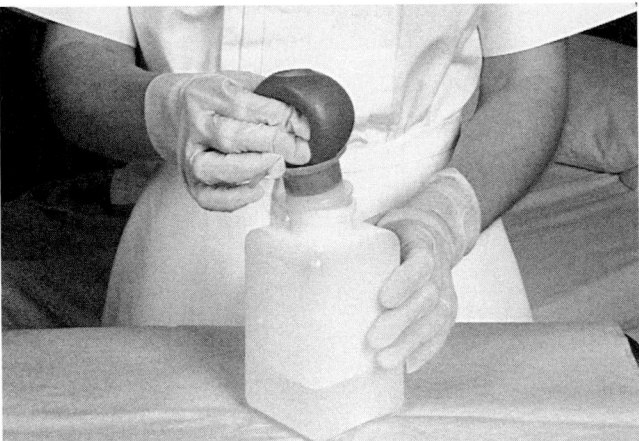

Step 3: Aspirating irrigant into syringe.

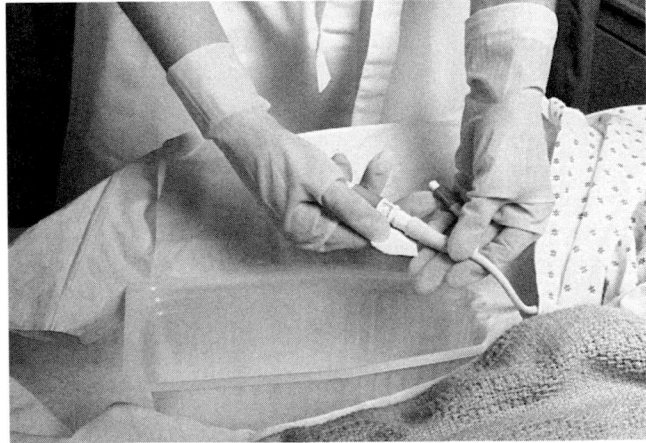

Step 4: Disinfecting the aspiration port.

5 Disconnect the catheter and drainage tube. Place the sterile cover over the drainage tip and secure drainage tubing on the bed. Hold catheter tubing 2.5 cm (1 inch) from its open end.	This avoids contaminating the sterile drainage system with microorganisms.
6 Position the sterile basin beneath the catheter. Insert the tip of the Asepto syringe into the catheter and gently irrigate with solution.	Gentle irrigation is less traumatic to the lining of the bladder.

(Continued)

Action	**Rationale**

7 Remove the syringe, keeping the bulb compressed, and allow drainage to return by gravity flow into the basin. If there is no return, gently aspirate the solution from the catheter. Continue with irrigation as ordered by the physician.

Gravity aids the drainage of urine and irrigant from the bladder. Irrigation maintains patency of the urinary drainage system.

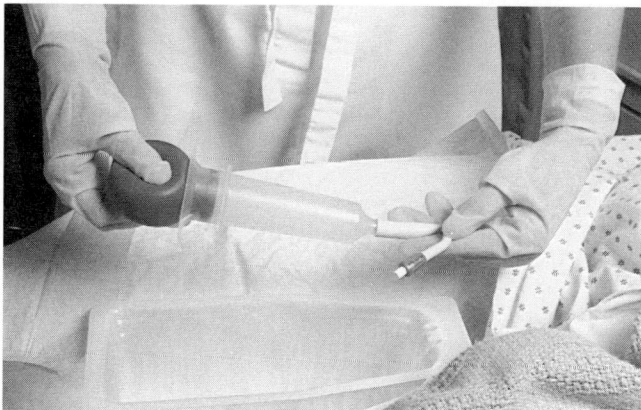

Step 6: Gently instilling solution.

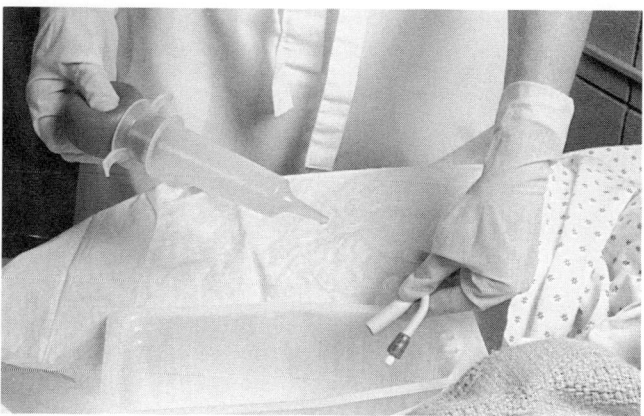

Step 7: Remove syringe keeping bulb compressed and allow drainage to return via gravity flow into basin.

8 Reattach the drainage tube to the catheter, being careful not to contaminate the system. Secure with tape or a Velcro leg strap.

This prevents entry of microorganisms. The tape or the Velcro leg strap discourages separation of the catheter and the tubing.

9 Document the client's response to the procedure and the quality and amount of drainage on the client's chart.

This provides accurate documentation of the procedure.

10 Remove the equipment and make the client comfortable. Wash your hands.

Handwashing deters the spread of microorganisms.

P R O C E D U R E   33-5
Giving Continuous Bladder Irrigation

Equipment

Sterile irrigating solution (at room temperature or warmed to body temperature), usually 2000-ml size bags	Sterile tubing with drip chamber and clamp for connection to irrigating solution	IV pole Three-way Foley catheter in place in client's bladder	Foley drainage set-up (tubing and collection bag) Bath blanket

(Continued)

Action

1 Explain the procedure and its purpose to the client.

2 Assemble the equipment.

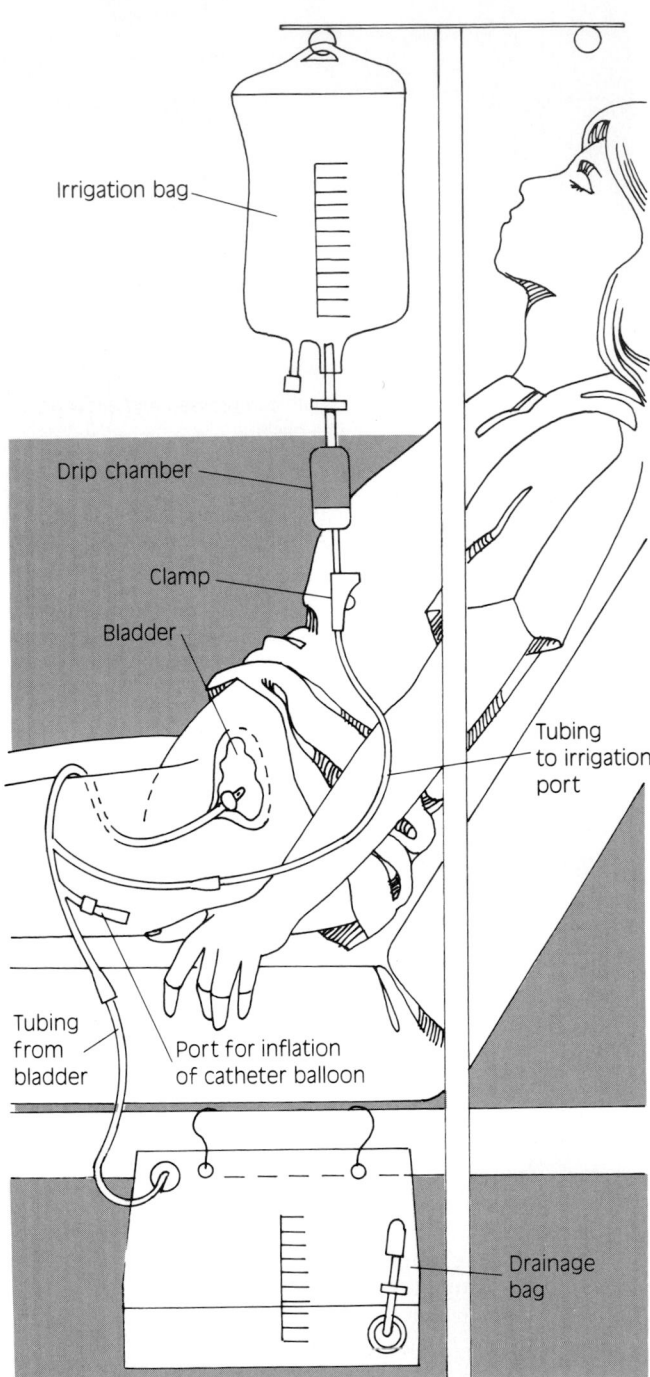

Irrigation bag

Drip chamber

Clamp

Bladder

Tubing to irrigation port

Tubing from bladder

Port for inflation of catheter balloon

Drainage bag

Continuous irrigation.

3 Wash your hands.

Rationale

An explanation encourages client cooperation and reduces apprehension.

Organization facilitates performance of tasks.

Handwashing deters the spread of microorganisms.

(Continued)

Action	Rationale

Action

4 Provide for privacy by closing the curtains or door and draping the client with the bath blanket.

5 Prepare the sterile irrigation bag for use as directed by the manufacturer. Secure the clamp and attach the sterile tubing with drip chamber to the container. Hang the bag on IV pole 2½ to 3 feet above the level of the client's bladder. Release the clamp and remove the protective cover on the end of the tubing without contaminating it. Allow the solution to flush the tubing and remove air. Reclamp.

Rationale

The procedure may be embarrassing for the client.

Irrigation solution continuously bathes the lining of the bladder and keeps the catheter patent. Flushing the tubing prior to irrigation clears air from the tubing that might cause bladder distention.

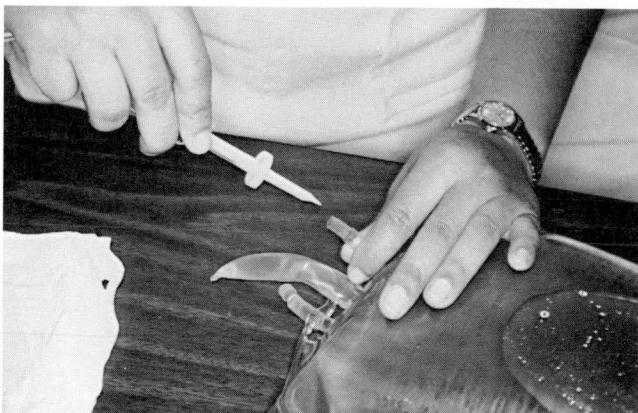

Step 5: Attach sterile tubing with drip chamber to container of irrigation solution.

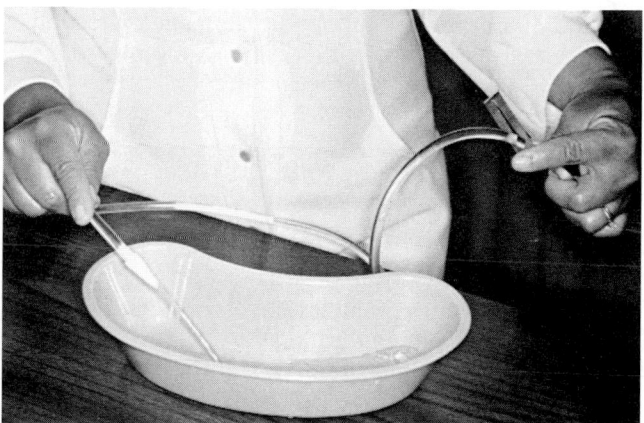

Step 5: Allow solution to flush tubing and remove air.

6 Using sterile technique, attach the irrigation tubing to the irrigation port of the three-way Foley catheter. If a closed system is used, tubing may already be connected to the irrigation port on the catheter.

Sterile technique prevents the spread of microorganisms into the bladder.

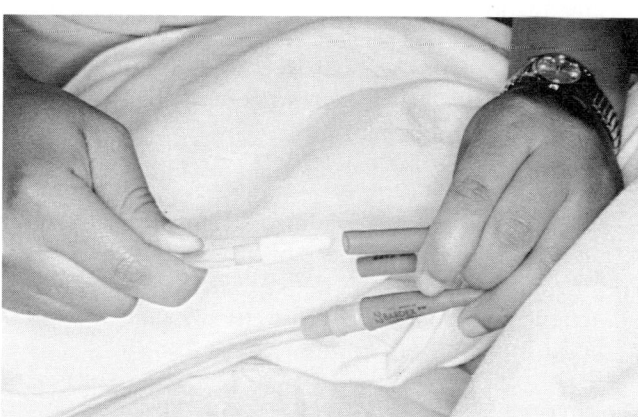

Step 6: Using sterile technique, attach irrigation tubing to irrigation port of three-way Foley catheter.

7 Release the clamp on the irrigation tubing and regulate the flow according to the physician's order.

This allows for continual gentle irrigation without causing discomfort to the client.

(Continued)

Action	**Rationale**
8 As irrigation is completed, clamp the tubing. Do not allow the drip chamber to empty. Disconnect the empty bag and attach a full irrigation bag. Continue as ordered by the physician.	This eliminates the need to separate tubing from the catheter and clear air from the tubing. Opening the drainage system provides access for introduction of microorganisms.
9 Assess the client's response to the procedure and the quality and amount of drainage. Document on the client's chart.	This provides accurate documentation of the procedure.
10 Record the amount of irrigant used on the intake and output record. Empty the drainage collection bag as each new container is hung and record.	This ensures accurate recording of urine output.
11 Wash your hands.	Handwashing deters the spread of microorganisms.

amounts, cranberry juice, and ascorbic acid are helpful in acidifying urine.

• Help the client take a tub or shower bath when permitted. The catheter should be clamped temporarily if the collecting container is higher than the bladder at any time. In a tub, with the catheter clamped, the container can be hung over the side of the tub. Care should be taken so that the catheter does not remain clamped after the bath. In a shower, the container can be attached to the client's leg, in which case clamping the tube is usually unnecessary.

• Plan to change indwelling catheters only as necessary. If rolling the drainage tubing between the hands frees the tubing of sandy particles, it is time to change the catheter. The usual length of time between catheter changes varies and can be anywhere from 5 days to 2 weeks. The less often a catheter is changed, the less the likelihood that an infection will develop.

Teaching Clients.   Clients who have indwelling catheters should be taught how the system functions and how they can assist with their care. Teaching points include keeping the tubing free of kinks, maintaining a constant downward flow of the urine, maintaining an adequate fluid intake, and reporting promptly if any unusual symptoms develop.

Removing the Indwelling Catheter.   The indwelling catheter and the aftercare of the client should include the following nursing measures:

• Be sure the balloon is deflated before attempting to remove the catheter! This is done by inserting a syringe into the balloon valve and aspirating the fluid initially used to inflate the balloon. Carefully check the size of the balloon so you know how much fluid to remove before proceeding. Do *not* cut the tubing with scissors.

• Have the client take several deep breaths to relax while gently removing the catheter. Wrap the catheter in a towel or disposable, waterproof drape.

• Clean the area at the meatus thoroughly with antiseptic swabs after the catheter is removed.

• See to it that the client's fluid intake is generous, and record the client's intake and output. Instruct the client to void into the bedpan or urinal.

• Inform the client that it may take a little while for the bladder to reestablish voluntary control and that an "accident" is not unusual.

• Tell the client there may be a slight burning sensation the first time or two the client voids after the catheter is removed.

• Observe the urine carefully for any signs of abnormality.

• Record and report any unusual signs, such as discomfort, a burning sensation when voiding, bleeding, and changes in vital signs, especially the client's temperature. Be alert to any signs of infection, and report them *promptly.*

Teaching Self-Catheterization

Medical asepsis practices are used by persons who self-catheterize. There is less danger of nosocomial urinary tract infection when the procedure is done at home rather than in a hospital. Research has shown that the technique is safe. The procedure for self-catheterization is essentially the same as the one the nurse uses to catheterize a client. The following are some differences, which should be emphasized when teaching self-catheterization.

- The client voids first and then inserts the catheter for residual urine.
- The male client uses either a standing or sitting position. The female client sits on a toilet.
- A good light is important, especially for the female client.
- The female client can locate the meatus more easily with the use of a mirror.
- The client should press down with the abdominal muscles to remove as much urine from the bladder as possible before removing the catheter.
- The time interval between catheterizations will vary. At first, every 2 or 3 hours may be necessary, but the time interval can gradually be increased.
- The client must wash reusable equipment well in soap or detergent and water, and rinse, dry, and store it in a clean, covered container.
- A minimum of 1500 ml of fluid a day is recommended for adults.

Applying a Condom Catheter

When voluntary control of urination is not possible for male clients, an alternative to an indwelling Foley catheter is the **condom catheter**. This is a soft and pliable plastic or rubberized material device that is applied externally to the penis. It is connected to tubing and a leg bag during the day and a drainage bag at night and thus allows the person to be dressed and to participate in activities without problem. Instructions for applying a condom catheter are given in Procedure 33-6.

Nursing care includes vigilant skin care to prevent excoriation. The condom should be removed daily and the penis washed with soap and water, carefully dried, and inspected for irritation. The manufacturer's instructions for applying the condom should be followed because there are several variations. In all cases, care must be taken to fasten the condom securely enough to prevent leakage yet not so tightly as to constrict the blood vessels in the area. The tip of the tubing should be kept 2.5 cm to 5 cm beyond the tip of the penis to prevent irritation to the sensitive glans. Maintaining free urinary drainage is another nursing priority as tubing may become kinked. To prevent urine from excoriating the glans, the tubing collecting urine from the condom should be positioned to draw urine away from the penis.

Assisting with Urinary Diversions

Obstructions or malignancies in the urinary tract may require some persons to have the urinary flow diverted surgically. They may have an abdominal opening for urinary excretion, such as the **ileal conduit**, a connection of the ureters to the ileum with a stoma on the abdominal wall. Figure 33-8 is a schematic drawing of an ileal conduit. A **stoma** is an artificial opening for waste excretion located on the body surface. Other types of surgery for urinary diversion are also performed, and except for the

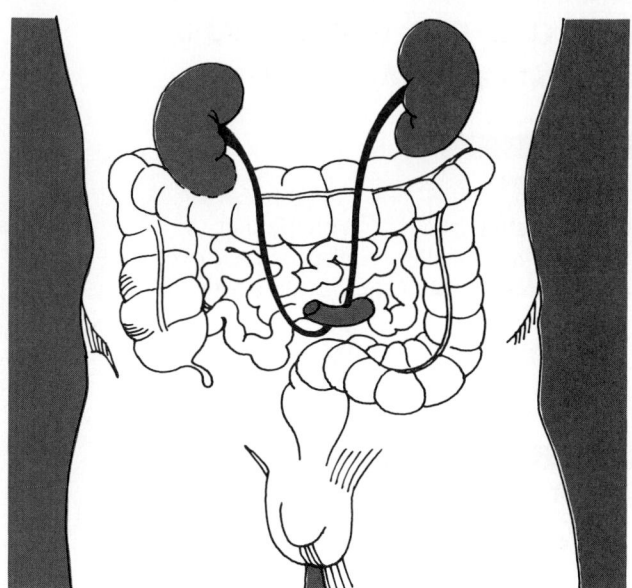

FIGURE 33-8
Location of an ileal conduit. Note that the ureters are brought to the ileum of the small intestine and a stoma is made where the urine is excreted. (Redrawn after Types of Ostomies. Copyright © 1979, Hollister Incorporated. All rights reserved)

location of the stoma, the nursing care is similar. Such diversions are generally permanent, and the person wears an external appliance to collect the urine since voluntary control over elimination of the urine from the stoma is not possible.

The person who has an ileal conduit must adapt to an altered body image and generally needs assistance in coping. The time required for adaptation varies, and the adjustment can often be promoted by numerous sources of support, such as family, friends, nurses, physicians, and persons with a similar health problem. Most of all, the person needs to understand that an active, useful life is compatible with a urinary diversion.

Appliances to Collect Urine. Typically, the external appliance is a soft, rubber or plastic pouch, either reusable or disposable. The upper part of the pouch generally has a firm faceplate, several inches in diameter, which has an opening the size of the stoma. Some faceplates are detachable from the pouch, others are not. The plate surface is firmly secured around the stoma opening with a moisture-proof adherent so that no urine leakage can occur. Many persons also use an elasticized belt worn around the waist for added support. The lower end of the pouch may have a drainage valve, which is used for emptying the pouch.

The pouch should be emptied before it becomes heavy with the weight of urine and causes the seal to loosen. This means emptying the appliance several times a day for most persons. Urine-collection receptacles designed to be placed under the bed are available for attachment to the appliance at night.

(Text continues on p. 887.)

PROCEDURE 33-6
Applying a Condom Catheter

Equipment

Condom sheath in appropriate size
Basin of warm water and soap
Washcloth and towel

Bath blanket
Disposable gloves (optional)

Elastic strip or Velcro strap
Reusable leg bag with drainage tubing or urinary drainage set-up

Action

1 Explain the procedure to the client.

2 Assemble the equipment. Prepare urinary drainage set-up or reusable leg bag for attachment to the condom sheath.

Rationale

This provides reassurance and promotes client cooperation.

This provides for an organized approach to the task.

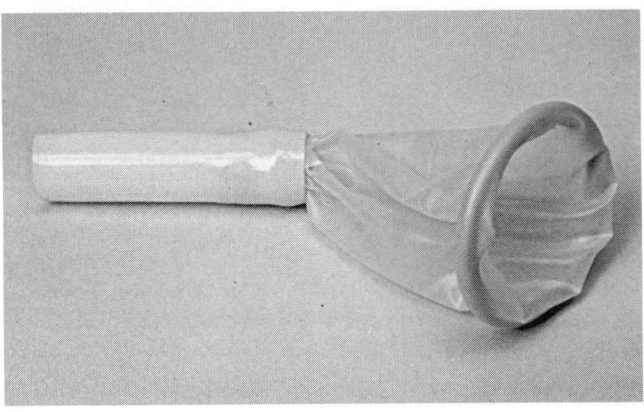

Condom sheath.

3 Wash your hands.

4 Assist the client to the supine position. Close the curtain or door. Use the bath blanket and sheet to expose only the client's genital area.

5 Don disposable gloves. Wash the genital area with soap and water, rinse, and dry thoroughly.

6 Roll the condom sheath outward onto itself. Grasp the penis firmly with your nondominant hand. Apply the condom sheath by rolling it onto the penis with your dominant hand. Leave 2.5-cm to 5-cm (1 to 2 inches) space between the tip of the penis and the end of the condom sheath.

7 Apply the elastic or Velcro strap in a snug but not tight manner. Do not allow the elastic or Velcro to come in contact with the skin.

8 Connect the condom sheath to the drainage set-up. Avoid kinking or twisting of the drainage tubing.

Handwashing deters the spread of microorganisms.

This provides privacy for the client.

Washing removes urine, secretions, and microorganisms. The penis must be clean and dry to minimize skin irritation.

Rolling the condom sheath outward allows for easier application. The space prevents irritation to the tip of the penis and allows for free drainage of urine.

The elastic or Velcro strap should secure the condom sheath but not interfere with blood circulation to the penis.

The collection device keeps the client dry. Kinked tubing encourages backflow of urine.

(Continued)

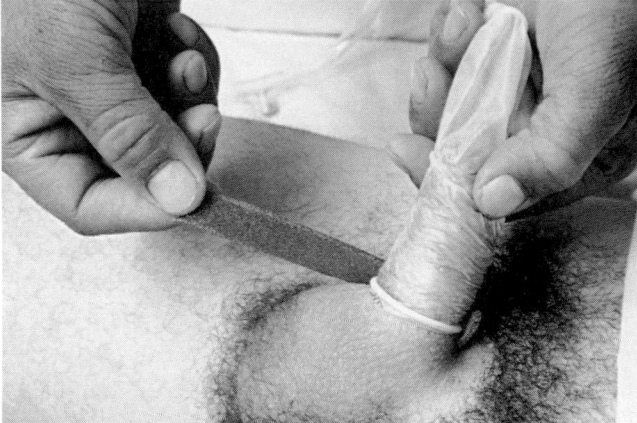

Step 7: Application of a Velcro strap at the base of the condom sheath.

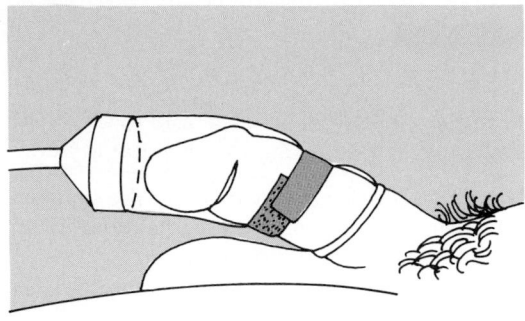

Step 8: Drawing of extra space at end of sheath and smoothing tubing to drainage unit.

9 Remove the equipment. Place the client in a comfortable, safe position. Wash your hands.

This provides a safe, comfortable setting for the client. Handwashing deters the spread of microorganisms.

10 Assess the client's response and record observations on the client's chart.

This provides accurate documentation and observation of urinary output.

PROCEDURE 33-7
Changing a Stoma Appliance on an Ileal Conduit

Equipment

Basin with warm water, soap, towel, washcloth or cotton balls	Sterile 2 × 2 gauze squares	Ostomy belt (optional)
Graduated container	Ostomy bag cut to the correct stomal size (with adhesive-backed faceplate, if available)	Adhesive cement (optional for reusable pouches)
Skin protectant or barrier		

Action

Rationale

1 Explain the procedure and encourage the client to observe or participate if possible. Provide for privacy.

Observing or assisting with procedure encourages self-acceptance.

2 Assemble the equipment.

Organization facilitates performance of task.

3 Wash your hands.

Handwashing deters the spread of microorganisms.

(Continued)

Action

Rationale

4 Have the client sit or stand if able to assist with procedure or assume supine position in bed.

These positions result in less abdominal folds and facilitate removal and application of the device.

5 Empty the pouch being worn into the graduated container (before removing if it is reusable and not attached to straight drainage).

Having the pouch empty before handling it reduces the likelihood of spilling the excretions. The physician may have ordered recording of intake and output.

6 Remove the pouch faceplate from the skin very gently.

The seal between the surface of the faceplate and the skin must be broken before the faceplate can be removed. Harsh handling of the appliance can cause damage to the skin and impair the development of a secure seal in the future.

7 Discard the pouch appropriately if disposable or wash reusable pouch in luke-warm soap and water and allow to air dry.

Thorough cleaning and airing of the appliance reduce odor and deterioration. For aesthetic and infection-control purposes, used appliances should be discarded appropriately.

8 Cleanse the skin around the stoma with soap and water or a commercial cleaner using washcloth or cotton balls. Make sure that you remove all of old adhesive from the skin.

Cleaning the skin removes excretions and old adhesive and skin protectant. Excretions or a build-up of other substances can cause irritation and damage to the skin.

9 Pat dry gently. Make sure the skin around the stoma is thoroughly dry. Assess the stoma and the condition of the surrounding skin.

Careful drying prevents trauma to the skin and stoma. An intact, properly applied urinary collection device protects skin integrity. Any change in the color and size of the stoma may indicate circulatory problems.

10 Place a gauze square or two over the stoma opening.

Continuous drainage must be absorbed to keep the skin dry during the appliance change.

11 Apply a skin protectant to a 2-inch radius around the stoma, and allow it to dry completely, which takes about 30 seconds.

The skin needs protection from the excoriating effect of the excretion and appliance adhesive. Allowing the protectant to dry completely enhances its effectiveness.

12 If necessary, enlarge the size of the faceplate opening to fit the stoma.

The appliance should fit snugly around the stoma, with only $1/16$ to $1/8$ inch of skin visible around the opening. A faceplate opening that is too small can cause trauma to the stoma. Exposed skin will be irritated by urine if the opening is too large.

13 Apply adhesive to the faceplate or remove the protective covering from the disposable faceplate, carefully position the appliance, and press it in place, moving from the center outward. Remove the gauze squares from the stoma before applying the pouch.

The appliance is effective only if it is properly positioned and securely adhered. Commercial deodorants may be used if odor is a problem.

14 Secure the optional belt to the appliance and around the client.

An elasticized belt helps support the appliance for some persons.

15 Remove or discard the equipment and assess the client's response to the procedure. Wash your hands.

The client's response may indicate acceptance of the ostomy as well as the need for health teaching. Handwashing deters the spread of microorganisms.

16 Record the appearance of the stoma and the surrounding skin as well as the client's reaction to the procedure.

A careful record is important for planning the client's care.

Changing the Urinary Appliance. The frequency of changing the appliance varies with the type being used. The appliance should be changed at a time following low fluid intake, such as early morning. Urine production will be less at this time, which makes changing the appliance easier. Procedure 33-7 describes how to change an appliance worn over an ileal conduit.

Teaching the Client. In general, nursing care is directed toward client education and the achievement of optimal self-care. As responsibility for self-care is assumed, the client should be taught to make the necessary observations, to be aware of indications of problems, and to recognize when to seek assistance. In order for these goals to be met, the client needs to be able to do the following:
- Explain the cause for the urinary diversion and the rationale for treatment
- Demonstrate self-care behaviors that effectively manage the diversion
- Describe follow-up care and existing support resources
- Report where supplies may be obtained in the community
- Verbalize related fears and concerns
- Demonstrate positive body image

The assistance of an enterostomal therapist (ET) can be invaluable in helping the client to achieve these outcomes. The client may be referred to the United Ostomy Association (see Appendix C) for further information and helpful periodicals. Detailed discussion of other aspects of the care of the person with a urinary diversion can be found in clinical texts.

EVALUATING

The nurse evaluates the effectiveness of a plan of care to promote healthy urinary functioning by checking whether the client has met the individualized client goals specified in the plan. In general, nursing care is considered effective if the client expresses satisfaction with the regular voiding pattern and is able to
- Produce a sufficient quantity of urine to maintain fluid, electrolyte, and acid–base balance
- Empty the bladder completely at regular intervals without discomfort
- Develop a plan to modify any factors contributing to present urinary problems or that might adversely affect urinary functioning in the future
- Correct unhealthy urinary habits such as delaying voiding, drinking insufficient water, or abusing diuretics

NURSING PROCESS in Clinical Practice

Once a urinary problem is detected, the nurse implements each phase of the nursing process to ensure correct identification and treatment of the problem. To identify and manage the urinary problem correctly, the nurse must possess the knowledge and clinical skills described earlier in this chapter. Following in outline format are the focused assessment priorities, client goals, nursing interventions, and evaluative criteria for common nursing diagnoses.

> *Altered patterns of urinary elimination related to dysuria*
>
> *Altered patterns of urinary elimination related to maturational enuresis*
>
> *Urinary incontinence (five types with varying etiologies)*
>
> *Urinary retention related to varying etiologies*
>
> *Potential for nosocomial infection related to indwelling Foley catheter*

Altered Patterns of Urinary Elimination Related to Dysuria

Dysuria or difficult urination is most often associated with a sensation of pain or burning. Clients report feeling the need to void but having great difficulty and pain in starting the stream. Dysuria is common in women and is associated with lower urinary tract infections and irritation of the urethral meatus following sexual intercourse or caused by use of bath and feminine hygiene products.

Assessment
- Interview the client for report of painful or burning sensation while voiding and presence of fever, chills, nausea, or flank pain.
- Identify potential causative factors:
    - Infection
    - Sexual activity one to two days prior to symptoms
    - Liquid detergent or bubble bath in bath water
- Examine urine for cloudiness, foul odor, hematuria, and proteinuria.

Client Goals
- Client reports absence of pain or burning during urination.
- Client describes appropriate self-care measures to prevent recurrence.

Interventions

- Instruct the client about the probable cause of the dysuria and reassure the client that the distressing symptoms will be relieved with treatment.
- Teach perineal care to include wiping from front to back after voiding and the need to cleanse the peri-anal region with soap and water after defecation and intercourse. Female clients should also be instructed to void before and after intercourse to flush the lower urinary tract of bacteria. Because the urethra in the female is short and close to the vagina and anus, bacteria from these areas can easily migrate to the urethral meatus and ascend up the urinary tract.
- Encourage a fluid intake of 2000 ml to 3000 ml to dilute infected urine and to flush the system.
- If indicated, assist the client to alter urinary ph by dietary manipulation. Large quantities of water and cranberry juice may acidify the urine and be helpful in reducing bacterial growth. If urine alkalization is warranted to soothe an irritated bladder, eating more vegetables and fruits may be helpful.
- Sitz baths promote relaxation of tense muscles and facilitate healing of an irritated urethral meatus.
- Administer prescribed medications to treat the pathology underlying dysuria.

Evaluative Criteria

Client meets above goals.

Altered Patterns of Urinary Elimination Related to Maturational Enuresis

Enuresis is involuntary urination after an age when continence should be present. *Nocturnal enuresis* is bed-wetting that occurs while a person is sleeping, and *diurnal enuresis* occurs when a person is awake. In *primary enuresis* the child has never had a long period of dryness; in *secondary enuresis* the pattern of bed wetting follows a period of dryness of weeks or months. An identifiable stress such as the birth of a sibling or parental divorce often precedes the onset of secondary enuresis. It is helpful for parents to understand that enuresis is primarily a maturational problem that usually ceases between 6 and 8 years of age.

Assessment

- Interview the child and parents to determine
  Pattern of bed wetting and precipitating factors (if present)
  Response of family members to the child
  History of toilet-training
  Familial history of enuresis
- Assess bladder capacity by measuring voided specimen after the child has been instructed to delay

voiding as long
cordings. Small

Client Goals

- Child develops d
  ination.
- Parents respond c

Interventions

- Instruct the parent
  rational problem th
  assistance and that
  can have harmful ef
- Share with the chilc
  wet and that this pr
- If both the parents a
  sponsibility/reinforc
  keep a calendar of d
  for rewards.
- If the child has small
  daytime bladder stret
  postpone voiding afte
- If the child is a sound
  time and have the chi
  retiring.
- If the child gets too ab
  spond to a full bladder
  sense a full bladder an
  ping to void. Reinforce
- Explore with the family
- Assist the family to eval
  conditioning therapy in
  and other therapies.

Evaluative Criteria

Clients meet above goals.

Urinary Incontinence

Urinary incontinence is the in
bladder after the age of toile
proximately 17% of the adult p
age (Thomas et al, 1980) and t
is a special problem for the e
ence decreasing control over
find it more difficult to reach
because of mobility problems
undressing. Farrar (1984) note
urinary incontinence among r
reaches 50%. This proportion
counts. The discomfort, odor,
urine-soaked clothing can grea
self-concept and cause the pers
outcast. Urinary incontinence ca
providers to be negatively dispos

Action	Rationale
4 Have the client sit or stand if able to assist with procedure or assume supine position in bed.	These positions result in less abdominal folds and facilitate removal and application of the device.
5 Empty the pouch being worn into the graduated container (before removing if it is reusable and not attached to straight drainage).	Having the pouch empty before handling it reduces the likelihood of spilling the excretions. The physician may have ordered recording of intake and output.
6 Remove the pouch faceplate from the skin very gently.	The seal between the surface of the faceplate and the skin must be broken before the faceplate can be removed. Harsh handling of the appliance can cause damage to the skin and impair the development of a secure seal in the future.
7 Discard the pouch appropriately if disposable or wash reusable pouch in luke-warm soap and water and allow to air dry.	Thorough cleaning and airing of the appliance reduce odor and deterioration. For aesthetic and infection-control purposes, used appliances should be discarded appropriately.
8 Cleanse the skin around the stoma with soap and water or a commercial cleaner using washcloth or cotton balls. Make sure that you remove all of old adhesive from the skin.	Cleaning the skin removes excretions and old adhesive and skin protectant. Excretions or a build-up of other substances can cause irritation and damage to the skin.
9 Pat dry gently. Make sure the skin around the stoma is thoroughly dry. Assess the stoma and the condition of the surrounding skin.	Careful drying prevents trauma to the skin and stoma. An intact, properly applied urinary collection device protects skin integrity. Any change in the color and size of the stoma may indicate circulatory problems.
10 Place a gauze square or two over the stoma opening.	Continuous drainage must be absorbed to keep the skin dry during the appliance change.
11 Apply a skin protectant to a 2-inch radius around the stoma, and allow it to dry completely, which takes about 30 seconds.	The skin needs protection from the excoriating effect of the excretion and appliance adhesive. Allowing the protectant to dry completely enhances its effectiveness.
12 If necessary, enlarge the size of the faceplate opening to fit the stoma.	The appliance should fit snugly around the stoma, with only $1/16$ to $1/8$ inch of skin visible around the opening. A faceplate opening that is too small can cause trauma to the stoma. Exposed skin will be irritated by urine if the opening is too large.
13 Apply adhesive to the faceplate or remove the protective covering from the disposable faceplate, carefully position the appliance, and press it in place, moving from the center outward. Remove the gauze squares from the stoma before applying the pouch.	The appliance is effective only if it is properly positioned and securely adhered. Commercial deodorants may be used if odor is a problem.
14 Secure the optional belt to the appliance and around the client.	An elasticized belt helps support the appliance for some persons.
15 Remove or discard the equipment and assess the client's response to the procedure. Wash your hands.	The client's response may indicate acceptance of the ostomy as well as the need for health teaching. Handwashing deters the spread of microorganisms.
16 Record the appearance of the stoma and the surrounding skin as well as the client's reaction to the procedure.	A careful record is important for planning the client's care.

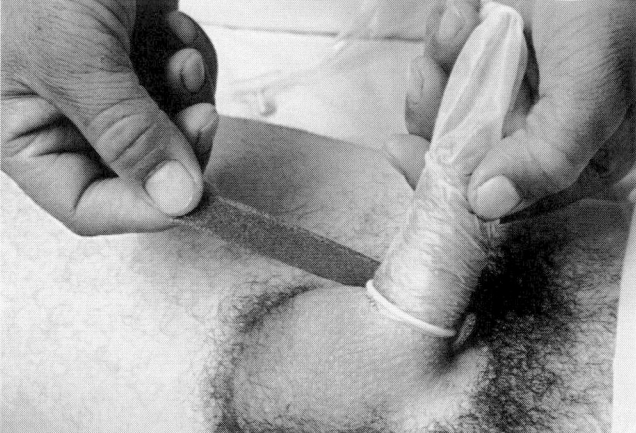

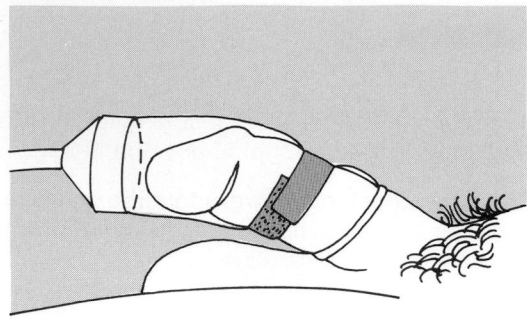

Step 7: Application of a Velcro strap at the base of the condom sheath.

Step 8: Drawing of extra space at end of sheath and smoothing tubing to drainage unit.

9 Remove the equipment. Place the client in a comfortable, safe position. Wash your hands.

This provides a safe, comfortable setting for the client. Handwashing deters the spread of microorganisms.

10 Assess the client's response and record observations on the client's chart.

This provides accurate documentation and observation of urinary output.

P R O C E D U R E   33-7
Changing a Stoma Appliance on an Ileal Conduit

Equipment

Basin with warm water, soap, towel, washcloth or cotton balls	Sterile 2 × 2 gauze squares	Ostomy belt (optional)
Graduated container	Ostomy bag cut to the correct stomal size (with adhesive-backed faceplate, if available)	Adhesive cement (optional for reusable pouches)
Skin protectant or barrier		

Action

Rationale

1 Explain the procedure and encourage the client to observe or participate if possible. Provide for privacy.

Observing or assisting with procedure encourages self-acceptance.

2 Assemble the equipment.

Organization facilitates performance of task.

3 Wash your hands.

Handwashing deters the spread of microorganisms.

(Continued)

Changing the Urinary Appliance. The frequency of changing the appliance varies with the type being used. The appliance should be changed at a time following low fluid intake, such as early morning. Urine production will be less at this time, which makes changing the appliance easier. Procedure 33-7 describes how to change an appliance worn over an ileal conduit.

Teaching the Client. In general, nursing care is directed toward client education and the achievement of optimal self-care. As responsibility for self-care is assumed, the client should be taught to make the necessary observations, to be aware of indications of problems, and to recognize when to seek assistance. In order for these goals to be met, the client needs to be able to do the following:

- Explain the cause for the urinary diversion and the rationale for treatment
- Demonstrate self-care behaviors that effectively manage the diversion
- Describe follow-up care and existing support resources
- Report where supplies may be obtained in the community
- Verbalize related fears and concerns
- Demonstrate positive body image

The assistance of an enterostomal therapist (ET) can be invaluable in helping the client to achieve these outcomes. The client may be referred to the United Ostomy Association (see Appendix C) for further information and helpful periodicals. Detailed discussion of other aspects of the care of the person with a urinary diversion can be found in clinical texts.

EVALUATING

The nurse evaluates the effectiveness of a plan of care to promote healthy urinary functioning by checking whether the client has met the individualized client goals specified in the plan. In general, nursing care is considered effective if the client expresses satisfaction with the regular voiding pattern and is able to

- Produce a sufficient quantity of urine to maintain fluid, electrolyte, and acid–base balance
- Empty the bladder completely at regular intervals without discomfort
- Develop a plan to modify any factors contributing to present urinary problems or that might adversely affect urinary functioning in the future
- Correct unhealthy urinary habits such as delaying voiding, drinking insufficient water, or abusing diuretics

NURSING PROCESS *in Clinical Practice*

Once a urinary problem is detected, the nurse implements each phase of the nursing process to ensure correct identification and treatment of the problem. To identify and manage the urinary problem correctly, the nurse must possess the knowledge and clinical skills described earlier in this chapter. Following in outline format are the focused assessment priorities, client goals, nursing interventions, and evaluative criteria for common nursing diagnoses.

- ***Altered patterns of urinary elimination related to dysuria***
  Altered patterns of urinary elimination related to maturational enuresis
  Urinary incontinence (five types with varying etiologies)
  Urinary retention related to varying etiologies
  Potential for nosocomial infection related to indwelling Foley catheter

Altered Patterns of Urinary Elimination Related to Dysuria

Dysuria or difficult urination is most often associated with a sensation of pain or burning. Clients report feeling the need to void but having great difficulty and pain in starting the stream. Dysuria is common in women and is associated with lower urinary tract infections and irritation of the urethral meatus following sexual intercourse or caused by use of bath and feminine hygiene products.

Assessment

- Interview the client for report of painful or burning sensation while voiding and presence of fever, chills, nausea, or flank pain.
- Identify potential causative factors:
  Infection
  Sexual activity one to two days prior to symptoms
  Liquid detergent or bubble bath in bath water
- Examine urine for cloudiness, foul odor, hematuria, and proteinuria.

Client Goals

- Client reports absence of pain or burning during urination.
- Client describes appropriate self-care measures to prevent recurrence.

Interventions

- Instruct the client about the probable cause of the dysuria and reassure the client that the distressing symptoms will be relieved with treatment.
- Teach perineal care to include wiping from front to back after voiding and the need to cleanse the perianal region with soap and water after defecation and intercourse. Female clients should also be instructed to void before and after intercourse to flush the lower urinary tract of bacteria. Because the urethra in the female is short and close to the vagina and anus, bacteria from these areas can easily migrate to the urethral meatus and ascend up the urinary tract.
- Encourage a fluid intake of 2000 ml to 3000 ml to dilute infected urine and to flush the system.
- If indicated, assist the client to alter urinary *p*h by dietary manipulation. Large quantities of water and cranberry juice may acidify the urine and be helpful in reducing bacterial growth. If urine alkalization is warranted to soothe an irritated bladder, eating more vegetables and fruits may be helpful.
- Sitz baths promote relaxation of tense muscles and facilitate healing of an irritated urethral meatus.
- Administer prescribed medications to treat the pathology underlying dysuria.

Evaluative Criteria

Client meets above goals.

Altered Patterns of Urinary Elimination Related to Maturational Enuresis

Enuresis is involuntary urination after an age when continence should be present. *Nocturnal enuresis* is bedwetting that occurs while a person is sleeping, and *diurnal enuresis* occurs when a person is awake. In *primary enuresis* the child has never had a long period of dryness; in *secondary enuresis* the pattern of bed wetting follows a period of dryness of weeks or months. An identifiable stress such as the birth of a sibling or parental divorce often precedes the onset of secondary enuresis. It is helpful for parents to understand that enuresis is primarily a maturational problem that usually ceases between 6 and 8 years of age.

Assessment

- Interview the child and parents to determine
    Pattern of bed wetting and precipitating factors (if present)
    Response of family members to the child
    History of toilet-training
    Familial history of enuresis
- Assess bladder capacity by measuring voided specimen after the child has been instructed to delay

voiding as long as possible. Use at least three recordings. Small bladder capacity is less than 300 ml.

Client Goals

- Child develops day and nighttime control over urination.
- Parents respond constructively to child.

Interventions

- Instruct the parents that enuresis is usually a maturational problem that the child will outgrow with assistance and that punishing or shaming the child can have harmful effects.
- Share with the child that many other children bed wet and that this problem will be outgrown.
- If both the parents and child are motivated, use responsibility/reinforcement therapy. The child can keep a calendar of dry days and nights and contract for rewards.
- If the child has small bladder capacity, encourage daytime bladder stretching by helping the child to postpone voiding after drinking fluids.
- If the child is a sound sleeper, limit fluids at bedtime and have the child void immediately before retiring.
- If the child gets too absorbed in daytime play to respond to a full bladder, teach the child how to sense a full bladder and the importance of stopping to void. Reinforce dry days.
- Explore with the family various laundry aids.
- Assist the family to evaluate the pros and cons of conditioning therapy involving an alarm system and other therapies.

Evaluative Criteria

Clients meet above goals.

Urinary Incontinence

Urinary incontinence is the inability to retain urine in the bladder after the age of toilet-training. It occurs in approximately 17% of the adult population over 65 years of age (Thomas et al, 1980) and throughout the life span. It is a special problem for the elderly, who often experience decreasing control over micturition and who may find it more difficult to reach a toilet in time to void because of mobility problems or dexterity problems in undressing. Farrar (1984) notes that the prevalence of urinary incontinence among nursing home residents reaches 50%. This proportion is alarming on two accounts. The discomfort, odor, and embarrassment of urine-soaked clothing can greatly diminish a person's self-concept and cause the person to feel like a social outcast. Urinary incontinence can also cause health-care providers to be negatively disposed toward clients.

In 1986 the North American Nursing Diagnosis Association defined five types of incontinence:

- **Functional incontinence**: The state in which an individual experiences an involuntry, unpredictable passage of urine
- **Reflex incontinence**: The state in which an individual experiences an involuntary loss of urine, occurring at somewhat predictable intervals when a specific bladder volume is reached
- **Stress incontinence**: The state in which an individual experiences a loss of urine of less than 50 ml occurring with increased abdominal pressure
- **Total incontinence**: The state in which an individual experiences a continuous and unpredictable loss of urine
- **Urge incontinence**: The state in which an individual experiences involuntary passage of urine occurring soon after a strong sense of urgency to void

Common etiologies for each type are listed in Table 33-3.

Assessment

- Establish a data base to identify the type and severity of incontinence and the effect it is having on daily living. Specht (1986) recommends attention to the following:

  Incontinence pattern: frequency, precipitating factors, degree of control

  Physical mobility, muscle tone, manual dexterity, balance, transfer capability, and vision

  Attitude toward self: self-esteem, perception of aging

  Mental status: orientation, ability to be aware of bladder cues, memory, interest and ability in learning, amount of sensory stimulation available

  Medications being taken, particularly diuretics, sedatives, tranquilizers, and tricyclic antidepressants

  Medical treatments: catheterization, surgery, intravenous fluids or prescribed fluid intake regimen, prescribed bed rest

  Food and fluid intake schedule in relationship to activity and sleep patterns

  Clothing: usual clothing worn (winter and summer) and time needed to remove them in preparation for urinating

  Environment: location of toilet or commode, use of urinal or cans, distance of bathroom from normal daytime and sleeping areas, stairs to bathroom, lighting, effects on availability of bathroom because others also use it

  Social activities and personal support: presence or absence of others who care about the person, events or activities the person wishes to participate in

- Identify high-risk populations. According to Specht (1986), the risk of incontinence that is nonpathologic in origin is increased by the following:

  Constipation and fecal impaction

  Untreated vaginal infections, urinary tract infections

  Slowing gait, insecure balance

  Clothing that requires much time and manipulation for removal

  Malnutrition, reduced fluid intake, and associated weakness

  Use of diuretics, tranquilizers, sedatives, or tricyclic antidepressants

  A view of oneself as old, powerless, neglected

  Failure to maintain physical activity, body flexibility, perineal exercises

  Taking to one's bed

- Those at greatest risk for not managing daily living with incontinence are those who

  Have no control over urinary flow

  Have accompanying physical disability

  Have cognitive deficits or psychiatric problems

  Lack money for supplies and services

  Experience recurrent urinary tract infections

  Do not wish to participate in an active treatment program

  Accept the dysfunction as a normal part of old age

  Have no primary caregiver to assist with treatments or maintain the hygiene of clothing and environment

  Wish to maintain an active social and travel schedule

Client Goals

The client will

- Eliminate or reduce incontinent episodes
- Explain the cause of incontinence and the rationale for treatment
- Participate in a bladder-training or reconditioning program
- Utilize appropriate incontinent aids (if indicated)
- Maintain skin integrity
- Demonstrate positive body image
- Participate in desired social activities

Interventions

As soon as medical evaluation of the client's problem has been made, nursing measures should be directed toward helping to restore normal functioning.

- Explain that efforts will be made to help the client. This is important to the client.
- Encourage a generous fluid intake, as much as 1800 ml to 2400 ml daily. Incontinent clients often voluntarily limit fluid intake in an effort to decrease urinary output. These clients need to be

helped to understand the relationship between adequate fluid intake and total body functioning.

- Encourage the client routinely to make an effort to void shortly after taking fluids. Voluntary efforts either to control or start voiding may be sufficiently stimulating to help restore function for some clients.
- Take chronically ill and elderly incontinent clients to the bathroom or offer a bedpan or urinal every 2 to 3 hours. This practice sometimes helps start at least some control over incontinence.
- Teach perineal exercises if possible. These exercises consist of contracting the muscles as though urination is to be halted. This is followed by relaxing muscles in the area, as though about to start to void. The exercises can be done 10 to 15 times daily and help strengthen muscles that control voiding.
- Use hygienic measures to keep the incontinent client dry, clean, and comfortable. Often, great skill is required to prevent discomfort caused by wet clothing and linens. The ammonia in the urine and lying on wet linen can quickly irritate the skin and soon lead to the development of bedsores.
- Try an external appliance for incontinent male clients, as indicated. Various types of appliances are available. These devices fit over the penis and are secured by straps. A collection bag is usually attached to the client's leg to permit the client to be up and about.
- Use absorbent pads and waterproof garments for female clients. Absorbent, waterproof briefs are now available for incontinent clients and are proving to be especially effective for women. External appliances have not been found to be particularly comfortable or effective for incontinent women.
- Demonstrate tact and understanding while caring for an incontinent client. Offering emotional support and allowing the client to talk about the problem and to assist with decisions about personal care are often helpful.
- Refer the client to HIP (Help for Incontinent People), a nonprofit client advocacy group to educate the public about urinary incontinence (HIP, PO Box 544, Union, SC 29379).

As a last resort, an indwelling catheter or intermittent clean catheterization may be necessary when other measures prove inadequate.

Under certain conditions, voluntary control of voiding is permanently impaired, but the reflex act of micturition remains intact. Clients with this condition may benefit from a formal bladder training program. This is a lengthy and difficult process for some persons and is impossible for others. It requires the effort and cooperation of the client and health personnel.

The nurse should keep in mind that management of the emotional problems of clients with urinary incontinence is often as important for the nurse as management of the physical problems.

Evaluative Criteria
Client meets above goals.

Urinary Retention Related to Varying Etiologies

Retention occurs when urine is produced normally but is not excreted from the bladder. The bladder continues to fill and may distend to hold 3000 ml to 4000 ml of urine. Normally in adults the micturition reflex is triggered when the bladder holds 250 ml to 450 ml of urine. Retention is suspected when clients report

- Difficulty voiding despite urge to void
- Frequent small voidings (less than 50 ml)
- Discomfort in the pubic area
- Urinary output that is much less than fluid intake

Palpation and percussion above the symphysis pubis are used to assess bladder distention. The abdomen swells as the bladder rises above the level of the symphysis pubis. The height of the bladder can be determined by palpating with light pressure on the abdomen. Physicians may order a client catheterized for **residual urine** to determine if urine is being retained in the bladder after voiding. Normally all but 1 ml to 3 ml of urine is excreted from the bladder with each voiding. The client is catheterized after voiding and both the amount of urine voided and that collected by catheterization are recorded.

Retention is often temporary, commonly following surgery involving the lower abdomen, pelvis, bladder, or urethra, especially if ambulation is delayed or fluid intake is minimal. Any mechanical obstruction, such as swelling at the meatus, which often occurs following childbirth, or an enlarged prostate in men, may cause retention. The cause may also be psychic or due to certain disease conditions. Injuries to the spinal cord may cause permanent retention. Urine that pools in the bladder predisposes the client to urinary tract infection.

Assessment
- Strict fluid intake and output; record time and amount of voidings.
- Note complaints of pain in the pubic area, swelling, urgency, frequency, dysuria.
- Palpate and percuss above the symphysis pubis.
- Catheterize for residual urine if indicated (ordered).

Client Goals
- Client will verbalize the importance of emptying the bladder as soon as possible.
- Client's bladder will empty completely as evidenced by

  Quantity of urine voided (24-hour output approximately equal to fluid intake)

  Normal pattern of voiding reestablished (each voiding > 50 ml)

  Flattened pubic area

  Absence of complaints

- Client will demonstrate no signs of urinary tract infection.

Interventions

- Utilize nursing measures to stimulate micturition:
    Provide privacy.
    Help client to assume natural position.
    Offer warm fluids to drink.
    Warm the bedpan.
    Run tap water within client's hearing.
    Pour warm water over the perineal area.
    Place client's hands in warm water.
    Manually press on the client's abdomen.
- Administer prescribed analgesics if appropriate to promote comfort.
- If independent nursing measures fail to produce bladder emptying, a physician must be contacted:
- Bethanechol chloride (Urecholine), a parasympathomimetic agent that stimulates micturition, may be prescribed.
- Catheterization may be ordered. Nursing measures should be exhausted before resorting to catheterizing clients with retention because of the danger of urinary tract infection.

Evaluative Criteria

Client meets above goals.

Potential for Nosocomial Infection Related to Indwelling Foley Catheter

Urinary tract infections are second only to respiratory tract infections in frequency of occurrence. Of special importance to nurses is that urinary tract infections are the most common type of hospital-acquired (nosocomial) infections in the United States and Canada. In a study by Platt and associates (1982) on mortality associated with nosocomial urinary tract infection, 131 patients acquired 136 urinary tract infections during 1,474 bladder catheterizations. Findings of this study noted a threefold increase in death rate among patients with acquired nosocomial urinary tract infections.

Catheterization predisposes to urinary tract infection for the following reasons:

- The introduction of the catheter through the urethra provides a direct route for microorganisms to travel up the urinary tract to the bladder.
- Catheter-induced local irritation to the urethra or bladder predisposes to infection.
- The catheter interferes with the most important defense against bacterial urinary tract infection, the unobstructed flow of urine throughout the urinary tract and regular, complete evacuation of the bladder.
- Clients requiring catheterization often have diseases or other conditions that interfere with the body's immune system, thereby decreasing the efficiency of the urinary tract's reaction to bacteriuria.

In summary, clients being catheterized are a highly vulnerable population and demand vigilant nursing care to prevent urinary tract infection. Breaks in aseptic technique may result in serious and even fatal consequences.

Assessment

- Note client complaints of frequency, urgency, dysuria, nocturia.
- Palpate the suprapubic area for tenderness.
- Urinalysis: urine may be dark yellow or pinkish red or cloudy with or without sediment, bacteriuria, and hematuria.
- Urine culture and sensitivity: greater than 100,000/ml bacterial colonies; sensitivity disks indicate bacterial sensitivity, intermediate sensitivity, or resistance to a given antibiotic agent.
- With worsening urinary tract infections, fever, chills, nausea and vomiting, and malaise may be present.
- Note that approximately one half of patients with significant bacteriuria are asymptomatic. This is especially true for the elderly.

Client Goals

- Client's urine culture is negative.
- Client demonstrates no signs of urinary tract infection.

Interventions

Prevention

- Force fluids to 2500 ml to 3000 ml/day.
- Teach client appropriate hygiene (careful cleansing of perineal area after each voiding and bowel movement; wiping front to back).
- Observe urine for color, odor, amount, and frequency.
- Utilize strict asepsis with catheter insertion and maintenance unless clean technique is indicated. (Intermittent clean catheterization is recommended for long-term maintenance at home when a catheter is required for bladder emptying. The reduced number and types of bacteria present in the home environment decrease the likelihood of nosocomial infection.)

Treatment

- Obtain urine for urinalysis and urine culture and sensitivity.
- Administer antimicrobial medication as ordered. Encourage client to continue medication for the entire period prescribed (usually 10 days).
- Ensure adequate hydration by oral or IV route.
- Monitor intake and output.
- Maintain thorough perineal hygiene.

Evaluative Criteria

Client meets above goals.

C A S E   S T U D Y

Mrs. Jaspers is an 83-year-old alert, white woman whose husband of 59 years died 6 months ago. Although Mrs. Jaspers was adamant about wanting to live independently in her own home, arthritis severely restricted her movement and ability to manage. Following a hospitalization for pneumonia, she was transferred to a nursing home 1 month ago. Admitting medical diagnoses included hypertension, osteoarthritis, and depression.

Assessment Findings

A comprehensive nursing assessment of Mrs. Jaspers performed 1 month after her admission to the nursing home included the following notations:

- Continent of urine on admission
- At present, incontinent of urine 1 to 2 times/day; often found wet in the morning; states it is "too much bother to get into the bathroom"
- Sits in chair in room unless encouraged and assisted to walk although capable of independent ambulation with care; progressive muscle atrophy and joint stiffness
- No identifiable pathology underlies incontinence.
- Medications include a diuretic for her hypertension and a tricyclic antidepressant.
- Reddened skin in the perineal area

Nursing Diagnoses

Functional incontinence related to difficult transition to nursing home and mobility deficit
Impairment of skin integrity related to functional incontinence

Planning

Since Mrs. Jaspers is alert, the nurse works collaboratively with her to develop a plan designed to reestablish urinary continence. The nurse enters the planning phase understanding the relationship between Mrs. Jaspers' urinary continence and her physical well-being and self-esteem. After discussion, Mrs. Jaspers indicates minimal acceptance of the following client goals.

Short-Term Goals

By next monthly assessment, 5/1, client will
- Verbalize the importance of getting to bathroom toilet when she first feels the need to void
- Demonstrate the ability to walk independently to the bathroom (using cane) to toilet herself
- Demonstrate satisfactory perineal hygiene
- Decrease urinary incontinent episodes to less than 3 to 4 per week

By next monthly assessment, 5/1, client's reddened perineal area will be healed.

Long-Term Goals

Client will maintain urinary continence after eliminating incontinent episodes.

See the care plan for details of the nursing strategies utilized to achieve these goals.

Implementation

In implementing the care plan the nurse needs the following specialized abilities:
- Strong assessment skills (interviewing and physical assessment) to carefully identify the problem and its etiology
- Knowledge of pathologic and nonpathologic basis for urinary incontinence and successful treatment strategies
- Interpersonal skills to communicate to Mrs. Jaspers empathy for her situation and the hope that with help better outcomes are a real possibility
- Teaching, counseling, and caregiver skills to empower Mrs. Jaspers to value and reestablish urinary continence
- Interpersonal and leadership skills to motivate the nursing staff to help Mrs. Jaspers reestablish urinary continence
- Accountability and patience

Documentation

Sample documentation of nursing interventions follows. The first example is a typical entry on the client record using the traditional note format.

4/3/86   This AM after an incontinent episode Mrs. Jaspers began to talk about how hard it is to get adjusted to living here and commented "I feel like just giving up." We talked about the importance of being as independent as possible and the dangers of becoming passively dependent. Nursing teaching/counseling included values of independently adhering to usual toileting schedule and importance of perineal hygiene. Two hours later after lunch Mrs. Jaspers walked to bathroom and toileted herself. Progress with urinary continence will continue to be monitored. Ability definitely present but encouragement needed.

C. Taylor, RN

A sample SOAP note follows next.
4/24/86   11 AM #1 Functional incontinence related to difficult transition to nursing home and mobility deficit.
S: "I'm too weak today to walk to the bathroom. Why don't you put one of those pads on me that some of the other residents wear?"

O: Incontinent of urine after 2 days of complete dryness

A: Is capable of voluntary control of urination; temporary regression

P: Diagnostic: Continue to explore her desire to be independent and today's reason for regressive behavior.

    Educative: Reinforce importance of urinary continence; communicate this is the staff's expectation of her, and verbally reinforce next period of dryness.

Evaluation

Short-term goal achievement is evaluated at next monthly assessment. See the nursing care plan for related evaluative statements and revisions of the plan of care. Long-term goal achievement is an ongoing evaluation.

N U R S I N G   C A R E   P L A N   for Mrs. Jaspers

Nursing Diagnosis: Functional incontinence related to difficult transition to nursing home and mobility deficit as manifested by incontinence of urine 1 to 2 times/day; feeling toileting is too much bother; mobility deficits secondary to osteoarthritis; taking a diuretic and antidepressant.

Long-Term Goal: Client maintains urinary continence after eliminating incontinent episodes.

Goals	Nursing Actions	Rationale	Evaluative Statement
By next monthly assessment 5/1 client will: 1. Verbalize the importance of getting to bathroom/toilet when she first feels the need to void	• Assess the value client attaches to voluntary control of urination and urinary continence; counsel appropriately. • Teach the importance of complete bladder emptying at regular intervals and the harmful effects of ignoring the urge to void. • Assess client's normal voiding habits at home and assist her to reestablish these. Initial reminders to toilet herself may be necessary.	Unless the client is committed to the plan of care, goal achievement is impossible. Client understanding of the etiologies and harmful effects of urinary incontinence may motivate desire for reestablishment of voluntary control. Respect for the client's normal voiding schedule and patterns communicates nursing's sincere concern for the individual; encourages client achievement of goals.	5/1 Goal partially met: client has commented on the importance of regular toileting but still finds this "too much trouble" some days. *Revision:* Reinforce value. *D. Mora, RN*
2. Demonstrate the ability to walk independently to the bathroom (using cane) to toilet self	• Assess the client's ability to toilet self independently. Work consistently with her to increase activity tolerance: encourage short walks throughout the day to increase mobility. • Refer to occupational therapy for assistance with diagnosis and treatment if necessary. • Communicate clearly that the client is expected to use the toilet to urinate. Refrain from using incontinent briefs	One response to experiencing the multiple losses associated with aging is to surrender all control and become increasingly dependent. Non–pathology-based incontinence is less likely to occur if the daily living of the individual keeps her more mobile, flexible, oriented, and motivated. An older person who seeks to take control and has a positive self-image will tend to be more continent.	5/1 Goal met: Client can safely walk to bathroom using cane and toilet herself when she wants to.

(Continued)

N U R S I N G   C A R E   P L A N (Continued)

Goals	Nursing Actions	Rationale	Evaluative Statement
	or pads. Talk with family about client having sufficient undergarments to allow changes as needed until control is reestablished.	The specialized skills of the occupational therapist may facilitate relearning toileting skills. Understanding that the staff *expects* continence and is committed to working with the client to achieve it is a powerful client motivator.	
3. Demonstrate satisfactory perineal hygiene	• Assess client's motivation and ability to be clean, dry, and comfortable. • Teach perineal hygiene.	Client may not understand how easily skin irritation can occur and danger of decubitus ulcers.	5/1 Goal not met. Client repeatedly neglects AM perineal care. *Revision:* Reteach both the importance and procedure of perineal care. Assess each AM.
4. Decrease urinary incontinent episodes to less than 3 to 4 per week	• Communicate to client that the nurses *care* about her reestablishing urinary continence and believe she can do this. Use verbal reinforcement to reward "dry" days. • Chart incontinent episodes and monitor progress; discuss this with client.	A common feeling of recently institutionalized elderly is *abandonment* and the sense that no one cares; response: "Why should I?" Communicating that the client's progress toward goal achievement is valued by the nurses is an excellent encouragement to continue progress.	5/1 Goal met. Client in last week was completely dry for four of seven days. Recorded four incontinent episodes.

Nursing Diagnosis:	Impairment of skin integrity related to functional incontinence as manifested by reddened perineal area (skin still intact)

Goals	Nursing Actions	Rationale	Evaluative Statement
By next monthly assessment 5/1 client's reddended perineal area will be healed	• Assess skin for breakdown each AM and PM and after each incontinent episode. • Teach the client the importance of washing this area carefully with soap and water each AM and after incontinent episodes. Teach the importance of always cleansing and wiping the perineum from front to back to prevent autoinfection. Until incontinent episodes are eliminated a protective waterproof ointment may be indicated.	Perineal care is often neglected or assigned to the least trained personnel in care settings. The woman who is doing self-care may neglect it entirely or use incorrect technique. Skin irritation not detected and treated early may progress to serious decubitus ulcers.	5/1 Goal partially met. Perineal area is less inflamed. *Revision:* Continue to monitor perineal hygiene. No need for protective ointment.

(Continued)

NURSING CARE PLAN (Continued)

Goals	Nursing Actions	Rationale	Evaluative Statement
	• Cotton underwear should be worn. Nylon pantyhose, girdles, tight-fitting pants should be avoided.		

KEY POINTS

■ Urinary elimination, a natural process in which the body excretes waste products and material that exceeds bodily needs, is usually taken for granted. When urinary problems arise, the nurse realizes that many clients consider urination a private act and may become embarrassed when they either need to discuss urination or require assistance with elimination and implements nursing interventions accordingly.

■ Healthy urinary elimination presupposes well-functioning kidneys, ureters, urinary bladder, and urethra. Problems in any of these areas can affect both the amount and quality of the urine formed and the manner in which it is expelled from the body.

■ Other factors affecting urination include growth and development, food and fluid intake, life-style variables, psychologic variables, activity and muscle tone, pathologic conditions, and medications.

■ A comprehensive assessment of the urinary system includes the collection of data about voiding patterns and urinary problems and the physical assessment of the kidneys, bladder, urethral meatus, skin integrity, and urine. These findings may need to be correlated with the results of diagnostic tests and procedures for examining urine and the urinary tract.

■ Identification of client health problems is often aided by the nurse's careful monitoring of fluid intake and output, collection of urine specimens, and testing of urine specimens for abnormalities.

■ Nursing diagnoses may be written specifically addressing problems in urinary functioning (incontinence, pattern alteration, and retention) and identifying the effect urinary problems have on other areas of human functioning (e.g., anxiety, comfort, skin integrity).

■ Nursing attention to the client's usual voiding schedule, need for privacy, natural position while voiding, and hygiene habits will help ensure the client's comfort and satisfactory urine output. Other measures facilitating normal urination include promoting an optimal fluid intake, strengthening tone in the perineal and abdominal muscles, and employing specific measures (e.g., running tap water) to initiate voiding.

■ The client with cognitive, sensory, motor, neurologic, or endurance deficits may need nursing assistance with the toilet, bedpan, commode, or urinal. Family members may also need to be taught how to assist the client with elimination needs.

■ Urinary catheterization may be indicated to relieve urinary retention, obtain select urine specimens, measure residual urine, or empty the bladder before and during surgery and before certain diagnostic procedures. Catheterization is considered the most prominent cause of nosocomial infections and should be avoided whenever possible.

■ Obstructions or malignancies in the urinary tract may require some persons to have the urinary flow diverted surgically. In the ileal conduit the ureters are connected to the ileum and a stoma is created on the abdominal wall. Nursing care is directed toward client education and the achievement of optimal self-care.

BIBLIOGRAPHY

Beaman E: I'll never take bladder catheters for granted again. RN 48(12):30–32, 1985

Birdsall C: How do you teach female self-catheterization? Am J Nurs 85(11):1226–1227, 1985

Brogna L, Lukaszawski ML: Nursing management: The continent urostomy. Journal of Enterostomal Therapy 13(4):139–147, 1986

Burke JP et al: Nosocomial bacteriuria: Estimating the potential by closed sterile urinary drainage. Infect Control 7(2):96–99, 1986

Conti MT, Eutropius L: Preventing UTIs: What works? Am J Nurs 87(3):307–309, 1987

Faller NA et al: The artificial urinary sphincter. Journal of Enterostomal Therapy 12(1):7–14, 1985

Farrar DJ: Urodynamics in the elderly. In Mundy AR, Stephenson T, Wein AJ: Urodynamics: Principles, Practice, and Application. Edinburgh, Churchill-Livingstone, 1984

Greengold BA, Ouslander JG: Bladder retraining: Program for elderly patients with post-indwelling catheterization. Journal of Gerontological Nursing 12(6):31–35, 1986

Hart JA: The urethral catheter—A review of its implication in urinary tract infection. Int Nurs Stud 22(1):57–70, 1985

Henderson JS et al: Age as a variable in an exercise program for the treatment of simple urinary stress incontinence. Journal of Obstetric, Gynecologic, and Neonatal Nursing 16(4):266–272, 1987

Hurley M (ed): Classification of Nursing Diagnoses: Proceedings of the Sixth Conference. St Louis, CV Mosby, 1986

Kneip-Hardy MJ, Votava K, Stubbings MJ: Managing indwelling catheters in the home. Geriatric Nursing 6(5):280–285, 1985

McConnell EA: Assessing the bladder for bladder distention. Nursing '85 15(11):44–46, 1985

Moore K: Childhood enuresis: A nursing approach. The Canadian Nurse 80(3):38–42, 1984

Petillo MH: The patient with a urinary stoma: Nursing management and patient education. Nurs Clin North Am 22(2):263–279, 1987

Platt R, Polk BF, Murdock B, Rosner B: Mortality associated with nosocomial urinary tract infection. N Engl J Med 307(11):637–642, 1982

Robb SS: Urinary incontinence verification in elderly men . . . amount and frequency. Nurs Res 34(5):278–282, 1985

Roe B: Catheter care: An overview. Int J Nurs Stud 22(1):45–56, 1985

Ruge CA: Catheter related U.T.I.s: What's the best way to prevent them? Nursing '87 17(12):50–51, 1987

Specht J: Genitourinary problems. In Carnevali D, Patrick M (eds): Nursing Management for the Elderly, 2nd ed, pp 447–466. Philadelphia, JB Lippincott, 1986

Thomas TM, Plymat KR, Blannin J, Meade TW: Prevalence of urinary incontinence. Br Med J 281:1243–1245, 1980

Urine self-testing: What your patient needs to know . . . glucose levels. Nursing Life 5(4):31–32, 1985

Voith AM: A conceptual framework for nursing diagnoses: Alterations in Urinary Elimination. Rehabilitation Nursing 11(1):18–21, 1986

Voith AM, Smith DG: Validation of the nursing diagnosis of urinary retention. Nurs Clin North Am 20(4):723–729, 1985

Wheatley JK: Causes and treatment of bladder incontinence. Compr Ther 9(8):27, 1983

Whitman S, Kursh ED: Curbing incontinence. Journal of Gerontological Nursing 13(4):35–40, 1987

Wilde MH: Living with a Foley. Am J Nurs 86(10):1121–1123, 1986

Yu LC: Incontinence stress index: Measuring psychological impact. Journal of Gerontological Nursing 13(7):18–25, 1987

Oxygenation

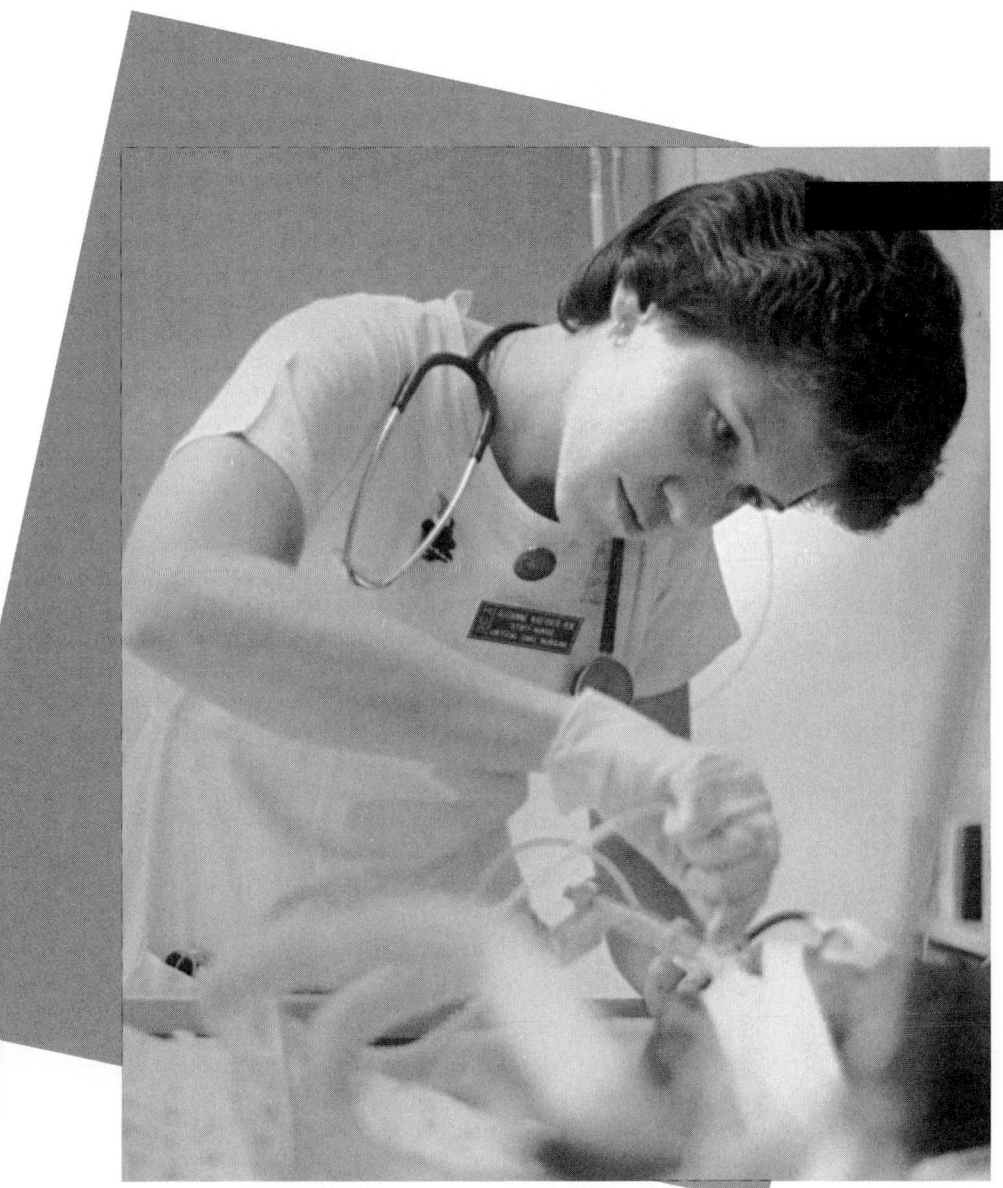

OBJECTIVES

After studying this chapter, the learner should be able to

Define key terms used in the chapter.

Describe the principles of respiratory physiology.

Describe age-related differences that influence care of the client with respiratory problems.

Identify six factors that influence respiratory function.

Perform a comprehensive respiratory assessment using appropriate interview questions and physical assessment skills.

Develop nursing diagnoses that correctly identify problems that may be treated by independent nursing interventions.

Describe 11 nursing strategies to promote adequate respiratory functioning, identifying their rationale.

Plan, implement, and evaluate nursing care related to select nursing diagnoses involving respiratory problems.

Most people take respiratory functioning for granted, but adequate respiratory functioning is necessary for life. Living cells require oxygen. The air passages must remain patent (*i.e.,* open) for oxygen to enter the system. Any condition that interferes with normal functioning must be reduced or eliminated to prevent pulmonary distress which could lead to death.

Normal functioning depends on essentially three factors:

- The integrity of the airway system to transport air to and from the lungs
- Properly functioning alveolar system in the lungs to oxygenate venous blood and to remove carbon dioxide from the blood.
- A properly functioning cardiovascular system to carry nutrients and wastes to and from body cells.

Study of this chapter will provide the nurse with knowledge of the physiology, general purpose, and general factors affecting respiratory functioning. Practical suggestions for performing a comprehensive respiratory assessment are given. Sample interview questions for both a general and focused respiratory history are presented along with information and collecting data from the nursing examination. The incorporation of results from laboratory and radiology studies is addressed in the assessment. After analyzing the data it is important to make decisions as to whether the respiratory data lead to the problem statement, are indicative of another problem, or are the possible cause of a problem. Numerous examples of nursing diagnoses are given. Client goals and specific nursing strategies for implementation are described. In the section entitled "Nursing Process in Clinical Practice," focused assessment planning, implementation and evaluation guides are offered for selected nursing diagnoses related to alteration in respiratory functioning: impaired gas exchange, ineffective breathing pattern, and ineffective airway clearance. These guides and the concluding case study illustrate how the nurse's knowledge of respiratory functioning is combined with skilled nursing interventions to successfully resolve respiratory problems.

KEY TERMS

atelectasis
bronchodilator
bronchoscope
bronchoscopy
congestion
cupping
cystologic study
fremitus
endoscopy
expectorant
expiratory reserve volume
forced vital capacity
functional residual capacity
hemoptysis
hyperventilation
hypoventilation
hypoxia
inspiratory reserve volume
laryngoscope
laryngoscopy

lozenge
nonproductive cough
percussion
perfusion
phlegm
postural drainage
productive cough
radiography
rales
residual volume
rhonchi
skin test
spirometer
suppressant
sympathomimetic agent
tidal volume
total lung capacity
thoracentesis
ventilation
vibration
vital capacity

PHYSIOLOGY OF RESPIRATION

A brief review of basic anatomy and physiology will aid the reader in understanding assessment findings and rationale for nursing interventions (see Fig 34-1).

The main organs of respiration, the lungs, are located within the thoracic cavity. The right lung has three lobes, and the left has two lobes. Each lobe is further subdivided into segments or lobules. The right lung has ten bronchopulmonary segments; the left has eight. The lungs extend from the base at the level of the diaphragm to the apex (top) which is above the first rib. The heart "sits" between the right and left lung. The lungs are comprised of elastic tissue which is capable of stretching

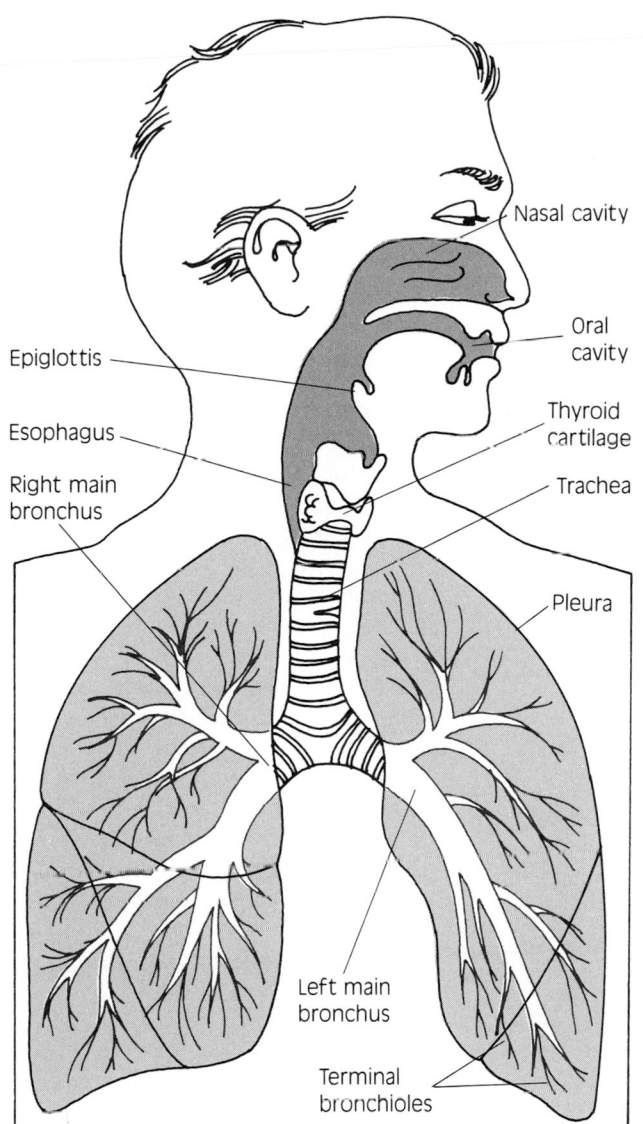

F I G U R E   34-1
The organs of the respiratory tract.

or recoiling. Normally, the elastic fibers are partially stretched at all times, partially filling the thoracic cavity.

The pleurae is a two-layered membrane: the visceral pleura covers the lungs, and the parietal pleura lines the thoracic cavity. These two are continuous with one another and form a closed sac. There is normally a "potential" space between them, not an actual space. Pleural fluid between the membranes acts as a lubricant and as an adhesive agent to hold the lungs in an expanded position. Pressure within the pleural space is always subatmospheric (*i.e.*, negative). This constant intrapleural negative pressure is essential for normal ventilation.

The airway system provides a pathway for the transport and exchange of oxygen and carbon dioxide. The upper airway is composed of the nose, pharynx, larynx, and epiglottis. Its main function is to warm, filter, and humidify inspired air. The lower airway, known as the tracheobronchial tree, includes the trachea, right and left main-stem bronchus, segmental bronchi, and terminal bronchioles. The major functions are: conduction of air, mucociliary clearance, and production of pulmonary surfactant. Cilia, microscopic hairlike projections, propel sheets of mucus toward the upper airway so the mucus can be removed (by cough) after it has trapped cells, particles, and infectious debris. Surfactant, a detergent-like phospholipid, reduces surface tension of the fluid lining the alveoli. When surfactant production is reduced, the lung becomes stiff and the alveoli collapse.

The actual lung is composed of alveoli, small air sacs at the end of the terminal bronchioles (Fig 34-2). These structures are the site of gas exchange. The average adult has over 300 million alveoli.

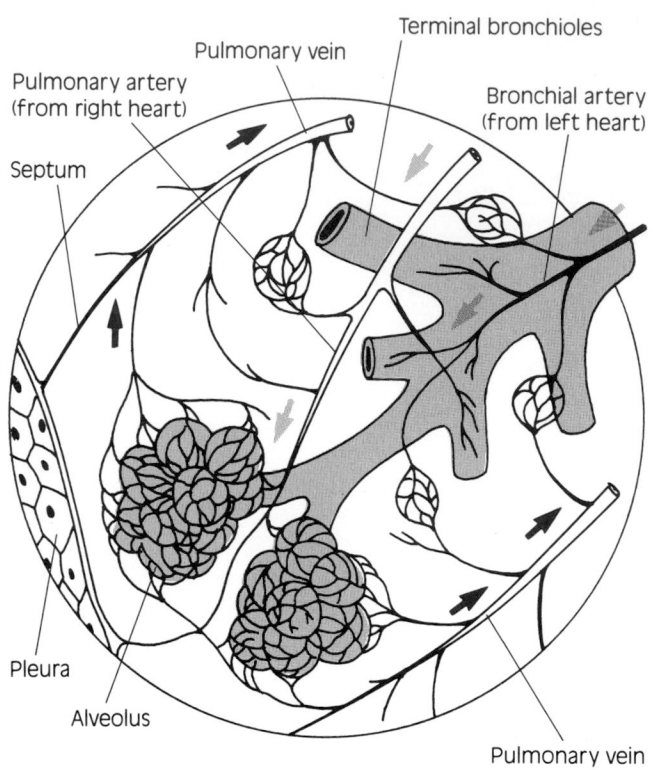

F I G U R E   34-2
Alveoli and the intrapulmonary circulatory system where gas exchange takes place.

The lungs and circulation act together to bring gases to body tissues for gas exchange. Movement of oxygen into the lungs by way of the airway system during inspiration and removing carbon dioxide by the airway system during exhalation is **ventilation**. Respiration occurs at the terminal alveolar capillary system where there is an exchange of gases between the air and blood (Fig 34-3). Diffusion refers to the movement of oxygen and carbon dioxide between the air (in the alveoli) and the blood (in the capillaries). The appropriate gas moves passively from an area of higher concentration to an area of lesser concentration.

The process of ventilation has two phases. Inhalation, the active phase, involves movement of muscles and thorax to bring air into the lungs. Exhalation, the passive phase, is the movement of air out of the lungs. The medulla in the brain stem immediately above the spinal cord is the respiratory center. It is stimulated by the increased concentration of carbon dioxide and hydrogen ions and, to a lesser degree, by the decreased amount of oxygen in the arterial blood. Chemoreceptors in the aortic arch and carotid bodies are also sensitive to the same arterial blood gas levels and can activate the medulla. Stimulation of the medulla increases the rate and depth of vntilation so carbon dioxide and hydrogen are blown off and oxygen levels are increased. The medulla sends an impulse down the spinal cord to the respi-

ratory muscles to stimulate a contraction leading to inhalation. If the system is intact, the diaphragm, the major respiratory muscle, contracts and descends into the abdomen. The thoracic cavity enlarges. Lungs expand in response to pressure changes in the intrapleural space and the lung. Inhalation ceases when atmospheric air pressure and pulmonary air pressure are equal. Exhalation occurs, and the lungs return to their resting position.

General Principles of Respiration

The following basic principles guide action in promoting respiratory functioning:

All living cells require oxygen, which the body cannot store. The body must at all times maintain a properly functioning respiratory system. Environmental oxygen, usually readily available under normal conditions, must be accessible to the body. Environmental oxygen may be in short supply, such as at high altitudes, where oxygen concentration in the air is low, and in the presence of toxic fumes, in which the air has reduced concentrations of oxygen.

The air passageways must remain patent for respiration to occur. Respiratory gases are transported from the nose to the alveoli and are then returned. Obstruction in any part of the normal passageways will impede respiration. Obstruction can occur from a foreign substance, such as a piece of food, a coin, a toy, or liquids, as in the case of the drowning victim. Obstruction can also arise from tissues or secretions within the body (*e.g.,*

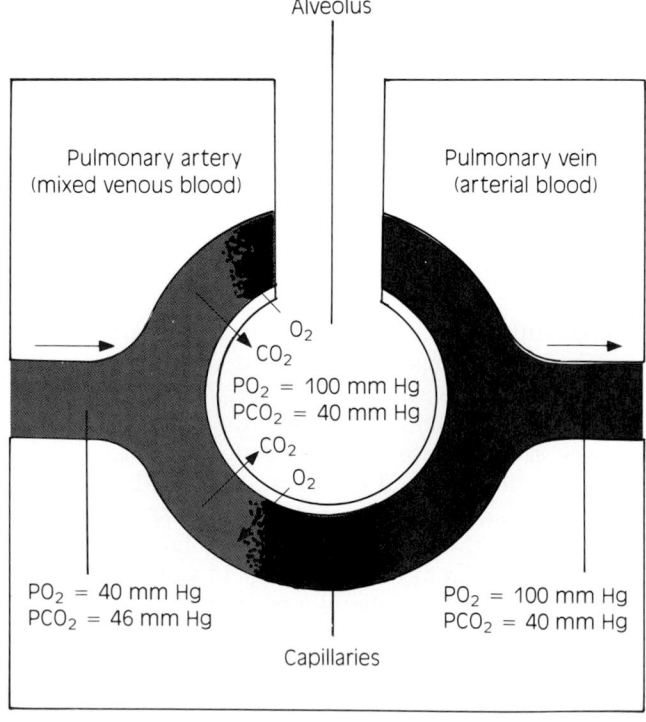

F I G U R E   34-3
Diagram of gas exchange in the alveolus.

excessive or thickened secretions, tumor growths, or edema in the respiratory tract). A decrease in the size of air passages due to constriction or to poor sitting, standing, and lying positions can impede respiration.

Muscle movements provide the physical force essential for respiration. The diaphragm and the intercostal muscles are responsible for normal inspiration and expiration (Fig 34-4). Accessory muscles of the abdomen, neck, and back are used to maintain respiratory movements at times when breathing is difficult. The condition of the body's musculature can affect the process of respiration. For example a depression of the respiratory center and pulmonary congestion with inadequate respiratory efforts are conditions that interfere with the normal movement of air into and out of the lungs.

The pressure changes resulting from expansion and contraction of the thoracic cavity produce pulmonary gas exchanges. Incomplete lung expansion or lung collapse, known as **atelectasis**, prevents the pressure changes and the exchange of gas by diffusion in the lungs. Atelectatic areas of the lung cannot fulfill a function of respiration. Examples of conditions that predispose to atelectasis include obstructions of the airway by foreign bodies, mucus, constricted airways, external compression by tumors or enlarged blood vessels, and immobility.

Adequate fluid intake is essential to respiratory functioning. Fluid is necessary for the production of watery mucus normally present in the respiratory tract and for ciliary action. This covering of mucus also protects the underlying tissues from irritation and infection. A few milliliters of fluid between the pleural surfaces allow the lungs to move easily along the chest wall as they expand and contract. In its absence, filling and emptying of the lungs are difficult.

Ventilation depends on the extent of perfusion in the area. **Ventilation** is the movement of air in and out of the lungs. **Perfusion** is the passing of fluid, in this case, the blood, through tissue. The amount of blood flow through the lungs is a factor in the amount of oxygen and other gases that are exchanged. The amount of blood present in any given area of lung tissue depends partially on whether the person is sitting, standing, or lying down. The perfusion of lung tissue also depends on activity. Greater activity results in increased cellular oxygen need and cardiac output and, consequently, in increased blood return to the lungs. In addition, perfusion depends on an adequate blood supply and proper cardiovascular functioning to carry oxygen and carbon dioxide to and from the lung tissues.

Oxygen and carbon dioxide must move through the alveoli and be carried to and from body cells by the blood. Oxygen is carried two ways in the body. It is dissolved in plasma, but because oxygen is not very soluble in liquids, little oxygen is carried in this way. The hemoglobin in red blood cells has a strong affinity for oxygen, and, therefore, most oxygen is carried in the body by red blood cells in the form of oxyhemoglobin. Hemoglobin carries carbon dioxide easily. Any abnormality in the alveoli or in the blood's constituents influences proper internal respirations.

There must be an exchange of oxygen and carbon dioxide between the blood and body cells. Conditions that influence the passage of oxygen and carbon dioxide through cell walls adversely affect internal respiration. Certain metabolic abnormalities can alter normal gas exchange at cell walls.

If a problem exists in any part of the respiratory process, **hypoxia**, an inadequate amount of oxygen available to cells, may occur. The most common symptoms of hypoxia are dyspnea, an elevated blood pressure with a small pulse pressure, increased respiratory and pulse rates, paleness, and cyanosis. Anxiety and restlessness are also common signs of hypoxia. Hypoxia is often caused by **hypoventilation**, a decreased rate or depth of air movement into the lungs. The effects of chronic hypoxia are detected in all body systems and include altered thought processes, headaches, chest pain, enlarged heart, anorexia, constipation, decreased urinary output, decreased libido, weakness of extremity muscles, and muscle pain. At the other extreme is **hyperventilation**, the increased rate and depth of ventilation above the body's normal metabolic requirements. This is discussed in more detail in the section entitled "Diagnosing."

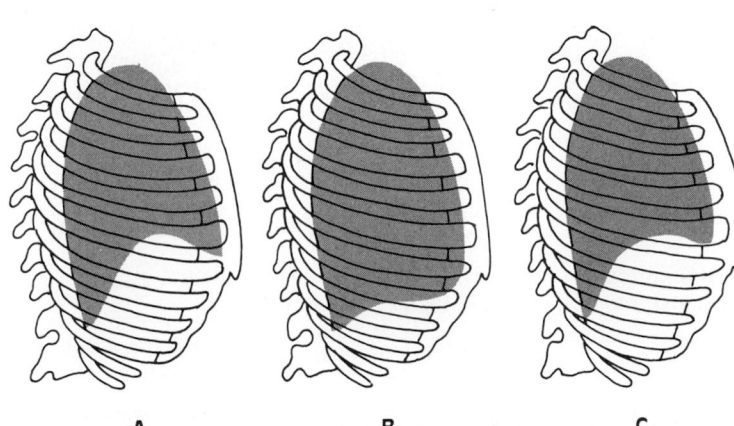

A   **B**   **C**

FIGURE 34-4

(A) With maximum expiration, the elevated diaphragm and depressed ribs shorten the length of the thoracic cavity and decrease the anteroposterior diameter. (B) At maximum inspiration, the diaphragm descends, lengthening the thoracic cavity and elevating the sternum and ribs to increase the anteroposterior diameter of the chest cavity. (C) End of normal expiration.

Developmental Variations

Birth necessitates many adaptations in the newborn. The most blatant of these changes occur with the lungs, as they change from fluid-filled organs to air-filled structures. In the normal infant the chest is small, the airways are short, and aspiration is a potential problem. The respiratory rate is more rapid in the infant than in any other age group (Table 34-1). As alveoli increase in number and size, adequate oxygenation is accomplished at lower respiratory rates. Respiratory rates stabilize in young adulthood.

Respiratory activity is abdominal in the infant. The infant's chest wall is so thin that ribs, sternum, and xyphoid space process are easily noted due to little musculature. The infant has a rounded chest wall where anterior–posterior diameter (*i.e.,* the measurement from the front to back of the thorax) equals transverse diameter. Occasional fine crackles at the end of deep inspiration noted upon auscultation in the infant's thorax are normal.

In the preschool and school-age child, some subcutaneous fat is deposited on the chest wall so landmarks are less prominent than in the infant. Muscular development is also more noticeable. Transverse diameter and anterior–posterior diameter ratio reaches adult configurations of one to two by age 6 years. The preschool child's eustachian tubes, bronchi, and bronchials are elongated and less angular so the number of "routine" colds and infections decreases until they enter school. Also, young children usually have not had the opportunity to develop antibodies for the variety of viruses and bacteria encountered. Good handwashing techniques and "tissue etiquette" are practices to be encouraged. Most children at this age will experience colds or upper respiratory infections but some will have more serious problems of otitis media, bronchitis, and pneumonia. At the end of late childhood and during adulthood the immune system is sufficiently seasoned to protect the person from most infections.

There are specific physical changes in elderly persons that are unrelated to any pathology. Bony landmarks are more prominent due to the loss of subcutaneous fat. Kyphosis (curvature of the spine) contributes to the older person's appearance of leaning forward. Barrel chest deformity may result in a widening of the anterior–posterior diameter. In the absence of any abnormal findings with the physical examination, this is known as senile emphysema. The tissues and airways of the respiratory tract (including alveoli) become more rigid with age. Power of respiratory and abdominal muscles is reduced so the diaphragm moves less efficiently. These alterations increase the risk of disease, especially pneumonia.

FACTORS AFFECTING RESPIRATORY FUNCTIONING

A variety of factors affect adequate respiratory functioning. Six important factors are included here.

Levels of Health. Persons with renal or cardiac disorders often demonstrate a compromise in respiratory functioning due to fluid overload. Persons with chronic illnesses often have muscle wasting and poor muscle tone, including those of the respiratory system. (Developmental variations are discussed in the previous section of this chapter.)

T A B L E   34-1
Developmental Variations in the Life Cycle

	Infant (0–1 year)	Early Childhood (1–5 years)	Late Childhood (6–12 years)	Aged Adult (65+ years)
Respiratory rate	30–60	20–40	15–25	16–20
Respiratory pattern	Abdominal breathing, irregular in rate and depth	Abdominal breathing, irregular	Thoracic breathing, regular	Thoracic, regular
Chest wall	Thin, little muscle, ribs and sternum easily seen	Same as infant's but with more subcutaneous fat	Further subcutaneous fat deposited, structures less prominent	Thin, structures very prominent
Breath sounds	Loud, harsh crackles at end of deep inspiration	Loud, harsh expiration longer than inspiration	Clear inspiration is longer than expiration	Clear
Shape of thorax	Round	Elliptical	Elliptical	Barrel shaped or elliptical

Development. Physical changes such as scoliosis (curvature of the spine) will influence breathing patterns so air trapping occurs. There is a statistically significant correlation between obesity and chronic bronchitis. Obese people are often short of breath with activity and thus participate in little exercise. The alveoli at the base of the lungs are rarely stimulated to expand fully.

Narcotics and Analgesics. These chemical agents depress the medullary respiratory center so that the rate and depth of respirations are decreased. This is especially noted with the use of morphine and meperidine (Demerol). One must be alert to the potential of respiratory arrest when administering any narcotic or sedative.

Life-style. Sedentary activity patterns do not encourage the expansion of alveoli and the development of pulmonary exercise patterns (deep breathing). Persons who exercise on a routine basis three to six times per week (*e.g.,* aerobics, walking, swimming) are better able to respond to stressors to respiratory health. Cigarette smoking (active and passive) is a major contributor to lung disease and respiratory distress.

Environment. It is impossible to pinpoint all effects of air pollution, but researchers have demonstrated a statistically high correlation between air pollution and cancer and lung diseases. The person with adequate respiratory functioning exposed to air pollution will experience stinging of eyes, coughing, choking, headache, and dizziness. Persons who have experienced an alteration in respiratory functioning in the past are often unable to continue self-care activities in a polluted environment.

Psychologic Health. Individuals responding to stress might demonstrate excessive sighing or hyperventilation breathing patterns. Generalized anxiety has been implicated by some scientists in establishing enough bronchospasm to produce an episode of bronchial asthma. It should be noted that those experiencing an alteration in respiratory functioning will develop some anxiety as a result of a physical disorder.

NURSE AS ROLE MODEL

Nurses working with clients to initiate changes in health habits affecting respiration must also examine themselves as a factor in the success of the plan. Clients use nurses as role models in achieving healthy life-styles. Nurses dealing with stresses from professional and personal aspects of their own lives sometimes channel their energies into destructive behaviors. If the nurse wishes

P R O M O T I N G   W E L L N E S S

Oxygenation

Use the assessment checklist to determine how well you are meeting oxygenation needs. Then develop a prescription for self-care by choosing appropriate behaviors from the list of suggestions.

Assessment Checklist

almost always	some times	almost never	
☐	☐	☐	1. I breathe easily, without discomfort or feeling "short of breath."
☐	☐	☐	2. I exercise regularly.
☐	☐	☐	3. I maintain normal weight for my height and body frame.
☐	☐	☐	4. I live in an enviromnent free of pollution.
☐	☐	☐	5. I avoid substances (tobacco, chemicals) that cause respiratory problems.

Self-Care Behaviors

1. Follow a regular exercise program with 30 min–45 min of moderate activity three to four times a week.
2. Maintain normal body weight.
3. Obtain medical evaluation for chest pain, problems with breathing, chronic cough with sputum or blood.
4. Avoid smoking cigarettes, cigars, or pipes.
5. Avoid chemical substances that cause respiratory depression.
6. Maintain a pollution-free environment (as much as possible).
7. Support federal and community efforts to keep the air free of pollution.

to encourage optimal respiratory functioning, he or she must demonstrate behaviors that support a healthy lifestyle. With this goal in mind the nurse will

- Maintain adequate fluid intake and proper nutrition
- Use deep breathing exercises
- Evaluate self use of nicotine
- Incorporate a plan to reduce smoking and then stop smoking with a specific target date
- Reduce activity patterns (*i.e.,* rest at home) in the presence of infection
- Create a pollution-reduced environment by avoiding use of strong perfumes, aftershaves, or other scents
- Arrange to have a tuberculin test (PPD) done annually
- Schedule three to four periods of exercise per week

ASSESSING RESPIRATORY FUNCTIONING

The health history is an essential component of assessing respiratory functioning. Either the client or the accompanying person can provide information. The nursing examination combined with laboratory findings can provide information to identify client's strengths, the nature of the problem, its course, related signs and symptoms, onset, frequency, and effect on activities of daily living. The nurse decides, based on the findings, what problems can be treated independently by nursing. Other problems are referred to the physician for decisions on treatment.

Elements of a Respiratory Assessment

Usual patterns of respiration
"How would you describe your breathing patterns?"
"Do you have allergies?"
"Do you smoke?"
"Do you live with a smoker or are there smokers in your workplace?"

Recent changes
"Have you noticed any changes in your breathing pattern (out of breath, cough, pain)?"
"Do you have chest pain?"

Cough
"How much and how often do you cough?"
"Is the cough related to the time of day or any activity?"
"What is it like (dry, bubbly, hoarse)?"
"Do you have a history of allergies?"
"Do you ever wheeze?"
"Are you exposed to dust? Fumes?"
"Where do you work? What kind of work?"
"How are you treating the cough?"

Sputum
"Do you ever cough up and spit out a mucousy substance?"
"How much do you spit out and do you associate it with anything (time of day, environment)?"
"What color is it? Is it ever blood tinged?"
"What is its odor?"

Chest Pain
"On a scale of 0 to 5, how severe is the pain?"
"Where is the pain?"
"Is the pain worse with inspiration? Expiration? Cough?"
"Does the pain radiate?"
"What measures are you using to relieve the pain?"

Dyspnea
"Is it constant or remittent or related to any activity?"
"How do different positions affect it?"
"How does it affect your daily activities?"
"Is any part of your body bluish during the breathing problems?"
"What do you do during and after the breathing attack?"
"Have you ever been told that you have asthma? Emphysema? Tuberculosis? Heart disease?"
"Do you think the problem is getting worse or staying the same?"

Fever
"Have you had pneumonia recently?"
"Do you have any contact with persons who have tuberculosis?"
"Do you have night sweats?"
"Are others in your household well or ill?"
"Have you traveled anywhere recently?"
"What medications are you using?"
"Have you been exposed to any pollutants?"

Nursing History

The nursing history, an important clinical tool in the early steps of the nursing process, always includes a respiratory component. The information gained provides data as to why a client needs nursing care and what kind of care is required to maintain a sufficient intake of air. Interview questions are used to identify current or potential health deviations, client actions for meeting this need and their effects, contributing factors, use of aids to improve intake of air, and effect on current life-style and relationship with others.

Prior to starting the interview, ascertain that the client and accompanying persons are comfortable. If the client is in any respiratory distress, appropriate actions should be initiated to relieve symptoms. The accompanying persons can answer questions to provide a data base. The nurse can expand this when the client is able to provide information. If the clinical condition of the client indicates that no emergency interventions are necessary, a comprehensive history can be obtained.

When a health deviation is noted during the data collection, the nurse needs to collect as much descriptive information as possible, verifying whether the status of the problem changed suddenly or slowly. Sample questions are given in the accompanying box.

Nursing Examination

The basic examination of the lungs and respiratory status are discussed in Chapter 24. The nurse proceeds in a well-organized manner with a sequence of inspection, palpation, percussion, and auscultation.

Inspection. Observation of the chest normally shows that the contour is slightly convex with no sternal depression. The anterior–posterior diameter should be less than the transverse diameter. Any abnormalities in thoracic structure should be described or sketched (see Fig 24-34 for examples). The contour of the intercostal spaces should be flat or depressed. Movement of the chest should be symmetric. The skin at the thorax should be warm and dry and exhibit even distribution of color with no cyanosis or pallor. Note any scars; origin would have been recorded in the history under previous surgery or accidents. Observe the respiratory rate and rhythm for 1 full minute. Normally, respirations are quiet and nonlabored. Any flaring of nostrils, intercostal restriction, tachypnea, or bradypnea suggests a health deviation which necessitates further evaluation.

Palpation. The tracheas should be equidistant from each clavicle. Skin temperature should be the same as the rest of the body. Respiratory excursion is measured by placing one's hand on the client's posterior thorax at the tenth rib with both thumbs almost touching the vertebrae. While the client takes a few deep breaths, the nurse's thumbs should move 5 to 8 cm symmetrically at maximal inspiration (see Fig 24-36). To assess vocal **fremitus** (the capacity to feel sound on the chest wall), the nurse should place his or her palm surface to the client's chest wall, avoiding bony areas (*e.g.*, scapulae); the nurse should detect equal vibrations as the client says some multisyllable word (*e.g.*, ninety-nine). Bilaterally equal mild fremitus should be detected with the greatest intensity noted at anterior and posterior base of neck and along trachea and large bronchi (see Fig 24-36). Increased fremitus is noted in clients with pneumonia, since solid tissue conducts sound well. Conversely, clients with chronic obstructive pulmonary disease (COPD) have decreased fremitus, because air does not conduct sound well. The presence or absence of crepitation, masses, edema, or tenderness should be noted.

Percussion. Percussion is performed posteriorly as the client pulls shoulders forward; examination proceeds down the client's back, comparing one side to the other. Anterior and lateral thorax can be examined with the client in a supine position. The nurse must listen to intensity and quality of each sound as the chest wall and underlying structures are set in motion. Resonance, a loud hollow, low-pitched sound, is heard over the normal lung. Emphysematous lungs produce a very loud, very low, booming sound called hyperresonance. A flat sound is detected over bone or heavy muscle. A dull sound with medium pitch and intensity is percussed on the liver (fifth intercostal space at the right midclavicular line). Tympany is a high-pitched, loud, drumlike sound produced over the stomach. Dullness over the lung field occurs when fluid or solid tissue replaces normal lung tissue in the pleural space and requires further investigation.

Auscultation. The nurse should move from apex to base with the stethoscope comparing one side with the other side. Normal breath sounds are of three types: vesicular (low pitch, soft expiration, and heard over most of lung); bronchial (high pitch and loud expiration and heard over trachea and peripheral lung); and bronchovesicular (medium pitch and medium expiration and heard over upper anterior chest and intercostal area). (See Fig 24-38). The client should breathe through his opened mouth slowly. Nasal breathing produces false abnormal breath sounds. Hyperventilation is conducive to syncope and client distress. If any abnormal breath sound is detected, the nurse should instruct the client to cough and should auscultate again for at least two breaths. A recording of location, change in breath sounds after coughing, and phase of respiration (*e.g.*, expiration) in which abnormal sound was heard is imperative.

Adventitious sounds can be divided into two categories: rales (or crackles) and rhonchi. **Rales** are noncontinuous sounds produced by a delayed reopening of deflated airways. Rales can be further grouped into fine, medium, and course rales. Fine rales, high-pitched crackling sounds heard toward the end of inspiration, indicate congestion. Medium rales are a lower-pitched, moist sound heard halfway through inspiration. Clients with pneumonia or pulmonary edema exhibit these and cannot clear them by coughing. Coarse rales are loud, bubbly noises heard during inspiration and also are not cleared by coughing. **Rhonchi** are continuous, musical sounds audible in expiration or inspiration or both. Rhonchi reflect obstruction in an air passage due to secretions or edema. They can sometimes be cleared with coughing. Sibilant rhonchi or wheezes originate in the smaller bronchi or bronchioles and are often detected in asthmatics. Sonorous rhonchi are coarser sounds (like a snore) which originate in the larger bronchi or trachea. Clients with COPD often exhibit these.

Pleural friction rub, a dry grating sound, is caused by inflamation of pleural surfaces. It is usually heard on inspiration and expiration and is unaltered by coughing.

The beginning practitioner should be able to discuss normal and abnormal breath sounds. (Review Chap 24.) A detailed description of any abnormal findings without applying a specific label will still aid in any planning of care.

Common Methods to Assess Respiratory Functioning

In addition to the nursing history and physical examination, various laboratory and radiologic tests described in Table 34-2 provide further assessment data which can aid in the formation of nursing diagnoses. These tests are not distinctive of a particular disease but they do reflect how well the respiratory system is functioning.

DIAGNOSING

After the assessment is completed and the data are examined, the nurse concludes either that there is no problem at this time or that there is an actual or potential respiratory problem which is amenable to independent or interdependent nursing action. Nursing diagnoses indicating alterations in respiratory functions are

Ineffective airway clearance
Ineffective breathing patterns
Impaired gas exchange

(These three nursing diagnoses are discussed in detail at the end of this chapter in the section entitled "Nursing Process in Clinical Practice.")

Common etiologies for these diagnoses are: inability to maintain proper position, pain or fear of pain, viscous secretions, fatigue, decreased level of consciousness, lack of knowledge, smoking, allergy, mechanical

obstruction, medications, and decreased elasticity of lungs.

Examples of these diagnoses, etiologic factors, and defining characteristics are given in Table 34-3.

Alteration in respiratory functioning may affect other areas of human functioning. Examples of other nursing diagnoses resulting from alterations in respiratory functioning are

Activity intolerance related to shortness of breath
Anxiety related to feeling of suffocation
Altered comfort (acute pain) related to pleurisy
Impaired verbal communication related to endotracheal intubation
Ineffective individual coping related to frequent hospitalization due to acute symptoms of COPD
Diversional activity deficit related to loss of ability to perform specific activities due to shortness of breath
Fear related to disabling respiratory illness
Grieving related to loss of normal respiratory functioning
Altered health maintenance related to smoking
Noncompliance with _____ (*e.g.,* performance of daily respiratory exercises) related to side-effects of therapy
Altered nutrition, less than body requirements related to difficulty breathing
Altered oral mucous membrane related to presence of endotrachial tube
Powerlessness related to inability for self-care due to COPD
Disturbance in self-concept related to loss of "normal" respiratory functions
Sleep pattern disturbance related to orthopnea and bronchodilators
Social isolation related to inability to walk to usual "people places"

Each nursing statement identifies what is wrong with the client and suggests client goals. The etiology of the problem directs nursing interventions. The nurse, analyzing the assessment data must decide if the alteration in respiratory functioning

1. Is the problem
2. Is contributing to a different problem
3. Is a sign or symptom of a problem

Altered respiratory functioning can fit into all three categories. Let's examine how ineffective airway clearance in a 17-year-old asthmatic baseball player who is waiting to hear from the college of his choice plays a role in three different nursing diagnoses.

1. Ineffective airway clearance related to pollen exposure, exercise, and stress of questionable college admission. The airway clearance *is the problem* statement. Nursing interventions will be directed to reducing exposure to pollens, specific stressors, and timing or degree of exercise. The outcome will be that the client achieves effective airway clearance.

(Text continues on p. 910.)

T A B L E   34-2

Common Methods to Assess Respiratory Functioning

Purpose	Normal Values	Nursing Implications

Spirometry measures lung capacity, volumes, and flow rates with the use of an instrument called a **spirometer.**

Purpose	Normal Values	Nursing Implications
Spirometry helps evaluate the pulmonary status and the efficacy of treatment. Corrections are made for age, sex, weight, and height.	**Tidal Volume (TV):** The amount of air inspired and expired in a normal respiration. Normal is 500 ml. **Inspiratory Reserve Volume (IRV):** The amount of air that can be inspired beyond tidal volume. Normal is 3500 ml to 4300 ml. **Expiratory Reserve Volume (ERV):** The amount of air that can be exhaled beyond tidal volume. Normal is 1200 ml to 1500 ml. **Residual Volume (RV):** The amount of air remaining in the lungs after a maximal expiration. Normal is 1200 ml to 1500 ml. **Vital Capacity (VC):** The maximal amount of air that can be exhaled following a maximal inhalation. Normal is 4000 ml to 4800 ml. **Forced Vital Capacity (FVC):** The maximal amount of air that can be inhaled followed by a fast maximal forced exhalation with greatest effort. FVC differs from VC in that VC does not require a forced inhalation, and the person exhales normally. Normal is 4800 ml. **Functional Residual Capacity (FRC):** FRC is equal to the expiratory reserve volume plus the residual volume. Normal is 2400 ml to 3000 ml. A normal range is 75% to 125% of normal FRC. **Total Lung Capacity (TLC):** The tidal volume plus the residual volume. Normal is 5500 ml.	The client's understanding and cooperation are important to successful study. Explanations should include teaching the client to wear a nose clip and a mouthpiece for breathing. Suffocation will not occur. The examination is not painful but it is fatiguing. The client should wear comfortable clothing. Tight clothing, such as a girdle or belt, may restrict breathing. Drugs affecting the respiratory tract, such as bronchodilators, are withheld prior to the examination so that test results reflect the client's present status. There is no special aftercare, but the client may need extra rest.

Arterial blood gas and *p*H analysis examine arterial blood to determine the pressure exerted by oxygen and carbon dioxide in the blood and the blood's *p*H.

Purpose	Normal Values	Nursing Implications
A blood sample is used to measure gas components in arterial blood and the *p*H of blood. It reflects quality of ventilation and perfusion.	The pressure of carbon dioxide (pCO_2) is normally 35 mm Hg to 45 mm Hg. The pressure of oxygen (pO_2) is normally 80 mm Hg to 100 mm Hg. The *p*H is normally between 7.35 and 7.45.	The procedure for obtaining arterial blood is uncomfortable, more so than an injection into a vein, muscle, or subcutaneous tissue, and the client should be prepared for this. The arm is usually used to obtain a blood sample. The radial artery or an artery in the inner aspect of the elbow is used. Occasionally, the femoral artery is entered. A pressure dressing is applied at the entry site for 3 minutes and watched for evidence of bleeding.

Cystologic study of respiratory secretions involves a study of sputum and cells it contains.

Purpose	Normal Values	Nursing Implications
A cystologic study is done primarily to study cells that may be malignant, deter-	Sputum is free of abnormal cells and of pus, blood, and bacteria.	Sputum is best obtained in the morning, before breakfast, after secretions have accumulated in the respiratory tract during the

(Continued)

Purpose	Normal Values	Nursing Implications
ɪnine organisms causing infection, and identify blood or pus in the sputum.		night. Usually, specimens are collected on 3 successive days. It is best to have the client brush his teeth and rinse his mouth so that saliva and oral debris do not contaminate the specimen. The client should be taught that sputum is matter ejected from the lower respiratory tract through the mouth and that saliva is an unsatisfactory specimen. The client should be instructed to inhale deeply and cough deeply on exhalation. About a teaspoon of sputum is needed for a specimen. The sputum should be coughed directly into a sterile specimen container, which is then covered with a sterile lid, properly labeled, and sent to the laboratory A note should be made on the client's record about the character of the sputum, including amount, appearance, and odor. If a specimen cannot be obtained, mechanical suctioning or stomach aspiration may be used.

Endoscopy is the direct visualization of a body cavity. A **bronchoscope** is used to examine the bronchi and a **laryngoscope** is used to examine the larynx. These are lighted, tubular instruments.

Purpose	Normal Values	Nursing Implications
Respiratory endoscopy is used to view lesions, obtain a biopsy, improve drainage, remove foreign substances, and drain abscesses.	No obstructions are normally found in respiratory passageways, and tissues appear normal.	An informed consent is necessary for endoscopy. Endoscopic examinations are uncomfortable for most clients, especially the bronchoscopy, and the client should be prepared for this. The client should be without food or fluid for 4 hr–6 hr prior to endoscopy to avoid the risk of aspirating stomach contents. An analgesic, sedative, or tranquilizer is generally given about 1/2 hr before endoscopy. The client should be taught that there may be gagging when local anesthesia is applied to the throat and there is a feeling that one cannot swallow or breathe. However, the airway remains open. Aftercare includes withholding fluids and food, usually for an hour or two, until the client can swallow and cough. Vital signs should be checked for signs of atelectasis and pneumonitis. Warm gargles may be used to relieve irritation in the pharynx. The client should be observed for **hemoptysis,** which is sputum containing blood, and for excessive bleeding, especially if a biopsy has been obtained.

(Continued)

Purpose	Normal Values	Nursing Implications
		If contrast media were used during the examination, the client should be helped and encouraged to cough to rid the bronchial tree of the material.

Skin tests determine antigen–antibody reactions.

| In intradermal tests, antigens, those to which the client may have been previously exposed, are injected into the superficial layer of skin with a needle and syringe or a sterile four-pronged lancet to evaluate immune response. Patch and scratch tests, applied to hairless portions of the client's body, are used to evaluate the immune system's ability to respond to known allergens. | Negative reactions indicate a lack of sensitivity. Positive reactions, which indicate a positive antigen–antibody reaction, are discussed in clinical texts. | Check the client's history for hypersensitivity to any of the test antigens. If positive, notify physician prior to performing tests. These skin tests are not usually performed with infants because of their immature immune system. If the client is an outpatient, instruct him to return at the appropriate time to have the test results read. Do not perform tests in areas with acne, dermatitis, or excessive hair. On the chart, record the test, time, date, method, and site of administration. After reading the results, document the reaction noting amount of erythema or induration. |

Radiography is an x-ray examination of the lungs and thoracic cavity.

| X-ray examinations of the lungs are done to help diagnose pulmonary diseases and to determine the progress of development of disease. | The bony thoracic and soft tissues have normal positions, symmetry, and shape. | There is no special preparation for flat films of the chest, and the examinations are without discomfort. The client should be taught that clothing and jewelry from the waist up must be removed and that the client will be asked to hold his breath when the x-ray film is taken. |

Lung scan is the recording on a photographic plate of the emissions of radioactive waves from a substance injected into a vein as it circulates through the lung.

| A perfusion scan (Q scan) is done to measure integrity of pulmonary blood vessels and evaluate blood flow abnormalities (e.g., pulmonary emboli). A ventilation scan (V scan) is done to detect ventilation abnormalities (especially in clients with emphysema). Both scans used together provide greater and more accurate diagnostic information than either test used solely. | Q scan shows no increased uptake of radioactive drug. V scan shows no abnormalities. | Explain procedure to client. In a Q scan the radiologist injects radiopharmaceutical into a peripheral vein. Scan of chest is done in x-ray department. Client will lie under the camera for 20 min–40 min. Ventilation scan is done after the perfusion scan. Scan is completed in x-ray department after client inhales radioactive gas by mask and then exhales it out of the lungs to room air. In 8 hr the radioactive isotope disintegrates and is cleared from the circulation. |

Thoracentesis is an aspiration of fluid or air from the pleural space (see Chap 41).

| Thoracentesis provides a fluid sample for diagnostic purposes or a tissue sample for biopsy. It is also used to relieve pulmonary com- | This sample should be negative for blood, bacteria, viruses, or abnormal cells. | Informed consent is necessary. Remind client that pressure, not pain, is felt after the local anesthetic is injected. Vital signs and breath sounds are checked prior to and following the procedure. |

(Continued)

T A B L E   34-2
Common Methods to Assess Respiratory Functioning   (Continued)

Purpose	Normal Values	Nursing Implications
pression and respiratory distress in clients with a variety of disorders.		Expose the entire chest for the procedure, and shave aspiration site. This sterile procedure necessitates the client to lay on the unaffected side or to sit with the overbed table supporting the head and arms. After the catheter is removed, the site is covered with a sterile dressing and observed for any drainage. Chest x-ray is usually done as part of the procedure to verify no complications. Documentation of amount of fluid, color, viscosity, and client response should appear in the nursing notes.

2. Activity intolerance related to ineffective airway clearance during and after baseball games, fatigue, and stress. Here the activity intolerance is the problem statement and ineffective airway clearance is just ne of the many factors *contributing to the problem.* All the nursing interventions will be directed to improving the tolerance for activity.
3. Ineffective individual coping related to stress of career choices and stress of performance during baseball games as demonstrated by recent increase in episodes of asthmatic attacks. In this case the ineffective airway clearance is a *symptom* of the client's real problem, ineffective coping. Nursing interventions will be directed to reducing stressors. When client is able to improve the use of his coping

skills, the expected outcome is that the number of asthma attacks will decrease.

Each nursing diagnosis is unique to the situation, and the etiology varies with each client. The nurse, with the client, decides which problem is the priority. With creativity and patience, the nurse arrives at a nursing diagnosis that clearly directs nursing interventions and client goals. However, there might be interventions initiated by another member of the health-care team for the nurse to follow (*e.g.,* the prescription for administering medications). This would be the dependent aspect of nursing practice. The interdependent aspect refers to problems in which the nurse and other health-care team members collaborate to treat (*e.g.,* nurses monitoring side-effects of prescribed medications).

T A B L E   34-3
Sample Nursing Diagnoses for Common Respiratory Problems

Title	Etiologic or Contributing Factors	Sample Defining Characteristics
Ineffective airway clearance	Thick yellow secretions, fever, fatigue, dehydration, poor nutrition.	"I never feel as though I am getting enough air". Seventy-year-old man with a 20-year history of COPD, recent development of pneumonia. He is pale with circumoral cyanosis. His respiratory rate is 40 per minute and shallow. Rhonchi are auscultated bilaterally. He does not sit quietly in chair or on bed. He cannot walk length of room without coughing episode which produces little sputum.
Impaired gas exchange	Smokes one pack per day. Works with asbestos in auto factory. Has had a cold for 7 days.	Cyanotic 50-year-old male. Using pursed-lip breathing while sitting on emergency room stretcher. Sitting hunched forward with overbed table supporting arms. Altered blood gases show respiratory acidosis. Admits to shortness of breath, nausea, and ankle edema for 1 week.
Ineffective breathing pattern	Anxious about results of cardiac catheterization and possible cardiac surgery.	Hyperventilating, tachypnea (40 min). "I have a tingling feeling in my fingers."

PLANNING: CLIENT GOALS

Whenever nurses care for clients with an alteration in respiratory functioning, nursing measures are supportive of the following general client goals:

- Client demonstrates improved gas exchange in his lungs by an absence of cyanosis or chest pain.
- Client relates causative factors, if known, and relates adaptive method of coping with the factors.
- Client preserves pulmonary function by maintaining optimal level of activity.
- Client demonstrates self-care behaviors which provide relief from symptoms and prevent further pulmonary problems.

When the client's physical, psychosocial, and spiritual conditions contribute to alterations in respiratory function, individualized client goals are developed with the client's input. For example: "By March 15 the client will be able to walk up one flight of steps at home without dyspnea."

IMPLEMENTING

Establishing a Trusting Nurse–Client Relationship

Most persons with a deviation in respiratory functioning experience anxiety as a result of symptoms and an actual or potential loss of independence. The nurse needs to create an environment that is likely to reduce anxieties. Immediate discomfort should be treated. Use of effective listening skills and accurate observation validates a caring attitude. Nurses must seek to understand clients' life experiences and habits without prejudging them. Clients often bring a fear of stigma into a professional relationship (especially with detrimental health habits), and this will impede the application of nursing interventions. The client who believes the nurse is genuinely concerned about him or her and the family will be more willing to work toward achieving mutually desirable goals.

Promoting Proper Breathing

Deep Breathing

Habits of breathing that are not conducive to maximal respiratory functioning are common in well and ill persons. Some people develop a pattern of shallow breathing or walk with a "caved in" chest wall. Ill persons, for any number of reasons, may limit respiratory efforts. Hypoventilation occurs when there is a decreased amount of air entering and leaving the lungs. Deep-breathing exercises to produce hyperventilation, a condition in which there is more than the normal amount of air entering and leaving the lungs, are often used to overcome hypoventilation.

The nurse will instruct the client to make each breath deep enough to move the bottom ribs. Unless there is a nasal condition that prohibits or prevents normal breathing, the client should start slow, deep ventilations nasally and expire slowly through the mouth. Breathing through the nose warms, filters, and humidifies the air. Respiratory status, motivation, and general clinical condition will dictate the timing of this exercise, done hourly while awake or four times daily.

In incentive spirometry (Fig. 34-5) the client takes a deep breath and observes the results of his efforts registered on the spirometry equipment as he sustains that maximal inspiration. (The mechanical device is three balls that rise in each cylinder. The electronic device has numbers or squares which are illuminated when the client inhales deeply.) Instructions are necessary prior to its use. This intervention offers immediate positive reinforcement to the client for his breathing efforts.

Breathing Exercises

Breathing exercises are designed to aid the client to achieve more efficient and controlled ventilations, to decrease the work of breathing, and to correct respiratory defects.

Abdominal or Diaphragmatic Breathing. Many people with COPD have a tendency to breathe in a shallow, rapid, and exhausting pattern. This type of upper chest breathing can be changed to diaphragmatic breathing,

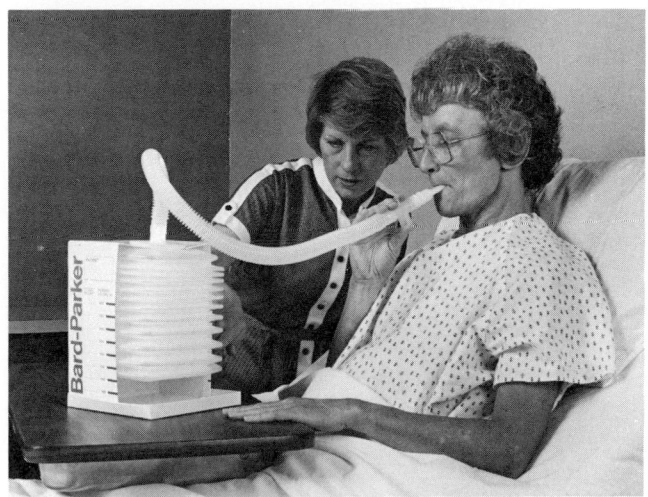

F I G U R E 34-5
The client is being taught how to use the incentive spirometer. When the client inhales, the accordion-pleated cylinder in the spirometer rises as it collapses. The goal is to cause as much collapse of the cylinder as possible while inhaling deeply.

R E S E A R C H   I N   N U R S I N G   *Making a Difference*

Oxygenation

All body cells require oxygen in order to function, and supplying the body with oxygen is fundamental to life. Both of the following studies have important implications for tailoring client care to promote efficient gas exchange. Because today's health care system is characterized by decreased lengths of stay, nursing is challenged to develop strategies to facilitate recovery without compromising care.

Related Research

Winslow EH, Lane LD, Gaffney FA: Oxygen uptake and cardiovascular responses in control: Adults and acute myocardial infarction patients during bathing. Nurs Res 34(3):164–169, 1985

Teaching energy conservation measures to post myocardial infarction patients has long been a widely practiced nursing intervention. Yet the actual "metabolic cost" of many activities of daily living have yet to be measured scientifically. This research team obtained data on three different bathing procedures (shower, bath, basin) by measuring the amount of cardiac stress that the different bathing methods cause. During the three bathing procedures, oxygen consumption was less than three times that of resting levels, and the clients had lower VO2 during bathing than the control subjects. This was related to the fact that the clients took their time while bathing and sat down to dry themselves off while the control subjects stood up. Peak heart rates and dysrhythmias did not differ significantly among the three types of baths. These researchers conclude that clients with cardiac problems can take tub baths or showers earlier on in their hospitalization.

Janson-Bjerklie S, Kohlman Carrieri V, Hudes M: The sensations of pulmonary dyspnea. Nurs Res 35(3):154–159, 1986

The purpose of this study was to describe the sensation of dyspnea in different pulmonary disease categories: emphysema, bronchitis, asthma, vascular and restrictive disease. This study focused particularly on factors precipitating dyspnea, predictable indicators of dyspnea, physical and emotional sensations perceived during acute episodes, and symptoms that could be observed by others. The frequency of symptoms was similar among the various diseases, but the intensity of dyspnea varied significantly. Variables related to dyspnea were disease group, social support, and attendance at a "better breather" class.

Summary

Apparently clients with cardiac disease pace themselves when carrying out activities requiring a high oxygen demand. Although further study is needed, it appears that activity restriction of clients with cardiac disease should not be standardized. Rather, nursing care involves monitoring cardiac status with varying activities and, thus, promoting individualized progress. Nurses caring for clients with respiratory dysfunction should help their clients learn more about what triggers acute episodes of dyspnea. Clients can then be taught preventive strategies of avoiding the respiratory irritant. In summary, care of clients with oxygen needs should be individualized.

---

reducing the rate, increasing the tidal volume, and reducing the functional residual capacity. The client is instructed to place one hand on the stomach and the other on the middle of the chest. He now should breathe in slowly through the nose, letting the abdomen protrude as far as it will go. Next, he should breathe out through pursed lips while contracting the abdominal muscles. One hand should be pressing inward and upward on the abdomen. These steps should be repeated for 1 minute followed by rest for 2 minutes. The breathing pattern should be practiced several times during the day, and eventually it will become automatic.

Pursed Lip Breathing.   Clients who experience dyspnea and feelings of panic often obtain control of the respiration by using pursed lip breathing. This exercise trains the muscles to prolong exhalation, increasing airway pressure during expiration and loosening the amount of airway trapping and resistance. To do this the client inhales through the nose while counting to three and exhales slowly and evenly against pursed lips while tightening the abdominal muscles. During exhalation, the client counts to seven. To purse the lips, the client should position the lips as though he were sucking through a straw or whistling. While walking, the client

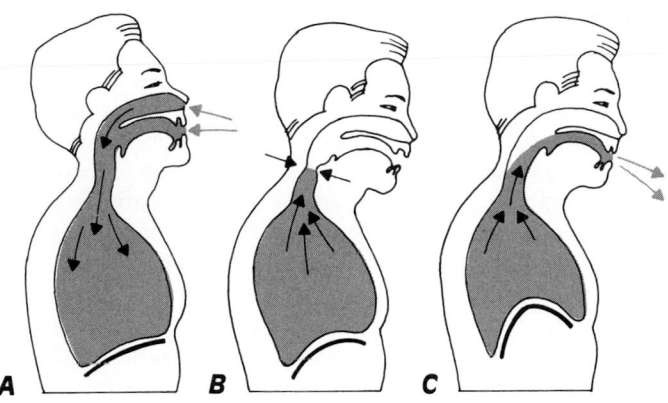

FIGURE 34-6
(A) A cough begins with a deep inspiration, distending the trachea and hyperinflating the lungs. (B) After inspiration, the glottis closes while intercostal and abdominal muscles contract forcibly. (C) When intrathoracic pressure reaches a high level, the glottis opens slightly, the diaphragm is pushed up, producing an explosive movement of air.

should inhale while walking two steps and then exhale through pursed lips while taking the next four steps and then repeat the cycle.

Prior to teaching these techniques, the nurse should practice them alone and then with a partner.

Promoting and Controlling Coughing

The presence of excessive fluids or secretions in an organ or body tissue is called **congestion**, and a person with secretions or fluid in his lungs is said to have congested lungs. If his cough is dry, he is said to be congested with a **nonproductive cough**. If his cough produces respiratory tract secretions, he is referred to as being congested with a **productive cough**. Thick respiratory secretions are sometimes called **phlegm**. A client who is coughing with no congestion or secretions produced is described as being noncongested with a nonproductive cough.

The Cough Mechanism. The cough mechanism (Fig. 34-6) consists of an initial irritation: a deep inspiration; a quick, tight closure of the glottis together with a forceful contraction of the expiratory intercostal muscles; and the upward push of the diaphragm. This causes an explosive movement of air from the lower to the upper respiratory tract. To be effective, a cough should have enough muscle contraction to force air to be expelled and to propel a liquid or a solid on its way out of the respiratory tract. This is most effective when the client is sitting upright with feet flat on the floor. A cough is a cleaning mechanism of the body. It is a means of helping to keep the airway clear of secretions and other debris.

Voluntary Coughing. When a cough does not occur as a result of reflex stimulation of the cough-sensitive areas, it can be induced voluntarily. Teaching the client to cough voluntarily is an important aspect of pre- and postoperative care. Although the teaching of deep breathing and coughing is relatively easy, experience has shown that is difficult to have the client follow through and do them on his own. Frequent reminders throughout the day are necessary for many clients. Having a specific schedule on the nursing care plan is advised. Coughing early in the morning after rising removes phlegm that accumulated during the night. Coughing prior to meals improves the taste of food and oxygenation. At bedtime, coughing will remove any build-up of phlegm and will improve sleep patterns. For the client who is unable to cough voluntarily, manual stimulation over the trachea and prolonged exhalation can be helpful. If neither of these methods is successful, mechanical endotracheal suctioning with a catheter is used sometimes.

Involuntary Coughing. Involuntary coughing often accompanies respiratory tract infections and irritations. It helps clear the airway if it is productive, but it is fatiguing and irritating when it is nonproductive. Medication may control involuntary coughing. Observations of the characteristics of breathing and coughing are necessary to determine the appropriate type of medication.

Cough Suppressants. Suppressants are drugs that depress a body function, in this case, the cough reflex. Codeine, which is present in many cough preparations, is generally considered the preferred cough suppressant ingredient. However, codeine can be addictive. Because of possible abuse, many states require a physician's prescription for its use. Dextromethorphan hydrobromide is considered by some authorities to be as effective as codeine, and it is not addictive. Diphenhydramine hydrochloride, a potent antihistamine, is an effective cough suppressant. However, drowsiness (also common in other antihistamines) is a side-effect of its use. Therefore, it may not be safe to use when the person must remain alert, as when driving a car.

An irritating nonproductive cough in persons without congestion may be appropriately treated with suppressants. Inappropriate suppression of the cough in a person with respiratory congestion can result in harmful retention of the secretions.

Expectorants. Expectorants are drugs that facilitate the removal of respiratory tract secretions by reducing the secretion viscosity. Clients with extremely tenacious secretions may need the secretions liquefied so the cough can be effective. In that way, the nonproductive cough of a person with lung congestion can become productive. An expectorant used by a person who does not have congestion is inappropriate. Ammonium chloride, terpin hydrate, and ipecac have been widely used as expectorants in cough preparations. Adequate fluid intake and air humidification are considered effective expectorants by some authorities.

Lozenges.

Mild nonproductive coughs in persons without congestion can often be relieved by lozenges. A **lozenge** is a small, solid medication intended to be held in the mouth until it dissolves. Lozenges generally control coughs by the local anesthetic effect of benzocaine. The local anesthetic can act on sensory and motor nerves by controlling the primary irritation and by inhibiting afferent and efferent impulses.

Teaching About Cough Preparations.

Because cough preparations are so readily available and persons who purchase them are usually eager for relief, the consumer sometimes takes excessive amounts of more than one type. The nurse can offer health teaching about the appropriate choice of expectorants and suppressants. Also, the nurse should teach other misuses of cough mixtures. For example, cough syrups with a high sugar or alcohol content can disturb the metabolic balance of persons with diabetes mellitus. Preparations containing antihistamines have an anticholinergic action, which can cause serious problems for persons with glaucoma, or cause urinary retention in men with prostate enlargement. Other cough preparations can be detrimental to persons with hypertension and with thyroid and cardiac diseases. In addition, prolonged use of self-prescribed cough preparations can conceal more serious health problems.

Promoting Comfort

Positioning.

Helping an incapacitated client assume a position that allows free movement of the diaphragm and expansion of the chest wall promotes ease of respiration. For example, sitting in a slumped position, which permits the abdominal contents to push upward on the diaphragm, results in less lung expansion during inspiration. Persons with dyspnea and orthonea are most comfortable in a high Fowler's position because the accessory muscles can then be used easily to promote respiration.

Maintaining Adequate Fluid Intake.

Secretions can be kept thin by having the client drink 2 qt to 3 qt (1.9 L–2.9 L) of clear fluid daily. The client's fluid intake should be increased to the maximum that his health state will tolerate. The client who has an elevated temperature, who is breathing through his mouth, who is coughing, or who is losing excessive body fluids in other ways should have special attention focused on his intake. If there is incidence of right side heart failure, fluid intake should not exceed 1.5 qt (1.4 L) daily. Milk products (milk, ice cream, yogurt, cheese, and so forth) work to thicken secretions and congestion. Clear fluids include water, apple juice, broths, and Jello.

Providing Humidified Air.

When air humidity is low, artificial means for humidifying inspired air may be advisable. The inspiration of dry air removes the normal moisture in the respiratory passages, which is essential for protection from irritation and infection. Room humidifiers may be helpful for some patients. Electric vaporizers that produce steam or cool mist are available. Authorities believe the therapeutic value of one over the other has not been demonstrated. A cool-mist vaporizer does not present dangers with burns because it does not generate heat or hot water. However, it can provide the medium for pathogen growth if not cleaned adequately. The steam vaporizer does not present this problem.

Percussing.

Cupping (Fig. 34-7) is the manual percussion of lung areas to loosen pulmonary secretions so that they can be expectorated with greater ease. Percussion by cupping with the client supine/prone is carried out as follows:

1. Cup the hand by holding it in a rigid, dome-shaped position.
2. Strike rhythmically over the lobes of the lungs to be drained while keeping your wrists, elbows, and shoulders relaxed. Move the cupped hands from the client's lower ribs to the shoulders in back, and from the lower ribs to the top of the chest in front.
3. Listen for a hollow sound while percussing. The client should experience no pain. You are probably not cupping the hand enough and are slapping the client's skin if the sound is not hollow and the client is uncomfortable.
4. Do not percuss on bare skin. The client may wear a gown or underclothing.
5. Do not percuss below the ribs or over the spine or breasts because of the danger of tissue damage.

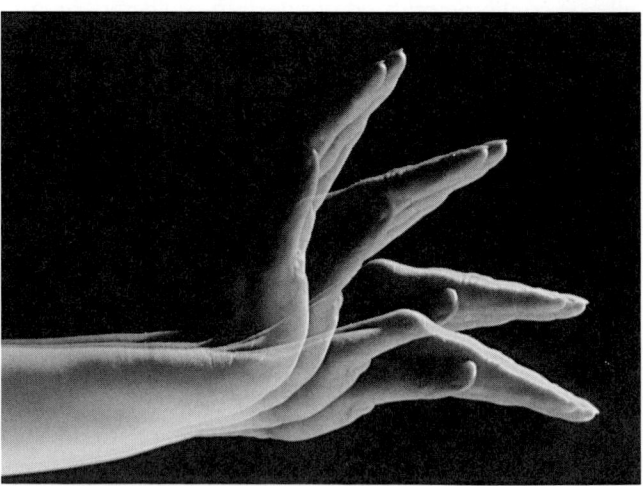

F I G U R E   34-7
The cupping position and action of the hand in manual percussion of lung area.

6. Use percussion for 30 to 60 seconds over an area several times a day, but up to 3 to 5 minutes for clients with very tenacious secretions.

The client may learn to percuss anterior surfaces of his chest wall. Family members are often taught to percuss posterior surfaces. Also, mechanical devices are available for percussion on the chest wall.

Vibrating. Vibration involves the nurse's rhythmic contraction and relaxation of the arm and shoulder muscles while holding the hands flat on the client's chest wall. The purpose is to help loosen respiratory secretions so that they can be expectorated with ease. Vibration (Fig. 34-8) is carried out as follows:

1. Place your hands flat on the client's chest wall, where vibration is desired, and hold the hands side by side with the fingers extended and together. Some authorities prefer placing one hand on top of the other.
2. Ask the client to inhale deeply and then exhale slowly.
3. While the client exhales, vibrate the chest wall by contracting and relaxing your arm and shoulder muscles rhythmically and quickly.
4. Stop vibration on the client's inhalations.
5. Do not vibrate over the client's breasts, spine, sternum, and lower rib cage.
6. Use vibration for several minutes several times a day.
7. Plan to deliver a vibration frequency of about 200 per minute.

Family members can be taught to use vibration on the client's chest wall. Also, mechanical devices are available for vibrating the chest wall.

Providing Postural Drainage. In postural drainage, gravity is used to drain secretions from the lungs. The person is positioned in a way that promotes the drainage of secretions from smaller pulmonary branches into larger ones, where they can be removed by drainage or coughing (see Fig. 34-9). Postural drainage is often preceded by vibration, percussion, or both. Postural drainage is carried out as follows:

1. Have tissues and an emesis basin close at hand for the client to use when coughing and expectorating secretions.
2. Place the client in an appropriate position to promote drainage from the lobes of the lungs, as follows:
    - Use a high Fowler's position to drain the apical sections of the upper lobes of the lungs.
    - Place the client in a lying position, half on his abdomen and half on his side, right and left, to drain the posterior sections of the upper lobes of the lungs.
    - Place the client lying on his left side with a pillow under the chest wall to drain the right lobe of the lung.

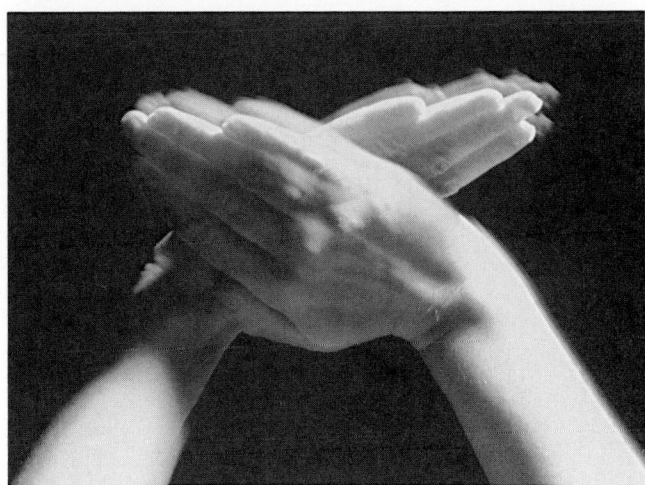

FIGURE 34-8
The position and action of the hands to use vibration to loosen respiratory secretions in the lungs.

- Place the client in Trendelenburg's position to drain the lower lobes of the lungs.
3. Carry out postural drainage two to four times a day for 20 to 30 minutes. Discontinue the drainage if the client begins to feel weak or faint.
4. Delay postural drainage after meals for 1 to 2 hours to avoid vomiting.

Maintaining Good Nutrition. Persons who are working hard at breathing often do not have energy for eating. Assessment of nutritional status is determined by measuring client's height, weight, upper arm circumference, serum protein levels, and nitrogen balance. Special attention and deliberate planning should be directed to adequate intake of proteins, vitamins, and minerals. Six small meals should be distributed over the course of the day instead of the usual three meals. Meals should be arranged 1 hour to 2 hours after breathing treatments and exercises.

Meeting Respiratory Needs with Medications. Although treating clients with medications is a dependent nursing intervention, monitoring client response and side-effects to medication is an independent nursing action. Table 34-4 shows some common medications for respiratory functioning, side-effects, and nursing implications.

Teaching Clients to Maintain Pollution-Free Environments

In addition to applying the previously discussed interventions, the client also needs to assess the environment and make adjustments where possible to factors that impair respiratory functioning. The client must actively plan to prevent exposure to pollutants. This might in-

(Text continues on p. 917.)

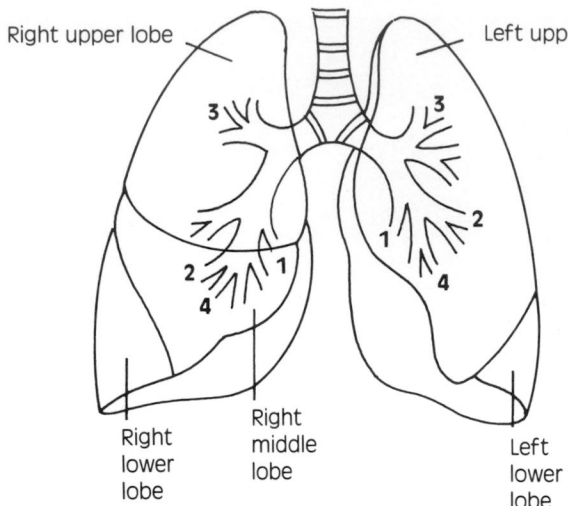

Right upper lobe

Left upper lobe

Right lower lobe

Right middle lobe

Left lower lobe

F I G U R E 34-9

Postural drainage. Shown are four positions that use the force of gravity to assist the drainage of secretions from the smaller bronchial airways into the main bronchi and trachea so the client is able to cough them up.

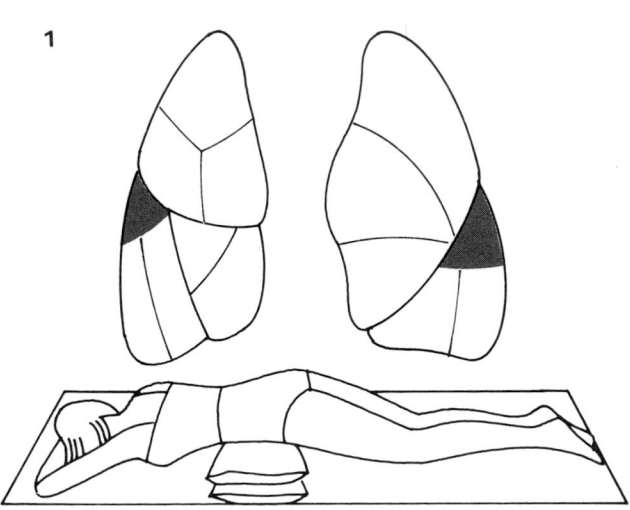

1

Lower lobes, superior segments

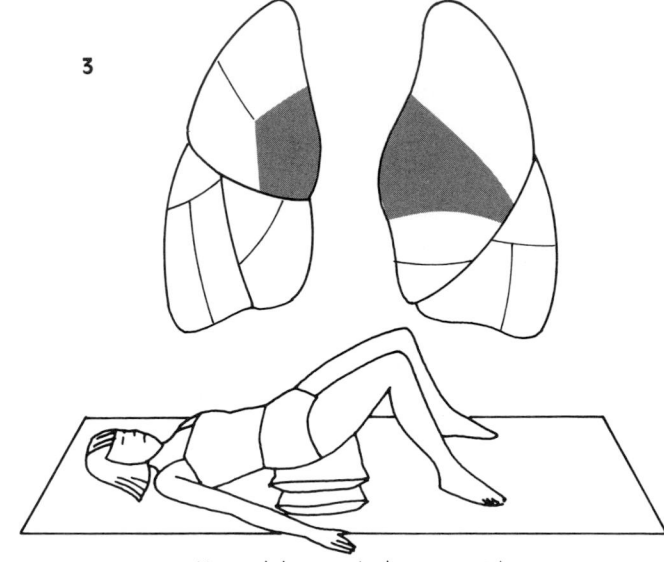

3

Upper lobes, anterior segment

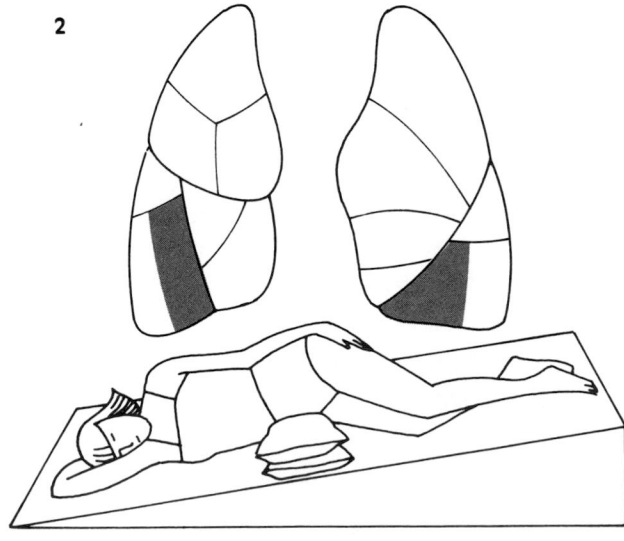

2

Lower lobes, anterior basal segment

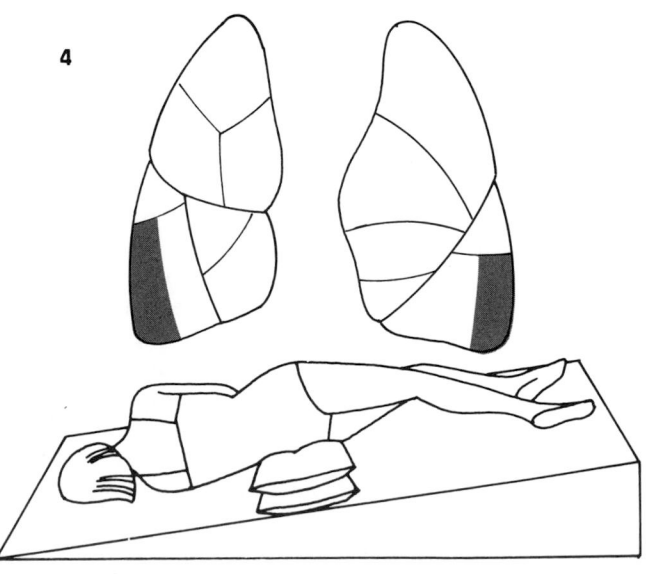

4

Lower lobes, lateral basal segment

TABLE **34-4**
Medications Used in Respiratory Functioning

Medication	Activity	Route	Side-Effects	Nursing Implications
epinephrine	Relaxes muscles that line bronchi and bronchioles	IV, SQ	Tremors, anxiety, insomnia, headache, palpitations, elevated BP, vomiting	Position client upright to prevent aspiration if vomiting occurs. Monitor heart rate, respirations, breath sounds, and BP every 15 min. May repeat medication within 15 min with an order.
isoproterenol (Isuprel)	Bronchodilator	Inhaler	Same as with epinephrine but milder	Monitor heart rate. Demonstrate proper use of inhaler. Warn client not to exceed prescribed frequency of doses.
metaproterenol (Alupent)	Bronchodilator	PO, inhalation	Same as epinephrine	Same as with epinephrine
theophylline (aminophylline)	Bronchodilator	PO, IV, rectally	Nausea, vomiting, rapid heart rate, diuresis, irritability, vertigo, convulsions	Monitor vital signs closely. Force fluids as clinical status allows. Monitor serum theophylline levels, especially if client does not respond to drug or severe side-effects develop.
Corticosteroids (ACTH, prednisone)	Reduces inflammation	PO, IV	Fluid retention, hypertension, mood swings, weight gain, gastritis, hyperglycemia	Reduce sodium intake. Make client and family aware of potential for labile emotions. Weigh daily in morning. Monitor BP and blood sugar. Warn client to follow administration directions accurately.
Antihistamines	Blocks histamine and relieves congestion of an allergic origin	PO	Drowsiness, anorexia, constipation, dry mouth, blurred vision, urinary retention	Warn client to use only with physician advice in presence of bronchial asthma. Do not mix with alcohol, tranquilizers, or sedatives. Client should avoid driving or using machinery. Observe clients for prolonged bleeding if they are using warfarin anticoagulants.
cromolyn sodium (Intal)	Prevents the release of histamines, serotonin, prostaglandin by the mast cell in an antigen–antibody reaction in asthma.	Inhaler	Cough	Remind client this is used to prevent asthma attacks, not to treat acute episodes. This drug contains lactose and will cause diarrhea in lactose-deficient clients. Inform client that this is effective only if taken on a routine basis (two to four times per day).

volve a job change, use of protective equipment, enforcement of existing laws by government agencies or subcontracting jobs. Dusting and vacuuming of work and home must be done minimally twice per week. If it is the client who must perform the tasks, a mask will prevent some symptoms of respiratory distress. Exposure to industrial or occupational hazards (*e.g.,* paint, varnish, gaseous fumes, and asbestos) must be restricted.

In the United States and Canada, fine pollutants which pose a hazard to health are monitored closely. They are carbon monoxide, sulfur dioxide, total suspended particulates, ozone, and nitrogen dioxide. On days when pollutant levels are significantly elevated, morbidity and mortality rates among people with preexisting pulmonary disease are greatly increased. Thus, on those days when pollution alerts are announced, the client with an alteration in respiratory functions should decrease activity level and stay inside using air conditioners, electronic air cleaner, or air filters. If pollen alters respiratory functions, the same principles apply.

Cigarette smoking is the most important risk factor in pulmonary disease. The inhalation of cigarette smoke increases airway resistance, reduces ciliary action, increases mucus production, causes thickening of the alveolar-capillary membrane, and causes bronchial walls to thicken and lose their elasticity. These effects are observed in the smoker and the nonsmoker (child and adult) who lives with the smoker. Habitual smokers find great difficulty in quitting or reducing smoking and need much encouragement. The American Lung Association and the American Heart Association offer many free educational materials to aid and support the client who is trying to stop smoking. Their addresses and phone numbers are listed in local telephone directories. Nurses are in a prime position to present accurate information regarding the deleterious effects of smoking and to encourage the decision to stop smoking or never to start smoking.

Providing Supplemental Oxygen

The amount of oxygen the client uses for inspiration can be increased by providing a supplemental supply. The provision of therapeutic oxygen is called oxygen therapy, and is usually prescribed by the physician. Oxygen therapy can frighten clients. Explanations from the nurse regarding procedures and purpose play a major role in reducing this fear. The client should be encouraged to discuss anxieties. If oxygen is given in an emergency, explanations concurrent with administration are appropriate.

Sources of Oxygen

Therapeutic oxygen is supplied from a wall outlet or a portable cylinder. The wall outlet source can be prepared for use quickly. The oxygen is supplied from a cental source through a pipeline, usually at 50 to 60 pounds per square inch of pressure. A specially designed flowmeter (Fig. 34-10) is attached to the outlet and opens it. A valve makes regulation of oxygen flow possible.

Oxygen can also be dispersed under pressure in steel cylinders or tanks. The tank is delivered with a protective cap to prevent accidental force against the cylinder outlet. When a standard, large-sized cylinder is full, its contents are under more than 2000 psi of pressure. The force behind an accidentally partially opened outlet could cause the tank to take off like an uncontrolled, dangerous jet. Smaller cylinders are available for emergency, ambulatory, and home use. The principles and precautions are the same for all size cylinders.

To release oxygen safely and at a desirable rate, a regulator is used. The regulator has two gauges. The one nearest the tank shows the pressure or amount of oxygen

in the tank. The other gauge indicates the number of liters per minute of oxygen being released. (Figure 34-11 shows an oxygen tank with its regulator.)

The oxygen cylinder and the regulator must be handled cautiously. The oxygen cylinder should be transported carefully, preferably strapped onto a wheeled carrier to avoid possible falling and breaking the outlet. The cylinder should be stabilized securely in a properly fitting stand.

Because of the possibility of dust and other particles becoming lodged in the outlet of the tank and being forced in the regulator, the tank is primed with two hands before a regulator is applied. The handle of the tank is turned slightly counterclockwise. This releases a small amount of oxygen and flushes out the outlet. The cylinder is closed again by turning the handle clockwise. The force with which the oxygen is released from this opening causes a loud, hissing sound which startles most people. Thus, clients and visitors need to be prepared for the noise with an appropriate explanation. It is recommended that tanks be primed away from the bedside.

Oxygen Flow Rate

The flow rate of oxygen, measured in liters per minute, is used to regulate the amount of oxygen available to the client. The rate varies depending on the condition of the client and the route of administration of the oxygen. The flow rate does not necessarily reflect the oxygen concentration actually inspired by the client because there is leaking and mixing with atmospheric air. More precise doses are usually prescribed in terms of percent of inspired oxygen. To regulate oxygen concentration accu-

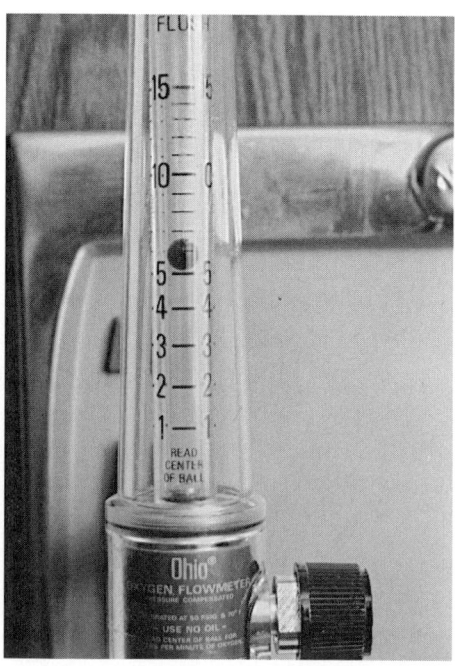

F I G U R E   34-10
Flowmeter of a piped-in oxygen-delivery system.

rately, analysis of samples of the air mixture the client is actually inhaling is recommended every 4 hours. Several types of commercial oxygen analyzers are available.

A physician prescribes the rate of oxygen administration. The nurse must monitor closely the flow rate for clients with chronic lung conditions, such as emphysema. Normally, excessive levels of carbon dioxide in the blood stimulate respirations. However, the chemoreceptors of clients with chronic lung disease become insensitive to carbon dioxide and respond to hypoxia to stimulate breathing. If excessive oxygen is given, the stimulus to breathe is removed and the client may stop breathing completely. Most clients with chronic lung disease can tolerate oxygen with a nasal cannula at 2 liters per minute but arterial blood gas analysis should be monitored closely.

Humidifying Oxygen

Unless oxygen is humidified, there is excessive drying of the mucous membranes lining the respiratory tract. Distilled water, normal saline, or a medicated solution may be used to humidify oxygen. Oxygen passes through these solutions with little loss. There is an exception: certain masks may be used that humidify oxygen before it is inhaled with moisture from the client's exhalations. This will be discussed later in this section.

Precautions For Oxygen Administration

Oxygen, which constitutes 20% of normal air, is a tasteless, odorless, colorless gas. It supports combustion. To prevent fires and injuries, the following precautions must be taken:

- Avoid open flames in the client's room.
- Place "No Smoking" signs in conspicuous places in the client's room. Instruct client and visitors on the hazard of smoking with oxygen in use.
- Check to see that electric equipment used in the room, such as electric bell cords, razors, radios, and suctioning equipment, is in good working order and emits no sparks.
- Avoid wearing and using synthetic fabrics which build up static electricity.
- Avoid using oils in the area. Oil can ignite spontaneously in the presence of oxygen.

Oxygen Administration

Oxygen can be administered by nasal cannula, nasal catheter, transtracheal oxygen, simple mask, partial rebreather mask, nonrebreathing mask, and Venturi mask and tent.

Nasal Cannula. A nasal cannula, also called nasal prongs, is probably the most commonly used aid to breathing. The cannula is a disposable, plastic device with two protruding prongs for insertion into the nostrils connected to an oxygen source with a humidifier and

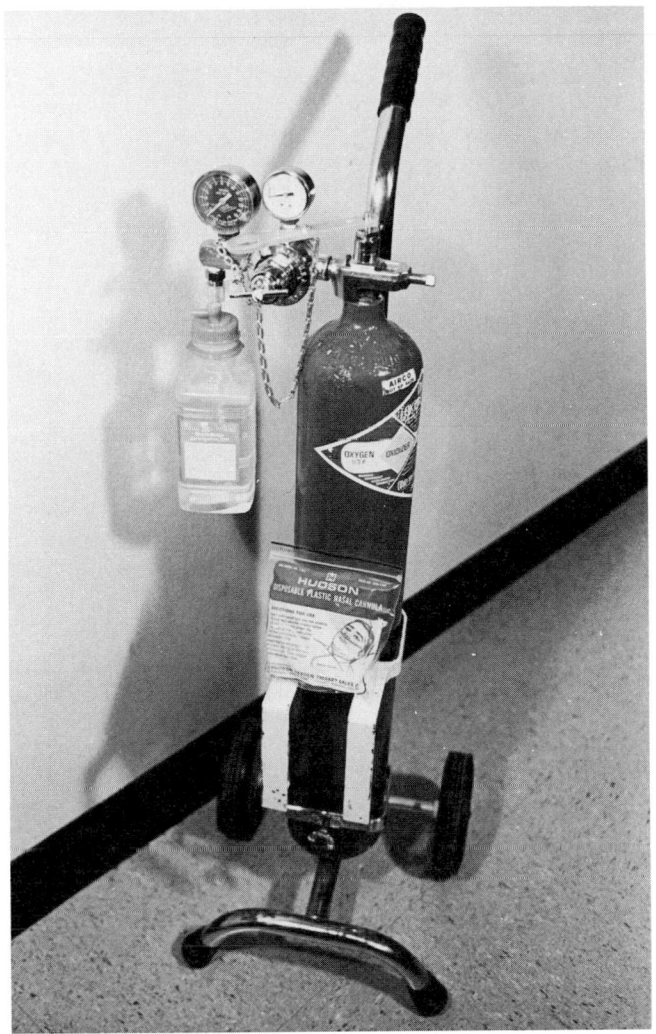

FIGURE 34-11
A small cylinder of oxygen is in readiness for an emergency or transfer situations. The regulator and humidifier bottle are attached and ready to use.

flowmeter. The cannula does not impede eating or speaking. Procedure 34-1 explains oxygen administration by nasal cannula.

Nasal Catheter. A nasal, or oropharyngeal, catheter (Fig. 34-12) is another efficient means for administering oxygen. It is inserted into the throat through one nostril and must be changed to the other nostril every 8 hours. Gastric distention often occurs because the gas flow can be misdirected into the stomach.

Transtrachial Oxygen Delivery. Clients using continuous supplemental oxygen therapy have another alternative: transtracheal oxygen delivery. A small catheter is inserted percutaneously into the trachea under local anesthesia. Clients usually report improved mobility, comfort, appearance, and lower cost with this delivery system.

(Text continues on p. 921.)

PROCEDURE 34-1
Administering Oxygen by Nasal Cannula

Equipment

Flowmeter connected to oxygen supply

Humidifier with sterile distilled water

Nasal cannula and tubing

Gauze to pad tubing over ears (optional)

Action	**Rationale**
1 Explain procedure to client and review safety precautions necessary when oxygen is in use. Place "No Smoking" signs in appropriate areas.	Oxygen supports combustion.

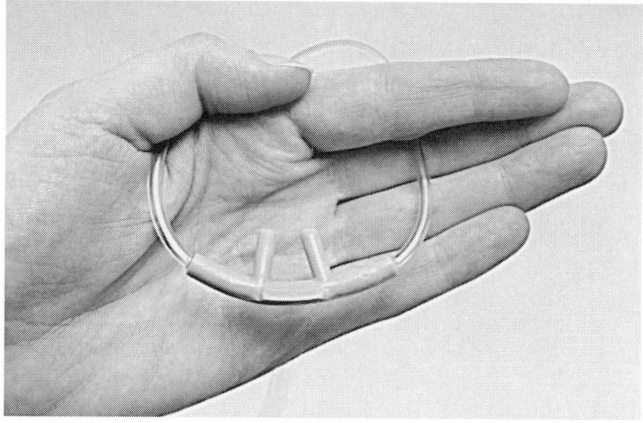

Nasal cannula.

2 Wash your hands.

Handwashing deters the spread of microorganisms.

3 Connect the nasal cannula to the oxygen set-up with humidification. Adjust the flow rate as ordered by physician. Check that oxygen is flowing out of prongs.

Oxygen forced through a water reservoir is humidified before it is delivered to the client, thus preventing dehydration of the mucous membranes.

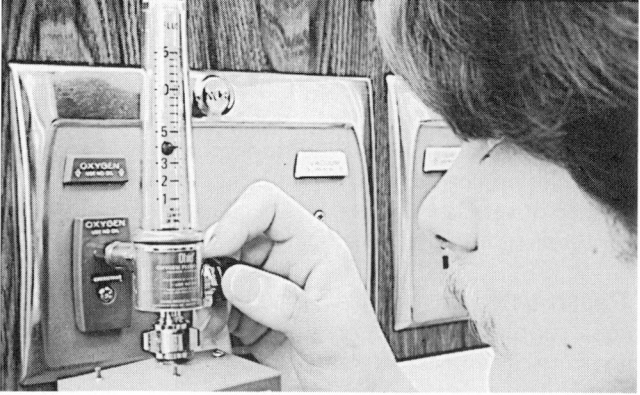

Step 3: Adjusting flow rate.

(Continued)

Action

4 Place the prongs in the client's nostrils. See figure. Adjust according to type of equipment:

  a. Over and behind each ear with adjuster comfortably under chin or

  b. Around the client's head

Rationale

Correct placement of the prongs and fastener facilitates oxygen administration and comfort for the client.

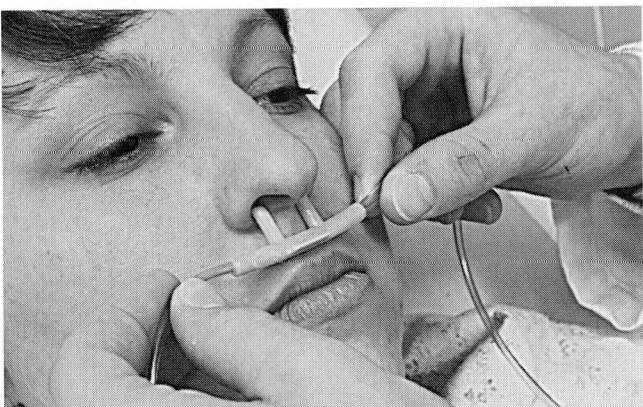

Step 4: Placing cannula prongs in nostrils.

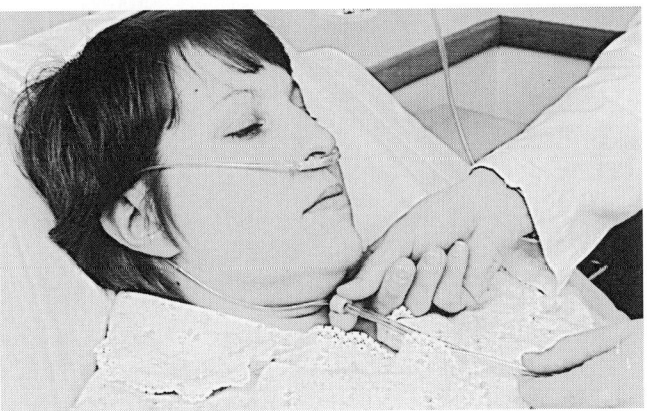

Step 4: Adjusting for comfort.

5 Use gauze pads at ears beneath the tubing as necessary.

Pads reduce irritation and pressure and protect the skin.

6 Encourage client to breathe through his nose with his mouth closed.

Provides for optimal delivery of oxygen to client

7 Wash your hands.

Handwashing deters the spread of microorganisms.

8 Assess and chart client's response to therapy.

Client's respirations, color, and so forth indicate effectiveness of oxygen therapy.

9 Remove and clean the cannula and nares at least every 8 hr or according to agency recommendations. Check nares for evidence of irritation or bleeding.

The continued presence of the cannula causes irritation and dryness of the mucuous membranes. Lubricant counteracts the drying effects of oxygen.

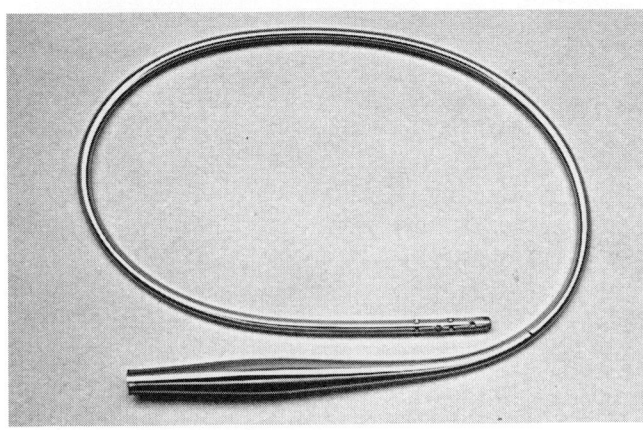

F I G U R E   34-12
A nasal catheter for administering oxygen.

Face Masks. Disposable and reusable face masks are available in plastic and rubber. The mask should be fitted carefully to the client's face to avoid leakage of oxygen. It should be comfortably snug but not tight against the client's face. The most commonly used types of masks include the simple face mask, the partial rebreather mask, the nonrebreather mask, the total rebreathing mask, and the Venturi mask. Procedure 34-2 describes actions and rationale in using face masks.

The *simple oxygen mask* connects to oxygen tubing, a humidifier, and a flowmeter, just as the nasal cannula does. At a flow rate of 6 to 10 liters per minute, the mask delivers 35% to 60% oxygen. This mask has vents on its sides which allow room air to leak in at many places, thereby diluting the source oxygen. Often it is used when an increased delivery of oxygen is needed for short

(Text continues on p. 923.)

Administering Oxygen by Mask

Equipment

Flowmeter con-
nected to oxy-
gen supply
Humidifier with
sterile distilled
water

Face mask specified
by physician

Gauze to pad elastic
band (optional)

Action	Rationale
1 Explain procedure to client and review safety pre-cautions necessary when oxygen is in use. Place "No Smoking" signs in appropriate areas.	Oxygen supports combustion. Explanation alleviates anxiety.
2 Wash your hands.	Handwashing deters the spread of microorganisms.
3 Attach the face mask to the oxygen set-up with hu-midification. Start the flow of oxygen at the speci-fied rate.	Oxygen forced through a water reservoir is humidified before it is delivered to the client, thus preventing de-hydration of the mucous membranes.
4 Position the face mask over the client's nose and mouth. Adjust it with the elastic strap so that the mask fits snugly but comfortably on the face.	A loose or poorly fitting mask will result in oxygen loss and decreased therapeutic value. Masks may cause feel-ing of suffocation, and client needs frequent attention and reassurance.
5 Use gauze pads to reduce irritation on the client's ears and scalp.	Pads reduce irritation and pressure and protect the skin.
6 Wash your hands.	Handwashing deters the spread of microorganisms.
7 Remove the mask and dry the skin every 2 hr–3 hr if the oxygen is running continuously. Do not powder around the mask.	The tight-fitting mask and moisture from condensation can irritate the skin on the face. There is danger of in-haling powder if it is placed on the mask.
8 Assess and chart client's response to therapy.	Client's respiratory rate and pattern, color, and so forth indicate effectiveness of oxygen therapy.

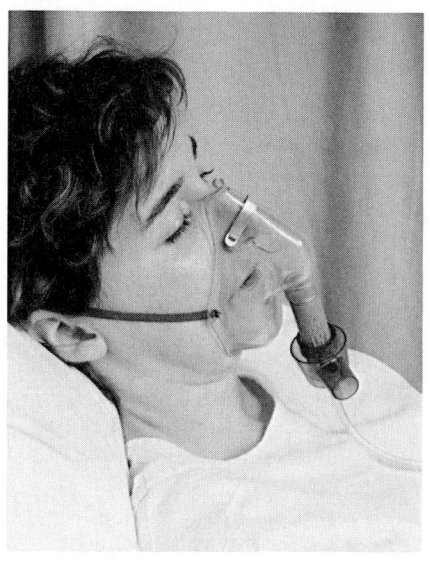

Venturi mask.

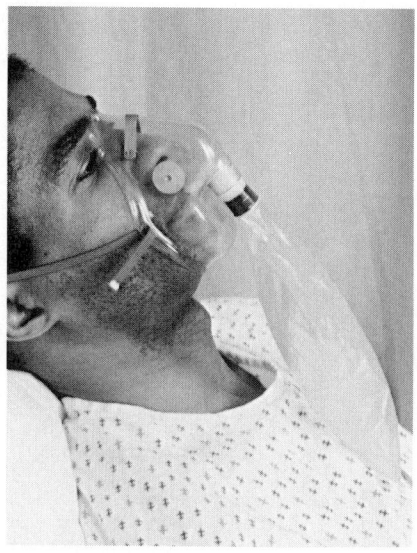

Nonrebreather mask.

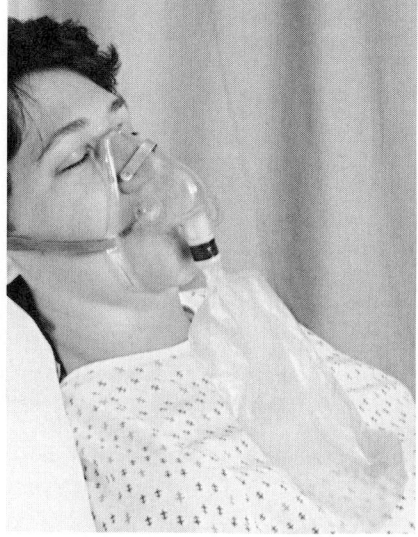

Partial rebreather mask.

periods (*i.e.,* less than 12 hours). This mask should cover the nose and the mouth if the client breathes through the mouth.

The *partial rebreather mask* is equipped with a reservoir bag for the collection of the first parts of the client's exhaled air. The air is mixed with 100% oxygen for the next inhalation. The client rebreathes approximately one third of the expired air from the reservoir bag. The remaining exhaled air exits through vents. The use of this type of mask permits the conservation of oxygen. This bag should deflate slightly with inspiration. If it deflates completely, the flow rate should be increased until only a slight deflation is noted.

The *nonrebreather mask* provides the highest concentration of oxygen with a mask to a spontaneously breathing client. It offers the most precise method of administration. It is similar to the partial rebreather mask except two one-way valves prevent conservation of exhaled air. The reservoir bag is filled with oxygen which enters the mask on inspiration. Exhaled air escapes 'through side vents. This mask can also be used to administer other gases.

The *total rebreathing mask* also has a reservoir bag, but it has no opening to the atmosphere. The exhaled carbon dioxide is absorbed by a chemical, and the reservoir bag supplies other gases. This type of mask may also be used for the administration of oxygen and anesthetic gases.

The *Venturi mask* gets its name from the Venturi effect which allows the mask to deliver exact concentrations of oxygen. This mask has a large tube with an oxygen inlet. As the tube narrows, the pressure drops, causing air to be sucked in through side ports. These ports are adjusted according to the prescription for oxygen concentration. It is a nursing responsibility to make sure the ports are always open. If these are occluded by linens, clothing, or a client rolling on it, the oxygen delivered might be at an unsafe concentration.

Oxygen Tent. Finally, oxygen can be administered via a tent, a light, portable structure made of clear plastic and attached to a motor-driven unit. The motor helps to circulate and cool the air in the tent. The cooling device functions on the same principles as an electric refrigeration unit. A thermostat in the unit keeps the tent at the temperature considered most comfortable for the client. The tent fits over the top part of the bed so that the client's head and thorax are in the tent. It has side openings through which nursing care can be administered. Today, it is commonly used with pediatric clients who need a cool and highly humidified air flow (*e.g.,* clients with pneumonia). The tent does not allow the maintenance of a satisfactory or precise oxygen concentration and thus, is usually not used outside of pediatrics. See Procedure 34-3.

Using Artificial Airways

Oropharyngeal and Nasopharyngeal Airways

An oropharyngeal or nasopharyngeal airway is a semicircular tube of plastic or rubber inserted into the back of the pharynx through the mouth or nose in the spontaneously breathing client. It is used to keep the tongue clear of the airway and to permit suctioning of secretions. It is often used for postoperative clients until they regain consciousness.

Endotracheal Tube

An endotracheal tube (Fig. 34-13) is an plastic airway inserted through the nose or the mouth into the trachea by a physician or anesthetist. It is used to administer oxygen by mechanical ventilator, to suction secretions easily, or to bypass upper airway obstructions (*e.g.,* tongue or tracheal edema). The cuffed endotracheal tube is commonly used to prevent air leakage and bronchial aspiration of foreign material. The nurse must take special precautions against excessive and prolonged inflation of the cuff to avoid tracheal edema and necrosis. Periodic deflation of the cuff should be scheduled in consultation with the physician and included in the nursing care plan based on institutional protocols.

Tracheostomy

A tracheostomy is an artificial opening made into the trachea. The curved tube inserted into this opening is made of plastic or metal. It measures 5 cm to 7.5 cm (2 inches–3 inches) in length. Some tracheostomy tubes have two cannulas. The outer cannula remains in place in the trachea while the inner cannula is removed for cleaning. A tracheostomy tube is insrted for a variety of reasons (*e.g.,* to replace an endotracheal tube, to provide a method to mechanically ventilate, to bypass an upper airway obstruction, or to remove tracheobronchial secretions). It is inserted in the operating room or intensive care unit under sterile conditions using local anesthesia. The tracheostomy tube is held in place by tapes fastened around the client's neck. Usually, a sterile, square piece of gauze is placed between the skin and

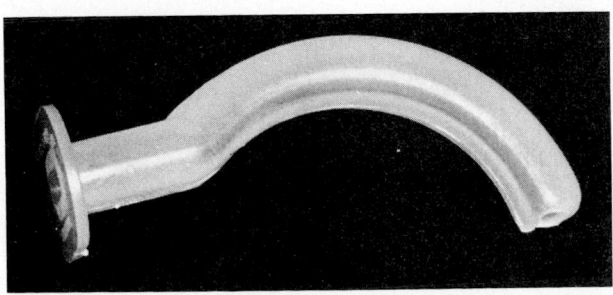

F I G U R E **34-13**
The plastic disposable airway is inserted through the mouth and is shaped to follow the contour of the mouth and upper respiratory tract. When placed properly, the airway holds the tongue so that it cannot drop back and into the throat. It can be suctioned easily if secretions accumulate.

PROCEDURE 34-3
Administering Oxygen by Tent

Equipment

Oxygen tent with tubing, flow regulator, and oxygen analyzer
Oxygen source

Humidifier
Sterile distilled water

Bath blankets
Ice

Action	Rationale
1 Explain procedure to client and family.	Reassures client and facilitates cooperation.
2 Gather equipment.	Provides for organized approach to task.
3 Wash your hands.	Handwashing deters the spread of microorganisms.
4 Use bath blanket to cover plastic mattress. Place second bath blanket over bottom sheet.	Bath blanket minimizes potential for static electricity from plastic mattress. Additional bath blanket is used to provide warmth and absorb moisture.
5 Prepare tent and position over bed. Attach to oxygen source.	Tent allows oxygen to be delivered in a confined environment.
6 Fill ice trough or start refrigeration component.	Ice or refrigeration unit cools the air in the tent.
7 Fill nebulizer or humidifier to recommended level with sterile distilled water. Turn on flowmeter and adjust oxygen flow to deliver required amount. Use oxygen analyzer now and recheck at least every 4 hr.	Humidification of oxygen prevents excessive drying of the respiratory tract. Oxygen analyzer measures oxygen concentration.
8 Place client in tent. Observe all safety precautions.	Oxygen supports combustion.
9 Secure tent between folded top sheet and under mattress.	Oxygen is heavier than air. If tent is not secure, oxygen content may be decreased.
10 Wash your hands.	Handwashing deters the spread of microorganisms.
11 Open tent as little as possible by organizing nursing care.	Maintains oxygen content in tent
12 Assess client at frequent intervals (vital signs, color, response to therapy). Monitor equipment on a frequent basis.	Oxygen toxicity may develop in response to exposure to a high concentration of oxygen.
13 Change gown and linens as necessary. Edges of tent may be loosened, and tent may be secured with bath blanket under client's chin when performing hygienic care or other procedures.	Provides warmth and comfort
14 Record type of therapy and client's response.	Provides accurate documentation of procedure

outer wings of the tube before the tube is tied. This tracheostomy dressing must be kept dry to prevent infection and skin irritation. The tracheostomy can be temporary or permanent.

The lower part of many tracheostomy tubes has inflatable cuffs. The distended cuff seals the opening around the tube against air leakage and entrance of foreign bodies. Care should be exercised to avoid overinflation of the cuff and to schedule routine deflation to avoid tracheal edema or necrosis of the mucous membranes. In some cases the cuff may be deflated every hour. Cuffs that mechanically deflate and inflate regularly prevent these complications. However, it remains a nursing responsibility to monitor equipment function and client condition. There are also low-pressure cuffs which exert minimum pressure on the tracheal mucosa. This type usually does not require periodic deflation.

The tracheostomy tube must remain free from foreign objects and nonsterile materials. Cotton balls, loose threads from dressings, needles, and other small objects must be kept away from the opening. Suctioning to remove secretions is completed under sterile technique described in Chapter 25. The frequency of suctioning varies with the amount of secretions present, but it should be done often enough to keep ventilation effective and as effortless as possible.

The tracheostomized client is unable to speak. His care should include consideration of his impaired ability to communicate. Communication tools (*e.g.,* writing board, letters, vocabulary cards) should be kept close at hand along with the call light or bell. To prevent anxiety, this client requires reassurance and frequent explanations and anticipation of needs.

Suctioning

If the client is unable to remove secretions with coughing after the application of artificial airways, secretions can be aspirated with a suctioning device (see Procedure 34-4). Suctioning irritates the mucosa and removes oxygen from the respiratory tract. Thus, the client must be hyperoxygenated prior to suctioning. Tracheal suctioning, also called deep suctioning, may be performed by passing a sterile catheter through the mouth (orotracheal), through the nose (nasotracheal), through an endotracheal tube or through a tracheostomy tube. Procedure 34-5 describes suctioning the tracheostomy. When performed correctly, suctioning provides comfort, relieves respiratory distress, and is painless. When performed incorrectly, it can increase anxiety and pain and cause respiratory arrest. Possible complications include infection, cardiac arrhythmias, hypoxia, mucosa trauma, and death. The suctioning catheter should be small enough not to occlude the airway being suctioned but large enough to remove secretions. Several sizes of soft, plastic, clear catheters are available.

The nurse should wear gloves on both hands to prevent infection. The client's color; heart rate; and secretion color, amount, and consistency should be monitored continuously. If cyanosis, excessively slow or rapid heart rate, or suddenly bloody secretions are noted, the nurse should stop suctioning immediately. The client should be ventilated with oxygen, and the physician should be notified.

Assisting Ventilation

Mechanical ventilators are used to assist or completely control ventilation. These machines are used with critically ill clients in conjunction with endotracheal or tra-cheostomy tubes. (The reader is referred to the general literature and other clinical texts which discuss their use in great detail.)

Another mechanical device used to assist ventilation is intermittent positive-pressure breathing (IPPB). This is a method of providing a specific amount of air, oxygen, and aerosolized medication under increased pressure to the respiratory tract when other simpler approaches have proved ineffective. IPPB forces deeper inspiration by positive-pressure inhalation and then permits passive exhalation. The amount of pressure varies with each client.

The physician prescribes this therapy, and it is delivered by the respiratory therapist or the nurse. Treatments are provided with the client in an upright position when he first rises and at bedtime. Often, it is also done twice during the day depending on the needs of the client. IPPB usually induces coughing, and the nurse should encourage the client to expectorate as much of the secretions as is possible. The client receiving IPPB inhales the mist through a mouthpiece or a face mask. Prior to each treatment, the nurse should remind the client to inhale slowly and deeply to allow the lungs to be filled. The client should exhale as completely as is possible before the next inspiration. Avoid treatment immediately preceding or following meals to prevent vomiting or depressed appetite.

Ambu Bag and Mask

In emergency situations the ambu bag (Fig. 34-14) is used to assist ventilation for clients whose respirations have ceased. With the client's head tilted back, jaw pulled forward, and airway cleared, the mask is held tightly over the client's nose and mouth. The operator's other hand compresses the bag at a rate that approximates normal respiratory rate (*e.g.,* 16 to 20 breaths per minute in the adult). The one-way valve in the mask allows exhaled air to escape. Artificial ventilation can be sustained until spontaneous breathing starts, until other mechanical assistance is available, or until death is confirmed. The bag is self-inflating.

(Text continues on p. 931.)

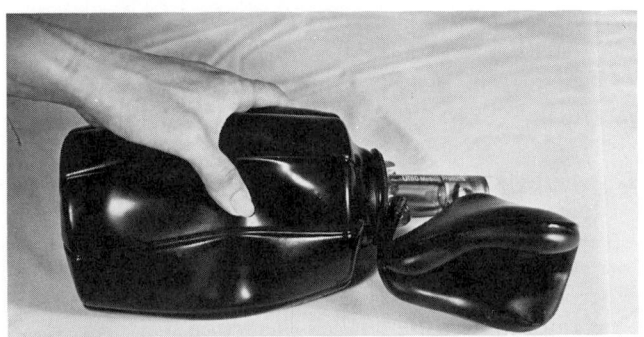

F I G U R E   **34-14**
The self-inflating bag and mask is used for assisting ventilation in emergency situations.

PROCEDURE 34-4
Suctioning the Nasopharyngeal and Oropharyngeal Areas

Equipment

Portable or wall suction unit with tubing	Sterile suction catheter with Y-port	Sterile water or saline	Sterile gloves
		Sterile disposable container	Towel or waterproof pad

Action | **Rationale**

1 Explain procedure to client.

Provides reassurance and promotes cooperation

2 Assemble equipment.

Provides for organized approach

3 Wash your hands.

Handwashing deters spread of microorganisms.

4 Adjust bed to comfortable working position. Lower side rail closer to you. Place the client in a semi-Fowler's position if conscious. An unconscious client should be placed in the lateral position facing you.

Having the client in a sitting position helps him to cough and makes breathing easier. Gravity also facilitates the insertion of the catheter. Lateral position prevents the airway from becoming obstructed and promotes drainage of secretions.

5 Place towel or waterproof pad across client's chest.

Protects bed linens

6 Turn suction to appropriate pressure:

Negative pressure must be at a safe level or pneumothorax may occur.

   a. Wall unit
      Adult 110 mm Hg–150 mm Hg
      Child 95 mm Hg–110 mm Hg
      Infant 50 mm Hg–95 mm Hg

   b. Portable unit
      Adult 10 mm Hg–15 mm Hg
      Child 5 mm Hg–10 mm Hg
      Infant 2 mm Hg–5 mm Hg

7 Open sterile suction package. Set up sterile container touching only the outside surface, and pour sterile saline or water into it.

Sterile normal saline or water is used to lubricate the outside of the catheter, thus minimizing irritation of mucosa as it is being introduced.

8 Put a sterile glove on the hand that will handle the catheter.

Handling the sterile catheter with a hand wearing a sterile glove helps prevent introducing organisms into the respiratory tract.

9 With sterile gloved hand, pick up sterile catheter and connect to suction tubing which is held with unsterile hand.

Sterilization can be maintained.

10 Moisten the catheter by dipping it into the container of sterile saline. Occlude Y-tube to check suction.

Lubricating the inside of the catheter with saline helps move secretions in the catheter.

11 Estimate the distance from the earlobe to the nostril, and place thumb and forefinger of gloved hand at that point on the catheter.

Ensures that catheter remains in pharynx rather than trachea

12 Gently insert the catheter with the suction off by leaving the vent on the Y-connector open. Slip the catheter gently along the floor of an unobstructed nostril toward the trachea to suction the nasopharynx. Or, insert the catheter along the side of the mouth toward the trachea to suction the oropharynx. Never apply suction as the catheter is introduced.

Using suction while inserting the catheter can cause trauma to the mucosa and removes oxygen from the respiratory tract. Coughing is induced when the trachea is touched. This helps the client raise secretions.

(Continued)

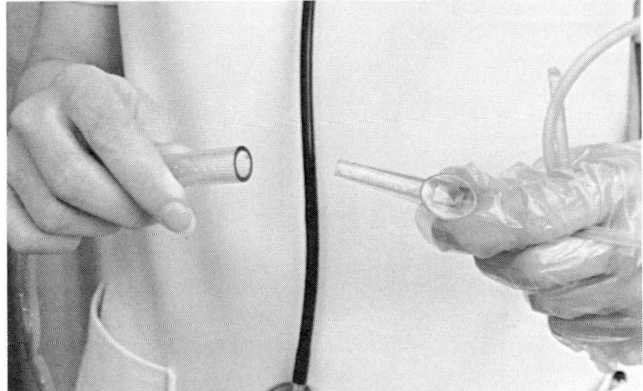

Step 9: Connecting catheter to suction tube.

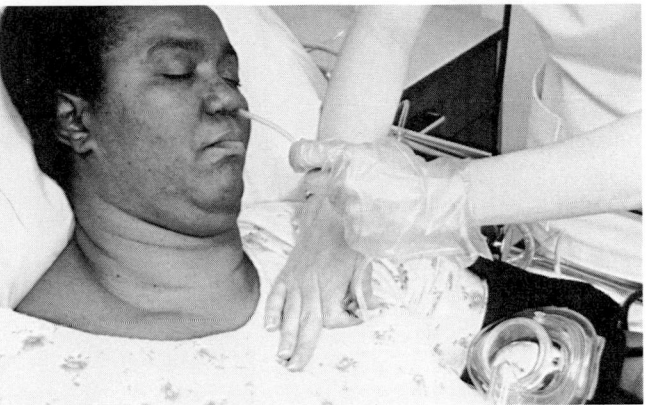

Step 12: Inserting catheter.

13 Apply suction by occluding the suctioning port with your thumb and gently rotate the catheter as it is being withdrawn. Do not allow the suctioning to continue for more than 10 sec–15 sec at a time.

Turning the catheter as it is withdrawn helps clean all surfaces of the respiratory passageways. Suctioning the client for longer than 10 sec–15 sec robs the respiratory tract of oxygen, which may result in hypoxia.

14 Flush the catheter with saline and repeat suctioning as needed and according to client's toleration of procedure.

Flushing cleans and clears catheter and lubricates it for next insertion.

15 Allow at least 20-sec–30-sec interval if additional suctioning is needed. The nares should be alternated when repeated suctioning is required. Do not force catheter through the nares. Encourage client to cough and deep breathe between suctionings.

Normal breathing between suctioning helps compensate for any hypoxia induced by the previous suctioning.

16 When suctioning is completed, remove sterile glove inside out and dispose of glove, catheter, and container with solution in proper receptacle. Wash your hands.

Prevents transmission of microorganisms

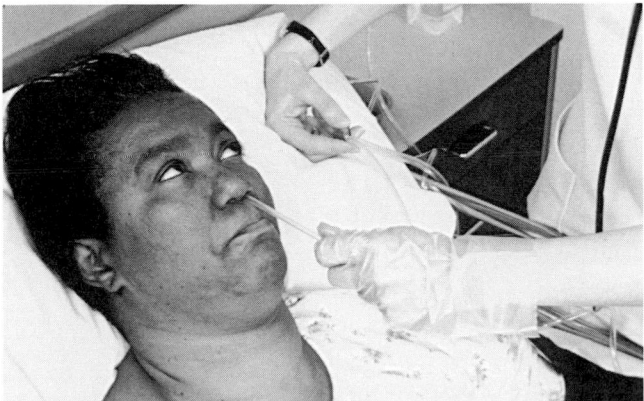

Step 13: Occluding port and rotating catheter while withdrawing.

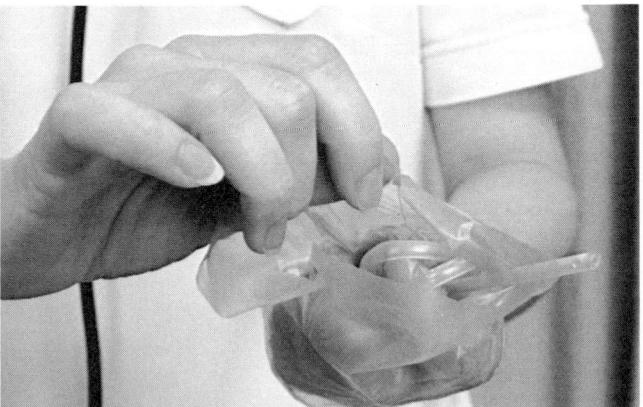

Step 16: Removing glove over catheter.

17 Use auscultation to listen to chest and breathing sounds to assess the effectiveness of suctioning.

Listening to chest and breathing sounds helps determine whether the respiratory passageways are clear of secretions.

(Continued)

PROCEDURE 34-4
Suctioning the Nasopharyngeal and Oropharyngeal Areas (Continued)

Action	Rationale

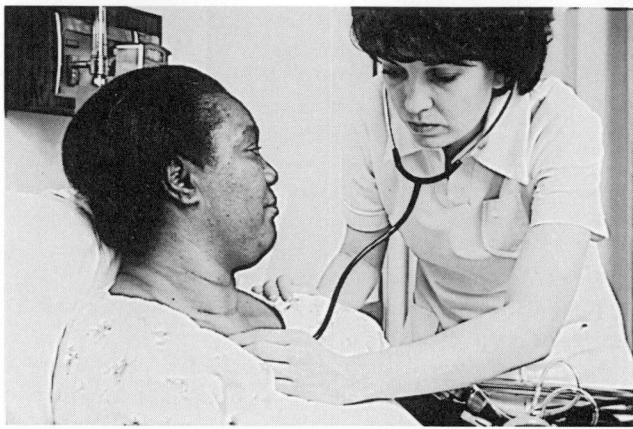

Step 17: Assessing effectiveness of suctioning.

18 Record the time of suctioning and the nature and amount of secretions. Also note the character of the client's respirations before and after the suctioning.

Records of nursing measures used help assess, evaluate, and coordinate care.

19 Offer oral hygiene after suctionings.

Respiratory secretions that are allowed to accumulate in the mouth are irritating to mucous membranes and unpleasant for the client.

PROCEDURE 34-5
Suctioning the Tracheostomy

Equipment

Portable or wall suction device with connecting tubing

Sterile suction kit containing the following or gather separately:

Sterile suction catheter of appropriate size with Y-port
Infants 6–8 F
Children 8–10 F
Adults 12–16 F
Sterile container
Sterile glove
Sterile normal saline

Clean towel or sterile drape (optional)

Action	Rationale

1 Explain procedure to client and reassure him that you will interrupt procedure if he indicates respiratory difficulty.

Facilitates cooperation and provides reassurance for client. Any procedure that compromises respiration is frightening for the client.

(Continued)

Action	**Rationale**

2 Gather equipment and provide privacy for client.

Provides for organized approach to task

3 Wash your hands.

Handwashing deters spread of microorganisms.

4 Assist the client to a semi-Fowler's or Fowler's position if conscious. An unconscious client should be placed in the lateral position facing you.

Sitting position helps client to cough and breathe easier. This position also uses gravity to aid in the insertion of catheter. Lateral position prevents the airway from becoming obstructed and promotes drainage of secretions.

5 Turn suction to appropriate pressure:

Negative pressure must be at safe level or damage to tracheal mucosa may occur.

  a. Wall unit
     Adult 110 mm Hg–150 mm Hg
     Child 95 mm Hg–110 mm Hg
     Infant 50 mm Hb.

  b. Portable unit
     Adult 10 mm Hg–15 mm Hg
     Child 5 mm Hg–10 mm Hg
     Infant 2 mm Hg–5 mm Hg

6 Place clean towel, if being used, across client's chest.

Protects client and bed linens

7 Open sterile kit or set up equipment and prepare to suction:

  a. Place sterile drape, if available, across client's chest.

Protects client and bed linens

  b. Open sterile container and place on bedside table or overbed table without contaminating inner surface. Pour sterile saline into it.

Maintains sterile set-up

  c. Preoxygenate client for several breaths.

Prevents hypoxia during suctioning

  d. Don sterile glove on dominant hand and pick up folded sterile suction catheter. Remove wrapper around catheter with nondominant unsterile hand and discard.

Maintains sterility of procedure

  e. Connect sterile suction catheter to suction tubing which is held with unsterile hand.

Sterile technique helps prevent introducing organisms into the respiratory tract.

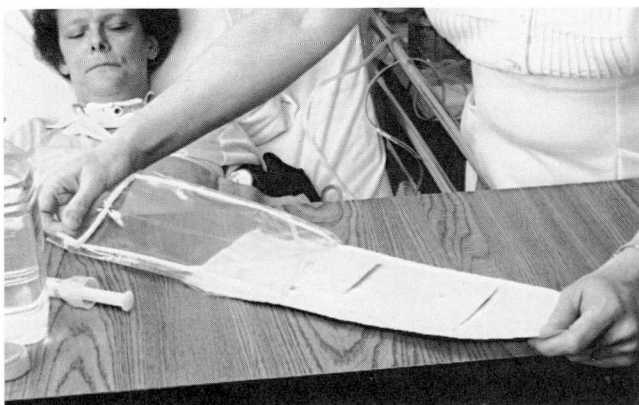

Step 7: Opening sterile kit.

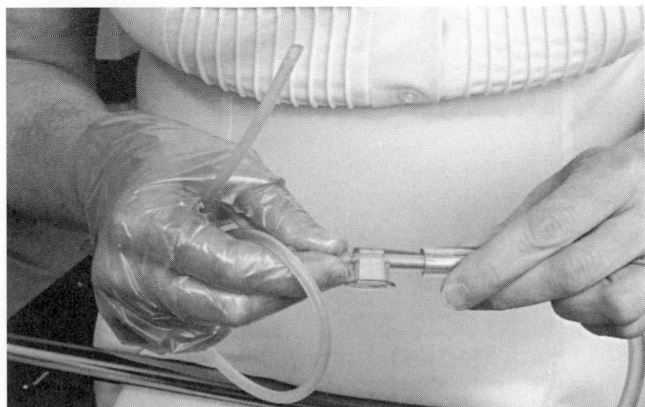

Step 7e: Connecting catheter to suction tube.

(Continued)

Suctioning the Tracheostomy (Continued)

Action

8 Moisten the catheter by dipping it into the container of sterile saline. Occlude the Y-port to check suction.

9 Remove oxygen delivery set-up with unsterile hand.

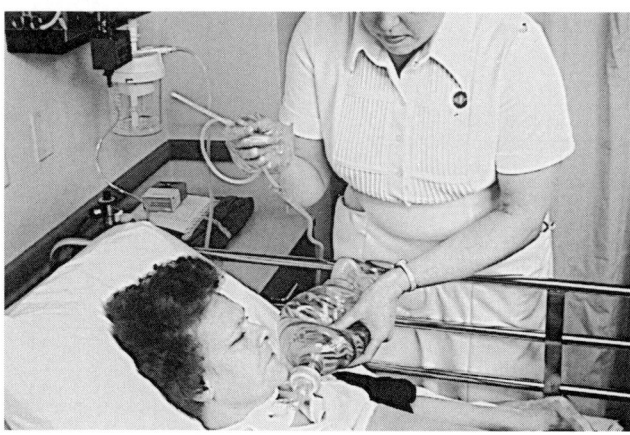

10 Using sterile hand, gently and quickly insert catheter into the trachea. Advance about 10 cm–12.5 cm (4 in–5 in) or until client coughs. *Do not occlude Y-port when inserting catheter.*

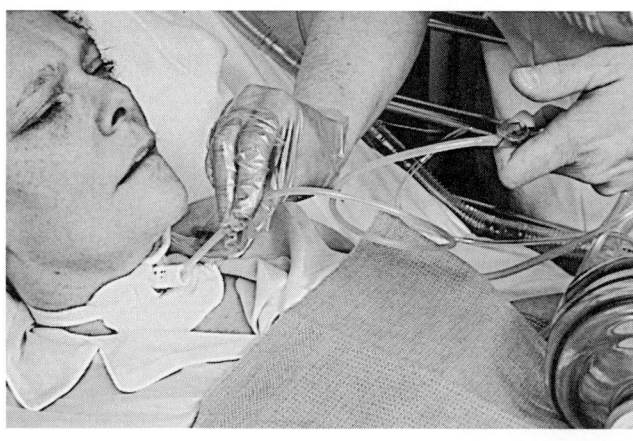

11 Apply intermittent suction by occluding Y-port with thumb of unsterile hand. Gently rotate catheter with thumb and index finger of gloved hand as it is being withdrawn. Do not allow suctioning to continue for more than 10 sec. Encourage client to cough and deep breathe between suctionings.

12 Flush the catheter with saline and repeat suctioning as needed and according to client's toleration of procedure. Allow client to rest at least 1 min between suctionings, and replace oxygen delivery set-up if necessary.

Rationale

Lubricating the inside of catheter with saline helps move secretions in the catheter.

Exposes tracheostomy tube

Step 9: Removing oxygen delivery.

Using suction when inserting catheter can cause trauma to mucosa and removes oxygen from the respiratory tract.

Step 10: Inserting catheter with Y-port open.

Turning the catheter while withdrawing it helps clean surfaces of respiratory tract and prevents injury to tracheal mucosa. Suctioning for longer than 10 sec may result in hypoxia.

Flushing cleans and clears catheter and lubricates it for next insertion. Allowing time interval and replacing oxygen delivery set-up helps compensate for hypoxia induced by the previous suctioning.

(Continued)

13 When procedure is completed, turn off suction and disconnect catheter from suction tubing. Remove sterile glove inside out and dispose of glove, catheter, and container with solution in proper receptacle. Wash hands.

Prevents transmission of microorganisms

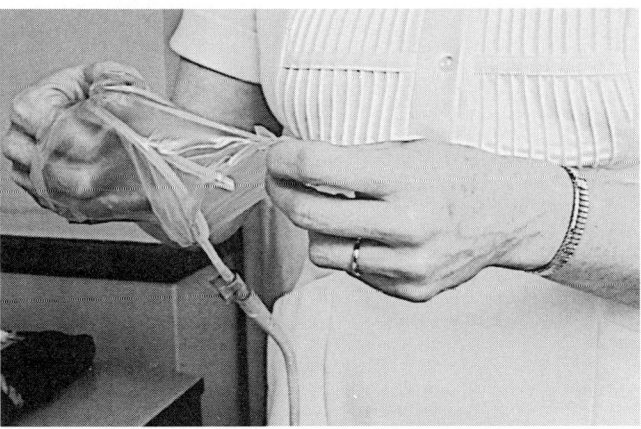

Step 13: Removing glove over catheter for disposal.

14 Adjust client's position. Auscultate chest to evaluate breath sounds.

Helps determine if respiratory passageways are cleared of secretions

15 Record the time of suctioning and the nature and amount of secretions. Also note the character of client's respirations before and after suctioning.

Provides accurate documentation and provides for comprehensive care

16 Offer oral hygiene.

Respiratory secretions that accumulate are irritating to mucous membranes and unpleasant for the client.

Most bag and mask ventilators can accommodate an oxygen tube to increase the oxygen supply to the client. Many also have an adapter so they can be directly connected to a tracheostomy or endotracheal tube for manual ventilation of an intubated client.

Clearing an Obstructed Airway

Foreign body obstruction of the airway usually occurs during eating. In adults, meat is the most common cause. In children, any variety of foods or objects have obstructed the upper airway. A semiconscious or unconscious client can develop airway obstruction because the tongue covers the pharynx as it falls back, obstructing the upper airway. The tongue is the most common cause of airway obstruction.

Foreign bodies can cause either partial airway obstruction or complete airway obstruction. In partial airway obstruction with good air exchange, the client can cough forcefully. This person should be allowed and encouraged to cough and breathe spontaneously. At this time, the nurse should not interfere with his efforts to expel the object.

Good air exchange can progress to poor air exchange, indicated by weak, ineffective cough, high-pitched noises while inhaling, increased breathing difficulties, and cyanosis. This should be managed the same way as complete airway obstruction.

With complete airway obstruction, the victim is unable to speak, cough, or talk. The client may demonstrate the universal distress signal (*i.e.,* clutching his throat with both hands). Immediate action is necessary or the client will become unconscious as the brain becomes hypoxic. Once complete airway obstruction has been established, the Heimlich maneuver (abdominal thrusts) should be provided. Application of this procedure for the conscious and unconscious adult is described in Procedure 34-6.

(Text continues on p. 934.)

Clearing An Obstructed Airway

Conscious Adult

Action

1 Assess victim. Ask "Are you choking?" Determine if he can speak or cough.

2 If victim is obstructed, initiate abdominal thrusts (Heimlich maneuver):

    a. Stand behind victim.

    b. Wrap arms around victim's waist.

    c. Make a fist with one hand with thumb outside of fist. Place thumb side of fist against victim's abdomen above navel and well below xiphoid process.

    d. Grasp fist with the other hand, and press upward with quick, firm thrusts.

    e. Continue distinct thrusts until foreign body is expelled or victim becomes unconscious.

Rationale

Inability to speak or cough indicates that airway is obstructed.

Firm abdominal thrusts force exhalation of air through the vitim's airway and aid in dislodging obstruction.

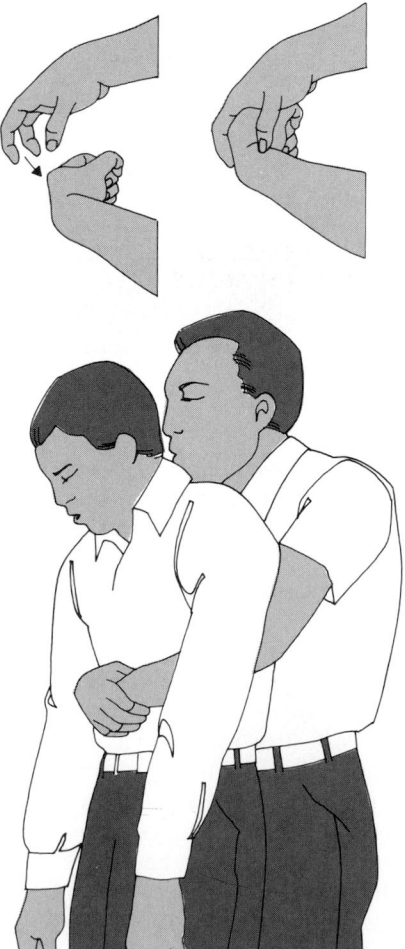

Step 2: Rescuer positioning to perform abdominal thrusts on conscious adult.

(Continued)

Action

1 Assess victim's unresponsiveness. Gently shake shoulder and ask "Are you ok?" Call for help.

2 Position victim on back on a flat, firm surface. Support head and neck and turn as a unit.

3 Tilt victim's head backward by placing hand on forehead. Place fingers of other hand underneath victim's jaw and lift upward and forward.

4 Determine breathlessness by placing ear over victim's mouth and observing chest.

5 Attempt ventilation if breathless. Seal victim's mouth and nose properly. If resistance is met, reposition victim's head and attempt to ventilate again. If anyone responds to call for help, send them to activate EMS system.

6 Initiate abdominal thrusts (Heimlich maneuver):

   a. Straddle victim's thighs.

   b. Place heel of one hand against victim's abdomen above navel and well below xiphoid process.

   c. Place second hand directly on top of first hand.

   d. Press upward with quick, firm thrusts.

   e. Perform 6 to 10 distinct abdominal thrusts.

Rationale

Determines need for CPR

Firm surface provides for maximum effect from abdominal thrusts.

Opens the airway

If victim is breathing, expired air can be heard and felt on cheek as well as observed as chest rises and falls.

If airway is not positioned properly or is obstructed, resistance will be felt when ventilating. Air will not enter lungs, and chest will not rise.

Firm abdominal thrusts force exhalation of air through the victim's airway and aid in dislodging obstruction.

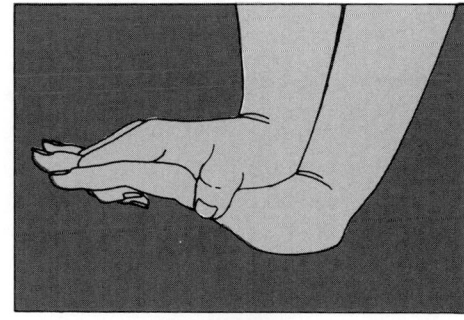

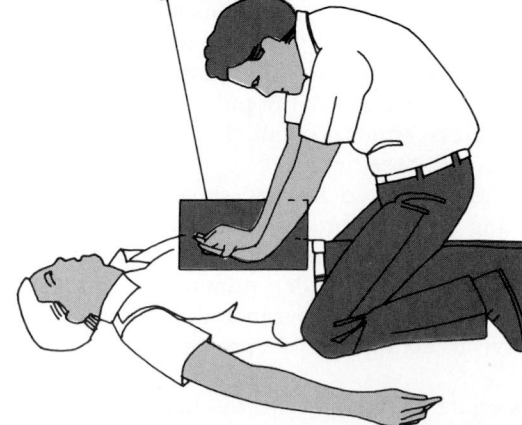

Step 6: Rescuer positioning for abdominal thrusts on unconscious adult.

7 Perform finger sweep using jaw lift to open mouth.

Finger sweep will detect expelled foreign body and remove it thus preventing foreign body from being forced back into airway.

(Continued)

Action

8 Attempt ventilation again using proper maneuver. If unable to ventilate, repeat sequence of thrusts, finger sweep, and ventilations until successful.

9 If successful in ventilation, continue with normal resuscitation procedure; pulse check, chest compression, and breathing.

Rationale

Forceful ventilation in unconscious victim may bypass obstruction and enable aeration of lungs.

Once airway is open, the need for continued intervention must be established.

Special Considerations

1 Use chest thrusts rather than abdominal thrusts on a pregnant woman or very obese victim. Place fist on middle portion of sternum and thrust backward.

Administering Cardiopulmonary Resuscitation

Cardiopulmonary resuscitation (CPR) is the combination of mouth-to-mouth breathing, which supplies oxygen to the lungs, and chest compressions, which circulate blood. It is often described as the ABCs of basic life support:

> *A is for airway.* Tip the head and check for breathing. The respiratory tract must be opened so air can enter.
>
> *B is for breathing.* If the victim does not start to breathe spontaneously after the airway is opened, give two slow, full breaths.
>
> *C is for circulation.* Check the pulse. If the victim is pulseless, artificial circulation must be started with breathing.

CPR should be started for any situation in which either breathing alone or breathing and heart beat are absent. The brain is very sensitive to hypoxia and will sustain irreversible damage after 4 minutes to 6 minutes of no oxygen. The faster CPR is initiated, the greater the chance of survival. Actions for CPR are described in Procedure 34-7.

The procedure for CPR by two rescuers is provided in Procedure 34-8. When there are two rescuers, they may switch positions during CPR to relieve fatigue. There should be no break in the rhythm and regularity of rescue breathing and cardiac compressions during this switch in positions. The technique for administering CPR to children and infants differs slightly from adult CPR. These techniques are discussed in depth in the Basic Life Support Course, which all health professionals should take prior to administering care in the health field.

Most professional organizations recommend and support widespread efforts to teach CPR to lay persons and all health professionals. Mannequins for practice can be obtained from the American Heart Association, the National Red Cross, and health agencies. It is a professional responsibility to maintain proficiency in CPR skills. This necessitates periodic practice with mannequins (adult and infant). CPR should be administered quickly and accurately, without hesitation, when an emergency arises.

EVALUATING

Evaluation is an ongoing and deliberate part of the nursing process which involves the nurse, client, family, and other health-care team members. It includes a comparison of the client's health status and the previously defined goals and an examination of the client's projected progress in meeting those goals. All involved in the evaluation process need to identify effective interventions and to identify reasons for any failures in achieving goals. Adjustments in the nursing care plan must be accordingly.

(Text continues on p. 938.)

Administering Cardiopulmonary Resuscitation on An Adult (One Rescuer)

Action

1 Assess victim's unresponsiveness. Gently shake shoulder and ask "Are you ok?" Call for help.

2 Position victim on back on a flat, firm surface. Support victim's head and neck and turn as a unit.

3 Tilt victim's head backwards by placing hand on forehead. Place fingers of other hand underneath victim's jaw and lift upward and forward.

4 Determine breathlessness by placing ear over victim's mouth and observing chest.

5 Remove dentures if they are loose; if snug, leave them in place.

6 Keeping head tilted backwards, pinch the victim's nose shut with thumb and fingers of hand that is on forehead. Seal your lips tightly around victim's mouth. Ventilate two times at 1 sec–1.5 sec per inspiration. Observe victim's chest rise and lift face away from victim between breaths.

7 Determine pulselessness by feeling for carotid pulse on near side of victim while maintaining head tilt with other hand (5 sec–10 sec). Send anyone who responds to call for help to activate EMS system.

Rationale

Determines need for CPR

Firm surface provides for maximum compression and proper positioning.

Opens the airway

If victim is breathing, expired air can be heard and felt on cheek as well as observed as chest rises and falls.

Loose dentures may block the airway. If they are snug, they help seal the mouth.

Pinching the nose shut allows maximum ventilation with no escape of air through nostrils. Force of breathing needs to be sufficient so that chest visibly rises when air is forced into victim's mouth and falls with victim's passive exhalation.

Carotid artery is large, centrally located, and ordinarily readily accessible. Five- to ten-second pause is needed to adequately assess for pulselessness.

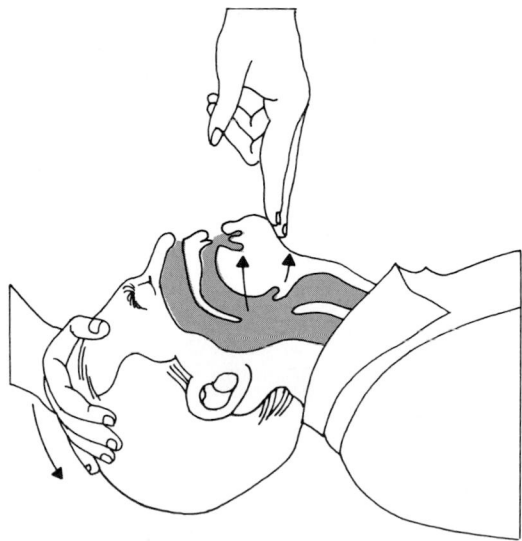

Step 3: Establishing open airway.

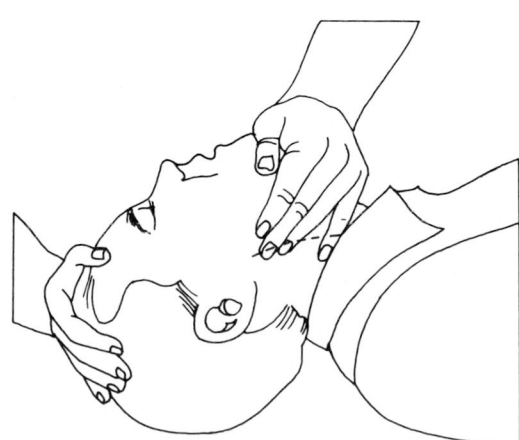

Step 7: Assessing carotid pulse.

8 Begin chest compressions if pulse is absent:

    a. Kneel by victim's shoulders.

Facilitates proper position

(Continued)

Action

b. Locate the xiphoid process on sternum by following the lower rib to notch on sternum where rib meets. Measure 4 cm–5 cm (1.5 in–2 in) above the xiphoid process, about the width of two fingers.

c. Place heel of one hand on this point and position the heel of other hand on top of first hand. Preferably, the fingers should interlock. Bring your shoulders over your hands and keep your elbows locked and arms straight.

d. Use body weight to depress victim's sternum about 4 cm–5 cm (1.5 in–2 in). Relax pressure immediately but keep hands on sternum during up stroke.

Rationale

Proper hand position keeps pressure off the xiphoid process and prevents injury to underlying organs and ribs.

Interlocking the fingers helps keep them off the victim's ribs, where pressure may cause fractures of the ribs. This position, with the elbows and arms straight, allows for best exertion of pressure on the sternum over the heart.

The depression of the sternum with pressure causes the heart to be compressed against the vertebral column forcing blood into the aorta and pulmonary arteries. Relaxation of pressure allows the heart to expand and refill. Keeping the hands in place over the sternum helps administer regular and even compressions.

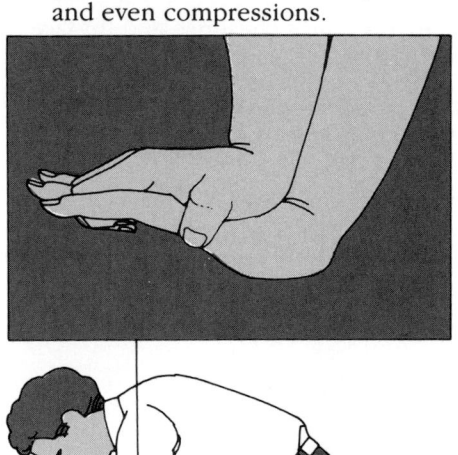

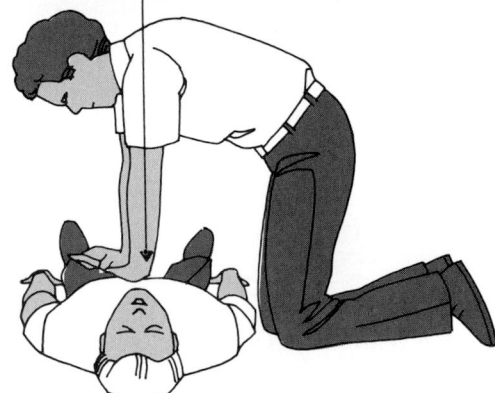

Step 8b & c: Locating site for compression.

Step 8c & d: Rescuer positioning and action of compression.

e. Compress at the rate of 80 to 100 per min (15 every 9 sec–11 sec).

9 Do 4 cycles of 15 compressions and 2 ventilations. Observe chest rise on ventilations (1 sec–1.5 sec per inspiration).

10 Reassess cardiopulmonary status. Feel for carotid pulse (5 sec).

This compression rate maintains adequate blood pressure and flow to maintain cell integrity.

Provides for maintenance of adequate blood flow and oxygenation

Determines pulselessness

(Continued)

Action

11 If pulse is absent, continue CPR. Ventilate twice (1 sec–1.5 sec per inspiration) and then resume compression/ventilation cycles. Feel for carotid pulse every few minutes.

Rationale

Continuation of compression/ventilation rate is necessary to sustain life.

Special Considerations

1 Second rescuer should announce to first rescuer, "I know CPR. Can I help?" Second rescuer then does pulse check (step 10) and continues with step 11. First rescuer should assess adequacy of second rescuer's ventilations (observe chest rise) and compressions (check pulse).

PROCEDURE 34-8
Administering Cardiopulmonary Resuscitation on an Adult (Two Rescuers)

Action

1 Rescuer who will ventilate initiates airway assessments. Sequence continues as for one rescuer (steps 1–6).

2 After pulselessness is determined, first rescuer states, "No pulse."

3 Compressor gets into position, locates anatomical landmarks and begins chest compressions. Correct ratio of compressions to ventilations is 5 to 1 with a compression rate of 80 to 100 per min. Stop compressing for each ventilation. Continue for a minimum of 10 cycles.

4 Compressor calls for switch when fatigued and gives clear signal. Compressor completes fifth compression, and ventilator completes ventilation after fifth compression. Rescuers switch simultaneously. Person who becomes ventilator does 5-second pulse check, states, "No pulse" (if pulse absent), and ventilates once. Person who becomes compressor then begins compressions at a 5 to 1 ratio.

Rationale

Determines need for CPR

This indicates clearly to second rescuer to initiate compression sequence.

The rate of 10 to 15 regularly spaced breaths per minute is considered necessary to supply the victim with sufficient oxygen to maintain cell integrity.

It is important to carry out CPR without interruption to ensure adequate flow of oxygenated blood to maintain cell integrity.

N U R S I N G   P R O C E S S   *in Clinical Practice*

The nurse uses all phases of the nursing process when identifying and treating alterations in respiratory functioning. The nurse's knowledge and application of clinical skills described earlier in the chapter play a major role in treating respiratory problems. This section addresses assessment priorities, client goals, nursing interventions, and evaluation criteria for those common types of respiratory problems treated by nurses: impaired gas exchange, ineffective breathing patterns, and ineffective airway clearance. In the case study that follows, nursing care is described for a young child with an alteration in respiratory functioning.

Impaired Gas Exchange

Impaired gas exchange is the state in which the person experiences an actual or potential decreased passage of gas (oxygen or carbon dioxide) between the alveoli of the lungs and the vascular system (Carpenito, 1987).

Assessment
- Use interview questions directed to the client and significant other persons to determine exactly what is the problem.
- Determine if the client's perception of the impaired gas exchange corresponds to actual physiologic changes.
- Explore the client's life-style, physical and mental health for contributing factors.
- Examine the client for signs of impaired gas exchange (*e.g.,* tachypnea, abnormal breath sounds, cough, neck vein distention, or barrel chest).
- Check lab and radiology data for more information (chest x-ray, arterial blood gas results, hemoglobin, protein levels, and so forth).
- Observe client's technique when dealing with actual or perceived impaired gas exchange.
- Assess client's effectiveness in dealing with impaired gas exchange.

Client Goals
The client will:
- Identify causes of the impaired gas exchange
- Incorporate adequate pulmonary hygiene techniques into the daily routine
- Institute life-style changes to eliminate factors contributing to impaired gas exchange
- Seek treatment for early signs of infection
- Use breathing techniques with ease to decrease the work of breathing

Interventions
- Instruct client to cough properly and deep breathe four times a day (½ hour prior to meals and at bedtime).
- Demonstrate and encourage client use of diaphragmatic breathing and pursed-lip breathing.
- Encourage good oral hygiene.
- Arrange (or encourage home manager to arrange) four to five small meals per day.
- Assist client to drink 2 to 3 qt of clear fluid each day. Keep a container of favorite juice at client's side.
- Incorporate a period of regular exercise into each day.
- Encourage client to socialize with others (friends, respiratory support group, church, and so forth)
- Use simple explanations (written and verbal) on medications, their actions, dose, timing, and side-effects.
- Explore with client and others who live with him or her, methods to reduce pollution in home or work environment.
- Use air conditioner on high pollution days.
- Avoid using respiratory irritants.
- If the client smokes, discuss the idea of reducing smoking with the goal of stopping the smoking habit.

Evaluative Criteria
Client meets the above goals.

Ineffective Breathing Patterns

This is a state in which the person experiences an actual or potential loss of adequate ventilation related to an altered breathing pattern (Carpenito, 1987).

Assessment
- Use interview questions directed to the client and significant other persons to determine the nature of the problem, its probable cause, and its effect on life-style.
- Examine client and assess respiratory rate, rhythm, symptoms of anxiety or pain.

Client Goals
The client will:
- Demonstrate effective respiratory rate and rhythm
- Identify possible contributing factors
- Evaluate adaptive coping mechanisms when dealing with stress and/or anxiety

Interventions
- Demonstrate conscious controlled breathing and encourage client to use it during periods of anxiety or activity.
- Maintain a "safe" environment. Same nurses always work with this client. Maintain eye contact during conversation.

- If fear is the cause, encourage client to ventilate concerns. Reduce cause of fear, if feasible.
- If there is a strong emotional component, discuss with client the development of effective coping skills with professional counseling.
- If pain is present, use appropriate methods for comfort (*e.g.,* position, analgesics, blankets, and so forth).

Evaluative Criteria
Client meets above goals.

Ineffective Airway Clearance

This is a state in which the person experiences a real or potential threat to the passage of air through the respiratory tract related to partial or complete airway obstruction (Carpenito, 1987).

Assessment
- Use interview questions directed to client or significant other persons to determine nature of the problem and its suspected cause.
- Examine the client and assess for signs of airway obstruction (*e.g.,* abnormal or absent breath sounds, inability to move secretions, cyanosis, restlessness, ineffective cough, nasal flaring).
- Evaluate laboratory studies (*e.g.,* arterial blood gases, tidal volume, vital capacity).
- Assess client's coughing techniques and other pulmonary hygiene practices.
- Verify client's ability to maintain a position that prevents aspiration and allows for complete opening of the airway.

Client Goals
The client will:
- Maintain good body alignment to ensure effective air exchange
- Maintain a fluid intake so secretions are thin
- Demonstrate appropriate use of controlled coughing and diaphragmatic breathing techniques
- Follow medication regimen accurately and be able to state drug actions, dose, and side-effects

Interventions
- Auscultate client's breath sounds every 4 hours.
- Encourage client to cough effectively or suction every 2 hours to 4 hours.
- Keep client's head up at at least 45 degrees or maintain side-lying position to maintain an open airway.
- Splint incisions (if any) for support. Treat pain with analgesics as needed.
- Force favorite fluids (2 qt–3 qt) unless cardiac or renal disturbances prevent this intake.
- Arrange periods of rest around activity (*e.g.,* 8 AM: After the walk down the hall, the client can sleep for 1 hour).
- Use praise liberally to encourage efforts and work.
- Review (orally and in writing) medications, their dose, actions, side-effects, and possible interactions.
- Let the client and caregiver know about support groups in the area.
- Encourage family to contact the American Lung Association for free pamphlets.

Evaluative Criteria
Client has met the above goals.

C A S E   S T U D Y

Freddie is a 1-year-old alert, well-developed child who has been a patient on the pediatric unit for 3 days with status asthmaticus. He has had two other admissions for acute asthma which responded quickly to intravenuous and inhalation bronchodilators. During this hospitalization either his mother, who is a teacher, or his father, a psychologist, has stayed with him. Other relatives are caring for Freddie's 5-year-old brother and his 9-year-old sister.

Freddie interacts happily with staff as long as a parent is within sight. Gross and fine motor coordination are appropriate for age. Vocabulary consists of 25 words. History is from mother who is a reliable source. Child has had a clear nasal discharge with slight, intermittent, nonproductive cough for 3 days with no change in appetite or activity pattern. On day of admission, he attended the day-care center as usual. After being there for 3 hours, his cough became more frequent and respirations

became more labored. The caregivers were not alarmed because he continued to eat, drink, nap, and play in usual pattern. Mother states that when she arrived in the afternoon to pick up the boys, she discovered this child to be using his intercostal and neck muscles excessively with every breath. His respirations were 50 per minute, labored and accompanied by a grunt. By the time she arrived home, he was pale and fitful and was crying weakly. Respirations were 60 per minute and circumoral, and peripheral cyanosis was noted. The pediatrician advised lung evaluation in the emergency department. While there, three subcutaneous injections of epinephrine were administered 5 minutes apart. The child did not respond satisfactorily so he was admitted for intraveneous aminophylline and steroid administration.

In addition to the history of asthma, Freddie is allergic to eggs and peanuts and has eczema on his face, arms, legs, and upper back. His current medications include Alupent every 8 hours, Lidex skin cream, and Poly-Vi-Sol vitamins 0.5 cc daily. No one in the family smokes. The caregivers at the day-care center smoke outside the building. The day-care center is clean and had the rugs shampooed the night prior to this child's illness. This child had no sputum production or fever. Immunizations are current.

Assessment Findings

    Respiratory rate: 44 per minute
    Irregular rhythm
    Excessive use of accessory muscles
    Nonproductive, frequent cough
    Rhonchi and expiratory wheeze noted
    Pale, no cyanosis
    Blood pressure: 100/60; heart rate: 120 per minute
    Restless child who naps for only 20 to 30 minutes
        at intervals day and night
    ABGs: normal values
    Chest x-ray: normal
    Poor appetite, vomiting one to two times daily
    Up early in morning
    Sweat test: negative for cystic fibrosis

Nursing Diagnosis

Alteration in respiratory functioning: ineffective airway clearance related to exposure to unknown allergies, bronchospasm, overproduction of thick mucus.

Planning

Freddie's parents state that they are willing to do anything to improve his current respiratory state and to prevent further need for hospitalization. During the staff conference the head nurse, two staff nurses and Freddie's mother developed several short-term goals:
Within the next 48 hours this child will:
1. Have less rhonchi throughout thorax
2. Have no vomiting and no aspiration
3. Eat six small meals and drink at least three 8-oz bottles per 24 hours
4. Have optimal movement of air in and out of lungs
Long-term goals include:
1. The family will go home in 5 days and state that they feel comfortable in providing medications and inhalation to this child.

Implementation

In activating this care plan, the professional nurse needs the following specialized abilities:
- Strong assessment skills
- Understanding of normal respiratory functioning and health deviations
- Knowledge of multiple factors that contribute to health deviations and their severity
- Knowledge of which deviations can be independently treated by nurse
- Interpersonal communication skills necessary to work with clients of all ages and their families

- Teaching and counseling skills to help the family understand the relationship between environment (dust, stuffed animals, pets, pollution, and so forth) and the development of the client's respiratory difficulties and to initiate the necessary changes
- Interpersonal and leadership skills to motivate the nursing staff to value the family's long- and short-term goals and to work with the entire health-care team (physicians, dietary, respiratory therapy)
- Accountability

Documentation

Sample documentation follows in the traditional note format:
    12/1/88   Family/staff conference to discuss Freddie's respiratory disturbance initiated by primary nurse's concern. Present were: Freddie's mother, MJ (primary nurse), TK (head nurse), TR (head of respiratory department), MM and LQ (staff nurses). Primary nurse presented findings from assessment and nursing examination. Discussion centered on strategies to: (1) control airway edema and reduce wheezes; (2) reduce coughing episodes and control vomiting; (3) prevent further bronchospasms and edema resulting from exposure to allergens in environment. See care plan. Client progress will be evaluated in 4 days during nursing grand rounds, 12/5/88.

Mary Jones, RN

SOAP Documentation:
    12/1/88 9 AM #2
S: "My son's chest is still very congested, and he is still wheezing. When will he be well enough to go home? Will he be all right when we go home?"
O: Rhonchi and expiratory wheezes noted throughout anterior and posterior thorax, vomiting food and mucus after breakfast every morning, aminophylline infusing intravenously, steroids, acetaminophen, and antibiotic administered orally as ordered.
A: Ineffective airway clearance related to exposure to allergens, bronchospasm, and overproduction of mucus.
P: 1. Control airway edema and reduce wheezes and rhonchi.
    2. Reduce coughing episodes and control vomiting.
    3. Prevent further bronchospasm resulting from exposure to allergens in environment.
E: Reevaluate respiratory status at nursing ground rounds on 12/5/88.

Mary Jones, RN

Evaluation

Short-term goal achievement is evaluated at the next scheduled assessment. Long-term goal achievement is a lengthier process.

NURSING CARE PLAN for Freddie

Nursing Diagnosis: Ineffective airway clearance related to exposure to allergens, viral infection, broncho-spasm, overproduction of mucus.

Long-Term Goal: This family will return home in 5 days expressing confidence in administering oral and inhalation medications.

Goals	Nursing Actions	Rationale	Evaluative Statement
By 12/5 Freddie will have rare episodes of coughing and no vomiting.	1. Hold meals until inhalation treatments are done. 2. Avoid milk products. 3. Offer clear juices every 3 hr in a bottle or cup. 4. Perform percussion during AM and PM bath.	Bronchodilators stimulate coughing and often cause vomiting if given after meals. Milk accelerates the production of mucus.	12/4, Freddie has not vomited in 2 days and has 2-hour intervals between coughing episodes.
By 12/3 parents will remove dust-collecting toys.	1. Give parents allergy pamphlets from American Lung Association. 2. Review with both parents methods to reduce exposure to possible allergens at home. 3. Encourage parents to examine day-care environment. Explore options with them.	Constant exposure to allergens (dust, mold, mildew, and so forth) and irritants (perfume, smog, cleaners, and so forth) will produce bronchospasm and will stimulate copious mucus production. Medications are most effective when allergens are removed.	12/2, Parents removed furry toys from hospital room.

KEY POINTS

■ The functioning units of the respiratory system are the alveoli where the actual exchange of oxygen and carbon dioxide between the lung and circulation occurs. Airways conduct available gases during inhalation and exhalation phases of ventilation.

■ There are normal variations in respiratory functioning unique to specific ages which allow appropriate oxygenation to meet cellular needs. These differences involve chest shape, breath sounds, and presence of landmarks. In addition to age, other factors affect adequate respiratory functioning including: level of health, growth and development, environment, and psychologic health. Persons with health deviations in respiratory functioning can initiate changes to improve the work of breathing.

■ The health history is an essential component of respiratory function assessment. The client's physical examination with laboratory findings can provide information to identify the nature of the problem,

its course, related signs and symptoms, onset and frequency, and effect on everyday living.

■ Nursing diagnoses can be written to address inadequate breathing patterns, ineffective airway clearance, and impaired gas exchange. Nursing diagnoses also can be written to address how altered respiratory functioning has an effect on other areas of human functioning (*e.g.,* anxiety).

■ Nursing interventions to promote adequate respiratory functioning include promoting effective breathing and coughing exercises, maintaining adequate fluid intake, maintaining good nutrition, promoting comfort by positioning, providing supplemental oxygen, using medications to promote adequate respiratory functioning, and educating clients to maintain a pollution-free environment.

■ Evaluation is ongoing. The health-care team and the client examine progress toward achieving the established goals. The plan is modified based on client's response to nursing actions.

BIBLIOGRAPHY

Bowers A, Thompsin J: Clinical Manual of Health Assessment. St Louis, CV Mosby, 1984

Brunner L, Suddarth D: Medical–Surgical Nursing, 6th ed. Philadelphia, JB Lippincott, 1988

Carpenito L: Nursing Diagnosis: Application to Clinical Practice. 2nd ed. Philadelphia, JB Lippincott, 1987

Fuchs P: Oxygen delivery systems. Nursing 80 34–43, Dec 1980

Hoffman LA, Wesmiller SW: Home oxygen: Transtracheal and other options. Am J Nurs 88(4):464–469, 1988

Jones, Lepley, Baker: Health Assessment Across the Lifespan

Luckman J, Sorenson K: Medical–Surgical Nursing, 3rd ed. Philadelphia, WB Saunders, 1987

Openbrier DR, Hoffman LA, Wesmiller SW: Home oxygen therapy: Evaluation and prescription. Am J Nurs 88(4):464–469, 1988

Orem D: Nursing: Concepts of Practice. New York, McGraw-Hill, 1980

Pety T: Drug strategies for airflow obstruction. Am J Nurs 180–184, Feb 1987

Stevens SA, Becker KL: How to perform picture-perfect respiratory assessment. Nursing 18(1):57–63, 1988

Telkior S, Cramer M, Telkior A: Clinical Implications of Laboratory Tests. St Louis, CV Mosby, 1983

_____: Transtracheal oxygen: The nose knows the difference. Am J Nurs 421–422, April 1987

Fluid, Electrolyte, and Acid–Base Balance

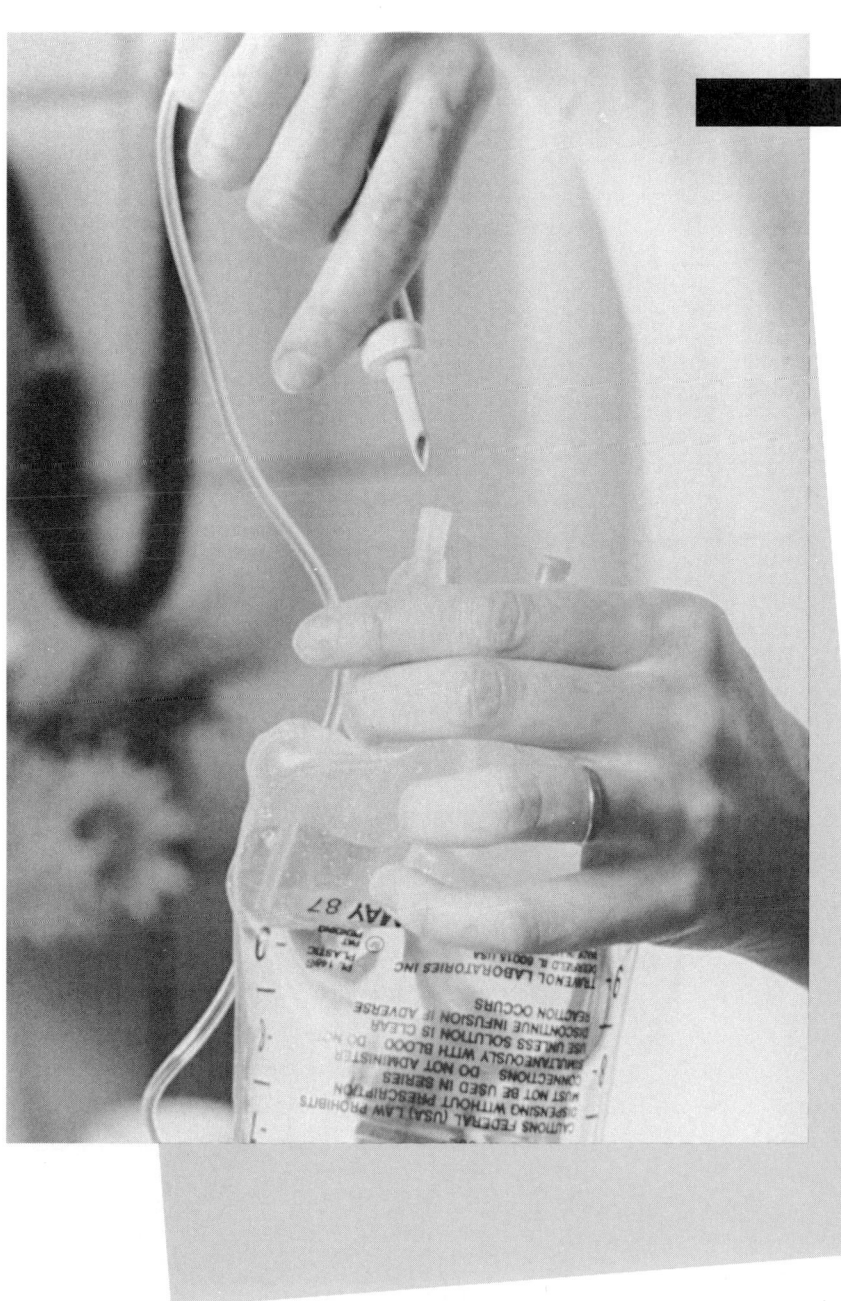

OBJECTIVES

After studying this chapter, the learner should be able to

Define key terms used in the chapter.

Describe the functions of body fluids, the two main compartments where fluids are located in the body, and factors that affect variations in fluid compartments.

Describe the functions, sources and losses, and regulation of main electrolytes of the body.

Explain the principles of osmosis, diffusion, active transport, and filtration.

Describe how thirst and the organs of homeostasis function to maintain fluid homeostasis.

Describe the role of buffer systems, and respiratory and renal mechanisms in achieving acid–base balance.

Identify the etiologies, defining characteristics, and treatment modalities for common fluid, electrolyte, and acid–base disturbances.

Perform a fluid, electrolyte, and acid–base balance assessment.

Describe the role of dietary modification, modification of fluid intake, medication administration, intravenous therapy, blood replacement, and total parenteral nutrition in resolving fluid, electrolyte, and acid–base imbalances.

Plan, implement, and evaluate nursing care related to select nursing diagnoses involving fluid, electrolyte, and acid–base imbalances.

KEY TERMS

acid
acidosis
active transport
agglutinin
alkali
alkalosis
anion
antibody
antigen
base
blood transfusion
buffer
cation
cellular fluid
colloid osmotic pressure
crossmatching
dehydration
diffusion
donor
edema
electrolyte
embolus
extracellular fluid
filtration
filtration pressure
fluid volume deficit
fluid volume excess
hydration
hydrostatic pressure
hypercalcemia
hyperkalemia
hypermagnesemia
hypernatremia
hyperphosphatemia
hypervolemia

hypocalcemia
hypokalemia
hypomagnesemia
hyponatremia
hypophosphatemia
insensible water loss
interstitial fluid
intracellular fluid
intravascular fluid
intravenous fluid
ion
ionization
metabolic acidosis
metabolic alkalosis
milliequivalent
milliliter
nonelectrolyte
oncotic pressure
osmolality
osmoreceptors
osmosis
osteomalacia
pH
phlebitis
respiratory acidosis
respiratory alkalosis
Rh
solute
solvent
speed shock
third-space fluid shift
total body water
total parenteral nutrition
typing

Water may comprise anywhere from 45% to 75% of a healthy person's body weight; the importance of fluid balance to health is readily apparent. Under usual conditions virtually every organ and system in the body helps in some way to maintain fluid balance. Nurses routinely encounter in their practice clients with serious and even life-threatening fluid, electrolyte, and acid–base balance disturbances. One of nursing's most important roles is the prevention of these disturbances in high-risk populations by vigilant nursing care.

Study of this chapter will provide the student with basic knowledge of the principles of fluid, electrolyte, and acid–base balance; and the etiologies, defining characteristics, and nursing interventions for common disturbances. Sample interview questions for performing a fluid balance nursing history are presented along with information on specific physical assessment measures and laboratory studies. Numerous examples of nursing diagnoses are offered. Client goals and specific nursing strategies for promoting fluid balance are described. These include dietary modification; modification of fluid intake; medication administration; and assisting with intravenous therapy, blood replacement, and total parenteral nutrition. In the section entitled "Nursing Process in Clinical Practice" focused assessment, planning, implementation, and evaluation guides are offered for surgical and oncology clients with fluid balance nursing diagnoses. These guides and the concluding case study illustrate how the nurse's knowledge of fluid, electrolyte, and acid–base balance is combined with skilled nursing interventions and caring to successfully resolve fluid balance problems.

PHYSIOLOGY

Body Fluids

Water is the primary body fluid and is the most important nutrient of life. Whereas life can be sustained for many days without food, it can be sustained for only a few days without water.

The following are the primary functions of water in the body:

- It serves as a medium for transporting nutrients to cells and wastes from cells.
- It serves as a medium to transport such substances as hormones, enzymes, blood platelets, and red and white blood cells.
- It is important for cellular metabolism and proper cellular chemical functioning.
- It is the solvent for electrolytes and nonelectrolytes.
- It helps maintain normal body temperature.
- It helps digestion and promotes elimination.
- It is necessary for the manufacture of the body's secretions.

Body Fluid Compartments

The two main compartments, or spaces, where fluids are located in the body are the intracellular fluid and extracellular fluid. **Intracellular fluid** (ICF) is the fluid within the cell. It comprises approximately 40% of an adult's body weight or 70% of the total body water. The **extracellular fluid** (ECF) is all the fluid outside of cell walls. It comprises approximately 20% of an adult's body weight or 30% of total body water. The extracellular fluid includes intravascular and interstitial fluids. **Intravascular fluid** or plasma is the liquid constituent of blood, (*i.e.,* fluid found within the vascular system). **Interstitial fluid** is the fluid in which tissue cells are bathed; it includes lymph. The term **total body water** or fluid (TBW or TBF) refers to the total amount of water in the body expressed as a percentage of body weight. Figure 35-1 illustrates a breakdown of total body fluid. Figure 35-2 is a microscopic visualization of body fluid distribution.

Variations in Fluid Content

In a healthy person, total body water comprises approximately 45% to 75% of the body's weight. Variations depend on such factors as the person's age, lean body mass, and sex. Table 35-1 illustrates age-related changes in total body water and in the various water compartments of the body. An infant, especially one born prematurely, has considerably more body fluid than an elderly person. Infants also have relatively more extracellular fluid than adults. Because extracellular fluid is more easily lost

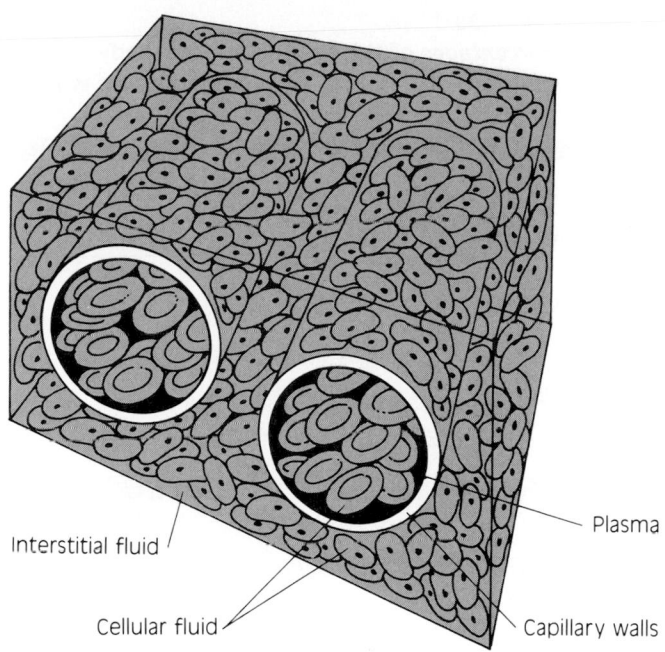

F I G U R E   35-2
Microscopic visualization of body fluid distribution.

from the body than intracellular fluid, infants are more prone to fluid volume deficits.

Total body water also depends on the build of a person. Because fat tissues contain a small amount of water while lean tissue is rich in water, the more obese the person, the smaller the percentage of total body water when compared with body weight. In an obese male, total body water can be as little as 50% of body weight; in an obese female, total body water can be as little as 42% of body weight. Because females tend to have proportionally more body fat than males, they also have less body fluid than males. Similarly, the decreasing percentage of body fluid in elderly persons is related to the decrease in lean body mass in favor of fat.

Electrolytes

Certain compounds in solution dissociate to form ions by the process of **ionization**. An ion is an atom or molecule carrying an electric charge in solution. Substances capable of breaking into electrically charged ions when dissolved in a solution are called **electrolytes**. Some ions develop a positive charge and are called **cations**. Others develop a negative charge and are called **anions**.

If molecules in the body's chemical compounds remain intact, they are called **nonelectrolytes**. In the human body, urea and glucose are nonelectrolytes.

Solvents are liquids that hold a substance in solution; **solutes** are substances that are dissolved in a solution. Water is the solvent in the body that makes up solutions with solutes. The solutes are electrolytes and nonelectrolytes.

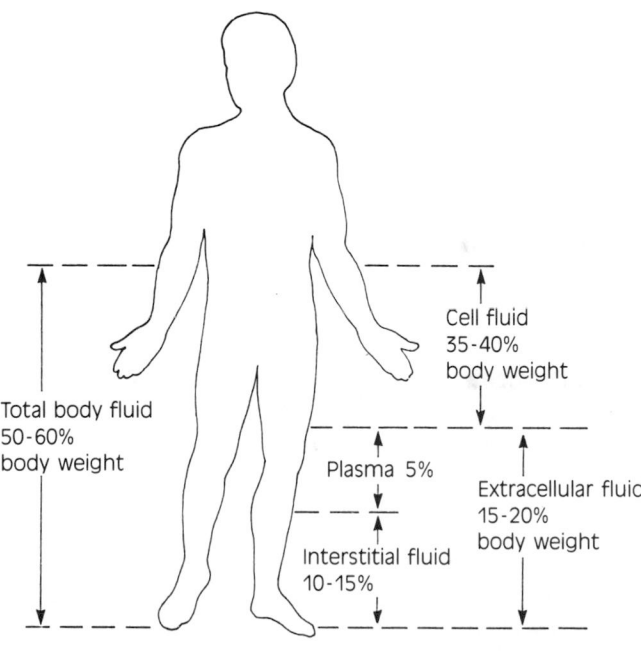

F I G U R E   35-1
Total body fluid represents 50% to 60% of body weight of a normal adult.

Total body fluid
50-60%
body weight

Cell fluid
35-40%
body weight

Plasma 5%

Extracellular fluid
15-20%
body weight

Interstitial fluid
10-15%

Average Percentages of Water in Relation to Body Weight in Persons of Different Ages in the Various Water Compartments of the Body

Water Compartment	Infant (%)	Adult (%)		Elderly Person (%)
		Man	Woman	
Extracellular				
Intravascular	4	4	5	5
Interstitial	25	11	10	15
Intracellular	48	45	35	25
TOTAL BODY WATER	77	60	50	45

Measurement of Electrolytes

The unit of measure used to describe electrolytes is expressed in terms of their chemical combining power, or chemical activity. Because the weight of an ion is not related to its combining power, a standard without regard for weight has been developed to compare the chemical activity of electrolytes.

The standard used to describe the chemical activity of electrolytes is the chemical activity of 1 milligram of hydrogen. The milliequivalent, abbreviated mEq, is used in the United States as the unit of measure to describe the chemical activity of an electrolyte. One **milliequivalent** is chemically equivalent to the activity of 1 milligram (abbreviated mg) of hydrogen. Stated inversely, 1 mg of hydrogen exerts 1 mEq of chemical activity. This is true whether the comparison with hydrogen is made with a cation or an anion. Hence, 1 mEq of any cation is equivalent to 1 mEq of any anion.

Using the milliequivalent system, the total cations in the body are normally equal to the total anions. In healthy persons, the milliequivalents per liter for electrolytes in the body vary within a relatively narrow range. When electrolytes are not in normal balance, the person is in a state of risk or jeopardy.

Regulation of Electrolytes

The chief functions of electrolytes include regulation of water distribution, regulation of acid–base balance, transmission of nerve impulses, clotting of blood, and generation of adenosine triphosphate (ATP) (Adams and Ackerman, 1987).

There are many different kinds of electrolytes in the body. This section summarizes information about the most prevalent ones. Electrolyte disturbances are discussed later in the chapter.

Sodium (Na⁺). The cation sodium is the chief electrolyte of extracellular fluid. It moves easily between intravascular and interstitial spaces and moves across cell

membranes by active transport. Many chemical reactions in the body are influenced by sodium, particularly in nervous-tissue cells and muscle-tissue cells.

Functions

- Maintains the isotonicity and volume of body fluids
  Controls water distribution throughout the body
  Is the primary regulator of extracellular fluid volume
  Also influences cellular fluid volume
- Participates in the generation and transmission of nerve impulses
- Is an essential electrolyte in the sodium–potassium pump

Sources/Losses

- Average daily requirements for sodium are not known precisely, but in North America, the average adult intake is estimated to be between 2 g and 7 g, an amount that more than adequately meets the body's needs.
- Sodium is found in many foods, particularly bacon, ham, sausages, catsup, mustard, relishes, processed cheese, canned vegetables, bread, cereals, and salted snack foods. It is found in table salt (sodium chloride), which is approximately 46% sodium.
- Sodium excesses are eliminated primarily by the kidneys; small amounts are lost in feces and perspiration.

Regulation

- Sodium normally is maintained in the body within a relatively narrow range, and deviations quickly result in a serious health problem. For this reason, health practitioners often speak of the "primacy of sodium."
- Salt intake regulates sodium concentrations.
- Sodium is conserved through reabsorption in the kidneys, a process stimulated by aldosterone.
- The normal extracellular concentration of sodium is 137 to 147 mEq/liter (mmol/liter).

Potassium (K⁺). Potassium is the major cation of intracellular fluid. Potassium and sodium work reciprocally. For example, an excessive intake of sodium results in an excretion of potassium, and vice versa.

Functions

- Is the chief regulator of cellular enzyme activity and cellular water content
- Plays a vital role in such processes as the transmission of electric impulses, particularly in nerve, heart, skeletal, intestinal, and lung tissue; protein and carbohydrate metabolism; and cellular building
- Assists in regulation of acid–base balance by cellular exchange with H⁺

Sources/Losses

- Average daily requirements for potassium are not known precisely, but about 2.5 g daily is ordinarily adequate.

RESEARCH IN NURSING *Making a Difference*

Fluid and Electrolyte Balance

Monitoring and maintaining fluid and electrolyte balance in clients is a major component of nursing care. Particularly in the acute care settings clients are at risk for imbalances which can be life threatening. Unfortunately, very little research has been carried out by nurses with respect to fluid and electrolyte status.

Related Research

Phillips K, Holm K, Wu AC: Contemporary table salt practices and blood pressure. Am J Public Health 75(4):405–406, 1985
Amounts of sodium intake are a concern not just for hypertensive clients but also for the general public. The purpose of this study was to relate the use of table salt and blood pressure, thus replicat-

ing a study done in 1954. The present study showed that there has been a trend toward reducing table salt usage since 1954; however, blood pressure levels are higher among the low-salt users. This finding suggests that subjects may be altering their salt intake in an effort to self-treat their higher blood pressures.

This study exemplifies the effects of one electrolyte on the body and the implications for healthy life-style adjustment. Nurses carry out routine interventions toward monitoring fluid and electrolyte status such as daily intake and output records, client weights, and monitoring lab values. These nursing actions need to be researched to learn more effective ways of maintaining clients in a state of balance.

- A well-balanced diet contains adequate quantities of potassium. Leading food sources include bananas, peaches, figs, dates, apricots, oranges, prunes, melons, raisins, broccoli, and potatoes. Meat and dairy products contain good amounts of potassium.
- Potassium is excreted primarily by the kidneys. The kidneys have no effective method of conserving potassium. Therefore, deficits develop readily if excreted in excess without being replaced simultaneously.
- Gastrointestinal secretions contain potassium in large quantities. Some is also found in perspiration and saliva.

Regulation
- Cellular K^+ is conserved by the sodium pump when Na^+ is excluded.
- The kidneys conserve K^+ when cellular K^+ is decreased.
- Aldosterone secretion triggers K^+ excretion in urine.
- The normal range for serum potassium is 4 to 5.6 mEq/liter.

Calcium (Ca^{++}). Calcium is the most abundant electrolyte in the body. Up to 99% of the total amount of calcium in the body is found in bones and teeth in ionized form. It works intimately with phosphorus.

Functions
- Is necessary for nerve-impulse transmission, blood clotting, and muscle contraction
- Is needed for vitamin B_{12} absorption and for its use by body cells

- Acts as a catalyst for many cell chemical activities
- Is necessary for strong bones and teeth
- Establishes thickness and strength of cell membranes

Sources/Losses
- The average daily requirement for calcium is about 1 g for adults. Higher amounts are required, according to body weight, for children and for pregnant and lactating women.
- It is found in milk, cheese, and dried beans. Some calcium is present in meats and vegetables.
- Utilization of calcium is stimulated by vitamin D.
- It leaves bones and teeth to maintain normal blood-calcium levels, if necessary.
- It is excreted in urine, feces, bile, digestive secretions, and perspiration.

Regulation
- When extracellular fluid calcium levels decrease, the parathyroid glands increase the secretion of parathyroid hormone (PTH) which acts on bones to increase the release of calcium into the blood, and acts on the kidney tubules and the intestinal mucosa to increase the reabsorption of calcium from the kidneys and the intestine.
- A high serum phosphate concentration causes a secondary depression of serum calcium; a low serum phosphate concentration may cause a secondary elevation of serum calcium.
- Calcitonin, a hormone secreted by the thyroid gland, has an opposite effect on calcium than PTH.

Increases in calcitonin reduce serum calcium concentration.

Magnesium (Mg⁺⁺). Most of the cation magnesium is found within body cells. It is present in heart, bone, nerve, and muscle tissues. Magnesium is the second most important cation of intracellular fluid.

Functions
- It is important for the metabolism of carbohydrates and proteins.
- It is important for many vital reactions related to the body's enzymes.
- It serves to help maintain electric activity in nervous membranes and muscle membranes.

Sources/Losses
- The average daily adult requirement for magnesium is about 500 mg; children require larger amounts.
- Magnesium is found in most foods but especially in vegetables, nuts, fish, whole grains, peas, and beans.

Regulation
- Magnesium levels in the body are largely controlled by the kidneys.
- Plasma concentrations of magnesium range from 1.4 to 2.3 mEq/liter.

Chloride (Cl⁻). Chloride, the chief extracellular anion, is found in blood, interstitial fluid, and lymph and in very small amounts in intracellular fluid.

Functions
- Acts with sodium to maintain the osmotic pressure of the blood
- Plays a role in the body's acid–base balance
- Is important in buffering action when oxygen and carbon dioxide exchange in red blood cells
- Is essential for the production of hydrochloric acid in gastric juices

Sources/Losses
- Average daily requirements of chloride are not known, but its intake is usually the same as sodium.
- It is found in foods high in sodium, in dairy products and meat.

Regulation
- It is normally paired with sodium, and excreted and conserved with sodium by the kidneys.
- Chloride deficits lead to potassium deficits, and vice versa.
- Normal serum chloride levels range from 98 to 106 mEq/liter (mmol/liter).

Bicarbonate (HCO₃⁻). The bicarbonate molecule is an anion. It is the major chemical base buffer within the body and is found in both extracellular and intracellular fluid.

Function
- Is essential for acid–base balance; bicarbonate and carbonic acid constitute the body's primary buffer system.

Regulation
- Bicarbonate levels are regulated primarily by the kidneys.
- Bicarbonate is ordinarily readily available as a result of carbon dioxide formation in the process of metabolism.
- In plasma, bicarbonate varies indirectly with intracellular potassium.
- Normal bicarbonate levels range between 25 and 29 mEq/liter (mmol/liter).

Phosphate (PO₄⁻). The phosphate ion is the major anion in body cells. It is a buffer anion in both intracellular and extracellular fluid.

Functions
- Helps maintain acid–base balance
- Has important chemical reactions in the body. For example, phosphorus is necessary for many B vitamins to be effective, helps promote nerve and muscle action, and plays a role in carbohydrate metabolism.
- It is important for cell division and for the transmission of hereditary traits.

Sources/Losses
- Average daily requirements for phosphorus are similar to those of calcium.
- It is found in most foods but especially in beef, pork, and dried peas and beans.
- It is metabolized in the same manner as calcium.

Regulation
- Phosphate is regulated by the parathyroid hormone and by activated vitamin D.
- Calcium and phosphate are inversely proportional; an increase in one results in a decrease in the other.
- The normal range of phosphate is 1.7 to 2.6 mEq/liter (mmol/liter).

Additional Electrolytes. The anion sulfate is found primarily within cells and is associated with cellular protein. Excesses are excreted by the kidneys. The organic-acid anions are normally intermediary in cell metabolism. The major one in the body is lactic acid. The protein anion functions in the process of diffusion to move substances to and from the capillaries. Plasma proteins include albumin, globulin, and fibrinogen.

Other electrolytes are required for proper cell functioning, but they are found only in traces in the body. One example is chromium. A well-balanced diet will ordinarily ensure an adequate supply of trace substances in the body.

Fluids in various compartments of the body differ from one another in terms of their constituents. For ex-

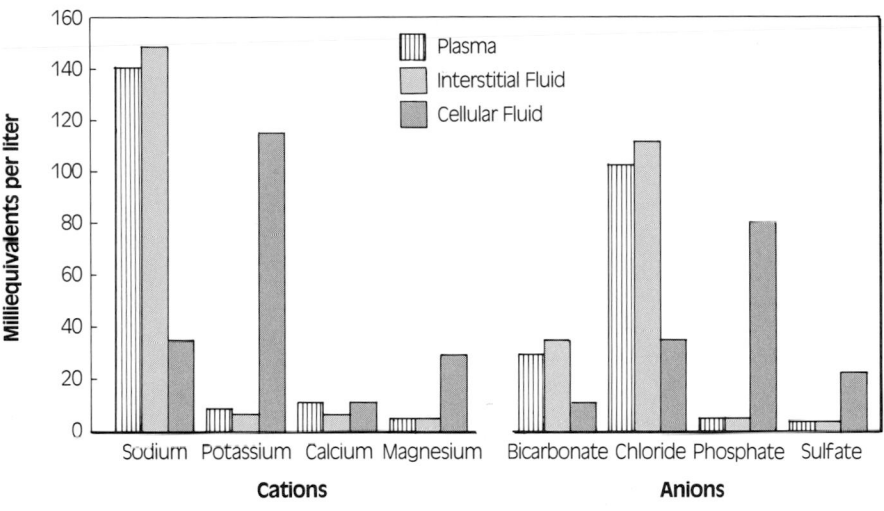

FIGURE 35-3
Electrolyte composition of normal body fluids.

ample, intracellular fluid has higher concentrations of certain electrolytes than extracellular fluid. Figure 35-3 illustrates differences in the electrolyte composition of body fluids according to the compartments in which the fluids are found.

Fluid and Electrolyte Movement

Extracellular fluid takes nourishment to each body cell and receives each cell's waste products. These exchanges, which normally result in fluid balance and homeostasis, are essential to life. The most common routes for transporting materials to and from intracellular compartments are osmosis, diffusion, active transport, and filtration.

Osmosis. The membranes of the body's cells are semipermeable. This makes it possible for water, a pure solvent, to be transported through cell walls.

Osmosis is the most important method of transporting body fluids. Water shifts, and hence, fluid balance, depend heavily on this mode of transport.

Through the process of **osmosis**, the solvent water passes from an area of lesser solute concentration to an area of greater solute concentration until equilibrium is established. As a result, the volume of more concentrated solution will increase, and the volume of the weaker solution will decrease. The greater the difference in the concentration of the two solutions on each side of a semipermeable membrane, the greater the osmotic pressure.

Diffusion. Diffusion is the tendency of solutes to move freely throughout a solvent. The solute moves from an area of higher concentration to an area of lower concentration (*i.e.,* "downhill") until equilibrium is established. Gases move about by diffusion. For example, if an open pan of water is left in a room, evaporation occurs as the water molecules disperse themselves evenly about the room. Oxygen and carbon dioxide exchange in the lung's alveoli and capillaries occurs by diffusion.

Active Transport. Active transport is a process that requires energy for the movement of substances through a cell wall, from an area of lesser concentration to an area of higher concentration. Adenosine triphosphate (ATP), released from a cell, makes it possible for certain substances to acquire energy needed to pass through a cell wall. Although the process is not entirely understood, the energy requirement is affected by characteristics of the cell membrane, specific enzymes, and concentrations of ions. This process explains the so-called pump mechanism and is illustrated in Figure 35-4 using sodium and potassium as examples. If diffusion can be called "coasting downhill," active transport can be called "pumping uphill." The following substances are believed to use active transport: amino acids; glucose, but in certain places only, such as in the kidneys and intestines; and ions of sodium, chloride, potassium, hydrogen, phosphate, calcium, and magnesium.

Filtration. Filtration is the passage of a fluid through a permeable membrane. Passage is from an area of high pressure to one of lower pressure.

Certain substances—those with high molecular weights, such as the plasma proteins—exert **colloid osmotic pressure** or **oncotic pressure**, which is exerted by plasma proteins on permeable membranes in the body. **Hydrostatic pressure** is force exerted by a fluid against the container wall. Blood hydrostatic pressure is the pressure of plasma and blood cells in the capillaries: it depends primarily on arterial blood pressure on the arteriolar side of capillaries, and on venous blood pressure on the venular side of capillaries. **Filtration pressure** is the difference between colloid osmotic pressure and blood hydrostatic pressure.

These pressures are significant to understand how fluid leaves arterioles, enters the interstitial compartment, and eventually returns again to the venules. The

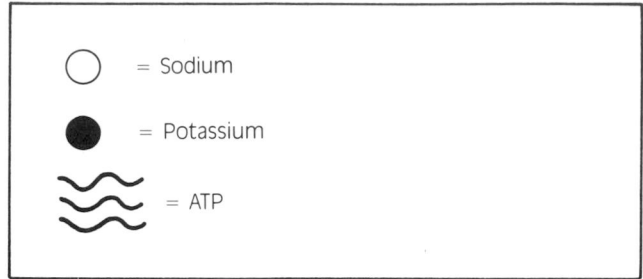

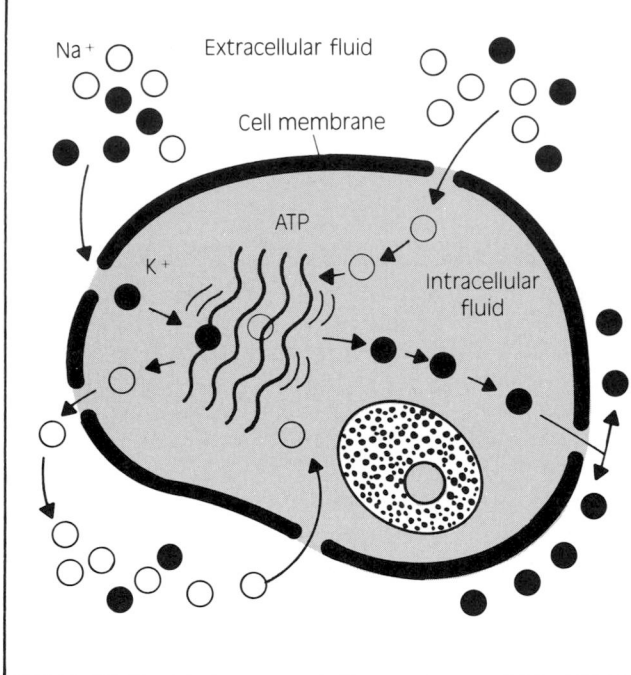

F I G U R E   35-4
Active transport. Sodium that diffuses into the cell through a pore in the cell membrane is actively pumped out of the cell by a carrier system, represented by the wavy lines. Similarly, potassium that diffuses out of the cell is actively replaced by the carrier system.

filtration pressure is positive in the arterioles and, hence, helps force or filter fluids into interstitial spaces; it is negative in the venules and, hence, helps fluid enter at the venules. This is illustrated in Figure 35-5.

Filtration is also involved in the proper functioning of the glomeruli of the kidneys.

Fluid Balance

Authorities indicate that a range of 1500 ml to 3500 ml daily is the desirable amount of fluid intake and loss in adults. The majority of persons have a 2500-ml average intake and loss per day. While these figures are helpful as guidelines, a person's balance between his actual intake and loss must be considered when assessing nursing needs. A person's intake should normally be approximately balanced by his output or fluid loss. A general rule is that in the healthy adult, the output of urine nor-

mally approximates the ingestion of liquids; and the water from food and oxidation is balanced by the water loss through the feces, the skin, and the respiratory process. The intake should be within the desirable average

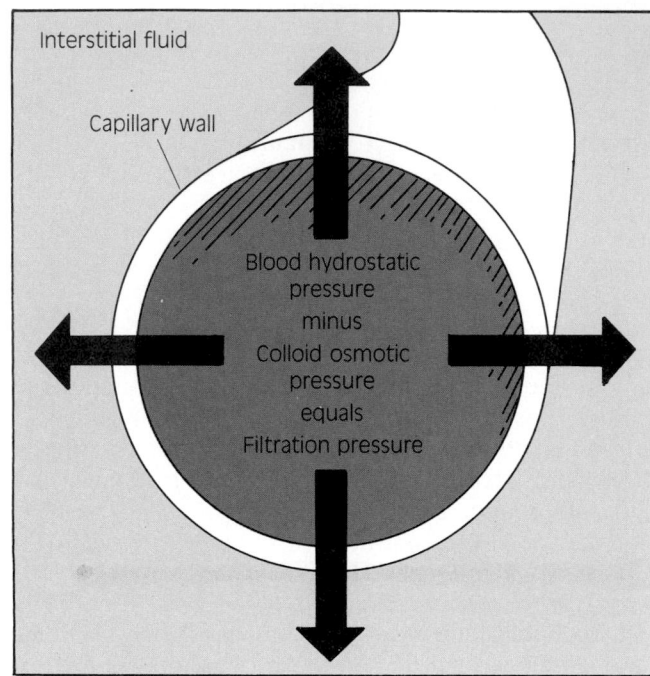

Arteriole: The pressure within the arteriole is **positive** and hence, fluid is forced into interstitial fluid.

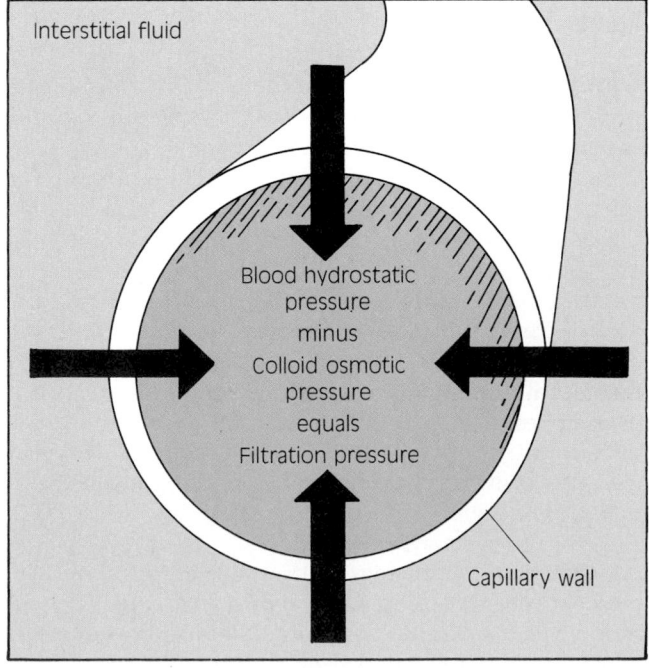

Venule: The pressure within the venule is **negative** and hence, fluid is forced into the venule.

F I G U R E   35-5
Filtration, which is the tendency of solutes to move from an area of higher pressure to an area of lower pressure.

range. The intake–output balance may not always exist in a single 24-hour period but should normally be achieved within 2 to 3 days.

Fluid Sources. Water is derived from several sources for the body.

Ingested Liquids. This source makes up the largest amount of water normally taken into the body. Fluid intake is primarily regulated by the thirst mechanism. Located within the hypothalamus, the thirst control center is stimulated by intracellular dehydration and decreased blood volume.

Water in Food. This is the second largest source of water for the body. The amount ingested depends on dietary items. For example, melons and citrus fruit are high in water content while cereal and dried fruits have a relatively low water content.

Water from Metabolic Oxidation. Water is an end product of the oxidation that occurs during the metabolism of food substances. This source also varies with different types of nutrients. For example, metabolism of 100 g of fat produces 107 g of water while 100 g of carbohydrate will yield 55 g of water, and 100 g of protein will produce 40 g of water. Therefore, a person whose diet is high in fat will have a proportionately greater amount of water resulting from his metabolic processes than a person whose diet is high in protein.

Fluid Losses. Water is lost from the body through the kidneys and intestinal tract, and through the skin as perspiration. Water is also lost in insensible ways. **Insensible water loss** is nonperceptible. For example, in addition to perspiration, which is perceptible, an invisible amount of water is lost from the skin constantly through evaporation. Insensible loss from the lungs is moisture exhaled through the breath.

Water losses vary according to the person and his circumstances.

Figure 35-6 illustrates fluid intake and output balance in healthy adults. Deviations from normal ranges for balance of water intake and output should alert the nurse to impending problems and possibly preventable imbalances.

Homeostatic Mechanisms. Fluid homeostasis normally functions automatically and effectively. Almost every organ and system in the body helps in some way to maintain fluid homeostasis. The following are the primary organs of homeostasis. Functions are highlighted in Table 35-2. Fluid balance is threatened when any organ fails to function properly.

Kidneys. The kidneys are frequently referred to as the master chemists of the body. They normally filter 170 liters of plasma daily in the adult while excreting only 1.5 liters of urine. They selectively retain electrolytes

and water and excrete wastes and excesses. Renal failure results in serious fluid and electrolyte problems.

Cardiovascular System. The cardiovascular system is responsible for pumping and carrying nutrients and water throughout the body.

Lungs. The lungs regulate oxygen and carbon dioxide levels of the blood. The regulation of the carbon dioxide level is especially crucial in maintaining acid–base balance, and is explained later in this chapter.

Adrenal Glands. The adrenal glands secrete aldosterone, which is known as the great sodium conserver of the body. The hormone also helps save chloride and water, and causes potassium to be excreted as indicated.

Pituitary Gland. The posterior lobe of the pituitary gland stores antidiuretic hormone (ADH), which is manufactured in the hypothalamus. Neurons called **osmoreceptors** are sensitive to changes in the concentra-

(Text continues on p. 953.)

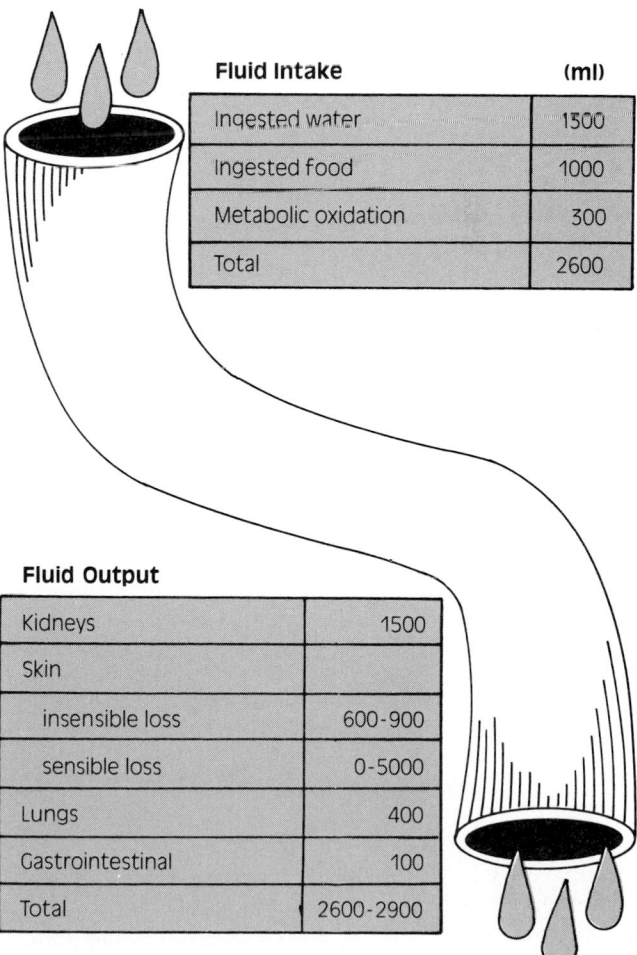

Fluid Intake	(ml)
Ingested water	1500
Ingested food	1000
Metabolic oxidation	300
Total	2600

Fluid Output

Kidneys	1500
Skin	
insensible loss	600-900
sensible loss	0-5000
Lungs	400
Gastrointestinal	100
Total	2600-2900

F I G U R E 35-6
In health, fluid intake and fluid losses are approximately equal. The amounts indicated are average adult daily fluid sources and losses.

T A B L E **35-2**

Homeostatic Mechanisms that Maintain the Composition and Volume of Body Fluid Within Narrow Limits of Normal

Organs of Homeostasis	Functions
Kidneys	• Regulate extracellular fluid volume and osmolality by selective retention and excretion of body fluids • Regulate electrolyte levels in the extracellular fluid by selective retention of needed substances and excretion of unneeded substances • Regulate *p*H of extracellular fluid by excretion or retention of hydrogen ions • Excrete metabolic wastes (primarily acids) and toxic substances
Heart and blood vessels	• Circulate blood through the kidneys under sufficient pressure for urine to form (pumping action of the heart) • React to hypovolemia by stimulating fluid retention (stretch receptors in the atria and blood vessels)

Lungs	• Eliminate about 13,000 mEq of hydrogen ions (H^+) daily, as opposed to only 40 mEq to 80 mEq excreted daily by the kidneys
	• Act promptly to correct metabolic acid–base disturbances; regulate H^+ concentration (pH) by controlling the level of carbon dioxide (CO_2) in the extracellular fluid as follows:
	  1. Metabolic alkalosis causes compensatory hypoventilation, resulting in CO_2 retention (increases acidity of the extracellular fluid).
	  2. Metabolic acidosis causes compensatory hyperventilation, resulting in CO_2 excretion (decreases acidity of the extracellular fluid).
	• Remove approximately 300 ml of water daily through exhalation (insensible water loss) in the normal adult

Adrenal glands	• Regulate blood volume and sodium and potassium balance by secreting aldosterone, a mineral corticoid secreted by the adrenal cortex
	  1. A drop of the extracellular sodium level, a rise in the extracellular potassium level, or a decrease in blood volume triggers aldosterone secretion which causes sodium retention (and thus water retention) and potassium loss.
	  2. Decreased secretion of aldosterone causes sodium and water loss and potassium retention.
	Cortisol, another adrenocortical hormone, has only a fraction of the potency of aldosterone. However, secretion of cortisol in large quantities can produce sodium and water retention and potassium deficit.

Pituitary gland	• Stores and releases the antidiuretic hormone (ADH) which makes the body retain water; functions of ADH include
	  1. Maintains osmotic pressure of the cells by controlling renal water retention or excretion
	    a. When osmotic pressure of the ECF is greater than that of the cells (as in hypernatremia—excess sodium—or hyperglycemia), ADH secretion is increased, causing renal retention of water.
	    b. When osmotic pressure of the ECF is less than that of the cells (as in hyponatremia), ADH secretion is decreased, causing renal excretion of water.
	  2. Controls blood volume (less influential than aldosterone)
	    a. When blood volume is decreased, an increased secretion of ADH results in water conservation.
	    b. When blood volume is increased, a decreased secretion of ADH results in water loss.

Parathyroid glands	• Regulate calcium (Ca 2^+) and phosphate (HPO_4 2^-) balance by means of parathyroid hormone (PTH); PTH influences bone resorption, calcium absorption from the intestines, and calcium reabsorption from the renal tubules.
	  1. Increased secretion of PTH causes
	    a. Elevated serum calcium concentration
	    b. Lowered serum phosphate concentration
	  2. Conversely, decreased secretion of PTH causes
	    a. Lowered serum calcium concentration
	    b. Elevated serum phosphate concentration

(Data from Metheny NM: Fluid and Electrolyte Balance. Philadelphia, JB Lippincott, 1987, pp 8–10.)

tion of extracellular fluid and send appropriate impulses accordingly to release ADH.

Thyroid Gland. Thyroxin, released by the thyroid gland, increases blood flow in the body. This in turn increases renal circulation, which results in increased glomerular filtration and urinary output.

Parathyroid Glands. The parathyroid glands secrete parathormone, which regulates the level of calcium in extracellular fluid.

Gastrointestinal Tract. The gastrointestinal tract absorbs water and nutrients that enter the body through this route.

Nervous System. The nervous system acts as a switchboard and inhibits and stimulates mechanisms that influence fluid balance. It functions chiefly as the regulator of sodium and water intake and excretion. The thirst center is located in the hypothalamus.

Acid–Base Balance

Body fluids must maintain a normal acid–base balance to sustain health and life. Acidity or alkalinity of a solution is determined by its concentration of hydrogen (H^+) ions and hydroxyl (OH^-) ions. An **acid** is a substance containing hydrogen ions that can be liberated or released. An alkali is a **base**, which is a substance that can accept or trap a hydrogen ion. The following equations illustrate:

Equation: An acid releases hydrogen, as follows:

$$H_2CO_3 \rightarrow H^+ + HCO_3^-$$

Carbonic acid releases hydrogen ion to form a bicarbonate base

Equation: A base traps hydrogen, as follows:

$$HCO_3^- + H^+ \rightarrow H_2CO_3$$

Bicarbonate base traps hydrogen ion to form carbonic acid

Equation: A base traps hydrogen, as follows:

$$OH^- + H^+ \rightarrow H_2O$$

Hydroxyl ion from a base traps hydrogen ion to form water

The unit of measure used to describe acid–base balance is *p*H, which is an expression of hydrogen-ion concentration and the resulting acidity of a substance. The *p*H scale ranges from 1 to 14. Neutrality of a solution is 7; an example is pure water. Because *p*H is based on a negative logarithm, as the hydrogen ions increase and a solution becomes more acid, the *p*H becomes less than 7. When the concentration of the hydroxyl ions exceeds the concentration of hydrogen ions, the solution is alkaline and the *p*H is greater than 7. Gastric secretions that are strongly acidic have an approximate *p*H of 1 to 1.3, while strongly alkaline pancreatic secretions have an approximate *p*H of 10.

Normal blood plasma is slightly alkaline and has a normal *p*H range of 7.35 to 7.45. When the normal *p*H range is exceeded in either direction, the person develops signs and symptoms of illness, and if the condition goes on unabated, death will result. **Acidosis** is the condition characterized by a proportionate excess of hydrogen ions in extracellular fluid in which the *p*H falls below 7.35. **Alkalosis** occurs when there is a proportionate lack of hydrogen ions and the *p*H exceeds 7.45. Figure 35-7 illustrates normal *p*H, acidosis, and alkalosis, and also the points at which death can be expected to occur.

The narrow range of normal *p*H is achieved by three major homeostatic regulators of hydrogen ions: buffer systems, respiratory mechanisms, and renal mecha-

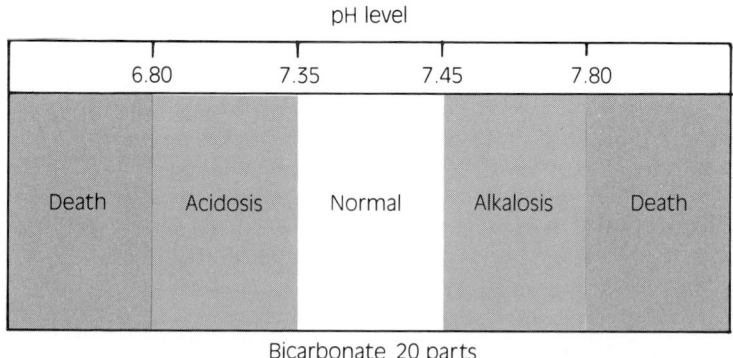

FIGURE 35-7

Acid–base balance. Note that acidosis is used to describe the condition when pH is between 6.80 and 7.35. When the fluid acidity falls below 7, the person is gravely ill or dying.

nisms. A **buffer** is a substance that prevents body fluids from becoming overly acidic or alkaline. The body has three buffer systems: the carbonic acid–sodium bicarbonate buffer system, the phosphate buffer system, and the protein buffer system.

Buffer Systems

Carbonic Acid–Sodium Bicarbonate Buffer System.
The most important buffer system of the body is the carbonic acid–sodium bicarbonate system. This system buffers up to 90% of the H^+ of the extracellular fluid. The following two equations illustrate the system.

Equation: A strong acid plus sodium bicarbonate yields a weak acid, as follows:

$$HCl + NaHCO_3 \rightarrow NaCl + H_2CO_3$$

Strong hydrochloric acid / added to / sodium bicarbonate base / yields / salt and / weak carbonic acid

Equation: A strong base plus a weak acid yields a weak base, as follows:

$$NaOH + H_2CO_3 \rightarrow NaHCO_3 + H_2O$$

Strong sodium hydroxide base / added to / carbonic acid buffer / yields / weak sodium bicarbonate base / and water

The ratio of carbonic acid to the base bicarbonate is important for acid–base balance. Normal extracellular fluid has a ratio of 20 parts bicarbonate to 1 part carbonic acid. The exact quantities are unimportant for acid–base balance as long as they remain in a 20 to 1 ratio.

Phosphate Buffer System.
Phosphate salts are formed in the kidneys by exchanging a sodium ion for a hydrogen ion in the conversion of alkaline sodium phosphate (Na_2HPO_4) to acid sodium phosphate (NaH_2PO_4). The acid sodium phosphate is then excreted. This occurs in the following way:

Equation: The conversion of sodium phosphate to acid sodium phosphate occurs as follows:

$$Na_2HPO_4 + H^+ \rightarrow NaH_2PO_4 + Na^+$$

Alkaline sodium phosphate / and hydrogen / yields / acid sodium phosphate / and sodium

Protein Buffer System.
The third buffer system is a mixture of plasma proteins and the globin portion of hemoglobin in red blood cells. Because plasma proteins and hemoglobin possess groups that can combine with or liberate hydrogen ions, they tend to minimize changes in *p*H and serve as excellent buffering agents over a wide range of *p*H values. The following equations illustrate the oxygenation of hemoglobin as it proceeds in conjunction with the bicarbonate buffer system.

Equation: The high oxygen pressure in the lungs forces oxygen into hemoglobin converting it to oxyhemoglobin:

$$HHb + O_2 \rightarrow HbO_2 + H^+$$

Hemoglobin in red cell / and / oxygen from air / yields / oxyhemoglobin goes in red cell to tissues / and / hydrogen ion in red cell

Equation: The hydrogen ions are promptly neutralized by bicarbonate ions producing carbonic acid:

$$H^+ + HCO_3^- \rightarrow H_2CO_3$$

Hydrogen ion just made / and / bicarbonate ion in red cell and from tissues / yields / carbonic acid in red cell

Equation: Carbonic acid decomposes to water and carbon dioxide which departs by exhaling:

$$H_2CO_3 \rightarrow H_2O + CO_2$$

Carbonic acid just made in red cell / yields / water / and / carbon dioxide leaves lungs in exhaled air

Respiratory Control of H⁺ Balance

The lungs are the primary controller of the body's carbonic-acid supply. They have a huge surface area from which CO_2 can readily diffuse and they can bring about rapid changes in H^+ when needed. Carbon dioxide is constantly produced by cellular metabolism and enters the extracellular fluid. As it does, the carbon dioxide and water are acted upon by the enzyme carbonic anhydrase to produce carbonic acid. The following equations illustrate how carbonic acid is produced and broken down.

Equation: The production of carbonic acid occurs as follows:

$$CO_2 + H_2O \xrightarrow{\text{(carbonic anhydrase)}} H_2CO_3$$

Carbon dioxide / and / water / yields / carbonic acid

Equation: The breakdown of carbonic acid occurs as follows:

$$H_2CO_3 \xrightarrow{\text{(carbonic anhydrase)}} H_2O + CO_2$$

Carbonic acid / yields / water / and / carbon dioxide

Carbon dioxide is excreted by exhalation. As the amount of carbon dioxide in the blood increases, the sensitive respiratory center in the medulla is stimulated and increases the rate and depth of respirations to eliminate more carbon dioxide. When the blood level of carbon dioxide is below normal, the center decreases the rate and depth of respirations to retain the carbon dioxide so that carbonic acid can be formed and the delicate balance maintained. This total respiratory process also occurs frequently and nearly as rapidly as the buffering action in the carbonic acid–sodium bicarbonate system.

Renal Control of H⁺ Balance

The concentration of bicarbonate in the plasma is regulated by the kidneys through the production of ammonia (NH_3), the excretion of hydrogen ions, and by forming additional bicarbonate as needed. The kidneys regulate hydrogen and bicarbonate ions in the following ways.

Equation: The reabsorption of bicarbonate becomes possible when a sodium ion combines with bicarbonate to form sodium bicarbonate, which is taken up in the kidney tubules, as follows:

$$Na^+ \ + \ HCO_3^- \ \rightarrow \ NaHCO_3$$
Sodium and bicarbonate yields   sodium bicarbonate

Equation: As a result of amino acid metabolism, ammonia (NH_3) is formed in the kidney tubules, where it unites with hydrogen to form an ammonium ion (NH_4^+), which, in turn, unites with chloride (Cl^-) to form ammonium chloride (NH_4Cl) for excretion, as follows:

$$NH_3 \ + \ H^+ \ \rightarrow \ NH_4^+$$
Ammonia and hydrogen yields ammonium

$$NH_4^+ \ + \ Cl^- \ \rightarrow \ NH_4Cl$$
Ammonium and chloride yields ammonium chloride

Acid–base regulation by the kidneys occurs more slowly than by the carbonic acid–sodium bicarbonate system or by respiratory regulation. It may take up to 3 days for fluid pH to be restored by the kidneys. The pH of urine varies, depending on the ions that are being excreted, but generally it is in the 4.5 to 8.2 range.

DISTURBANCES IN FLUID, ELECTROLYTE, AND ACID–BASE BALANCE

Nurses commonly encounter disturbances in fluid, electrolyte, and acid–base balance while caring for acutely or chronically ill clients. While many of these disturbances are interrelated and may occur together they will be presented singly for the purpose of study.

Fluid Imbalances

Fluid imbalances occur when the body's compensatory mechanisms are not able to maintain a homeostatic state. Fluid imbalances may relate to either volume or distribution of water or electrolytes.

Fluid Volume Deficit (FVD).
Fluid volume deficit is a deficiency in the amount of both water and electrolytes in the extracellular fluid, but the water and electrolyte proportions remain near normal. The state is commonly known as hypovolemia. Both osmotic- and hydrostatic-pressure changes force the interstitial fluid into the intravascular space. As the interstitial space is depleted, its fluid becomes hypertonic, and cellular fluid is then drawn into the interstitial space, leaving cells without adequate fluid to function properly.

Dehydration is sometimes used as a synonym for hypovolemia, but this is technically inaccurate. **Dehydration** refers only to a decreased volume of water, but water is not decreased without electrolyte changes also. **Hydration** is the union of a substance with water and is often used to indicate that there is normal water volume in the body.

Fluid volume deficits result from the loss of body fluids, especially if fluid intake is simultaneously decreased. Table 35-3 summarizes fluid volume deficit, common problems, and general nursing interventions. Specific interventions are presented later in this chapter.

The very young and the elderly and those fatigued or weakened by illness are particularly susceptible to hypovolemia. A weight loss of 5% for adults and 10% for infants can occur rapidly. A 5% weight loss is considered to be pronounced fluid deficit, and an 8% loss or more is considered severe. A 15% weight loss owing to fluid deficiency usually threatens life.

Third-space fluid shift refers to a distributional shift of body fluids into body spaces such as the pleural, peritoneal, pericardial, or joint cavities, the bowel, or into the interstitial space (plasma-to-interstitial shift). Once trapped in these spaces the fluid is not easily exchanged with extracellular fluid and a deficit in extracellular fluid volume is created. Treatment is directed toward correction of the cause of the third-space shift.

Fluid Volume Excess (FVE).
Excessive retention of water and sodium in extracellular fluid in near-normal proportions results in a condition termed **fluid volume excess**. It is also called **hypervolemia**. Overhydration is commonly used as a synonym for hypervolemia, but strictly speaking, this is inaccurate. **Overhydration** refers only to above-normal amounts of water in extracellular spaces. Malfunction of the kidneys, causing an inability to excrete the excesses, is the most common cause. When water is retained in excessive amounts, so is sodium.

Because of the increased extracellular osmotic pressure from the retained sodium, fluid is pulled from the cells to equalize the tonicity. By the time the intracellular and extracellular spaces are isotonic to each other, an excess of both water and sodium are in the extracellular fluid, while the cells are nearly depleted. The excessive extracellular fluid may accumulate in tissue spaces; this is known as **edema**. Edema is most frequently seen around the eyes, fingers, ankles, and sacral space (Fig. 35-8). It may result in a weight gain in excess of 5%. When the excess fluid remains in the intravascular space, the concentration of solids in the blood is decreased.

Interstitial-to-plasma shift is the movement of fluid from the space surrounding the cells to the blood. This shift, also called hypervolemia, is a compensatory response to volume or osmotic-pressure changes of the intravascular fluid.

While the body attempts to maintain normal balance in all fluid spaces, if circumstances demand, the intravascular fluid is usually protected at the expense of intersti-

(Text continues on p. 957.)

T A B L E   35-3
Fluid Volume Disturbances: Etiologic Factors, Defining Characteristics, and Nursing Interventions

Etiologic Factors	*Defining Characteristics*	*Nursing Interventions*

Summary of Fluid Volume Deficit

Etiologic Factors	Defining Characteristics	Nursing Interventions

Loss of water and electrolytes, as in
• Vomiting
• Diarrhea
• Excessive laxative use
• Fistulas
• GI suction
• Polyuria
• Fever
• Excessive sweating
• Third-space fluid shifts
 	
Decreased intake, as in:
• Anorexia
• Nausea
• Inability to gain access to fluids
• Inability to swallow fluids
• Depression
	Weight loss over short period of time (except in third-space losses)
	• 2% (mild deficit, such as 2.4 lb in 120-lb person or 1 kg in a 54.5-kg person)
	• 5% (moderate deficit, such as 6 lb in 120-lb person or 2.1 kg in a 54.5-kg person)
	• 8% or > (severe deficit, such as 10 lb or > in 120-lb person or 4.5 kg or more in a 54.5-kg person)
	
	Decreased skin and tongue turgor
	
	Dry mucous membranes
	
	Urine output < 30 ml/hr in adult
	
	Postural hypotension (systolic pressure drops by more than 10 mm Hg when client moves from lying to standing or sitting position
	
	Weak, rapid pulse
	
	Slow-filling peripheral veins
	
	Decreased body temperature, such as 95° F–98° F (35° C–36.7° C) unless infection is present
	
	CVP less than 4 cm of water in vena cava
	
	BUN elevated out of proportion to serum creatinine
	
	Urinary SG high
	
	Hematocrit elevated
	
	Flat neck veins in supine position
	Marked oliguria, late
	Altered sensorium
	Cold extremities, late
		1. Assess for presence, or worsening of FVD (see defining characteristics).
		2. Give oral fluids if indicated.
		  • Consider the client's "likes" and "dislikes" when offering fluids.
		  • Consider the type of fluid the client has lost and replace appropriately.
		  • If the client is reluctant to drink because of oral discomfort, select fluids that are nonirritating to the mucosa, and provide frequent mouth care (offer saline gargles and apply lubricant to lips).
		  • Offer fluids at frequent intervals.
		  • Explain the need for fluid replacement to the client and attempt to gain his cooperation.
		  • Administer p.r.n. medications if nausea is present to provide relief before fluids are offered.
		3. Consider the following interventions for clients with impaired swallowing:
		  • Assess gag reflex and ability to swallow water before offering solid foods; have a suction apparatus on hand.
		  • Position the client in an upright position with head and neck flexed slightly forward during feeding (tilting the head backward during swallowing predisposes to aspiration because this position opens the airway).
		  • Provide thick fluids or semisolid foods (such as puddings or gelatin). These are more easily swallowed because of their consistency and weight than are thin liquids.
		4. If the client is unable to eat and drink, discuss possibility of tube feedings with the physician.
		5. Consult with the physician for parenteral fluid directives if the client is unable to consume fluids by the enteral route.
		6. Monitor response to fluid intake, either orally or parenterally. If therapy is adequate, one should observe:
		  • Increased urinary volume, toward 40 ml–60 ml/hr in adult
		  • If previously hypotensive, increased BP toward normal
		  • Return of pulse rate to baseline
		  • Improved sensorium and sense of vitality
		  • Improved skin and tongue turgor
		  • Decreased dryness of oral mucosa
		  • Increased CVP, toward normal
		  • Normal, or no worse, breath sounds
		  • Decreased urinary specific gravity (SG) as urinary volume increases
		  • Increased body weight, toward pre-illness level

(Continued)

Etiologic Factors	Defining Characteristics	Nursing Interventions

Summary of Fluid Volume Deficit (continued)

7. Monitor clients with tendency for abnormal fluid retention (such as renal or cardiac problems) for signs of overload during aggressive fluid replacement.
8. Turn client frequently; apply moisturizing agents to skin and massage bony prominences to avoid skin breakdown.
9. Give frequent oral care.

Summary of Fluid Volume Excess

Etiologic Factors	Defining Characteristics	Nursing Interventions
Compromised regulatory mechanisms: • Renal failure • Congestive heart failure • Cirrhosis of liver • Cushing's syndrome Overzealous administration of sodium-containing IV fluids Excessive ingestion of sodium-containing substances in diet or sodium-containing medications	Weight gain over short period of time: • 2% (mild excess, such as 2.4-lb gain in 120-lb person or 1 kg in a 54.5-kg person) • 5% (moderate excess, such as 6-lb gain in 120-lb person or 2.7 kg in a 54.5-kg person) • 8% or > (severe excess, such as 10-lb gain or > in 120-lb person or 4.5 kg or more in a 54.5-kg person) Peripheral edema (excess of fluid in interstitial space) Distended neck veins Distended peripheral veins Slow-emptying peripheral veins CVP > 11 cm of water in vena cava Moist rales in lungs Polyuria (if renal function is normal) Ascites, pleural effusion (when FVE is severe, fluid transudates into body cavities) Decreased BUN (due to plasma dilution) Decreased hematocrit (also due to plasma dilution) Bounding, full pulse Pulmonary edema, if severe	1. Assess for the presence, or worsening of FVE. 2. Encourage adherence to sodium-restricted diet, if prescribed. Assist dietitian in diet instruction. 3. Instruct clients requiring sodium restriction to avoid over-the-counter drugs without first checking with the health-care adviser. 4. When fluid retention persists despite adherence to dietary sodium intake, consider hidden sources of sodium, such as water supply or use of water softeners. 5. When indicated, encourage rest periods. Lying down favors diuresis of edema fluid. 6. Monitor the client's response to diuretics. Discuss significant findings with physician. 7. Monitor rate of parenteral fluids and the client's response. Discuss significant findings with physician. 8. Teach self-monitoring of weight and intake and output measurements to clients with chronic fluid retention (such as those with congestive heart failure, renal disease, or cirrhosis of liver). 9. Monitor for worsening of underlying cause of FVE. 10. If dyspnea and orthopnea are present, position the client in semi-Fowler's position to favor lung expansion. 11. Turn and position the client frequently; be aware that edematous tissue is more prone to skin breakdown than is normal tissue.

(Data from Metheny NM: Fluid and Electrolyte Balance. Philadelphia, JB Lippincott, 1987, pp 42–45, 49–51.)

tial and intracellular fluids. Table 35-3 summarizes fluid volume excess, examples of common problems likely to produce them, and common nursing interventions. Specific nursing interventions for these problems are presented later in this chapter.

Electrolyte Imbalances

When clients present with deficits or excesses of sodium, potassium, calcium, magnesium, or phosphate, special nursing care is required. Table 35-4 highlights etiologic factors, defining characteristics, nursing interventions for common electrolyte imbalances, and specific nursing strategies to prevent these problems.

Hyponatremia and Hypernatremia. Hyponatremia refers to a sodium deficit in the extracellular fluid. Osmotic pressure changes result in extracellular fluid moving into the cells. When this occurs, a typical sign is fingerprints over the sternum, that is, an examiner's fin-

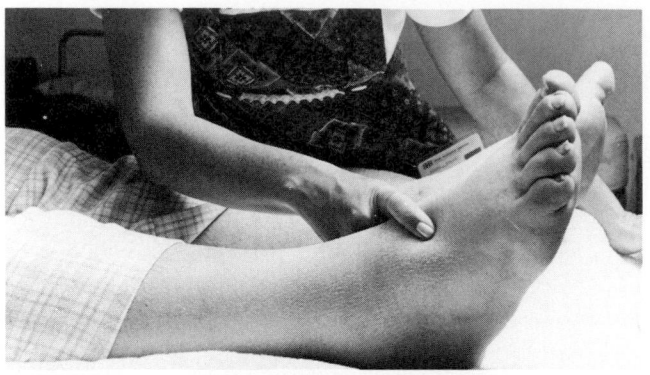

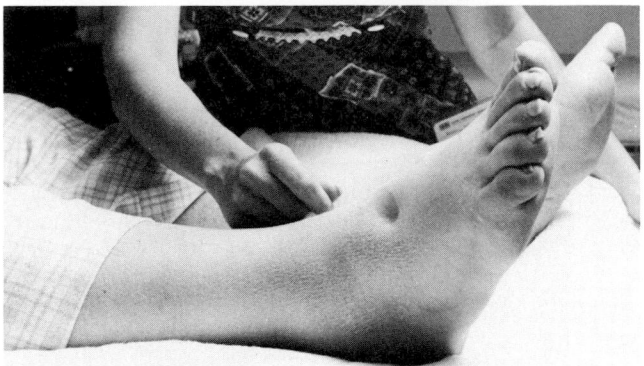

F I G U R E   35-8
(Top) The nurse depresses an area near the ankle of the client where edema is present. (Bottom) Note the indentation of edematous tissues after the nurse releases pressure.

gerprints tend to remain on the patient's skin over the sternum when pressure is applied with the fingers. The phenomenon results from tissue plasticity as fluid moves into cells in excess amounts. **Hypernatremia** refers to a surplus of sodium in extracellular fluid. Because of the increased extracellular osmotic pressure, fluids move from the cells, leaving them without sufficient fluid.

Hypokalemia and Hyperkalemia.   Hypokalemia refers to a potassium deficit in the extracellular fluid. When the extracellular potassium level falls, potassium moves from the cell, creating an intracellular potassium deficiency. Sodium and hydrogen ions are then retained by the cells to maintain isotonic fluids. These electrolyte shifts not only influence normal cellular functioning but also influence the *p*H of extracellular fluid. Muscle tissues are generally the first to demonstrate a potassium deficiency. **Hyperkalemia** refers to an excess of potassium in extracellular fluid. Although this condition occurs less frequently than hypokalemia, it can be very hazardous. The transmission of stimuli through heart muscle is slowed or prevented, and cardiac arrest will eventually occur if hyperkalemia is not corrected.

Hypocalcemia and Hypercalcemia.   Hypocalcemia refers to a calcium deficit in extracellular fluid. If the condition is prolonged, calcium will be taken from the

bones. This results in **osteomalacia**, which is characterized by soft and pliable bones. **Hypercalcemia** refers to an excess of calcium in extracellular fluid. Hypercalcemia presents an emergency situation because the condition often leads to cardiac arrest.

Hypomagnesemia and Hypermagnesemia.   **Hypomagnesemia** refers to a magnesium deficit. The body's potassium level also drops because the kidneys tend to excrete more potassium when magnesium supplies are poor. As a result, hypomagnesemia and hypokalemia very often occur together. A magnesium deficit is ordinarily treated with the administration of magnesium sulfate. **Hypermagnesemia** refers to a magnesium excess. It is a rare condition, but it does occur when the kidneys fail to excrete magnesium and when excessive amounts are used therapeutically.

Hypophosphatemia and Hyperphosphatemia.   **Hypophosphatemia** refers to a below normal serum concentration of inorganic phosphorus. While this may indicate phosphorus deficiency multiple factors may lower serum phosphate levels while total body phosphorus stores are normal. **Hyperphosphatemia** refers to above normal serum concentrations of inorganic phosphorus.

Acid–Base Imbalances

Acid–base imbalances can be assessed by using laboratory plasma findings. The *p*H of plasma indicates balance or impending acidosis or alkalosis. But, in addition, a study of the blood's oxygen and carbon dioxide gases is important. The partial pressures of these gases, or their tensions, are determined by the use of a nomogram, which reflects the chemical and physical activities of the two gases. The partial pressure of carbon dioxide is abbreviated pCO_2; for oxygen, it is pO_2. When the pO_2 is low, hemoglobin carries less than normal amounts of oxygen; when the pO_2 is high, the hemoglobin carries more oxygen. The pCO_2 is influenced almost entirely by respiratory activity. When pCO_2 is low, carbonic acid leaves the body in excessive amounts; when the pCO_2 is high, there are excessive amounts of carbonic acid in the body. The following equations illustrate.

Equation: When the pCO_2 exceeds normal, carbonic acid has increased, as follows:

$$CO_2 + H_2O \rightarrow H_2CO_3$$

Equation: When the pCO_2 is below normal, carbon dioxide leaves the body in excessive amounts, as follows:

$$H_2CO_3 \rightarrow CO_2 + H_2O$$

The measure of *p*H, pCO_2, and pO_2 is almost universally carried out in clinical laboratories at 37°C using arterial whole blood. Many blood gas instruments have microprocessors which can calculate bicarbonate, CO_2 content, base excess, and oxygen saturation. Alterna-

(Text continues on p. 966.)

T A B L E 35-4
Electrolyte Disturbances: Etiologic Factors, Defining Characteristics, and Nursing Interventions

Etiologic Factors	Defining Characteristics	Nursing Interventions
Hyponatremia		
Loss of sodium, as in: • Loss of GI fluids • Use of diuretics • Adrenal insufficiency • Salt-losing nephritis • Osmotic diuresis Gains of water, as in: • Excessive administration of D_5W • Psychogenic polydipsia • Excessive water administration with hypotonic tube feedings Disease states associated with SIADH: • Oat-cell carcinoma of lung • Carcinoma of duodenum or pancreas • Head trauma • Stroke • Pulmonary disorders (abscesses, pneumonia, tuberculosis) Pharmacologic agents that may impair renal water excretion, such as: • Nicotine • Morphine • Barbiturates • Acetaminophen	Anorexia Nausea Vomiting Lethargy Confusion Muscle cramps Fingerprinting over sternum Muscular twitching Seizures Coma Papilledema Hemiparesis Serum Na < 135 mEq/liter (mmol/liter) Serum osmolality < 285 mOsm/kg (nmol/kg) Urinary Na level varies with cause of hyponatremia	1. Identify clients at risk for hyponatremia. 2. Monitor fluid losses and gains. Look for loss of sodium-containing fluids, particularly in conjunction with low-sodium intake. 3. Monitor for presence of gastrointestinal symptoms, such as anorexia, nausea, vomiting, and abdominal cramping. 4. Monitor for central nervous system changes, such as lethargy, confusion, muscular twitching, and convulsions. Be aware that more severe neurologic signs are associated with very low sodium levels that have fallen rapidly due to water overloading. 5. Monitor laboratory data for serum sodium levels less than normal. 6. Check specific gravity of urine. 7. With clients able to consume a general diet, encourage foods and fluids with a high sodium content. For example, broth made with one beef cube contains approximately 900 mg of sodium; 8 oz (250 ml) of canned tomato juice contain about 700 mg of sodium. 8. Be familiar with the sodium content of commonly used parenteral fluids. Monitor clients with cardiovascular disease receiving sodium-containing fluids closely for signs of circulatory overload, such as moist rales in the lungs. 9. Use extreme caution when administering hypertonic saline solutions (3% or 5% NaCl). Be aware that these fluids can be *lethal* if infused carelessly. 10. Avoid giving large water supplements to clients receiving isotonic tube feedings, particularly if routes of abnormal sodium loss are present or water is being retained abnormally. 11. Monitor clients with decreased adrenal function for signs of acute adrenocortical insufficiency (adrenal crisis) when they are exposed to severe stress (such as surgery, trauma, emotional upset, excessive heat, or prolonged medical illness). Look for extreme weakness, acute onset of nausea and vomiting, hypotension, confusion, and even shock.
Hypernatremia		
Deprivation of water, most common in those unable to perceive or respond to thirst Hypertonic tube feedings with inadequate water supplements Increased insensible water loss (as in hyperventilation)	Thirst Elevated body temperature Tongue dry and swollen, sticky mucous membranes Severe hypernatremia: • Disorientation • Hallucinations • Lethargy when undisturbed • Irritable and hyper-reactive when stimulated	1. Identify clients at risk for hypernatremia. 2. Monitor fluid losses and gains. Look for abnormal losses of water or low water intake, and for large gains of sodium as might occur with ingestion of proprietary drugs with a high sodium content (such as Alka-Seltzer). Also, consider that prescription drugs may have a high sodium content. And, of course, one should look for excessive intake of high sodium foods. 3. Monitor for changes in behavior, such as restlessness, disorientation, and lethargy.

(Continued)

Electrolyte Disturbances: Etiologic Factors, Defining Characteristics, and Nursing Interventions   (Continued)

Etiological Factors	Defining Characteristics	Nursing Interventions
Hypernatremia (continued)		
Watery diarrhea	• Focal or grand mal seizures, coma	4. Look for excessive thirst and elevated body temperature. If present, evaluate in relation to other signs.
Ingestion of salt in unusual amounts	Serum Na > 145 mEq/liter (mmol/liter)	5. Monitor serum sodium levels as indicated.
Excessive parenteral administration of sodium-containing solutions: • Hypertonic saline (3% or 5% NaCl) • 7.5% sodium bicarbonate • Isotonic saline	Serum osmolality > 295 mOsm/kg (mmol/kg) Urinary SG > 1.015, provided water loss is from nonrenal route	6. Prevent hypernatremia in debilitated clients unable to perceive or respond to thirst by offering them fluids at regular intervals. If fluid intake remains inadequate, consult with the physician to plan an alternate route for intake, either by tube feedings or by the parenteral route.
Profuse sweating		7. If tube feedings are used, give sufficient water to keep the serum sodium and the blood urea nitrogen (BUN) level within normal limits. Be aware that the higher the osmolality of the feeding, the greater the need for water supplements.
Diabetes insipidus		
Heatstroke		8. Monitor the client's response to corrective parenteral fluids by reviewing serial sodium levels and by observing for changes in neurologic signs. With gradual decrease in the serum sodium level, the neurologic signs should improve, not worsen. Be aware that the serum sodium should be dropped gradually.
Drowning in sea water		
Hypertonic saline accidentally introduced into maternal circulation during therapeutic abortion		
Hypokalemia		
Diarrhea	Fatigue	1. Be aware of clients at risk for hypokalemia and monitor for its occurrence. Hypokalemia can be life-threatening; it is important to detect it early.
Vomiting or gastric suction	Anorexia, nausea, and vomiting	2. Assess digitalized clients at-risk for hypokalemia especially closely for symptoms of digitalis toxicity because hypokalemia potentiates the action of digitalis. Be aware that the physician usually prefers to keep the serum potassium level > 3.5 mEq/liter in digitalized clients.
Potassium-losing diuretics (such as furosemide and thiazides)	Muscle weakness	
Steroid administration	Decreased bowel motility (intestinal ileus)	3. Take measures to prevent hypokalemia when possible. a. Prevention may take the form of encouraging extra potassium intake for at-risk client (when the diet allows).
Carbenicillin, sodium penicillin, amphotericin B	Cardiac arrhythmias Increased sensitivity to digitalis toxicity	b. When hypokalemia is due to abuse of laxatives or diuretics, education of the client may help alleviate the problem.
Hyperaldosteronism	Polyuria, nocturia, dilute urine (if hypokalemia is prolonged)	4. Administer oral potassium supplements when prescribed.
Hyperalimentation	Mild hyperglycemia	
Poor intake, as in anorexia nervosa, alcoholism, potassium-free parenteral fluids	Postural hypotension Serum K < 3.5 mEq/liter (mmol/liter)	5. Be aware that clients may not need potassium supplements if they are using salt substitutes because these substances usually contain sizable amounts of potassium. Educate clients regarding the use of salt substitutes.
Osmotic diuresis (as occurs in uncontrolled diabetes mellitus or mannitol adm.)	Paresthesias or tender muscles ECG changes: Flattened T waves ST segment depression	6. Be thoroughly familiar with the critical facts related to administering potassium intravenously.
Renal tubular acidosis		7. Be aware that any client experiencing life-threatening symptoms, such as arrhythmias or paralysis, requires urgent replacement of potassium.
Cushing's syndrome		

(Continued)

Etiological Factors	Defining Characteristics	Nursing Interventions

Hyperkalemia (continued)

Pseudohyperkalemia:
- Tight tourniquet
- Hemolysis of sample
- Leukocytosis
- Thrombocytosis

Decreased potassium excretion:
- Oliguric renal failure
- Potassium-conserving diuretics
- Hypoaldosteronism

High potassium intake, especially in presence of renal insufficiency:
- Improper use of oral potassium supplements
- Rapid or excessive administration of IV potassium
- Rapid transfusion of aged blood
- High-dose potassium penicillin
- Foods high in potassium (such as dried apricots)

Shift of potassium out of cells:
- Acidosis
- Tissue trauma
- Malignant cell lysis

Vague muscular weakness is usually first sign

Cardiac arrhythmias, bradycardia, and heart block can occur

Paresthesias of face, tongue, feet, and hands

Flaccid muscle paralysis (spreads from legs to trunk and arms; respiratory muscles may be affected)

Gastrointestinal symptoms such as nausea, intermittent intestinal colic, or diarrhea may occur

ECG changes:
tall, peaked T waves, widened QRS complex, progressing to sine waves

Serum K > 5.5 mEq/liter (mmol/liter)

---

1. Be aware of clients at risk for hyperkalemia and monitor for its occurrence. Hyperkalemia is life-threatening; it is imperative to detect it early.
2. Take measures to prevent hyperkalemia when possible by following guidelines for administering potassium safely, both intravenously and orally.
   a. Follow rules for safe administration of potassium.
   b. Avoid administration of potassium-conserving diuretics, potassium supplements, or salt substitutes to clients with renal insufficiency.
   c. Caution clients to use salt substitutes sparingly if they are taking other supplementary forms of potassium or are taking potassium-conserving diuretics (such as spironolactone, triamterene, and amiloride).
   d. Caution hyperkalemic clients to avoid foods high in potassium content. Some of these are coffee, cocoa, tea, dried fruits, dried beans, whole-grain breads, and milk desserts. Meat and eggs also contain substantial amounts of potassium. (Foods with minimal potassium content include butter, margarine, cranberry juice or sauce, ginger ale, gumdrops or jellybeans, lollypops, root beer, sugar or honey.)
3. To avoid false reports of hyperkalemia, take the following precautions:
   a. Avoid prolonged use of tourniquet while drawing blood sample
   b. Do not allow client to exercise extremity immediately before drawing blood sample
   c. Take blood sample to laboratory as soon as possible (serum must be separated from cells within 1 hr after collection)
   d. Avoid drawing blood specimen from a site above an infusion of potassium solution (or any solution for that matter).
4. Be familiar with usual treatment regimens for hyperkalemia and factors related to their safe implementation.

Hypocalcemia

Surgical hypoparathyroidism (may follow thyroid surgery or radical neck surgery for cancer)

Malabsorption

Vitamin D deficiency

Acute pancreatitis

Excessive administration of citrated blood

Primary hypoparathyroidism

Numbness, tingling of fingers, circumoral region, and toes

Cramps in muscles of extremities

Hyperactive deep-tendon reflexes (such as patellar and triceps)

Trousseau's sign

Chvostek's sign

Mental changes, such as confusion and alterations in mood and memory

---

1. Be aware of clients at risk for hypocalcemia and monitor for its occurrence.
2. Be prepared to take seizure precautions when hypocalcemia is severe.
3. Monitor condition of airway closely because laryngeal stridor can occur.
4. Take safety precautions if confusion is present.
5. Be aware of factors related to the safe administration of calcium replacement salts.
6. Educate persons in high-risk groups for osteoporosis (especially postmenopausal women not on estrogen therapy) as to the need for dietary calcium intake. If adequate amounts are not consumed in the diet (as is often the case), calcium supplements should be considered.

(Continued)

T A B L E   35-4

Electrolyte Disturbances: Etiologic Factors, Defining Characteristics, and Nursing Interventions   (Continued)

Etiological Factors	Defining Characteristics	Nursing Interventions

Hypocalcemia (continued)

Etiological Factors	Defining Characteristics	Nursing Interventions
Alkalotic states (decreased ionized calcium) Hyperphosphatemia Medullary carcinoma of thyroid Hypoalbuminemia (as in cirrhosis, nephrotic syndrome, and starvation) Hypomagnesemia Decreased ultraviolet exposure	Convulsions (usually generalized but may be focal) Spasm of laryngeal muscles Cardiac manifestations; ECG shows prolonged Q–T interval Spasms of muscles in abdomen (can simulate acute abdominal emergency) Total serum calcium level below 8.5 mg/dl (2.12 mmol/liter) or ionized level below normal (<50%) Sulkowitch's test shows light precipitation	a. Most sources recommend that the calcium intake for these individuals be 1000 mg–1500 mg each day. Of course, the best way for healthy persons to ensure an adequate calcium intake is to eat a wide variety of foods from the four food groups daily. b. As stated above, calcium supplements may be necessary for persons unable to consume enough calcium in the diet, such as those who do not tolerate milk or dairy products well. Numerous preparations are obtainable over-the-counter and consumers need advice in selecting suitable products. It appears that calcium is best absorbed when taken in divided doses, rather than all at once. Also, it is suggested that some of the calcium be taken at bedtime because calcium loss accelerates during sleep. (Antacids containing aluminum may increase bone loss and their use is discouraged in persons having bone health problems; among these products are Rolaids, Tempo, DiGel, Gaviscon, Gelusil, and Mylanta.) c. Some postmenopausal women are advised by their physicians to take estrogen. For those who cannot take estrogen, synthetically produced calcitonin is now available by prescription. d. Encourage persons with a tendency to form renal stones to consult their physicians before greatly increasing their calcium intake. Also, it is important to encourage these persons to drink no less than 2 to 3 quarts of fluid a day to protect against stone formation. 7. Educate persons at risk for osteoporosis about the value of regular physical exercise in decreasing bone loss. 8. In order to prevent osteoporosis in later years, educate young women about the need for a normal diet to ensure adequate calcium intake. Also, discuss the calcium-losing aspects of alcohol and nicotine use.

Hypercalcemia

Etiological Factors	Defining Characteristics	Nursing Interventions
Hyperparathyroidism Malignant neoplastic disease: • Solid tumors with metastases (breast, prostate, and malignant melanomas) • Solid tumors without bony metastases (lung, head and neck, and renal tumors) • Hematologic tumors (lymphoma, acute leukemia, and myeloma)	Muscular weakness Tiredness, listlessness, lethargy Constipation Anorexia, nausea, and vomiting Decreased memory span, decreased attention span, and confusion Polyuria and polydipsia Renal stones	1. Be aware of clients at risk for hypercalcemia and monitor for its presence. 2. Increase client mobilization when feasible; recall that immobilization favors hypercalcemia. 3. Encourage the oral intake of sufficient fluids to keep the client well hydrated. Sodium-containing fluids should be given, unless contraindicated by other conditions, since sodium favors calcium excretion. 4. Discourage excessive consumption of milk products and other high-calcium foods. 5. Encourage adequate bulk in the diet to offset the tendency for constipation.

(Continued)

Etiological Factors	Defining Characteristics	Nursing Interventions

Hypercalcemia (continued)

Prolonged immobilization
 	
Large doses of vitamin D
 	
Overuse of calcium-containing antacids or calcium supplements
 	
Thiazide diuretics
 	
Milk–alkali syndrome
	Neurotic behavior progressing to frank psychoses may occur (reversible with correction of hypercalcemia)
	
	Cardiac arrest may occur in hypercalcemic crisis
	
	ECG shows shortened Q–T interval
	
	Bone changes seen on film in chronic hypercalcemia
	
	Itching and ocular changes (band keratopathy)
	
	Serum calcium > 10.5 mg/dl (2.62 mmol/liter)
	
	Sulkowitch's test shows dense precipitation
		6. Take safety precautions if confusion or other mental symptoms of hypercalcemia are present. Explain to the client and family that the mental changes associated with hypercalcemia are reversible with treatment.
		7. Be aware that cardiac arrest can occur in clients with severe hypercalcemia; be prepared to deal with this emergency situation.
		8. Be aware that bones may fracture more easily in clients with chronic hypercalcemia because bone resorption has been excessive, weakening the bony structure. Transfer clients cautiously.
		9. Educate home-bound oncology clients with a predisposition for hypercalcemia, and their families, to be alert for symptoms that occur with this condition and to report them to the health-care providers before they become severe.
		10. Be alert for signs of digitalis toxicity when hypercalcemia occurs in digitalized clients.
		11. Help prevent formation of calcium renal stones in clients with long-standing hypercalcemia or immobilization by
		  a. Forcing fluids to maintain a dilute urine, thus avoiding supersaturation of precipitates.
		  b. Encouraging fluids that yield an acid-ash (such as prune or cranberry juice) because a urinary *p*H less than 6.5 favors calcium deposits.
		  c. Preventing urinary stasis by turning the immobilized client frequently, elevating the head of the bed, and having the client sit up if this can be tolerated.
		  d. Encouraging weight-bearing and ambulation as soon as possible.

Hypomagnesemia

Chronic alcoholism, particularly during withdrawal Intestinal malabsorption syndromes Diarrhea Nasogastric suction Aggressive refeeding after starvation (as in TPN) without adequate Mg replacement Prolonged administration of magnesium-free maintenance IV fluids Diabetic ketoacidosis	Neuromuscular irritability: • Increased reflexes • Coarse tremors • Positive Chvostek's and Trousseau's signs • Convulsions Cardiac manifestations: • Tachyarrhythmias • Increased susceptibility to digitalis toxicity • ECG changes in severe cases: P–R and Q–T interval prolongation, widened QRS complex, ST segment depression, and T-wave inversion Mental changes: • Disorientation in memory • Mood changes • Intense confusion • Hallucinations	1. Be aware of clients at risk for hypomagnesemia and monitor for its presence. 2. Assess digitalized clients at risk for hypomagnesemia especially closely for symptoms of digitalis toxicity because a deficit of magnesium predisposes to toxicity. 3. Be prepared to take seizure precautions when hypomagnesemia is severe. 4. Monitor condition of airway, because laryngeal stridor can occur. 5. Take safety precautions if confusion is present. 6. Be familiar with magnesium replacement salts and factors related to their safe administration. 7. Be aware that magnesium-depleted clients may experience difficulty in swallowing. 8. When magnesium deficit is due to abuse of diuretics or laxatives, educating the client may help alleviate the problem.

(Continued)

T A B L E   35-4

Electrolyte Disturbances: Etiologic Factors, Defining Characteristics, and Nursing Interventions   (Continued)

Etiological Factors	Defining Characteristics	Nursing Interventions

Hypomagnesemia (continued)

Hyperaldosteronism (either primary, or secondary, as in congestive heart failure or cirrhosis)

Drugs:
- Diuretics
- Aminoglycoside antibiotics (such as gentamicin)
- Cisplatin
- Excessive doses of vitamin D or calcium supplements
- Citrate preservative in blood products

Pancreatitis

Thyrotoxicosis

Hyperparathyroidism

Others:
  Burns, sepsis, and hypothermia

Serum magnesium level < 1.5 mEq/liter or 1.8 mg/dl (0.8 mmol/liter). Usually symptoms don't appear until serum magnesium is < 1 mEq/liter (0.8 mmol/liter).

Hypocalcemia and hypokalemia frequently occur with severe hypomagnesemia.

9. Be aware that most commonly used intravenous fluids have either no magnesium or a relatively small amount. When indicated, discuss need for magnesium replacement with physician.
10. For clients experiencing abnormal magnesium losses, but able to consume a general diet, encourage the intake of magnesium-rich foods (such as green vegetables, nuts and legumes, and fruits such as bananas, oranges, and grapefruits).

Hypermagnesemia

Renal failure (particularly when magnesium-containing medications are administered)

Adrenal insufficiency

Excessive magnesium administration during treatment of eclampsia

Hemodialysis with excessively hard water or with a dialysate inadvertently high in magnesium content

Untreated ketoacidosis

Early signs (serum magnesium level of 3 mEq–5 mEq/liter or 1.5 mmol–2.5 mmol/liter)
- Flushing and a sense of skin warmth (due to peripheral vasodilation)
- Hypotension (due to blockage of sympathetic ganglia as well as to a direct effect on smooth muscle)
- Nausea and vomiting

Drowsiness, hypoactive reflexes, and muscular weakness (can occur at a serum magnesium level of 5 mEq–7 mEq/liter or 2.5 mmol–3.5 mmol/liter)

Depresses respirations (can occur at a serum magnesium level of 10 mEq/liter or 5 mmol/liter)

Coma (can occur at a serum magnesium level of 12 mEq–15 mEq/liter 6 mmol–7.5 mmol/liter)

1. Be aware of clients at risk for hypermagnesemia and assess for its presence. When hypermagnesemia is suspected, assess the following parameters:
   - Vital signs: Look for low blood pressure and shallow respirations with periods of apnea
   - Patellar reflexes: If absent, notify physician because this usually implies a serum magnesium level greater than 7 mEq/liter (3.5 mmol/liter). If allowed to progress, cardiac or respiratory arrest could occur.
   - Level of consciousness: Look for drowsiness, lethargy, and coma.
2. Do not give magnesium-containing medications to client with renal failure or compromised renal function. (Be particularly careful in following "standing orders" for bowel preparation for x-ray because some of these include the use of magnesium citrate.)
3. Caution clients with renal disease to check with their health-care providers before taking over-the-counter medications.
4. Be aware of factors related to safe parenteral administration of magnesium salts.

(Continued)

Etiological Factors	Defining Characteristics	Nursing Interventions

Hypermagnesemia (continued)

| | Cardiac abnormalities:
• Sinus bradycardia, prolonged P–R, QRS, and Q–T intervals (at serum magnesium levels of 7.1 mEq–10.0 mEq/liter or 3.5–5 mmol/liter)
• Heart block and cardiac arrest in diastole (can occur at a serum magnesium level of 15 mEq–20 mEq/liter or 7.5 mmol–10 mmol/liter)

Weak or absent cry in newborn | |

Hypophosphatemia

| Glucose administration

Refeeding after starvation

Hyperalimentation

Alcohol withdrawal

Diabetic ketoacidosis

Respiratory alkalosis

Phosphate-binding ant acids

Recovery phase after severe burns | Paresthesias

Muscle weakness (perhaps manifested as decreased strength of hand grasp and difficulty speaking)

Muscle pain and tenderness

Mental changes, such as apprehension, confusion, delirium, and coma

Cardiomyopathy

Acute respiratory failure (perhaps related to chest muscle weakness)

Seizures

Decreased tissue oxygenation

Joint stiffness

Serum phosphate < 2.5 mg/dl (0.8 mmol/liter) | 1. Identify clients at risk for hypophosphatemia.
    • Particularly at risk are extremely malnourished clients being started on TPN or large caloric intake by tube feeding (refeeding syndrome in starving clients).
    • Also at great risk are alcoholic clients undergoing withdrawal therapy and initial treatment with intravenous fluids.
    • Similarly at great risk are clients with diabetic ketoacidosis during the early treatment period with insulin and intravenous fluids.
2. Monitor clients at risk for the presence of hypophosphatemia. *See Defining Characteristics.*
3. Be aware that severely hypophosphatemic clients are thought to be at greater risk for infection because of changes in white blood cells.
4. Administer intravenous phosphate products cautiously. Be aware that they should be administered slowly in dilute infusion solutions to avoid phosphate intoxication. Frequent monitoring of serum phosphorus levels is required to guide therapy.
5. Be aware that in adults the usual maintenance dose of phosphorus is 10 mM to 15 mM per liter of TPN solution. However, maintenance doses may not be sufficient if the client is in a high anabolic state. Allowances must also be made for existing phosphorus deficit.
6. Be aware of the need to introduce hyperalimentation *gradually* in clients who are malnourished. Gradual introduction of the feeding solution is less apt to be associated with rapid shifts of phosphate into the cells. Monitor rates of TPN flow frequently.
7. Be aware that sudden increase in the serum phosphorus level can cause hypocalcemia. For this reason, serum calcium levels should be monitored. Watch for twitching around the mouth, laryngospasm, positive Chvostek's sign, paresthesias, arrhythmias, and hypotension. |

(Continued)

T A B L E   35-4

Electrolyte Disturbances: Etiologic Factors, Defining Characteristics, and Nursing Interventions   **(Continued)**

Etiological Factors	Defining Characteristics	Nursing Interventions
Hypophosphatemia (continued)		
		8. Because it is possible to give too much phosphorus when administering phosphate solutions, monitor for signs of hyperphosphatemia and of the salt in which it is administered.
		9. Monitor for diarrhea in clients taking oral phosphorus supplements; consult with physician if it persists or becomes severe.
		10. Mix powdered oral phosphorus supplements with chilled or iced water to make them more palatable. Also, palatability may be increased by refrigerating the solution made from the powder.
Hyperphosphatemia		
Renal failure	Short-term consequences: symptoms of tetany, such as tingling of fingertips and around mouth, numbness, and muscle spasms	1. Identify clients at risk for hyperphosphatemia.
Chemotherapy, particularly for acute lymphoblastic leukemia and lymphoma		2. Monitor for signs of tetany, such as tingling sensations in the fingertips and around the mouth, and presence of muscle cramps or positive Chvostek's and Trousseau's signs in at-risk clients. Be aware that these symptoms are probably due to hypocalcemia induced by the high phosphate level and are most likely to occur in clients who have taken in a high phosphate load.
Large intake of milk, as in treatment of peptic ulcer	Long-term consequences: precipitation of calcium phosphate in nonosseous sites, such as the kidney, joints, arteries, skin, or cornea.	3. Be aware that soft-tissue calcification can be a long-term complication of a chronically elevated serum phosphate level. Calcification may occur in sites such as the kidney, arteries, joints, and cornea. Monitor for signs of these complications.
Use of cow's milk in infants	Serum phosphate > 4.5 mg/dl (1.4 mmol/liter)	4. Administer prescribed oral and intravenous phosphate supplements cautiously and monitor serum phosphorus levels periodically during their use.
Excessive intake of phosphate-containing laxatives		5. When appropriate, instruct clients that use of phosphate-containing laxatives may result in acute phosphate poisoning.
Overzealous administration of phosphorus supplements, orally or intravenously		6. Be aware that phosphate-containing enemas can result in hyperphosphatemia if used injudiciously, particularly in children and those with slow bowel emptying. Instruct clients accordingly.
Excessive use of Fleet's phosphosoda as enema solution, particularly in children and persons with slow bowel elimination		7. When a low-phosphorus diet is prescribed, instruct clients to avoid foods high in phosphorus content. Such foods include hard cheese or cream, nuts and nut products, whole grain cereals (such as bran and oatmeal), dried fruits, dried vegetables, special meats such as kidneys and sardines and sweetbreads, and desserts made with milk).
Large vitamin D intake (increases phosphorus absorption)		
Hypoparathyroidism		
Hyperthyroidism		

(Data from Metheny NM: Fluid and Electrolyte Balance. Philadelphia, JB Lippincott, 1987, Chaps 4–8.)

tively, these values can be determined from nomograms or figures. Laboratory levels for arterial blood gases are given later in this chapter.

Acid–base imbalances occur when the carbonic acid or bicarbonate levels become disproportionate. When there is a single primary cause, these disturbances are known as respiratory acidosis or alkalosis and metabolic acidosis or alkalosis, which are defined and described below. These disturbances are a result of an upset in acid–base balance, as follows:

- A respiratory disturbance alters the carbonic-acid portion:

  Respiratory acidosis and alkalosis are the results of respiratory phenomena.

  Compensation occurs to restore balance in the kidneys by either trying to conserve or excrete more bicarbonate.

- A metabolic disturbance alters the bicarbonate portion:

  Metabolic acidosis and alkalosis are almost entirely the result of metabolic processes.

  The primary organs for compensation to restore balance are the lungs, which either try to conserve or excrete more carbon dioxide, which is available in weakly ionized carbonic acid.

Table 35-5 summarizes acid–base imbalances. Complicated clinical situations may occur when respiratory and metabolic imbalances coexist.

Respiratory Acidosis.

Respiratory acidosis is a primary excess of carbonic acid in the extracellular fluid. Any decrease in alveolar ventilation that results in retention of carbon dioxide can cause respiratory acidosis. Because the lungs are the source of the problem, they are unable to participate in compensation. As the carbonic acid content increases, the kidneys attempt to retain more bicarbonate and increase their hydrogen excretion. Thus,

Respiratory acidosis = high pCO_2 owing to alveolar hypoventilation.

Respiratory Alkalosis.

Respiratory alkalosis is a primary deficit of carbonic acid in the extracellular fluid. It is the result of increased alveolar ventilation and, therefore, a decrease in carbon dioxide. An increase in respiratory rate and depth causes the carbon dioxide loss because the carbon dioxide is excreted faster than normal.

Because of the deficit of carbon dioxide, which is a respiratory stimulant, depression or cessation of respirations eventually occurs. Because the lungs are the source of the problem, they are unable to participate in compensation. Therefore, the kidneys attempt to alleviate the imbalance by increasing the bicarbonate excretion and by retaining more hydrogen. Thus,

Respiratory alkalosis = low pCO_2 owing to alveolar hyperventilation.

Metabolic Acidosis.

Metabolic acidosis is a proportionate deficit of bicarbonate in the extracellular fluid. The deficit can occur as the result of an increase in acid components or an excessive loss of bicarbonate. The lungs attempt to increase the carbon dioxide excretion by increasing the rate and depth of respirations. The kidneys attempt to compensate by retaining bicarbonate and by excreting more hydrogen. If the body is unable to achieve normal balance, the person may lose consciousness as metabolic acidosis increases, and death will eventually result. Thus,

Metabolic acidosis = low bicarbonate. Nonvolatile acid is present to use up HCO_3^- in disproportionate amounts or HCO_3^- is lost in disproportionate amounts.

Metabolic Alkalosis.

Metabolic alkalosis is a primary excess of bicarbonate in the extracellular fluid. This may be the result of excessive acid losses or increased base ingestion or retention. The body attempts to compensate by retaining carbon dioxide. The respirations become slow and shallow, and periods of no breathing may occur. The kidneys attempt to excrete potassium and sodium with the excessive bicarbonate, and retain hydrogen in carbonic acid. Thus,

Metabolic alkalosis = high bicarbonate. Nonvolatile acid is lost and is not using up HCO_3^- or HCO_3^- is gained in disproportionate amounts.

NURSE AS ROLE MODEL

Nurses wishing to be a role model of self-care behaviors that promote fluid, electrolyte, and acid–base balance should meet the following goals:

The nurse will

- Daily ingest the quantity and type of fluids (to include six to eight glasses of water) that promote healthy hydration and urinary functioning
- Evaluate use of fad diets, diuretics, laxatives, and alcohol, identifying potential risks to health
- Identify situations of high risk for fluid and electrolyte imbalance and intervene appropriately

ASSESSING

The pathophysiology underlying both acute and chronic illness, trauma, and select therapeutic interventions may all place a client at high risk for fluid, electrolyte, and acid–base imbalances. Once present these imbalances can seriously compromise the client's health status and may prove life threatening. Nursing assessment is directed toward

- Identification of clients at high risk for fluid, electrolyte, and acid–base imbalance
- Determination that a specific imbalance is present, identification of nature of imbalance, severity, etiology, and defining characteristics
- Determination of the effectiveness of the plan of care

Important assessment parameters include the nursing history and nursing examination, record of fluid intake and output, daily weight, and laboratory studies.

(Text continues on p. 970.)

Etiologic Factors	Defining Characteristics	Treatment

Respiratory Acidosis (Carbonic Acid Excess)

Acute respiratory acidosis:
- Acute pulmonary edema
- Aspiration of a foreign body
- Atelectasis
- Pneumothorax, hemothorax
- Overdosage of sedatives or anesthetic
- Position on OR table that interferes with respirations
- Cardiac arrest
- Severe pneumonia
- Laryngospasm
- Mechanical ventilation improperly regulated

Chronic respiratory acidosis:
- Emphysema
- Cystic fibrosis
- Advanced multiple sclerosis
- Bronchiectasis
- Bronchial asthma

Factors favoring hypoventilation:
- Obesity
- Tight abdominal binders or dressings
- Postoperative pain (as in high abdominal or chest incisions)
- Abdominal distention from cirrhosis or bowel obstruction

Acute respiratory acidosis:
- Feeling of fullness in the head ($PaCO_2$ causes cerebrovascular vasodilatation and increased cerebral blood flow, particularly when higher than 60 mm Hg)
- Mental cloudiness
- Dizziness
- Palpitations
- Muscular twitching
- Convulsions
- Warm, flushed skin
- Unconsciousness
- Ventricular fibrillation may be first sign in anesthetized patient (related to hyperkalemia)
- ABGs:
  - $pH < 7.35$
  - $PaCO_2 > 42$ mm Hg (primary)
  - HCO_3^- normal or only slightly elevated

Chronic respiratory acidosis:
- Weakness
- Dull headache
- Symptoms of underlying disease process
- ABGs:
  - $pH < 7.35$ or within lower limits of normal
  - $PaCO_2 > 42$ mm Hg (primary)
  - $HCO_3^- > 26$ mEq/liter (mmol/liter) (compensatory)

Treatment is directed at improving ventilation; exact measures vary with the cause of inadequate ventilation. Pharmacologic agents are used as indicated. For example, bronchodilators help reduce bronchial spasm; antibiotics are used for respiratory infections. Pulmonary hygiene measures are employed, when necessary, to rid the respiratory tract of mucus and purulent drainage. Adequate hydration (2–3 liters/day) is indicated to keep the mucous membranes moist and thereby facilitate removal of secretions. Supplemental oxygen is used as necessary.

A mechanical respirator, used cautiously, may improve pulmonary ventilation. One must remember that overzealous use of a mechanical respirator may cause such rapid excretion of carbon dioxide that the kidneys will be unable to eliminate excess bicarbonate with sufficient rapidity to prevent alkalosis and convulsions. For this reason, the elevated $PaCO_2$ must be decreased slowly.

Respiratory Alkalosis (Carbonic Acid Deficit)

Extreme anxiety (most common cause)

Hypoxemia

High fever

Early salicylate intoxication (stimulates respiratory center)

Gram-negative bacteremia

Central nervous system lesions involving respiratory center

Pulmonary emboli

Thyrotoxicosis

Excessive ventilation by mechanical ventilators

Pregnancy (high progesterone level sensitizes the respiratory center to CO_2: physiologic)

Lightheadedness (a low $PaCO_2$ causes cerebral vasoconstriction and thus decreased cerebral blood flow)

Inability to concentrate

Those of decreased calcium ionization (numbness and tingling of extremities and circumoral paresthesia; more likely to occur if respiratory alkalosis develops rapidly)

Hyperventilation syndrome:
- Tinnitus
- Palpitations
- Sweating
- Dry mouth
- Tremulousness
- Precordial pain (tightness)
- Nausea and vomiting
- Epigastric pain
- Blurred vision
- Convulsions and loss of consciousness (may be partly due to cerebral ischemia, caused by cerebral vasoconstriction)

If the cause of respiratory alkalosis is anxiety, the client should be made aware that the abnormal breathing practice is responsible for the symptoms accompanying this condition. Instruct the client to breathe more slowly (to cause accumulation of carbon dioxide) or to breathe in a closed system (such as a paper bag) is helpful. Usually a sedative is required to relieve ventilation in very anxious patients. (If alkalosis is severe enough to cause fainting, the increased ventilation will cease and respirations will revert to normal.)

Treatment for other causes of respiratory alkalosis is directed at correcting the underlying problem.

(Continued)

Respiratory Alkalosis
(Carbonic Acid Deficit) (continued)

ABGs:
- $pH > 7.45$
- $PaCO_2 < 38$ mm Hg (primary)
- $HCO_3^- < 22$ mEq/liter (mmol/liter) (compensatory)

Metabolic Acidosis
(Base Bicarbonate Deficit)

Normal anion gap:
- Diarrhea
- Intestinal fistulas
- Ureterosigmoidostomy
- Hyperalimentation
- Acidifying drugs (such as ammonium chloride)
- Renal tubular acidosis (RTA)

High anion gap:
- Diabetic ketoacidosis
- Starvational ketoacidosis
- Lactic acidosis
- Renal failure
- Ingestion of toxins (such as salicylates, ethylene glycol, and methanol)

Headache

Confusion

Drowsiness

Increased respiratory rate and depth (may not become clinically evident until HCO_3^- is quite low)

Nausea and vomiting

Peripheral vasodilatation (may be present, causing warm, flushed skin)

Decreased cardiac output when pH falls below 7; bradycardia may develop

- ABGs:
  - Fall in pH (<7.35)
  - $HCO_3 < 22$ mEq/liter (mmol/liter) (primary)
  - $PaCO_2 < 38$ mm Hg (compensation by lungs)
  - Base excess (BE) always negative

Hyperkalemia is frequently present (except in RTA, diarrhea, and use of acetazolamide)

Treatment is directed toward correcting the metabolic defect. If the cause of the problem is excessive intake of chloride, treatment obviously focuses on eliminating the source. When necessary, bicarbonate is administered.

Metabolic Alkalosis
(Base Bicarbonate Excess)

Vomiting or gastric suction

Hypokalemia

Hyperaldosteronism

Cushing's syndrome

Potassium-losing diuretics (*e.g.,* thiazides, furosemide, ethacrynic acid)

Alkali ingestion (bicarbonate-containing antacids)

Parenteral $NaHCO_3$ administration for cardiopulmonary resuscitation

Abrupt relief of chronic respiratory acidosis

Those related to decreased calcium ionization, such as
- Dizziness
- Tingling of fingers and toes
- Circumoral paresthesia
- Carpopedal spasm
- Hypertonic muscles

Depressed respiration (compensatory action by lungs)

- ABGs:
  - $pH > 7.45$
  - Bicarbonate > 26 mEq/liter (mmol/liter) (primary)
  - $PaCO_2 > 42$ mm Hg (compensatory)
  - Base excess (BE) always positive

Hypokalemia often present

Serum Cl relatively lower than Na

Treatment is aimed at reversal of the underlying disorder. Sufficient chloride must be supplied for the kidney to absorb sodium with chloride (allowing the excretion of excess bicarbonate). Treatment also includes restoration of normal fluid volume by administration of sodium chloride fluids (because continued volume depletion serves to maintain the alkalosis).

(Data from Metheny NM: Fluid and Electrolyte Balance. Philadelphia, JB Lippincott, 1987, Chap 9.)

Elements of a Fluid, Electrolyte, and Acid–Base Balance History

1. Usual pattern of fluid intake
   "Describe the amount and types of fluids you usually drink in a 24-hr period. Have there been any recent changes?"
   • Types of fluids ingested and amounts
2. Usual pattern of fluid elimination
   "Describe your usual voiding/urination habits. Any recent changes in frequency or amount?"
   • Characteristics of urine and amount
   "Is your body losing fluids in any other major way?"
   • Vomiting
   • Diarrhea
   • Excessive perspiration
   • Fistula
3. Client's evaluation of hydration status
   "Do you think there is an approximate balance between your fluid intake and output?"
   "Have you noticed any signs that your body is experiencing too much or too little hydration

(difficulty breathing, edema, dry skin and mucous membranes, thirst)?"
4. History of disease process or injury state that might disrupt fluid and electrolyte balance (*e.g.,* diabetes mellitus, cancer, burns)
5. History of medications or treatments that might disrupt fluid and electrolyte balance (*e.g.,* steroids, diuretics, total parenteral nutrition, dialysis)
6. Fluid, electrolyte, and acid–base imbalances/contributing factors
   "Are you aware of any specific fluid, electrolyte, or acid–base problems you may be experiencing?"
   • Nature
   • Onset of problem and frequency
   • Causes
   • Severity
   • Symptoms
   • Interventions attempted and results

Nursing History

Each comprehensive nursing history should include questions that allow the nurse to assess the client's fluid, electrolyte, and acid–base balance. The accompanying box includes interview questions helpful in identifying the client's usual pattern of fluid intake and elimination and the client's evaluation of his hydration status and awareness of particular problems. Interview questions should also assist in the identification of clients at high risk for imbalances. Risk factors include

- The pathophysiology underlying both acute and chronic illness (*e.g.,* diabetes mellitus, congestive heart failure, renal failure)
- Abnormal losses of body fluids (*e.g.,* prolonged or severe vomiting and diarrhea, draining wounds, fistulas). See Table 35-6 for a listing of imbalances resulting from fluid loss of specific body fluids.
- Burns and trauma
- Therapies with the potential to disrupt fluid and electrolyte balance (*e.g.,* medications such as diuretics and steroids, treatments such as intravenous therapy and total parenteral nutrition)

Nursing Examination

Metheny (1987) recommends that the nurse pays attention to the following parameters when assessing a client's fluid and electrolyte status: comparison of total intake and output of fluids, urine volume and concentration, skin and tongue turgor, degree of moisture in oral cavity, body weight, thirst, tearing and salivation, appear-

ance and temperature of skin, facial appearance, edema, vital signs, neck and hand vein filling, central venous pressure, and neuromuscular irritability. When suspecting imbalance of particular electrolytes knowledge of their defining characteristics should guide the assessment (see Table 35-4). Table 35-7 presents select nursing considerations for each of these parameters, findings in a healthy adult, and significant findings.

Measuring Fluid Intake and Output

When either the physician or nurse orders that a client's fluid intake and output be continuously measured, the client, his family, and all caregivers should be alert to the need to measure all fluids entering and leaving the body —to the extent that this is possible. The client's condition will dictate how strict the intake and output measurement is to be. Adherence to the following guidelines will help eliminate common errors in measuring fluid intake and output:

- As soon as measured intake and output is ordered for the client, the client and family are instructed that the nurse needs a record of all fluids entering the body and all fluid output. A simple explanation of why this is being done is offered as well as specific instructions as to how the client can help to keep his record accurate. Some clients may need to be reminded during nursing rounds each morning that this measurement will continue.
- The client's plan of care and nursing Kardex are used to communicate to nursing personnel the need to measure fluid intake and output. A sign posted in the client's room and bedside form for

recording intake and output are helpful reminders for both the client and nurses.

- The client's fluid intake includes:

a. All fluids and foods that are liquid at room temperature (ice cream, Jell-O, and so forth).

  1. Use the agency's designation of specific volumes for common food containers (*e.g.,* juice glass = 90 ml; milk carton = 240 ml).

  2. Remind the client that sips of water or other fluids in between meals need to be recorded; small disposable calibrated cups at the bedside facilitate accurate measurement.

  3. Remember that liquid medications or water taken with pills may significantly increase the fluid intake of some clients.

b. All parenteral fluids

c. Other fluids taken into the body: subcutaneous fluids, fluids instilled into drainage tubes, enema solutions

- The client's fluid output includes

a. Urine; vomitus; diarrhea; drainage from fistulas, wounds and ulcers; and drainage from suctioning devices. Calibrated measuring devices should be readily available for accurate measurement. Disposable, calibrated urine collection containers which fit under the toilet seat are available for ambulatory clients. Urine or liquid feces in diapers or bed clothes, vomitus on clothing or bed linens, wound drainage saturating dressings, and so forth, need to be estimated.

b. Heavy perspiration should be noted on the output record especially when the client's clothing or bed linens are soaked.

c. Hyperventilation (water vapor loss) should also be noted on the output record.

- Both intake and output should be measured whenever possible, rather than estimated. Output measurement is described in Chapter 33. Failure to record intake or output when it is measured may result in it being forgotten.

- Intake and output totals are generally recorded for each 8-hour shift and totaled each 24 hours. At the conclusion of each shift the alert client should be questioned about his intake and output.

Daily Weights

Because of the numerous sources of inaccuracies in fluid intake and output measurement (Pflaum, 1979), the recording of a client's daily weight may offer a more accurate depiction of his fluid balance status. Guidelines for accurate weight measurement include weighing the client (1) at the same time each day, preferably in the morning before breakfast and after the first morning void; (2) with the same or similar clothing; and (3) on the same scale.

Laboratory Studies

Laboratory tests are helpful in determining whether fluid, electrolyte, and acid–base balance exists. Standard tests include the following (tables of normal values are given in Appendix B):

Complete Blood Count (CBC). This basic screening test provides a determination of the total number of red blood cells (RBC) and values for hemoglobin and hematocrit. Significant values include

- Increased hematocrit values: Found in severe dehydration and shock (when hemoconcentration rises considerably)
- Decreased hematocrit: Found with acute, massive blood loss, and with hemolytic reaction following transfusion of incompatible blood
- Increased levels of hemoglobin: Found in hemoconcentration of the blood
- Decreased levels of hemoglobin: Found with severe hemorrhage and following a hemolytic reaction

TABLE 35-6
Imbalances Resulting from Fluid Loss of Specific Body Fluid

Fluid Lost	Imbalances Likely to Occur
Gastric juice	Extracellular fluid-volume deficit Metabolic alkalosis Sodium deficit Potassium deficit Tetany (if metabolic alkalosis is present) Ketosis of starvation Magnesium deficit
Intestinal juice	Extracellular fluid-volume deficit Metabolic acidosis Sodium deficit Potassium deficit
Bile	Sodium deficit Metabolic acidosis
Pancreatic juice	Metabolic acidosis Sodium deficit Calcium deficit Extracellular fluid-volume deficit
Sensible perspiration	Extracellular fluid-volume deficit Sodium deficit
Insensible water loss	Water deficit (dehydration) Sodium excess
Wound exudate	Protein deficit Sodium deficit Extracellular fluid-volume deficit
Ascites	Protein deficit Sodium deficit Plasma-to-interstitial-fluid shift Extracellular fluid-volume deficit

(Text continues on p. 977.)

T A B L E   35-7

Parameters to Be Considered in Clinical Assessment for Fluid, Electrolyte, and Acid–Base Balance

Assessment Parameters	Nursing Considerations	Findings in Healthy Adult	Significant Findings
Comparison of total intake and output of fluids	• Records may be initiated by the nurse for any client with a real or potential water or electrolyte problem. • Intake should include all fluids taken into the body (oral fluids, foods that are liquid at room temperature, intravenous fluids, subcutaneous fluids, fluids instilled into drainage tubes as irrigants, tube feeding solutions and water, even enema solutions in clients requiring strict fluid intake recording) • Output should include urine, vomitus, diarrhea, drainage from fistulas, and drainage from suction apparatus. Perspiration and drainage from lesions should be noted and estimated. Prolonged hyperventilation should also be noted as it is an important route of water vapor loss.	• Fluid intake approximately equals fluid output—when averaged over 2–3 days. • Range of 1500 ml–3500 ml fluid intake and loss; 2000 ml is average adult intake and loss per day. • Output of urine normally approximates the ingestion of liquids; water from food and oxidation is balanced by the water loss through feces, the skin, and the respiratory process.	• When the total intake is substantially less than the total output, the client is in danger of fluid volume deficit. • When the total intake is substantially more than the total output, the client is in danger of fluid volume excess.
Urine volume and concentration	• Measure all fluid losses according to routes. • Use a device calibrated for small volumes of urine when hourly urine volumes need to be measured. • Account for factors that can alter urinary output: 1. Amount of fluid intake 2. Losses from skin, lungs, and gastrointestinal tract 3. Amount of waste products for excretions 4. Renal concentrating ability 5. Blood volume 6. Hormonal influences (primarily aldosterone and ADH)	• Normal urinary output is about 1 ml per kilogram of body weight per hour (for the average adult: 1500 ml/24 hr which is equivalent to approximately 40 ml–80 ml/hr). • Stress may diminish the 24-hr urine volume in the adult to 750 ml–1000 ml (or 30 ml–50 ml/hr) because of increased aldosterone and ADH secretion. • The range of specific gravity is from 1.003 to 1.035. Urine osmolality ranges between 500 mOsm and 800 mOsm/kg (mmol/kg).	• A low urine volume with a high specific gravity indicates fluid volume deficit. • A low urine volume with a low specific gravity indicates renal disease. • A high urine volume suggests fluid volume excess. • Urine volume is increased in conditions with high solute loads, such as diabetes mellitus, high protein tube feedings, and fever. • Hypovolemia causes decreased renal perfusion and thus, oliguria; hypervolemia causes increased urinary volume if the kidneys are functioning normally.
Body weight	• Because of the common inaccurancies in recording intake and output, body weight is believed to be a more accurate indicator of fluid gained and lost. • Guidelines for weighing clients: 1. Use the same scale each time.	A client's dry weight should remain relatively stable.	• Rapid variations in weight closely reflect changes in body fluid volume. • A rapid loss of body weight will occur when the total fluid intake is less than the total fluid output. 1. Rapid loss of 2% total body weight (TBW) indicates mild fluid volume deficit. 2. Rapid loss of 5% TBW indicates moderate fluid volume deficit.

(Continued)

Assessment Parameters	Nursing Considerations	Findings in Healthy Adult	Significant Findings
	2. Measure weight at the same time each day: in the morning before breakfast and after voiding. 3. Be sure the client is wearing the same, or similar clothing (clothing should be dry). 4. If the client is unable to stand on a small, portable scale, use a bed scale. • A client may have a severe fluid volume deficit even though body weight is essentially unchanged when there is a third-space loss of body fluid.		3. Rapid loss of 8% or more of TBW indicates severe fluid volume deficit. • A rapid gain of body weight will occur when the total fluid intake is greater than the total fluid output. 1. Rapid gain of 2% TBW indicates mild fluid volume excess. 2. Rapid gain of 5% TBW indicates moderate fluid volume excess. 3. Rapid gain of 8% or more of TBW indicates severe fluid volume excess. • A rapid gain or loss of 1 kg (2.2 lb) of body weight is approximately equivalent to the gain or loss of 1 liter of fluid.
Skin turgor (elasticity)	• Pinch the client's skin over the sternum, inner aspect of the thighs, or forehead. • Some prefer to test skin turgor in children over the abdominal area and on the medial aspect of the thighs. • Skin turgor can vary with age, nutritional state, and even race and complexion. Observations are most meaningful if done sequentially prior to the development of a fluid balance abnormality.	• Pinched skin will immediately fall back to its normal position when released. • Reduced skin turgor is common in older clients (those more than 55 to 60 years of age) due to a primary decrease in skin elasticity.	• In a person with a fluid volume deficit, the skin flattens more slowly after the pinch is released; the skin may remain elevated for many seconds. • Severe malnutrition, particularly in infants, can cause depressed skin turgor even in the absence of fluid depletion.
Tongue turgor	• Unlike skin turgor, tongue turgor is not affected appreciably by age and thus is a useful assessment for all age groups.	Tongue has one longitudinal furrow.	• In the person with fluid volume deficit there are additional longitudinal furrows and the tongue is smaller. • Sodium excess causes the tongue to look red and swollen.
Moisture and oral cavity	• A dry mouth may be the result of fluid volume deficit or of mouth breathing. When in doubt the nurse should run a finger along the oral cavity and feel the membrane where the cheek and gum meet; dryness in this area indicates a true fluid volume deficit.	Moist mucous membranes in oral cavity.	• Dryness of the membrane where the cheek and gum meet indicates fluid volume deficit. • Dry sticky mucous membranes are noted in sodium excess. (The oral cavity feels like "flypaper.")
Tearing and salivation		Tearing and salivation decrease normally with age.	The absence of tearing and salivation in a child is a sign of fluid volume deficit; it becomes obvious with a fluid loss of 5% of TBW.

(Continued)

T A B L E 35-7

Parameters to Be Considered in Clinical Assessment for Fluid, Electrolyte, and Acid–Base Balance *(Continued)*

Assessment Parameters	Nursing Considerations	Findings in Healthy Adult	Significant Findings
Appearance of skin and skin temperature			• Metabolic acidosis can cause warm, flushed skin (due to peripheral vasodilatation). • Severe fluid volume deficit causes the skin to be pale and cool (due to vasoconstriction, which occurs to compensate for hypovolemia).
Facial appearance			• A person with a severe fluid volume deficit has a pinched, drawn, facial expression. • A fluid volume deficit of 10% of body weight causes decreased intraocular pressure causing the eyes to appear sunken and to feel soft to the touch.
Edema (excessive accumulation of interstitial fluid)	• Pitting edema (phenomenon manifested by a small depression that remains after one's finger is pressed over an edematous area and then removed) may be indicated by using plus signs to indicate the amount, ranging from +1 (barely perceptible edema) to +4 (severe edema). See Figure 35-8. • Measurement of an extremity or body part with a millimeter tape, in the same area each day, is a more exact method of measurement. • An excess of interstitial fluid may accumulate predominantly in the lower extremities of ambulatory clients and in the presacral region of bedridden clients. • The presence of periorbital (around the eyes) edema or pedal edema should prompt one to look for edema in other parts of the body.	No edema	• Clinically edema is not usually apparent in the adult until the retention of 5 lb–10 lb of excess fluid occurs. • Pitting edema is not evident until at least a 10% increase in weight has occurred. • Formation of edema may be localized (as in thrombophlebitis) or generalized (as in heart failure, cirrhosis of liver, or nephrotic syndrome). Edema of congestive heart failure, liver cirrhosis, or nephrotic syndrome is the result of sodium retention. • There is no peripheral edema with only water retention (as occurs with excessive secretion of ADH). Instead there is a cellular swelling which can be detected by pressing one's finger over the sternum and producing a visible fingerprint.
Body temperature	• Because fever increases the loss of body fluids it is important that temperature elevations be detected early and appropriate interventions be taken. • Body temperature and other vital signs should be assessed at the nurse's discretion.	Baseline temperature: diurnal variations	• There is an elevation of body temperature in hypernatremia (dehydration) probably related to lack of available fluid for sweating. Also, dehydration has a direct effect on the hypothalamus. • There is a decrease in body temperature in fluid volume deficit, when uncomplicated by infection (probably as a result of decreased metabolism).

(Continued)

Assessment Parameters	Nursing Considerations	Findings in Healthy Adult	Significant Findings

			• Fever increases the loss of body fluids
			  1. Increased metabolism produces more metabolic wastes and increases urinary output.
			  2. Fever also causes hyperpnea, an increase in breathing which results in extra water vapor loss through the lungs).
			• A temperature elevation between 101°F (38.3°C) and 103°F (39.4 C) increases the 24-hr fluid requirement by at least 500 ml, and a temperature above 103°F increases it by at least 1000 ml.

Pulse		Baseline pulse rate, rhythm, and volume	• Tachycardia is usually the earliest sign of the decreased vascular volume associated with fluid volume deficit. It may also be associated with deficits of magnesium or potassium. • Excesses of magnesium or potassium can cause decreased heart rate. • Irregular pulse rates also occur with potassium imbalances and magnesium deficit. • Pulse volume is decreased in fluid volume deficit and increased in fluid volume excess.
Respirations		Baseline respiratory rate, rhythm, and qualities	• Deep, rapid respirations may be a compensatory mechanism for metabolic acidosis or a primary disorder causing respiratory alkalosis. • Slow, shallow respirations may be a compensatory mechanism for metabolic alkalosis or a primary disorder causing respiratory acidosis. • Weakness or paralysis of respiratory muscles is likely in severe hypo- or hyperkalemia and in severe magnesium excess. • Moist rales, in the absence of cardiopulmonary disease, indicate fluid volume excess.
Blood pressure	Whenever a fluid imbalance is suspected, check the client's blood pressure while he is lying down, sitting, and standing.	Baseline blood pressure	• A fall in systolic pressure exceeding 10 mm Hg from the lying to the sitting or standing position (postural hypotension) usually indicates fluid volume deficit. • Hypotension may occur with magnesium excess (first occurring at a level of 3 mEq–5 mEq/liter or 1.5 mmol–2.5 mmol/liter).

(Continued)

T A B L E 35-7

Parameters to Be Considered in Clinical Assessment for Fluid, Electrolyte, and Acid–Base Balance (Continued)

Assessment Parameters	Nursing Considerations	Findings in Healthy Adult	Significant Findings
			• Hypertension can occur with magnesium deficit and with fluid volume excess.

Neck veins/central venous pressure	• The jugular veins provide a built-in manometer for following changes in central venous pressure (CVP).
	• To estimate central venous pressure, the nurse
	  1. Positions the client in a semi-Fowler's position (head of bed elevated to a 30- to 45-degree angle), keeping the neck straight
	  2. Removes any of the client's clothing that could constrict the neck or upper chest
	  3. Provides adequate lighting to visualize effectively the external jugular veins on each side of the neck
	  4. Measures the levels to which the veins are distended on the neck or above the level of the manubrium
	• More accurate assessments of blood volume are obtained by measuring central venous pressure with a manometer or by hemodynamic monitoring with a device that measures pressures in both sides of the heart.
		• Normally, when the client is supine, the external jugular veins fill to the anterior border of the sternocleidomastoid muscle. With the client positioned sitting at a 45-degree angle, the venous distentions normally should not extend higher than 2 cm above the sternal angle.
		• Pressure in the right atrium is usually 0 cm to 4 cm of water; pressure in the vena cava is approximately 4 cm to 11 cm of water.
			• A low CVP may indicate
			  1. Decreased blood volume
			  2. Drug-induced vasodilatation (causing pooling of blood in peripheral veins).
			• A high CVP may indicate
			  1. Increased blood volume
			  2. Heart failure
			  3. Vasoconstriction

Neuromuscular irritability	• When imbalances in calcium, magnesium, and sodium are suspected it is important to assess clients for increased or decreased neuromuscular irritability • To test for *Chvostek's sign* the facial nerve should be percussed about 2 cm anterior to the earlobe.	Negative response	Clients with hypocalcemia or hypomagnesemia will respond positively with a unilateral twitching of the facial muscles, including the eyelid and lips.
	• To test for *Trousseau's sign,* place a blood pressure cuff on the arm and inflate above systolic pressure for 3 min.	Negative response	A positive response is the development of carpal spasm.
	• A deep tendon reflex is elicited by briskly tapping a partially stretched tendon with a rubber percussion hammer, preferably over the tendon insertion of the muscle. The broad head of the hammer is	The response in the prospective muscle is a sudden contraction (2+).	Deep tendon reflexes may be hyperactive in the presence of hypocalcemia, hypomagnesemia, hypernatremia, and alkalosis.

(Continued)

Assessment Parameters	Nursing Considerations	Findings in Healthy Adult	Significant Findings

	used to stroke easily accessible tendons and the pointed end for less accessible tendons.
	• The muscle being tested should be slightly stretched and the client should be relaxed.
	• Reflexes usually graded on a 0 to +4 scale
	    0 = no response
	    1+ = somewhat diminished, but present
	    2+ = normal
	    3+ = brisker than average and possibly but not necessarily indicative of disease
	    4+ = hyperactive
			Deep tendon reflexes may be hypoactive in the presence of hypercalcemia, hypermagnesemia, hyponatremia, hypokalemia, and acidosis.

• Behavior • Sensation • Fatigue level	Because these changes are often vague they are best evaluated in context with specific imbalances.		

(Data from Metheny NM: Fluid and Electrolyte Balance. Philadelphia, JB Lippincott, 1987, pp 12–26.)

Serum Electrolytes. This screening test performed routinely upon hospital admission provides information on plasma levels of select electrolytes. Commonly determined are plasma levels of sodium, potassium, chloride, and bicarbonate ions.

Urine pH and Specific Gravity. Both the urine pH and specific gravity may be obtained by dipstick measurement on a fresh voided specimen or through laboratory analysis. The urine pH expresses the strength of the urine as a dilute acid or a base solution and measures the free hydrogen ion (H^+) concentration of the urine. Specific gravity is a means by which the kidney's ability to concentrate urine is measured. The range of specific gravity depends on the state of hydration and varies with urine volume and the load of solutes to be excreted. Normal values range from 1.003 to 1.035 (concentrated urine: 1.025–1.030+; dilute urine: 1.001–1.010).

Arterial Blood Gases (ABGs). Arterial blood gases are obtained to determine the adequacy of oxygenation and ventilation and to assess acid–base status. Blood gas analysis provides values for pH, pCO_2, HCO_3^-, pO_2, and oxygen saturation. When interpreting blood gases,

1. Determine if the pH is alkalotic (>7.45) or acidotic (<7.35).
2. Next check the pCO_2 (respiratory parameter) and HCO_3^- (metabolic parameter) to identify the cause of the pH change. Acidosis is caused by high carbon dioxide levels (hypoventilation) or low bicarbonate levels. Alkalosis is caused by low carbon dioxide levels (hyperventilation) or high bicarbonate levels.
   a. In respiratory acid–base imbalances, the pH and pCO_2 values are inversely abnormal.
   b. In metabolic acid–base imbalances, the pH and HCO_3^- values are both high or both low

Respiratory acidosis	$\downarrow pH$ <7.35	$\uparrow PCO_2$	normal HCO_3^-
Metabolic acidosis	$\downarrow pH$ <7.35	normal PCO_2	$\downarrow HCO_3^-$
Respiratory alkalosis	$\uparrow pH$ >7.45	$\downarrow PCO_2$	normal HCO_3^-
Metabolic alkalosis	$\uparrow pH$ >7.45	normal PCO_2	$\uparrow HCO_3^-$

3. Determine if the body is compensating for the pH change.

Examples

pH	7.25	Decreased	Metabolic acidosis (both the pH and HCO_3^- are decreased); decreased pCO_2 indicates respiratory compensatory attempt—hyperventilation
pCO_2	31	Decreased	
HCO_3^-	12	Decreased	
pH	7.16	Decreased	Respiratory acidosis (pH is decreased whereas
pCO_2	70	Increased	

HCO₃⁻ 31	Decreased	pCO₂ is increased; *i.e.,* inversely abnormal); decreased HCO₃⁻ indicates renal compensatory attempt

HCO_3^- 31 Decreased pCO_2 is increased; *i.e.,* inversely abnormal); decreased HCO_3^- indicates renal compensatory attempt

DIAGNOSING

When assessment data point to fluid and electrolyte problems amenable to nursing therapy they receive one of three diagnostic labels:

Alteration in fluid volume: Excess
Alteration in fluid volume: Actual deficit
Alteration in fluid volume: Potential deficit

Excess fluid volume may result from greatly increased fluid intake, or more frequently from decreased excretion such as occurs in progressive renal disease and with certain cancers. Fluid volume deficits may result from decreased intake, increased excretion of fluids, fluid shifts, and from the special need for fluids and electrolytes created by strenuous exercise, extreme heat or dryness, and conditions that increase the metabolic rate (fever). Table 35-8 presents contributing factors and defining characteristics for these diagnoses.

The nurse's analysis of assessment data may also lead to the diagnosis of specific electrolyte or acid–base disturbances that are termed collaborative problems because they require joint intervention by nursing and medicine (see Tables 35-4 and 35-5).

Disturbances in fluid, electrolyte, and acid–base balance may affect many other areas of human functioning. Sample diagnoses follow:

T A B L E   35-8
Nursing Diagnoses for Common Fluid and Electrolyte Problems

Title	Etiologic or Contributing Factors	Sample Defining Characteristics
Fluid volume excess	Pathophysiologic factors: renal failure, decreased cardiac output, liver disease, abnormal fluid accumulations, hormonal problems	• "I've noticed that my wedding ring is tight . . . also my clothes don't fit as well as they used to. I guess I've gained some weight." • Reports dyspnea with exertion, feeling weak and fatigued • Pitting edema in feet, ankles, lower legs • Taut, shiny skin • Jugular venous distention
	Situational factors: excessive intravenous infusion	• Bounding pulse, increased from baseline • Shallow, rapid respirations, rales • Increased blood pressure
	Nutritional factors: excessive sodium intake, low protein intake	• 10-lb (4.5-kg) weight gain over last month • Fluid intake greater than output • "Sometimes I can't catch my breath and I feel like my heart is pounding away." • "I feel bloated."
Fluid volume deficit	Decreased fluid intake: imposed fluid restrictions, inability to obtain or swallow fluids (debilitation, oral pain), depression	• "After I got the flu I got so weak I couldn't get out of bed. . . . I think I was out of it for a couple of days." • Increased pulse and respirations • Dry oral mucosa, cracked lips, furrowed tongue • Scanty urine ouput
	Abnormal fluid loss: vomiting; diarrhea; abnormal drainage; excessive use of laxatives, enemas, diuretics; blood loss; diaphoresis; burns	• "I'm thirsty all the time." • "I've been vomiting and I have diarrhea—several times a day." • Weight loss: 5 lb (2–3 kg) • Urine is concentrated (specific gravity: 1.035). • Fluid output greater than fluid intake • Neck veins collapsed when lying flat • Decreased skin turgor
	Increased need for fluids: strenuous exercise, extreme heat or dryness, fever (increased metabolic rate)	• Skin is warm to touch, moist, and flushed • Increased temperature, pulse, respirations • Decreased blood pressure

Activity intolerance related to dyspnea upon exertion

Anxiety related to pulmonary edema

Ineffective breathing pattern related to compensatory mechanism by lungs (hypo- or hyperventilation)

Decreased cardiac output related to decreased blood volume, shock

Altered comfort related to fluid restrictions, edema

Potential for injury related to neuromuscular irritability, cardiac arrhythmia

Knowledge deficit: potential harmful effects of abuses of dieting, alcohol, diuretics, laxatives and enemas related to no previous experience

Altered oral mucous membrane related to dehydration

Impaired skin integrity related to dehydration, edema

Altered thought processes related to cerebral edema, mental confusion/disorientation, convulsions

Altered tissue perfusion related to decreased cardiac output

Altered pattern of urinary elimination related to decreased kidney perfusion secondary to decreased plasma volume

PLANNING: CLIENT GOALS

Nursing care for any client is supportive of the following client goals:

The healthy adult client will

- Maintain an approximate balance between fluid intake and fluid output (average about 2500 ml fluid intake and output over 3 days)
- Maintain a urine specific gravity within normal range (1.010–1.025)
- Practice self-care behaviors to promote fluid, electrolyte, and acid–base balance—maintain adequate intake of fluid and electrolytes; respond appropriately to body's signals of impending fluid, electrolyte, or acid–base imbalance.

When an imbalance exists, the client will relate relief of symptoms (specify) after implementation of treatment regimen (*e.g.,* 1 month after decreasing sodium intake client reports 4 lb [1.8 kg] weight loss).

IMPLEMENTING

Nursing interventions to prevent or correct fluid, electrolyte, and acid–base imbalances include dietary modi-

fication, modification of fluid intake, medication administration, intravenous therapy, blood and blood products replacement, and total parenteral nutrition.

Preventing Fluid Imbalances

An adequate fluid intake and a well-balanced, nutritious diet with appropriate adjustments throughout the life cycle are basic essentials to promote fluid balance. The following are some of the basic items the nurse needs to consider to help prevent fluid imbalances:

- Be familiar with common events in life that lead to fluid imbalances, and observe the client carefully.
- Note the client's present fluid and food intake, and learn what his previous eating and drinking patterns have been. Learn whether the client has used fad diets, which may lead to imbalances.
- Note whether thirst is excessive or whether the client experiences little or no thirst. Thirst is a subjective sensation and an important factor in determining water intake and, eventually, output through the kidneys. Thirst is poorly understood, although both psychologic and physiologic factors appear to be involved.
- Be aware of excessive losses of fluids from the body, and attempt to prevent losses when possible. Vomiting, pronounced perspiration, diarrhea, draining wounds, and excessive urinary output, for example, may cause excessive losses.
- Consider ways in which the client's medical regimen may lead to imbalances. For example, many drugs to stimulate urine formation increase the elimination of potassium. If food supplements high in potassium are not included in the diet or if drug therapy is not started, hypokalemia often follows. Adrenocorticosteroids may lead to sodium and water retention and to excessive potassium excretion.
- Learn whether the client has been "treating" himself and, as a result, threatening fluid balance. Common practices that threaten fluid balance include the indiscriminate use of enemas, laxatives, antacids, and over-the-counter drugs to promote urination.
- Consider conditions that induce destructive effects on the body as threats to fluid balance. Examples include immobilization, trauma, burns, surgical procedures, and exposure to toxic agents.
- Teach clients to observe for fluid imbalances and to report them promptly. Examples include rapid weight gains and losses; swollen fingers, feet, and ankles; puffy eyelids; muscle weakness; change in skin sensations; and scanty or profuse urine production.
- Help clients and their families understand the significance of maintaining fluid balance and preventing imbalances.

Developing a Dietary Plan

Simple dietary changes may help to resolve fluid and electrolyte disturbances. After doing a nutritional assessment to identify actual or potential imbalances and food preferences, the nurse can initiate teaching. It is important to involve both the client and the person who prepares meals in the development of the nutritional plan. The plan should include foods that will both help to resolve the fluid or electrolyte imbalance and are acceptable to the client. For example, for fluid volume deficit, increase foods with high water content (*e.g.,* citrus fruit, melons, celery); hypokalemia, increase foods with high potassium content (*e.g.,* bananas, citrus fruits, apricots, melons, broccoli, potatoes); hypernatremia, avoid foods high in sodium (*e.g.,* processed cheese, lunch meats, canned soups and vegetables, salted snack foods); eliminate use of table salt.

When given a list of foods, the client should be able to identify those that can be eaten freely or moderately as well as those that should be avoided. Both the client and person responsible for food preparation should be able to describe a 24-hour diet plan compatible with the recommended modifications.

Modifying Fluid Intake

Depending on the nature of the fluid or electrolyte imbalance, a client's fluids may need to be increased, decreased, or modified in terms of types of fluids ingested. The nurse is responsible for

- Identifying the appropriate fluid modification (with certain illnesses the physician may order fluid directives [*e.g.,* "Restrict fluids to 1000 ml/ day."])
- Determining if the client (1) understands the rationale for the fluid modification, (2) is motivated to comply with the modification, and (3) is capable of compliance (*e.g.,* a bedridden client who needs to increase his fluid intake cannot do this independently).
- Developing and implementing a plan of care based on the above information. For example, three clients with the same tendency to retain fluids may need very different nursing care. One has never learned that the high-sodium beverages she frequently drinks are contributing to her problem. One teaching session may be sufficient to resolve her fluid imbalance. A second client has a history of poor self-care behaviors. Intelligent and the recipient of much health education in the past, this client has no need for further teaching. Nursing time will best be invested in counseling and exploring why the client fails to value his health sufficiently to comply with the treatment regimen. Until the client values the proposed fluid modification, compliance will probably be poor. Finally, the third client is a frail elderly woman with pneumonia and a history of congestive heart failure who is dependent on the nursing staff for care. Her fluid intake will be determined by the fluids offered her by the nursing staff.

Increasing Fluids

An above-average intake of fluids is prescribed for certain clients. The usual order reads, "force fluids," and indicates the amount of fluid the client is to have in each 24-hour period. The plan of care should specify (1) the amount of fluid to be ingested in 24 hours (for hospitalized clients shift totals are helpful, *e.g.,* 7–3: 1200 ml, 3–11: 900 ml, 11–7: 300 ml), and (2) the client's food preferences. Fluids should be chosen that best provide the calories and electrolytes needed by the client.

A variety of techniques is recommended to help the client take more than average amounts of fluids:

- Explain to the client in language he can understand, the specific goal of taking the daily amount of fluid prescribed for him. This helps promote motivation and is more meaningful than simply telling the client to increase his fluid intake.
- Set short-term or interim goals with the client. Examples include a glass of water every hour, a particular beverage by the time a television program is finished, or a pitcher of water by lunchtime. Most clients will try to reach goals that they help to set, even when they do not feel thirsty.
- Plan to offer a proportionately larger amount of fluid during the early hours of the client's waking day. The client is usually able to take fluids relatively easily after having few or no fluids during sleeping hours.
- Try to avoid making it necessary to offer large amounts of fluid before sleep. This helps prevent disturbing rest because the client needs to urinate.
- Encourage as wide a variety of liquids as possible to make larger intake more interesting and palatable. If clients dislike taking fluids (a common problem with children) or have swallowing difficulties, offering Jello, popsicles, water ice, and so forth may meet with more success.
- Keep fluids readily available for the client. It is distressing to see persons who are unable to secure their own fluids left with an unfilled water pitcher, an empty glass, a full pitcher out of reach, or a pitcher too heavy to lift.
- Serve fluids at the appropriate temperature. For example, the client is likely to drink more when iced liquids are iced and cold, and coffee and tea when they are hot but not so hot that the client is likely to burn himself.
- Use attractive, clean, and easily handled cups and glasses, a practice that helps to encourage the client's desire to take fluids.

- Have the client assist in keeping a record of his intake when this is possible. This often serves as a motivating factor to increase fluid intake.
- Provide support, understanding, and encouragement because forcing fluid intake for the person experiencing no thirst can be very uncomfortable.

Increasing the fluid intake of clients is among the most common nursing care objective. Often, creativity and considerable patience by the nurse are necessary to reach desired goals. Fluids may also be replaced through nasogastric, gastrostomy, or jejunostomy tubes (see Chap 31).

Restricting Fluids

Restricting the client's fluid intake is sometimes necessary. The usual order reads, "restrict fluids," and indicates the amount of fluid the client is to have in each 24-hour period.

A variety of techniques is recommended to help the client who is to have a restricted fluid intake:

- Explain to the client, in language he can understand, the specific goal of taking the daily amount of fluid prescribed for him. This often helps promote motivation and is more meaningful to the client than simply telling him to restrict his fluid intake.
- With the client, space the time at which fluids will be served. Usually, it is best to offer fluids between meals because food often helps to relieve some feelings of thirst.
- Set short-term or interim goals for offering fluids at 1-hour or 2-hour intervals when this seems helpful and when the client can cooperate.
- Serve ice chips instead of water from time to time. When they melt, the water is approximately one half of its volume when frozen.
- Use small glasses or cups so that the container appears to contain more fluid than it actually does. Large containers partially full make the amount of fluid seem smaller than it actually is.
- Provide oral hygiene at regular intervals so that the client's mouth remains clean. Lubricate his lips and mucous membranes as indicated.
- Allow the client to rinse his mouth with water when he can cooperate without swallowing this fluid and exceeding his intake limit.
- Avoid offering the client dry, salty, or sweet foods and fluids, because they tend to increase thirst.
- Avoid offering the client hard candy or gum. They were often thought to relieve thirst by stimulating salivation. The sugar content increases oral tonicity and temporarily draws fluids to the mouth membranes. After about 15 to 30 minutes, the membranes are even more dry than before. Sugarless gum may be offered to some clients.
- Divert the client's attention from thirst by involving

him in various activities to the degree that he is able to participate.
- Keep fluids not intended for the client out of his sight.
- Have the client assist in keeping a record of his intake when this is possible. This may serve as a motivating factor to limit fluid intake.
- Provide understanding, support, and encouragement because limiting fluid intake for the person experiencing thirst is very uncomfortable.

Administering Medications

Clients with fluid, electrolyte, and acid–base imbalances are often prescribed medications as part of the therapeutic regimen. Nurses need to be knowledgeable about the therapeutic effects of mineral–electrolyte preparations and diuretics as well as alert for adverse effects of other medications such as steroids and hormone replacements.

Mineral–Electrolyte Preparations. Mineral–electrolyte preparations are frequently prescribed to correct electrolyte imbalances. Nursing responsibilities include

- Accurate administration consistent with manufacturer's guidelines (*e.g.,* dilute oral potassium supplements to disguise the unpleasant taste and decrease gastric irritation; monitor arterial blood gases for increased *p*H after each 50 mEq to 100 mEq of sodium bicarbonate to avoid overtreatment and metabolic alkalosis).
- Knowledge of the intended therapeutic effect and evaluation (*e.g.,* with magnesium sulfate look for decreased restlessness and irritability, decreased muscle tremors, and control of convulsions).
- Observation for adverse effects (*e.g.,* with sodium chloride injection observe for hypernatremia and circulatory overload).
- Observation for drug interactions (*e.g.,* drugs that increase the effects of minerals and electrolytes include acidifying agents, alkalinizing agents, cation exchange resin, iron salts, and potassium salts).
- Teaching the clients appropriate self-care behaviors.

Diuretics. Diuretics are drugs that increase renal excretion of water, sodium, and other electrolytes. While helpful in treating clients with fluid volume excess they have the potential to cause dehydration and serious electrolyte deficiencies. Clients need careful monitoring and education while on diuretic therapy.

Administering Intravenous Therapy

A relatively common form of therapy for handling fluid disturbances is the use of various solutions infused intravenously. The physician is responsible for prescribing the kind and amount of solution to be used. The nurse is

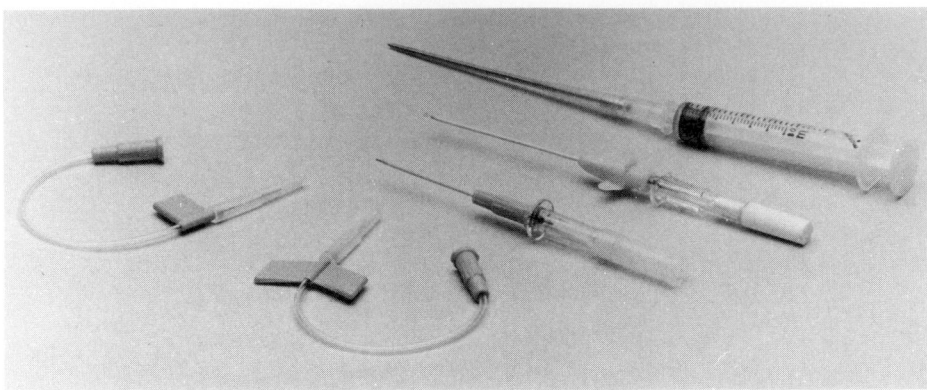

F I G U R E   35-9
Various types of intravenous infusion needles. On the left are the single- and double-winged (butterflies) infusion needles. Three types of around-needle intracatheters are illustrated on the right.

responsible for initiating, monitoring, and discontinuing the therapy. As is true with other therapeutic agents, the nurse should understand the client's need for intravenous therapy, the type of solution being used, its desired effect, and untoward reactions that may occur. Contents of selected water and electrolyte solutions with comments about their use are presented in Table 35-9.

Equipment. Sterile technique is observed when a vein is entered. Disposable infusion tubing and needles are used to help eliminate many possible sources of contamination and to reduce the cost of aftercare of equipment.

Equipment varies according to the manufacturer. The nurse is responsible for being familiar with the equipment used in the agency where he or she cares for clients. Typically, solutions for infusions are dispensed in either 1-liter or 500-ml glass or plastic bottles or in plastic bags. The plastic bags collapse under atmospheric pressure as the solution enters the client's vein. Rigid containers, such as glass bottles, cannot collapse. Therefore, they have an air vent that allows air to replace fluid as it enters the client's vein. Small 50-ml and 100-ml solution bags are available to administer medications intravenously.

Tubing is attached to the solution container. The rate of flow is manually controlled by a clamp or constricting device on the tubing. A device called a dripmeter or dripchamber connects the solution bottle and tubing and permits the number of drops per minute of solution to be determined.

Figure 35-9 illustrates a variety of needles and catheters commonly used for the intravenous infusion. Intravenous catheters, increasingly being used for intravenous therapy, are plastic tubes that have been mounted on a needle or are threaded through a needle for insertion. Single- or double-winged infusion needles (butterflies) are short-beveled, thin-walled needles with plastic flaps. They are used extensively because of the ease in handling and stabilizing them. The flaps, or wings, are brought together tightly in the nurse's fingers and are used to hold the needle securely as it is being inserted.

Other common equipment is listed in Procedure 35-1.

Site Selection. Suitability of veins for intravenous infusions varies with individual circumstances. Selection should be determined after considering several factors.

Accessibility of a Vein

• Determine the most desirable accessible vein. The lower cephalic vein, accessory cephalic vein, and the basilic vein are good sites for infusion. The superficial veins on the dorsal aspect of the hand can also be used successfully for some persons. Figure 35-10 illustrates common infusion sites on the arm and hand. Either arm may be used for intravenous therapy. If the client is right-handed and both arms appear to be equally usable, usually the left arm is selected in order to free the right arm for the client's use.

• Determine accessibility based on the client's condition. For example, a person with severe burns on both forearms will not have vessels available in these areas.

• Avoid the antecubital veins for long-term infusions. They are not a good choice for infusion because of the need to limit flexion of the client's arm for an extended period of time. Because there is danger of dislocation of the needle and of vein trauma even with slight movement, damage to these vessels may limit later use of the lower arms and the hand veins that are distal to it. These vessels are quite satisfactory for blood withdrawal or for small amounts of intravenous medication administration.

• Avoid veins in the leg, unless other sites are not accessible, because of the danger of stagnation of peripheral circulation and possible serious complications.

• Avoid veins in surgical areas. For example, infusions in the arm should not be given on the same side as recent extensive breast surgery because of vascular disturbances in the area.

• Select scalp veins for infants because of their accessibility and because of relative ease of preventing dislocation of the needle.

Condition of the Vein

• Determine the condition of the vein. Thin-walled and scarred veins, especially in some elderly

(Text continues on p. 989.)

T A B L E 35-9

Contents of Selected Water and Electrolyte Solutions With Comments About Their Use

Solution	Comments
0.9% NaCl (isotonic saline): NA$^+$ 154 mEq/liter Cl$^-$ 154 mEq/liter	An isotonic solution that expands plasma volume—used in hypovolemic states Supplies an excess of Na$^+$ and Cl$^-$—can cause fluid volume excess and hyperchloremic acidosis if used in excessive volumes (particularly in clients with compromised renal function) Sometimes used to correct mild metabolic alkalosis Sometimes used to correct mild Na$^+$ deficit Not desirable as a routine maintenance solution because it provides only Na$^+$ and Cl$^-$ (and these are provided in excessive amounts)
0.45% NaCl (half-strength saline): Na$^+$ 77 mEq/liter Cl$^-$ 77 mEq/liter	A hypotonic solution that provides Na$^+$, Cl$^-$, and free water Free water is desirable to aid the kidneys in elimination of solute. Na$^+$ and Cl$^-$ are provided, allowing the kidneys to select needed amounts of these electrolytes. Lacking in other electrolytes needed for daily replacement
0.3% NaCl (third-strength saline): Na$^+$ 51 mEq/liter Cl$^-$ 51 mEq/liter	A hypotonic solution that provides Na$^+$, Cl$^-$, and free water Often used to treat hypernatremia (because this solution contains a small amount of Na$^+$, it dilutes the plasma sodium while not allowing it to drop too rapidly)
3% NaCl: Na$^+$ 513 mEq/liter Cl$^-$ 513 mEq/liter	Grossly hypertonic solutions used *only* to treat severe hyponatremia These are *dangerous* solutions.
5% NaCl: Na$^+$ 855 mEq/liter Cl$^-$ 855 mEq/liter	
Lactated Ringer's solution (Hartmann's solution): Na$^+$ 130 mEq/liter K$^+$ 4 mEq/liter Ca^{++} 3 mEq/liter Cl$^-$ 109 mEq/liter Lactate (metabolized to bicarbonate) 28 mEq/liter	An isotonic solution that contains multiple electrolytes in roughly the same concentration as found in plasma (note that this solution is lacking in Mg^{2+}) Used in the treatment of hypovolemia, burns, and fluid lost as bile or diarrhea Useful in treating *mild* metabolic acidosis Does not supply free water for renal excretory purposes; excessive use without provision for free water (as with D$_5$W or hypotonic electrolyte solutions) can cause elevation of the serum sodium level in persons not deficient in sodium
5% dextrose in water (D$_5$W): No electrolytes 50 g of dextrose	Supplies approximately 170 cal/liter and free water to aid in renal excretion of solutes Should not be used in excessive volumes in the early postoperative period (when ADH secretion is increased due to stress reaction) Some authorities caution against the administration of electrolyte-free solutions in head-injured clients.
Isotonic multiple electrolyte solutions: Plasma-Lyte (Travenol) Isolyte E (McGaw) Na$^+$ 140 mEq/liter K$^+$ 10 mEq/liter Ca^{2+} 5 mEq/liter Mg^{2+} 3 mEq/liter Cl$^-$ 103 mEq/liter HCO$_3^-$ 55 mEq/liter (or equivalent)	Isotonic solution with electrolyte content similar to plasma except that it has twice as much K$^+$ and a higher HCO$_3^-$ content Sometimes used to replace intestinal fluid losses
Potassium chloride: 0.2% in dextrose 5% K$^+$ 27 mEq/liter Cl$^-$ 27 mEq/liter Glucose 50 g	Both solutions provide KCl, water and calories

(Continued)

Contents of Selected Water and Electrolyte Solutions With Comments About Their Use   (Continued)

Solution	Comments
0.3% in dextrose 5% K^+ 40 mEq/liter Cl^- 40 mEq/liter Glucose 50 g	
Gastric replacement solution: Electrolyte No. 3 (Travenol) Isolyte G (McGaw) Ionosol G (Abbott) Na^+ 63 mEq/liter K^+ 17 mEq/liter NH_4^+ 70 mEq/liter Cl^- 150 mEq/liter	An isotonic solution used to replace gastric fluid lost in vomiting or gastric suction pH is acidic (3.3–3.7)—irritating to vein Give in large peripheral veins with good blood flow to protect venous wall from irritation Contraindicated in presence of hepatic or renal failure
Duodenal replacement solution: Na^+ 138 mEq/liter K^+ 12 mEq/liter HCO_3^- 50 mEq/liter (or equivalent) Cl^- 100 mEq/liter	Used to replace water and electrolytes lost as a result of intestinal suction, drainage, or fistulas K^+ concentration is similar to that in intestinal secretions.
Sodium bicarbonate, 1.5%: Na^+ 178 mEq/liter HCO_3 178 mEq/liter	Isotonic solution used to treat severe metabolic acidosis Due to high Na^+ content, observe for fluid overload in clients with renal or cardiac impairment Observe for signs of hypocalcemia (which may be induced with rapid alkalinization of plasma)
Sodium lactate solution, 1/6 molar: Na^+ 167 mEq/liter Lactate 167 mEq/liter	Used to correct severe metabolic acidosis (lactate is metabolized to bicarbonate in 1 hr–2 hr by the liver) Calcium salts may be needed to correct symptomatic hypocalcemia that may occur with rapid alkalinization of plasma Not used in clients with liver disease, because lactate cannot be converted to bicarbonate in such individuals; also, not used in clients with oxygen lack (unable to adequately convert lactate to bicarbonate)
Ammonium chloride, 2.14%: NH_4^+ 400 mEq/liter Cl^- 400 mEq/liter	An acidifying solution used to correct severe metabolic alkalosis Due to high ammonia content, must be administered cautiously to clients with compromised hepatic function
Electrolyte no. 48: Na^+ 25 mEq/liter K^+ 20 mEq/liter Mg^{2+} 3 mEq/liter Cl^- 22 mEq/liter PO_4^{2+} 3 mEq/liter HCO_3 23 mEq/liter (or equivalent)	A pediatric hypotonic maintenance solution Supplies numerous electrolytes plus free water Note high K^+ content
Electrolyte no. 75: Na^+ 40 mEq/liter K^+ 35 mEq/liter Cl^- 40 mEq/liter PO_4^{2+} 15 mEq/liter HCO_3 20 mEq/liter (or equivalent)	Hypotonic maintenance solution Supplies numerous electrolytes plus free water

(Metheny NM: Fluid and Electrolyte Balance. Philadelphia, JB Lippincott, 1987, pp 146–147)

A commonly used IV solution in Canada is called "2/3–1/3." It is 3.3% dextrose and 0.3% sodium chloride (each mL contains 3.3 g dextrose and 300 mg sodium chloride). It is available also with KCl added and used for fluid, nutrient, and electrolyte replenishment.

P R O C E D U R E 35-1
Starting an Intravenous Infusion

Equipment

IV solution	Tourniquet	Infusion control pump, if required
IV infusion set	Antiseptic swabs	
IV tubing	IV pole	Dressings with Betadine or other antiseptic ointment
Needle (Angiocatheter, Intracath, Standard needle, butterfly)	Tape	
		Armboard, if needed
		Clean disposable gloves

Action

1 Gather all equipment and bring to bedside. Check IV solution and medication additives with physician's order.

2 Explain procedure to client.

3 Wash your hands.

4 Prepare IV solution and tubing:

  a. Maintain aseptic technique when opening sterile packages and IV solution.

  b. Clamp tubing, uncap spike, and insert into entry site on bag or bottle as manufacturer directs.

  c. Squeeze drip chamber and allow it to fill at least half way.

Rationale

Having equipment available saves time and facilitates accomplishment of task. Ensures that client receives the correct IV solution and medication as ordered by physician.

Explanation allays client's anxiety.

Handwashing deters the spread of microorganisms.

Prevents spread of microorganisms

Punctures the seal in the intravenous bag or bottle

Suction effect causes fluid to move into drip chamber. Also prevents air from moving down the tubing.

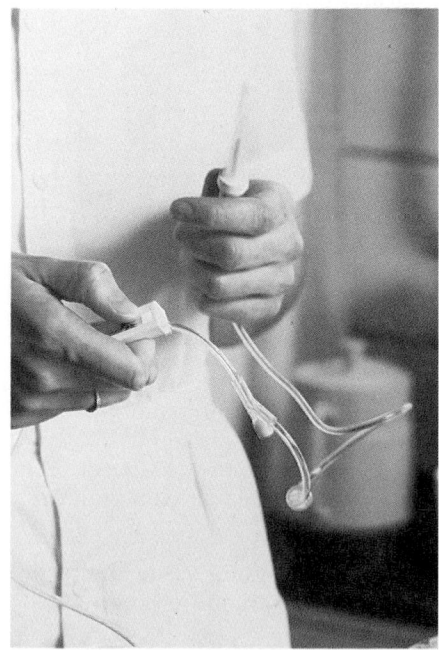
Step 4b: Clamping tubing.

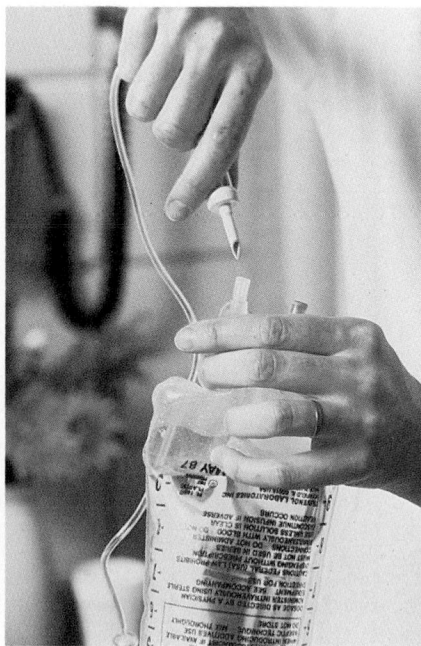
Step 4b: Inserting spike.

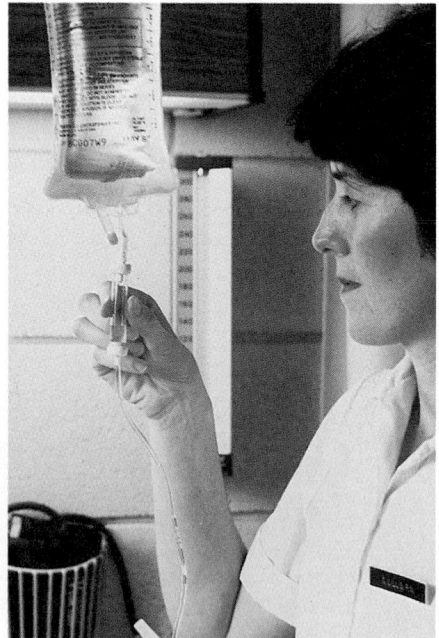
Step 4c: Squeezing drip chamber.

(Continued)

Action

    d. Remove cap at end of tubing, release clamp, and allow fluid to move through tubing. Allow fluid to flow until all air bubbles have disappeared. Close clamp and recap end of tubing maintaining sterility of set-up.

    e. If an infusion control pump is to be used, follow manufacturer's instructions for inserting tubing and setting infusion rate.

5 Have the client in a low Fowler's position in bed.

6 Select an appropriate site and palpate accessible veins.

7 If the site is hairy and agency policy permits, shave a 2-inch area around the intended site of entry.

8 Apply a tourniquet five inches–six inches above the venipuncture site to obstruct venous blood flow and distend the vein. Direct the ends of the tourniquet away from the site of entry. Check to be sure that the radial pulse is still present.

9 Ask the client to open and close his fist. Observe and palpate for a suitable vein. Try the following techniques if a vein cannot be felt:

    a. Release the tourniquet and have the client lower his arm below the level of the heart to fill the veins. Reapply tourniquet and gently tap over the intended vein to help distend it.

    b. Remove tourniquet and place warm compresses over the intended vein for 10 min–15 min.

10 Don clean, disposable gloves.

11 Cleanse the entry site with an antiseptic solution. Use a circular motion to move from the center outward for several inches.

12 Use the nondominant hand, placed about 1 inch or 2 inches below entry site, to hold the skin taut against the vein.

Rationale

Removes air from tubing which can, in larger amounts, act as an air embolus

Ensures correct flow rate and proper use of equipment

The supine position permits either arm to be used and allows for good body alignment. The low Fowler's position is usually most comfortable for the client.

The selection of an appropriate site decreases discomfort for the client and possible damage to body tissues.

It is difficult to clean the site of entry in the presence of hair because hair can harbor microorganisms. Adhesive tape will adhere better and may be removed more easily if hair is removed from site.

Interrupting the blood flow to the heart causes the vein to distend. Interruption of the arterial flow will impede venous filling. Distended veins are easy to see, palpate, and enter. The end of the tourniquet could contaminate the area of injection if directed toward the site of entry.

Contraction of the muscles of the forearm forces blood into the veins, thereby distending them further. Lowering the arm below the level of the heart, tapping the vein, and applying warmth help distend veins by filling them with blood.

Care must be used when handling any blood or body fluids to prevent transmission of HIV and other bloodborne infections.

Cleansing that begins at the site of entry and moves outward in a circular motion carries organisms away from the site of entry. Organisms on the skin can be introduced into the tissues or the bloodstream with the needle.

Pressure on the vein and surrounding tissues helps prevent movement of the vein as the needle is being inserted.

(Continued)

Action	**Rationale**

13 Enter the skin gently with the needle held in dominant hand, bevel side up, at a 30-degree to 45-degree angle, and when the needle is through the skin, lower the needle until it is nearly parallel to the skin. While following the course of the vein, advance the needle or catheter into the vein. A sensation of "give" can be felt when the needle enters the vein.

This allows needle to enter the vein with minimal trauma and deters passage of the needle through the vein.

14 When blood returns through the lumen of the needle, advance the needle further into the vein. The exact technique depends on the type of needle used. With an angiocatheter, the needle is removed leaving the catheter in place.

The tourniquet causes increased venous pressure resulting in automatic backflow. Having the needle placed well into the vein helps to prevent dislodgement of the needle.

15 Quickly remove protective cap from the intravenous tubing and attach the tubing to the catheter or needle. Stabilize the catheter or needle with nondominant hand and release the tourniquet with your other hand.

Bleeding is minimized and patency of the vein is maintained if the connection is made smoothly between the catheter and tubing.

16 Start the flow of solution promptly by releasing the clamp on the tubing. Examine the tissue around the entry site for signs of infiltration.

Blood will clot readily if intravenous flow is not maintained. If needle accidentally slips out of vein, solution will accumulate and infiltrate into surrounding tissue.

17 Support the needle with small piece of gauze under the hub, if necessary, to keep the needle properly positioned in the vein.

The pressure of the wall of the vein against the bevel of the needle will interrupt the rate of flow of the solution. The wall of the vein can be easily punctured by the needle.

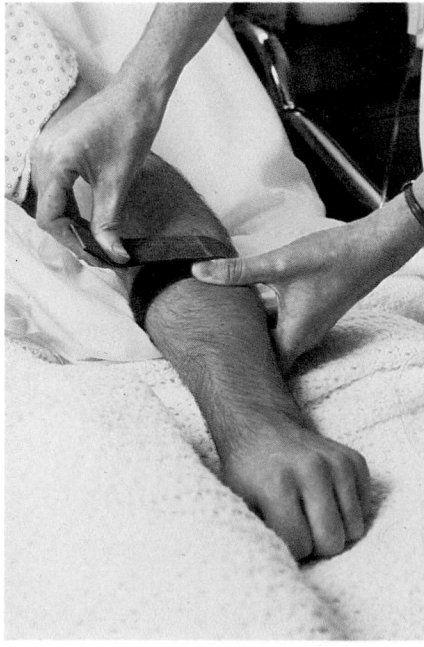
Step 8: Applying tourniquet.

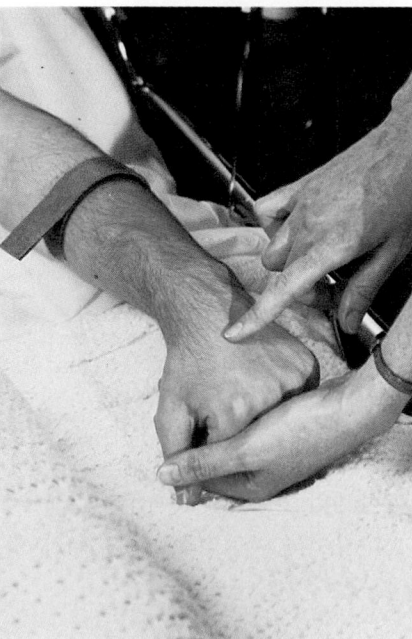
Step 9: Palpating vein.

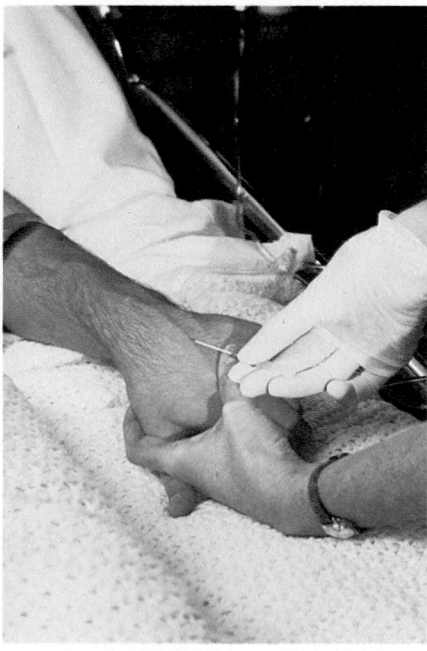
Step 13: Entering vein.

(Continued)

Action

Rationale

18 An antiseptic ointment may be applied to the needle's site of entry with a sterile dressing according to agency policy. Remove soiled gloves and discard appropriately.

Dressing and antiseptic ointment reduce skin contamination and protect against infection.

19 Loop the tubing near the site of entry, and anchor with tape to prevent pull on the needle, as illustrated in figure.

The smooth structure of the vein does not offer resistance to the movement of the needle. The weight of the tubing is sufficient to pull the needle out of the vein if it is not well anchored.

20 Mark the date, time, and type and size of the needle used for the infusion on the tape anchoring the tubing.

Personnel working with the infusion will know what type of needle is being used and when it was inserted. Protects client and intravenous site from infection.

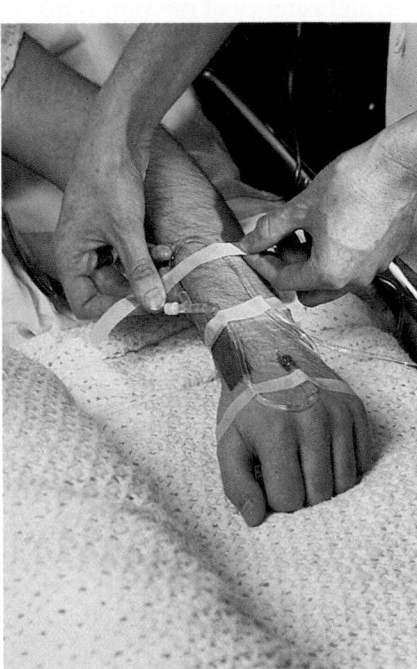

Step 19: Looping and anchoring tubing.

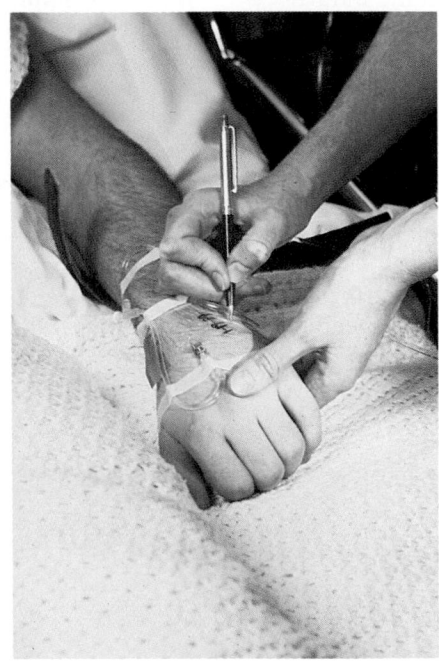

Step 20: Marking pertinent information on tape.

21 Anchor arm to an armboard for support, if necessary.

An armboard protects against change in the position of the vein and acts as a reminder to the client to minimize movements of his arm.

22 Adjust the rate of solution flow according to the amount prescribed or follow manufacturer's directions for adjusting flow rate on infusion pump.

The physician prescribes the rate of flow.

23 Remove all equipment and dispose in proper manner. Wash hands.

Deters the spread of microorganisms.

24 Document the procedure and client's response. Chart time, site, device used, and solution.

Provides accurate documentation and ensures continuity of care.

25 Return to check flow rate and observe for infiltration ½ hr after starting infusion.

Documents client's response to infusion.

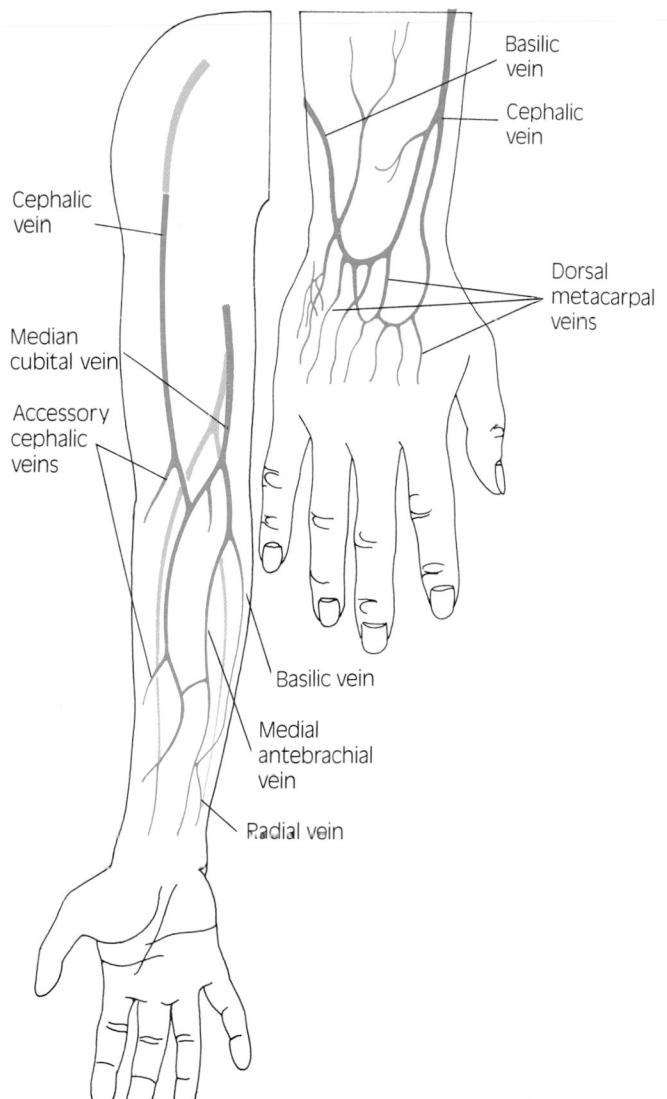

Cephalic
vein

Median
cubital vein

Accessory
cephalic
veins

Basilic
vein

Cephalic
vein

Dorsal
metacarpal
veins

Basilic vein

Medial
antebrachial
vein

Radial vein

F I G U R E **35-10**
Infusion sites on the ventral and dorsal aspects of the lower arm and hand.

clients, make continued infusion a problem. Experience will help the nurse acquire skill in palpating veins to determine their general condition.

Type of Fluid to be Infused

- Select a vein appropriate for the solution. Hypertonic solutions, those containing irritating medications, those administered at a rapid rate, and those with a high viscosity should be given in a large vein to minimize vessel trauma and to facilitate the rate of flow.

Anticipated Duration of Infusion

- Select a site where restriction in movement is kept to a minimum.
- Change sites every 48 hours if possible, starting with sites as distal as possible and moving in a

proximal direction on the alternate arms.

The following considerations are also important in the selection of a site:

- Select a vein large enough to accommodate the needle that will be used.
- Select a site that is naturally splinted by bone, such as the back of the hand or the forearm.
- Select a site distal to the heart, and move proximally, as necessary, to find an appropriate injection site.
- Select a site while moving toward the heart, and away from a damaged vein.

Starting an Intravenous Infusion. Before the infusion is started, a final check should be made of the solution to make sure that it is clear and contains no particles or precipitates. This check is especially important when substances have been added to the solution, because some additives create precipitates. Inline filters to help reduce the risk of contamination are commercially available to filter the solution immediately before it enters the client's vein.

The nurse should wash hands well before starting the infusion because of the threat of infections posed by intravenous therapy. Centers for Disease Control (CDC) guidelines recommend that gloves be worn as a preventive measure against AIDS.

Techniques for starting an intravenous infusion are described in Procedure 35-1.

Regulating and Monitoring. The nurse is responsible for maintaining the proper flow rate while assuring the comfort and safety of the client. The physician prescribes the flow rate. The amount of solution to be infused within a specified period of time is indicated. The rate is then determined on the basis of drops of solution to be infused every minute. This is called the drip rate.

The drop factor, or drops per milliliter of solution, is determined by the size of the opening in the infusion apparatus. It varies with the company producing the product. Most health agencies use the products of a single company. The most common drop factors are 10, 15, 20, and 60 drops per milliliter. Sixty drops per milliliter is used most often when small fluid volumes are important, such as with infants and small children. Adapters may be added to common infusion tubings to reduce the size of the drops.

A method for determining flow rate is given in Procedure 35-2.

A time tape can be placed on the container of solution to provide a quick reference for the nurse to monitor the rate at which the solution is entering the client. The tape gives an hourly indication of where the fluid level should be, based on the nurse's calculation of the drip rate. A time tape is illustrated in Figure 35-11.

Many factors can alter the rate of flow of an intravenous infusion, such as the height of the container in relation to the client, the client's blood pressure, the

(Text continues on p. 992.)

PROCEDURE 35-2
Regulating IV Flow Rate

Action	**Rationale**
1 Check physician's order for IV solution.	Ensures that correct solution is being given with the correct medications and determines the exact time period for administration of IV
2 Check patency of IV line and needle.	Any interference with patency will influence IV flow rate.
3 Verify drop factor (number of drops in 1 ml) of the equipment in use.	Drop factor of the equipment varies according to manufacturer and will be displayed on outer package. Equipment labeled microdrop or minidrip is standard and delivers 60 gtt/ml, but macrodrip delivery systems vary. Some of the more common types of equipment according to manufacturer are

Travenol Macrodrip   10 gtt/ml
Abbott Macrodrip   15 gtt/ml
McGaw Macrodrip   15 gtt/ml

4 Calculate the flow rate:

a. *Standard formula*

$$\text{gtt/min} = \frac{\text{volume (ml)} \times \text{drop factor (gtt/ml)}}{\text{time (in minutes)}}$$

Standard formula for calculating IV flow rate produces the correct number of gtt/min.

EXAMPLE— Administer 1000 ml 5% D/W over 10 hours (set delivers 60 gtt/1 ml).

$$\text{gtt/min} = \frac{1000 \text{ ml} \times 60}{600 \ (60 \text{ min} \times 10 \text{ hr})}$$

$$= \frac{60{,}000}{600}$$

$$= 100 \text{ gtt/min}$$

b. *Short formula using milliliters per hour*

$$\text{gtt/min} = \frac{\text{milliliters per hour} \times \text{drop factor (gtt/ml)}}{\text{time (60 minutes)}}$$

Short formula results in calculations using smaller numbers by using milliliters per hour. This is particularly useful for calculating drip rates when infusing piggyback IV medication.

EXAMPLE— Administer 1000 ml 5% D/W over 10 hours (set delivers 60 gtt/1 ml).

Find milliliters per hour by dividing 1000 ml by 10 hr:

$$\frac{1000}{10} = 100 \text{ ml/hr}$$

$$\text{gtt/min} = \frac{100 \text{ ml} \times 60}{60 \text{ min}}$$

$$= \frac{6{,}000}{60}$$

$$= 100 \text{ gtt/min}$$

5 Count drops per minute in drip chamber (# of gtts/15-sec interval × 4 = gtts/min). Hold watch beside drip chamber.

Holding watch next to drip chamber allows eyes to focus on drops and second hand on watch to provide accurate count.

(Continued)

Action

6 Adjust IV clamp as needed and recount drops per minute.

7 Mark IV container according to agency policy and manufacturer's recommendations. Use a time tape or label to measure amount to be infused at timed intervals.

8 Monitor IV flow rate at frequent intervals. Document client's response to infusion at prescribed rate.

Rationale

Regulates flow rate into drip chamber.

Allows for comparison of volume actually infused with scheduled infusion rate.

Provides for observation of IV infusion and ensures accurate documentation of client's response to IV infusion.

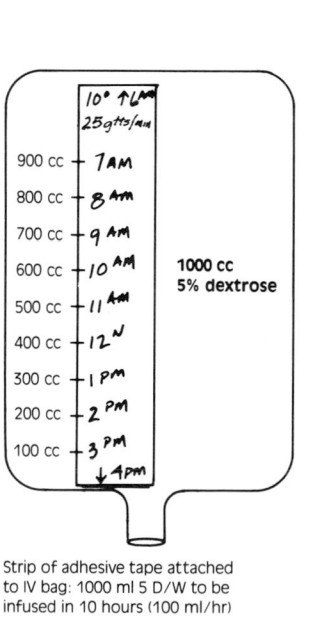

10° ↑6ᴬᴹ
25gtts/ᴬᴹ

900 cc — 7 AM
800 cc — 8 ᴬᴹ
700 cc — 9 ᴬᴹ
600 cc — 10 ᴬᴹ
500 cc — 11 ᴬᴹ
400 cc — 12 ᴺ
300 cc — 1 ᴾᴹ
200 cc — 2 ᴾᴹ
100 cc — 3 ᴾᴹ
↓ 4ᴾᴹ

1000 cc
5% dextrose

Strip of adhesive tape attached to IV bag: 1000 ml 5 D/W to be infused in 10 hours (100 ml/hr)

Commercially prepared IV label: 1000 cc 5 D/W + 20 mEg KCL to be infused in 8 hours (125 ml/hr)

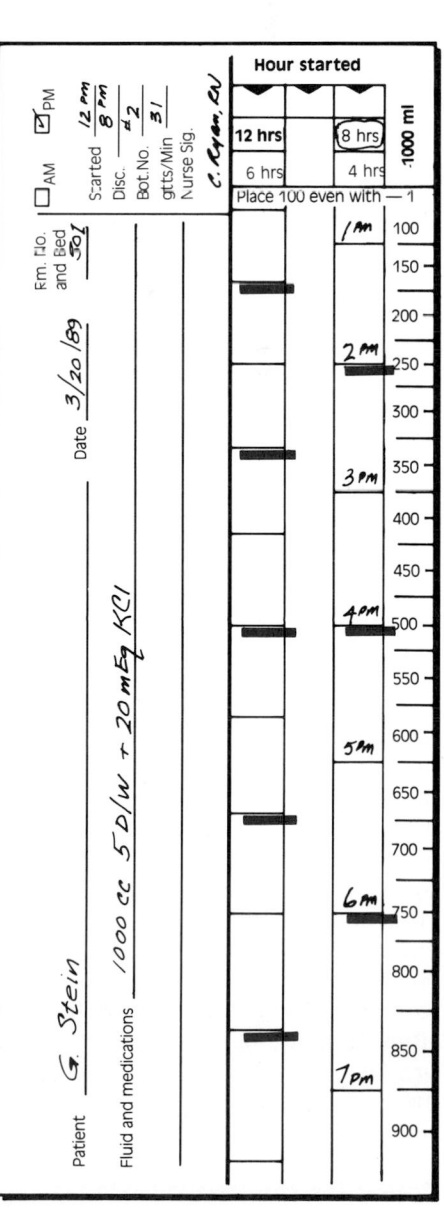

FIGURE 35-11

Time tapes. Use of time tapes enables the nurse to quickly evaluate if the intravenous solution is infusing according to schedule and to regulate the drip rate if needed.

client's position, the patency of the intravenous needle or catheter, infiltration, and a knot or kink in the tubing. The nurse can periodically check the infusion and determine quickly by glancing at the time tape if the solution is being infused at the proper hourly rate. If it is not, the nurse again regulates the flow. Because the client's movements, disturbances of the regulation mechanism, or change in the height of the infusion bottle or bed can alter the flow rate, even after it is regulated, the nurse needs to continue to check on the infusion at regular intervals. It has been reported that standard intravenous administration sets lose up to one half of their initial flow rate during the first hour of infusion because of tubing flexibility, and therefore the rate needs adjustment.

Maintenance of the flow rate is important because of the implications relative to the client's fluid balance. Too slow a flow may result in either the occurrence of deficits because the input is not balancing the loss, or in delaying the restoration of the balance. Infusing intravenous fluid too rapidly can overtax the body's capacities to adjust to the increase in the water volume or the electrolytes it contains. Nurses who allow infusions to get behind schedule and increase the rate to catch up may be seriously insulting the client's compensatory mechanisms and jeopardizing the client's well-being.

Several devices that limit the amount of fluid to be infused at any one time are available on the market. There are also battery-operated rate meters which quickly calculate the milliliter-per-hour flow rate of a solution as it is infusing. Some agencies use infusion pumps that automatically regulate the flow rate at preset limits and notify the nurse by an alarm system when the solution level of the bottle is getting low. Some models also sound an alarm when there is air in the tubing. These pumps bring solution to the vein by exerting positive pressure, either on the fluid or on the intravenous tubing. Syringe pumps are also available. They deliver small amounts of fluid, 100 ml or less, and are particularly useful with children. There are portable models on the market also, which are handy for the ambulatory patient. An infusion pump is shown in Figure 35-12.

Changing Solution and Tubing.
If more than one bottle of solution is ordered for the client, the nurse attaches the additional bottles. The method by which this is done depends on the procedure of the agency. Some intravenous equipment is designed to simplify the procedure by making it possible to attach additional bottles with a tandemlike arrangement. Because infusions often are continued after the responsibility for a client's care changes from one nurse to another, it is a good practice to agree on one common method for managing infusions. Without such uniformity, serious errors can occur, or valuable time is lost in checking and rechecking. One method for changing the solution and tubing is presented in Procedure 35-3.

Caring for the Infusion Site.
Scrupulous care of the infusion site should be observed to help control contam-

ination and to help prevent the introduction of microorganisms into the bloodstream. Regular dressing changes and tubing replacements are important means of preventing infection. Hospital policy should be followed in relation to changing dressings and tubing.

It is best to change the needle or catheter and the site of entry to a vein every 48 to 72 hours. The longer the needle remains in place, the greater the chances of complications, such as infection and phlebitis. Under certain circumstances, the nurse must use discretion in deciding how often to change the infusion site. For example, the client who is receiving long-term chemotherapy quickly runs out of suitable veins. Procedures 35-4 and 35-5 explain how to monitor an IV site and how to change an IV dressing.

A controversial aspect of the care of the site of insertion concerns irrigation of the needle. An irrigation is sometimes used when the needle begins to clog with blood and the client does not have other good sites for starting another infusion. *The procedure should not be used unless agency policy recommends it.*

Complications.
The client can be an important source of information regarding the possibility of complications associated with intravenous therapy. If the client is un-

(Text continues on p. 999.)

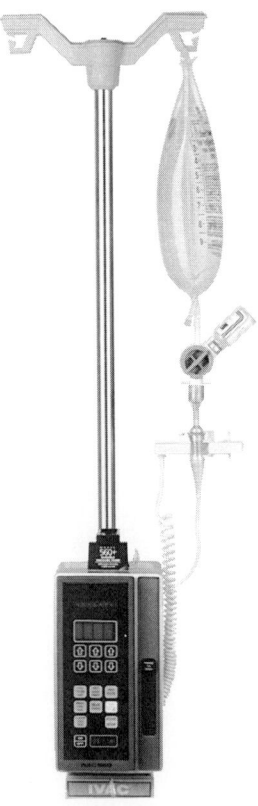

FIGURE 35-12

This is an example of an infusion pump. It is a positive-pressure pump that automatically regulates the flow rate. The alarm on this model is activated by an empty fluid container, an occluded tubing, or an unobtainable drop rate. (Ivac Corporation, San Diego, California)

PROCEDURE   35-3
Changing IV Solution and Tubing

Equipment

For solution change
   IV solution as or-
   dered by physi-
   cian

For tubing change
   Administration set
   Sterile gauze
   Tape or label
   Sterile dressings
     and antiseptic
     solutions/oint-
     ments (accord-
     ing to agency
     recommenda-
     tions)
   Clean disposable
     gloves

Action

1 Gather all equipment and bring to bedside. Check IV solution and medication additives with physician's order.

2 Explain procedure to client.

3 Wash your hands.

Rationale

Having equipment available saves time and facilitates accomplishment of task. Ensures that client receives the correct IV solution and medication as ordered by physician.

Explanation allays client's anxiety.

Handwashing deters the spread of microorganisms.

To Change IV Solution

4 Carefully remove protective cover from new solution container and expose entry site.

5 Close clamp on tubing.

6 Lift container off IV pole and invert it. Quickly remove the spike from the old IV container being careful not to contaminate it.

7 Steady new container and insert spike. Hang on IV pole.

8 Reopen clamp on tubing and adjust flow.

9 Label container according to agency policy. Record on intake/output record and document on chart according to agency policy. Discard used equipment in proper manner. Wash your hands.

Maintains sterility of IV solution

Stops the flow of IV fluid during change of solution

Maintains sterility of IV set-up

Allows for uninterrupted flow of new solution

Regulates flow rate into drip chamber

Ensures accurate continuation and administration of correct IV solution. Handwashing deters the spread of microorganisms.

To Change IV Tubing and Solution

10 Follow steps 1 through 4.

11 Open the administration set and remove protective covering from infusion spike. Using sterile technique insert into new container.

Maintains sterility of IV set-up

(Continued)

Changing IV Solution and Tubing (Continued)

Action

Rationale

To Change IV Tubing and Solution (continued)

12 Close clamp on new tubing. Hang IV container on pole and squeeze drip chamber to fill at least half way.

Gravity and suction effect cause fluid to move into drip chamber. Also prevents air from moving down the tubing.

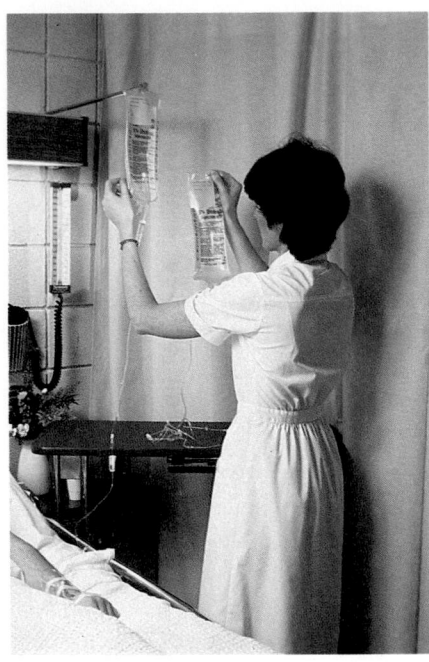

Step 12: Hanging new bag and tubing.

13 Remove cap at end of tubing, release clamp, and allow fluid to move through tubing until all air bubbles have disappeared. Close clamp and recap end of tubing maintaining sterility of set-up.

Removes air from tubing which can, in larger amounts, act as an air embolus

14 Loosen tape at IV insertion site. Don clean, disposable gloves. Carefully remove dressing and tape.

Care must be used when blood contact is possible. This prevents transmission of HIV and other blood-borne infections. Removing dressing provides access to needle hub necessary for tubing change.

15 Place sterile gauze square under needle hub.

Absorbs any leakage when tubing is disconnected from needle

16 Place new IV tubing close to client's IV site and slightly loosen protective cap.

Facilitates removal of cap and attachment to needle hub

17 Clamp the old IV tubing. Steady the needle hub with nondominant hand until change is completed. Remove tubing with dominant hand using a twisting motion.

Stabilizes needle and prevents inadvertently dislodging it

(Continued)

To Change IV Tubing and Solution (continued)

18 Set old tubing aside. While maintaining sterility, carefully remove cap and insert sterile end of tubing into the needle hub. Twist to secure it. Remove soiled gloves.

Maintains sterility of IV set-up

19 Open the clamp.

Allows solution to flow to client

20 Reapply sterile dressing to site according to agency protocol. See Procedure 35-5.

Deters entry of microorganisms at site

21 Regulate the IV flow according to physician's order. See Procedure 35-2.

Ensures that client receives IV solution at the prescribed rate

22 Attach to IV tubing tape or label that states date, time, and your initials. Label container and record procedure according to agency policy. Discard used equipment in proper manner and wash hands.

Documents IV tubing change. Handwashing deters the spread of microorganisms.

23 Record client's response to IV infusion.

Ensures accurate documentation of client's response

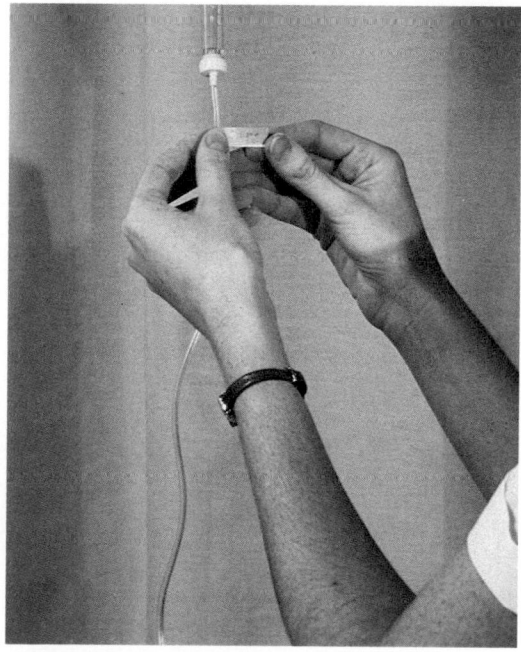

Step 22: Labeling IV tubing.

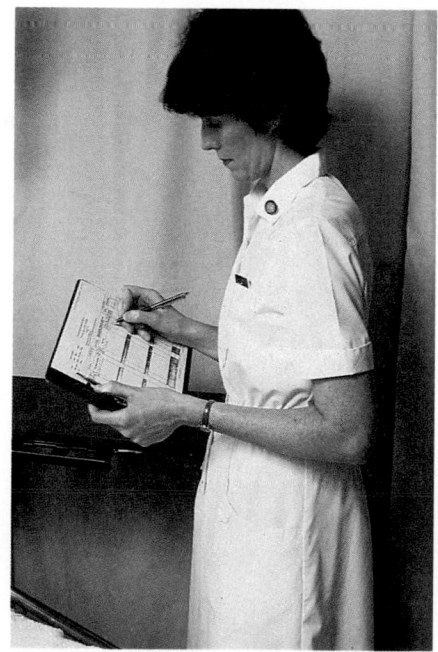

Step 23: Recording client's response to infusion.

Monitoring An IV Site and Infusion

Action

1 Monitor IV infusion at least once every hour. More frequent checks may be necessary if medication is being infused:

   a. Check physician's order for IV solution.

   b. Check drip chamber and time drops if IV is not regulated by an infusion control device.

Rationale

Promotes safe administration of IV fluids and medication. Too rapid administration of medications can result in the development of speed shock.

   Ensures that correct solution is being given at the correct rate and in the proper sequence with the correct medications

   Ensures that flow rate is correct

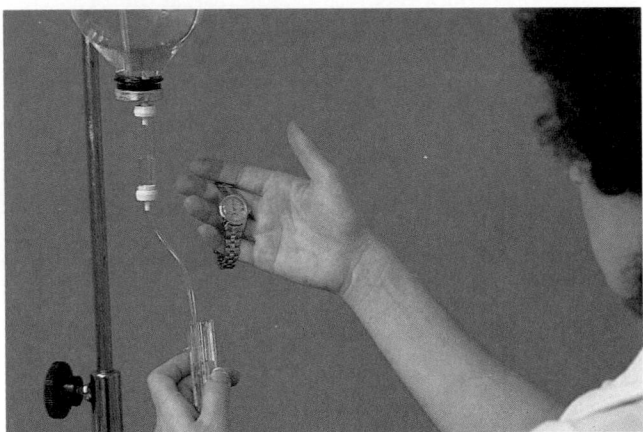

Step 1b: Timing drops.

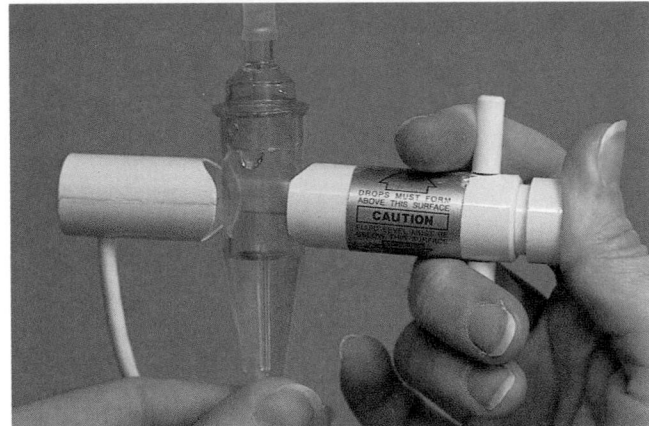

Step 1b: Placing electronic eye for infusion control device.

   c. Check tubing for anything that might interfere with flow. Be sure that clamp is in the open position. Observe dressing for leakage of IV solution.

   d. Observe settings, alarm, and indicator lights on infusion control device if one is being used.

Any kink or pressure on tubing may interfere with flow. Leakage may occur at connection of tubing with hub of needle or catheter and allow for loss of IV solution.

Ensures that infusion control device is functioning and that alarm is in "On" position

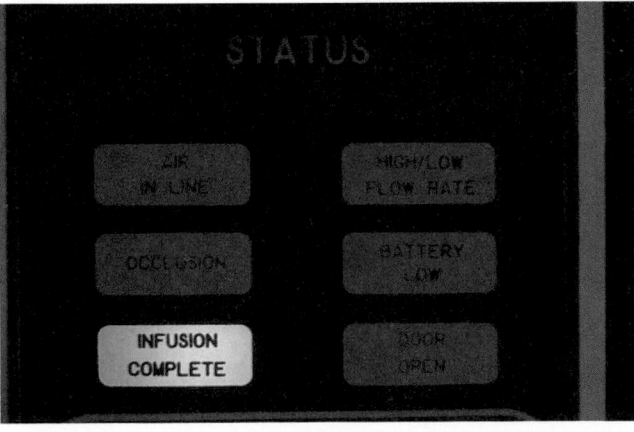

Step 1d: Checking indicator lights on infusion control device.

(Continued)

2 Inspect site for swelling, pain, coolness, or pallor at site of insertion which may indicate *infiltration* of IV. This necessitates removing IV and restarting at another site. Another method of validating whether IV is infiltrated involves applying a tourniquet above the insertion site. If IV needle is in the vein the solution will stop flowing.

Needle may become dislodged from vein, and IV solution may flow into subcutaneous tissue.

3 Inspect site for redness, swelling, heat, and pain at the IV site which may indicate *phlebitis* is present. IV will need to be discontinued and restarted at another site. Notify physician if you suspect that phlebitis may have occurred.

Chemical irritation or mechanical trauma cause injury to the vein and can lead to the development of phlebitis.

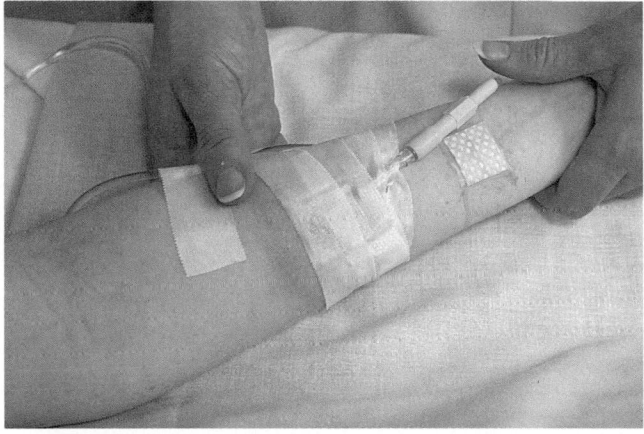

Step 3: Example of inflammation surrounding infusion site.

4 Check for local or systemic manifestations that indicate an *infection* is present at the site. IV will be discontinued and physician notified. Never disconnect IV tubing when putting on client's hospital gown.

Poor aseptic technique may allow bacteria to enter the needle or catheter insertion site or tubing connection.

5 Be alert for additional complications of IV therapy.

a. *Circulatory overload* can result in signs of cardiac failure and pulmonary edema. Monitor intake and output during IV therapy.

Infusing too much IV solution results in an increased volume of circulating fluid.

b. *Bleeding* at the site is most likely to occur when the IV is discontinued.

Bleeding may be caused by anticoagulant medication.

6 If possible, instruct client to call for assistance if any discomfort is noted at site, solution container is nearly empty, or flow has changed in any way.

Facilitates cooperation of client and safe administration of IV solution

7 Document IV infusion, any complications of therapy, and client's reaction to therapy.

Provides accurate documentation and ensures continuity of care

PROCEDURE 35-5
Changing an IV Dressing

Equipment

Sterile gauze (2 × 2 or 4 × 4) or transparent polyurethane dressing

Betadine solution or swabs

Adhesive remover

Povidone-iodine ointment (or other antiseptic ointment recommended by agency)

Alcohol swabs
Tape
Clean disposable gloves

Action	Rationale
1 Assess client's need for dressing change.	Agency policy determines interval for dressing change (every 24 hr–72 hr). The presence of moisture or a nonadhering dressing increases risk of bacterial contamination at the site.
2 Gather equipment and bring to bedside.	Having equipment available saves time and facilitates the performance of the task.
3 Explain procedure to client.	Explanation allays client's anxiety.
4 Wash your hands. Don clean disposable gloves.	Handwashing deters the spread of microorganisms. Gloves prevent transmission of HIV and other blood-borne infections.
5 Carefully remove old dressing but leave tape that anchors IV needle or catheter in place. Discard in proper manner.	Prevents dislodging of IV needle or catheter.
6 Assess IV site for presence of inflammation or infiltration. Discontinue and relocate the IV if noted.	Inflammation or infiltration causes trauma to tissues and necessitates removal of the IV needle or catheter.
7 Loosen tape and gently remove, being careful to steady catheter or needle hub with one hand.	Stabilizes needle and prevents inadvertently dislodging it.
8 Use adhesive remover to initiate cleansing procedure at site.	Removes adhesive residue and facilitates attachment of new dressing.
9 Cleanse the entry site with Betadine solution. Use a circular motion to move from the center outward. Follow with alcohol cleansing.	Cleansing in a circular motion while moving outward carries organisms away from the entry site. Use of antiseptic solutions reduces the number of microorganisms on the skin surface.
10 Reapply tape strip to needle or catheter at entry site.	Anchors needle or catheter to prevent dislodgement
11 Apply povidone-iodine ointment to the entry site if agency policy recommends this.	Antiseptic ointment reduces skin contamination and protects against infection.
12 Apply sterile gauze or transparent polyurethane dressing over entry site. Remove gloves and dispose properly.	Protects site and deters contamination with microorganisms.
13 Secure IV tubing with additional tape if necessary. Label dressing with date, time of change, and initials. Check that IV flow is accurate and system is patent.	Documents IV dressing change.
14 Discard equipment properly and wash hands.	Protects against spread of microorganisms
15 Record client's response to dressing change and observation of site.	Provides accurate documentation and ensures continuity of care

comfortable, the nurse should check to see that the infusion is entering the vein as intended, that the flow rate is not too rapid, and that the client's position is satisfactory. Anxiety over the implications of an infusion can also cause discomfort for the client.

Local complications such as infiltration, phlebitis, and thrombophlebitis occur more frequently than systemic complications. Systemic complications (fluid overload, embolus, infection), however, are more serious and may be life-threatening. Table 35-10 defines these complications, noting common causes, signs and symptoms, and pertinent nursing considerations.

Discontinuing the Infusion.

When the amount of solution the physician has ordered has been infused, the nurse assumes responsibility for discontinuing the infusion. It is helpful before discontinuing the infusion to see if the client is still ordered intravenous medications. In this case while the continuous infusion solutions are discontinued the needle or catheter is "capped" with a heparin lock which allows access to a vein for intermittent medications. If the needle or catheter are to be removed the adhesive strips and sterile dressing are removed, the needle or catheter is removed in line with the vein, and pressure is immediately applied to the site. If the client is able to do so, he may be asked to hold the pressure for a minute or more.

If the client's arm or leg has been immobilized for several hours or longer, the nurse should manipulate it carefully in an attempt to put the joint through range of motion and passively move the muscles of the area.

The following information is recorded when the infusion has been completed:

The date and time the infusion was completed
The kind and amount of solution infused
The name of the person discontinuing the infusion
Symptoms of any untoward reactions
Signs of the desired effects of the infusion

Replacing Blood and Blood Products

A **blood transfusion** is the infusion of whole blood or a blood component such as plasma, packed red blood cells, or platelets, from a healthy person into a recipient's vein. The person receiving the blood is called the recipient. The person giving the blood is called the **donor.** Blood may be given by either direct or indirect transfusion. In an *indirect transfusion,* blood is infused after it has been collected from a donor and processed; this is the method used most commonly. The technique is similar to that for giving an intravenous infusion. In a *direct transfusion,* the blood is infused as it is being taken from a donor. This method is rarely used, except in emergencies, and will not be discussed here.

Typing and Crossmatching.

Before blood can be given to a person, it must be determined that the blood of the donor and that of the recipient are compatible. If they are not, clumping and hemolysis of the recipient's blood cells will result. The laboratory examination to determine a person's blood type is called **typing**. The process of determining compatibility between blood specimens is known as **crossmatching**.

Blood Types.

The four main blood groups in the ABO system of blood typing are A, B, AB, and O. Some of these groups are broken down into still more subgroups.

Blood type is an inherited trait and is determined by the type of antigens and antibodies present in the blood. An **antigen** is a substance that causes the formation of antibodies. An **antibody** is a protein substance developed in the body in response to the presence of an antigen that has in some way gained access to the body. An **agglutinin** is an antibody that causes a clumping of specific antigens. People who have type-A blood have an A antigen in their red blood cells; those with type-B blood have B antigens in their cells; those in the AB group have A and B antigens; and persons with type-O blood have neither A or B antigens in their red blood cells. Persons in each blood group have the agglutinins to the red cell antigens that they lack. Group-A persons have the agglutinin for B; group-AB persons have no agglutinins for A and B, while group-O persons have both A and B agglutinins in their blood serum. Assume a person with type-O blood is transfused with blood from either a person with group-A or group-B blood. There would be destruction of the recipient's red cells since his anti-A or anti-B agglutinins would react with the A or B antigens in the donor's red cells. From this example, it can be seen why group-AB persons are often called universal recipients, because persons in this blood group have no agglutinins for either A or B antigens, and group O persons are often called universal donors because they have neither A nor B antigens.

Rh Factor.

The **Rh** factor is an inherited antigen in human blood. There are five antigens in the Rh system, but the one designated D is of first concern. A person whose blood contains a D antigen is called Rh positive; an Rh-negative person lacks D. It is important that an Rh-negative person receive blood from another Rh-negative person. If Rh-positive blood is injected into an Rh-negative person, the recipient will develop anti-Rh agglutinins. Subsequent transfusion with Rh-positive blood may cause serious reactions with clumping and hemolysis of red blood cells.

The Rh factor is of special importance during pregnancy because Rh incompatability between mother and fetus is often the problem when an infant has hemolytic disease.

Selection of Blood Donors.

The selection of blood donors must be done with care. Not only must the

(Text continues on p. 1001.)

T A B L E   35-10

Complications Associated with Intravenous Infusions

Name and Definition	Causes	Signs and Symptoms	Nursing Considerations
Infiltration: The escape of fluid into the subcutaneous tissue	• Dislodged needle • Penetrated vessel wall	Swelling; pallor; coldness; or pain around the infusion site; significant decrease in the flow rate	• Check the infusion site often for symptoms. • Discontinue the infusion if symptoms occur. • Restart the infusion at a different site. • Limit the movement of the extremity with the IV.
Phlebitis: An inflammation of a vein	• Mechanical trauma from needle or catheter • Chemical trauma from solution • Septic (due to contamination)	Local, acute tenderness; redness; warmth; and slight edema of the vein above the insertion site	• Discontinue the infusion immediately. • Apply warm, moist compresses to the affected site. • Avoid further use of the vein. • Restart the infusion in another vein.
Thrombus: A blood clot	• Tissue trauma from needle or catheter	Symptoms similar to phlebitis Intravenous fluid flow may cease if clot obstructs needle	• Stop the infusion immediately. • Apply warm compresses as ordered by the physician. • Restart the IV at another site. • *Do not rub or massage the affected area.*
Speed shock: The body's reaction to a substance that is injected into the circulatory system too rapidly	• Too rapid a rate of fluid infusion into circulation	Pounding headache; fainting; rapid pulse rate; apprehension; chills; back pains; and dyspnea	• If symptoms develop, discontinue the infusion immediately. • Report symptoms of speed shock to the physician immediately. • Monitor vital signs if symptoms develop. • Use the proper IV tubing. A microdrip (60 gtts/ml) should be used on all pediatric clients. • Carefully monitor the rate of fluid flow. • Check the rate frequently for accuracy. A time tape is useful for this purpose.
Fluid overload: The condition caused when too large a volume of fluid infuses into the circulatory system	• Too large a volume of fluid infused into circulation	Engorged neck veins; increased blood pressure; and difficulty in breathing (dyspnea)	• If symptoms develop, slow the rate of infusion. • Notify the physician immediately. • Monitor vital signs. • Carefully monitor the rate of fluid flow. • Check the rate frequently for accuracy.
Embolus: A foreign body or air in the circulatory system	• Thrombus dislodges and circulates in the blood • Air enters the vein through the infusion line	Dependent on whether the embolism causes an obstruction or infarction in the circulatory system	• Check the site regularly to identify signs of phlebitis. • Do not allow air to enter the infusion line. • Treat phlebitis with the utmost caution. • Report any sudden pain or breathing difficulty immediately.
Infection: An invasion of pathogenic organisms into the body	• Nonsterile technique used in starting infusion • Improper care of infusion site • Contaminated IV solution	Fever; malaise; and pain, swelling, inflammation, or discharge at IV insertion site	• Use scrupulous aseptic technique when starting an infusion. • Change the dressing over the site regularly. • Change IV tubing every 24 hr if agency policy permits. • Always wash hands before working with the IV.

donor's blood be accurately typed, but it is also important to determine whether or not the donor is free from diseases, such as AIDS and type-A or type-B hepatitis. The virus causing these diseases can be transmitted to the recipient. Persons who have allergies usually are not used; nor those with a history of a chronic disease, such as tuberculosis. As a further precaution, some blood banks will not accept blood from a donor who has been immunized recently because of a possible allergic reaction to the blood.

The donor is examined carefully at the time of donation and is permitted to give blood only if heart and chest sounds, blood count, temperature, pulse and respiratory rates, and blood pressure are within normal ranges.

In the early 1980s a number of persons contacted AIDS after receiving contaminated blood. Although careful screening of both donors and donated blood has greatly decreased the likelihood of this happening, both blood donors and recipients continue to have many questions regarding safety. *There is no way that donors may contract AIDS or any other disease by giving blood* because single-use sterile set-ups are used for each donor. Some clients who know in advance that they will need blood are now requesting to be allowed to have family members or themselves (autologous transfusion) donate the blood. This practice is growing in popularity.

Blood Extracts. Some persons do not need all of the constituents of whole blood. For example, one may need red blood cells but not the blood plasma and its constituents. Red blood cells in concentrated form are called packed red blood cells and may be used in the following situations: a client with anemia suffering with a low red blood cell count; a client with cardiovascular failure, in order to increase his blood volume and red blood cells while avoiding cardiovascular overload; and a client with gastrointestinal bleeding, to maintain adequate hemoglobin levels without increasing blood pressure, which would likely lead to more bleeding.

In other situations, only plasma is required, such as when plasma protein or the blood's clotting factor is in low supply. Human serum or plasma is particularly useful in emergencies for immediate restoration of fluid because serum presents no compatibility problems and time need not be lost seeking donors and matching blood. It is also an excellent blood-volume expander when time is of essence, an example being for the person who is severely burned and losing plasma rapidly from burn areas.

Components of plasma that are used therapeutically include human albumin (hypovolemic shock, albuminemia, liver failure), cryoprecipitates (bleeding due to hemophilia or disseminated intravascular coagulation [DIC]), and gamma globulins—the antibody-containing part of plasma (gamma globulin deficiencies).

Dextran is a plasma extender or substitute. It is most commonly used for clients with hypovolemic shock and for priming pump oxygenators for clients having heart surgery.

Initiating the Transfusion. The procedure for starting a blood transfusion (Procedure 35-6) is basically the same as for an intravenous solution. If possible, larger veins should be selected because no smaller needle than a 19-gauge needle should be used. This size is necessary because of the viscosity of blood.

Transfusion Reactions. When preparing and administering the transfusion, the nurse should take every precaution to prevent the occurrence of transfusion reactions through scrupulous technique. Table 35-11 describes some potential transfusion reactions. A nurse should stay with the client for at least 5 to 10 minutes after starting a blood transfusion and then check him every 15 minutes while the client receives blood. A transfusion reaction can be very serious!

Giving Total Parenteral Nutrition

Hypertonic solutions consisting of dextrose, amino acids, and select electrolytes and minerals may be infused using a central vein by a procedure known as **total parenteral nutrition** (TPN). Used in cases of severe malnutrition, TPN is directed to

- Reestablishing and maintaining positive nitrogen balance
- Weight gain and maintenance
- Correction of metabolic complications

This procedure and the related nursing responsibilities are described in Chapter 31.

EVALUATING

When evaluating the effectiveness of the plan of care aimed at promoting healthy fluid, electrolyte, and acid–base balance the nurse pays attention to the following parameters:

- Are the client's drinking and eating patterns supplying the fluid and electrolytes he needs? Are food and fluid likes and dislikes interfering with the implementation of the plan of care? Is the client having any difficulties with oral fluids, tube feedings, intravenous therapy, or total parenteral nutrition?
- Is the client's urine output approximately equal to the fluid intake? Does the client void at least once each shift (except when sleeping)? Do urine characteristics (color, odor, specific gravity) indicate healthy functioning of the kidneys and excretion of fluids?

(Text continues on p. 1005.)

PROCEDURE 35-6
Administering a Blood Transfusion

Equipment

Blood product
Blood administra-
tion set (tubing
with inline filter
and Y for saline
administration)

0.9% Normal saline
IV pole

Intravenous line
with a #18 or
#19 needle or
catheter

Action

1 Determine if client knows reason for transfusion.
Ask if the client has had a transfusion or transfusion
reaction in the past.

2 Explain procedure to client. Check for signed consent for transfusion if required by agency. Advise
client to report any chills, itching, rash, or unusual
symptoms.

3 Wash your hands.

4 Hang container of 0.9% normal saline with blood
administration set to initiate IV infusion and follow
administration of blood.

Rationale

Directs teaching prior to beginning transfusion.

Provides reassurance and facilitates cooperation.
Prompt reporting of any reaction to transfusion necessitates stopping immediately.

Handwashing deters the spread of microorganisms.

Dextrose may lead to clumping of red blood cells and
hemolysis. Filter in blood administration set removes
particulate material formed during storage of blood.

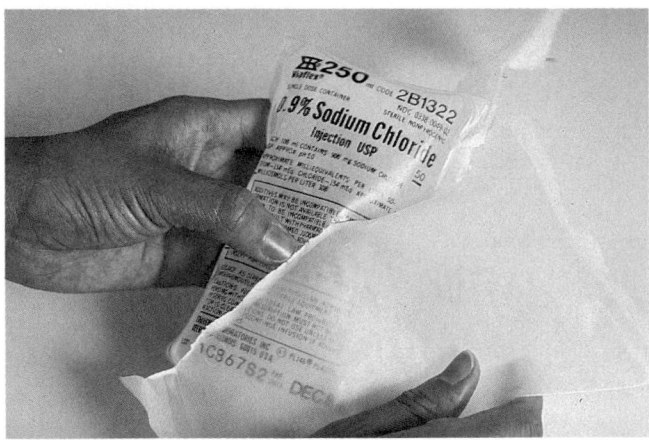

Normal saline container.

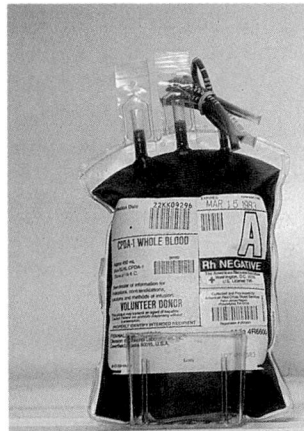

Unit of packed red blood cells.

5 Start intravenous with #18 or #19 catheter if not already present. See Procedure 35-1. Keep IV open
by starting flow of normal saline.

6 Obtain blood product from blood bank according
to agency policy.

7 Complete identification and checks as required by
agency:

    a. Identification number

    b. Blood group and type

Large-bore needle or catheter is necessary for infusion
of blood products. The lumen must be large enough
not to cause damage to red blood cells.

Blood must be stored in refrigerated unit at carefully
controlled temperature (4°C).

Some agencies require two registered nurses to verify
information:

    Verifies that unit numbers match

    Verifies that ABO group and Rh type are the same

(Continued)

    c. Expiration date

    Safe storage of blood is limited to 35 days before red blood cells begin to deteriorate.

    d. Client's name

    Never administer blood to a client without a name band.

    e. Inspect blood for clots

    If clots are present, blood should be returned to blood bank.

8 Take baseline set of vital signs prior to beginning transfusion.

Any change in vital signs during the transfusion may indicate a reaction.

9 Start infusion of the blood product:

    a. Prime in-line filter with blood.

    Necessary if blood is to flow properly

    b. Start administration slowly.

    Transfusion reactions typically occur during this period, and a slow rate will minimize the volume of red blood cells infused. If there have been no adverse effects during this time, the infusion rate is increased.

    c. Check vital signs every 5 min for first 15 min.

    If complications occur, they can be observed, and the blood can be stopped immediately.

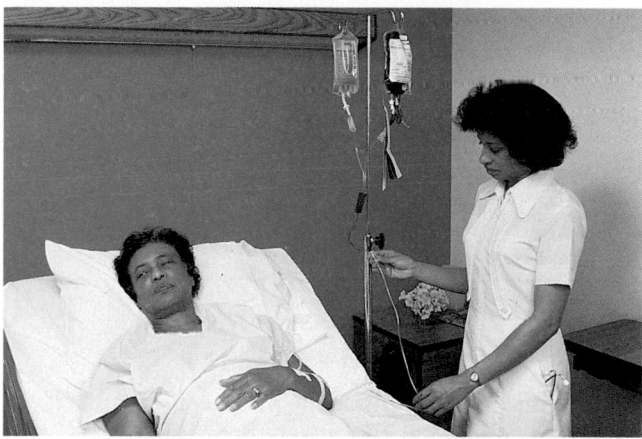

Step 9a: Priming the in-line filter.

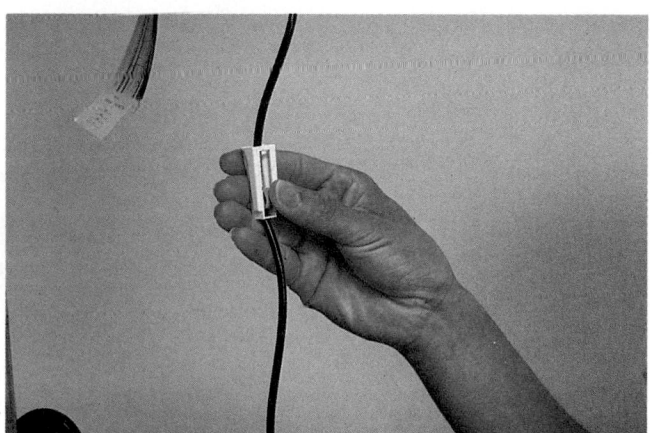

Step 9b: Starting infusion of blood slowly.

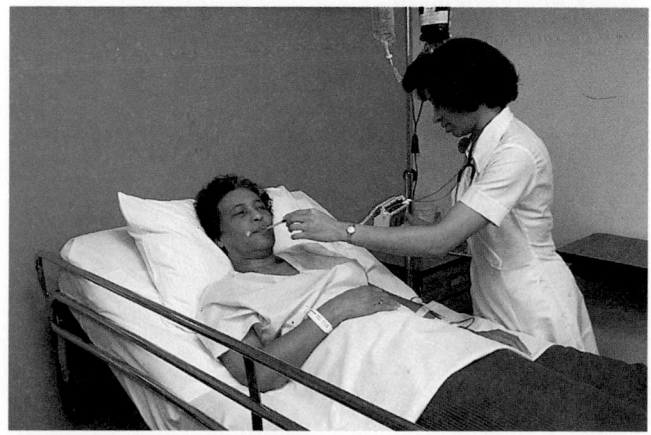

Step 9c: Checking vital signs.

(Continued)

Action	Rationale
d. Observe client for flushing dyspnea, itching, hives, or rash.	May be early indication of a transfusion reaction.
e. Use a blood warming device, if indicated, especially with rapid transfusions through a central venous pressure catheter.	Rapid administration of cold blood can result in cardiac arrhythmias.
10 Maintain the prescribed flow rate as ordered and assess frequently for transfusion reaction. Stop blood transfusion and allow saline to flow if you suspect a reaction. Notify physician and blood bank.	Rate must be carefully controlled, and client's reaction must be monitored on a frequent basis.
11 When transfusion is complete, infuse 0.9% normal saline.	Saline prevents hemolysis of red blood cells and clears remainder of blood in IV line.
12 Record administration of blood and client's reaction as ordered by agency. Return blood transfusion bag to blood bank according to agency policy.	Provides for accurate documentation of client's response to blood transfusion.

T A B L E   35-11
Transfusion Reactions

Reaction	Signs and Symptoms	Nursing Activity
Allergic reaction: Allergy to transfused blood	Hives, itching Anaphylaxis	• Stop transfusion immediately and KVO with normal saline. • Notify physician stat. • Administer antihistamine parenterally as necessary.
Febrile reaction: Fever develops during infusion	Fever and chills Headache Malaise	• Stop transfusion immediately and KVO with normal saline. • Notify physician. • Treat symptoms.
Hemolytic transfusion reaction: incompatibility of blood product	Immediate onset Facial flushing Fever, chills Headache Low back pain Shock	• Stop infusion immediately and KVO with normal saline. • Notify physician stat. • Obtain blood samples from site. • Obtain first voided urine. • Treat shock if present. • Send unit, tubing and filter to lab.
Circulatory overload: Too much blood administered	Dyspnea Dry cough Pulmonary edema	• Slow or stop infusion. • Monitor vital signs. • Notify physician.
Bacterial reaction: Bacteria present in blood	Fever Hypertension Dry, flushed skin Abdominal pain	• Stop infusion immediately. • Monitor vital signs. • Notify physician. • Administer antibiotics stat.

- Are abnormal sources of fluid loss (vomiting, diarrhea, draining wounds, fistula, and so forth) responding to treatment? Are these losses effectively being replaced by the designated therapy? Are the signs of fluid volume deficit improving?
- Do the client's weight and record of fluid intake and output indicate fluid balance?
- Are the signs and symptoms which initially manifested fluid, electrolyte, or acid–base imbalances absent or improved? Has therapy created any troublesome new signs or symptoms?

- Is the client now able to manage his own care (*i.e.,* practice self-care behaviors to maintain fluid, electrolyte, and acid–base balance)? Can the client describe appropriate responses to potential future problems?

This evaluation should be ongoing as the plan of care is implemented. As the client achieves short-term goals these should be noted and reinforced. Before nursing care is terminated the client (and family) should be able to independently promote fluid, electrolyte, and acid–base balance.

NURSING PROCESS *in Clinical Practice*

When identifying and treating fluid, electrolyte, and acid–base balance problems categorized as nursing diagnoses the nurse uses each phase of the nursing process. Quality care is dependent on the nurse's possession of the knowledge and clinical skills described earlier in this chapter. In this section the special fluid, electrolyte, and acid–base balance needs of two target populations will be explored: surgical clients and oncology clients. Both groups of clients are at increased risk for fluid, electrolyte, and acid–base balance problems.

In the case study that follows, nursing care is described for a client with a fluid volume deficit related to prolonged diarrhea.

The Surgical Client

Clients undergoing surgery are at high risk for fluid, electrolyte, and acid–base balance problems pre-, intra-, and postoperatively because of
- The pathology that underlies the need for surgery
- Aggressive diagnostic testing
- The stress of anesthesia and surgery
- Postoperative treatment
- Effects of surgery
Potential nursing diagnoses include

Preoperative
Fluid volume deficit related to fluid restrictions for diagnostic tests or pathology that results in decreased fluid intake (anorexia, intestinal obstruction) or abnormal fluid losses (vomiting, draining fistula)

Intraoperative
Fluid volume deficit related to bleeding, which if severe may cause shock and acute renal failure or actual fluid loss and third-space fluid shift during surgical procedure

Postoperative
Fluid volume deficit related to vomiting, gastric suction, or oral fluid restriction secondary to ileus following abdominal surgery

Fluid volume excess related to increased antidiuretic hormone (ADH) secondary to surgery and anesthesia, aldosterone secretion, or overadministration of isotonic electrolyte solutions

Alteration in acid–base balance (metabolic alkalosis) related to vomiting or gastric suction

Alteration in acid–base balance (respiratory acidosis) related to hypoventilation during surgery and to shallow respiration from pain and splinting after surgery

Alteration in sodium balance (hyponatremia) related to excessive ADH activity

Assessment

Preoperative
- Obtain baseline vital signs, body weight.
- Review laboratory data to ensure normal electrolytes and a hematocrit at 33% or higher (because transport of oxygen to cells depends on an adequate hemoglobin level). Notify physicians of any abnormalities so these can be corrected prior to surgery.
- Use intake and output records (and daily weights if fluid balance problems are suspected) and assessment of urine characteristics to assess fluid balance.
- Check for malnutrition (muscles with a wasted appearance—decreased strength, pale skin that breaks down easily, listlessness and apathy, dull, dry hair that falls out easily).

Postoperative
- Monitor vital signs according to agency policy and client's condition.
Tachycardia and hypotension may indicate severe fluid volume deficit. Changes in respirations and abnormal breath sounds are key indicators of acid–base and fluid volume disturbances.
- Maintain accurate intake and output record which includes *intraoperative* fluid intake and output. Ensure in adults an hourly urine output of 30 ml to

50 ml. Factors that contribute to decreased urinary volume in the postoperative period include

Stress reaction (healthy physiologic response to surgery)

Hypovolemia resulting from fluid loss incurred in surgery

Preoperative dehydration

Subtle accumulation of fluid at the surgical site

Disturbance in myocardial function causing decreased blood flow to the kidneys

Renal failure, a serious cause of postoperative oliguria (Metheny, 1987).

- Assess for signs of electrolyte imbalance (see Table 35-4).

Client Goals

The client will

- Enter surgery in fluid balance as evidenced by
  1. Stable body weight
  2. Urine output of 30 ml to 50 ml/hour
  3. Urine specific gravity of 1.010 to 1.025.
- Enter surgery in electrolyte balance as evidenced by normal laboratory values for sodium, chloride, potassium, and bicarbonate

Postoperatively the client will

- Maintain approximately equal fluid intake and output
- Maintain urine output of 30 ml to 50 ml/hour
- Maintain stable body weight
- Maintain stable vital signs
- Be free of signs indicating fluid, electrolyte, or acid–base disturbance

Interventions

The best intervention for fluid, electrolyte, and acid–base disturbances is *prevention.*

- Prior to client's surgery offer oral foods and fluids that the client likes and that are most likely to result in fluid, electrolyte, and nutritional balance.
- Bring any suspected abnormality to the physician's attention and execute orders for fluid or electrolyte replacement, strategies to reduce excesses, and so forth.
- Assist in identifying contributive factors and reduce or eliminate these if possible.
- Administer intravenous fluids as prescribed and maintain accurate drip rates to prevent under- or overinfusion.
- As soon as the client is able to tolerate oral fluids (check for swallowing reflex and bowel sounds), begin oral fluid replacement with fluids the client prefers.
- In clients with severe fluid imbalances an indwelling Foley catheter may need to be inserted so that hourly urine outputs can be monitored.

Evaluative Criteria

Client meets above goals.

The Oncology Client

Fifty to seventy-five percent of all clients with cancer experience problems with fluid and electrolyte regulation (Dorr and Frita, 1980). These problems are related to

- Faulty regulation or availability of calcium, uric acid, sodium, potassium, phosphate
- Altered hormonal regulation (malignant tumors may produce hormones that interfere with water and electrolyte balance: antidiuretic hormone, parathyroid hormone, osteoclastic activating factor, adrenocorticotropic hormone)
- Third-space fluid accumulation related to malignant effusions into the peritoneal, pericardial, or pleural compartments, or to edema resulting from blocked lymphatic drainage or venous return
- Treatment-related imbalances (Metheny, 1987).

Sample nursing diagnoses for the client with cancer include

Fluid volume deficit related to anorexia and vomiting (may be secondary to chemotherapy or radiation therapy), prolonged gastric suction, or third-space fluid shifts into the peritoneal, pericardial, or pleural compartments

Fluid volume excess: edema related to obstruction of lymphatic drainage or venous return secondary to tumor pressure

Common electrolyte disturbances include:

Hypercalcemia related to increased osteoclastic activity of select tumors or treatment with estrogens, progestins, and so forth

Hypocalcemia related to decreased intake and absorption of calcium or increased utilization of calcium for healing of bony lesions

Hyponatremia related to certain tumors releasing an ADH-like substance or salt loss from the gastrointestinal tract (vomiting, draining fistula)

Hyperkalemia related to rapid cell destruction following successful treatment of large tumors

Assessment

- Assess for the signs and symptoms that accompany electrolyte disturbances associated with specific tumors and treatment modalities.
- Weigh clients daily or weekly for signs of fluid deficit or excess. Fluid volume deficit is characterized by decreased skin turgor, decreased urinary output, concentrated urine, and postural hypotension. Clients with third-space fluid shifts have an *increase* in total body fluid, thus no decrease in weight, although clinically their condition is described as fluid volume deficit.
- Be alert for signs of third space fluid shifts:
  Peritoneal—increased abdominal girth
  Pleural—difficulty breathing

- Assess for signs of dependent edema; check the feet and ankles of persons who sit or stand for long periods of time and the back and sacral area of the bedridden client.
- Assess for the development of weeping edema (leakage of fluid through the pores).

Client Goals
The client will:
- Take in sufficient fluids (oral if possible) to maintain fluid balance as evidenced by
  - Normal skin turgor
  - Moist mucous membranes
  - Stable body weight
  - Baseline blood pressure
- Report (demonstrate) relief of symptoms of dehydration, third-space fluid shifts, edema, or other electrolyte disturbances
- Exhibit decreased dependent edema
- Describe self-care behaviors to prevent future fluid and electrolyte disturbances

Interventions
Interventions will vary according to the nature of the fluid, electrolyte, or acid–base disturbance. To prevent problems the client should be encouraged to drink sufficient fluids (about 2500 ml for the adult) and to eat nutritious meals.

- Clients with anorexia may need to be taught how to choose times when their systems will best tolerate food and fluids to ingest high-calorie liquids with key electrolytes.
- Clients with abnormal fluid losses may need to be taught the importance of fluid replacement.
- Clients with fluid volume deficits resulting from third-space fluid shifts may require intravenous fluid replacement—however, this will also increase the volume of fluids trapped in the third space (*e.g.,* pleural cavity) and increase the client's discomfort. The client needs to be carefully monitored for signs of fluid overload during the administration of intravenous fluids.
- Clients with dependent edema require frequent position changes and a skin care program to prevent skin breakdown. Special mattresses are helpful.
- See Tables 35-3, 35-4, and 35-5 for nursing interventions to treat specific fluid, electrolyte, and acid–base balance disturbances.

Evaluative Criteria
Client meets above goals.

CASE STUDY

Gerry Stein is a 22-year-old Jewish male who is a senior in the pre-med program at a large state university. Although his grades were poor his first year in college he is now an honors student and plans to take the MCATs in 2 weeks. His overwhelming ambition is to be accepted into a prestigious medical school and to become a psychiatrist. He presents at the campus health clinic.

Assessment Findings
A comprehensive nursing assessment of Mr. Stein yields the following data:
- History of problems with diarrhea since his junior year in high school; treatment: Kaopectate and limiting his food and fluid intake; believes diarrhea is stress related; no medical evaluation to date
- Has had two to three loose bowel movements per day for the last week with urgency and occasional incontinence; believes this is related to anxiety about performance on MCATs and need for good grades; always thirsty but afraid to drink much; urine output is decreased and he noted it is darker in color and has a stronger odor
- Nursing examination: T—99.8°F (37.6°C), P—92, R—18, BP—100/60; skin and mucous membranes are pale and dry; weight is 4 lb less than usual (present weight: 170 lb).

Nursing Diagnosis
Mr. Stein will receive a thorough medical work-up to rule out irritable bowel syndrome and inflammatory disorders of the bowel. Meanwhile several nursing diagnoses are identified and a plan of care is developed. Among the diagnoses is
> Fluid volume deficit related to prolonged diarrhea and decreased fluid intake

Planning
Mr. Stein expresses serious concern about his ability to continue to cope with the diarrhea, "Up until now my problem has been manageable." He understands the importance of fluid and electrolyte balance and is highly motivated to practice any new self-care behaviors that will help to decrease the diarrhea so he can get on with his studies. He is supportive of the following short-term goals:
> By the next week's visit 3/24, the client will
1. Describe two effective means he has used to cope with stress
2. Report that his diarrhea is eliminated or decreased to one to two episodes per day
3. Demonstrate improved fluid and electrolyte balance as evidenced by
   a. Maintenance of present weight (170 lb)

b. Moist mucous membranes

c. Report of increased urinary output

Long-term goal

Client will demonstrate signs of fluid and electrolyte balance.

Implementation

In implementing the plan of care the nurse needs the following specialized abilities:

- Strong assessment skills and knowledge of causative factors of diarrhea and means to eliminate them—and knowledge of the etiologies, defining characteristics, and treatment of fluid and electrolyte imbalances
- Interpersonal skills to facilitate the nurse's ability to empathize with Mr. Stein regarding his stressors and to communicate realistic hope that his situation can be improved as well as competence and caring as the nursing plan is implemented
- Knowledge of effective stress management techniques
- Teaching and counseling skills to assist Mr. Stein to develop the self-care behaviors that will enable him to live with his chronic condition with minimal discomfort and complications
- Accountability

Documentation

Sample documentation of the client's first return visit follows in traditional note format:

3/24/89   Mr. Stein returned to the clinic reporting that his diarrhea is decreased to one to two episodes per day and that he has an appointment with a gastroenterolo-

gist. He believes that modifying his diet, increasing rest periods, and medications (loperamide hydrochloride to control diarrhea and methylcellulose to increase the consistency of stool) were of great help. He still doesn't know how he can reduce his stress level. Nursing examination revealed: T—98.9°F (37.1°C), P—88, R—18, BP—110/60; weight—169 lb; skin and mucous membranes less dry than on previous visit. States he has not noted much change in urine output but possibly less concentrated.

C. Ryan, RN

SOAP documentation:

3/24/89   6 PM #2 fluid volume deficit related to prolonged diarrhea and decreased fluid intake.

S: "I certainly feel better. I still have one or two loose BMs a day but I'm drinking more and seem less dry." Reports no noticeable change in urine output but urine "may be" less concentrated.

O: 98.8°F (37.1°C), 88, 18, 110/60; 1-lb weight loss (170 to 169 lb); skin and mucous membranes less dry

A: Fluid volume deficit responding to treatment

P: Continue plan of care, reinforce follow-up with gastroenterologist

C. Ryan, RN

Evaluation

Short-term goal achievement is evaluated weekly, see Nursing Care Plan for evaluative statements and revisions of the plan of care. Long-term goal achievement is an ongoing evaluation by client.

N U R S I N G   C A R E   P L A N   *for Mr. Stein*

Nursing Diagnosis:	Fluid volume deficit related to prolonged diarrhea and decreased fluid intake as evidenced by 4-lb weight loss, dry skin and mucous membrane, and report of decreased urine output and concentrated urine.
Long-Term Goal:	Client will continue to demonstrate signs of fluid and electrolyte balance.

Goals	**Nursing Actions**	**Rationale**	**Evaluative Statement**
By the next week's visit 3/24, the client will: 1. Describe two effective means he has used to cope with stress	1. Explore with the client (a) what he finds most stressing at present, (b) the control he believes he has over these stressors, and (c) the adequacy of his past and present stress management strategies.	Because the diarrhea seems stress related it is critical to assist the client to both eliminate or reduce stress where possible and learn to cope better with unavoidable stress (identify and eliminate causative factors).	3/24 Goal not met. Client reports little progress in coping with stress. With MCATs 1 week away he feels more tense than ever before. Reports no time to explore stress management techniques. *Revision:* Goal is appro-

(Continued)

N U R S I N G   C A R E   P L A N (Continued)

Goals	Nursing Actions	Rationale	Evaluative Statement
	2. Assess for other factors contributing to diarrhea and fluid volume deficit. 3. Teach relationship between stress and bouts of diarrhea. 4. Stress management counseling. Refer to counseling center on campus.		priate. Encourage visit to counseling center if not before MCATs then as soon as possible afterward. *C Ryan, RN*
2. Report that his diarrhea is eliminated or decreased to one to two episodes per day	1. Teach client to link causative factors with diarrhea and to note anything that brings relief or assists in establishment of usual pattern of defecation. 2. Make sure client understands diet: chemically and mechanically non-irritating diet high in calories, protein, and minerals; exclude foods such as cocoa, chocolate, alcohol, cold or carbonated beverages, citrus juices; try frequent, small meals. 3. Teach client proper use of prescribed medications: loperamide hydrochloride to control diarrhea and methylcellulose to increase consistency of stool.	Helps client to assume charge of his own condition and to reinforce preventive strategies and successful relief measures Reduces bowel irritation and decreases peristalsis. Food and fluid replacement are needed. Some clients fear eating because it stimulates the gastrocolic reflex and may result in a stool. Antidiarrheal preparation	3/24 Goal met. Client reports diarrhea decreased to one to two episodes per day. *Recommendation:* Advise client that it is important to keep appointment with gastroenterologist because relief may only be temporary. *C Ryan, RN*
3. Demonstrate improved fluid and electrolyte balance as evidenced by: a. Maintenance of present weight (170 lb) b. Moist mucous membranes c. Report of increased urinary output	1. Explore with client workable plan for oral replacement of fluids—despite his fear to drink because in the past consumption of fluids led to new episodes of diarrhea. 2. Have client note which calorie and electrolyte (sodium and potassium) rich fluids he can tolerate. Increase fluid intake to maintain a normal urine specific gravity.	Increased fluid intake is necessary to compensate for excessive loss in diarrhea and to reestablish fluid balance.	3/24 Goal partially met. Client reports diarrhea decreased to once or twice a day. Two days there was no diarrhea. Weight—169 lb. Mucous membranes are moist. Urine output is increased. *C Ryan, RN*

(Continued)

N U R S I N G   C A R E   P L A N   (Continued)

Goals	Nursing Actions	Rationale	Evaluative Statement
	3. Instruct client to weigh himself every other day and to note changes in the volume or appearance of his urine. 4. Teach client defining characteristics of electrolyte imbalances associated with prolonged diarrhea: hyponatremia and hypokalemia.	All other things being equal, weight loss is a good indicator of continued fluid volume deficit. Other signs include decreased urinary output and high specific gravity. Excreted stool pulls electrolytes with it, especially sodium and potassium.	

K E Y   P O I N T S

- Whereas life can be sustained for many days without food, it can be sustained for only a few days without water.

- There are two major compartments for body fluids: (1) intracellular fluid (ICF) which is the fluid within cells and (2) extracellular fluid (ECF), located outside of body cells, which includes intravascular fluid (plasma) and interstitial fluid (fluid in which tissue cells are bathed).

- A person's age, lean body mass, and sex can all influence the distribution of body fluids in the different compartments. Because lean tissue has higher water content than fat, thin persons, females, and younger persons tend to have higher percentages of total body water in relation to body weight than obese, male, and older persons because of their increased lean body mass.

- Sodium and chloride are the principal ions of ECF; potassium and phosphate are principal ions of ICF.

- The most common routes for transporting fluid and electrolytes among the body compartments are osmosis, diffusion, active transport, and filtration.

- In a healthy adult, fluid intake and loss should average approximately 2500 ml over 2 to 3 days. The output of urine generally approximates the ingestion of liquids; water from food and oxidation is balanced by the water loss through the feces, the skin, and the respiratory process.

- Deficiencies in the amount of both water and electrolytes in ECF in near-normal proportions are termed fluid volume deficits. Excessive retention of water and electrolytes in ECF is termed fluid volume excess.

- To prevent the serious complications that can result from untreated electrolyte imbalances, nurses must be familiar with the etiologies, defining characteristics, and treatment of imbalances of sodium, potassium, calcium, magnesium, and phosphate.

- Normal blood plasma is slightly alkaline and has a normal pH range of 7.35 to 7.45. Slight deviations in either direction (acid–base imbalances) if untreated may result in death.

- The narrow range of normal pH is achieved by complex buffer systems (bicarbonate, phosphate, protein) and specific respiratory and renal mechanisms.

- Failure of acid–base regulating mechanisms may result in respiratory or metabolic disturbances which can be acidosis or alkalosis.

- Risk factors for fluid, electrolyte, and acid–base imbalances include (1) pathologies involving homeostatic regulators of fluid balance (*e.g.,* diabetes mellitus, congestive heart failure, renal failure); (2) abnormal losses of body fluids; (3) burns and trauma; and (4) therapies with the potential to disrupt fluid and electrolyte balance (*e.g.,* medications such as diuretics and steroids, intravenous therapy, total parenteral nutrition).

- Pertinent assessment measures include maintaining accurate intake and output records, recording daily weights, observing for the signs and symptoms that characterize specific imbalances, and monitoring results of laboratory studies.

- Nursing diagnoses may be developed in which the fluid imbalance is (1) the problem statement: fluid volume deficit or excess, or (2) the etiology: alteration in comfort related to edema, impaired oral mucous membrane related to dehydration.

■ Nursing interventions are directed to maintaining a client's fluid, electrolyte, and acid–base balance; to *preventing* disturbances; and to correcting imbalances.

■ When fluids are being encouraged or restricted it is important that both the nursing staff and client understand the target amount of fluid to be taken each shift and that the client's fluid preferences be respected.

■ Nurses administering intravenous fluids should accurately prepare the prescribed solution; understand the desired effect of treatment and possible adverse responses; and assume responsibility for

initiating, monitoring, and, when ordered, discontinuing the therapy.

■ Complications associated with intravenous infusions include infiltration, phlebitis, thrombus, speed shock, fluid overload, embolus, and infection.

■ Administering blood transfusions requires a careful pretransfusion assessment of the client, accurate identification and matching of the blood to be transfused with its intended recipient, and ongoing monitoring of the client throughout the transfusion for transfusion reactions. These include hemolytic, febrile, allergic, and hypervolemic reactions.

■ In total parenteral nutrition, hypertonic solutions of dextrose, amino acids, and select electrolytes and minerals—capable of reestablishing positive nitrogen balance and weight gain—are infused using a central vein.

BIBLIOGRAPHY

Abbott P, Schlacht, K: Pediatric IVs: A special challenge. Canadian Nurse 80(10):24–26, 1984

Adams Ackerman: 1987

Beckwith N: Fundamentals of fluid resuscitation. Nursing Life 7(3):49–55, 1987

Birdsall C: Clinical savvy: How do you avoid transfusion complications? Am J Nurs 85(3):312, 1985

Calloway C: When the problem involves magnesium, calcium, or phosphate. RN 30–35, May 1987

Committee on Transfusion Practices, American Association of Blood Banks: The latest protocol for blood transfusions. Nursing 16(10):34–42, 1986

Cyganski JM, Donahue JM, Heaton JS: The case for the heparin flush. Am J Nurs 87(6):796–797, 1987

Dunn DL, Lenihan SF: The case for the saline flush. Am J Nurs 87(6):798–799, 1987

Dorr R, Frita W: Cancer Chemotherapy Handbook. New York, Elsevier North-Holland, 1980

Feldstein A: Detect phlebitis and infiltration before they harm your patient. Nursing 16(1):44–47, 1986

Folk-Lightly M: Solving the puzzle of patients' fluid imbalances. Nursing 14(2):34–41, 1984

Gahart BL: Intravenous Medications, 4th ed. St Louis, CV Mosby, 1985

Girard NJ, Morgan RG, Orr MD: Autologous salvage of blood. AORN J 47(2):492–503, 1988

Goldberger E: A Primer of Water, Electrolyte and Acid–Base Syndromes, 6th ed. Philadelphia, Lea & Febiger, 1980

Intermed Communications: Monitoring Fluids and Electrolytes Precisely. Nursing Skillbook Series. Horsham, PA, Intermed Communications, 1981

Intermed Communications: Managing IV Therapy. Nursing 80 Photobook Series. Horsham, PA, Intermed Communications, 1980

Irwin M: "Encourage oral intake"—yes, but how? Am J Nurs 87(1):100, 102, 104, 106, 1987

Landier WC, et al: How to administer blood component to children. MCN 12(3):178–184, 1987

MacLaughlin JE: Intravenous containers—variability in measurement. Canadian Nurse 77(8):29–31, 1981

Martof M: Fluid balance, part 1. Journal of Nephrology Nursing 2(1):10–18, 1985

Martof M: Electrolyte balance, part 2. Journal of Nephrology Nursing 2(2):49–55, 1985

Metheny NM: Fluid and Electrolyte Balance. Philadelphia, JB Lippincott, 1987

Metheny NM, Snively W: Nurse's Handbook of Fluid Balance, 4th ed. Philadelphia, JB Lippincott, 1983

Millam DA: Tips for improving your venipuncture techniques. Nursing 17(6):46–49, 1987

Millam DA: Performing I.V. procedures like an expert: 10 questions about I.V. therapy—and the revealing answers. Nursing Life 6(1):33–40, 1986

Patrick ML, Woods SL, Craven RF, et al: Medical–Surgical Nursing. Philadelphia, JB Lippincott, 1986

Peck N: Perfecting your I.V. therapy techniques. Nursing, part 1: 15(5):38–43; part 2: 15(6):48–51; part 3: 15(7):32–35, 1985

Pflaum S: Investigation of intake-output as a means of assessing body fluid balance. Heart Lung 8(3):495–498, 1979

Romanski SO: Interpreting ABGs in four easy steps. Nursing 16(9):58–64, 1986

Schwartz MW: Potassium imbalances. Am J Nurs 87(10):1292, 1987

The SI Manual in Health Care, 2nd edition. Ottawa, Canada, Ontario Ministry of Health, 1982

Weldy NJ: Body Fluids and Electrolytes: A Programmed Presentation. St Louis, CV Mosby, 1987

UNIT

VIII

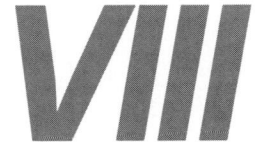

Promoting Healthy Psychosocial Responses

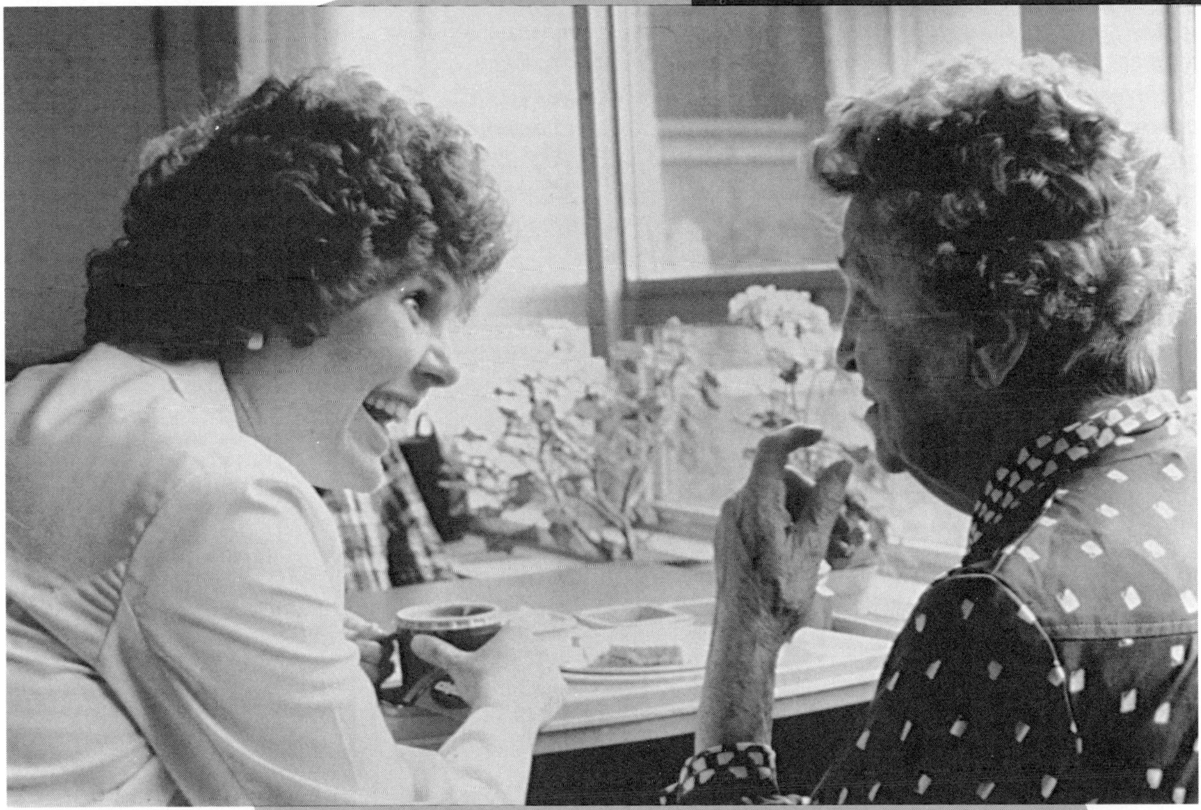

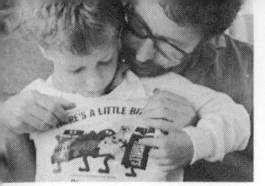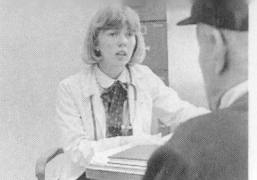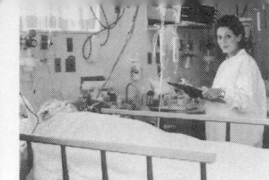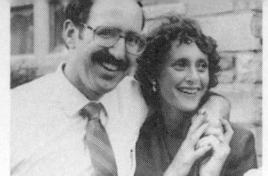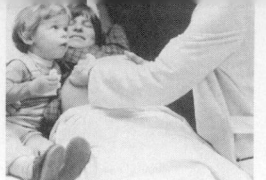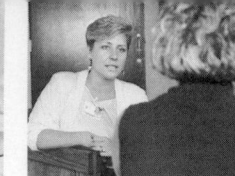

*E*ach individual person is a composite of interrelated physiologic and psychosocial dimensions; alterations in one dimension affect all of the others. Unit VIII discusses psychosocial considerations in holistic client care, focusing on self-concept, sensory stimulation, sexuality, and spirituality.

One's self-concept can serve as a positive strength, or if altered, can interfere with meeting other needs. Nursing interventions to maintain, strengthen, or change self-concept are basic to all aspects of client care.

Intact and functioning senses are necessary for life, normal growth and development, and pleasurable experiences. Alterations in any of the senses require caring, knowledgeable, and individualized nursing interventions to meet needs and prevent further overload or deprivation.

Sexuality and spirituality are important components of human functioning. These dimensions are an integral part of each person's identity and are critical elements in holistic client care. To facilitate sexual and spiritual wellness, nurses must develop self-awareness in these areas and become comfortable with values

and practices different from their own. Nursing interventions and therapeutic interpersonal skills are used to elicit concerns, identify needs, implement teaching, make referrals, and demonstrate empathic acceptance and caring.

Unit VIII provides the knowledge base for promoting healthy psychosocial responses in clients. Using the nursing process, interventions can be planned and implemented to meet needs and support strengths in both health and illness.

Self-Concept

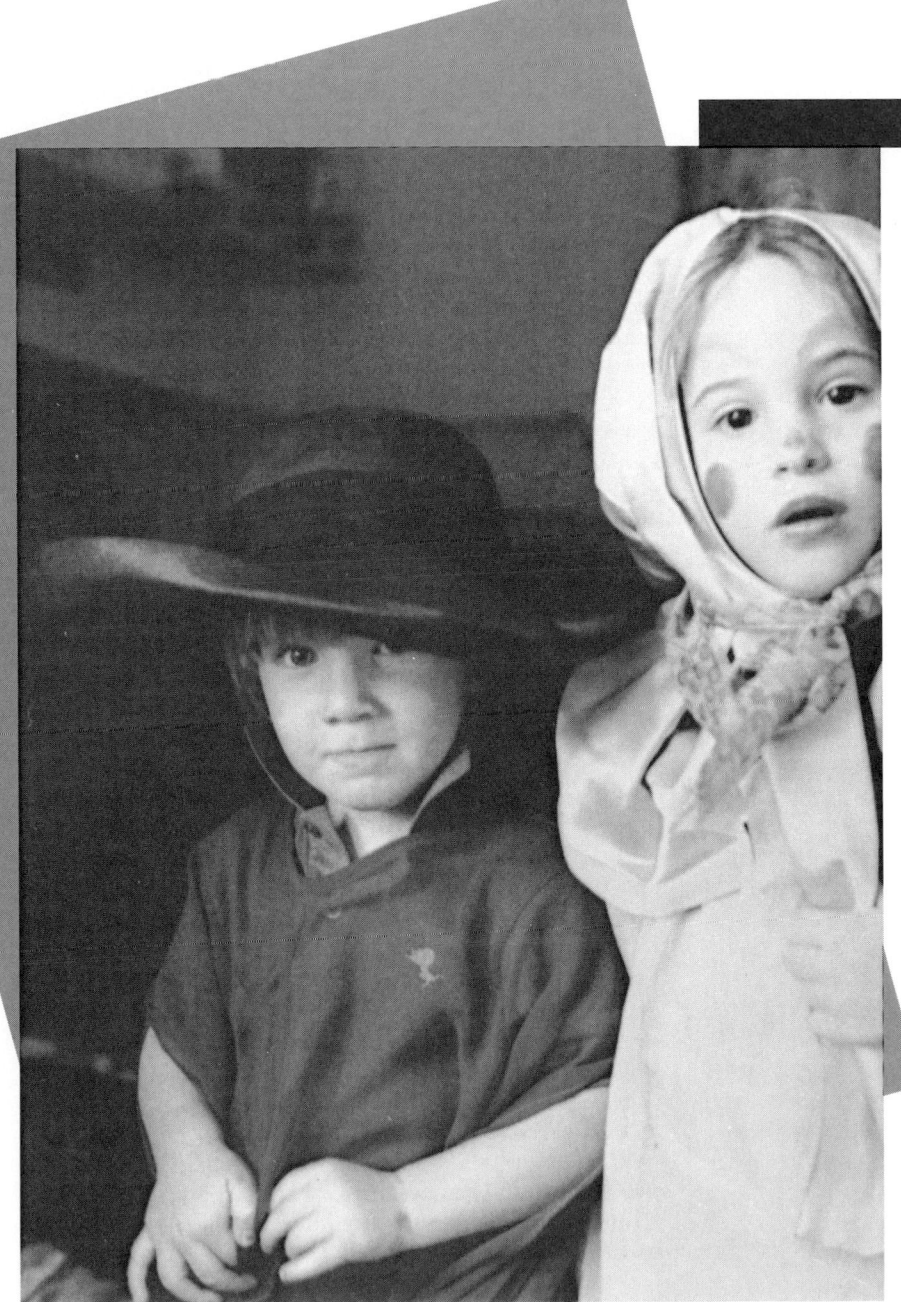

After studying this chapter, the learner should be able to

Define key terms used in the chapter.

Identify three dimensions of self-concept: self-knowledge, self-expectation, self-evaluation (self-esteem)

Describe three major steps in the development of self-concept.

Differentiate positive and negative self-concept and high and low self-esteem.

Identify six variables that influence self-concept.

Use appropriate interview questions and observations to assess a client's self-concept: self-knowledge (body image, client strengths), expectations, self-esteem (significance, role competence, virtue, power).

Develop nursing diagnoses to correctly identify disturbances in self-concept (body image, self-esteem, role performance, self-identity).

Describe nursing strategies that are effective in resolving self-concept problems.

Plan, implement, and evaluate nursing care related to select nursing diagnoses for disturbances in self-concept.

As persons move through the hierarchy of human needs to a higher level, needs for self-esteem and self-actualization occur as discussed in Chapter 7. **Self-esteem** is the need to feel good about one's self and to believe that others also hold one in high regard. **Self-actualization** is the need to reach one's potential through full development of one's unique capability. A critical component of both of these needs is self-concept. One's self-image or self-concept has the power to either encourage or thwart personal growth.

Persons who think of themselves as "born losers" most likely will not be motivated to learn self-care behaviors in response to illness or trauma. Nursing efforts aimed at teaching such persons will be doomed to failure until the client values self enough to want to invest energy in self-care. On the other hand, clients may desperately want to modify their self-concept and self-care behaviors and have no idea how to do it. Nursing assistance can help them explore factors in self-esteem. The experience of illness, diagnostic testing, and treatment can severely threaten the self-concept of a client. Nurses sensitive to the self-concept needs of clients can use each nurse–client interaction to enhance the client's sense of self and to assist the client in resolving self-concept disturbances.

Study of this chapter provides the student with knowledge of the (1) dimensions of self-concept, (2) formation of self-concept, (3) defense mechanisms, and (4) key factors affecting self-concept. Practical interview guides are offered for assessing self-concept. Strategies for enhancing the self-esteem of the nurse are given also. Numerous examples of nursing diagnoses are given with specific nursing strategies for assisting clients to meet the self-concept goals described. In the section entitled "Nursing Process in Clinical Practice," focused assessment, planning, implementation, and evaluation guides are offered for the nursing diagnoses: disturbance in body image and negative self-concept. These guides and the concluding case study illustrate how the nurse's knowledge of self-concept may be combined with skilled nursing interventions and caring to successfully resolve disturbances in self-concept.

K E Y　T E R M S

body image	self-concept
competence	self-esteem
defense mechanisms	significance
ideal self	social self
power	virtue
self-actualization	

OVERVIEW OF SELF-CONCEPT

Dimensions of Self-Concept

Self-concept is the mental image or picture of self. All the feelings, beliefs, and values associated with "I" or "me" comprise self-concept. Included in the notion of self-concept are the following:

Body image: How I experience my body
Subjective self: How I see myself, who I think I am
Ideal self: Self I would like to be or feel I should be
Social self: Way I feel others see me (Atwater, 1987)

The dimensions of self-knowledge, self-expectations, and self-evaluation describe self-concept (Calhoun and Acocella, 1983). Persons with a positive self-concept have broad and diversified knowledge of the self, realistic expectations, and high self-esteem.

Self-Knowledge: "Who am I?"

A person's self-knowledge includes basic facts (age, race, occupation), which place him in social groups, and a listing of qualities or traits, which describe typical behaviors, feelings, moods, and other characteristics (generous, hot-headed, ambitious, intelligent, sexy). Although some labels cannot be changed, (*e.g.,* sex, age and race), most are unstable and subjective.

Self-Expectations: "Who or what do I want to be?"

Expectations for the self flow from the ideal self, the self I want to be or think I should be. These expectations often develop early in childhood and are based on the image of a role model. These expectations may be healthy or unhealthy. Many contemporary thinkers are expressing concern that many children today identify as their heroes rock stars or pimps, prostitutes, and drug dealers rather than parents, government leaders, or other professional persons.

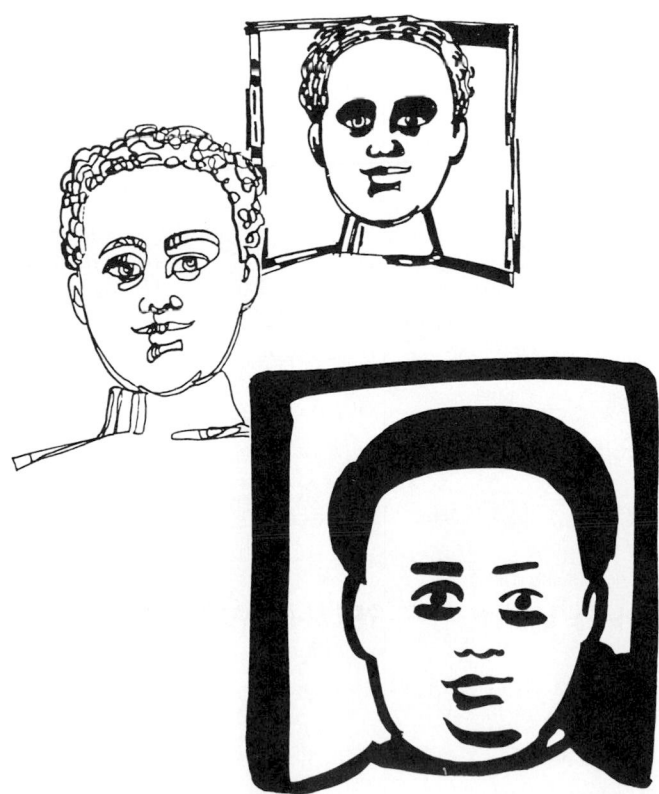

FIGURE 36-1

The dimensions of self-knowledge, self-expectation, and self-evaluation describe our self-concept. The artist characterizes himself visually in a self-portrait. We all describe and present our concept of self in our actions and associations, as well as in our self-descriptions.

Self-Evaluation: "How well do I like me?"

Self-esteem is the evaluative component of the self-concept, sometimes termed self-respect, self-approval, or self-worth. According to Maslow (1954, p 90), all persons "have a need or desire for a stable, firmly based, usually high evaluation of themselves, for self-respect or self-esteem, and for the esteem of others." Accordingly he identified two subsets of esteem needs: self-esteem needs (strength, achievement, mastery and competence, confidence in the face of the world, independence, and freedom) and respect needs or the need for "esteem from others" (status, dominance, recognition, attention, importance, and appreciation).

Coopersmith (1967) identified the four bases of self-esteem as (1) **significance**—the way a person feels he is loved and approved of by the people important to him; (2) **competence**—the way tasks that are considered important are performed; (3) **virtue**—the attainment of moral-ethical standards; and (4) **power**—the extent to which a person influences his own and others' lives. According to Coopersmith, persons with high, medium, and low self-esteem differ in their expectations of the future, in their affective reactions, and in their basic styles of adapting to environmental demands. Persons with high self-esteem are accustomed to being well received and successful. They are able to approach people, tasks, and new situations freely, with confidence in their ability to interact and to get along with people and to respond successfully to life's challenges.

Formation of Self-Concept

A person is not born with a self-concept. Rather it is a social creation which develops as a result of interactions with others. Steps in the formation of self-concept include:

1. An infant learns that the physical self is different from the environment. If basic needs are met and warmth and affection are experienced, the child begins life with positive feelings about self.
2. The child next internalizes (incorporates into self) other person's attitudes toward self. Parents play the most influential role here with the influence of peers being second.
3. Finally, the child or adult internalizes the standards of society.

Coleman, Morris, and Glaros (1987, pp 75–79) identify the following psychologic conditions which foster healthy development of the self in children:

- Emotional warmth and acceptance
- Effective structure and discipline

    Clearly defined standards and limits, so that children understand what goals, procedures, and conduct are approved

    Adequately defined roles for both older and younger members of the family

    Established methods of handling children that produce the desired behavior, discourage

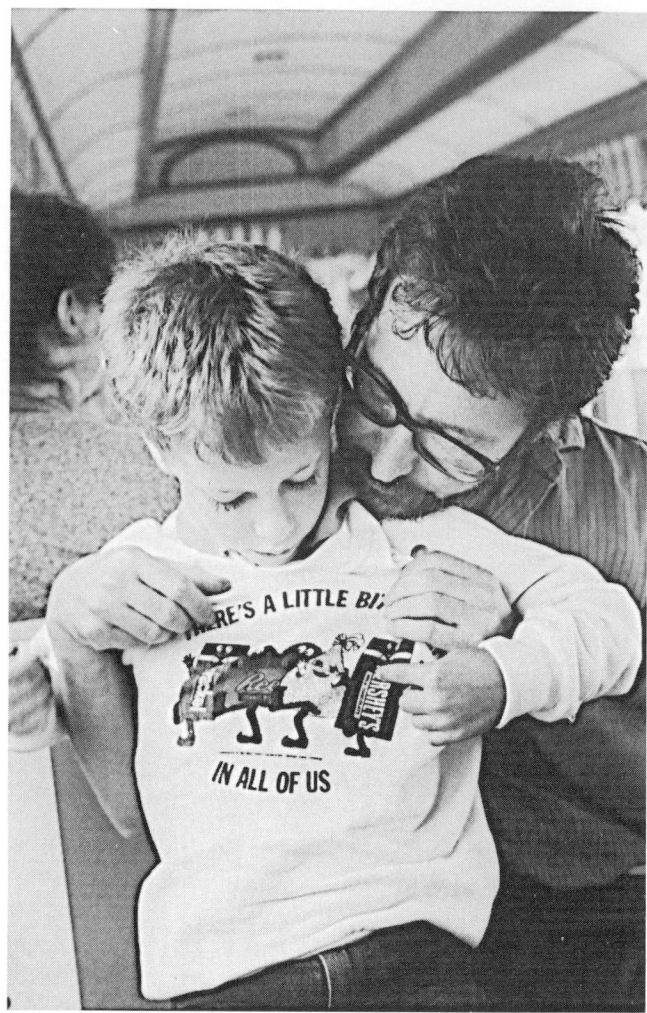

F I G U R E   36-2
The child internalizes other persons' attitudes toward him. His self-esteem is based on his feelings of being loved and approved of. Parents play the most influential role in the formation of the child's self-concept.

misbehavior, and deal with infractions
when they occur
• Encouragement of competence and self-confidence
• Helping children meet challenges
• Appropriate role models
• A stimulating and responsive environment
Formation of self-concept is further understood in the developmental theories, especially in Erikson's stages of development, Piaget's cognitive developmental stages, and Havighurts's developmental tasks (see Chaps 10 and 11).

Threats to Self-Concept

Anxiety is a threat to self-concept. According to psychoanalysts, the ego uses many different methods to protect itself from anxiety. Among these methods are coping and defense mechanisms. (Anxiety and coping and defense mechanisms are discussed briefly in Chap 9.)

FACTORS AFFECTING SELF-CONCEPT

Almost any life experience can influence a person's self-concept. Key factors include developmental considerations, culture, internal and external resources, history of success and failure, stressors, and illness or trauma.

Developmental Considerations.   As a person matures the criteria that mark the experiences necessary for a positive self-concept change. (See the preceding discussion of formation of self-concept.) While the infant needs a supportive environment in which all human needs are met, the growing child needs the freedom to explore and develop the ability to meet more and more personal needs. Table 36-1 highlights developmental changes affecting self-concept, related nursing implications, and potential self-concept disturbances.

Culture.   As a child internalizes the values of parents and peers, culture begins to influence a sense of self. If the culture is relatively stable little tension may be experienced between what culture expects of the child and what the child expects of self. When parents, peers, and the adult world confront the child with different cultural

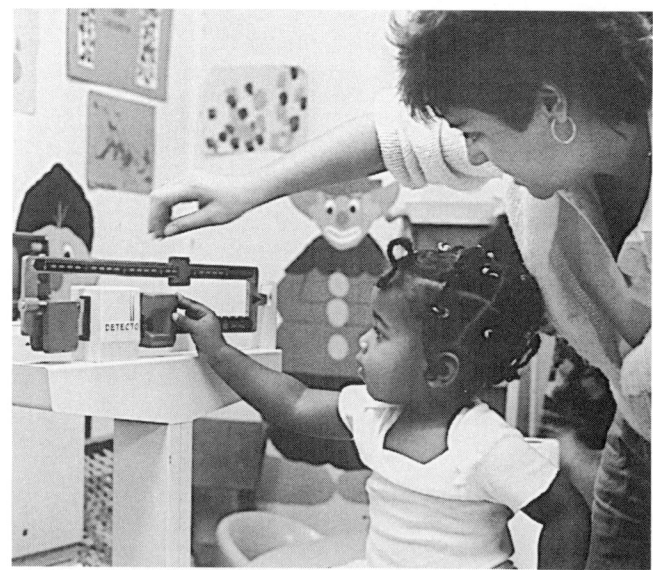

F I G U R E   36-3
Conditions fostering healthy development of the self in children include emotional warmth and acceptance, effective structure and discipline, encouragement of competence, self-confidence, and ability to meet challenges, appropriate role models, and a stimulating and responsive environment. (Photo by Gates Rhodes, courtesy of the School of Nursing, University of Pennsylvania)

TABLE 36-1
Developmental Changes Affecting Self-Concept

Developmental Period	Changes Affecting Self-Concept	Implications for Nursing	Disturbances in Self-Concept May Be Caused by:
Infancy	• No self-concept at birth • Beginning differentiation of self and nonself	• Teach parents the critical importance of providing consistent and affectionate parenting • Assess if the parents have reasonable expectations of the infant: sleeping, eating, other awake behaviors	• Unmet basic human needs • Lack of adequate body and sensory stimulation • Parents' unacceptance of the infant's appearance or behavior
Childhood	• An intact body is very important to the young child who fears bodily mutilation • During middle childhood a sense of being trusted and loved, of being competent and trustworthy develops • Differences between self and others are strong	• If invasive procedures are indicated, explain simply to the child what is being done and offer the child support • Assess the parents' ability to provide the type of developmental environment in which the child's self-concept can evolve positively	• Dysfunctional family • Too much or too little structure • Sensory perceptual impairments
Adolescence	• Development of secondary sex characteristics; rapid body changes • Emphasis on sexual identity • Parental influences on self-concept are often rejected; peers become more important; movement is toward development of own identity	• Assess adolescent's self-knowledge and understanding of bodily changes • Counsel adolescent re: mature and healthy use of independence he craves • Anticipatory guidelines regarding hazards to life, health, human functioning	• Inability to accept body • Inability to resolve competing pulls to be both a child and an adult • Unhealthy peer pressure
Adulthood	• Society places emphasis on intactness of body, fitness, energy, sexuality, style, sophistication, beauty • Very important to meet role expectations well	• Assess how realistic the adult's expectations are and the incentive they provide for growth and development • Assist client to deal constructively with negative influences in self-image • Preretirement counseling	• Inability to fulfill conflicting role expectations • Failure to accept role responsibility (e.g., parenting responsibilities) • Unreasonable expectations • Irreversible body change related to trauma, illness • Unsatisfying job • Failure to develop new goals to give meaning and purpose to life
Later years	• Declining physical and possibly mental abilities	• Assess how the older person is adjusting to effects of aging • Counsel regarding meaningful use of time • Explore resources	• Loss of significant work (retirement); feelings of uselessness • Death of spouse, significant others • Diminished physical attractiveness, strength, overall health • Multiple stressors • Fear of dependency

expectations, the sense of self may be confused. For example, an adolescent may realize his parents live by the work ethic and believe it is necessary to rise early every day and put in a full day's work. His peer group have few demands placed on them and encourage him to "hang-out" with them. His vocational aptitudes, meanwhile, are leading him to consider a music career in a rock group which will keep him out late many nights doing something his parents do not classify as "work."

Internal and External Resources. The personal strengths a person recognizes, develops, and uses are powerful but subjective determinants of self-concept. One person may use humor as both an effective coping mechanism and as a successful interpersonal tool. Another person uses humor to avoid facing conflict and feels bad about being known as a joker or clown. External resources such as a network of support persons, adequate finances, organizational supports, and so forth, are also subjective determinants of self-concept. Generally, the more resources a person has and uses wisely the better the feelings about self.

History of Success and Failure.
A person with a history of repeated failure (school, friendships, work, marriage) may perceive himself as a failure and actually perpetuate this image by unconsciously instructing others to treat him this way. He may come to fear success and actually find it easier to fail even though he does not like himself this way. Thus failure influences his self-concept negatively, and his self-concept instructs him to continue to fail. On the other hand, one successful experience conditions a person to strive for the next success and a positive self-concept is forged to expect success.

Stressors.
Life stressors (marriage, divorce, an exam, a new job, a gray hair, a fire) may call forth a personal response and mobilize an individual's talents which results in good feelings about oneself. Stressors may also evoke maladaptive responses which diminish the self-concept. Examples of these include withdrawal, depression, extreme anxiety, and substance abuse. How the person perceives the stressor (threat, challenge, defeat) and his ability to mobilize personal strengths and other resources is determined largely by his self-concept which is then influenced by the response he chooses.

Aging, Illness, or Trauma.
Because most persons take a healthy body for granted, the diminishment of physical attractiveness or functioning, the suggestion of disease, or sudden impact of trauma may pose serious threats to the self. Persons vary greatly in their response to aging, illness, and trauma.

NURSE AS ROLE MODEL

Before nurses can successfully identify and resolve self-esteem disturbances in clients they must be comfortable with themselves and possess a certain measure of self-esteem. Important goals for the nurse's personal esteem are the following:

- Identify basic unmet human needs, exploring positive means to meet these needs
- Schedule time into every day to meet personal needs
- Assess the effect of feedback from significant others on self-esteem
- Describe personal strengths accurately
- Develop a realistic plan to achieve goals for personal growth and development

Specific strategies for developing self-esteem in relationship to one's professional practice follow (Fig. 36-4):

P R O M O T I N G   W E L L N E S S

Self-Concept

Use the assessment checklist to determine how well you are meeting your need for positive self-concept. Then develop a prescription for self-care by choosing appropriate behaviors from the list of suggestions.

Assessment Checklist

almost always	some times	almost never	
☒	☐	☐	1. I have established appropriate expectations and goals for myself.
☒	☐	☐	2. I have effective and satisfying relationships with others.
☐	☒	☐	3. I cope effectively with change and loss.
☐	☒	☐	4. I accept and feel good about myself.

Self-Care Behaviors

1. Accept normal variations in physical appearance and capabilities.
2. Use problem-solving and decision-making strategies to define expectations and set goals.
3. Set priorities and accept that no one person can be all things to all people.
4. Forget past mistakes; carrying around "excess baggage" is not healthy.
5. Emphasize strengths and abilities in self.
6. Take an active part in group activities in school, work, church, and/or the community.
7. Volunteer time, talents, or services.
8. Avoid alcohol or drugs.
9. Live life one day at a time.

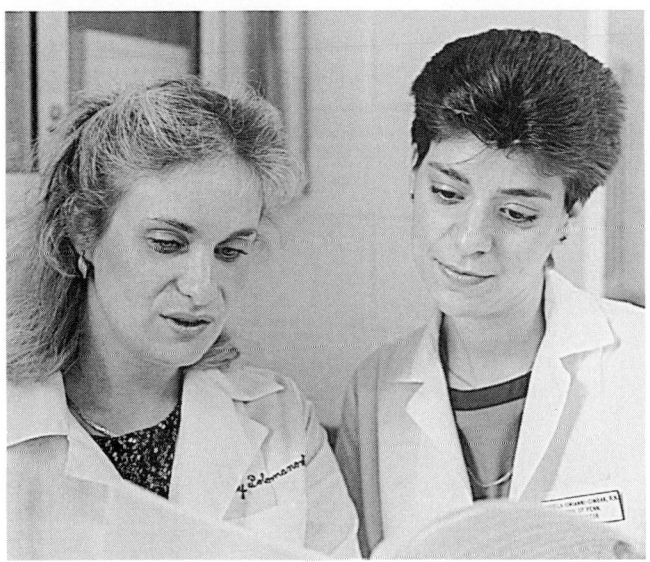

FIGURE 36-4
Two strategies for developing one's own professional self-esteem as a nurse are to recognize that it is okay to ask about what you do not know or are uncertain about and, in doing so, to develop team self-esteem. (Photo by Gates Rhodes, courtesy of the School of Nursing, University of Pennsylvania)

1. *Dispel the myth that it is necessary to know all there is to know about nursing to be a "good nurse."* At no one point in time does any nurse ever have it all together. Acceptance of the need to learn new theories or new procedures frees you from having to practice defensively (*i.e.,* pretend to be on top of every new development) and is a great stimulus for professional growth and development.
2. *Realistically evaluate strengths and weaknesses.* Build a periodic review into your practice and be *fair* in your self-evaluation. "I think I'm giving better care than ever before and I know my clients are appreciative, but I'm sensing a lot of tension between myself and a couple of the other nurses. . . ."
3. *Accentuate the positive.* Many of us have a knack for forgetting the 99 things we did well and focusing on our one error. Errors need to be taken seriously and evaluated but not to the exclusion of overlooking positive accomplishments.
4. *Develop a conscious plan for changing weaknesses into strengths.* Professional growth and development depend on strong motivation to become better at what you do. "Realizing that I never know what to say when a client receives bad news I can try to avoid these clients or consciously plan to develop better interpersonal skills." Nurses are tremendous resources for each other. Tapping into one another's strengths is a great way to build one another's self-esteem. "You always seem to know the right thing to say or do with clients. Do you

mind if I observe for a while and then 'try on' some of your behaviors?"
5. *Work to develop "team self-esteem."* A basic interpersonal principle that seems to work well in practice is to offer to others what you want yourself. Because our sense of self is strongly influenced by the feedback we receive from others, positive reinforcement of our strengths and sincere offers to help us correct deficiencies are needed by everyone.
6. *Actively demonstrate your commitment to nursing and concern about nursing's public image.* To feel good about yourself, you need to be able to experience pride in your profession. Active participation in professional organizations can offer many personal rewards—not the least of which is enthusiasm and pride in being a nurse.

ASSESSING SELF-CONCEPT

The nurse assessing self-concept focuses on the client's self-knowledge, self-expectations, and self-evaluation (self-esteem). A general assessment of self-concept should be included in every comprehensive nursing assessment. It is as important to identify and label a client's positive self-concept as it is to note problems. Positive self-concept can be used as a key strength when working with clients to achieve other health goals. Clients experiencing (1) illness or trauma that results in body disfigurement or altered functioning or (2) life crises that arrest development and thwart the achievement of life goals are at high risk for problems related to self-concept and should be assessed more carefully. If problems surface during the interview, a more thorough assessment should be carried out. The box on page 1022 highlights elements common to any self-concept assessment. The discussion that follows offers specific interviewing guides for each element in the assessment.

It is important for the nurse conducting this assessment to realize the limitations of self-reporting. A client may give what he believes are the desired or "socially acceptable" responses to interview questions. "Why, of course I like myself. I'm a pretty good person. Yes, I have friends." For this reason the nurse must evaluate the client's responses in relation to observations made about the client and what is known about the client from other sources. The other box on page 1022 outlines behaviors often associated with low self-concept. When the nursing assessment reveals a clustering of these behaviors it is important to discuss this with the client. This is especially true when there is a discrepancy between the client's words and behavior. "You've told me that you feel in control of your situation right now and are committed to the treatment plan, but I notice you've broken three therapy appointments this month and you did mention that you are drinking more heavily. . . ."

Elements Common to a Self-Concept Assessment

1. Self-knowledge
   "How would you describe yourself to others?"
   • Personal characteristics and traits
   • Body image
   • Strengths

2. Expectations
   "Who would you like to be?"
   "Who or what has influenced your self-expectations?"
   "Are these expectations realistic?"

3. Self-esteem
   "Do you like who you are?"

    a. Significance
   "Does it bother you when you feel unloved or when others fail to appreciate you?"
    b. Competence
   "How do you feel about your ability to do all the things your roles demand of you (spouse, parent, employee)?"
    c. Virtue
   "Are you satisfied with the way you are able to live according to your moral-ethical standards?"
    d. Power
   "To what extent do you feel able to control your life?"

Self-Knowledge

When assessing self-concept, the first information needed is the client's description of self. "How would you describe yourself to others?" The nurse pays special attention to the labels used by the client and the order in which they appear. Calhoun and Acocella (1983, p 63) recommend the following exercise:

Defining Characteristics of Low Self-Concept

Refusal to touch or look at a body part
Refusal to look into a mirror
Unwillingness to discuss a limitation, deformity, or disfigurement
Refusal to accept rehabilitation efforts
Inappropriate attempts to direct own treatment
Denial of the existence of a deformity or disfigurement
Increasing dependence on others
Signs of grieving: weeping, despair, anger
Refusal to participate in own care or take responsibility for self-care (self-neglect)
Self-destructive behavior (alcohol, drug abuse)
Displaying hostility toward the healthy
Withdrawal from social contacts
Changing usual patterns of responsibility
Showing change in ability to estimate relationship of body to environment

(Carpenito LJ: Nursing Diagnosis: Application to clinical practice, 2nd ed. Philadelphia, JB Lippincott, 1987, p 515)

As an exercise in understanding how people organize knowledge about themselves, make a list of ten labels that you feel identify you (for example, "student," "Italian-American," "opera fan," "premed major"). Put the most important label first and then list the others in order of decreasing importance. (What if the order were reversed?) To what extent do you think your way of organizing information about yourself affects your behavior?

Body Image. When body image disturbances are suspected the nurse can specifically ask the client how he would describe his body to another person. When illness or trauma has resulted in a temporary or permanent alteration in body image the nurse should assess (1) the nature of the threat, (2) the meaning the client attaches to the threat, (3) the adequacy of the client's coping strategies, and (4) the resources and supports available to the client.

Client Strengths. Many clients focus naturally on their deficiencies; asking pointed questions about personal strengths can help a client identify positive factors.
   "What are some of your personal strengths . . . qualities you are proud of . . . things you do well?"
   "What special talents or abilities do you have?"
   "What has helped you cope in the past when things were tough?"

Self-Expectations

A person's ideal self may differ dramatically from the present sense of self and positively or negatively influence behavior and personal development. After assessing self-knowledge the nurse next questions the client about self-expectations.

"You've told me something about who you are, how you view yourself now. Tell me who you would like to be in the future."

"What life goals are important to you?"

"Where do you see yourself five years from now? Ten years?"

"Are these expectations realistic?"

"Are your expectations stemming from who you would *like* to be or from who you think you *should* be?"

"Who or what has influenced your self-expectations?"

The nurse is assessing if the client possesses life goals that are positively motivating personal development. Unrealistic expectations need to be identified, and their source needs to be explored with the client. For example,

"You seem to feel that it is necessary to be all things to all people—no matter what this costs you. How might this belief have developed? Is it helpful to you?"

"What I'm hearing is that your performance must always be perfect, that while you allow others to make mistakes you cannot allow yourself this luxury . . . tell me more about this."

"Then unless you graduate at the top of your class you will not be satisfied? Why is this so important? Is this type of achievement realistic with your abilities? What will this success both benefit and cost you?"

"You state you have no goals for the future . . . when you wake up each morning what gets you out of bed? What keeps you moving?"

Self-Evaluation or Self-Esteem

Once a client has shared perceptions of self, the nurse questions if he likes himself, if he is pleased with his expectations and the progress he is making to realize them.

"Tell me what you like about yourself."

"What would you change about yourself if you could?"

Using Makay and Gaw's (1975) graphic description of self-esteem as the "discrepancy between the 'real self' (what we think we really are) and the 'ideal self' (what we think we would like to be or think we should be)," the nurse can obtain a quick indication of a client's self-esteem by having the client plot two points on a line: "real self" and "ideal self" (Fig. 36-5). The greater the discrepancy, the lower the self-esteem; the smaller the discrepancy, the higher the self-esteem.

If this exercise indicates the need for a more detailed assessment the nurse next explores the concepts of significance, competence, virtue, and power.

Significance

"Are there persons in your life with whom you share a close relationship?"

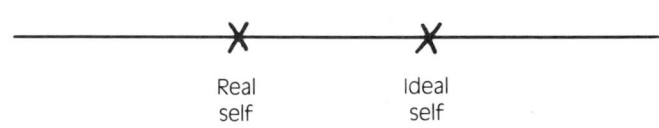

High self-esteem

Real self — Ideal self

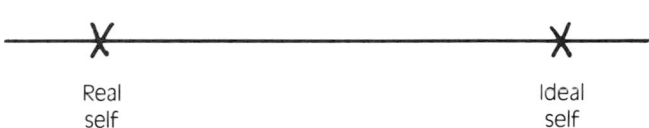

Low self-esteem

Real self — Ideal self

F I G U R E   36-5
The client who perceives his real self as relatively close to his ideal self has high self-esteem. The client who perceives his real self as far from his ideal self has low self-esteem.

"Many persons have 'people' problems, are your relationships causing you any problems right now?"

"To what extent do you feel loved and approved of by the key persons in your life?"

"Does it bother you when you feel unloved or when others fail to appreciate you?"

"In what ways do you let family members and friends know that you like them or are proud of their accomplishments?"

Competence

"What major roles describe you: son, daughter, spouse, parent, employer/employee, student, club member, etc.?"

"How important is it to you to be "good" in each of these roles?"

"Tell me how successful you think you are in each of these roles."

"What roles or expectations would you change if you could?"

"If you feel 'incompetent' or less than successful in some of these roles, why? What is preventing you from being more successful? What can you do about this? How might I help you?"

Virtue

"Tell me something about the moral-ethical principles that govern your life."

"How must you live in order to describe yourself as a 'good' person?"

"How do you feel about your ability to live this way?"

"Describe any difficulties you experience in living up to your moral principles which you would like to discuss."

"In what ways can the nurses help you to better live according to your moral standards?"

Power

"How important is it to you to 'be in control' of your life (health)?"

"To what extent did you feel 'in control' of your life (health) prior to this illness (trauma, crisis, etc.)?"

"To what extent do you feel 'in control' of your life (health) *at the present moment?*"

"What is it that makes you feel *not in control?*"

"How might you change this? How can nurses help you to develop/gain more control?"

DIAGNOSING

Specific disturbances in self-concept that can be treated by independent nursing interventions receive one of four nursing diagnostic labels:

Disturbance in body image
Disturbance in self-esteem
Disturbance in role performance
Disturbance in personal identity

Common etiologies and defining characteristics for these diagnoses are found in Table 36-2.

When assessment data point to an alteration in self-concept, the nurse's first task is to determine if the altered self-concept is the problem, the cause of the problem (etiology), or merely a sign that a problem exists. Self-concept data seem to fit well in all three categories. It is important that an accurate determination be made because this will direct the goals developed for the client and related nursing interventions.

For example, three different diagnoses might be written for a 25-year-old woman who is recently divorced.

1. *Disturbance in self-esteem* related to perceived failure in role of wife (recent divorce) as manifested by neglect of personal appearance and inability to accept positive reinforcement.

Assessment data point to a disturbance in self-esteem as the priority problem. Nursing energies will be directed to helping the client evaluate herself positively despite the stress of the divorce.

2. Alteration in health maintenance related to *decreased self-esteem* as manifested by failure to follow through on referrals (support group, stress-management class, and so forth); "Why bother? Nothing ever works for me anyway."

Here low self-esteem is contributing to the client's problem of failing to follow through with health-seeking behaviors. Nursing energies will be best directed to improving the client's use of health resources; one of the means used will be to help her to value herself enough to choose healthy behaviors.

3. Ineffective individual coping related to inability to accept recent divorce *as manifested by low self-esteem statements: "I never should have gotten married—my mother said I'd be a rotten wife." "I know I can't make it on my own." "Why did he do this to me?"*

Here low self-esteem statements are the cues that led to the identification of the problem statement. One of the criteria used to evaluate nursing intervention to increase the client's coping skills will be a reduction in or elimination of low self-esteem statements.

Because disturbances in self-concept have the potential to affect so many other areas of human functioning they may serve as etiologies for numerous problem statements. Examples of these follow:

Impaired adjustment related to change in health status (increasing dependency, need for ongoing medical evaluation and treatment, etc.

Anxiety related to irreversible change in body image (*e.g.,* amputation, mastectomy, burn), delayed development of secondary sex characteristics (body image), discrepancy between real and ideal self (self-esteem), perceived incompetence in important roles, loss of key roles (child or spouse dies, separation, retirement, graduation)

Ineffective individual coping related to inability to identify personal strengths, low self-esteem, "I know I can't manage this," role conflict

Anticipatory or dysfunctional grieving related to change in body image, loss of key role(s)

Altered health maintenance related to low self-esteem, "why bother."

Hopelessness related to low self-esteem, overwhelming role demands, belief that nothing will change (destiny is controlled externally)

Knowledge deficit: how to help children develop high self-esteem related to lack of experience with parenting

Noncompliance related to low self-esteem

Altered parenting related to disturbance in role performance (rejection of parent role)

Post-trauma response related to disturbance in personal identity

Self-care deficit related to learned helplessness, low self-esteem, "I can't"

Sensory-perceptual alteration related to disturbance in personal identity (ability to distinguish between self and nonself)

Altered sexuality patterns related to changed body image, disturbance in self-concept

Impaired social interaction or social isolation related to low self-esteem, disturbance in personal identity

Altered thought processes related to disturbance in personal identity

Potential for violence to self related to disturbance in self-concept, overwhelmed by failure to live according to moral-ethical standards

(Text continues on p. 1026.)

T A B L E 36-2

Nursing Diagnoses for Common Disturbances in Self-Concept

Problem	Etiologic Factors	Sample Defining Characteristics
Disturbance in body image	Irreversible changes in body image: amputation, mastectomy, hysterectomy, colostomy, scars, burns, disfiguring skin disorder	"Look at me. Nothing can ever be the same again. I feel less whole. When I look in the mirror all I see is my (stump, missing breast, scar). I know when others look at me they feel repulsed or at the very least pity me."
	Effects of treatment (*e.g.,* braces, casts)	Thirteen-year-old female adolescent with scoliosis wearing a Milwaukee Brace (covers pelvic area and has rods in the front and back which extend up to the chin): "I feel dumb in this thing . . . it's bad enough that my back is crooked but this makes me look like a freak. Besides, it's hot. Must I wear it to school?"
	Difficulty accepting development of secondary sex characteristics or delayed development of same	Fifteen-year-old male adolescent, sophomore in high school, height 5'1", weight 88 lb; "When am I going to grow up and start looking like the other guys in my class?" No pubic hair, penis, testes, and scrotum are the same size and proportion as in childhood.
	Extreme thinness or obesity	• Twenty-year-old woman, height 5'7"; weight 98 lb; works out for 30 min three times a day in addition to 100 sit-ups/day; "When I look in the mirror I see fat!" • Twenty-year-old woman, height 5'7"; weight 200 lb; "I hate my body . . . I've been fat all my life and I'm always on a diet. Why can't I be like everyone else?"
Disturbance in self-esteem	Feeling unloved or unapproved of by significant others	Twelve-year-old son of parents in the process of getting a divorce: "No matter what I do to make my dad like me he acts like I don't exist. When he's home he fights with mom, but mostly he's away. I wouldn't even care if he yelled at me so long as he noticed me. I wonder why he doesn't like me?"
	Feelings of incompetence	Forty-two-year-old car salesman, with company for 18 years: "What's wrong with me? I do my job, I'm also never absent, I have a good sales record, but I keep getting passed over for promotions. I think I'm too old to move to a different company but I don't want to just sell cars for someone else for the rest of my life!"
	Failure to live according to personal moral ethical code	Thirty-three-year-old single female computer programmer: "I should have known I'd get pregnant—I deserve it. I knew I was wrong to go to bed with this guy. Basically I've tried to live the way I think I should all my life up until now. What if something's wrong with the baby because of my sin?"
	Powerlessness	Sixty-seven-year-old alert widow with degenerative joint disease: "It may be hard for me to move around now but darn it—there's nothing wrong with my mind. The kids think they are helping me by making all my decisions but they aren't. I'm not a doddering old lady in a nursing home."
Disturbance in role performance	Rejection of role	Twenty-two-year-old mother 2 days after the birth of her second son (first son is 15 months old): "I don't know who my husband got to watch our son. I never wanted to be a mother anyway. My husband and I have never had any time for ourselves—and things aren't going to get any better."
	Role conflict Role fatigue Multiple life stressors	Twenty-one-year-old, full-time junior nursing student who failed a major exam; is married and the mother of an 18-month-old daughter; works every other weekend in a hospital as an EKG technician: "I'm trying so hard to get my grades up, but I don't know what else I can do. My husband seems to be losing patience with me more and more and I sometimes feel awful about neglecting my daughter. I'd stop working but we need the money. I want nursing so bad but I'm getting awfully tired."

(Continued)

T A B L E   36-2
Nursing Diagnoses for Common Disturbances in Self-Concept   (Continued)

Problem	Etiologic Factors	Sample Defining Characteristics
	Changing personal resources (physical heatlh, mental abilities, motivation)	Fifty-year-old college chemistry teacher begins exhibiting signs of early Alzheimer's disease; forgets where she is and what she is doing; began rambling in class and saying things that made no sense—much to the class's amusement. Later cried and called herself "stupid."
Disturbance in personal identity	Unresolved crisis	Eighty-eight-year-old male who lost his wife 6 months ago; wife took care of all his needs; sits alone in house all day, "We always did everything together. I wish I had died first. What shall I do?"
	Declining physical, mental, or sensory abilities	• Above male 3 months after admission to long-term care institution, medical diagnosis "rule out depression/dementia"; has become increasingly withdrawn, never initiates conversation; responses to questions are sometimes inappropriate: "What do you mean, what's my name? Who cares? I want to go home to my wife."
	Rejection of membership in minority group	Fifteen-year-old Cambodian girl recently emigrated to the United States with family in constant conflict with parents as she rejects her family's culture in hopes of fitting in with peer group. "Sometimes I feel like I no longer know who I am or how I should act. I feel lonely inside and afraid."

PLANNING: CLIENT GOALS

Whenever nurses care for clients, nursing measures need to be supportive of the following client goals:
   The client will:
   • Describe self realistically, identifying both strengths and deficiencies
   • Verbalize realistic expectations for self based on who he would like to be
   • Verbalize that self is liked or at least "ok"
   • Communicate his feelings and needs in a way that is comfortable and effective in meeting needs
   • Nurture relationships in which needs for love and worth are mutually met (significance)
   • Assume role-related responsibilities with confidence (competence)
   • Express satisfaction with ability to live according to one's moral-ethical standards (virtue)
   • Demonstrate confidence in ability to accomplish what is desired (power)
Client goals for specific disturbances in self-concept are presented later in this chapter.

IMPLEMENTING

Nursing interventions to assist clients to develop and maintain a positive self-concept may vary tremendously from one client to another. Nurses must be comfortable with their own self-image before they can address image problems in clients. Specific nursing strategies addressed in this section include helping clients identify and use personal strengths, helping high-risk clients maintain a sense of self, changing the self-concept, and working with parents and educators to develop self-esteem in children and adolescents.

Helping Clients Identify and Use Personal Strengths

When confronted with a major stressor many persons forget that they have a previous history of successful coping and numerous personal strengths. Clients at high risk for "giving up" are those with low self-esteem or multiple stressors perceived as being overwhelming.
   While attributing strength to a client sounds like something a nurse would do naturally, nurses frequently fall into the trap of "doing for" clients (*i.e.,* solving their problems, rather than helping them to identify and tap their personal power and strengths). Moreover, clients continually instruct nurses as to how they should be perceived, and some clients successfully communicate a manipulative helplessness which encourages the nurse's taking charge. An appropriate nursing response in this case is: "I wonder why you want me to speak with your physician about treatment alternatives. I am sure you would feel much better hearing this information first-hand. If you'd like I will stay here while you talk with the physician."

Clients experiencing powerlessness may need help recognizing their strengths. Examples of personal strengths include healthy functioning body, cognitive abilities, emotional strengths, communication strengths, other interpersonal skills, sense of life meaning and purpose, belief system which is a strength, social support network, meaningful work, hobbies, other interests, education, life experience, and past history of effective coping. A good sense of humor, belief in a loving God, healthy nutritional state, ability to make decisions, and sense of self-worth are all personal strengths which better equip a person to respond to life's challenges.

Specific strategies nurses can use to help clients identify and use personal strengths include
- Encouraging clients to identify their strengths
- Replacing self-negation with positive thinking
- Noticing and reinforcing client strengths
- Encouraging clients to will for themselves the strengths they desire and to try them on

Helping High-Risk Clients Maintain a Sense of Self

Persons who are acutely ill are often separated not only from their strengths but also from any real sense of self. One client, a college president who was recovering from serious complications following surgery for ovarian cancer, shared the following:

> When I was very sick, I felt utterly weak and devoid of any personal strength. During this time how I felt about myself was totally dependent upon how the doctors and nurses approached me. My esteem was at their mercy. If they came into my room and did something to me without talking to me or talked as if I were not present, then I felt like a nonperson, unworthy of their care. But if they approached me gently and caringly and spoke with me, then I felt like a human being again, worthy of human respect and care. Once I started feeling stronger, then I could fight feelings of depersonalization. But when I was really sick, I was totally dependent on others for my feelings of worth.

Nurses can help clients maintain a sense of self and worth by
- Speaking respectfully to the client and addressing the client by name whenever the client's room is entered
- Offering the client a simple explanation before initiating any procedure
- Moving the client's body respectfully if the client is unable to do this
- Respecting the client's privacy and sensitivities

This type of caring does not require additional nursing time or energy. It does require from the nurse continual reaffirmation that nursing is a person-centered profession and that nothing is more important at any moment of a nurse's workday than the person being served.

Changing the Self-Concept

The time is ripe for change when a client realizes that a negative self-concept is hindering personal development. A nurse working in a setting that allows long-term nurse–client relationships may intervene to assist the client in modifying self-concept. At the outset it must be remembered that the self-concept is firmly entrenched and that by nature it resists change. Calhoun and Acocella (1983) recommend the following process of change: (1) describing the problem and (2) functional analysis of the problem. Steps in this process are elaborated in the box on the next page.

Working with Parents and Educators to Develop Self-Esteem in Children and Adolescents

Nurses who work in practice settings where they have access to groups of parents or teachers can offer specific guidelines for creating developmental environments that build high self-esteem.

Children are most likely to develop high self-esteem when parents
- Frequently communicate "unconditional regard" for the child (use body language and words to let the child know he or she is *liked*)
- Communicate a range of acceptable behaviors
- Challenge the child to explore strengths and limitations
- Celebrate the child's competencies and accomplishments
- Assist the child to respond to mistakes responsibly and to learn from them

Since some parents and educators may not have experienced these helps to personal growth themselves, it is beneficial for the nurse to role model these behaviors when interacting with children.

Dinkmeyer (1970) called on educators to arrange learning experiences in ways that strengthen a child's self-esteem and enable the child to meet social, emotional, and academic needs. Dinkmeyer recommends that the learning atmosphere be characterized by
- A mutual respect and trust by teacher and child
- A focus on mutual alignment of purposes by teacher and child
- A feeling on the part of students that they belong to the group
- An environment where it is safe for the child to look at inner needs, hopes, and wishes
- An opportunity to express needs which, if not articulated and clarified, hamper the learning process
- An emphasis on the importance of self-evaluation in contrast to evaluation by others
- A climate marked by identification, recognition, acceptance, and appreciation of individual differences
- An emphasis on growth from dependence to independence

Self-Analysis

A. Describing the problem:
1. Choose a problem as your target behavior, whether physical, behavioral, or psychological. (Note: For a first analysis, a physical or behavioral problem may be easiest to analyze.)
2. Decide on a method of description.
   a. Physical measurement.
   b. Self-report.
   c. Performance measure.
3. Apply the three basic rules of description.
   a. Simplicity: If you're worried about a big, general problem, focus on a simple unit of it.
   b. Objectivity: Stick to aspects of the problem that you can observe and measure.
   c. Specificity: Spell out the details of your problem.
4. Follow these additional suggestions for writing a description.
   a. Limit yourself to describing the problem only as it occurs in one specific situation.
   b. Show your description to someone else to see if he or she can get a clear picture of the problem; fill in missing details if necessary.
   c. Keep records through self-monitoring; use a mirror or tape recorder if needed.

d. Plot your recorded behavior on a graph.

B. Functional analysis of the problem:
1. Look for correlations between your problem behavior and other variables.
   a. Try to identify positive or negative correlations.
   b. If correlations are difficult to find, examine events that occur before, during, or after the target behavior.
   c. Watch out for third variables and circular relationships.
2. Selecting the most likely correlation, develop a hypothesis, specifying the independent variable (the cause) that is affecting the dependent variable (the target behavior).
3. Test your hypothesis:
   a. Make a specific plan as to how you will change the independent variable
   b. Set a target for improvement in the dependent variable.
   c. Change the independent variable.
   d. Examine changes in the dependent variable.
   e. If there is no change or only a very small change, repeat steps B2 and B3, using a different variable. Continue doing this until you see some lasting change in your problem behavior.

(From PSYCHOLOGY OF ADJUSTMENT AND HUMAN RELATIONSHIPS, Second Edition, by J.F. Calhoun and J.R. Acocella. Copyright © 1983, 1978 by Random House, Inc. Reprinted by permission of the publisher.)

• Situations in which limits are most often a result of natural and logical consequences and not merely reflection of the personal needs of the teacher*

Important learning tasks for children include understanding and accepting oneself and understanding feelings; others; independence; goals and purposeful behavior; mastery, competence, and resourcefulness; emotional maturity; and choices and consequences.

EVALUATING

Nurses who are sensitive to the relationship between self-concept and general well-being will consistently evaluate the effect the plan of nursing care has on the client's self-concept. For example, while educating a

* List reprinted by permission of American Guidance Service, Circle Pines, MN 55014. *Developing Understanding of Self & Others* (DUSO-1) by Don Dinkmeyer, Sr. Copyright 1970. Rights reserved.

client with hypertension for whom life-style counseling was recommended the nurse may detect that the client is feeling extremely guilty about his smoking, dietary habits, and lack of exercise. "Why should I even try to change any of these things now. I made myself sick so I may as well live with the punishment." If the plan of care is to be effective the nurse must first help this client value himself and his health sufficiently to want to take care of himself.

When the plan of care includes specific interventions to assist clients with disturbances in body image, self-esteem, role performance, and personal identity, then the nurse listens carefully to the client's self-report and observes client behaviors to see if the disturbances are being resolved. Basically the client should be

• Comfortable with body image and able to use it effectively to meet human needs
• Able to describe self positively
• Able to meet realistic role expectations without undue anxiety and fatigue
• Capable of interacting appropriately with environment while recognizing self to be a separate and distinct entity

N U R S I N G P R O C E S S *in Clinical Practice*

When identifying and treating disturbances in self-concept categorized as nursing diagnoses the nurse uses each phase of the nursing process. Quality care is dependent on the nurse's possession of the knowledge and skills described earlier in this chapter. What follows in outline format are the assessment priorities, client goals, nursing interventions, and evaluative criteria for two common types of self-concept disturbances treated by nurses: disturbances in body image and negative self-concept related to faulty thinking (distortions and denials, faulty categorizing, and inappropriate standards).

In the case study that follows the development of these diagnoses, nursing care is described for a woman with low self-esteem.

Disturbance in Self-Concept: Body Image

Disturbances in body image are common given today's emphasis on physical appearance. In one 2,000-person survey conducted in 1985, 34% of the men and 38% of the women disagreed with the statement "I like my looks just the way they are" (Cash, Winstead, and Janda, 1986). In general persons who like their appearance, fitness, health, and sexual attractiveness tend to feel happier and more adjusted.

Disturbances in body image result from multiple causes. As a child gains control over body parts and functioning, this control is integrated into the self. Anything that threatens this control is perceived as a threat to the self. A child being prepared for surgery may become hysterical when asked to put on a hospital gown and remove all personal clothing including underpants. This action may leave the body too vulnerable in the child's eye. Similarly, an injection or any other penetrating device may threaten the child's sense of self. For adults, loss of control of body parts and functioning is especially traumatic. Normal aging, loss of breast or uterus, loss of memory, mobility or sexual functioning—are all significant stressors. McCloskey (1976) describes the concept of "spread" which occurs when a person's attitude about a part of his body spreads to his entire concept of himself. McCloskey notes two major types of boundary disturbances.

1. Body wall changes but the client "keeps" the old body boundary (may explain the phantom pain some clients feel in amputated limbs). *Example:* Woman with a history of obesity (210 lb) who is now a size 14 continues to buy clothes that would look good on an obese person and to think herself overweight.
2. Client changes a body boundary even though his body wall remains intact. *Example:* A client whose left side is paralyzed following a stroke may refuse to believe that this side is still a part of his body—

despite efforts to make him conscious of it—because he cannot feel it or move it.

Assessment
- Once a body image disturbance is suspected, carefully interview and observe the client to identify (1) the nature of the threat to the person's body image (functional significance of the part involved, importance of physical appearance, and visibility of the part involved), (2) the meaning the client attaches to the threat, (3) the adequacy of the client's coping abilities, (4) response of family members and significant others, and (5) help available to the client and his family (McCloskey, 1976).
- Assess the client's response to the deformity or limitation including changes in independence-dependence patterns and in socialization and communication (Carpenito, 1987).
  1. Response to deformity or limitation
     Adaptive responses: Exhibits signs of grief and mourning (shock, disbelief, denial, anger, guilt, acceptance)
     Maladaptive responses: Continues to deny and to deal with the deformity or limitation, engages in self-destructive behavior, talks about feelings of worthlessness or insecurity, equates deformity or limitation with whole person, shows a change in ability to estimate relationship of body to environment
  2. Independence-dependence patterns
     Adaptive responses: Assumes responsibility for care (makes decisions); develops new self-care behaviors; uses available resources; interacts in a mutually supportive way with family
     Maladaptive responses: Assigns responsibility for his care to others; becomes increasingly dependent or stubbornly refuses necessary help
  3. Socialization and communication
     Adaptive responses: Maintains usual social patterns; communicates needs and accepts offers of help; serves as support for others
     Maladaptive responses: Isolates himself; exhibits superficial self-confidence; unable to express needs (becomes hostile, ashamed, frustrated, depressed)

Client Goals
The client will
- Describe his body positively, integrating the change in body part or functioning into his self-concept

- Verbalize or demonstrate acceptance of irreversible body changes
- Develop new abilities to compensate for irreversible losses
- Use his body effectively to meet basic human needs
- Demonstrate by appearance and self-care behaviors (hygiene, exercise, nutrition) a respect for his body
- Maintain maximal independence while accepting necessary help
- Continue pre-existing social patterns

Interventions

Interventions for body image disturbances will vary according to the nature of the disturbance. Interventions may include any combination of the following:

- Establish a trusting relationship with the client. Allow the client to openly share his feelings. Sitting quietly by the client for a few minutes with a few words like "How are things?" or "Gee it must be hard to lie there after all you've been through . . ." communicates to the client your willingness and readiness to share his experience.
- Support the client through the various stages of loss, grief, and mourning (shock, disbelief, denial, anger, guilt, acceptance) remembering that there is no one "right way" to proceed through these stages. Rather clients may move fluidly in and out of various stages, sometimes returning to earlier stages. Some clients may need to learn that it is "ok" to cry, to be angry, to be "down."
- Use play therapy with children so they can describe their feelings and work through their grief using the nonthreatening medium of dolls or animals.
- Role model for the client a healthy acceptance of the client's body. Be careful that facial expressions, words, or body positioning do not communicate to the client disgust, fear, or rejection.
- While communicating support to the client who is slow to develop and use appropriate self-care behaviors, firmly insist that the client participate in his care to the extent that he is able. Whenever possible provide the client with honest answers to his questions or put him in touch with the appropriate person to give the answers.
- Strengthen the decision-making ability of the client by honestly exploring alternatives; help the client to imagine living with the consequences of different courses of action.
- Reinforce the client's personal strengths and help the client and family to identify all possible resources.
- Assess the response of the client's significant others and intervene if they are negatively influencing the client.

Evaluative Criteria

Client meets above goals.

Negative Self-Concept

Many of the clients nurses interact with, especially on a long-term basis, may be interested in modifying some aspect of a negative self-concept which is related to faulty thinking. Common analogies of negative self-concepts include: distortions and denials; faulty categorizing and inappropriate standards; perfectionism, conventionality, "What the other guy thinks" (Calhoun and Acocella, 1983).

Distortions and Denials

A woman who was taught early in life that a woman's place is in the home may systematically have distorted or denied any talents or feelings which she thought were inconsistent with being a full-time wife and mother. For example, if she enjoyed math and did well in her math courses in high school, rather than feel good about this she might think it abnormal and consciously limit her study of math. If a guidance counselor recommended college to her she might "laugh-off" the suggestion.
Nursing diagnosis: Negative (limited) self-concept related to a long history of distorting and denying her abilities and desires.

Faulty Categorizing

A positive self-concept is characterized by a broad image of the self. The more labels we can attach to ourselves the more self-information we are able to assimilate and make part of us. An adolescent who repeatedly hears from her father that she is "no good" and who consistently characterizes herself this way may reject genuine affirmations of her positive qualities and strengths from other family member, her peers, teachers, and so forth. Moreover, she may choose to act in ways that reinforce her image of being "no good."
Nursing diagnosis: Negative self-concept related to inability to recognize and "own" positive qualities, strengths ("I'm no good").

Old Standards

At the root of the negative self-concepts of some clients may be an unrealistic ideal-self. With all the emphasis in today's society on "being number 1," many persons hold *perfectionistic standards* which they will never be able to meet. In describing their self-expectations these clients may reveal that they must always get an A to feel good about themselves, or always be the center of everyone's attention and love. Anything less is viewed as failure.

Conventionality offers another set of problems for the person who uncritically accepts all his culture dictates. When his feelings or preferred actions conflict with society's standards then he concludes that something must be wrong with him. Because sick-role behaviors are dictated by many cultures the person who finds he cannot "suffer in silence" or conversely, cannot express his pain or grief vocally, may feel alienated from his culture. An older person whose family is considering nursing home placement may find this more difficult to accept if his culture is one in which family members traditionally respect and care for aged members at home.

What the Other Guy Thinks is the third faulty standard. Allowing others to define ideal behavior sets up a person for constant failure because it is impossible to please everyone. The young executive who tries to live up to the expectations of her boss, peer group at work, husband and children, and college friends, is bound to lose herself in the process.

Nursing diagnosis: Negative self-concept related to unrealistic self-expectations (perfectionism, conventionality, "What the other guy thinks").

Assessment

- Assess how accurately the client is able to describe himself; note in particular the use of negative labels and their significance for the client.
- Determine if the client is motivated to modify the self-concept. Does he see a relationship between a negative self-concept and self-defeating thoughts, feelings, and behaviors?
- Teach the client to choose a day on which he will write down every self-critical thought that enters his mind. At the end of the day the list should be reviewed and three questions asked: 1. What is the standard (perfectionism, conventionality, other people's judgments) on which this self-criticism is based? 2. From whom do you think you picked up this standard? 3. Do you really subscribe to the standard wholeheartedly? (Calhoun and Acocella, 1983, p 110)

Client Goals

The client will
- Describe the relationship between self-concept and behavior
- Identify faulty thinking which reinforces a negative self-concept (distortions and denials, faulty categorizing, inappropriate standards)
- Integrate positive self-knowledge into self-concept
- Report feeling better about himself

Interventions

- See the box entitled Changing the Self-concept.
- Once the client has identified faulty thinking patterns (negative self-talk) which reinforce the negative self-concept, teach him to "red flag" this behavior as soon as he is aware of it happening. The goal is to replace the negative self-talk with talk that will develop a more positive self-image.
- Help the person explore the positive dimension of himself that he wishes to develop and incorporate this new knowledge into the self-concept.

Changing the Self-Concept

A. Analyzing the problem:
  1. Isolate the basic problem label.
  2. Describe your problem in situational terms.
  3. Search for correlations, watching out especially for negative self-talk.
  4. Review the background of your problem to check for such causes as:
    a. Distortions and denials.
    b. Faulty categorizing.
    c. Perfectionism.
    d. Conventionality.
    e. Other people's judgments.
B. Changing the self-concept:
  1. Set a goal.
  2. Gather new information about this aspect of yourself.
  3. Engage in cognitive restructuring:
    a. Listen to your old self-talk.
    b. Talk back to this old self-talk, cross-examining it to get at the reality.
    c. Act on your back-talk, substituting new behavior to accompany your new, more rational self-talk

(From PSYCHOLOGY OF ADJUSTMENT AND HUMAN RELATIONSHIPS, Second Edition, by J.F. Calhoun and J.R. Acocella. Copyright © 1983, 1978 by Random House, Inc. Reprinted by permission of the publisher.)

Example: Twenty-year-old new mother who perceives herself as "a failure in everything I try"; states husband feels childrearing is the woman's responsibility and she is terrified.

Immediate goal: Develop confidence in parenting skills, see herself as a good mother

1. Explore and reinforce the client's personal qualities and strengths which will help her to reach her goal.

   "You look like a natural mother when you hold your baby, some women are afraid at the beginning to even hold their infants."

   "That's good that you are talking with your baby. Babies quickly sense how a parent feels about them."

2. Teach the client how to substitute positive self-talk for negative self-talk.

   Negative self-talk (mother during feeding): "She's awfully fussy tonight I mustn't be doing this right. . . . It was probably dumb luck that she took to breast so well this morning. . . .

New positive self-talk: ". . . but she fed so well this morning and the nurse said her weight is good. I wonder what else might be making her fussy . . . maybe she's wet. . . ."

Evaluative Criteria
Client meets above goals.

C A S E   S T U D Y

Melissa Motsky is a 31-year-old married woman, mother of three children (ages 12, 10, and 8), and junior level nursing student. She works every other weekend as a nurse's aide. She has just received a letter from the nursing division head informing her that she is in academic jeopardy and will fail out of the program unless her grades improve. She presents this to her advisor.

Assessment Findings

After talking with Mrs. Motsky who keeps calling herself a failure and who begins to cry as she describes her situation at home, her faculty advisor suspects a serious self-esteem problem and helps her to list factors contributing to her present sense of failure and low self-esteem. The following list is generated:

Significance

−   Receives little understanding, affection, approval from husband. "I stay with him because of the kids. I started back to school because I had to get out of the house and want to make something of myself. He doesn't understand this."

+   "Children are very supportive but get impatient when I have to study and can't spend time with them."

Competence

−   Feels a failure in all the roles that are important to her: wife, mother, and, now, student. "I jeopardized everything to go back to school—if I fail, it's all over for me. There just isn't enough time or energy to do anything well."

+   "They do love me at work though, which makes me feel like nursing is what I should be doing."

Virtue

+   "I do still try and live according to my beliefs and feel ok about this. I treat others as I'd like to be treated."

−   "I've always believed that hard work pays off and that if you were faithful to your duty you'd be rewarded by the 'good life'—I'm begin-

ning to doubt that. Maybe I'm a fool for trying so hard."

Power

−   "I always believed I could do anything I put my heart and soul into. But I can't seem to change my marriage and if I fail out of school that will be the end of all my dreams."

Key indicators of low self-esteem which also surfaced in the interview include overeating (10-lb weight gain over last year), difficulty sleeping, fatigue, new sensitivity to criticism, and expressions of feeling unloved, alone, and no longer able to manage. Personal strengths include history of "can-do" mentality, high motivation to succeed, and past history of success as mother and nurse's aide.

Nursing Diagnosis

Disturbance in self-esteem related to decreased sense of significance, competence, virtue, and power. Many nursing diagnoses could be developed for Mrs. Motsky. This was given high priority because her nursing advisor felt it to be a key to other problems.

Planning

Mrs. Motsky is eager to try anything that will help her to feel better about herself and enable her to perform better academically. "I'd like to start feeling like myself again." She cautions her advisor that she doesn't have much time to devote to this because she obviously needs to spend every spare minute studying. In response to her advisor's question, "What personal goals would you like to achieve in the next month," she suggests the following:

11/2   By this time next month I will demonstrate increased self-esteem as evidenced by:

• Expression of positive statements about myself
• Report of ability to receive negative feedback from family, school and so forth, without "falling apart"
• Passing grade on next quarterly exam
• Ability to verbalize that the way I am living my life is "ok"
• Report of two recent instances when my power was effective in accomplishing what I desired.

Long-term goal: I will consistently maintain sufficient self-esteem to successfully develop and achieve new life goals.

See plan of care developed to aid Mrs. Motsky in accomplishing her goals.

Implementation

In order to assist Mrs. Motsky in meeting her goals the nurse needs the following specialized abilities:

- Belief that a person's self-esteem influences all aspects of her functioning and a commitment to addressing this human need (*i.e.,* holistic orientation)
- Empathy for the multiple role expectations the client is experiencing and ability to identify and mobilize the client's inner strengths so that a *realistic* plan can be developed to assist the client to *satisfactorily* meet necessary role expectations
- Knowledge of etiologies and defining characteristics for disturbances in self-esteem and specific nursing strategies to enhance self-esteem
- Interpersonal skills to communicate to client that she is important, cared about, competent, good, and that she possesses within herself the power/strength to turn her situation around
- Ability to correctly decide that it is wise to encourage this student to continue in the nursing program whereas another student of lesser ability would be assisted to reevaluate her career goals
- Teaching, counseling, and advocacy skills
- Accountability (ability and willingness to encourage student and follow-up on her progress; "celebrate" goal achievement or make realistic plans if student should fail out of program).

Documentation

Sample documentation of Mrs. Motsky's initial visit to her advisor follows in the traditional note format:
10/2/89.   Melissa Motsky presented today after receiving academic jeopardy letter. She is strongly motivated to complete nursing program successfully and seems to have the ability to do this. Multiple life stressors at the present: lack of support from husband, need to "mother" three children (12, 10, 8), part-time nurse's aide job (necessary for financial reasons), and current academic jeopardy (test grades 68, 74), are all contributing to her low self-esteem and overwhelming sense of being a failure. We together developed a plan of care which will hopefully help her to do better academically as well begin to feel better about herself. See attached. She will return 11/2/89 at 10:00 AM for follow-up.

C Taylor, RN

SOAP documentation:
10/2/89
Academic jeopardy—Melissa Motsky
12:30 PM

S: "I jeopardized everything to go back to school—if I fail, it's all over for me."
Reports lack of support from husband, grief that she doesn't have enough time for children, failure of personal work ethic "hard work pays off," and sense of powerlessness.

O: Nursing II quarterly exam grades: 68, 74; weight gain of 10 lb over last year; facial and body expressions of fatigue, profuse tears

A: Disturbance in self-esteem related to decreased sense of significance, competence, virtue, and power

P: See attached plan of care.

C Taylor, RN

Evaluation

Short-term goal achievement will be evaluated informally as student is met at school and formally at the next month's conference. Long-term goal achievement is an ongoing personal evaluation.

N U R S I N G   C A R E   P L A N   *for Mrs. Motsky*

Nursing Diagnosis:	Disturbance in self-esteem related to decreased sense of significance, competence, virtue, and power as manifested by expressions of being a failure, powerlessness, fatigue, tears, weight gain, low academic performance (test grades 68, 74).
Long-Term Goal:	Client will consistently maintain sufficient self-esteem to successfully develop and achieve new life goals.

Goals	Nursing Actions	Rationale	Evaluative Statement
By this time next month (11/2) client will demonstrate increased self-esteem by:	Assist client to rediscover and "own" personal strengths: identify personal qualities and	Clients can lose touch with their strengths— especially when multiple stressors seem to create	11/3 Goal partially met. Client's statements are of the "This is good, *but* . . ." variety. "I think I'm

(Continued)

N U R S I N G   C A R E   P L A N (Continued)

Goals	Nursing Actions	Rationale	Evaluative Statement
1. Expression of positive statements about herself	strengths which have pleased her in the past and explore why this has changed; recommend that she make at least one positive statement about herself each morning and evening. Consistently interact with the client as if she had the power to "weather" the crisis successfully (*i.e.,* "will" strength to her). Role-model positive self-concept behaviors	impossible demands Once the client senses that an "authority" believes in her power and expects her to use it, she may internalize this knowledge and act on it.	doing better in school but I don't know if it will continue." *Recommendation:* Continue to identify and reinforce personal strengths. *C Taylor, RN*
2. Report ability to receive negative feedback without "falling apart"	Explore with client to what degree she allows the opinions of others to influence her self-concept. Teach how the self-concept "filters" life experiences; thus, if I feel that I am a failure, I may interpret the words and behaviors of others as confirming this—even though that was not their intention. Explore with the client ways she can enhance her self-concept independently of others (*e.g.,* take time each day for herself). Teach the client how to analyze feedback constructively and respond appropriately; *cancel negative thinking*. For example, client receives care plan back with many corrections and notation "sloppy work." *Maladaptive response:* "She hates me. See, this proves I'll never be a good nurse. I wasted my time even doing this." *Adaptive response:* "I spent as much time as I had on this . . . now let me see what I did wrong.	Significance, sense of being loved and approved of by significant others, is a critical component of self-esteem. Principle of self-consistency: once I am "down" I may reinforce this by distorting what I feel, hear, experience. Encourage client to draw on personal strengths: "wasting" time on self communicates that self is valuable. Important to break cycle of negative thinking which reinforces negative self-concept	11/3 Goal partially met. Client reports being able to handle everything except "put downs" from her husband. *Recommendation:* Explore origin of power she has given to her husband to influence her sense of self and what she wants to do about this. *C Taylor, RN*

(Continued)

NURSING CARE PLAN (Continued)

Goals	Nursing Actions	Rationale	Evaluative Statement
	Maybe I should make an appointment with my instructor so she can show me how to improve."		
3. Passing grade on next quarterly exam	Explore study skills with client; recommend study group. Discuss importance of how she *perceives* present situation: if present failures are equated with *defeat* she may be unable to mobilize her resources to succeed; if present failures represent *challenge* it may call forth her best efforts and result in success. Discuss importance of breaking cycle of failure leading to another failure.	Meaning given to present stressor can dramatically affect response to it and condition one for success or failure If this short-term goal is met it will set the stage for future successes and contribute to positive self-concept	11/3 Goal met. Grade: 82 *C Taylor, RN*
4. Ability to verbalize that the way client is living her life is "ok"	Assist client to examine her moral-ethical standards; explore sources of these standards and if the client feels comfortable with them. Identify unrealistic standards; client may need "permission" to be human. Refer if appropriate for counseling.	Moral-ethical standards may be uncritically internalized and place the client in conflict. Unrealistic standards (perfectionism, conventionality) may constantly undermine the client's self-esteem. Support groups on campus (counseling centers, ministries) may be able to meet client's needs.	11/3 Goal met. Client stated: "I guess I'm living the best way I know how right now. If things are meant to be different someone is going to have to show me how." *Recommendation:* Reinforce self-acceptance. *C Taylor, RN*
5. Report of two recent instances when personal power was effective in accomplishing desired goals	Identify and affirm client's use of personal power to accomplish goals.	A negative self-concept may deny or distort personal successes; outside intervention may be necessary to bring these to consciousness.	11/3 Goal met . . . with difficulty. Needed considerable prompting to identify successful use of her personal power. Was ready to attribute passing grade to luck rather than her own efforts. *Recommendation:* Have client record daily her use of personal power and results. *C Taylor, RN*

KEY POINTS

- Self-concept is the mental image or picture of self. It has the power to encourage or thwart personal growth and development.

- Included in the notion self-concept are body-image, how I experience my body; subjective self, how I see myself; ideal self, the self I want to be; and social self, way I feel others see me.

- It is helpful to explore the self-concept by assessing self-knowledge, self-expectations, and self-evaluation or self-esteem. Self-esteem is a measure of a person's satisfaction with his significance, competence, virtue, and power.

- Self-concept is a social creation. An infant, born without a self-concept, develops positive feelings about self if basic needs are met and warmth and affection are experienced.

- A positive self-concept is characterized by stable and diversified self-knowledge, realistic self-expectations and positive self-evaluation and acceptance of self.

- High self-esteem is characterized by positive expectations of the future, ability to approach others freely because of a history of being well received and successful, and ability to approach new tasks and situations freely—confident of own ability to "get along."

- Defense mechanisms are unconscious processes the self uses to protect itself from stress, threats to self-esteem, and other dangers.

- Life experiences both affect and are affected by a person's self-concept. Key factors influencing self-concept are developmental state, culture, internal and external resources, history of success and failure, stressors and illness or trauma.

- The nurse who wishes to effectively meet the self-concept needs of clients needs to be comfortable with self, his or her abilities, and his or her needs before the nurse can interact therapeutically with clients. It is important for the nurse to role-model positive self-concept behaviors.

- Because a client may offer the responses the interviewer wants rather than what is really felt, client responses should be evaluated in relation to observations the nurse makes of the client's behaviors.

- Nursing diagnoses may be written specifically addressing disturbances in self-concept: negative self-concept, disturbances in body-image, self-esteem, role competence, and self-identity, or identifying the effect these disturbances have on other areas of human functioning (*e.g.*, coping, health maintenance, powerlessness).

BIBLIOGRAPHY

Antonucci TC, Jackson JS: Physical health and self-esteem. Family and Community Health 6(2):1–9, 1983

Atwater E: Psychology of Adjustment, 3rd ed. Englewood Cliffs, NJ, Prentice-Hall, 1987

Baird SE: Development of a nursing assessment tool to diagnose altered body image in immobilized patients. Orthopedic Patients 4(1):47–54, 1985

Calhoun JF, Acocella JR: Psychology of Adjustment and Human Relationships, 2nd ed. New York, Random House, 1983

Carpenito: 1987

Cash TF, Winstead BA, Janda LH: The great American shape-up. Psychology Today April, 1986, p 33

Cline VB: How to Make Your Child a Winner. Walker & Co, 1980

Coleman JC, Morris CG, Glaros AG: Contemporary Psychology and Effective Behavior, 6th ed. Glenview, IL, Scott, Foresman and Company, 1987

Coopersmith S: The Antecedents of Self-Esteem. San Francisco, WH Freeman, 1967

Critelli JW: Personal Growth and Effective Behavior. New York, Holt, Rinehart, & Winston, 1987

Crouch MA, Straub V: Enhancement of self-esteem in adults. Family and Community Health 6(2):65–78, 1983

Darling-Fisher CS: Impairment of body image. In Jacobs MM, Geels W (eds): Signs and Symptoms in Nursing. Philadelphia, JB Lippincott, 1985

Dinkmeyer D: Developing Understanding of Self and Others. Manual DUSO-D1. Circle Pines, MN, American Guidance Service, 1970

Gilbert R: The evaluation of self-esteem. Family and Community Health 6(2):29–49, 1983

Horowitz LG: The self-care motivation model: Theory and practice in healthy human development. J Sch Health 55(2):57–61, 1985

Janelli LM: The realities of body image. Journal of Gerontological Nursing 12(10):23–27, 1986

Long KA, Hamlin CM: Use of the Piers-Haris self-concept scale with Indian children: Cultural considerations. Nurs Res 37(1):42–46, 1988

Makay, Gaw: 1975

Maslow A: Motivation and Personality. New York, Harper & Row, 1954

McCloskey: 1976

Meisenhelder JB: Self-esteem in women: The influence of employment and perception of husband's appraisals. Image 18(1):8–14, 1986

Muhlenkamp AF, Sayles JA: Self-esteem, social support, and positive health practices. Nurs Res 35(6):334–338, 1986

Norris J, Kunes-Connell M: Self-esteem disturbance. Nurs Clin North Am 20(4):745–761, 1985

Otto H: The human potentialities of nurses and patients. Nurs Outlook 13(8):32–35, 1965

Pensiero M, Adams M: Dress and self-esteem. Journal of Gerontological Nursing 13(10):11–17, 1987

Reasoner RW: Enhancement of self-esteem in children and adolescents. Family and Community Health 6(2):51–64, 1983

Rutkowski BL: 6 steps to building your confidence. Nursing Life 6(1):26–29, 1986

Sanford LT, Donovan ME: Women and Self-Esteem. New York, Penguin Books, 1984

Stanwyck DJ: Self-esteem through the life span. Family and Community Health 6(8):11–28, 1983

Taylor Sr C: The need for self-esteem. In Yura H, Walsh MB (eds): Human Needs 2 and the Nursing Process. Norwalk, CT, Appleton-Century-Crofts, 1982

Whall AL: Self-esteem and the mental health of older adults. Journal of Gerontological Nursing 13(4):41–42, 1987

White JH, et al: Femininity, image, femininism, and a decision to seek treatment in obese women. Health Care of Women International 7(6):455–467, 1986

Williamson ML: The nursing diagnosis of body image disturbance in adolescents dissatisfied with their physical characteristics. Holistic Nursing Practice 1(4):52–59, 1987

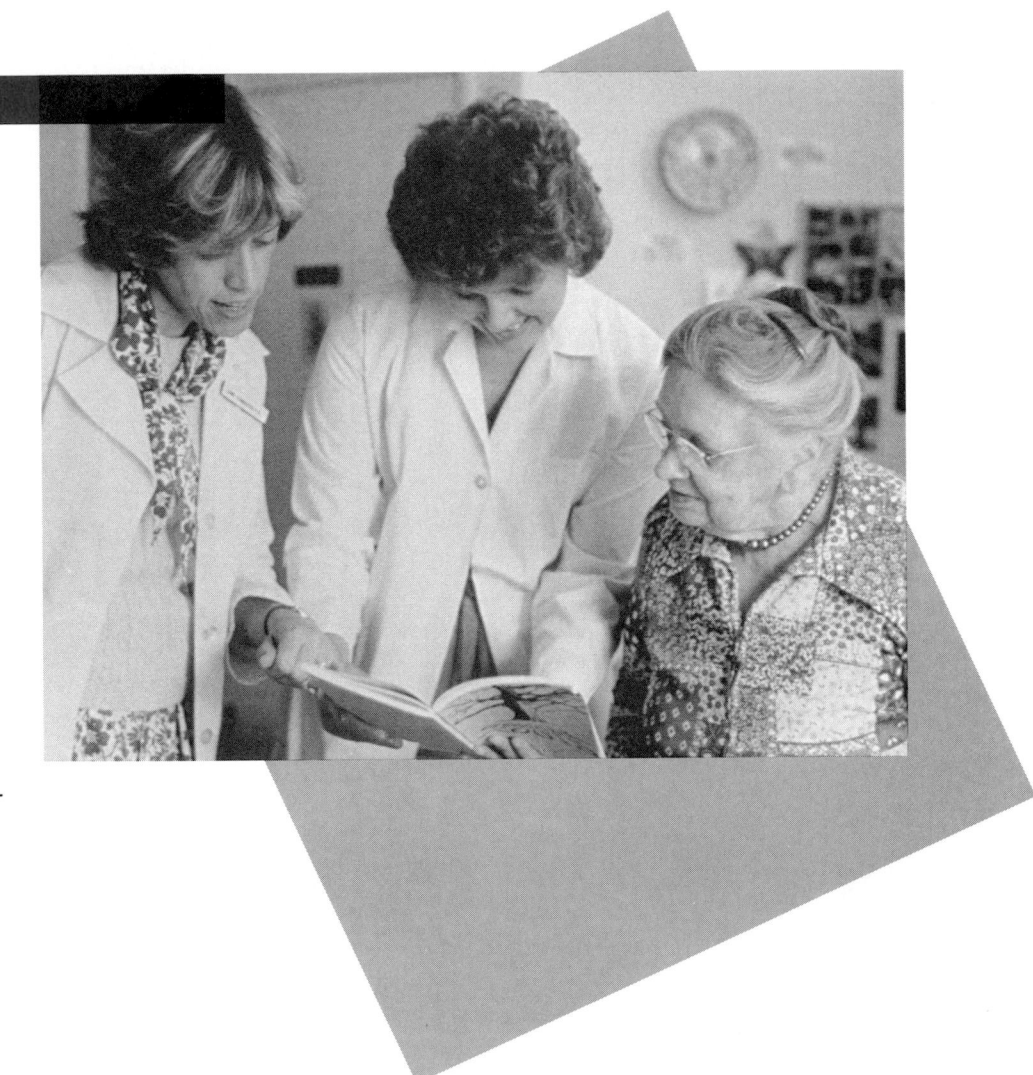

37 Sensory Stimulation

OBJECTIVES

After studying this chapter, the learner should be able to

Define key terms in the chapter.

Describe the four conditions that must be met in each sensory experience.

Explain the role of the reticular activating system in sensory experience.

Identify etiologies and perceptual, cognitive, and emotional responses to sensory deprivation and sensory overload.

Perform a comprehensive assessment of sensory functioning utilizing appropriate interview questions and physical assessment skills.

Develop nursing diagnosis that correctly indentify sensory–perceptual alterations that may be treated by independent nursing intervention.

Describe specific nursing strategies to prevent sensory alterations, to stimulate the senses, and to assist clients with sensory difficulties.

Develop a plan of nursing care to assist clients meet individualized sensory–perceptual goals.

Implement individualized nursing strategies that successfully resolve the client's individualized sensory–perceptual alterations.

Evaluate the plan of nursing care using specified criteria.

A person's senses are vital to survival, growth and development, and experience of bodily pleasure.

- Being able to smell smoke and interpret this as potentially life threatening, I can protect myself from fire.
- Seeing a client smile when I walk into her room and hearing her say "I couldn't have gone through this week without you" bolsters my professional confidence and self-esteem and encourages me to offer quality nursing to others.
- Feeling someone's gentle hands stroke my body I luxuriate in feelings of care, pleasure, and sensual delight.

Intrinsic to each of these experiences is intact sensory functioning.

Many of the clients nurses encounter have impaired sensory functioning, which places them at high risk of injury and altered growth and development and decreases their well-being. Moreover, the stress of illness or trauma and the need for diagnosis and treatment may quickly result in sensory deprivation or overload with serious disturbances in visual, perceptual, cognitive, or emotional functioning.

Study of this chapter provides the student with knowledge of (1) the process of sensation, (2) the role of the arousal mechanism, (3) sensory alterations, and (4) factors affecting sensory stimulation. Practical suggestions are given for performing an assessment of sensory functioning. Examples are given of nursing diagnoses identifying specific sensory–perceptual alterations, as are many diagnoses describing the effects of altered sensory functioning on other areas of human functioning. Client goals for preventing and managing sensory alterations are described. Specialized nursing interventions for vision- or hearing-impaired, confused, or unconscious clients are presented. In the section Nursing Process in Clinical Practice, focused assessment, planning, implementation, and evaluation guides are offered for select nursing diagnoses of sensory deprivation related to inadequate parenting, to the effects of aging, and to unfamiliar culture.

KEY TERMS

arousal
auditory
gustatory
kinesthesia
olfactory
perception
reception
reticular activating system
sensoristasis

sensory deprivation
sensory overload
sensory–perceptual alterations
stimulus
tactile
visceral
visual

THE SENSORY EXPERIENCE

Components and Conditions

The two components of any sensory experience are **reception** and **perception**. *Sensory reception* is the process of receiving data about the internal or external environment through the senses. The senses by which individuals maintain contact with the external environment are vision (**visual**), hearing (**auditory**), smell (**olfactory**), taste (**gustatory**), and touch (**tactile**). The kinesthetic and visceral senses arise internally from muscles and hollow organs, respectively, and are the basic orienting systems. (**Kinesthesia** refers to awareness of positioning of body parts and body movement, and **visceral** pertains to inner organs.) *Sensory perception* is the conscious process of selecting, organizing, and interpreting data from the senses into meaningful information. Perception is influenced by the intensity, size, change, or representation of stimuli, as well as by past experiences, knowledge, and attitudes.

For a person to receive data necessary to experience the world, four conditions must be met:

- A **stimulus**, an agent, act, or other influence capable of initiating a response by the nervous system, must be present.
- A *receptor* or *sense organ* must receive the stimulus and convert it to a nerve impulse.
- The nerve impulse must be *conducted* along a nervous pathway from the receptor or sense organ to the brain.
- A particular area in the brain must receive and *translate* the impulse into a sensation. (Tortora and Anagnostakos, 1981, p 358)

Arousal Mechanism

To receive stimuli and respond appropriately, the brain must be alert or aroused. The **reticular activating system** (RAS), located in the core of the brain stem, mediates **arousal**. According to Schultz (1965), the arousal state of the RAS is a general drive state, which he called **sensoristasis**. Nerve impules from all the sensory tracts reach the RAS, which then selectively allows certain impulses to reach the cerebral cortex and be perceived. With its many ascending and descending connections to other areas of the brain, the RAS serves to monitor and regulate incoming sensory stimuli and thereby maintain, enhance, or inhibit cortical arousal.

A stimulus must be variable or irregular to evoke a response. The body quickly adapts to constant stimuli; thus the repeated stimulus of a continuing noise such as city traffic or a noxious odor eventually goes unnoticed. This phenomenon is termed *adaptation*. Impulses that are not acted on when received may be used at a later date. The memory process involves the storage of that material. For example, thought and memory are used when a new sensory experience occurs and the organism uses a response based on previous knowledge and experience.

Sensory Alterations

When admitted to a health agency, the client is confronted with stimuli that are different in quality and quantity to the accustomed stimuli. For example, the client confined to bed rest may receive many fewer stimuli, whereas the client undergoing multiple diagnostic tests may receive a greater than normal level of sensory input. These and other typical experiences are likely to result in the client's having sensory alterations. Behavioral changes in hospitalized clients have been reduced since more attention is being paid to the use of color and

sound and increased privacy and social interaction. Table 37-1 provides an overview of sensory deprivation and sensory overload with related nursing interventions.

Sensory Deprivation

Sensory deprivation results when a person experiences decreased sensory input or input that is monotonous, unpatterned, or meaningless. With decreased sensory input the RAS is no longer able to project a normal level of activation to the brain and the individual may hallucinate simply to maintain an optimal level of arousal (MacKinnon-Kesler, 1983). Factors placing a client at high risk for sensory deprivation include

- An environment with decreased or monotonous stimuli (institutionalized clients, clients confined to a small living area at home, clients on bed rest or in isolation, and so on)
- Impaired ability to receive environmental stimuli (clients with sensory alterations: impaired vision or hearing; clients with bandages or casts that interfere with vision, hearing, or tactile stimulation; clients with affective disorders who "close-out" the environment, and so on)
- Inability to process environmental stimuli (clients with spinal cord injuries or brain damage, clients who are confused or disoriented, clients taking prescribed or recreational drugs that affect the central nervous system)

Effects of sensory deprivation include perceptual, cognitive, and emotional disturbances:

- *Perceptual responses:* Inaccurate perception of sights, sounds, tastes, smells, and body position, coordination, and equilibrium; mild to gross distortions ranging from daydreams to hallucinations
- *Cognitive responses:* Inability to control the direction of thought content; decreased attention span and ability to concentrate; difficulty with memory, problem solving, and task performance
- *Emotional responses:* Inappropriate emotional responses: apathy, anxiety, fear, anger, belligerence, panic, depression; rapid mood changes

See Table 37-1 for additional information.

Sensory Overload

Sensory overload is the condition that results when a person experiences so much sensory stimuli that the brain is unable meaningfully to respond to or ignore the stimuli. The person feels out of control and may exhibit all of the manifestations observed in sensory deprivation. The amount and quality of stimuli necessary to produce overload may differ greatly from one individual to another and are influenced by factors such as age, culture, personality, and life-style.

In some clients, especially those coming from a quiet environment with unvarying stimuli, the experience of being hospitalized quickly results in sensory overload. In such clients, the brain is assaulted by the

(Text continues on p. 1043.)

T A B L E   37-1
Overview of Sensory Deprivation and Sensory Overload

Sensory Deprivation	Insufficient quantity or quality of stimuli; may result from decreased sensory input or monotonous, unpatterned, and unmeaningful input

Defining Characteristics	Contributing Factors	Clients at Risk	Nursing Interventions
Physical behaviors: drowsiness, excessive yawning; *escape behaviors*—eating, exercising, sleeping, running away to escape the deprived environment	*Decreased environmental stimuli:* institutionalized environment; separation from significant others, such as from work and usual sources of stimuli; treatments that decrease access to stimuli, such as bed rest or isolation	Institutionalized clients, especially those in long-term care settings	Maintain sufficient level of arousal by increasing sensory stimuli from all sensory modalities:
Changes in perception: unusual body sensations, preoccupation with somatic complaints (dry mouth, palpitations, difficulty breathing, nausea), change in body image, illusions and hallucinations	*Impaired ability to recieve environmental stimuli:* impaired vision, hearing, taste, smell, touch resulting from treatments such as bandages or body casts that interfere with reception of stimuli, or as a result of depression and other affective disorders	Clients with communicable diseases (*e.g.,* AIDS)	• Instruct the client in self-stimulation methods: counting, singing, reading, reciting poetry. • Structure meaningful tangible stimuli into client's external environment; include a variety of people, ideas, sensations; a pet may provide excellent stimulation.
Changes in cognitive behavior: decreased attention span, inability to concentrate, decreased problem solving and task performance	*Inability to process environmental stimuli:* spinal cord injuries, brain damage, confusion, dementia, medications that depress the central nervous system	Clients confined to bed Clients with sensory alterations (*e.g.,* impaired vision or hearing, or clients with eye patches or body casts) Clients who are depressed Clients from a different culture Clients with a disturbance of the nervous system	• *Visual stimulation* Colorful sheets, pajamas, robes Colorful uniform tops for the nurse Face-to-face human contact Clocks, calendars, wrist watches Pictures, flowers, greeting card • *Auditory stimulation* Call person by name. Conversation that communicates caring as well as orients client Reading to the client Television, radio • *Gustatory and olfactory stimulation* Attention to oral hygiene and properly fitting dentures Food of different textures, colors, temperatures served attractively Smelling food before eating it and recalling pleasurable aromas from the past Seasoning foods or having favorite foods brought from home • *Tactile stimulation* Back rubs Turning and repositioning Passive range-of-motion exercises Hair brushing, combing, washing Foot soaks Hugs Touching of arms or shoulders • *Cognitive input* Orient client to environment. Encourage client participation in self-care. Discuss current events or client's occupation, hobbies, or interests.
Changes in affective behavior: crying, increased irritability and annoyance over small matters, confusion, panic, depression			

(Continued)

Sensory Deprivation	Insufficient quantity or quality of stimuli; may result from decreased sensory input or monotonous, unpatterned, and unmeaningful input

Defining Characteristics	Contributing Factors	Clients at Risk	Nursing Interventions
			Reinforce reality without arguing with a client who is hallucinating. "No, I don't see a man standing there but the linen hamper may be confusing you." • *Emotional input.* Encourage client to share fears, concerns, and perceptions; reassure client that illusions and misperceptions do occur with sensory deprivation. • Since it can be difficult to distinguish the behavioral manifestations of sensory deprivation from sensory overload, introduce more stimulation cautiously. If the added stimulation only increases the client's maladaptive behaviors, consider reducing sensory input because the client may be experiencing sensory overload.

Sensory Overload	Excessive stimuli over which an individual feels little control; brain is unable meaningfully to respond to or ignore stimuli

Similar to those observed in sensory deprivation Elderly clients and clients who have suffered a stroke are more likely to experience confusion or agitation. Young clients are more likely to seek the comfort of their parents' embrace to block out sensory overload.	*Increased internal stimuli:* pain, pressure and discomfort of intrusive tubes (*e.g.,* IVs, catheters, endotracheal tubes, nasogastric tubes), worry about state of health or need to make treatment decisions *Increased external stimuli:* unfamiliar healthcare environment, such as lights, noises, sounds, odors, movement, and constant presence of strangers many of whom touch the body; intrusive procedures such as diagnostic tests and treatments; scratchy linens *Inability perceptually to disregard or selectively ignore some stimuli:* Nervous system disturbances, medications such as caffeine that stimulate the central nervous system arousal mechanism	Any acutely or chronically ill client Clients in pain Clients with intrusive monitoring or treatment equipment Hospitalized clients, especially those in critical care settings Clients with disturbances of the nervous system	• Provide a consistent, predictable pattern of stimulation to help the client develop a sense of control over the environment. • Offer simple explanations before procedures, tests, and examinations. • Establish a schedule with the client for routine care such as eating, bathing, turning, positioning, coughing, and exercise. • Speak calmly with the client and move slowly; communicate confidence. • Explore with the client what stimuli are most distressing and develop a plan to reduce or eliminate these (*e.g.,* incoming phone calls, visitors); ear plugs or pain medication may be indicated. • Be careful not to cause sensory deprivation.

(Adapted in part from Lee KA: Sensory overload, sensory deprivation, and sleep deprivation. In Patrick ML, Woods SL, Craven RF, Rokosky JS, Bruno PM: Medical-Surgical Nursing, pp 103–107. Philadelphia, JB Lippincott, 1986)

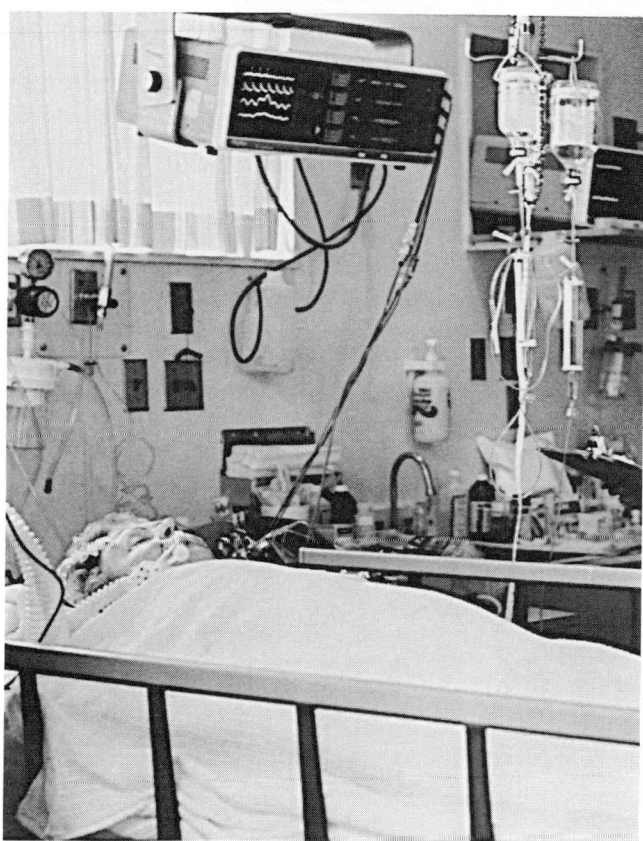

F I G U R E 37-1
Illness, pain, and medication stress the individual's capacity to process normal sensory stimuli and the hospital environment of strange sights, sounds, odors, and people can cause symptoms of sensory overload in some clients. (Photo by Gates Rhodes, courtesy of the School of Nursing, University of Pennsylvania)

constant presence of strangers who not only demand to be spoken to but who also touch and poke at the body; by the strange sights, odors, sounds, and feels of the unfamiliar environment; by the constant presence of pain or discomfort from dressings, IVs, drainage tubes, or endotracheal tubes; and by the ever-present worries about the meaning and course of the illness. Nursing assistance is directed to reducing distressing stimuli and helping the client to gain control over the environment (see Table 37-1).

FACTORS AFFECTING SENSORY STIMULATION

There appears to be considerable variation in the amount of stimuli different individuals consider optimal. Factors influencing the amount and quality of stimuli needed to maintain cortical arousal include developmental considerations, culture, personality/life-style, stress, and illness/medications.

Developmental Considerations. Different types of sensory stimulation are needed for growth as sensory receptors and organs and the nervous system mature. Although the newborn is capable of rudimentary perceptual discriminations at birth, many neural pathways are immature and must be stimulated to develop, become refined, and function adequately. Appropriate stimulation includes soothing, holding, rocking and changes of position (tactile and kinesthetic sensations), singing and being talked to (auditory sensations), and changing patterns of light and shade, such as through the use of mobiles and bright objects (visual sensations).

Developmentally appropriate play develops the child's muscles and coordination, provides an outlet for surplus physical energy, develops communication skills, furnishes sources of learning, acts as a stimulant to creativity, develops social skills, teaches sex roles, provides an outlet for the release of emotional energy, and develops self-insights (Waechter et al, 1985).

Sensory functioning may progressively decline throughout adulthood as the result of aging or chronic illness. The adult may experience the need to compensate for the loss of one type of stimulation by increasing other sources of sensory stimuli.

Culture. An individual's culture may dictate the amount of sensory stimulation considered "normal." For example, the amount of touching a child experiences in a Puerto Rican family may be very different from that experienced by a child in a German family. Similarly, male and female roles may be culturally defined and while the male is expected to respond to the challenge of out-of-the-home sensory stimuli, the female who attempts to do so may be scorned if her place is considered to be in the home. Ethnic norms, religious norms, income group norms, and the norms of subgroups within a culture all influence the amount of sensory stimulation sought by an individual and perceived as meaningful.

Personality/Life-style. Apart from a person's culture, different personality types demand different levels of stimulation. One person may thrive on a steady stream of fast-paced changes and excitement whereas another may feel best when daily routines are rigidly structured and life sends no challenges necessitating changes. Life-style choices can dramatically influence the quantity and quality of stimuli received by an individual. The nurse who elects to work in the emergency room of a large city hospital is exposed to vastly different stimuli than the nurse working on a small unit in a residential long-term care setting.

Stress. Increased sensory stimulation may be sought during periods of low stress simply to maintain cortical arousal. During high-stress periods, multiple stressors may already be overloading the sensory system and decreased sensory stimulation is desired. The stress of physical illness, pain, hospitalization, testing, surgery, and treatment may provide more stimulation than an individual can process and respond to without assistance.

Illness/Medication. Illness can affect the reception of sensory stimuli (*e.g.,* diminution of the sense of touch associated with diabetes and cerebrovascular disease) and their transmission and perception (*e.g.,* neurologic disorders, dementias). Medications that alert or depress the central nervous system may interfere with the perception of sensory stimuli. Finally, certain medications may contribute to impaired sensory functioning by decreasing reception (*e.g.,* captopril, an antihypertensive, can cause taste alteration; aspirin can cause tinnitus, ringing in the ear).

NURSE AS ROLE MODEL

Sensitivity to the important role sensory functioning plays in a person's well-being guides the nurse to promote personal well-being. Awareness of one's own sensory functioning and the stimulation in one's own life is a stepping stone to providing proper stimulation to clients. The nurse works to achieve the following goals:
The nurse will
- Evaluate the quantity and quality of sensory stimuli present in both the home and work
- Identify stimuli important to self-development as a person (mental, physical, and spiritual health) and as a professional nurse
- Manipulate the environment to decrease distressing stimuli and increase positive stimuli
- Practice nursing conscious of the need to promote optimal sensory functioning in clients

ASSESSING SENSORY FUNCTIONING

When assessing a client for sensory disturbances the nurse interviews the client and examines the client for sensory deficits and manifestations of sensory deprivation or overload. Examination of the client's environment is included in the assessment to determine whether it is providing adequate sensory stimulation for

---

Elements in a Sensory Functioning Assessment

Stimulation
"Does your present environment stimulate you? For example, do you have problems sleeping? If so, why?"
"Are you bored? Why?"
"Are you able to read? Watch television? Knit? Why not?"
"Are there other people in your home during the day? Do you spend much time together? How do you spend the time?"
"Who visits you while you are in the hospital?"
Assess the following:
- Reduction in the patterns or meaningfulness of stimulation in each sensory modality
- Changes in stimulation other than decreases (*e.g.,* new or unusual stimulation)
- Developmental appropriateness of stimulation

Reception
"Does anything interfere with the functioning of your senses?"
"Describe any corrective devices you use for sensory impairments."
Assess the following:
- Vision
- Hearing
- Taste
- Smell
- Touch

- Awareness of body position
- Visceral awareness

Transmission–Perception–Reaction
"Are you aware of any problems with your nervous system?"
"Have you found it difficult to communicate verbally?"
Assess the following:
- Consciousness
- Orientation
- Appropriateness of responses
- Ability to perform usual self-care activities
- Ability to follow simple commands
- Decision-making abilities
- Pathology affecting central nervous system
- Prescribed or recreational drugs that affect the central nervous system

Behavioral Manifestations of Sensory Deprivation or Overload
- Perceptual responses: mild to gross sensory distortions (illusions, hallucinations)
- Cognitive responses: thought disorganization, slowness of thought, decreased attention/concentration, difficulty with problem solving and task performance
- Emotional responses: rapid mood changes, anxiety, panic

healthy development. The assessment may be structured using stimulation, reception, transmission, perception, and reaction, the components of the sensory experience. Since clients may adapt to sensory impairments it may be helpful to include someone the client knows well (spouse, parent) in the assessment to see if they have noticed behavioral characteristics in the client that suggest a sensory disturbance (*e.g.,* "I've noticed he turns the TV volume much louder than ever before").

Stimulation

Specific assessments and focused questions are given as suggestions for use in assessing sensory function.

"Do you have problems sleeping? If so, why?"

"Are you bored? Why?"

"Are you able to read? Watch television? Knit? Why not?"

"Are there other people in your house during the day? Do you spend much time together? How do you spend the time?"

"Who visits you while you are in the hospital?"

Assess if there have been any recent changes in sensory stimulation, for example, reduction of stimulation from one or more sensory modalities ("Since my husband died no one touches me anymore. It sounds crazy but I'm hungry to be touched!") or new or unusual stimulation ("Ever since my granddaughter moved in with me my house is always noisy. I can't stand the constant noise and her smoking."). Assess if the type of stimulation present is developmentally appropriate.

High-risk clients for problems related to stimulation include children in nonstimulating environments, the elderly, terminally ill clients, clients on bed rest, clients in isolation, and clients requiring intensive nursing in a critical care setting.

Reception

- Assess for anything that may interfere with sensory reception. "Does anything interfere with the functioning of your senses? Vision? Hearing? Taste? Smell? Touch? Awareness of body position or movement? Awareness of internal body?" Note pathology and effects of treatment (*e.g.,* medications affecting hearing).

  "Describe any corrective devices you use for sensory impairments (glasses, contacts, hearing aids)."

- Assess for visual disturbances.

  "Please read my name tag (or this page of print)." Note if the client can correctly identify objects directly in front of the eyes as well as those requiring peripheral vision. Note eye rubbing, squinting, movements indicating faulty vision (bumping into furniture, overreaching or underreaching for objects), changes in the appearance of the eye (cataracts, swelling) and complaints of eye pain, spots, halos, or other visual disturbances.

- Assess for auditory disturbances.

  "Repeat the words that I will speak softly close to each ear." Note if the client is able to hear equally well from both ears, distinguish voices, locate the direction of a sound, if the client needs to face the person speaking and relies on lip reading, if the client's responses to questions include blank looks, many nods, smiling, or inappropriate responses indicating faulty hearing. Note complaints of ringing or buzzing in ears.

- Assess for gustatory (taste) disturbances.

  "Close your eyes, stick out your tongue, and tell me if what I place on your tongue is sweet, sour, bitter, or salty."

  "Have you been experiencing any strange tastes (bitter, metallic) or aftertastes lately?" Note if the client is able to differentiate sweet, sour, bitter, or salty tastes or reports unusual, persistent taste sensations. Note deficient oral hygiene, ill-fitting dentures, braces, or anything else that might contribute to gustatory disturbances.

- Assess for olfactory (smell) disturbances.

  "Close your eyes and tell me what you smell."

  "Have you smelled odors lately that others cannot smell or have you been especially sensitive to odors?" Note if the client can correctly identify common odors (coffee, vanilla) or has noticed increased sensitivity to odors.

- Assess for tactile (touch) disturbances.

  "Close your eyes and tell me when you feel something (brush skin with cotton ball), if what you feel is dull or sharp (use both ends of safety pin), hot or cold (use items from food tray). Now, keep your eyes closed and tell me what I am placing in your hand (coin, cotton ball, paper clip)." Note if the client can correctly sense touch and distinguish sharp and dull, hot and cold, and different shapes. Note if the client reports decreased sensation in any part of the body; numbness, pins and needles, tingling; or abnormal sensitivity to pain or touch. Note if the client withdraws from being touched.

- Assess for kinesthetic and visceral disturbances.

  "Have you noticed any changes in the way you perceive your body?"

  "Do you feel any unusual pressure or pain inside your body?"

  Note if the client seems unsure of his body parts or body position and if he experiences new internal sensations (fullness, pressure, pain).

High-risk clients for reception problems include persons with visual, auditory, or other sensory impairments.

Transmission–Perception–Reaction

"Are you aware of any problems with your nervous system?" Note if the client follows usual pattern of wakefulness and sleep; if the client is easily aroused; oriented to time, place, and person; able to respond appropriately to stimuli; able to follow simple commands; and capable of decision making and demonstrating usual self-care abilities. Note any pathology affecting the central nervous system (Alzheimer's disease, increased intracranial pressure, stroke). Note if the client is taking any prescribed or recreational drug that stimulates or depresses the central nervous system.

High-risk clients for transmission–perception–reaction problems include confused clients and clients with nervous system impairments.

Defining Characteristics of Sensory Deprivation and Overload

Complete the assessment of the client's sensory functioning by assessing for specific indicators of sensory deprivation or overload (see Table 37-1), including boredom, inactivity, slowness of thought, daydreaming, increased sleeping, thought disorganization, anxiety, panic, illusions, or hallucinations (Schiefer, 1982). It is important to know the client's usual state to be able to identify changes stemming from sensory deprivation or overload.

Nursing Examination

Physical examinations related to the senses are discussed in Chapter 24. Ear and eye tests, whether performed by a physician or the nurse, should be taken into consideration when planning care. Problems with the neurologic system indicate the necessity of further assessment of the sensory experience.

DIAGNOSING

When assessment data point to sensory disturbances that can be treated independently by nursing interventions, nursing diagnoses are developed and labeled **sensory/perceptual alterations**. These alterations may be further specified as visual, auditory, gustatory, olfactory, tactile, or kinesthetic. *Sensory deprivation* and *sensory overload* may also be used to further specify the sensory–perceptual alteration and in some cases may be the etiology.

Common etiologies for sensory-perceptual alterations include

Altered environmental stimuli, excessive or insufficient

Altered sensory reception, transmission or integration

Chemical alterations, endogenous (electrolytes) or exogenous (drugs, etc.)

Psychological stress
(Harley, 1986)

Sample nursing diagnoses in which the sensory–perceptual alteration is the problem are listed in Table 37-2.

Since sensory–perceptual alterations affect many other areas of human functioning, they serve as etiologies for multiple problem statements. Examples of these follow:

Activity intolerance related to impaired balance and coordination (kinesthetic alteration)

Anxiety related to paranoia stemming from hearing impairment, sensory deprivation (specify setting), sensory overload

Impaired verbal communication related to difficulty receiving, transmitting, and perceiving sensory stimuli

Ineffective individual coping related to sensory overload (multiple stressors)

Diversional activity deficit related to impaired vision or hearing

Altered growth and development related to non-stimulating home environment

Potential for injury related to decreased or impaired sensation (specify visual, auditory, tactile, kinesthetic)

Knowledge deficit: means to compensate for sensory impairment (blindness, deafness, etc.) related to lack of previous experience with this problem, unavailability of resources

Knowledge deficit: providing a developmentally stimulating environment related to lack of experience with children's growth and development

Impaired physical mobility related to impaired balance and coordination (kinesthetic alteration)

Altered parenting: failure to provide stimuli for growth related to lack of knowledge, decreased motivation to provide for child's growth and development

Powerlessness related to inability to interact meaningfully with environment

Self-care deficit related to visual impairment, auditory impairment, tactile impairment

Disturbance in body image related to kinesthetic impairment (distorted sense of body parts), sensory deprivation

Disturbance in self-esteem related to sensory–perceptual alterations (specify visual, auditory, etc.)

Disturbance in role performance related to sensory–perceptual alteration (blindness, deafness, etc.)

(Text continues on p. 1048.)

TABLE 37-2
Nursing Diagnoses for Common Sensory–Perceptual Alterations

Title	Etiologic or Contributing Factors	Sample Defining Characteristics
Sensory–perceptual alteration: sensory deficit/excess		
Visual	Eye patches following surgery	"I never realized before how sight-dependent I am. I don't know what time of day it is now unless I have the radio on or smell food coming in."
		"It's frightening not to know who is in my room and what they are doing."
		Client observed sitting in room with blank facial expression; frequently comments on how bored she is and how slowly time is passing; hesitant to move about room without assistance although she has been oriented repeatedly
Auditory	Effects of aging	"You're right. I don't always hear what people are saying anymore so I try not to get involved in conversations. If people insist on talking, I just nod and hope I'm giving the right response."
		Able to hear moderately spoken word close to right ear; cannot hear same from left ear; often startled when someone approaches from left side
		Sits close to TV and radio; loud volume, no history of hearing testing
Gustatory/olfactory	Chemotherapy	"I always seem to have a bitter taste in my mouth now and can't stomach certain foods at all that I used to enjoy, like beef, tomatoes, coffee . . . I also can't take sweets and I used to be a real sweets junkie."
		"Sometimes the very smell of certain foods or even the thought of eating nauseates me."
		Client has been receiving vincristine (cancer chemotherapeutic agent) for last three months; some nausea and vomiting; history of poor oral hygiene
Tactile	Psychologic stress	"I don't know why I feel this way, but I'm hypersensitive to any touch. If anyone even brushes against me I feel burning pain. Even the weight of my clothes against my skin bothers me. I'm trying to move my body as little as possible and keep it protected—but that's obviously impossible when even a breeze assaults me."
		Client observed holding body stiffly looking like she doesn't know what to do with her arms and legs; dressed only in a loose-fitting sundress; reports that she sits at home all day afraid to go out
Kinesthetic	Clinitron bed therapy	"I've been in this bed for two weeks now and I've lost all sense of my body . . . it's a curious weightless feeling that I have . . . sort of like floating in Jello. I'm no longer sure where my body begins and ends, and when I try to lift an arm or leg I feel like I'm in slow motion. I hope I'll be able to walk when I get out of here."
Sensory–perceptual alteration: sensory deprivation	Isolation	"One of the worst things that has happened to me since I found out I had AIDS is that everyone is afraid of me—and no one touches me. I'm so lonely. I've always needed a lot of people around."

(Continued)

Title	Etiologic or Contributing Factors	Sample Defining Characteristics
		"Here in the hospital I think I'm going crazy. I can't leave this room. Everyone who comes in looks the same dressed in those yellow gowns. Lately I've seen some bizarre things that I know can't be real. I look at the clock and it turns into a swirling sun with a sad face that keeps coming closer and closer to me and I'm terrified I'll burn up if it gets too close. That's crazy isn't it? I'm really losing it now."
		Disturbed sleep for last two weeks; during the day yawns excessively and catnaps; limited attention span; states he is unable to concentrate on anything.
Sensory–perceptual alteration: sensory overload	Trauma of rape and aftercare	"When is everyone going to stop touching me? First he wouldn't stop. Now everyone here is poking at me, looking at me, asking me hundreds of questions . . . Why did I have to report this and come to the hospital? Oh please leave me alone. Get out of here everyone. . . .''

Disturbance in personal identity related to sensory deprivation or overload

Sexual dysfunction related to decreased sensation

Impairment of skin integrity related to absent tactile sensation (injury)

Sleep pattern disturbance related to sensory deprivation or overload

Impaired social interaction related to inability to receive and process interactional stimuli

Social isolation related to visual or auditory impairment

Alteration in thought processes (specify: illusions, hallucinations, decreased attention or concentration, etc.) related to sensory deprivation or overload

PLANNING: CLIENT GOALS

In whatever setting nurses encounter and care for clients, optimal sensory stimulation is a priority and nursing care is supportive of the following client goals:
The client will
- Live in a developmentally stimulating and safe environment
- Exhibit a level of arousal that enables the brain to receive and meaningfully organize patterns of stimulation
- Demonstrate intact functioning of the senses: vision, hearing, taste, smell, touch, kinesthetic and visceral awareness
- Maintain orientation to time, place, and person
- Respond appropriately (verbally and nonverbally) to sensory stimuli while executing self-care activities

Clients with impaired sensory functioning require individualized goals similar to the following:
The client will
- Report feeling safe and in control of the environment
- Describe different types of meaningful stimuli present in the environment
- Demonstrate (describe) appropriate self-care behaviors for visual impairment, hearing impairment, or other sensory impairment
- Verbalize acceptance of the sensory deficit

IMPLEMENTING

The nurse can assist clients to improve sensory functioning by teaching clients and significant others means to stimulate the senses, teaching clients with intact and impaired senses appropriate self-care behaviors, and interacting therapeutically with impaired clients. In this section the nursing interventions described are preventing sensory alteration, stimulating the senses, meeting the needs of the visually impaired, meeting the needs of the hearing impaired, communicating with a confused person, and communicating with an unconscious person.

Preventing Sensory Alteration and Stimulating the Senses

The most effective means by which sensory alteration can be managed is prevention. The key to prevention is, with the client's help, to create a functional and meaningful environment while keeping limitations in mind. The creation of such an environment requires careful observation, analysis, and creative planning.

RESEARCH IN NURSING *Making a Difference*

Sensory Stimulation

Maintaining an appropriate level of sensory stimulation is a major nursing challenge. Sensitivity to overload or deprivation requires an acute awareness of the environmental factors that contribute to the phenomenon. This problem is continuously addressed by nurses in acute-care settings, where the noise and activity levels affect the client's sensory system.

Related Research

Hilton B: Noise in acute patient care areas. Res Nurs Health 8:283–291, 1985

Hilton conducted this study to collect baseline data about sound in patient care areas. Variables examined were sound sources, sound levels, client perceptions of sound levels, effects of sound, and what sounds could be modified. The following data were significant: (1) smaller hospitals are quieter than larger hospitals; (2) sound levels dropped at night on several units but remained high in the recovery room and intensive care unit of the large hospitals; (3) levels of talking by staff, patients, and visitors in all units were louder than necessary; and (4) clients in the recovery room had strong negative feelings about the noise level, while clients on other units were satisfied with sound levels. Recommendations include consideration of equipment

sound level prior to purchase and inservice education to promote noise level reduction.

Salyer J, Stuart B: Nurse–patient interaction in the intensive care unit. Heart Lung 14(1):20–24, 1985

This study was done to determine if there was a lack of therapeutic communication between alert, intubated clients and nurses who work in intensive care settings. The researchers found that clients seldom initiated interaction with nurses, and that nurses are commonly silent during administration of client care. Based on the conclusion that some nurses were unable to recognize or accept client communication needs, it is suggested that data from the study will help nurses strengthen communication skills and become more aware of nonverbal cues.

Summary

Nursing research has shown that sensory overload and deprivation produce anxiety and stress, impeding healing. Prevention requires sensitive and individualized attention. Further research needs to examine the role of environmental sound level as the cause or prevention of feelings of isolation and alienation in the hospital setting. Additionally, research has demonstrated that communication needs of clients must be identified and met by nurses as they give care, especially in critical care areas.

Numerous nursing measures can be considered in planning care. Appropriate measures for implementing will depend on the circumstances (Table 37-3). Well-being is promoted by offering care that provides rest and comfort (see Chaps 29 and 30). Client discomfort should be controlled whenever possible. The nurse should be aware of the need for sensory aids and prostheses, such as eyeglasses, contact lenses, hearing aids, dentures, canes, and artificial limbs, and these should be made available as needed. Physical activity and exercise, which help maintain normal sensory perceptions and decrease the likelihood of sensory alteration, should be encouraged (exercises are discussed in Chap 28).

Stimulate as many senses as possible. Varied sights, sounds, smells, body positions, and textures can be helpful in providing a variety of sensations. Be aware of cultural factors and take them into consideration when offering nursing care. This is especially important when caring for clients from cultures other than your own.

Explain procedures to the client because a more informed client is better able to handle fears, frustration,

and confusion. Explanations also help prevent the client from feeling that space and body are invaded. Individuals experiencing perceptual and thought distortions should have the opportunity to acknowledge that fact. The opportunity to discuss such experiences and be reassured that they are normal and usually temporary generally eases anxiety.

Teaching is a significant nursing responsibility. The nurse can aid clients in sensory self-stimulation and guide parents in stimulation of their infants and children. Table 37-3 gives helpful suggestions for teaching clients about sensory stimulation.

Meeting the Needs of the Visually Impaired

When caring for a client with a sensory deficit it is important for the nurse to check with the physician if the problem is temporary, permanent, partial, or complete and the degree to which the problem is likely to affect

(Text continues on p. 1051.)

T A B L E   37-3
Suggestions for Stimulating the Senses

Sense	Client	Nurse
Vision	Surround yourself with different colors and with an environment that changes (walk through a mall, sit by a window where you see people come and go).	Wear visually stimulating and comforting colors. Keep meaningful visual stimuli such as photos, greeting cards, toys, or flowers near client. Position clients with impaired mobility where they can see out a window or watch local traffic on the unit.
	Develop a sensitivity to changes in nature (weather patterns, dawn to night cycle, changing seasons, changes in a plant or animal).	
	Use visual devices to keep oriented (watches, calendars, newspaper, TV).	
	Use crossword puzzles and games to stimulate mental activities.	
	Create favorite scenes in your mind, paying attention to tiny details.	
Hearing	Decrease or eliminate distressing auditory stimuli (change bedroom, talk with family members about noise of stereos and other such equipment, use earplugs, use headphones to listen to soft music).	Speak in a warm and pleasant tone and communicate caring to the client.
	Develop sensitivity to different sounds (music, chirping birds, night sounds, different voices).	Use your voice to orient client to environment and current situation (*e.g.,* procedure, treatment).
	Use the telephone to maintain contact with family and friends.	Avoid speaking about the client to others within the client's hearing.
	Use TV, radio, cassettes to keep current and to stimulate mental activities.	Remember that clients overhearing snatches of conversation outside their room often presume it is about *them!*
	Recall favorite sounds of the past with the situations in which they were heard.	Decrease extraneous noise (intercom, movement of carts, loud converstions of staff); use carpets and sound-absorbing material whenever possible.
Taste	Experiment with foods of different tastes (seasonings), colors, temperature, and textures; realize that as taste buds age, things will no longer taste the same.	Consult with the dietitian about preparing meals with varied taste sensations; serve meals attractively.
	Practice thorough oral hygiene and have regular dental examinations.	Perform routine oral hygiene for clients who are unable to do this for themselves.
	Recall foods that tasted especially good in the past and the events surrounding these tastes (*e.g.,* grandmother baking cookies or homemade bread).	
Smell	Consciously savor smells that are pleasant; decrease or eliminate noxious odors.	Keep the client's room well ventilated, utilizing opportunities when the client is out of the room to air it out.
	Recall pleasant aromas or smells from the past and the events surrounding them (*e.g.,* smell of the ocean as the vacation house was neared, smell of fresh pine in the house at Christmas, the body scent of a loved person or animal).	Remove dressings, drainage, and any equipment with odors from the client's room as quickly as possible.
		Encourage clients to focus on pleasant or familiar smells, such as coffee, newspaper, or flowers.
		Avoid wearing heavy perfumes.
Touch	Consciously surround yourself with different textures and let yourself feel and enjoy them (scratchy afghan; a puppy's moist, wet tongue; soft petal of a flower; smooth silk scarf; mug of hot chocolate).	Include different textures in the client's environment (silky pillow sham from home, soft sheepskin, wooley blanket).

(Continued)

Sense	Client	Nurse
	Allow these textures to evoke memories of past tactile experiences (granddaughter's hug may bring back memories of hugs from own children, scrap of fabric may recall a prom dress or wedding gown or baby blanket).	Respect the client's need and desire to be touched or not touched (touch the client's forearm or shoulder, hug the client).
	Recognize need to be touched and tell someone "I need a hug today!"	Utilize physical care (bath time, foot soaks, hair care, back massages, turning and positioning, passive range of motion) to provide tactile stimulation.
	Receive tactile stimulation from a pet.	Limit intrusive procedures and times when the client needs to be uncomfortably manipulated.
General Nursing Strategies in the Hospital or Other Residential Care Setting		Encourage the client to participate in activities that require exploration of the environment (exercise, feeling, tasting, touching, moving, listening).
		Use conversation to explore areas of interest to the client.
		Encourage the client to share feelings.
		Familiarize the environment by encouraging the client to wear own clothes and keep personal items nearby.
		Suggest the use of self-stimulation techniques—humming, singing, whistling, reciting, memory review, and problem solving.

the client's everyday functioning. The nurse cannot develop a realistic teaching plan without this information.

The nurse's first priority is to teach clients self-care behaviors to maintain vision and prevent blindness. Lindberg and Kruszewski (1983) offer the following suggestions:
- Avoid rubbing eyes.
- Avoid eyestrain.
- Avoid damage from ultraviolet rays.
- Protect eyes from foreign bodies.
- Keep eyeglasses clean, protected, adjusted.
- Avoid nonprescription eyedrops and seek attention for symptom.
- Avoid cleaning eyes or contact lenses with soiled articles.
- Use caution with aerosol sprays.
- Use caution with ammonia, lye, and so on.
- Visit your physician frequently if you are prone to eye problems.
- Know the danger signals that indicate serious eye problems: persistent eye redness; pain or discomfort, especially after injury; visual disturbances; crossing eyes; growth on or near the eyes; discharge or increased tearing; or pupil irregularities.

The following guidelines are recommended for communicating with persons who are visually impaired:
- Acknowledge your presence in the client's room. Identify yourself by name.
- Speak in a normal tone of voice. Remember that the blind person will be unable to pick up most nonverbal cues during communication.

- Explain the reason for touching the person before doing so.
- Keep the call light or bell within easy reach of the person and place the bed in the lowest position.
- Orient the person to sounds in the environment.
- Orient the person to the arrangement of the room and its furnishings. Clear pathways for the person and do not rearrange furnishings. Clarify this fact with housekeeping personnel also.
- Assist with ambulation by walking slightly ahead of the person, allowing the person to grasp your arm.
- Stay in the person's field of vision if the person has partial or reduced peripheral vision.
- Provide diversions using other senses.
- Indicate to the person when the conversation has ended and when you are leaving the room.

Meeting the Needs of the Hearing Impaired

Temporary hearing losses are most often *conductive* in nature, that is, they are due to a problem with the external or middle ear (wax build-up, foreign body obstruction, infection). *Sensorineural hearing losses* are caused by inner ear or central nervous system problems and may not be totally correctable. Health teaching to prevent hearing problems includes the following recommendations:
- Avoid excessive noises.
- Avoid inserting sharp objects into ears.

- Avoid excessive cleaning of ears.
- Avoid practices that can cause infection; treat infection early.
- Know the symptoms of hearing loss: asking frequently that statements be repeated, inability to hear at a distance, need to see the person who is talking, leaning forward or turning an ear toward the speaker, answering inappropriately, talking too loudly, inability to carry on a phone conversation, strained facial expression (Lindberg and Kruszewski, 1983, pp 307, 312)

The following are recommended guidelines for communicating with persons with hearing deficits:

- Orient the person to your presence before initiating conversation. This may be done by moving so you can be seen or by *gently* touching the person.
- Decrease background noises (TV, radio) if possible before you speak.
- Position yourself so the light is on your face and the person can see your lips and expressions.
- Talk directly to the person while facing the person or angle the chair so that your voice reaches the ear that hears best. If the person is able to speech-read, use simple sentences and speak in a quiet, natural manner and pace. Be aware of nonverbal communication.
- Do not chew gum, cover your mouth, or turn away when talking with the person.
- Demonstrate or pantomime ideas you wish to express, as appropriate.
- Use sign language or finger spelling, as appropriate.
- Write any ideas that you cannot convey to the person in another manner.

Communicating With a Confused Person

The client who lacks the mental ability to process environmental stimuli may be aware of this inability and find it frustrating. This client needs the nurse's support to make adjustments to this limitation. Other clients may be oblivious to the deficiency. In both instances the nurse must protect the safety of the client while providing optimal sensory stimulation. Nursing interventions include

- Using frequent face-to-face human contact to communicate the social process (use touch when appropriate, walking arm in arm, hug, back rub)
- Speaking calmly, simply, and directly to the client and allowing sufficient time for the client to think before responding
- Orienting and reorienting the client to the environment and filling the client's personal space with as many personal objects as possible
- Using conversation, watches, clocks, calendar, newspaper, TV, radio, and other such devices to orient the client to time, place, and person
- Clearly communicating that the client is expected to perform all self-care activities of which the client is capable

- Keeping the emphasis on client strengths rather than on deficiencies and verbally reinforcing strengths
- Offering the client simple explanations for care, new activities, and so on
- Varying environmental stimuli gradually while keeping the environment structured enough that the client feels "comfortable" and "at home"
- Using objects from the client's past (baseball, picture of a train, photo) to spark reminiscences and discussions
- Reinforcing reality if the client is delusional

Communicating With an Unconscious Person

The following are recommended guidelines for communicating with an unconscious client:

- Be careful of what is said in the person's presence. Hearing is believed to be the last sense lost in the unconscious person, and therefore the person is often likely to hear what is being said, even though there does not appear to be a response.
- Assume the person can hear you. Talk with the person in a normal tone of voice about things you would ordinarily discuss.
- Speak to the person before touching. Remember that touch can be a very effective means of communication with the unconscious person.
- Keep environmental noises at as low a level as possible. This helps the person focus on the communication.

EVALUATING

While implementing a plan of nursing care designed to decrease excessive sensory stimuli or increase meaningful stimuli the nurse evaluates the effectiveness of the plan by observing for a decrease in the behavioral manifestations of sensory deprivation or overload. It may be concluded that the plan of care is working if a client who had begun to withdraw and spend most of the day lying in bed with a blank facial expression appears more alert and begins to initiate conversations and to take an interest in personal care. The nurse also evaluates the client's ability to interact appropriately with the environment while practicing necessary self-care behaviors. The client's achievement of the individualized goals specified in the plan of care is evaluated at set times.

The nurse also evaluates the client's need for nursing versus ability to manage the plan of care independently. Ideally the client and family learn to manipulate the environment to promote optimal sensory stimulation for growth and development. Clients with specific sensory impairments are evaluated for their knowledge of the impairment, acceptance, management of the treatment regimen, and ability to perform usual self-care activities

N U R S I N G   P R O C E S S   *in Clinical Practice*

The nurse uses each phase of the nursing process when identifying and treating sensory–perceptual alterations categorized as nursing diagnoses. Quality care depends on the nurse's knowledge and clinical skills as described earlier in this chapter. Following in outline format are the assessment priorities, client goals, nursing interventions, and evaluation criteria for two common types of age-related sensory deprivation problems:

> *Sensory perceptual alteration: sensory deprivation related to parent's inability to provide a developmentally stimulating environment*
>
> *Sensory perceptual alteration: chronic sensory deprivation related to effects of aging and institutionalization*

In the case study that follows the development of these diagnoses, nursing care is described for a non–English-speaking client who is experiencing mixed sensory deprivation and overload on admission to the maternity unit in a large teaching hospital.

Sensory Deprivation Related to Inadequate Parenting

Studies have shown that sensory organs and nerve fibers need early sensory stimulation to develop normally both structurally and functionally. Waechter, Phillips, and Holaday (1985) support the hypothesis of "sensitive periods," which holds that the quantity or quality of desired learning is diminished after the passing of the optimal time period. Parents may fail to provide a developmentally stimulating environment for their child for many reasons:

- Lack of knowledge of the child's growth and development needs
- Lack of motivation to promote the child's development
- Inadequate resources: parenting skills, finances, and so on

Assessment

- Utilize well-baby/child visits to monitor the child's development (gross motor behavior, fine motor, adaptive, language, personal–social).
- Assess if the child is receiving the stimulation and interactional experiences with the environment necessary to develop optimally. For example, if an infant is slow to crawl, see if parents and caretakers are providing supervised time to explore the environment on the floor versus leaving the infant in a baby chair, swing, or some other device all day. Similarly, if a child's expressions are dull and the child's language development is slow, assess the quality of human interaction/communication the child is receiving.
- Assess if the child's sensory–perceptual abilities are intact; identify sensory impairments and make appropriate referrals.
- If a lack of environmental stimulation is suspected, assess for possible etiologies: parents' lack of knowledge, motivation, skill, or resources; inadequate child care outside the home; other such factors.

Client Goals

The child will

- Appear alert and interested in the environment
- Demonstrate improved sensory stimulation by achieving targeted developmental milestones (specify these)

The parents will

- Identify the relationship between sensory stimulation and the child's development
- Suggest reasons for the child's limited sensory experiences to date
- Describe a realistic and developmentally appropriate plan to increase visual, auditory, olfactory, gustatory, and tactile stimulation for the child
- Verbalize commitment to the above plan

Interventions

Interventions should be tailored to the etiology of the problem. If the parents are eager to participate in the plan of care and simply lack knowledge

- Offer suggestions for increasing environmental stimulation and role model appropriate interactional behaviors.

> *Visual:* Vary colors in the child's environment, increase access to out-of-the-home stimulation (parks, stores, fire engines, and other such stimuli), offer the child books with interesting pictures, limit television.
>
> *Auditory:* Talk with and sing or hum to the child, read stories to the child, have the child join a storytelling group at the library, teach the child to become sensitive to nature's sounds or other sounds in the environment.
>
> *Olfactory:* Allow the child to identify and distinguish different odors; role model for the child savoring special aromas (pizza coming out of the oven).
>
> *Gustatory:* Encourage the child to experiment with foods of different tastes, shapes, colors, textures, and temperatures; recognize that children enjoy finger foods, foods that are crispy, chewy, or bubbly.
>
> *Tactile:* Increase body contact with the child by means of games and sports as well as through demonstrative affection (hugs,

holding child in lap, stroking face, and so on); if possible, allow the child to select a pet.
- Discuss with the parents developmentally appropriate play activities for children that will enable the child to learn social behavior, develop cognitive abilities, develop gross and fine motor skills, and work through emotional conflicts.
- Refer parents to parenting education group.

If the parents lack the motivation to provide a developmentally stimulating environment for the child, intensive counseling is indicated with follow-up to ensure that the child is receiving adequate care. Counseling should explore the parents' experiences as children, the meaning the child holds for the parents, and the probability that the parents will learn and be motivated to use adequate parenting skills. If parents are resistant to counseling and child neglect is suspected, the nurse is legally responsible to report the family for evaluation.

If lack of resources is contributing to the parents' difficulty in stimulating the child's development, available resources are explored. A referral to social service may be indicated.

Evaluative Criteria
The child and parents meet above goals.

Chronic Sensory Deprivation Related to Effects of Aging

Although the phenomenon of acute sensory deprivation has been carefully studied by nurses and other researchers, less attention has been paid to chronic sensory deprivation, a condition experienced by many of the elderly. The elderly person who has multiple sensory deficits or who lives in a deprived environment is a prime candidate for chronic sensory deprivation. Symptoms of this disorder will most likely be gradual in onset and are all too often mistaken for senility (Gioiella and Bevil, 1985).

Assessment
To define the extent of the problem and its etiologies, Gioiella and Bevil recommend careful data collection in the following areas: (1) sensory status; (2) level of mobility; (3) preferred stimulation level; (4) sensory, perceptual, and social environment; (5) mental status; (6) behavioral changes; and (7) personal resources. Using assessment guidelines presented earlier in this chapter, the nurse assesses the elderly person's vision, hearing, taste, smell, touch, and kinesthetic and visceral awareness. It is critical to understand that some older persons have a need to deny sensory impairment and may evolve remarkable compensatory abilities. Behavioral changes (*e.g.,* withdrawal or the paranoia that many hearing-impaired elderly demonstrate) may be the best indicator of an underlying sensory problem.

Sensory Status
The senses of vision, hearing, and touch (and to a lesser degree taste and smell) all decline with age. Moreover, many of the chronic illnesses experienced by the elderly impair sensory functioning. Common sensory problems include vision problems such as cataracts, presbyopia (condition of aging in which decreased elasticity of the lens hinders accommodation to close vision), glaucoma, and macular degeneration; hearing problems such as presbycusis (age-related hearing loss in which there is decreased ability to distinguish higher frequencies); diminution of touch with diabetes and cerebrovascular disease; and altered body sense or awareness associated with restricted mobility and arthritis, cardiovascular and respiratory diseases, and neurologic disorders involving some degree of paralysis.

Level of Mobility
The less mobile an elderly client is, the more dependent the client is on the immediate environment and the more likely to experience sensory deprivation in an impoverished environment. The nurse needs to determine the client's physical ability to ambulate; the need for supportive devices (braces, canes, walkers, wheelchairs, railings, ramps); the client's motivation to be mobile; the presence of external factors hindering mobility ("I'm afraid if I go out of the house I'll be mugged"); and the need for support services (physical therapy, walking partner, transportation assistance, planned reinforcement).

Preferred Stimulation
Individuals vary greatly in the amount of stimulation they need. One older woman sitting quietly may be enjoying reminiscences that effectively stimulate the brain whereas another woman may be utterly bored and becoming disoriented.

Sensory, Perceptual, and Social Environment
The client's environment is assessed to determine if it presents a sufficient *variety* of meaningful sensory, cognitive, and emotional stimulation. Determine if each sense is being stimulated, if the client's mental abilities are being challenged, and if different emotions are being evoked. In caring families there often is a tendency to "do for" the older person, which may be counterproductive. The older person who has no need to meet everyday demands may feel useless and lose abilities not being used.

Mental Status
Changes in mental status or behavior may be the first indication of sensory deprivation. Assess for disorientation to time, place, or person; altered ability to concentrate or problem solve; and perceptual changes such as illusions or hallucinations.

Behavioral Changes

Significant behavioral changes include personality changes such as boredom and apathy, restlessness, withdrawal, and paranoia; alterations in sleep–wake patterns; decreased attention to personal hygiene and appearance; change in responses to others and communication patterns; and rapid mood swings.

Personal Resources

It is important to assess how well the client has coped with stresses in the past and the adequacy of supports available to the client at the present time.

Client Goals

The client will

- Demonstrate orientation to time, place, and person
- Demonstrate interest in everyday self-care activities
- Demonstrate a decrease in the perceptual, cognitive, and emotional responses indicating sensory deprivation (specify)
- Actively participate in a plan to increase sensory stimulation
  The client's caretakers (family, nursing staff) will
- Identify factors contributing to sensory deprivation
- Develop a realistic plan to increase sensory, cognitive, and emotional stimulation

Interventions

- Make every effort to correct client's sensory impairments (*e.g.,* medical evaluation and treatment of sensory deficits; correct use and care of glasses, contact lenses, hearing aids, ambulation aids).
- Make sure that the client has adequate periods of

rest and that daytime activities prevent boredom and catnapping. Discourage the use of sedatives. Assess the central nervous system effect of any other medications the client is taking.
- Implement the plan to increase sensory stimulation (see Table 37-3). Homebound or institutionalized elderly may benefit greatly from visits by children. Pet therapy is an excellent source of stimulation. Simple activities like rolling a colorful, large, soft ball among four people seated at a table can effectively stimulate multiple senses (vision, hearing, touch, kinesthetic) for confused clients. Exercise classes for the elderly also provide excellent stimulation.
- Make a concerted effort to increase the client's mobility and encourage changes in the environment. Utilize family and community resources to get the homebound client out of the house. Implement a plan to assist institutionalized clients to visit other parts of the institution, to get outside, and to participate in scheduled social events. Volunteers may be extremely helpful once committed to a plan of action.
- When interacting with the elderly client, communicate that the client is important and valued and make your expectations known.
- Avoid endorsing confusion. Gently reorient the client to reality whenever delusional statements are made.
- Keep the environment safe for the client.

Evaluative Criteria

Client and caretakers meet above goals.

C A S E   S T U D Y

Two days ago, Mrs. Philomela Palikias delivered by cesarean birth a 32-week old, small-for-gestational-age infant girl weighing 3 lb 8 oz. Because of her size and respiratory distress, the infant was placed in the neonatal intensive care unit. Postpartal assessments indicate that Mrs. Palikias's physical progress is satisfactory. However, the nurses are concerned about her mental status. Mrs. Palikias arrived in the United States 3 months ago with her husband. Both speak only Greek and neither has family in the United States.

Assessment Findings

Recorded in the client's progress notes the evening of her second postpartal day is the following nursing assessment.
12/4/89 9 PM Client refused to get out of bed again this evening—demonstrates no interest in seeing baby; to date has not ambulated to neonatal intensive care unit. Refusing to learn/participate in self-care activities: ex-

pressing breast milk, performing perineal care. Nurses throughout the day reported sudden mood changes: apathy, frustration–panic, and hostility. Unable to find someone who speaks Greek to serve as translator. Husband does not speak English but appears very concerned about his wife.

N. Gable, RN

Nursing Diagnosis

> Sensory–perceptual alteration: mixed sensory deprivation and overload related to unfamiliar hospital environment (different culture) and stress of cesarean birth and infant's prematurity

Planning

The nurse recognizes that the client's behaviors are most likely related to her

- Being in a strange environment in which she cannot communicate

- Lacking familiar supports
- Being bombarded by new stimuli: cesarean birth; discomfort and pain; fear about the baby; fear about her parenting skills; strangers handling her body for reasons she does not understand; unfamiliar sights, sounds, smells, tastes, and touches of the hospital environment; unfamiliar feel of her own body (postsurgery and deliver), and so on

The nurse's first move is to search the hospital (and outside community if necessary) to find an interpreter to explain to Mrs. Palikias what is happening. With the assistance of the interpreter the nurse and client agree on the following short-term goals:

Prior to discharge the client will
- Demonstrate increased "comfort" in the hospital environment (absence of mood swings, apathy, frustration–panic, hostility)
- Resume usual self-care activities
- Demonstrate interest in her baby by visiting the neonatal intensive care unit, holding the baby, expressing her milk, and so on

The long-term goal for the client is to develop communication strategies that will enable her to control the amount and quality of sensory stimulation she receives from her environment.

Implementation

The nurse needs the following specialized abilities in implementing the plan of care:
- Knowledge of and respect for different cultures and their influence on health and human functioning
- Ability to empathize with a young woman experiencing multiple stressors (sensory overload) with few customary supports
- Strong interpersonal skills and creative ability to communicate well to non–English-speaking client using body language, services of interpreter, and so on
- Strong assessment skills and knowledge of factors contributing to sensory alterations and of nursing interventions to prevent and treat sensory alterations
- Knowledge and clinical skills of maternity nursing
- Ability to communicate to client that what she is experiencing is understandable and that help is available
- Teachng and counseling skills to prepare the client to assume new mothering role with confidence

- Ability and willingness to "go the extra mile" with this client to make sure she is not lost in the system and discharged without receiving the assistance she needs
- Interpersonal and leadership skills to help the nursing staff view this client as a challenge and together to be committed to her plan of care
- Human caring, compassion, strong sense of accountability for delivering quality care

Documentation

Sample documentation of the first session with the interpreter follows in the traditional note format:

12/5/89 10:00 AM First session with interpreter and client at 9:00 AM. Client's face brightened as soon as she heard someone speak to her in Greek. Basically, client shared she didn't care too much about what was happening to her but she was terrified about the baby and afraid of what everyone was doing to the baby. Directed interpreter to orient client to her environment, daily routine, and neonatal intensive care unit. Client appeared very anxious when she first saw baby but looked content when able to hold her. Scheduled teaching session for tomorrow AM when interpreter will come for 1 hour. Client resting comfortably at present.

R. Traner, RN

The following is an example of SOAP documentation;

12/5/89 9:00 PM #4 Sensory–perceptual alteration: mixed sensory deprivation and overload related to unfamiliar hospital environment and stress of cesarean birth and infant's prematurity

S:

O: Cried after husband left this evening; refused post-partal check; turned away from nurses

A: Still feels overwhelmed by newness of all that is happening to her and tries to "shut out" what she can't handle

P: Continue to intervene with help of interpreter; focus on helping client develop more control over her situation; proceed at slow pace; referral to social service for follow-up care

N. Gable, RN

Evaluation

Short-term goal achievement is evaluated each shift. See the care plan for related evaluative statements. Long-term goal achievement is ongoing.

N U R S I N G   C A R E   P L A N   *for Mrs. Palikias*

Nursing Diagnosis: Sensory–perceptual alteration: mixed sensory deprivation and overload related to unfamiliar hospital environment (different culture) and stress of cesarean birth and infant's prematurity

(Continued)

NURSING CARE PLAN (Continued)

Signs and Symptoms: No interest in baby or self-care activities; limited ability to concentrate on new tasks (pericare, expressing breast milk); sudden mood changes—apathy, frustration–panic, hostility

Long-Term Goal: Client will develop communication strategies that will enable her to control the amount and quality of sensory stimulation she receives from the environment.

Goals	Nursing Actions	Rationale	Evaluative Statement
Prior to discharge the client will: 1. Demonstrate increased "comfort" in the hospital environment (decreased or absent mood swings: apathy, frustration–panic, hostility)	• Secure assistance of an interpreter and work with the interpreter to Orient the client to her surroundings (explaining reasons for equipment, procedures, treatment) Determine the client's needs Reassure the client that what she is experiencing is "normal" given her recent stresses (moving to new country, cesarean birth of first child, infant's prematurity) • Have the interpreter teach the nurse several Greek words and make recommendations about how the client can personalize her environment. • See if the interpreter can explain usual customs regarding childbirth and aftercare in Greece. • Limit the number of nurses and other persons interacting with the client. Attempt to have the same nurse each shift caring for her so that a trusting nurse–client relationship can be developed. • Schedule care to allow for uninterrupted periods of sleep and rest.	Sensory deprivation results from *meaningless,* unpatterned stimuli; once the client understands her environment she can respond to it appropriately. Clients experiencing strange perceptual, cognitive, and affective responses to sensory deprivation/overload often fear they are going "crazy" and hesitate to share their feelings. Contributing to sensory deprivation is the absence of *familiar* sounds (native language), sights, tastes, or scents. Having the husband provide usual food, music, and other familiar items may reduce sensory deprivation. Sleep deprivation contributes to other sensory alterations.	12/6/89 Goal met. Client is quiet but no longer apathetic, fearful, or hostile. Moving about in hospital with more confidence. *N. Gable, RN*
2. Resume independent self-care activities	• Utilize services of interpreter to teach client importance of ambulating and becoming independent again in self-care measures.		12/6/89 Goal partially met. Client is ambulating but she resists pericare and is fearful when expressing breast milk.

(Continued)

N U R S I N G   C A R E   P L A N   (Continued)

Goals	Nursing Actions	Rationale	Evaluative Statement
	• Have interpreter write simple directions for follow-up care, times when baby may be visited after client is discharged, and so on. Share these instructions with the client's husband. • See if husband has bilingual friends or work acquaintances who might be willing to help the client when she gets home until she has established a comfortable routine of care for the baby and is knowledgeable about community resources.	Cognitive responses to sensory deprivation/overload include decreased attention span/concentration and problem-solving ability. Written instructions, husband's knowledge will reinforce the client's learning. Careful discharge planning is necessary to ensure that the client can manage new parenting responsibilities in an unfamiliar country.	*Recommendation:* continue teaching with assistance of interpreter. *N. Gable, RN*
3. Demonstrate interest in her baby by visiting the neonatal intensive care unit, holding the baby, expressing her milk, and other such activities.	• Learn and respect cultural norms for new mothering behaviors. • Assist the client to ambulate to unit to see the baby; if interpreter is available, have the person explain equipment surrounding the baby and answer the client's questions about the baby.	The client may be refusing to visit the unit to protect herself from barrage of frightening stimuli (sensory overload); the goal is for her to become familiar with the unit so she will be able to focus on bonding with her daughter.	12/6/89 Goal met. Client now visiting baby in the unit on her own. *N. Gable, RN*

K E Y   P O I N T S

■ The senses of vision, hearing, smell, taste, and touch keep an individual in contact with the external environment. The kinesthetic and visceral senses arise from muscles and hollow organs, respectively, and orient the individual to the internal environment.

■ The brain must be alert or aroused to receive stimuli and respond appropriately. The reticular activating system, with its many ascending and descending connections to other areas of the brain, monitors and regulates incoming sensory stimuli and thus maintains, enhances, or inhibits cortical arousal.

■ Sensory alterations occur when a person experiences decreased sensory input or input that is monotonous, unpatterned, or meaningless (sensory deprivation); or excessive sensory input such that the brain is unable to respond meaningfully (sensory overload).

■ Responses to both sensory deprivation and overload include perceptual changes (mild to gross distortions or hallucinations), cognitive changes (decreased attention and concentration, decreased problem-solving ability), and affective changes (apathy, anxiety, fear, panic, anger, depression or rapid mood swings).

■ Clients at high risk for sensory deprivation include those experiencing decreased environmental stimuli (homebound or institutionalized clients, clients on bed rest or in isolation) and those with impaired ability to receive or process environmental stimuli (clients with sensory deficits, clients from a different culture, clients with certain affective disorders and disturbances of the nervous system, clients with bandages or casts that interfere with sense reception, clients taking medications that affect the central nervous system).

■ Clients at high risk for sensory overload include acutely ill clients, clients in critical care settings, clients in pain, clients with intrusive and discomforting monitoring or treatment equipment, and clients with disturbances of the nervous system.

■ Factors affecting sensory stimulation include age, culture, personality/life style, stress, illness, and medication.

■ A comprehensive nursing assessment of sensory functioning includes an examination of the client for sensory deficits and manifestations of sensory deprivation or overload and an examination of the client's environment to see if it is providing adequate sensory stimulation for healthy development.

■ Nursing diagnoses may be written specifically addressing sensory–perceptual alterations (visual, auditory, olfactory, gustatory, tactile, sensory deprivation, sensory overload) or identifying the effect sensory–perceptual alterations have in other areas of human functioning (verbal communication, self-care, social interaction, thought processes).

■ Small modifications in a client's environment and in the nurse's pattern of interacting may be all that is needed to prevent sensory alterations.

■ Sensory deprivation during a child's formative years may yield permanent results because sensory organs and nerve fibers need early sensory stimulation to develop normally both structurally and functionally. Parents may fail to provide a developmentally stimulating environment for their child because of lack of knowledge, decreased motivation, or inadequate resources.

■ The elderly person who has multiple sensory deficits or who lives in a nonstimulating environment is at high risk for chronic sensory deprivation. Symptoms of this disorder are frequently mistaken for senility.

BIBLIOGRAPHY

Anderson J: Sensory intervention with the preterm infant in the neonatal intensive care unit. Am J Occup Ther 40(1):19–26, 1986

Bolin RH: Sensory deprivation: An overview. Nurs Forum 13(3):240–258, 1974

Brown IA: The widespread influence of olfaction. J Neurosurg Nurs 17(5):273–279, 1985

Burnside IM: Touching is talking. Am J Nurs 73(12):2060–2063, 1973

DeForest J, Porter A: Cuddlers: A volunteer infant stimulation program. Canadian Nurse 77(4):38–40, 1981

Gioiella E, Bevil C: Nursing Care of the Aging Client. Norwalk, CT, Appleton-Century-Crofts, 1985

Koniak-Griffin D, Ludington-Hol SM: Developmental and temperament outcomes of sensory stimulation in healthy infants. Nurs Res 37(2):70–76, 1988

Lindberg JB, Kruszewski AZ: Special senses and the environment. In Lindberg J, Hunter M, Kruszewski A: Introduction to Person-Centered Nursing, pp 297–315. Philadelphia, JB Lippincott, 1983

MacKinnon-Kesler S: Maximizing your ICU patient's sensory and perceptual environment. Canadian Nurse 79(5):41–45, 1983

Morganett BA: Nature hikes for nursing home residents. Geriatric Nursing 8(4):178–179, 1987

Norris CM: Primitive pleasure as the basic human state. Advances in Nursing Science 8(1):25–43, 1985

Rose MA: Sensory loss stimulation use in nursing education. Journal of Gerontological Nuring 12(7):22–24, 1986

Schiefer Sr CC: The need for effective perception. In Yura H, Walsh M (eds): Human Needs 2 and the Nursing Process, pp 155–203. Norwalk, CT, Appleton-Century-Crofts, 1982

Schultz D: Sensory Restriction: Effects on Behavior. New York, Academic Press, 1965

Suedfeld P: Stressful levels of environmental stimulation. Issues in Mental Health Nursing 7(1/4):83–104, 1985

Topics in Clinical Nursing 6(4): entire issue, 1985

Waechter E, Phillips J, Holaday B: Nursing Care of Children, 10th ed. Philadelphia, JB Lippincott, 1985

Wyness MA: Perceptual dysfunction: Nursing assessment and management. J Neurosurg Nurs 17(2):105–110, 1985

Zegeer LJ: The effects of sensory changes in older persons. J Neurosurg Nurs 18(6):325–332, 1986

38 Sexuality

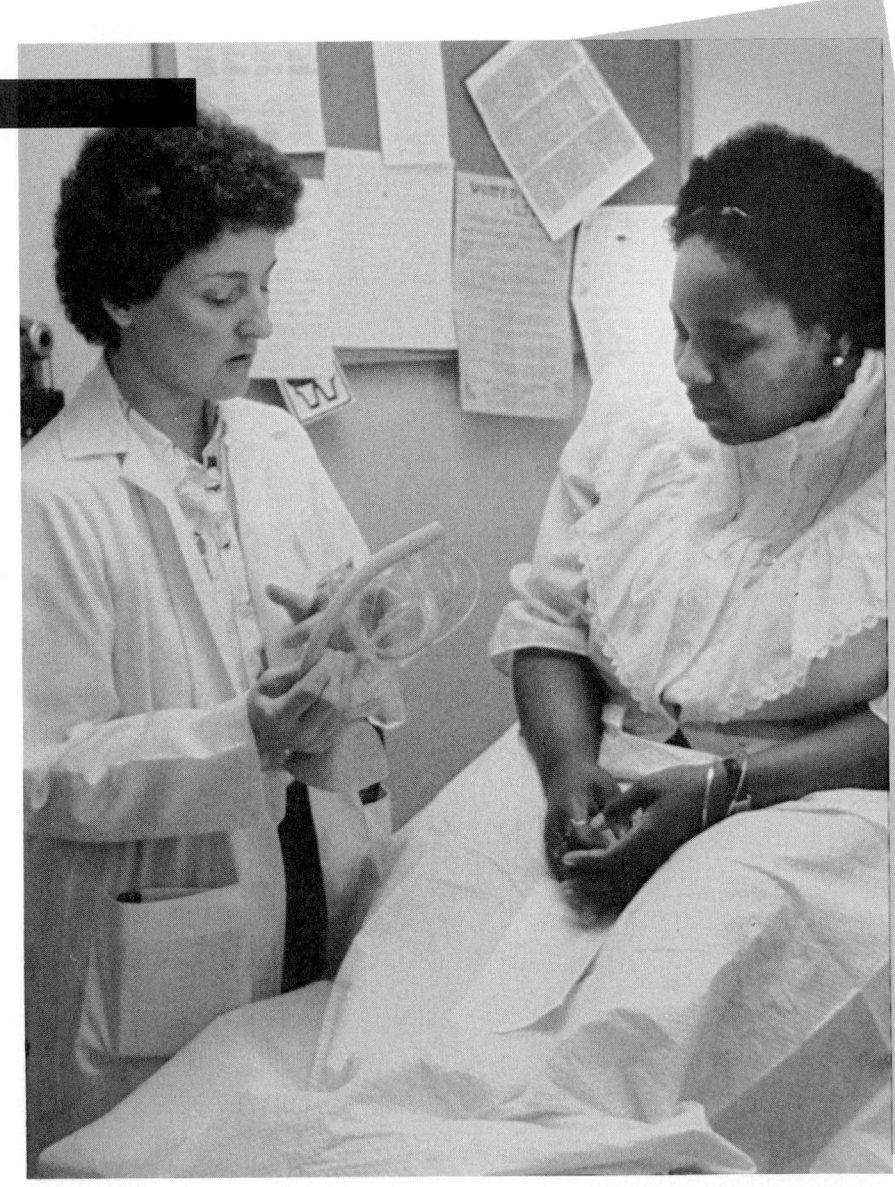

OBJECTIVES

After studying this chapter, the learner should be able to

Define key terms used in the chapter.

Describe male and female reproductive anatomy and physiology.

Describe the sexual response cycle and differentiate between male and female responses.

Identify and describe factors that affect an individual's sexuality.

Perform a sexual assessment utilizing suggested interview questions and appropriate physical assessment skills.

Describe types of sexual dysfunctions and assessment priorities for each one.

Develop nursing diagnoses identifying a problem with sexuality that may be remedied by independent nursing actions.

Describe five areas in which the nurse can provide the client with education to promote knowledge of sexuality.

Plan, implement, and evaluate nursing care related to select nursing diagnoses involving problems of sexuality.

When people visit a health-care facility they bring all aspects of their individuality with them. This includes sexuality, which permeates a person's life both in illness and in wellness. **Sexuality** is the degree to which a person exhibits and experiences maleness or femaleness physically, emotionally, and mentally. Sexuality is not only defined by a person's genitalia, but also by attitudes and feelings. It can also be defined as learned behaviors in how a person reacts to his or her own sexuality and by how one behaves in relationships with others. Finally, sexuality is an integral part of a person's identity and is present in one's demeanor through actions, communications, and physical appearances. A person's sexuality is therefore a concern in professional nursing care.

This chapter discusses reproductive anatomy and physiology, the sexual response cycle, and factors that affect sexuality. Information in performing a sexual history as part of a comprehensive client history is presented as well as interview questions that specifically address a client with a sexual dysfunction. Nursing priorities with regard to assessment of the reproductive system are presented along with the progressive steps of the examination. Analysis of assessment data is discussed with examples of corresponding nursing diagnoses. Planning and setting goals help the nurse and client develop appropriate interventions. The section Nursing Process in Clinical Practice provides the nurse with a format that utilizes assessment data, planning, interventions, and evaluations for nursing diagnoses that pertain to concerns with sexuality (Sexual dysfunction: inhibited sexual desire; Altered sexuality patterns: change in sexual expression; Knowledge deficit: contraceptive methods; and Disturbance in body image: surgical removal of a breast). The case study and care plan provide the nurse with examples of how the information presented in the chapter can be utilized in a clinical setting to nurture and promote aspects of sexuality in clients.

KEY TERMS

abstinence
bisexuality
coitus
coitus interruptus
contraception
cunnilingus
dyspareunia
ejaculation
erectile failure
erection
erogenous zones
fellatio
fetishism
foreplay
gay
heterosexuality
homosexuality
impotence
Kegel exercise
lesbian
masochism
mastectomy
masturbation
menarche
menopause
menses
nocturnal emission
orgasm
orgasmic dysfunction
ovulation
ovum
pregnancy
premature ejaculation
rape
retarded ejaculation
sadism
sadomasochism
semen
sexual dysfunction
sexual intercourse
sexuality
sexually transmitted disease (STD)
sodomy
sperm
spermicides
sterilization
transsexual
transvestism
vaginismus
virginity

PHYSIOLOGY

Female

The female genitalia are represented by both internal and external structures. The external genitalia are illustrated in Figure 24-51. The appearance of these structures varies slightly among individuals.

External Genitalia

The *mons pubis* is actually a pad of fatty tissue that lies over the part of the bony pelvis called the *symphysis pubis*. In the physically mature female, the mons pubis is covered with coarse hair called *pubic hair*. It contains many nerve endings that make the mons pubis sensitive to touch and pressure. The *labia majora* consist of two rounded folds of fatty tissue. The outer lips separate downward from the mons pubis and meet again below the vaginal introitus. The labia majora contain a multitude of sebaecous and sweat glands. They respond to touch during sexual activity. The *labia minora* are the smaller lips located within the labia majora. They are thin and sensitive structures and are pale pink in color. When stimulated by touch, the labia minora may turn a darker pink or even red due to the presence of many blood vessels. The labia minora have no hair and are smooth in texture.

The *clitoris* is found above the urinary meatus at the joining of the labia minora, called the *clitoral hood.* The clitoris is a small button-like structure similar to the male penis in its reaction to stimuli. The clitoris contains erectile tissue, blood vessels, and nerves. It is extremely sensitive. The opening of the vagina lies between the urinary meatus and the anus. It may contain a structure called the *hymen,* which is a thick membrane with no apparent function. At one time the hymen was thought to represent **virginity**; however, this is erroneous. Remnants or "tags" of the hymen may be noted at the vaginal introitus in both sexually active and inactive women.

Internal Genitalia

The internal genitalia—the ovaries, fallopian tubes, uterus, and vagina (Fig. 38-1)—are located deep within the pelvis of the female. The female body normally contains two ovaries, one on each side of the body. The ovaries closely resemble an almond in size and shape. At the time of a female child's birth, each ovary contains approximately 200,000 to 400,000 follicles. This number steadily decreases until puberty, when 100,000 to 200,000 follicles remain, and the number continues to decline over the reproductive years (McCary and McCary, 1982). The process of ovulation is discussed later in this chapter. The ovaries also secrete the hormones estrogen and progesterone.

The *fallopian tubes* are very slender structures that extend from either side of the uterus and end in a fringed fashion near each ovary. Their function is to transport a mature ovum from an ovary to the uterus. Fertilization of the ovum by a sperm usually takes place in the tube. The fertilized ovum then travels the rest of the way to the uterus where it implants. An unfertilized ovum travels the same path but does not implant. It is eventually expelled from the body during the menses. Because the lumen of each tube is so narrow, it can easily be damaged by the effects of infection and surgery.

The *uterus* is a pear-shaped organ approximately 3 inches long located between the urinary bladder and the rectum. Its primary purpose is to house and nurture a **pregnancy**. The uterus is composed of three layers: the outermost layer, the *perimetrium,* is composed of elastic tissue; the middle layer, the *myometrium,* is very muscular; and the innermost layer, the *endometrium,* is composed of tissue that will thicken and slough off with the menses. The *cervix* is the structure at the lower portion of the uterus that connects the uterus and the vagina. The cervix is usually closed. However, during the birth process it will dilate and thin out extensively to permit the birth of a baby. The cervix is a smooth, pink-colored

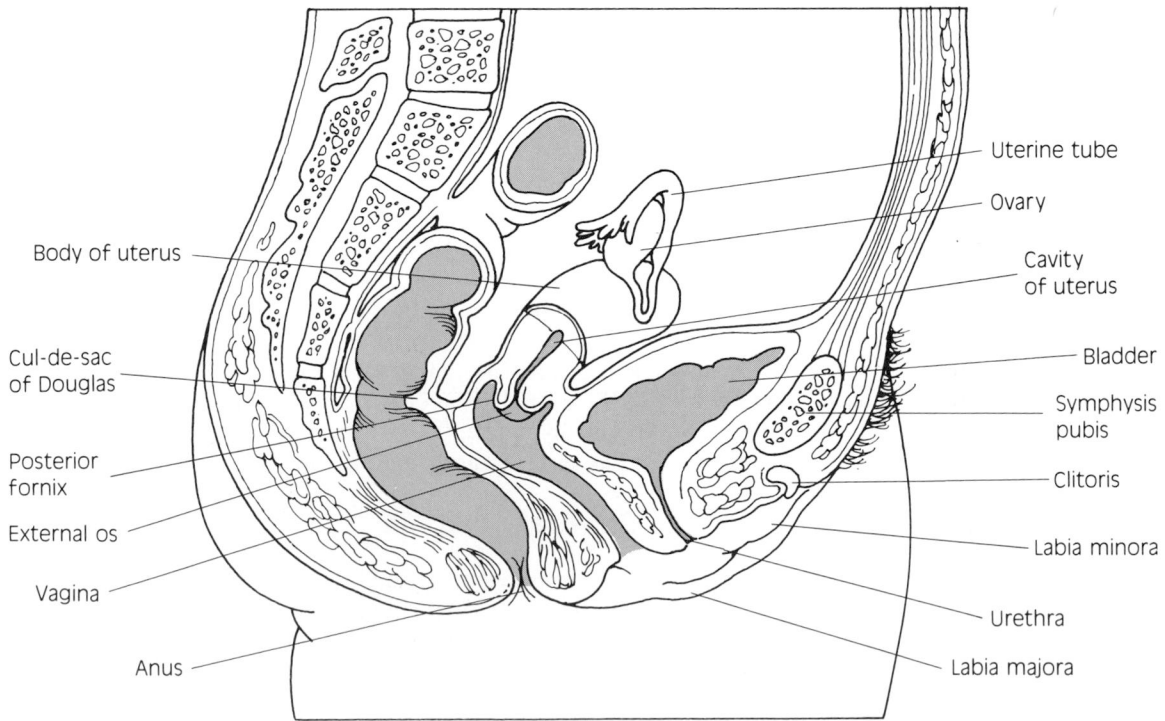

Body of uterus

Cul-de-sac of Douglas

Posterior fornix

External os

Vagina

Anus

Uterine tube

Ovary

Cavity of uterus

Bladder

Symphysis pubis

Clitoris

Labia minora

Urethra

Labia majora

F I G U R E   38-1
Sagittal section of the female reproductive organs.

structure that possesses few nerve endings. When touched, the sensation resembles that of touching the end of one's nose.

The *vagina* is a tubular, hollow organ that lies between the urinary urethra and the rectum. Its size and shape are very individual among women. The walls of the vagina are composed of rugated or ribbed tissue. The vagina serves three purposes: a receptacle for the penis during sexual intercourse, a birth canal for the passage of a baby, and an exit for menstrual flow from the uterus. During sexual activity, the walls of the vagina "sweat" or secrete a thin watery material, sometimes in copious amounts. This lubrication is necessary for the comfortable placement and movement of the penis in the vagina.

Breasts

Although the *breasts* are not considered part of the internal or external genitalia, they are an important aspect of the female's physical sexuality. The breasts are composed of fatty and glandular tissues and the nipples. Their size and shape vary widely among women. The nipples are pale to deep pink in color. Caressing of the breasts can be very pleasurable during sexual activity and many women can be brought to orgasm by this action alone (McCary and McCary, 1982).

Menstrual Cycle

Menstruation is a cycle during which the body prepares for the presence of a fertilized **ovum**. Each cycle is approximately 28 days in length but may vary from as short as 21 days to as long as 40 days. The first menstrual period, called **menarche**, is experienced around age 12 years. Again, the age of menarche is very individual and may occur at age 8 years to age 17 years. **Menopause**, the cessation of a woman's menstrual activity, occurs between the ages of 45 to 55 years. The woman may experience irregular menses over a period of time before menstruation comes to an end.

The menstrual cycle is controlled by a series of reactions that rely on feedback from the ovaries to the pituitary gland. Actually two cycles occur simultaneously, one in the ovaries and one in the uterus (Fig. 38-2).

In the ovaries, the phase from day 4 to day 14 is called the *follicular phase*. During this phase, a number of follicles will mature but only one will produce a mature ovum. At the same time, in the uterus, the endometrium is becoming thick and velvety in preparation for receiving a fertilized egg. This phase in the uterus is called the *proliferation phase*. **Ovulation** occurs on day 14. The mature ovum ruptures from the follicle and the surface of the ovary and is swept into the fallopian tube. If sperm are present, the ovum will be fertilized at this time. Some women can detect ovulation by the presence of a sharp, cramping pain over the ovulating ovary. This pain is called *mittelschmerz,* or middle pain, because it occurs in the middle of the cycle. From day 15 to day 28, the phase in the ovaries is called the *luteal phase*. The

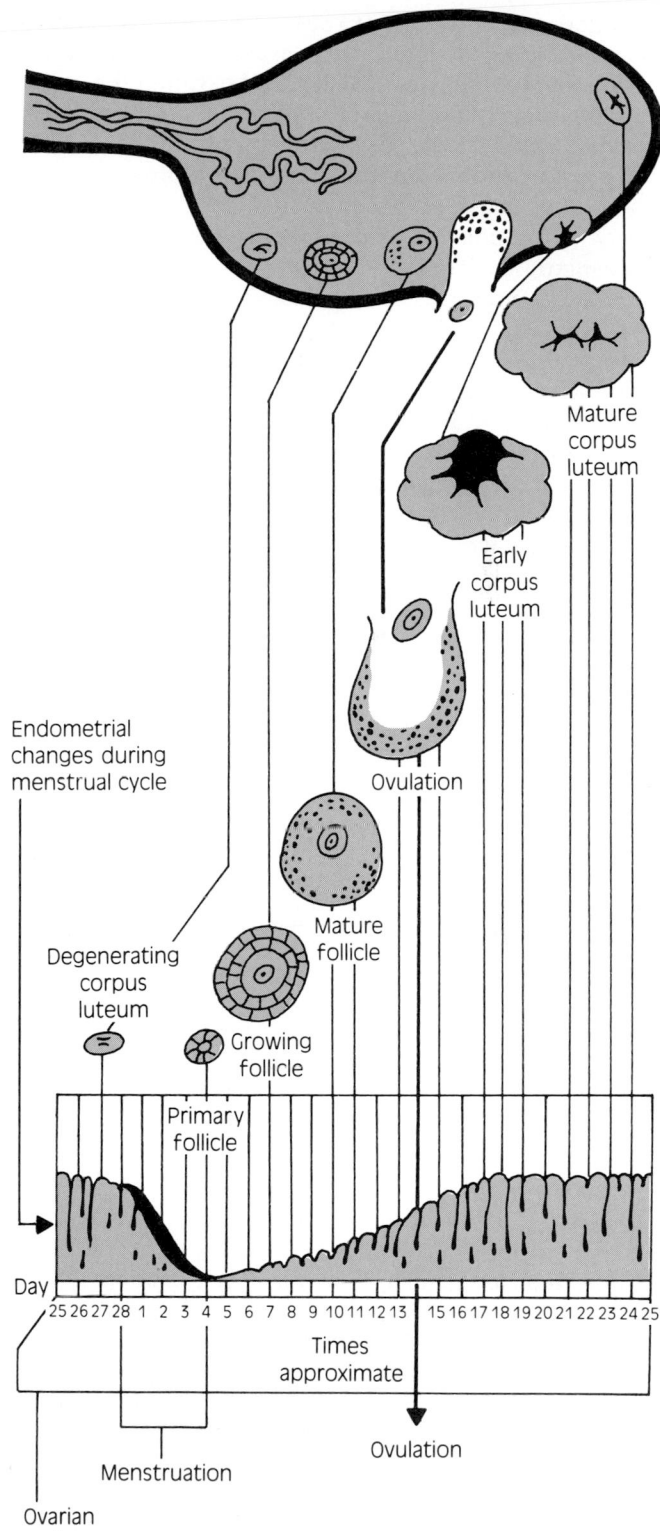

FIGURE 38-2
Schematic representation of one ovarian cycle and the corresponding changes in the endometrium.

leftover empty follicle fills up with a yellow pigment and is then called the *corpus luteum,* or yellow body. The purpose of the corpus luteum is to produce hormones that will encourage a fertilized egg to grow. If fertilization does not occur, the corpus luteum begins to disintegrate. During the luteal phase in the ovaries, the uterus also undergoes changes. This phase is called the *secretory phase.* The endometrial lining becomes very thick. However, in the absence of a fertilized egg, the corpus luteum dies and the endometrial lining disintegrates. At day 28, the **menses**, or the menstrual flow, will begin as a result of the uterus shedding the useless portion of its endometrium.

The menses lasts for 3 to 7 days, the average length of flow being 5 days. The menstrual discharge is a bloody fluid that also contains endometrial debris, mucus, and enzymes. It is odorless until exposed to the air, when a light, fleshy, pungent odor may be noticed by the woman. Deodorized pads and tampons do little to minimize odor and can cause a chemical irritation to the vulva and vagina. Good hygiene and regular bathing are much more effective during the menses to prevent odor. Normal blood loss averages between 30 ml and 80 ml. Pads and tampons should be changed frequently to prevent odor and irritation from wetness. Usually the flow is the heaviest and is bright red in color on the first day or two of the menses, gradually tapering off in amount to light brown staining. Many women experience some degree of discomfort either premenstrually or at the time of the menses.

There is no scientific rationale supporting abstinence from sexual activity during the menses. Many women enjoy sex during the menses due to the increase in vascularity in the pelvic region, which heightens enjoyment. Men may also enjoy the warm wetness the menstrual flow provides to the vagina. If the flow is heavy, a diaphragm can be used to hold back the flow until sexual activity ceases or a towel can be placed under the woman's buttocks to protect bedding. Women who experience abdominal cramping during the menses, or dysmenorrhea, find that sexual activity and orgasm relieve their discomfort.

Male

Unlike female genitalia, the male genitalia are found primarily outside the body. These structures are illustrated in Figure 24-53. The *testes,* which are approximately the size of walnuts, feel smooth and are freely movable within the scrotum. Normally two testes are present. The testes produce **sperm** and the hormones necessary for the maintenance of male sex characteristics. The primary hormone secreted by the testes is testosterone, which is responsible for a man's deep voice, beard growth, and body hair.

The *scrotum* is the loose bag-like structure that houses the testes. The scrotum hangs between a man's upper thighs. The area around the base of the penis and the scrotum is covered with pubic hair. The looseness of the scrotum is intentional to provide expansion and contraction. When exposed to cool temperatures, the scrotum contracts and draws the testes closer to the body for

warmth. In warm temperatures, the scrotum will become very loose and allow the testes to hang further away from the heat of the body. The testes are sensitive organs and can suffer discomfort, sometimes extreme, if handled roughly or jostled about. It is important that a man wear a properly fitted athletic support, or "jock-strap," when engaged in strenuous physical activity. However, the continuous use of a support can cause the temperature within the scrotum to rise and the delicate sperm to die because of constant exposure to high temperatures. Snug-fitting garments such as tight blue jeans can have the same effect on a man's fertility. The scrotum can be a source of sexual pleasure when lightly stroked, fondled, or caressed during sexual activity.

Tubules from the testes drain into the *epididymis,* which in turn drains into the *vas deferens* and *ejaculatory ducts.* These ducts then drain directly into the urethra. It is believed that the vas deferens acts as a reservoir for sperm between ejaculations.

The seminal vesicles, prostate gland, and Cowper's glands produce a liquid called *seminal plasma.* The seminal plasma and the sperm collectively make up the **semen**. The plasma aids in the transport of sperm and also provides energizing nutrients for the sperm. It contains a form of sugar (fructose), mucus, salts, water, base buffers, and coagulators to aid the sperm in their journey. Semen is a thick, creamy white fluid with the consistency of mucus or egg whites. The normal amount of semen per ejaculate is 2 ml to 6 ml. A fertile man will dispel 120 to 160 million sperm per ejaculate. Cowper's glands produce small droplets of fluid during sexual activity that neutralize the acidity of the male urethra and aid in the transport of sperm. This fluid may contain sperm. Therefore, contraceptive measures, if used, must be taken before this fluid can be introduced into the woman's vagina.

The penis is a tubular structure located above the scrotum. It functions to eliminate urine from the bladder, to ejaculate semen and impregnate a woman, and as a sex organ for sexual pleasure. It is composed of the shaft and the glans. In the uncircumcised male, the glans is covered by loose skin (*foreskin*) that can be retracted. In the circumcised male, the foreskin has been surgically removed and the glans is exposed. Penis size and shape vary among individuals. Normally the penis is soft and flaccid and 2.5 inches to 4 inches in length (McCary and McCary, 1982). The dimensions of the penis in no way dictate the man's ability to perform effectively during sexual activity. When an **erection** occurs, the blood vessels in the shaft of the penis become congested and the penis becomes "hard" and erect. The size of the penis during an erection may increase to 5.5 inches to 7 inches in total length. The penis, particularly the glans or head of the penis, is extremely sensitive to stimulation. Stroking and handling of the shaft of the penis are also pleasurable during sexual activity. Stimulation to prompt the penis to an erection is varied. A full bladder on awakening in the morning can cause an erection. Fantasy, memories of a past sexual encounter, and accidental brushing by an attractive stranger can all lead to an erection. An erection in the male does not always signify desire for sexual activity. Exposure of the male client by the nurse during a bed bath may cause an erection. An erection is a normal physiologic response and not something the man can voluntarily control. The erection will cease if no further stimulation is added.

Ejaculation is the expulsion of semen by the rhythmic contractions of the penis. The penis engages in short, jerky movements that produce a spurt of semen with each motion. The period of ejaculation is very short and the penis becomes flaccid after ejaculation. Many males, particularly adolescent boys, may experience a phenomenon known as **nocturnal emission** or "wet dream." These ejaculatory episodes occur during sleep without physical stimulation. They are perfectly normal and do not represent any sort of deviation.

Male breasts contain little real breast tissue. Male breasts may be stimulated during sexual activity. Although the area of sensitivity is usually limited to the nipple and areola, its stimulation can be as pleasurable an experience for the male as it is for a female.

SEXUAL RESPONSE CYCLE

The physiologic responses to sexual activity of female and male are more similar than different (Fig. 38-3). Also, body response is essentially the same regardless of the source of stimulation; that is, fantasy, masturbation, and sexual intercourse between two individuals can all bring about the same body reactions. The sexual response cycle is not limited to the genital organs but is a total body response that causes many physiologic changes throughout the body. Masters and Johnson, two researchers best known for their work on sexual re-

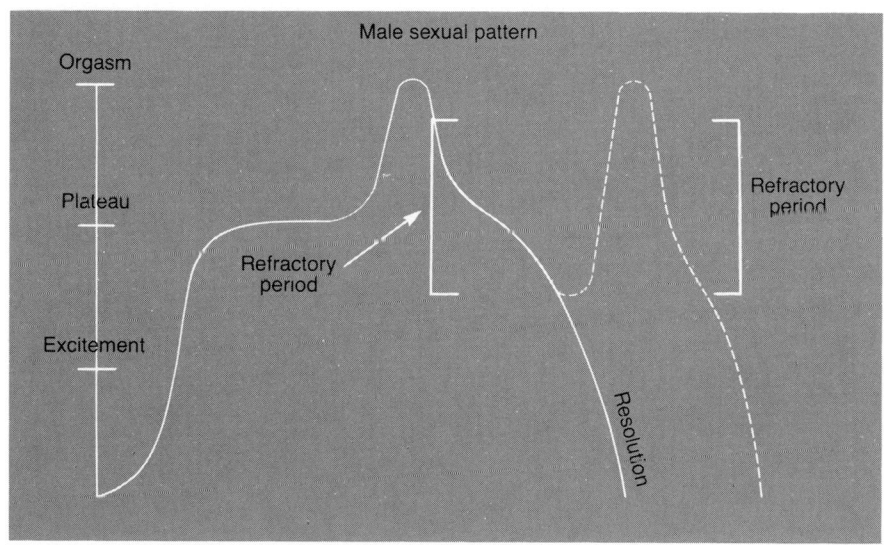

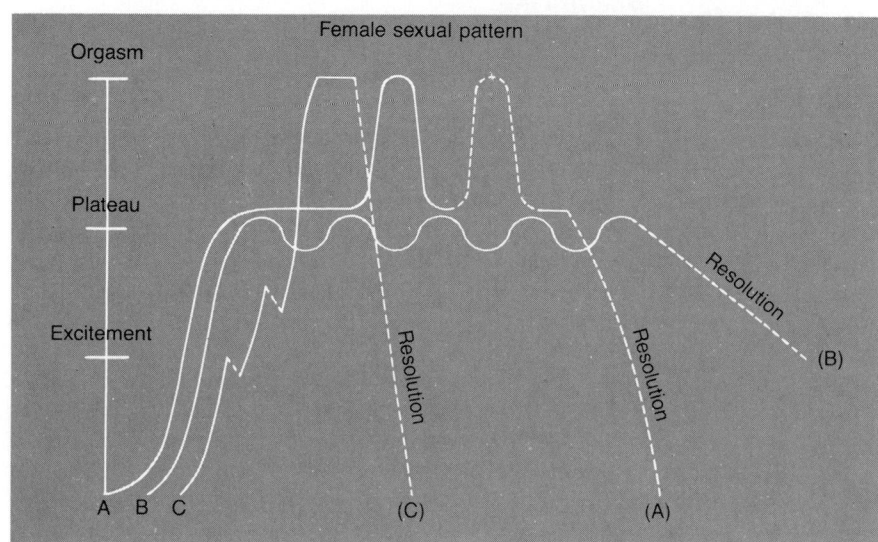

FIGURE 38-3

Male and female sexual response patterns. There are three female patterns shown. (A) Steady progression to plateau stage is followed by intense orgasm; subsequent orgasms may occur; resolution is slower. (B) Slower progression to plateau stage is followed by minor surges toward orgasm causing prolonged pleasurable feelings without definitive orgasm; resolution is slowest. (C) Rapid progression to plateau stage with some peaks and dips; one intense orgasm follows with rapid resolution. This most closely resembles the male pattern. (Reeder SJ, Martin LL: Maternity Nursing, 16th ed. Philadelphia, JB Lippincott, 1987)

sponse (Woods, 1984), divided the response cycle into the four phases of *excitement, plateau, orgasm,* and *resolution,* with a smooth progression from one phase to the next. Although only physiologic response is discussed here, the reader should keep in mind that the emotional and mental involvement of sexual response contributes a great deal to the pleasure and satisfaction of sexual activity.

The human body contains many **erogenous zones**, which are areas that when stimulated cause sexual arousal and desire. The genitals are an obvious source of sexual pleasure for both men and women, but other areas of the body are also considered erogenous zones. The skin of the body is the largest erogenous zone. Other areas include the ears, lips, thighs, and breasts. Some people can reach orgasm simply by stimulation of erogenous zones other than the genitals. The most important body organ for sexual arousal and stimulation is the brain. It allows individuals freedom to enjoy a sexual experience but also may prevent satisfaction by inhibitions, doubts, and guilt.

Excitement

The excitement phase is initiated by erotic stimulation and arousal. Some of the physiologic changes common in both men and women include increase in heart rate and blood pressure and the appearance of a pink flush to the skin. This sex flush, which is more evident in women than in men, spreads over the face, neck, back, and upper torso of the body. Congestion of the genitals with increased blood flow begins in the excitement phase and causes even more arousal. The length of the excitement phase varies greatly among individuals and even from one experience to another. Women usually enjoy a more prolonged period of stimulation than do men.

During the excitement phase the breasts of the woman swell and the nipples become erect and hard to the touch. Lubrication of the vagina seeps to the outside of the body along the vulvar creases and makes stimulation of the genitals more pleasurable by decreasing friction. The upper two thirds or so of the vagina enlarge and expand. The clitoris enlarges and appears to emerge slightly from the clitoral hood. The labia also enlarge and separate and turn a deep rosy red in color with arousal.

The first obvious sign of arousal in the man is an erection of the penis caused by increased pelvic congestion of blood. The scrotum noticeably elevates, thickens, and enlarges. The skin of the penis and scrotum turns a deep reddish-purple in response to congestion and arousal. Male nipples may also harden and become erect.

Plateau

The intensity of the plateau phase is greater than that of excitement, but not enough to begin orgasm. Desire and arousal continue to build and intensify. The length of time of this phase varies from a few minutes to 15 to 20 minutes. In the female, the clitoris retracts and disappears under the clitoral hood. It is thought that the clitoris performs in this mysterious way as the body's protection against overstimulation. In the male, secretions from Cowper's glands may appear at the glans of the penis during the plateau phase.

Orgasm

The term **orgasm** defines the climax and sexual explosion of the tension built over the preceding phases. Orgasm lasts a matter of seconds, but it is an extremely intense reaction. Characteristic of the orgasm phase are the involuntary spasmodic contractions of the genital organs. The number of contractions felt by the individual depends on the intensity of the orgasm.

The orgasm phase in the female begins with a heightened feeling of physical pleasure followed by overwhelming release and involuntary contractions of the genitals. Loss of muscular control can also be seen in spastic contractions and twitching of the arms and legs. The number of contractions can be as few as four or as many as 15 to 20. Areas of the body that contract spasmodically are the uterus, anal sphincter, rectum, and urethral sphincter. It is now believed that women achieve orgasm in a variety of ways. While some women can achieve orgasm by penile thrusting in the vagina alone, most women need clitoral stimulation to reach orgasm.

Involuntary spasmodic contractions of the genitals occur in the male during orgasm. These take place in the penis, epididymis, vas deferens, and rectum. The male orgasm is most often accompanied by ejaculation of semen from the urinary meatus of the penis. It is not necessary for ejaculation and orgasm to occur simultaneously. Rather, it is a coincidence that the two events usually happen at the same time.

Resolution

The resolution phase is characterized by a return to normal body functioning present before the excitement phase. Feelings of relaxation, fatigue, and fulfillment are common. Some people may also have a need to be held, fondled, and caressed. Physical demonstrations of affection may initiate the sexual response cycle once again. The human female has no real need to recover from sexual activity. That is, the woman is physiologically capable of immediate response to sexual stimulation. Because of this, many women can achieve multiple orgasms. The man experiences a period of time during which he is incapable of sexual response, called the *refractory period.* The length of the refractory period is individual. It may last a few minutes or even days before the man's body will respond readily to continued sexual stimulation.

SEXUAL EXPRESSION

The methods by which a person or persons gain satisfaction through sexual stimulation are varied. Also, a number of factors are involved in the degree to which a sexual experience is enjoyable. Touch, smell, sight, sounds, eelings, thoughts, and fantasy can all contribute to sexual fulfillment in any form of expression chosen by individuals. Feelings of love for another person are also closely associated with desire. Fantasies can greatly aid sexual stimulation and are quite normal.

Masturbation

Masturbation is a technique of sexual expression in which an individual practices self-stimulation. Many myths and misinformation surround the issue of masturbation. Masturbation is a means of learning what is preferred by a person during stimulation and what feels good. Men masturbate by holding and stroking the shaft of the penis. Women find manual stimulation of the clitoris enjoyable, although variations of technique are numerous. People masturbate regardless of sex, age, or marital status. People who do not masturbate usually abstain because of a sense of guilt or wrongness associated with self-stimulation. Masturbation is not dirty and will not lead to blindness, nor will it cause insanity.

Sexual Intercourse

Sexual intercourse between a man and a woman is the most common image that comes to mind when sexuality is mentioned. Unlike other animals, human beings must learn how to engage in sexual intercourse (McCary and McCary1982). The act of intercourse, or **coitus**, usually begins by stimulation of the senses in some way, followed by a period of activity known as **foreplay**. Petting is part of foreplay and can be simple stroking of the breasts, arms, back, and neck without genital involvement or may lead to mutual masturbation and orgasm. Many adolescents engage in petting without further sexual involvement. However, the progressive steps of intercourse are merely shades of gray. An adolescent couple may find themselves involved in the sexual act without any preparation or forewarning.

Penetration. The act of placing the penis in the vagina, or *penetration,* can be accomplished by various positions. The most common position in Western cultures is the "missionary" position, which places the woman horizontally under the man. (This position was named *missionary* by the Polynesians because it was the preferred position utilized for intercourse by religious missionaries [McCary and McCary, 1982].) Other positions may be more stimulating and comfortable. Clitoral stimulation is difficult to achieve in the missionary position.

Lying side by side, female on top, and rear entry are some examples of coital positions that make clitoral stimulation more successful. Some people are so inhibited they need permission to engage in alternate sexual positions.

When the penis is pushed into the vagina, the man will begin rhythmic thrusting movements of his hips to stroke the penis back and forth along the vaginal walls. The woman may match her partner's hip movements with movements of her own body. These movements continue until orgasm is attained by both people. Simultaneous orgasms, or both people attaining orgasm at the same moment, are difficult to achieve. Preoccupation with attaining simultaneous orgasms may disrupt the ultimate intimacy and satisfaction possible during the coital experience.

The period of time after coitus is just as significant as the events leading up to it. Caressing, hugging, and kissing actually deepen the intimacy shared by the couple and should be nurtured and not rushed.

Variant Forms

Stimulation by using the mouth and tongue on the genitals may be used during foreplay or as a method to reach orgasm. **Cunnilingus** is stimulation of the female genitals by licking and sucking the clitoris and surrounding structures. **Fellatio** is stimulation of the male genitals by licking and sucking the penis and surrounding structures. These techniques may be used singularly or simultaneously.

Sodomy, the act of introducing the penis into the rectum, is still considered illegal in some areas. Once a finger or the penis is placed in the rectum, it should not be introduced into the vagina without thorough cleansing, because many organisms present in the rectum can cause subsequent vaginal infections. Care should be exercised to avoid injury to the delicate rectal mucosa and lubrication is essential for comfort.

Sadism refers to the practice of gaining sexual pleasure while inflicting abuse on another person. **Masochism** refers to gaining sexual pleasure from the humiliation of being abused. When practiced together, the act is called **sadomasochism. Fetishism**, usually practiced by a male, is sexual arousal with the aid of an inanimate object not generally associated with sexual activity. Items such as shoes, leather, rubber, and women's undergarments may be used.

Transvestism is sexual arousal of a man when he wears clothing normally worn by a woman. Most transvestites are heterosexual and many are married with children. Transvestites usually have a great need to keep their habit a secret from others and indulge in cross dressing in private or choose to wear women's undergarments that are not easily detectable.

The extent to which people practice variants of sexual expression may range from totally harmless to compulsive in nature. Nurses must be able to provide care to these individuals as they do to any other consumers of health care.

FACTORS AFFECTING SEXUALITY

Many factors influence and affect a person's sexuality and thus differentiate personal feelings regarding sexuality. That is, the brain rather than the genitals plays the most significant role in how people perceive themselves as sexual beings.

Developmental Considerations

The process of human development affects the psychosocial, emotional, and biologic aspects of life, and these in turn affect an individual's sexuality. Sexuality is the only distinguishing trait present at conception. From birth onward, gender, or sex, will influence behavior throughout life. See Table 38-1 for a summary of sexuality throughout the life span and nursing implications for each stage.

Culture

The manner in which sexuality is perceived by a society of people will in turn influence the individual. Every culture has its own norms regarding sexual behavior. To some degree, culture dictates the duration of sexual intercourse, methods of sexual stimulation, and sexual positions. In some cultures, women may be expected merely to tolerate sex, whereas in others the woman's participation is encouraged.

Religion

Organized religion has had a generally negative effect on expression of sexuality. Many forms of sexual expression other than male–female coitus are considered unnatural by some religions. Also, over time the concept of virginity came to be synonymous with purity and sex became synonymous with sin. Double standards and rigid regulations have inflicted a considerable amount of guilt and anxiety on many individuals. A number of sexual dysfunctions can be related to the individual's an-

(Text continues on p. 1070.)

R E S E A R C H   I N   N U R S I N G   Making a Difference

Sexuality

A strong sense of self, based on acceptance of all facets of self, is vital for psychosocial security. One of the facets of self needing definition is sexuality. The state of being masculine or feminine and the understanding of its implications begin in childhood and continue through old age. Sexuality influences the perception of self in relationships with others and also affects attitudes experienced during each transitional stage of development.

Related Research

Glazebrook C, Munjas B: Sex roles and depression. Journal of Psychosocial Nursing 24(12):8–12, 1986

This study explored the changing of traditional sex roles resulting from the women's movement and the relationship of depression to sex role. A correlation was found between sex role strain and depression in both men and women.

Uphold C, Susman E: Child-rearing, marital, recreational, and work role integration and climacteric symptoms in midlife women. Res Nurs Health 8:73–81, 1985

This study investigated the relationships between female midlife roles and the frequency and severity of symptoms reported at menopause. Results indicated that women who fulfill more roles are less likely to experience menopausal symptoms, and that adjustment to the marital role and an active recreational role are the best indicators for mild menopausal symptoms.

Woods N, Most A, Longnecker G: Major life events, daily stressors and perimenstrual symptoms. Nurs Res 34(7):263–267, 1985

The purpose of this study was to determine the relationship of major life events and daily stressors to perimenstrual symptoms. Most significant to symptoms were daily stressors (as compared to major life events) and a generally stressful life (as compared to episodes of stress).

Summary

The implications of nursing research are numerous. Nurses must be introspective and explore their own concept of self to reach their potential and develop a strong sense of sexuality. They must accept men and women at any given point of sexual development and help them reach goals of individual adaptability and self-knowledge.

T A B L E 38-1
Developmental Aspects of Sexuality Through the Life Span

Stage	Characteristics	Nursing Implications and Teaching Guidelines
Infancy—birth to 18 months	• Needs affection and tactile stimulation • Boys have penile erections and girls have orgasmic potential. • Gradually can differentiate self from others • Obtain pleasure from touching genitals • Dressed according to gender • Toys are gender related	• Avoid early weaning to prevent oral deprivation. • Encourage parents to provide ample physical touch, deprivation of which may cause physical and mental underdevelopment. • Self-manipulation of genitals is normal behavior; avoid denoting this as ''bad.'' • Avoid confusion of sex by consistent use of male or female role reinforcement.
Toddler—age 1–3 years	• Establishes control over bowels and bladder • Both sexes enjoy fondling genitals. • Able to identify own gender • Develops vocabulary related to anatomy	• Allow toddler to designate his/her readiness to toilet-training. Strict measures may lead to compulsive behaviors later. • Punishment of genital fondling may lead to guilt and shame regarding sexual behavior later in life. • Use proper terms for body parts.
Preschool—age 4–6 years	• By age 6, sexuality has been internalized and preference for sexual partners determined. • Methods of play and dress are in accordance with gender. • Enjoys exploring body parts of self and playmates • Engages in masturbation	• Parents may cause anxiety in the child by intolerance of inconsistency of sex-role behavior • Negative overreaction by parents of child's masturbating behavior can lead to a belief that the genitals and sex are bad and dirty.
School-age—age 6–10 years	• There is attachment to the parent of the opposite sex. • Tendency toward having same-sex friends • Curiosity about sex and sharing of fears • Increasing self-awareness	• Same-sex preference for relationships is not related to heterosexual or homosexual tendencies. • Give child the information desired in a clear, factual form. May look to peers for information that may be incorrect.
Preadolescence—age 10–13 years	• Puberty begins for most boys and girls with development of secondary sex characteristics. • Menarche takes place. • May test behavioral limits	• Information is necessary regarding body changes to alleviate fears. This information should be given to the young person before pubertal changes begin. • Parents need to find a satisfactory middle ground for role-setting. Rules that are either too rigid or too lenient can interfere with the development of self-confidence and internal value system. • Treat body image changes with a positive attitude to prevent poor self-image.
Adolescence—age 13–19 years	• Begins to develop opposite-sex relationships • Sexual fantasies are common. • Masturbation is common. • May begin to partake in sexual activity with light to heavy petting • Girls concerned with reputations and self-image • Boys preoccupied with competitiveness of sexual activity • Incidence of adolescent pregnancies is increasing.	• Parents share their beliefs and moral value systems with their children. • Teenagers may share their feelings with parents. If not taken seriously, may lead to lack of trust and communication gap. • Teens need information regarding contraceptive measures and the potential for contracting sexually transmitted diseases (STDs).

(Continued)

T A B L E   38-1
Developmental Aspects of Sexuality Through the Life Span   (Continued)

Stage	Characteristics	Nursing Implications and Teaching Guidelines
Young adulthood—age 20–35 years	• Premarital sex is common. • Although many young adults choose cohabitation instead of marriage, most marry and begin families before age 30. • Knowledge regarding sexual response and activity increases pleasure of relationship. • May experiment with various sexual expressions • Develops own value system and respects values of other people • Many couples share financial responsibilities as well as household tasks.	• Encourage communication between partners regarding sexual needs and differences. • Teach use of contraceptive measures and encourage use to prevent unwanted pregnancies. • Counsel against promiscuous behavior to guard against STDs and loss of trust of partner. • Daily communication is necessary to vent stresses and work out difficulties.
Adulthood—age 35–55 years	• Bodily changes as a result of menopause • Couples focus on quality rather than quantity of sexual experiences. • Divorce is common. • Grown children begin their own lives and sexual experiences. • Sexual satisfaction may actually increase due to loss of fear of pregnancy.	• Both men and women need positive reinforcement of what is good about themselves and their relationships. • Teach parents that empty nest syndrome (feelings of loss caused by children leaving) is common. Accentuate positive aspects of this situation. • Encourage couple to use this period as one of renewal for themselves.
Late adulthood and elderly—age 55 years and over	• Orgasms may become shorter and less intense in both men and women. • Vaginal secretions decrease and period of resolution in men lengthens. • May feel need to conform to stereotypes regarding the aging process and cease sexual activity • Fear of loss of sexual abilities	• Sexual activity need not be hindered by age. • Teach couples that adaptation to bodily changes is possible with use of comfortable positions for intercourse and increased time for stimulation. • Teach alternatives to coitus, such as caressing, hugging, and stroking, when coitus is not possible due to illness or disability. • Couples who have been consistently sexually active throughout their lives may continue their intimate relationship for as long as they desire.

guish over the negative connotation of sex as dictated by some religious groups. On the other hand, groups such as the United Methodists have recognized the importance of a solid sex education within the realm of the church (McCary and McCary, 1982).

Ethics

Healthy sexuality depends on freedom from guilt and anxiety. What one person believes is wrong may be perfectly natural and correct to another. Some individuals, however, may feel that certain forms of sexual expression are bizarre and the people that participate in them are perverted. If the sexual expression is performed by consenting adults, is not harmful to them, and is practiced in privacy, it is not considered a deviant behavior (McCary and McCary, 1982). Individuals should personally decide with which aspects of sexual expression they are comfortable. Frequently, all an individual needs to alleviate guilt and consequently enhance sexual satisfaction is permission from a health-care provider to engage in a different form of expression.

Life-Style

Modern life-styles greatly affect sexuality and its expression. Both men and women are exposed to stress, and many are under considerable strain to perform and function in the work place as well as at home. Stressors may be external, such as job and financial demands, or internal, such as a competitive nature. These varied responsibilities place a time restraint on communication between a couple, as well as on the energy level and motivation for sexual satisfaction. Although some couples view sexual activity as a release from the stressors of everyday life, the majority place sex far from the top of the list of things to do. It is crucial to a relationship's survival that a couple set aside priority time if not for love-making, then for intimate quiet contact.

Sexual Orientation

Most adults develop a sexual orientation resulting from childhood experiences (Table 38-1). Sexual orientation refers to the preferred sex of the partner of an individual. *Homosexual* people prefer sexual activity with a person of the same sex. *Heterosexual* people prefer sexual activity with a person of the opposite sex. Heterosexuality and homosexuality can be placed at opposite ends of a continuum with many variations in between. **Bisexuality** refers to a person who finds pleasure with both opposite-sex or the same-sex partner. Homosexual or heterosexual people may have bisexual relationships at times.

Heterosexuality. Heterosexuality is the most common form of sexual orientation among human beings, and coitus between a man and woman is their most common form of sexual expression. Although some people feel coitus should only take place in a marital relationship, it also occurs premaritally, extramaritally, and postmaritally.

Premarital sex is the practice of coitus before marriage. The standard for sexual **abstinence** before marriage has been a cultural and religious norm in many societies for centuries. Abstinence and virginity have been perceived as more important for women to maintain than for men. This double standard appears to be changing as increasing numbers of women report having premarital sexual relations, especially in Western societies. Extramarital sexual relationships are usually a symptom of a troubled marriage and rarely the cause of the failure of a strong one. Extramarital relationships are often the product of stress-filled lives and sexual dissatisfaction at home and are destructive to a marriage relationship.

Homosexuality. Homosexuality occurs in both males and females. The term **gay** is synonymous with male homosexual. A **lesbian** is a female homosexual. The sexual behaviors of the heterosexual and the homosexual are the same except for penile–vaginal penetration. The primary difference between a heterosexual and a homosexual is in the gender of the preferred sex partner and not in a particular type of behavior.

Homosexuality has been considered an illness or deviant behavior, but in 1974 the American Psychiatric Association removed homosexuality from the category of mental illness. While this move and certain research findings eliminated some of the stigma attached to homosexuality, society as a whole has made slow progress in accepting the gay movement.

Transsexuality. A transsexual is a person of a certain biologic sex with the feelings of the opposite sex. In other words, the person feels trapped within the body of the wrong sex. The reason, or etiology, behind this is unknown, although many factors are believed to be involved. For many transsexuals the solution for this agonizing problem is to change their bodies to match their inner feelings through surgery and hormone therapy.

Health State

A healthy body, mind, and emotions are necessary for sexual wellness. Any trauma or stress that interferes with an individual's ability to perform daily functions will certainly also affect the expression of sexuality. Illness is no exception.

Chronic Pain. Many chronic illnesses are accompanied by constant pain and an individual with persistent pain may not desire any sexual contact. However, the desire for human warmth and contact does not cease because of pain (Cash, 1984). Altered or modified positions for coitus are sometimes necessary, and these are discussed in more detail later in this section.

Diabetes Mellitus. Diabetes mellitus is a hormonal disease in which the body is deficient in the amount of insulin secreted by the pancreas. Although almost all hormonal disorders affect sexuality in some way, diabetes is the most prevalent and well known. Erectile dysfunction, or impotence, is a great concern among diabetic men. Treatment to date depends largely on the degree of erectile ability lost. Some men may be candidates for a penile prosthesis, which was developed in 1973. The prosthesis is surgically implanted below the base of the penis and inflation of the device produces an erection when sexual activity is desired (Googe and Mook, 1983).

It is not uncommon for diabetic women to experience loss of ability for orgasm (orgasmic dysfunction). Difficulty experiencing arousal and loss of vaginal lubrication have also been reported (Woods, 1984). Frequent *Monilia* infections of the vagina are also common and cause discomfort during coitus.

Cardiovascular Disease. Cardiovascular disease is prevalent in North America. It is known that the sexual response cycle can greatly increase the demands of the heart and other structures. A person with a cardiovascular disease may experience much anxiety over the effect the illness will have on sexuality and sexual functioning.

Hypertension. The most significant difficulty a hypertensive person faces regarding sexuality is that the medication used to control the disease frequently causes a change in sexual functioning (see Table 38-3). These sexual dysfunctions may be relieved by modifying the dose of the medication or switching to a different medication.

Myocardial Infarction (Heart Attack). The primary goal after a myocardial infarction (MI) is to allow the heart ample time to heal. Activities of daily living, including sexual activity, should be resumed gradually and stressors such as overexertion, alcohol consumption, and emotional upheavals should be avoided. In an uncomplicated MI, sexual activity may begin around the third week of recovery, beginning with masturbation to partial erection in the male. Generally this activity is gradually increased until three months after the MI when sexual intercourse may be resumed (Woods, 1984). A comfortable position should be assumed that places the least stress on the affected partner.

Diseases of the Joints and Mobility. Joint diseases and disorders affect young and old people. Pain, fatigue, stiffness, and loss of range of motion can accompany any of the dozens of known diseases of the joints. The disease itself does not affect sexual functioning, although the manifestation of it can cause discomfort and anxiety.

Surgery and Body Image. Surgery is performed to remove diseased tissue and repair body organs. It usually requires an incision with resulting scars. The most devastating kinds of surgery are those used to remove cancerous tissue and surrounding structures. The client is almost always distressed over a diagnosis of cancer and possible death. After surgery, people need to cope and adjust to major alterations to their bodies. Changes in body image also affect a person's self-perception as a sexual being.

Mastectomy is a surgical procedure to remove a breast and its surrounding tissue. Following such surgery, a woman's return to sexual functioning depends on many factors, such as support of her partner, the value placed on the breast by the man or woman, and fear of discomfort during sexual activity.

An *ostomy* is a surgical opening placed on the outside of the body to allow for the passage of secretions and elimination into a closed drainage bag. The grief over the loss of the natural means to eliminate waste, such as urine or feces, accompanies learning to live with an obvious artificial device. Many people are anxious as to how this apparatus will affect their sexual lives and how accepting sexual partners will be of it.

Spinal Cord Injuries. Thousands of people are victims of spinal cord injuries each year as a result of various types of accidents. This type of injury almost always results in some degree of permanent disability. These people face multiple adaptations in normal living styles, including those related to mobility, bowel and bladder control, sexual functioning, and role expectations. The extent of remaining sexual response after a spinal cord injury depends primarily on the level and extent of the injury. Ejaculation and orgasm are most likely to remain with low spinal injuries. Women are more likely to experience orgasm than men but complain more about the lack of physical sensations during the excitement phase than do men. Many people find that other erogenous zones become more easily stimulated after the injury.

Mental Illness. Various psychologic and physical disorders can cause mental illness. The mind plays a powerful role in sexuality and any disruption of its functioning will no doubt cause a disturbance in some way to sexual functioning. Even a disorder such as mild depression can affect desire and sexual functioning. Sometimes it is difficult for the partner of a client who has developed a mental illness to continue the sexual relationship. People afflicted with Alzheimer's disease can lose the memory of any contact with a partner or spouse. At times, clients with mental illness "act out" in a sexual manner, such as touching themselves or discarding their clothing at inappropriate times and places.

Sexually Transmitted Diseases. The term **sexually transmitted disease (STD)** is currently used to describe diseases that are almost always transmitted through direct sexual contact. The number of cases and varieties of STDs has increased over the years and many are now at epidemic proportions. STDs are hard to control because the partner or partners also need treatment. This is usually difficult if the partner is promiscuous or a one-time contact. It is now believed that to have sexual contact with one person is also to have sexual contact with everyone else that person has had contact with in the past. The only clear way to avoid exposure to an STD is for a virginal person to have sexual contact with another virgin. Some STDs can be treated easily and effectively whereas others have longstanding implications. For instance, women may suffer severe consequences from an STD by developing pelvic inflammatory disease (PID). The resulting adhesions from PID cause much damage to delicate reproductive structures and may lead to infertility. Furthermore, other STDs are deadly because there is no cure and no effective treatment. Acquired immunodeficiency syndrome (AIDS) is an example of a deadly STD. Table 38-2 lists the more common types of STDs and their signs and symptoms and corresponding treatment.

Medications

Medications are used to halt a disease, cure an illness, and promote and stabilize body functions. Some medications are necessary to prevent severe illness and even death. Most medications have some side-effects that may

(Text continues on p. 1074.)

T A B L E   38-2
Sexually Transmitted Diseases

Disease	Signs and Symptoms	Treatment
Acquired immunodeficiency syndrome (AIDS)	• HTLV III virus • Positive ELISA and western blot tests • Incidence high in IV drug users and homosexual and bisexual men • Fatigue, diarrhea, weight loss, enlarged lymph nodes, fever, anorexia, and night sweats	• No cure or effective treatment • All treatment directed toward opportunistic diseases and symptomatic relief
Cervical intraepithelial neo- plasia (CIN) Cervical cancer	• Abnormal Pap smears • Women with multiple sex partners, women who began sexual activity before age 18, and women whose partners have multiple female partners • Asymptomatic • Possible vaginal bleeding or spotting	• Depends on extent and stage of dysplasia • Surgical removal of cervix and other surrounding struc- tures if severe; cryosurgery and laser treatment also used
Chlamydia trachomatis Nongonococcal urethritis (NGU) *Chlamydia*	• The most prevalent STD to date • Gram-negative bacteria • Vaginal discharge, burning on urination, urinary fre- quency, dysuria, and urethral soreness • Many women are asymptomatic.	• Tetracycline 500 mg by mouth qid for 7 days, or erythromycin 500 mg by mouth qid for 7 days for both partners
Cytomegalovirus (CMV)	• A virus similar to herpes • May be asymptomatic or may be confused with an- other disease such as pneumonia, mononucleosis, or hepatitis	• No specific treatment; aimed at relief of symptoms; may be passed *in utero* and affect newborn
Gardnerella vaginalis Nonspecific vaginitis Hemophilus *Gardnerella*	• Gram-negative bacteria • Foul-smelling thin grayish-white vaginal discharge • Male partners are asymptomatic	• Flagyl (metronidazole) 500 mg by mouth bid for 7 days for both partners; alcohol must not be consumed while taking medication.
Neisseria gonorrhoeae, "The clap" or "the drip" Gonorrhea	• Gram-negative bacteria • Both men and women may be asymptomatic • Symptoms in men: purulent penile discharge, dys- uria, frequency of urination • Symptoms in women: dysuria, abnormal menses, va- ginal discharge, pelvic inflammatory disease • Symptoms of pharyngitis if oral sex practiced • May be accompanied by chlamydia infection • Detected by gonorrhea culture of cervix or penile discharge from men • Exposed newborns at birth at risk for blindness and pneumonia • Untreated gonorrhea can result in infertility, skin rash with lesions, and acute arthritis.	• All partners must be treated Tetracycline 500 mg by mouth qid for 7 days *plus* Aqueous procaine penicillin G 4.8 million units IM *plus* Probenecid 1 g by mouth • Cultures should be repeated in 1 week post treatment.
Herpes simplex virus type 1 and 2 "Cold sores" *Herpes*	• A DNA virus • Lesions develop mostly in oral and genital areas. • Appear as single or multiple painful vesicles, which rupture and form ulcer-like lesions; these form scabs as they heal. • First infections last approximately 10–14 days while subsequent infections are shorter in duration. • Recurrences are usually preceded by prodromal symptoms of tingling and fullness.	• No cure. • The antiviral drug acyclovir is useful in treatment: acyclovir 200 mg by mouth 5 times per day. • Areas of lesions should be kept clean and dry. • Utilize analgesics to reduce pain as well as topical anes- thetics. • Avoid sexual contact while le- sions are present. • May be transmitted to new- born at birth

(Continued)

T A B L E   38-2
Sexually Transmitted Diseases   (Continued)

Disease	Signs and Symptoms	Treatment
Human papilloma virus Condylomata acuminata Genital warts Venereal warts	• A DNA virus • Pale, soft, papillary lesions found around the internal and external genitalia, and perianal and rectal areas of the body; vary in size • Profuse watery vaginal discharge, dyspareunia, intense pruritus, and vulvar irritation • Women with HPV are at risk for developing cervical cancer. • Male partner may or may not have lesions.	• Treat male partner if he has lesions. • Podophyllum 10%–25% in tincture of benzoin may be applied to external lesions. Wash off in 1–4 hours. Repeat treatment until lesions are gone. • Cryosurgery and carbon dioxide laser surgery may also be used. • Use condoms or abstain from sex.
Treponema pallidum Syphilis	• A spirochete detected through serologic blood test (VDRL, RPR, STS) • Three stages to disease if left untreated *Primary*—single painless genital lesion 10 days to 3 months after exposure *Secondary*—Generalized skin rash, enlarged lymph nodes, fever that may appear 2–4 weeks after appearance of primary lesion; may last for several years *Latent*—Usually no clinical symptoms present for as long as 20 years; may continue to involve and damage neurologic and cardiovascular organs; dementia, confusion, paralysis, and paresis may occur.	• Treatment of both partners • Benzathine penicillin G 2.4 million units IM if of less than 1 year's duration; increase dosage and length of treatment if unknown duration of disease or longer than 1 year. • Repeat serology studies. • Avoid sexual contact or use condoms.
Trichomoniasis "Trich" *Trichomonas vaginalis*	• Protozoan with flagella • Identified on wet-mount microscopic examination of vaginal discharge • May be identified on Pap smear • Males usually asymptomatic • Foul-smelling vaginal discharge, thin, foamy, and green in color, causes itching of vulva and vagina, burning on urination and dyspareunia; "strawberry" cervix may be seen on speculum examination.	• Treat both partners. • Flagyl (metronidazole) 2 g by mouth at one time; avoid alcohol consumption. • Avoid sex or use condoms.

(Data from Baldwin K, Goodwin K: The Papanicolaou smear. Journal of Nurse-Midwifery 30(6):327–331, 1985; Bourcier K, Seidler A: Chlamydia and condylomata acuminata: An update for the nurse practitioner. Journal of Obstetric, Gynecologic and Neonatal Nursing 16(1):17–21, 1987; Fromer M: Ethical Issues in Sexuality and Reproduction. St Louis, CV Mosby, 1983; Hatcher R et al: Contraceptive Technology. New York, Irvington, 1986; and Hill L, Smith M: Self-Care Nursing. Englewood Cliffs, NJ, Prentice-Hall, 1985)

affect sexual functioning. Illegal drugs are used by some people because of their ability presumably to heighten the sexual experience. These drugs can have serious and even deadly side-effects of their own. Table 38-3 lists some of the categories of medications and their possible effects on sexual functioning.

NURSE AS ROLE MODEL

A nurse's attitudes, biases, and prejudice regarding sexuality are readily transmitted to clients through the nurse's actions, manner of speech, avoidance of certain circumstances, and types of discussion. The level of knowledge

a nurse has about sexual issues can inhibit or promote discussion of sexual health. The nurse who does not have a sound knowledge base of reproductive anatomy and physiology, sexual response, sexual expression, and other issues surrounding sexuality will be unable effectively to assess, teach, or counsel the client with sexual concerns. The nurse must also feel comfortable with self as a sexual being.

Nursing aims to enhance interactions with clients promote individual sexual wellness are as follows:
The nurse will be able to
• Define individual sexuality
• Assess degree of comfort with sexual issues
• Feel comfortable as a sexual being
• Develop self-awareness regarding sexual topics

Sexuality

Use the assessment checklist to determine how well you are meeting your sexuality needs. Then develop a prescription for self-care by choosing appropriate behaviors from the list of suggestions.

Assessment Checklist

almost always	some times	almost never	
☐	☐	☐	1. I feel good about my sexual identity.
☐	☐	☐	2. I have satisfying relationships with others.
☐	☐	☐	3. I accept sexual needs as a normal part of life.
☐	☐	☐	4. I am comfortable with physical actions that indicate love and belonging (such as touching and hugging).

Self-Care Behaviors

1. Avoid stereotyping "typical" gender roles.
2. Learn the biologic aspects of sexual functioning.
3. Ask questions about sexual needs and sexual activity when necessary.
4. Enjoy close relationships with others who love you.
5. Give a hug to someone you love.
6. Accept touch from others as a sign of caring and affection.
7. Practice "safer sex" (*e.g.,* use of contraceptives, condoms, and choice of partner).
8. Recognize how age, illness, or disability influences sexual needs and expression.

- Develop communication skills that promote discussion of sexual concerns with clients
- Practice responsible sexual expression

ASSESSING

Sexual History

The comprehensive health history should include information regarding a client's reproductive and sexual health, depending on the circumstances in which the client is receiving care. As a rule, three general categories of clients should have a sexual history recorded by the nurse:

- Any inpatient or outpatient client who is receiving care for pregnancy, STD, infertility, or contraception
- Any client who is currently experiencing a sexual dysfunction or problem
- Any client whose illness will affect sexual functioning and behavior in any way

Information is best obtained from the client by beginning with nonthreatening questions and progressing to more sensitive concerns. Clients usually have no difficulty answering questions regarding their bodies and general reproductive issues such as "When did your menstrual periods first begin?"

Clients should understand why the nurse needs information about their intimate sexual functioning.

Nurses should explain to clients that this information may be very helpful in assisting them in the plan of care. The sexual history is a vital portion of the reproductive history. It also assists the nurse in identifying any sexual problems or concerns. It is an excellent opportunity for the nurse to teach by helping the client confront fears and allay myths. There are four general levels of sexual history suggested by Watts (1979):

- Level 1: as part of a health history—obtained by a nurse
- Level 2: sexual history—obtained by a nurse with education and training in sexuality
- Level 3: sexual problem history—obtained by a sex therapist
- Level 4: psychiatric/psychosocial history—obtained by a psychiatric nurse clinician

Each level acquires more specific information from the client regarding sexual health and also requires the interviewer to have more sophisticated preparation and skills. The professional nurse usually performs a sexual history on level 1.

The nurse sets the tone or atmosphere for the interview. The nurse's attitudes will greatly affect the client's response to the sexual history, and clients will be more cooperative if they sense the nurse's security and ease during the interview. Privacy is essential for the sexual history; doors should be closed and no interruptions allowed. Sit close to the client and speak in a quiet, relaxed, objective tone of voice. Use eye contact and open body posture. The client needs to know what will hap-

T A B L E   38-3
Medications and Their Effects on Sexual Functioning

Drug	Effect on Sexual Functioning
Amyl nitrite	Peripheral vasodilator used in the past for treating angina; has become popular as sex enhancer among male homosexuals in particular; when inhaled at time of orgasm the resulting vasodilation is felt to cause an intensified orgasmic release. Loss of erection, hypotension and faintness may occur.
Anticonvulsants	Dilantin (phenytoin) has sedative effects, which may decrease desire and reduce sexual response.

Antidepressants
  Tricyclic compounds
  Monoamine oxidase inhibitors
  Lithium carbonate
	Similar to antihypertensive drugs; male impotence is significant.
	Male impotence and ejaculatory dysfunction in 25%–30% of men
	Decreases serum testosterone in men. Some antidepressants have been found to cause prolonged painful erections known as *priapism*. One such drug is trazodone.

Antihistamines	May have sedative effect that decreases desire; may also cause decreased vaginal lubrication

Antihypertensives
  Methyldopa
  Clonidine
  Reserpine
	May decrease desire in both male and female clients
	Erectile failure in 24% of men; no adverse effect on female clients
	Decreased desire in women; erectile and ejaculation dysfunctions in men

Antipsychotics	Causes decreased desire in 10%–20% of clients; may also cause erection and ejaculatory dysfunctions Small amount of the antipsychotic drug may be found in the semen. The partner may experience resulting genital rash. Wear condoms while on therapy.
Antispasmodics	These drugs relax smooth muscle; male impotence may occur.
Barbiturates	In low initial doses sexual pleasure may be increased due to loss of inhibitions. However, long-term use commonly causes decreased desire and orgasmic dysfunction. Male impotence is not uncommon.
Cocaine	Reported to increase quality of sexual experience. Chronic use, however, results in sexual dysfunction and loss of desire in both men and women.
Ethyl alcohol	In moderate amounts decreases inhibitions and consequently improves sexual functioning. Continued consumption decreases sexual functioning. Chronic alcoholics are impotent and often sterile. Testicular damage and permanent dysfunction are common. Female alcoholics experience decreased desire and orgasmic dysfunction.
Marijuana	Release of inhibitions may cause feeling of increased sexual functioning. Marijuana users have increased incidence of decreased desire and male impotence.
Narcotics	Serious impairment of sexual functioning with increased dependence. Erectile and ejaculatory dysfunctions common in men. Testosterone levels and amount of semen decreased. High incidence of decreased desire occurs in both men and women.

(Data from Fuentes R et al: Sexual side effects. What to tell your patients, what not to say. RN 46(2):34–41, 1983; and Woods NF: Human Sexuality in Health and Illness. St Louis, CV Mosby, 1984)

pen to this information and who will have access to it. The nurse needs to explain to the client that no one will have access to this information unless it is significant to the client's care. Reproductive health information should be obtained from the client first, followed by the client's sexual health history. The best approach is to begin with general open-ended questions and progress to more specific ones. The nurse should use the lan-

guage used by the client. If not, clients may be reluctant to tell the caregiver that they do not understand certain terms for fear of appearing ignorant or foolish. For example, the client may choose the term *come* to mean climax or orgasm.

It is useful to begin questions with "many people like" or "many people feel." This gives clients security in knowing they are not alone in how they feel and are

Elements of a Sexual History

Women

    Date of menarche
    Date of last menstrual period (LMP)
    Duration and length of flow in days
    Number of pregnancies, living children,
        miscarriages, and abortions
    Method of birth control currently used
    Known sexually transmitted disease past or
        present

Men

    Describe urinary function
    Number of children fathered
    Method of birth control used
    Known sexually transmitted disease past or
        present

encouraged to talk about their problems or concerns. An example of this type of questioning is the following: "Many people feel that it's helpful to discuss your concerns about sex with your partner. What do you think about this?"

A brief sexual history may include the following three questions:

    Has [*anything*] interfered with your being a husband or father/wife or mother?
    Has [*anything*] changed the way you feel about yourself as a man/woman?
    Has [*anything*] changed your ability to function sexually?
    (Woods, 1984, p 88)

(The disease, surgery, medication, or other appropriate term is used in place of the word *anything*.) The answers to these questions provide much information about the client.

Annon (Reamy, 1984) has described one method of obtaining information from a client with a sexual problem. This method elicits information in a short period of time.

- Description of the problem: "How would you describe the problem?"
- Onset and cause of the problem: "What do you think caused the problem or what was happening when you first noticed it?"
- Past attempts at resolution: "What have you tried in the past to correct the problem?"
- Goals of the client: "What do you wish to accomplish?"

A narrative form of recording a sexual history is generally used because it allows the interviewer to document the data in many of the client's own words. If a client is seeking help for a sexual problem, a more specific format will be utilized in recording information obtained by a skilled therapist.

Sexual Dysfunction

The term **sexual dysfunction** refers to a problem that prevents an individual or couple from engaging in or enjoying satisfactory sexual intercourse and orgasm. Dysfunctions may occur as a result of physiologic malfunctions, conflicts with cultural norms, interpersonal problems, or any combination of these. Anxieties and fears concerning the sexual act are most always present. Clients with severe sexual dysfunctions require intensive professional therapy from a qualified sex therapist. It is hypothesized that sexual dysfunctioning is a problem of considerable magnitude. A few of the major dysfunctions are briefly discussed here and in Table 38-4.

Male Sexual Dysfunctions. Erectile failure, also called **impotence**, is the inability of a man to attain or maintain an erection to such an extent that he cannot have satisfactory intercourse. Common causes of impotence include various illnesses, treatments for these illnesses, and personal anxieties.

Premature ejaculation is the condition when a man consistently reaches ejaculation or orgasm before or very soon after entering the vagina. The result is that his partner usually does not have time to reach sexual satisfaction. Causes of the problem are rarely physical in nature.

Retarded ejaculation, also called *ejaculatory incompetence,* refers to a man's inability to ejaculate into the vagina or to suffer with delayed intravaginal ejaculation. The causes of this problem are similar to those of impotence. When it occurs after having experienced normal ejaculations, the cause is most probably due to interpersonal problems.

Female Sexual Dysfunctions. *Inhibited sexual desire* consists of an inhibition in sexual arousal so that congestion and vaginal lubrication are absent or minimal. Causative factors may be anxiety, negative emotions, fear, interpersonal problems, or physical factors.

Orgasmic dysfunction is defined as the inability of a woman to reach orgasm. The causes are similar to those of inhibited sexual desire.

Dyspareunia is painful intercourse. Although it is most often described by women, some men may also suffer from this disorder. The cause is usually physical in nature, although psychologic problems such as fear and anxiety can cause pain in some women.

Vaginismus is a rare condition in which the vaginal opening closes tightly and prevents penile penetration. Vaginismus is due to involuntary spastic contractions of muscles at and around the vaginal opening and the levator ani muscles. The cause of vaginismus may be physical or psychologic, or both.

(Text continues on p. 1079.)

T A B L E   38-4
Sexual Dysfunction and Nursing Assessment

Sexual Dysfunction	Assessment Priorities
Male	
Erectile failure (impotence)	• History of diabetes, spinal cord trauma, cardiovascular disease, surgical procedure, alcoholism • Use of certain medications such as antihypertensives, antidepressants, or illicit drugs • Determine degree of mental depression that may be present • Obtain specific information regarding the degree of impotence, length of time of disorder, continuing life factors
Premature ejaculation	• Assess what client defines as his dysfunction and ability to control ejaculation. • Assess any causative relationship factors, such as anxiety, guilt, lack of time, new partner, and so on.
Retarded ejaculation	• History of neurologic disorders, Parkinson's disease, or use of certain medications • Same assessment priorities as for premature ejaculation, above
Female	
Inhibited sexual desire	• Use of oral contraceptives or other hormonal therapy, use of alcohol or certain medications • History of sexual abuse, rape or incest, depression, or other sexual dysfunctions • Assess any other contributing or relationship factors.
Orgasmic dysfunction	• Assess knowledge level regarding sexual response cycle and anatomy. • Assess communication pattern between the client and her partner. • Assess usual sexual pattern and behavior between client and her partner. • Assess any other contributing factors.
Dyspareunia	• History of diabetes, hormonal imbalance, vaginal infection, endometriosis, urethritis, cervicitis, or rectal lesions • Use of antihistamines, alcohol, tranquilizers, or illicit drugs • Assess client's ability for vaginal lubrication during sexual act. • Assess client's use of coital positions. • Assess use of cosmetic or chemical irritants to genitals such as deodorant tampons, contraceptive creams, or jellies or condoms. • Physical assessment of internal and external genitalia • Assess any other contributing factors.
Vaginismus	• Assess knowledge regarding anatomy and sexual response. • Assess pattern of sexual activity: how often, level of arousal, orgasm. • Assess presence of other sexual dysfunctions. • History of sexual abuse, trauma, or rape • Assess client's feelings regarding her partner. • Assess any other causative factors, such as fear of pregnancy, anxiety, guilt. • Physical assessment of internal and external genitalia

Nursing Examination

Physical examination of the reproductive or genitourinary system for either male or female clients is necessary under the following circumstances:

- As part of a routine physical examination
- Annual women's health care, including Pap smear
- Suspicion of an STD
- Suspicion of pregnancy
- Work-up for infertility
- Unusual lump, discharge, or unusual appearance of the genital organs noticed by the client
- Request for birth control
- Change in urinary function

The examiner may routinely perform a complete physical examination along with assessment of the reproductive system if the client has not had contact with the health-care system within a year or if assessment findings of a complete examination would be useful in diagnosing an ailment or complaint of the client.

The nurse should initially ask whether the client has experienced this type of examination in the past if this information is not evident by the client's records. Depending on the client's knowledge base, the nurse should explain the progressive steps of the examination and what the client may feel during the examination. This will give the client some feeling of control and security during the examination. The nurse's responsibilities during an examination of the reproductive system are

- To provide information to the client regarding the examination
- To teach the client
- To provide support for the client during the examination
- To assist the examiner, if appropriate, with any procedures or laboratory studies

Female

Examination of body parts that are considered private and not usually viewed by others is embarrassing for some women. Many physical examinations are performed by nurse practitioners in women's health facilities. However, the majority of examiners are male physicians. It is the responsibility of the nurse present at such an examination to anticipate anxiety and discomfort on the part of the client. Preparation for the examination and discussion of the examination are covered in Chapter 24. Breast examination is discussed in Chapter 24 also. The breast examination provides an excellent opportunity to assess the woman's knowledge of breast self-examination and to teach her how to examine her breasts properly. Breast self-examination is discussed later in this chapter.

The woman should be informed before the examiner touches her. This information greatly diminishes a woman's reflex to "jump" when her external genitalia are initially palpated and consequently will prevent tightening of the pelvic muscles. Her relaxation will eliminate much of the discomfort of the examination.

The vaginal speculum, as illustrated in Figure 24-1, is a two-bladed instrument used to open the vagina and to inspect the cervix and vaginal walls. Its use can cause discomfort if the client is not assisted to relax or if the wrong size speculum is used. It is helpful to show the speculum to the woman and explain its function beforehand. A Papanicolau test (Pap smear) is performed of the cervix, and cultures may be taken while the speculum is in place. The speculum is slowly withdrawn from the vagina while the examiner notes the condition of the vaginal walls.

A bimanual examination is performed to assess internal structures. The examiner introduces the index and middle fingers of one hand into the client's vagina while the other hand lies on the client's lower abdomen. The cervix is palpated for movement, tenderness, and consistency. The areas around the cervix are also palpated. The uterus is examined by palpation between the internal and external hands for size, shape, contour, and consistency and for the presence of lumps or lesions.

The client is assisted to a sitting position by instructing her first to push back on the examining table from the stirrups to avoid straining the back. A running commentary about assessment findings by the examiner is necessary throughout the examination to teach the woman about her body as well as to assist her to relax and remove the mystery of a pelvic examination.

Male

The examination of the male genitalia is described in Chapter 24. Examination of the man's breast should always be included in the nursing examination. Although cancer of the male breast is rare, it can occur. The breast tissue and underlying muscle mass are palpated for lesions and the nipples are assessed for presence of discharge.

The external male genitalia should be examined with gloved hands. The perineum and anal sphincter are best inspected with the client lying on his side with the knees bent. The prostate gland is palpated through the rectum. The client can be assisted in this portion of the examination if he is asked to bear down against the examiner's finger as it is placed within the rectum.

The male client should be given the same consideration during the genitourinary examination as the female client. All procedures should be explained and the client's involvement in the examination encouraged.

DIAGNOSING

Before a nursing diagnosis can be made regarding a sexual problem, the assessment data collected by the nurse must be carefully reviewed to determine if the situation can be corrected by independent nursing interventions.

Although many problems of sexuality experienced by a client in a health-care situation are amenable to nursing action, some require the expertise of other specialties. For example, an impotent diabetic client who would benefit from a penile implant needs medical consultation. A client with a serious sexual dysfunction or who practices a destructive sexual expression needs intensive therapy by a clinical psychologist, sex therapist, or counselor. Appropriate referrals by the nurse should follow the identification of such problems. Either of the two diagnoses Sexual dysfunction or Altered sexuality patterns is used to describe problems of sexuality amenable to nursing intervention.

Sexual dysfunction may be specified by erectile failure (impotence), premature ejaculation, retarded ejaculation, inhibited sexual desire, orgasmic dysfunction, vaginismus, or dyspareunia. Common etiologies for sexual dysfunction include effects of medication (specify), effects of alcohol consumption, effects of disease process (specify), history of abuse (specify rape, incest), feelings of depression, guilt, anxiety, fear of rejection, miscommunication with partner, fear of pain, effects of birth control method (specify), lack of knowledge, or effects of surgical procedure (specify). The nursing diagnosis Altered sexuality patterns can be further specified by loss of desire (to abstinence), increased desire (to promiscuity), or change in sexual expression. Common etiologies for Altered sexuality patterns include stress (life-style, job, family, finances, marital conflict), isolation from partner, effects of pregnancy (specify), feelings of depression, loss of privacy, loss of communication with partner, relationship change (new partner), effects of disease process (sexual position, frequency, mode of expression), change in body image, change in self-concept, or loss of partner.

A representative sample of some nursing diagnoses concerning sexuality is given in Table 38-5.

Changes in sexuality can affect other areas of human functioning. In the following nursing diagnoses, problems of sexuality are the etiology of another problem:

Impaired adjustment related to loss of sexual partner, loss of sexual body part

Anxiety related to fear of pregnancy, loss of sexual functioning or desire, effects of disease process on sexual functioning

Alteration in comfort (pain) related to sexual position, penile penetration, effects of genital surgery, lack of vaginal lubrication

Ineffective individual coping related to effects of body image on sexual expression, change in sexual partner

Fear related to pain during sexual intercourse, history of sexual abuse

Anticipatory grieving related to loss of sexual functioning, effects of surgical excision of genital body part

Altered growth and development related to sexual exploitation or abuse, sexual guilt, effects of

hormonal imbalance, lack of information about sexuality

Knowledge deficit (specify: contraceptive methods, spread of STDs, sexual response, genital anatomy, modes of sexual expression, self-examination, effects of disease and/or medications) related to misinformation, sexual myths, lack of interest in learning, cognitive limitation

Impaired mobility related to position during sexual intercourse

Disturbance in body image (specify: surgical excision of genital body part, loss of or gain of body weight) related to fear of rejection

Impaired social interaction related to effects of marital separation or divorce

Social isolation related to fear of contraction of STD, fear of sexual encounter

Alteration in thought processes related to obsession with sexual fantasies

PLANNING: CLIENT GOALS

It is important for nurses to value sexuality as an important aspect of who the client is and how the client is identified as a unique human being. Specific client goals to promote sexual wellness will be determined.

- The client will define individual sexuality.
- The client will establish open patterns of communication with significant others.
- The client will develop self-awareness and body awareness.
- The client will practice responsible sexual expression (*e.g.,* by 5/1, the client will utilize rubber condoms with all sexual encounters).

Specific client goals will depend on the nature of the client's problem or concern. Client goals should be client oriented, that is, something the client desires to do or has the ability to accomplish. For example, it is not enough to advise a method of birth control; rather, the nurse needs to know which method the client is motivated and able to use.

IMPLEMENTING

Establishing a Trusting Nurse–Client Relationship

It is impossible to address or help a client's sexuality if trust has not developed between the nurse and the client. The nurse needs to project an objective, nonthreatening, and nonjudgmental attitude and an aura of confidentiality. The nurse's anticipating client concerns and needs through awareness of the client's behav-

T A B L E 38-5
Nursing Diagnoses for Problems Affecting Sexuality

Title	Etiologic or Contributing Factors	Sample Defining Characteristics
Sexual dysfunction: erectile failure	Use of antihypertensive medication	• 45-year-old man with 3-year history of hypertension • Maintained normotensive on reserpine 0.25 mg daily • "I have had trouble keeping an erection. My wife and I haven't made love in months. We don't talk about it anymore. I guess that part of my life is over." • Client appears resigned and saddened.
Sexual dysfunction: dyspareunia	Effects of menopausal process	• 54-year-old female whose last menses was 1 year ago. • "Whenever my husband and I make love my vagina burns and stings." • States decrease in vaginal lubrication over past several months.
Altered sexuality patterns: change in sexual expression	Loss of privacy due to hospitalization	• 23-year-old man hospitalized for past 6 weeks with injuries resulting from car crash; has been in traction for fractured right femur. • "I can't take this place anymore! Everyone barges in here whenever they want to—nobody cares about my feelings—a guy can't even act like a guy around here. I wish I could be alone with my wife for a while with no interruptions."
Altered sexuality patterns: Loss of desire	Change in body image due to body-altering surgery	• Surgery for bowel cancer with construction of permanent colostomy 1 month ago. • "I know the colostomy was necessary to save my life, but it is so disgusting. I'll never be able to have a relationship with my husband again. It's a real turn-off to me—just imagine what he'll think—how can I expect him to want to make love to a freak?"
Alteration in comfort: pain	Abduction of hips in sexual positioning	• 60-year-old woman with history of osteoarthritis for 6 years. • "The act of intercourse hurts my hips so bad that I'm in pain the whole next day. I don't want to stop having intercourse with my husband, but I'm going to have to if this pain gets worse." • Client states that the missionary position is the only position utilized during sex with her husband throughout their 40-year marriage.

ior and verbal and nonverbal cues also helps the client trust the nurse later on with information of an intimate nature. It is important to establish respect for the individual and empathy before sexual topics are discussed. An empathetic nurse takes into consideration all of an individual's circumstances and life experiences and views them from a therapeutic, not a pitying approach. Only when the nurse is accepted as a trusted caring person will the client relay details of private life, including concerns of a sexual nature.

Teaching the Client

The majority of nursing interventions regarding a client's sexuality encompass teaching to promote wellness. Major goals of client teaching are a change in knowledge, a change in client attitude, or a change in behaviors. In some situations, clients need assistance in defin-

ing or redefining their sexuality and its importance to their lives. Offering information, dispelling fears, and providing positive reinforcement are some ways nurses can assist clients to increase their knowledge about their bodies and sexual functioning. Clients may need assistance in modifying behaviors or learning new skills to increase the quality of sexual health and functioning.

Sexual Myths and Body Awareness

Many people believe things about sex that they have heard from family, friends, or as part of their culture that are simply not true or not founded on scientific data. The nurse may refute sexual myths (Table 38-6) and teach factual information during the assessment or while providing care.

Clients may need assistance in becoming familiar with what they believe and feel about their sexual selves.

(Text continues on p. 1083.)

T A B L E   38-6
Sexual Myths and Facts to Refute Them

Myths	Facts
Each person is born with a certain amount of sexual drive, which if overdrawn in youth leaves little reserve for later years.	Actually the correlation between sexual activity and length of time it persists throughout life is just the opposite. The more consistently sexually active a person is, the longer the activity continues into the later years of life.
The need for expressing one's sexuality becomes less important in the later half of one's life.	Physiologically, sexual desire and ability do not decrease markedly after middle age. The expression of one's sexuality, as an integral part of development, follows the overall pattern of health and physical performance.
Sexual abstinence is necessary in training for sports.	Physiologically the achievement of orgasm is rarely more demanding than most activities encountered in daily life. The desire for sleep that often follows is most commonly due to factors other than physical exhaustion from sexual activities. There is *no* scientific evidence that sex "weakens" a person.
Excessive sexual activity can lead to mental illness.	The biologic significance of human sexuality is of no greater impact on total development than any other necessary biologic function. There is no scientific basis for believing that one will develop a mental or physical illness with excessive or no sexual activity.
Wet dreams are indicators of sexual disorders.	Erotic dreams that culminate in orgasms are normal common physiologic phenomena in at least 85% of all men. They can occur at any age after puberty. Some women also report in clinical studies that their sexual dreams culminate in orgasm. In women, this phenomenon is believed to increase with advancing age.
Because of the anatomic nature of the sex organs, women are passive and men are aggressive.	Physiologic studies disprove this myth by showing the woman to be far from passive. Maximum gratification requires each partner to be both passive and aggressive in participating mutually and cooperatively.
It is "unnatural" for a woman to have as strong a desire for sex as a man—for women should not enjoy sex as much as men.	These myths have been reinforced by a society that has traditionally taught women that they are to suppress sexual desires to gain love, security, and society's respect, based on the assumption that it is the "basic nature" of women to be submissive, dependent, and subordinate. Physiologic studies indicate that, in some respects, the woman's sex drive is not only as strong but may be even stronger than that of the man.
Women who have multiple orgasms or who readily come to climax are nymphomaniacs or promiscuous.	Physiologic studies at this time suggest that we do not know women's sexual potential; these studies indicate that there is a wide range of intensity and duration of orgasmic experience and the potential for multiple or frequent orgasms within a brief period of time is not at all uncommon. Therefore, women normally may have greater orgasmic capacity than men with regard to duration and frequency of orgasm.
There is a difference between vaginal orgasm and clitoral orgasm.	Physiologic misunderstanding has produced the myth of separate clitoral and vaginal orgasms rather than their interrelationships. Female orgasm is normally initiated by clitoral stimulation, but since it is a total body response there are marked variations in intensity and timing. There is no reason to believe that the female response to the sex act is due to a vaginal rather than a clitoral orgasm.
A mature sexual relationship requires the man and woman to achieve simultaneous orgasm.	While simultaneous orgasm may be desirable, it is an unrealistic goal. Often it is possible only under the most ideal circumstances and is not a determinant of sexual achievement or of satisfaction (except to someone who accepts this as dogma).
It is dangerous to have intercourse during menstruation.	Since the source of the menstrual flow is from the uterus rather than the vagina, there is no basis for concern about tissue damage to the vagina. Actually the desire for sex increases during the menses due to increased pelvic vasocongestion. There is no physiologic basis for abstinence during the menses.

(Continued)

Myths	Facts
The larger penis has greater possibilities for producing orgasm in the woman.	Physiologically, there is practically no relationship between the size of a man's penis and his ability to satisfy a woman sexually. Furthermore, there is very little correlation between penile size and body size and their relationship to sexual potency.
The face-to-face coital position is the proper, moral, and healthy one.	Recent knowledge of human sexual practices dispels this myth with the recognition that there is no normal or single most acceptable sexual position. Whatever position offers the most pleasure and is acceptable to both partners is correct for them. Any variation is normal, healthy, and proper if it satisfies both partners.
The ability to achieve orgasm is an indicator of a person's sexual responsiveness.	Achievement of a satisfactory sexual response is the result of numerous physical, psychologic, and cultural influences. Too often the physical fact of orgasm (or lack of orgasm) is taken to be symbolic of sexual responsiveness and seen out of context of the entire relationship between man and woman.

The nurse can be helpful in a situation where a client has difficulty accepting or developing his or her sexuality by promoting self-confidence and a good self-concept in the client. When clients feel comfortable about themselves and their sensual feelings they can begin to focus on how they feel about their sexual functioning and specific sexual expressions.

Getting to know one's physical body is very important to healthy sexual development. Every man and woman, sexually active or not, needs to be aware of the appearance of his or her individual genitalia. Some people, because of their background, feel ashamed and repulsed by their bodies. Others feel that touching the body is dirty and may feel guilt and anxiety in stimulating themselves. Clients will need assistance in improving body awareness if any of these issues are present. Clients become accustomed to looking at their bodies by looking at nonthreatening anatomy first and then proceeding to the genitals. This can be done in the shower or with the use of a mirror. Knowing what looks normal can be of great importance in reporting the development of an unusual appearance later on. After clients have developed some degree of comfort in looking at their bodies, they can progress to experiencing touch. Again, clients should progress from nonthreatening parts of the body until the genitals can be touched without stress.

A good exercise for women in developing body awareness is the use of **Kegel exercises**. These exercises promote good vaginal tone by localizing and strengthening the *pubococcygeal* muscle. A woman can locate this muscle by stopping a stream of urine midway through urination. This maneuver can be repeated at any time of the day in any circumstance because its performance is not detectable. Women who practice Kegel exercises have found that sexual satisfaction is greatly improved.

Self-Examination

It is important for both men and women to learn to examine themselves through inspection and palpation of sexual body parts. Many conditions, some life threatening, can be detected when self-examination is performed. Early detection of cancer is crucial to its control and cure. The presence of some STDs may also be detected by self-examination.

Breast Self-Examination. The importance of breast self-examination (BSE) lies in its routine monthly performance, which helps the person to become familiar with what is normal. BSE should be performed after each menses or once a month for a postmenopausal woman. Any contact with a female client in the health-care delivery system should include assessment of her knowledge and practice of BSE.

The steps in performing BSE are shown in Figure 38-4 and are as follow:

1. Stand before a mirror with hands on hips to inspect the breasts. Look for the presence of indentations, dimpling, or odd position of a nipple. Any discharge from a nipple is abnormal unless the woman is nursing. Changes in size or shape of breasts should be reported.
2. Lie on the bed with a small pillow under the shoulder on the side of the breast to be examined, with the arm over the head. Using the opposite hand, palpate the breast starting at the very outer edge of the breast and using small circular motions of the flat portions of the fingers. Work inward in a clockwise manner toward the nipple. The nipple should be gently squeezed to detect the presence of any discharge. This procedure should be repeated for the opposite breast. Any unusual lump

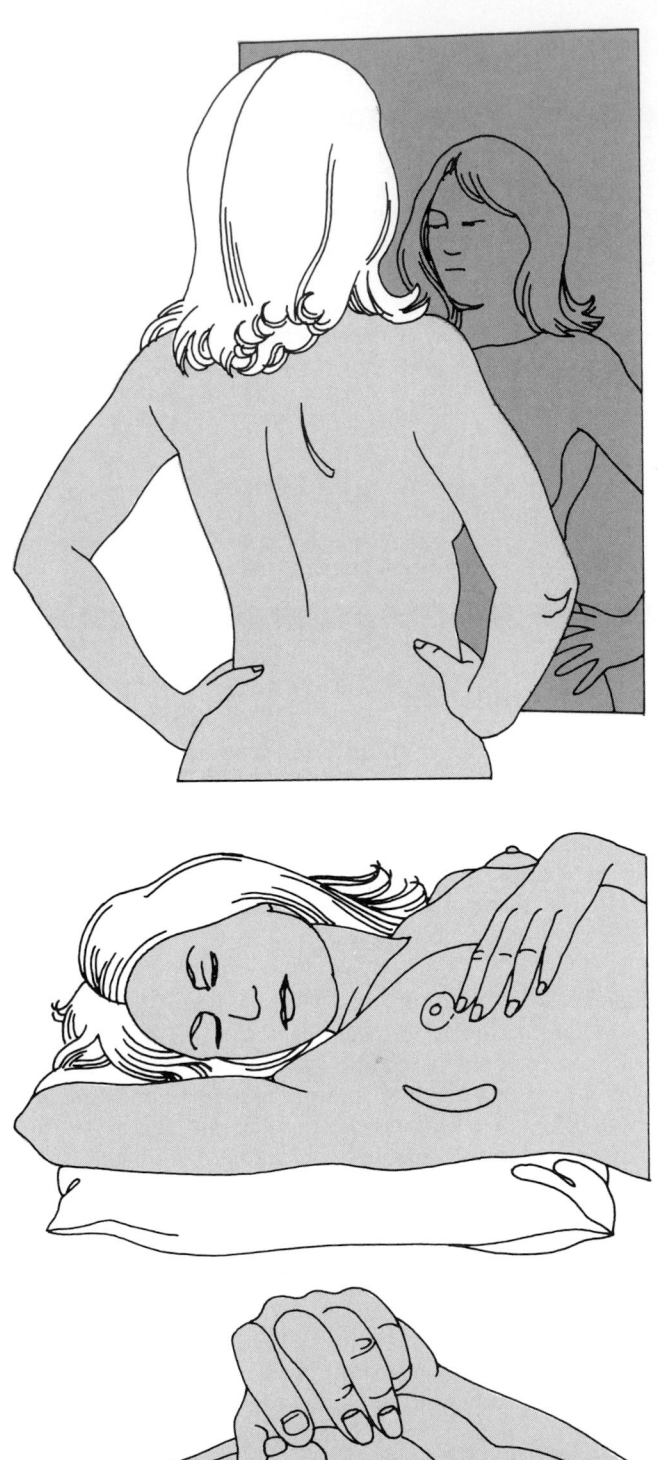

or tenderness should be reported to a health-care professional.

Testicular Self-Examination.   Male clients need to be taught to perform monthly assessment of the testicles. Although testicular cancer is not widespread, it can be easily detected and prognosis is good if found early. A good time to examine the testes is during a shower, when the scrotum becomes warm and loose. Men should also be taught the importance of examining their breasts.

The steps in testicular self-examination are shown in Figure 38-5 and are as follow:

1. The thumb and the fingers of each hand are used to palpate each testicle simultaneously. The client should systematically palpate the testes for the presence of lumps or differences in texture. The testes should feel smooth.
2. The epididymis is palpated above each testicle. The epididymis will feel soft and not as smooth as a testicle.
3. The spermatic cord, or vas deferens, extends upward from the scrotum toward the base of the penis and should be palpated for firmness and smoothness in texture.

Contraception

Clients choose **contraception** for many reasons and may contact health-care providers for information on birth control or contraceptive methods. Some people utilize contraception for the orderly spacing of pregnancies in a family. Others use a contraceptive method to prevent pregnancy from occurring until a family is desired. Some people choose a permanent method to prevent the possibility of pregnancy from ever occurring.

The best method available to prevent a pregnancy is sexual abstinence. However, for the majority of people this is not an acceptable method. All of the contraceptive methods currently available (Fig. 38-6) have distinct advantages and disadvantages. It is the responsibility of the nurse to understand and explain thoroughly the available methods so the client can choose one that will best meet the client's unique situation and needs.

Natural Family Planning.   Natural family planning methods are available to everyone but using them effec-

---

F I G U R E   38-4
Breast self-examination (BSE) is to be performed once a month. It is begun with inspection using a mirror. Attention is given to contours of the breast and to the skin. Pressing down on the hips serves to tense pectoralis major muscles to inspect for any retraction of the skin. Palpatory examination is performed in a supine position with the side to be examined elevated on a pillow or blanket. Self-examination is completed with a squeeze of the nipple to detect abnormal discharge.

tively requires motivation and an understanding of male and female reproductive anatomy and physiology. The methods of coitus interruptus, rhythm or calendar method, basal body temperature, and Billings method are utilized simultaneously in some way to achieve satisfactory results for the client and the partner. **Coitus Interruptus**, one of the oldest and most widely used methods, is the withdrawal of the penis from the vagina before ejaculation. Its drawbacks include the possibility of the presence of sperm in Cowper's gland secretions before ejaculation and the stress it places on the man's sexual experience. The *rhythm* or calendar method is based on a woman's monthly menstrual cycle in determining safe and unsafe days. It is not an appropriate method for a woman with irregular cycles. The unsafe days are regarded as periods for sexual abstinence because these days are optimal for conception. The *basal body temperature* method is based on the body's response to hormones and ovulation. The woman takes and records her temperature on awakening every morning. A sudden drop in temperature indicates ovulation. This method restricts sexual activity to the second half of the menstrual cycle after ovulation has occurred. The *Billing's* method is based on the changes in the cervical mucus throughout the menstrual cycle. As ovulation occurs, the mucus changes considerably in consistency, becoming sticky, clear, and slippery like an egg white. This method requires the woman to be aware of and have the ability to assess her cervical mucus.

Barrier Methods. The barrier methods include the condom, diaphragm, cervical cap, and vaginal sponge used in combination with a spermicidal agent. The *diaphragm* has been used in various forms since ancient times. It is currently marketed as a large dome-shaped device made of latex rubber that mechanically prevents semen from coming into contact with the cervix. It is also used to hold a quantity of spermicidal jelly in place against the cervix. The diaphragm is placed in the vagina before sexual activity. It fits between the pelvic notch at the front of the vagina to behind the cervix at the back. It should not be detected by either the woman or her partner when correctly situated in the vagina. A diaphragm must be individually fitted at a pelvic examination. The woman needs to be familiar with her body and able to handle her genitals for diaphragm placement and removal. The diaphragm must be worn during each episode of sexual activity and consistently used with a spermicidal agent.

The *condom* or "rubber" is used by men, although it is appropriate for a woman to have them available for her partner's use. The condom is rolled over the erect penis and collects the semen after ejaculation takes place. The condom is readily and conveniently available over the counter. The condom has had a surge of popularity with

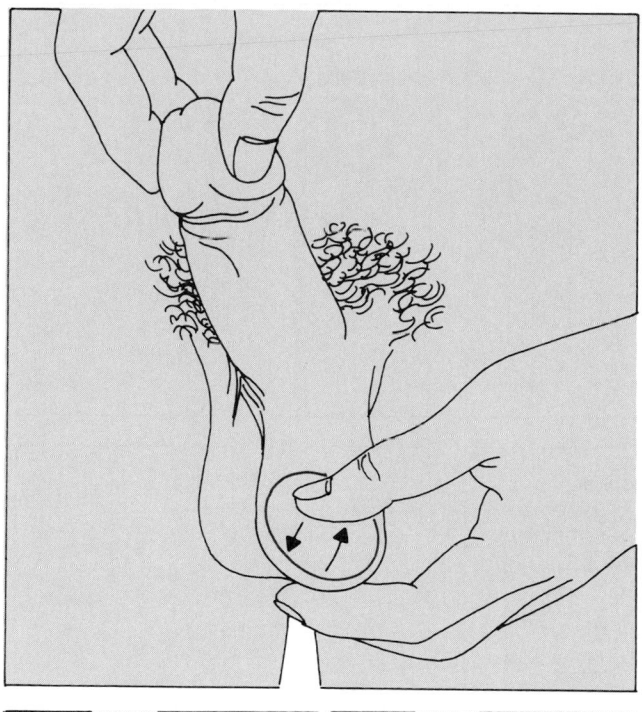

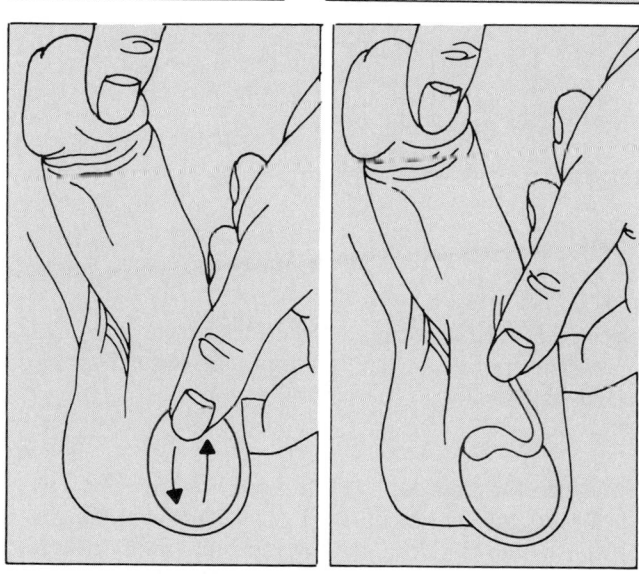

F I G U R E   38-5

Testicular self-examination (TSE) is to be performed once a month. A convenient time is after a warm bath or shower when the scrotum is relaxed. Both hands are used to palpate the testis; the normal testicle is smooth and uniform in consistency. (A) With the index and middle finger under the testis and the thumb on top, roll the testis gently in a horizontal plane between the thumb and fingers, feeling for any evidence of a small lump or abnormality. (B) Follow the same procedure for palpation in the "vertical" plane. (C) Locate the epididymis (cordlike structure on the top and back of the testicle that stores and transports sperm). Repeat the examination for the other testis; it is normal to find one testis larger than the other. Any evidence of a small, pea-size lump should be checked by a physician. It may be due to an infection or a tumor growth.

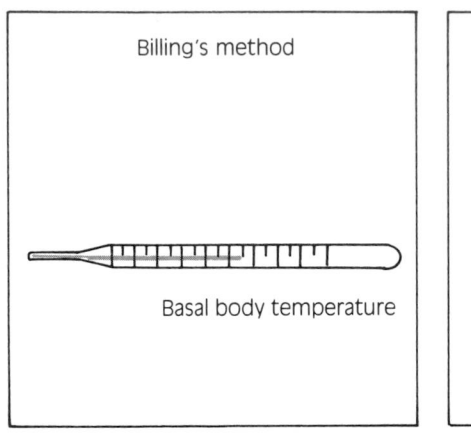

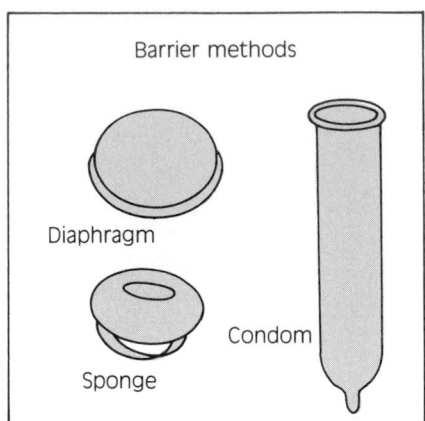

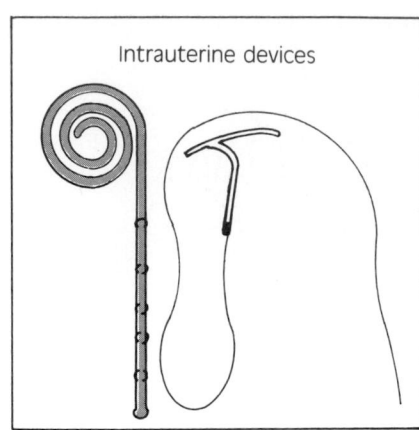

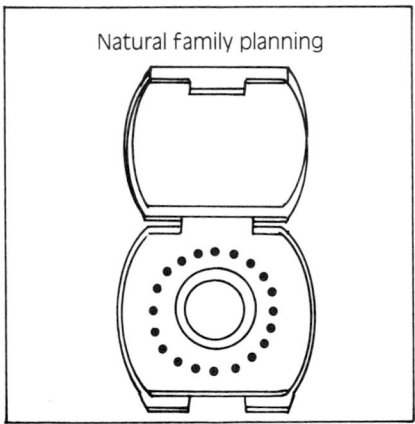

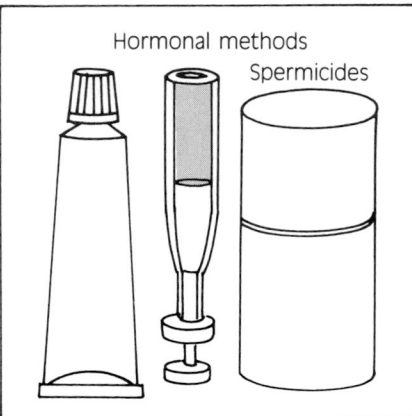

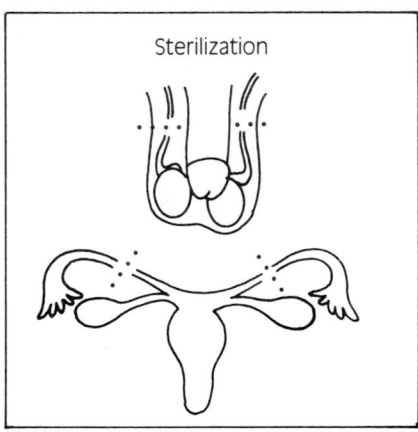

F I G U R E   38-6
Various methods of contraception.

the recent increased incidence of AIDS and other STDs among single people.

The *cervical cap* is not universally available at present. Its mechanism of action is similar to that of the diaphragm. The cervical cap is a thimble-shaped rubber device that is placed over the cervix and may be left there for up to 3 days at a time. Not all women can wear a cervical cap due to individual anatomic differences. There is some evidence to suggest that the cervical cap can cause cervical inflammation and increase risk of pelvic infection.

Spermicides are used with barrier methods but can also be used alone. Spermicides come in creams, jellies, foams, and suppositories. Although readily available, spermicides are not as effective alone as when combined with another method, such as a diaphragm or a condom.

The *vaginal sponge* is a barrier method that contains a spermicide. It has been available over the counter for several years. The sponge not only acts as a barrier between the semen and the cervix but also serves as a reservoir to hold semen. The vaginal sponge does carry some risk of toxic shock syndrome and is contraindicated for use in women who have a past history of toxic shock. It is important for women who use the vaginal

sponge to follow package directions carefully and to remove the sponge within 24 hours. The vaginal sponge is about as effective as the diaphragm.

Intrauterine Device. The intrauterine device (IUD) is an object that is placed by a physician or nurse practitioner within the uterus to prevent implantation of fertilized ovum. The precise mechanism by which it works is not known. Although it has a high effectiveness rate and requires little care or motivation on the part of the client, the IUD has many serious side-effects and resulting complications. It is an excellent method for women who have completed their families but are not ready or willing to take the final step toward sterilization. Owing to the litigation resulting from complications caused by the IUD, it has been taken off the market by most IUD-producing pharmaceutical companies. Although the IUD may reappear in the future, all women who currently have an IUD in place should seek assistance from a health-care provider to have it removed. Women wearing a Progestasert IUD should check for the presence of the string in the vagina after every menses and should have the IUD replaced every year.

Hormonal Methods.

Hormonal methods are based on the feedback mechanism of hormones of the menstrual cycle. Synthetic estrogens and progestin chemical compounds are utilized in the form of a pill, shot, or implant to prevent ovulation.

The *oral contraceptive* ("the pill") is the most common contraceptive method and the most popular method for women in their twenties. Most of the harmful side-effects and dangers associated with taking the pill are related to the estrogen component. However, most pills currently available contain a small dose of 35 μg of estrogen. The pill has many beneficial noncontraceptive effects. It has been shown to protect women against the development of breast, ovarian, and endometrial cancer (Dickerson, 1983). Taken consistently and as prescribed, the pill is almost 100% effective in guarding against pregnancy. However, the cost may be prohibitive to some women. The woman must also be motivated to take a pill every day at the same time. A health history and physical examination by a health-care provider are necessary to obtain a prescription for oral contraceptives. Some women should not take the pill in the presence of certain physiologic disorders or diseases.

Sterilization.

Although male and female sterilization methods can be surgically reversed, the results are not always satisfactory and the methods should therefore be regarded as permanent and irreversible. Sexual desire and ability are not affected by sterilization.

Sterilization in the woman is accomplished by surgically severing the fallopian tubes. This procedure is known as a *tubal ligation* and prevents travel of the ovum down the tube. Today, it is usually performed on an outpatient basis. Some physicians can also perform the tubal ligation under local anesthesia. Postoperative care and recovery time are required after a tubal ligation.

Sterilization in the man is accomplished by surgically severing the vas deferens, which prevents sperm from entering the semen. The *vasectomy* is usually performed in a physician's office under local anesthesia. It is important that the man know that he and his partner must use an alternate form of contraception until he has produced two semen analyses with zero sperm. It usually takes approximately 4 to 6 weeks for all stored sperm to be eliminated from the ductal system of the male.

Coping With Special Sexual Needs

The nurse can do much for clients to facilitate coping with sexual concerns generated by diseases and their treatments. Anticipatory guidance and information should be offered to the client. The importance of open communication with the partner should be stressed. The nurse should include the partner in teaching. Discussion about possible sexual positions is useful and can aid in eliminating pain during coitus. The client can utilize drawings in selecting possible sexual positions. The client will also find that intercourse may be more comfortable if pain medication is taken before beginning any sexual activity.

When teaching clients about medications it is important to include known possible sexual alterations to prevent future anxiety and also depression. Clients should alert their physicians if these side-effects are experienced. Often a drug dosage can be modified or the drug changed if sexual functioning is affected. Otherwise, clients may opt to discontinue the medication on their own rather than sacrifice optimal sexual functioning, if this is an important aspect of life.

Nurses also need to be aware of the special concerns and issues surrounding the care of a homosexual client. Homosexuals have the same right to health care as do heterosexuals. The homosexual has the right to information and the right to confidentiality just like anyone else.

Responsible Sexual Expression

Clients need to know how best to gain satisfactory sexual experiences and yet behave responsibly in their activities. Responsible sexuality encompasses these major areas: the form of sexual expression, the prevention of unwanted pregnancy, the prevention of spread of STDs, and sex education.

The form of sexual expression used by clients should not inflict unwanted harm on themselves or others. When the sexual expression encroaches on the rights of others, it is not healthy or desirable. Sexual acts that violate another's rights are usually considered to be acts of aggression or hostility rather than stemming from sexual need or desire. Acts of **rape** in particular are motivated by the need to dominate and humiliate the victim.

The prevention of an unwanted pregnancy must be a conscious decision. Anyone considering the possibility of a sexual encounter should seek out a contraceptive method either from a health-care provider or from the pharmacy; it is too late to think about contraception during sexual intercourse. To practice responsible sexuality, the contraceptive method must be used consistently and according to instructions.

The incidence of the various STDs is widespread. The only absolute method to avoid an STD is to remain a virgin until marriage, to marry a person who is a virgin, and henceforth never to have sex with anyone else. When this is not practical, other practices that can decrease a person's exposure to STDs are the following:

- The client should limit the number of sexual partners. The risk of an STD rises with the addition of each new partner.
- If a partner has symptoms of an STD, the client should abstain from any sexual activity.
- If the client is in doubt about possible exposure, he or she should report to a health-care facility for examination.

- If the client does contract an STD, all partners should be notified and advised to seek treatment.
- The use of condoms is now advocated for protection against STDs as well as against pregnancy. The client should keep a box of condoms on hand if monogamy is not practiced within the relationship.

Sex education is critical to healthy sexual development and safe sexual behaviors (McCary and McCary, 1982). Information received from peers and friends is almost always inadequate and erroneous. Parents should be taught to answer children's questions immediately and accurately.

Meeting Sexuality Needs of the Hospitalized Client

A hospital experience puts a strain on a person's individuality and sexual self. Illness may delete feelings of sexual desire. Therefore, it can be a good sign of a client's improving health if sexual interaction is desired with the partner. This necessitates anticipatory guidance on the part of the nurse, for many clients may hesitate to make such a request for fear of being ridiculed. Often a client merely desires the privacy to hold and caress the partner. The intimacy of this act often fulfills feelings of longing to be needed and loved.

There are many ways nurses can advocate for a client's sexual needs. Some may seem very obvious and commonplace, whereas others may necessitate nurses coming to terms with their own sexuality (see the box entitled Advocating Clients' Sexual Needs).

Counseling the Client Regarding Sexuality

Not all clients with sexual concerns need intensive therapy. Some clients benefit greatly by the presence of another to listen to verbally expressed concerns. Voicing their concerns allows clients the opportunity to put information into perspective and gain a clearer focus on what the problem really is and how to solve it. Nurses counseling clients need to refrain from offering their own advice because what is right for one person may be very wrong for another. Also, offering false reassurances

---

Advocating Clients' Sexual Needs

- All clients should be accepted as sexual beings with the right to be treated with dignity and with sensitivity to their feelings.
- All clients have the right to some degree of privacy regardless of the circumstances surrounding their hospitalization.

    Anticipate the client's desire for privacy by the simple act of drawing a curtain or closing a door.

    Clients should be given the option of wearing their own bed clothes to promote sexual identity.
- Potentially shaming situations for the client should be anticipated.

    Give information regarding what the procedure is and why it needs to be done, and acknowledge that the client's embarassment is normal and understandable.
- Health-care providers should not simply take for granted that clients do not mind intrusive or embarassing procedures performed on their bodies and private parts.
- Clients have a right to question the physician regarding sexual needs or future sexual functioning.

    Anticipate these questions for the client. Ask clients if they have any concerns regarding sexuality that can be answered by the nurse.

    Nurses can interface with the physician to obtain information required by the client.
- The atmosphere within the hospital unit needs to allow for sexual expression between clients and their partners.
- Confidentiality is a right of every hospitalized client.

    Do not promise confidentiality if that promise cannot be kept.

    Allow no one access to the client's personal records who is not directly involved in the client's care.

    Allow no information regarding clients to escape into idle conversation.
- All clients should be referred to formally as Mr., Mrs., Miss, Ms.
- Visitors, including a visiting spouse, should be referred to as people with genders, rather than as ''the visitor.''
- Clients should be allowed to keep some personal possessions if it is practical to do so.

Model for Counseling Clients with Sexual Problems (PLISSIT)

P—*Permission giving:* The nurse may make a suggestion that the client can use. Permission giving is not the same as advice. Permission giving implies giving the client freedom to choose to do something that the authority figure (such as a nurse) deems to be a positive alternative. It may be something the client wanted to do all along. For example

Client: "Aren't some sexual positions perverted?"

Nurse: "Many people enjoy using different positions for sex. Some positions are more pleasurable to some couples than others. You and your partner have the right to use any position for sex that you desire."

LI—*Limited information:* Specific factual information is required by the client. It often involves some aspect of anatomy and physiology or the specifics of certain sexual expressions.

SS—*Specific suggestions:* Clients need very specific instructions regarding a useful technique. Many clients have a sexual dysfunction for which they are seeking intervention and correction.

IT—*Intensive therapy:* Utilized primarily by therapists, it involves issues such as marriage, self-concept, and sexual desire, to name a few. If the first three levels of counseling presented were unsuccessful, intensive therapy is indicated.

such as "It will be all right" is nonproductive. Rather, the nurse needs to adopt an objective, empathetic, and receptive attitude to facilitate an open communication between nurse and client.

Annon (Hatcher, 1986) developed a model, termed PLISSIT, for counseling to be used by therapists and nontherapists for clients with sexual problems. The four stages to this model, each increasing in intensity with the seriousness of the client's problem, are listed in the box entitled Model for Counseling Clients With Sexual Problems (PLISSIT).

EVALUATING

To evaluate the plan of care for the client's sexuality needs the nurse will need to utilize information from the client for the majority of client goals. It is not realistic or appropriate for the nurse to evaluate the client by observation of expression of client sexuality. However, the nurse can evaluate how the client is progressing toward sexuality-oriented goals by appearance, level of self-confidence, and manner. For example, a client who has expressed feelings of anxiety in the past over a sexual concern should be observably more confident and free of anxiety if client goals are being met. The nurse will also need to question the client regarding progress toward goals. Some goals will need to be steppinr goals, for not all client problems will be easily resolved with one-time intervention and direction.

One line of questioning when evaluating a client's progress is as follows: "In what ways have you been able to achieve (orgasm, increased desire, comfortable intercourse, erection)?" "What methods seemed most effective? Which were not?" "What do you think should be the next step?" The nurse should determine from this interaction with the client if something more needs to be accomplished. It is not enough to assume that since a set of goals have been met the client is satisfied with the results.

NURSING PROCESS *in Clinical Practice*

The nurse uses each phase of the nursing process when identifying and treating problems of sexuality categorized as nursing diagnoses. Quality care depends on the nurse's possession of the knowledge and clinical skills described earlier in this chapter. Numerous nursing diagnoses can be written to address problems of sexuality depending on specific client assessment data. The four nursing diagnoses chosen for review here are examples of the types of diagnoses that can be developed. The

following outlines the assessment priorities, client goals, nursing interventions, and evaluative criteria for sexual concerns treated by nurses.

Sexual dysfunction: inhibited sexual desire
Altered sexuality patterns: change in sexual expression
Knowledge deficit: contraceptive methods
Disturbance in self-concept: body image, related to surgical removal of a breast

In the case study that follows the development of these concerns of sexuality, nursing care is described for an adolescent client with a knowledge deficit.

Sexual Dysfunction: Inhibited Sexual Desire

For information on inhibited sexual desire, the reader is referred to the section of this chapter on sexual dysfunctions. It is important to identify the causative factors of inhibited desire. This is difficult due to the often complex nature of the problem. Therefore, an accurate and thorough assessment is crucial.

Assessment
- Assess the client's past ability for sexual arousal to determine if this is a new problem or a chronic one.
- Assess the client's interest for sexual activity.
- Assess for other contributing factors such as change in relationship or stressors (life-style, finances, job, children).
- Assess medications the client is currently taking (prescription, nonprescription, alcohol consumption).
- Assess the client's physical and mental status for presence of guilt, fear, anxiety, depression, fatigue.
- Assess the client's relationship with the current partner and also the quality of communication patterns.
- Utilize Annon's set of questions during interviewing to determine specific data related to the problem (see sexual history).

Client Goals
The client will
- Report an increase in sexual desire
- Identify factors in life-style that may be affecting desire
- Promote changes in life-style to relieve factors contributing to decreased desire
- Initiate open communication pattern with partner

Nursing Interventions
The nursing interventions utilized for assisting the client to develop an increase in sexual desire actually stem from the causative factors involved in creating the problem initially. A thorough assessment is critical to identify these causative factors. The interventions listed below specifically address inhibited sexual desire caused by stressful life-style.
- Assist the client to identify the specific stressor.
- Assist the client to determine if the stressor can be modified or controlled.
- Plan sexual activity for the time of day when stressors are minimized. (It may be helpful to block a 1- or 2-hour time period out on specific days on a calendar.)

- Advise the client to initiate honest dialogue with the partner regarding the plan.
- Utilize the blocked-out time period for stroking and relaxing to focus in on partner.
- Stress that sexual intercourse need not always be the goal of this exercise and not to feel stressed if it does not, since this would defeat the purpose of the exercise.

Evaluative Criteria
- The client meets above goals.
- Refer the couple to the appropriate resource for more intensive therapy if inhibited desire persists.

Altered Sexuality Patterns

Altered sexuality patterns is a broad diagnosis with many interpretations for utilization in nursing practice. Loss of desire, increased desire, and change in sexual expression are three dimensions of the problem that are defined more specifically below:

1. Loss of desire may also be interpreted as loss of opportunity or involuntary abstinence. The problem can be further specified by any number of causative factors.
2. Increased desire may also be interpreted as preoccupation with sexual activity. An example would be the beginning of a new sexual relationship. Although this in itself is rarely a problem for the individual, it could be if the desire leads to promiscuous or nondiscriminating behaviors.
3. A change in sexual expression may be a problem if it is involuntarily imposed on the client and the partner. Any disease process, the aging process, isolation from the partner, or life stressors can change the mode of sexual expression for the couple. Change in sexual expression is discussed in more detail in this section.

A disruption in a client's usual mode of sexual expression can cause stress and anxiety in the client's relationship. Although nursing actions cannot change medical conditions or reverse pathophysiology, nurses can assist clients to adapt to the changes in their lives.

Assessment
Assessment is important because it helps the nurse identify the specific etiologic factors that are amenable to nursing action. The reader is referred to the section Diagnosing, above, for a list of possible etiologic factors. As an example of the nursing process in clinical practice, the effects of disease process on sexual expression will be utilized.
- Utilize the three interview questions regarding relationships, feelings of sexuality, and sexual functioning to determine the significance of the problem (see Sexual History, earlier in this chapter).

- Assess past sexual behaviors such as frequency, sexual positions, favored methods of foreplay, use of oral–genital sex, or sexual intercourse.
- Assess importance of each activity and what will remain the same or constant.
- Assess what has or will change for the client and partner as a result of the disease or surgery.
- Assess communication patterns between the client and partner.

Client Goals

The client will

- Identify positive aspects of the current sexual relationship
- Identify at least three viable alternatives to altered sexuality pattern
- Express satisfaction with change in sexual expression

Nursing Interventions

Nursing measures are needed to assist the client to discover possible alternatives to the change in sexual expression that will prove satisfying to the client and the partner.

If the preferred sexual position has been altered

- Allow the client to voice any preferences regarding alternative sexual positions.
- Give the client permission to utilize alternative sexual positions.
- Teach the client regarding the use of alternative positions: use charts or diagrams, and give specific instructions.

If frequency of sexual activity has been altered

- Review past frequency of sexual activity.
- Identify options for increasing frequency (*i.e.,* increase desire, increase opportunity, increase privacy).
- Take pain medication, if indicated, before any sexual activity.

If method of sexual activity has been altered

- Review with the client and partner their feelings regarding the use of oral–genital stimulation and mutual masturbation.
- Give the client permission to utilize alternative modes of sexual expression.
- Give the client specific information regarding the use of alternative activities.
- Encourage open communication between the client and partner to express their satisfaction or dissatisfaction with the activated plan of care.

Evaluative Criteria

- The client meets above goals.
- Any client who does not meet the above client goals or whose problem is severe should be referred to an appropriate resource for further intensive therapy.

Knowledge Deficit

Many areas of knowledge deficit can be identified and treated by nurses. Some examples as they pertain to sexuality are reproductive anatomy and physiology, sexual response cycle, modes of sexual expression, self-examination, spread of STDs, contraceptive methods, and effect of disease and medications on sexual functioning.

To illustrate how the nursing process in clinical practice can be utilized for a knowledge deficit of a sexual concern, knowledge deficit about contraceptive methods will be used as an example here. For a discussion of the various contraceptive methods currently available, the reader is referred to the pertinent section of this chapter.

Assessment

- Determine past use of contraceptive methods.
- Assess effectiveness and satisfaction with past methods.
- Assess the client's current knowledge of contraceptive methods.
- Assess frequency of the client's sexual activity.
- Identify any methods that are unacceptable to the client.
- Assess motivation of the client to use certain methods.
- Assess the client's level of comfort with manipulation of genital body parts.
- Obtain complete client history and perform a physical examination if indicated.

Client Goals

The client will

- Choose a contraceptive method that the client is motivated to use
- List the adverse effects or danger signs associated with the contraceptive method
- List the steps needed to use the contraceptive method effectively
- Utilize the contraceptive with every act of sexual intercourse
- Choose a back-up method
- Report back to the health-care setting for follow-up as directed

Nursing Interventions

- Describe in terms at the client's level of understanding each contraceptive method for which the client needs information (give objective information in matter-of-fact manner to avoid bias by nurse).
- Describe the effectiveness of each method and side-effects or possible complications.
- Instruct the client in the use of a chosen method giving step-by-step instructions.
- Advise the client in the importance of having a back-up method on hand.

- Instruct the client in the use of the back-up method.
- Have the client obtain a physical examination if indicated by the chosen contraceptive method (*e.g.,* the pill).
- Instruct the client to report back in a specified time period for follow-up of utilization of method if indicated (follow-up visits to a health-care facility are important, particularly if a client elects to use the pill).

Evaluative Criteria

Client meets above goals.

Disturbance in Self-Concept: Body Image, Related to Breast Removal

Any change in one's physical body will need to be integrated into one's mental image of that body. Because the body plays such a large part in the expression of sexuality, any disturbance in body image will no doubt have some effect on the expression of sexuality for the client.

In this section, a disturbance in body image as the result of the loss of a breast will be illustrated. As stated previously, the effect of mastectomy on a woman's sexuality depends largely on how much significance she places on her breasts. Also, some women find stimulation of their breasts during foreplay a very satisfying component of sexual activity. Some men place a great deal of sexual emphasis on women's breasts as well.

The fears experienced by some women after surgery include the fear of rejection by society and fear of rejection by the sexual partner. A woman may fel she has been mutilated and is defective as a woman and sex partner. Some women may choose to hide the surgical site from their partners by undressing in the dark or by wearing a bra to bed. Although a stable marriage should not be threatened by illness and surgery, many marriages cannot bear the stress of the trauma of a mastectomy because of other contributing factors. The fear of causing revulsion in her partner and the possibility of the partner ending the relationship also cause much anxiety to the postoperative mastectomy client.

Assessment

Assessment should include review of preoperative relationship factors between the woman and her partner because these will be helpful in determining the causative factors of disturbed body image and provide clues for effective nursing intervention.

- Assess the client's feelings regarding herself as a wife, woman, and sexual partner (use the interview questions listed in the section Sexual History, earlier in this chapter).
- Assess the client's fears regarding change in her femininity, sexual relationship, and images of herself as a person.
- Assess the client's concerns regarding the illness, treatment, and prognosis.
- Assess the value placed on the lost breast by the client.
- Assess the client's support system, including family and close friends.

Client Goals

The client will

- List positive aspects of her body
- List positive aspects of sexual relationship
- Maintain open communication patterns with her partner
- Enhance physical appearance and positive features with use of feminine clothing, make-up, and breast prosthesis if desired
- Report satisfactory sexual activity
- Verbalize integration of mastectomy into body image

Nursing Interventions

- Support the client as she examines her thoughts and feelings regarding her lost breast.
- Encourage the client to talk openly with her partner regarding her feelings and fears.
- Provide positive reinforcement by identifying the client's positive aspects.
- Instruct the client that as she recovers from surgery, desire for sexual closeness will return.
- Advise the client to strive to continue previous behaviors with partner.
- Inform the client that much is available today in the way of attractive clothing to minimize the effects of mastectomy.
- Give the client information as desired regarding breast prosthesis and reconstructive surgery.
- Contact Reach for Recovery or other support persons to assist client in adaptation to mastectomy.

Evaluative Criteria

- The client meets above goals.
- Refer the client to the appropriate resource for intensive therapy if goals are not achieved.

C A S E   S T U D Y

Pete is a 13-year-old adolescent boy attending the area health clinic. He is very nervous as he explains to the nurse his need for health care. He has noticed "sticky white stuff" around his penis and bed clothes on arising some mornings and fears he may be ill. Pete has also expressed concern over his lack of knowledge regarding sexuality. He has heard a lot of stories from his friends but does not feel he can talk to his parents because the subject has never been broached at home. Also, although Pete is a virgin, he is beginning to feel pressured by his friends, who boast of many sexual experiences.

Assessment Findings

After spending time in conversation with Pete the nurse gathered the following data:

- Pete is experiencing nocturnal emissions and has little scientific knowledge about their source.
- Pete is anxious over the stories regarding sex he has heard from his friends.
- There is no communication or dialogue at home with parents about issues of sexuality.
- Pete is having feelings of insecurity and anxiety over his present virginal status which he feels he should change.
- Peer pressure from friends is also a concern.

Nursing Diagnosis

Knowledge deficit: adolescent sexuality concerns related to misinformation

Planning

The nurse will work together with Pete to develop a plan of care to correct misinformation and relieve his anxiety. Planning will be directed toward correcting myths and supplying Pete with accurate information. Since Pete has a negligible knowledge base on sexuality, the plan of care should allow for ongoing sessions to augment the initial information (see the nursing care plan). The nurse should outline this plan with Pete to be certain it is acceptable to him.

Short-Term Goals

By the end of the teaching session on 8/1, the client will

- Describe the nature of nocturnal emissions
- Differentiate sexual myths from sound knowledge
- List the positive aspects of abstinence
- Describe the use of rubber condoms
- Express a decrease in anxiety

Although Pete did not express an interest in contraception at this initial interview, he should have some knowledge regarding condoms before he leaves. It is possible that he may not return to the clinic for future teaching and may not receive this information before he becomes sexually active.

Long-Term Goals

The client will develop a knowledge base of sexuality according to his stage of growth and development and level of understanding.

Implementation

In implementing the care plan, the nurse needs the following specialized abilities:

- Strong assessment skills of interviewing a client with concerns of sexuality
- Interpersonal communication skills to build rapport with an adolescent client
- Nonjudgmental attitude to avoid bias, which would impede trusting nurse–client relationship
- Strong knowledge base of human sexuality, including anatomy and physiology, growth and development, sexual myths, and current issues of sexuality
- Teaching skills to provide client with necessary information and skills
- Counseling skills to diffuse client anxiety over sexual growth and development
- Sense of own sexuality and comfort with sexual issues

Documentation

An example of a traditional note follows:

8/1/87 Consultation with 13-year-old client regarding anxiety over cause and source of nocturnal emissions. Client also expressed concern about sexual myths he has heard from friends. Stated that much peer pressure exists to become sexually active. Client admits to possessing little knowledge regarding sexual issues. Feels he cannot discuss sexuality with parents, as it is not a topic that has been brought up in the past at home. Will conduct initial teaching session with client to provide information and decrease anxiety about priority concerns. Client is agreeable to return to clinic for at least three more teaching sessions to further expand knowledge base of sexuality.

R. Gordon, RN.

SOAP documentation is as follows:

8/1/87 Knowledge deficit: adolescent sexuality concerns related to misinformation

S: "I'm afraid I might have a disease because of the sticky white stuff I find on my penis in the morning. . . . All I know about sex is what I hear from the guys."

O: Concern over source and cause of nocturnal emission. No information about sexuality discussed at home. Client's information received from friends. Feels pressure from peers to become sexually active.

A: Healthy 13-year-old male desiring information on sexuality

P: Begin initial teaching session today on
1. Nocturnal emissions
2. Sexual myths
3. Sexual abstinence and use of rubber condoms
Will plan three more teaching sessions of sexuality issues.

R. Gordon, RN

Evaluation

Short-term goals are evaluated after the initial session. Long-term goal will be evaluated as an ongoing process after each future teaching session.

N U R S I N G   C A R E   P L A N   *for Pete*

Nursing Diagnosis: Knowledge deficit: adolescent sexuality concerns related to misinformation

Long-Term Goal: Client will develop sound knowledge base of sexuality according to his stage of growth and development and level of understanding to decrease anxiety.

Goals	Nursing Actions	Rationale	Evaluative Statement
By end of teaching session, the client will 1. Describe the nature of nocturnal emissions	• Assess client's present knowledge base on nocturnal emission and the source of his information. • Teach the client that nocturnal emissions or "wet dreams" are normal in men of all ages and that they are particularly common in the teen years. • Nocturnal emissions occur during sleep as the result of erotic dreams. The "white sticky stuff" is the result of ejaculation of semen from the penis. • This is an involuntary action over which the male has no control.	It is necessary to discover what the client does know and to build on that knowledge. Use terms that the client has used and language at the level of the client's understanding. It is important to include that nocturnal emissions are normal and common and not the result of disease.	8/1 Goal met. Client able to describe the source of nocturnal emissions.
2. Differentiate sexual myths from sound knowledge	• Assess what client has heard from peers regarding sexual information. Myth 1: "A large penis is better for sex than a small one." True: No relationship exists between the size of a penis and the man's ability to perform sexually. When a penis becomes "hard" or erect, it reaches sufficient size to engage in sexual intercourse. Myth 2: "Jerking off causes blindness. It is a dirty habit." True: Masturbation or self-stimulation is a natural and healthy outlet for sexual urges. Men	The nurse can then specifically address the myths to which the client has been exposed. The nurse gives the client permission to engage in a sexual activity of a masturbatory nature.	8/1 Goal met. Client was able to differentiate between truth and sexual issues and what is myth.

(Continued)

NURSING CARE PLAN (Continued)

Goals	Nursing Actions	Rationale	Evaluative Statement
	and women of all ages masturbate. Masturbation can also teach the person what feels good and what does not. Every person has the right to "jerk off" or masturbate if he or she wishes to do so. Myth 3: "It looks bad for a guy to be a virgin—everybody's doing it." True: No one, whether male or female, should feel pressured into sexual activity at any age. Engaging in sexual activity carries with it a great deal of responsibility and concerns of pregnancy and spread of STDs. No one needs to know of another person's status if the person chooses not to discuss it.	The nurse gives the client permission to abstain from sexual activity and not to feel pressured by friends. Almost 39% of teens have had sex by age 16 years.	
3. List the positive aspects of abstinence from a sexual relationship.	• Assessment includes previous discussion of sexual myths and knowledge. • The positive aspects of abstinence include the following: 　Engagement in any sexual activity should be a personal decision and not the result of pressure from friends. 　Abstinence will guarantee protection from pregnancy. 　Abstinence will guarantee protection against most STDs.	Giving the client all the information necessary will allow him to make an informed decision. Many young people feel they are immune to the consequences of their actions. Therefore, it is important to stress that pregnancy and STDs are very probable results of sexual intercourse.	8/1 Goal partially met. Client able to verbally list all positive aspects of abstinence but is still undecided. *Revision:* Reinforce to client that this is a personal decision that he can make for himself with a good knowledge base. Also, he does not have to make a firm decision for or against abstinence immediately. He should take time to think about this information.

(Continued)

N U R S I N G   C A R E   P L A N (continued)

Goals	Nursing Actions	Rationale	Evaluative Statement
	It is difficult to understand and undertake all the implications of a sexual relationship during the teen years. A successful sexual relationship requires intimacy, love, and sharing. It should not only be an outlet for sexual feelings.		
	People can show affection for each other without sexual involvement.		
	Every person has the right to say "no."	The nurse gives the client permission to refuse an activity in which he is not sure he wishes to engage. (Howard, 1985)	
4. Describe the use of rubber condoms	• Assess what the client knows about rubber condoms and their use.	Since client is undecided over whether to initiate a sexual relationship in the future, it is prudent to give him information to protect against pregnancy and STDs.	8/1 Goal met. Client successfully listed the steps in using a condom.
	• Rubber condoms are available over the counter in drug stores. Prices will vary according to type and style.	Client should know where to purchase condoms and the variety available.	
	• Teach client the steps in using rubber condoms. Condom should be rolled onto the penis as soon as it becomes erect.	Protects against sperm from secretions from Cowper's glands	
	If condom does not have a nipple receptacle end, leave a small space at end of condom to collect semen.	Provides a pocket to collect semen and prevents breakage	
	Immediately after ejaculation, remove penis and condom from vagina by holding onto base of condom.	Prevents spillage of semen into the vagina	
	Discard condom.	Condoms are not meant to be used over. A new condom is used for each act of intercourse.	

(Continued)

NURSING CARE PLAN (Continued)

Goals	Nursing Actions	Rationale	Evaluative Statement
	Use a condom with every act of intercourse. Spermicides used with condom increase effectiveness. The rubber condom used with spermicide is effective against pregnancy and the spread of STDs.	To be as effective as possible, the condom should be used with every act of intercourse. The woman using a spermicide foam in the vagina increases effectiveness.	
5. Express a decrease in anxiety	• Assess client's anxiety level by verbal and nonverbal behavior.	Client was anxious when he came into clinic. It is important to evaluate level of anxiety before he leaves. If he is still anxious, reassessment should occur because plan of care may have been unsuccessful.	8/1 Goal met. Client expressed relief that he is normal. Would like to bring a friend to next session. Future teaching sessions to include these topics identified by client: STDs, particularly AIDS Pregnancy—occurrence and prevention Sexual expression Further discussion of sexual myths

---

KEY POINTS

- Sexuality is a human component that is not adequately understood.

- Sexuality defines maleness and femaleness and is evident in behaviors, physical appearances, and relationships with others.

- Nurses are concerned with clients' sexuality because individuals bring with them to a health-care setting all aspects of what makes them human.

- A sound knowledge base of female and male reproductive anatomy and physiology, the sexual response cycle, and factors that affect sexuality is important for the nurse to be an effective teacher, counselor, and advocate in dealing with clients with sexual concerns.

- Factors that affect sexuality include developmental stage, culture, religion, etics, life-style, sexual orientation, health state, and medications.

- Obtaining a comprehensive history and performing a physical assessment are paramount before nursing care can be planned for a client with a sexual concern. However, the collection of a sexual history is not appropriate in all health-care situations. Clients who should have at least a brief sexual history recorded are clients with concerns of a reproductive nature, clients experiencing a sexual dysfunction, and clients whose illness or treatment will affect their sexual functioning.

- The physical assessment of reproductive anatomy can be stressful and uncomfortable for both male and female clients. Because the major portion of female genitalia is internal, the examination is invasive and may be frightening. The nurse should provide support and information before and during the pelvic examination to create a positive experience for the woman.

- Problems associated with sexuality are rarely simple and clear-cut due to the integral nature of sexuality. Clients may need assistance to talk through their concerns before definitive nursing diagnoses can be formulated.

- Nursing diagnoses can be written specifically to address Altered sexuality patterns and Sexual dysfunctions. The effect of sexual concerns on other areas of human functioning can also be identified (*e.g.,* disturbance in body image, anxiety, impaired adjustment).

■ Nurses who are good role models in promoting healthy sexuality have developed a definition of their own sexuality, have developed a self-awareness of their beliefs, and possess a knowledge base of sexual topics and issues.

■ Nursing interventions that promote healthy sexuality include establishing a trusting nurse–client relationship, advocating for hospitalized clients' sexual needs, counseling clients regarding sexual concerns, and teaching clients about sexuality-related subjects. Client education, which includes topics of self-examination, contraceptive methods, and responsible sexual expression, can be implemented in many health-care situations.

B I B L I O G R A P H Y

Abrums M: Health care for women. Journal of Obstetric, Gynecological and Neonatal Nursing 15(3):250–255, 1986

Baldwin K, Goodwin K: The Papanicolaou smear. Journal of Nurse-Midwifery 30(6):327–331, 1985

Berkoritz I: Healthy development of sexuality in adolescents: The school's contribution. Medical Aspects of Human Sexuality 19(10):34–49, 1985

Bernhard L, Dan A: Redefining sexuality from women's own experiences. Nurs Clin North Am 21(1):125–135, 1986

Bourcier K, Seidler A: Chlamydia and condylomata acuminata: An update for the nurse practitioner. Journal of Obstetric, Gynecologic and Neonatal Nursing 16(1):17–21, 1987

Cash J: Sexuality and chronic pain. Am J Nurs 84(11):1417, 1984

Dickerson J: Oral contraceptives: A closer look. Am J Nurs 83(10):1393–1398, 1983

Fromer M: Ethical Issues in Sexuality and Reproduction. St Louis, CV Mosby, 1983

Fuentes R et al: Sexual side effects. What to tell your patients, what not to say. RN 46(2):34–41, 1983

Garvey M: Decreased libido in depression. Medical Aspects of Human Sexuality 19(2):30–34, 1985

Googe M, Mook TM: The inflatable penile prosthesis: New developments. Am J Nurs 83(7):1044–1047, 1983

Hammond D: Screening for sexual dysfunction. Clin Obstet Gynecol 27(3):732–737, 1984

Hatcher R et al: Contraceptive Technology. New York, Irvington, 1986

Hill L, Smith N: Self-Care Nursing. Englewood Cliffs, NJ, Prentice-Hall, 1985

Howard M: How the family physician can help young teenagers postpone sexual involvement. Medical Aspects of Human Sexuality 19(6):76–87, 1985

Kisker E: Teenagers talk about sex, pregnancy, and contraception. Fam Plann Perspect 17(2):83–90, 1985

Leppert P: Adolescent anxiety at first pelvic examination. Medical Aspects of Human Sexuality 19(7):24–32, 1985

McCary J, McCary S: Human Sexuality, 4th ed. Belmont, CA, Wadsworth Publishing, 1982

Penninger J et al: After the ostomy: Helping the patient reclaim his sexuality. RN 48(4):46–50, 1985

Pollard M, Barker E: Straight talk on sex for the older patient. RN 48(2):17–18, 1985

Reamy K: Sexual counseling for the nontherapist. Clin Obstet Gynecol 27(3):781–788, 1984

Renshaw D: Sex, age, and values. J Am Geriatr Soc 33(9):635–643, 1985

Rosenfield A: Contraception: Where are we in 1985? Contemporary Ob/GYN 27(2):79–91, 1985

Semmens J, Semmens E: Sexual function and the menopause. Clin Obstet Gynecol 27(3):717–723, 1984

Watts R: Dimensions of sexual health. Am J Nurs 79(9):1568–1572, 1979

Weisberg M: Physiology of female sexual function. Clin Obstet Gynecol 27(3):697–706, 1984

Willard M, Heaberg G, Pack J: The educational pelvic examination. Women's responses to a new approach. Journal of Obstetric, Gynecologic and Neonatal Nursing 15(2):135–139, 1986

Woods NF: Human Sexuality in Health and Illness. St Louis, CV Mosby, 1984

Yost M: When your patient's problem is sexual dysfunction. Contemporary OB/GYN 28(2):171–185, 1986

Spirituality

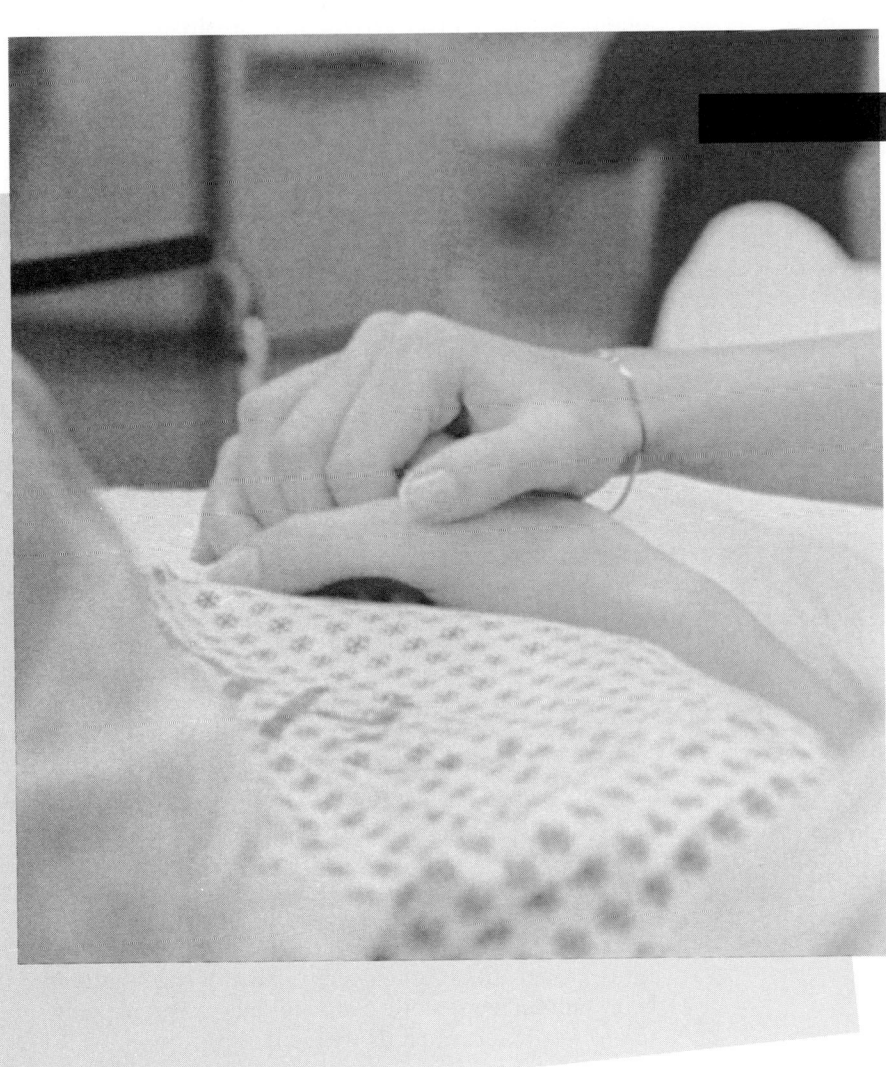

After studying this chapter, the learner should be able to

Define key terms used in the chapter.

Identify three spiritual needs believed to be common to all persons.

Describe the influences of spirituality on everyday living, health, and illness.

Differentiate life-affirming influences of religious beliefs from life-denying influences.

Distinguish the spiritual beliefs and practices of the major religions practiced in the United States and Canada: Protestantism, Catholicism, Judaism.

Identify five factors that influence spirituality.

Perform a nursing assessment of spiritual health, utilizing appropriate interview questions and observation skills.

Develop nursing diagnoses that correctly identify spiritual problems.

Describe seven nursing strategies to promote spiritual health and state their rationale.

Plan, implement, and evaluate nursing care related to select nursing diagnoses involving spiritual problems.

K E Y   T E R M S

agnostic   spiritual beliefs
atheist   spiritual distress
faith   spiritual needs
religion   spirituality

The "spirit" dimension of the human person was recognized in ancient cultures. "The dual roles of priest and physician were generally held by one individual, and thus the functions and dictates of religion (pertaining to the spirit) and medicine (pertaining to the body) were closely interwoven" (O'Brien, 1982, p 85). Over the years, however, medicine and religion evolved separately. Not until the holistic health movement took root was the human person once again viewed as an integrated whole of body, mind, and spirit and health-care practitioners began again to probe the relationships among physical, psychologic, and spiritual health.

Nursing has always been a strongly holistic tradition and nurses have practiced nursing sensitive to the physical, psychosocial, and spiritual needs of persons. According to Fish and Shelly (1978), there are three **spiritual needs** underlying all religious traditions and common to all persons: (1) need for meaning and purpose, (2) need for love and relatedness, and (3) need for forgiveness. Although nurses may differ in their beliefs about how involved they should become in meeting clients' spiritual needs, it is impossible to nurse individuals well while ignoring the spiritual dimensions of health. Nurses can assist clients to meet spiritual needs with the following measures: (1) assist the client to begin or continue a meaningful relationship with God in the face of stress or pain; (2) support the client in reestablishing ties with religious traditions and methods of worship; or (3) help the client to discover and express a sense of purpose in the present hospitalization and future recovery of course of illness (Salladay, 1987).

Study of this chapter provides the student with a knowledge base of spirituality. Practical suggestions for performing a spiritual assessment are given, along with specific interview questions. Sample nursing diagnoses are developed for common problems of spiritual distress (spiritual pain, alienation, anxiety, guilt, anger, loss, and despair). Related client and nurse goals and specific nursing strategies for promoting spiritual health are described. In the section Nursing Process in Clinical Practice, focused assessment, planning, implementation, and evaluation guides are offered for clients experiencing spiritual distress related to challenged beliefs and value systems. These guides and the concluding case study illustrate how the nurse's knowledge of spirituality may be combined with skilled nursing interventions and caring to resolve spiritual distress successfully.

SPIRITUALITY AND FAITH

Although the terms *spirituality, religion,* and *faith* are used interchangeably by some, there are distinctions. Spirituality can be defined as anything that pertains to a person's relationship with a nonmaterial life force or higher power. Whereas one person describes spirituality in terms of coming to know, love, and serve God, another speaks of transcending the limits of body and experiencing a universal energy. Spirituality may include **religion**, which refers to an organized system of beliefs about a higher power. Religions are often characterized by set forms of worship, spiritual practices, and codes of conduct. Thus a person may be deeply spiritual yet not profess a "religion." The fact that persons do not belong to an organized religion should not be interpreted by the nurse to mean that they have no spiritual needs. **Faith** generally refers to a confident belief in something for which there is no proof or material evidence. It can involve a person, idea, or thing, and it is usually followed by action related to the ideals or values of that belief.

An **atheist** is a person who denies the existence of a God, while an **agnostic** is one who holds that nothing is known about the existence of a God. The agnostic and the atheist are guided by philosophies of living that do not include a religious faith. They deserve respect for what they choose to believe, just as do those who accept a particular religious creed.

Spirituality and Everyday Living

Spiritual beliefs and practices are associated with all aspects of a person's life, including health and illness. Aspects of a person's life commonly influenced by spirituality and religion include relationships with others, daily living habits, required and prohibited behaviors, and the general frame of reference for thinking about oneself and the world.

"Life-affirming influences enhance life, give meaning and purpose to existence, strengthen one's feelings of self-worth, encourage self-actualization, and are health-giving and life-sustaining. Life-denying influences restrict or enclose life patterns, limit experiences and associations, place burdens of guilt on individuals, encourage feelings of unworthiness, and are generally health-denying and life-inhibiting" (Larue, 1981).

Spirituality, Health, and Illness

Spiritual beliefs are of special importance to nurses because of the many ways they can influence a client's level of health and self-care behaviors.

Guide to Daily Living Habits. Certain practices generally associated with health care may have religious significance for a client. For example, many religions prescribe dietary requirements and restrictions. Acceptable birth-control practices are determined by some religious faiths, as are some types of medical treatments.

Source of Support. It is common for many persons to seek support from their religious faith during times of stress. This support is often vital to the acceptance of an illness, especially if the illness brings with it a prolonged period of convalescence or indicates a questionable outcome. Prayer, devotional reading, and other religious practices often do for the person spiritually what protective exercises do for the body physically.

Source of Strength and Healing. The values derived from religious faith cannot be enumerated or evaluated easily. However, the effects attributable to faith are constantly in evidence to health workers. Persons have been known to endure extreme physical distress because of strong faith. Clients' families have taken on almost unbelievable rehabilitative tasks because they had faith in the eventual positive results of their effort.

Source of Conflict. There are times when religious beliefs conflict with prevalent health-care practices. For example, the doctrine of the Jehovah's Witnesses prohibits blood transfusions. In the Islamic religion, humans are regarded as largely helpless in controlling their environment, and illness is accepted as their fate rather than something against which action might be taken. Some Navajo Indians use a lengthy religious ceremony to "cure" certain diseases, such as tuberculosis. For some people, illness is viewed as punishment for sin and therefore inevitable.

Such beliefs may require the health worker to modify a treatment plan to accommodate the person's religion. In some instances, acknowledgment of the client's religious convictions and efforts by health practitioners to accommodate the client's beliefs can result in quality health care without violating the person's religious practices. In other situations, an objective explanation of alternative treatments and the predicted consequences of each may help the client determine acceptable therapy. Whatever the person's decision about health care, the nurse should remember that each person is unique and has a right to pursue his or her own convictions, even though they may differ from those of the health-care provider.

Religious Faiths

For easier discussion, in this chapter the term *spiritual adviser* is used to discuss the clergy person, counselor, or shepherd of followers of each religion. While it is impractical to discuss all faiths in this text, the nurse should be aware that all beliefs have a direct influence on health care. Examples of these are found in the accompanying box. Some areas of the United States and Canada have citizens of Chinese, Korean, Japanese, and Indian descent, and there has been a recent influx of people from Southeast Asia, so the nurse may come into contact with religious beliefs not mentioned here. Hinduism, Buddhism, Shintoism, Confucianism, and Islam are major world religions. Many blacks have embraced Islam as their religion. The nurse having contact with a

Spiritual Beliefs and Medical Procedures

Amniocentesis
Acceptable to most major religious traditions. Amniocentesis solely for the purposes of abortion is not accepted by the Roman Catholic tradition or by Orthodox Judaism.

Anatomical Donations
Generally allowed in most religious traditions—a special problem for Hindus

Artificial Insemination
Prohibited in Orthodox Judaism and Roman Catholicism except when the donor would be the natural father

Autopsies
Most major religions allow autopsies. They are prohibited by Hinduism. Conservative and Orthodox Judaism oppose routine autopsy as being a sacrilege, but permit autopsies that will yield knowledge that may save another person's life.

Birth Control vs Contraception
Non-orthodox Judaism accepts that parents should decide the number of children desired and the means to be used in spacing the births of their children, provided they have had two children, if they can. Islam accepts contraception in certain circumstances, that is, to avoid material hardships, to protect the health of the mother, and so on. Artificial birth control is not acceptable to Roman Catholics and Orthodox Jews. Roman Catholicism accepts and encourages natural family planning. Protestants generally find birth control acceptable.

Blood Transfusions
On religious grounds, Jehovah's Witnesses oppose any transfusion of blood or blood products as being a use of blood forbidden by God. Otherwise blood transfusions are accepted by various denominations.

Burial vs Cremation
Cremation is forbidden in Orthodox and Conservative Judaism. Cremation is accepted in a Roman Catholic tradition when it does not imply denial of the resurrection of the body, for example, fear of being buried alive or the need to transport the remains a long distance.

Circumcision
Generally there is no objection to the medical procedure of circumcision. Judaism recognizes circumcision as a sacred ritual to be performed on the eighth day after birth. If performed by a surgeon, it may be followed by a ritual ceremony.

Dietary Laws
Many Seventh Day Adventists are lacto-vegetarians. Some eat meat except for pork and certain shell fish. Observant Jews will not eat shell fish or any food containing milk products and meat products mixed together. Also, meat must be "kosher," that is, only certain animals qualify and must be ritually slaughtered.

Euthanasia
The direct taking of human life or the direct means to hasten the end of human life are considered wrong by most traditions. The use of extraordinary means that may only prolong the dying process are not encouraged.

Fetal Disposal
All religious traditions reverence the human body. Most faiths call for a dignified burial of the fetus.

Fetal Experimentation
Many religious traditions consider the fetus to be a person or a potential person and therefore to be treated as a client would be treated. Experimentation that would be of direct benefit may be acceptable. Judaism does not permit experimentation on a living fetus; however, experimentation on a dead fetus is permitted providing proper respect is shown.

Healing Processes
The major religious traditions accept the unity of the human person. Therefore, prayer and medical treatment are both accepted as important parts of the healing process. Christian Scientists may refuse any or some medical treatment.

Immunization
Some groups have refused immunization on religious grounds, for example, Christian Science and Amish, and have been legally exempted.

Infertility Tests
In most Protestant denominations the administration of infertility tests is governed by the standard medical procedure, the well-being of the client, and the sanctity of the client's conscience. Roman Catholics and Orthodox Jews generally accept an infertility test for medical reasons. In semen examination the specimen is obtained by means other than masturbation.

Living Will
The client or legal guardian has the right to refuse any or all medical treatment. A living will merely expresses the wishes of the client.

Spiritual Beliefs and Medical Procedures (continued)

Narcotics
Major religions agree narcotics are acceptable when prescribed by a competent medical authority for pain and suffering.

Organ Transplants
In most Protestant and Roman Catholic traditions organ transplants are generally accepted. Organ transplants would be accepted by most segments of the Jewish community except for certain Orthodox groups.

Right to Die vs Prolongation of Life
Many moral philosophers and theologians feel allowing people to refuse lifesaving treatment drives a wedge that opens the way to active euthanasia. This must be balanced against the generally recognized right of a person to refuse means that are extraordinarily expensive or painful to prolong life.

Sabbath Observances
In regard to the sick, the restoration to health takes precedence over the observance of the sabbath in Judaism and Christianity. Orthodox Judaism limits sabbath violation to acts that would save another's life. Seventh Day Adventists encourage an atmosphere of quiet for the patient from sunset Friday to sunset Saturday.

Sacraments
In the Roman Catholic Church sick people are encouraged to receive Holy Communion and the sacrament of anointing of the sick. Anointing of the sick is administered only once during an illness. Since anointing of the sick is a sacrament of the living, it is never administered after the client has expired. The Episcopalian tradition also sees the religious sacraments as part of the healing process. The United Church of Christ, the United Presbyterian Church, and the Seventh Day Adventists Church encourage reception of baptism and communion during illness, for those not previously baptized.

Sterilization
Compulsory sterilization laws exist in many countries and in 21 states of the United States. They are aimed chiefly at mentally incompetent persons. Some Catholic theologians have defended punitive sterilization while many oppose it. Some Protestant theologians, for example, Fletcher and Ramsay, suggest there might be limited cases in which punitive sterilization is justifiable. Officially the Roman Catholic church accepts only therapeutic sterilization. Sterilization procedures are permitted in Judaism only when medically indicated.

(Printed with permission of the Philadelphia County Medical Society, Philadelphia, PA. The Committee on Medicine and Religion of the Philadelphia County Medical Society compiled this list to assist physicians, medical students, nurses, and other hospital personnel in the understanding of their clients religious beliefs and practices. They recognize a broad spectrum of views within each religious group or denomination but have attempted to present the most widely accepted practices after consultation with religious leaders and theological statements. Refusal of diagnostic studies, treatment, or surgery by a client or family may need to be reviewed with the knowledge of religious beliefs and practices. Wisdom and understanding will allow us to respect the religious beliefs of our clients and ensure quality medical care.)

person of a faith that is unfamiliar should acknowledge this fact. Through reading and discussion with the person, family, and spiritual adviser, the nurse can learn about the basic tenets of the faith and how they may affect health care.

The religions practiced most commonly in the United States and Canada are Protestantism, Catholicism, and Judaism. They are summarized below.

Judaism

There are three forms of Judaism: Reform, Conservative, and Orthodox. Reform Judaism is more liberal than the other two in its beliefs, whereas Orthodox Judaism is the most traditional of the three. Conservative Judaism finds its place more or less between Reform and Orthodox Judaism.

For the observant Jewish client, treatments and procedures should not be scheduled on the Sabbath and important holy days, provided this will not harm the client.

The spiritual adviser of the Jewish faith is the rabbi. Figure 39-1 illustrates a rabbi's visit with an elderly client in a geriatric center.

Dietary Practices. Because dietary practices vary in Judaism and also occasionally among Jews practicing the same form of Judaism, the nurse should consult with the client, a family member, or a rabbi, especially before making modifications if dietary practices interfere with a medical regimen. Jewish law permits dietary modifications under certain circumstances.

The dietitian should be aware of dietary practices and holy day observances. The nurse must identify observant Jewish clients for proper diets. Basically, the practice includes eating only kosher foods, not mixing meat and milk dishes at the same meal, and cooking and

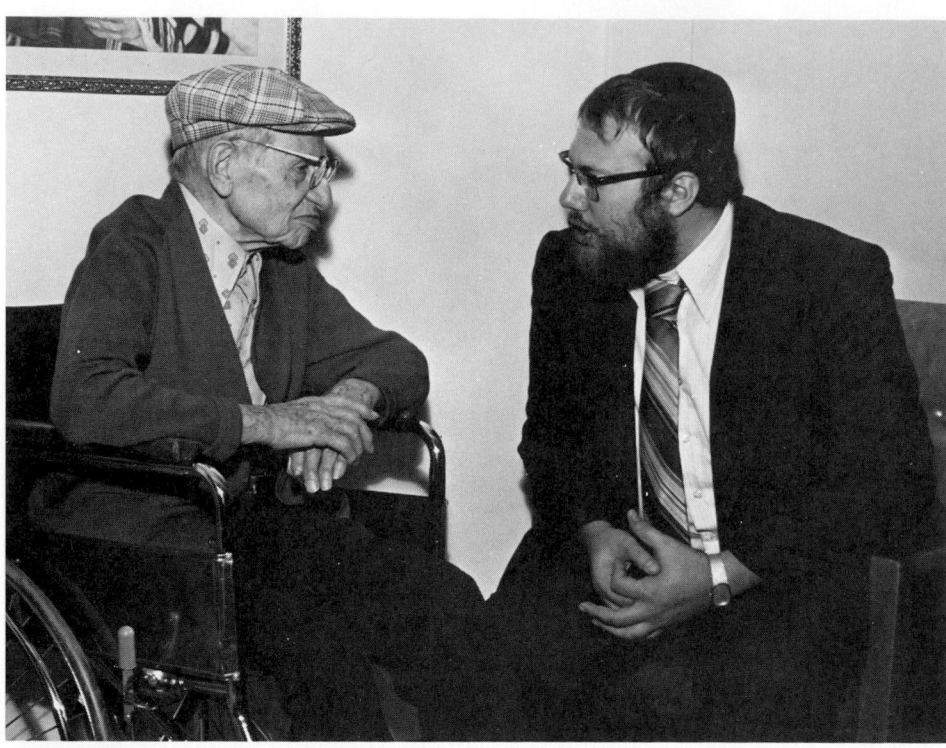

F I G U R E 39-1
The rabbi's visit is important for this gentleman, who is a resident in a geriatric center.

serving food on specific kosher dishes or on paper plates if kosher dishes are not available or practical.

Circumcision. Male Jewish infants are required to be circumcised on the eighth day after birth. However, the rite may be postponed for as long as necessary if the infant's health does not permit it at that time.

Death and Preparation for Burial. There are appropriate prayers for the dying client. If the client and family so desire, a service of confession and prayer may be observed as death approaches. Preferably, the rabbi is present for this—if not the client's own rabbi, then one associated with the health agency.

A client who has died may be washed and covered with a clean cloth. If there is no kin to claim the body, a rabbi should be contacted immediately.

Christianity

In the United States and Canada, most Christians are Roman Catholic or Protestant. The spiritual adviser in the

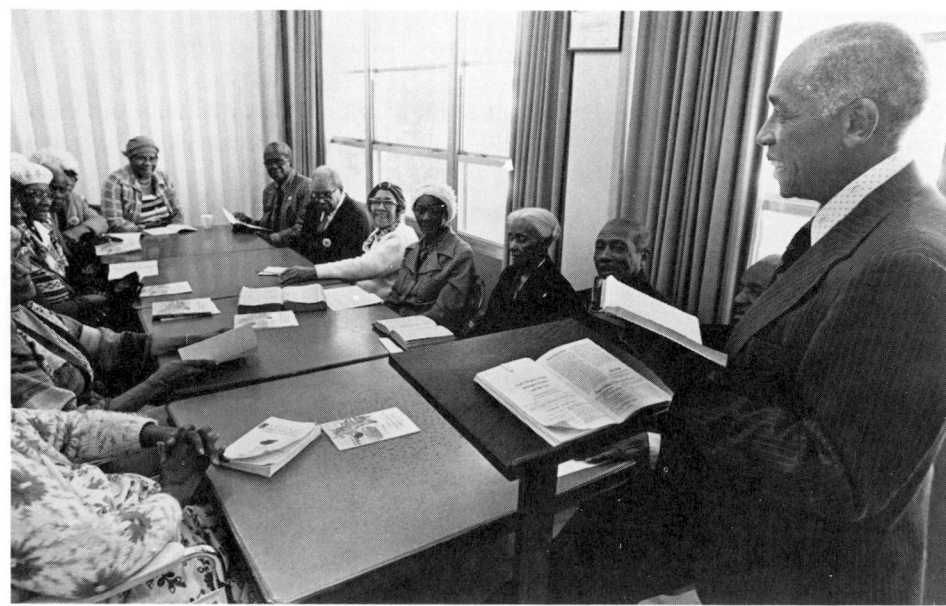

F I G U R E 39-2
A group of retired persons gather for their weekly Bible study.

Roman Catholic faith is the priest. Protestant spiritual advisers are called minister, pastor, or preacher (Fig. 39-2).

Most Christians observe Sunday as a day for worship. An exception is the Seventh Day Adventist, who sets aside Saturday for worship. Dietary practices are observed by some Christians. The nurse should check with the individual client for preference.

Roman Catholicism.   When caring for Roman Catholic clients, the nurse will find it necessary to be acquainted with the sacraments of baptism, reconciliation, holy communion, and the anointing of the sick.

Sacrament of Baptism.   Since a nurse may be present during the delivery of a child or the miscarriage of a living fetus, it is imperative to understand that for a Catholic family any child in danger of death must be baptized. If a priest is not available, the nurse or physician, preferably Catholic, should administer the sacrament of baptism. If a Catholic is not available, anyone having the use of reason may baptize the infant. It is necessary that the person conferring the sacrament use the proper form and have belief in the sacrament and the intention of doing what the Catholic Church desires. The procedure is as follows: while pouring plain water over the infant's forehead so that it flows on the skin, say, "I baptize you in the name of the Father, and of the Son, and of the Holy Spirit." The fact that the sacrament of baptism was conferred should be recorded on the infant's chart and in the chaplain's baptismal roster if there is one in the health agency.

Sacrament of Reconciliation.   The sacrament of reconciliation involves the confessing of one's sins against God and fellow man and asking for forgiveness. It is often called *penance* or *confession.* The priest hears the person's confession and offers assistance and counseling to help the penitent avoid future sins

Sacrament of Holy Eucharist or Holy Communion.
Holy Communion is the most revered of all sacraments of the Catholic faith. Most Catholics in danger of death desire to receive communion if possible. As necessary, confession precedes communion. To prepare to receive communion, Catholics, except those in danger of death, may wish to fast from solid food for 1 hour. A person is not required to fast from water or medications.

Sacrament of the Anointing of the Sick.   The sacrament of the anointing of the sick encourages that the sacrament be administered to ill persons who are not in immediate danger of death, any person who must undergo surgery for a reason that has caused the person to be seriously or critically ill, or to those whose life forces are growing weaker simply because of age, even though death may be remote.

Protestantism.   The Protestant faith embraces a large number of denominations. While certain doctrines are common to most of these denominations, there are individual practices and interpretations that give each a distinct pattern. Some denominations employ certain sacraments that are similar to those in the Catholic faith, and others reject the concept of sacraments and observe baptism and communion as ordinances that are means of grace but not of salvation. Others, such as the Friends (Quakers), reject both ordinances and sacraments.

Sacrament or Ordinance of Baptism.   Some Protestant faiths hold that baptism should be performed in infancy. The Baptists, the Disciples of Christ, and some others believe that the ordinance of baptism should not be administered before the person reaches the age of accountability. If a child of Protestant parents is in danger of dying, the nurse should ask whether the parents wish to have the child baptized. If a Protestant minister is not available, the child may be baptized as follows: a baptized nurse who has understanding of and

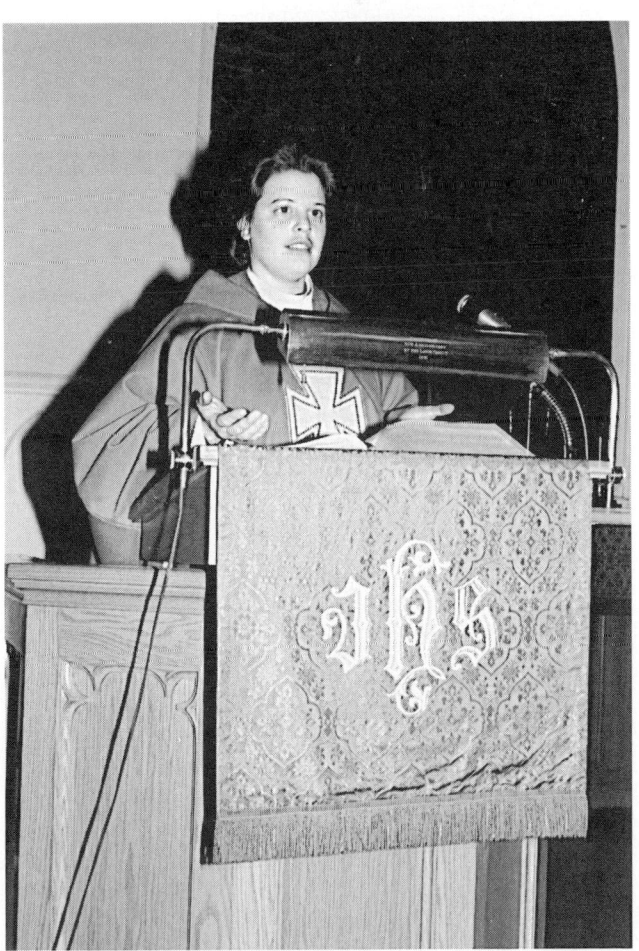

F I G U R E   39-3
The protestant faith embraces a large number of denominations. Some doctrines are common to most of these denominations but individual practices and interpretations give each a distinct pattern. This group has chosen a female spiritual leader. (Photo by Isadore Faven)

belief in the act that is being performed may baptize the baby by pouring water continuously over the child's forehead and saying the following words, "I baptize you in the name of the Father, and of the Son, and of the Holy Spirit. Amen." The baptism is recorded on the child's chart by the person performing it and the parents are informed.

Sacrament or Ordinance of Communion. Many Protestant clients request communion prior to surgery or during a period of illness.

FACTORS AFFECTING SPIRITUALITY

Among the many factors that can influence a person's spirituality the most important are developmental considerations, family, ethnic background, formal religion, and life events.

Developmental Considerations. Since spirituality has to do with the nonmaterial realm of being, a child must have some capacity for abstract thought before beginning to understand "spiritual self" and explore a rela-

tionship with a higher power. This is not to say that spirituality is meaningless for children.

David Heller (1985) interviewed 40 children, ages 4 to 12 years, affiliated with one of four major religions—Judaism, Catholicism, Protestantism, or Hinduism—and discovered that the children had very definite perceptions of God and preferred forms of prayer or spiritual exercises, which differed according to the age, sex, religion, and personality of the child. Central themes in all the children's descriptions of God included

- Notion of a God who works through human intimacy and the interconnectedness of lives
- Belief that God is involved in self-change and growth, transformations that make the world fresh, alive, and meaningful
- Attributing to God tremendous and expansive power and then showing considerable anxiety in the face of this power
- Image of light

As the child matures, life experiences usually influence and mature spiritual beliefs. With advancing years the tendency to think about life after death prompts some individuals to reexamine and reaffirm their spiritual beliefs.

R E S E A R C H   I N   N U R S I N G   *Making a Difference*

Spirituality

The importance of spirituality to client well-being has been widely accepted within the nursing community. Spirituality is a broad term relating to many areas of client care. Developmental theorists include spirituality in describing concepts of personal integrity and self-actualization. Investigators have researched spirituality from such varying perspectives as religiousness, folk beliefs, and crisis.

Related Research

Francis M: Concerns of terminally ill adult Hindu cancer patients. Cancer Nursing 9(4):164–171, 1986

In this study, Francis investigated concerns of terminally ill Hindu adults. Persons with cancer were chosen for the study because of the existential concerns common to this medical diagnosis. Identified areas of concern were physiologic, illness-related, social, personal, and spiritual. Clients expressed their faith in God and reported receiving strength and reducing stress through prayer. Recommendations for nursing derived from this study are to carry out a spiritual assessment of clients and to provide time and space for prayers.

Reed P: Religiousness among terminally ill and healthy adults. Res Nurs Health 9(1):35–41, 1986

Reed compared terminally ill adults with healthy adults for differences in religiousness and well-being, based on the hypothesis that those adults who were terminally ill would report greater religiousness. Results supported this hypothesis, with terminally ill females reporting the greatest level of religiousness. No differences in levels of well-being were found between groups. It appears that both religion and well-being have varying levels of importance for specific groups of clients.

Summary

Spirituality is an area that deserves further research by nurses. Whether assisting clients toward higher levels of self-actualization or supporting families during the grieving process, spirituality has important implications for nursing practice in enhancing wellness. Studies indicate that the role of spirituality differs based on a person's cultural background, gender, age, and medical diagnosis. Further research could help isolate target groups desiring spiritual support and also facilitate the development of appropriate nursing assessment tools and care plans.

Family. A child's parents play a key role in the development of the child's spirituality. What is important is not so much what parents teach a child about God and religion, but rather what the child learns about God, life, and self from parents' behavior. Since the family is the first world the child experiences, a world view will be colored by experiences with parents and siblings.

Ethnic Background. Religious traditions differ among ethnic groups. There are clear distinctions between Eastern and Western spiritual traditions as well as among those of individual ethnic groups such as the Native Americans. A person's culture and formal religion has much to do with whether the basic approach to religion will be "doing something," "being someone," or "continually striving for harmony."

Formal Religion. Each of the major religions discussed earlier in this chapter has several characteristics in common:
- Basis of authority or source of power
- A portion of scripture or sacred word
- An ethical code that defines right and wrong
- A psychology and identity so that its adherents fit into a group and the world is defined by the religion
- Aspirations or expectations
- Some ideas about what follows death
  (Murray and Zentner, 1985, p 475)

Life Events. Both positive and negative life experiences can influence spirituality and in turn are influenced by the meaning a person's spiritual beliefs attribute to them. For example, if two women who believe in a loving God both lose a child in a car accident, one may bitterly deny God's existence and stop going to church whereas the other may spend more time in prayer asking God to help her understand and accept her loss. Similarly, a chain of successful life experiences (marriage, degree, promotion) may cause one person to assume success and experience no need for God whereas for another it occasions deep gratitude and rejoicing.

NURSE AS ROLE MODEL

As mentioned in the introduction to this chapter, there are three spiritual needs common to all persons: (1) need for meaning and purpose, (2) need for love and relatedness, and (3) need for forgiveness (Fish and Shelly, 1978). These needs are common to nurses, whether they observe an established religion, believe in a spiritual essence, or recognize a field of power. As the nurse develops plans to be a spiritual role model to clients, the nurse develops goals for self. The nurse will:
- Hold spiritual beliefs that meet her need for meaning and purpose, love and relatedness, forgiveness
- Derive from these beliefs strength for everyday living, especially when confronting in her professional practice pain, suffering, and death
- Set aside regular periods of time to nurture her spiritual self
- Demonstrate in her interactions with others peace, inner strength, warmth, joy, caring, creativity
- Respect the spiritual beliefs and practices of others even when they are different from her own
- Increase her knowledge of how the spiritual beliefs of her clients influence their life-styles, re-

PROMOTING WELLNESS

Spirituality

Use the assessment checklist to determine how well you are meeting spirituality needs. Then develop a prescription for self-care by choosing appropriate behaviors from the list of suggestions.

Assessment Checklist

always always	some times	almost never	
☐	☐	☐	1. I am comfortable with my spiritual beliefs and values.
☐	☐	☐	2. My beliefs meet my needs for love and belonging, meaning and purpose.
☐	☐	☐	3. I respect the belief systems of others.

Self-Care Behaviors
1. Explore personal values and beliefs of self and others
2. Explore practices that are spiritually supportive.
3. Respect the belief systems of others.
4. Practice loving relationships with self and others.
5. Seek spiritual assistance to help cope with stress, crisis, or loss.

sponses to illness, health care choices, and treatment options
- Demonstrate sensitivity to the spiritual needs of clients
- Develop successful nursing strategies to assist clients in spiritual distress

ASSESSING SPIRITUALITY

Nursing History

Since a person's spirituality and religious beliefs have the potential to influence every aspect of being, an assessment of the client's spirituality should be included in each comprehensive nursing history. Helpful assessment guides are offered by Fish and Shelly (1978), Stoll (1979), and O'Brien (1982). Data are gathered about the client's spiritual beliefs and practices, the effect of these beliefs on everyday living, spiritual distress, and spiritual needs. Sample questions are listed in the box entitled Elements of Spiritual Assessment.

The following questions are from O'Brien's "Spiritual Assessment Guide" (1982, p 102):

Spiritual pain: Do you ever feel hurt or pain associated with the spiritual or religious beliefs which you hold? Do you feel pain related to uncertainty or nonbelief?

Spiritual alienation: Do you frequently feel "far away" from God? Does it seem that He is remote and far removed from your everyday life?

Spiritual anxiety: Are you afraid that God might not take care of your needs? That He might not "be there" when you need Him?

Spiritual guilt: Have you ever done things which God would be angry at you for? Are you feeling badly about things which you have done or failed to do in your life?

Spiritual anger: Are you angry at God for allowing you to be ill? Do you ever feel like blaming God for your illness? Do you think God is unfair to you?

Spiritual loss: Do you ever feel that you have lost God's love? That you have broken or weakened your relationship with God? Has God turned His back on you?

Spiritual despair: Do you ever feel that there is no hope of having God's love? Of pleasing Him? That God doesn't love you anymore?

If the client shares a spiritual problem, remember to use interview questions to determine (1) the specific nature of the problem, (2) its probable causes, (3) related signs and symptoms, (4) when it first began and how often it occurs, (5) how it affects everyday living, (6) the severity of the problem and whether it can be treated independently by nursing or needs to be referred, and (7) how well the client is coping with the problem.

Elements of Spiritual Assessment

- Spiritual beliefs
  "Are there particular spiritual or religious beliefs that are important to you?"
  - Spiritual or religious beliefs
  - Recent changes in these beliefs
  - Ways illness (injury, life crisis) has challenged beliefs
- Spiritual practices
  "Describe your usual spiritual practices and anything interfering with your ability to perform them."
  - Usual spiritual practices
  - Factors interfering with these practices
  - Aids necessary for these practices (prayer shawl, Bible, rosary, ikon)
- Relationship between spiritual beliefs and everyday living
  "Describe ways your spiritual beliefs affect everyday living."
  - Life-affirming vs life-denying influences
    - Daily schedule
    - Diet
    - Sense of self and the world

  - Interactions with health-care system
  - Treatment options
- Spiritual deficit/distress
  "Are your spiritual beliefs causing you any distress at the present time?"

Spiritual pain	Spiritual anger
Spiritual alienation	Spiritual loss
Spiritual anxiety	Spiritual despair
Spiritual guilt	

- Spiritual needs
  "In what ways can I and the other nurses help you to meet your spiritual needs?"
  - Need for meaning and purpose
  - Need for love and relatedness
  - Need for forgiveness
  - Desired nursing interventions
  - Need for referral to religious counselor
- Significant behavioral observations
  - Sudden changes in spiritual practices
  - Mood changes
  - Sudden interest in spiritual matters
  - Sleep disturbances

Nursing Observation

Since many clients may find it difficult to talk about their spiritual beliefs and problems, the nurse also observes the client's behavior for signs of spiritual distress. A family member or close friend may share significant observations.

> "He's been awfully moody since his heart attack . . . I can't believe the change in him."

> "I've never seen my father so depressed. He's never in his life been away from the Synagogue at Passover. I don't know how to help him."

Significant behavioral observations include sudden changes in spiritual practices (rejection, neglect, fanatical devotion), mood changes (frequent crying, depression, apathy, anger), sudden interest in spiritual matters (reading religious books or watching religious programs on television, visits to clergymen), and disturbed sleep. A nurse who observes these behaviors should follow up with appropriate interview questions. Often problems with spiritual distress do not surface until well after a client's admission history and examination. Effective questions include

> "You've been lying there so quietly . . . what are you thinking about?"

> "After all you've been through you must have done a good bit of soul searching. . . . Experiences like these are enough to shake anyone's faith—how is yours holding up?"

DIAGNOSING

When assessment data point to a spiritual problem that can be treated by independent nursing intervention it receives the label **spiritual distress**. This may be further specified as spiritual pain, alienation, anxiety, guilt, anger, loss, or despair (O'Brien, 1982). Common etiologies for spiritual distress include inability to reconcile present life situation (*e.g.,* illness, death of loved person, divorce) with spiritual beliefs ("God is all-powerful, all-loving, all-wise and he cares about me") or separation from religious community/supports. Sample nursing diagnoses of spiritual distress are presented in Table 39-1. Spiritual distress may affect other areas of human functioning. In the following nursing diagnoses, spiritual distress is the etiology of another problem.

Impaired adjustment to illness related to inability to reconcile illness with spiritual beliefs

Ineffective coping related to loss of religion as primary support (feels abandoned by God)

Fear related to feeling unprepared for death and afterlife experience

Dysfunctional grieving related to belief that religion is meaningless: despair

Hopelessness related to belief that no one cares—including God

Powerlessness related to feeling victimized by a tyrannical and arbitrary God

Disturbance in self-esteem related to failure to live according to dictates of religion

Sexual dysfunction related to values conflict

Sleep pattern disturbance related to spiritual distress

Potential for violence to self related to feeling that life is meaningless: despair

PLANNING: CLIENT GOALS

Nurses, sensitive to the role spiritual beliefs play in influencing both a person's thoughts about self and the world and interactions with the world, value spiritual health. Their interactions with any client who values spirituality are supportive of the following client goals:

- The client will identify spiritual beliefs that meet needs for (1) meaning and purpose, (2) love and relatedness, and (3) forgiveness.
- The client will derive from these beliefs strength, hope, and comfort when facing the challenge of illness, injury, or other life crisis.
- The client will develop "spiritual practices" that nurture communion with inner self, with God, and with the world.
- The client will express satisfaction with the compatibility of spiritual beliefs and everyday living.

Goals for clients in spiritual distress need to be individualized and may include some of the following:

- The client will explore the origin of spiritual beliefs and practices.
- The client will identify factors in life that challenge spiritual beliefs.
- The client will explore alternatives given these challenges: deny, modify, or reaffirm beliefs; develop new beliefs.
- The client will identify spiritual supports (*e.g.,* spiritual reading, faith, community).
- The client will report a decrease in spiritual distress following successful intervention.

IMPLEMENTING

There are a variety of interventions available to the nurse who wishes to help clients meet spiritual needs. Like other nursing skills, these interventions need to be practiced before the nurse is able to use them confidently, competently, and at the right moment. In this section the following nursing interventions are presented: offering supportive presence, facilitating the client's practice of religion, nurturing spirituality, praying with a client, spiritual counseling, referring a client to a religious counselor, and resolving conflicts between spiritual beliefs and treatment.

T A B L E 39-1
Nursing Diagnoses for Common Problems of Spiritual Distress

Title	Etiologic or Contributing Factors	Sample Defining Characteristics
Spiritual Distress		
Spiritual pain	Inability to accept death of son	A 46-year-old woman, agnostic, only son died 6 months ago (lung cancer)
		"I've often wondered throughout my life if there is a God—thought maybe if I had tried harder I'd have recognized him. Now I don't care if God exists or not because if he allows this I don't want to know him."
		"My son was my whole life; there's nothing left for me to live for."
		Lost 10 lb in 6 months since son died; leaves home only when necessary to purchase food, go to bank, and other routine activities.
Spiritual alienation	Separated from "faith community"	A 72-year-old Orthodox Jewish man, recently admitted to Protestant nursing home following 3-week hospitalization for stroke
		"I guess Yahweh has written me off; first the stroke that killed half my body and then I'm abandoned here where I can't even observe the Sabbath."
		"I want to go home."
Spiritual anxiety	Challenged belief and value system	A 37-year-old previously healthy male executive recovering from massive myocardial infarction
		"My parents were strict Methodists but when I left home for college I stopped going to church . . . never gave it much thought . . . there was always something else to do. I started going again but it never meant much."
		"I haven't exactly done anything awful but I've also not been a saint and I find myself wondering if there is a God what does he think of me."
		"Funny, I guess I thought I'd live forever. I sure never thought about dying and what happens after that."
		Often observed lying quietly in bed awake; asked to see minister
Spiritual guilt	Failure to live according to religious rules	A 23-year-old, single, Baptist woman being treated for premenstrual syndrome
		"I was raised in a strict Baptist home but had to leave . . . I needed more room to be me. I like life here at the university but there's a restlessness in me I can't describe. I've dated several men, one or two I really liked, but I always do something to mess up the relationship. It would kill my mother if she knew I lived with Gary for three months."
		"What it really comes down to is my own sense of betraying myself, my family, and my religion. Who am I anyway?"
Spiritual anger	Inability to accept illness	A 38-year-old homosexual man recently diagnosed with AIDS
		"My parents are fundamentalists . . . all I ever heard at home was how much Jesus loves me . . . all the while my mom was beating the daylights out of me . . . Does he love me? Does he love me so much that he had my parents throw me out when I finally told them I was gay? Does he love me so much that I got AIDS and now no one comes near me?"
		Facial features are tight; body held rigidly; speech is sharp, appears angry with God, the world, himself.
Spiritual loss	Terminal illness; anticipatory grieving; inability to find comfort in religion	A 40-year-old mother of three sons who was diagnosed with ovarian cancer 18 months ago; at present in advanced stage of disease
		"I've tried hard to do it all right . . . I read my Bible, prayed every day, went to church each Sunday, loved my husband and kids . . . why is this all happening to me? Why must I lose it all? Where is God now that I need him? Some mornings I wish I could shoot myself and end it all—instead another day drags on. Who can help me?"

(Continued)

Title	Etiologic or Contributing Factors	Sample Defining Characteristics

Spiritual Distress (continued)

		Cries frequently, no longer interested in everyday activities of family, no interest in praying, told family not to have pastor call anymore. "No one can help now."
Spiritual despair	Feeling that no one (not even God) cares	A 92-year-old frail widow who lives alone in a 2-room apartment; crippled with arthritis; has two married sons she has not seen for years.
		Says to community nurse who visits every week, "No one should have to live like this. If it weren't for the neighbor who comes on Saturday with a few groceries and you I'd be dead. I guess that would be for the best. It's been a long time since I felt like my living or dying would matter to anyone. Since I'm 92 now I guess even God doesn't want me. Couldn't you do something to put me out of my misery?"

Offering Supportive Presence

A nurse's gift of supportive presence must underlie all other types of intervention to meet spiritual needs. Supportive presence communicates value and respect. Chapter 20 presents basic communication skills helpful in establishing this type of presence.

The client who senses that the nurse is sincerely concerned and committed to helping meet human needs is better able to participate in the plan of care. Clients who experience respect and affirmation from other human beings find it easier to hold spiritual beliefs that meet their needs for meaning and purpose, love and relatedness, and forgiveness.

Facilitating the Client's Practice of Religion

The nurse can assist the hospitalized client in meeting spiritual needs. The following are means of helping the client continue normal spiritual practices in the unfamiliar environment of the hospital or care center:

- Familiarize the client with religious services and materials available within the institution.
- Respect the client's need for privacy or quiet during periods of prayer.
- Assist the client to obtain devotional objects and protect them from loss or damage.
- Arrange for the client wishing to receive the sacraments to do so.
- Attempt to meet the client's religious dietary restrictions.
- Arrange for the client's minister, priest, or rabbi to visit if the client wishes this.

If the client has a conflict between spiritual beliefs and the proposed medical therapy the nurse can assist the client in discussing this with the physician.

Nurturing Spirituality

Some clients experiencing a need to get in touch with their "spiritual self" and to nurture their spiritual development may look to the nurse for direction. The person who lives life enmeshed in the action and noises of today's society may feel strangely uncomfortable when illness forces self-introspection. The nurse can be helpful in recommending means to develop a relationship with one's inner world and manifest spiritual energy in one's outer world (Hill and Smith, 1985). (See the box entitled Nurturing Spirituality.)

Praying With a Client

Clients accustomed to regular periods of prayer but who feel too ill to pray as they would like or who enjoy praying with others may ask the nurse to pray with them or hope that the nurse will suggest this. Since there are many forms of prayer—quiet reflection, silent communion with God or higher power, reading or recitation of formal prayers, silent or loud calling on God or conversation with God, reading the Bible—the nurse can take the lead from the client by asking, "How would you like us to pray?" The religious background of the client is considered along with the type of prayers that have been meaningful in the past. It is also helpful to ask the client if there is a particular prayer request.

The nurse unaccustomed to praying aloud or in public may find it helpful to have a Bible passage or formal prayer readily available. The prayer may also be a simple expression aloud of the client's needs and hopes. A sample follows:

Lord God, our Creator and Healer, I entrust Mrs. Smith and her family to your loving care . . . bring

Nurturing Spirituality

Ways to Develop a Relationship With One's Inner World

- Prayer
- Reflection or "quiet listening to one's essence"
- Communion with nature through walks in the park, woods, beach
- Enjoyment of music, drama, art, dance
- Inner dialogues with oneself or with a higher being
- Dream analysis

Ways to Manifest Spiritual Energy in One's Outer World

- Loving relationships with others
- Service to others in need
- Forgiveness of others
- Empathy, compassion, and hope
- Laughter, joyous expressions
- Participation in church services and activities and social gatherings

(Adapted from Hill L, Smith N: Self-Care Nursing. Englewood Cliffs, NJ, Prentice-Hall, 1985)

peace to her mind and health and strength to her body. . . . Be with her (*as her treatment begins today, as she goes for surgery, and so on*). . . . We remember all your blessings to us in the past and thank you. . . . We are confident of your help now as we claim your promises."

It is important not to use prayer to block communication with the client. Praying before a client feels ready to pray may communicate to the client a lack of interest in the client's feelings. Since prayer often evokes deep feelings, the nurse should be prepared to spend time with the client after sharing prayer to respond to these feelings (Fish and Shelly, 1978).

Spiritual Counseling

The client who feels that the nurse is sensitive to spiritual needs and comfortable in his or her own spirituality may choose to share spiritual concerns with the nurse rather than with a religious counselor. The nurse who feels able to counsel the client may assist the client to

- Articulate spiritual beliefs
- Explore the origin of the client's spiritual beliefs and practices
- Identify life factors that challenge the client's spiritual beliefs (cause spiritual distress)
- Explore alternatives given these challenges: modify

life-style; deny, modify, or reaffirm beliefs; develop new beliefs
- Develop spiritual beliefs that meet needs for meaning and purpose, care and relatedness, forgiveness

To be an effective spiritual counselor, the nurse must be open to different spiritual beliefs and forms of spiritual expression and supportive of the client's efforts to nurture spiritual growth.

Referring a Client to a Religious Counselor

Nursing's responsibility is to identify when the client wishes to see a religious counselor and then to make the appropriate referral. Options include contacting the client's own spiritual adviser, contacting the institution's pastoral ministry department (if this exists), and utilizing the institution's referral list of clergy in the local community. At times a representative of the client's own religion may not be able to visit but a clergy person from another faith may be both able to help and welcomed by the client.

The nurse can assist the religious counselor by making the counselor feel welcome, answering questions about the client, directing the counselor to the client, and making sure that the client is ready to receive the counselor. Preparations of the client's room for the visit may vary, but the following are generally recommended practices:

- The room should be orderly and free of unnecessary equipment and items.
- There should be a seat for the religious counselor at the bedside or near the client so that both can be comfortable during the visit.
- The top of the bedside table should be free of items and covered with a clean, white cover if a sacrament is to be administered.
- The bed curtains should be drawn to provide privacy if the client is in a unit with other clients and is unable to be moved to a more private setting.

Some clients and spiritual advisers may value the nurse's participation in prayers, rituals, or the administration of sacraments. When a nursing diagnosis of spiritual distress is made, the nurse and the religious counselor can often collaborate on the plan of care and reinforce one another's efforts to assist the client to meet goals.

Resolving Conflicts Between Spiritual Beliefs and Treatments

Both the client and members of the client's family may experience conflict between a particular spiritual belief or religious law and proposed medical treatment or health option. The client may want the nurse's assistance when conferring with the spiritual adviser about a particular procedure. The nurse's role is to assist the client in obtaining the information needed to make an informed decision and to support the *client's* decision making. Since what the nurse says and the way it is said may powerfully influence the client's decision, it is important for the nurse to maintain objectivity.

EVALUATING

The nurse working with a client and family to achieve specified goals to meet spiritual needs can utilize each client interaction to evaluate the plan of care. Necessary to the evaluation are sensitivity to what the client is saying and not saying and observation of the client when alone as well as when interacting with the family and nurses.

In general, the nurse evaluates the client's ability to
- Find meaning and purpose in the client's present condition
- Interact honestly with family, friends, and others who meet the client's need for love and relatedness
- Derive strength and peace from the client's spiritual beliefs
- Reconcile any interpersonal differences causing the client anguish (religious belief or law in conflict with medical therapy)

The nurse helps the client to determine if spiritual beliefs are generally life-affirming or life-denying and if there is harmony between these beliefs and the client's everyday life experiences.

NURSING PROCESS *in Clinical Practice*

The nurse uses each phase of the nursing process when identifying and treating spiritual problems categorized as nursing diagnoses. Quality care depends on the nurse's possession of the knowledge and skills described earlier in this chapter. Following in outline format are the assessment priorities, client goals, nursing interventions, and evaluative criteria for a common spiritual problem encountered by nurses: spiritual distress. In the case study, nursing care is described for a middle-aged male client who has not practiced any formal religion recently and who is concerned about his relationship with God following a heart attack.

Spiritual Distress

Spiritual distress may result when an individual is unable to meet one or more of the basic spiritual needs for meaning and purpose, for love and relatedness, or for forgiveness (Fish and Shelly, 1978). Possible etiologies for these spiritual deficits include the following:

Deficit: meaning and purpose
Inability to reconcile spiritual beliefs with illness, pain, suffering, impending death
No prior need to explore life or its meaning and purpose

Deficit: love and relatedness
Human relationships to date have been painful.
Belief that people are "bad" and best dealt with as little as possible
Belief that God is a distant and uncaring superpower

Deficit: forgiveness
Inability to forgive oneself or others for human failings
Belief that God is a harsh taskmaster who desires nothing less than perfection

When identifying spiritual deficits, it is important to remember that individuals have different spiritual needs and meet them differently. The meaning one person attributes to life may be very different from that of another. It must be sufficient that it enables the individual to face each day with renewed energy for living in pursuit of some good.

Assessment
- Utilize interview questions and observations of the client's behavior to identify defining characteristics of each spiritual deficit.
  Meaning and purpose: (1) statements reflecting sense of despair, hopelessness, powerlessness ("What's the use?" "Nothing matters any more. . ." "Why should I bother?"); (2) apathy, indifference, listlessness, lethargy; (3) decreased energy for daily living and for healing
  Love and relatedness: (1) statements indicating loneliness, desire for meaningful relationships with God and people; (2) statements describing God and humans as overwhelmingly negative (evil, hurtful, distant, indifferent, uncaring); (3) decreased ability to interact with others (withdrawal, behaviors that alienate others); (4) absence of visitors for hospitalized client
  Forgiveness: (1) statements reflecting dissatisfaction with self, shame, guilt, desire for forgiveness, belief that one's failings are unforgivable; (2) belief that God is punishing; (3) anger, depression, cynicism; (4) confessions of failings to others

- Identify attempts client has made or is making to resolve these deficits and their effectiveness.
- Assess the need for referral to a spiritual adviser.

Client Goals

The client will
- Identify some spiritual belief that gives meaning and purpose to everyday life
- Move toward a healthy acceptance of the present situation: illness, pain, suffering, impending death
- Develop mutually caring relationships
- Verbalize satisfaction with relationship with God (if this is important)
- Express peaceful acceptance of limitations and failings
- Express ability to forgive others and to live in the present
- Demonstrate an "interior state of peace and joy; freedom from abnormal anxiety, guilt, or a feeling of sinfulness; and a sense of security and direction in the pursuit of one's life goals and activities" (O'Brien, 1982, p 98)

Interventions

Deficit: Meaning and Purpose
- Explore with the client (1) what has given the client's life meaning and purpose up to the present, (2) sources of meaning for other persons, and (3) possible meanings for the client's present experience of illness, pain, suffering, or impending death.
- Refer the client to a spiritual adviser if the client wishes this.
- Explore with the client spiritual practices from which strength and hope might be derived (*e.g.*, prayer or reading scripture or other spiritual books).
- Recommend that the client read spiritual biographies or Harold Kuschner's book *Why Bad Things Happen to Good People* (available in paperback in most book stores).

- Refer the client to the appropriate support groups (*e.g.*, self-help groups for persons with stroke, cancer, and so on).

Deficit: Love and Relatedness
- Treat the client at all times with respect, empathy, and genuine caring.
- Encourage the client to talk about relationships with others and to identify the origin of negative beliefs about persons.
- Encourage conversation about God as the client knows and experiences God (if God is part of the client's spiritual beliefs). If appropriate, introduce or reinforce the belief that God is a loving and personal God who is concerned about the client.
- Whenever possible encourage and facilitate visits from the client's family, friends, and spiritual adviser.

Deficit: Forgiveness
- Offer a supportive presence to the client that demonstrates your acceptance of the client.
- Explore with the client the importance of *learning* to accept oneself and others, including both strengths and limitations.
- Explore negative images of God and others that make it difficult for the client to seek forgiveness and to believe that the client is forgiven.
- Explore the client's self-expectations and assist the client to determine how realistic these are.
- Allow the client to verbalize shame, guilt, and anger and counsel about the importance of expressing negative emotions in healthy ways. Refer the client to a spiritual adviser if appropriate.
- Offer the client examples of how feelings of unforgiving toward others can end up hurting only the one who cannot forgive.

Evaluative Criteria

Client meets above goals.

C A S E   S T U D Y

Mr. Gargan is a 38-year-old divorced man on a step-down unit following treatment for a myocardial infarction. He owns a small car dealership. His religion is listed as Protestant. Frequently unable to sleep at night, Mr. Gargan often talks with the night nurse and once asked "Did you ever give much thought to whether or not there is a God?" Sensing much concern behind this question, the nurse asks specific questions to determine if the client has spiritual needs that are not being met.

Assessment Findings

12/26/89 2 AM Client again unable to sleep and initiated discussion about God. States was raised in a Lutheran home where everyone went to church on Sunday and tried to live according to God's commandments. Upon leaving home he stopped going to church (was never a value for his wife) and simply has not given much thought to religion—too busy running his business. Until *now* has not experienced any need for God. "But when I think how close I was to dying and that I've no idea what to expect after death—I'm actually scared. Do others feel this way?" Wants to explore religious beliefs —feels lack in his life. Said he would like to talk with hospital minister—will arrange for tomorrow. *E. Nolan, RN*

Nursing Diagnosis

Spiritual Distress: anxiety related to concerns about relationship with God

Planning

Mr. Gargan expresses his concerns about religion hesitantly and admits it isn't easy for him to talk about religious matters. He also states that he hasn't been able to think about much else ever since his heart attack. The following short-term goals are suggested to him and he quickly endorses them. "I need to make some peace with God and really don't know how much time I have, so the sooner we start the better."

Short-Term Goals

Prior to discharge, the client will
- Identify his religious beliefs
- Reconcile his life up until the present with God
- Verbalize that his spiritual beliefs have become a source of strength and peace rather than anxiety
- Increase night sleep to at least 6 hours

Long-Term Goal

The client's spiritual beliefs will effectively meet his needs for meaning and purpose, love and belonging, and forgiveness. See the care plan designed to accomplish the above goals.

Implementation

Successful implementation of the plan of care will require the following specialized nursing abilities:
- Holistic orientation to nursing, which values physical, psychologic, and spiritual health
- Sensitivity to the spiritual needs of clients and the ability and willingness to address these needs
- Respect for and knowledge of different spiritual beliefs (traditions) and the means persons use to meet spiritual needs
- Ability to offer the client a supportive nursing presence, including listening skills, empathy, vulnerability, humility, and commitment, as he struggles with his spiritual anxiety
- Willingness to refer the client to a spiritual adviser and to work collaboratively with this person
- Interpersonal and leadership skills to motivate the entire nursing staff to value spiritual health and to

better understand its role in facilitating cardiac rehabilitation

Documentation

Following is a sample SOAP documentation written when the problem was first detected:

12/26/89
2 AM

S: "I need to make some peace with God and really don't know how much time I have . . ." Reports was raised in Lutheran home but has not practiced any formal religion for most of his adult life—up until now no need for God

O: Frequently unable to fall asleep at night—often observed lying quietly in bed with face tense

A: Spiritual distress: anxiety related to concerns about his relationship with God

P: 1. Add above diagnosis to problem list.
   2. Refer to hospital minister in AM.
   3. See plan of care.

E. Nolan, RN

Sample documentation of nursing interaction with the client following the first visit of the hospital minister in traditional note format follows:

12/27/89 3 PM B. Hanks, Protestant minister, here to see client at 1 PM. Afterwards client said he felt "a whole lot better." Reported minister had assured him that many people in the hospital with a serious illness go through exactly what he is experiencing now—and this thought seemed to decrease much of his anxiousness. Minister had reinforced nurse's suggestion that he explore his religious beliefs and he has already jotted down some thoughts. "I knew you fixed bodies in hospitals but didn't know you fix souls, too." Client looking forward to minister's visit tomorrow.

G. Paris, RN

Evaluation

Short-term goal achievement is continuously evaluated prior to client's discharge. See the nursing care plan for evaluative statements. The client is taught how to evaluate the long-term goal since this will require ongoing evaluation.

NURSING CARE PLAN for Mr. Gargan

Nursing Diagnosis: Spiritual distress: anxiety related to concerns about relationship with God

Long-Term Goal: The client's spiritual beliefs will effectively meet his needs for meaning and purpose, love and belonging, forgiveness.

Goals	Nursing Actions	Rationale	Evaluative Statement
Prior to discharge the client will 1. Identify his religious beliefs	• Assist the client to (1) identify the spiritual beliefs he had as a child and the origin of these	Life experiences may challenge religious beliefs that were uncritically held as a child.	12/30/89 Goal partially met. Client states he has a much clearer concept of God and no longer fears

(Continued)

N U R S I N G   C A R E   P L A N *(Continued)*

Goals	Nursing Actions	Rationale	Evaluative Statement
	beliefs; (2) evaluate these beliefs in terms of his life experiences; and (3) reaffirm, modify, or reject these beliefs or develop new spiritual beliefs.		that God will reject him for ignoring him for so long . . . but feels he also has a lot to learn. *E. Nolan, RN*
	• Assist the client to assess whether his newly articulated spiritual beliefs are life-affirming or life-denying and the degree to which they meet his needs for meaning and purpose, love and relatedness, and forgiveness.	Since spiritual beliefs can exert positive (life-affirming) and negative (life-denying) influences on a person's life, individuals should have some criteria to use when evaluating their beliefs.	
	• Refer the client to the hospital minister for assistance with the above.		
2. Reconcile his life up until the present with God	• Reassure the client that many persons get involved in day-to-day living to the extent that they forget about God and that in some religions persons believe that God uses illness and other stressors to invite people to rethink their spiritual beliefs. In these traditions God is often pictured with "open arms" waiting to welcome a child "Home."	Guilt often inhibits persons from seeking and experiencing the forgiveness they desire. Images of a stern and unyielding God ready to strike down transgressors may contribute to a client's spiritual distress. Many persons have unrealistic self-expectations.	12/30/89 Goal met. "This minister has really helped. I wish I had talked to him a long time ago. I've carried so much guilt about my divorce and some other things— thought God would never forgive me. I feel so much more at peace now." *E. Nolan, RN*
	• Refer the client to a spiritual advisor for help in experiencing forgiveness if he mentions guilt feelings.		
	• Communicate to the client the importance of people accepting themselves—with all their strengths and weaknesses.		
3. Verbalize that his spiritual beliefs have become a source of strength and peace rather than anxiety	Same as above		12/30/89 Goal met. "It's good to be able to feel more peaceful about whatever the future brings. I'm anxious to get out of here because there's a lot I want to do with God's help." *E. Nolan, RN*

(Continued)

N U R S I N G   C A R E   P L A N   (Continued)

Goals	Nursing Actions	Rationale	Evaluative Statement
4. Increase night sleep to at least 6 undisturbed hours	• Nurse on the 11 to 7 shift to check on client at beginning of shift to make sure he is comfortable and ready for sleep. • Use power of suggestion to enhance sleep. "I'm sure when I check back you'll be sound asleep." • If sleep remains disturbed, try relaxation exercises or guided imagery (see Chap 9).	As spiritual anxiety decreases, sleep should improve. If sleep does not improve, need to explore other contributing factors and interventions.	12/30/89 Goal met. Client slept last night from midnight to 6 AM. Will continue to monitor. *E. Nolan, RN*

K E Y   P O I N T S

■ The tradition of nursing has always been strongly holistic and nurses have practiced nursing sensitive to the physical, psychosocial, and spiritual needs of clients.

■ Spiritual needs underlying all religious traditions and common to all persons include need for meaning and purpose, need for love and relatedness, and need for forgiveness.

■ Spiritual beliefs and practices are associated with all aspects of a person's life, including health and illness, relationships with others, daily living habits, required and prohibited behaviors, and the general frame of reference for thinking about oneself and the world may all be influenced by spiritual beliefs.

■ Spiritual beliefs during illness may be an important source of support, strength, and healing but may also be a source of anxiety when they conflict with proposed medical therapy.

■ It is important for the nurse to be knowledgeable about and respect the spiritual beliefs of clients.

■ The nurse who demonstrates peace, inner strength, warmth, joy, caring, and creativity in interactions with others will be most effective when assisting clients to meet spiritual needs.

■ A comprehensive nursing assessment of spirituality addresses spiritual beliefs and practices, relationship between spiritual beliefs and everyday living, indicators of spiritual distress, and unmet spiritual needs.

■ Nursing diagnoses may be written that specifically address spiritual distress (spiritual pain, alienation, anxiety, guilt, anger, loss, or despair) or that identify the effect of spiritual distress on other areas of human functioning (ineffective coping, dysfunctional grieving, hopelessness, powerlessness, disturbance in self-esteem).

■ Nursing interventions that promote spiritual health include offering a supportive presence, facilitating the client's practice of religion, nurturing spirituality, praying with a client, spiritual counseling, referring a client to a religious counselor, and assisting clients to resolve conflicts between spiritual beliefs and treatment.

B I B L I O G R A P H Y

Brittain JN, Boozer J: Spiritual care: Integration into a collegiate nursing curriculum. J Nurs Educ 26(4):155–159, 1987

Brooke V: The spiritual well-being of the elderly. Geriatric Nursing 8(4):194–195, 1987

Burkhardt MA et al: Dealing with spiritual concerns of clients in the community. Journal of Community Health Nursing 2(4):191–198, 1985

Burnard P: Spiritual distress and the nursing response: Theoretical considerations and counselling skills. J Adv Nurs 12(3):377–382, 1987

Byrne Sr M: A zest for life! Journal of Gerontological Nursing 11(4):30–33, 1985

Carson VB et al: The effect of didactic teaching on spiritual attitudes. Image 18(4):161–164, 1986

Ellerhorst-Ryan J: Selecting an instrument to measure spiritual distress. Oncology Nursing Forum 12(2):93–94, 99, 1985

Ellis D: Whatever happened to the spiritual dimension? Canadian Nurse 76(9):42–43, 1980

Ferszt GG: When your patient needs spiritual comfort. Nursing 18(4):48–49, 1988

Fish S, Shelly J: Spiritual Care: The Nurse's Role. Downer's Grove, IL, InterVarsity Press, 1978

Heller D: The children's God. Psychology Today 19(12):22–27, 1985

Hill L, Smith N: Self-Care Nursing. Englewood Cliffs, NJ, Prentice-Hall, 1985

Larue GA: Religion and the aged. In Burnside IM: Nursing and the Aged, pp 642–650. New York, McGraw-Hill, 1981

Miller JF, Powers MJ: Development of an instrument to measure hope. Nurs Res 37(1):6–10, 1988

Murray RB, Zentner JP: Nursing Concepts for Health Promotion, 3rd ed. Englewood Cliffs, NJ, Prentice-Hall, 1985

O'Brien ME: The need for spiritual integrity. In Yura H, Walsh M (eds): Human Needs 2 and the Nursing Process, pp 81–115. Norwalk, CT, Appleton-Century-Crofts, 1982

Peck MS: The Road Less Traveled. A Touchstone Book. New York, Simon & Schuster, 1978

Peterson EA: The physical . . . the spiritual . . . can you meet all your patients needs? Journal of Gerontological Nursing 11(10):23–27, 1985

Pumphrey JB: Recognizing your patient's spiritual needs. Nursing 8(12):64–69, 1977

Reed PG: Religiousness among terminally ill and healthy adults. Res Nurs Health 9(1):35–41, 1986

Rew L: Exercises for spiritual growth. Journal of Holistic Nursing 4(1):20–22, 1986

Salladay SA: Spiritual care of clients. Nursing and Humanities Newsletter, Society for Health and Human Values 5(3):8–9, 1987

Schwarzbaum L: Women and God. Glamour 84(5):300–303, May, 1986

Sodestrom KE et al: Patients' spiritual coping strategies: A study of nurse and patient perspectives. Oncology Nursing Forum 14(2):41–46, 1987

Soeken KL, Martinson IM: Study measures nurse' attitudes about providing spiritual care. Health Progress 67(3):52–55, 1986

Stoll RI: Guidelines for spiritual assessment. Am J Nurs 79(9):1574–1577, 1979

UNIT

IX

Promoting Optimal Health in Special Situations

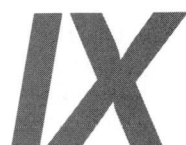

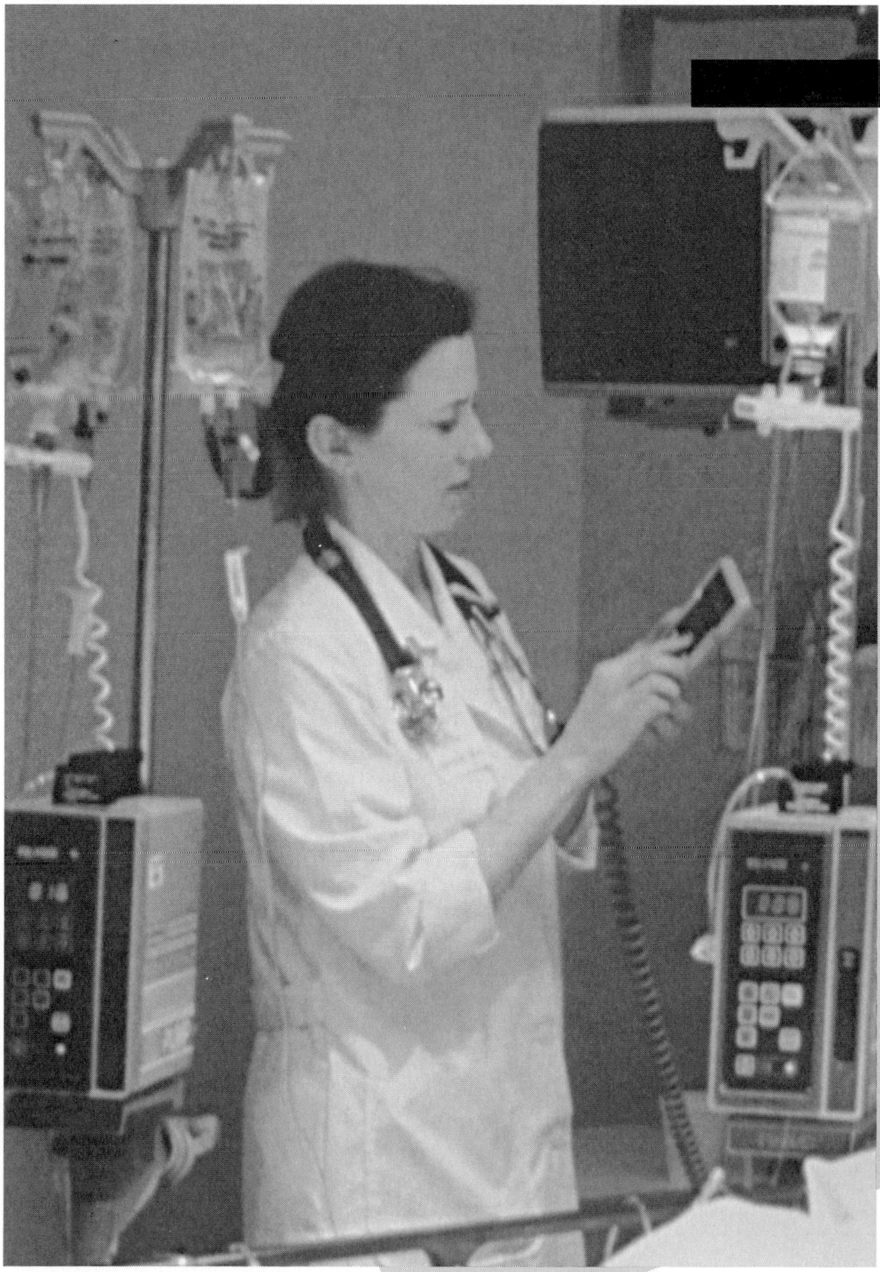

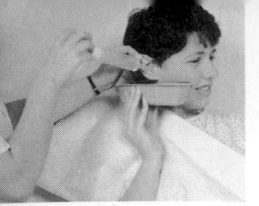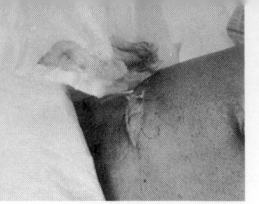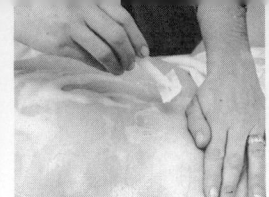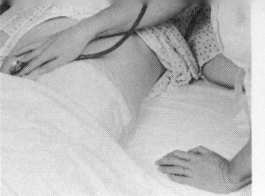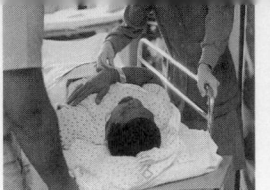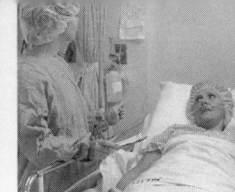

*T*hrough use of the nursing process, nurses give holistic care to promote wellness, prevent illness, restore health, and facilitate coping. These broad aims of holistic nursing are integrated when nursing care is focused on promoting optimal health in special situations. Unit IX discusses the nurse's role in situations that occur commonly in health-care settings: medication administration, diagnostic procedures, wound care, and care of the client having surgery. In each situation, the nurse uses knowledge and skill to carry out client care in a variety of roles. As caregiver, the nurse assesses, plans, implements, and evaluates nursing interventions to meet holistic physical and psychosocial needs and to provide safety and comfort. As communicator and teacher, the nurse provides psychologic support and meets knowledge deficits to facilitate coping, maximize strengths, and ensure client and family understanding and continuity of care. The nurse also serves as a client advocate and follows legal guidelines.

The situations discussed in this unit are typical of the interdependent (or collaborative) aspects of nursing and medicine. The physician orders the medications, diagnostic tests, or surgical care; the nurse implements actions to provide client safety and knowledge and to facilitate optimal function or recovery. Although procedures and protocols are often used in these situations, nursing interventions are individualized to the unique needs of each person requiring care.

Unit IX provides the content and special skills necessary for knowledgeable, safe, and individualized nursing care when administering medications, assisting with diagnostic procedures, caring for wounds, and caring for the client having surgery.

Medications

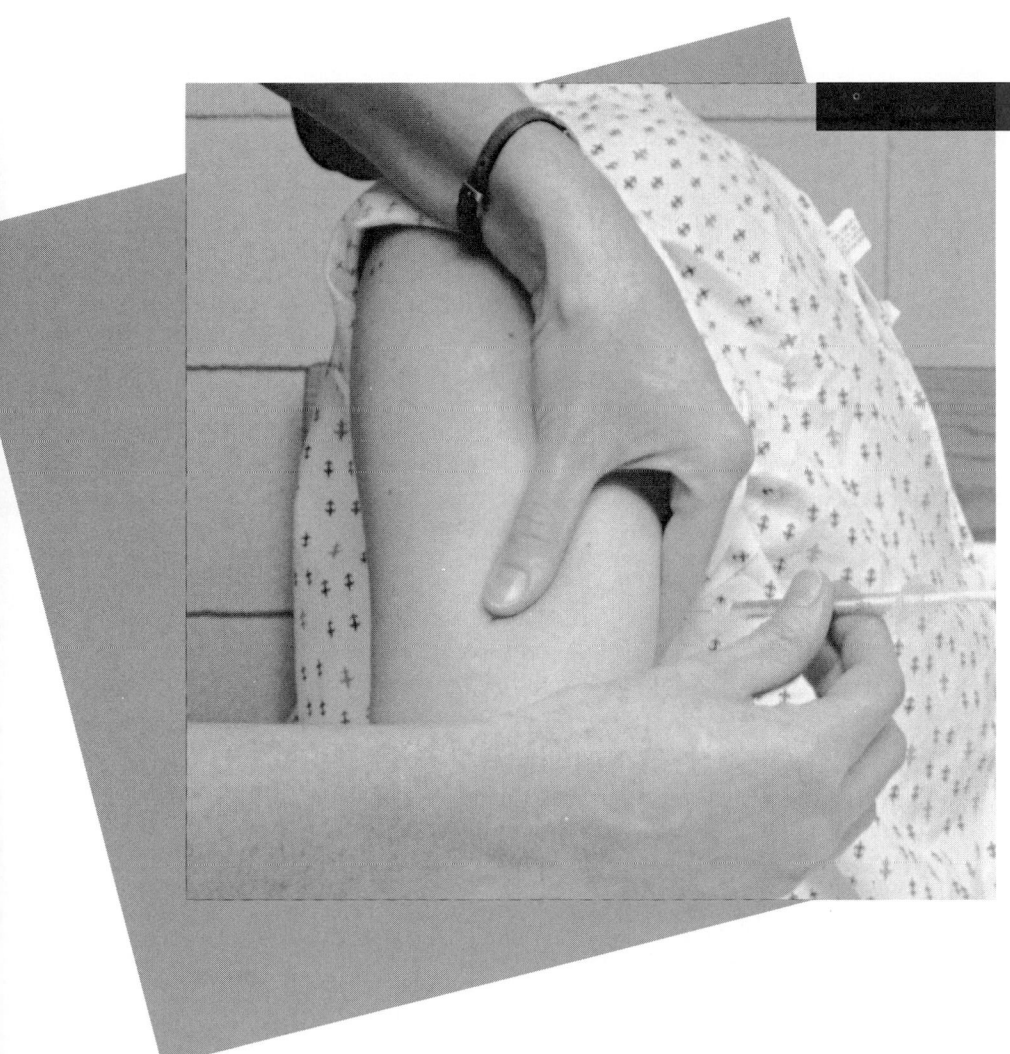

OBJECTIVES

After studying this chapter, the learner should be able to

Define key terms used in the chapter.

Discuss drug legislation in the United States and Canada.

Describe drug names, types of preparation, and types of drug orders.

Identify drug classifications and actions.

Discuss adverse effects of drugs, including allergy, tolerance, cumulative effect, idiosyncratic effect, and interactions.

Obtain client information necessary to establish a medication history.

Calculate drug dosages, using the various systems of equivalents.

Describe principles used to safely prepare and administer medications, orally, parenterally, topically, and by inhalation.

Develop teaching plans to meet client needs specific to medication administration.

Medication administration is a basic nursing function, involving skillful technique and consideration of the client's development. Medications are prepared and administered with safety in mind. The nurse administering medications is expected to have a knowledge base concerning drugs, including drug names, preparations, classifications, adverse effects, and physiologic factors affecting drug action.

The nursing process can be applied to the fundamental nursing skill of medication administration. Assessment entails a comprehensive medication history as well as ongoing assessments of the client's response during and after drug therapy. Nursing diagnoses are developed from the assessment data. Client-centered outcomes are evaluated after implementation of the plan of care, tailored to the client's needs.

A **drug** or a **medication** is any substance that modifies body functions when taken into the living organism. The study that deals with chemicals affecting the body's functioning is called **pharmacology**. A *pharmacist* is a person licensed to prepare and dispense drugs. The physician is legally responsible for prescribing medications. Legislation in some states grants nurse practitioners this privilege also. The physician or nurse practitioner conveys the medication plans to others by an order called a **prescription**. After the medication is prepared by the pharmacist, the nurse administers the medication to the client.

Some medications are given frequently and the nurse becomes familiar with the facts concerning these drugs. Other medications may not be given by the nurse often and the nurse needs to seek information before administering the drugs. Information about specific drugs is more appropriately discussed in pharmacology texts. Many references are available to nurses to help them develop a personal medication data base.

KEY TERMS

absorption	inunction
ampule	irrigation
anaphylactic reaction	medication
antagonist effect	medication order
body surface area	metabolism
bolus	official name
chemical name	parenteral
cumulative effect	pharmacodynamics
diluent	pharmacokinetics
distribution	pharmacology
drug	piggyback
drug allergy	prefilled cartridge
drug tolerance	prescription
excretion	receptor
generic name	reconstitution
heparin lock	stock supply
iatrogenic disease	subcutaneous
idiosyncratic effect	synergistic effect
individual supply	topical application
inhalation	trade name
injections	unit dose
instillation	vial
intradermal	Z-track
intramuscular	
intravenous	

DRUG LEGISLATION

United States

In 1906 the Pure Food and Drug Act designated the United States Pharmacopeia (USP) and the National Formulary (NF) as official standards of drugs and empowered the federal government to enforce these standards. This legislation was updated in 1938 by the Federal Food, Drug and Cosmetic Act. The Food and Drug Administration is responsible for enforcing this law. Extensive testing of new drugs is required before they may be marketed for use. An amendment to the Federal Food, Drug and Cosmetic Act in 1952 distinguished prescription (legend) drugs from nonprescription (over-the-counter) drugs and provided directions for dispensing prescription drugs.

The Comprehensive Drug Abuse Prevention and Control Act, also known as the Controlled Substances

Act, was passed in 1970. This law was designed to regulate the distribution of narcotics and other drugs of abuse. Such drugs have been categorized according to their therapeutic usefulness and potential for abuse. Government programs for the prevention and treatment of drug abuse were established.

Canada

Drug legislation in Canada includes the Canadian Food and Drug Act, passed in 1953, which addresses regulations for the manufacture and sale of drug substances. This law has been amended often. According to the Act, drugs must comply with standards outlined in specific pharmacopeias and formularies (British Pharmacopeia, Canadian Formulary). The regulations of the Canadian Narcotic Control Act, enacted in 1961, restrict the sale, possession, and use of opiates, coca, and marijuana. Amendments made since 1961 include restrictions on methadone. Only authorized persons can possess narcotics. Enforcement of this law has been the charge of the Royal Canadian Mounted Police.

INTRODUCTION TO PHARMACOLOGY

Drug Preparations

Nomenclature

One drug can have several names. The **chemical name** is a very precise description of the drug's chemical composition, identifying the drug's atomic and molecular structure. This name is of significance to the pharmacist. The **generic name** is the name assigned by the manufacturer who first develops the drug. Often the generic name is derived from the chemical name. The **official name** is the name by which the drug is identified in the official publication, *United States Pharmacopeia and National Formulary* (*USP and NF*). The **trade name**, also referred to as the *brand name* or *proprietary name,* is selected by the drug company selling the drug and is copyrighted. A drug can have several trade names when produced by different manufacturers.

Nurses should be familiar with a drug's generic and trade names. For example, acetaminophen (generic name) is known by such trade names as Tylenol, Tempra, and Liquiprin.

Types of Preparations

Drugs are available in many forms, or preparations. The form in which the drug is prepared may determine the route of administration. Some drugs may be prepared in only one form to be administered by a certain route. Others may be supplied in several preparations, which allow it to be given through various routes. One type of preparation may be desirable in a given situation. For example, a liquid preparation of a medication would be indicated for young children who are not able to swallow solid preparations such as tablets. Drug preparations are available for oral, topical, and injectable administration. Table 40-1 describes drug preparations commonly used by the nurse.

Classifications

How does the nurse organize the vast amount of information about medications? Where does the nurse begin the study of medications? It is recommended that the nurse focus on drug classifications.

Drugs can be classified from different perspectives. For example, drugs may be classified by body systems (*e.g.,* drugs affecting the respiratory system, drugs affecting the cardiovascular system), by the symptom relieved by the drug, or by the clinical indication for the drug (*e.g.,* analgesic, antibiotic).

Mechanism of Drug Action

Pharmacodynamics

Drugs act at the cellular level to achieve their desired effects. The process by which drugs alter cell physiology is called **pharmacodynamics** (Spencer, 1986, p 56). One mechanism of drug action is a drug–receptor interaction in which the drug interacts with one or more cellular structures to alter cell function. These specialized structures are called **receptor** sites. The drug fits the receptor as a key fits a lock. Drugs may also combine with enzymes to achieve the desired effect, which is referred to as a *drug–enzyme interaction.* Some drugs act on the cell membrane or alter the cellular environment.

Pharmacokinetics

Pharmacokinetics is the study of the movement of drug molecules in the body in relation to the drug's absorption, distribution, metabolism, and excretion.

Absorption.   **Absorption** is the process by which a drug is transferred from its site of entry into the body to the bloodstream. Absorption of a drug is influenced by several factors:
- Route of administration: Injected medications usually are more rapidly absorbed than are oral medications.
- Drug solubility: Liquid medications are absorbed more rapidly than solid preparations: Liquid preparations do not have to be dissolved in the gastrointestinal fluids. Most drugs are weak acids and bases. When in solution, drugs are a mixture of ionized and un-ionized forms. The un-ionized form is more readily absorbed.

T A B L E   40-1
Common Types of Drug Preparations

Preparation	Description
Capsule	Powder or gel form of an active drug enclosed in a gelatinous container
Elixir	Medication in a clear liquid containing water, alcohol, sweeteners, and flavor
Liniment	Medication mixed with alcohol, oil, or soap, which is rubbed on the skin
Lotion	Drug particles in a solution for topical use
Lozenge	Small oval, round, or oblong preparation containing a drug in a flavored or sweetened base, which dissolves in the mouth and releases the medication; also called a *troche*
Ointment	Semisolid preparation containing a drug to be applied externally; also called an *unction*
Pill	Mixture of a powdered drug with a cohesive material; may be round or oval in shape
Powder	Single or mixture of finely ground drugs
Solution	A drug dissolved in another substance (*e.g.,* in an aqueous solution the drug has been dissolved in water)
Suppository	An easily melted medicated preparation in a firm base such as gelatin that is inserted into the body (rectum, vagina, urethra)
Suspension	Finely divided, undissolved particles in a liquid medium; should be shaken before use
Syrup	Medication combined in a water and sugar solution
Tablet	Small, solid dosage of medication, compressed or molded; may be any color, size, or shape. Enteric-coated tablets are coated with a substance that is insoluble in gastric acids. This reduces gastric irritation by the drug.

- *p*H: The form in which the drug is found depends on the *p*H of the environment. Acidic drugs are well absorbed in the stomach. Drugs that are basic remain ionized or insoluble in an acid environment. These drugs are not absorbed before reaching the small intestine.
- Local conditions at the site of administration: The more extensive the absorbing surface, the greater the absorption of the drug and the more rapid the effect. A client with burns would have poor absorption from an intramuscular injection. Food in the stomach can delay the absorption of some medications or enhance the rate of absorption of other drugs. Drug absorption can be manipulated with sustained-release preparations or enteric-coated preparations. Enteric-coated preparations are resistive to the digestive action of the stomach.
- Drug dosage: A loading dose is higher than body capacity. A maintenance dose is a lower dosage that becomes the usual or daily dosage. Clients receiving digoxin or phenobarbital may receive loading doses when therapy is initiated.

Distribution.   After a drug has been absorbed into the bloodstream, it is distributed throughout the body. The drug accumulates in specific tissues for its action. Distribution depends on the rate of perfusion and capillary permeability to the drug. Certain other factors may also influence distribution. The drug may bind to plasma proteins, which causes unequal distribution and may prevent the drug from reaching its intended site of action. The blood–brain barrier is poorly permeable to water-soluble drugs. Some drugs fail to penetrate the tissues of the central nervous system as readily as others. The placenta, on the other hand, is not a selective barrier to the distribution of drugs. Drugs move across the placenta readily and many produce harmful effects on the unborn fetus.

Metabolism.   Metabolism, or biotransformation, is the breakdown of the drug to an inactive form. The liver is the primary site for drug metabolism. A variety of processes and enzymes are involved in metabolism. The reader is referred to a pharmacology text for a further explanation of metabolism.

Excretion.   After the drug is broken down to an inactive form, **excretion** of the drug from the body occurs. Most drugs are excreted by the kidneys. The lungs are the primary route for the excretion of gaseous substances such as inhalation anesthesia. Many drugs are excreted through the intestines. The sweat, salivary, and mammary glands are also routes of drug excretion.

Factors Affecting Drug Action

Certain variables are known to influence the action or effect of a medication.

Developmental Considerations. A child's dose for medication is smaller than an adult's dose. Infants especially are very responsive to medications because of the immaturity of their organs. The elderly are responsive to medications because their bodies have experienced physiologic changes associated with the aging process, including decreases in gastric motility, acid production, and blood flow, which affect drug absorption. Small body size, reduced weight, and reduced body water also alter distribution, as do decreases in cardiac output and organ perfusion. Decreased plasma binding increases the possibility of drug toxicity. Liver function declines with advancing age and changes in hepatic enzymes involved in drug metabolism. Blood flow to the liver decreases secondary to a decrease in cardiac output. Drugs are excreted more slowly from the body as a result of changes in kidney function. Receptor sensitivity is altered in the elderly and sensitivity to certain drugs increases in the elderly person.

Weight. Expected responses to drugs are based largely on those reactions occurring when given to healthy adults (18–65 years, 150 lb). The nurse should be aware of the usual dosage for a particular medication. Drug dosages for children are calculated by weight or body surface area.

Sex. This variable refers to the difference in the distribution of body fat and fluids in men and women. During pregnancy drugs are generally contraindicated because of their possible adverse effects on the fetus.

Genetic Factors. Differences in the responses of clients receiving the same medication may be attributed to genetic differences. Enzyme deficiencies or metabolic disturbances can alter the way the body handles the medication.

Psychologic Factors. The client's expectations of the medication affect the response to the medication, as for instance in studies of drug effects where some clients receive a "placebo." A placebo is a pharmacologically inactive substance. In clinical drug trials, one group of clients receives the active drug, while another group receives a placebo to study the drug's effects. Some clients have the same response with the placebo as with the active drug.

Pathology. The presence of disease can affect the action of the drug. The liver is the primary organ for drug

breakdown. Pathologic conditions involving the liver may slow down the process of metabolism.

Environment. The environment surrounding the client may influence the response to medications. Sensory deprivation and overload may affect drug responses. The relative oxygen deprivation at high altitudes may increase sensitivity to some drugs (Hahn et al., 1986, p 64). The client receiving pain medication or a sedative in an active environment may not be able to benefit fully from the effects of the medication.

Time of Administration. Generally the presence of food in the stomach delays the absorption of orally administered medications. Some medications should be given with food to prevent gastric irritation, and the nurse should consider this when establishing a client's medication schedule. Human rhythms and cycles may also influence drug action.

Adverse Drug Effects

Therapeutic effect is the desired effect of the medication; it is the reason the drug was administered. However, drugs may react unpredictably, be harmful, and sometimes have unexplainable response. Side-effects are effects that are not intended or desired. There are several known adverse drug effects.

Iatrogenic disease is disease caused unintentionally by drug therapy. **Drug allergy** occurs in an individual who has been previously exposed to the drug and has developed antibodies. Drug allergies can be manifested in a variety of symptoms ranging from minor to serious. The reaction can occur immediately after the client received the medication or be delayed for hours to days. Some of the signs and symptoms of a drug allergy are skin rash, urticaria, fever, diarrhea, nausea, and vomiting. A life-threatening immediate reaction is called an **anaphylactic reaction** and results in respiratory distress, sudden severe bronchospasm, and cardiovascular collapse. It is treated with epinephrine, bronchodilators, and antihistamines.

Drug tolerance is said to exist when the body becomes accustomed to a particular drug over a period of time. Larger doses of the drug must be given to the client to produce the same effects. A **cumulative effect** occurs when the body cannot metabolize one dose of a drug before another dose is administered. The drug is taken in more frequently than it is excreted and each new dose increases the total quantity in the body than is excreted in the same amount of time. An **idiosyncratic effect** is any abnormal or peculiar response to a drug that may manifest itself by overresponse, underresponse, or response different from the expected outcome. Elderly clients often have unpredictable or erratic responses to medications. Idiosyncratic effects are thought to be the result of genetic enzyme deficiencies that lead to an abnormal mechanism for drug breakdown.

In a *drug interaction,* the combined effect of two or more drugs acting simultaneously produces either an effect less than that of each drug alone (**antagonist effect**) or greater than that of each drug alone (**synergistic effect**). Alcohol and barbiturates taken together create a synergistic effect.

ASSESSING: THE MEDICATION HISTORY

Assessment of the client receiving medications begins during a nursing history, one component of which is the medication history. During the interview, the nurse's questions can be adapted or elaborated to meet the client's needs and level of understanding. The nurse should avoid use of medical jargon that the client may not understand. Familiar terms the client or family recognize should be chosen. For instance, the client may refer to a diuretic as the "water pill" or an anticoagulant as a "blood thinner."

Areas to be included in the medication history are listed in the accompanying box.

Assessment is an ongoing process. The nurse not only assesses the client with regard to medications during the nursing history but continues the assessment of the client during and following medication administration. A discussion of how the nurse would measure the client's response to medications is included in the evaluation section later in this chapter.

PREPARING FOR MEDICATION ADMINISTRATION

Medication Orders

No medication may be given to a client without a **medication order** from a physician. Each health agency has a policy specifying the manner in which the physician writes an order. In most instances, orders are written on a form specifically designed for the physician's order. This becomes part of the client's permanent record.

Safe practice dictates that the nurse follow only a written order. A written order by the physician is least likely to result in error or misunderstanding. Under certain circumstances, such as in an emergency, a verbal order from the physician may be given to a registered nurse or pharmacist. The legal implications for dispensing and administering an agent without a written order vary, and the nurse is cautioned to be familiar with the exact agency policy whenever called upon to administer

---

Elements of a Medication History

- *Previous and current drug use*—Prescriptions, self-prescribed over-the-counter medications, nonmedicinal drugs (*e.g.,* alcohol and caffeine, home remedies). What medications is the client presently taking? What is the reason for taking the medication(s)? What medications has the client taken during the past year and for what reasons?
- *Medication schedule*—At what times does the client take medications? Are there any special considerations when the client takes medications, such as crushing medication and mixing it with soft foods?
- *Response to medications*—Have the medications had the expected effects? Has the client ever experienced any adverse drug reactions? The nurse may need to describe known adverse drug effects. The client may not be aware of having experienced an adverse drug reaction. Is there any family history of adverse drug reactions? Is the client aware of any allergies to medications?
- *Attitude toward drugs and use of drugs*—What are the client's feelings about taking medications? Why does the client take medication(s)?
- *Compliance to regimen*—Does the client understand the reason for taking medication? Does the client adhere to the medication schedule? Are there any problems preventing the client from adhering to the regimen?
- *Storage*—Where are medications stored in the client's home? How long does the client keep medications in the home? If the nurse is making a home visit, an inspection of the storage area would be appropriate.

---

therapeutic agents. The legal implications of verbal orders are discussed in Chapter 6.

Usual hospital policy dictates that when a client is admitted, unless specific orders to the contrary are written, all drugs that the physician may have ordered while the client was at home are discontinued. This may prove to be a problem when a client brings medications from home to the hospital. To avoid the possibility of having the client continue taking the home medications while receiving the same ones or others under new orders, all medications should be sent home with the family or removed from the client's unit and placed in safekeeping. This will require an explanation to the client and family of how the client's drug plan will be implemented. However, in some inpatient facilities, clients keep their medications at their bedside and learn or continue to administer them as they would at home. It is felt that this approach helps promote the independence of clients. The nurse should be aware when clients are allowed to take their own medications while hospitalized and should know each agent's purpose and possible undesirable side-effects. Also, a notation should be made on the client's plan of care so that everyone knows the client has medications at the bedside.

When a client has had surgery or is transferred to another clinical service or another health agency, it is general practice that all orders related to drugs are discontinued, and new orders are written. To keep physicians aware of orders in effect, some hospitals specify a day of the week when orders are to be rewritten or they will be automatically discontinued.

Types of Orders

There are several types of orders that the physician may write.

A *standing order* is one that is carried out as specified until it is canceled by another order. Many physicians whose practices are limited to a particular clinical area have a specified set of written orders for all their hospitalized clients. These are also referred to as *standing orders*. Occasionally, a physician writes a standing order and its cancellation simultaneously, that is, the physician specifies that a certain order is to be carried out for a stated number of days or times. After the stated period has passed, the order is canceled automatically.

The physician may write an *"as needed" (prn) order* for medication. The client receives medication when it is requested or is needed. A prn order is commonly written for postoperative pain medication.

Another type of order is called a *single order*, that is, the directive is carried out only once at a time specified by the physician. Medication to be administered immediately prior to surgery is an example of a single order.

A *stat order* is also a single order but one that is carried out at once. A stat order for epinephrine or an antihistamine would be carried out immediately for a client experiencing an anaphylactic drug reaction.

Parts of the Medication Order

The medication order consists of seven parts:
- Client's name
- Date and time the order is written
- Name of drug to be administered
- Dosage of the drug
- Route by which the drug is to be administered
- Frequency of administration of the drug
- Signature of person writing the order

Client's Name. The client's full name is used. The middle name or initial should be included to avoid con-

fusion with other clients. In most agencies, the client's full name, the hospital number, and the physician's name are mechanically imprinted on all sheets on the client's chart, including the physician's order sheet.

Date and Time the Order Is Written. The date the order is written is given. In some situations, the time the order is written is also included. Since the nursing staffs in inpatient agencies change several times during each 24-hour period, the date and the time help to prevent errors of oversight as different nurses take charge of a unit. When an order is to be followed for a specified number of days, the date and the time are important in order that the discontinuation date and time can be determined accurately. The time that an order for a narcotic remains valid is determined by law. Therefore, the date and time the order is written are essential for determining when the order for a narcotic becomes invalid.

Name of Drug to Be Administered. The name of the drug is stated in the order, either by the brand name or the generic name. Certain brand names are well known, but the practice of using the generic name is generally considered safest and is required by some health agencies.

If the nurse is unfamiliar with a drug, there are several sources for obtaining information. The *United States Pharmacopeia and National Formulary* (*USP and NF*) is the official source in the United States. In Canada, the *Compendium of Pharmaceutical Specialties* (*CPS*) is published with information written by the pharmaceutical companies. Most other countries have similar references that describe official therapeutic agents. Many agencies also provide their own book listing the official drugs commonly used by the agency. The *Physician's Desk Reference* (*PDR*) is another source of information. It is published by Medical Economics, Inc. from information supplied by pharmaceutical companies. In addition, the nurse may obtain information about drugs from the hospital pharmacist, the physician, and any of several texts written specifically for the nursing role in the management of drug therapy.

Dosage of the Drug. The dosage of a drug can be stated in either the apothecary or metric system. The metric system has been adopted internationally. A very similar system (le Système international d'unités), abbreviated as SI, is used in Canada. It includes familiar metric units with some differences (*e.g.,* the base unit of weight is the kilogram, not the gram, and temperature is measured in Celsius). In SI, the spelling of liter is litre.

Apothecary measurements are being used less frequently. Self-administered drugs are frequently labeled in household measurements to facilitate administration. Most agencies post a table of common equivalent dosages for persons who have learned to use one system and find that the agency in which they work uses the other

T A B L E 40-2
Common Abbreviations for Measures

Abbreviation	Unabbreviated Form
ℨ	Dram
gt	Drop
gtt	Drops
gr	Grain
g	Gram
mg or mgm	Milligram
ml or mL	Milliliter
m or min	Minim
℥	Ounce
tbsp	Tablespoon
tsp	Teaspoon

system. Although these tables are convenient and useful, the nurse should be prepared to convert from one system to the other, since such tables are not available in every situation. The nurse should also be familiar with common equivalent measurements when using household equipment, such as teaspoons, tablespoons, and so on, since usually the home is not equipped with special measuring devices. The most common equivalents can be found in Appendix A.

Certain standard abbreviations are used to indicate drug amounts and the nurse should know the common abbreviations before administering drugs. Table 40-2 lists some of the most commonly used abbreviations.

Route by Which the Drug Is to Be Administered.
The route to be used when administering a medication is stated clearly because some drugs can be given in more than one way and some may be used safely only through one route. Table 40-3 describes common routes by which medications are administered.

Frequency of Administration of the Drug. The time and frequency with which a drug is to be administered usually are stated in standard abbreviations in the medication order. Common abbreviations used in writing prescriptions, including time and frequency, are listed in Table 40-4.

The nursing service department of inpatient facilities usually determines the hours at which routine drugs are given. For example, if certain drugs are to be given every 4 hours, the nursing service policy indicates the times. Every 4-hour administration may be at the times of 1200, 1600, 2000, 2400, 0400, and 0800 hours. Another agency may use the hours 1300, 1700, 2100, 0100, 0500, and 0900. If a drug is ordered to be given before or after meals, the time will depend on the hours at which meals are served.

If a drug is to be given only once or twice a day, the decision as to which hours to use will depend on the nature of the drug and the client's plan of care. When-

T A B L E 40-3
Routes for Administering Drugs

Route	How Drug Is Administered	Term Used to Describe Route
Given by mouth	Having patient swallow drug	Oral administration
Given via respiratory tract	Having patient inhale drug	Inhalation
Given by injection	Injecting drug into	Administration by injection
	Subcutaneous tissue	Subcutaneous injection
	Muscle tissue	Intramuscular injection
	Corium (under epidermis)	Intradermal injection
	Vein	Intravenous injection
	Artery	Intra-arterial injection
	Heart tissue	Intracardial injection
	Peritoneal cavity	Intraperitoneal injection
	Spinal canal	Intraspinal injection
	Bone	Intraosseous injection
Given by placing on skin or mucous membrane	Inserting drug into	
	Vagina	Vaginal administration
	Rectum	Rectal administration
	Placing drug under tongue	Sublingual administration
	Placing drug between cheek and gum	Buccal administration
	Rubbing drug into skin	Inunction
	Placing drug into direct contact with mucous membrane	Instillation
	Flushing mucous membrane with drug in solution	Irrigation

T A B L E   40-4
Common Abbreviations Used in Prescribing Medications

Abbreviation	Meaning
aa	Of each
ac	Before meals
ad lib	As desired
aq	Water
bid	Twice a day
c̄	With
cap	Capsule
DC	Discontinue
elix	Elixir
hs	At bedtime; hour of sleep
IM	Intramuscular
IV	Intravenous
IVPB	IV piggyback
KVO	Keep vein open
OD	Right eye
od	Every day
OS	Left eye
OU	Each eye
pc	After meals
PO	By mouth
per	By
prn	As needed; when necessary
q	Every
qd	Every day
qh	Every hour
q2h	Every 2 hours
qid	4 times a day
qod	Every other day
qs	Quantity sufficient
Rx	Take
s̄	Without
SC	Subcutaneous
stat	Immediately
supp	Suppository
susp	Suspension
tid	3 times a day
tinct	Tincture
ung	Ointment

ever possible, the client's choice of time should be considered.

Drugs should be administered punctually as ordered. However, a nurse administering drugs to several clients cannot give all of them exactly on the hour indicated. Agency policies vary, but a common one is that drugs should be administered within a half hour before or after the indicated hour. Thus, a drug to be administered at 9 AM can be administered any time between 8:30 AM and 9:30 AM, using this policy. This policy does not apply to all drugs. A preoperative medication ordered to be given at 7:30 AM should be administered at that hour since the time was planned in relation to the time surgery is to begin. This also holds true when clients are given drugs prior to certain diagnostic procedures and stat orders.

Signature of Person Writing the Order.   The signature of the person writing the order follows the order. The signature is of importance for legal reasons because the authority to prescribe drugs is defined by state laws. Also, if there is a question about the order, the signature indicates who should be contacted.

Questioning the Medication Order

The nurse is legally responsible for drugs administered. Any drug order suspected to be in error should be questioned. The suspected error may be in any part of the order. The legal implications are serious in a situation in which there is an error in a drug order and in which the nurse could be expected, based on knowledge and experience, to have noted and reported the error.

On occasion, the nurse may not feel there is an error in the order but may not understand why the medication has been prescribed. In such instances, the nurse should ask in order to understand how the order relates to the client's plan of care.

A drug to which the client is allergic may be inadvertently prescribed. The client may describe past adverse reactions with the drug. It is general practice to indicate any drug allergies clearly on the client's chart. The drug should not be given, and the order should be questioned when, in the nurse's judgment, the client is allergic to a drug. An allergic reaction can be life-threatening to the client.

A nurse may have difficulty reading an order. Guessing is gross carelessness. Rechecking with the person who wrote the order is the only safe procedure.

The nurse has the right to refuse to administer any medication that, based on knowledge and experience, may be harmful to the client. Although this situation rarely occurs, the nurse needs to understand that the client's safety is a primary objective in the administration of medications.

Checking the Medication Order

Agency policy specifies the manner in which the medication order is checked. Various systems are used. Nurses should be familiar with the system used in the agency where they care for clients and should implement it correctly to minimize errors in administering therapeutic agents.

Some agencies use a card system. In many institutions the order is copied onto the client's medication record, often called a *Kardex*. Increasing numbers of health-care facilities are computerizing client records, including medication records. The nurse is responsible for checking that the transcription of the medication order is correct by comparing it with the original order.

Medication Supply Systems

Medications are supplied in a number of ways. With a **stock supply** system, large quantities of medications are kept on the nursing unit. With an **individual supply** system, each client is supplied with the medication needed for a period of time. The nurse is responsible for accurately measuring the drug dosage from the medication containers. In the **unit dose** system, the pharmacist simplifies medication preparation by packaging and labeling each dose of medication for a 24-hour period. In some inpatient facilities, clients self-administer medications.

Most nursing units use a medication cart for the administration of medications. The medication cart contains individual drawers into which the medications for each client are placed. The drawer is labeled with the client's name. The nurse moves the cart from room to room when dispensing medications. A medication cart is displayed in Figure 40-1.

Dosage Calculations
Systems of Measurement

Nurses need to be proficient in the use of weights and measures and systems of measurement to calculate drug

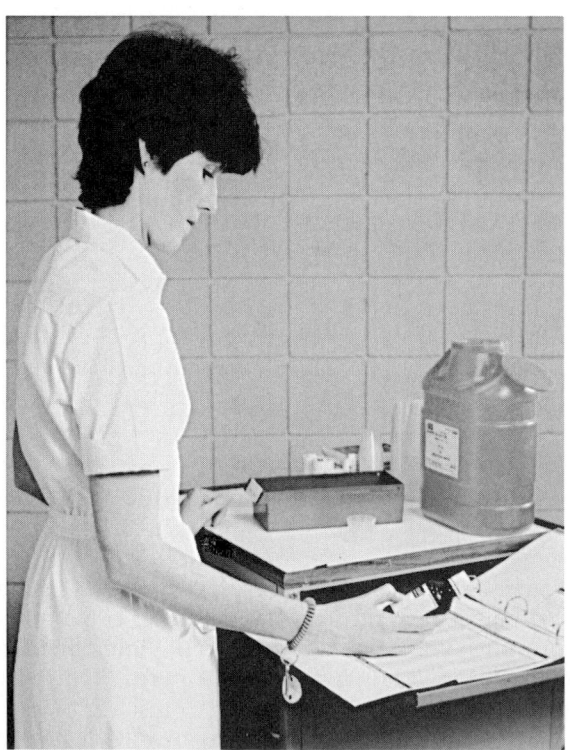

F I G U R E   40-1
The mobile medications cart and the Kardex are taken to the client's room when medications are given. Each client's medications are stored in a separate drawer. The nurse carefully checks the medication she will give with the Kardex to avoid errors. The cart is stored between uses in a locked room near the nurses' station.

dosages and prepare medications for administration. Currently there are three systems of measurement in use for administering medications: the metric system, the apothecary system, and the household system.

Metric System. The metric system is the most widely accepted and convenient system. The official system used in Canada is the SI, which is similar to the metric system. The basic units of measurement are the meter (linear), the liter (volume), and the gram (weight). The metric system is a decimal system, in which each unit can be divided into multiples of ten (10, 100, 1000). To do calculations in the metric system, the decimal point is moved to the right or left. In the preparation of medications, the nurse will most likely use the following metric units:

Weight
1 kilogram = 1000 grams
1 gram = 1000 milligrams
1 milligram = 1000 micrograms

Volume
1 liter = 1000 milliliters or cubic centimeters

Converting Dosages. It may be necessary to convert drug dosages to a different unit in the metric system. To convert a larger unit into a smaller unit, move the decimal point to the right (the new number will be larger than the original). To convert a smaller unit into a larger unit, move the decimal point to the left. The new number will be smaller than the original.

> Example
>
> 0.5 g = ? mg
>
> Move decimal point three places to right.
>
> Answer = 500 mg
>
> 900 mg = ? g
>
> Move decimal point three places to the left.
>
> Answer = 0.9 g

Apothecary System. The apothecary system is less convenient and precise than the metric system. It is currently used for only a few drugs. The basic unit of weight is the grain. The minim, dram, ounce, pint, and quart are used for volume. In the apothecary system, Roman numerals are used to express numbers (grains X) and quantities less than one are written in fraction form (grains ¼).

Household System. The household system is the least accurate system of measurement. It is not widely used except in home settings. Teaspoon, tablespoon, teacup, and glass are commonly used household measures.

Equivalents of Measurement. All three systems of measurement are in use in the United States. The nurse may be called upon to convert dosages from one system to another. It is then extremely important that the nurse know and be able to calculate commonly used equivalents as listed in Appendix A.

Formulas for Computing Drug Dosage

Sometimes drugs are prepared and supplied in the amount ordered by the physician and the nurse can see that no calculation is necessary when checking the medication label. At other times, drugs are not prepared and supplied in the exact quantities called for in the medication order and the nurse must do a dosage calculation to determine what quantity of medication the client is to receive.

There are several formulas that can be used to calculate drug dosages. One such formula consists of ratios to set up a proportion and can be used to calculate dosages for solid and liquid preparations. A ratio shows the relationship between numbers. A proportion contains two ratios. The nurse is usually seeking the quantity of on-hand medication that is equal to the desired dosage (the dosage ordered). The formula is as follows:

$$\frac{\text{Dose on hand}}{\text{Quantity on hand}} = \frac{\text{dose desired}}{\text{X (quantity desired)}}$$

The dosages must be in the same unit of measurement. This applies to the quantities as well. Dosages are on the top line of the proportion and quantities on the bottom line. After the numbers are placed in the proportion, the nurse cross-multiplies to find the desired quantity.

Example. Amoxicillin 625 mg PO is ordered. It is supplied as a liquid preparation containing 250 mg in 5 ml. How much would the nurse administer?

$$\frac{250 \text{ mg}}{5 \text{ ml}} = \frac{625 \text{ mg}}{\text{X ml}}$$

Cross-multiply

$$3125 = 250X$$

$$X = 12.5 \text{ ml}$$

Example. Phenobarbital grains i PO is ordered. It is available in 30-mg tablets. How many tablets would the nurse administer?

There are two systems of measurement in this problem. The nurse checks the list of equivalents to learn 60 mg is equivalent to grains i.

$$\frac{30 \text{ mg}}{1 \text{ tablet}} = \frac{60 \text{ mg}}{\text{X tablets}}$$

$$60 = 30X$$

$$X = 2 \text{ tablets}$$

Another formula that can be used to calculate drug dosages is

$$\frac{\text{Dose desired}}{\text{Dose on hand}} \times \text{quantity on hand}$$

$$= \text{desired quantity}$$

This formula can be used for both liquid dosages and fractions of tablets.

Pediatric Calculations

Pediatric dosages are calculated according to the child's weight or **body surface area**.

The *body surface area formula* provides the most accuracy in calculating pediatric dosages since it considers weight and height. To find a child's body surface area the West nomogram for body surface area (Fig. 40-2) is used. The child's height is located by a point in the left-hand column and the weight is located by a point in the right-hand column. The two points are connected with a line. The point at which the line crosses the surface area column is the child's body surface area (BSA). The formula for calculating the child's dose is

$$\frac{\text{BSA (child)}}{\text{BSA (adult)}} \times \text{adult dose} = \text{child's dose}$$

The average adult BSA is 1.7 square meters.

A common formula based on the child's weight is *Clark's rule,* which assumes that the average adult weighs 150 pounds. The formula is as follows:

$$\text{Usual adult dose}$$

$$\times \frac{\text{weight of child in pounds}}{150} = \text{child's dose}$$

Accepted pediatric dosages according to mg/kg/24-hour period for many drugs are listed in medication references.

Using Safety Measures While Preparing Drugs

Safety is of the utmost importance in preparing and implementing drug administration. The nurse observes the *three checks* and the *five rights* when administering medications.

- *Three checks.* The label on the medication container should be checked three times during medication preparation. The label is read (1) when the nurse reaches for the container, (2) immediately prior to pouring the medication, and (3) when replacing the container to the drawer or shelf.
- *Five rights.* The *five rights* help ensure accuracy when administering medications. The nurse gives the (1) *right medication* to the (2) *right client* in the (3) *right dosage* through the (4) *right route* at the (5) *right time.* In some literature seven rights are listed.

The importance of the three checks and the five rights cannot be overemphasized. The safe nurse does

Nomogram for Estimating Surface Area of Infants and Young Children

Height		Surface Area	Weight	
feet	centimeters	in square meters	pounds	kilograms

F I G U R E   40-2

West nomogram for calculating body surface area. (From Behman R. E. and Vaughan, V. C. Nelson Textbook of Pediatrics, 12th edition. Philadelphia, W. B. Saunders Co. 1983. Reprinted by permission)

not allow automatic habits of preparing medications to replace constant thinking, purposeful action, and repeated checking for accuracy.

Maintaining a Safe Environment

An environment that promotes safety and good working habits contributes to accuracy in the preparation of drugs for administration. It is important that good lighting be available when preparing drugs. Also, the nurse preparing drugs should work alone. This practice helps prevent distractions and interruptions, which may lead to errors.

After the nurse begins to prepare drugs for administration, they should not be left. If it is imperative to leave for a short time, the drugs that have been prepared should be placed carefully in a locked area. The nurse who prepares the medication also administers the drug

and records the drug administration. When the nurse is not working at the medication cart, it should be locked.

Caring for Narcotics Safely

Narcotics are kept in a double-locked drawer, box, or room. This precaution is observed as a safety measure. Narcotics may be ordered only by physicians registered with the Department of Justice, Bureau of Narcotics and Dangerous Drugs, or as specified by the Narcotic Control Act and Regulations (Canada). According to federal law, a record must be kept for each narcotic that is administered. Health agencies provide forms for keeping such records, and these forms are kept with the narcotics. Although the forms differ, the following information generally is required: the name of the client receiving the narcotic, the amount of the narcotic used, the hour the narcotic was given, the name of the physician who prescribed the narcotic, and the name of the nurse who administered the narcotic. It is common practice to check narcotics daily at specified intervals. In hospitals checking is usually done at each change of shift. The amount of narcotics on hand is counted, and each used narcotic must be accounted for on the narcotic record. A narcotic count that does not check must be reported immediately. The law requires these special precautions in the use of narcotics in order to aid in the control of drug abuse. The nurse administering narcotics has an important responsibility to see that the federal law is observed. If for any reason a narcotic prepared for administration has to be discarded, it is best to have a second person act as a witness and have that person sign the narcotic sheet also.

Identifying the Client

The nurse prepares medications, considering safety at all times, as discussed in the previous sections. Positive identification of the client is essential to safe drug administration. Before the nurse administers the drug, it is essential to check carefully to see that the right drug is given to the right client. Clients in inpatient health agencies generally wear identification bracelets. In Figure 40-3, the nurse is identifying the client by checking the identification bracelet. Also, the client should be asked to state his or her name if possible. It is generally considered unsafe to call the client by name because the client may respond even when the nurse has used an improper name.

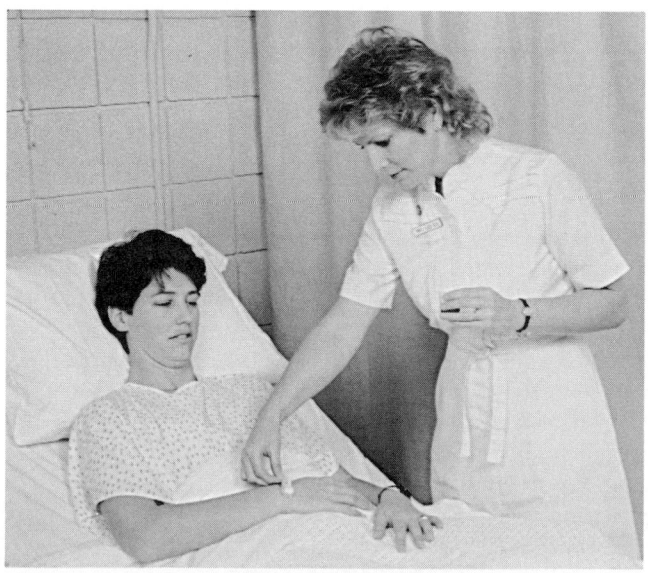

F I G U R E 40-3
An essential step is to check the client's identification bracelet carefully before administering medications to ensure that the right medication is given to the right person.

ADMINISTERING A MEDICATION

The nurse should remain with the client and see that the medication is taken. If the client receives several drugs, offer them separately so that if one is refused or dropped, positive identification can be made and the drug recorded or replaced. Never leave medications at the bedside for the client to take later. This is unsafe practice because the client may forget to take the medication or someone else may take the medication. The nurse records medication administration as soon as possible after the client takes the medication. Some agencies allow clients to self-administer certain drugs to promote the client's independence. The nurse should be familiar with agency policy on this matter.

Administering Oral Medications

Drugs given orally are intended for absorption in the stomach and small intestine. The oral route is the most frequent route of administration. It is usually the most convenient and comfortable and generally the safest for the client. Following oral administration, drug action has a slower onset and a more prolonged but less potent effect.

There are certain situations when oral medications would not be administered, such as when the client has impaired swallowing, is unconscious, is to receive nothing by mouth, or is vomiting.

Oral medications are available in two forms: solid preparations and liquid preparations. Solid preparations include tablets, capsules, and pills. Some tablets are scored for easy breaking if a partial quantity is needed. Enteric-coated tablets are covered with a hard surface that impedes absorption until the tablet has left the stomach. Absorption takes place in the small intestine because the active ingredient of the drug is irritating to the stomach mucosa. Enteric-coated tablets should not be chewed or crushed.

Liquid preparations include elixirs, spirits, suspensions, and syrups. Some are water-based solutions and others are alcohol-based solutions. Liquid preparations should be prepared with an appropriate measuring device. Disposable, calibrated cups are available for the preparation of liquid medications. When liquids are being poured from a bottle, they should be poured from the side of the bottle opposite the label. This prevents drops from running onto the label, making it difficult to read. Hold the container and the bottle at eye level, and place the thumb nail on the line on the container that indicates the proper dosage. Because of surface tension, a meniscus (a curved convex surface) forms on the liquid in the measuring container. The liquid should be measured at the *bottom* of this meniscus.

Extractors are available on the market to remove liquids from a bottle. The extractor resembles a syringe and fits tightly into the bottle neck. The medication is withdrawn and then placed in a medication cup. The extractor has markings on it so that proper dosage can be determined as the liquid is withdrawn. For certain clients who find it difficult to take liquids from a cup, the medication can be placed in the mouth directly from the extractor or from a syringe. The extractor or syringe should be placed between the gum and cheek, and the liquid given to the client slowly. These techniques help prevent the client from choking and aspirating the medication.

If a label becomes difficult to read or accidentally comes off the container, it should be returned to the pharmacy. A medication should never be given from a bottle without a label or with a label that cannot be read with accuracy. Because of the danger of error, medications should not be returned to their bottle. Therefore, care should be exercised to pour carefully to prevent unnecessary loss. Medications should not be transferred from one pharmacy container to another. Many medication bottles now have an identification code number on them. If similar medications were mixed and a client had a reaction, it would be difficult to identify which drug was responsible. A medication with an unexpected precipitate should not be used, nor should one that has changed color.

Procedure 40-1 describes the techniques for preparing and administering oral medications.

Special Techniques

Certain drugs given orally discolor the teeth or tend to damage the enamel. Such medications are mixed well with water or some other liquid vehicle; the client takes it through a drinking straw, and water is taken following administration. This practice reduces the strength of the drug that comes in contact with the teeth. Dilute hydrochloric acid is an example of a drug that damages the enamel of the teeth and should be given well-diluted and with a drinking straw.

Some clients object to the taste of certain medications. The following techniques are suggested to disguise or mask the objectionable taste:

- Sometimes it is necessary to crush a medication or add it to food so the client can swallow it. Some drugs cannot be crushed (*e.g.,* enteric-coated and sustained-release capsules).
- Allow the client to suck on a small piece of ice for a few minutes before taking the medication. The ice numbs the taste buds, and the objectionable taste is less discernable.
- Store oily medications in the refrigerator. Cold oil is less aromatic than oil at room temperature.
- Place the medication in a syringe, and place the syringe well back on the tongue, being careful not to cause the client to gag. This places the medication on the part of the tongue where taste buds are few.
- Offer oral hygiene immediately after giving a medication with an objectionable taste.

- Give the medication with generous amounts of water or other liquids, if permitted. This dilutes the medication and its taste.

Children

- Nurses will find administration of medications to infants and children challenging as well as frustrating at times.
- Children under 5 years of age have difficulty swallowing tablets and capsules. Most medications are available in a liquid form.
- Use a dropper to give infants or very small children liquid medications while holding them in a sitting or semisitting position. Place the medication between the gum and cheek to prevent possible aspiration. This same technique can be used for the adult who has trouble swallowing.
- Crush uncoated tablets or empty a soft capsule, and mix the medication with soft foods, such as potatoes or cereal, for clients who are likely to aspirate liquids. Proper absorption may not occur if coated tablets or hard capsules are added to food.
- Explain to the child when a medication has an objectionable taste if the child is old enough to understand. Failing to warn the child is likely to decrease the child's trust in the nurse.
- Care should be taken when selecting the food to be mixed with the medication. The item should not be an essential part of the child's diet such as formula or the child's favorite food. The child may refuse a food associated with medications.
- Praise the child for a job well done after he or she swallows the medication.

Elderly Clients

- Allow extra time to administer medications to an elderly client because reflexes are often slowed and understanding of the treatment may be decreased.
- Elderly clients may experience some difficulty swallowing medications and may find it easier to take their medications when crushed or given in a liquid form. Swallowing can be initiated by massaging the laryngeal prominence or the area just below the chin prominence. The pressure from the gentle massage creates the desire to swallow.
- Reevaluation of drug dosage is necessary with the elderly client. Weight and age should be used as criteria for dosage.
- The nurse would assist the elderly client to set up a home medication schedule.

Administering Medications Through a Nasogastric Tube

Occasionally, a client with a nasogastric tube receives a medication through the tube. The insertion of the tube is described in Chapter 31. The following are suggestions for giving medications through the tube:

(Text continues on p. 1138.)

PROCEDURE 40-1
Administering Oral Medications

Equipment

Medication Kardex, cards, or record form	Medication cups (disposable)	Water or juice
Medication cart or tray	Straws	

Action

1 Gather equipment. Check each medication order against the original physician's order according to agency policy. Clarify any inconsistencies. Check the client's chart for allergies.

2 Know the actions, special nursing considerations, and side-effects of medications to be administered.

3 Wash your hands.

4 Move the medication cart to the outside of the client's room or prepare for administration in the medication area.

5 Unlock the medication cart or drawer.

6 Prepare medications for one client at a time.

7 Select the proper medication from the drawer or stock and compare with the Kardex or order. Check expiration dates and perform calculations if necessary:

   a. Place unit-dose-packaged medications in a disposable cup. *Do not open wrapper* until at bedside. Keep narcotics and medications that require special nursing assessments in a separate container.

   b. When removing tablets or capsules from a bottle, pour the necessary number into the bottle cap and then place the tablets in a medication cap. Break only scored tablets, if necessary, to obtain proper dosage.

   c. Hold liquid medication bottles with the label against the palm of your hand. Use the appropriate measuring device when pouring liquids, and read the amount of medication at the bottom of the meniscus at eye level. Wipe the lip of the bottle with a paper towel.

8 Recheck each medication package, card, or preparation with the order as it is poured.

9 When all medications for one client have been prepared, recheck once again with the medication order before taking them to client.

Rationale

This comparison helps identify errors that may have occurred when orders were transcribed. The physician's order is the legal record of medication orders for each agency.

This knowledge aids the nurse in evaluating the therapeutic effect of the medication in relation to the client's diagnosis.

Handwashing prevents the spread of microorganisms.

Organization facilitates error-free administration and saves time.

Locking of the cart or drawer safeguards each client's medication supply.

This prevents errors in medication administration.

Comparison of medication to physician's order reduces errors in medication administration. Verify calculations with another nurse if necessary. This is the *first* safety check.

The label is needed for an additional safety check. Prerequisites to giving certain medications may include monitoring of certain vital signs.

Pouring tablets or capsules into the nurse's hand is unsanitary.

Accuracy is possible when the appropriate measuring device is used and then read accurately. Liquid that may drip onto the label makes the label difficult to read.

This is a *second* check to guard against a medication error.

This is a *third* check to ensure accuracy and to prevent errors.

(Continued)

Administering Oral Medications   (Continued)

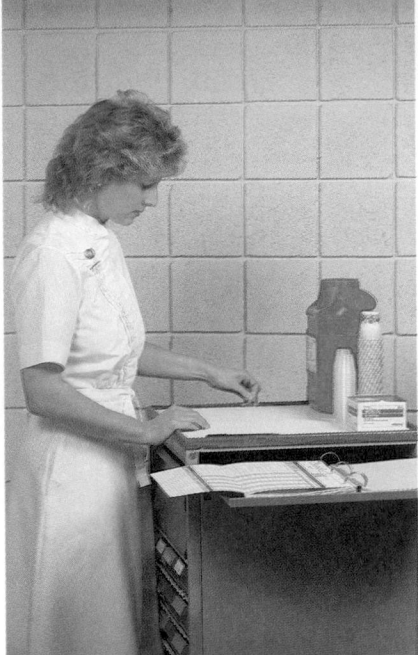

Step 5: Unlocking medications cart.

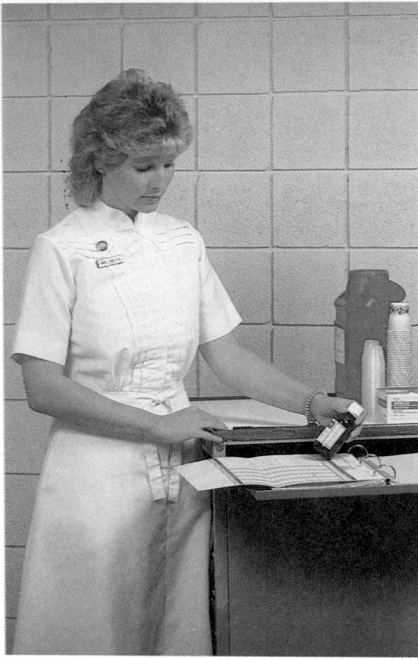

Step 7: Comparing medication with Kar-
dex/order.

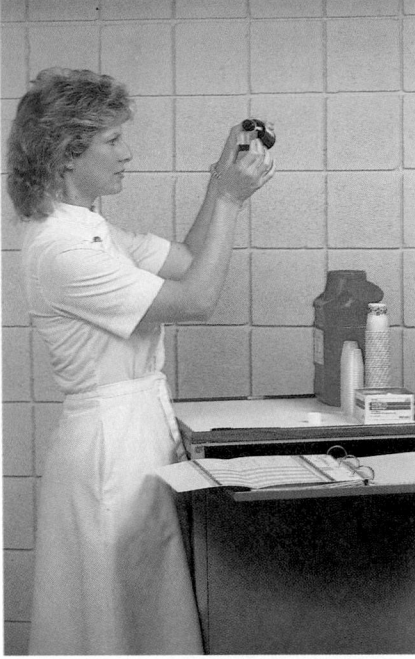

Step 7c: Measuring at eye level.

Action	Rationale
10 Transport medications to the client's bedside carefully, and keep the medications in sight at all times.	Careful handling and close observation prevent accidental or deliberate disarrangement of medications.
11 See that the client receives medications at the correct time.	Check agency policy, which may allow for administration within a period of 30 minutes before or 30 minutes after designated time.
12 Identify the client carefully. There are three correct ways to do this:	Identifying the client is the nurse's responsibility to guard against error.
a. Check the name on the client's identification band.	This is the most reliable method. Replace the identification band if it is missing or inaccurate in any way.
b. Ask the client his or her name.	This requires a response from the client, but illness and strange surroundings often cause clients to be confused.
c. Verify the client's identification with a staff member who knows the client.	This is another way to double check identity. Do not use the name on the door or over the bed because these may frequently be inaccurate.
13 Complete necessary assessments before administration of medications. Explain the purpose and action of each medication to the client.	Assessment is a prerequisite to administration of medications.
14 Assist the client to an upright or lateral position.	Swallowing is facilitated by proper positioning.
15 Administer medications:	
a. Offer water or other permitted fluids with pills, capsules, tablets, and some liquid medications.	Liquids facilitate swallowing of solid drugs. Some liquid drugs are intended to adhere to the pharyngeal area, in which case liquid is not offered with the medication.

(Continued)

Action	**Rationale**

b. Ask the client's preference regarding medications to be taken by hand or in a cup and one at a time or all at once.

This encourages the client's participation in taking the medications.

c. If the capsule or tablet falls to the floor it must be discarded and a new one administered.

This prevents contamination.

d. Record any fluid intake if intake/output is ordered.

This provides for accurate documentation.

16 Remain with the client until each medication is swallowed. Unless the nurse has seen the client swallow the drug, it cannot be recorded that the drug was administered.

The client's chart is a legal record. Only with a physician's order can medications be left at the bedside.

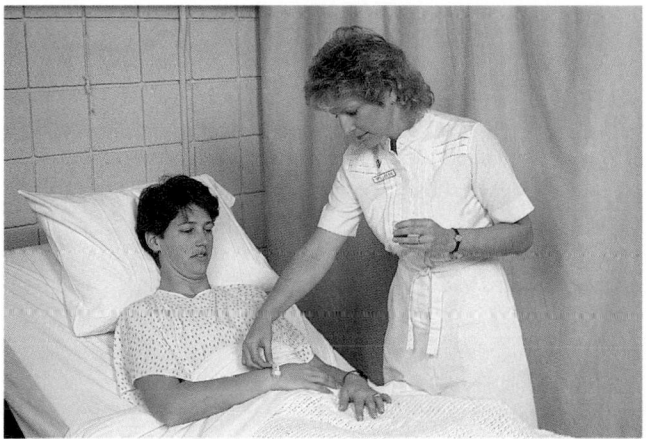

Step 12a: Checking identity.

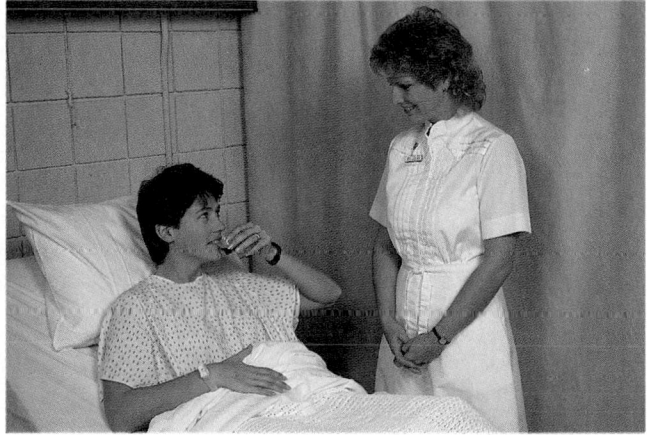

Step 16: Observing client swallowing medication. (Photos © Ken Kasper)

17 Wash your hands.

Handwashing prevents the spread of microorganisms.

18 Record each medication given on the medication chart or record using the required format.

Prompt recording avoids the possibility of accidentally repeating the administration of the drug.

a. If the drug was refused or omitted, record this in the appropriate area on the medication record.

This verifies the reason medication was omitted.

b. Recording of administration of a narcotic requires additional documentation on a narcotic record stating drug count and other specific information.

Controlled substance laws necessitate careful recording of narcotic use.

19 Check on the client within 30 minutes to verify response to medication.

This provides opportunity for further documentation and additional assessment.

Age Considerations

Special devices are available in a pharmacy to ensure accurate dosage calculations for small children and infants.

(Continued)

Home Care Considerations

Encourage the client to discard outdated prescription medications.

Discuss safe storage of medications when there are children and pets in the environment.

Devices are available to help the client remember to take medications as scheduled. These may be simple charts or appliances that can be made in the home or more elaborate devices that can be purchased in a pharmacy or from the manufacturer.

Special Considerations

If the client questions a medication order or states that the medication is different from the usual dose, *always* recheck and clarify with the original order before giving medication.

If the client has altered level of consciousness or impaired swallowing, check with the physician to clarify the route of administration or alternative forms of medication.

Use a straw to swallow a liquid medication that may have a harmful effect on the teeth or mucous membranes.

- Use liquid medications or crushed medications combined with liquid. Solid medications are not given because they are likely to obstruct the tube.
- Bring the liquid medication to room temperature. Cold liquids are uncomfortable for the client.
- Remove the clamp from the tube and use recommended procedure to check for tube placement in the stomach *prior* to administering the drug.
- Pour the medication into a syringe barrel or funnel attached to the tube *after* determining tube placement and patency.
- Flush the tube with 30 ml to 50 ml of water immediately after giving the medication. This flushes the tube of medication and helps maintain patency of the tube.
- Position the client in a semisitting position on the right side after removing the syringe barrel or funnel and after reclamping the nasogastric tube. This positioning helps the stomach to empty and helps prevent regurgitation. If the medication is to remain in the stomach for a period of time, position the client on the left side.

Administering Medications Sublingually

Certain drugs, sublingual nitroglycerin being typical, are administered *sublingually;* that is, a tablet is placed under the client's tongue. This area is rich in superficial blood vessels, which allows the drug to be absorbed relatively rapidly into the bloodstream for quick systemic effects. This type of medication should not be swallowed but held under the tongue where complete absorption will occur.

Administering Parenteral Medications

The term *enteral* means within the intestines, and **parenteral** means outside the intestines or alimentary canal. Many persons use the term parenteral to refer to injection routes only, although technically the term includes other routes as well, such as agents given by inhalation, those placed on the skin, and most of those placed on the mucous membrane.

Table 40-3 defines terms used to describe various types of **injections**. As shown, medications may be injected into an artery, the peritoneum, heart tissues, the spinal canal, and bones. Techniques for injecting medications into these areas are discussed in clinical texts. In most instances, physicians are responsible for these procedures, and the nurse acts as an assistant.

Absorption occurs more rapidly with injection than it does when other routes are used. Absorption is also more nearly complete; therefore, the results are more predictable, and the desired dosage can be determined with greater accuracy. Giving drugs by injection is necessary if the drug is available in no other form. Injections are particularly desirable for clients who are irrational, unconscious, or having gastrointestinal disturbances. The injection of drugs is also used in emergencies because absorption and desired results occur rapidly.

Needles and Syringes

Needles are available in various lengths and gauges with different sized bevels. Figure 40-4 shows the parts of a needle. Needle lengths vary from ½ inch to 2 inches. The length of the needle will be determined by the route of administration. The gauge is determined by the width of the needle. Needle gauges are numbered 18 through 27. As the diameter of the needle increases, the gauge number decreases. An 18-gauge needle is larger than a 27-gauge needle. The bevel of the needle is its sloped edge, designed to make a narrow, slit-like opening that closes quickly.

Syringes are supplied in a variety of sizes. Most are plastic and disposable. Some syringes are supplied with the needle attached, whereas others are not, in which case the nurse selects an appropriate needle. The parts of a syringe are pictured in Figure 40-4.

The nurse chooses the equipment needed for an injection based on the following criteria:

- Route of administration. A longer needle is required for an intramuscular injection than for an intradermal or subcutaneous injection.

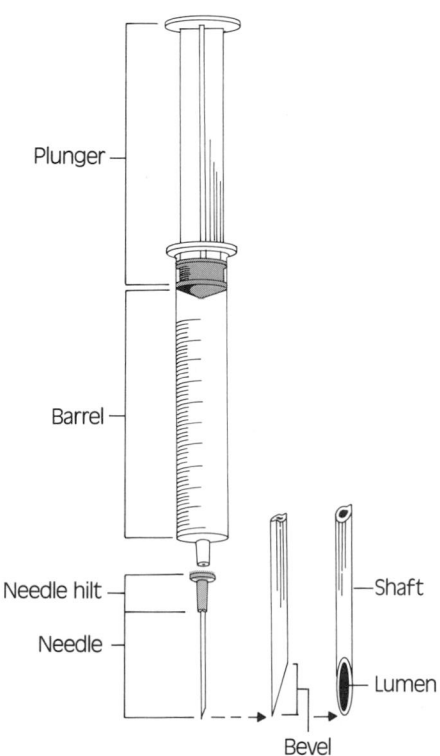

FIGURE 40-4
Parts of a needle and syringe.

Plunger

Barrel

Needle hilt

Needle

Shaft

Lumen

Bevel

- Viscosity of the solution. Some medications are more viscous than others and require a large-lumen needle to inject the drug.
- Quantity to be administered. The larger the amount of medication to be injected, the greater the capacity of the syringe.
- Body size. An obese person requires a longer needle to reach muscular tissue than a thin person.
- Type of medication. There are special syringes for certain uses. An example is the insulin syringe used to inject insulin. Some medications, such as iron–dextran injection (Imferon), are irritating to subcutaneous tissue. Therefore, a longer needle should be used to ensure proper placement of the medication in the muscle tissue.

After use, needles and syringes are destroyed and placed in designated containers to prevent risk of puncture with contaminated equipment and to prevent reuse.

Techniques of surgical asepsis must be strictly followed for parenteral injections to help avoid introducing organisms into the body. The parts of the syringe and needle that must be kept sterile during the procedure of preparing and administering an injection are the inside of the barrel, the part of the plunger that enters the barrel, the tip of the barrel, and the needle, except for the needle's hub.

Surgical asepsis applies to cleansing the skin for an injection. The skin is cleansed with alcohol or povidone–iodine (Betadine) in a circular motion from the center of the designated site outward. The skin is then considered clean enough to pierce with a sterile needle.

Preparing Medications for Administration by Injection

Drugs for administration by injection are packaged in several ways. Those that deteriorate in solution usually are dispensed as powders and are placed in solution immediately prior to injection. If drugs remain stable in solution, they are usually dispensed in ampules, bottles, or vials in an aqueous or oily solution or suspension.

Drugs may be dispensed in single-dose, glass *ampules;* single-dose, rubber-capped *vials;* multiple-dose, rubber-capped *vials;* and *prefilled cartridges.* Figure 40-5 illustrates several types of ampules and vials, as well as a prefilled cartridge.

Ampules. An **ampule** is a glass flask containing a single dose of medication for parenteral administration. There is no way to prevent airborne contamination of any unused portion of medication once the ampule is opened. If all of the medication is not used, the remainder must be discarded. Medication can be removed from an ampule by breaking the thin neck. The ampule can be inverted or placed on a flat surface to draw the solution into the syringe. Care must be taken not to contaminate the needle by touching the rim of the ampule. Procedure 40-2 illustrates how to prepare medication from an ampule.

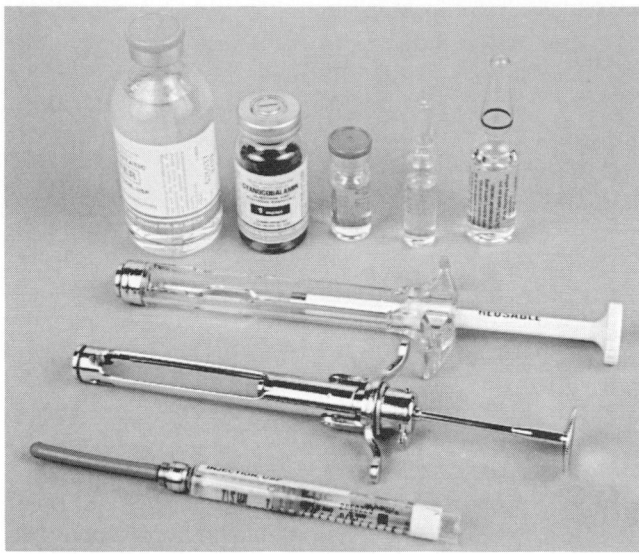

F I G U R E   40-5
Ampules and prefilled vials.

Vials. As Figure 40-5 illustrates, a **vial** is a glass bottle with a self-sealing stopper through which medication is removed. For safety in transporting and storing, the single-dose, rubber-capped vial usually is covered with a soft, metal cap that can be removed easily. The rubber part that is then exposed is the means of entrance into the vial.

Some drugs are dispensed in vials containing several or multiple doses. This means that the nurse can remove several doses from the same container. To remove medication from a vial, the nurse injects air into the vial, which facilitates removal of medication from the vial. The amount of air is the same as the desired quantity of solution. Procedure 40-3 describes and illustrates removing medication from a vial.

Prefilled Cartridges.
When medications are supplied in prefilled cartridges, the nurse inserts the cartridge into a holder. The **prefilled cartridge** provides a single dose of medication. The holder is reusable. Prior to giving the injection, the nurse checks the dosage in the cartridge and clears the cartridge of excess air. **Tubex** and **Carpuject** are two types of prefilled cartridges currently available.

Mixing Medications in One Syringe

Preparation of medications in one syringe depends on how the medication is supplied. When using a single-dose vial and a multiple-dose vial, air is injected into both vials and the medication in the multiple-dose is drawn into the syringe first. This prevents contamination of the contents of the multiple-dose vial with the medi-

cation in the single-dose vial. The nurse must ensure that the two drugs are compatible.

The steps to follow when preparing medications from two multiple-dose vials in one syringe are as follow:
1. Inject air into vial A, keeping the needle from touching the medication.
2. Inject air into vial B and withdraw the quantity of medication needed.
3. Change the needle. This prevents contamination of vial A from the contents of vial B.
4. Carefully withdraw needed quantity of medication from vial A. The two medications are now combined in the syringe. Excess medication must not be reinjected into vial A because this may cause an imbalance in the two dosages.

This procedure is illustrated in Figure 40-6.

When preparing medications from an ampule and a vial, the medication in the vial is prepared first. The medication in the ampule is drawn up after the medication in the vial.

It is important for the nurse to be aware of drug incompatibilities when preparing medications in one syringe. Certain medications such as diazepam (Valium) are incompatible with other drugs when combined in the same syringe. Other drugs are provisionally compatible and should be administered within 15 minutes of preparation (Coblio, 1981, p 48). Incompatible drugs may become cloudy or form a precipitate in the syringe. Such medications are discarded and re-prepared in separate syringes. A drug compatibility table should be available to nurses preparing medications.

Mixing Insulins in One Syringe

Insulin is a naturally occurring hormone produced by the islets of Langerhans in the pancreas and enables cells to utilize carbohydrates. Clients with diabetes mellitus produce no insulin or produce insulin in insufficient amounts. There are several types of insulin available for use by clients with diabetes mellitus. Insulins vary in the onset and duration of action and are classified as short-acting, intermediate-acting, and long-acting. Some insulins have a modifying protein that slows absorption. The modifying proteins are globin and protamine (NPH, globin zinc, protamine zinc).

Insulin dosages are calculated in units. The scale commonly used today is U-100, which is based on 100 units of insulin contained in 1 ml of solution. An insulin syringe is calibrated in units also. Before administering insulin, the nurse should check the dosage with the physician's orders. Many clients with diabetes mellitus are regulated with a combination of two insulins (*e.g.,* regular and NPH insulins).

Procedure 40-4 gives the steps for combining two types of insulins in the same syringe.

The importance of rotating injection sites for insulin

(Text continues on p. 1144.)

PROCEDURE 40-2
Removing Medication from an Ampule

Equipment

Ampule of medication

Medication card or Kardex

Sterile syringe and needle (size depends on medication being administered and client)

Alcohol swab or gauze pad

Action

1 Gather equipment. Check the medication order against the original physician's order according to agency policy.

2 Wash your hands.

3 Tap the stem of the ampule or twist your wrist quickly while holding the ampule vertically.

4 Wrap a small gauze pad or dry alcohol swab around the neck of the ampule.

5 Use a snapping motion to break off the top of the ampule along the prescored line at its neck. Always break away from your body.

Rationale

This comparison helps identify errors that may have occurred when orders were transcribed.

Handwashing deters the spread of microorganisms.

This facilitates movement of medication in the stem to the body of the ampule.

This protects the nurse's fingers from the glass as the ampule is broken.

This protects the nurse's face and fingers from any shattered glass fragments.

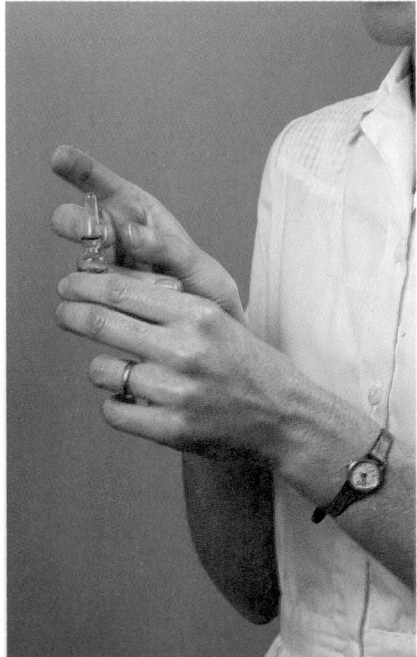

Step 3: Tapping stem of ampule.

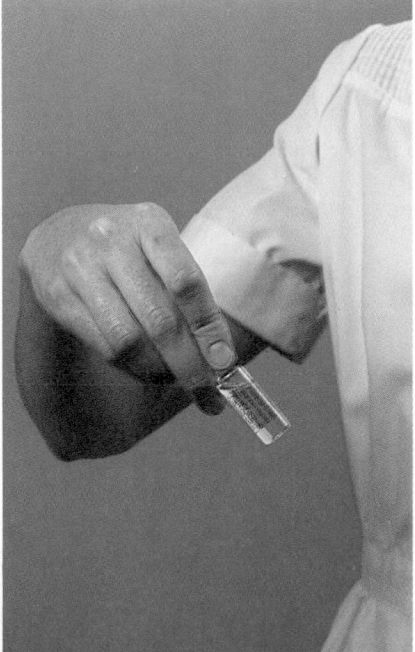

Step 3: Twisting motion of wrist while holding ampule.

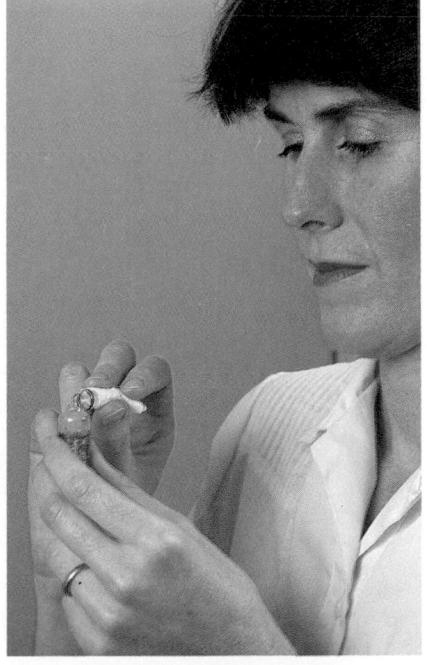

Step 5: Snapping off top of ampule.

6 Remove the cap from the needle by pulling it straight off. Insert the needle into the ampule, being careful not to touch the rim.

The rim of the ampule is considered contaminated.

(Continued)

Action

Rationale

7 Withdraw medication in the amount ordered. Do not inject any air into solutions. Use either of the following methods:

   a. Insert the tip of the needle into the ampule, which is *upright* on a flat surface, and withdraw fluid into the syringe.

The contents of the ampule are not under pressure; therefore, air is unnecessary and will cause the contents to overflow.

   b. Insert the tip of the needle into the ampule and *invert* the ampule. Keep the needle centered and not touching the sides of the ampule. Remove the prescribed amount of medication.

Surface tension holds the fluid in the ampule when inverted. If the needle touches the sides or is removed and then reinserted into the ampule, surface tension will be broken and fluid will run out.

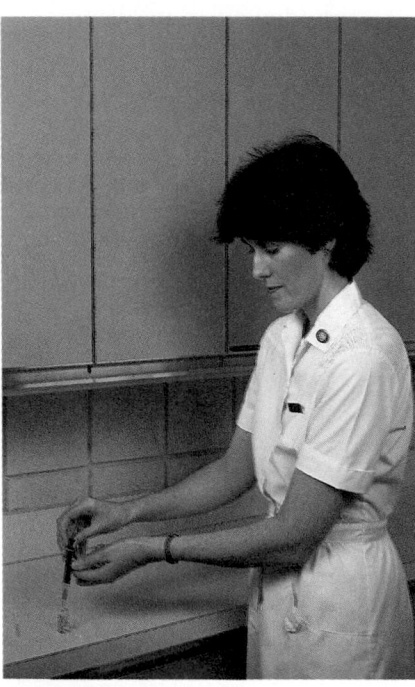

Step 7a: Withdrawing medication from upright ampule.

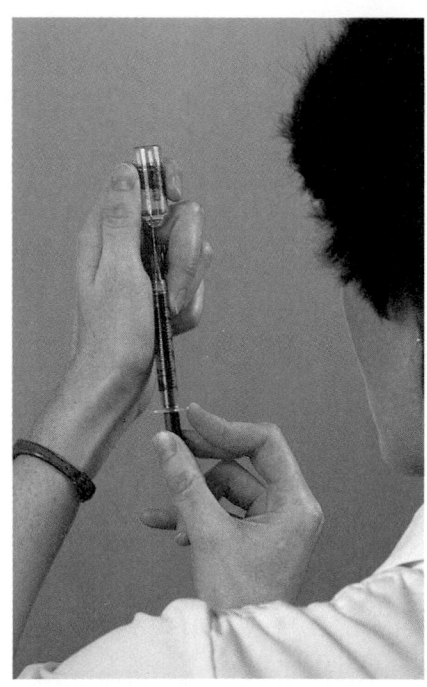

Step 7b: Withdrawing medication from inverted ampule. (Photos © Ken Kasper)

8 Do not expel any air bubbles that may form into the solution. Wait until the needle has been withdrawn to tap the syringe and expel the air carefully. Check the amount of medication in the syringe and discard any surplus.

Ejecting air into the solution will increase pressure in the ampule and can force the medication to spill out over the ampule.

9 Discard the ampule in a suitable container after comparing with the medication card or kardex.

If all of the medication has not been removed from the ampule, it must be discarded because there is no way to maintain sterility of contents in an opened ampule.

10 Cap the needle on the syringe.

This prevents contamination of the needle and protects the nurse against inadvertent sticks by the needle.

11 Wash your hands.

Handwashing deters the spread of microorganisms.

P R O C E D U R E 40-3
Removing Medication from a Vial

Equipment

Vial of medication
Medication card or
Kardex

Sterile syringe and
needle (size de-
pends on medi-
cation being ad-
ministered and
client)

Alcohol swab

Action

1 Gather equipment. Check medication order against the original physician's order according to agency policy.

2 Wash your hands.

3 Remove the metal or plastic cap on the vial that protects the rubber stopper.

4 Swab the rubber top with the alcohol swab.

5 Remove the cap from the needle by pulling it straight off.

6 Pierce the rubber stopper in the center with the needle tip and inject the measured air into the space above the solution. (Do not inject air into the solution). The vial may be positioned upright on a flat surface or inverted. See figure.

Rationale

This comparison helps identify errors that may have occurred when orders were transcribed.

Handwashing deters the spread of microorganisms.

The metal cap prevents contamination of the rubber top.

Alcohol removes surface bacteria contamination. This is not necessary the first time the rubber stopper is entered but subsequent reentries into the vial require the use of alcohol cleansing.

Before fluid is removed, injection of equal amount of air is required to prevent the formation of a partial vacuum, because a vial is a sealed container. If not enough air is injected, the negative pressure makes it difficult to withdraw the medication.

Air bubbled through the solution could result in withdrawal of an inaccurate amount of medication.

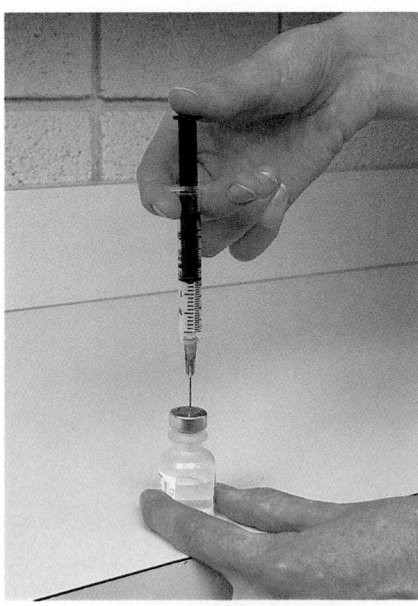
Step 6a: Injecting air with vial upright.

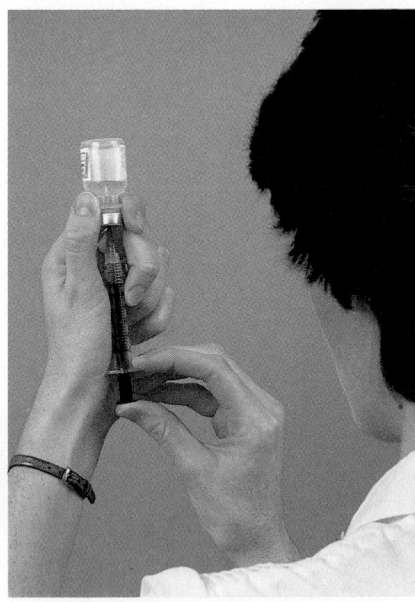
Step 6b: Injecting air with vial inverted and needle above solution.

Action

7 Invert the vial and withdraw the needle tip slightly so that it is below the fluid level.

8 Draw up the prescribed amount of medication while holding the syringe at eye level and vertically.

9 If any air bubbles accumulate in the syringe, tap the barrel of the syringe sharply and move the needle past the fluid into the air space to reinject the air bubble into the vial. Return the needle tip to the solution and continue withdrawal of the medication.

Rationale

This prevents air from being aspirated into the syringe.

Holding the syringe at eye level facilitates accurate reading, and the vertical position makes removal of air bubbles from the syringe easy.

Removal of air bubbles is necessary to ensure accurate dose of medication.

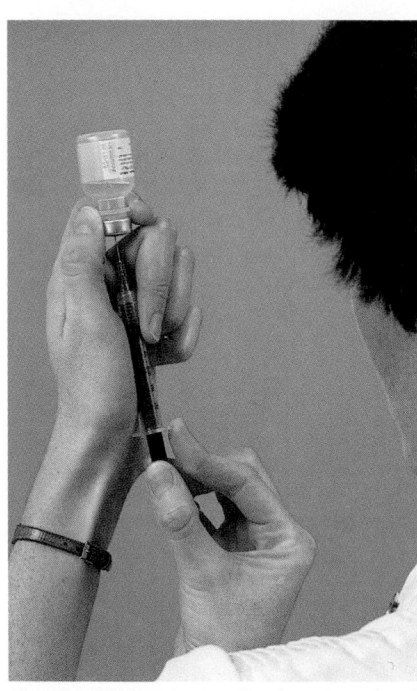
Step 8: Withdrawing medication at eye level.

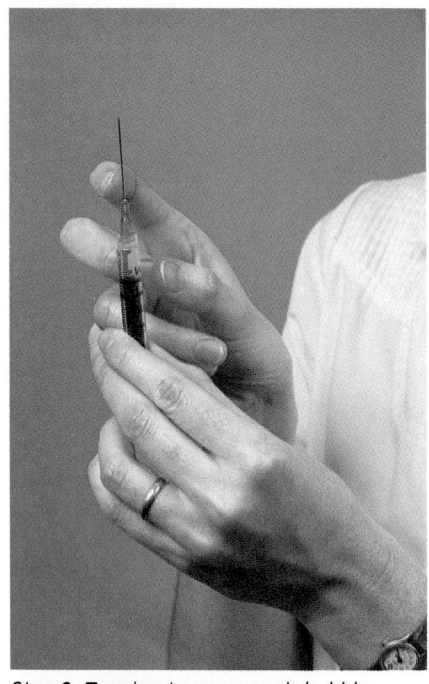
Step 9: Tapping to remove air bubbles.
(Photos © Ken Kasper)

10 Once the correct dose is withdrawn, remove the needle from the vial and cap it. If a multiple-dose vial is being used, store the vial containing the remaining medication according to agency policy.

11 Wash your hands.

Since the vial is sealed, the medication inside remains sterile and can be used for future injections.

Handwashing deters the spread of microorganisms.

administration cannot be overemphasized. A discussion of injection sites is included under Administering Medications Subcutaneously, below. Insulin should be stored in a cool place. It can be warmed prior to administration by rolling the vial between the palms of the hands. Some insulins are stable at room temperature.

50 units
air
injected

10 units
air
injected

NPH

Vial A

Regular

Vial B

Step 1

Step 2

Vial B

Regular

Vial A

NPH

10 units
regular
insulin
withdrawn

50 units
NPH
insulin
withdrawn

Step 3

Step 4

F I G U R E   40-6
Mixing medications in one syringe.

Reconstitution of Powdered Medications

Several drugs, including many antibiotics, are supplied as powders in vials. A liquid or **diluent** must be added to the powder before it is administered as a solution. The technique of adding a diluent to a powdered drug is called **reconstitution**. Information needed for reconstitution and dosage calculation can usually be located on the label of the vial. The nurse must know the amount and type of diluent to be added to the powder. Common diluents are sterile water for injection and 0.9% sodium chloride injection. After the diluent is added to the solution, the nurse reads the label further to determine the concentration of drug per milliliter of solution. This is essential to the dosage computation. If all of the medication is not used at the time of reconstitution, the nurse refers to the vial label for storage instructions. Additional sources of information about reconstitution of medications are package inserts and the pharmacist. Figure 40-7 displays a package insert and the label of a vial containing a powdered drug.

Administering Medications Intradermally

The **intradermal** route has the longest absorption time of all parenteral routes. For this reason, intradermal injections are used for diagnostic purposes, such as the tuberculin test and tests to determine sensitivity to various substances. The advantage of the intradermal route for these tests is that the body's reaction to substances is easily visible, and degrees of reaction are discernible by comparative study.

Intradermal injections are placed just below the epidermis. Sites commonly used are the inner surface of the forearm, dorsal aspect of the upper arm, and the upper

(Text continues on p. 1149.)

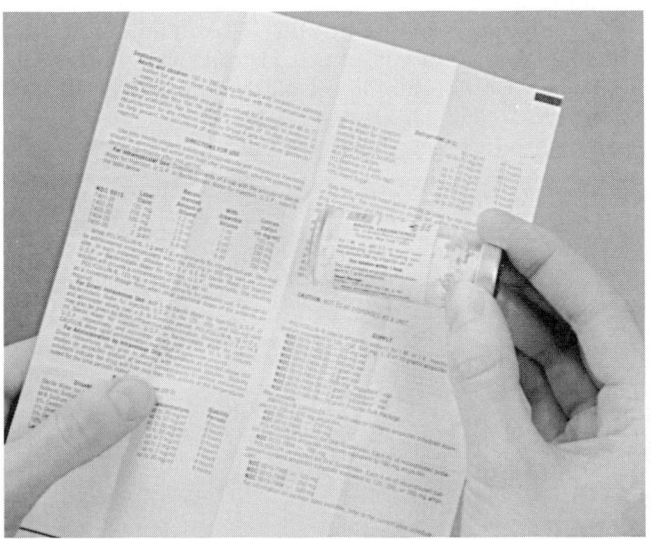

F I G U R E   40-7
Package insert and label for instructions on reconstituting powdered medications. (Photo © Ken Kasper)

Mixing Insulins in One Syringe

Equipment

Two vials of insulin
Medication card or
Kardex

Sterile insulin sy-
ringe with 25-
gauge or 27-
gauge needle

Alcohol swabs

Action

1 Gather equipment. Check medication order against the original physician's order according to agency policy.

2 Wash your hands.

3 If necessary, remove the metal cap that protects the rubber stopper on each vial.

4 If insulin is a suspension, rotate the vial between the palms of your hands to mix prior to withdrawal.

5 Cleanse the rubber tops with alcohol swabs.

6 Remove cap from needle. Inject air into the modified insulin preparation (*e.g.,* NPH insulin). Use an amount of air equal to the amount of medication to be withdrawn. Do not allow the needle to touch the medication in the vial. Remove the needle.

7 Inject air into the clear insulin without additional protein (*e.g.,* regular insulin). Use an amount of air equal to the amount of medication to be withdrawn. Do not bubble the air through the medication.

Rationale

This comparison helps identify errors that may have occurred when orders were transcribed.

Handwashing deters the spread of microorganisms.

The metal cap prevents contamination of the rubber top.

Shaking vials creates froth that may interfere with withdrawal of accurate dose. Regular insulin is clear because it does not contain any modifying agents to slow its absorption.

Alcohol removes surface bacteria contamination. This is not necessary the first time a metal cap is removed but subsequent reentries into the vial require use of alcohol cleansing.

Regular, or short-acting, insulin should never be contaminated with NPH or any insulin modified with added protein. Placing air in the NPH insulin first without allowing the needle to contact the insulin ensures that regular insulin will not be contaminated with the additional protein in the NPH.

An equal amount of air must be injected into the vacuum to allow easy withdrawal of medication.

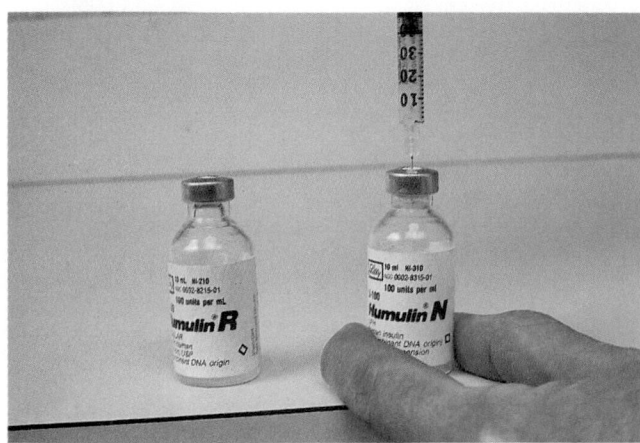

Step 6: Injecting air into modified insulin preparation.

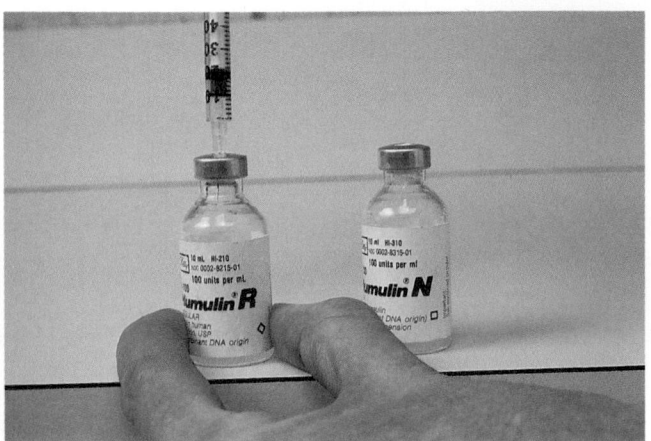

Step 7: Injecting air into clear insulin.

(Continued)

Action	Rationale
8 Invert the vial of clear insulin and aspirate the amount prescribed. Remove the needle from the vial.	Regular insulin that contains no additional protein is not contaminated by insulin containing globulin or protamine.
9 Cleanse the rubber top of the modified insulin vial. Insert the needle into this vial, invert it, and withdraw the medication. Cap the needle.	Previous addition of air eliminates need to create positive pressure.

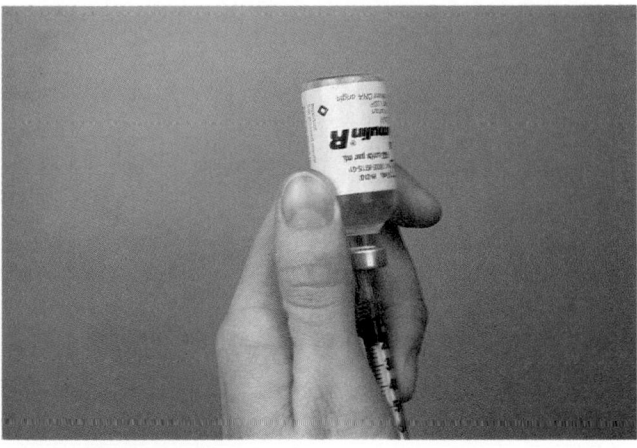

Step 8: Withdrawing clear insulin.

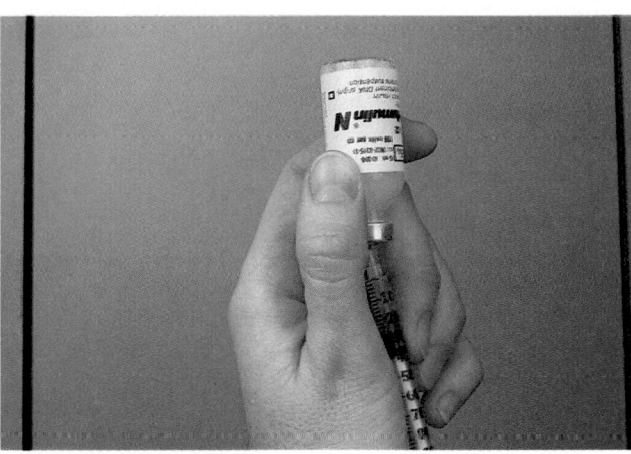

Step 9: Withdrawing modified insulin. (Photos © Ken Kasper)

10 Store the vials according to agency recommendations.	Insulin need not be refrigerated but must be protected from temperature extremes.
11 Wash your hands.	Handwashing deters the spread of microorganisms.

P R O C E D U R E   40-5
Administering an Intradermal Injection

Equipment

Medication	Sterile syringe and	Acetone and 2 × 2
Medication card or	needle (size de-	sterile gauze
Kardex	pends on medi-	square (op-
	cation being ad-	tional)
	ministered and	
	client)	
	Alcohol swab	

(Continued)

Administering an Intradermal Injection   (Continued)

Action

1 Assemble equipment and check the physician's order.

2 Explain the procedure to the client.

3 Wash your hands.

4 If necessary, withdraw medication from an ampule or vial as described in Procedures 40-2 and 40-3.

5 Select an area on the inner aspect of the forearm. The upper chest or upper back beneath the scapulae are also sites for intradermal injections.

6 Cleanse the area with an alcohol swab while wiping with a firm, circular motion and moving outward from the injection site. Allow the skin to dry. If the skin is oily, cleanse the area with a pledget moistened with acetone.

7 Use the nondominant hand to spread the skin taut over the injection site.

8 Remove the needle cap with the nondominant hand by pulling straight off.

9 Place the needle almost flat against the client's skin, bevel side up, and insert the needle into the skin so that the point of the needle can be seen through the skin. Insert the needle only about ⅛ inch.

10 Slowly inject the agent while watching for a small wheal or blister to appear. If none appears, withdraw the needle slightly.

Rationale

This ensures that the client receives the right medication at the right time by the proper route. Many intradermal drugs are potent allergens and may cause a significant reaction if given in an incorrect dosage.

Explanation encourages cooperation and reduces apprehension.

Handwashing deters the spread of microorganisms.

The forearm is a convenient and easy location for introducing an agent intradermally.

Pathogens on the skin can be forced into the tissues by the needle. Introducing alcohol into tissues irritates the tissues and is uncomfortable for the client. Acetone is effective for removing oily substances from the skin.

Taut skin provides an easy entrance into intradermal tissue.

This protects the needle from contact with microorganisms.

Intradermal tissue will be entered when the needle is held as nearly parallel to the skin as possible and is inserted about ⅛ inch.

If a small wheal or blister appears, the agent is in intradermal tissue.

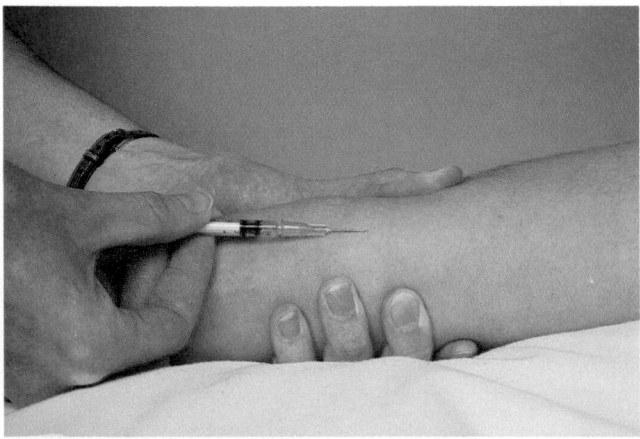

Step 9: Inserting needle almost level with skin.

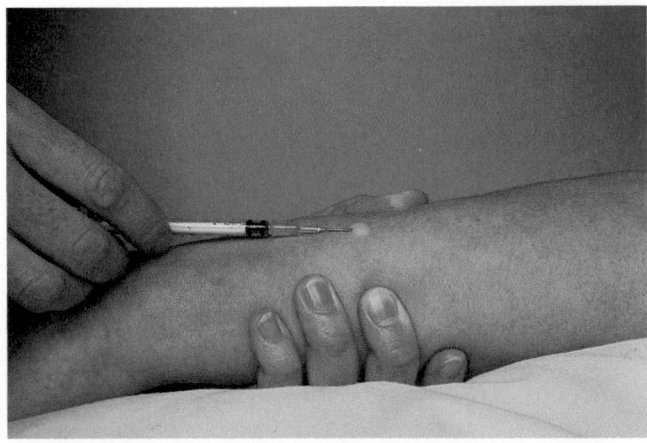

Step 10: Observing for wheal while injecting medication. (Photos © Ken Kasper)

11 Withdraw the needle quickly at the same angle that it was inserted.

Withdrawing the needle quickly and at the angle at which it entered the skin minimizes tissue damage and discomfort for the client.

12 Do not massage the area after removing the needle.

Massaging the area where an intradermal injection is given may interfere with test results by spreading medication to underlying subcutaneous tissue.

13 Do not recap the used needle. Discard the needle and syringe in the appropriate receptacle.

Proper disposal of the needle protects the nurse from accidental injection. Most accidental puncture wounds occur when recapping needles.

14 Assist the client to a position of comfort.

This provides for the well-being of the client.

15 Wash your hands.

Handwashing deters the spread of microorganisms.

16 Chart the administration of the medication.

Accurate documentation is necessary to prevent medication error.

17 Observe the area for signs of a reaction at ordered intervals, usually at 24- to 72-hour periods. Inform the client of this inspection. In some agencies, a circle may be drawn on the skin around the injection site.

This easily identifies the site of the intradermal injection and allows for careful observation of the exact area.

back. Equipment used for an intradermal injection includes a tuberculin syringe calibrated in tenths and hundredths of a milliliter. The dosage given intradermally is very small, usually less than 0.5 ml. A ½-inch, 25- to 27-gauge needle is used.

To administer an intradermal injection, the site is cleansed with alcohol in a circular motion from the center of the site outward. The nurse holds the client's skin taut with the nondominant hand and the syringe in the dominant hand with palm down to enable the needle to be inserted bevel upward at a 5- to 15-degree angle. The needle is inserted until the bevel is no longer visible and the medication is injected. A small raised area or wheal should be present at the injection site. The site is not massaged after injection to prevent hastened absorption. The site of injection is recorded. The client should receive instructions about care and observation of the site and follow-up. Procedure 40-5 outlines and illustrates the procedure for administering an intradermal injection.

Administering Medications Subcutaneously

Subcutaneous tissue lies between the epidermis and the muscle. Because there is subcutaneous tissue all over the body, various sites are used for subcutaneous injections. These sites are the outer aspect of the upper arm, anterior aspects of the thigh, lower abdominal wall, and upper back. Figure 40-8 illustrates sites on the body where subcutaneous injections can be given. This route is used to administer insulin, heparin, and certain immunizations.

Equipment used for a subcutaneous injection depends on the medication to be given. For instance, insulin is prepared with an insulin syringe. Heparin is prepared with a tuberculin syringe or supplied in a prefilled cartridge. A 25-gauge, ½-inch to 1-inch needle would be used for this route. Ordinarily, no more than 1 ml of solution is given subcutaneously. Giving larger amounts adds to the client's discomfort and may predispose to poor absorption.

The skin is cleansed for a subcutaneous injection in the same manner as for an intradermal injection. The nurse chooses the angle of needle insertion based on the amount of subcutaneous tissue present and the length of the needle. For a large client, the nurse stretches the skin taut. Holding the syringe palm upward the nurse inserts the ⅝-inch needle bevel upward at a 45-degree angle. When the client is a small child or an emaciated adult, the nurse bunches the skin at the injection site. Holding

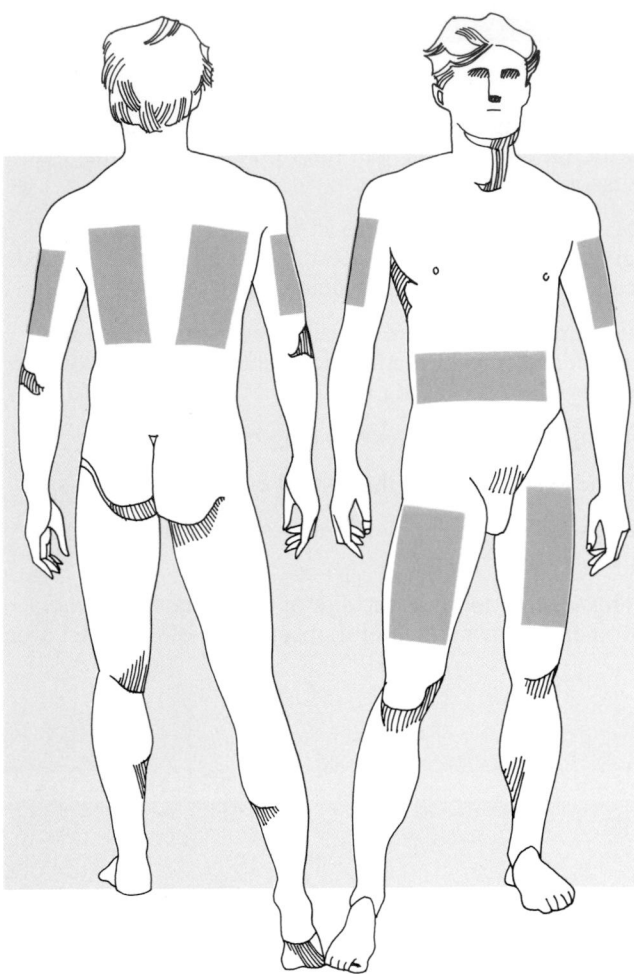

F I G U R E   40-8
Sites on the body where subcutaneous injections can be given.

the syringe palm downward, the ½-inch needle is inserted at a 90-degree angle, bevel upward.

After the needle is in place, the nurse gently pulls back on the plunger to determine that the needle has not entered a blood vessel. If blood enters the barrel of the syringe, the needle is removed and a new site is selected. If no blood enters the barrel of the syringe, the medication is injected into the client. Aspiration of the plunger is not recommended with administration of subcutaneous heparin because this act can result in hematoma formation. The site is gently massaged, except in the case of heparin and insulin because massaging the site can increase the rate of absorption of these agents. The site of administration is recorded in the client's record. Procedure 40-6 illustrates the procedure for administering medications subcutaneously.

It is necessary to rotate sites if the client is to receive frequent injections. This helps prevent irritation and permits complete absorption of the medication. Clients who receive injections repeatedly in one site are likely to develop an area of hardened and tender tissue. A marked diagram incorporated into the client's plan of care is

helpful for noting alternative sites. It is futile to rely on memory. Not even the client will always be able to recall the site of the previous injection. Techniques for reducing discomfort in subcutaneous administrations are listed following the discussion Administering Medications Intramuscularly.

Administering Medications Intramuscularly

The **intramuscular** route often is used for drugs that are irritating, since there are few nerve endings in deep muscle tissue. If a sore or inflamed muscle is entered, the muscle may act as a trigger area, and severe referred pain often results. It is best to palpate a muscle prior to injection. A site should be selected that does not feel tender to the client and where the tissue does not contract and become firm and tense.

Absorption occurs as in subcutaneous administration but more rapidly because of the greater vascularity of muscle tissue. The amount of 3 ml is considered the maximum to be given in one site.

Intramuscular Injection Sites.   An important point in the administration of an intramuscular injection is the selection of a safe site, one that is away from large nerves, bones, and blood vessels. When care is not taken, common complications include abscesses, necrosis and skin slough, nerve injuries, lingering pain, and periostitis.

The sites for injecting intramuscular medications should be rotated when therapy requires repeated injections. The sites described in this chapter may all be used on a rotating basis. Whatever pattern of rotating sites is used, a description of it should appear in the client's nursing care plan.

Dorsogluteal Site.   The dorsogluteal site, located in the buttock, is a common site for administering intramuscular injections. The site can be located by two methods. The first method uses anatomic landmarks to locate the dorsogluteal site. The posterior superior iliac spine and the greater trochanter are palpated. An imaginary line is drawn between the posterior superior iliac spine and the greater trochanter. The injection site is lateral and slightly superior to the midpoint of the line, as illustrated in Figure 40-9.

A second method of locating the dorsogluteal site is to divide the buttock into four quadrants using the crest of the ileum and gluteal fold as the superior and inferior boundaries, respectively, between which an imaginary vertical line is drawn. An imaginary horizontal line is drawn from the medial fold to the lateral aspect of the buttock. The injection is given in the *upper outer* quadrant. Site selection using this method is depicted in Figure 40-10.

If the site is identified correctly, the nurse will avoid damage to the sciatic nerve. Palpation of anatomic landmarks ensures that the nurse has identified the injection

(Text continues on p. 1154.)

PROCEDURE 40-6
Administering a Subcutaneous Injection

Equipment

Medication
Medication card or
    Kardex

A sterile syringe and
    needle (size de-
    pends on medi-
    cation being ad-
    ministered and
    client)

Alcohol swabs

Action	Rationale
1 Assemble equipment and check the physician's order.	This ensures that the client receives the right medication at the right time by the proper route.
2 Explain the procedure to the client.	An explanation encourages client cooperation and reduces apprehension.
3 Wash your hands.	Handwashing deters the spread of microorganisms.
4 If necessary, withdraw medication from an ampule or vial as described in Procedures 40-2 and 40-3.	
5 Add air to the syringe according to agency policy (0.1 ml of air is usually added to a heparin injection).	The air bubble will force medication out of the needle.
6 Identify the client carefully. See Procedure 40-1, Step 12. Close curtain to provide privacy.	It is the nurse's responsibility to guard against error.
7 Have the client assume a position appropriate for the site selected:	Injection into a tense muscle causes discomfort.
a. Outer aspect of upper arm—the client's arm should be relaxed and at the side of the body.	
b. Anterior thighs—the client may sit or lie with the leg relaxed.	
c. Abdomen—the client may lie in a semirecumbent position.	
d. Scapular area—the client may be prone, on side, or assume a sitting position.	
8 Locate the site of choice according to directions given in this chapter and ensure that the area is not tender and is free of lumps or nodules.	Good visualization is necessary to establish the correct location of the site and avoid damage to tissues. Nodules or lumps may indicate a previous injection site where absorption was inadequate.
9 Clean the area of skin around the injection site with an alcohol swab. Use a firm, circular motion while moving outward from the injection site. Allow the antiseptic to dry. Leave the alcohol swab in a clean area for reuse when withdrawing the needle.	Friction helps clean the skin. A clean area is contaminated when a soiled object is rubbed over its surface.
10 Remove the needle cap with the nondominant hand, pulling it straight off.	This protects the needle from contact with microorganisms.

(Continued)

Action

11 Grasp and bunch the area surrounding the injection site or spread the skin at the site.

12 Hold the syringe in the dominant hand between the thumb and forefinger. Inject the needle quickly at an angle of 45 degrees to 90 degrees, depending on the amount and turgor of the tissue and the length of the needle as illustrated.

Rationale

This provides for easy, less painful entry into the subcutaneous tissue. The decision to pinch or spread tissue at the injection site depends on the size of the client. If the client is obese, skin needs to be bunched to allow the needle to penetrate below the fatty layer in the subcutaneous tissue.

Subcutaneous tissue is abundant in well-nourished, well-hydrated persons and sparse in emaciated, dehydrated, or very thin persons.

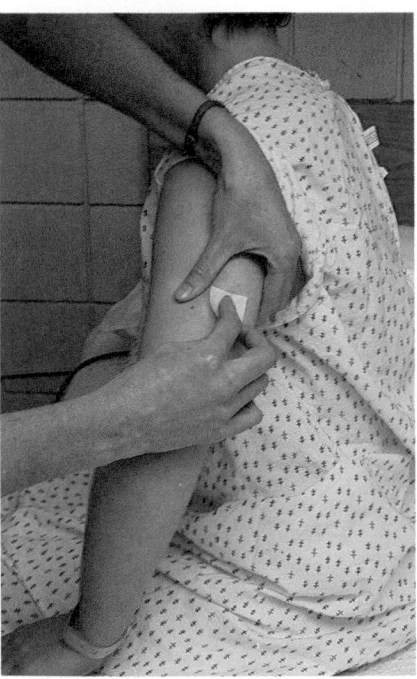

Step 9: Cleaning injection site.

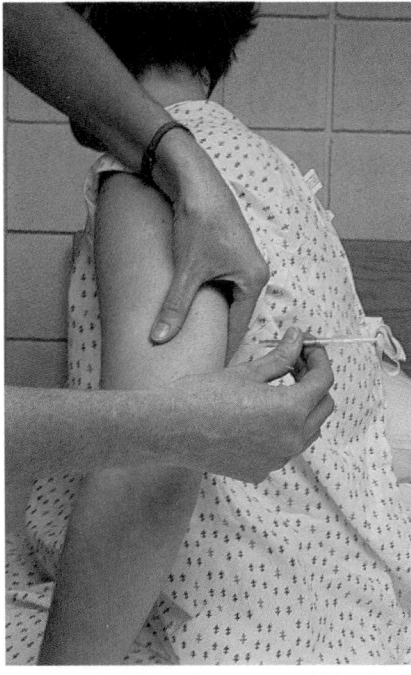

Step 11: Bunching tissue around injection site.

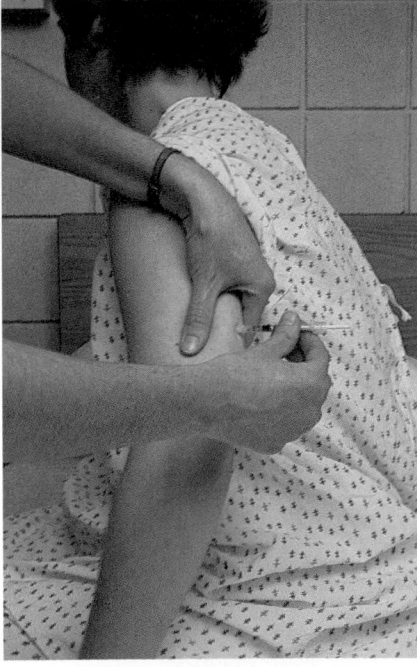

Step 12: Inserting needle.

13 After the needle is in place, release the grasp on the tissue and immediately move your nondominant hand to steady the lower end of the syringe. Slide your dominant hand to the tip of the barrel.

14 Aspirate by pulling back gently on the plunger of the syringe to determine whether the needle is in a blood vessel. If blood appears, the needle should be withdrawn and discarded, and a new syringe with new medication prepared. (Most agencies recommend that a subcutaneous heparin injection should not be aspirated.)

15 If no blood appears, inject the solution slowly.

Injecting the solution into compressed tissues results in pressure against nerve fibers and creates discomfort. The nondominant hand secures the syringe and allows for smooth aspiration.

Discomfort and possibly a serious reaction may occur if a drug intended for subcutaneous use is injected into a vein. Heparin, an anticoagulant, may cause bruising if aspirated.

Rapid injection of the solution creates pressure in the tissues, resulting in discomfort.

(Continued)

Action

16 Withdraw the needle quickly at the same angle that it was inserted, as illustrated.

Rationale

Slow withdrawal of the needle pulls the tissues and causes discomfort. Applying countertraction around the injection site helps prevent pulling on the tissue as the needle is withdrawn. Removing the needle at the same angle it was inserted minimizes tissue damage and discomfort for the client.

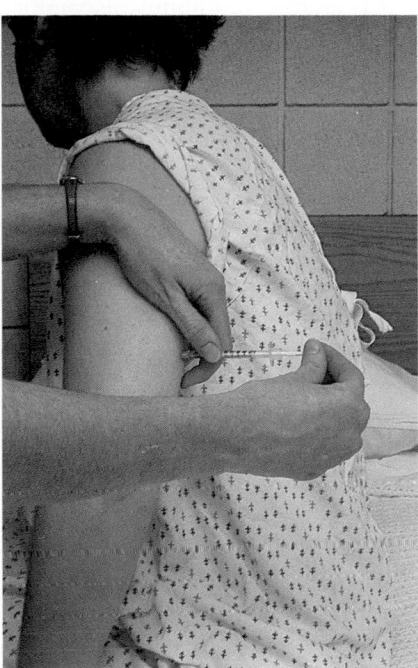

Step 14: Aspirating.

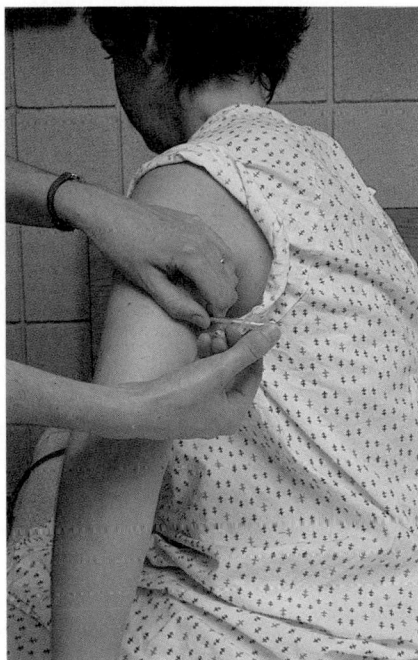

Step 15: Injecting medication.

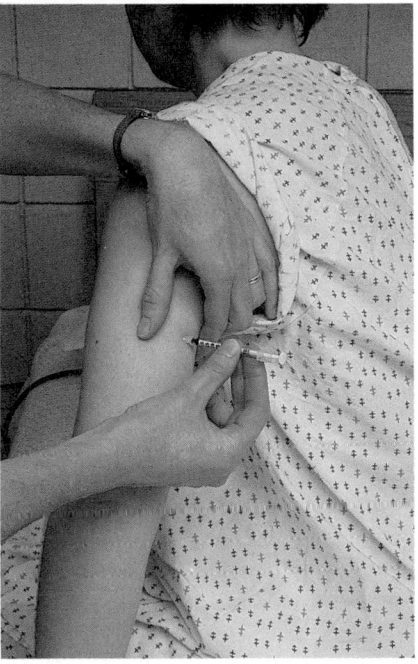

Step 16: Withdrawing needle. (Photos © Ken Kasper)

17 Massage the area gently with the alcohol swab. (Do not massage a subcutaneous heparin injection site.)

Massaging helps distribute the solution and hastens its absorption. Massaging the site of a heparin injection causes additional bruising.

18 Do not recap the used needle. Discard the needle and syringe in the appropriate receptacle.

Proper disposal of the needle protects the nurse from accidental injection. Most accidental puncture wounds occur when recapping needles.

19 Assist the client to a position of comfort.

This provides for the well-being of the client.

20 Wash your hands.

Handwashing deters the spread of microorganisms.

21 Chart the administration of the medication.

Accurate documentation is necessary to prevent medication error.

22 Evaluate the response of the client to medication within an appropriate time frame.

Reaction to medication given by the parenteral route may occur within 15 to 30 minutes after injection.

Special Considerations

If a diabetic client is visually impaired, several insulin syringes may be preloaded and stored in the refrigerator for future use.

A poster or body log may be used to indicate sites for systematic rotation of insulin injections as well as to record the location of injections.

Refer the diabetic client to the American Diabetic Association for additional information and assistance.

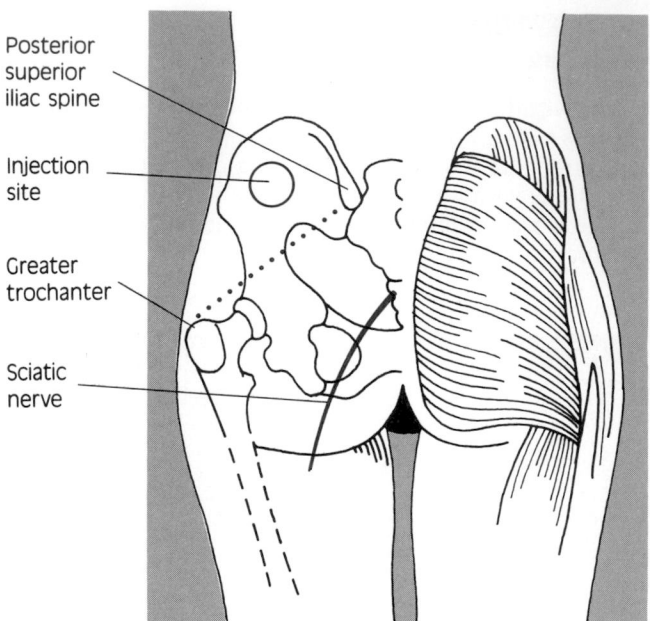

F I G U R E   40-9
The dorsogluteal site for administering an intramuscular injection is lateral and slightly superior to the midpoint of a line drawn from the trocanter to the posterior superior iliac spine.

site. The gluteal muscles are developed by walking and therefore the dorsogluteal site is not to be used for children under 3 years of age because their gluteal muscles are too small.

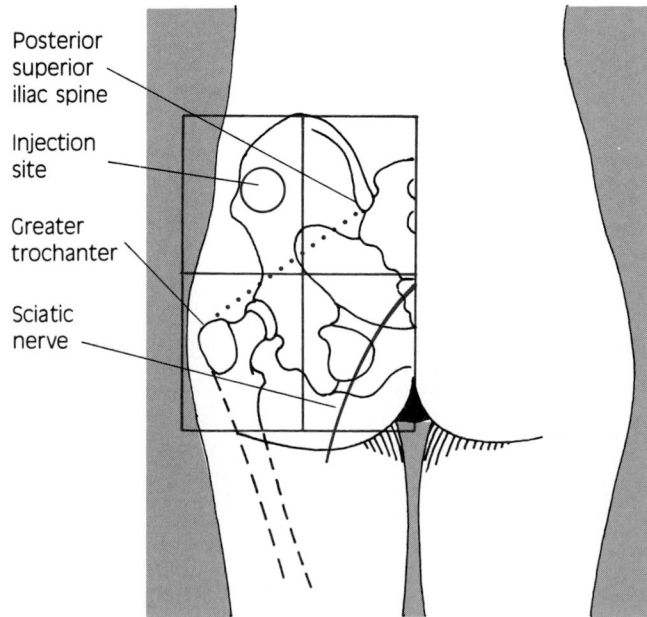

F I G U R E   40-10
A second method of locating the dorsogluteal site is to divide the buttock into 4 quadrants. The injection is given in the upper outer quadrant.

The site is so important that no injection into the buttock should be given without good visualization of the entire area and careful mapping to locate the proper site. This necessitates adequate exposure by lowering the undergarments. Merely raising one side of underclothing permits only a partial visualization of the area. It is recommended that the client be in a prone position with the toes pointed inward, or the side-lying position with the upper knee flexed and the upper leg in front of the lower leg. These positions help promote maximum muscle relaxation and therefore minimum discomfort. When the client is in a standing position, the gluteus muscle is usually tense.

Ventrogluteal Site.   The ventrogluteal site involves the gluteus medius and gluteus minimus muscles in the hip area. The ventrogluteal site is recommended for both adults and children. There are no large nerves or blood vessels in the injection area, it is removed from bone tissue, the area is clean because fecal contamination is rare at this site, and the client can be on the back, abdomen, or side for the injection. To relax the gluteal muscle, the client may flex the knees while lying on the back, point the toes inward while lying in the prone position, and flex the top leg in front of the lower leg in the side-lying position. Although any of the three posi-

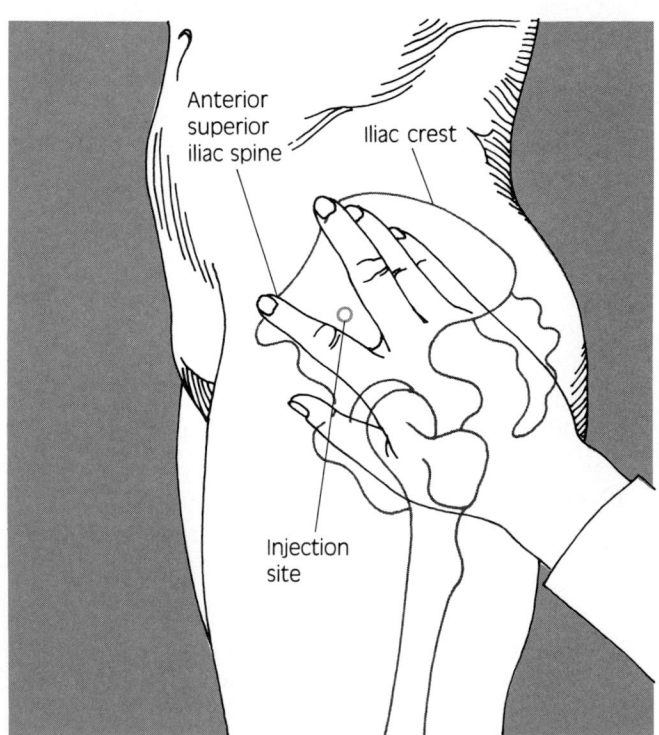

F I G U R E   40-11
The ventrogluteal site is located by placing the palm of the hand on the greater trochanter and the index finger toward the anterior superior iliac spine. The middle finger is then spread posteriorly away from the index finger as far as possible. The V or triangle is formed by this maneuver. The injection is made in the middle of the triangle.

tions just described may be used when injecting the ventrogluteal site, nurses increasingly prefer the side-lying position.

To locate the ventrogluteal site, the nurse places the palm of the hand over the greater trochanter, with the fingers facing the client's head. The right hand is used for the client's left hip and the left hand is used for the right hip to identify landmarks. The index finger is placed on the anterior superior iliac spine and the middle finger extends dorsally, palpating the crest of the ileum. A triangle is formed. The injection is made in the center of the triangle. Figure 40-11 illustrates injecting the ventrogluteal site.

Vastus Lateralis Site. The vastus lateralis muscle is being recommended more frequently for the injection of medications. It is a thick muscle, and there is little or no danger of serious injury. There are no large nerves or vessels in close proximity, and it does not cover a joint. The muscle covers the anterolateral aspect of the thigh. It is bounded by the midanterior thigh on the front of the

leg and by the midlateral thigh on the side. The thigh is divided into thirds horizontally and vertically. The injection is given in the *outer middle* third. This space provides a large number of injection sites. The syringe is held parallel to the surface of the bed. Figure 40-12 illustrates the location of this site. The vastus lateralis site is particularly desirable for infants and children whose gluteal muscles are poorly developed.

Rectus Femoris Site. The rectus femoris muscle is on the anterior part of the thigh. The site is used only when others are contraindicated, since many clients find it uncomfortable. However, some clients who must inject themselves at home use this site because of its convenience. The muscle is included in the sketch of the thigh in Figure 40-13.

Deltoid Muscle Site. The deltoid muscle is located in the lateral aspect of the upper arm. It is not often used because it is a small muscle. The deltoid muscle is not capable of absorbing large amounts of solution. Damage

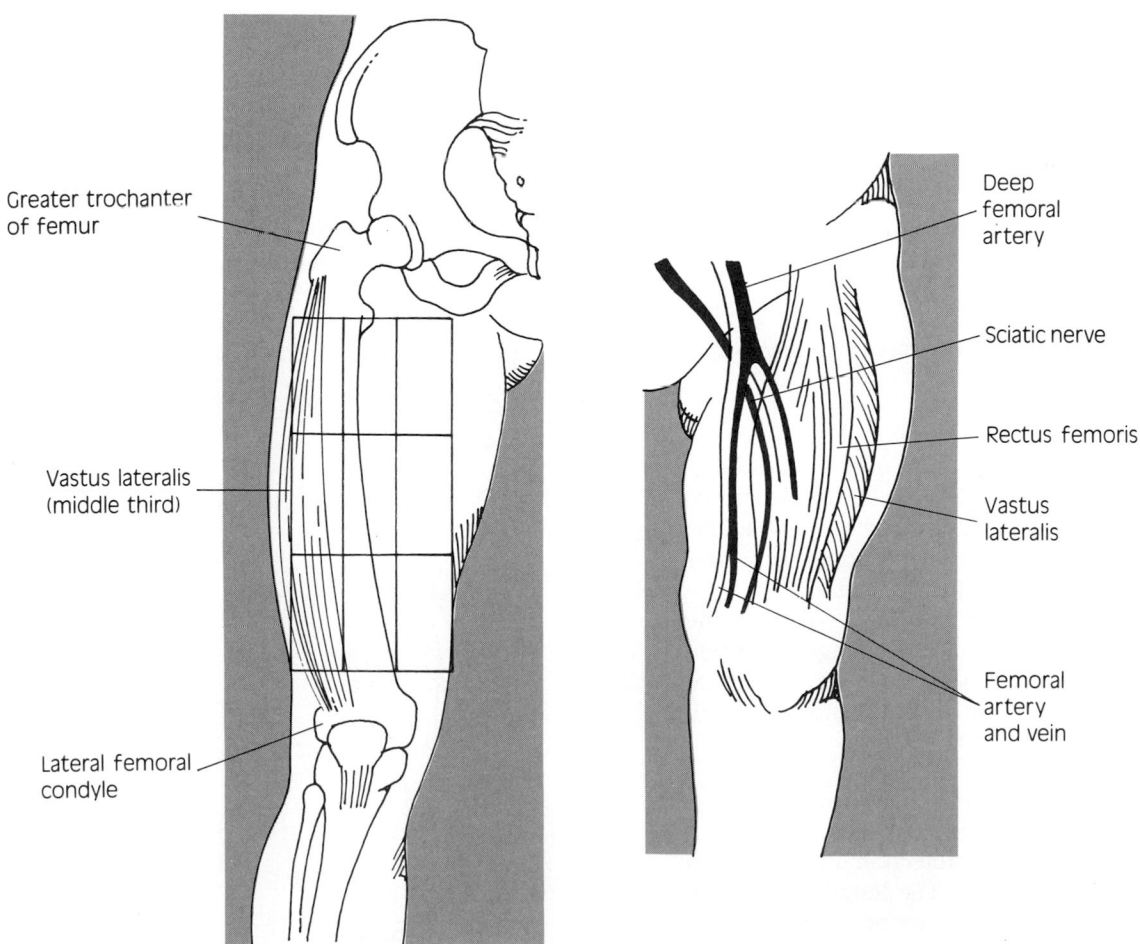

Greater trochanter of femur

Vastus lateralis (middle third)

Lateral femoral condyle

Deep femoral artery

Sciatic nerve

Rectus femoris

Vastus lateralis

Femoral artery and vein

FIGURE 40-12

The vastus lateralis site for intramuscular injections is identified by dividing the thigh into thirds horizontally and vertically. The injection is given in the outer middle third.

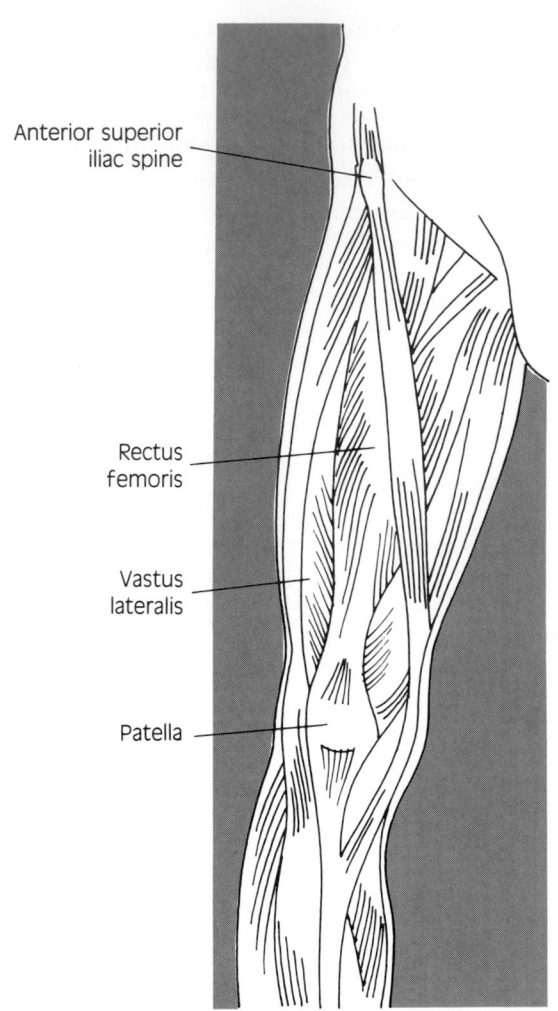

F I G U R E   40-13
The rectus femoris site for intramuscular injections is used only when others are contraindicated.

should be exchanged for a longer one. Evidence does not suggest that a short needle minimizes discomfort or that a longer one adds to discomfort. The characteristic of the client's anatomy should dictate needle length. The most important consideration is to use a needle with a tip that will reach deep into the muscle.

Just before injecting a medication intramuscularly, a small air bubble, approximately 0.2 ml to 0.3 ml, may be added to the syringe after the solution to be administered has been accurately measured. Figure 40-15 illustrates the air bubble in the syringe. This air bubble helps expel solution that is trapped in the shaft of the needle. Solution that remains in the needle shaft after the medication is injected is in danger of being pulled up through the tissues as the needle is withdrawn. If the drug is an irritating one, this causes discomfort to the client and may result in tissue damage. The air bubble also helps trap the injected solution in intramuscular tissue. There is no danger of air embolism with this procedure.

To administer an intramuscular injection, the nurse cleans the site, spreads the skin taut with the nondominant hand, and inserts the needle in a dart-like manner at a 90-degree angle into the skin. The nurse aspirates the plunger and injects the medication if the needle is not in a blood vessel. The site is gently massaged after the injection and recorded in the client's record. The proce-

to the radial nerve and artery is a risk of the deltoid site. Intramuscular injections into the deltoid muscle should be limited to 1 ml of solution and used only for adults. The deltoid muscle is not developed enough in infants and children to absorb medication adequately.

The deltoid muscle can be located by palpating the lower edge of the acromion process. A triangle is formed at the midpoint in line with the axilla on the lateral aspect of the upper arm. Figure 40-14 illustrates the deltoid site.

Injection Procedure.   Not more than 3 ml should be injected into a single injection site. Equipment commonly used for an intramuscular injection includes 20- to 22-gauge, 1- to 1½-inch needles. The length of the needle should be selected with care before administering any intramuscular injection. The prepackaged loaded syringes usually have a needle that is 1 inch in length. However, if there is any question about whether the belly of the target muscle will be reached, the needle

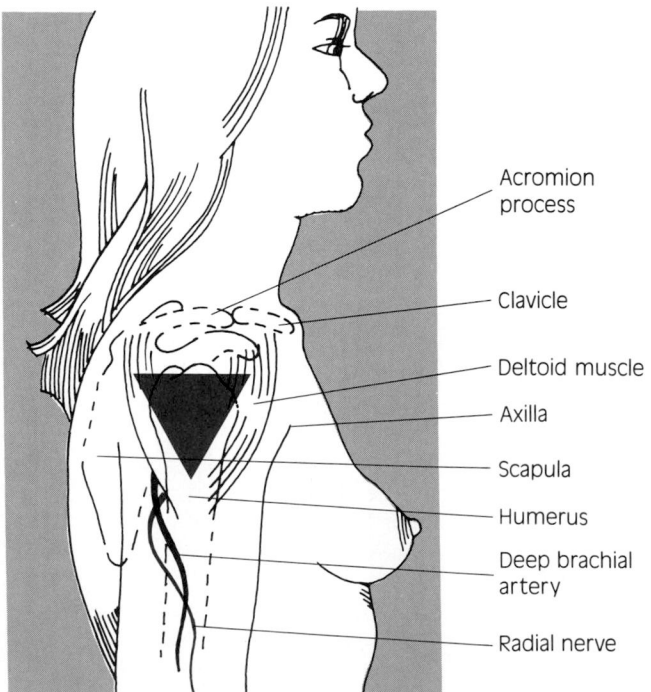

F I G U R E   40-14
The deltoid muscle site for intramuscular injections is located by palpating the lower edge of the acromion process. At the midpoint, in line with the axilla on the lateral aspect of the upper arm, a triangle is formed.

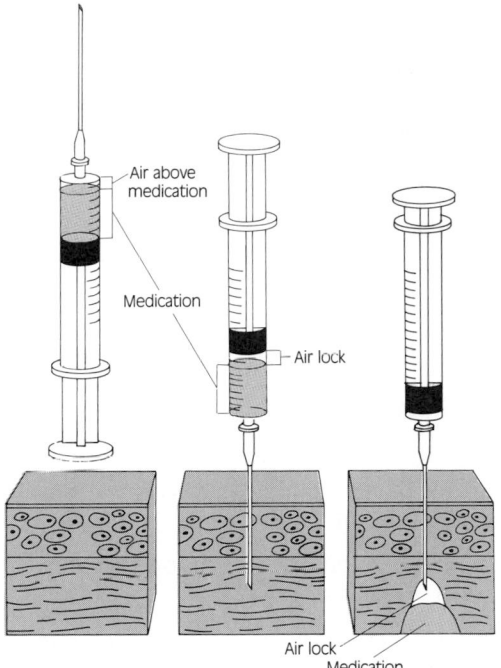

F I G U R E   40-15
An air bubble added to the syringe after the medication has been accurately measured helps expel solution that is trapped in the shaft of the needle when the injection is given. It also helps trap the injected solution in the intramuscular tissue.

dure for administering an intramuscular injection is outlined in Procedure 40-7.

Z-track Technique. The **Z-track** or zigzag technique is used to administer medications that are highly irritating to subcutaneous tissues, for example, iron—dextran injection (Imferon). An air lock of 0.2 ml to 0.3 ml is created after the medication is prepared in the syringe. A clean needle is attached to the syringe to prevent the injection of medication on the needle into superficial tissues. The needle should be a minimum of 1½ inches long; for obese persons, a 3-inch needle may be required so that there is no danger of injecting the medication into subcutaneous tissue. The dorsogluteal or vastus lateralis sites can be used for this procedure. The skin is pulled to one side, about 1 inch laterally, and held in this position with the left hand for a right-handed person. The needle is inserted and aspirated for blood. The solution is injected. The needle is allowed to remain in place for 10 seconds after injecting the medication to prevent seepage of the solution into the needle tract. The needle is withdrawn and the displaced tissue is allowed to return to its normal position. Light, steady pressure is applied over the site. The area may be massaged unless the manufacturer's directions on the drug label state that massage is contraindicated. The procedure for administering a **Z**-track injection is outlined in Figure 40-17.

Reducing Discomfort in Subcutaneous and Intramuscular Administrations

The following are recommended techniques to help reduce discomfort when injecting medications subcutaneously and intramuscularly:

- Select a needle of the smallest gauge that is appropriate for the site and solution to be injected.
- Be sure the needle is free of medication that may irritate superficial tissues as the needle is inserted. Recommended procedure is to use two needles, one to remove the medication from the vial or ampule and a second one to inject the medication.
- Inject the medication into relaxed musculature. There is more pressure and discomfort when the medication is injected into a contracted muscle. Have the client lie on the abdomen while rotating the legs to point the toes inward. Or, when in the side-lying position, have the client flex the upper knee and place it in front of the lower leg. These positions relax the gluteal muscle.

(Text continues on p. 1160.)

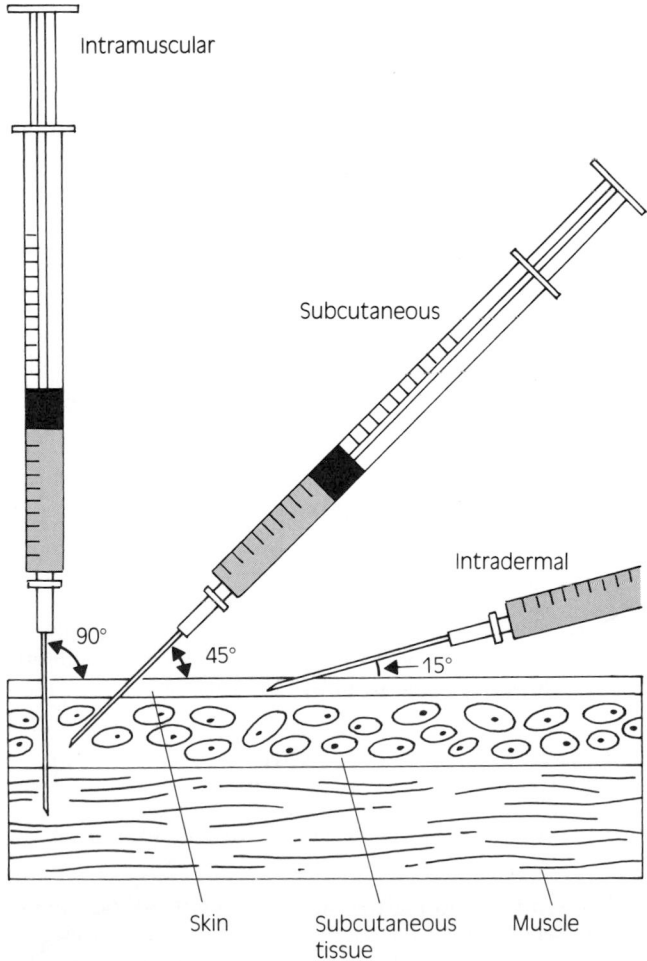

F I G U R E   40-16
Comparison of the angles of insertion for intramuscular, subcutaneous, and intradermal injections.

Administering an Intramuscular Injection

Equipment

Medication
Medication card or
   Kardex

Sterile syringe and
   needle (size de-
   pends on medi-
   cation being ad-
   ministered and
   client)

Alcohol swab

Action

1 Assemble equipment and check the physician's order.

2 Explain the procedure to the client.

3 Wash your hands.

4 If necessary, withdraw medication from an ampule or vial as described in Procedures 40-2 and 40-3.

5 Add 0.2 ml of air to the syringe.

6 Provide for privacy. Have the client assume a position appropriate for the site selected.

   a. Dorsogluteal—the client may lie prone with toes pointing inward or on the side with the upper leg flexed and placed in front of the lower leg.

   b. Ventrogluteal—the client may lie on the back or side with the hip and knee flexed.

   c. Vastus lateralis—the client may lie on the back or assume a sitting position.

   d. Deltoid—the client may sit or lie with arm relaxed.

7 Locate the site of choice according to directions given in this chapter and ensure that the area is not tender and is free of lumps or nodules.

8 Clean the area thoroughly with an alcohol swab, using friction.

9 Remove the needle cap by pulling it straight off.

10 Spread the skin at the site using your nondominant hand.

11 Hold the syringe in your dominant hand between the thumb and forefinger. Quickly dart the needle into the tissue at a 90-degree angle.

Rationale

This ensures that the client receives the right medication at the right time by the proper route.

Explanation encourages cooperation and alleviates apprehension.

Handwashing deters the spread of microorganisms.

The air bubble will force medication out of the needle shaft and helps trap it in the muscle tissue. Some experts question this practice and feel that it interferes with administration of an accurate dose.

Injection into a tense muscle causes discomfort.

Good visualization is necessary to establish the correct location of the site and avoid damage to tissues. Nodules or lumps may indicate a previous injection site where absorption was inadequate.

Pathogens present on the skin can be forced into the tissues by the needle.

This protects the needle from contact with microorganisms.

This makes the tissue taut and minimizes discomfort.

A quick injection is less painful. Inserting the needle at a 90-degree angle facilitates entry into muscle tissue.

(Continued)

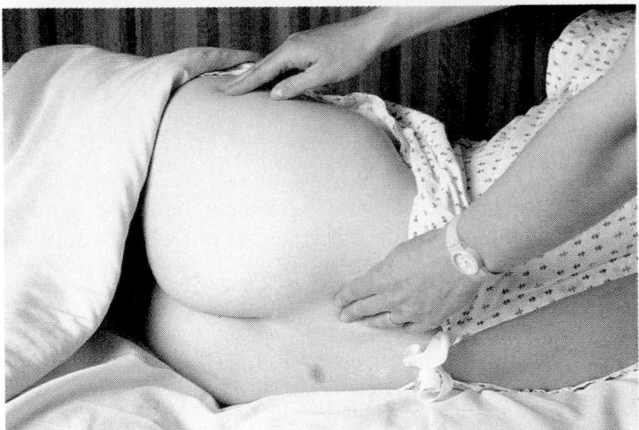

Step 7: Identifying landmarks for dorsogluteal injection site.

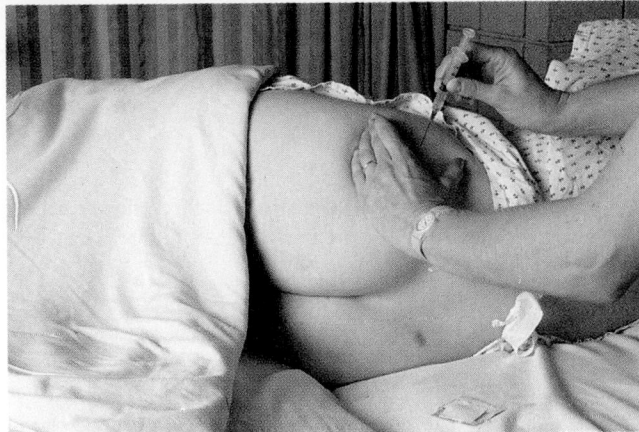

Steps 10 & 11: Spreading skin at site and darting needle in at 90-degree angle.

Action

12 As soon as the needle is in place, move your non-dominant hand to hold the lower end of the syringe. Slide your dominant hand to the tip of the barrel.

13 Aspirate by slowly pulling back on the plunger to determine whether the needle is in a blood vessel. If blood is aspirated, discard the needle, syringe, and medication, prepare a new sterile set-up, and inject another site.

Rationale

This acts to steady the syringe and allows for smooth aspiration.

Discomfort and possibly a serious reaction may occur if a drug intended for intramuscular use is injected into a vein.

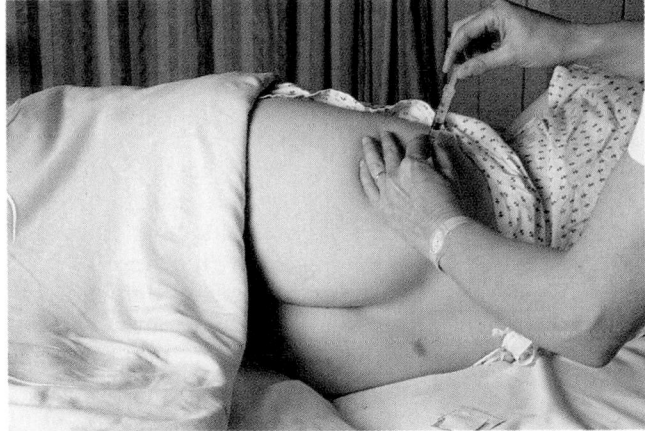

Step 13: Aspirating.

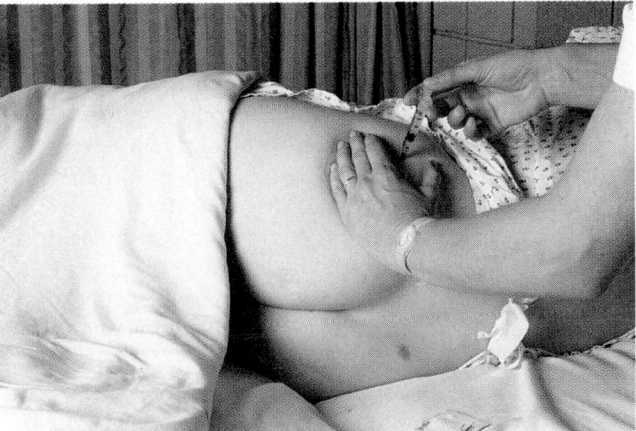

Step 14: Injecting.

14 If no blood is aspirated, inject the solution slowly, followed by the air bubble.

15 Remove the needle quickly.

16 Massage the injection site with the alcohol swab using gentle pressure.

Injecting slowly helps reduce discomfort by allowing time for the solution to disperse in the tissues.

Slow removal of the needle pulls tissues and may cause discomfort.

Massaging helps distribute the solution and hastens its absorption by increasing blood flow to the area.

(Continued)

Action	Rationale
17 Do not recap the used needle. Discard the needle and syringe in the appropriate receptacle.	Proper disposal of the needle protects the nurse from accidental injection. Most accidental puncture wounds occur when recapping needles.
18 Assist the client to a position of comfort.	This provides for the well-being of the client.
19 Wash your hands.	Handwashing deters the spread of microorganisms.
20 Chart the administration of the medication.	Accurate documentation is necessary to prevent medication error.
21 Evaluate the response of the client to the medication within an appropriate time frame.	Reaction to medication given by the parenteral route may occur within 15 to 30 minutes after injection.

- Do not inject areas that feel hard on palpation or feel tender to the client.
- Insert the needle with a dart-like motion without hesitation, and remove it quickly at the same angle at which it was inserted. These techniques help reduce discomfort and tissue irritation.
- Do not administer more solution in one injection than is recommended for the site. Injecting more solution creates excess pressure in the area and increases discomfort.
- Inject the solution slowly so that it may be dispersed more easily into the surrounding tissue.
- Hold an alcohol pad against the skin while removing the needle from the tissue. This minimizes pull on the skin, which causes discomfort.
- Massage the area after injection, unless this technique is contraindicated. Massage helps spread the solution into surrounding tissues and hastens absorption by increasing circulation to the area.
- Allow the client who is fearful of injections to talk about the fears. Answer the client's questions truthfully, and explain the nature and purpose of the injection. Taking the time to offer support will often allay fears that ordinarily add to the discomfort of the procedure for the client.
- Rotate the sites when the client is to receive repeated injections. Injections in the same site may cause undue discomfort, irritation, or abscesses in tissues.

Administering Medications Intravenously

Medications administered intravenously have an immediate effect. The **intravenous** route is the most dangerous route of administration. Because the drug is placed directly into the bloodstream, it cannot be recalled nor can its actions be slowed. Intravenous administration would be the route chosen in an emergency situation when immediate absorption is required. However, there are many clinical situations in which drugs are administered intravenously when an emergency does not exist. Procedure 35-1 describes the basic technique for administering an intravenous infusion.

There are several ways to administer medications intravenously. Medications may be added to the client's infusion solution. The recommended procedure is for the pharmacist to add the prescribed drug to a large volume of intravenous solution, but sometimes the drug is added in the nursing unit, in which case sterile technique must be maintained. Steps for adding medications to intravenous solutions are given in Procedure 40-8.

When medication is administered by continuous infusion, the client receives it slowly and over a long period of time. Although this can sometimes be an advantage when it is desirable to give the medication slowly, it is a disadvantage when it is necessary for the client to receive the drug more quickly. Also, if for some reason all of the solution cannot be infused, the client will not receive the prescribed amount of the medication. The client receiving medication by a continuous intravenous infusion should be checked for possible adverse effects at least every hour.

A medication can be administered as an intravenous **bolus**. A bolus dose of medication is a single injection of a concentrated solution administered directly into an intravenous line (see Procedure 40-9).

Medications can be administered by intermittent intravenous infusion. The drug is mixed with a small amount of the intravenous solution, such as 50 ml to 100

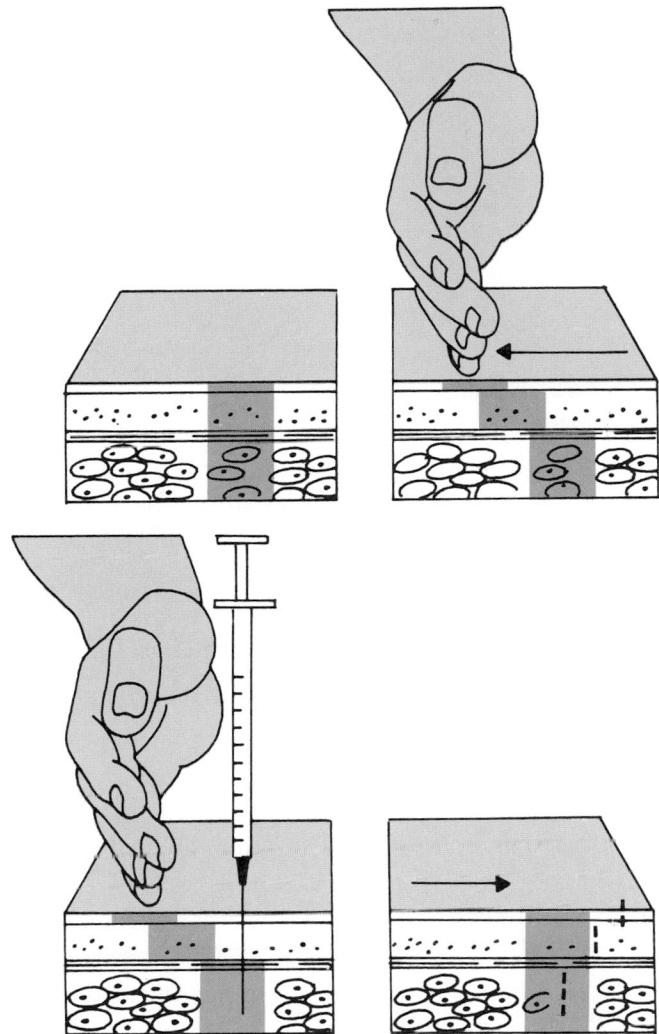

F I G U R E   40-17
The Z-track or zig-zag technique is used to administer medications that are irritating to subcutaneous tissue. The skin is pulled to one side, blood aspirated, and the solution injected. When the needle is withdrawn and the displaced tissue is allowed to return to its normal position, the solution is prevented from escaping from the muscle tissue.

small amount of solution and administered through the client's intravenous line (see Procedure 40-11). This type of equipment is also used for infusing solutions into children and elderly clients when the volume of fluid infused must be carefully monitored.

A **heparin lock** is used for a client who requires intermittent intravenous medication but not a continuous intravenous infusion. The needle may be either an intra-catheter with a resealable injection pad or a winged infusion needle with a short catheter, the end of which has an injection pad. A heparin lock with a winged infusion needle is illustrated in Figure 40-18. After the needle is in place in the client's vein, the needle and tubing are anchored to the client's arm so that the needle remains in place until the client no longer requires the repeated medication intravenously.

A heparin lock allows the client more freedom than a continuous intravenous infusion. The client is connected to the intravenous line when it is time to receive the medication and disconnected when the medication is completed. The heparin lock is flushed with a dilute heparin solution to check for intravenous placement and patency prior to medication administration. The intermittent infusion is not started until the nurse confirms intravenous placement. The heparin lock is flushed after the infusion is completed to clear the vein of any medication and to prevent clot formation in the needle. The procedure for flushing a heparin lock is discussed in Procedure 40-12. The intravenous site is assessed for complications discussed in Chapter 35. If infiltration or phlebitis occurs, the heparin lock is removed and replaced in a new site.

Intermittent intravenous medication may be administered through a catheter placed in the subclavian vein. Medications are prepared under laminar flow in a sterile environment if they are to be administered through a central intravenous line such as a Hickman catheter. Aseptic technique is observed when the nurse administers medications through a central intravenous line. All connections are cleaned with povidone—iodine (Betadine) for its antiseptic properties.

(Text continues on p. 1170.)

ml, and administered at the prescribed interval, for example, every 4 hours. The client with an intravenous line in place receives the solution containing the medication in a tandem manner. This is often called the **piggyback** method (Procedure 40-10). The piggyback solution is connected to the main intravenous line at the injection port. The main intravenous solution is lowered while the medication infuses. The piggyback solution is usually regulated to infuse in 30 to 60 minutes. When the piggyback solution is completed, it is clamped off and the primary intravenous solution is adjusted to its usual height and flow rate.

Medications can be placed in a controlled-volume administration set (Soluset, Buretrol) for intermittent intravenous infusion. The medication is diluted with a

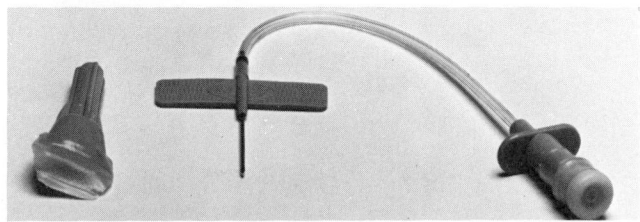

F I G U R E   40-18
A heparin lock. The needle sheath has been removed. The flaps on either side of the needle are flexible and make the needle easy to handle and anchor. There is a sterile plug at the end of the tubing. When it is removed, a syringe containing a drug in solution can be attached, and the medication is then injected.

PROCEDURE 40-8
Adding Medications to an IV Solution Container

Equipment

Medication prepared in a syringe with a 19- to 21-gauge needle

Alcohol swab

IV fluid container (bag or bottle)

Label to be attached to the IV container

Action

1 Gather all equipment and bring to the client's bedside. Check the medication order with the physician's order.

2 Explain the procedure to the client.

3 Wash your hands.

4 Identify the client by checking the band on the client's wrist and asking the client his or her name.

5 Add the medication to the IV solution that is infusing:

   a. Check that the volume in the bag or bottle is adequate.

   b. Close the IV clamp.

   c. Clean the medication port with an alcohol swab.

   d. Steady the container, uncap the needle, and insert the needle into the port. Inject the medication.

Rationale

Having equipment available saves time and facilitates performance of the task. Checking the orders ensures that the client receives the correct medication at the correct time and in the right manner.

Explanation allays the client's anxiety.

Handwashing deters the spread of microorganisms.

This ensures that medication is given to the right person.

The volume should be sufficient to dilute the drug.

This prevents backflow directly to the client of improperly diluted medication.

This deters entry of microorganisms when the needle punctures the port.

This ensures that the needle enters the container and medication can be dispersed into the solution.

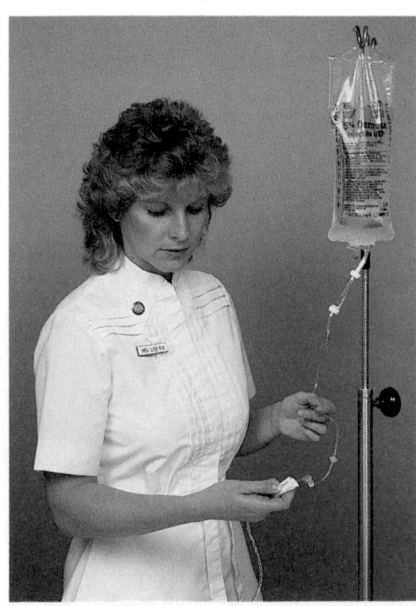

Step 5b: Closing IV clamp.

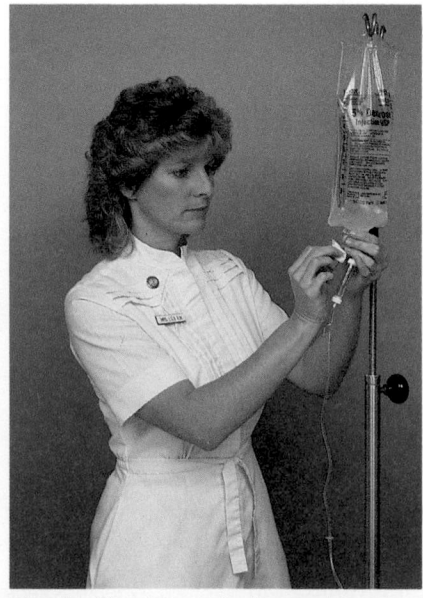

Step 5c: Cleaning medication port.

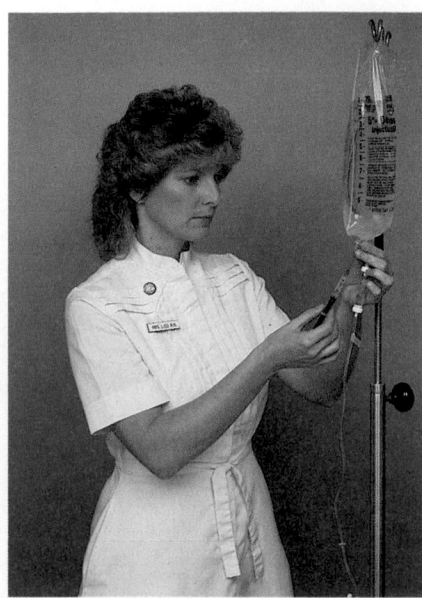

Step 5d: Injecting medication.

(Continued)

e. Remove the container from the IV pole and gently rotate the solution.

This mixes the medication with the solution.

f. Rehang the container, open the clamp, and readjust the flow rate.

This ensures the infusion of the IV with medication at the prescribed rate.

g. Attach the label to the container so that the dosage of medication that has been added is apparent.

This confirms that the prescribed dose of medication has been added to the IV solution.

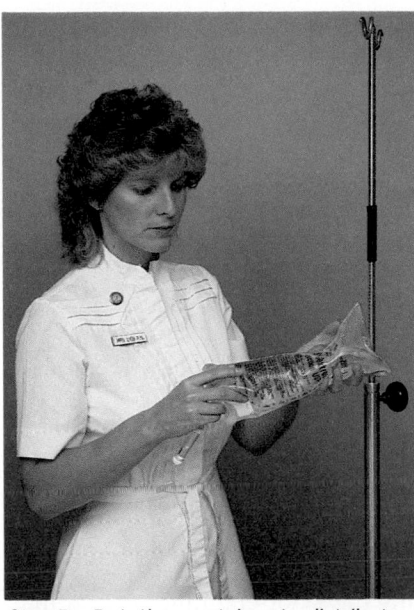

Step 5e: Rotating container to distribute medication.

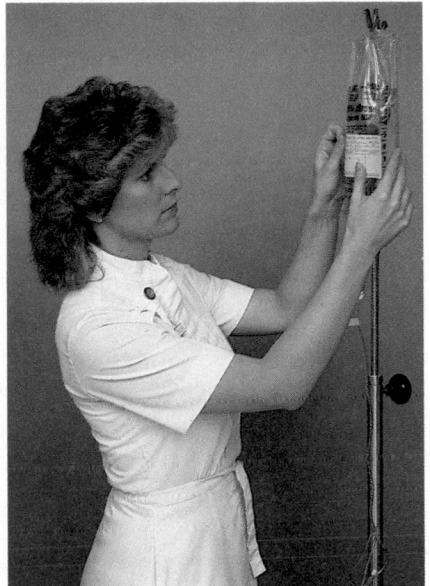

Step 5g: Labeling container to show medication. (Photos © Ken Kasper)

6 Add the medication to the IV solution prior to infusion:

a. Carefully remove any protective cover and locate the injection port. Cleanse with an alcohol swab.

This deters entry of microorganisms when the needle punctures the port.

b. Uncap the needle and insert into the port. Inject the medication.

This ensures that the needle enters the container and that medication can be dispersed into the solution.

c. Withdraw the needle and insert the spike into the proper entry site on the bag or bottle.

This punctures the seal in the IV bag or bottle.

d. With tubing clamped, gently rotate the IV solution in the bag or bottle. Hang the IV.

This mixes medication with the solution.

e. Attach the label to the container so that the dosage of medication that has been added is apparent.

This confirms that the prescribed dose of medication has been added to the IV solution.

7 Dispose of equipment according to agency policy.

This prevents inadvertent injury from the equipment.

8 Wash your hands.

Handwashing deters the spread of microorganisms.

9 Chart the addition of medication to the IV solution.

Accurate documentation is necessary to prevent medication errors.

10 Evaluate the client's response to medication within the appropriate time frame.

Clients require careful observation because medications given by the IV route may have a rapid effect.

Adding a Bolus IV Medication to an Existing IV

Equipment

Medication prepared in a syringe with 23- to 25-gauge, 1-inch needle

Alcohol swab

Watch with second hand

Action	Rationale
1 Gather the equipment and bring to the client's bedside. Check the medication order with the physician's order.	Having the equipment available saves time and facilitates performance of the task. Checking the orders ensures that the client receives the correct medication at the correct time and in the right manner.
2 Explain the procedure to the client.	Explanation allays the client's anxiety.
3 Wash your hands.	Handwashing deters the spread of microorganisms.
4 Identify the client by checking the band on the client's wrist and asking the client his or her name.	This ensures that the medication is given to the right person.
5 Assess the IV site for the presence of inflammation or infiltration.	IV medication must be given directly into a vein for safe administration.
6 Select the injection port on the tubing that is closest to the venipuncture site. Clean the port with an alcohol swab.	Using the port closest to the needle insertion site minimizes dilution of the medication. Cleansing with alcohol deters entry of microorganisms when the needle punctures the port.
7 Uncap the syringe. Steady the port with your nondominant hand while inserting the needle into the center of the port.	This supports the injection port and lessens the risk of accidentally dislodging the IV or entering the port incorrectly.
8 Move your nondominant hand to the section of IV tubing just beyond the injection port. Fold the tubing between your fingers to temporarily stop the flow of the IV solution.	This minimizes the dilution of IV medication with IV solution.
9 Pull back slightly on the plunger just until blood appears in the tubing.	This ensures injection of medication into a vein.
10 Inject the medication at the prescribed rate.	This delivers the correct amount of medication at the proper interval.

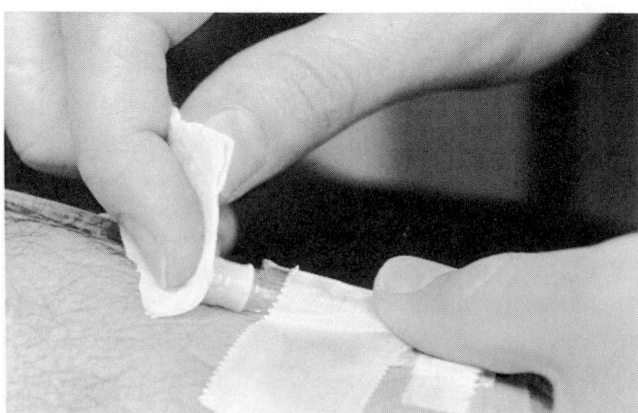

Step 6: Cleaning injection port.

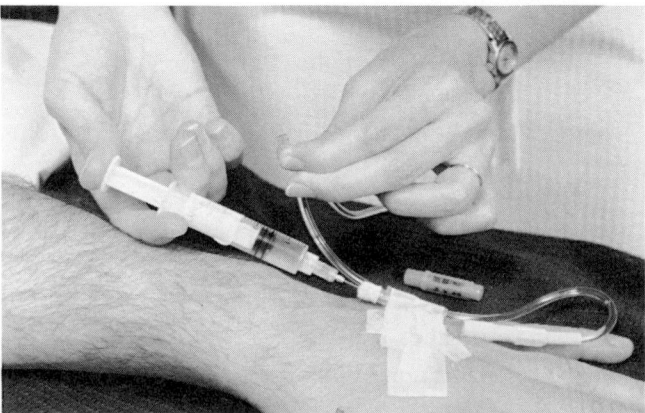

Step 10: Injecting medication while interrupting IV flow.

(Continued)

Action

11 Remove the needle. Do not cap it. Release the tubing and allow the IV to flow at the proper rate.	This prevents accidental needle stick.
12 Dispose of the needle and syringe in the proper receptacle.	Proper disposal of the needle prevents accidental injury and spread of microorganisms.
13 Wash your hands.	Handwashing deters the spread of microorganisms.
14 Chart the administration of the medication.	Accurate documentation is necessary to prevent medication errors.
15 Evaluate the client's response to the medication within the appropriate time frame.	The client requires careful observation because medications given by an IV bolus injection may have a rapid effect.

PROCEDURE 40-10
Administering Medications by IV Piggyback

Equipment

Medication preparation in labeled piggyback set (50 ml–100 ml)	Sterile needle (21- to 23-gauge)	Tape
Secondary infusion tubing (microdrip or macrodrip)	Alcohol swab	

Action

Rationale

1 Gather all equipment and bring to the client's bedside. Check the medication order against the original physician's order according to agency policy.	Having equipment available saves time and facilitates performance of the task. Checking the orders ensures that the client receives the correct medication at the correct time and in the right manner.
2 Explain the procedure to the client.	Explanation allays the client's anxiety.
3 Wash your hands.	Handwashing deters the spread of microorganisms.
4 Assess the IV site for the presence of inflammation or infiltration.	IV medications must be given directly into a vein for safe administration.
5 Attach the infusion tubing to the piggyback set containing diluted medication. Open the clamp and prime the tubing (see Step 5, Procedure 40-8). Close the clamp. Connect the capped sterile needle to the sterile end of the tubing.	This removes air from the tubing and preserves the sterility of the set-up.
6 Hang the piggyback container on the IV pole, positioning it at same level or higher than the primary IV according to the manufacturer's recommendations.	The position of the container influences the flow of the IV fluid into the primary set-up.

(Continued)

Administering Medications by IV Piggyback   (Continued)

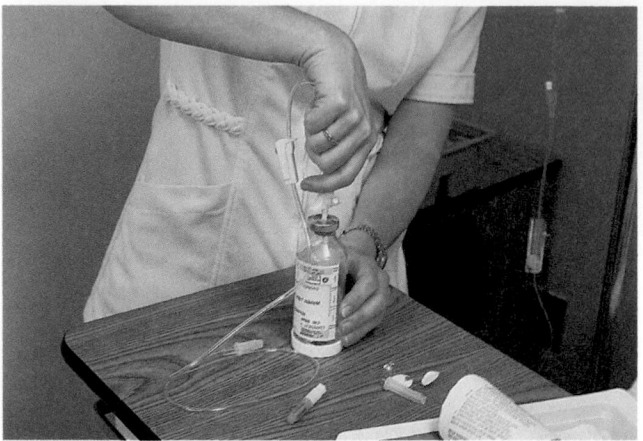

Step 5: Attaching infusion tubing to piggyback set containing medication.

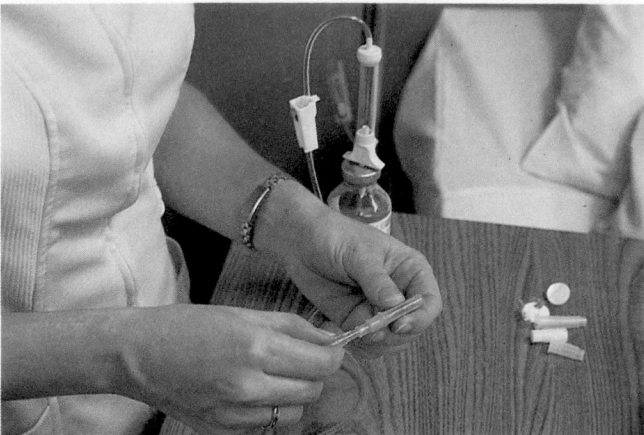

Step 5: Connecting capped sterile needle to tubing.

Action

7 Identify the client by checking the identification band on the client's wrist and asking the client his or her name.

8 Use an alcohol swab to cleanse the secondary IV port.

9 Remove the cap and insert the needle into the secondary port. Use a strip of tape to secure the secondary set tubing to the primary infusion tubing.

Rationale

This ensures that the medication is given to the right person.

This deters entry of microorganisms when the needle punctures the port.

The tape stabilizes the needle in the infusion port and prevents it from slipping out.

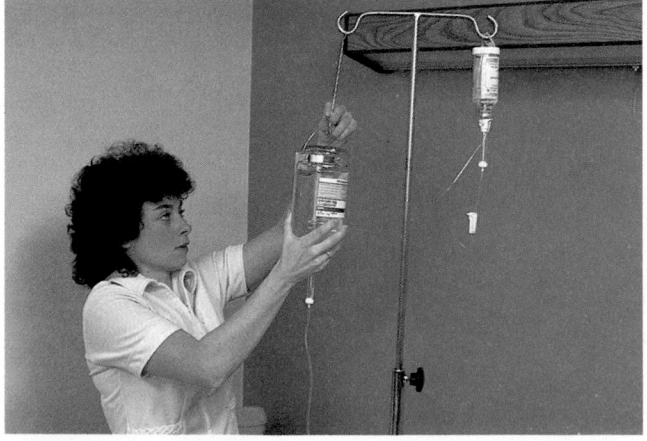

Step 6: Hanging on IV pole.

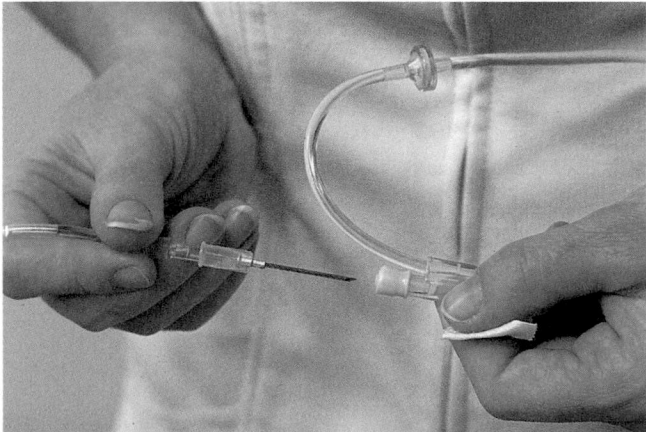

Step 9: Inserting needle into secondary port.

10 Open the clamp on the piggyback set and regulate the flow at the prescribed delivery rate. Monitor the medication infusion at periodic intervals.

11 Clamp the tubing on the piggyback set when the solution is infused. Follow agency policy regarding disposal of equipment.

Delivery over a 30- to 60-minute interval is a safe method of administering IV medication.

This reduces the risk of contaminating the primary IV set-up.

(Continued)

Action	Rationale
12 Readjust the flow rate of the primary IV.	Piggyback medication administration may interrupt the normal flow rate of the primary IV. Readjustment of the rate may be necessary.
13 Wash your hands.	Handwashing deters the spread of microorganisms.
14 Chart the administration of medication after it has been infused.	Accurate documentation is necessary to prevent medication errors.
15 Evaluate the client's response to medication within the appropriate time frame.	The client requires careful observation because medications given by the IV route may have a rapid effect.

P R O C E D U R E 40-11
Administering IV Medications by Volume-Control Administration Set

Equipment

Volume-control administration set (50 ml–100 ml)	Syringe with 20- or 21-gauge needle attached	Medication label
Medication (in vial or ampule)	Alcohol swab	

Action	Rationale
1 Gather all equipment and bring to the client's bedside. Check the medication order against the original physician's order according to agency policy.	Having equipment available saves time and facilitates performance of the task. Checking of the orders ensures that the client receives the correct medication at the correct time and in the right manner.
2 Explain the procedure to the client.	Explanation allays the client's anxiety.
3 Wash your hands.	Handwashing deters the spread of microorganisms.
4 Assess the IV site for the presence of inflammation or infiltration.	IV medications must be given directly into a vein for safe administration.
5 Withdraw medication from the vial or ampule into the prepared syringe. See Procedure 40-2 or 40-3.	The correct dose is prepared for dilution in the IV solution.
6 Identify the client by checking the identification band on the client's wrist and asking the client his or her name.	This ensures that medication is given to the right person.
7 Open the clamp between the IV solution and the volume-control administration set or secondary set-up. Follow the manufacturer's instructions and fill with the desired amount of IV solution. Close the clamp.	This dilutes the medication in the minimal amount of solution. Reclamping prevents the continued addition of fluid to the volume to be mixed with the medication.

(Continued)

Action

Rationale

8 Use an alcohol swab to cleanse the injection port on the secondary set-up.

This deters entry of microorganisms when the needle punctures the port.

9 Remove the cap and insert the needle into the port while holding the syringe steady. Inject the medication. Mix gently with IV solution.

This ensures that the medication is evenly mixed with solution.

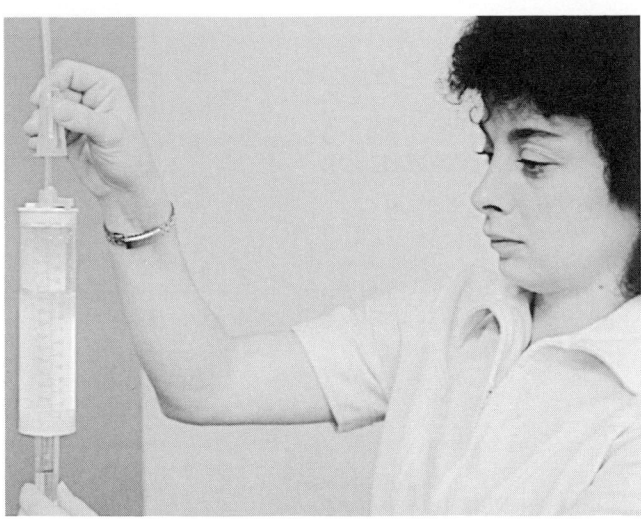

Step 7: Filling volume control set.

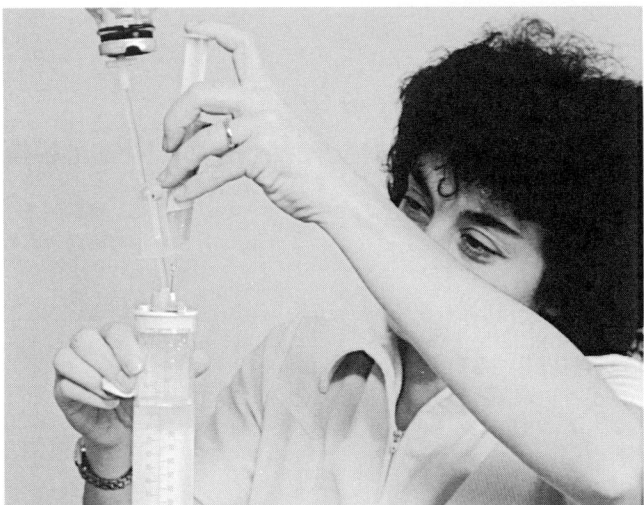

Step 9: Injecting medication.

10 Open the clamp below the secondary set-up and regulate at the prescribed delivery rate. Monitor the medication infusion at periodic intervals.

Delivery over a 30- to 60-minute interval is a safe method of administering IV medication.

11 Attach the label to the volume-control device.

This prevents medication error.

12 Place the syringe with the uncapped needle in the designated container.

Proper disposal of the needle prevents inadvertent needle stick.

13 Wash your hands.

Handwashing deters the spread of microorganisms.

14 Chart the administration of the medication after it has been infused.

Accurate documentation is necessary to prevent medication errors.

15 Evaluate the client's response to the medication within the appropriate time frame.

The client requires careful observation because medications given via the IV route may have a rapid effect.

PROCEDURE 40-12
Introducing Drugs Through a Heparin Lock and the Heparin Flush

Equipment

Medication
Medication card or
  Kardex

Sterile syringe and
  needle (25-
  gauge) with 1
  ml of diluted
  heparin flush
  solution
  (usually 1:1000
  solution of hep-
  arin sodium)
Sterile syringe and
  needle (25-
  gauge) with 2
  ml of sterile sa-
  line and extra
  25-gauge needle

Watch with second
  hand or digital
  readout
Alcohol swabs

Action

1 Assemble equipment and check the physician's order.

2 Explain the procedure to the client.

3 Wash your hands.

4 Withdraw heparin flush solution and sterile saline from the appropriate vials into the syringes.

5 Clean the rubber diaphragm of the heparin lock with an alcohol swab.

6 Remove the needle cap by pulling it straight off.

7 Stabilize the heparin lock port with your nondominant hand and insert the needle of the syringe containing 2 ml of sterile normal saline into the injection port.

Rationale

This ensures that the client receives the right medication at the right time by the proper route.

Explanation alleviates the client's apprehension about IV drug administration.

Handwashing deters the spread of microorganisms.

Proper technique maintains sterility of syringes and solutions.

Cleansing removes surface bacteria at the heparin lock entry site.

This protects the needle from contact with microorganisms.

This allows for careful insertion of the needle into the center circle of the heparin device.

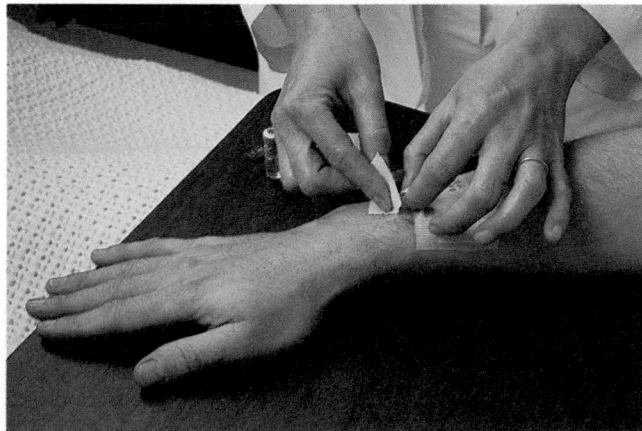

Step 5: Cleaning diaphragm of heparin lock port.

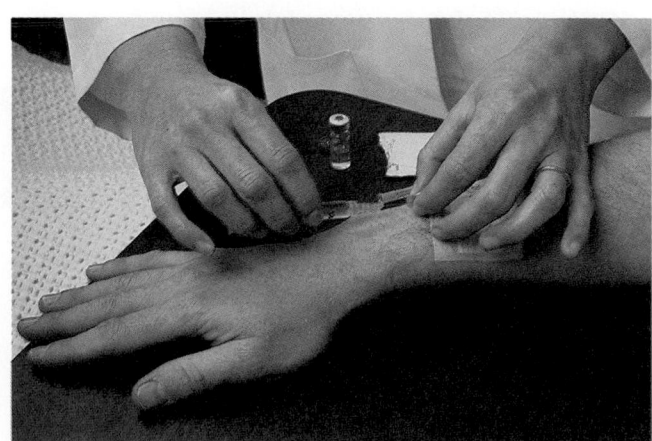

Step 7: Stabilizing heparin lock port and inserting syringe needle.
(Photos © Ken Kasper)

(Continued) **1169**

Action	**Rationale**
8 Aspirate gently and inject 1 ml of saline. (Agency policy may omit use of saline flush prior to administration of medication.) If the lock is clogged it will have to be changed. Do not force saline through a clogged lock.	Blood return indicates that the heparin lock is still patent and in the vein.
9 Remove the needle and discard it in the appropriate receptacle. Replace with an additional sterile 25-gauge needle.	Proper disposal of the needle protects the nurse from an accidental needle stick.
10 If medication is to be given through a heparin lock, check the drug package for the correct injection rate of the bolus of medication. Cleanse the port with an alcohol swab and insert the needle of the syringe with the medication into the port. Inject the medication, using a watch to verify correct injection rate.	After patency has been established and the site has been cleansed, the medication can be administered. A slow rate of infusion allows the nurse to assess for adverse reactions to the drug.
11 Remove the medication syringe and needle. Insert the needle of the syringe containing saline and flush the reservoir with the remaining 1 ml of sterile saline. Remove the syringe and needle and discard in the appropriate receptacle.	Saline clears the line of medication.
12 Cleanse the port of the heparin lock with an alcohol swab. Insert the needle of the syringe containing 1 ml of heparinized saline and instill the solution into the lock device. Remove the syringe and needle and discard in the appropriate receptacle.	Injecting heparin ensures the patency of the lock between injections by preventing the formation of blood clots in the needle. Usually 1 ml fills the heparin lock catheter.
13 Wash your hands.	Handwashing deters the spread of microorganisms.
14 The injection site and heparin lock should be checked at least every 8 hours and a small amount of heparinized saline administered if medication is not given at least that often.	This ensures the patency of the system for continuing injections.
15 The heparin lock should be changed at least every 48 hours. A clogged lock should be changed immediately.	Changing a heparin lock regularly and having it free of clotted blood reduces dangers of infection and emboli in the circulating blood.
16 Chart the administration of the heparin flush or medication.	Accurate documentation is necessary to prevent medication error.

Administering Topical Medications

When a drug is applied directly to a body site, it is called a **topical application**. Other terms sometimes used include the *dermal* and *mucosal route*.

Topical applications usually are intended for direct action on a particular site, although some systemic effect may also occur. The action depends on the type of tissue and on the nature of the agent.

If the site of application is readily accessible, such as the skin, an agent can be placed on it easily. If it is a cavity, such as the nose, or is enclosed, such as the eye, it is necessary to use a mechanical applicator for introducing the drug.

Skin Applications

The skin is a mechanical and chemical barrier protecting the underlying tissues. It is a sense organ, having receptors that respond to touch, pain, pressure, and temperature. It functions to help in excretion, regulation of the body's temperature, and the storage of such essentials to the body as water, salts, and glucose.

When a drug is incorporated in an agent, such as an ointment, and is rubbed into the skin for absorption, the procedure is referred to as an **inunction**. On normal skin, drugs are absorbed into the lining of the sebaceous glands. Absorption is hindered because of the protective outer layer of the skin, which makes penetration difficult, and because of the fatty substances that protect the lining of the glands. Absorption can be enhanced by cleaning the skin well with soap or detergent and water prior to administration and then rubbing the medicated preparation into the skin. Absorption also can be improved by using the drug in a vehicle, such as an ointment, or a volatile vehicle as used in many of the liniments that will mix with the fat in the gland lining. The following are typical preparations applied to skin areas, and their primary purposes:

- *Powders:* To promote drying of the skin and to prevent friction on the skin
- *Ointments:* To provide prolonged contact of a medication on the skin and to soften the skin
- *Creams and oils:* To lubricate and soften the skin and to prevent drying of the skin
- *Lotions:* To protect and soothe the skin
- *Counterirritants:* To relieve discomfort
- *Astringents and alcohol:* To cool and dry the skin

The following are recommended nursing measures for applying medications to the skin:

- Be sure the skin is dry and clean before applying anything on it. Most often, previous preparations are removed before applying additional medication, except in the case of lotions used for soothing the skin.
- Cleanse the skin with detergent or soap and water before administering a preparation to the skin. This technique removes substances from the skin that will delay absorption of the drug and prevents debris from interfering with the desired actions.
- Apply local heat to the area, when indicated. This measure promotes absorption by improving blood circulation to the area.
- Shake lotions, which are suspensions of powder, before using so that the active ingredient reaches the skin in desired amounts. Apply lotions with cotton balls or gauze.
- Thoroughly massage creams and ointments into intact skin, or, if this is contraindicated, pat them onto the skin with the fingers.
- Warm the preparation in the hands or fingers if a large part of the body is to be covered, such as the back. This technique helps prevent the client from feeling chilly.
- Keep powders away from the nose and mouth to prevent the client from inhaling them. If they are applied on or near the face, apply them while the client exhales.
- Follow the manufacturer's directions regarding use of gloves for skin applications.
- Apply nitroglycerin ointment as prescribed in centimeters or inches, measuring the ordered amount on a special paper or plastic applicator.
- Always wear gloves when applying nitroglycerin ointment to the skin because some of the medication can be absorbed through the skin of your fingers.
- Wear gloves, as indicated, especially when the client has a disease condition that is infectious.

Eye Instillations and Irrigations

The receptors for the sense of sight are located in the eye. The outer layer of the eyeball is called the *sclera.* The cornea is the transparent part of the sclera in the front of the eyeball. The sclera is fibrous and tough, but the cornea is injured easily by trauma. For this reason, applications to the eye are rarely placed directly onto the eyeball.

Since direct application cannot be made onto the sensitive cornea, applications intended to act on the eye or the lids are placed onto, or instilled or irrigated into, the lower conjunctival sac.

The eye is a delicate organ, highly susceptible to infection and injury. Although the eye is never free of microorganisms, the secretions of the conjunctiva have a protective action against many pathogens. For maximum safety for the client, equipment, solutions, and ointments introduced into the conjunctival sac should be sterile. If this is not possible, the most careful measures of medical asepsis should be followed.

Eyedrops. Instillation of eyedrops is done for their local effects, such as for dilatation or constriction of the pupil when examining the eye or for treating an infection. The type and the amount of solution depend on the purpose of the instillation.

Exposing the lower conjunctival sac is necessary for eye instillations. It is important to work carefully and gently to prevent injuring the conjunctiva and the eyeball when exposing the sac. This is particularly important when the lids are swollen, inflamed, or tender. The following techniques are used to expose the lower conjunctival sac and instill eyedrops:

- Offer the client paper tissues to remove solution and tears that may spill from the eye during the procedure.
- Cleanse the eyelids and eyelashes of any drainage with cotton balls or gauze pledgets moistened with normal saline because debris can be carried into

the eye when the conjunctival sac is exposed. Use each cotton ball for only one stroke, moving from the inner toward the outer canthus to prevent carrying debris to the lacrimal ducts.

- Tilt the client's head back slightly if sitting, or place the client's head over a pillow if lying down. The head may be turned slightly to the affected side to prevent solution or tears from flowing toward the opposite eye.
- Draw up only sufficient solution required for the eyedrops. Hold the dropper with the bulb higher than the dropper. Allowing solution to enter the bulb by holding the bulb lower than the dropper may result in contaminating the solution with particles in the bulb. Unused solution should not be returned to a stock bottle.
- Have the client look up while focusing on something on the ceiling.
- Place the thumb or two fingers near the margin of the lower eyelid immediately below the eyelashes, and exert pressure downward over the bony prominence of the cheek. The lower conjunctival sac is exposed as the lower lid is pulled down.
- Hold the dropper close to the eye, but avoid touching the eyelids or lashes, which may startle the client and cause blinking. Also, avoid touching the eyeball with the dropper because this could easily injure the eye.
- Allow the prescribed number of drops to fall in the lower conjunctival sac. Do not allow drops to fall onto the cornea because of the danger of injuring it and the unpleasant sensation it causes the client.
- Release the lower lid after the eyedrops are instilled. Ask the client to gently close the eyes.
- Apply gentle pressure over the inner canthus to prevent the eyedrops from flowing into the tear duct. This minimizes the risk of systemic effects from the medication.

Figure 40-19 illustrates a nurse exposing the lower conjunctival sac and instilling eyedrops.

Ointments.   Various types of medications in an ointment form may be prescribed for the eye. These ointments are usually used in the presence of a local infection or irritation. Eye ointments are dispensed in a tube. A small amount of ointment is distributed along the exposed lower conjunctival sac after the eyelids and eyelashes have been cleansed. About ½ inch of ointment is squeezed from the tube along the exposed sac. Following the application, the eyes should be closed. The warmth helps to liquify the ointment. Also, the client should be instructed to move the eye because this helps to spread ointment under the lids and over the surface of the eyeball.

Eye Irrigation.   An eye **irrigation** is done frequently to remove secretions from the eye. In an emergency, an eye irrigation can be done to remove chemicals that may burn the eye. Copious amounts of tap water should be

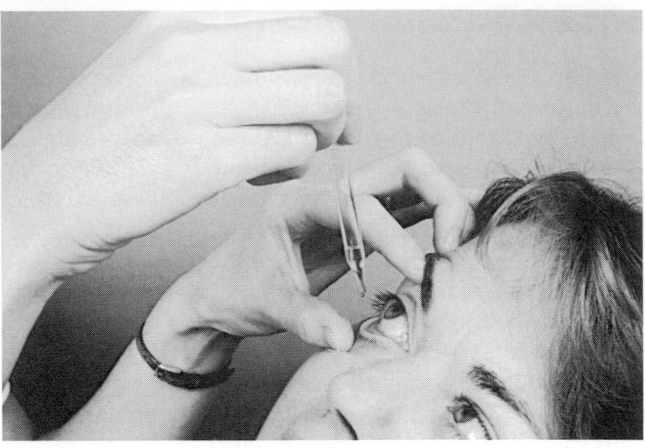

F I G U R E   40-19
The nurse exposes the lower conjunctiva of the eye, where she will place eyedrops by having the patient look up and by applying pressure downward over the bony prominence of the cheek. (Photo © Ken Kasper)

used to remove chemicals such as acid. The irrigation should continue for at least 15 minutes, and then professional help should be sought.

The techniques for administering a conjunctival irrigation are described in Procedure 40-13.

Ear Instillations and Irrigations

The ear contains the receptors for hearing and for equilibrium. It consists of the external ear, the middle ear, and the inner ear. The external ear consists of the auricle or pinna and the exterior auditory canal. The auditory canal serves as a passageway for sound waves. Drugs or irrigations are instilled into the auditory canal.

Drugs in solution are placed in the auditory canal for their local effect. They are used to soften wax, relieve pain, apply local anesthesia, destroy organisms, or destroy an insect lodged in the canal, which can cause almost intolerable discomfort.

The tympanic membrane separates the external ear from the middle ear. Normally, it is intact and closes the entrance to the middle ear completely. If it is ruptured or has been opened by surgical intervention, the middle ear and the inner ear have a direct passage to the external ear. When this occurs, instillations and irrigations should be done with the greatest of care to prevent forcing materials from the outer ear into the middle ear and the inner ear. Sterile technique is used to prevent infection.

Ear Drops.   The following techniques are recommended to place drops in the external auditory canal:

- Warm the solution to be instilled to body temperature to minimize discomfort for the client.
- Cleanse the external ear of drainage with cotton balls moistened with normal saline, as necessary.
- Place the client on the unaffected side in bed, or, if ambulatory, have the client sit with the head well tilted to the side so that the affected ear is upper-

PROCEDURE 40-13
Administering an Eye Irrigation

Equipment

Sterile irrigating so-
lution (warmed
to 37°C
[98.6°F])
Sterile irrigation set
(sterile con-
tainer and irri-
gating or bulb
syringe)
Cotton balls

Emesis basin or irri-
gation basin
Disposable gloves
(optional)

Waterproof pad
Towel

Action

1 Explain procedure to client.

2 Assemble equipment.

3 Wash your hands.

4 Have the client sit or lie with the head tilted toward the side of the affected eye. Protect the client
and the bed with a waterproof pad.

5 Don disposable gloves if infection is present. Clean
the lids and the lashes with a cotton ball moistened
with normal saline or the solution ordered for the
irrigation. Wipe from the inner canthus to the outer
canthus. Discard the cotton ball after each wipe.

6 Place the curved basin at the cheek on the side of
the affected eye to receive the irrigating solution. If
sitting up, ask the client to support the basin.

7 Expose the lower conjunctival sac and hold the
upper lid open with your nondominant hand.

Rationale

Explanation facilitates cooperation and provides reassurance for the client.

This provides for an organized approach to the task.

Handwashing deters the spread of microorganisms.

Gravity will aid the flow of solution away from the unaffected eye and from the inner canthus of the affected
eye toward the outer canthus.

Materials lodged on the lids or in the lashes may be
washed into the eye. This cleansing motion protects
the nasolacrimal duct and the other eye.

Gravity will aid the flow of solution.

The solution is directed onto the lower conjunctival sac
because the cornea is very sensitive and easily injured.
This also prevents reflex blinking.

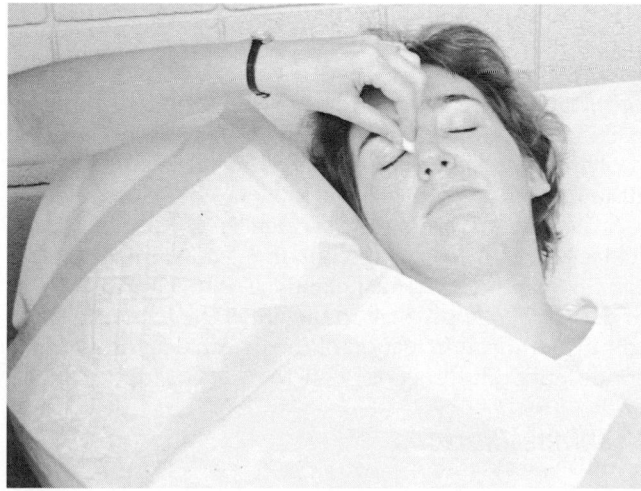

Step 5: Cleansing lids and lashes from inside of eye to outside.

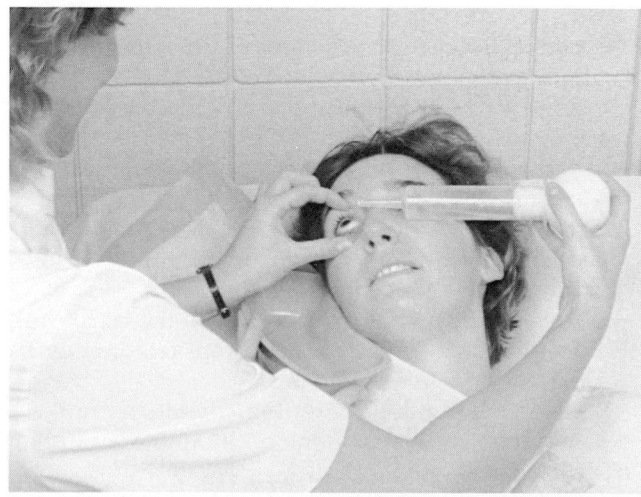

Step 7: Preparing to irrigate the eye. (Photos © Ken Kasper)

(Continued)

Action	**Rationale**
8 Hold the irrigator about 2.5 cm (1 inch) from the eye. Direct the flow of the solution from the inner canthus to the outer canthus along the conjunctival sac.	This minimizes the risk of injury to the cornea. Solution directed toward the outer canthus helps prevent the spread of contamination from the eye to the lacrimal sac, the lacrimal duct, and the nose.
9 Irrigate until the solution is clear or all of the solution has been used. Use only sufficient force gently to remove secretions from the conjunctiva. Avoid touching any part of the eye with the irrigating tip.	Directing solutions with force may cause injury to the tissues of the eye, as well as to the conjunctiva. Touching the eye is uncomfortable for the client.
10 Have the client close the eye periodically during the procedure.	Movement of the eye when the lids are closed helps move secretions from the upper conjunctival sac to the lower.
11 Dry the area after the irrigation with cotton balls or a gauze sponge. Offer a towel to the client if the face and neck are wet.	Leaving the skin moist after an irrigation is uncomfortable for the client.
12 Wash your hands.	Handwashing deters the spread of microorganisms.
13 Chart the irrigation, appearance of the eye, drainage, and the client's response.	This provides accurate documentation.

most. This positioning prevents the drops from escaping from the ear.

- Draw up the amount of solution needed in the dropper. Draw up only the amount needed. Excess medication should not be returned to a stock bottle.
- Straighten the auditory canal by pulling on the cartilaginous portion of the pinna up and back in an adult, and down and back if the client is an infant or a child under 3 years of age. In an adult, the auditory canal is directed inward, forward, and down. In the child, the canal is chiefly cartilaginous and almost straight, with the floor of the auditory canal resting on the tympanic membrane. Pulling on the pinna as described helps straighten the canal properly for ear instillation.
- Hold the dropper in the ear with its tip above the auditory canal. For an infant or an irrational or restless client, protect the dropper with a piece of soft tubing to help prevent injury to the ear.
- Allow the drops to fall on the side of the canal. It is uncomfortable for the client if drops fall directly onto the tympanic membrane.
- Release the pinna after instilling the drops, and have the client maintain the position to prevent the escape of the medication.
- Gently press on the tragus a few times to help move the medication from the canal toward the tympanic membrane.

- Insert a loose, cotton wick when continuous application of the medication in the canal is desired. The wick should be removed 30 minutes after insertion. A tightly packed wick is contraindicated because it interferes with outward movement of secretions and may cause excessive pressure.
- Wait 5 minutes before instilling drops in the second ear, if ordered.

Figure 40-20 illustrates a nurse about to instill drops in the ear of an adult. Figure 40-21 illustrates the instillation of ear drops for a child.

Ear Irrigations. Irrigations of the external auditory canal are ordinarily done for cleansing purposes or for applying heat to the area. Usually, normal saline is used, although an antiseptic solution may be indicated for local action. An irrigation syringe is used in most instances. Or, an irrigating container with tubing and an ear tip may be used, especially if the purpose of the irrigation is to apply heat to the area. The techniques for administering an irrigation of the external auditory canal are described in Procedure 40-14.

Nasal Instillations

Besides serving as the olfactory organ, the nose also functions as an airway to the lower respiratory tract and protects the tract by cleaning and warming the air that is

PROCEDURE 40-14
Administering an Ear Irrigation

Equipment

Prescribed irrigating solution (warmed to 37°C [98.6°F])

Irrigation set (container and irrigating or bulb syringe)

Emesis basin

Cotton-tipped applicators

Cotton balls

Waterproof pad

Action

1 Explain the procedure to the client.

2 Assemble the equipment. Protect the client and bed linens with a moisture-proof pad.

3 Wash your hands.

4 Have the client sit up or lie with the head tilted toward the side of the affected ear. Have the client support a basin under the ear to receive the irrigating solution.

5 Clean the pinna and the meatus at the auditory canal as necessary with the applicators dipped in normal saline or the irrigating solution.

6 Fill the bulb syringe with solution. If an irrigating container is used, allow air to escape from the tubing.

7 Straighten the auditory canal by pulling the pinna down and back for an infant and up and back for an adult.

8 Direct a steady, slow stream of solution against the roof of the auditory canal, using only sufficient force to remove secretions. Do not occlude the auditory canal with the irrigating nozzle. Allow solution to flow out unimpeded.

Rationale

Explanation facilitates cooperation and provides reassurance for the client.

This provides for an organized approach to the task.

Handwashing deters the spread of microorganisms.

Gravity causes the irrigating solution to flow from the ear to the basin.

Materials lodged on the pinna and at the meatus may be washed into the ear.

Air forced into the ear canal is noisy and therefore unpleasant for the client.

Straightening the ear canal aids in allowing solution to reach all areas of the canal easily.

Solution directed at the roof of the canal aids in preventing injury to the tympanic membrane. Continuous in-and-out flow of the irrigating solution helps prevent pressure in the canal.

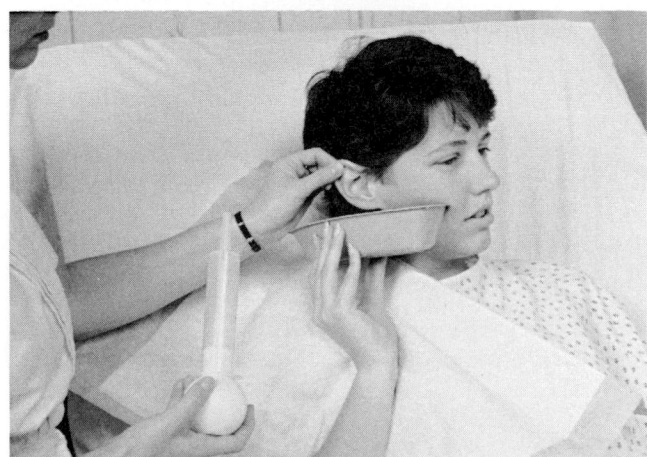

Step 7: Straightening the auditory canal.

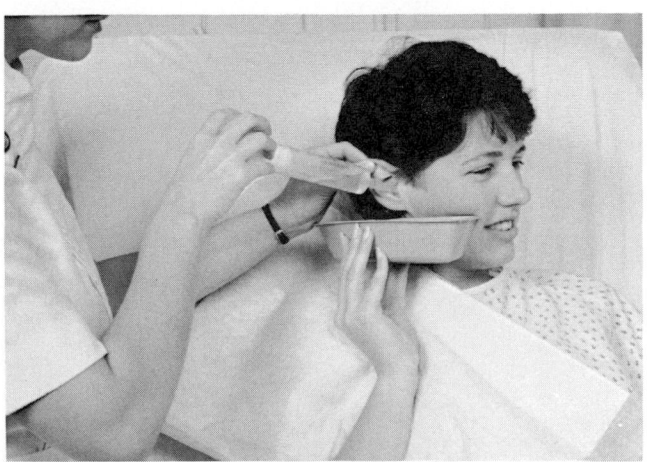

Step 8: Instilling irrigation fluid. (Photos © Ken Kasper)

(Continued)

Action

9 When the irrigation is completed, place a cotton ball loosely in the auditory meatus and have the client lie on the side of the affected ear on a towel or an absorbent pad.

10 Wash your hands.

11 Chart the irrigation, the appearance of the drainage, and the client's response.

12 Return in 10 to 15 minutes and remove the cotton ball and assess drainage.

Rationale

The cotton ball absorbs excess fluid and gravity allows the remaining solution in the canal to escape from the ear.

Handwashing deters the spread of microorganisms.

This provides accurate documentation.

Drainage or pain may indicate injury to the tympanic membrane.

taken in by inspiration. Cilia project on most of the surfaces of the nasal mucous membrane and are important in helping to remove particles of dirt and dust from the inspired air. The nose also serves as a resonator when speaking and singing.

Nasal instillations are used to treat sinus infections and nasal congestion. Medications having a systemic effect such as vasopressin may also be prepared as a nasal instillation. Normally, the nose is not a sterile cavity. However, because of its connection with the sinuses, medical asepsis should be observed carefully when using nasal instillations. The following are recommended techniques to instill nose drops:

- Provide the client with paper tissues for the expectoration of secretions.
- Have the client sit up with head tilted well back. Or, if the client is lying down, tilt the head back over a pillow. These positions allow the solution to flow well back into the nares.
- Draw sufficient solution into the dropper for both nares. Excessive solution should not be returned to a stock bottle.
- Hold up the tip of the nose and place the dropper just inside the nares, about one third of an inch. Instill the prescribed number of drops in one naris and then into the other. Protect the dropper with a

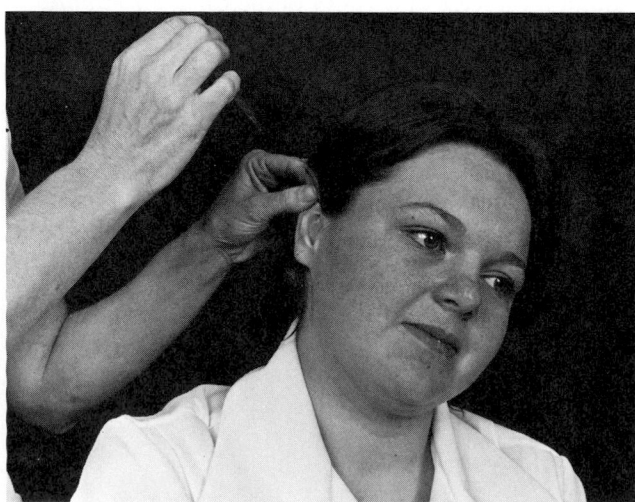

F I G U R E   40-20
The nurse pulls the pinna of the ear up and back in order to straighten the ear canal in this adult patient. She then will place eardrops on the side of the canal.

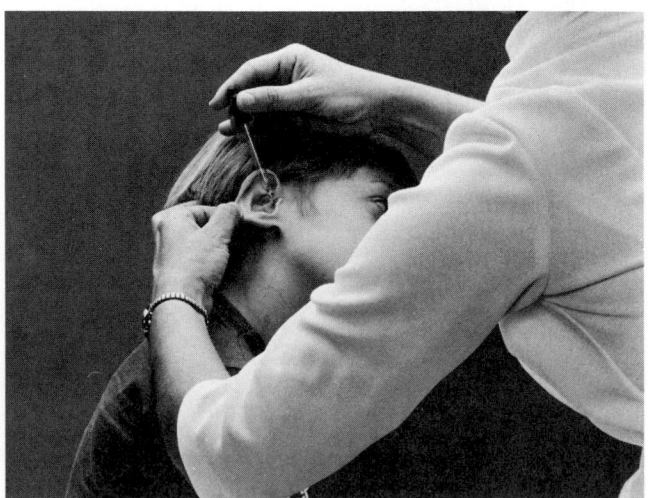

F I G U R E   40-21
The nurse pulls the pinna of the ear down and back in order to straighten the auditory canal in the child. She will then place the eardrops on the side of the canal.

piece of soft tubing when the client is an infant or small child.

- Avoid touching the nares with the dropper because it may cause the client to sneeze.
- Have the client remain in position with the head tilted back for a few minutes to prevent the escape of the solution.

Figure 40-22 illustrates a nurse instilling nose drops.

Solutions that are instilled by drops may also be applied to the nasal mucous membrane by using a spray. A small atomizer generally is used. The end of the nose is held up, and the tip of the nozzle is placed just inside the naris and directed backward. Only sufficient force to bring the spray into contact with the membrane is used. Too much force may drive the solution and contamination into the sinuses and eustachian tubes.

Vaginal Applications

A healthy vagina contains few pathogens but many non-pathogenic organisms. The nonpathogens are important because they protect the vagina from the invasion of pathogens. The normal secretions in the vagina are acidic in reaction and further serve to protect the vagina from microbial invasion. Therefore, the normal mucous membrane is its own best protection.

Creams can be applied intravaginally, using a narrow, tubular applicator with an attached plunger. Suppositories that melt when exposed to body heat are also prepared for vaginal insertion. Suppositories should normally be refrigerated for storage.

The client should be asked to void prior to inserting the medication. The client is positioned lying on her back with the knees flexed. Privacy should be maintained with draping. Adequate light should be available to visualize the vaginal opening.

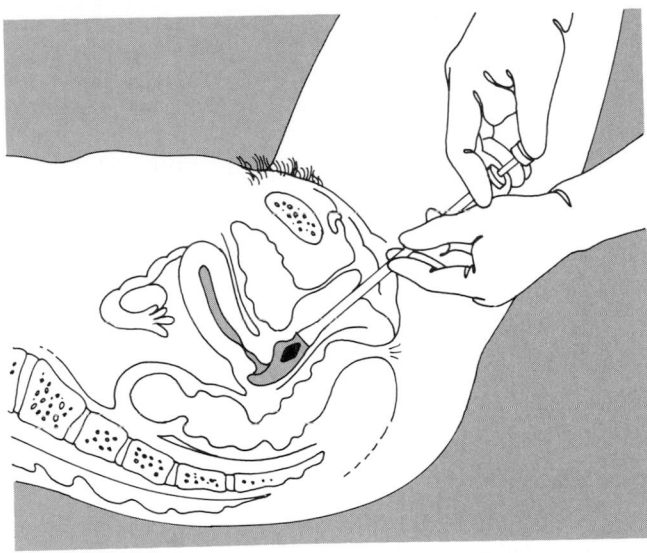

F I G U R E 40-23
Cream or suppository vaginal preparations should be inserted well into the vagina using an applicator or a gloved hand.

The following are recommended techniques for introducing a suppository or cream into the vagina:

- Fill a vaginal applicator with the prescribed amount of cream. Or, have a suppository ready.
- Lubricate the applicator with water, as necessary. A suppository may be lubricated with a water-soluble gel. Ordinarily, lubrication is unnecessary but may be used to reduce friction while inserting the applicator or suppository.
- Wear disposable gloves.
- Use clean aseptic technique to administer the medication.
- Spread the labia well with the fingers, and cleanse the area at the vaginal orifice with cotton balls and warm water to remove discharge, as necessary. With each cotton ball, use a single stroke moving from above the orifice downward toward the sacrum. These techniques prevent contamination of the vaginal orifice with debris surrounding the anus.
- Introduce the applicator gently in a rolling manner while directing it downward and backward to follow the normal contour of the vagina for its full length. Push the plunger to its full length, and then gently remove the applicator with the plunger depressed. After the applicator is properly positioned, the labia may be allowed to fall in place to free the nurse's hand for manipulating the plunger. Insert a suppository with gloved fingers well into the vagina.
- Ask the client to remain in the supine position for 5 to 10 minutes after insertion.
- Offer the client a perineal pad to collect excess drainage.
- Instruct proper techniques to the client who wishes to administer vaginal suppositories and creams herself.

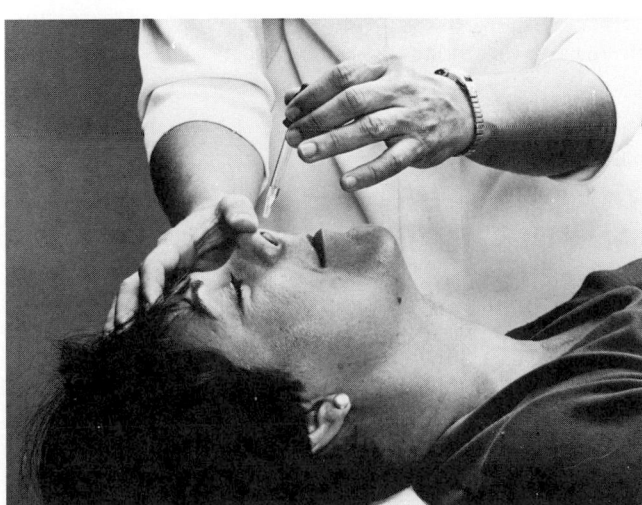

F I G U R E 40-22
The nurse is preparing to instill nose drops. Note that the patient's head is tilted back to facilitate proper placement of the medication.

Rectal Instillations

Rectal suppositories are used primarily for their local action, such as a laxative and fecal softener. However, systemic effects are also achieved with rectal suppositories. Acetaminophen suppositories are utilized for an antipyretic effect, and many antiemetics are available in suppository form to relieve nausea and vomiting.

The following are recommended techniques for inserting a rectal suppository:

- Use a finger cot or a glove to protect your fingers while inserting the suppository.
- Have the client lie on either side, and pie-fold top linens over the client.
- Lubricate the suppository and your fingertips to reduce irritation on intestinal mucosa while inserting the suppository.
- Separate the buttocks, and then have the client relax by breathing through the mouth while the suppository is inserted.
- Introduce the suppository well beyond the internal sphincter so that the suppository is in the rectum, approximately 4 inches for adults and 2 inches for infants and children.
- Ask the client to remain in this position for 5 minutes. If the suppository has been given for a laxative effect, the client should be instructed to retain the suppository until the urge to defecate is experienced, usually 30 minutes after insertion.

Administering Medications by Inhalation

The lungs are richly supplied with blood and have a large surface area. These characteristics allow drugs to

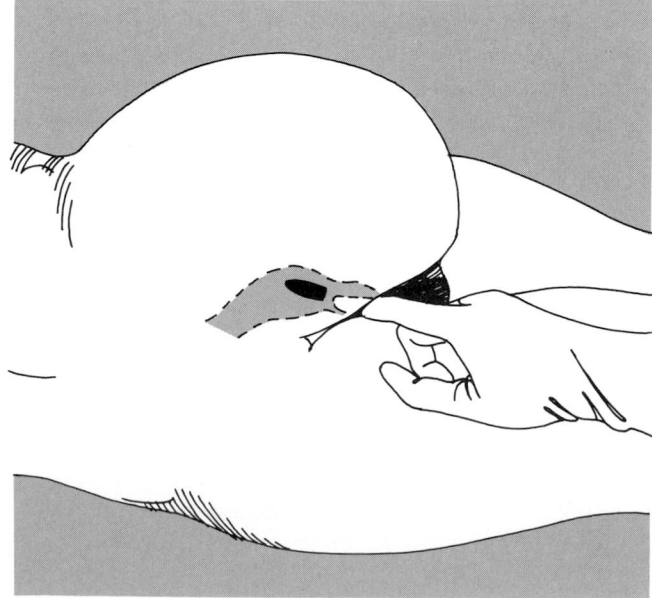

F I G U R E   40-24
Rectal suppositories should be introduced through the anus well beyond the internal sphincter.

be absorbed from the lower respiratory tract. The smaller the particles of inhaled medication, the lower in the respiratory tract the medication tends to travel. A disadvantage of using this route is that the drug dosage is difficult to establish.

Drugs classified as bronchodilators and decongestants are frequently administered by **inhalation**. They act to decrease resistance to air flow by providing an enlarged passageway. Decongestants are local vasoconstrictors. Bronchodilators promote relaxation of musculature in the tracheobronchial tree. The relaxed passages produce less resistance to air flow and provide an opened respiratory passageway. Bronchodilators are further discussed in Chapter 34.

Drugs for inhalation may be administered by a hand atomizer or nebulizer. These work to cause increased pressure in the unit, which forces solution into a specially constructed strictured device. The force with which the solution is made to move through the stricture and to leave the container is sufficient to break the large droplets of medication into a mist.

Nebulization can also be accomplished by using the force of an oxygen stream or compressed air passed through the fluid in a nebulizer or an atomizer. This method is valuable for clients who require inhalation of a drug several times a day when the hand atomizer or nebulizer is fatiguing. The oxygen stream is also useful in the production of vapors when high humidity is needed continuously for long periods of time. One of the most common means of administering a nebulized drug using air pressure is the intermittent positive-pressure breathing machine, which is discussed in Chapter 34.

A popular nebulizer now on the market is one that supplies premeasured amounts of medication each time the nebulizer releases the drug in solution. This equipment helps control the amount of medication the client receives and minimizes the dangers of overdosing when ordinary hand nebulizers are used. Figure 40-25 illustrates and describes this nebulizer.

DOCUMENTING MEDICATION ADMINISTRATION

The medication record is a legal document. Recording each dose of medication as soon as possible after it is given leaves a documented record that can be consulted if there is any question as to whether the client received the medication. The nurse should not record medications before they are given. If the medications are not given, the medication record would show the client received the medication when in fact that was not true.

Different forms are utilized for recording medications. However, the name of the medication, dosage, route of administration, time given, and the nurse's initials are always noted on the form. The site used for an

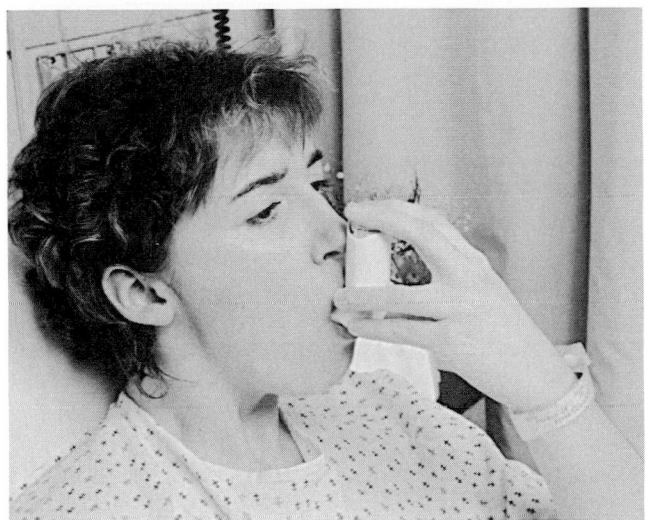

FIGURE 40-25
Inhaler. A bottle of medication is attached to a mouthpiece. After the client exhales, the mouthpiece is gripped with the lips, and while the client takes a deep inhalation slowly, the bottle is firmly pushed down on the mouthpiece to release one dose of medication. (Photo © Ken Kasper)

injection should be recorded. The nurse's full signature must appear on the form for initial identification. Other specific client information may be required. For instance, the pulse rate may be recorded when administering some cardiac drugs, or a description of the effects on the client's pain when administering analgesics.

Omitted Drugs. Drugs may be omitted intentionally or inadvertently. The omission and the reason for it are documented on the client's record. Drugs may be omitted intentionally for the following reasons:

- The client is to have a diagnostic test and is to fast prior to the test. Oral drugs are usually omitted or their administration is delayed, depending on the physician's wishes.
- The problem for which the medication is intended no longer exists. For example, a laxative has been ordered for a client. However, the client has a bowel movement and no longer needs the laxative. The laxative is then omitted.
- The client is suspected of having an allergy to the medication. Any suspected allergy should be reported to the physician.

Inadvertent omission of a drug should be reported as soon as it is detected to determine whether a dose should be administered at that time. For example, a certain medication given daily might be administered in the afternoon when it is discovered that it had been inadvertently omitted in the morning.

Refused Drugs. If the client refuses a drug that is considered essential to the therapeutic regimen, the nurse should report this promptly. Frequently, the nurse can play an important role in determining the reason for the refusal and can help the client accept needed drugs. However, if reasonable efforts fail to accomplish this, it is unwise to continue urging the client who adamantly refuses a medication. Clients have the right to refuse therapy, and the nurse should recognize and respect that right. Refusals to take prescribed drugs and the manner in which the situation was managed should be described on the client's record and reported according to agency policy.

Medication Errors. The conscientious nurse takes every precaution to avoid errors when administering therapeutic agents. However, humans are subject to occasional poor judgment, and errors unfortunately may occur.

Nursing actions that may result in medication errors include the following:

- The nurse does not know why a medication is to be given or is not familiar with the drug.
- The nurse does not identify the client by checking the identification bracelet and asking the client to say his or her name.
- The nurse does not check with the prescribing physician when the medication order is unclear.
- The nurse carelessly puts down medications before administering them.
- The nurse inaccurately reads labels on medication containers.
- The nurse incorrectly calculates drug dosages.

Prompt acknowledgment of errors can often minimize their possible detrimental effects. The following steps are recommended when a medication error occurs.

- Check the client's condition immediately when the error is noted.
- Notify the physician to discuss possible courses of action, which depend on the client's condition.
- Write a description of the error on the client's permanent record, including remedial steps that were taken.
- Complete a special form for reporting errors, as dictated by agency policy. These forms, frequently called *accident, incident,* or *unusual occurrence reports,* require a full explanation of the situation and the steps that were taken following its commission. For legal reasons, it is essential that errors be described fully and accurately.

TEACHING CLIENTS ABOUT MEDICATIONS

In many cases, clients continue a prescribed medication regimen at home following discharge from the hospital.

(Text continues on p. 1181.)

CROZER-CHESTER MEDICAL CENTER
MEDICATION ADMINISTRATION + PARENTERAL THERAPY RECORD

FORM NS-MAR-1

Legend for Injection Sites

Allergies: Operative Date:
                    Procedure:

Penicillin

RA- Right Arm   RT- Right Thigh
LA- Left Arm   LT- Left Thigh
RB- Right Buttock   R.Abd- Right Abdomen
LB- Left Buttock   L.Abd- Left Abdomen

STANDING ORDERS (MEDICATION ORDERED PER ROUTINE SCHEDULE OR WITH SPECIFIC NUMBER OF DOSES)

ORDER DATE & RN INIT.	EXP. DATE & TIME	MEDICATION, DOSAGE, FREQUENCY, ROUTE	HOURS	11/29 INJ. SITE	INIT.	11/30 INJ. SITE	INIT.	12/1 INJ. SITE	INIT.	12/2	12/3	12/4	12/5	12/6	12/7	12/8
11/29/89 SM		Digoxin 0.25 mg po QD	10A		AC / AR =88		AC / AR =92		CL / AR = 86							
11/29/89 SM		Lasix 20 mg QD po	10A		AC		AC		CL							
11/29/89 SM		Trental 400 mg TIO Po	10A		AC		AC		CL							
			2P		AC		AC		CL							
			6P		PR		PR		PR							
11/29/89 SM		Slow Ktt po QD	10A		AC		AC		(CL)							
11/29/89 SM		Serax 15 mg Po q. 8°	6A		SP		SP		MS							
			2P		AC		AC		CL							
			10P		PR		PR		PR							
11/29/89 SM		Procardia 20 mg po TIO	10A		AC		AC		CL							
			2P		AC		AC		CL							
			6P		PR		PR		PR							

SINGLE ORDERS (STAT, PRE-OP, ONE TIME DOSE, ON CALL, DIAGNOSTIC PREP)

ORDER DATE & RN INIT.	MEDICATION, DOSAGE, ROUTE	TO BE GIVEN DATE	TIME	INJ. SITE	RN INIT.	ORDER DATE & RN INIT.	MEDICATION, DOSAGE, ROUTE	TO BE GIVEN DATE	TIME	INJ. SITE	RN INIT.
11/29 PR	Dalmane 15 mg po now	11/29	11P	–	PR						
11/30	Dulcolax Tab. iii po at 6 pm	11/30	6P		PR						

F I G U R E   40-26
Example of a medication record.

PRN MEDICATIONS (ENTER DATE, TIME GIVEN, INJECTION SITE AND RN INITIALS)																
ORDER DATE & RN INIT.	EXP. DATE & TIME	MEDICATION, DOSES, FREQUENCY, ROUTE		DOSES GIVEN												
11/29/89 SM		Tylox tab ii po q 3° prn	DATE	11/29	11/30											
			TIME	1q	3A											
			INJ.SITE													
			RN INIT.	AC	SP											
11/29/89 SM		Maalox 30cc po q 6° prn	DATE													
			TIME													
			INJ.SITE													
			RN INIT.													
			DATE													
			TIME													
			INJ.SITE													
			RN INIT.													
			DATE													
			TIME													
			INJ.SITE													
			RN INIT.													
			DATE													
			TIME													
			INJ.SITE													
			RN INIT.													
			DATE													
			TIME													
			INJ.SITE													
			RN INIT.													
			DATE													
			TIME													
			INJ.SITE													
			RN INIT.													

PATIENT NAME:

PARENTERAL THERAPY			DOCUMENTATION FOR MEDICATION WITHHELD			
ORDER DATE & RN INIT.	I.V. SOLUTIONS	SCHEDULE	DATE	TIME	MEDICATION	REASON FOR WITHHOLDING
11/29/89 SM	1000 cc D5W	q 8°	12/1	10A	Slow K tab ii	patient refused

RN IDENTIFICATION								
INIT.	SIGNATURE	INIT.	SIGNATURE	INIT.	SIGNATURE
AC	A. Christopher RN				
PR	P Rogers RN				
SP	S. Pointer RN				
CL	C. Lewis RN				

A factor affecting the client's compliance to the medication regimen at home is education about the prescribed medications. Teaching should be tailored to the client's level of understanding. Written instructions can be used as a reference for the client. The client should know the name of the drug, dosage, route of administration, and frequency. A frequent cause of errors in the self-administration of medications is a lack of understanding about the dose and the frequency for taking the medication. The nurse should help the client establish a medication schedule that best fits the prescribed frequency of medications and the client's life-style. Clients can be taught to establish a medication routine by taking medications at the same times each day.

Medication Do's and Don't's for Clients

Do read and follow directions for use.

Do be cautious when using a drug for the first time.

Do dispose of old prescription drugs and outdated OTC medications.

Do seek professional advice before combining drugs.

Do seek professional advice when symptoms persist or return.

Do get medical check-ups regularly.

Don't be casual about taking drugs.

Don't take drugs you don't need.

Don't overbuy and keep drugs for long periods.

Don't combine drugs carelessly.

Don't continue taking OTC drugs if symptoms persist.

Don't take prescription drugs not prescribed specifically for you.

Techniques of medication administration should be explained to the client and family. Prior to discharge from a health-care facility, the client should practice the necessary techniques under the supervision of a nurse to acquire sufficient skill for safe administration. Many clients have learned to give themselves injections, as well as many other medications when the teaching has been well planned and the client is able and willing to learn.

The client should understand the desired effects of medications and their possible adverse effects. The client should also be taught the symptoms of toxic drug effects and the exact course of action to take if symptoms occur.

The nurse must stress the importance of taking medications as prescribed and for as long as prescribed. A common error made by clients is simply omitting a drug, either through carelessness or because they believe that missing a dose is not important. The client should be instructed not to alter the dosage without consulting the physician. Medications should not be discontinued when symptoms disappear. Drugs used to maintain health, such as those to control high blood pressure, need to be continued as ordered to avoid recurrence of symptoms.

Clients should be taught the importance of safe storage of medications. Keeping medications out of the reach of children can prevent accidental poisoning.

Caution the client not to share prescribed medications with other family members or with friends and neighbors. Inappropriate use of another person's drugs can have serious consequences.

Nurses have a teaching responsibility to society in relation to the abuse of any drug. Teaching may be done on an individual basis or on a family or community level. Drug abuse is a major public health concern worldwide, according to authorities on the subject, especially among teenagers and young adults. Not only is continued public and individual education indicated, but nurses are also expected to teach by setting high standards for their own behavior and the use of drugs.

Important Do's and Don't's that should be noted when teaching clients about medications are listed in the accompanying box.

EVALUATING THE CLIENT'S RESPONSE TO MEDICATIONS

Drug effectiveness can be assessed in several ways. Clinical observation is the first method. Subjective data from the client (*e.g.,* "My pain has disappeared") can be collected. Objective data (*e.g.,* the client's vital signs) help the nurse evaluate medication effectiveness. The alert nurse assesses the client for adverse drug effects.

Measurement of drug levels in body fluids provides data about the client's response to a particular medication. For many drugs, including digoxin, theophylline, anticonvulsants, and aminoglycoside antibiotics, monitoring blood levels is an important component of therapy. The client is tested to determine if the drug level in the blood is within the therapeutic range. Drug dosages may be adjusted as a result of the serum drug level.

Monitoring systems can also assist the nurse in evaluating drug effectiveness. For the client with an arrhythmia, a cardiac monitor would show a change in heart rhythm.

K E Y   P O I N T S

■ Medications have several names. The nurse should be aware of a drug's generic and trade names. Drugs can be classified by body system and by the symptom they relieve (clinical indication).

■ Drugs are available in many forms. Some drugs are supplied in a number of preparations; others are available in only one form.

■ Factors influencing drug absorption include route of administration, local conditions at the site of administration, drug solubility, pH, and drug dosage.

■ Variables influencing the action of medications are age, weight, sex, genetic factors, psychologic factors, illness, environment, and time of administration.

- Known adverse drug effects include iatrogenic disease, drug allergy, drug tolerance, cumulative effect, idiosyncratic reaction, and drug interactions.

- Assessment of clients receiving medications includes obtaining a comprehensive medication history.

- Components of a medication order are client's name, date and time order is written, name of the drug, dosage, route, frequency, and signature of the prescriber. The nurse questions any unclear medication order before the order is implemented.

- Pediatric dosages are calculated by the child's weight or body surface area.

- The nurse observes the *five rights* and *three checks* in medication preparation and administration. The nurse who prepares a medication administers the medication. The medication area is locked when not in use.

- The nurse identifies the client correctly before administering a medication and remains with the client until the medication is taken. The nurse records the medication on the client's record as soon as possible after administration.

- Selection of equipment for a parenteral injection is based on the route of administration, the viscosity of the drug, quantity to be administered, type of medication, and client's body size.

- Sterile equipment is used to prepare a drug for injection.

- Modified insulin should never be subjected to a vial of unmodified insulin when preparing two insulins to be mixed in the same syringe.

- Proper site selection for an intramuscular injection should include palpation of anatomic landmarks. The **Z**-track method for an intramuscular injection is used to administer medications that are irritating to the subcutaneous tissues.

- Intravenous medications can be administered as a continuous infusion, bolus, or intermittently. A bolus dose and an intermittent infusion may be administered through the primary intravenous line or through a heparin lock. The nurse checks the placement of a heparin lock prior to administering any medication.

- Topical medications are applied to the skin and mucous membranes primarily for their local effects, although some systemic effects may occur.

BIBLIOGRAPHY

Anderson K, Poole C: Self-administered medication on a postpartum unit. Am J Nurs 83(6):1178–1180, 1983

Birdsell G, Uretsky S: How do I administer medication by NG? Am J Nurs 84(10):1259–1260, 1284, 1984

Chaplin G, Shull H, Welk P: How safe is the air-bubble technique for I.M. injections? Nursing '85 15(9):559, 1985

Coblio NA: Don't combine those drugs! Nursing '81 11(8):48–49, 1981

Frank T, Fischer RG: What are some of the most common reasons for medication errors? Pediatric Nursing 10(4):294, 1984

Gever LM: Administering drugs through the skin. Nursing '82 12(3):88, 1982

Gioiella EC, Bevil CW: Nursing Care of the Aging Client: Promoting Healthy Adaptation. Norwalk, CT, Appleton-Century-Crofts, 1985

Hahn AB, Oestreich SJ, Barkin RL: Pharmacology in Nursing, 16th ed. St Louis, CV Mosby, 1986

Hayes JE: Normal changes in aging and nursing implications of drug therapy. Nurs Clin North Am 17(2):253–262, 1982

Hegsted LN, Hayek W: Essential Drug Dosage Calculations. Bowie, MD, Brady Communications, 1983

Howry LB, Bindler RM, Tso Y: Pediatric Medications. Philadelphia, JB Lippincott, 1981

Hudson MF: Drugs and the older adult: Take special care. Nursing '84 14(8):47–54, 1984

Jerrett MD: Taking the ouch out of injections. Canadian Nurse 79(1):24–27, 1983

Malseed RT: Pharmacology: Drug Therapy and Nursing Considerations, 2nd ed. Philadelphia, JB Lippincott, 1985

McConnell EA: The subtle art of *really* good injections. RN 45(2):25–34, 1982

Moree NA: Nurses speak out on patients and drug regimens. Am J Nurs 85(1):51–54, 1985

Nurses' drug alert: When should plasma drug concentrations be monitored? Am J Nurs 85(1):63, 1985

Shepherd MJ, Swearington PL: Z-track injections. Am J Nurs 84(6):746–747, 1984

Spencer RT et al: Clinical Pharmacology and Nursing Management, 2nd ed. Philadelphia, JB Lippincott, 1986

Thatcher G: Insulin injections: The case against random rotation. Am J Nurs 85(8):690–692, 1985

Whaley LF, Wong DL: Nursing Care of Infants and Children, 2nd ed. St Louis, CV Mosby, 1983

Wong DL: Significance of dead space in syringes. Am J Nurs 82(8):1237, 1982

41 Diagnostic Procedures

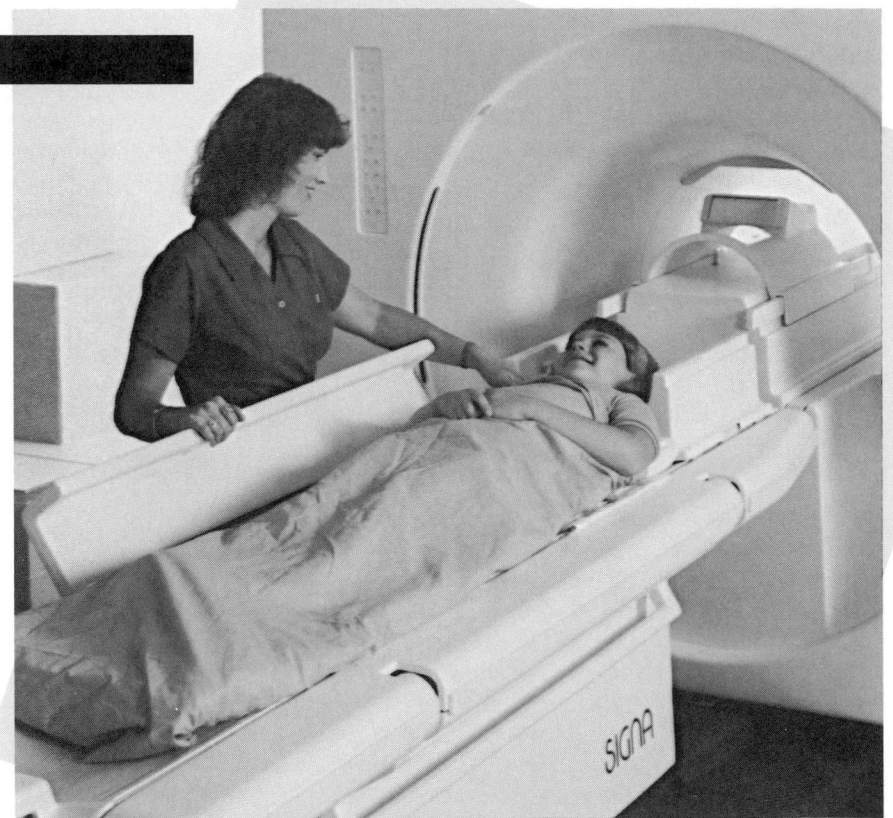

OBJECTIVES

After studying this chapter, the learner should be able to

Define key terms used in the chapter.

Describe various diagnostic tests and their purpose.

Describe nursing responsibilities for a client prior to, during, and following a diagnostic test.

Discuss the importance of psychologic preparation and support to clients having diagnostic tests.

Diagnostic tests are a valuable adjunct to the treatment regimen and provide a variety of information about the client's state of health. Most clients will undergo some type of diagnostic evaluation during their life time of health-care experiences. Decisions concerning which diagnostic tests to schedule are made by the physician when problems are noted during the history or physical examination or because of a problem stated by the client.

In this chapter, basic responsibilities of the nurse assisting with all diagnostic tests are discussed first. Major tests are then summarized. Further information can be obtained from *A Manual of Laboratory Diagnostic Tests* by Frances Fischbach. Some tests mentioned here are described fully in clinical chapters.

NURSING RESPONSIBILITIES

The nurse assumes a variety of roles and responsibilities when a client requires a diagnostic test. Emphasis on assessing each client's particular needs as well as their response to the testing procedure individualizes nursing care and initiates the nursing process. Results of the diagnostic tests also add to the knowledge base as the nurse accumulates information, formulates nursing diagnoses, and plans nursing care.

The following section discusses the nurse's basic responsibilities before, during, and after the testing. However, the definitive protocol may depend on the institution.

Prior to the Test

Preparing a client for a diagnostic test requires a multi-faceted approach by the nurse. Agency policy dictates the need for a permit, the requirements for scheduling the test, necessary equipment that must be available, and the physical preparation of the client for the test. The nurse's responsibility may encompass all these areas but must also focus on the psychologic preparation of the client for the examination. Nursing interventions that communicate caring, support, and an awareness of individual needs can ease the client's fear and help immeasurably.

Obtaining Consent. The physician is responsible for obtaining a signed consent form prior to any diagnostic test. The client has the legal right to know what the test involves, any risks or complications that might directly result from the test, and any other available options. An awareness of all these factors indicates that the client is informed about the procedure and the client's signature affirms consent. The general consent a client signs on admission to the agency may be sufficient to indicate consent for some diagnostic examinations whereas other invasive procedures may require that the client sign an additional consent form prior to the test.

KEY TERMS

ascites
atrioventricular (AV) node
barium enema
biopsy
bronchoscopy
cholecystogram
computed tomography
colonoscopy
cystoscopy
depolarize
electrocardiogram
electrocardiograph
electroencephalogram
electroencephalograph
endoscope
endoscopic retrograde cho-langiopancreatography (ERCP)
esophagogastroduodeno-scopy
fasting state
fluoroscopy
intravenous pyelogram
leads

liver biopsy
lumbar puncture
magnetic resonance imag-ing (MRI)
paracentesis
polarity
proctosigmoidoscopy
Purkinje system
radiography
radioisotope
radiopaque
repolarize
roentgen ray
sinoatrial (SA) node
spinal tap
thoracentesis
transducer
ultrasonography
ultrasound waves
upper gastrointestinal (GI) series
urinalysis
x-ray

Scheduling Tests. The nurse may be responsible for scheduling diagnostic tests or special procedures with another hospital department. In addition to a thorough understanding of the procedure, it is important for the nurse to know the proper sequence when multiple tests have been ordered. An intravenous pyelogram, for example, must be scheduled prior to any barium studies because barium takes three to four days to be excreted and may interfere with visualization of the kidneys. Knowledge coupled with practice and experience helps the nurse to collaborate effectively and plan for a diagnostic test. This effort saves the health-care consumer time and money, minimizes anxiety and trauma, and may eliminate the need to have a test repeated.

Preparing the Client. The nursing care plan should incorporate physical and psychologic preparation of the client before any diagnostic testing. Generally, the nurse follows written protocols for physical preparation of the client but may feel less confident meeting emotional needs. Both are vital toward promoting cooperation and securing reliable test results.

Physical Preparation. Physical preparation may be simple or extensive, depending on the type of diagnostic study. Some tests require only a simple explanation beforehand whereas more involved measures such as dietary restrictions, enemas, and sedation may be necessary before other procedures. The preparation may occur in a hospital setting or, if the test is performed on an outpatient basis, in the client's home, in a clinic setting, or in a physician's office. Instruction pamphlets are helpful, particularly if the client is responsible for self-preparation and is probably anxious about the upcoming test and its results.

As a client advocate, the nurse must monitor all test preparations to ensure that the client is not in a prolonged fasting state if tests are scheduled one after the other. It is also important to clarify which, if any, of the client's medications should be continued despite the test preparation.

Psychologic Preparation. Preparing a client emotionally and intellectually for a diagnostic examination presents a challenging opportunity for the nurse. Uncertainty associated with the preparations for the test, misgivings about pain or the test itself, and anxiety about the results or future treatment are stress-provoking experiences for the client. The nurse needs to recall personal experiences and rely on interpersonal communication skills to help the client deal with these fears.

Explanations by the nurse need to take into account the client's level of understanding and previous experience with the testing situation. Some clients desire explicit information about all facets of the examination and may request details on what they can expect to see, hear, and feel during the study. Simple clarification of the physician's explanation or a brief discussion may be appropriate for other clients. If the client is receptive, any available visual resources such as pamphlets or films may provide additional reinforcement.

It is helpful for the nurse to observe as many diagnostic procedures as possible to describe them more accurately to others. A client whose expectations match the actual testing experience is apt to be less anxious, more cooperative, and better able to withstand the demands of any diagnostic procedure.

Assembling Equipment. Responsibility for assembling equipment for a diagnostic test will vary depending on the setting. The nurse is usually responsible for gathering supplies and equipment when the examination is performed at the client's bedside or in a nearby treatment room. It is important for the nurse to take into account the physician's preference for any special instruments as well as the orderly arrangement of all supplies. If the procedure is sterile, the nurse maintains surgical asepsis. It is vital that protective equipment is available (gloves, gown, mask, and goggles) and frequent handwashing done if any contact with blood or body fluids is expected to prevent transmission of HIV and other blood-borne organisms.

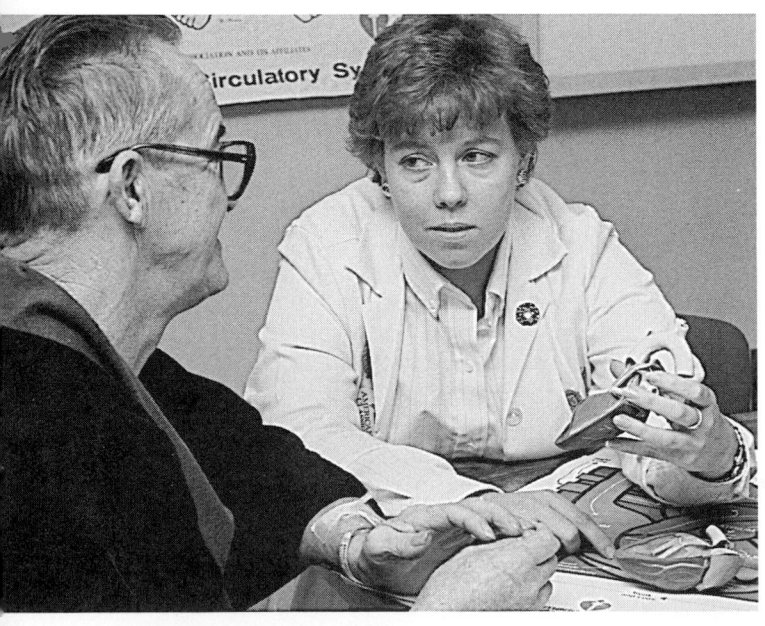

F I G U R E   41-1
Preparing a client emotionally and intellectually for a diagnostic procedure may require a simple clarification of the physician's explanation or explicit information about all facets of the test. (Photo by Don Walker, courtesy of Thomas Jefferson University Hospital)

During the Test

Whether actually assisting with the procedure or evaluating the client's response to it, the nurse's primary role during the test is that of client advocate. The client is the focus for nursing assessments and support and the nurse can communicate concern and support in a variety of ways. Holding the client's hand, helping the client to maintain an awkward position during the test, or reinforcing a direction or explanation demonstrate the compassionate care that belongs uniquely to nursing.

Collecting Baseline Data. Baseline data are necessary to evaluate the client's response to the testing process. Any deviation from normal may indicate an unfavorable reaction. The nurse is responsible for informing the physician of any manifestation that may threaten the client's life and that has caused difficulty in the past (*e.g.,* hives and itching associated with a previous dye injection). Such reactions may necessitate additional interventions before the test or its postponement and possible cancellation.

Undue anxiety should be noted so that the physician is aware of the client's fear and may take steps to minimize it prior to the start of the diagnostic procedure.

Evaluating the Client. If the nurse is present during the diagnostic study, assessment of the client is apt to focus on physical reaction and emotional state during the procedure. Any untoward response must be reported immediately to the physician. The nurse needs to be alert for any significant deviation from baseline vital signs, nausea or vomiting, pallor, unusual pain, or excessive anxiety. The physician may opt to intervene medically or pause to comfort and evaluate the client. It may be that the nurse is most qualified to observe any alteration in the client's condition based on prior knowledge from assessments and interviews.

Supporting the Client. Supportive measures are particularly meaningful to the client during a diagnostic test. The nurse respects the client's sense of privacy and provides a drape or cover to ensure warmth. The nurse may have occasion to use touch therapeutically by assisting the client to hold steady in an uncomfortable position. Holding a client's hand may help provide comfort during a particularly tense or painful moment. It may be the nurse who reinforces or repeats directions to the client during the test (*e.g.,* take a deep breath, cough, hold that position steady) or prepares the client to expect a certain sensation. A nurse who is particularly sensitive to the client's needs is able to support him emotionally as well as physically throughout the test in an individualized, compassionate manner.

Assisting the Examiner. The nurse who is assisting with the diagnostic procedure may be responsible for handing equipment to the physician and providing additional supplies as needed in addition to maintaining a sterile field and using whatever protective equipment is required. The client's safety is a paramount concern and the nurse may need to apply restraints and use side rails

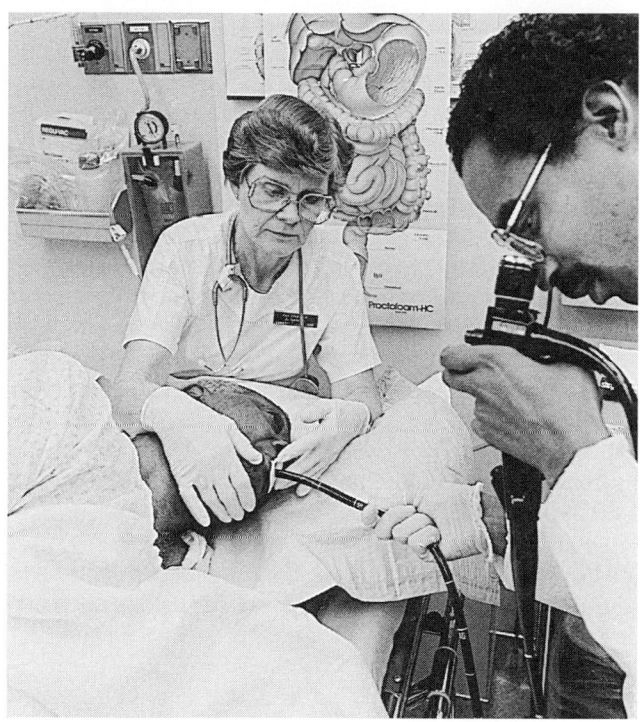

F I G U R E 41-2
Diagnostic procedures can be a very uncomfortable and frightening experience for the client. Supportive measures taken by the nurse are particularly meaningful to the client. (Photo by Kathy Sloane, courtesy of Merrit Hospital)

appropriately during the test. If a specimen is obtained, the nurse needs to prepare and label it correctly before it is transported to the laboratory.

After the Test

The nurse's first priority after the test is the client's comfort. Assessments may be ordered at regular intervals and the nurse must be aware of baseline data for comparison with observations and vital signs obtained after the diagnostic study. The type of equipment used and the nature of the laboratory specimen determine the techniques for proper disposal. All nursing assessments and interventions must be documented to ensure that the client's response to the diagnostic procedure is accurately recorded.

Assessing the Client. The type of test and the condition of the client determine the interval and type of nursing assessments following a diagnostic test. It is appropriate to assess the client immediately after the procedure. Baseline data should be available for comparison and may indicate the onset of any adverse reactions. Some tests require very frequent assessments that are recorded on a flowsheet at the client's bedside. It is imperative that the nurse is familiar with the diagnostic procedure in order to recognize any clinically significant deviations in the client's health status.

Assisting the Client. In addition to being aware of clinical implications after the study, the nurse is concerned about the client's comfort. Supportive measures that provide warmth, relieve pain, or provide direction and explanation are effective nursing interventions. The client may be relieved that the test has been completed but still anxious and apprehensive about test results and future therapy. The client may want to discuss the test experience or may have questions about the results. The physician needs to be notified if the client is unusually apprehensive about the consequences of the test. Specific instructions after the test (*e.g.,* concerning position or dietary status) need to be explained clearly to the client and any concerned support persons. It is important that the client understand that the frequent nursing assessments are routine rather than an indication of a clinical problem.

Preparing Specimens and Caring for Equipment.

Any specimens obtained during a test must be properly identified and delivered to the appropriate laboratory. The label should include the client's name, identification number, date, and nature of the specimen. Care must be taken to avoid contact with any potentially infective blood or body fluids and the label should indicate any hazards. The nurse also needs to be cautious about accidentally discarding the specimen with any used equipment. This action would require that the procedure be repeated.

Equipment that is reusable needs to be rinsed of blood and body fluids and prepared for sterilization. The nurse should wear disposable gloves for protection when handling any used equipment. Disposable equipment needs to be discarded in the proper receptacle. If necessary, replace any supplies and return the room to its former condition.

Documenting the Procedure. After a procedure is completed, the nurse needs to record the date and time, the type of diagnostic study, whether a specimen was obtained, and the client's response. Additional documentation may be necessary to record ongoing observations and nursing interventions. The diagnostic testing experience needs to be incorporated into the nursing care plan and used to plan individualized nursing interventions.

DIAGNOSTIC TESTS

Aspiration Procedures

Certain diagnostic studies involve insertion of a needle or similar instrument into a body organ or cavity. Fluid or tissue may be aspirated, prepared, labeled properly, and sent to the laboratory for examination. The tests may be performed at the client's bedside or other designated examination area.

Liver Biopsy

Overview. A liver biopsy is the needle aspiration of a sample of liver tissue. The specimen is then examined to determine if liver disease is present. The procedure is brief and may be performed at the client's bedside. A local anesthetic is administered prior to the test.

Since liver disease may be associated with some blood-clotting deficiencies, a prothrombin time and platelet count must always be checked before the test is performed. Food and fluids are restricted for at least 2 hours beforehand. Baseline vital signs must be recorded. Since it is an invasive test, a permit is required.

The client assumes a supine position with the right hand placed under the head. To immobilize the chest wall and prevent injury to the liver, the client is asked to hold his breath for approximately 10 seconds after an exhalation. Using sterile technique the physician inserts the needle between two of the right lower ribs or below the right rib cage, obtains the biopsy specimen, and removes the needle. Instructions to the client to resume

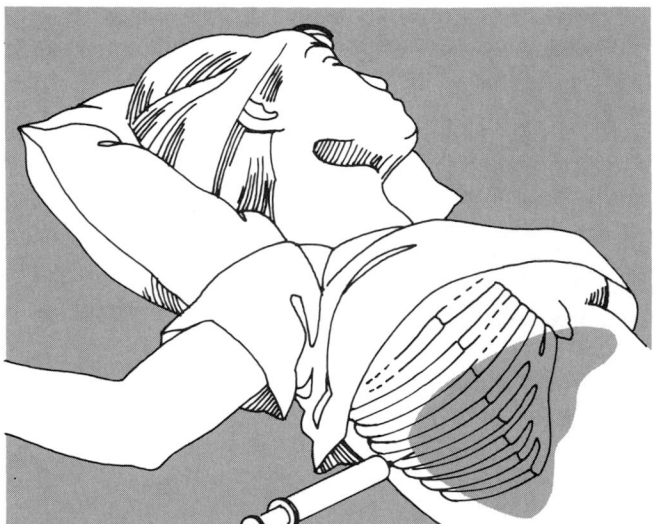

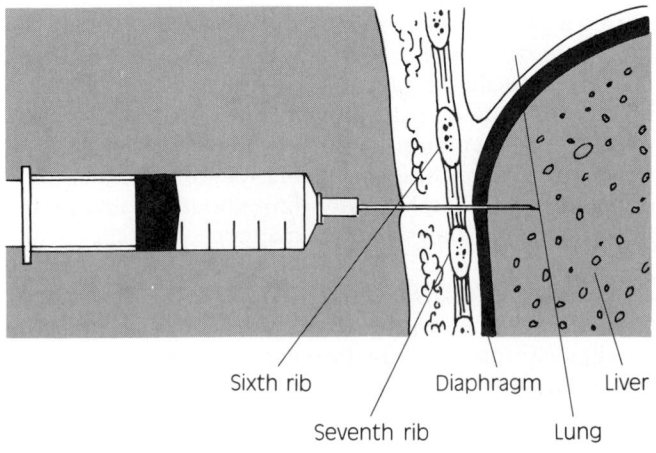

Sixth rib   Diaphragm   Liver

Seventh rib   Lung

F I G U R E   41-3
The position of the client and the site for a liver biopsy.

breathing and application of a pressure dressing complete the procedure.

Nursing Responsibilities. The nurse assumes responsibility for collecting baseline data and reviewing pertinent laboratory reports. Any abnormalities must be reported to the physician. Explanations to the client include details of the procedure as well as the instructions and rationale for holding the breath during the needle insertion and biopsy.

After the procedure the client requires careful assessment and observation. The client is assisted to lie on the right side with a pillow or folded towel under the needle insertion site. This position must be maintained for several hours. Vital signs must be monitored at frequent intervals (*e.g.*, every 15 minutes the first hour, every 30 minutes for the next 2 hours, and every 4 hours until they are stable). The nurse needs to be alert for complications such as hemorrhage, peritonitis if bile escapes from the liver, or pneumothorax. Normal diet may be resumed.

If the nurse is responsible for delivery of the specimen, it must be labeled correctly and quickly transported to the appropriate laboratory.

Lumbar Puncture

Overview. A **lumbar puncture**, or **spinal tap**, is the insertion of a needle into the subarachnoid space in the spinal canal. This test is usually done in the hospital for selected clients and is generally performed by a physician with the nurse assisting. It is a sterile procedure and requires the use of a local anesthetic.

Cerebrospinal fluid, which normally fills the ventricles of the brain, the subarachnoid space, and the central canal of the spinal cord, is clear and transparent. It may be necessary to enter the subarachnoid space for several reasons: to obtain a specimen of the fluid for analysis and for culture; to establish any alterations in the usual pressure of the cerebrospinal fluid; to relieve pressure; to inject drugs; or to inject dyes for x-ray visualization. Normal laboratory values for cerebrospinal fluid (CSF) are included in Appendix B.

Prior to the lumbar puncture, the client needs an explanation of the procedure and reassurance to allay any fears that paralysis may result. The usual site of needle entry is between the third and fourth lumbar vertebrae, which is below the level where the spinal cord ends. Occasionally a client may express concern about experiencing a postspinal headache but this is less likely to occur when the client cooperates with instructions during and after the test. Since this is an invasive procedure, a consent form must be signed by the client or a responsible family member.

In order to spread the vertebrae and to provide the widest possible space for easier insertion of the needle, the client is positioned on the side with the knees flexed and the head bent forward with the chin touching the chest. This hyperextends the spine. A small pillow may

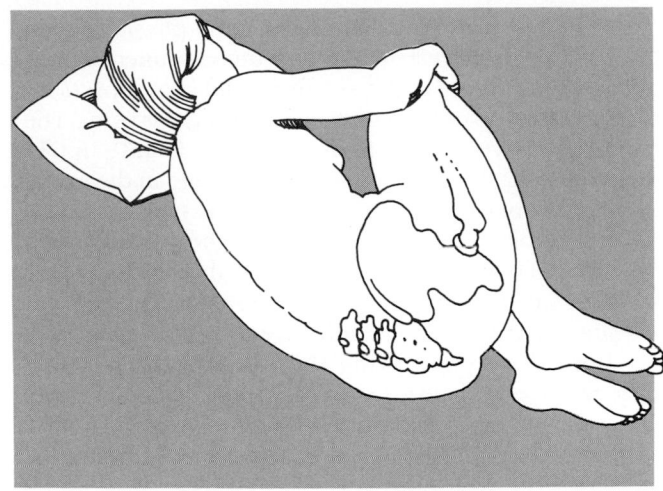

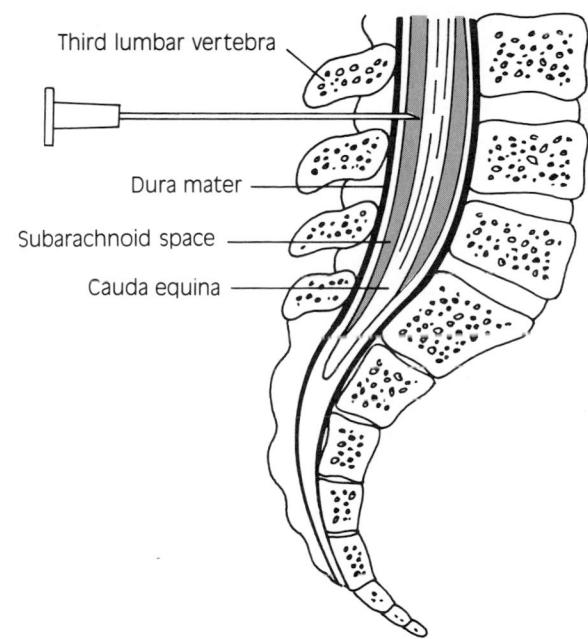

F I G U R E   41-4
The position of the client and the site for a lumbar puncture.

be placed under the client's head and between the knees for comfort. Some clients may be unable to assume or maintain this position without assistance. Others may have difficulty in understanding or may be disoriented and will need repeated assurances of what is being done. It is important to explain to the client the need to remain motionless and to breathe normally during the procedure. Moving about or hyperventilating makes insertion of the needle more difficult and may interfere with accurate pressure readings.

Nursing Responsibilities. During the procedure the nurse observes the client's reaction carefully. The client's color, pulse rate, and respiratory rate are noted and reported to the physician immediately if they deviate from normal.

The nurse may be asked to assist the physician with the Queckenstedt test. While the lumbar puncture needle is resting freely in the subarachnoid space, pressure is applied to one or both of the client's jugular veins. The nurse assists with this compression. An increase in CSF pressure is the normal response; a blockage in the spinal canal prevents the normal rise in pressure readings. When the procedure is completed, the needle is removed, and compression is applied to the site for a short while. A small, sterile piece of gauze may be applied to the site and fastened with adhesive.

Immediately following the procedure, the client may be placed in the recumbent position, preferably without a pillow. Fluids usually are offered. This is intended to avoid postspinal headache. Some experts believe that the headache is due to the tear in the dura mater made by the needle, which allows for seepage of small amounts of CSF. Differences of opinion exist about the effectiveness of positioning in avoiding the occurrence of the headache. The nurse should follow established agency protocol. If a headache does occur, the client usually is treated symptomatically.

The client's general physical reaction to the procedure is observed. This is of particular importance if the procedure was carried out to relieve pressure. Any unusual reactions, such as twitching, vomiting, or slow pulse, are reported to the physician promptly.

Paracentesis

Overview. The withdrawal of fluid from the peritoneal cavity is called an *abdominal paracentesis*. The word **paracentesis** means the withdrawal of fluid from any body cavity, but it is common practice to use the term when referring to the removal of fluid from the peritoneal cavity. The technique is used to obtain abdominal fluid for analysis to determine whether or not malignant tumor cells are present. A paracentesis also has therapeutic value because it helps relieve symptoms caused by **ascites**, which is an accumulation of fluid in the peritoneal cavity.

Since the peritoneal cavity is normally a sterile cavity, surgical asepsis is observed for the procedure. Normally, the pressure in the peritoneal cavity is no greater than atmospheric pressure, but when fluid is present the pressure is greater. Gravity will aid in the removal of fluid, so the fluid will drain freely until pressure is equal.

A sterile trocar and cannula are used to enter the peritoneal cavity near the midline of the abdomen, approximately halfway between the umbilicus and the pubis. The physician anesthetizes the site of entry, incises the skin, and introduces the trocar and the cannula. When the trocar is in place, the physician pulls back on the cannula to see if fluid will drain. If it does, the drainage tube is attached. The specimens will be obtained and should be carefully labeled. If a plastic catheter is used, it is threaded through at this time. The nurse places the distal end of the tubing in a clean container for drainage. If fluid is draining too rapidly, the container should be

elevated on a stool. Rapid drainage may produce symptoms of shock.

Nursing Responsibilities. The client is weighed and abdominal girth measured prior to and after the procedure. Baseline vital signs must be recorded. The client should be encouraged to void before the procedure begins because if the urinary bladder is full, there is danger of puncturing it with the trocar. The physician should be notified if the client is unable to void; the physician may order the client to be catheterized.

Since gravity is used to assist the drainage, the client is placed in a sitting position. The client may be supported in the sitting position in bed, placed at the side of the bed or the treatment table with the feet supported on a chair, or may sit on a chair during the procedure (Fig. 41-5). The client should be covered adequately for warmth and to prevent unnecessary exposure.

During and after the procedure, the nurse observes the client for untoward reactions associated with electrolyte imbalance. The client's color, blood pressure, pulse, and respiratory rate are noted. Fainting may occur. The nurse notes the type and the amount of drainage present. After the needle has been withdrawn and the incision sutured, the nurse should place a sterile, heavy dressing over the site of incision because leakage usually occurs. The dressing is changed as necessary. The client

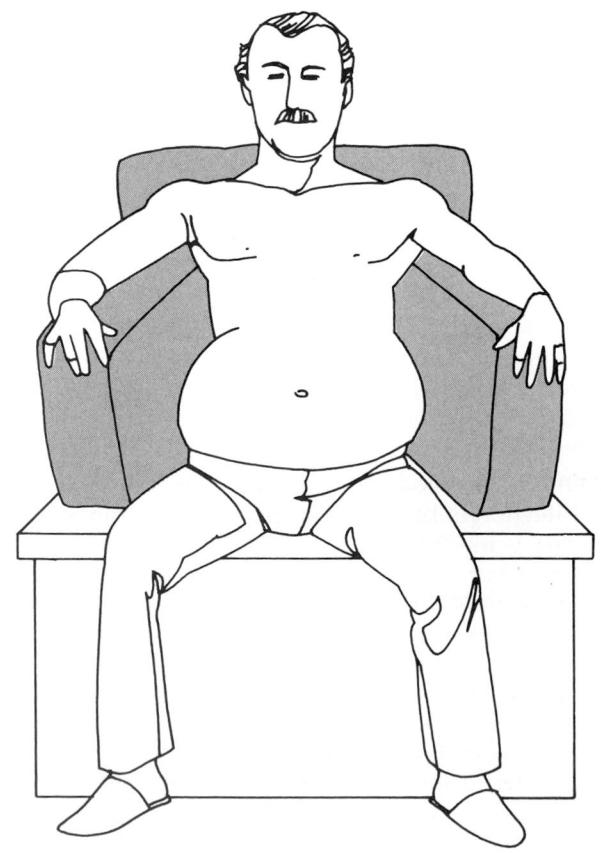

F I G U R E   41-5
Position of the client for paracentesis.

often is more comfortable if an abdominal binder is used for support following the procedure.

Thoracentesis

Overview. A **thoracentesis** is the entering and aspirating of fluid from the pleural cavity. The pleural cavity is a *potential* cavity, since normally it is not distended with fluid or air. Its walls are normally separated by a small amount of lubricating fluid to keep them from adhering. The physician generally performs the thoracentesis at the bedside with the nurse assisting. The client is required to sign a permit for this procedure.

A thoracentesis may be performed to obtain and analyze a specimen for diagnostic purposes or to remove fluid that has accumulated in the pleural cavity and caused respiratory difficulty and discomfort. Because the cavity being entered is sterile, surgical asepsis is used.

One way to remove fluid or air from the pleural cavity is to aspirate it with a syringe. Another method for removing fluid is to drain the fluid into a bottle in which a partial vacuum has been created. A small, plastic catheter may be threaded through the needle, allowing the needle to be withdrawn. This catheter reduces the possibility of puncturing the lung. When this method is used, the tubing connecting the needle and the bottle should be sterile. It is convenient to use a calibrated bottle for the drainage to determine readily the amount of fluid that has been removed. Normally, the pressure in the pleural cavity is less than atmospheric pressure and equipment for suction may be necessary to remove the fluid.

The skin is prepared over the area where the physician indicates the needle will be inserted. The exact location depends on the area where fluid is present and where the physician can best aspirate it. After a local anesthetic is administered, the needle is inserted between the ribs through the intercostal muscles and fascia and into the pleura.

The nurse usually is asked to assist with the collection of specimens. When the procedure is completed, the needle or plastic catheter is removed and a small, sterile dressing is placed over the entry site.

Nursing Responsibilities. The nurse is responsible for the collection of baseline data prior to the examination. The client must be instructed not to cough or breathe deeply during the test. It is imperative that the client remain as still as possible to diminish the risk of accidental injury to the lung.

Usually, this procedure is carried out when the client is sitting on a chair or on the edge of a treatment table or bed with the feet supported on a chair. Figure 41-6 illustrates this position. The client may lie on the side if unable to sit up. Usually, the client is placed on the affected side with the hand of that side resting on the opposite shoulder.

During the procedure, the nurse observes the client for reactions. The client's color, pulse rate, and respira-

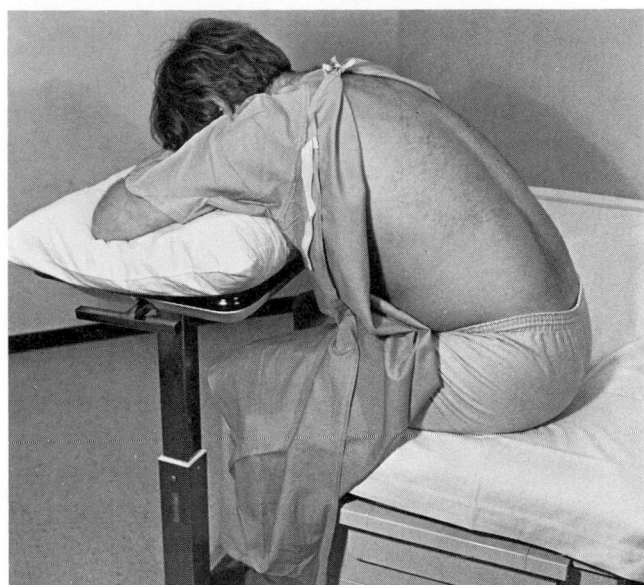

FIGURE 41-6
Position of the client for thoracentesis.

tory rate are observed, and any deviation from the norm is reported to the physician immediately. Fainting, nausea, and vomiting may occur.

Following the procedure, the client should be observed for changes in respirations. If a large amount of fluid is removed, respirations usually will be eased. If the lung has been punctured inadvertently, respiratory distress becomes acute. If blood appears in the sputum or the client has severe coughing, the physician should be notified promptly.

Electrical Impulse Procedures

Electrical impulses can be recorded on a graph and displayed on an oscilloscope screen. An **electrocardiograph** records the electrical impulses of the heart and an **electroencephalograph** records the electrical impulses of the brain. Both studies use a machine with electrodes attached to the body over the appropriate area to monitor electrical activity.

Electrocardiography

Overview. The electrocardiograph findings are important for studying heart function. The graphic record produced by the electrocardiograph is called the **electrocardiogram**, commonly abbreviated ECG or EKG.

The electrical activity in the heart is received through electrodes placed on the skin on various places on the body. The placement patterns of electrodes are called **leads**. The same cardiac activity is monitored on each lead, but the waves on the electrocardiogram look somewhat different, depending on the electrode's placement. The trained observer recognizes normal and abnormal findings for each placement of electrodes. Figure 41-7 illustrates a client having an electrocardiogram.

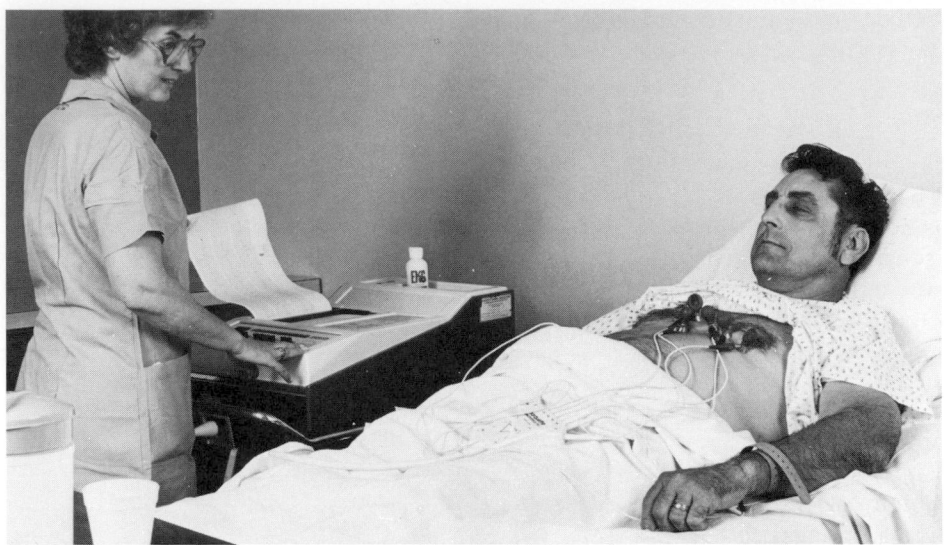

F I G U R E   41-7
Electrodes are placed on the arms, legs, and chest of the client having an electrocardiogram done. The nurse runs the electrocardiograph while observing the client.

Heart muscle cells are electrically charged, or polarized, in a state of rest. When cells are electrically stimulated, they **depolarize**, or lose their charge, and contraction follows. The cells repolarize during the resting phase that follows contraction. **Repolarize** means to restore **polarity** or regain an electrical charge. Depolarization and repolarization are electrical happenings that are recorded by the electrocardiogram.

When atrial depolarization occurs, the atria contract. Atrial repolarization occurs when the atria are at rest. When ventricular depolarization occurs, the ventricles contract. Ventricular repolarization occurs during ventricular rest.

The electrical activity that causes the heartbeat originates in the **sinoatrial (SA) node** (pacemaker), which is located in the upper part of the right atrium. Electrical

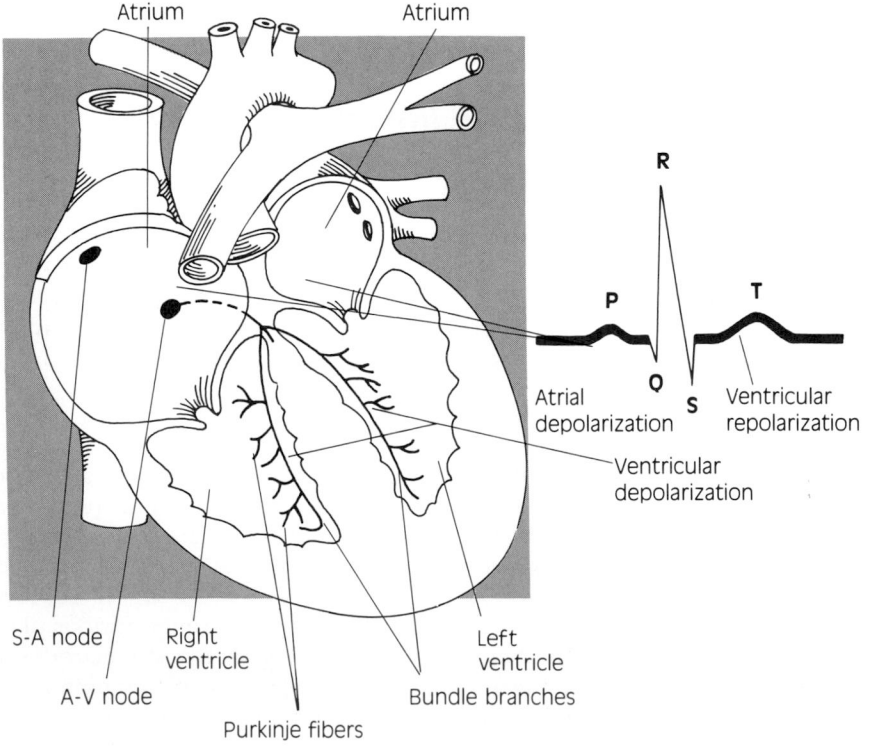

F I G U R E   41-8
How electrical phenomena occurring in the normal heart appear on the electrocardiogram.

currents radiate quickly throughout the atria from the SA node and stimulate contraction. A second node, the **atrioventricular (AV) node**, picks up the current. The node is situated at the base of the atrial septum. The AV node divides into two bundle branches, and each in turn gives rise to multiple smaller branches that interlace throughout the ventricles. This interlacing system is called the **Purkinje system**. Figure 41-8 illustrates the structures through which electrical current travels through the heart.

Figure 41-8 also illustrates the association between the electrical system in the heart and the ECG waves produced on the electrocardiogram. Note that the waves on the electrocardiogram are lettered. The P wave occurs when electrical charges, originating in the SA node, cause the atria to depolarize and contract. The wave of Q, R, and S occurs when the electrical charges result in ventricular depolarization and contraction. Wave T represents relaxation of the ventricles, during which time ventricular repolarization occurs. Repolarization of the atria occurs during the QRS segment, but it is not usually as visible on the electrocardiogram as ventricular repolarization is. The sum total of P, Q, R, S, and T represents the cardiac cycle. Another way of describing the cardiac cycle is that it consists of atrial and ventricular depolarization and repolarization.

The ruled paper for an ECG is calibrated to assist in reading it. The paper is ruled in 1-mm squares with heavier lines every 5 mm, as Figure 41-9 illustrates. The horizontal lines represent the measurement of voltage and the vertical lines measure time. When the heart is diseased, the waves may be abnormal in size, form, or position. The time interval between waves also has diagnostic significance.

Nursing Responsibilities. The client having an electrocardiogram for the first time needs an explanation of the purpose and technique being used. The client should be told that the electrodes are applied to the chest and extremities and that it is necessary to lie quietly while the tracing is being recorded. It should be clearly explained that the electrodes pick up the electrical impulses coming from the heart and that they are recorded on the paper. Electricity will not be transferred to the body. Some persons misunderstand the use of the word *electrical* and are fearful that they will receive an electrical shock. This fear needs to be allayed. There is no sensation of discomfort from the electrocardiograph.

Constant monitoring of the heart action is common in clients who are seriously ill. ECGs are displayed on a video screen, as well as recorded on ECG paper for a permanent record. As the physical condition improves, the client is disconnected from the monitor and attached to a device that permits movement around and allows some activity while still being monitored. A compact recording device, such as a Holter monitor, allows the client a certain amount of mobility but requires that the client record activities during the specified time period. These actions are correlated with the events on the ECG. The nurse may need to assist the client with this recording to ensure that all pertinent activities are documented and available for comparison with the ECG tracing. In addition, monitoring is now possible for persons not in a health agency who are carrying out normal activities of daily living. The electronic devices extend the health practitioner's ability to secure complete data about the client.

Electroencephalography

Overview. The electroencephalograph is an instrument that receives and records electrical currents in the brain. The recording is known as an **electroencephalogram**, or EEG. From 19 to 25 electrodes in the form of small disks are attached to the scalp with paste. The procedure does not cause any pain or discomfort for the client.

The EEG is a valuable tool that aids in the diagnosis of epilepsy and various other cerebrovascular diseases. An EEG recording that is flat is also used as an indication of brain death.

During the test, the technician carefully observes the client and notes any activity (*e.g.,* talking, blinking, or swallowing) that may cause an artificial movement on the tracing. This provides for a more accurate analysis of the client's brain wave patterns. A baseline recording is standard procedure. As part of the test the client may be asked to breathe deeply and rapidly for a short period of

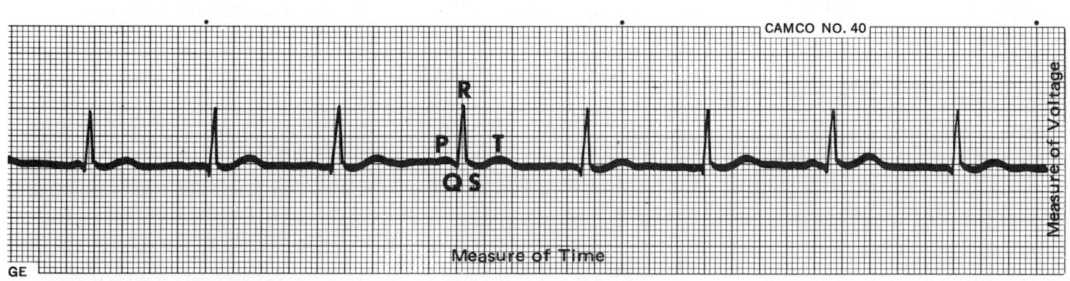

FIGURE **41-9**

The calibrated paper used for the electrocardiogram illustrates time and voltage measures. (Sharp LN, Rabin B: Nursing in the Coronary Care Unit. Philadelphia, JB Lippincott. 1970)

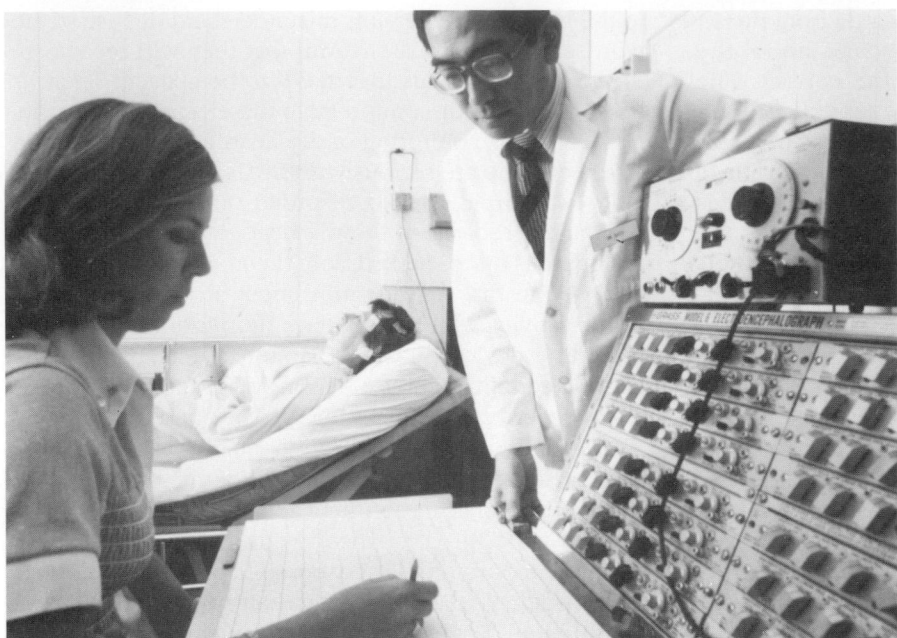

F I G U R E   41-10
Neurologist and EEG technician checking the client's electroencephalograph, which is a valuable diagnostic instrument in epilepsy and neurologic disorders. (Courtesy of National Institute of Neurological and Communication Disorders and Stroke)

time or view a series of flashing lights. These activities may activate a seizure pattern, which will be recorded on the EEG tracing.

Nursing Responsibilities. The client undergoing an EEG needs a thorough explanation of the procedure and reassurance that no electricity will be transferred to the body. Certain medications may be withheld for 24 to 48 hours before the test. There are no restrictions on food and fluid intake. Following the study, the nurse may need to assist the client to shampoo the hair in order to remove the paste residue from the scalp.

Endoscopic Procedures

Overview. Endoscopic studies allow for direct visual examination of various body cavities and organs by means of a hollow, lighted tube, called an **endoscope**. The endoscope may be flexible or rigid. Endoscopic examinations provide valuable diagnostic information and may be used to obtain tissue specimens for **biopsy** or microscopic examination. Another therapeutic reason for endoscopic examination is removal of a foreign body. Common endoscopic studies include the following:

Bronchoscopy—Visual examination of the trachea and bronchi
Esophagogastroduodenoscopy—Visual examination of the esophagus, stomach, and duodenum (also called *gastroscopy*)
Proctosigmoidoscopy—Visual examination of the rectum, rectosigmoid junction, and lower sigmoid colon
Colonoscopy—Visual examination of the entire large intestine
Cystoscopy—Visual examination of the bladder, urethra, and urethral orifices

Nursing Responsibilities. The client needs an explanation of the procedure and must sign a consent prior to the procedure. Preparations vary according to the area being studied but may also include dietary restrictions and laxatives or enemas. A local anesthetic may be administered as well as an analgesic or tranquilizer/sedative, which may be given by injection.

Following the examination, the client's vital signs need to be checked at frequent intervals. The nurse needs to evaluate the client's ability to cough or swallow if the endoscopic study involved the use of a local anesthetic on the trachea or esophagus. The client needs to be monitored for pain and hemorrhage after the test because perforation with the endoscope is a possible complication (see also Table 34-2).

Laboratory Procedures

Laboratory test results are invaluable as the physician attempts to diagnose and treat the client. Attention to detail when preparing the client, collecting specimens, and transporting them to the laboratory contributes to reliable test results. A vigilant, conscientious approach by the nurse is ultimately beneficial to the client.

Blood Specimens

Overview. Blood is one of the most significant body fluids that conveys information about the person's health state. The majority of physical examinations include some type of blood analysis. A multitude of laboratory tests can be done with blood specimens. Blood specimens are generally collected by laboratory personnel.

Nursing Responsibilities. The role of the nurse is generally one of explaining to the client what will happen and what preparation is necessary for the examination. Many blood specimens are secured while the client is in the **fasting state** (*i.e.,* abstaining from food or fluid intake, or both). The period of fasting will vary with the tests to be done and laboratory techniques used. Whether in the home or in a health agency, clients need careful explanation about the fasting period.

The nurse should be familiar with the more common normal blood values to be able to recognize deviations. Blood examination results provide data about the client that help plan for effective nursing care. Normal adult values for some of the more common laboratory blood tests are given in Appendix B.

When securing specimens for laboratory examination, the nurse is responsible for the correct labeling of specimens before they are transported to the laboratory. An inaccurate or unmarked specimen can be more hazardous than no specimen at all. A request for the type of examination desired should accompany the specimen.

Care must be used when handling any blood or body fluids to prevent transmission of HIV and other blood-borne infections. Precautions always include thorough handwashing and the use of gloves. Gown, mask, or protective eye covering may also be recommended.

Urine Specimens

Overview. A **urinalysis** is the laboratory examination of a urine specimen. Analysis of the urine is another common way of securing data about a person's health state.

Most laboratories prefer a specimen of several hundred milliliters collected soon after arising from sleep. Special urine collection techniques are discussed in Chapter 33.

Nursing Responsibilities. The nurse is often responsible for instructing the client about urine collection techniques or for obtaining a sample of urine from the client. A cooperative client can be instructed to put the specimen into a clean or, in some instances, a sterile container. Care should be taken that the outside of the container is not contaminated. Precautions similar to those used when handling blood are appropriate with all body fluids.

As with common blood test results, the nurse should be able to recognize deviations from normal in the urinalysis. Normal adult laboratory analysis values for urine are presented in Appendix B.

Secretion Specimens

Overview. Specimens of body secretions are collected for microscopic examination or to introduce them into a culture medium to grow any microorganisms that are present. Body secretions from the throat, vagina, penis, rectum, and wounds or lesions are most often collected for these purposes. A sterile, long-handled applicator or swab and a sterile container or tube with an enclosed

ampule of culture medium are generally used. The sterile cotton-tipped end of the applicator should be placed directly into the area where the specimen is desired and rotated to make certain secretions adhere to the applicator. The applicator is then carefully placed directly into the test tube and handled according to the laboratory policy. This may involve crushing the ampule of medium to allow the swab tip to be covered by the fluid and carefully capping the container prior to labeling it. Precautions should be taken so that the applicator is not contaminated before or after securing the secretion specimen. Nor should the secretions be allowed to contaminate the other surfaces. The specimen should be taken to the laboratory immediately for examination. Allowing the specimen to stand for a prolonged period may encourage the overgrowth of other microorganisms.

Nursing Responsibilities. The nurse is frequently responsible for the collection of specimens of body secretions. Explanation to the client and careful documentation of the type of specimen, location it was collected from, and date and time are vital nursing interventions. Precautions when handling body fluids or secretions must be enforced.

Radiography Procedures

Radiography is the use of x-rays to secure data about health status. An **x-ray** or **roentgen ray** is a high-energy electromagnetic wave capable of penetrating solid matter and acting on photographic film. X-ray films are commonly taken to determine the size, shape, and functioning of some organs, the characteristics of bones, and the detection of masses.

A radiopaque contrast substance may be used to secure more detailed viewing of some organs. **Radiopaque** means impenetrable by x-rays. The radiopaque substance, often containing barium or iodine, produces a contrasting shadow on x-ray films as compared to tissues that are penetrated by the x-rays.

Radiology procedures are performed in various health-care settings and on many of the body systems. Certain procedures such as ultrasonography are frequently used in conjunction with radiography or nuclear medicine studies and are discussed with these procedures.

Contrast Radiologic Studies

Overview. An **upper gastrointestinal (GI) series** is the x-ray visualization of the esophagus, stomach, and duodenum. The client is usually in a fasting state and is asked to drink a radiopaque barium preparation immediately prior to the x-ray examination. The radiopaque substance outlines the organs for visualization. **Fluoroscopy**, which is the radiologic visualization of the motion of an organ as the radiopaque substance moves through it, may also be used. An upper GI series with fluoroscopy is not uncomfortable, although the radiopaque substance does not taste particularly good. Many persons say it tastes like flavored chalk. Following the test, a mild laxative is usually ordered to allow for evacuation of any residual barium. More details of this test and the following are given in Chapter 32.

A **barium enema** allows for the x-ray visualization of the large intestine. A barium solution is instilled through the anus to distend the rectum and colon. In addition to fasting, preparation for the barium enema generally includes cleansing of the colon with laxatives and enemas. The technique for giving enemas is discussed in Chapter 32. Laxatives and enemas may also be used to cleanse the intestine of residual barium following the examination. The client should be prepared for the fact that a barium enema is a rather uncomfortable and tiring procedure and also told to expect that fecal material may be white from the barium for several days following the examination.

A gallbladder x-ray film or oral **cholecystogram** is the x-ray visualization of the gallbladder. An iodine radiopaque substance is taken orally, absorbed by the liver, and concentrated in the gallbladder. Preparations generally include some dietary modification on the day preceding the examination, followed by taking pills containing the contrast material during the evening. A cholecystogram should be scheduled prior to any barium studies because barium may interfere with visualization.

The procedure should cause no discomfort, although occasionally some persons may experience side-effects from the contrast material. Any history of allergic reactions to dye must be clearly noted on the chart on admission. An intravenous cholangiogram uses contrast material given intravenously. The examination is similar to the oral cholecystogram.

An **intravenous pyelogram**, or IVP as it is commonly called, is the x-ray visualization of the kidney's ability to excrete urine. An IVP should be scheduled prior to any barium studies because barium takes 3 to 4 days to be excreted and may interfere with visualization of the kidneys. A radiopaque dye is injected intravenously, and films are taken at timed intervals to determine the amount of dye excreted by the kidneys. Preparations for an IVP usually include a laxative or enema and having the person urinate before the examination. Normally, there should be no discomfort. However, some persons are sensitive to the dye and may have allergic reactions to it, and this information must be clearly noted on the chart on admission.

Endoscopic retrograde cholangiopancreatography (ERCP) is the x-ray visualization of the pancreatic ducts as well as the liver and biliary tree by means of injection of a contrast medium. This procedure involves passage of an endoscope into the duodenum so the contrast material can be directly introduced through the endoscope and into the pancreatic duct and hepatobiliary tree. ERCP is used to aid in the diagnosis of pancreatic disease and to evaluate the cause of a type of jaundice. It is an

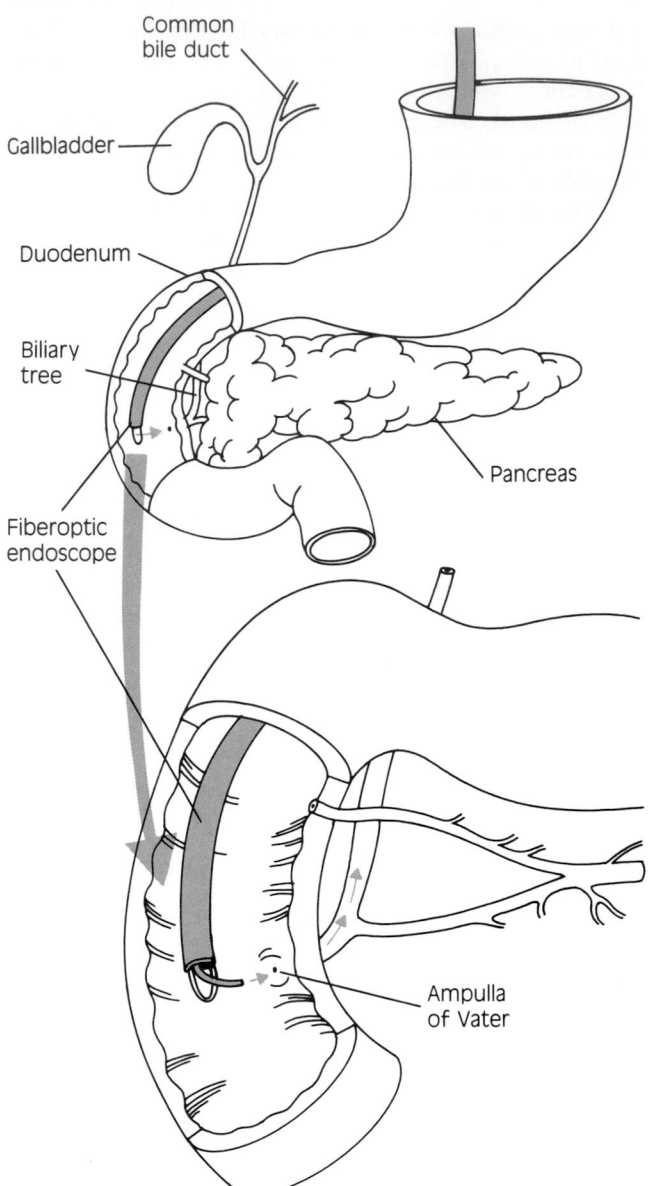

F I G U R E   41-11
Endoscopic retrograde cholangiopancreatography (ERCP) uses both radiography and endoscopy to examine the pancreatic ducts and hepatobiliary tree. An endoscope is passed through the esophagus, stomach, and duodenum to the ampulla of Vater. A contrast medium is introduced by inserting a cannula through the endoscope.

invasive procedure and requires that the client sign a permit. The client must be in a fasting state. A local anesthetic is used to assist in passage of the endoscope. Any previous allergic reaction to a contrast medium needs to be reported to the physician.

Lung scan is discussed in Table 34-2.

Nursing Responsibilities.   The role of the nurse in the diagnostic use of x-rays is generally to teach and to prepare persons as necessary. The physician's order for the specific study and agency protocol will determine the type of preparation before the procedure. Food and fluid restrictions will vary and must be communicated and reinforced with the client and concerned support persons. The nurse is responsible for monitoring the client's condition and recording observations when the diagnostic procedure is completed.

Computed Tomography

Overview. Computed tomography, also referred to as a *CT scan,* is a noninvasive x-ray procedure. It is a method by which a body part can be scanned from different angles with an x-ray beam and a computer that calculates varying tissue densities and records a cross sectional image on paper. The radiologist can distinguish structures by their shape, size, symmetry, color, and position. An iodine contrast dye may need to be given intravenously during the test to enhance tissue contrast. Since iodine preparations may cause nausea and vomiting, food and fluids are usually withheld for 3 to 4 hours prior to the test. The client must lie absolutely still during the examination. Some people occasionally experience a claustrophobic sensation when the head or body is placed inside the CT machine.

Nursing Responsibilities. The client requires an explanation of any reactions that may occur related to the dye injection (warm sensation and flushing of the face, nausea, vomiting, salty taste in the mouth). Any history of allergic reaction or hypersensitivity to shellfish, iodine, or any contrast dye is vital information and needs to be reported to the physician. All metal objects need to be removed from the body area being scanned. The nurse should explain that the test itself is brief (15 to 30 minutes) and reassure the client that exposure to radiation is no more than that experienced in conventional x-ray studies.

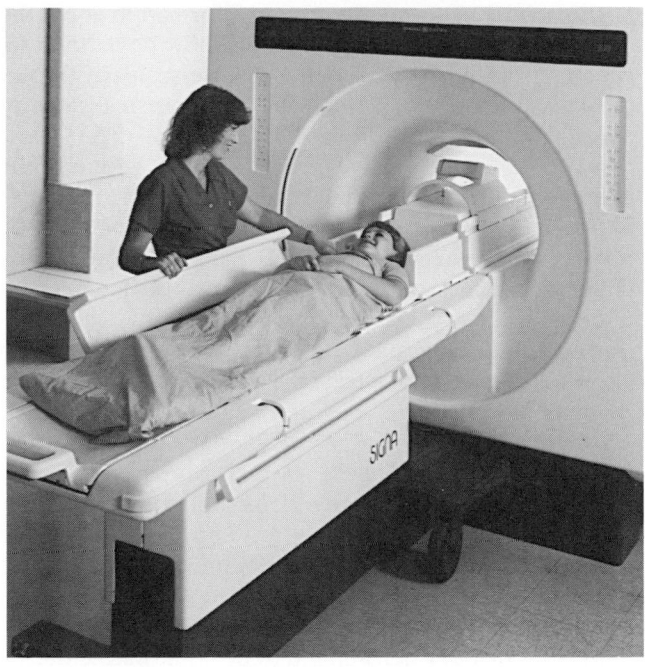

FIGURE 41-12
The magnetic resonance imaging (MRI) scanning machine can provide unique diagnostic information in a noninvasive technique, but requires the client be placed head first in the supine position into a narrow tunnel-like space within the machine. The nurse must prepare the client with the knowledge that the procedure may be a claustrophobic experience. Keeping eyes closed during the procedure sometimes lessens the discomforting sensation. (Courtesy of GE Medical Systems)

Magnetic Resonance Imaging

Overview. Magnetic resonance imaging (MRI) is an advanced scanning technique that uses magnetism and radiowaves to produce cross-sectional images of body tissues on a computer screen. Although very costly, the

COMPUTER APPLICATIONS IN NURSING

Computerized Diagnostic Tests

Computed tomography (CT) provides a computerized image of an organ or body part. The test is considered to be noninvasive, but one form does require the injection (into a peripheral vein) of a radiopaque substance.

CT scans are used for the diagnosis and monitoring of
- Brain tumors, lesions, and injuries
- Spinal lesions and abnormalities
- Effects of intracranial and spinal surgery

- Effects of x-ray or chemotherapy for intracranial tumors
- Tumors, abscesses, hematomas, or infections of the liver, spleen, or pancreas
- Abnormalities of the paranasal sinus
- Abnormalities of the eye and bony orbit
- Renal pathology or transplant
- The retroperitoneum

New uses of CT scans are being discovered and utilized in all areas of medical diagnosis and treatment.

MRI machine can provide unique information about the chemical make-up of tissues. It can show deviations between normal and diseased blood vessels, clearly display the heart's pumping action, and distinguish lesions or masses in fluid-filled soft tissues.

MRI is a noninvasive procedure that requires the client to be placed head first in the supine position into a narrow tunnel-like machine. All metal objects must be removed, and because the MRI uses magnetism, any client with a surgically implanted metal device may not undergo the study. Only clients in stable physical condition are eligible because the confined structure does not allow for recording of vital signs or monitoring of cardiac rhythms.

Nursing Responsibilities. A well-prepared client is better able to withstand the claustrophobic experience of an MRI scan. Suggestions to keep the eyes closed during the test sometimes prove helpful. The client also needs to be aware of the necessity to lie still while enclosed in the machine. It is important that the client empty the bladder beforehand to be comfortable during the procedure.

The technician maintains communication with the client during the test through nonmetallic earphones. The client should also be told that the machine makes a monotonous, steady noise when operating. No special observations are necessary when the test is completed.

Radioisotope Scanning

Overview. A **radioisotope** is a radioactive chemical. When used for diagnostic examination, a substance containing a small amount of radioisotope is administered orally or by injection. The particular substance is selected according to its ability to localize in the target organ. Blocking agents are sometimes given to prevent its absorption by other organs. The heart, vessels, brain, spinal canal, lungs, thyroid, and abdominal organs are examined in this way. The size, shape, and function of organs and the presence of abnormal masses can be determined. A mechanism called a *scanner* detects emission of the radioactive waves and records them on a photographic plate.

Nursing Responsibilities. Preparation for radioisotope scanning should include reassurance that the amount of radioisotope normally used is minute and produces no more radiation than that of a single x-ray. Some people fear that they will become dangerously radioactive. The client should also be prepared for the fact that lengthy placement in an awkward position may be necessary during the test. No discomfort should normally be experienced except for that caused by injection and the positioning.

Ultrasonography

Overview. **Ultrasonography** is a noninvasive procedure that involves the use of ultrasound to produce an image or photograph of an organ or tissue. This procedure is also referred to as an *echogram*. The kidneys, liver, spleen, pancreas, gallbladder, thyroid, heart, eyes, lymph nodes, aorta, and female reproductive organs can be examined in this way. **Ultrasound waves** are extremely high-frequency and inaudible sound waves. The ultrasound waves penetrate and bounce back, or echo, according to the density of the tissue. A **transducer**, an instrument that converts energy from one form to another, produces the ultrasound waves and converts the reflected waves into electrical energy. The electrical energy then produces an image on a viewing screen. The person will be asked to remain quiet while the transducer, which is approximately 2.5 cm (1 inch) in diameter, is applied to the lubricated skin and moved about over the area to be examined.

Nursing Responsibilities. Generally, no special preparations are necessary, except for abdominal ultrasonography, which requires food and fluid restrictions. There is no discomfort with this procedure. It is helpful if the client is aware of the need to remain motionless during the test.

K E Y   P O I N T S

- Diagnostic tests ordered by the physician provide valuable information about the client's state of health.

- Nursing responsibilities associated with diagnostic tests may include obtaining the consent, scheduling the test, physical and emotional preparation of the client, nursing care after the test, disposal of equipment, and proper care of any specimen.

- A liver biopsy involves the needle aspiration of a sample of liver tissue to determine the presence of a disease process.

- A lumbar puncture involves withdrawal of fluid from the subarachnoid space in the spinal canal to obtain a specimen for culture and analysis, to relieve pressure or check for alterations in the usual pressure of cerebrospinal fluid, or to inject drugs or dyes for x-ray visualization.

- With a thoracentesis, fluid is aspirated from the pleural cavity, and a paracentesis involves aspiration of fluid from the peritoneal cavity.

- An electrocardiogram (ECG) is a recording of the electrical impulses of the heart, and an electroencephalogram (EEG) is a recording of the electrical activity of the brain.

- An endoscopic study provides valuable diagnostic information obtained by direct visual examination of an organ or cavity and also allows for microscopic examination of tissue specimens taken from the site.

- Laboratory analysis of blood, urine, and secretion specimens is a common way of securing data about a person's health state. Minimal client preparation is involved.

- Radiologic studies, or x-rays, are valuable diagnostic tests for determining size, shape, and functioning of some organs, the characteristics of bones, and the detection of masses.

- Computed tomography produces a cross-sectional image of a body part that reflects various tissue densities.

- Magnetic resonance imaging (MRI) uses magnetism and radiowaves to produce cross-sectional images of body tissues on a computer screen.

- Radioisotope scanning requires the oral intake or injection of a small amount of radioisotope that when localized in a target organ aids in the determination of the size, shape, and function of the organ and the presence of an abnormal mass.

- An ultrasound study is a recording of the pattern of sound waves as they are reflected off body tissues.

BIBLIOGRAPHY

Antman EM: Ambulatory ECG monitoring: Clinical applications of Holter recording. Consultant 25(6):96–97, 100–101, 104–105, 1985

Diagnostics. Springhouse, PA, Intermed Communications, 1983

Fay MF et al: Intraoperative monitoring: The EEG monitor can be a window to the brain. AORN J 41(6):1046–1049, 1985

Fischbach FT: A Manual of Laboratory Diagnostic Tests, 3rd ed. Philadelphia, JB Lippincott, 1988

Hadley A: The anxieties of endoscopy. Nursing Mirror 158(4):26–28, 1984

Hurwitz M: Intraoperative ultrasound. AORN J 38(6):979–984, 1983

Kee J: Laboratory and Diagnostic Tests with Nursing Implications. East Norwalk, CT, Appleton-Century-Crofts, 1983

Keller H et al: Assessing the risk of disease with multiple lab variables. Diagn Med 6(8):50–52, 54, 56–60, 1983

Kleinman MS: Flexible fiberoptic sigmoidoscopy. Hosp Pract 19(6):106N-O, 106S-T, 1984

Marchette L, Holloman F: A first hand report on the new body scanners. RN 48(11):28–31, 1985

Peternel E: A high-tech approach to a GI problem . . . endoscopic retrograde cholangiopancreatograph—ERCP . . . gallstones. RN 48(6):44–47, 1985

Proyer AC: A comparison of blood cultures withdrawn from the arterial line and by venipuncture. Heart Lung 13(4):411–415, 1984

Purcell JA et al: Using the ECG to detect MI. Am J Nurs 84(5):627–642, 1984

Questions and answers about the CT scan exam . . . patient education aid. Patient Care 19(7):185, 1985

Sugabaker PH: Endoscopy in cancer diagnosis and management. Hosp Pract 19(11):111–122, 1984

Wieck L et al: Illustrated Manual of Nursing Techniques, 3rd ed. Philadelphia, JB Lippincott, 1986

Wilson C: The diagnostic work-up for the patient with inflammatory bowel disease. Nurs Clin North Am 19(1):51–59, 1984

Care of Wounds

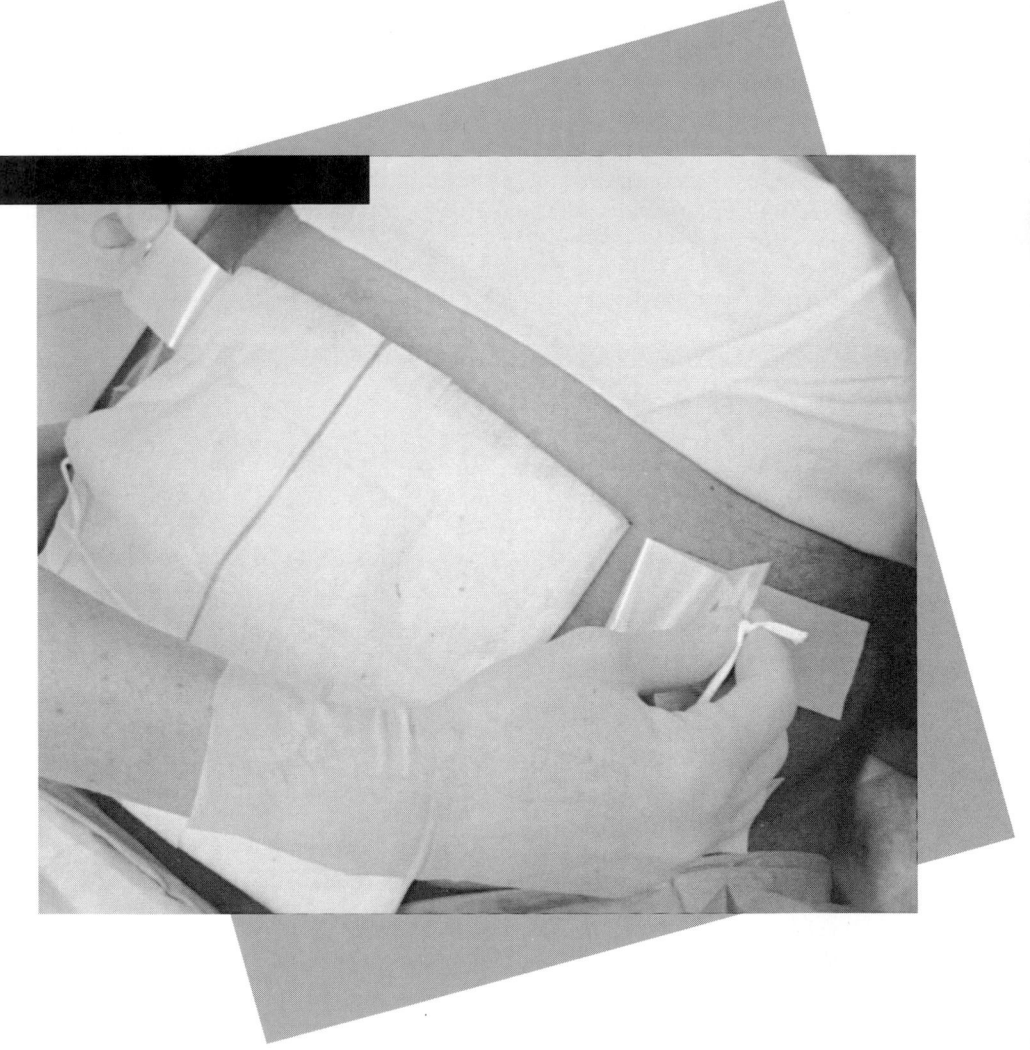

OBJECTIVES

After completing this chapter, the learner should be able to

Define key terms used in the chapter.

Describe the physical and psychologic effects of trauma to the body, with resultant wounds.

Discuss the processes involved in wound healing.

Describe wound complications, integrating factors affecting wound healing.

Summarize emergency wound assessment and care.

Describe the effects of the application of heat or cold.

Use the nursing process to knowledgably derive an individualized plan of care for the client with a wound, including the application of dressings and heat or cold.

The skin, the largest organ of the body, serves many functions: protective, sensory, regulatory, and self-concept. Trauma to the skin, either accidental or intentional, results in an alteration in skin integrity, which may impair basic need attainment and predisposes an individual to the risk of further alterations in health.

A **wound** is an alteration in the integrity of the skin, and the care of the client with a wound is an aspect of nursing care that requires knowledge and skill. Nurses use the nursing process to assess potential and actual problems; make nursing diagnoses; and plan, implement, and evaluate appropriate interventions to facilitate healing, prevent further injury or illness, and support coping with changes in self-concept and body image.

Study of this chapter provides the student with knowledge of wounds and wound healing, including the wound healing process and factors affecting wound healing. Guidelines, rationale, and procedures for wound care (dressings, heat and cold applications) are provided. The use of the nursing process includes selected nursing diagnoses for both the client with a wound and the client receiving heat or cold applications. A sample care plan for one nursing diagnosis is included at the end of the chapter to illustrate the application of the nursing process in the clinical setting.

PHYSIOLOGY OF THE SKIN

The skin, or integument, is the largest organ of the body, and serves a variety of functions in response to both the internal and external environments. Because an interruption of skin integrity is a risk factor for altered health, a knowledge base of normal structures and functions is necessary in using the nursing process to give care to clients with wounds.

Structure. The skin is made up of two layers, the *epidermis* and the *dermis* (Fig. 27-1). The epidermis has two parts: a layer of dead squamous cells covering a layer of cells containing melanin. There are no blood vessels in this outer layer of skin. The dermis, connected to the epidermis, is composed of collagen fibers which support the epidermis, and contains nerves, blood vessels, sweat glands, sebaceous glands, and hair follicles. Assessment of the skin, with a description of each component, is included in Chapter 24, *Nursing Assessment.*

Functions. The functions of the skin are
- Provide protection for underlying tissues from the external environment. The potential for injury or infection is increased when the skin is undernourished, aged, traumatized, overly dry, or wet for long periods of time; or when a physical illness is present.
- Control body temperature by the processes of radiation, conduction, convection, or evaporation (as described in Chap 23)

KEY TERMS

abrasion
abscess
bandage
binder
capillarity
closed wound
compress
contusion
dehiscence
dressing
evisceration
exudate
granulation tissue
incision
laceration

many-tailed binder
open wound
pack
puncture
purulent
retention sutures
sanguineous
scar
scultetus binder
serous
sitz bath
skin sutures
stab wound
wound

- Provide sensory perception of pain, touch, heat, or cold
- Assist in the maintenance of the fluid and electrolyte balance of the body. Excessive sweating or drainage from the body results in the loss of water and salt (see Chap 35).
- Use sunlight to synthesize vitamin D, necessary to calcium and phosphorus metabolism
- Communicate feelings, and to serve as a major component in self-concept and body-image

This chapter, focusing on the care of wounds, is most concerned with the protective, sensory, and psychosocial functions of the skin.

BODY'S REACTION TO TRAUMA

Wounds

The nurse cares for wounds, but only as one aspect of the nursing care given to the *client* with the wound. Using the nursing process, an individualized plan of care is developed to assess, identify and prevent complications, to implement and evaluate skills essential to wound care, and to provide the necessary physical and emotional support so that healing, adaptation, and self-care are facilitated.

Types of Wounds

A wound is a disruption in the normal integrity of the skin and underlying tissues. This trauma may be accidental or intentional, and wounds may be open or closed, clean or contaminated, superficial or deep. Table 42-1 lists the types, causes, descriptions, and implications of different types of wounds. Many wounds combine several descriptors; for example an intentional wound to remove the appendix is usually a clean, open wound. In comparison, following an automobile accident, a person may have an unintentional, open, laceration considered to be contaminated. Understanding the definitions and types of wounds prepares the nurse for wound care through assessing risk factors, implementing wound care, and evaluating wound healing.

General Principles of Tissue Healing

The following principles are used to guide action in promoting tissue healing. The healthy body has an innate capacity to protect and restore itself. Increasing the blood supply to the damaged area, walling off and removing cellular and foreign debris, and initiating cellular development are parts of the body's healing process. The healing process occurs normally, without assistance, although some care measures can help support the process. For example, keeping the injured area free of debris by proper cleaning helps promote tissue healing,

as does positioning the wounded area to promote circulation to the part.

The body's ability to handle tissue trauma is influenced by the extent of the damage and by the person's general state of health. The capacity to deal adequately with an injury is limited when a healthy person sustains a very massive injury, when the person has a chronic disease, or when the patient is very young or very old. The promotion of wellness to improve resistance to an insult to the body is partially directed toward maintaining adequate body reserves to deal with traumatic experiences.

The body's response to injury is more effective if proper nutrition has been maintained. Undernourished clients have difficulty in mounting their cell-mediated defense system associated with T-lymphocyte activity. These clients may demonstrate diminished immune response to an antigen. Some leukocytic functions are diminished in the presence of protein deficiency. Undernourished clients, then, are at higher risk for developing a wound infection. Although the role of fatty acids in wound healing is still not understood, it is known that certain quantities of glucose are necessary to meet the energy requirements of wound healing.

A variety of vitamins and minerals and trace elements are needed for efficient wound healing. Vitamin A is necessary for collagen synthesis and epithelialization. Vitamin B complex serves as a cofactor of enzyme reactions needed for wound healing. Vitamin C is needed for collagen synthesis, capillary formation, and resistance to infection. Vitamin K is needed for the synthesis of prothrombin. Zinc, copper, and iron assist in collagen synthesis. Manganese serves as an enzyme activator (Flynn and Rovee, 1982).

The body responds systematically to trauma in any of its parts. Local physical responses to an injury cannot be separated from an overall body reaction. For example, an injured foot or hand or an abdominal incision can cause a variety of systematic reactions, which include an increased body temperature, increased heart and respiratory rates, anorexia or nausea and vomiting, skeletal-muscle tension throughout the body, and harmful hormonal changes. Adequate rest, relief of emotional stress, and sufficient nutrients and fluids are particularly important for the person undergoing a response to trauma.

The blood transports substances to and from injured tissue. An adequate blood supply is essential for the body's normal response to any injury. The blood brings increased amounts of leukocytes, erythrocytes, and platelets to the site of injury. Antibodies are also carried by the plasma. Increased circulation to the injured part provides for the removal of toxins and debris and allows for nutrients, oxygen, and other cell-building materials to be supplied. Areas of the body that have a good blood supply, such as the head and the neck, tend to heal faster than areas in which the blood supply is not as great, such as the distal part of an extremity.

Intact skin and mucous membranes serve as first lines of defense against microorganisms. A break in the

T A B L E   **42-1**
Types of Wounds

Types	Causes	Description/Implications
Broad Classification		
Intentional wound	Planned therapy, such as surgical incisions, radiation, or use of a needle or trochar (IV therapy, spinal tap, thoracentesis)	Carried out under surgical asepsis, using sterile supplies and skin preparation. Wound edges clean, bleeding controlled, decreased risk of infection; healing facilitated. In unsterile environment contamination may occur. Wound edges usually jagged with bleeding and multiple tissue trauma. High risk for infection and prolonged healing.
Unintentional wound	Unexpected trauma, such as from accidents, forceable injury (*i.e.,* stabbings, gun shots), and burns	
Skin Integrity Definition		
Closed wound	Body is subjected to a blow, force, or strain (such as a fall, assault, or car wreck).	Skin is not broken, but soft tissue is damaged and internal injury and hemorrhage may occur.
Open wound	Trauma that is either intentional or unintentional	Skin surface is broken, providing portal of entry for microorganisms. May also have bleeding, tissue damage, and increased risk of infection.
Wound Descriptors		
Contusion (bruise)	Blow from a hard object	A closed wound, results in soft-tissue damage and ruptured blood vessels; causes swelling and pain. If internal organs are contused, serious effects may result.
Incision	Made with a sharp instrument or needle	See intentional (open) wound.
Abrasion	An accidental injury or fall that scrapes or rubs off the skin surface; or an intentional dermatologic procedure	An open wound; involves only the skin; is painful.
Laceration	Accidental trauma	Tissues are torn, and wound edges are ragged. Depth of wound varies, and affects risk of complications. Often caused by an unclean object, increasing risk of infection.
Puncture	Made by a sharp instrument or object that penetrates the skin and underlying tissue	May be intentional, or unintentional (see above)
Possibility and Degree of Contamination		
Clean	Surgical incision or closed wound	Contains no pathogenic organisms. Surgery did not enter the respiratory, gastrointestinal, or genitourinary systems.
Clean–contaminated	A specific surgery	Surgery enters the respiratory, gastrointestinal or genitourinary system. Increased risk of infection.
Contaminated	Open accidental wounds, surgery with a major break in asepsis, or surgery with major contamination from the gastrointestinal system	Tissue becomes inflamed. High risk of infection.
Infected	A wound with demonstrated pathogens; an old, traumatic wound; or a surgical incision into an infected area	Wound demonstrates inflammation, heat, purulent drainage, skin separation.

continuity of the skin or mucous membranes increases the likelihood of a wound infection. Surgical asepsis is used in caring for an open wound to minimize the possibility of pathogens entering the site. Precautions are also taken for persons with closed wounds because the resistance of the damaged tissue is lowered and there is a possibility of pathogenic organisms being present. Careful handwashing before caring for a wound is probably the single most effective method for preventing wound infections.

Normal healing is promoted when the wound is free of foreign bodies, including bacteria. Healing will generally not start until foreign bodies are removed from the wound. Excessive exudate; dead or damaged tissue cells; pathogenic organisms; or embedded fragments of bone, metal, glass, or other substances can all act as foreign bodies. The body's own rejection mechanisms generally

are sufficient to remove many foreign substances. However, sometimes mechanical means may be employed to assist the process. There are situations in which the body walls off a collection of pus or another foreign body, and healing occurs around it. This localized collection of pus is called an **abscess**. Usually it can be expected that the person will develop symptoms at the unhealed site, although they may be delayed in their appearance.

Wound Healing

Wounds heal by one of three processes: primary, secondary, or tertiary intention (Fig. 42-1). Most surgical incisions and small sutured lacerations heal by *primary* intention. The wound is a clean, straight line, with little loss of tissue, and all wound edges are well approxi-

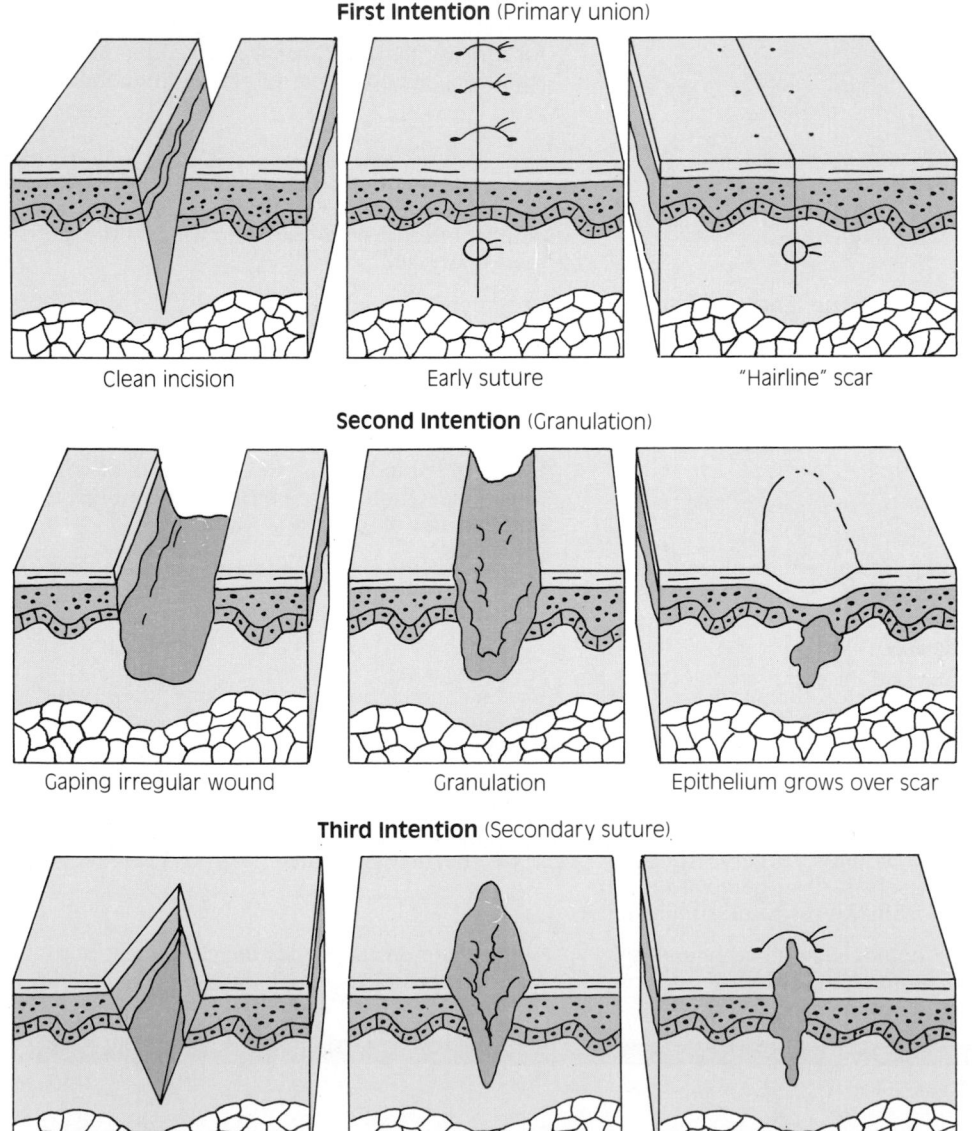

First Intention (Primary union)

Clean incision   Early suture   "Hairline" scar

Second Intention (Granulation)

Gaping irregular wound   Granulation   Epithelium grows over scar

Third Intention (Secondary suture)

Wound   Granulation   Closure with wide scar

F I G U R E   42-1
Chronologic course of wound healing.

mated with sutures. These wounds normally heal rapidly with minimal scarring.

Healing by *secondary* intention takes place in large wounds that have considerable tissue loss so that the edges cannot be approximated. Healing by secondary intention is accomplished through filling in the wound with granulation tissue. Because the wounds are more open, there is a greater chance of infection, healing time is longer, and more scarring takes place.

Healing by *tertiary* intention occurs when there is an increased period of time between the occurrence of the wound and suturing of the wound. This delay allows access for pathogens, so there is an increased possibility of infection. There also is a greater inflammatory reaction and (in comparison to healing by primary intention) more granulation tissue.

An injury to tissues results in two major responses: the stress response and the inflammatory response. All wounds follow the same phases in healing, although differences occur in the length of time required for each phase of the healing process and in the extent of granulation tissue formed. The four phases in wound healing (Phipps et al, 1987) will be described as they occur in the surgical wound, because this is the one most commonly requiring nursing care.

Phase I. Phase I takes place from the time of the incision to the second day following surgery. The inflammatory response is immediate and prepares the tissues for wound healing; this defensive reaction is the local response of the body to injury. As a major stressor, injury initiates the general adaptation syndrome (GAS) and the local adaptation syndrome (LAS). (These responses to stress are described in Chap 9, Stress and Adaptation.) The response of the tissues in phase I is the initial stage of the LAS. During this stage there is first an immediate and brief constriction of blood vessels in the injured area, allowing blood clotting to seal the wound. This is followed by vasodilatation, allowing increased blood flow to the area, permitting white blood cells (leukocytes) to invade the area and engulf bacteria and debris. Fibroplasts also migrate from the bloodstream into the wound, depositing fibrin that stretches through the clot. A thin layer of epithelial cells forms across the wound, and blood flow across the wound tissues is reinstituted.

In this phase, the client will demonstrate the generalized body responses of mildly elevated body temperature, leukocytosis, and generalized malaise.

Phase II. Phase II takes place from the third day after surgery to day 14. Leukocytes begin to decrease, and collagen fibers are deposited in the tissue spaces. Epithelial layers are regenerated by the end of the first week. This new tissue, called **granulation tissue**, is highly vascular and reddish in color, and bleeds easily. The client will begin to look and feel better during this time period.

Phase III. Phase III lasts from approximately the end of the second week to the sixth week after surgery. Throughout this time period, collagen continues to be deposited, and blood flow across the wound decreases and finally stops. The wound looks like a broad, pink, raised scar.

Phase IV. Phase IV, the final phase, lasts from several months to 1 year after surgery. The wound contracts and shrinks, and eventually becomes a flat, thin, white line. This **scar** is avascular collagen tissue that will not sweat, grow hair, or tan in sunlight.

Wound Drainage

During the first two phases of wound healing, the inflammatory response results in exudate that escapes from the wound. **Exudate** is composed of fluid and cells that escape from blood vessels and are deposited in or on tissue surfaces. This exudate is called *wound drainage* and is described as *serous* or *sanguineous;* or, if infected, *purulent.* Further descriptions follow:

Serous: composed primarily of the clear serous portion of the blood, and from serous membranes; serous drainage is clear and watery.

Sanguineous: consists of large numbers of red blood cells and looks like blood. Bright red sanguineous drainage is indicative of fresh bleeding while darker drainage indicates older bleeding.

Purulent: made up of white blood cells, liquefied dead tissue debris, and both dead and live bacteria. Purulent drainage is thick, often has a musty or foul odor, and has varying colors depending on the causative organism(s).

Drainage may be a mixture of these three types; surgical wounds most commonly have a mixture of serum and red blood cells, called *serosanguineous* drainage.

Wound Complications

Although all wounds follow the previously described wound healing process, certain factors can either delay or facilitate tissue repair and healing. Factors having positive effects have already been discussed; factors affecting wound healing negatively are age, circulation/oxygenation, wound condition, and client level of wellness.

Factors Affecting Wound Healing

Developmental Considerations. Children and healthy adults heal more rapidly than do elderly persons, who have physiologic changes resulting in diminished fibroblastic activity and circulation. Elderly persons are also more likely to have one or more chronic illnesses, with pathologic changes that impede the healing process.

Circulation/Oxygenation. A number of physical conditions can affect wound healing. Obesity, with the presence of large amounts of subcutaneous and tissue fat (having fewer blood vessels), may impede wound healing because fatty tissue is difficult to suture, more prone to infection, and takes longer to heal. Circulation may be impaired in elderly persons and in persons with peripheral vascular disease, cardiovascular disorders, hypertension, or diabetes mellitus. Oxygenation of tissues is decreased in persons with anemia and in individuals who smoke.

Wound Condition. As previously described, wounds that are large, contaminated, infected, or retain foreign bodies either heal very slowly or fail to heal at all. Wounds with several of these conditions are especially prone to complications.

Client Wellness. Clients who have inadequate nutrition, are on steroid drugs, or require postoperative radiation have a high risk of delayed healing and wound complications. Additionally, the presence of a chronic physical illness or severe emotional stress can negatively affect wound healing. In some instances, it is necessary to improve nutritional status or treat underlying conditions before surgery is done.

Specific Wound Complications.

Wound complications increase postoperative morbidity and mortality as well as total hospital care costs. Wound complications include wound infections, wound hemorrhages, and dehiscence and evisceration.

Wound Infections. Bacterial invasion can occur at the time of trauma, during surgery, or postoperatively. The likelihood of infection is related, to a degree, to the type and location of surgery performed and to the cause of the wound (Cruse and Foord, 1980). It is generally accepted that a wound is infected if it drains purulent material, whether or not a positive culture specimen has been obtained (Simmons, 1982). Infection may become apparent 2 to 7 days postoperatively. Therefore, in some cases, infection may appear after the client has been discharged from the hospital. Symptoms of wound infection, besides purulent drainage, may include pain, redness, swelling, fever, and increased white blood cell count (Flynn and Rovee, 1982). Nursing care of infected wounds is discussed later in this chapter in the section entitled "Changing Dressings in Special Situations."

Wound Hemorrhages. Hemorrhage may indicate a slipped suture, a dislodged clot because of stress at the operative site, infection, or the erosion of a blood vessel by a foreign body (such as a drain). Postoperative wounds require careful nursing assessment so that hemorrhage is detected early. Hypovolemia may not be immediately evident. Therefore, dressings should be checked frequently during the first 48 hours after surgery

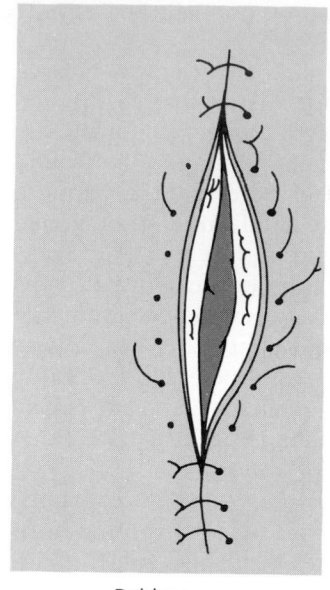 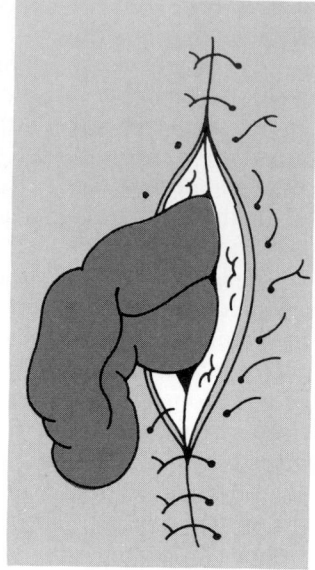

Dehiscence   Evisceration

F I G U R E   42-2
Wound complications.

and no less frequently than every 8 hours thereafter. Close attention should be given to excessive thirst, increased pulse and respiratory rates, and generalized weakness. These may be early signs of hemorrhage. If excessive bleeding does occur, additional sterile pressure dressings or packings may be necessary, fluid replacement will probably be essential, and surgical intervention may be required (Flynn and Rovee, 1982).

Dehiscence and Evisceration. Dehiscence and evisceration are the most serious postoperative wound complications. **Dehiscence** is the partial or total disruption of wound layers. **Evisceration** is the protrusion of viscera through the incisional area. (See Fig. 42-2.) These are frightening occurrences for both client and the nurse. Astute nursing assessment can help identify the predisposing signs of these events. An appreciable increase in the flow of serosanguineous fluid into the wound dressings between the fifth and twelfth postoperative days is a clue to impending dehiscence (Flynn and Rovee, 1982). Wound disruption is often preceded by a sudden straining such as coughing, sneezing, or vomiting. It is not uncommon for the client to comment that something has suddenly given way (Cooper and Schumann, 1979). If dehiscence or evisceration occurs, the wound area should be covered with sterile towels soaked in saline, and the physician should be notified immediately. Both these situations are emergencies that require prompt preparation for surgical repair (Flynn and Rovee, 1982).

Psychologic Effects of Wounds

Trauma, with resultant wounds, causes psychologic stress as well as physical injury. Because the skin functions as a sensory organ and plays a major role in the way we communicate with others and feel about ourselves, wounds require adaptation in the emotional as well as the physical dimensions of the traumatized person. Although stress and adaptation are highly individualized, there are actual and potential emotional stressors common to all clients with wounds. These stressors include pain, anxiety, fear, and alterations in self-concept.

Pain. Pain is a part of almost any trauma, from a small cut on the finger to a large abdominal incision made during surgery on the bowel. Although pain can be considered to be a physical complication, there is a large psychologic component as well. Pain from wounds is often increased by activities such as ambulating, coughing, moving in bed, and dressing changes. The actual pain may be made worse for the client by anticipatory apprehension of such activities. Nursing interventions to reduce pain through skill and explanations can greatly reduce emotional stress.

Anxiety and Fear. Anxiety and fear are common responses to a wound. Clients are apprehensive about the wound strength, how much privacy will be lost as the wound is cared for, and how they and others will react to the sights and smells of the wound. They may actually fear the sight of blood or the sight of what they consider mutilation of their body. As nurses care for clients with wounds, it is important to be accepting and empathic, encourage ventilation of feelings, answer questions accurately and honestly, and avoid excessive exposure of body parts when giving wound care.

Alterations in Self-Concept. The self-concept of each person is that of a whole entity. When the skin and tissues are traumatized, that concept is changed, and the person must adapt and reformulate the concept of self. Wounds and scars that are visible to others, especially on the face, can leave the client with feelings of being conspicuous, ugly, and of less worth. Large scars, such as those remaining from removal of a breast or colostomy openings, can seriously impact sexuality, social relationships, and body image. When developing a plan of care, nurses must include interventions to resolve these concerns; referral to support groups or counselors may be necessary to facilitate coping and acceptance—by both the client and family—of changes in body structure or function.

WOUND CARE

This section of the chapter will discuss the nurse's role in the care of wounds, including the use of all phases of the nursing process in the clinical setting. A case study and sample care plan for one common nursing diagnosis will be included at the end of the chapter to illustrate the application of knowledge and skills presented.

Assessing the Wound

Trauma to tissues can occur unexpectedly through a wide variety of accidental injuries, or can be planned, as in surgical intervention. Nurses need to know how to assess clients and their wounds in both emergency and structured settings, and to make appropriate interventions to meet client needs specific to the setting. This section will discuss the assessment and first aid for wounds from unplanned trauma as well as the assessment of surgical wounds.

Emergency Wound Assessment and Care

Nurses must assess accidental wounds and make decisions about care and treatment. Family members, neighbors, and friends will cut themselves, fall, be bitten by pets, or be injured in any number of possible accidents. Following are general guidelines for assessing and treating wounds in emergency situations, Table 42-2 gives specific guidelines for different types of accidental wounds.

The following are general guidelines for first aid of wounds (Fritz, 1982):

1. Assess the general condition of the person to be sure there is an open and intact airway, spontaneous respirations, and strong pulses. Assessment of the client's status *must* be the priority; after ensuring that the client is stable, assess the wound.
2. Assess the severity of the wound; if major trauma is apparent, call an ambulance, or have someone else make the call while you remain with the injured person.
3. Control bleeding by applying direct pressure over the wound.
4. Apply ice (in a covered plastic bag) to control swelling and reduce pain.
5. Assess for injuries associated with the trauma (*i.e.*, fractures, internal bleeding, spinal cord injuries, head trauma).
6. Clean and cover the wound with a clean dressing (sterile, if possible).
7. For anything other than minor wounds, refer or take the person to the emergency room (ER) or emergency care facility. Immediate treatment reduces the risk of infection and allows healing with less scar formation. A tetanus toxoid injection may also be necessary if the person has not had one in the last 5 years.
8. Teach the person to immediately report redness, swelling, purulent or increased drainage, or continued pain.

T A B L E 42-2
Emergency Assessments and Care of Specific Wounds

Type	Assessing/Interventions
Abrasion	Assess extent and depth.
	Flush the wound under running water, then wash with soap and water to remove dirt.
	Leave small wounds open; cover larger wounds with a light dressing.
Laceration	Assess the length, depth, location, and effect on function of body part.
	Control bleeding by applying pressure with sterile or clean material.
	Clean wound with soap and water, removing embedded dirt.
	Cover the wound with adhesive strips or a dressing to hold wound edges together.
	Take the person to the ER if the wound is severe or requires suturing.
Puncture	Assess cause (may need tetanus or rabies injections).
	Let wound bleed for several minutes to help flush out dirt or saliva.
	Clean with soap and water.
	Cover with a light dressing.
	Take the person to the ER.
Impaled object	Assess for treatment priorities (refer to general guidelines) and call an ambulance.
	Do not remove the object.
	Control bleeding by pressure around the object.
	Stay with the person.
Amputated digits or limbs	Assess wound, blood loss, vital signs; call ambulance.
	Control bleeding by direct pressure to wound or to appropriate pressure points.
	Cover the wound with a dry, clean or sterile pressure dressing.
	Elevate the extremity (*e.g.,* for amputated fingers, place arm on client's chest) and keep the client supine.
	Place the amputated body part in a sealed plastic bag; place this bag in an ice-filled plastic bag or container. (New microsurgery techniques can be used to attach severed digits or extremities.)
	Immediately transport *both* the person and the amputated part to the ER.

(Data from Fritz C: Emergency! First aid for wounds. Nursing 82 October: 68–75, 1982)

Assessing the Surgical Wound

Surgical wounds are defined here as wounds that result from intentional surgical therapy, or wounds that were unintentional but have been treated (cleaned and sutured). Wounds are assessed by inspection (sight and smell) and palpation, and are assessed for appearance, drainage, and pain. Included in the assessment are drains or tubes, sutures, and signs of possible complications, as previously described.

Appearance. Included in assessing the appearance of a wound are the approximation of wound edges, color of the wound and surrounding area, drains or tubes, sutures, and signs of dehiscence or evisceration. The wound edges should be clean and well approximated, with a crust along the wound edges. Normally, the edges of the wound will initially be reddened and slightly swollen, but by the end of about a week the skin should be closer to normal in appearance, and the wound edges should be healed together. Skin surrounding the wound may at first be bruised, but this too will return to normal as blood is reabsorbed. If an infection is present, the wound will be swollen, have increased reddness, and feel hot to touch. If dehiscence is impending or present, the wound edges will be separated.

Skin sutures may be black silk, synthetic material, metal staples, fine wire, or metal skin clips, and are used to hold tissue and skin together. Retention sutures are used to provide extra support for obese clients and for wounds with increased risk of dehiscence (Fig. 42-3). Most skin sutures are removed in 7 to 10 days. Silk and synthetic sutures are removed with a suture removal set (Fig. 42-4); staples are removed with a special staple remover. The steps in removing sutures and staples are summarized in the box on the next page. Following the removal of skin sutures, Steri-Strips are sometimes applied across the healed wound to give additional support as the wound continues to heal. The status of skin sutures is included in wound assessment.

Drains and tubes are inserted into or near a wound when it is anticipated that a collection of fluid in a closed area will delay healing. After a surgical procedure, the physician places one end of the tube or drain in or near the area to be drained, and passes the other end through the skin, either directly through the incision, or through

a separate opening called a stab wound. Drains and tubes may or may not be sutured in; drains placed directly through the wound (for example, a Penrose drain) usually have a large safety pin in the part outside the wound to prevent slipping back into the incised area and are not sutured (Fig. 42-5). Tubes that are connected to suction or that have a built-in reservoir to maintain constant low suction are usually sutured to the skin (for example, a Jackson-Pratt drainage tube or a Hemovac). It is important to know what type of drain or tube was inserted during surgery so that accurate assessment can be made. The patency and placement of tubes or drains are included in wound assessment. Table 42-3 describes the purpose and common use of selected drains and tubes.

Drainage. The amount, color, odor, and consistency of wound drainage is also assessed. The amount and color will depend on the wound location and size, with larger wounds having more drainage. Wound drainage, as pre-

Types of sutures

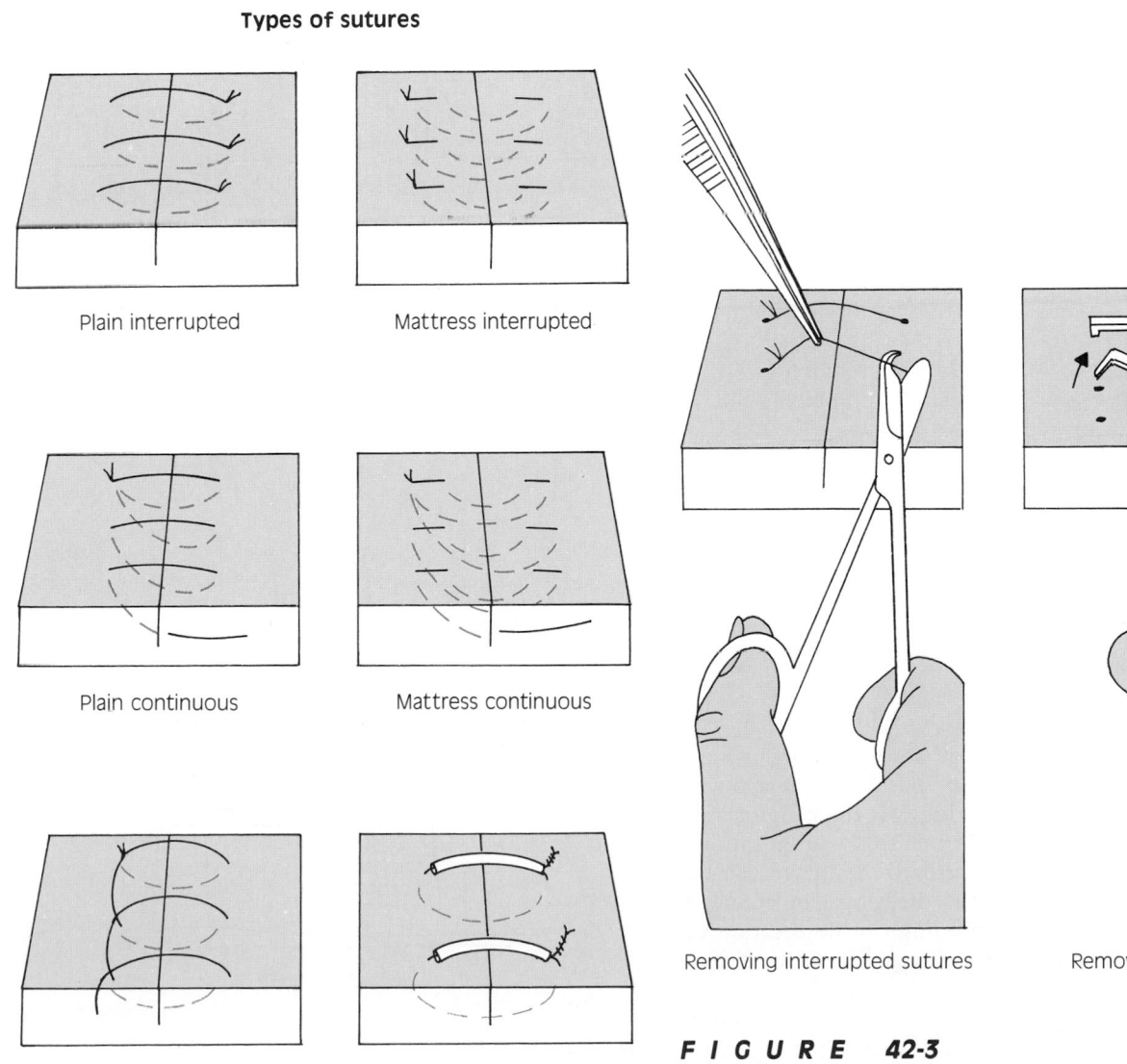

Plain interrupted

Mattress interrupted

Plain continuous

Mattress continuous

Blanket continuous

Retention

Removing interrupted sutures

Removing staples

FIGURE **42-3**
Types of sutures and techniques for removal.

Removal of Staples and Sutures

The removal of staples or sutures may be done by the physician, or by a nurse with a physician's order. Agency protocol should be followed, but general guidelines are:

Removing Sutures

- Explain the procedure to the client.
- Remove the dressing, and cleanse the incision from the center of the wound outward.
- Grasp the knot of the first suture with the sterile forceps, and gently lift it.
- Using sterile suture scissors, cut one side of the suture below the knot, close to the skin.
- Grasp the knot and pull the cut suture through the skin (be sure to only pull through the portion that has been inside the tissue).
- Remove every other suture first to be sure wound is healed; if so remove remaining sutures as ordered.
- Replace dressing, if necessary.

Removing Staples

- Explain the procedure to the client.
- Remove the dressing, and cleanse the incision from the center of the wound outward.
- Place the sterile staple remover, as directed on the package, gently under the staple.
- Firmly close the remover to straighten the staple ends (do not lift upward while disengaging staple).
- Continue as for suture removal, removing every other staple first, and then replacing dressing as ordered.
  Some physicians will order that Steri-Strips be applied to the healed incision after removal of sutures or staples to give additional support to the wound as it continues to heal. Follow agency protocol and physician preference as to placement of these tapes.

increased or purulent, signals delayed healing or an infection. Incisional pain is usually most severe for the first 2 to 3 days, and then progressively becomes milder. Incisional pain that remains severe beyond the expected time can indicate infection, an abscess, or delayed healing.

Related Assessments. In addition to assessments of the wound, the nurse also assesses the general condition of the client and the results of laboratory tests. *Infection* may cause generalized malaise, increased pain, anorexia, and an elevated body temperature and pulse rate; laboratory data will include an elevated white blood count (WBC) and, if a wound culture is done, a causative or-

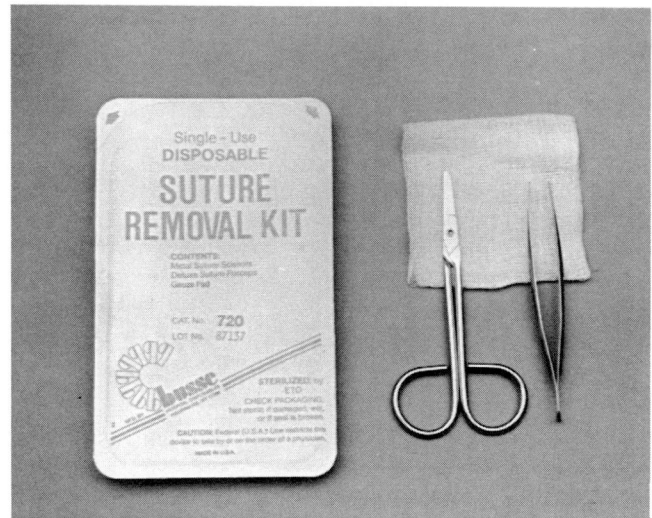

F I G U R E   42-4
Suture removal kit. (Photo © Ken Kasper)

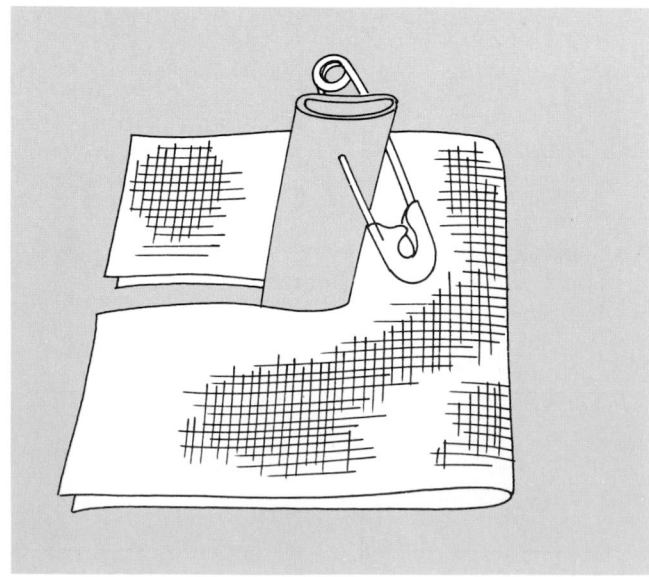

F I G U R E   42-5
Penrose drain.

viously described, may be serous, serosanguineous, sanguineous, or if infected, purulent. Purulent drainage will usually have a musty or foul odor; it is thick and is yellow, green, or brown in color. Frankly sanguineous drainage is indicative of hemorrhage. Drainage can be assessed on the wound, on the dressings, in drainage bottles or reservoirs, or, depending on the location of the wound and the amount of drainage, under the client.

Pain.   When assessing a wound, the nurse should gently palpate the surrounding area. Pain with palpation, especially when accompanied by a flow of drainage that is

TABLE 42-3
Common Types of Drains

Type	Purpose	Example
Penrose	Provides sinus tract	After incision and drainage of abscess, in abdominal surgery
T-tube	For bile drainage	After gallbladder surgery
Jackson-Pratt (J-P)	Decrease dead space by collecting drainage	After breast removal, abdominal surgery
Hemovac	Decrease dead space by collecting drainage	After abdominal, orthopedic surgery
Gauze, iodoform gauze, NuGauze	Allow healing from base of wound	Infected wounds, after removal of hemorrhoids

ganism. *Hemorrhage* would be further identified by restlessness, anxiety, a drop in systolic blood pressure, increased pulse and respirations, decreased urinary output, and a decrease in hemoglobin and hematocrit levels.

Diagnosing

Nursing diagnoses made to identify human responses to alterations in health status as a result of a wound are written to guide nursing interventions that support wound healing and prevent complications. Additionally, holistic assessments and nursing care focus on the *client* with the wound, and identify problems in other functions or dimensions affected by the presence of the wound.

In formulating nursing diagnoses for the client with a wound, the nurse must consider the assessment and nursing history information that support the specific diagnosis. Data used would include

- Physical status of the client, including age, presence or absence of other illnesses, health habits, and obesity
- Cause of the wound
- Location, size, and severity of the wound
- Support systems available
- Social and work history of the client

Included below are examples of nursing diagnoses developed to describe problems experienced by the client with a wound:

Alterations in skin integrity related to midline abdominal incision.

Alterations in skin integrity related to purulent wound drainage.

Alterations in comfort: left flank incisional pain.

Altered sexuality patterns related to presence of burn scars.

Anxiety related to effects of radical mastectomy to relationship with husband.

Disturbance in self-concept related to traumatic injuries and lacerations of face.

Fear related to previous painful dressing changes.

Knowledge deficit: care of wound on right thigh.

Potential for infection related to malnutrition and contaminated wound.

Self-care deficit: bathing: related to presence of large flank incision and multiple drains.

Planning

Although many nursing diagnoses can be identified as appropriate for the client with a wound, there are so many different types of wounds that planning is highly individualized and specific. With the major goals of promoting health, preventing further injury or illness, and facilitating coping, nursing care for any client with a wound is focused on the following client goals:

- The client will demonstrate progressive healing of the wound, as evidenced by
  1. Wound edges closing together
  2. Reduced swelling and redness of wound edges
  3. Reduction in amount and color of drainage
  4. Decreased wound pain
- The client will remain free of infection, with normal temperature and WBC; absence of wound swelling, odor, purulent drainage; and no increase in pain.
- The client will practice self-care behaviors to promote healing
  1. Wash hands appropriately
  2. Keep hands away from wound, wound drainage, dressing
  3. Maintain fluid intake at appropriate levels
  4. Select and eat a balanced diet, as ordered.
- The client will verbalize and demonstrate wound and dressing care.

In caring for the client with a wound, the nurse carries out interventions to promote wound healing, prevent further injury or alteration in skin integrity, prevent infection, promote physical and emotional comfort, and facilitate coping.

Implementing

There are two methods of caring for wounds: the open method, in which no dressing is used to cover the wound, and the closed method, in which a **dressing** is used as a protective cover over a wound.

Dressings have advantages and disadvantages. The advantages are listed in the box; the disadvantages are that dressings can rub or stick to the wound, causing further superficial injury. Dressings can also create a warm, damp, and dark environment—all components conducive to the growth of organisms, with resultant infection. The majority of wounds are covered with a dressing, and nurses are responsible for most dressing changes. This section of the chapter will discuss supplies needed for dressing changes, guidelines for prevention of infection, and procedures for changing selected types of dressings.

Gathering Supplies for Dressings

Before changing a dressing, the nurse should gather needed supplies. These may be separate items or may be packaged in a sterile dressing tray. Some hospital units have special dressing carts, with all dressing supplies located in one area. The supplies needed will vary with the type, location, and amount of drainage of the wound; the nursing care plan should include specifics about each client's dressing procedure and supplies. Materials and supplies will include cleansing agents, materials to cover the wound (the dressing), and materials used to secure the dressing and support the wound.

Cleansing Agents. Many possible antiseptic cleansing agents can be used to cleanse the wound. Some commonly used are Betadine, 70% alcohol, 3% hydrogen peroxide, and sterile normal saline. Some authorities question the use of any agent other than saline because of the caustic effect on skin, tissues, and granulating tissue of the other agents (Rodeheaver, 1982). However, the choice of cleansing agent will largely depend on agency protocol and physician preference.

Dressing Supplies. The number and types of dressings used will depend on the location and size of the wound, as well as the amount and type of drainage. In discussing dressings, supplies will be defined as they are used from the incision outward. An incision line is often covered with sterile Vaseline gauze, or a special gauze called Telfa. Telfa has a shiny outer surface which is applied to the wound and allows drainage to pass through and be absorbed by the center (or outer) absorbent layer. Both these protective dressings prevent outer dressings from adhering to the wound and causing further injury when removed.

Gauze dressings are commonly used to cover wounds (Fig. 42-6). These dressings come in various sizes (2 × 2 inches, 4 × 4 inches, 4 × 8 inches) and are commercially packaged as single units or in packs. Special gauze dressings (*e.g.,* Soft-Wick) are precut halfway to fit around drains or tubes. Larger dressings, (8 × 10s, ABDs, Surgipads) are placed over the smaller gauzes and serve to absorb drainage and protect the wound from contamination or injury.

There are also transparent dressings (*e.g.,* Op-Site) that are applied directly over a small wound or tube; these are occlusive, decreasing the possibility of contamination while allowing visualization of the wound. This type of dressing is often used over IV sites, subclavian catheter insertion sites, and healing wounds.

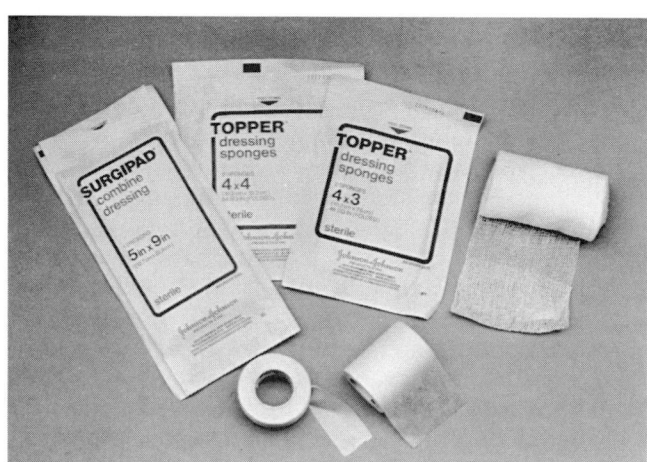

F I G U R E   42-6
Various types of gauze dressings and tape (Photo © Ken Kasper).

TABLE 42-4
Types of Tape

Type	Purpose
Adhesive (can cause occlusion, allergy, skin maceration, shearing)	Used for strength, support, and economy • To secure dressings and splints • To strap joints to prevent athletic injuries • To immobilize or stabilize body parts • To provide pressure • To approximate wound edges
Paper, plastic, acetate	Increased comfort, decreased allergic and skin problems • To close small wounds • To secure dressings
Microfoam	Used for compression or pressure dressings

Tape. There are many different kinds of tape, in a variety of widths ranging from ½ inch to 4 inches (although 1-inch wide tape is the most commonly used). Table 42-4 summarizes the types and purposes of different tapes.

Bandages and Binders. Bandages are strips of cloth, gauze (*e.g.,* roller gauze, Kerlix, Kling), or elasticized material (*e.g.,* Ace bandages) used to wrap a body part. These bandages come packaged in rolls and are of various widths, ranging from 1 inch to 6 inches. Bandages are used to secure dressings, apply pressure, and support the wound; they are especially useful in injuries of the extremities.

Binders are designed for a specific body part, and include slings, abdominal binders, chest binders, and T-binders. Binders may be made of cloth (flannel, muslin) or of an elasticized material that fastens together with Velcro.

Applying Bandages and Binders

General Principles. A bandage or binder promotes healing by preventing damage to wounds and skin by holding dressings on a wound, and by offering the patient comfort and security. The following principles guide action for applying bandages and binders:

Unclean bandages and binders may cause infection if applied over a wound or skin abrasion. This fact guides what may be rather obvious action: bandages and binders should be kept clean and free of contamination. Medical asepsis is observed when applying bandages and binders. Skin abrasions and wounds are first covered with sterile dressings before clean bandages and binders are applied to protect the wound from trauma and contamination. Certain bandages and binders may be reused, but should be changed if they become soiled or wet.

Prolonged heat and moisture on the skin may cause epithelial cells to deteriorate. This principle indicates that the area to be covered should be cleaned and dried throughly before applying a bandage or a binder. An unnecessarily thick or extensive bandage should be avoided so that the part being covered does not become excessively warm. Porous materials are preferable to nonporous materials to allow air to circulate and perspiration to evaporate.

Placing and supporting the body part to be bandaged in the normal functioning position prevents deformities and discomfort and enhances circulation of blood to the body part. Bandages and binders usually restrict some motion and often are intended to immobilize a part of the body. Therefore, it is important that the body part involved first be placed comfortably in the position of normal functioning.

Blood flow through tissues is decreased by applying excessive pressure on blood vessels. The healing process is impaired, and tissue cells may die if the blood supply is inadequate to remove wastes and bring nourishment to the body part involved. The bandage or the binder is applied with sufficient pressure to provide the amount of immobilization or support desired, to remain in place, and to secure a dressing if one is present. However, pressure should not be so great that circulation of blood in the body part involved is impeded. Leaving a small portion of an extremity exposed, such as the fingers or toes, allows the nurse to assess for proper circulation in the bandaged area. Leaving a considerable portion of the end of an extremity exposed is likely to impede circulation if swelling in the exposed area occurs. For example, the heel should not be exposed when bandaging the foot and leg.

The tension of each bandage turn should be equal, and unnecessary and uneven overlapping of turns should be avoided. These techniques help prevent undue and uneven pressure on tissues. Bony prominences over which bandages and binders must be placed are padded. Hollows in the body contour may be filled with padding to provide comfort and to help maintain equal pressure from the bandage or binder. An extremity should be bandaged toward the trunk to promote venous return and impaired circulation in the distal part. After a bandage or binder has been applied, the body part is assessed frequently for signs of impaired circulation. In addition to being dangerous, a bandage applied too tightly is uncomfortable for the patient.

Pins and knots, often used to secure a bandage or a binder, are placed well away from the wound, a pressure point, or a tender and inflamed area. Pins and knots, as well as seams in a bandage or binder, cause undue and uneven pressure. They also cause discomfort for the patient if located incorrectly.

A well-applied bandage or binder will be comfortable for the patient, durable, neat, and clean. This is important for the patient's emotional security as well as for promoting the best possible physiologic functioning of the body.

Applying Bandages (Fig. 42-7)

Applying Roller Bandages.   A roller bandage is a continuous strip of material wound on itself to form a cylinder or roll. Plain gauze, elastic webbing, and stretchable roller bandages are made in various widths and lengths.

When the bandaging is begun, the free end is held in place with one hand while the other hand passes the roll around the body part. After the bandage is anchored, the roll is passed or rolled around the body part, taking care that equal tension is being exerted with each turn. It is easier to keep tension equal by unwinding the bandage gradually and only as it is required.

Basic Turns for Applying Roller Bandages.

Circular Turn.   When using the circular turn, the bandage is wrapped around the body part with complete overlapping of the previous bandage turn. It is used primarily for anchoring a bandage where it is begun and where it is terminated.

Spiral Turn.   When using the spiral turn, the bandage ascends in spiral fashion so that each turn overlaps the preceding one by one-half or two-thirds the width of the bandage. The spiral turn is useful when the body part being bandaged is cylindrical, such as the area around the wrist, the fingers, and the trunk.

Spiral-Reverse Turn.   A spiral-reverse turn is a spiral turn in which reverses are made halfway through each turn. Spiral-reverse turns are particularly effective for bandaging a cone-shaped body part, such as the thigh, the leg, or the forearm.

Figure-of-Eight Turn.   The figure-of-eight turn consists of making oblique overlapping turns that ascend and descend alternately. Each turn crosses the one preceding it so that it appears like the figure eight. It is effective for use around joints, such as the knee, the elbow, the ankle, and the wrist. It provides a snug bandage and therefore is used often for immobilization.

Spica.   The spica consists of ascending and descending turns that overlap and cross each other to form an angle. It is particularly useful for bandaging the thumb, the breast, the shoulder, the groin, and the hip.

Recurrent Bandage.   Sometimes this type of bandage is called a stump bandage. It is used for fingers and for the stump of an amputated limb. After a few circular turns to anchor the bandage, the initial end of the bandage is placed in the center of the body part being bandaged, well back from the tip to be covered. The body is passed back and forth over the tip, first on the one side and then on the other side of the center piece of bandage. Figure 42-7 illustrates applying a recurrent bandage to a stump and using the figure-of-eight turn to finish the bandage. Recurrent bandages are also used effectively for head bandages.

Whichever turn is being used, care should be taken to provide even overlapping of one-half to two-thirds the width of each bandage, except for the circular turn. All surfaces of the skin should be covered by the finished bandage to prevent pinching the skin between turns of the bandage. The bandage is completed well away from the wound or inflamed and tender areas. The terminal end of the bandage may be secured with adhesive, special clamps, or with a safety pin, being careful to avoid undue pressure.

Removing Roller Bandages.   It is best to cut a roller bandage with a bandage scissors to prevent excessive manipulation of the part. Cutting should be done on the side opposite the injury or the wound, from one end to the other, so that the bandage can be folded open for its entire length. If it is a bandage that will be reused, it may be unwound by keeping the loose end together and passing it as a ball from one hand to the other while unwinding it.

Applying Binders

T-Binders.   A T-binder is so named because it looks like the letter T. T-binders are particularly effective for securing dressings on the rectum, perineum, and in the groin. The single T-binder is used for female patients and the double T-binder is used for male patients. The belt is passed around the waist and secured with safety pins. The single or the double tails are passed between the legs and pinned to the belt.

Many-Tailed Binders.   Many-tailed binders are also called **scultetus binders**. The binder consists of a rectangular piece of fabric, which has tails, each about 5 cm (2 inches) wide, attached to the side of the rectangular piece. They support the abdomen or hold dressings on it or on the chest. When a scultetus binder is applied to the abdomen, the patient lies on his back and on the center of the binder. The lower end of the binder is placed well down on the hips, but not so low that it will interfere with the use of a bedpan or with walking. The tails are

(Text continues on p. 1217.)

Roller Bandages

Circular Turn

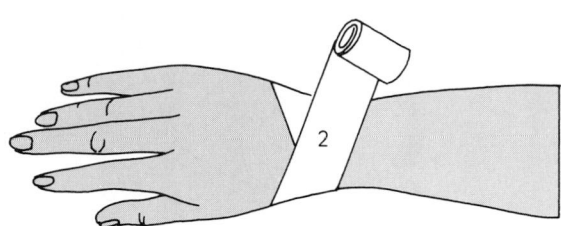

How the circular turn is started to anchor a
roller bandage.

Spiral-Reverse Turn

Spiral Turn

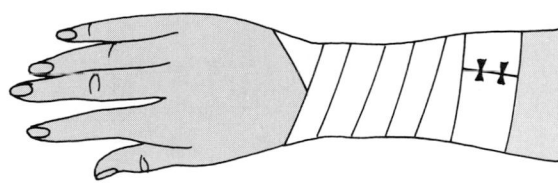

A spiral turn, which was performed after the
bandage was anchored.

Figure-Eight

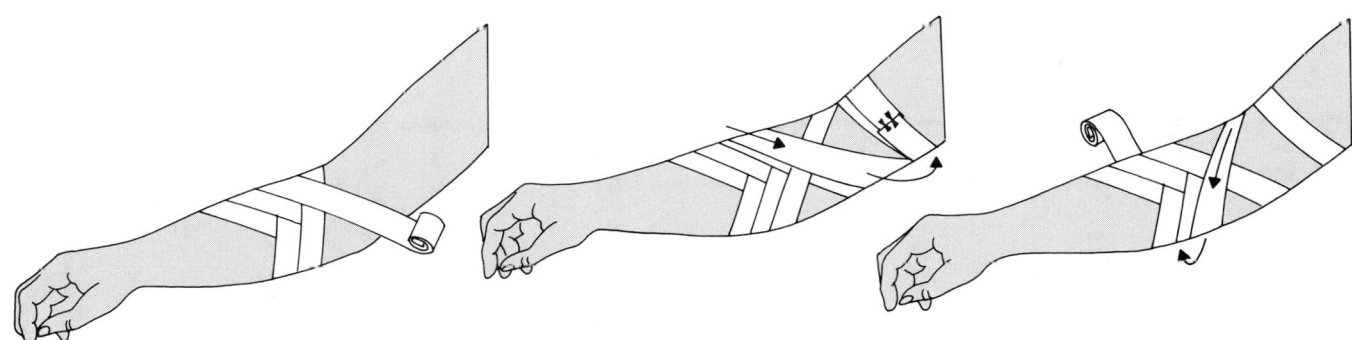

Spica

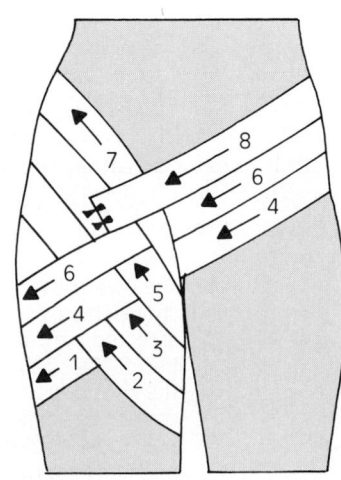
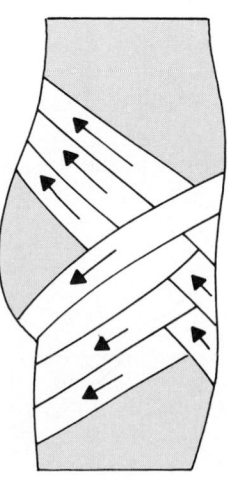

F I G U R E   42-7
Techniques for applying various types of bandages. (Continued on next page.)

Recurrent—Stump Bandage

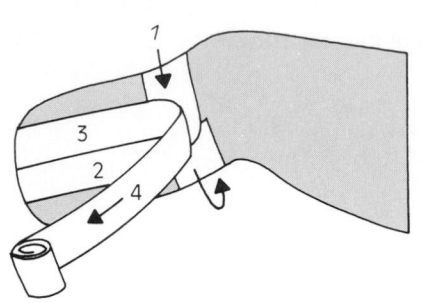 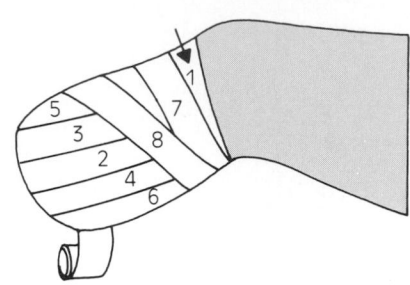 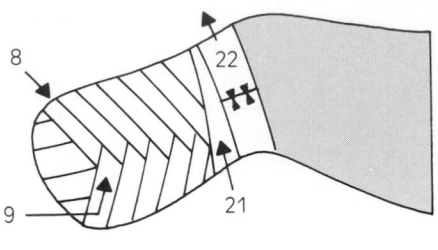

Binders

T-binders

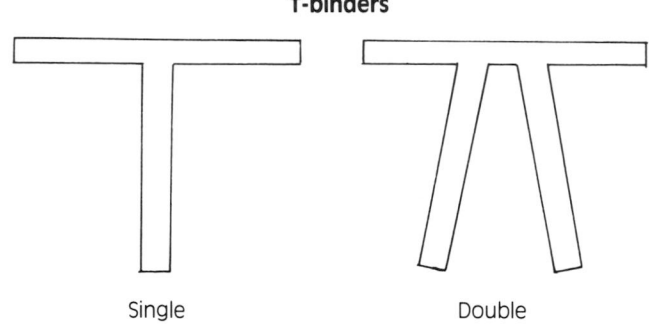

Single   Double

Many-Tailed Binders

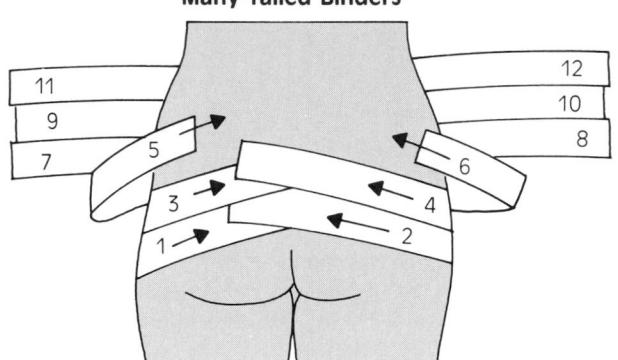

Slings

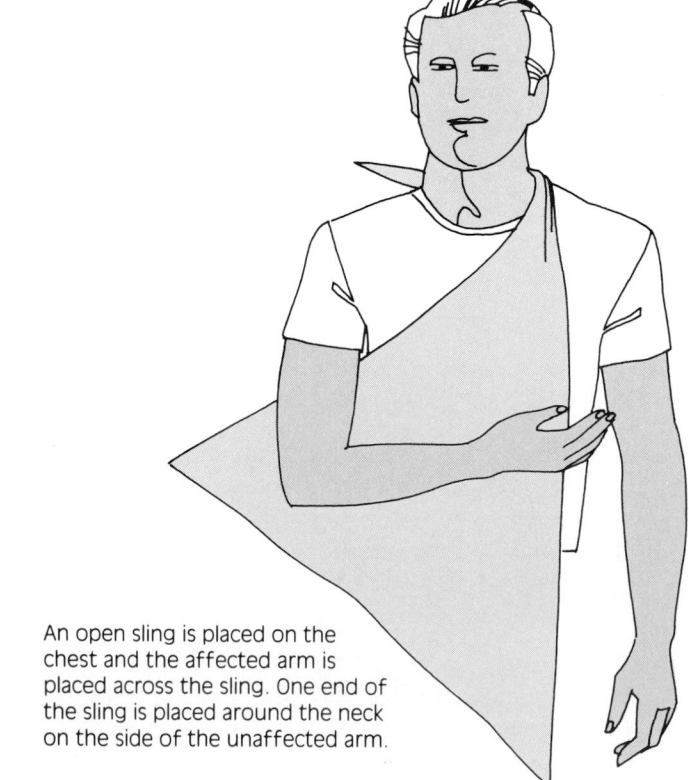

An open sling is placed on the chest and the affected arm is placed across the sling. One end of the sling is placed around the neck on the side of the unaffected arm.

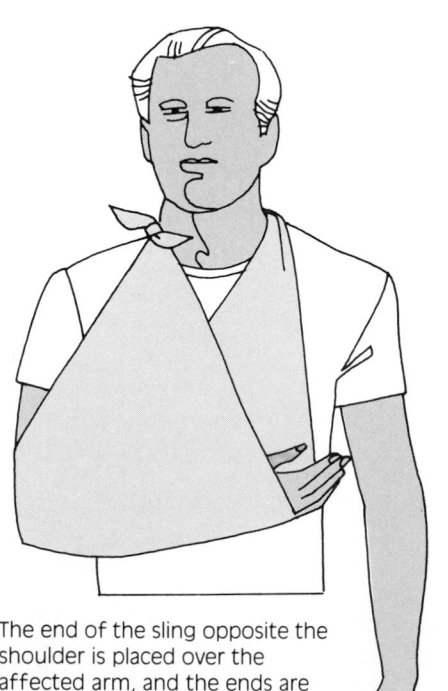

The end of the sling opposite the shoulder is placed over the affected arm, and the ends are tied at the side of the neck so that the knot does not rub over the cervical vertebra. The material at the elbow is folded neatly and may be secured with a pin placed behind the sling so that it is out of sight.

F I G U R E   42-7   (continued)

brought out to either side on the patient's body with the bottom tail in position to wrap around the lower part of the abdomen first. A tail from each side is brought up and placed obliquely over the abdomen until all tails are in place. The last tails are fastened with safety pins.

Sling. A sling is used for the support of an upper extremity. Health-care agencies generally have commercial strap slings or sleeve slings available for use. In the home, a large piece of cloth folded into a triangle can be used as a sling.

Straight Binders. A straight binder is a straight piece of material, usually about 15 cm to 20 cm (6 inches to 8 inches) wide and long enough to more than circle the torso. It generally is used for the chest and the abdomen. Straight binders may be pinned or may fasten with Velcro. A straight binder for the chest often is provided with shoulder straps so that it will not slip down on the trunk and may require tucks to fit the contours of the body.

A binder around the chest wall should not be applied so tightly that it interferes with the patient's breathing.

Changing the Dressing

The nurse should prepare the client for the dressing change by explaining, before the procedure is started, what will be done. Proper screening should be used to provide privacy. The client should be assisted to assume a position that is comfortable for him and convenient for the person changing the dressing. The area is exposed while maintaining proper draping.

It is important to use appropriate aseptic techniques when changing the dressing. It is especially important to wash hands thoroughly before and after changing dressings and follow Centers for Disease Control (CDC) guidelines. Among the most common causes of nosocomial wound infections is carelessness in observing medical and surgical asepsis techniques when changing dressings.

Cleaning a Wound and Applying a Clean Dressing.
The wound is cleaned and the dressing changed as described in Procedure 42-1.

Very often, the nurse is afforded an excellent opportunity for teaching while changing the client's dressing. Teaching becomes especially important when the client will be changing his own dressings after discharge from a health agency. He can be encouraged to help to the extent possible, beginning with such assistance as preparing adhesive strips.

A client may be disturbed by the sight of his wound. The nurse should listen carefully to what the patient is saying and observe for nonverbal communication as well. In some instances, the client may not wish to look at his wound. This is apt to occur when a client has a wound that involves a change in normal body functions or appearance, such as a wound resulting from the removal of a breast, the amputation of an extremity, or the placement of a tube in a draining wound. Patience and emotional support help the client become accustomed to the sight of the wound in time.

Frequency of Changing Dressings. The frequency with which dressings should be changed cannot be stated categorically. It depends on the amount of drainage, the physician's preference, and the nature of the wound. It is customary for the physician to perform the first dressing change following surgery. The first dressing change is usually performed in 24 hours to 48 hours after surgery (Neuberger and Reckling, 1985). Thereafter, nurses change the dressings on an as-needed basis or daily. Frequency for dressing changes should be noted on the client's nursing care plan.

Documenting Wound Care

The nurse is responsible for caring for a wound and for noting factors that may be interfering with the process of healing.

The nurse documents assessments and interventions each time wound care is given and describes the appearance of the wound. If drainage is present, the kind and amount are described. If the client has a complicated dressing, details for caring for the wound should be described in the care plan. Often, the client has preferences for when dressings are changed and how they can be best arranged. Patients often become distressed if one nurse uses one method and another nurse uses a different one, even if both employ proper technique.

Documentation Example. 9/24 0900 Midline abdominal incision cleansed with 0.9%. NS and new dressing applied. Wound edges well approximated, crust formed along wound, edges slightly reddened and swollen. Skin sutures intact. Penrose drain present in lower ⅓ of incision. Moderate amount of serosanguineous drainage present on old dressings.

A. Sprengel, RN

Removing Staples and Sutures

Sutures are removed when enough tensile strength has developed to hold the wound edges together during healing. This varies from client to client, depending on age, nutritional status, and location of the wound. Silk sutures should be removed in 6 to 8 days to prevent suture marks even though collagen formation and remodeling will take at least 21 days altogether. That means the scar may still stretch and widen after the silk sutures have been removed. Special subcutaneous techniques have now been developed to reduce this problem. Small wound closure strips of adhesive (Steri-Strips) may now be applied directly to the wound to help hold it together. Unless otherwise directed, the nurse

(Text continues on p. 1220.)

Cleaning a Wound and Applying Clean Dressing

Equipment

Sterile gloves

Gauze dressings or squares

Sterile dressing set or suture set (contains scissors and forceps)

Cleansing solution

Clean disposable gloves

Sterile basin (optional)

Sterile drape (optional)

Plastic bag for soiled dressings

Waterproof pad

Bath blanket

Tape or ties

Surgi-pads or ABDs

Additional dressing supplies as needed or ordered (antiseptic ointments, extra dressings)

Acetone or adhesive remover (optional)

Sterile normal saline (optional)

Action	Rationale
1 Explain procedure to client.	An explanation encourages client cooperation and reduces apprehension.
2 Gather equipment.	Provides for organized approach to task
3 Wash your hands.	Handwashing deters spread of microorganisms.
4 Check physician's order for dressing change. Note if drain is present.	Clarifies type of dressing
5 Close door or curtain. Use bath blanket as needed when exposing area to be redressed. Position waterproof pad under client if desired.	Provides for privacy and warmth
6 Assist client to comfortable position that provides easy access to wound area.	Provides for comfort
7 Place opened, cuffed plastic bag near working area.	Soiled dressings may be placed in disposal bag without contaminating outside surfaces of bag.
8 Loosen tape on dressing. Use adhesive remover if necessary.	It is easier to loosen tape before putting on gloves.
9 Don clean disposable glove, and remove soiled dressings carefully. Check position of drains before removing dressing. If dressing is not wet-to-dry application and is adhering to skin surface, it may be moistened by pouring a small amount of sterile saline onto it. Keep soiled side of dressing away from client's view.	Protects nurse from handling contaminated dressings. Cautious removal of dressing is more comfortable for client and ensures drain will not be removed if one is present. Sterile saline provides for easier removal of dressing.
10 Assess amount, type, and odor of drainage.	Documents wound healing process or presence of infection
11 Discard dressings in plastic disposal bag. Pull off glove inside out, and drop it in bag.	Prevents spread of microorganisms by contaminated dressings
12 Using aseptic technique, open sterile dressings and supplies on work area.	Supplies are within easy reach, and sterility is maintained.
13 Open sterile cleansing solution, and pour over gauze sponges in plastic container or over sponges placed in sterile basin.	Maintains sterility of dressings and solution

(Continued)

Action	**Rationale**
14 Don sterile gloves. See Procedure 25-2.	Maintains surgical asepsis
15 Cleanse wound or surgical incision. Use sterile forceps if desired	
a. Clean from top to bottom or from center outward.	Clean from least to most contaminated area.
b. Use one gauze square for each wipe discarding each square by dropping into plastic bag. Do not touch bag with forceps.	Previously cleaned area is not recontaminated.
c. Clean around drain, if present, moving from center outward in a circular motion. Use one gauze square for each circular motion.	Move from least to most contaminated area.
d. Dry wound using gauze sponge and same motion.	Moisture provides medium for growth of microorganisms.
e. Apply antiseptic ointment if ordered.	May retard growth of microorganisms and improve healing process
16 Apply a layer of dry, sterile dressings over wound. Use sterile forceps if desired.	Primary dressing serves as a wick for drainage.
17 Cut sterile 4 × 4 gauze square to place under and around drain if one is present (see Fig. 42-5).	Absorbs drainage and protects surrounding skin area
18 Apply second gauze layer to wound site.	Provides for increased absorption of drainage
19 Place Surgi-pad or ABD dressing over wound as outermost layer.	Protects wound from microorganisms in environment

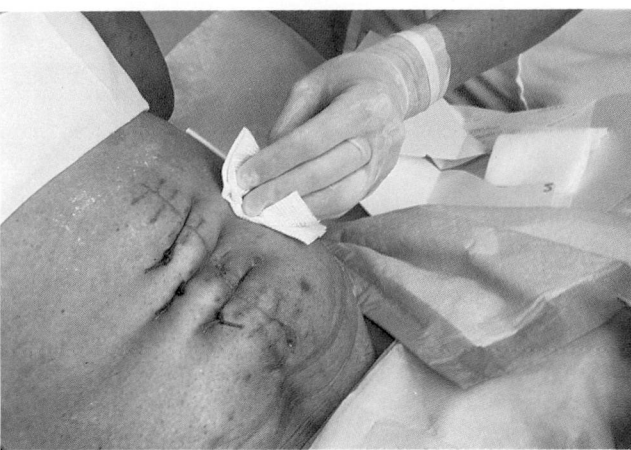

Step 15: Cleansing a surgical incision.

Step 19: Applying Montgomery straps over outer layer of dressing.

Action	**Rationale**
20 Remove gloves from inside out, and discard them in plastic waste bag. Apply tape or tie existing tapes to secure dressings.	Tape is easier to apply after gloves have been removed.
21 Wash hands. Remove all equipment, and make client comfortable.	Prevents spread of microorganisms
22 Check dressing and wound site every shift. Record dressing change, appearance of wound, and describe any drainage in chart.	Provides accurate documentation of procedure

Age Considerations

To keep a dressing intact or to prevent contamination of wound and supplies on an infant or small child, it may be necessary to restrain the child's hand. An old stocking or piece of stockinette may be used to encircle child's hand and then may be secured to the bed or crib with a tie or safety pin. Care must be taken not to compromise circulation to that extremity.

Home Care Considerations

Reinforce need for thorough handwashing before and after dressing change.
Have plastic bag available for safe disposal of soiled dressings and equipment.
Boil any nondisposable equipment (*e.g.,* forceps) for 10 minutes to ensure sterility after washing carefully in warm soapy water.
Inform client about availability of disposable wound care supplies.

Special Considerations

Client must be instructed that any break or interruption in the suture line may require immediate intervention and the surgeon should be notified immediately. Instruct client and family about significant changes that need to be reported to the nurse or physician.
Encourage splinting of wound during activity (coughing, sneezing, sudden movement, or change in position).

should not remove these Steri-Strips during wound care (Neuberger and Reckling, 1985). The guidelines for removing sutures and staples are included in the section on assessing the wound.

Changing a Dressing for a Draining Wound

The basic care of a draining wound is similar to the care of a wound with little or no drainage. The following are additional techniques that are important in caring for a draining wound:

Promoting Comfort.   If wound care is an uncomfortable procedure for the client, it is best to administer a prescribed analgesic or sedative 30 minutes to 45 minutes prior to changing the dressing. It is also preferable to change the dressing midway between meals so that the patient's appetite and mealtimes are not disturbed.

Maintaining Skin Integrity.   A protective ointment or paste may be applied to cleaned skin surrounding the draining wound. This protection acts to prevent skin irritation and excoriation from wound drainage. Protecting the skin is particularly important when it is anticipated that the drainage period may be prolonged or when the person's skin is especially susceptible to irritation. The protective ointment or paste should be removed regularly, at least daily, and the skin should be cleaned thoroughly. It is best to remove the protective material with a minimal amount of rubbing to prevent injury to epithelial cells caused by friction. It is recommended that the first layer of dressing material applied directly to a draining wound be nonabsorbent but hydrophilic (*i.e.,* capable of carrying moisture). This type of material allows drainage from the wound to pass from the first dressing without absorption to overlying absorbent layers of dressing. The advantage of such a dressing is that it does not hold the drainage in direct contact with the wound to cause maceration and reinfection. Also, the material tends not to stick to the wound, a characteristic that makes changing a dressing less uncomfortable for the client. Material to absorb and collect drainage is then placed on the first layer of nonabsorbent material.

The property of surface tension exhibited by liquids and the forces of cohesion and adhesion cause a column of liquid to rise in a fine tube or on a hair. This is called capillary action or **capillarity**. For example, absorbent cotton allows for greater capillarity than untreated cotton. Therefore, cotton-lined gauze sponges soak up more liquid than unlined sponges. Loosely packed gauze, the threads of which act as numerous wicks, enhances capillarity and will allow for drainage to be directed upward and away from its source. Fluffed and loosely packed dressings, then, are more absorbent than tightly packed dressings and will carry drainage up and away from the wound. The number of gauze sponges used in the dressing depends on the amount of drainage. The top of the dressing may further be protected by surgical or abdominal pads, which are thick, absorbent pads that help to absorb profuse drainage.

Because a draining wound requires more frequent changes of dressing than a wound without drainage, it is recommended that Montgomery straps (Fig. 42-8) be used to secure the dressing. These straps do not require changing with each dressing, as tape strips do. Montgomery straps can be made or are available commercially. The adhesive end of the strap is placed on the skin well away from the wound. The end of the strap near the wound remains free because the adhesive side is turned back upon itself. Gauze or woven strips passed through eyelets are tied over the wound to secure the dressing. When the dressing is changed, the strips are untied and turned back to allow for wound care. After the fresh

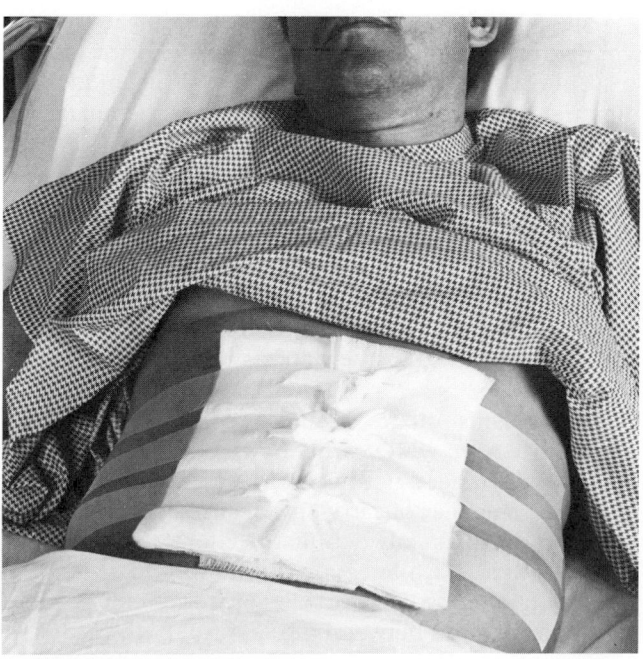

FIGURE 42-8
Montgomery straps make it possible to care for a wound without removing adhesive strips with each dressing change.

dressing is applied, the straps are retied to hold the dressing in place.

Preventing Infection and Promoting Healing. In caring for wounds, the nurse uses principles of both medical and surgical asepsis. The Centers for Disease Control (CDC) makes the following general recommendations for preventing infection of a wound:

- Always wash hands before and after caring for a wound.
- Use sterile gloves or sterile forceps to touch a wound until the wound is sealed.
- Change dressings on both open and closed wounds when wet.
- Take a culture of any suspect drainage.

In addition, the CDC (1988) makes these recommendations to prevent transmission of human immunodeficiency virus (HIV), the causative agent of acquired immunodeficiency syndrome (AIDS), in health-care settings: (only recommendations specific to wound care are included here)

Blood and body-fluid precautions should be consistently used for all clients.

- Wear gloves when touching blood, body fluids containing visible blood, or nonintact skin of all clients, and when handling items or surfaces soiled with blood or body fluids.
- Wash hands thoroughly after removing gloves, and if contaminated with blood or body fluids containing visible blood.
- Take precautions to prevent injuries by needles, sharp instruments, or sharp devices.
- Do not give direct client care if you have open or weeping lesions or dermatitis.
- If procedures commonly cause droplets or splashing of blood or body fluids to which universal precautions apply, wear gloves, surgical masks, protective eyewear, and gloves as appropriate.

Contamination occurs through a moist medium. Microorganisms can move from the external surface through the dressing to the wound if a dressing remains in place until it is saturated. In like manner, microorganisms can move from the wound to the outer surface of a saturated dressing. For this reason, dressings should not be allowed to become saturated. They should either be replaced with fresh dressings or reinforced before drainage causes saturation.

A rubber plastic tubular drain (Penrose), a sump tube, or a catheter is sometimes placed in a wound to promote exudate drainage. Care must be used so that these devices are not dislodged while dressings are changed. A Penrose drain may be ordered to be shortened each day. This can be done by grasping the end of the drain with sterile forceps, pulling it out a short distance while using a twisting motion, and cutting off the end of the drain with sterile scissors. A sterile safety pin (or Klip) often is placed at the end of the drain so that it cannot slip down into the wound.

Closed drainage systems are now being used more

often in place of incisional drains like the Penrose drain. Some studies show that the infection rate is cut nearly in half when drains are placed only when necessary and through a separate stab wound rather than in the incision itself.

Closed drainage systems consist of a drain connected to an electric suction machine or a portable closed drainage suction system (Fig. 42-9).

Portable closed drainage systems have directions for their use printed on the container itself. The nurse should avoid touching the open port when emptying the drainage. Reflux of drainage from a contaminated port could contaminate the wound itself. The use of a closed drainage system eliminates a potential source of microorganisms. The frequent dressing changes needed with the open Penrose drain (which empties directly onto a dressing) are no longer necessary (Neuberger and Reckling, 1985). Closed drainage systems also allow accurate measurement of drainage.

Collecting a Wound Culture.   If assessment of the wound and the drainage indicates a possible infection, a specimen of the drainage is obtained and sent to the laboratory for culture and sensitivity as outlined in Procedure 42-2.

Irrigating and Packing a Wound.   An irrigation consists of directing a flow of solution over traumatized tissues. The purposes of an irrigation include cleaning the area of pathogens and other debris, and applying local heat or an antiseptic to the area.

Generally, nonsterile solutions are used if the wound is closed. Sterile equipment and solutions are required for irrigating an open wound, even in the presence of an existing infection.

The type and amount of solution vary with the condition of the wound. Sterile normal saline, an antiseptic, or an antibiotic solution is used. Hydrogen peroxide may be the solution of choice because its oxygen-releasing ability has an cleans effectively. A sterile, large-volume syringe is generally used to hold the solution. Packing is placed in wounds to allow granulation tissue and healing by secondary intention to take place.

The techniques for administering a wound irrigation and inserting packing are described in Procedure 42-3.

Changing Dressings in Special Situations

Infected Wounds.   CDC guidelines for minor abscesses, infected decubitus ulcers, and minor skin or wound infections (which are *not* infections caused by *Staphylococcus aureus,* beta-hemolytic streptococcus, and *Clostridium perfringens*) include:

- Masks are not indicated.
- Use gowns if soiling is likely.
- Use gloves to touch infected materials.
- Wash hands after touching the client or potentially contaminated articles. Wash hands before taking care of another client.
- Discard and bag contaminated materials separately and label them before sending them for decontamination (Neuberger and Reckling, 1985).

The CDC also recommends special techniques for the care of extensive wounds with purulent drainage. In particular, wounds infected with *Staphylococcus aureus,* beta-hemolytic streptococcus, and *Clostridiun perfringens* (gas gangrene) require the use of these special techniques. When information about the causative organism is unknown, the CDC advises the use of these techniques for all infected and extensive wounds.

The following special precautions should be taken when caring for extensive wounds with purulent drainage:

- Wash hands prior to wound care.
- Wear a gown while caring for the client's wound. This gown need not necessarily be sterile unless there is danger of carrying organisms on a clean gown to an already debilitated client.
- Wear a mask while caring for the wound.
- Be prepared to use two pairs of sterile gloves, and change gloves between the removal of the old dressing and the application of the new dressing.
- Wash the hands thoroughly between glove changes. An antimicrobial soap is recommended by many health agencies.

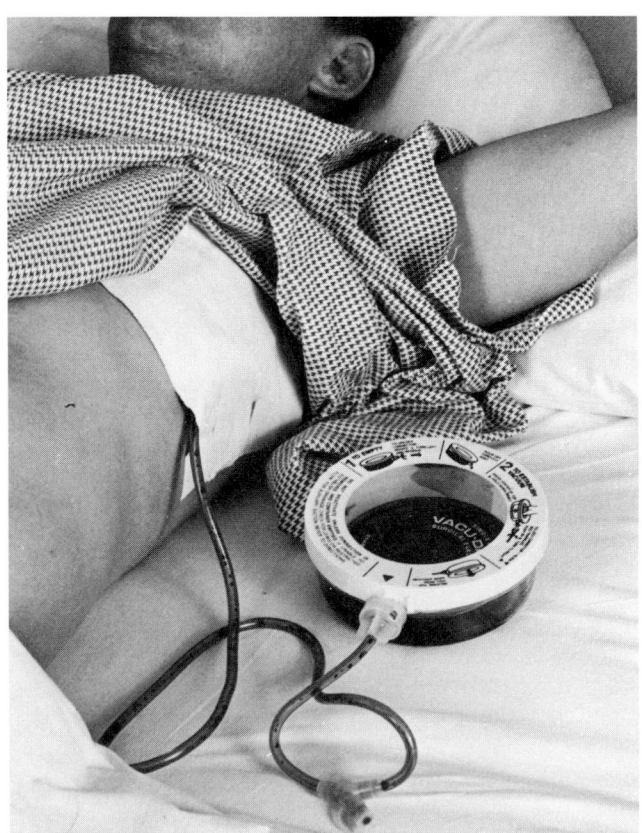

F I G U R E   42-9
The portable suction apparatus shown here helps remove drainage from the site of a wound.

(Text continues on p. 1226.)

PROCEDURE 42-2
Collecting a Wound Culture

Equipment

Sterile Culturette
 tube with en-
 closed swab (or
 culture tube
 with individual
 swabs)

Sterile gloves
Clean disposable
 gloves
Plastic bag for soiled
 dressing

Label for Culturette
 tube
Laboratory requisi-
 tion with rubber
 band or plastic
 bag

Action	Rationale
1 Explain procedure to client.	An explanation encourages client cooperation and reduces apprehension.
2 Gather equipment.	Provides for organized approach to task
3 Wash your hands.	Handwashing deters the spread of microorganisms.
4 Don clean disposable gloves. Remove dressing and assess wound and drainage. See Procedure 42-1, steps 5–11.	Protects nurse from handling contaminated dressings
5 Using aseptic technique, don sterile gloves and cleanse wound. See Procedure 42-1, step 15. Remove sterile gloves.	Removes previous drainage and skin flora
6 Twist cap to loosen swab in Culturette tube, or open separate swab and remove cap from culture tube keeping inside uncontaminated.	Supplies are within easy reach, and sterility is maintained.
7 Don clean glove or new sterile glove, if necessary.	Use of Culturette does not require any immediate contact with skin or wound. If contact with wound is necessary to collect specimen, wear sterile glove on that hand.
8 Carefully insert swab into drainage and roll gently. Use another swab if collecting specimen from another site.	Cotton tip absorbs wound drainage. Prevents cross-contamination of wound.
9 Place swab in Culturette tube being careful not to touch outside of container. Twist cap to secure.	Prevents outside of container from contamination with microorganisms
10 If using Culturette tube, crush ampule of medium at bottom of tube.	Allows swab with drainage to be surrounded by culture medium

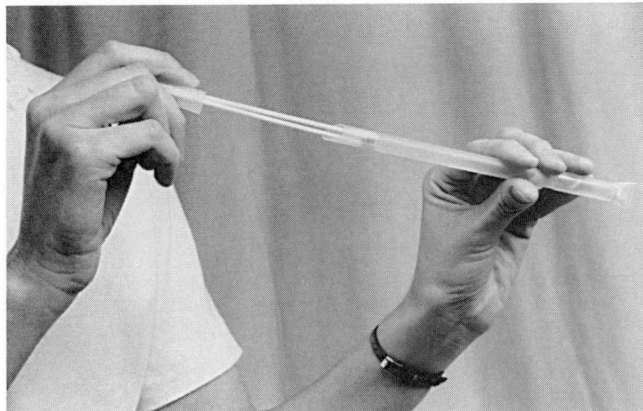

Step 9: Placing swab in a Culturette tube

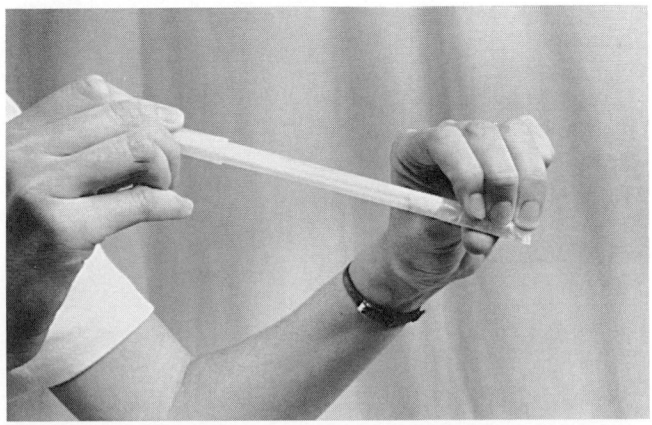

Step 10: Crushing ampule of medium at bottom of tube. (Photos © Ken Kasper)

(Continued) **1223**

Action	**Rationale**
11 Remove gloves from inside out, and discard them in plastic waste bag.	Prevents spread of microorganisms
12 Wash your hands.	Handwashing deters the spread of microorganisms.
13 Apply clean dressing to wound. See Procedure 42-1, steps 16–20.	Provides for absorption of drainage from wound
14 Wash your hands. Remove all equipment, and make client comfortable.	Handwashing deters the spread of microorganisms.
15 Label specimen container appropriately (client's name, date, time, nature of specimen). Attach laboratory requisition to tube with rubber band or place tube in plastic bag with requisition attached. Send to laboratory within 20 minutes.	Ensures proper identification of specimen. Overgrowth of other organisms can interfere with test results if specimen remains at room temperature for extended period of time.
16 Record collection of specimen, appearance of wound, and description of drainage in chart.	Provides accurate documentation of procedure

PROCEDURE 42-3
Irrigating a Sterile Wound and Inserting Packing

Equipment

Sterile irrigation set (basin, container for irrigant, irrigating syringe)

Prescribed irrigating solution (warmed to body temperature or 34°–37°C)

Sterile soft catheter (optional)

Sterile gloves

Clean disposable gloves

Sterile dressing set or suture set (contains scissors and forceps)

Waterproof pad

Sterile gauze and surgi-pads or ABDs (for dressing change)

Plastic bag for soiled dressings

Packing gauze (as specified by physician)

Gown (optional)

Bath blanket

Tape

Action	**Rationale**
1 Explain procedure to client. Check physician's order for irrigation and packing of wound.	Explanation facilitates client cooperation. Clarifies procedure and type of supplies required.
2 Gather equipment.	Provides for organized approach to task
3 Wash your hands.	Handwashing deters the spread of microorganisms.

(Continued)

Action	**Rationale**

4 Close door or curtain. Use bath blanket as needed when exposing wound site.

Provides for privacy and warmth

5 Position client so irrigating solution will flow from upper end of wound toward lower end. Place waterproof pad under client.

Gravity directs flow of liquid from least contaminated to most contaminated area. Waterproof pad protects client and bed linens.

6 Warm sterile irrigating solution to body temperature.

Warmed solution is more comfortable for client and promotes vasodilation.

7 Place opened, cuffed plastic bag near working area. Don gown if recommended.

Soiled dressings and packing may be placed in disposal bag without contaminating outside surfaces of bag. Gown protects uniform from contamination should splashing occur.

8 Loosen tape on dressing, and put on clean glove to remove soiled dressings and packing.

Protects nurse from handling contaminated dressings

9 Assess amount, type, and odor of drainage. Observe condition of wound.

Provides information about wound healing process or presence of infection

10 Discard dressings in plastic disposal bag. Remove glove inside out, and drop it in bag.

Prevents spread of microorganisms via contaminated dressings.

11 Using aseptic technique, open sterile dressings and supplies on work area.

Supplies are within easy reach and sterility is maintained.

Step 9: Assessing wound drainage.

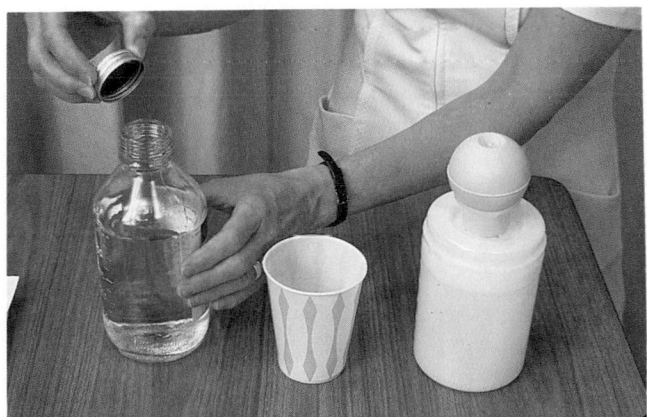

Step 11: Preparing sterile irrigating solution.

12 Pour warmed sterile irrigating solution into sterile container. Amount may vary from 200 ml–500 ml depending on size of wound.

Facilitates wound irrigation.

13 Put sterile glove on dominant hand. See Procedure 25-2.

Maintains surgical asepsis

14 Position the sterile basin below the wound to collect irrigation fluid with nondominant clean hand.

Facilitates irrigation and protects client and bed linens from contaminated fluid

15 Use dominant gloved hand to fill syringe with irrigant. Gently direct a stream of solution into wound keeping tip of syringe 1 inch (2.5 cm) above upper tip of wound. If using a catheter tip on syringe, insert it gently into wound to point of resistance.

Debris and contaminated solution flow from least contaminated to most contaminated area. Catheter allows introduction of irrigant into wound with small opening or one that is deep.

(Continued)

Irrigating a Sterile Wound and Inserting Packing   (Continued)

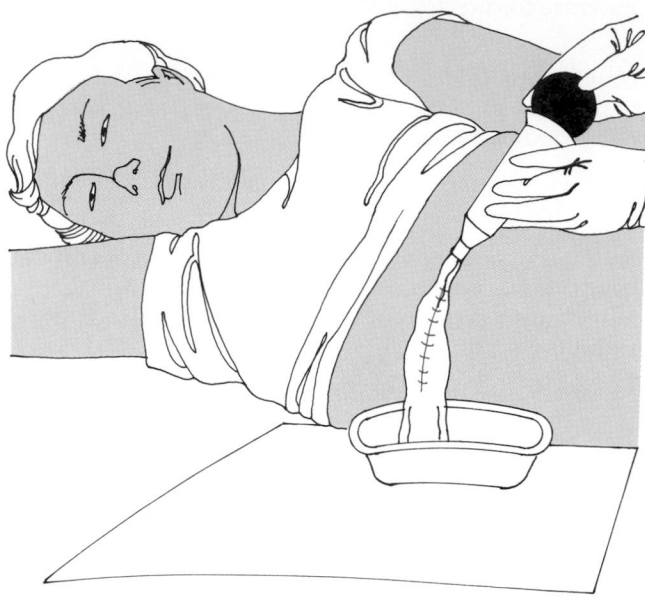

Step 15: Irrigating wound.

Action

16 Continue irrigation until solution returns clear. Try to maintain a steady flow of solution.

17 Use sterile forceps to gently insert sterile packing into wound. Be careful not to pack wound excessively. Cut packing with sterile scissors if necessary. Allow small strip of packing to protrude from small and deep wound for easier removal.

18 Dry area around wound with a sterile gauze sponge.

19 Apply layers of sterile dressing.

20 Remove gloves, and discard them in plastic waste bag. Apply tape to secure dressings.

21 Wash hands. Remove all equipment, and make client comfortable.

22 Check dressing and wound site every shift. Record dressing change, insertion of packing, appearance of wound, and describe any drainage in chart.

Rationale

Irrigation removes exudate and debris.

Packing may be used to absorb drainage and promote healing. Excessive packing of wound may impede blood flow and delay healing process.

Moisture provides medium for growth of microorganisms.

Absorbs drainage and protects surrounding skin area

Tape is easier to apply after gloves have been removed.

Prevents spread of microorganisms

Provides accurate documentation of procedure

• Use a no-touch technique when handling soiled dressings. Lift soiled dressings with a clamp or forceps. This is to eliminate any possible contamination of the hands.

• Place soiled dressings in a moisture-proof bag, which is then closed securely, double-bagged, and incinerated without being opened.

• Be sure to wash the hands again thoroughly after completing wound care. If organisms accumulate

on the hands because proper technique was broken, the organisms are not only likely to be carried to others, but they may eventually become resident flora on the nurse's hands.

Wet-to-Dry Dressings.   Some authorities suggest that covering a wound with a moist or ointment-saturated dressing protects the new epithelium when the dressing is changed. Others believe that these wounds appear to become clean faster than those treated with a dry dressing, simply because the dressing is changed more frequently.

Wet-to-dry dressings may be used to debride an open wound. A sterile saline or povidone-iodine soaked dressing is applied, allowed to dry, and removed. This allows the drying dressing to adhere so the dead wound tissue will stick to it when it is removed. If the dressing is moistened before its removal, however, the purpose of debridement is lost. It should be noted also that a dried dressing may indiscriminately pull off new, healing epidermis along with the dead tissue.

Along with providing protection, covering a wound also provides a moist, dark environment in which microorganisms can grow. A wet-to-dry dressing, then, has to be changed frequently to prevent an accumulation of microorganisms and drainage. The frequency of the wet-to-dry dressing change depends on the topical medication being used and on the amount of drainage (Neuberger and Reckling, 1985).

Semipermeable Membrane Dressings. Semipermeable membrane dressings are being used increasingly with decubitus ulcer wounds (pressure sores) and with intravenous insertion sites. These transparent membranes are permeable to air but are impermeable to liquids. Their advantages include less frequent dressing changes (approximately every 5 days to 7 days), ease of wound observation, and mechanical protection of the wound.

Disadvantages include expense and the difficulty of sterile application because the dressings tend to stick to themselves during application. When using this type of dressing, the site should be cleaned well and allowed to air-dry before the dressing is applied. The site should be inspected daily, and the dressing should be changed if it is not intact or if it has lost its intended seal around the wound (Neuberger and Reckling, 1985).

Evaluating

Evaluating the effectiveness of the nursing care plan is based on the client goals. The plan of care for the client with a wound will be effective if the client has a healed wound, has remained free of infection, and can carry out wound and dressing care by himself, if needed.

HEAT AND COLD APPLICATIONS

Hot and cold agents are applied to an area of a client's body to bring about a local or systemic change in body temperature for a variety of therapeutic purposes. Physiologic responses to heat and cold are modified by the method and duration of application, the degree of heat and cold applied, the age and physical condition of the client, and the amount of body surface covered by the application. This section of the chapter will discuss the

effects of heat and cold, and will use the phases of the nursing process to define the responsibilities of the nurse in caring for the client receiving applications of heat or cold.

Physiologic Responses to Heat and Cold

Heat and cold cause both local and systemic effects. Body temperature is regulated by cells in the hypothalamus in response to signals from thermal (heat and cold) receptors located close to the surface of the skin. Stimulation of these receptors sends sensory messages to cells of the anterior hypothalamus to dissipate heat (by such mechanisms as vasodilation and sweating) or to the cells of the posterior hypothalamus to conserve heat (by vasoconstriction and shivering). Pain receptors, also located near the surface of the skin, are activated if external temperatures are too hot or too cold.

Local Effects of Heat

The many benefits of heat are summarized in Table 42-5. Heat causes vasodilation of peripheral blood vessels, a mechanism that helps dissipate heat from the body to the environment. Vasodilation also increases blood flow to a body part that is injured or has altered function. In turn,

TABLE 42-5
Benefits of Heat and Cold

Heat	Cold
Relaxes muscles	Relaxes muscle
Decreases pain	Decreases pain
Increases circulation	Decreases circulation
Relieves congestion	Reduces swelling
Raises body temperature, prevents infection	Prevents edema
Promotes healing	Reduces temperature
Has sedative effect	Retards bacterial growth
Reduces need for medication	Acts as local anesthetic; decreases need for analgesics
Reduces joint stress, reduces need for anti-inflammatory agents	Decreases oxygen supply to area
Promotes resolution of superficial infections, reduces need for antibiotics	Decreases metabolism
Relieves dysmenorrhea	

(Spencer RT, et al: Clinical Pharmacology and Nursing Management, 3rd ed. Philadelphia, JB Lippincott, 1989)

oxygen and nutrients are increased to the area, and venous congestion is decreased. Reduced viscosity of blood and increased capillary permeability improves the delivery of leukocytes and nutrients while also facilitating the removal of wastes and prolonging clotting time. These actions, combined with increased tissue metabolism, accelerate the inflammatory response to promote healing. Heat reduces muscle tension to promote relaxation and helps relieve muscle spasms and joint stiffness. It decreases the viscosity of the synovial fluid in joint spaces. Heat also reduces pain through vasodilation, and the relaxation effect.

Because of these local physiologic effects, heat in various forms is used to treat infections, surgical wounds, inflamed tissue, arthritis, joint and muscle pain, dysmenorrhea, and ischemia of peripheral tissue.

Local Effects of Cold

In general, the effects of cold are opposite those of heat. The benefits of cold are listed in Table 42-5. Cold causes vasoconstriction of peripheral blood vessels, reducing blood flow to tissue. Decreased metabolic needs and capillary permeability combined with increased coagulation of blood at the wound site facilitates the control of bleeding and reduces edema formation. Cold also reduces muscle spasm, alters tissue sensitivity (producing numbness), and promotes comfort by relieving pain.

Cold, for these effects, is used after direct trauma (especially in closed wounds, trauma to muscles and bones, and burns) and in the treatment of arthritis.

Other Effects of Heat and Cold

The *systemic effects* of extensive heat are increased cardiac output, sweating, increased pulse rate, and a decreased blood pressure. Application of heat to a large body area increases the blood flow to that area while decreasing it to another part of the body. Extensive cold produces systemic effects of increased blood pressure, shivering, and "goose bumps." Another generalized response is found when the effects of heat or cold in one body part are also found in another area of the body; for example the application of heat to the right leg results in vasodilatation in both legs.

The *rebound phenomena* is important to the therapeutic value of heat and cold, and to the safety of clients receiving such therapy. Heat produces maximum vasodilitation in 20 minutes to 30 minutes; if heat is continued beyond that time period, tissue congestion and vasoconstriction occur (for unknown reasons). With cold, maximum vasoconstriction occurs when the skin reaches 60°F (15°C); then vasodilation begins. If hot and cold applications are applied for long time periods, burns (from heat) and freezing (from cold) can occur, and the intended purpose of the application will not be realized.

The ability of the body to *adapt* to heat and cold is also an important consideration in this type of therapy. Heat and cold skin receptors are initially strongly stimu-

lated by sudden changes in temperature. For the first few seconds after being stimulated, the stimulation decreases rapidly, and then more slowly for the next 30 minutes, as the receptors adapt to the temperature. A hot application, even if the temperature remains constant, will not feel as warm after adaptation has taken place. Clients must be taught that increasing the temperature or lengthening the time of application can cause serious tissue damage.

Assessing

Before initiating heat or cold applications, the nurse must assess the physical and mental status of the client, the condition of the body area to be treated with heat or cold, and the condition of the equipment to be used. Those factors that influence the tolerance of heat and cold need to be carefully considered, and are the base for the following questions:

- How long will the heat or cold be applied? As previously discussed, prolonged exposure causes increased tolerance and rebound effects are undesirable.
- What body part is involved? Some body areas are more sensitive to thermal changes: the neck, the perineum, and the inner aspect of the forearm and wrist.
- Is the skin intact? Open tissue or abraded skin is more sensitive to thermal changes.
- How large is the area? Applications of heat or cold to large areas of the body cause systemic responses, and lower tolerance of change of temperature.
- What is the client's age? Infants, children, and the elderly tolerate temperature changes less well than do adults.
- What is the client's physical condition? Clients with certain alterations in health will have reduced response or tolerance of thermal changes, increasing the risk of injury.

Assessing Physical and Mental Status.   Assessing the physical status of the client includes a health history and physical assessment. A history of cardiovascular or peripheral vascular impairment, sensory impairment, and alterations in mental status (such as confusion or decreased level of consciousness) indicate caution with the use of heat or cold because of the danger of tissue damage. Heat should not be applied to an open wound immediately after the trauma; during hemorrhage; over noninflammatory edema; or to an acutely inflamed area, a localized malignant tumor, the testes, the abdomen of a pregnant female, or over metallic implants. Cold should not be used for open wounds or for clients with impaired peripheral circulation or allergy to cold.

Assessments would include response to stimuli (sharp and dull), color and appearance of body tissues, circulation (pulses, blanching sign, temperature and color), level of consciousness, and orientation.

Assessing the Area of Application.

Although heat or cold is commonly ordered to be applied to a specific body part, it is the nurse's responsibility to assess the area and evaluate the client's response to the applications. Baseline data derived from assessments are used to ensure safety and evaluate outcomes of therapy. The risk of damage to tissues is increased if the area is traumatized, has altered skin integrity (assess for open lesions, blisters, wounds, edema, bleeding, drainage), or has altered circulation (assess color, temperature, sensation). As with any assessment, bilateral body parts are compared for changes. Tissue that has decreased or absent pulses, is pale or cyanotic, and feels cold to touch has decreased circulation and is at high risk for injury, especially from cold.

Assessing the Condition of Equipment.

The nurse is responsible for checking the equipment used and maintaining client safety. Included is the condition of cords and plugs, heating or cooling elements, fluid leaks, and distribution and constancy of temperature.

Diagnosing

Heat and cold applications are initiated only with a physician's order; the role of the nurse is interdependent, specific to the ordered therapy. However, the response of the client to the heat or cold indicates possible nursing diagnoses. Collaborative problems include potential complications: hypothermia (specify body part), hyperthermia (specify body part), impaired circulation, tissue injury, and neurovascular deficits.

The following *nursing diagnoses* may be indicated (Carpenito, 1987):

Altered comfort: Pain related to large hematoma, left calf, requiring hot packs to right leg every 4 hours.

Knowledge deficit: Use of heating pad.

Potential for infection related to trauma of left hand with daily debridment and hot soaks.

Potential alteration in peripheral tissue perfusion related to cold applications and presence of altered peripheral circulation.

Potential for injury related to decreased thermal perception.

Planning

Heat and cold are used for a wide variety of therapeutic purposes that are an essential part of planning individualized client care and form the basis for client outcomes.

Indications for Heat Applications

Promote Wound Healing. Heat promotes wound healing in a variety of ways. The increased blood supply resulting from vasodilatation increases cell metabolism by bringing additional nutrients to the injured tissue and by increasing waste and toxin removal. These phenomena promote wound healing. The blood also brings increased numbers of leukocytes to defend against infection. Heat hastens the physical and chemical processes of suppuration, which is the formation of pus. The pus becomes localized in the infected area, where it is then carried away by the circulatory and lymph systems or drains from the wound rather than spreading to surrounding tissues. Drainage is thereby also increased with heat applications.

Relieve Pain. One of the most common uses of the local application of heat is to relieve pain. The exact mechanism is not clearly understood, although some believe heat decreases the perception of pain. Others theorize that in the presence of both heat and pain stimulation, the perception of either decreases.

Relieve Muscle Tension and Joint Stiffness. Although the effects of the local application of heat do not occur deeply in the body, heat has a muscle-relaxing effect and, therefore, promotes rest and relaxation. The exact mechanism is not clearly understood. Heat also decreases the viscosity of synovial fluid and allows improved joint range of motion.

Warm a Part of the Body. Heat may be applied locally to warm the body. For example, by placing warmth on cold feet, heat is transmitted to the body by conduction.

Reduce Edema. Heat facilitates the removal of excess fluid from the interstitial fluid spaces as blood supplies to the area are increased. As a result, increased absorption of fluid takes place in the capillaries. Excess fluid in the tissues is absorbed into the general circulation.

Indications for Cold Application

Relieve Pain. Cold applications are frequently used to limit the accumulation of fluid in the body's tissues. This occurs by the phenomenon of vasoconstriction and decreased circulation to the area so that excess fluid cannot gather in an injured area to increase pressure and pain. Pain and muscle spasms are also relieved by the anesthetic effects of cold. Cold is especially useful in traumatic injuries and burns.

Limit Inflammation and Suppuration. Cold causes vasoconstriction, a decrease in cell metabolism, and inhibited microbial activity. These mechanisms act to control an inflammatory process and suppuration.

Control Bleeding. Cold applications help control bleeding by vasoconstriction. Also, the decreased flow rate of blood and its increased viscosity promote blood clotting.

Client Goals

When applications of heat or cold are a part of a plan of care, the following outcomes are appropriate; specific outcomes should be chosen based on the purpose of the application.

- The client will verbalize increased comfort, as evidenced by decreased muscle spasms, increased ability to rest, decreased local inflammation, and decreased edema.
- The client will demonstrate signs of wound healing.
- The client will verbalize and demonstrate safe hot or cold application.

The nurse's aims, in applying heat and cold, are (1) promote wound healing, (2) facilitate comfort, (3) use knowledge and skill in carrying out the application, and (4) follow safety measures when providing heat or cold therapy.

Implementing

Heat and cold are applied to the body as both moist and dry applications, using many different forms and methods. Types of applications and their definitions are described in the box. Temperatures for heat and cold applications are given in Table 42-6.

Client Teaching.   As with any other procedure, the nurse explains the purpose and steps of the application, and the sensations that will be experienced. To promote safety, it is important to ask the client to report immediately any changes in sensation or discomfort, to provide a timer or clock, and to have the call light in reach. The client should be instructed not to move the application or adjust any controls.

Physician's Order.   An order is necessary for any type of heat or cold application. The order should include the type of application, body area to be treated, frequency of application, and the length of time for each application. Guidelines are given in this chapter for various applications; specific details may vary according to agency protocol.

Applying Heat

Heat is applied by both dry and moist methods. Hot water bottles, electric heating pads, Aqua K pads, or chemical heat packs provide local heat by conduction (see Procedure 42-4). Dry heat by radiation is provided by heat lamps or heat cradles. Moist heat, by conduction, is provided by hot compresses or packs, sitz baths, or soaks.

Dry Heat

Hot Water Bags/Bottles.   Hot water bags have disadvantages: they may leak, their weight often makes them uncomfortable for the client, and there is a danger of burns from improper use. However, they are relatively easy and inexpensive to use (see Procedure 42-4).

Electric Heating Pads.   The electric heating pad can be used to apply dry heat locally. It is easy to apply, provides constant and even heat, and is relatively safe to use. Nevertheless, improper use can result in injury. The following are recommended techniques for using an electric heating pad:

- Avoid pins to secure a heating pad. There is danger of electric shock if a pin touches a wire.
- Place a covering over the pad, preferably one that is moisture-proof. Prevent wet and moist conditions around the pad. Short circuiting the heating element may cause an electric shock to occur. The pad should not be covered too heavily. Heat may accumulate and burn the client when it cannot dissipate normally from the pad.
- Place a heating pad anteriorly or laterally to a body part—not under a portion of the body. If the heat-

T A B L E   42-6
Temperatures for Heat and Cold Applications

Description	Temperature Range	Example
Very Cold	Below 59°F (15°C)	Ice bags
Cold	59°F–65°F (15°C–18°C)	Cold pack
Cool	65°F–80°F (18°C–27°C)	Cold compress
Tepid	80°F–98°F (27°C–37°C)	Alcohol sponge bath
Warm	98°F–105°F (37°C–40°C)	Aqua-K pad
Hot	105°F–115°F (40°C–46°C)	Hot soak
Very Hot	Above 115°F (46°C)	Hot water bottle

Heat and Cold Applications

Dry Applications

Aquamatic (K-matic) pad: A rubber pad of tubular construction that can be filled with distilled water. An electric control unit heats the water and keeps it at an even temperature. This pad permits the maintenance of a constant temperature at the level prescribed by the physician; therefore, it is both safer and more effective than a hot water bottle or electric heating pad.

Cold chemical packs: A rubberized or plasticized flat bag containing a chemical substance that is frozen and used as a cold, dry application to the body surface. It must be covered with a protective covering before application.

Heat cradle: A metal cradle in which several electric sockets are installed for luminous bulbs; a means of providing radiant heat.

Heat lamp: A gooseneck lamp containing a 60-watt bulb, applied 18 inches to 24 inches from the body site. The heat lamp provides dry-heat radiation.

Ice bag or collar: A rubber or plastic device filled with ice chips and covered with a protective fabric before application to the client's body site. Vasoconstriction of peripheral vessels is caused by cold application.

Ice glove: A rubber glove filled with ice chips, placed in a light covering, and applied to a body surface. It is usually used in a postoperative oral surgery client and for relief of discomfort of the perineum after childbirth.

Moist Applications

Alcohol or cold sponge baths: A means by which reduction of body temperature occurs from evaporation. Cool water or a combination of cool water and alcohol is applied to the skin.

Compresses: Compresses may be either moist (gauze) dressings or washcloths. A compress usually is applied to smaller body areas and must be changed frequently. Compresses may be either hot or cold, sterile or unsterile, as designated by the physician.

1. Hot compresses use the principle of heat conduction and can be sterile or unsterile moist applications. Generally, gauze is soaked in the solution designated by the physician. The excess fluid is wrung out of the gauze to be applied. Sterile precautions are indicated when the compress is to be applied to an open wound or to an organ, such as the eye, to prevent the entrance of

microorganisms. An insulating, waterproof cloth is placed over the compress to aid in heat retention. Hot compresses hasten the suppurative process and improve circulation.

2. Cold or ice compresses are usually made of gauze or washcloths. The application of cold to open wounds or to lesions that may rupture requires sterile technique. Cold diminishes the formation and absorption of bacterial toxins. It also causes vasoconstriction, decreased tissue metabolism, and sensory anesthesia. It is used for contusions, sprains, strains, and for controlling hemorrhages. Cold compresses also may be used for an injured eye, headache, tooth extraction, or hemorrhoids. The material used for application is immersed in a basin (clean or sterile, as ordered) that contains pieces of ice and water or ordered solution. If sterile technique is used, the sterile solution bottle is set in the bowl of ice. Compresses should be changed frequently.

Packs: Packs are usually applied to an extensive area of body surface. They may be either cold or hot, sterile or unsterile, as designated in the order. Examples are as follows:

1. Hot pack (fomentation) is a piece of heated, moist towel that is applied to a client's skin to provide superficial heat. The effect of moderate heat is vasodilation, lessened viscosity of the blood, increased tissue metabolism, as well as relief of pain, congestion, inflammation, swelling, and muscle spasms. Application to open wounds or lesions that may rupture should be done using sterile technique. A heating device may be used to keep the pack warm. If the sterile procedure is ordered, the solution, towels, and dry covering must be sterile as well as the gloves or forceps used for wringing them dry.

2. A cool wet pack is composed of bath towels moistened in water cooled with a small amount of ice chips. After wringing, the towels are applied full length to cover the anterior and posterior trunk of the body and each extremity. The temperature of the water is maintained at 75°F. Ice bags may be placed at the axillae, groin, and head. The cool wet pack is used to reduce body temperature by evaporation. This procedure may be done under sterile conditions.

Heat and Cold Applications   (continued)

3. Ice packs are used occasionally to lower the temperature of a client's limb before surgery or to decrease swelling. It is a method of hypothermia that should be used with caution. Plastic bags of ice, which are covered with a pillowcase or towel, are placed on the specified area. Lower body temperatures are used for checking inflammation and suppuration by decreasing blood supply, slowing cellular metabolism, and inhibiting microbial activity. Extreme cold can destroy tissue if the length of application is excessive, however.

Soaks: A soak usually refers to the immersion of a part of the body, such as a foot or a hand, or may refer to wrapping the part with gauze and saturating it with fluid. The soak may be done under sterile conditions.

(Wieck L, King EE, Dyer M: Illustrated Manual of Nursing Techniques, 3rd ed, pp 419–420. Philadelphia, JB Lippincott, 1986)

---

ing pad is between the client and the mattress, there may be inadequate heat dissipation. This could cause the client or bed linens to be burned.

- Use a heating pad with a selector switch that cannot be turned up beyond a safe temperature. After heat has been applied and a certain amount of adaptation of heat receptors takes place, the patient often increases the heat when the switch is not permanently preset, because the pad does not seem sufficiently warm. Many persons have been burned by turning up the heat in an electric pad because they believed the pad was too cool.
- Assess the client's skin at regular intervals for the effects of excessive exposure to heat.
- Be sure to check agency protocol for use of heating pads; a release form may need to be signed.

Aqua K (Aquathermia) Pads. Aquathermia pads (Fig. 42-10) are commonly used in health-care agencies for a variety of health problems, including back pain, muscle spasms, thrombophlebitis, and mild inflammations. These devices are safer than a heating pad but still must be checked carefully. Guidelines for use are (also see Procedure 42-4):

- The temperature setting is usually set and locked before application.
- If the distilled water in the reservoir runs low, more is added at the top of the control unit. Tap water is not used.
- An application should only last 20 minutes to 30 minutes.
- Assess the client's skin frequently for signs of burning.

Heat Lamps. Heat lamps are used to provide dry heat to increase circulation to a small area, such as a decubitus ulcer. Heat lamps come with either infrared or regular 40- to 60-watt bulbs. The lamps (often gooseneck type) are placed 18 inches to 30 inches from the area to be treated, and are applied for 15 minutes to 20 minutes. Precautions with use are:

- Clean and dry the area before the treatment to prevent burning.
- Do not cover the lamp or place it under bedclothes.
- Assess the skin exposed to the heat every 5 minutes.

Heat Cradles. A heat cradle is a metal half-circle frame that encloses the body part to be treated with heat. A series of 25-watt bulbs, 16 inches to 18 inches from the client, provide heat over a larger area. The cradle may be

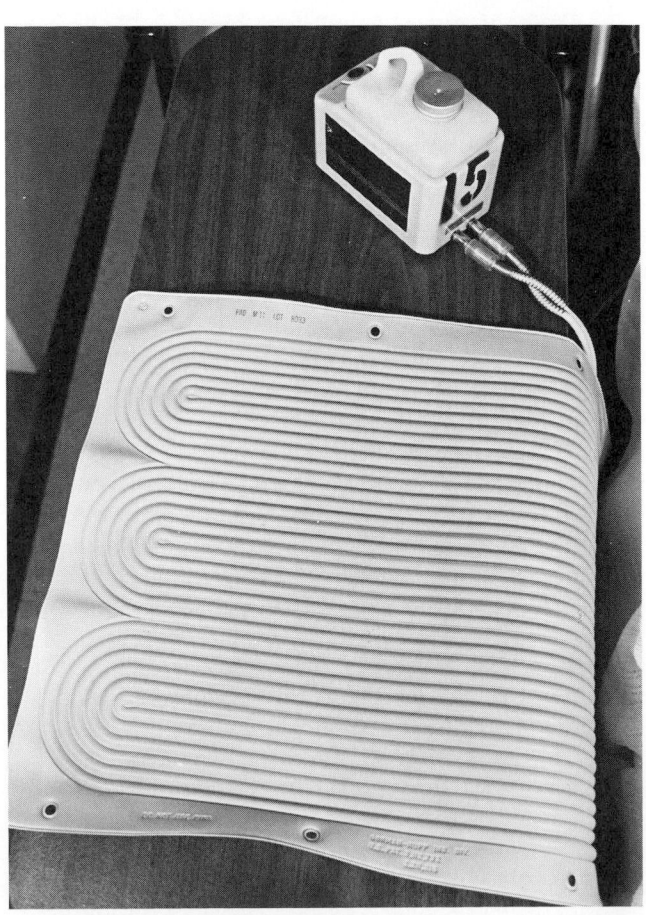

F I G U R E   42-10
The Aquathermal pad is an electric device that can be set to maintain water at a constant temperature and circulate it through the coils of the plastic pad. The pad can be used to provide dry heat, or it can be placed over a moist dressing to provide moist heat.

PROCEDURE 42-4
Applying an External Heating Device

Equipment

Hot water bag
  Cover for bag
  Water at the appropriate temperature:
  46.1°C–51.6°C
    (115°F–125°F)
    for older children and adults
  40.5°C–43.3°C
    (105°F–110°F)
    for infants, young children, elderly, diabetics, unconscious clients
Bath thermometer

Aquathermia pad
  Electrically controlled unit
  Distilled water
  Cover for pad
  Gauze bandage or tape (to secure pad)

Action	Rationale
1 Explain the procedure to the client.	Facilitates cooperation and provides reassurance for client
2 Assess condition of skin where heat is to be applied.	Impaired circulation may affect sensitivity to heat. Elderly persons and very young children have the least tolerance to applications of heat.
3 Assemble necessary equipment, and close door or curtain if privacy is desired.	Organization facilitates performance of task.
4 Wash your hands.	Handwashing deters the spread of microorganisms.

Hot Water Bag

Action	Rationale
5 Check temperature of water with bath thermometer or test on inner wrist. Rinse bag with water, empty, and then fill.	Provides for application of heat within the acceptable range for individual. Rinsing bag with warm water warms the rubber
6 Fill hot water bag one-half to two-thirds full.	Hot water bottle molds more easily to area and puts less pressure on site.
7 Expel remaining air from bag in one of two ways: place the bag on a flat surface, permit the water to come to the opening, and then close the bag; or, hold the bag up, twist the unfilled portion to remove the air, and then close the bag. Fasten top securely. Check for leaks.	Air reduces pliability of bag. Securing top prevents leakage of water and discomfort for client.
8 Cover bag with towel or other protector, and apply hot water bottle to prescribed area.	Protects skin from direct contact with rubber. Heat travels by conduction from one object to another.
9 Assess condition of skin and client's response to heat at frequent intervals. Do not exceed prescribed length of time for application of heat. Remove hot water bag if excessive swelling, redness, or pain occurs, and report to physician.	Maximum therapeutic effects from application of heat occur within 20 min–30 min. Extended use of heat (beyond 45 min) results in tissue congestion and vasoconstriction. This *rebound phenomenon* results in increased risk to client of burns from application of heat.

(Continued)

PROCEDURE 42-4
Applying an External Heating Device (Continued)

Action

10 After removal, record client's response, and dispose of equipment appropriately.

11 Wash your hands.

Aquathermia Pad

12 Check that distilled water is at appropriate level. Use key to adjust temperature at 40.5°C (105°F) if it has not already been preset. Plug in unit, and warm pad before use if manufacturer recommends.

13 Cover pad with pillowcase or other protector, and apply to prescribed area. Do not allow client to lie on pad if applying to back. Client should assume prone position and place aquathermia pad on back.

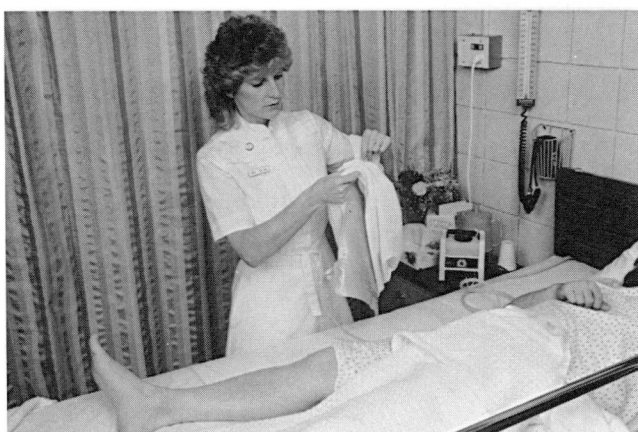

Step 13: Covering pad with pillowcase.

14 Secure with gauze bandage or tape. Never use safety pins to hold pad in place.

15 Same as steps 9, 10, and 11.

Rationale

Provides accurate documentation of procedure

Handwashing deters the spread of microorganisms.

Water temperature is regulated by key. Presetting the temperature eliminates risk of client adjusting the temperature.

Protects skin from direct contact with rubber or source of heat. Pressure reduces dissipation of heat.

Hold pad in position on client. Pins may puncture and damage the pad.

Same as steps 9, 10, and 11.

---

covered with a sheet. Treatments usually last 15 minutes. Precautions should be taken to prevent burning as for a heat lamp.

Hot Packs. Commercial hot packs provide a specified amount of dry heat for a specific time period. Instructions on the package describe how to activate the pack.

Moist Heat
Warm Moist Compresses. Sterile hot moist compresses are used to treat open wounds to promote circu-

lation and wound healing (especially if infected) and to reduce edema. To maintain heat, because moist heat evaporates and cools rapidly, the compresses must be changed frequently, covered with a heating agent (hot water bottle, heating pad, Aqua K pad), or covered with a plastic wrap. Procedure 42-5 describes the application of warm sterile compresses to an open wound.

Sitz Baths. As a means of applying tepid or hot water to the pelvic or rectal area, clients are often placed in a tub filled with sufficient water to reach the umbilicus. These baths are called **sitz baths**. Special tubs and

PROCEDURE 42-5
Applying Warm Sterile Compresses to an Open Wound

Equipment

Prescribed solution (warmed to approximately 40°C–43°C (105°F–110°F)

Sterile container for solution

Sterile gauze dressings or compresses

Sterile gloves

Clean disposable gloves

Waterproof pad

Dry bath towel

Bath blanket

Tape or ties

Aquathermia or external heating device (optional)

Sterile bath thermometer (if available, to check temperature of solution)

Action

1 Assess client for any circulatory impairment to area where compress is to be applied (numbness, tingling, impairment in temperature sensation, or cyanosis).

2 Check physician's order for warm compresses. Explain procedure to client.

3 Gather equipment.

4 Wash your hands.

5 Close door or curtain. Use bath blanket as needed when exposing area for application of warm compresses. Position waterproof pad under client.

6 Assist client to comfortable position that provides easy access to area.

7 Place opened, cuffed plastic bag near working area.

8 Prepare aquathermia pad or external heating device (optional).

9 Using sterile technique, open dressings and warmed solution. Pour solution into sterile container, and carefully drop gauze for compresses into sterile solution.

10 Don clean disposable glove, and remove any dressing carefully. Discard dressing in disposable plastic bag. Pull off soiled glove inside out, and drop it in bag.

11 Assess wound healing or presence of infection.

12 Don sterile gloves. See Procedure 25-2.

13 Retrieve sterile compress from warmed solution, and squeeze moisture from it. Apply carefully, and gently mold around wound. Be alert for client's response to heat.

Rationale

Circulatory impairment may interfere with client's ability to perceive heat and place him at risk of injury from the application of heat.

An explanation encourages client cooperation and reduces apprehension.

Provides for organized approach to task

Handwashing deters spread of microorganisms.

Provides for privacy and warmth

Provides for comfort and ease of application of compresses

Soiled dressings may be placed in disposal bag without contaminating outside surfaces of bag.

External heating device allows compress to retain heat for longer interval.

Sterile technique is used for warm moist compresses to an open wound.

Prevents spread of microorganisms by contaminated dressings

Documents condition of wound prior to application of compress

Maintains surgical asepsis

Excess moisture may contaminate surrounding area and is uncomfortable for client. Molding compress to skin promotes retention of warmth around wound site.

(Continued)

Applying Warm Sterile Compresses to an Open Wound (Continued)

Action	**Rationale**
14 Cover the gauze compresses with dry bath towel, and tie in place if necessary.	Towel provides additional insulation.

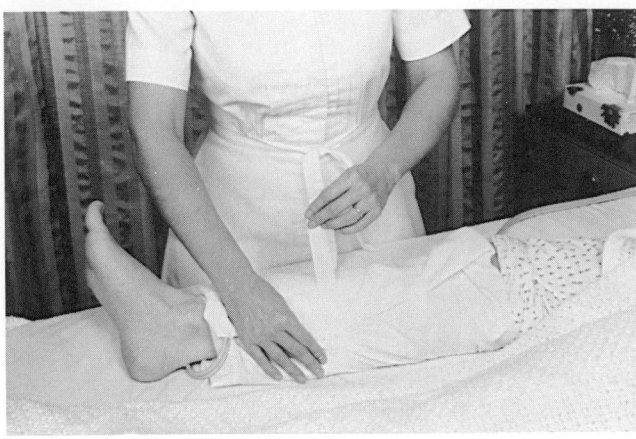

Step 15: Applying and securing pad in place (Photos © Ken Kasper)

Action	**Rationale**
15 Apply aquathermia pad or external heating device over towel (optional).	Controls temperature and extends therapeutic effect of compress
16 Monitor condition of skin and client's response to warm compress at frequent intervals.	Impaired circulation may affect sensitivity to heat.
17 After 30 min (or time ordered by physician), remove warm compress. Carefully observe condition of skin around wound and client's response to application of heat.	Maximum therapeutic effects of heat occur within 20 min–30 min. Extended use of heat (beyond 45 min) results in tissue congestion and vasoconstriction. This *rebound phenomenon* results in increased risk to client of burns from application of heat.
18 Apply sterile dressing to wound. See Procedure 42-1.	Protects wound from microorganisms in environment
19 Dispose of equipment appropriately. Wash hands.	Deters spread of microorganisms
20 Record client's response and condition of wound and surrounding skin area.	Provides accurate documentation of procedure

chairs or basins that fit onto the toilet seat are available, and are designed so that the client's buttocks fit into a rather deep seat that is filled with water of the desired temperature; the legs and the feet remain out of the water. The basins are disposable and economical for home or health agency use. A regular bathtub is not as satisfactory for a sitz bath because the heat causes generalized vasodilation, altering the effect desired.

The following are recommended techniques for administering a sitz bath:

- Test the water in a sitz bath with a thermometer before the client enters the tub. If the purpose of the sitz bath is to apply heat, water at a temperature of 43°C to 46°C (110°F to 115°F) for 15 minutes will produce relaxation of the parts involved after a short initial period of contraction. Warm water should not be used if considerable congestion is already present.
- If the purpose of the sitz bath is to produce relaxation or to help to promote healing in a wound by cleaning it of discharge and debris, then water at a temperature of 34°C to 37°C (94°F to 98°F) is used. Check agency protocols for correct temperature.

- Assist the client into the tub, and position properly. The client should be able to sit in the basin or tub with the feet flat on the floor. There should be no pressure on the sacrum or thighs.
- Wrap a bath blanket around the client's shoulders to protect the client from feeling chilly and from exposure.
- Observe the client closely for signs of weakness and fatigue. Discontinue the bath if the client has signs of faintness, skin pallor, a rapid pulse, and nausea.
- Test the water in the tub several times, and keep it at the desired temperature. Additional hot water may be added by pouring it slowly from a pitcher or by opening a hot water faucet a little bit. The water should be agitated by stirring it as hot water is added to prevent burning the client.
- Do not leave the client alone unless it is absolutely certain that it is safe to do so.
- Help the client out of the tub when the bath is completed. Normally, a sitz bath should last for 15 minutes to 30 minutes. Help the client dry, and cover the client adequately.

Warm Soaks. The immersion of a body area into warm water or a medicated solution is called a soak. The purposes of soaks vary: to increase blood supply to a locally infected area; to aid suppuration; to aid in cleaning large, sloughing wounds, such as burns; to improve circulation; and to apply medication to a locally infected area. A soak has the added advantage of making manipulation of a painful area much easier, because the body part is buoyed up by the weight of water it displaces.

- If a soak is prescribed for a large wound, such as might cover an entire arm or lower leg or even an area of the torso, a compromise with sterile technique usually is made. The container into which the body area is placed is sterilized before use if possible; if not, the container should be cleaned scrupulously. Tap water may be used for soaks, because it is accepted generally as being free from pathogens.
- Unless the temperature of the soak is prescribed otherwise, a range of 40.5°C to 43°C (105°F to 110°F) is considered as being physiologically effective and comfortable for the client.
- The container holding the fluid should be positioned so that the part to be immersed is comfortable and the client is in good body alignment.
- During the treatment, which is usually 15 minutes to 20 minutes per soak, the temperature should be kept as constant as possible. This may be done by discarding some of the fluid every 5 minutes and replacing it, or by adding solutions at a higher temperature while agitating the water. The client must remove the extremity from the soak while replacing or adding fluids.

Applying Cold

Dry Cold

Ice Bags. Ice bags have essentially the same disadvantages as hot water bags, but they are also a relatively easy and inexpensive way to apply cold to an area. The following are recommendations for the use of an ice bag:

- Fill the bag with small pieces of ice to about two-thirds full. This makes the bag light in weight. Ice chips, rather than cubes, make it easier to mold the bag to a body part.
- Remove air from the ice bag in the same manner as for removing air from a hot water bag.
- After securing the cap, test the ice bag for leaks and wipe off excess moisture.
- Place a cover on the ice bag to provide comfort and to absorb moisture that may accumulate on the outside of the bag.
- Apply an ice bag for 30 minutes, and then remove it for about an hour before reapplying it. This technique prevents the effects of prolonged exposure to cold.

Cold Packs. Commercially prepared ice bags are available in many health agencies. These bags are sealed containers filled with a nontoxic substance. The bags are frozen in the freezing compartment of a refrigerator. An advantage of these bags is that the frozen solution remains pliable and can be molded easily to fit a body part. Their cover consists of a ribbed, cotton sleeve so that the bag can be slipped onto an extremity. Or, the bag can simply be placed on a body part, such as the head. These bags cannot be reused.

Moist Cold

Cold Compresses. Moist, cold, local applications are called cold compresses. They might be used for an injured eye, headache, tooth extraction, and in some situations, for hemorrhoids. The texture and the thickness of the material used will depend on the area to which it is to be applied. For example, eye compresses could be prepared from surgical gauze compresses, which have a small amount of cotton filling. A washcloth makes an excellent compress for the head or the face.

The material used for the application is immersed in a clean basin, appropriate for the size of the compress, that contains pieces of ice and a small amount of water. The compress should be wrung thoroughly before it is applied to avoid dripping, which is uncomfortable for the client and may also wet the bed or clothing. The compresses should be changed frequently. The application should be continued for 20 minutes and repeated every 2 hours to 3 hours. Ice bags or commercial devices for keeping the compresses cold decrease the frequency with which the compresses must be changed.

Alcohol or Cold Sponge Bath. Alcohol or cold sponge baths are used to reduce body temperature. Plain water may be used, but alcohol added to water makes the temperature more easy to tolerate for most clients and removes heat from skin surfaces rapidly. Cold water very often produces a strong initial reactionary effect, which elevates the temperature even further. This is observed when the client shivers and has gooseflesh.

The following techniques are recommended for administering an alcohol or cold-water sponge bath:

- Prepare a water and alcohol solution at about 29.5°C to 32°C (85°F to 95°F). If plain water is used, prepare it at a temperature of about 29.5°C (85°F), but add ice chips to bring the temperature down while bathing the client until the water temperature reaches about 18°C (65°F).
- Protect the client's bed with moisture-proof material.
- Prepare several ice bags. One ice bag is placed on the client's head to promote comfort. Others are placed in the groin and axillary areas, where blood vessels are close to the skin surface. The ice bags help to cool the client further.
- Drape the client properly to prevent shivering as various parts of the body are exposed for bathing.
- Sponge the face and forehead, the neck, arms, and legs for 3 minutes to 5 minutes, and the back for 10 minutes. Usually, the anterior chest and abdomen are not sponged. Cover, but do not dry, each part as it is sponged. Evaporation of moisture on the skin further helps to reduce body temperature.
- Move on from one part of the body to another, and continue the bathing for 25 minutes to 30 minutes. If the bath is short in duration, the body does not adjust to the coolness. It then reacts to conserve heat, and the client's temperature may go even higher.
- Check the client's color and pulse during the bath. Discontinue bathing if the client is reacting unfavorably.
- Pat the client dry after the bath is completed. The friction of rubbing him dry may increase body temperature.
- Check the client's body temperature about ½ hour after the bath to evaluate the effectiveness of the cool bath.

Evaluating

The effectiveness of the plan of care is evaluated based on the established client goals. If the goals are met, the plan was effective.

CASE STUDY *

Joe Blue is a 65-year-old, 5-foot, 8-inch tall, white male weighing 70.9 kg. He is married and has two grown children and four grandchildren. He is a retired lumber-yard worker. He lives at home with his wife who is a borderline diabetic. This is his third admission for a recurrent umbilical hernia. Two months ago the hernia was repaired with a mesh graft, to which he developed an abdominal abscess. Mr. Blue was readmitted for surgical incision and drainage of the abscess on January 1. He returned from surgery with a 2-inch opened draining wound.

Assessment Findings

Upon assessing Mr. Blue on January 3, 2 days after surgery, the nurse noted the following data:

Generalized abdominal discomfort
Irritated, reddened, excoriated skin around wound edges

4 × 4s packed in 2-inch-diameter wound saturated with serosangineous and yellow-green purulent drainage
Temperature: 99.8°F; Respirations: 28; Pulse: 96; Blood pressure: 140/88
Skin slightly diaphoretic and pale. Weight: 156 lb (loss of 2 lb since admission)
Wife appears anxious and is at bedside holding client's hand. Mr. Blue states, "I just didn't have any appetite for breakfast."
Lab values: Hgb 15g; Hct: 43%; WBC: 13,000
Other medical diagnosis—mild COPD, lung sounds coarse, scattered rales on inspiration in lower bases bilaterally, clears somewhat with coughing

* Case study and nursing care plan were developed and written by Janet R. Weber, Department of Nursing, Southeast Missouri State University, Cape Givardeau, MO.

NURSING CARE PLAN *for Mr. Blue*

Nursing Diagnosis: Alteration in skin integrity related to abdominal wound drainage secondary to post-op incision and drainage of abscess.

Long-Term Goal: The client's abdominal wound will show progressive healing and absence of infection.

Short-Term Goals	Nursing Actions	Rationale	Evaluative Statement
1. By 1/6 the wound edges will show decreased swelling and redness and the surrounding skin will be less excoriated with no breakdown.	1. Change dressing every 4 hr using sterile technique. Irrigate wound with sterile saline and pack wound with saline-soaked 4×4s. Apply sterile abdominal dressing over 4×4s.	1. Sterile technique reduces potential infection of wound. Saline irrigation cleanses the wound and promotes healing which exudates would inhibit. An 8×10 abdominal dressing over 4×4s will protect wound and promote upward absorption of drainage. The soaked 4×4s will prevent dressing from clinging to dried wound drainage which would further irritate wound with each dressing change.	1. 1/6, wound edges clean and pink. No further excoriation noted. Serous light yellow drainage on 4×4s. No sanguineous drainage noted. Temperature 99°F.
2. Sanguineous and purulent yellow drainage will change to serous drainage by 1/6.	2. Apply Montgomery straps over client's wound dressing.		*J. Weber, RN*
3. Body temperature will be normal by 1/6.	3. Wear gown, gloves, and mask during dressing procedure. Use good handwashing technique before and after procedure.	2. Montgomery straps prevent skin damage and increase client's level of comfort by eliminating need for repeated removal of dressings and adhesives.	
4. The client's abdominal discomfort will decrease.	4. Assess drainage for amount, color, odor, and consistency with each dressing change.	3. Using CDC guidelines for care of wounds with purulent drainage decreases chances of contamination.	
	5. Assess temperature every 4 hr.	4. Early detection of further infection will allow for prompt intervention.	
	6. Give pain medication 30 min prior to dressing change to promote comfort.		

Long-Term Goal: The client will participate in self-care activities promoting wound healing and prevention of infection.

1. By 1/6 client will choose and eat a diet high in calories (40/kg/day) and high in protein (2.0 g/kg/day) and include: vitamins A, B, C, K and iron and zinc.	1. Teach client and wife the importance of proteins and vitamins in promoting wound healing.	1. A draining wound increases need for protein because exudate is high in protein. Protein replaces body mass lost during catabolism of cells from surgery and wound. This, in addition to bed rest, leads to a negative nitrogen balance. Increased cal-	1. 1/5, client and wife choosing appropriate foods from menu, yet client lacks appetite. Eats 1/2 of each tray. Fails to eat much meat and other protein sources. Fluid intake adequate: 2,000 ml–2,500 ml per day.
2. By 1/5 client will drink 2,000 ml of fluid per day.	2. Identify those foods high in protein and vitamins for client and wife (protein: meat, eggs, fish, milk, leafy vegetables).		*J. Weber, RN*

(Continued)

N U R S I N G   C A R E   P L A N *(Continued)*

Short-Term Goals	Nursing Actions	Rationale	Evaluative Statement
	3. Record intake and output, and teach client and wife how to participate in this. 4. Weigh client before breakfast each day. 5. Encourage 2,000 ml of fluids per day.	ories are needed to restore weight, spare protein, and replace losses during surgery and stress periods. Stress and catabolism cause the early postoperative client to lose an increased amount of nitrogen and weight. Weight loss is common postop, whereas, an immediate weight gain postop may indicate fluid retention (Metheny, 1983). 2. Vitamin A enhances wound healing and resistance to infection. Vitamin B_{12} promotes tissue synthesis; iron replaces that lost in blood loss; zinc promotes protein synthesis and wound healing. Vitamin C assists with synthesis of collagen, formation of capillaries, and resistance to infection. Vitamin K assists with synthesis of prothrombin (Flynn and Rovee, 1982). 3. Adequate hydration is necessary to replace losses through wound drainage and exudates and to maintain hydration.	
1. By 1/4 the client will turn, cough and deep breathe every 2 hr. 2. By 1/4 the client will ambulate to waiting room and back two times per day.	1. Teach client to splint abdomen and proper method of turning, coughing, and deep breathing every 2 hr. Assist client until he is able to do it by himself. 2. Increase ambulation length each time as tolerated by client.	1. Activity stimulates appetite and sleep—both necessary for wound healing. 2. Immobilization promotes a negative nitrogen balance and delays wound healing. 3. Activity increases circulation to the wound and promotes healing	1. By 1/4 client was turning, coughing, and deep breathing every 2 hr by himself during the day. He is ambulating two times a day full length of hall. *J. Weber, RN*

(Continued)

NURSING CARE PLAN (Continued)

Short-Term Goals	Nursing Actions	Rationale	Evaluative Statement
		by bringing increased leukocytes, oxygen, nutrients, antibodies, platelets, and erythrocytes to the damaged area. Increased circulation to the area also increases removal of toxins and debris.	
1. Client's wife will demonstrate proper changing of dressing by time of discharge. 2. Client will identify warning signs of wound infection by time of discharge.	1. Teach client and wife sterile procedure. Provide rationale for sterile dressing changes and avoidance of touching wound drainage. 2. Demonstrate procedure and allow time for return demonstration. 3. Teach the early warning signs of infection: increased temperature; pain; generalized malaise; purulent, foulsmelling drainage; hot and reddened skin around wound.	1. Wound healing is a lengthy process, and the client and family may be required to learn to care for the wound at home. 2. Allowing the client and family to participate in self care and promoting their understanding of the procedure and purpose may promote compliance and selfcare. 3. Early detection of infection allows for prompt intervention.	1. By 1/8 client was able to assist wife with dressing change, using sterile technique. 2. Both the wife and client identified the warning signs of wound infection. *J. Weber, RN*

KEY POINTS

- The skin, as the largest organ of the body, provides protection, sensation, and fluid balance; the skin also facilitates communication and self-concept.

- A wound is a disruption in the normal integrity of the skin and tissues and may be described using various terms.

- Wounds heal more rapidly in a person who has a healthy physical status, proper nutrition, and intentional (surgical) trauma.

- Wounds heal by primary, secondary, or tertiary intention. Both the stress response and the inflammatory response influence tissue healing from the initial trauma through scar formation.

- Wound healing is affected by age, circulation/oxygenation, wound condition, and client wellness.

- Wound complications are infection, hemorrhage, dehiscence, and evisceration.

- Common psychologic effects of wounds are pain, anxiety, fear, and altered self-concept.

- Wounds are assessed for appearance, skin sutures, drains, tubes, drainage, pain, and complications.

- Changing a dressing requires various supplies, may require bandages or binders, and is carried out using knowledge and skill.

- Heat and cold have local and systemic effects; both are used as therapeutic agents to treat traumatized body tissues.

- When assessing prior to the application of heat or cold, consideration is given to factors influencing tolerance, physical and mental status, the area to be treated, and the equipment to be used.

- Heat and cold may be applied in either dry or moist forms. Specific guidelines for performing procedures facilitate client safety and prevent tissue damage.

BIBLIOGRAPHY

Bauman B: Update your techniques for changing dressings: Dry to dry. Nursing 12(1):64–67, 1982

Brunner S, Suddarth DS: Textbook of Medical-Surgical Nursing, 5th ed. Philadelphia, JB Lippincott, 1988

Carpenito L: Nursing Diagnosis: Application to Clinical Practice, 2nd ed. Philadelphia, JB Lippincott, 1987

Centers for Disease Control: Recommendations for prevention of HIV transmission in health-care settings. MMWR 1987; Vol. 36 Suppl. 2S

Centers for Disease Control: Update: Universal precautions for prevention of transmission of human immunodeficiency virus, hepatitis B virus, and other bloodborne pathogens in health-care settings. MMWR 37:24, 1988

Cooper DM, Schumann D: Postsurgical nursing intervention as an adjunct to wound healing. Nurs Clin North Am 14(4):713–725, 1979

Cruse PJ, Foord R: The epidemiology of wound infection: A ten-year prospective study of 62,939 wounds. Surg Clin North Am 60:27–40, 1980

Dudek SG: Nutrition Handbook for Nursing Practice. Philadelphia, JB Lippincott, 1987

Flynn ME, Rovee DT: Promoting wound healing. Am J Nurs 82(10):1543–1558, 1982

Fritz C: Emergency! First aid for wounds. Nursing 82 October:68–75, 1982

Hotter AN: Physiologic aspects and clinical implications of wound healing. Heart Lung 11(6):522–540, 1982

Metheny NM: Fluid and Electrolyte Balance: Nursing Considerations. Philadelphia, JB Lippincott, 1987

Neuberger GB, Reckling JB: A new look at wound care. Nursing 15(2):34–42, 1985

O'Byrne C: Clinical detection and management of postoperative wound sepsis. Nurs Clin North Am 14(4):727–741, 1979

Patrick ML, et al: Medical-Surgical Nursing: Pathophysiological Concepts. Philadelphia, JB Lippincott, 1986

Phipps W, Long B, Woods N: Medical-Surgical Nursing: Concepts and Clinical Practice, 3rd ed. St Louis, CV Mosby, 1987

Recommendations for Prevention of HIV Transmission in Health-care Settings. U.S. Department of Health and Human Services, Centers for Disease Control, MMWR 36:55–75, 1987

Rodeheaver G, et al: Bacterial activity and toxicity of iodine-containing solutions in wounds. Arch Surg 117(February):181–186, 1982

Simmons BP: Guidelines for prevention of surgical wound infections: centers for Disease control Guidelines. Infect Control 3(2), 1982

Wieck L, King E, Dyer M: Ilustrated Manual of Nursing Techniques, 3rd ed. Philadelphia, JB Lippincott, 1986

Perioperative Nursing

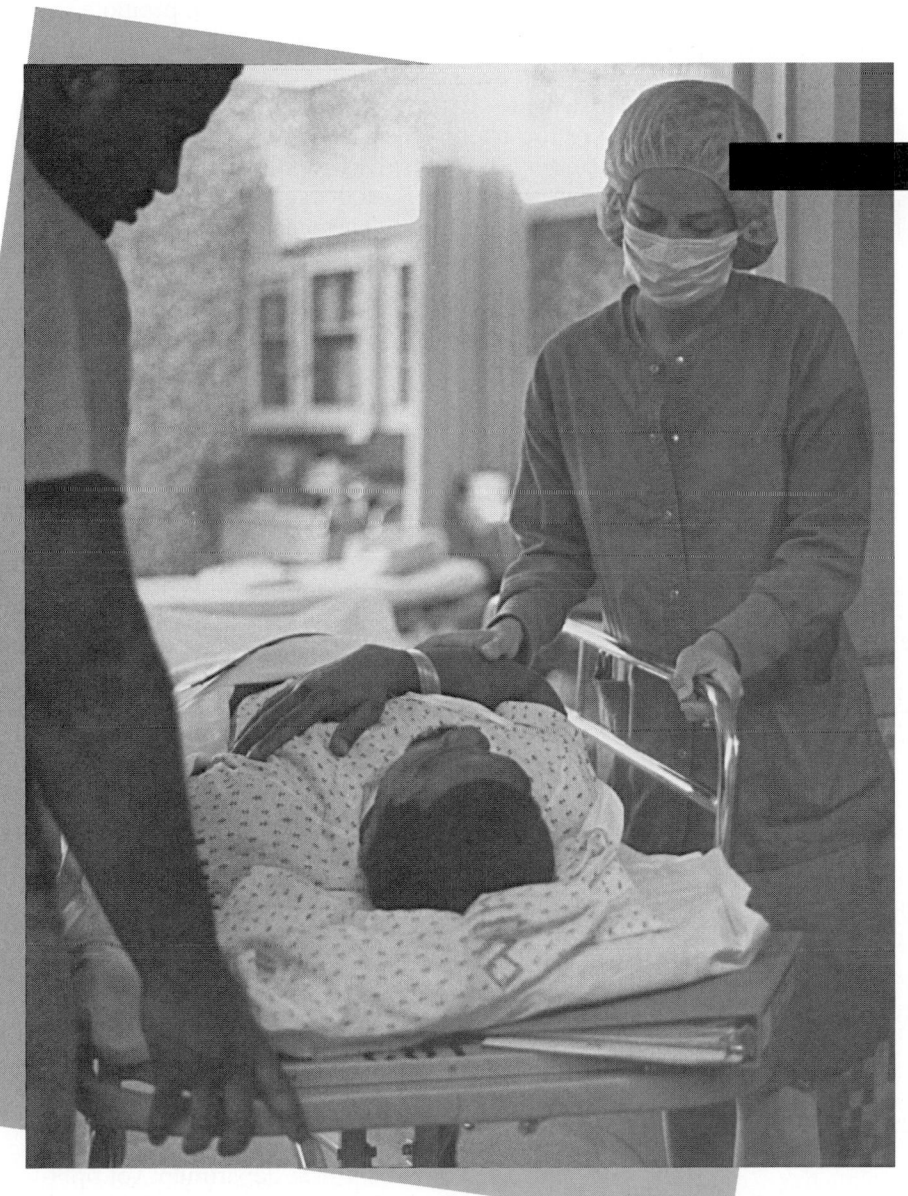

After studying this chapter, the learner should be able to

Define key terms used in the chapter.

Describe the surgical experience; including perioperative phases, categories of surgery, types of anesthesia, and informed consent.

Conduct a preoperative nursing history and nursing examination to identify client strengths as well as factors increasing surgical and postoperative complication risk.

Demonstrate preoperative exercises: deep-breathing, coughing, and leg exercises.

Prepare a client physically and psychologically for surgery.

Describe the nurse's role in the intraoperative phase.

Identify assessments specific to the prevention of complications in the immediate postoperative phase.

Plan and implement interventions for ongoing postoperative care to prevent complications, promote a return to health, and facilitate coping with alterations.

Use the nursing process to knowledgably develop an individualized plan of care for the surgical client during each phase of the perioperative period.

The treatment of illness or injury often involves surgical intervention, an invasive method of medical therapy. Surgery may be planned or unplanned, major or minor, and may involve any body part or system. Regardless of the cause or extent, surgery is a stressful event for the client and family, imposing physical and psychosocial alterations and adaptations. Skilled and knowledgeable nursing care is essential to the successful recovery of the surgical client; it is an area in which nurses give care based on physician's orders, but they also use all phases of the nursing process to provide independent nursing assessments and interventions necessary to promote the recovery of health, prevent further injury or illness, and facilitate coping.

This chapter discusses nursing care appropriate to preparing the client for surgery, supporting the client during surgery, and assisting with recovery after surgery. The nurse's role during each stage is described, using the phases of the nursing process. Selected nursing diagnoses are included, and the application of the nursing process in the clinical setting is described at the end of the chapter in a case study and care plan for the surgical client.

KEY TERMS

ambulatory surgery
atelectasis
circulating nurse
dehiscence
elective surgery
emergency surgery
evisceration
general anesthesia
hemorrhage
holding area
hypovolemic shock
informed consent
intraoperative phase

paralytic ileus
perioperative nursing
perioperative period
pneumonia
postanesthesia recovery
  room
postoperative phase
preoperative phase
pulmonary embolus
regional anesthesia
scrub nurse
shock
thrombophlebitis

THE SURGICAL EXPERIENCE

Regardless of the surgical intervention required, all clients progress through specific perioperative phases, have a defined surgical procedure, require anesthesia, and give their consent for surgery. This part of the chapter will describe those components of the surgical experience to serve as a knowledge base for the application of the nursing process when giving nursing care to the client having surgery.

Perioperative Period

The client having surgery progresses through several distinct phases, with the entire time frame labeled the **perioperative period**. **Perioperative nursing** is the name given to the wide variety of nursing activities carried out before, during, and after surgery. The three phases of the perioperative period are: the **preoperative phase** beginning with the decision that surgical intervention is necessary, and lasting until the client is transferred to the operating room table; the **intraoperative phase**, extending from admission to the surgical department (or operating room) to transfer to the recovery area; and the **postoperative phase**, lasting from admission to the recovery area to the complete recovery from surgery. The nursing process is used during each phase to meet physical and psychosocial needs and facilitate the client's return to health. Each of these phases, with related client needs and nursing activities, will be described in the remainder of the chapter.

T A B L E 43-1
Classification of Surgical Procedures

Classification	Purpose	Examples
Based on Urgency		
Elective: Delay of surgery has no ill effects; can be scheduled in advance based on client's choice	• To remove or repair a body part • To restore function • To improve health • To improve self-concept	Tonsillectomy, hernia repair, cataract extraction and lens implant, hemorrhoidectomy, hip prosthesis, scar revision, face lift, mammoplasty
Urgent: Usually done within 24hr–48 hr	• To remove or repair a body part • To preserve or restore health • To restore function • To prevent further tissue damage	Removal of gallbladder, coronary artery bypass, surgical removal of a malignant tumor, colon resection, amputation
Emergency: Done immediately	• To preserve life (plus purposes as listed above)	Control of hemorrhage, repair of trauma, perforated ulcer, intestinal obstruction, tracheostomy
Based on Degree of Risk		
Major: may be elective, urgent or emergency	• To preserve life • To remove or repair a body part • To restore function • To improve or maintain health	Carotid endarterectomy, cholecystectomy, nephrectomy, colostomy, hysterectomy, radical mastectomy, amputation, trauma repair
Minor: Primarily elective	• To restore function • To remove skin lesions • To correct deformities	Teeth extraction, removal of warts, skin biopsy, D and C, laparoscopy, cataract extraction, arthroscopy
Based on Purpose		
Diagnostic: May be major or minor	• To make or confirm a diagnosis	Breast biopsy, laparoscopy, bronchoscopy, exploratory laparotomy
Ablative: usually major	• To remove a diseased body part	Appendectomy, subtotal thyroidectomy, partial gastrectomy, colon resection, amputation
Palliative	• To relieve or reduce intensity of an illness; is not curative	Colostomy, nerve root resection, debridement of necrotic tissue
Reconstructive	• To restore function to traumatized or malfunctioning tissue • To improve self-concept	Scar revision, plastic surgery, skin graft, internal fixation of a fracture
Transplant	• To replace organs or structures that are diseased or malfunctioning	Kidney, liver, cornea, heart, joints
Constructive	• To restore function in congenital anomalies	Cleft palate repair, closure of atrial-septal defect

Classification of Surgical Procedures

Surgical procedures are usually categorized by the major classifications of urgency, risk, and purpose. Table 43-1 lists each classification, with purposes and selected examples for each. The classifications are described below.

Based on Urgency. Surgery may be classified as **elective surgery,** meaning it is preplanned and based on the client's choice; *urgent surgery,* in which the surgery is necessary for the client's health, but not an emergency; and **emergency surgery,** when surgery must be done immediately to preserve the client's life, body part, or body function.

Based on Degree of Risk. Surgery is classified as *major* or *minor* based on the degree of risk for the client. Minor surgery may be done in a physician's office, in an outpatient clinic, in "same-day surgery" settings, or in the operating room of a hospital. This classification means that the surgical procedure is usually brief, carries a low risk, and results in few complications. In contrast, major surgery always requires hospitalization, is usually prolonged, has a higher degree of risk, involves major body organs or life-threatening situations, and has the potential of postoperative complications.

Based on Purpose.   Descriptors used to classify surgical procedures based on purpose include *diagnostic, ablative, palliative, reconstructive, transplant,* and *constructive.*

Combinations.   Surgical procedures may combine several classifications and labels (*e.g.,* a client who has been in an automobile accident and has severe trauma and bleeding may require major, reconstructive, emergency surgery). It is important to remember that, no matter the defined degree of risk, any surgical procedure imposes physical and psychologic stress and is rarely considered "minor" by the individual.

Anesthesia

Anesthesia, depending on its classification as *general* or *regional* (Table 43-2), produces such states as narcosis (loss of consciousness), analgesia, relaxation, and loss of reflexes. General anesthesia produces all of these responses, while regional anesthesia does not cause narcosis, but does result in analgesia and reflex loss. Anesthetic agents are administered by a physician, an anesthesiologist (MD), or a nurse anesthetist.

General Anesthesia

General anesthesia occurs when drugs given by inhalation, intravenous, rectal, or oral routes to produce central nervous system depression, with the desired action being loss of consciousness, relaxation of skeletal muscles, and reduction of reflex action. The most common

route for general anesthetic agents is by inhalation; this route has the advantages of rapid excretion and reversal of effects (McConnell, 1987).

There are four stages of inhalation anesthesia; although these are distinct stages, the combination of anesthetic agents with narcotics or neuromuscular blocking agents may alter the transition from one stage to another. The stages are

Stage I: Beginning anesthesia—As the anesthetic agent is breathed in (by face mask or endotracheal tube), the client experiences feelings of warmth, detachment, numbness, dizziness, and ringing or buzzing in the ears. During this stage, the client is still conscious, and noises are exaggerated.

Stage II: Excitement—The smooth and rapid administration of anesthesia will help avoid this stage, characterized by uncontrolled movements, struggling, talking, laughing, crying, and so forth. The pupils dilate but respond to light, and the respirations are rapid and irregular. Because the client may have exaggerated reflexes and is especially reactive to stimuli, noise and touch should be avoided. To maintain safety during this stage (and throughout the surgical procedure), restraints are placed across the client prior to the induction of anesthesia.

Stage III: Surgical anesthesia—In this stage, the client is unconscious. The pupils constrict; the face is expressionless; and skin color may be flushed, pale, or slightly cyanotic. The pulse is strong, respirations are full and regular, blood pressure may slightly drop, and body temperature drops. This stage can be maintained for hours at a desired depth.

Stage IV: Overdose—This undesired stage is reached when too much anesthesia is given, or the client has an adverse reaction to the anesthetic agent. Paralysis of the diaphragm and respiratory arrest precede vasomotor collapse.

T A B L E   43-2
Major Classifications of Anesthetic Agents

Classification	Action	Routes of Administration	Effects
General	Blocks central awareness centers	Inhalation, intravenous, rectal, oral	Loss of consciousness, general loss of sensation, skeletal muscle relaxation, reduction of reflexes
Regional	Blocks transmission of all nerve impulses along nerve	Injection, nerve infiltration, extradural, spinal	Nerve sensation abolished over a specific body area
	Blocks transmission of nerve impulses at site of origin	Topical, local infiltration	Nerve sensation abolished over a limited body area

(McConnell EA: Clinical Considerations in Perioperative Nursing: Preventive Aspects of Care. Philadelphia, JB Lippincott, 1987)

Death will occur unless the anesthetic is discontinued and resuscitation with drugs and artificial respiration is instituted (McConnell, 1987; Brunner and Suddarth, 1988).

General anesthesia has advantages and disadvantages. The advantages are that it can be used for clients of any age and for any surgical procedure, leaving the client unaware of physical trauma. However, there are major risks of circulatory and respiratory depression.

Regional Anesthesia

The client receiving a regional anesthetic remains awake but loses sensation (and reflexes in some instances) in a specific area of the body. **Regional anesthesia** occurs when an anesthetic drug is injected or applied topically near a nerve or nerve pathway, inhibiting the transmission of sensory stimuli to central nervous system receptors (McConnell, 1987). Regional anesthesia may be by surface anesthetic, local infiltration, nerve blocks, or subdural or epidural blocks. These are defined as follows:

- Surface (topical) anesthesia is used on mucous membranes, open skin surfaces, wounds, and burns. Cocaine, 4% to 10% solution, is the most commonly used agent; others are lidocaine (Xylocaine) and benzocaine.
- Local infiltration with an agent such as lidocaine or tetracaine 0.1% is used in minor surgical procedures such as skin biopsy and suturing small wounds.
- Nerve blocks are done by injecting a local anesthetic around a nerve trunk supplying the area of surgery, such as the jaw, face, and extremities.
- Subdural blocks are used to provide spinal anesthesia. The injection of a local anesthetic into the subarachnoid space (through a lumbar puncture) causes sensory, motor, and autonomic blockage, and is used for surgery of the lower abdomen, perineum, and lower extremities. Side-effects of spinal anesthesia may include hypotension, headache, and urinary retention.

Informed Consent

Informed consent for treatment (surgery) means that information is given to a client about a procedure or treatment, and the client agrees to the procedure or treatment. Informed consent protects the client, the physician, and the health-care institution, and is a legal document. The information, given to the client in understandable words, includes

- Description of the procedure or treatment
- Name and qualifications of the person performing the procedure or treatment
- Explanation of the risks involved, including potential for damage, disfigurement, or death
- Explanation of alternative procedures or treatments

- Explanation of the possible effects of not having the procedure or treatment
- Information that the client has the right to refuse treatment, and that consent can be withdrawn

The responsibility for securing a client's informed consent lies with the person who will perform the treatment or procedure, usually the physician. The nurse, signing as witness, signifies that the client signed the consent form and was alert and aware of the act.

Consent forms are not legal if the client is considered a minor (specific guidelines for minors are written in states in the United States and provinces in Canada), confused, unconscious, sedated, or mentally incompetent. Consent may be given in those instances by a parent, spouse, next-of-kin, or legal guardian. In emergency situations, the physician may obtain consent over the telephone or by court order. More detailed information about informed consent is in Chapter 6, Legal Implications of Nursing. An example of an informed consent form is shown in Figure 43-1.

PREOPERATIVE NURSING CARE

Clients requiring surgical intervention and nursing care enter the health-care setting in a wide variety of situations, ranging from essentially healthy persons who have planned elective procedures to emergency admissions for treatment of trauma. Surgical clients may be any age, and at any point on the health–illness continuum. It is the nurse's responsibility to identify factors that affect risk from a surgical procedure, assess physical and psychosocial needs of the client and family, and establish a plan of care, based on appropriate nursing diagnoses, that includes interventions to meet needs and facilitate recovery as the client progresses through the perioperative period.

Assessing

McConnell (1987, p 23) accurately describes the importance of preoperative assessment: "The successful outcome of a client's perioperative experience begins with the preoperative assessment. Surgery is a planned assault on the body, and the preoperative assessment helps identify factors increasing the risk of that assault." Assessment of the surgical client includes a nursing history and nursing examination (physical assessment) to establish baseline data and identify risk factors and a determination of the need for teaching and psychosocial support of the client and family.

Nursing History

The nursing history assesses risk factors and strengths in the client's physical and psychosocial status. Information significant to the surgical experience includes a health

PRESBYTERIAN–UNIVERSITY OF PENNSYLVANIA MEDICAL CENTER

CONSENT TO OPERATION AND/OR PROCEDURE OR TREATMENT, ADMINISTRATION
OF ANESTHETICS AND RENDERING OF OTHER MEDICAL SERVICE

Patient _____ Age _____

Date _____ Time _____

   1. I AUTHORIZE and DIRECT _____ M.D., with the
Associates and Assistants of his choice to perform upon—

_____
                             ("Myself" or state name of patient)

The following operation and/or procedure or treatment _____

_____

_____

and if any unforeseen condition arises in the course of the operation calling in their judgment for other operations, diagnostic or therapeutic procedures including blood transfusions in addition to or different from those now contemplated, I further request and authorize them to do whatever is deemed advisable for my recovery, health and well-being.

   2. The nature, purpose, and possible risks and alternate methods of treatment have also been discussed and consequences of the proposed operation and/or procedure or treatment have been explained to me. I am aware that the practice of medicine and surgery is not an exact science and I acknowledge that no guarantee or assurance has been made to me as to the results.

   3. I consent to the administration of anesthesia and supportive measures by or under the direction of the Department of Anesthesiology of the Presbyterian–University of Pennsylvania Medical Center, and to the use of such anesthetics as the members of the Department deem advisable.

I have been advised of the alternative type of anesthesia, if any, and the possible consequences of the use of each type have been explained to me.

   4. I certify that I understand the above, acknowledge that the explanations referred to above have been made, and consent to the operation and/or procedure or treatment and the administration of anesthesia and supportive measures.

   5. I further understand that if I do not understand any aspect of this consent form that I may request and receive additional explanation and information.

   6. I agree that any tissue or other body parts removed will go to the Department of Pathology for pathological examination and photography and then be preserved or disposed of by that Department at their discretion unless otherwise stated.

                    SIGNATURE OF PATIENT _____

When patient is a minor or incompetent to give consent:
SIGNATURE of person authorized to consent for Patient:

_____

and Relationship to Patient _____

Witness to authenticity of signature _____

I have explained the procedure to the patient and/or nearest relative, along with possible risks, alternate methods of treatment and consequence of the procedure, and to the best of my knowledge the patient understands and comprehends and concurs with the performance of this procedure.

_____
            M.D.   Date

CONSENT TO OPERATION

F I G U R E   43-1
Example of an informed consent form.

history, life-style habits, and coping patterns/support systems, including client perceptions of self and surgery.

Health History.   Health History data identifying risk factors and individualized assessments are developmental level, medical history, medications, previous surgeries, and perceptions and knowledge of surgery to be done.

Developmental Considerations.   Infants and older adults are at a greater risk from surgery than are children and young and middle-aged adults. The infant has a lower total blood volume, making even a small loss of blood a serious consideration, because of the risk of dehydration and the inability to respond to the need for increased oxygen during surgery. The infant also has difficulty maintaining stable body temperature during surgery, because the shivering reflex is not well developed, making potential hypothermia or hyperthermia more likely.

Physiologic changes associated with aging (described in Chap 12) place the elderly client at risk for surgery. These changes, summarized in Table 43-3, decrease the ability of the older adult to respond to the stress of surgery, alter the response to pre- and postoperative medications and anesthesia, and prolong or alter wound healing processes. With an increasingly elderly population, assessment of physiologic changes is critical in providing knowledgeable, safe, holistic nursing care to the elderly surgical client.

Medical History.   The medical history provides information about past and present illnesses; pathologic changes associated with past and present illnesses increase surgical risk as well as the potential for postoperative complications. Preoperative assessments and documentation are necessary to provide a data base for individualized assessments and interventions in the intra- and postoperative phases of care. Selected examples and associated risks are:

Cardiovascular diseases (thrombocytopenia, hemophilia, recent myocardial infarction or cardiac surgery, congestive heart failure, arrhythmias) increase the potential for hemorrhage and hypovolemic shock, hypotension, venous stasis, thrombophlebitis, and overhydration with intravenous fluids.

Pulmonary disorders (pneumonia, bronchitis, asthma, chronic obstructive pulmonary diseases) increase the possibility of respiratory depression from anesthesia, as well as postoperative pneumonia, atelectasis, and alterations in acid–base balance.

Renal and liver function alterations influence the client's response to anesthesia, affect fluid–electrolyte and acid–base balance, alter the metabolism and excretion of drugs, and impair wound healing.

Metabolic disorders, especially diabetes mellitus, increase the potential of hypoglycemia or acidosis and impede wound healing.

T A B L E   43-3
Physiologic Changes with Aging that Increase Surgical Risk

System	Change	Preoperative Nursing Interventions
Cardiovascular	• Decreased cardiac output, heart rate, and cardiac reserve • Decreased peripheral circulation • Increased vascular rigidity	• Establish baseline data of vital signs • Assess peripheral pulses • Teach leg exercises, turning, and ambulating • Document normal activity levels and tolerance of fatigue
Respiratory	• Reduced vital capacity • Diminished cough reflex • Decreased oxygenation of blood	• Establish baseline data of respiratory depth, rate • Teach coughing and deep breathing exercises • Assess color of skin
Neurologic	• Sensory deficit • Decreased reaction time	• Orient to surroundings • Institute safety measures (*e.g.,* elevate side rails, use night-light) • Allow additional time for questions and teaching
Renal	• Decreased renal blood flow • Reduced bladder capacity	• Assess amount and times of voiding • Monitor fluid and electrolyte status • Institute intake and output
Integument	• Decreased vascularity • Dry, inelastic	• Assess skin status • Monitor fluid status • Monitor nutritional status

Medications. Use of drugs, whether prescribed or over-the-counter, can affect the client's reaction to and can increase the risk from the stress of surgery and the effects of the anesthetic agent. Medications are usually cancelled when a client goes to surgery, but it is important for the nurse to know the purposes and specific actions of drugs as well as physician's orders; specific medications may be given even when the client is going to surgery (*e.g.,* clients with heart or cardiovascular problems or diabetes mellitus).

Surgical risk is increased by drugs in the following categories:

Anticoagulants: May precipitate hemorrhage
Diuretics: May cause electrolyte imbalances, with resulting respiratory depression from anesthesia
Tranquilizers: May increase the hypotensive effect of anesthetic agents
Adrenal steroids: Long-term users may have cardiovascular collapse if the drug is abruptly withdrawn.
Antibiotics: The "mycin" group of antibiotics, when combined with certain muscle relaxants used during surgery, can cause respiratory paralysis.

Previous Surgery. Data about previous surgeries provide a knowledge base for meeting physical and psychologic needs throughout the perioperative period.

Physical implications of previous surgeries are important to the intra- and postoperative phases (*e.g.,* previous heart or lung surgery may require adaptations in anesthesia and positioning during surgery). Complications following prior surgery, such as pneumonia, thrombophlebitis, or wound infection, provide data to support careful postoperative monitoring.

The client's past experiences with surgery will also affect the plan of care established in the preoperative phase, especially if those experiences were negative. When the interview elicits negative feelings about the surgical experience, pain control, or nursing interventions carried out to prevent complications during previous surgeries, teaching and mutual goal setting and even more important.

Perceptions and Knowledge of Surgery. Included in the medical history review is the client's perceptions about and knowledge of the surgical procedure to be performed. Questions asked or statements made by the client provide a base for meeting psychologic and family needs when preparing the client for surgery.

Life-Style. The nursing history data about the client's life-style provides valuable information about surgical risk and postoperative recovery and rehabilitation. Areas especially important for the surgical client are nutrition, use of alcohol or nicotine, activities of daily living, and occupation.

Nutrition. Both malnutrition and obesity increase surgical risk. Surgery increases the body's need for nu-trients, necessary for normal tissue healing and resistance to infection. The client who is malnourished is at higher risk for alterations in fluid and electrolyte balance, delay in wound healing, and wound infection. The obese client is at increased risk for pulmonary, cardiovascular, and gastrointestinal problems. Fatty tissue is more difficult to suture and has less resistance to infection; postoperative complications of delayed wound healing, wound infection, and disruption in the integrity of the wound are more common (Brunner and Suddarth, 1988).

Use of Alcohol or Nicotine. Clients who habitually have a large alcohol intake will require larger doses of anesthetic agents and postoperative analgesics, increasing the risk of drug-related complications. Clients who smoke are at higher risk for respiratory complications following surgery; pulmonary secretions are retained by all clients during anesthesis, but the smoker, with already increased mucous secretions, has more difficulty clearing the respiratory passages after surgery. In addition, the tracheobronchial mucosa is chronically irritated in persons who smoke; anesthesia further increases this irritation.

Activities of Daily Living. Exercise and rest/sleep habits are important considerations in preventing postoperative complications and facilitating recovery. The client who has a well-established exercise program will have improved cardiovascular, respiratory, metabolic, and musculoskeletal function, thereby lowering the risks of surgery. Rest and sleep are essential to physical and emotional adaptation and recovery from the stress of surgery. Information from the nursing history will allow the nurse to individualize interventions to promote rest and sleep.

Occupation. Many surgical procedures require a delay in returning to a career or occupation or may necessitate a change in the way the client supports self and family. Knowledge of a client's usual work and concerns about returning to work prepare the nurse for necessary teaching and referrals.

Coping Patterns/Support Systems. Assessment of the psychologic, sociocultural, and spiritual dimensions of the client is as important as the physical history and examination. Surgery is a major psychologic stressor, affecting coping patterns, support systems, and sociocultural needs.

Coping Patterns. A surgical procedure, no matter whether planned or unexpected, major or minor, causes anxiety and fear. The nursing history interview is often a time when the nurse can use cues from verbal and nonverbal communication of the client and family to identify fears and concerns and to plan nursing interventions to provide information and emotional support necessary to the successful recovery from surgery.

Surgery is an unknown experience over which a person has no control; the resulting anxiety may be expressed in many ways, such as anger, withdrawal, apathy, confrontation, questioning. Therapeutic communication skills are essential in establishing a trusting nurse–client relationship necessary to identify and resolve fear. The causes of fear in the preoperative phase include:

Fear of the unknown: The client has fears about the surgery itself, the anesthesia, the diagnosis, the future, financial and family responsibilities, response to pain, possible disfigurement or disability.

Fear of pain or death: Common fears are that the anesthesia will not "put me to sleep," that death will occur during surgery, or that the client will not be able to handle postoperative pain.

Fear of changes in body image and self-concept: Surgical procedures often leave the client with permanent changes in body structure, function, or appearance. Commonly, clients fear alterations in physical attractiveness, social relationships, life-style, and sexuality.

It is important that the nurse encourage clients to identify and verbalize fears; often simply talking about fears helps diminish the magnitude that has built up. At the same time, incorrect knowledge can be identified and corrected, strengths can be identified, and teaching can be done. The reduction of fear is of major importance in preoperative preparation; emotional stress added to the physical stress of surgery increases surgical risk.

Support Systems.   Coping with stress can be facilitated through various support systems, identified during the assessment phase of preoperative nursing care. As much as possible, family members or significant others should be a part of the initial interview, and should be included in discussions of fears and concerns. Family members should be encouraged to be a part of the surgical experience, providing support before and after surgery.

By identifying spiritual beliefs in the nursing history, the nurse can support the client's spiritual needs through acceptance, participation in prayer, or referral to clergy or chaplain. Faith in a higher being provides support and helps decrease fears.

The need for other support systems can also be identified in the initial interview (*e.g.,* the client having a colostomy or mastectomy may have many questions answered and anxieties reduced by a preoperative visit from a person who has had the same operation and has adapted successfully).

The nursing history should elicit those ways in which a client provides self-support to reduce stress. These have been previously discussed in Chapter 9 and range from listening to music to actively practicing relaxation techniques.

Sociocultural Needs.   A person's perceptions of and reactions to the surgical experience are influenced by sociocultural factors, including family health beliefs and practices, economic factors, and cultural background.

As discussed in Chapter 2, each person is influenced by family health beliefs and practices. If the client requiring surgery grew up in a family that believes surgical intervention is the last possible option in treating illness, he or she may refuse to have surgery or may be convinced death will result. The resulting anxiety and physical condition make this particular client even more susceptible to surgical risk; a "self-fulfilling prophecy" has come true. Reactions to teaching, physical care, and pain are also influenced by family values (*e.g.,* the male client, reared with the belief that it is "unmanly" to acknowledge pain, will present a stoic acceptance of pain and will deny needed medications postoperatively).

Economic factors influence the point on the health–illness continuum at which a person seeks medical care or has elective surgery. Cultural influences on the surgical experience also impact the client's responses and perceptions. Cultural backgrounds may require nursing interventions individualized to meet needs in such areas as language spoken, foods eaten, family interactions and participation, personal space, and health beliefs and practices (*e.g.,* a client from a cultural background that believes bed rest is the most important treatment for illness or injury will have difficulty accepting the need for postoperative exercises and ambulation).

Nursing Examination

Assessment of the present physical status of the client done during the nursing examination provides data for interventions to decrease surgical risk and potential postoperative complications. Depending on the situation, the nursing examination is done as described in Chapter 24. Table 43-4 summarizes assessments specific to the surgical client.

Screening Tests

Various screening tests done in the preoperative phase provide objective data of normal body function, or if abnormal, provide data for medical interventions to improve physical status and thus decrease potential surgical complications. The nurse's role is to ensure the tests are ordered and done, results are recorded in the client's record prior to surgery, and abnormal findings are reported. Additionally, abnormal results provide data to support nursing diagnoses and collaborative problems. Usual screening tests are chest x-ray, electrocardiogram, complete blood count, electrolyte levels, and urinalysis. These tests are discussed in Chapter 25; normal findings for laboratory tests are found in Appendix A. Significant abnormal findings are an elevated white blood count (presence of infection), decreased hemoglobin and hematocrit (presence of bleeding, anemia), hyper- or hypokalemia (increased risk of cardiac problems), ele-

T A B L E   43-4
Preoperative Physical Assessments

Component	Assessment	Purpose
General survey	• Height • Weight • Vital signs • General appearance	• Indicates nutritional status, especially obesity and malnutrition • Provides baseline data for intra- and postoperative phases • May indicate fluid and electrolyte imbalances, or underlying infection • Reflects energy levels, physical and emotional status
Status of skin	• Oral cavity • Skin turgor • All skin surfaces, especially over bony prominences	• Indicates hydration levels • Significant in hydration status • Indicates potential for injury or decubitus ulcers during and after surgery
Respiratory status	• Respiratory depth, rate • Adventitious sounds on auscultation • Diameter and shape of thorax	• Any abnormalities found would indicate potential respiratory difficulties during surgery, or postoperative atelectasis or infection
Cardiovascular status	• Apical pulse: character, rate, rhythm • Peripheral pulses • Presence of edema	• Provides baseline data for intra- and postoperative phases • Abnormal findings indicate potential complications intra- and postoperatively, such as thrombophlebitis, emboli, congestive heart failure, arrhythmias
Abdominal status	• Size, shape, symmetry • Bowel sounds • Last bowel movement	• Provides baseline data for postoperative assessments
Neurologic status	• Level of consciousness • Mood • Motor and sensory function	• Provides baseline data for postoperative assessments • Especially important to postoperative assessments following spinal anesthesia

vated blood urea nitrogen or creatinine (possible renal failure), and abnormal urine constituents (indicating infection, fluid imbalances, renal failure).

Diagnosing

Nursing diagnoses for the client in the preoperative phase may be identified for a variety of actual or potential problems, based on the analysis of subjective and objective data obtained from the nursing history and nursing examination, as well as information from other health-team members and screening tests. Many diagnoses reflect assessment of potential risk and are made to provide interventions to meet client needs during the intra- and postoperative phases. Nursing care throughout the perioperative period must be consistent and documented; the preoperative nursing diagnoses are the base for consistent holistic care from admission through recovery.

Examples of nursing diagnoses pertaining to the preoperative phase are the following:

Anxiety related to effects of impending surgery on ability to function as head of household

Ineffective individual coping related to conflict between need for surgery and religious beliefs (Christian Scientist)

Fear related to surgery for treatment of ovarian cancer and an unknown future

Grieving related to perceived loss of body image resulting from scheduled amputation of left leg

Potential for infection related to obesity and surgical procedure to remove gallbladder

Knowledge deficit: Preoperative routines

Knowledge deficit: Postoperative exercises and activities

Potential ineffective airway clearance related to history of smoking and administration of anesthesia during surgery

Planning

Preoperative nursing care is affected by the length of the preoperative phase; clients admitted through the emergency room with the need for emergency surgery and clients having "same-day" surgery will not have time for comprehensive assessments or teaching, and adjustments must be made accordingly. However, for the client having elective surgery (with admission 24 hours to 48 hours before the scheduled surgery), expected client and nursing goals can be established. (Goals are established for all clients having surgery, but needs must be prioritized according to specific clients and situations.)

Client Goals

Planning for the entire perioperative period is included in the preoperative phase and includes the client, family, and nurse; goals must be mutually discussed and agreed upon. Although each plan of care is individualized, broad outcome standards for perioperative nursing, established by the Association of Operating Room Nurses (1982), are the following:

- Client demonstrates knowledge of the physiologic and psychologic responses to surgery.
- Client is free of infection.
- Client's skin integrity is maintained.
- Client is free of injury from surgical positioning.
- Client is free of injury from extraneous objects, or chemical, physical, and electric hazards.
- Client participates in the rehabilitation process.
  More specific client goals, as defined by McConnell (1987), are
- Client will be physically prepared for surgery.
- Client will be emotionally prepared for surgery.
- Client will correctly demonstrate how to turn, cough, deep breathe, and splint the incision.
- Client will verbalize understanding of postoperative pain control.
- Client will verbalize events of the intra- and post-operative phases.
- Client will maintain nutritional and fluid intake to meet needs.
  To help the client meet these goals, during the preoperative phase, the nurse
- Establishes a data base and plan of care to meet client needs throughout the perioperative period
- Identifies and meets client and family learning needs
- Identifies physical and psychosocial risk factors
- Provides interventions to maximize physical and emotional safety and security

Implementing

Preoperative nursing interventions provide the client with the necessary physical and psychologic preparation for surgery and the postoperative phase. This section of the chapter discusses implementing the plan of care to meet established client goals; Procedure 43-1 outlines the actions and rationales for preoperative client care.

Preparing the Client Psychologically

As discussed in the assessment section, surgery is almost always viewed as a life crisis and evokes feelings of anxiety and fear. Anxiety can be reduced and recovery can be facilitated by nursing actions that focus on therapeutic communications and client and family teaching.

Communicating. The nurse uses therapeutic communication skills and techniques, as described in Chapter 20, to establish a supportive and trusting nurse–client relationship and to facilitate psychologic safety and security. Guidelines for the nurse in meeting psychologic needs of the surgical client are

- Establish and maintain a therapeutic relationship, allowing the client to verbalize fears and concerns.
- Use active listening skills to identify and validate verbal and nonverbal responses indicative of anxiety and fear.
- Use touch, as appropriate, to demonstrate genuine empathy and caring.
- Be prepared to respond to common client questions about surgery. These include
  - Will I lose control of body functions while I'm having surgery?
  - How long will I be in the operating and recovery rooms?
  - Where will my family be?
  - Will I have pain when I wake up?
  - Will the anesthetic make me sick?
  - Will I need a blood transfusion?
  - How long will it be before I can eat?
  - What kind of scar will I have?
  - When will I be able to be sexually active?
  - When can I go back to work?

Remember that each client is a unique individual and will respond to the surgical experience in a unique way. One note of caution: the nontherapeutic use of false reassurance must be avoided. In an attempt to allay anxiety and fear, the nurse may be tempted to reassure that "everything will be alright" or "don't worry, you'll be fine." These responses deny the client's emotional needs, shut off therapeutic communications, and may not be true.

Teaching. Teaching postoperative activities is done in the preoperative phase and is the nurse's responsibility. Clients and families need to know about surgical events and sensations, how to manage pain, and how to perform the physical activities necessary to decrease postoperative complications and facilitate recovery. The teaching-learning process (Chap 21) is individualized to meet both specific and common client needs.

The timing of teaching is a significant consideration; teaching done too far in advance of surgery or when the client is very anxious will be less effective. In today's

(Text continues on p. 1256.)

Preoperative Client Care

Action

Rationale

General

1 Identify clients for whom surgery is a greater risk:

Allows for recognition of clients who may be prone to complications after surgery

   a. Very young and elderly clients

   b. Obese or malnourished clients

   c. Clients with fluid and electrolyte imbalances

   d. Clients in poor general health from chronic diseases and infectious processes

   e. Clients taking certain medications (*i.e.,* anticoagulants, antibiotics, diuretics, depressants, steroids)

   f. Clients who are extremely anxious

2 Review nursing data base, history, and physical examination. Check that baseline data are recorded.

Identifies clients who are surgical risks

3 Check that diagnostic testing has been completed and results are available.

May influence type of surgery and anesthetic as well as timing of surgery or need for additional consultation

4 Promote optimum nutritional and hydration status.

Promotes wound healing

5 Identify learning needs of client. Conduct preoperative teaching regarding the following:

Minimizes surgical risk and allays anxiety by preparing clients for postoperative period

   a. Coughing and deep-breathing exercises

   b. Management of pain after surgery

   c. Leg exercises and ambulation

   d. Postoperative equipment and monitoring devices

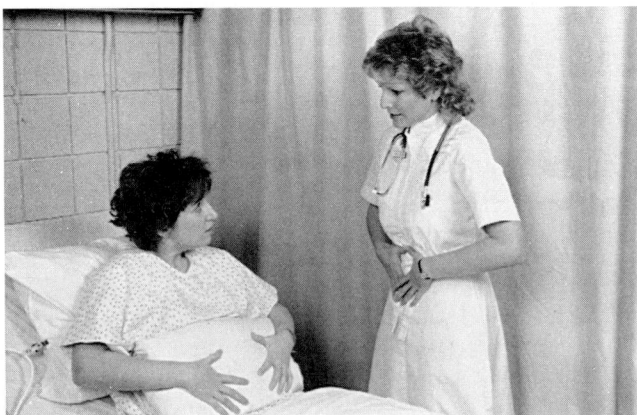

Step 5a: Teaching client to splint incision before coughing.

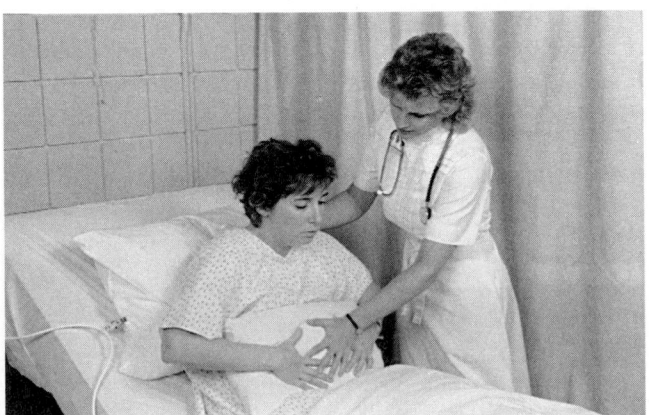

Step 5a: Teaching client to cough.

(Continued)

Action	**Rationale**

Day Before Surgery

6 Provide emotional support. Answer questions realistically. Provide spiritual assistance if requested.

Allays client's misconceptions and fears

7 Follow preoperative dietary restrictions.

Reduces risk of vomiting and aspiration during surgery. Anesthetic agents temporarily depress gastrointestinal function and processes.

8 Prepare for elimination needs during and after surgery.

Anesthetic agents and abdominal surgery interfere with normal elimination function. A urinary catheter inserted preoperatively minimizes risk of inadvertent trauma to bladder during surgery.

9 Shave and prepare the operative site if ordered by physician.

Reduces number of microorganisms present on skin

10 Attend to client's special hygiene needs (*i.e.,* use of antiseptic cleansing agents).

Decreases potential for infection

11 Provide for adequate rest.

Minimizes stress prior to surgery

Day of Surgery

12 Check that proper identification band is on client.

Ensures identity of client

13 Check that preoperative consent forms are signed and medical record is in order.

Fulfills legal requirement related to informed consent

14 Check vital signs. Notify physician of any pertinent changes (*i.e.,* rise or drop in blood pressure, elevated temperature, cough, symptoms of infection).

Provides baseline data for comparison

15 Provide hygiene and oral care. Remind client not to swallow water if NPO for surgery.

Promotes comfort

16 Continue nutritional and hydration preparation.

Prepares client for operative procedure

17 Remove cosmetics and prostheses (*e.g.,* contact lenses, false eyelashes, dentures, and so forth). Assess for loose teeth.

Interfere with assessment during surgery

18 Have client empty bladder and bowel prior to surgery.

Minimizes risk of injury or complications during and after surgery

19 Place valuables in appropriate area. Hospital safe is most appropriate place for valuables. They should not be placed in narcotics drawer.

Ensures safety of valuables and personal possessions

20 Attend to any special preoperative orders.

Prepares client for operative procedure

21 Complete preoperative checklist and record of client's preoperative preparation.

Ensures accurate documentation

22 Administer preoperative medication as ordered by physician.

Reduces anxiety, provides sedation, and diminishes salivary and bronchial secretions

health-care delivery system, clients often enter the hospital the day before or the day of surgery, and teaching must be adapted to this schedule. Many institutions provide teaching sessions before admission so that the client is prepared for surgery. Whether done prior to or after admission, a preoperative teaching checklist gives nurses organized and comprehensive guidelines for instruction.

Nursing research has indicated that the success of preoperative teaching varies with the timing of the teaching, the individual client and his support systems, the type of surgery, and group versus individual sessions (Voss, 1986). Preoperative teaching has proven to be beneficial in decreasing postoperative complications and in positively influencing recovery.

Surgical Events and Sensations.   Clients and their families need to know when surgery is scheduled, approximately how long surgery and recovery room care will last, and what will be done before, during, and after surgery (procedures, medications, equipment). If the surgery is elective, a tour of the operating room suite is helpful in reducing anxiety and fear of the unknown (although especially helpful for children, this is also very useful in teaching adult clients). The description of the surgical events also includes a description of the various members of the health-care team. An outline of surgical events is found in the box.

Clients also need to know what sensations they will be experiencing during the perioperative period. Although the sensations will differ depending on the type of surgery, teaching should include

- Feelings experienced from preoperative medications, such as a dry mouth and drowsiness
- Sensations that normally occur following surgery and anesthesia, such as a sore throat from an endotracheal tube, a gradual return of feeling and movement after spinal anesthesia, and a lower tolerance of activity with increased fatigue
- Sensations experienced after surgery, such as incisional pain, intravenous catheters and fluids, tight dressings, dry mouth, and drowsiness

Pain Management.   Pain is a normal part of the surgical experience and an area of major concern for the client and family. Guidelines for teaching the client about pain control are

- Medications to relieve pain will be ordered by the physician and administered by the nurse.
- Pain medications are usually ordered on an as-needed (PRN) basis, with a time restriction between doses (*e.g.,* every 3 or 4 hours). The client needs to ask for the medication and should do so before the pain is severe; if the medication does not control the pain, a different one can be ordered.
- Medications for pain are usually given by injection for the first few days (and as long as the client is

---

Sample Preoperative Teaching Checklist: Activities and Events

I. Preoperative phase
   A. Exercises and physical activities
      1. Deep-breathing
      2. Coughing
      3. Incentive spirometry
      4. Turning
      5. Leg exercises
   B. Pain management
      1. Meaning of PRN orders
      2. Timing for best effect
      3. Splinting incision
   C. Visit by anesthesiologist
   D. Physical preparation
      1. NPO
      2. Sleeping medication the night before
      3. Preoperative checklist (review items)
   E. Visitors and waiting room
   F. Transported to OR by stretcher
II. Intraoperative phase
   A. Holding area
      1. Skin preparation
      2. IV fluids
      3. Medications
   B. Operating room
      1. Operating room table
      2. Lights
      3. Restraints
      4. Sensations
      5. Staff
III. Postoperative phase
   A. Postanesthesia recovery area
      1. Frequent vital signs
      2. Dressings
      3. IVs
      4. Pain medications
      5. Family notification
      6. Sensations
      7. Staff
   B. Transfer to unit (on stretcher)
      1. Frequent vital signs
      2. Sensations
      3. Pain medications
      4. NPO, diet
      5. Exercises
      6. Ambulation
      7. Family visits

NPO); with food intake and decreasing pain levels, oral medications can be used.
- There is very little danger of addiction to pain medications when they are used in the postoperative management of pain.

- The use of relaxation techniques (such as deep breathing or guided imagery) will facilitate the effects of pain medications.
- Pain medications allow the client to manage pain and increase his ability to carry out activities and exercises necessary to recovery.

Physical Activities. The most common causes of postoperative complications are cardiovascular and pulmonary alterations, including atelectasis, pneumonia, thrombophlebitis, and emboli. Physical activities are taught in the preoperative period to reduce the potential of these complications. The following sections describe deep (diaphgramatic) breathing, coughing, incentive spirometry, and turning in bed. The client should be able to verbalize the purpose and demonstrate the activities before going to surgery. (This section will give the rationale for the activities; postoperative complications are discussed later in the chapter.)

Deep Breathing. During surgery, the cough reflex is suppressed, mucous accumulates in the tracheobronchial passageways, and the lungs do not fully ventilate. After surgery, respirations are often less effective as a result of the anesthesia, pain medications, and pain from the incision (*e.g.,* clients who have thoracic or high abdominal incisions are especially prone to shallow breathing because of incisional pain with deeper respirations). As a result, alveoli do not inflate and may collapse, and secretions are retained, increasing the potential for atelectasis and pulmonary infection.

Deep breathing exercises hyperventilate the alveoli and prevent their recollapse, improve lung expansion and volume, help expel anesthetic gases and mucus, and facilitate oxygenation of tissues.

Guidelines for teaching effective deep breathing exercises are (McConnell, 1987)

- Place the client in semi-Fowler's position, with support for the neck and shoulders.
- Ask the client to place his hands over his rib cage, so he can feel the chest rise as the lungs expand.
- Have the client
    Exhale gently and completely.
    Inhale through the nose gently and completely.
    Hold his breath and mentally count to three.
    Exhale as completely as possible through the mouth with lips pursed (as if whistling).
    Repeat three times.
- This exercise should be done every 1 hour to 2 hours, while awake, for the first 24 hours to 48 hours after surgery, and as necessary thereafter depending on risk factors and pulmonary status.

Coughing. Coughing facilitates the removal of retained mucus from the respiratory tract and usually is taught in conjunction with deep breathing. Coughing is painful; the client should be taught how to splint the incision (*i.e.,* to support the incision with a pillow or folded bath blanket, as illustrated in Procedure 43-1) and

to use the time period after pain medications to best advantage. Guidelines for teaching effective coughing are (McConnell, 1987)

- Place the client in a semi-Fowler's position, leaning forward.
- Provide a pillow or folded bath blanket to use in splinting the incision.
- Have the client
    Inhale and exhale deeply and slowly through the nose three times.
    Take a deep breath and hold it for 3 seconds.
    "Hack" out for three short breaths.
    With mouth open, take a quick breath.
    Cough deeply once or twice.
    Take another deep breath.
- Repeat the exercise every 2 hours, while awake.

Incentive Spirometry. An incentive spirometer, (see Fig. 34-5) is often ordered for clients having surgery, and its use should be practiced preoperatively. This device produces increased lung volume and inflation of alveoli; it also facilitates venous return. Client teaching includes

- Sit upright or elevate the head of the bed 45 degrees.
- Take two or three normal breaths, then insert the spirometer's mouthpiece into the mouth.
- Inhale through the mouth and hold the breath for 3 seconds to 5 seconds.
- Exhale slowly and fully.
- Repeat the sequence ten times during each waking hour for the first 5 days after surgery (except immediately before or after meals).

Leg Exercises. During surgery, venous blood return from the legs slows; some surgical positions may also decrease venous return. With circulatory stasis of the lower extremities, thrombophlebitis and resultant emboli are potential complications. Leg exercises increase venous return through flexion and contraction of the quadriceps and gastrocnemius muscles. Guidelines for leg exercises (illustrated in Fig. 43-2) are to have the client

- Alternately point toes toward his chin (dorsiflex) and toward the foot of the bed (plantar flex); then make a circle with his toes.
- Flex and extend the knees, pressing the knees down toward the mattress on extension.
- Raise and lower each leg with the leg straight.
- Repeat the exercises every 1 hour to 2 hours.

Leg exercises must be individualized to client needs and physical condition, physician preference, and agency protocol.

Turning in Bed. Turning in bed improves venous return, respiratory function, and gastrointestinal peristalsis. Although turning in bed sounds like a simple procedure, incisional pain will make it more difficult, and it should be practiced before surgery. To turn in bed, the client should raise one knee, reach across to grasp the side rail (on the side to be turned to), and roll over while pushing with the bent leg and pulling on the side rail. A small pillow is useful in splinting the incision while

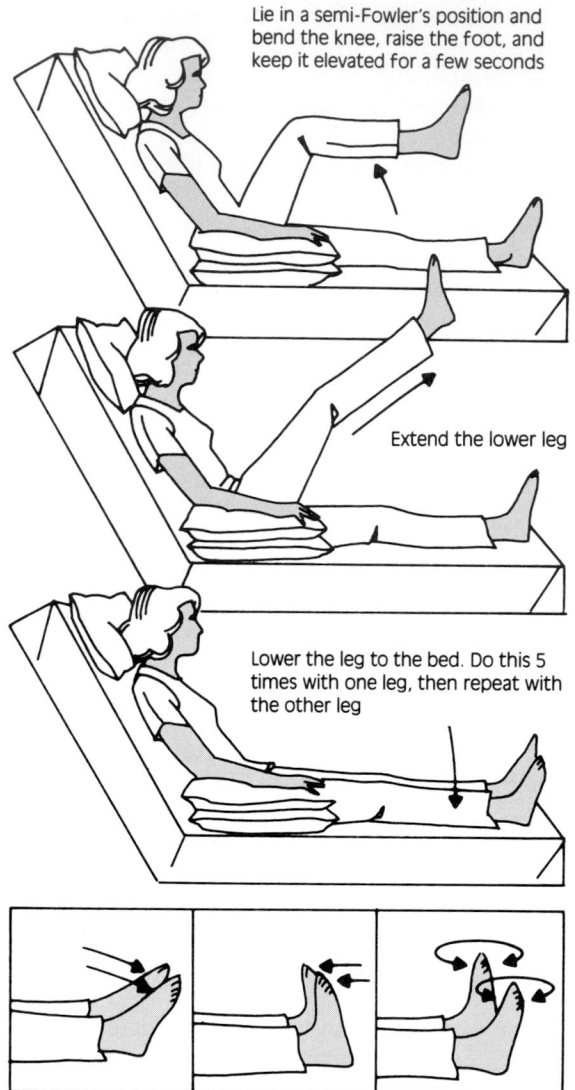

Lie in a semi-Fowler's position and bend the knee, raise the foot, and keep it elevated for a few seconds

Extend the lower leg

Lower the leg to the bed. Do this 5 times with one leg, then repeat with the other leg

A. Point the toes of both feet toward the foot of the bed. Relax both feet

B. Pull toes toward the chin. Relax both feet

C. Make circles with both ankles. First circle to the right, then to the left. Repeat 3 times, Relax feet

F I G U R E   43-2
Leg exercises to increase venous return.

turning. The client should turn from side to side every 2 hours.

Preparing the Client Physically

The physical preparation of the client for surgery may vary, depending on the client's physical status and special needs, the type of surgery to be done, and physician's orders. However, certain independent and interdependent nursing interventions are appropriate for all surgical clients in the areas of nutrition and fluids, hygiene and skin preparation, elimination, and rest and sleep. The nurse is also responsible for the preparation and safety of the client on the day of surgery.

Hygiene and Skin Preparation. Intact skin is the body's first line of defense against microorganisms, and an alteration in skin integrity (such as the surgical incision) provides a potential source of infection. Therefore, the skin is prepared to minimize skin contamination and decrease the risk of postoperative wound infection.

The skin is cleansed by scrubbing the operative site one or more times with an antibacterial soap or solution to remove bacteria. This can be done by the client while taking a bath or shower. Ideally, a shower is taken the evening before or morning of surgery. Shampooing the hair and cleaning fingernails also help reduce organisms.

The operative area is usually shaved before surgery, because hair serves as a reservoir for bacteria. This may be done by the nurse or by surgery personnel. Although shaving the skin was once done routinely the evening before surgery, it is now most often done immediately before the operation, often in the surgical holding area, based on findings that small cuts made by the razor serve as sites for bacterial growth; increased time for growth of bacteria increases potential for infection. The procedure for shaving the skin of the preoperative client is outlined in Procedures 43-2 and 43-3. Presurgical shaving is not always done; depilatory creams or hair clippers may be used to remove hair (and are recommended by the CDC). Agency protocol should be followed for timing, persons responsible, and method.

Elimination. Emptying the bowel of feces is no longer a routine procedure before surgery, but the nurse should use preoperative assessments to determine the need for an order for bowel elimination. If the client has not had a bowel movement for several days or has had preoperative barium diagnostic tests, an enema will help prevent postoperative constipation.

If the client is scheduled for surgery of the gastrointestinal tract, cleansing enemas are usually ordered. Peristalsis does not return for 24 hours to 48 hours after handling the bowel, so preoperative cleansing will help decrease postoperative constipation. An empty bowel also prevents contamination of the surgical area during surgery.

A Foley catheter may be ordered to be inserted prior to surgery, especially in clients having pelvic surgery, to prevent bladder distention or accidental injury. If the client does not have a Foley catheter, they void immediately before receiving preoperative medications to ensure an empty bladder during surgery.

Nutrition and Fluids. The diet order for the client having surgery will depend on the type of surgery and the type of anesthesia to be used. Clients having general anesthesia or major regional anesthesia are made NPO 8 hours to 12 hours before the surgery (often at midnight prior to next morning surgery) to prevent aspiration of gastric contents if the client should vomit while anesthetized. The nurse explains the reason to the client, re-

PROCEDURE 43-2
Shaving the Skin of the Preoperative Client (Dry Shave)

Equipment

Adequate lighting	Scissors	Antiseptic solution
Electric clippers		and applicator
		(if ordered)

Action | **Rationale**

1 Explain procedure to client. — Facilitates cooperation and provides reassurance for client

2 Assemble equipment. Expose the area to be shaved, and drape the client appropriately. — Having equipment in readiness saves time. Draping client provides for privacy.

3 Wash your hands. — Handwashing deters the spread of microorganisms.

4 Shave with the clippers. — Minimizes risk of abrasions on operative area

5 Move drape and continue until entire area is shaved. — Provides for client's privacy

6 Brush off remaining hair with towel. — Minimizes skin irritation and improves client's comfort

7 If antiseptic solution is ordered, use cotton-tipped applicators to clean in crevices (groin, umbilicus). — This is additional protection against microorganisms which may accumulate in crevices.

8 Discard equipment according to agency policy. Cleanse electric clippers by wiping with antiseptic solution. — Protects against injury from razor blade

9 Wash your hands. — Handwashing deters the spread of microorganisms.

10 Record completion of skin preparation. — Provides documentation for procedure

PROCEDURE 43-3
Shaving the Skin of the Preoperative Client (Wet Shave)

Equipment

Adequate lighting	Prep kit containing:
Bath blanket	Razor
	Sponge soaked
	with antiseptic
	soap
	Waterproof pad
	Basin
	Cotton-tipped ap-
	plicator
	Washcloth

(Continued)

Shaving the Skin of the Preoperative Client (Wet Shave)   (Continued)

Equipment

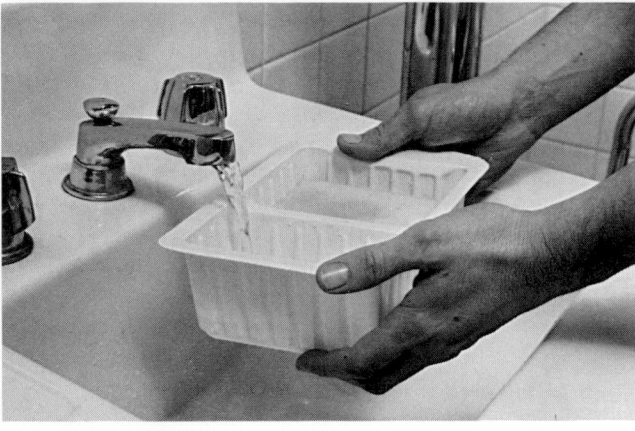

Wetting prepared prep kit.

Action

1 Follow steps 1, 2, and 3 of Procedure 43-2.

2 Place waterproof pad under area to be shaved.

3 Apply soap solution to small areas of the skin, and work up a lather.

4 Shave with one hand while gently stretching the skin taut with the other hand. Hold the razor between a 30-degree and a 45-degree angle, and take long, gentle strokes in the direction of hair growth. Rinse hair and soap from razor as necessary.

Rationale

Protects bed linens

Soap emulsifies normal fatty substances on the skin and loosens dirt so that water can penetrate and soften the hair.

Stretching the skin eliminates wrinkles and smooths the skin so that the nurse can accomplish a close shave. Gentle, long strokes with the razor held at a 30-degree to a 45-degree angle help prevent nicking and cutting the skin. Shaving in the direction of hair growth helps minimize skin irritation.

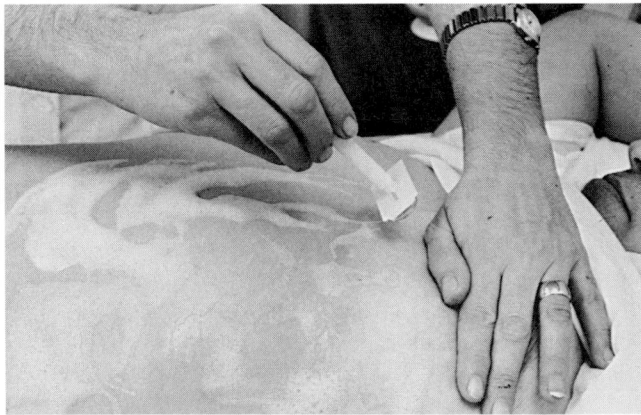

Step 4: Shaving area while gently stretching skin taut with other hand.

5 Continue moving drape until entire area is shaved. Replace razor if it becomes dull.

Provides for client's privacy. Sharp edge on razor reduces risk of injury.

(Continued)

Action	Rationale
6 Use washcloth and warm water to remove any excess soap and remaining hair. Dry carefully.	Minimizes irritation to skin
7 Stoop so that the eyes are at the level of the shaven area to check for isolated hairs that may have been missed by razor.	Looking at the area with the eyes at the level of the skin helps in checking whether all hair has been removed.
8 Report any cuts in skin to physician or charge person.	Cut in skin may be a potential source of infection.
9 Follow steps 8, 9, and 10 of Procedure 42-2.	

moves all food and fluids from the bedside, and places a sign over the bed so all health-team members and visitors will know about the restriction. If the client should eat or drink, the physician should be notified at once.

Clients need to be well nourished and hydrated before surgery to counterbalance fluid, blood, and electrolyte loss during surgery, and to facilitate tissue healing after surgery. Preoperative assessments provide a base for physical preparation for surgery, including the need for supplemental nutrition, fluids, or electrolytes. The client who is undernourished may require parenteral nutrition (Chap 31) and intravenous electrolyte replacements. If the client's screening tests show a hemoglobin of less than 10 g/dl and a hematocrit less than 33%, blood may be given preoperatively to maintain volume and increase oxygenation of tissue during surgery (McConnell, 1987).

Rest and Sleep. Rest and sleep are important components in reducing stress before surgery and in healing and recovery after surgery. The nurse can facilitate rest and sleep in the immediate preoperative period by meeting psychologic needs, carrying out teaching, providing a quiet environment, and administering the ordered bedtime sedative medication.

Physical Preparation: Day of Surgery

The preoperative checklist (Fig. 43-3) outlines the nurse's responsibilities on the day of surgery; these activities must be completed before the client is transported to surgery. Some of these activities have already been described (NPO, preoperative teaching, informed consent, skin preparation, screening tests, bladder elimination); other nursing responsibilities are

1. To take and record vital signs, both to serve as baseline data for the intraoperative phase, and to assess for and report any possible abnormal findings (such as an elevated temperature).
2. To prepare the client physically for the intraoperative phase.

- Have the client remove all personal clothing and put on an OR gown
- Remove all hairpins or hairpieces. This prevents injury to the client during surgery, as well as possible loss of hairpieces or wigs.
- Remove make-up and fingernail polish to allow intra- and postoperative assessment of skin and nailbeds for circulation and oxygenation of tissues.
- Remove all prostheses, such as dentures or partial plates, eyeglasses, contact lenses, and artificial limbs. Dentures may cause respiratory obstruction during anesthesia; other prostheses may be damaged or lost. Be sure items are stored safely while the client is in surgery.
- Remove jewelry. Jewelry is removed to prevent loss or injury from swelling during or after surgery; if the client prefers not to remove a wedding band, it can be securely taped to the finger (depending on the type of surgery, in some cases leaving jewelry on is not allowed). When jewelry is removed, it should be given to a family member or locked in a safe place.
- Leave on a hearing aid, and be certain that operating and recovery room nurses know the client has one.
- Be sure that the client's identification bracelet is in place to ensure accurate identity.
- If the client has allergies, be sure they are noted according to institutional policy (*e.g.,* on the front of the client's record or on an allergy bracelet)
3. To carry out any special procedures that are ordered, such as securing previous records, inserting a nasogastric tube, starting an IV, applying antiembolic stockings, or giving medications.
4. To give the preoperative medications that are ordered, either at a scheduled time, or "on call" (the operating room will call and tell the nurse to give the medication). Medications commonly ordered are

Pre-Op Surgical Checklist

Nurse's Name: _____

_____

_____

O.R.		Comments or Lab Values	Nurses' Initials
☐	PRE OP HYPO ORDERED		
☐	NPO AFTER MIDNIGHT OR AS ORDERED		
☐	I.D. BAND ON PATIENT		
☐	PRE-OP TEACHING DONE		
☐	SURGICAL PERMIT SIGNED		
☐	INFORMED CONSENT SIGNED (IOL OR LASER CASES)		
☐	OPERATIVE AREA SHAVE PREPPED		
☐	HISTORY AND PHYSICAL DICTATED		
☐	CBC REPORT ON CHART	HGB.	
		HCT.	
☐	URINALYSIS REPORT ON CHART		
☐	PROFILE REPORT ON CHART IF ORDERED	K+	
	(NORMAL RANGE K+ 3.5 to 5)		
☐	BLOOD SCREENED _____ TYPED & X MATCHED	Exp. Date # of Units Set Up	
☐	PT AND PTT	PT PTT	
☐	CHEST X-RAY REPORT ON CHART		
☐	EKG		
☐	T _____ P _____ R _____ BP _____		
☐	DENTURES OR PARTIAL PLATE REMOVED		
☐	CONTACT LENSES OR GLASSES REMOVED		
☐	JEWELRY REMOVED OR SECURED		
☐	HAIR PINS, MAKE UP AND NAIL POLISH REMOVED		
☐	HEARING AID TO O.R. WITH PATIENT		
☐	BATHED		
☐	O.R. GOWN ON PATIENT		
☐	VOIDED OR CATHETERIZED AND FOLEY EMPTIED		
☐	PRE-OP ANTIBIOTIC GIVEN IF ORDERED		
☐	PRE-OP MEDICATION GIVEN		
☐	ALLERGIES		
☐	FAMILY O.R. WAITING ROOM		
☐	OLD CHART TO O.R.		
☐	X-RAY FILMS FROM FLOOR TO O.R.		

Floor Nurse Sending Patient to O.R.: _____ O.R. Nurse Receiving Patient: _____

Arrival Time: _____

COMMENTS:

F I G U R E   43-3
Example of a preoperative check list.

- Sedatives and tranquilizers, such as pentobarbital (Nembutal), chloropromazine (Thorazine), or diazepam (Valium), to alleviate anxiety and facilitate anesthesia induction
- Anticholinergics, such as atropine and glycopyrrolate (Robinul), to decrease pulmonary and oral secretions, and also to prevent laryngospasm
- Narcotic analgesics, such as morphine and meperidine hydrochloride (Demerol), to facilitate client sedation and relaxation, and also to decrease the amount of anesthetic agent needed
- Neuroleptanalgesic agents (Innovar) to cause a general state of calmness and sleepiness
- H$_2$-receptor antihistaminics, such as cimetidine (Tagamet) and rantidine (Zantac), to decrease gastric acidity and volume, so that if vomiting and aspiration occur during surgery, there is less danger of aspiration pneumonia

5. To maintain client safety, by elevating side rails, lowering the bed to low position, and instructing the client to stay in bed.
6. To meet family (or other support person's) needs. The family may visit the morning of surgery and are told where the client will be taken after surgery (if a different location, such as the intensive care unit). The waiting area for the family is described, and the family is taken there after the client leaves for the operating room. The family is also told that the surgeon will come to the waiting room to tell them what happened in surgery.
7. To document, through checklists and narrative charting, the nursing interventions carried out.
8. To assist in moving the client from the bed to the operating room stretcher when it is time to transport the client to surgery, ensuring accurate identification.
9. To prepare the client's bed and room for postoperative care:
   - Making a surgical bed
   - Having necessary equipment and supplies in the room for postoperative care (equipment to measure vital signs, IV standard, and so forth)

Evaluating

The evaluation of the plan of care established for the preoperative phase is based on the established client goals. The plan is effective if the client is physically and emotionally prepared for surgery, can verbalize events and sensations of the perioperative period, and can demonstrate postoperative exercises and activities.

INTRAOPERATIVE NURSING CARE

The intraoperative phase of the perioperative period begins with admission of the client to the surgical area and lasts until the client is transferred to the recovery area. Although the surgeon has the dominant role during this phase, the nurse has specific responsibilities and roles in collaboratively meeting client needs. The nursing process uses the preoperative data and plan as a base.

The type of surgery scheduled will influence the assessments and interventions carried out by the nurse. For example, the role of the nurse when caring for the client having outpatient or "same day" surgery may be that of providing client care from admission through dismissal ("same day" surgery is described later in this chapter), while the role of the nurse for hospital-based surgery is usually specific to the phases (*i.e.,* one group of nurses provides care on the hospital unit pre- and postoperatively, another group practices operating room nursing, and still another group provides specific postanesthesia recovery room care). This section of the chapter will discuss the role of the nurse specific to intraoperative care.

Assessing

When the client is transferred to the surgical area, the first room they enter is usually the **holding area**. Nurses, in surgical scrub dress, assess the client's emotional and physical status and verify the information on the preoperative checklist. They may also carry out ordered immediate preoperative care, including skin preps, starting IV fluids (using a large gauge intercatheter), and giving preoperative medications. The client's response to procedures is assessed, and events of surgery are explained. When the operating room is prepared, a nurse from the OR arrives to transport the client to the operating room table.

In the operating room, the client is positioned on the operating table, anesthetized, and draped. The operating room nurse assesses the client and reviews preoperative data, paying particular attention to factors that increase surgical risk. The nurse also assesses the client during positioning and monitors supplies used to maintain safety for the client.

Diagnosing

Client problems in the intraoperative phase are primarily collaborative problems, although positioning can cause altered responses, with the following appropriate nursing diagnoses:

Potential for impairment of skin integrity related to surgical position

Potential for ineffective breathing pattern related to surgical position

Examples of collaborative problems (Carpenito, 1987) during the intraoperative phase are:

Potential complications: Neuromuscular damage, nosocomial infection, altered tissue perfusion

Planning

The planning phase of the nursing process focuses on preventing potential complications and client problems, and on ensuring client safety.

Client goals for the intraoperative phase are
- Client will remain free of neuromuscular damage.
- Client will maintain intact skin surfaces.
- Client will have symmetric breathing patterns.
- Client will be free of injury from burns, inaccurate count of supplies, or wound contamination.

During the intraoperative phase, the nurse performs the following:
- Assesses and monitors the client's physiologic response
- Positions the client to prevent injury or alterations in skin, respiratory, or neuromuscular function
- Maintains physical safety of the client
- Maintains aseptic technique

Implementing

During surgery, nurses function either as scrub nurses or circulating nurses. **Scrub nurses** assist the surgeon during the surgery and maintain surgical asepsis while draping and handling instruments and supplies. The **circulating nurse** assesses the client on admission to the OR; helps position the client on the operating table; helps with monitoring devices; gets additional supplies; and (at the end of the operation) counts the number of instruments, needles, and gauze sponges used during the operation to prevent the accidental loss of an item in the wound.

Positioning

The client is placed in a specific operative position after anesthesia has produced loss of consciousness and reflexes. The nurse must ensure client safety and comfort in positioning to prevent alterations in respiratory, vascular, and neuromuscular function. The potential of skin injury is avoided by lifting the client to a position, rather than rolling or pulling him, which can cause shearing force, in which two or more tissue layers slide on each other, stretching subcutaneous blood vessels, obstructing blood flow, and contributing to decubitus ulcers (Groah, 1983).

Although the various operative positions are not included here, the nurse needs to know what position was used and significant nursing considerations for that position. Two examples are

Trendelenburg's position: The downward displacement of the abdominal viscera decreases diaphragm movement and respiratory exchange; blood pools in the upper torso and blood pressure increases; hypotension can result with return to the supine position.

Lithotomy position: The placement of legs in stirrups causes pooling of blood in the lower extremities, increasing the potential of thrombo-

phlebitis. Pressure can also cause damage to the peroneal nerve, with resultant foot drop.

Draping

Drapes are used to establish a sterile field around the operative site, preventing the passage of microorganisms between sterile and nonsterile areas. The only area left exposed is the incision site. Plastic adhesive drapes may be used, forming a complete seal over the skin; with these skin color is visible, and the incision is made through the drape (McConnell, 1987).

Documenting

Throughout surgery, the nurse documents item counts, monitored data, positioning, medications, dressings, and so forth on the intraoperative record.

Transfer to the Postanesthesia Recovery Room

After the operation, the client is carefully moved from the operating room table to a stretcher. This is an especially critical time; sudden or rough handling can cause severe hypotension or potentially lethal cardiac or respiratory arrest (McConnell, 1987).

The client is then moved to the postanesthesia recovery (PAR) room, and relevant preoperative and postoperative assessments and interventions are communicated to the PAR nurses.

Evaluating

Evaluation of the effectiveness of the plan of care for the intraoperative phase is based on the established client goals. If goals are met, the plan was effective.

POSTOPERATIVE NURSING CARE

The postoperative phase can be divided into two stages: immediate care (usually provided in the PAR) and ongoing postoperative care, lasting from return to the unit through convalescence. Nursing assessments and interventions are consistent with those in the pre- and intraoperative phases and are carried out to maintain function, promote recovery, and facilitate coping with alterations in structure or function.

In this section, assessments and nursing interventions will be combined in discussing the immediate postoperative care; the phases of the nursing process will be used to describe ongoing postoperative care.

Immediate Postoperative Care

Nurses in the postanesthesia recovery (PAR) room assess and evaluate postoperative clients, with emphasis on preventing complications from anesthesia or the surgery (Drain and Christoph, 1987). Assessments are continuous and ongoing, using preoperative and intraoperative data as a basis for comparison. The assessments made in the PAR are respiratory status, cardiovascular status, central nervous system status, fluid status, wound status, and general condition. These assessments are made every 10 minutes to 15 minutes initially. The average recovery room stay is 2 hours or less.

Respiratory Status. Assessments of respiratory function are made by monitoring respiratory rate, rhythm, and depth; and by observing skin color. Cardiovascular and neurologic function assessments provide data about oxygenation. Assessments that indicate ineffective ventilation are

- Restlessness, apprehension
- Unequal chest expansion with use of accessory muscles
- Shallow, noisy respirations
- Cyanosis
- Rapid pulse

During the surgical procedure with general anesthesia, an artificial airway is inserted to maintain patent air passages. The airway is not removed until the laryngeal and pharyngeal reflexes return, allowing the client to control the tongue, cough, and swallow.

Respiratory obstruction is the most common PAR emergency. It may be due to secretion accumulation, obstruction by the tongue, laryngospasm (a sudden violent contraction of the vocal cords), or laryngeal edema. Assessments of respiratory obstruction include those previously outlined, plus wheezing or crowing sounds with respiratory effort.

Positioning, administering oxygen, and suctioning may all be used to maintain a patent airway and tissue oxygenation.

Cardiovascular Status. Evaluation of cardiovascular function includes assessing the blood pressure and pulses, skin color, respirations, and the wound.

Blood pressure findings are compared with baseline data from the preoperative period; hypotension may be the result of varied factors, including anesthetic agents, preoperative medications, position changes, blood loss, respiratory alterations, or peripheral blood pooling. Transient hypertension can also occur, due to anesthetic effects, respiratory insufficiency, the surgical procedure, or the excitement phase of recovery from anesthesia. Low blood pressure can be increased by oxygen administration, deep breathing, leg exercises, verbal stimulation (to help expel anesthetic gases and facilitate increasing level of consciousness) and maintaining accurate IV flow rates.

All pulses are assessed for bilateral equality, rhythm, rate, and character. Of special significance are assessments of abnormal function: arrhythmias, absence of pulses, and tachycardia. Tachycardia, an early symptom of shock, must be carefully evaluated. Other related as-

sessments are cyanosis, edema, skin temperature, and urinary output.

Central Nervous System Status. Anesthetics cause loss of consciousness and reflexes; the return of CNS function is assessed through response to stimuli and orientation. Reflexes return in reverse order, with the usual pattern being (1) unconsciousness, (2) response to touch and sounds, (3) drowsiness, (4) awake but not oriented, and (5) awake and oriented (McConnell, 1987). Nurses in the PAR verbally reorient the client frequently by touching and calling him or her by name.

Fluid Status. Fluid imbalance may be the result of factors such as preoperative fluid restriction, fluid loss during surgery, wound drainage, or stress (with retention of sodium and water).

Assessments of fluid status include skin turgor, vital signs, urinary output, wound drainage, and intravenous fluids; potential fluid volume deficit or excess is a risk.

Assessments of intravenous fluids include the type of fluid ordered, the rate, the needle insertion site, and the tubing.

Wound Status. The nurse in the PAR assesses the wound dressing for amount, consistency, and color of drainage, as well as for any tubes or drains and drainage by that route. It is also important to assess under the client for drainage.

Large amounts of bright red drainage, combined with other abnormal physical status assessments (restlessness, pallor, cold moist skin, decreasing blood pressure, increasing pulse and respirations) may indicate hemorrhage and hypovolemic shock. These symptoms should be reported immediately.

General Condition. Other assessments and interventions are made to ensure physical and emotional comfort and safety. If the client is having pain and his condition has stabilized, pain medications are given (usually by IV route). Most clients are cold and should be covered with blankets to keep them warm. Psychologic comfort is provided by constant reorientation and reassurance that the surgery is over. Physical safety is maintained by careful assessments, proper positioning, and use of side rails and restraints.

The client is dismissed from the PAR when physical status and level of consciousness are considered stable. The family is notified that the client is being transferred back to his room, and the PAR nurse makes a verbal report to the unit nurse about the assessments and interventions during the intraoperative and immediate postoperative phases.

Ongoing Postoperative Care

Nurses use the nursing process during all phases of perioperative care, with the focus being the special and unique needs of each client in each phase. Ongoing postoperative care is planned to facilitate recovery from surgery and to facilitate coping with alterations. The plan of care is based on individualized nursing diagnoses and includes promoting physical and psychologic health, preventing complications, and teaching self-care when the client returns home. Procedure 43-4 outlines postoperative client care.

Assessing

The nurse on the unit assists recovery room personnel in transferring the client to the bed in his room and, using data from the preoperative and intraoperative phases, makes an initial assessment. A postoperative checklist or flow sheet (Fig. 43-4) may be used. The initial assessment is often combined with the implementation of postoperative physician orders and includes

- Vital signs: Assess temperature, blood pressure, pulses, and respirations. Note alterations from postoperative and recovery room data, as well as symptoms of complications (as discussed in section entitled "Immediate Postoperative Care").
- Color and temperature of skin: Assess for warmth, pallor, cyanosis, diaphoresis.
- Level of consciousness: Assess orientation to time, place, and person as well as reaction to stimuli and ability to move extremities.
- Intravenous fluids: Assess type and amount of solution, rate, tubing, and infusion site.
- Wound: Assess dressing and dependent areas for drainage (color, amount, consistency). Assess drains and tubes and be sure they are intact, patent, and properly connected to drainage systems.
- Other tubes: Assess Foley catheter, gastrointestinal suction, and so forth for drainage, patency, and amount of output. Be sure dependent drainage bags are hanging properly and suction drainage is attached and functioning. If oxygen is ordered, ensure placement of ordered application and flow rate.
- Altered comfort level: Assess for pain (location, duration, intensity) and if present, determine if analgesics were given in the PAR. Assess for nausea and vomiting.
- Position and safety: Place the client in an ordered position (*e.g.,* following spinal anesthesia, client may have to remain flat for a specified period of time) or if the client is not fully conscious, place him in side-lying position. Elevate side rails and place bed in low position.
- Comfort: Cover with blanket, reorient to room as necessary, and allow family members to remain with client after initial assessment is completed.

Following assessment, document time of arrival and all assessments. Follow agency protocol for assessment routines: common time frames are every 15 minutes until stable, turn every 1 hour to 2 hours the first 24 hours, and every 4 hours thereafter.

Diagnosing

Nursing diagnoses in the postoperative phase may be made for actual or potential altered responses, or for collaborative problems to implement nursing actions necessary for monitoring and preventing postoperative complications. When making nursing diagnoses, the nurse uses assessment data and plans of care established before and during surgery, and includes the family.

Examples of postoperative nursing diagnoses are (Carpenito, 1987)

Potential for infection: Abdominal wound related to surgical incision's disruption of normal skin integrity

Potential alteration in respiratory function related to effects of anesthesia, high abdominal incision, and pain

Alteration in comfort: Acute pain related to flank incision

Alteration in family processes related to financial burden of surgical procedure and hospitalization

Potential volume deficit related to abnormal fluid loss from wound drainage and nasogastric suction

Disturbance in self-concept related to inability to carry out personal hygiene secondary to surgical intervention to remove breast and diagnosis of cancer

Impaired tissue integrity related to mechanical destruction (surgery to repair fractured hip)

Knowledge deficit: Discharge teaching for self-care following surgical procedure (wound care, activity restrictions)

Examples of postoperative collaborative problems are (Carpenito, 1987)

Potential complications: Hemorrhage, hypovolemic shock, urinary retention, thrombophlebitis, paralytic ileus, neurovascular deficits

Planning

The plan of care in the postoperative phase begins in the preoperative phase, when nursing activities to reduce stress and teach postoperative activities are carried out. From admission, the client and family are prepared for uneventful recovery and self-care on dismissal. Specific client goals will be individualized, based on risk factors, surgical procedure, and unique needs. Examples of postoperative goals are

- Client will carry out leg exercises every 2 hours to 4 hours as taught.
- Client will deep-breathe and cough effectively every 2 hours as taught.
- Client will verbalize decreasing levels of pain.
- Client will have a balanced intake and output.
- Client will regain normal bowel and bladder elimination.

Postoperative Care When Client Returns to Room

Immediate

Action	Rationale
1 Place client in safe position on side with face down and neck slightly extended. Note level of consciousness.	Prevents aspiration of vomitus and airway obstruction
2 Monitor and record vital signs frequently. Assessment order may vary, but usual frequency includes taking vital signs every 15 min the first hour, every 30 min the next 2 hr, every hour for 4 hr, and finally, every 4 hr.	Comparison with baseline preoperative vital signs may indicate impending shock or hemorrhage.
3 Provide for warmth. Assess skin color and condition.	Depressed level of functioning results in fall in body temperature.
4 Check dressings for color, odor, and amount of drainage, and feel under client for bleeding.	Hemorrhage and shock are life-threatening complications of surgery.

Step 4: Feeling under client for bleeding.

Action	Rationale
5 Verify that all tubes are patent and equipment is operative.	Ensures maintenance of vital functions
6 Maintain intravenous infusion at correct rate.	Provides nutrition and prevents dehydration and electrolyte imbalances
7 Provide for a safe environment. Keep bed in low position with side rails up. Have call bell within client's reach. Have "No Smoking" sign posted if client is receiving oxygen.	Prevents accidental injury
8 Relieve pain by administering medications ordered by physician. Check record to verify if analgesic medication was administered in recovery room.	Analgesics are used for relief of postoperative pain.
9 Record assessments and interventions on chart.	Provides for accurate documentation

(Continued)

General

Action	Rationale
10 Promote optimum respiratory function:	Anesthetic agents may depress respiratory function: Clients who have existing respiratory or cardiovascular disease, abdominal or chest incisions or who are obese, elderly, or in a poor state of nutrition are at greater risk of developing respiratory complications.
a. Coughing and deep breathing	
b. Incentive spirometry	
c. Early ambulation	
d. Frequent position change	
e. Administration of oxygen as ordered	
11 Maintain adequate circulation:	Preventive measures can improve venous return and circulatory status.
a. Maintenance of IV therapy	
b. Early ambulation	
c. Application of antiembolic stockings if ordered by physician	
d. Leg exercises and range-of-motion exercises if not contraindicated	
12 Assess urinary elimination status:	Anesthetic agents may temporarily depress bladder tone and response.
a. Promote voiding by offering bedpan at regular intervals	
b. Monitor catheter drainage if present	
c. Measure intake and output	
13 Promote optimal nutritional status and return of gastrointestinal function:	Anesthetic agents depress peristalsis and normal functioning of gastrointestinal tract.
a. Assess for return of peristalsis	

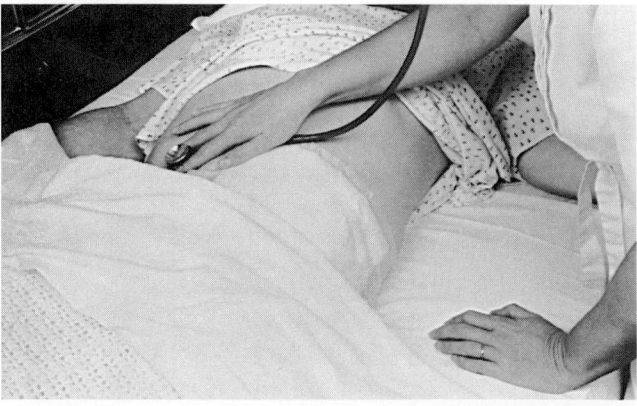

Step 13a: Assessing for return of peristalsis. (Photos © Ken Kasper)

(Continued)

Action

  b. Assist with diet progression

  c. Encourage fluid intake

  d. Monitor intake

  e. Medicate for nausea and vomiting as ordered by physician

14 Promote wound healing:

  a. Use surgical asepsis

  b. Assess condition of wound

  c. Assess any drainage

15 Provide for rest and comfort.

16 Provide emotional and spiritual support.

Rationale

Alterations in nutritional, circulatory, and metabolic status may predispose clients to infection and delayed healing.

Shortens recovery period and facilitates return to normal function

Facilitates individualized care and client's return to normal health

---

- Client will have a well-healed surgical incision.
- Client will remain free of infection.
- Client will verbalize any concerns about appearance of wound.
- Client will verbalize and demonstrate self wound care.
  The aims of nursing are
- Assess and monitor physical and emotional status of the client
- Promote physical and psychologic comfort and safety
- Prevent complications
- Facilitate coping with alterations in structure or function
- Promote a return to health and maximize wellness

Implementing

Many nursing activities implemented in the postoperative phase have been discussed in this chapter, or are fully discussed in other chapters; therefore, this section will focus on the nursing interventions implemented to meet the client goals of the plan of care. Nursing care will be presented in three broad areas: preventing complications, promoting a return to health, and facilitating coping with alterations.

Preventing Complications. A wide variety of factors increase the risk of postoperative complications. These have been described in the pre- and intraoperative sections of this chapter, and include age, health habits, physical condition, medical history, psychologic status, and surgical intervention (anesthesia, positioning, wound). Preoperative assessments and teaching are implemented to decrease the risk of postoperative complications; this section will describe the implementation of those activities, focusing on preventing respiratory, cardiovascular, and wound complications.

Preventing Cardiovascular Complications. Nursing interventions to prevent or monitor for cardiovascular complications are
- Assess and document vital signs as ordered, using preoperative assessments as a baseline.
- Provide covers as necessary to prevent chilling.
- Maintain fluid balance:
  - Maintain accurate intake and output.
  - Monitor rate and type of intravenous (IV) fluids.
  - Assess skin turgor and hydration of mucous membranes.
- Monitor amount, color, and consistency of wound drainage.
- Implement leg exercises and turning in bed every 2 hours.

Name _____

M.R. # _____

POST-OP
PROGRESS FLOW RECORD

DATE										
TIME										
BP										
PULSE										
RESPIRATIONS										
TEMPERATURE										
I.V.										
WOUND										
DRAIN (S)										
LOC										
PAIN										
NAUSEA										
FOLEY/ OTHER CATH OR VOIDING										
TURN, COUGH DEEP BREATHE										
MOVES ALL EXTREMITIES										
Initials										

Key _____   _____

640-044-830/0800751   _____   _____

F I G U R E   43-4
Example of a postoperative progress record.

- Assist with ambulation. (Ambulation usually begins the evening of surgery and increases as tolerated; blood pressure, pulse, and respirations monitor tolerance.)
- Apply and follow protocols for antiembolitic stockings, if ordered.
- Give anticoagulant medications as ordered.
- Assess and record Homans' sign every 8 hours.
- Avoid positioning that will impede venous return (*e.g.,* do not raise the knee gatch or place pillows under knees).

Specific cardiovascular complications are described in the following paragraphs.

Shock is the body's reaction to acute peripheral circulatory failure as the result of an alteration in circulatory control or to a loss of circulating fluid. The type of shock most commonly seen in the postoperative client is **hypovolemic shock**, which occurs with a decrease in blood volume. Common assessments of shock are hypotension; cold, clammy skin; a weak, thready and rapid pulse; deep rapid respirations; a decreased urinary output; thirst; and apprehension and restlessness. The primary purpose of care for the client in shock is to improve and maintain tissue perfusion by eliminating the cause of the shock. The following are recommended interventions in caring for the client in shock:

- Maintain airway.
- Place the client in a flat position with the legs elevated 45 degrees. (The Trendelenburg's or "shock" position is no longer recommended, because this position causes the diaphragm to ascend, reducing total lung volume and ventilation [Patrick, et al, 1986].)
- Be prepared to assist with fluid administration, as well as whole blood or its components.
- Administer oxygen therapy as indicated.
- Place extra covering on the client to maintain warmth.
- Administer medications as ordered.
- Monitor vital signs and general condition continuously.
- Provide psychologic support to the client and family.

Hemorrhage is an excessive blood loss, either internally or externally. Hemorrhage may lead to hypovolemic shock. Hemorrhage may occur from a slipped suture, a dislodged clot in the wound, or stress on the operative site; it may also be the result of pathophysiologic conditions or certain medications. Common assessments of hemorrhage are the early symptoms of restlessness and anxiety, frank bleeding, and the symptoms listed above for shock. The primary purposes of care for the client having a hemorrhage include stopping the bleeding and replacing blood volume. The following interventions are recommended when caring for the client who is hemorrhaging:

- Apply a pressure dressing to the bleeding site.
- Be prepared to have the client return to the operating room if bleeding cannot be stopped or is massive.
- Give nursing care as outlined for the client in shock.

Thrombophlebitis is an inflammation of a vein associated with thrombus (blood clot) formation. Thrombophlebitis is most commonly seen in the lower extremities in the postoperative client. Common assessments of thrombophlebitis are pain and cramping in the calf or thigh of the involved extremity, redness and swelling in the affected area, elevated temperature, and positive Homans' sign (pain with dorsiflexion of the foot). Care for the client with thrombophlebitis includes preventing a clot from breaking loose and becoming an embolus that travels to the lungs, heart, or brain; and preventing further clot formation. Interventions in caring for the client with thrombophlebitis are

- Administer anticoagulant medications as ordered.
- Maintain bed rest as ordered.
- Use high antiembolitic stockings, and follow protocols for care.
- Elevate the affected leg to heart level.
- Do *not* massage or rub the legs.
- Give analgesics and use external heat applications as ordered.
- Measure bilateral calf or thigh circumference every shift.
- Provide emotional support to the client and family.

An *embolus* is a blood clot or other foreign substance that is dislodged and travels through the bloodstream until it lodges in another smaller vessel. In postoperative clients, the embolus is often part of a thrombus that breaks free from a vein wall. If the embolus lodges in the pulmonary vessels, it is called a **pulmonary embolus**. Common assessments of a pulmonary embolus include dyspnea, chest pain, cough, cyanosis, rapid respirations, tachycardia, and anxiety. The primary purposes of care are to stabilize cardiovascular and respiratory function, and to prevent further emboli. The following are recommended interventions for the client with a pulmonary embolus:

- Maintain bed rest, with the client in semi-Fowler's position.
- Maintain fluid balance; especially assess and maintain IV fluid rates to prevent overhydration.
- Administer oxygen therapy as appropriate.
- Administer anticoagulant medications as ordered.
- Administer prescribed analgesic medications for pain; use caution with narcotic analgesics which depress respirations.
- Assess vital signs and general status frequently.
- Instruct the client to avoid Valsalva's maneuver (forced exhalation against a closed glottis, such as straining to have a bowel movement) to prevent increased intrathoracic pressure and possible increased emboli.
- Provide emotional support for client and family.

Preventing Respiratory Complications. Nursing interventions to prevent or monitor for respiratory complications are

- Assess and monitor vital signs, using preoperative assessments as a baseline.
- Implement deep breathing, coughing, incentive spirometry, and turning in bed every 2 hours.
- Ambulate as ordered.
- Maintain hydration.
- Avoid positioning that decreases ventilation.
- Carefully monitor responses to narcotic analgesics.

Specific respiratory complications are described in the following text.

Pneumonia is an inflammation of the alveoli as the result of an infectious process or presence of foreign material, which can occur postoperatively as a result of factors such as aspiration, infection, depressed cough reflex, and increased secretions from anesthesia, dehydration, and immobilization. Assessments common to pneumonia are an elevated temperature, chills, cough productive of purulent or rusty sputum, rales and rhonci, dyspnea, and chest pain. The purposes of care are to treat the underlying infection and maintain respiratory status, and to prevent the spread of microorganisms. The following are recommended interventions in caring for the client with pneumonia:

- Promote full aeration of the lungs by positioning the client in semi-Fowler's or Fowler's position.
- Administer oxygen therapy as indicated.
- Maintain nutritional and fluid status.
- Administer antibiotic medications as ordered.
- Administer expectorants and analgesics as ordered.
- Implement deep-breathing and coughing exercises every 2 hours.
- Maintain personal hygiene, including frequent oral hygiene.
- Teach proper disposal of tissues and sputum.
- Ensure rest and comfort.
- Provide emotional support to client and family.

Atelectasis is the incomplete expansion or collapse of alveoli with retained mucous, involving a portion of the lung and resulting in poor gas exchange. Assessments of atelectasis are decreased lung sounds over affected areas, dyspnea, cyanosis, rales, restlessness, and apprehension. The primary purposes of care for the client with atelectasis include to ensure oxygenation of tissues, preventing further atelectasis and expanding involved lung tissues. The following are recommended interventions in caring for the client with atelectasis:

- Position the client in semi-Fowler's position.
- Administer oxygen therapy as indicated.
- Implement deep breathing, coughing, and incentive spirometry every 2 hours.
- Implement leg exercises every 2 hours, and ambulate as ordered.
- Maintain hydration.
- Administer analgesics for pain as ordered.
- Provide emotional support to client and family.

Preventing Wound Complications. Nursing interventions to prevent or monitor for wound complications are

- Assess vital signs, especially monitoring elevated temperature.
- Maintain hydration.
- Maintain nutritional status; encourage diet selection high in carbohydrates, proteins, calories, and vitamins.
- Use medical asepsis (handwashing) protocols.
- Follow CDC guidelines for wound care (Chap 42).
- Maintain aseptic technique in dressing changes and care of tubes or drains.

Specific wound complications are **dehiscence** (separation of the layers of a surgical wound) and **evisceration** (disruption of a wound with protrusion of body organs). Both complications are described in Chapter 42.

Promoting a Return to Health. Nurses provide interventions in ongoing postoperative care to promote the return of clients' physical and psychologic functioning to as near a normal state as possible. The plan of care will include activities to meet elimination, fluid/electrolyte and nutrition, and rest/comfort needs.

Meeting Elimination Needs. Both urinary and bowel elimination can be altered by anesthesia, manipulation of organs during the surgical procedure, inactivity, and altered fluid and food intake during the perioperative period.

The return of normal *bowel elimination* is promoted by the following nursing interventions:

- Assess for the return of peristalsis.
  Auscultate bowel sounds every 4 hours when client is awake.
  Assess abdominal distention, especially if bowel sounds are not audible or are high-pitched (indicative of possible **paralytic ileus,** which is an absence of peristalsis).
  Assess client's ability to pass flatus or stool.
- Assist with movement in bed and ambulation (to help relieve gas pains, a common postoperative discomfort).
- Encourage food and fluid intake when ordered especially fruit juices and high-fiber foods.
- Maintain privacy when client is using the bedpan, commode, or bathroom.
- Administer colon tubes, suppositories, or enemas if ordered.

The return of normal *urinary elimination* if promoted by the following nursing interventions:

- Monitor intake and output.
- Assist with assumption of normal position to void.
  Place client in upright sitting position when using bedpan.
  Use bedside commode or assist client to bathroom, when able.
  Help male clients stand upright to void.

- Assess for distention of the bladder (palpate above the symphasis pubis) if the client does not void in 8 hours after surgery; or if the client voids frequently, with amounts of less than 50 ml.
- Maintain ordered rate of IV fluids.
- Encourage PO fluids, when ordered.
- Provide privacy when the client is using bedpan, commode, or bathroom.
- Carry out catherization procedure, if ordered.

Meeting Fluid/Electrolyte and Nutrition Needs. Fluid and nutrition needs can be met by the following nursing interventions:

- Monitor intake and output.
- Maintain IV fluids as ordered.
- Assess for dehydration and weight loss, if appropriate.
- Provide oral hygiene before meals and PRN.
- Monitor tolerance of ordered diet. (After surgery, diets usually progress from clear liquids to full liquids to soft to regular.)
- Maintain an environment conducive to good appetite (keep bedside articles clean and neat, eliminate odors).
- Encourage client to sit up in bed or chair for meals.
- Encourage family participation in meals.
- Remember that the presence of drains, gastric suction, fever, and IV therapy increases the risk of fluid and electrolyte imbalances in the surgical client.

Meeting Comfort and Rest Needs. Following surgery, comfort needs are often a priority for the client. Alterations in comfort are the result of many factors, including nausea and vomiting, hiccups, thirst, and surgical pain. Nursing interventions to meet comfort and rest needs are

Nausea and vomiting can be decreased by

- Maintaining a clean environment
- Providing oral hygiene PRN
- Avoiding large intake of food or fluids at one time, especially after being NPO
- Maintaining bowel elimination
- Assessing allergic response to antibiotics or analgesics
- Administering ordered medications

Thirst can be relieved by

- Providing oral hygiene PRN
- Offering sips of water or ice chips when NPO (if allowed)

Hiccups may be relieved by a variety of individualized interventions, including

- Having the client
    Take several swallows of water while holding his breath (if not NPO)
    Rebreathe into a paper bag
    Eat a teaspoon of granulated sugar

- Placing gentle pressure over the closed eyelids
- Administering ordered medications

Surgical pain may be managed by

- Assessing for pain, and offering ordered analgesics every 3 hours to 4 hours during the first 24 hours to 36 hours after surgery
- Reinforcing preoperative teaching about pain management
- Offering other comfort measures: position changes, back rubs, relaxation techniques

Comfort and rest are also facilitated by providing personal hygiene, keeping the bed linens and environment clean, providing quiet during rest periods and at night, and allowing family members to remain with the client.

Facilitating Coping with Alterations. Surgical incisions often alter physical appearance and normal physiologic function, leading to actual or potential alterations in self-concept and body image and threatening psychologic security. Changes in the way a person perceives himself can influence all of the human dimensions and area of human functioning: self-esteem, relationships with others, sexual identity, spiritual beliefs, sociocultural values, and independent conduct of activities of daily living and work.

Many surgical clients have the same reaction to loss of a body part as to a death (crisis is discussed in Chap 9; loss and grief are discussed in Chap 13). The response and the adaptation made by the client is influenced by multiple factors, including age, values and beliefs, sociocultural background, significance of the body part, visibility of the body part, time to prepare for the change, and support persons available. The nurse must be aware and accepting of the client's needs and must establish interventions to meet needs in coping with change. The nursing process is used to implement interventions, beginning with the client's decision to have surgery and continuing through convalescence. Nursing activities to facilitate coping are

- Accept each client as a unique individual.
- Identify, through verbal and nonverbal cues, clients who are at risk for alterations in self-concept (risk is increased if the client has little support from others, has a visible alteration, or has an alteration that will seriously affect functional ability).
- Allow time for clients and families to verbalize feelings about the alteration, and do not assume that all clients will have problems.
- Support strengths and effective coping mechanisms.
- Allow the client to be a part of goal setting and decision making throughout the surgical experience.
- Provide teaching and honest information to the client and family about all aspects of care.
- Work collaboratively with other members of the health team and provide referrals as necessary to meet physical, psychologic, and spiritual needs.

PRE-ADMISSION TEACHING/TESTING
PERI-OPERATIVE ASSESSMENT

PLANNED SURGERY & DATE:

DATE OF VISIT:

SURGICAL HISTORY:

Lab Ordered:

Abnormal Lab work called to

Dr. _____ on _____ Initials _____

ANESTHESIA HISTORY:

X-ray

SYSTEMS REVIEW: **Allergy:**

Dental:

Abnormal X-ray called to

CONTACT LENS/IOL:

Dr. _____ on _____ Initials _____

HEARING AID:

EKG

CARDIOVASCULAR

Rheumatic Fever: Murmur:

Hypertension: Infarction:

Abnormal EKG work called to

Date Last EKG:

Dr. _____ on _____ Initials _____

RESPIRATORY

PRE-OP TEACHING GUIDELINES

Pneumonia: TBC:

____ Pre-Op Injection   ____ Shave Prep

Asthma: Recent URI:

____ Transported to Holding Room   ____ Awake in Recovery Room

Date Last CXR:

____ Visitors To Waiting Room   ____ Oxygen Face Tent

____ I.V. Fluids   ____ Deep Breaths & Cough

HEMATOLOGY

____ Pneumatic Boots (Appr. Surg.)   ____ Frequent Check BP & P

Bleeding Tendency:

____ Leggins (Cysto or GYN)   ____ NPO after MN or Liq. Breakfast

GI

____ Taken to O.R.   ____ Cannot Drive Self Home

Recent Vomiting: Diarrhea:

____ Strap   ____ Jewelry, Make-up Left Home

Jaundice: Hepatitis:

____ BP Cuff, Monitor Pads   ____ Wear Loose Clothing

GYN

____ Bovie Pad   ____ Video _____

L.M.P.:   Para:

____ Hand-out/Packet _____

Gravida:

NOTES: _____

GU

UTI/Problems:

NEUROPSYCH

Syncope: Epilepsy:

MUSCULOSKELETAL

RECOVERY ROOM FOLLOW UP: _____

Neck or

Arthritis: Back Inj.:

R.O.M.:   Prothesis:

Skin Integrity:

METABOLIC

Diabetes:

POST-OP FOLLOW-UP: _____

Thyroid:

MEDICATIONS:

B/P _____ T. _____ P. _____ R. _____ WT. _____

HT. _____   **PHONE:** _____

F I G U R E   43-5

Example of an ambulatory surgery assessment record.

The final factor in facilitating coping is ensuring that when the client and family are discharged from the hospital or surgical clinic they know how to provide care at home. (Teaching activities, such as medication administration or wound care, is discussed in specific chapters of this text; discharge and home visits are fully described in Chap 26.)

Ambulatory Surgery

Ambulatory surgery is becoming more and more common, and information about this method of care is a part of any discussion of the surgical client. In 1980, 3.2 million surgical procedures were done on an outpatient basis, representing 17% of the total surgeries performed in the United States that year. Seventy percent of the acute care hospitals, clinics, and centers offer outpatient surgery, in units called *same day surgery* or *short procedure units*. Predictions are that 40% to 45% of all surgical procedures can be performed safely in ambulatory (outpatient) settings (Gruendemann, 1985). Outpatient surgery places an increased emphasis on conservation of resources and on cost effectiveness. The ambulatory surgery client does not remain hospitalized, but rather is discharged, when stable, from the setting where the surgery and postoperative recovery took place to home and self-care.

Preoperative nursing assessments and teaching are key elements in providing care for the ambulatory surgical client (Fig. 43-5). Preoperative teaching can often be combined with preoperative screening tests, usually done 2 to 5 days before the scheduled surgery. Preoperative teaching for the ambulatory surgical client should include

- Have the client list medications routinely taken.
- Instruct the client to inform the operating staff of any allergies.
- Give the client written instructions concerning limitations on eating or drinking prior to surgery, with specific instructions concerning what time to begin those limitations.
- Instruct the client to notify the surgeon's office if a cold or infection develops prior to surgery.
- Instruct the client to remove all nailpolish before coming to the ambulatory center.
- Instruct the client to wear clothing that buttons in the front (especially for facial, nasal, or hand surgery). For surgery on the hands, clothing with short sleeves is more convenient.
- Instruct the client to avoid wearing jewelry or bringing valuables.
- Tell the client the time to arrive in the setting, as well as the estimated time of the procedure.
- Inform the client that someone must be available to drive him home, because preoperative medications and anesthesia cause drowsiness (Horwitz, 1985; Voss, 1986).

Evaluating

As with any client, the plan of care for the surgical client is evaluated based on the established client goals. The plan has been effective if the client is discharged after surgery without complications, with a healing wound, and with knowledge and ability for self-care.

CASE STUDY*

Mrs. Grace Overman, a 67-year-old, white female, was admitted with right upper quadrant abdominal pain. On February 7, the client was diagnosed with cholelithiasis (gall stones). Mrs. Overman is a retired school teacher and lives alone. She has no history of previous physical or mental illnesses. On February 7, the nurse visits Mrs. Overman with Dr. Appleton, who informs her of the need for surgery. She requests a discharge for 5 days to attend her only granddaughter's wedding. After the Doctor leaves, the nurse returns to Mrs. Overman's room to assess her. She is crying and anxious. She states, "I've always taken care of myself, I just don't know what to think of all this, I've never needed surgery before." Mrs. Overman will be readmitted February 11 for surgery on February 12.

* Case study and nursing care plan were developed and written by Janet R. Weber, Department of Nursing, Southeast Missouri State University, Cape Girardeau, MO.

Physical Assessment

Height: 5'4"

Weight: 160 lb

Tissue turgor: good

Color: Fair with slight yellow cast; sclera—white.

Temperature: 98.8°F

Respirations: 28

Pulse: 98

Blood pressure: 150/90

Support Systems

The client has four married daughters and one single son who lives next door. She is very active in Lutheran church activities. Mrs. Overman's insurance coverage includes Blue Cross, Blue Shield, and Medicare.

N U R S I N G   C A R E   P L A N   *for Mrs. Overman*

Nursing Diagnosis: Knowledge deficit: perioperative surgical events

Long-Term Goal: The client will be emotionally prepared for surgery.

Short-Term Goals	Nursing Actions	Rationale	Evaluative Statements
The client will: 1. On 2/7, verbalize concerns related to surgery 2. Appear less anxious about surgery by 2/12, and her vital signs will be in her normal range of B/P—$\frac{130}{80}$, pulse—80, respirations—24, temperature—98.6. 3. Not be crying. 4. By 2/11, be able to explain purpose of surgery and surgical events to occur. 5. By 2/12, be able to verbalize purpose of surgery and surgical events to occur. 6. Visit with significant pastoral representative by 2/11.	1. Assess level of client's anxiety before initiating preoperative teaching. 2. Encourage client and family questions to uncover unknown fears and concerns. 3. Explain purpose of surgery and surgical events and postoperative events to occur to client and family. 4. Establish a therapeutic relationship with client by active listening and touch. 5. Suggest to client to inform church pastor of impending surgery.	1. Excessive fear and apprehension may trigger the adrenocortical stress reaction and produce changes in electrolyte metabolism, and necessitate postponing surgery. (Metheney, 1983). Thus, emotional stress increases one's surgical risks. Creating an environment where the client is comfortable in expressing thoughts and concerns decreases psychological stress. 2. The family and significant others can convey anxiety if they lack understanding and are anxious. Moderate to severe anxiety also decreases one's readiness to learn. 3. It is necessary to identify the client's concerns and fears to provide correct information and emotional support. Because surgery is an unknown experience, a variety of fears (*i.e.,* death, pain, alteration in body image) may exist, and anxiety may be expressed in different ways. Simply talking about fears may reduce them. 4. Assessing the activities client will engage in before surgery will help the nurse assess client's preoperative nutritional and physical status.	1. Client continued to ask questions about surgery and expressed fear of postoperative pain and immobility on 2/7. 2. Client verbalized need for surgery and surgical events to occur on 2/11. 3. 2/12, vital signs: B/P—$\frac{136}{80}$, pulse—88, respiration—24, temperature—98.4. Client's pastor visited. Family at bedside and client lying comfortably in bed visiting with them. Client and family voice no further questions about surgery. *J. Weber, RN*

(Continued)

NURSING CARE PLAN (Continued)

Short-Term Goals	Nursing Actions	Rationale	Evaluative Statements
		5. The family is an important support system to help client cope. Each person is influenced by family health beliefs and practices. 6. A relationship with a higher being may provide client support by providing hope, meaning, and purpose in life during times of crisis.	

Long-Term Goal: Client will understand nursing procedure and self-care activities necessary to prevent postoperative complications (infection, pneumonia, emboli, fluid and electrolyte imbalance).

Short-Term Goals	Nursing Actions	Rationale	Evaluative Statements

The client will:
1. On 2/7, identify importance of proper nutrition, exercise, and rest prior to surgery.
2. Verbalize perioperative events of surgery by 2/11.
3. Express understanding of postoperative pain control by 2/11.
4. Correctly demonstrate how to turn, cough, deep breathe, exercise legs, and splint incision by 2/11.
5. Verbalize understanding of purpose of foley catheter and T-tube.
	1. Inform client of the importance of proper nutrition, fluids, and exercise during preoperative teaching.
	2. Inform client of surgery schedule, approximate length of surgery, and recovery room care. Offer agency booklet, "You and your surgery."
	3. Request anesthesiologist visit by 2/11.
	4. Inform client of the cause of normal postanesthesia feelings of dry mouth, dizziness, sore throat, and fatigue.
	5. Complete preoperative checklist by teaching client purpose of the following:
	  a. NPO status and preoperative medication
	  b. Removal of jewelry, makeup, hairpieces
	  c. Side rails
	  d. Family waiting room
	  e. Foley catheter
	  f. T-tube
	6. Demonstrate necessary postoperative exercises to client and explain
		1. Correct information clarifies any erroneous beliefs and lets client know what to expect.
		2. Good nutrition prevents postoperative negative nitrogen balance. Decreased intake of protein and vitamin C delays wound healing and promotes infection. Activity stimulates appetite, circulation, and sleep, decreasing stress and promoting recovery.
		3. During surgery, cough reflex is suppressed, mucus accumulates, and lungs do not ventilate fully. A high abdominal incision prevents deep breathing owing to pain. Splinting incision aids in comfort and promotes lung expansion and oxygenation of tissues. This should be done once every 1–2 hr for 24–48 hr postoperatively.
		4. Effective coughing removes retained mucus.
			1. 2/7, client verbalized importance of proper nutrition, exercise, and rest prior to surgery.
			2. 2/11, client verbalized events of pre-, intra-, and postoperative events of surgery.
			3. By 2/11, client correctly demonstrated turning, coughing, deep breathing, leg exercises, incision splinting, and use of incentive spirometer correctly.
			
			J. Weber, RN

(Continued)

NURSING CARE PLAN (Continued)

Short-Term Goals	Nursing Actions	Rationale	Evaluative Statements
	how these activities prevent complications: a. Turning, coughing, and deep breathing b. Splinting of wound c. Leg exercises d. Incentive spirometer usage	5. Using an incentive spirometer inflates alveoli and promotes venous return. This is done 10 times during waking hours for first 5 days postoperatively. Avoid doing this before and after meals. 6. During surgery, venous return slows and may promote circulatory stasis. Leg exercises increase venous return and prevent thrombophlebitis and emboli. These should be done every 1–2 hr when client is awake. 7. Turning promotes ventilation, venous return, and gastrointestinal peristalsis, all physiologic processes that are slowed during surgery. 8. A Foley catheter prevents bladder distention. 9. Preoperative medications are given to alleviate anxiety, facilitate anesthesia induction, promote relaxation, and decrease pulmonary, oral, and gastric secretions. Elevation of side rails after administration of preoperative medications promotes patient safety.	

KEY POINTS

- Surgery is a stressful time for the client and family, imposing physical and psychosocial alterations and adaptations.

- The time before, during, and after surgery is named the perioperative period; it is divided into preoperative, intraoperative, and postoperative phases.

- Surgical procedures are categorized by urgency, risk, and purpose.

- Anesthesia may be general or regional. General anesthesia is given to induce narcosis, loss of reflexes, and relaxation of skeletal muscles; regional anesthesia produces sensory loss, but the client remains awake.

- Clients agree to surgery by signing an informed consent form.

- Preoperative assessment identifies physical and psychosocial risk factors and strengths.

- Preoperative nursing interventions to prepare the client for the intra- and postoperative phases include therapeutic communications, preoperative teaching, and physical preparation.

- Intraoperative nursing roles are either as a scrub nurse or a circulating nurse; each has specific client responsibilities.

- Immediate postoperative nursing care in the postanesthesia recovery area focuses on assessing and monitoring to prevent complications from anesthesia or surgery.

- Ongoing postoperative nursing care is planned to facilitate recovery from surgery and coping with alterations; both the client and the family are a part of care.

- Ambulatory surgery is provided on an outpatient basis; preoperative assessment and teaching are critical elements in safe surgery and recovery.

- The nursing process is used throughout the perioperative period to provide knowledgable, holistic, individualized client care.

BIBLIOGRAPHY

American Nurses' Association and Association of Operating Room Nurses: Standards of Perioperative Care. Kansas City, MO, The Association, 1982

Brunner L, Suddarth D: Textbook of Medical-Surgical Nursing, 6th ed. Philadelphia, JB Lippincott, 1988

Carpenito L: Nursing Diagnosis: Application to Clinical Practice, 2nd ed. Philadelphia, JB Lippincott, 1987

Drain C, Christoph S: The Recovery Room: A Critical Care Approach to Postanesthesia Nursing, 2nd ed. Philadelphia, JB Lippincott, 1987

Groah L: Operating Room Nursing: The Perioperative Role. Reston, VA, Reston Publishing, 1983

Gruendemann BJ: Guest editorial—Dare to excell in ambulatory surgery. AORN J 41(2):330–331, 333, 337, 1985

Horwitz: 1985

Lammers P: Ambulatory surgery: Competition creates challenges. AORN J 44(1):87–94, 1986

McConnell E: Clinical Considerations in Perioperative Nursing: Preventive Aspects of Care. Philadelphia, JB Lippincott, 1987

Montanari J: Documenting your postop assessment findings. Nursing 15(8):31–35, 1985

Patrick ML et al: Medical-Surgical Nursing: Pathophysiological Concepts. Philadelphia, JB Lippincott, 1986

Smallwood SB: Preparing children for surgery. AORN J 47(1):177–185, 1988

Voss SJ: Ambulatory surgery scheduling: Assuring a smooth patient flow. AORN J 43(5):1009–1012, 1986

Appendices

APPENDIX A
Equivalents

Metric Units

The metric system, developed by the French, uses the *meter* as the basic unit. The metric system is a decimal system, with prefixes that designate the various multiples or divisibles of 10. The most commonly used prefixes in medicine are

Milli, which means one one-thousandth (0.001)

Centi, which means one one-hundredth (0.01)

Kilo, which means one thousand (1,000)

These prefixes may be affixed to any of the three basic units of measurements, which are

Meter (m), the unit of length

Gram (g), the unit of weight

Liter (L), the unit of volume

Therefore

1 millimeter (mm) = 0.001 m

1 milligram (mg) = 0.001 g

1 milliliter (ml) = 0.001 L

1 kilometer (km) = 1,000 m

1 kilogram (kg) = 1,000 g

1 kiloliter (kl) = 1,000 L

Length

The meter (a little longer than a yard) and the kilometer (approximately 0.6 mile) are rarely used in medicine or nursing. The commonly used measure of length is 1 centimeter (cm) = 0.01 m = approximately 0.4 inch.

Volume

The most frequently used measures of volume are the *liter* and the *milliliter.* Some useful equivalents to know are

1,000 milliliters (ml) = 1 liter (L)

1,000 cubic centimeters (cc) = 1 liter (L)

1 milliliter (ml) = 1 cc

Weight

The gram designates the weight of 1 ml of distilled water at 4°C. The most frequently used units of weight are

1,000,000 micrograms (mcg or μg) = 1 gram (g)
1,000 micrograms (mcg) = 1 milligram (mg)
1,000 milligrams (mg) = 1 gram (g)
1,000 grams (g) = 1 kilogram (kg) = 2.2 pounds (lb)

Metric Units and Their Household Equivalents

Household measurement is inaccurate, with wide variations in the size of teaspoons, teacups, and so forth. The generally accepted household measures are

60 drops (gtt) = 1 teaspoon (tsp or t)
3 tsp = 1 tablespoon (Tbs or T)
12 Tbs = 1 teacup
16 Tbs = 1 glass (or a standard measuring cup)

Table A-1
Metric and Household Equivalents

Metric Unit	Household Unit
5 cc	1 tsp
15 cc	1 Tbs
180 cc	1 full teacup
240 cc	1 full glass

Apothecary Units

In the apothecary system
The unit of weight is the *grain*.
The unit of volume is the *minim*.
Of the many units of measure in the apothecary system, you should know the following units, abbreviations, and equivalents.

Weight

60 grains (gr) = 1 dram (dr or ʒ)
 8 drams (dr or ʒ) = 1 ounce (oz or ʒ)

Volume

60 minims (min) = 1 fluid dram (fl dr or fʒ)
 8 fl dr = 1 fluid ounce (fl oz or fʒ)
16 fl oz = 1 pint (pt)
 2 pt = 1 quart (qt)
 4 qt = 1 gallon (gal)

In the apothecary system, when the symbol or abbreviation is used, the quantity is written in lowercase Roman numerals and follows the symbol. Arabic numerals are used, however, in preference to large Roman numerals. For example

5 gr = gr v
8 dr = ʒ viii

The quantity one half may be indicated by the symbol ss.

1 ½ gr = gr iss
7 ½ gr = gr viiss

Other fractional parts are expressed as common fractions, for example, gr ¹/₂₅₀, gr ¹/₁₀.

When pint, quart, and gallon are written, the quantity is expressed in Arabic numerals, for example, 1½ pints or 7½ quarts.

Apothecary Units and Their Household Equivalents

1 drop = 1 minim (m i)
1 tsp = 1 dr (℥ i)
1 Tbs = ½ oz (℥ ss)
2 Tbs = 1 oz (℥ i)
1 teacup = 6 oz (℥ vi)
1 glass or measuring cup = 8 oz (℥ viii)
2 measuring cups = 1 pt

Table A-2
Most Commonly Used Approximate Equivalents

Metric	Apothecary	Household
0.06 g	gr i	
0.06 cc	min i	1 drop
1.0 g	gr xv	
1.0 cc	min xv	⅕ tsp
5 cc	(1 dr) ℥ i	1 tsp
15 cc	(½ oz) ℥ ss	1 Tbs
30 cc	(1 oz) ℥ i	2 Tbs
500 cc	(16 oz) ℥ 16	1 pt
1000 cc	(32 oz) ℥ 32	1 qt

There are many discrepancies among these approximate equivalents. For example, 30 cc is the accepted equivalent for 1 oz (29.57 cc is the exact equivalent); however, multiplying 5 cc per dram by 8 (℥ viii per ounce) results in an equivalent of 40 cc for 1 oz rather than the accepted equivalent of 30 cc = 1 oz.

Such discrepancies are inevitable when two systems are used whose equivalents are not exact. The discrepancies are within a 10% margin of error, however, which is usually acceptable in pharmacology.

Table A-3
Commonly Used Metric Units and Their Approximate Apothecary Equivalents

Metric		Apothecary
1 g	1,000 mg	gr xv
0.6 g	600 mg	gr x
0.5 g	500 mg	gr viiss
0.3 g	300 mg	gr v
0.2 g	200 mg	gr iii
0.1 g	100 mg	gr iss
0.06 g	60 mg	gr i

(Continued)

	Metric	Apothecary
0.05 g	50 mg	gr $^3/_4$
0.03 g	30 mg	gr $^1/_2$ or gr ss
0.02 g	20 mg	gr $^1/_3$
0.015 g	15 mg	gr $^1/_4$
0.016 g	16 mg	gr $^1/_4$
0.010 g	10 mg	gr $^1/_6$
0.008 g	8 mg	gr $^1/_8$
0.006 g	6 mg	gr $^1/_{10}$
0.005 g	5 mg	gr $^1/_{12}$
0.003 g	3 mg	gr $^1/_{20}$
0.002 g	2 mg	gr $^1/_{30}$
0.001 g	1 mg	gr $^1/_{60}$
	0.6 mg	gr $^1/_{100}$
	0.5 mg	gr $^1/_{120}$
	0.4 mg	gr $^1/_{150}$
	0.3 mg	gr $^1/_{200}$

A P P E N D I X   B
Normal Adult Laboratory Values*

Commonly Used Abbreviations

kg = kilogram
g = gram
mg = milligram
μg = microgram
$\mu\mu$g = micromicrogram
ng = nanogram
mEq = milliequivalent
L = liter
dl = 100 milliliters
ml = milliliter
cu mm = cubic millimeter
nM = nanomolar
mIU = milliInternational Unit
pg = picogram
mm = millimeter
μ = micron or micrometer
mm Hg = millimeters of mercury
mU = milliunit
μU = micronunit
IU = International Unit

* Laboratory values may vary according to techniques used in different laboratories.

Table B-1
Hematologic Values—Reference Ranges

Determination	Conventional	SI
Coagulation Factors		
Factor I (fibrinogen)	0.15 g–0.35 g/100 ml	4.0 μmol–10.0 μmol/L
Factor II (prothrombin)	60%–140%	0.60 μmol–1.40μmol/L
Factor V (accelerator globulin)	60%–140%	0.60 μmol–1.40 μmol/L
Factors VII to X (proconvertin to Stuart factor)	70%–130%	0.70 μmol–1.30 μmol/L
Factor X (Stuart factor)	60%–140%	0.70 μmol–1.30 μmol/L
Factor VIII (antihemophilic globulin)	50%–200%	0.50 μmol–2.0 μmol/L
Factor IX (plasma thromboplastic cofactor)	60%–140%	0.60 μmol–1.40 μmol/L
Factor XI (plasma thromboplastic antecedent)	60%–140%	0.60 μmol–1.40μmol/L
Factor XII (Hageman factor)	60%–140%	0.60 μmol–1.40 μmol/L
Coagulation Screening Tests		
Bleeding time (Simplate)	2 min–8 min	180 sec–540 sec
Prothrombin time	9.5 sec–12 sec	Less than 2 sec from control
Partial thromboplastin time (activated)	20 sec–45 sec	25 sec–37 sec
Whole blood clot lysis	No clot lysis in 24 hours	0/day
Fibrinolytic Studies		
Euglobin lysis	No lysis in 2 hours	0 (in 2 hours)
Thrombin time		Control + 5 sec
Complete Blood Count		
Hematocrit	Male: 42%–50%	Male: 0.42–0.52
	Female: 40%–48%	Female: 0.37–0.48
Hemoglobin	Male: 13 g–18 g/dl	Male: 8.1 mmol–11.2 mmol/L
	Female: 12 g–16 g/dl	Female: 7.4 mmol–9.9 mmol/L
Leukocyte count	5000–10,000/mm^3	4.3–10.8 $\times$ 10^9/L
Erythrocyte count	4.2 million–5.9 million/mm^3	4.2–5.9 $\times$ 10^{12}/L
Mean corpuscular volume (MCV)	80 μm^3–94 μm^3	80 fl–94 fl
Mean corpuscular hemoglobin (MCH)	27 pg–32 pg	1.7 fmol–2.0 fmol
Mean corpuscular hemoglobin concentration (MCHC)	33%–38%	19 mmol–22.8 mmol/L
Erythrocyte sedimentation rate (Zeta Centrifuge)	41%–54%	Male: 1 mm–13 mm/hour
		Female: 1 mm–20 mm/hour
Erythrocyte Enzymes		
Glucose-6-phosphate dehydrogenase	5 U–15 U/g Hb	5 U–15 U/g
Pyruvate kinase	13 U–17 U/g Hb	13 U–17 U/g
Ferritin (serum)	Females: 5 ng–100 ng/ml	
	Males: 10 ng–270 ng/ml	
Folic acid, RIA	4 ng–16 ng/ml	
Haptoglobin	50 mg–250 mg/dl	1.0 g–3.0 g/L
Hemoglobin Studies		
Electrophoresis for A$_2$ hemoglobin	1.5%–3.5%	0.015–0.035
Hemoglobin, met- and sulf-	0	0
Serum hemoglobin	2 mg–3 mg/100 ml	1.2 μmol–1.9 μmol/L
Lupus erythematosus (LE) preparation		
Heparin as anticoagulant	0	0
Defibrinated blood	0	0
Muramidase	Serum, 3 μg–7 μg/ml	3 mg–7 mg/L
	Urine, 0 μg–2 μg/ml	0–2 mg/L

(Continued)

Determination	Conventional	SI

Hemoglobin Studies (continued)

Determination	Conventional	SI
Osmotic fragility of erythrocyte	Increased if hemolysis occurs in over 0.5% NaCl; decreased if hemolysis is incomplete in 0.3% NaCl	
Peroxide hemolysis	Less than 10%	<0.10
Platelet count	100,000–400,000/mm³	150–350 × 10⁹/L

Platelet Function Tests

Determination	Conventional	SI
Clot retraction	50%–100%/2 hours	0.50–1.00/2 hours
Platelet aggregation	Full response to ADP, epinephrine, and collagen	1.0
Platelet factor 3	33 sec–57 sec	33 sec–57 sec
Reticulocyte count	0.5%–1.5% rcd cells	0.005–0.15
Vitamin B₁₂	90 pg–280 pg/ml (borderline: 70–90)	66 pmol–207 pmol/L (borderline: 52–66)

Table B-2
Blood, Plasma or Serum Values—Reference Ranges

Determination	Conventional	SI
Acetoacetate plus acetone	0.3 mg–2.0 mg/dl	3 mg–20 mg/L
Aldolase	1.3 mU–8.2 mU/ml	12 nmol–75 nmol s⁻¹/L
Alpha amino nitrogen	3.0 mg–5.5 mg/100 ml	2.1 mmol–3.9 mmol/L
Ammonia	80 µg–110 µg/100 ml	47 µmol–65 µmol/L
Ascorbic acid	0.4 mg–1.5 mg/100 ml	23 µmol–85 µmol/L
Bilirubin (van den Bergh test)	1 minute: 0.4 mg/100 ml	Up to 7 µmol/L
	Direct: 0.1 mg–0.2 mg/dl	Up to 17 µmol/L
	Total: 1.0 mg/100 ml	
	Indirect: 0.1 mg–1.0 mg/dl	
Blood volume	8.5%–9.0% of body weight in kg	80 ml–85 ml/kg
	Toxic level: 17 mEq/L	
Bromsulphalein (BSP)	Less than 5% retention 45 min after 5 mg/kg IV	<0.05 L
Calcium	8.5 mg–10.5 mg/100 ml	2.1 mmol–2.5 mmol/L
Carbon dioxide content	24 mEq–32 mEq/L	24 mmol–30 mmol/L
Carcinoembryonic antigen (CEA)	0.25 mg/ml	0–2.5 µg/L
Carotenoids	0.8 µg–4.0 µg/ml	1.5 µmol–7.4 µmol/L
Ceruloplasmin	27 mg–37 mg/100 ml	1.8 µmol–2.4 µmol/L
Chloride	95 mEq–105 mEq/L	100 mmol–106 mmol/L
Cholesterol	150 mg–250 mg/dl	3.10 mmol–5.69 mmol/L
Cholinesterase (pseudocholinesterase)	0.5 pH U or more/hour	0.5 arb unit or more
	0.7 pH U or more/hour for packed cells	
Copper	Total: 100 µg–200 µg/100 ml	16 µmol–31 µmol/L
Creatine phosphokinase (CPK)	Female: 50 mU–250 mU/ml	0.08 µmol–0.58 µmol s⁻¹/L
	Male: 50 mU–325 mU/ml	
Creatinine	0.7 mg–1.4 mg/100 ml	60 µmol–130 µmol/L
Ethanol	0.3%–0.4%, marked intoxication;	65 mmol–87 mmol/L
	0.4%–0.5%, alcoholic stupor;	87 mmol–109 mmol/L
	0.5% or over, alcoholic coma	>109 mmol/L

(Continued)

Table B-2

Blood, Plasma or Serum Values—Reference Ranges   (Continued)

Determination	Conventional	SI
Glucose	Fasting: 60 mg–110 mg/100 ml	3.9 mmol–5.6 mmol/L
Iron	65 μg–170 μg/100 ml (higher in males)	9.0 μmol–26.9 μmol/L
Iron-binding capacity	250 μg–410 μg/100 ml	44.8 μmol–73.4 μmol/L
Lactic acid	0.6 mEq–1.8 mEq/L	0.6 mmol–1.8 mmol/L
Lactic dehydrogenase isoenzymes	100 mU–225 mU/ml	1.00 μmol–2.00 μmol s^{-1}/L
Lead	50 μg/100 ml or less	Up to 2.4 μmol/L
Lipase	2 U/ml or less	Up to 2 arb units
Lipids, total	400 mg–1000 mg/dl	3.10 mmol–5.69 mmol/L
Magnesium	$\frac{1}{3}$ mEq–2.4 mEq/L	0.8 mmol–1.3 mmol/L
5' Nucleotidase	0.3 Bodansky U–3.2 Bodansky U	30 nmol–290 nmol s^{-1}/L
Osmolality	280 mOsm–300 mOsm/kg water	285 mmol–295 mmol/kg
Oxygen saturation (arterial)	95%–100%	0.96 L–1.00 L
Pco_2	35 mm Hg–45 mm Hg	4.7 kPg–6.0 kPg
pH	7.35–7.45	Same
Po_2	95 mm Hg–100 mm Hg (dependent on age while breathing room air) Above 500 mm Hg while on 100% O_2	10.0 kPa–13.3 kPa
Phenylalanine	0 mg–2 mg/100 ml	0–120 μmol/L
Phosphorus (inorganic)	3.0 mg–4.5 mg/100 ml	1.0 mmol–1.5 mmol/L
Potassium	3.8 mEq–5.0 mEq/L	3.5 mmol–5.0 mmol/L
Primidone (Mysoline)	Therapeutic level, 4 μg–12 μg/ml	18 μmol–55 μmol/L
Protein, total	6.0 g–8.0 g/100 ml	60 g–84 g/L
Albumin	3.5 g–5.0 g/100 ml	33 g–50 g/L
Globulin	1.5 g–3.0 g/100 ml	23 g–35 g/L
Electrophoresis	% of total protein	% of total protein
Albumin	3.3 g–5.0 g/dl	0.52–0.68
Globulin		
Alpha$_1$	0.2 g–0.4 g/dl	0.042–0.072
Alpha$_2$	0.6 g–1.0 g/dl	0.068–0.12
Beta	0.6 g–1.2 g/dl	0.093–0.15
Gamma	0.7 g–1.5 g/dl	0.13–0.23
	0.3 mg–0.7 mg/dl	0–0.11 mmol/L
Sodium	135 mEq–145 mEq/L	135 mmol–145 mmol/L
Sulfate	0.5 mg–1.5 mg/100 ml	0.05 mmol–1.2 mmol/L
Transaminase (SGOT) (aspartate amino-transferase)	7 U–40 U/ml	0.08 μmol–0.32 μmol s^{-1}/L
Urea nitrogen (BUN)	10 mg–20 mg/100 ml	2.9 mmol–8.9 mmol/L
Uric acid	2.5 mg–8.0 mg/100 ml	0.13 mmol–0.42 mmol/L
Vitamin A	50 μg–220 μg/dl	0.5 μmol–2.1 μmol/L

Table B-3

Urine Values—Reference Ranges

Determination	Conventional	SI
Acetone plus acetoacetate (quantitative)	0	0 mg/L
Alpha amino nitrogen	64 mg–199 mg/day; not over 1.5% of total nitrogen	4.6 mmol–14.2 mmol/day
Amylase	35 U–260 U/ml	24–76 arb units
Calcium	150 mg/day or less	3.8 mmol/day or less
Catecholamines	Epinephrine, 10%–40% Norepinephrine, 60%–90%	<55 nmol/day <590 nmol/day

(Continued)

Determination	Conventional	SI
Copper	20 μg–70 μg/day	0–1.6 μmol/day
Coproporphyrin	50 μg–300 μg/day	80 nmol–380 nmol/day
Creatine	0–200 mg/24 hours	<0.75 mmol/day
Cystine or cysteine	0	0
Follicle-stimulating hormone		
Follicular phase	5 IU–20 IU/day	Same
Mid cycle	15 IU–60 IU/day	
Luteal phase	5 IU–15 IU/day	
Menopausal	50 IU–100 IU/day	
Men	5 IU–25 IU/day	
Hemoglobin and myoglobin	0	
5-Hydroxyindole acetic acid	2 mg–9 mg/day (women lower than men)	10 μmol–45 μmol/day
Phenolsulfonphthalein (PSP)	At least 25% excreted by 15 min; 40% by 30 min; 60% by 120 min	0.25 L
Phosphorus (inorganic)	Varies with intake; average 1 g/day	32 mmol/day
Porphobilinogen	0	0
Protein, quantitative	<150 mg/24 hours	<0.15 g/day

Steroids 17-Ketosteroids (per day)	Age (years)	Male (mg)	Female (mg)	Male (μmol/day)	Female (μmol/day)
	10	1–4	1–4	3–14	3–14
	20	6–21	4–16	21–73	14–56
	30	8–26	4–14	28–90	14–49
	50	5–18	3–9	17–62	10–31
	70	2–10	1–7	7–35	3–24

Determination	Conventional	SI
17-Hydroxysteroids	3 mg–8 mg/day (women lower than men)	8 μmol–22 μmol/day as hydrocortisone
Sugar		
Quantitative glucose	0	0 mmol/L
Identification of reducing substances		
Fructose	0	0 mmol/L
Pentose	0	0 mmol/L
Titratable acidity	20 mEq–40 mEq/day	20 mmol–40 mmol/day
Urobilinogen	<0.25 mg/dl	To 1.0 arb unit
Uroporphyrin	Up to 50 μg in 24 hours	0 nmol/day
Vanilmandelic acid (VMA)	0.7 mg–6.8 mg/24 hours	Up to 45 μmol/day

Table B-4
Cerebrospinal Fluid Values—Reference Ranges

Determination	Conventional	SI
Bilirubin	0	0 μmol/L
Chloride	100 mEq–130 mEq/L	
Albumin	15.5 mg–32.0 mg/dl	0.295 g/L ± 2 SD (0.11–0.48)
IgG	0–6.6 mg/dl	0.043 g/L ± 2 SD (0–0.086)
Glucose	50 mg–75 mg/100 ml (30%–50% less than blood)	2.8 mmol–4.2 mmol/L
Pressure (initial)	70 mm H₂O–180 mm H₂O	70–80 arb units
Protein		
Lumbar	15 mg–45 mg/100 ml	0.15 g–0.45 g/L
Cisternal	15 mg–25 mg/100 ml	0.15 g–0.25 g/L
Ventricular	5 mg–15 mg/100 ml	0.05 g–0.15 g/L

Table B-5
Special Endocrine Tests—Reference Ranges

Steroid Hormones

Aldosterone	Excretion: 5 μg–19 μg/24 hours	14 nmol–53 nmol/day
Fasting, at rest, 210 mEq sodium diet	Supine: 48 ± 29 pg/ml	133 ± 80 pmol/L
	Upright: (2h) 65 ± 23 pg/ml	180 ± 64 pmol/L
Fasting, at rest, 110 mEq sodium diet	Supine: 107 ± 45 pg/ml	279 ± 125 pmol/L
	Upright: (2h) 239 ± 123 pg/ml	663 ± 341 pmol/L
Fasting, at rest, 10 mEq sodium diet	Supine: 175 ± 75 pg/ml	485 ± 208 pmol/L
	Upright: (2h) 532 ± 228 pg/ml	1476 ± 632 pmol/L
Cortisol		
Fasting	8 AM: 5 μg–25 μg/100 ml	0.14 μmol–0.69 μmol/L
At rest	8 PM: below 10 μg/100 ml	0–0.28 μmol/L
20 U ACTH	4-hour ACTH test: 30 μg–45 μg/100 ml	0.83 μmol–1.24 μmol/L
Dexamethasone at midnight	Overnight suppression test: below 5 μg/100 ml	<0.14 nmol/L
	Excretion: 20 μg–70 μg/24 hours	55 nmol–193 nmol/day
11-Deoxycortisol	Responsive: over 7.5 μg/100 ml (after metrapone)	>0.22 μmol/L
Testosterone	Adult male: 300 ng–1100 ng/100 ml	10.4 nmol–38.1 nmol/L
	Adolescent male: over 100 ng/100 ml	>3.5 nmol/L
	Females: 25 ng–90 ng/100 ml	0.87 nmol–3.12 nmol/L
Unbound testosterone	Adult male: 3.06 ng–24.0 ng/100 ml	106 pmol–832 pmol/L
	Adult female: 0.09 ng–1.28 ng/100 ml	3.1 pmol–44.4 pmol/L

Polypeptide Hormones

Adrenocorticotrophin (ACTH)	15 pg–70 pg/ml	3.3 pmol–15.4 pmol/L
Calcitonin	Undetectable in normals	0
	>100 pg/ml in medullary carcinoma	>29.3 pmol/L
Growth hormone		
Fasting, at rest	Below 5 ng/ml	<233 pmol/L
After exercise	Children: over 10 ng/ml	>465 pmol/L
	Male: below 5 ng/ml	<233 pmol/L
	Female: up to 30 ng/ml	0–1395 pmol/L
After glucose	Male: below 5 ng/ml	<233 pmol/L
	Female: below 10 mg/ml	0–465 pmol/L
Insulin		
Fasting	6 μU–26 μU/ml	43 pmol–187 pmol/L
During hypoglycemia	Below 20 μU/ml	<144 pmol/L
After glucose	Up to 150 μU/ml	0–1078 pmol/L
Luteinizing hormone	Male: 6 mU–18 mU/ml	6 U–18 U/L
Preovulatory or postovulatory	Female: 5 mU–22 mU/ml	5 U–22 U/L
Mid cycle peak	30 mU–250 mU/ml	30 U–250 U/L
Parathyroid hormone	<10 μl equiv/ml	<10 ml equiv/L
Prolactin	2 ng–15 ng/ml	0.08 nmol–6.0 nmol/L
Renin activity		
Normal diet	Supine: 1.1 ± 0.8 ng/ml/hour	0.9 ± 0.6 nmol/L/hour
	Upright: 1.9 ± 1.7 ng/ml/hour	1.5 ± 1.3 nmol/L/hour
Low-sodium diet	Supine: 2.7 ± 1.8 ng/ml/hour	2.1 ± 1.4 nmol/L/hour
	Upright: 6.6 ± 2.5 ng/ml/hour	5.1 ± 1.9 nmol/L/hour
Low-sodium diet	Diuretics: 10.0 ± 3.7 ng/ml/hour	7.7 ± 2.9 nmol/L/hour

(Continued)

Thyroid Hormones

Thyroid-stimulating hormone (TSH)	0.5 μU–3.5 μU/ml	0.5 mU–3.5 mU/L
Thyroxine-binding globulin capacity	15 μg–25 μg T_4/100 ml	193 mU–322 mU/L
Total triiodothyronine by radioimmun-oassay (T_3)	70 ng–190 ng/100 ml	1.08 nmol–2.92 nmol/L
Total thyroxine (T_4) by RIA	4 μg–12 μg/100 ml	52 nmol–154 nmol/L
T_3 resin uptake	25%–35%	0.25–0.35
Free thyroxine index (FT₄1)	1 ng–4 ng/100 ml	12.8 pmol–51.2 pmol/L

(Adapted from Brunner L, Suddarth D: The Lippincott Manual of Nursing Practice, 4th ed. Philadelphia, JB Lippincott Company, 1986. SI units used with permission: Office of Publications, World Health Organization, Geneva, Switzerland)

A P P E N D I X   C
Nursing Organizations

Aerospace Medical Association
Flight Nurse Section
Washington National Airport
Washington, DC 20001

Alpha Tau Delta
National Fraternity for Professional Nurses
489 Serento Circle
Thousand Oaks, CA 91360

American Association of Colleges of Nursing
Suite 430
11 DuPont Circle
Washington, DC 20036

American Association of Critical Care Nurses
One Civic Plaza
New Port Beach, CA 92660

American Association of Nephrology Nurses and Technicians
Box 56
N Woodbury Road
Pitman, NJ 08071

American Association of Neurological/Neurosurgical Nurses
Suite 1519
625 N Michigan Avenue
Chicago, IL 60611

American Association of Nurse Anesthetists
Suite 929
111 E Wacker Drive
Chicago, IL 60601

American College of Nurse Midwives
Suite 1120
1522 K Street NW
Washington, DC 20005

American Holistic Nurses' Association
PO Box 116
Telluride, CO 81435

American Indian Nurses Association
PO Box 1588
Norman, OK 73071

American Nurses Association
2420 Pershing Road
Kansas City, MO 64108

American Society for Nursing
Service Administrators
840 N Lakeshore Drive
Chicago, IL 60611

Association for Practitioners in Infection Control
23341 N Milwaukee Avenue
Half Day, IL 60069

Association of Operating Room Nurses
10170 E Mississippi Avenue
Denver, CO 80231

Association of Pediatric Oncology Nurses
PO Box 7999
San Francisco, CA 94120

Association of Rehabilitation Nurses
Suite 470
1701 Lake Avenue
Glenview, IL 60025

Canadian Association of Enterostomal Therapy
Royal Jubilee Hospital
Victoria, British Columbia
V8R 1J8

Canadian Association of Neurological and Neurosurgical Nurses
96 Palace Road
Kingston, Ontario
K7L 4T3

Canadian Council of Cardiovascular Nurses
1200–1 Nicholas Street
Ottawa, Ontario
K2P 1E2

Canadian Gerontological Nursing Association
Continuing Nursing Education
University of Saskatchewan
Saskatoon, Saskatchewan
S7W 0W0

Canadian Intravenous Nurses Association
200–4433 Sheppard Avenue East
Agincourt, Ontario
M1S 1V3

Canadian Nurses Respiratory Society
c/o Canadian Lung Association
908–75 Albert Street
Ottawa, Ontario
K1P 5E7

Canadian Orthopedic Nurses Association
43 Wellesley Street E
Toronto, Ontario
M4Y 1H1

National Organization for the Advancement of Associate Degree Nursing
    (NOAADN)
Amarillo College
PO Box 447
Amarillo, TX 79178

Emergency Department Nurses Association
Suite 1131
666 N Lakeshore Drive
Chicago, IL 60611

Gay Nurses' Alliance
PO Box 530
Back Bay Annex
Boston, MA 02117

International Association for Enterostomal Therapy
1701 Lake Avenue
Glenview, IL 60025

Internationl Council of Nurses
3, rue Ancien-Port 1201
Geneva, Switzerland

International Committee of Catholic Nurses
Square Vergota
43, B1040
Brussels, Belgium

North American Nursing Diagnosis Association
St Louis University
Department of Nursing
3525 Caroline Street
St Louis, MO 63104

National Association of Hispanic Nurses
4359 S. Rockdale
San Antonio, TX 78233

National Association of Pediatric Nurse Associates/Practitioners
Box 56
N Woodbury Road
Pitman, NJ 08071

National Black Nurses' Association, Inc.
425 Ohio Building
175 South Main Street
Akron, OH 44308

National Center for Nursing Ethics
PO Box 2237
Cincinnati, OH 45201

National Conference of Operating Room Nurses
c/o Operating Room
St Boniface General Hospital
Winnipeg, Manitoba
R2H 2A6

National League for Nursing
10 Columbus Circle
New York, NY 10019

National Male Nurses' Association
2308 State Street
Saginaw, MI 48502

National Nurses Society on Alcoholism
PO Box 7728
Indian Branch Creek
Shawnee Mission, KS 66207

National Student Nurses' Association
10 Columbus Circle
New York, NY 10019

Nurses Christian Fellowship
233 Langdon Street
Madison, WI 53703

Nursing Sisters Association of Canada
8500 Francis Road
Richmond, British Columbia
V6Y 1A6

Oncology Nursing Society
701 WAshington Road
Pittsburgh, PA 15228

Operating Room Nurses Association of Canada
c/o Montreal Children's Hospital
2300 Tupper Street
Montreal, Quebec
H3H 1P3

Orthopedic Nurses Association
Suite 501
1938 Peach Tree Road NW
Atlanta, GA 30309

Psychiatric Nurses Association of Canada
1854 Portage Avenue
Winnipeg, Manitoba
R3J 0G9

Registered Nurses of Canadian Indian Ancestry
500–275 Portage Avenue
Winnipeg, Manitoba
R3B 2B3

Sigma Theta Tau
National Honor Society of Nursing
1100 West Michigan Street
Indianapolis, IN 46223

World Health Organization
Avenue Appia 1211
Geneva 27, Switzerland

A P P E N D I X   D
Canadian Nutritional Tables

Table D-1
Average Energy Requirements

Age	Sex	Average Height (cm)†	Average Weight (kg)†	Requirements*					
				kcal/kg†‡	MJ/kg†	kcal/day§	MJ/day‖	kcal/cm#	MJ/cm‖
Months									
0–2	Both	55	4.5	120–100	0.50–0.42	500	2.0	9	0.04
3–5	Both	63	7.0	100–95	0.42–0.40	700	2.8	11	0.05
6–8	Both	69	8.5	95–97	0.40–0.41	800	3.4	11.5	0.05
9–11	Both	73	9.5	97–99	0.41	950	3.8	12.5	0.05
Years									
1	Both	82	11	101	0.42	1100	4.8	13.5	0.06
2–3	Both	95	14	94	0.39	1300	5.6	13.5	0.06
4–6	Both	107	18	100	0.42	1800	7.6	17	0.07
7–9	M	126	25	88	0.37	2200	9.2	17.5	0.07
	F	125	25	76	0.32	1900	8.0	15	0.06
10–12	M	141	34	73	0.30	2500	10.4	17.5	0.07
	F	143	36	61	0.25	2200	9.2	15.5	0.06
13–15	M	159	50	57	0.24	2800	12.0	17.5	0.07
	F	157	48	46	0.19	2200	9.2	14	0.06
16–18	M	172	62	51	0.21	3200	13.2	18.5	0.08
	F	160	53	40	0.17	2100	8.8	13	0.05
19–24	M	175	71	42	0.18	3000	12.4		
	F	160	58	36	0.15	2100	8.8		
25–49	M	172	74	36	0.15	2700	11.2		
	F	160	59	32	0.13	1900	8.0		
50–74	M	170	73	31	0.13	2300	9.6		
	F	158	63	29	0.12	1800	7.6		
75+	M	168	69	29	0.12	2000	8.4		
	F	155	64	23	0.10	1500	6.0		

* Requirements can be expected to vary within a range of ± 30%.

† Figures rounded to the closet whole number when ≥10 and to the closest 0.5 when <10.

‡ First and last figures are averages at the beginning and at the end of the 3-month period.

§ Figures rounded to the nearest 50 when <1000 and to the nearest 100 when ≥1000.

‖ Figures include 2 decimals if value is <1 and 1 decimal if ≥1.

Figures rounded to the nearest 0.5.

(Recommended Nutrient Intakes for Canadians. Ottawa, Canada, Bureau of Nutritional Sciences, 1983)

Table D-2

Summary of Nutritional Allowances of Water-Soluble and Fat-Soluble Vitamins

Vitamin C: 60 mg, males; 45 mg, females
Vitamin B_1: 0.3 mg/1000 calories or 0.36 mg/5000 kJ
Vitamin B_2: 0.50 mg/1000 calories or 0.60 mg/5000 kJ
Niacin: 7.2 niacin equivalents (NE)/1000 Kcal or 8.6 NE/5000 kJ
Vitamin B_6: 0.9 mg to 1.8 mg/day, males; 0.6 mg to 1.1 mg/day, females
Folic acid: 210 μg, males; 165 μg, females
Vitamin B_{12}: 2.0 μg
Pantothenic acid: 5 mg to 7 mg
Biotin: 1.5 μg/kg body weight
Vitamin A: 800 RE, females; 1000 retinol equivalents (RE), males
Vitamin D: 2.5 μg
Vitamin E: 6 μg to 10 μg, males
Vitamin K: 0.03 μg to 1.5 μg/kg body weight

> Information on sources, functions, signs and symptoms of deficiency and excess, and pharmacologic uses are given in Table 31-5.

> (Recommended Nutrient Intakes for Canadians. Ottawa, Canada, Bureau of Nutritional Sciences, Department of National Health and Welfare, 1983)

Table D-3

Summary of Nutritional Allowances of Macro and Micro Minerals

Calcium: 800 mg, males; 700 mg to 800 mg, females (under review in Canada)

Phosphorus: none specified. The average (composite) diet in 1972 was estimated to contain 1600 mg of phosphorus.

Magnesium: 240 mg, males; 190 mg, females

Sodium: 0.4 mEq (9 mg)/kg body weight

Potassium: 0.75 mEq (30 mg)/kg body weight

Chlorine: none given. *Nutrition Recommendations for Canadians* suggests minimizing salt intake.

Iron: 8 mg, males; 8 mg to 14 mg, females

Iodine: 160 μg

Zinc: 9 mg, males; 8 mg, females

Copper: approximately 2.0 mg

Manganese: approximately 2.5 mg

Fluorine: none specified

Chromium: 50 μg to 100 μg estimated safe and adequate intake

Selenium: 20 μg to 50 μg

Molybdenum: 120 μg to 240 μg safe and adequate intake

Cobalt: none established

> Information on sources, functions, and signs and symptoms of deficiency and excess are given in Table 31-6.

> (Data from Recommended Nutrient Intakes for Canadians. Ottawa, Canada, Bureau of Nutritional Sciences, Department of National Health and Welfare, 1983; and Canada's Food Guide Handbook, revised. Ottawa, Canada. Department of National Health and Welfare, 1982)

Table D-4
Summary Examples of Recommended Nutrient Intakes for Canadians

Age	Sex	Weight (kg)	Protein (g/day)	Fat-Soluble Vitamins			Water-Soluble Vitamins			Minerals				
				Vitamin A (RE/day)	Vitamin D (μg/day)	Vitamin E (mg/day)	Vitamin C (mg/day)	Folacin (μg/day)	Vitamin B$_{12}$ (μg/day)	Calcium (mg/day)	Magnesium (mg/day)	Iron (mg/day)	Iodine (μg/day)	Zinc (mg/day)
Months														
0–2	Both	4.5	11	400	10	3	20	50	0.3	350	30	0.4	25	2
3–5	Both	7.0	14	400	10	3	20	50	0.3	350	40	5	35	3
6–8	Both	8.5	17	400	10	3	20	50	0.3	400	50	7	40	3
9–11	Both	9.5	18	400	10	3	20	55	0.3	400	50	7	45	3
Years														
1	Both	11	19	400	10	3	20	65	0.3	500	55	6	55	4
2–3	Both	14	22	400	5	4	20	80	0.4	500	70	6	65	4
4–6	Both	18	26	500	5	5	25	90	0.5	600	90	6	85	5
7–9	M	25	30	700	2.5	7	35	125	0.8	700	110	7	110	6
	F	25	30	700	2.5	6	30	125	0.8	700	110	7	95	6
10–12	M	34	38	800	2.5	8	40	170	1.0	900	150	10	125	7
	F	36	40	800	2.5	7	40	180	1.0	1000	160	10	110	7
13–15	M	50	50	900	2.5	9	50	150	1.5	1100	210	12	160	9
	F	48	42	800	2.5	7	45	145	1.5	800	200	13	160	8
16–18	M	62	55	1000	2.5	10	55	185	1.9	900	250	10	160	9
	F	53	43	800	2.5	7	45	160	1.9	700	215	14	160	8
19–24	M	71	58	1000	2.5	10	60	210	2.0	800	240	8	160	9
	F	58	43	800	2.5	7	45	175	2.0	700	200	14	160	8
25–49	M	74	61	1000	2.5	9	60	220	2.0	800	250	8	160	9
	F	59	44	800	2.5	6	45	175	2.0	700	200	14	160	8

(Recommended Nutrient Intakes for Canadians. Ottawa, Canada, Bureau of Nutritional Sciences, Department of National Health and Welfare, 1983)

Glossary

Abduction: lateral movement of the body part away from the midline of the body

Abrasion: wound that results from scraping or rubbing off skin or mucous membrane

Abscess: localized collection of pus

Absorption: process by which drugs are transferred from the site of entry into the body to the bloodstream

Abstinence: refraining from sexual activity, particularly sexual intercourse; a method of birth control

Accommodation: (1) ability to adjust the eye to see at various distances; (2) process by which intellectual acts are changes to handle increasingly complex information

Accreditation: process by which an educational program is evaluated and then recognized as having met certain predetermined standards of education

Acid: substance containing a hydrogen ion that can be liberated or released

Acidosis: condition characterized by a proportionate excess of hydrogen ions in the extracellular fluid, in which the pH falls below 7.35

Acne: skin condition owing to inflammation and infection or sebaceous glands

Acquired immune deficiency syndrome (AIDS): fatal condition in which the body's immune system is rendered ineffective as a result of infection by the retrovirus HTLV-III

Active exercise: joint movement activated by the person

Active immunity: antibodies against harmful effects of microorganisms or toxins are self-produced

Active transport: movement of ions or molecules across cell membranes, usually against a pressure gradient, and with the expenditure of metabolic energy

Acupressure: application of pressure or massage, or both, to usual acupuncture sites

Acupuncture: technique that uses long, thin needles to prick specific parts of the body to produce insensitivity to pain

Acute illness: rapidly occurring illness that runs its course, allowing the person to return to their previous level of functioning

Acute pain: episode of pain that lasts for seconds to less than 6 months

Adaptation: continuous change and adjustment of living things to other living things and to environmental conditions

Addictive: substance to which a person develops a psychologic and physiologic dependency

Adduction: movement of a body part toward the midline of the body

Admitting: act of entering something into a system; department that enters a client into a health-care facility

Adolescence: period of development between childhood and adulthood, characterized by the onset of puberty

Adult day-care centers: centers providing day-care service (including recreation and nutrition) for older adults

Adventitious breath sounds: abnormal breath sound heard over the lungs

Advocacy: protection and support of another's rights

Aerobic exercise: exercise that promotes cardiovascular fitness; it increases blood flow, heart rate, and the metabolic demand for oxygen over a period of time

Affective learning: changes in attitudes, values, and feelings

Ageism: attitudes that stereotype the older adult on the basis of chronologic age

Agglutinin: antibody that causes a clumping of specific antigens

Agnostic: person who holds that nothing is known about the existence of a god

Albuminuria: albumin in the urine; indication of kidney disease

Alkali: substance that can accept or trap a hydrogen ion; synonym for base

Alkalosis: condition, characterized by a proportionate lack of hydrogen ions in the extracellular fluid concentration, in which the pH exceeds 7.45

Alopecia: baldness

Alternative care: general term used to identify various methods of non-hospital health care, including residential housing, day care, respite care, hospice, and extended care facilities

Alzheimer's disease: type of dementia in which discrete patches of brain tissue degenerate; this devastating disease eventually affects all body systems

Ambulatory care centers: health-care settings, either hospital or community-based, that provide a wide variety of services (medical, surgical, mental health, drug-related)

Ambulatory surgery: surgery performed on an outpatient basis, with admission and discharge the same day. Also known as same-day surgery or outpatient surgery.

Amino acid: basic building blocks used to manufacture protein and the end-products of protein digestion

Ampule: glass flask containing a single dose of medication for parenteral administration

Anaerobic exercise: exercise in which the supply of oxygen is less than the demand created by contracting muscles; oxygen debt results

Analgesic drug: pharmaceutical agent used to relieve pain

Anaphylactic reaction: severe reaction occurring immediately after exposure to a drug. Characterized by respiratory distress and vascular collapse.

Androgen: steroid hormone (*e.g.,* androsterone, testosterone) produced primarily by the testes in males, but also produced to a lesser extent by the adrenal glands in both sexes and the ovaries in the female

Andropause: midlife decrease in androgen levels in the male; the male remains capable of reproduction

Anion: ion that carries a negative electric charge

Ankylosis: fixation or immobilization of a joint

Anorexia: lack or loss of appetite for food

Anorexia nervosa: eating disorder characterized by the denial of appetite and bizarre eating habits

Anoxia: absence of oxygen

Antagonistic effect: combined effect of two or more drugs that produces less than the effect of each drug alone

Anterior fontanelle: diamond-shaped membrane-covered space remaining at the junction of the frontal and parietal bone sutures in a fetus or infant

Anthropometric: measurements of the body and body parts

Antibody: immunoglobin produced by the body in response to a specific antigen

Anticipatory guidance: identification of expected learning needs that commonly arise as a result of past or present health problems

Antigen: foreign material capable of inducing a specific immune response

Antipyretic: agent that reduces fever

Anuria: technically, no urine voided; 24-hour urine output is less than 100 ml; synonyms are complete kidney shutdown or renal failure

Anxiety: vague sense of impending doom or apprehension precipitated by new and unknown experiences

Apical-radial pulse rate: rates counted simultaneously for a full minute at the apex of the heart and at the radial artery

Apnea: absence of breathing

Approximate: to bring the two edges of a wound together (usually held together with suture materials)

Arousal: condition in which the cortical area of the brain receives and responds appropriately to stimuli

Arousal threshold: intensity of stimulus required to produce awakening

Arrhythmia: irregular pattern of heartbeats; synonym for dysrhythmia

Ascites: the accumulation of fluid in the peritoneal cavity

Asepsis: absence of disease-producing microorganisms; being free of infection

Assault: a threat, or an attempt, to make bodily contact with another person without that person's permission

Assertiveness: claiming and defending one's rights

Assessing: systematic and continuous collection, validation, and communication of client data

Assimilation: process by which a person interprets information to fit the present level of cognition

Asymmetry: lack of symmetry of parts or organs on opposite sides of the body

Atelectasis: incomplete expansion or collapse of the lungs

Atheist: person who denies the existence of a god

Atrioventricular node: tissue at the base of the atrial septum that normally picks up the electric current from the S–A node. Abbreviated A–V node.

Atrophy: decrease in the size of a body structure

Attitude: feeling or emotion, generally including a positive or negative judgment toward persons, objects, or ideas

Auditory: pertaining to hearing

Auscultation: listening for sounds within the body

Authoritative knowledge: knowledge that comes from an expert and is accepted as truth based on a perceived level of expertise

Autocratic leadership: leadership style in which the leader assumes complete control over the decisions and activities of the group

Autonomy: self-determination; being independent and self-governing

Bandage: piece of gauze or other material used to cover a wound

Barium enema: x-ray visualization of the large intestine following the introduction of barium into the lower intestine

Basal metabolism: amount of energy required to carry out involuntary activities of the body at rest

Base: substance that can accept or trap a hydrogen ion; synonym for alkali

Base of support: foundation that provides stability for an object

Basic human needs: something essential to the health and survival of humans; common to all persons

Battery: assault that is carried out

Bedsore: area of cellular necrosis caused by a lack of circulation to the involved area; synonym for pressure sore and decubitus ulcer

Beliefs: special class of intellectual attitudes based primarily on faith as opposed to fact

Beneficence: principle of doing good

Bereavement: state of grieving or going through the grief process

Bigeminal pulse: pulse rhythm in which every two pulsations is followed by a pause

Bilateral: pertaining to two sides of the body

Binder: type of bandage, usually designed to fit a large body area

Biopsy: removal of a piece of tissue for microscopic examination

Biot's respirations: respirations of the same depth followed by a period of apnea

Bisexuality: having sexual feelings for persons of both sexes

Blended family: two single-parent families joined together to form a new family unit

Blood pressure: force of blood against arterial walls

Blood transfusion: infusion of whole blood from a healthy person into a recipient

Body fluid: liquid part of the body consisting of both water and its solutes

Body image: how an individual experiences his body

Body mechanics: efficient use of the body as a machine and as a means of locomotion

Body water: liquid part of the body consisting of water only

Bolus: single injection of a concentrated solution administered intravenously

Bounding pulsation: pulse that reaches a higher level than normal, then disappears quickly

Bowel movement: emptying of the intestinal tract; synonym for defecation

Bowel training program: program that manipulates factors within a person's control (timing of defecation, exercise, diet) to produce a regular pattern of comfortable defecation with medication or enemas

Bradycardia: a slow heart rate

Bradypnea: abnormally slow rate of breathing

Brief pain: pain that passes quickly; synonym for transient pain

Bronchodilator: medication that relaxes contractions of smooth muscles of the bronchioles

Bronchoscope: lighted, tubular instrument used for visual examination of the bronchi

Bronchoscopy: visual examination of the trachea and bronchi

Bronchovesicular: normal breath sounds heard over the mainstem bronchus

Bruit: unusual sound, generally abnormal, heard in auscultation

Buffer: substance that prevents body fluid from becoming overly acid or alkaline

Bulimia: eating disorder characterized by episodes of gorging followed by purging; often occurs with anorexia nervosa

Burnout: behaviors exhibited as the result of prolonged occupational stress

Calorie: measure of heat, or energy. A *kilocalorie,* commonly referred to as a calorie, is defined as the amount of heat required to raise 1 kg of water 1°C.

Capillarity: process by which a liquid at the point of contact with a solid will rise; synonym for capillary action

Caput succedaneum: localized edema, congestion, and petechiae on the fetal and newborn scalp, crossing suture lines

Cardiac output: volume of blood pumped from the left ventricle per minute

Cardinal signs: body temperature, pulse and respiratory rates, and blood pressure; synonym for vital signs

Cardiogenic shock: shock owing to a decrease in cardiac output

Caries: cavitation of the teeth

Carrier: person or animal who is without signs of illness but who has pathogens on or within his body that can be transferred to others

Cathartic: medication that strongly increases gastrointestinal motility and promotes defecation

Catheter: tube for injecting or removing fluids

Cation: ion that carries a positive electric charge

Cellular fluid: fluid within the cell; synonym for intracellular fluid

Center of gravity: point at which the mass of an object is centered

Contracture: permanent contraction state of a muscle

Centers for Disease Control (CDC): U.S. government agency whose responsibilities include investigation, identification, prevention, and control of disease

Cerumen: heavy, brown secretion in the external canal of the ear which is secreted by the ceruminous glands

Ceruminous gland: gland found in the external auditory canal which secretes a substance called cerumen

Change: process of transforming, altering, or modifying something

Change agent: person who purpose-fully and systematically implements change

Change of shift report: communication method used by nurses completing care for a client to transmit client information to nurses about to assume responsibility for continuing care; may be exchanged verbally in a meeting or audiotaped

Chemical name: precise description of a drug's chemical composition

Cheyne-Stokes respirations: gradual increase and then gradual decrease in depth of respirations followed by a period of apnea

Chiropodist: one who treats foot disorders; synonym for podiatrist

Chiropody: health discipline that deals with the treatment of foot disorders; synonym for podiatry

Cholecystogram: x-ray examination of the gallbladder

Cholesterol: fat-like substance found only in animal tissues. Cholesterol is important for cell membrane structure, is a precursor of steroid hormones, and is a constituent of bile. High serum cholesterol levels are a risk factor in the development of atherosclerosis.

Chronic disorder: illness or condition for which there is no cure; it persists over an extended period of time (over 6 months) and often affects one's ability to meet basic needs

Chronic illness: irreversible illness that causes permanent physical impairment and requires long-term health care

Chronic pain: episode of pain that lasts for 6 months or longer. The pain may be intermittent or continuous.

Chyme: semifluid state that food is in when it leaves the stomach

Circadian rhythm: rhythm that completes a full cycle every 24 hours; synonym for diurnal rhythm

Circadian synchronization: condition existing when a person's sleep–wake patterns follow his or her inner biologic clock

Circulating nurse: a nurse, working in the operating room, who assesses the client, helps position the client for surgery, secures supplies, and maintains count of items used during surgery

Civil law: rule that regulates relationships among people; synonym for private law

Cleft lip: congenital fissure, or split, in lip

Cleft palate: congenital fissure, or split, in the roof of the mouth (*i.e.,* the palate).

Client: person requiring health care

Client goal: statement describing an expected client outcome

Closed wound: injury in which there is no break in the skin

Clubbing: rounding and swelling of nailbeds

Cognition: cerebral functioning; process of perceiving and understanding one's world

Cognitive learning: storing and recalling of new knowledge in the brain

Cohabiting family: persons who choose to live together for a variety of reasons; includes unmarried adults, communes, group marriages, and gay/lesbian relationships

Coitus: sexual activity in which the penis is placed in the vagina; synonym for sexual intercourse

Coitus interruptus: method of contraception; the penis is removed from the vagina before ejaculation

Cold: relative state meaning the absence of heat

Collaborative problem: actual or potential health problem which may occur from complications of disease, diagnostic studies, or the treatment regimen; the nurse works together with other members of the health-care team toward its resolution.

Colloid osmotic pressure: pressure exerted by plasma proteins on permeable membranes in the body; synonym for oncotic pressure

Colon: section of the large intestine from the cecum to the rectum

Colonization: harmless growth of microorganisms in or on the body

Colonoscopy: visual examination of the entire large intestine

Common law: law resulting from court decisions which is then followed when other cases involving similar circumstances and facts arise. Common law is as binding as civil law.

Communication: process of sharing information; process of generating and transmitting meanings

Compensation: substitution of what is perceived as a good for a perceived weakness

Competence: the way a person performs the tasks or role expectations that are important to him

Complaint: legal statement of the plaintiff's claim; once filed it initiates legal proceedings

Complete proteins: proteins that contain all the essential amino acids in sufficient quantities for protein synthesis to occur; also termed high biologic value proteins

Compliance: act of completing what is expected

Compress: several layers of moist, absorbent cloth or gauze folded to cover a small body area

Computerized tomography: scanning procedure which produces a cross-sectional image of a body part and reflects various tissue densities; also called CT scan

Concept: abstract images that are formed as impressions from the environment are organized into symbols of reality

Conceptual framework model: set of concepts, along with the statements that arrange the concepts into an understandable pattern

Concurrent audit: evaluation of nursing care and client outcomes conducted while the client is receiving care (uses direct observation of nursing care, client interview, and chart review)

Condom catheter: tube for draining urine which connects a device applied externally to the penis to a collection bag

Conduction: transfer of heat to another object during direct contact

Confidentiality: respecting privileged information

Congenital anomaly: absence of, deformity in, or excess of body parts present at birth and resulting from faulty in utero development or chromosomal abnormality

Congenital syphilis: syphilis, a sexually transmitted disease, acquired by an infant in utero from an infected mother. The disease is passed from mother to infant across the placenta.

Congestion: presence of excessive fluids or secretions in an organ or body tissue

Constant fever: body temperature that remains consistently elevated and fluctuates less than 2°C (3.5°F); sometimes called a continuing fever

Constipation: passage of dry, hard, fecal material

Continuing care retirement community: self-contained retirement agencies which provide services to the elderly, designed to serve residents as their needs change with illness and increasing age

Continuum: graduated scale

Contraception: prevention of conception or pregnancy; also used to describe methods used for birth control

Contractual agreement: pact made between two persons for the achievement of mutually set goals

Contralateral stimulation: stimulation to an area opposite the affected area

Contusion: wound in which the skin remains intact; often called a bruise

Convalescent period: stage of an infection that represents recovery from the infection

Convection: dissemination of heat by motion between areas of unequal density

Coping mechanism: patterns of behavior used to neutralize, deny, or counteract anxiety

Core temperature: temperature of internal areas of the body

Counseling: giving guidance; assisting with problem solving

Credentialing: general term that refers to ways in which professional competence is maintained

Crenation: process of losing fluid from a red blood cell, which eventually results in a shrunken, knobbed cell owing to loss of intracellular water

Crime: offense against persons or property. The act is considered to be against the government, referred to in a lawsuit as "the people," and the accused is prosecuted by the state.

Crisis: (1) point at which body temperature drops rapidly to normal; (2) occurs when coping and defense mechanisms are no longer effective, resulting in high levels of anxiety, disorganized behavior, and the inability to function normally

Crisis intervention: five-step problem-solving technique to promote adaptation and improve future coping

Crisis intervention centers: centers that provide counseling or psychotherapy to reduce stress and facilitate coping in persons in a life crisis

Criteria: specified behavior, for example, the measurable criteria in a client goal specifies how the client must perform the desired behavior

Crossmatching: act of determining the compatibility of two blood specimens

Cue: significant data that is helpful in making decisions

Culture: sum total of human behavior or social characteristics peculiar to a specific group and passed from generation to generation, or from one to another within the group

Culture shock: those feelings, usually negative, a person experiences when placed in a different culture

Cumulative effect: occurs when the body cannot metabolize a drug before additional doses are administered

Cunnilingus: kissing, sucking, and licking female genitalia, particularly the vulva, clitoris, and vaginal introitus

Cupping: manual percussion of lung areas to loosen pulmonary secretions

Cutaneous stimulation: pain relief modalities that utilize stimulation of the skin by massage, application of heat or cold, vibration, and pressure

Cyanosis: bluish coloring of the skin and mucous membranes

Cystoscopy: direct visual examination of the bladder, ureteral orifices, and urethra with a cystoscope

Cytologic study: study of cells and fluids from the body

Dandruff: condition characterized by itching and flaking of the scalp

Dangling: position in which the person sits on the edge of the bed with his legs and feet over the side of the bed

Data: information

Data base: all the pertinent client information that enables a comprehensive and effective plan of care

to be designed and implemented for the client

Data cluster: grouping of client data or cues that point to the existence of a client health problem

Death: termination of life and its related clinical signs

Debridement: the cleaning away of infected and devitalized tissue from a wound

Decubitus ulcer: area of cellular necrosis caused by a lack of circulation to the involved area. Synonym for *pressure sore* and *bedsore.*

Deductive reasoning: thinking in which a general or broad idea is examined, and then specific ideas or actions are considered

Defamation: wrongs of slander and libel; making derogatory remarks about one person to another

Defecation: emptying of the intestinal tract; synonym for bowel movement

Defendant: person accused of a tort or crime

Defense mechanisms: forms of self-deception; unconscious process the self uses to protect itself from anxiety or threats to self-esteem

Dehiscence: separation of the layers of a surgical wound; may be partial, superficial, or a complete disruption of the surgical wound

Dehydration: decreased water volume

Delta sleep: deep sleep, occurring during stage III and especially stage IV in NREM sleep

Dementia: organic impairment of intellectual functioning, gradually leading to interference with social or occupational functioning, memory, and often personality integration

Democratic leadership: leadership style characterized by a sense of equality between the leader and followers

Denial: refusal to acknowledge some truth; form of self-deception

Dentition: complement of natural teeth in place in the alveoli of the dental arch

Dependent intervention: nursing action carried out at the instruction or order of an authorized health-care professional other than a nurse

Dependent variables: factors in a research study that remain the same

Depilatory: agent that destroys hair shafts or mechanically removes hair

Depolarize: to destroy polarity

Deposition: legal testimonies; may be given by the plaintiff, defendants, fast witnesses, and expert witnesses

Dermis: underlying portion of the skin

Development: increase in the complexity of function and progression to skill advancement

Development theory: theory to describe the orderly and predictable process of the growth and development of humans, individualized by social, biologic, and environmental factors

Developmental crisis: predictable patterns of behavior and change occurring throughout the lifespan

Developmental delay: measure of development that lags behind the normal range for a given age

Developmental task: successful achievement of psychomotor, psychosocial, or cognitive skills at certain periods in life. Failure to obtain the developmental task can lead to unhappiness and difficulty with later tasks.

Diagnosis: analysis of client data to identify client strengths and health problems that independent nursing intervention can prevent or resolve

Diagnostic related groups (DRGs): classification of clients by major medical diagnoses for the purpose of standardizing health-care costs (see *prospective payment*).

Diarrhea: passage of liquid and unformed stools

Diastolic pressure: the least amount of pressure exerted on arterial walls, which occurs when the heart is at rest between ventricular contractions

Diffuse pain: pain that covers a large area

Diffusion: tendency of solutes to move freely throughout a solvent from an area of higher concentration to an area of lower concentration until equilibrium is established

Diluent: liquid used to reconstitute powdered medications

Direct transfusion: infusion of blood while it is being taken from the donor

Disaccharides: double sugars composed of two monosaccharides. The most common disaccharides are sucrose (table sugar), lactose (mild sugar), and maltose (grain sugar).

Discharge planning: systematic process for preparing the client to leave the health-care agency and for continuity of care

Discharge summary: description of where the client stands in relation to problems identified in the record at discharge; documents any special teaching or counseling the client received, including referrals

Disease: change in the body's structure or function

Disinfectant: substance, usually intended for use on inanimate objects, that destroys pathogens but generally not spores

Disinfection: process by which pathogens but not spores are destroyed

Displacement: substitution of more acceptable behavior for an unacceptable behavior

Distribution: movement of drugs by the circulatory system to the site of action

Diurnal enuresis: involuntary urination that occurs during wakefulness

Donor: person who donates blood to be given to another person

Dorsal position: position in which the client lies flat on his back with legs together

Dorsal recumbent position: position in which the client is placed on his back close to the edge of the bed with the legs separated and knees flexed

Dorsiflexion: backward bending of the hand or foot

Down's syndrome: congenital conditions characterized by physical malformations and some degree of mental retardation. It is caused by a defect in chromosome 21 and is also called trisomy 21 syndrome.

Dressing: protective covering placed over a wound

Drug: substance that modifies body functions when taken into the living organism; synonym for medication

Drug allergy: hypersensitivity caused by previous exposure to a medication. May occur immediately or may be delayed. Manifestations range from mild to severe.

Drug tolerance: the body becomes accustomed to a drug over a period of time. Larger doses are required to produce the desired effects.

Dry cough: forceful expiratory effort; also known as nonproductive cough

Dull pain: gnawing discomfort less intense and acute than sharp pain

Dyspareunia: painful coitus which occurs most often in women and rarely in men

Dyspnea: difficult breathing

Dysrhythmia: irregular pattern of heartbeats; synonym is arrhythmia

Dysuria: difficulty in voiding; may or may not be associated with pain. A feeling of warm local irritation occurring during voiding is called burning.

Ecchymosis: collection of blood in subcutaneous tissues which causes a purplish discoloration

Edema: accumulation of fluid in extracellular spaces

Ego integrity/despair: last stage of life according to Erikson, which begins around the age of 60 years. The stage is characterized as a time to review one's life and find wholeness and acceptance, or unresolved problems and missed opportunities.

Ejaculation: expulsion of semen from the penis resulting from stimulation from sexual arousal

Elective surgery: surgery that is recommended but can be omitted or delayed without catastrophe

Electrocardiogram: graphic record produced by the electrocardiograph; abbreviated EKG or ECG

Electrocardiograph: instrument that measures and records electric impulses of the heart

Electroencephalogram: graphic record produced by the electroencephalograph; abbreviated EEG

Electroencephalograph: instrument that measures and records electric impulses of the brain

Electrolyte: substance capable of breaking into ions and developing an electric charge when dissolved in solution

Electromyogram (EMG): instrument that records muscle tone

Electrooculogram (EOG): instrument that records eye movements

Embolism: blocking of an artery by a blood clot or by other foreign matter brought to the site by the blood flow

Embolus: foreign body or air in the circulatory system. The plural form is emboli.

Emergency surgery: surgery that must be performed immediately to save the person's life or a body organ

Emollient: agent that soothes and softens the part of the body to which it is applied; the term usually applies to agents affecting the surface of the body

Empathy: intellectually identifying with the way another person feels

"Empty nest" syndrome: feeling of loss after the last child has moved away from home

Endogenous: infection in which the causative organism comes from microbial life the person himself harbors

Endorphins: morphinelike substances released by the body which appear to alter the perception of pain

Endoscope: flexible or rigid lighted tube which allows direct visual examination of various body cavities and organs

Endoscopic retrograde cholangiopancreatography (ERCP): injection of a contrast medium through an endoscope for visualization of the pancreatic ducts and the hepatobiliary tree

Endoscopy: direct visualization of hollow organs of the body using an endoscope or flexible, lighted tube

Endurance: ability to sustain movement or to perform an activity overtime

Enema: introduction of solution into the lower intestinal tract

Enuresis: involuntary urination; most often used to refer to a child who involuntarily urinates during the night

Environment: condition of both internal and external physical factors affecting and influencing the growth and development of the person

Epidermis: superficial portion of the skin

Erect position: position in which the client stands

Erectile failure: condition in which a man is unable to attain or maintain an erection to such an extent that he cannot have satisfactory coitus; synonym for impotence

Erection: condition that results when erectile tissue of the penis fills with blood due to stimulation

Erogenous zones: areas of the body that when stimulated produce sexual desire and arousal

Esophagogastroduodenoscopy: visual examination of the esophagus, stomach, and duodenum; also called gastroscopy

Essential hypertension: abnormally elevated blood pressure with no known cause; synonym for primary hypertension

Ethics: system dealing with standards of behavior related to what is right and wrong

Ethnic group: minority groups that retain distinct customs, language, or social values as a result of a common heritage

Ethnocentrism: judgment of other people based on the standards and practices of one's own culture

Euphoria: unrealistic sense of well-being

Eupnea: normal respirations

Euthanasia: mercy killing or the deliberate termination of the life of a terminally ill person

Evaluating: measurement of the extent to which the client has achieved the goals specified in the plan of care. Factors that positively or negatively influenced goal achievement are identified, and the plan of care is terminated or revised.

Evaporation: conversion of liquid to a vapor

Evisceration: protrusion of viscera through an incisional area

Excretion: removal of a drug from the body

Excruciating pain: pain that could be described to range between 8 and 10 on a scale of 1 to 10; synonym for severe pain

Exhalation: act of breathing out; synonym is expiration

Exit from the reservoir: point of escape for organisms from a reservoir

Exogenous: infection in which the causative organism is acquired from other persons

Expectorant: drug that facilitates the removal of respiratory secretions

Expert witness: person having special training or experience who assists a judge and jury in their decision-making process

Expiration: act of breathing out; synonym for exhalation

Expiratory reserve volume (ERV): additional amount of air that can be exhaled beyond tidal volume

Extended care facility: type of care given after hospitalization of acute illness; includes residential care and intermediate or skilled nursing home care

Extended family: nuclear family and other related persons

Extension: state of being in a straight line

External respiration: act of lung ventilation, oxygen absorption, and carbon dioxide elimination

External rotation: body part turning on its axis away from the midline of the body

Extracellular fluid (ECF): fluid outside the cells; includes intravascular and interstitial fluids

Extraneous variables: unknown factors that affect research outcomes

Exudate: fluid and cells that escape from blood vessels of wounds (drainage)

Failure to thrive (FTT): physical and developmental retardation of infants or children resulting from physical and/or emotional neglect

Faith: spiritual dimensions of a person's life regardless of religious affiliation; confident belief in something for which there is no proof or material evidence

False imprisonment: unjustifiable retention or prevention of the movement of another person without proper consent

Fasting state: abstinence from food and fluids

Fatty acids: structural components of fats

Feces: intestinal waste products

Fellatio: kissing, sucking, and licking the male genitalia, particularly the scrotum and penis

Felony: crime punishable by imprisonment in a state or federal penitentiary for more than 1 year; crime of greater offense than a misdemeanor

Fertilization: process in reproduction by which the male sperm unites with the female ovum

Fetishism: practice of arousing sexual desires with inanimate objects

Fever: elevation above the upper limit of normal body temperature; synonym for pyrexia

Fiber: all dietary plant material that is not digestible by GI tract, enzymes, and secretions

Fidelity: keeping promises and commitments made to others

Fight-or-flight response: the body prepares itself against threat, to either resist (fight) or evade (flight) the danger

Filtration: passage of a fluid through a permeable membrane whose spaces do not allow certain solutes to pass. Passage is from an area of higher pressure to one of lower pressure.

Filtration pressure: difference between colloid osmotic pressure and blood hydrostatic pressure

Fingerprint: impression of an examiner's fingerprints on the skin made by applying pressure over the sternum

Fitness: degree of physical functioning characterized by physical strength, flexibility, endurance, and strong cardiovascular functioning

Flaccidity: decreased muscle tone; synonym for hypotonicity

Flatulence: excessive formation of gases in the gastrointestinal tract

Flatus: intestinal gas

Flexibility: ability to use a muscle through its entire range of motion

Flexion: state of being bent

Flowsheets: graphic record of abbreviated aspects of client's condition (*e.g.,* vital signs, routine aspects of care)

Fluid balance: state in which water and its solutes in the body are in normal proportions and concentrations and are in appropriate body compartments

Fluid imbalance: state in which water and its solutes in the body are in improper proportions and concentrations or are improperly located in body compartments

Fluid volume deficit: deficiency in the amount of both water and electrolytes in ECF; water and electrolyte proportions remain near normal

Fluid volume excess: excessive retention of water and sodium in ECF in near normal proportions

Fluoroscopy: radiologic visualization of motion without its being recorded on film

Flushing: red appearance of the skin

Foley catheter: tube introduced through the urethra into the bladder for the purpose of withdrawing urine

Fomite: inanimate object other than food that can absorb and transmit infectious material

Footdrop: complication resulting from extended plantar flexion

Forced vital capacity (FVC): maximal amount of air that can be inhaled followed by a fast maximal forced exhalation with the greatest effort

Foreplay: activity engaged in prior to sexual intercourse to further stimulate sexual arousal

Formal teaching: planned teaching done while following learner objectives

Fowler's position: semi-sitting position with the head of the bed raised 45 degrees to 60 degrees

Fraud: willful and purposeful misrepresentation that could cause, or has caused, loss or harm to persons or property

Fremitus: vibration of the chest wall that can be palpated during the physical examination

Frequency: increased incidence of voiding

Friction rub: crackling sounds heard in the chest cavity, caused by inflamed pleura rubbing against the chest wall

Full stage of infection: stage of an infection characterized by the presence of specific signs and symptoms

Functional health: level of health defined by one's ability to carry out usual and desired daily activities

Functional incontinence: state in which an individual experiences an involuntary, unpredictable passage of urine

Gastric gavage: introduction of nourishment into the stomach by mechanical means

Gastroenteritis: inflammation of the lining of the stomach and the intestine resulting from irritation, al-

lergic reaction to foods, or emotional upset

Gate control theory: theory that explains that excitatory pain stimuli carried by small-diameter nerve fibers can be blocked by inhibiting signals carried by large-diameter nerve fibers

Gay: commonly used term that is synonymous with homosexual

General adaptation syndrome (GAS): biochemical model of stress, describing the body's general response to stress

General anesthesia: anesthetic drugs produce narcosis, relaxation of skeletal muscles, and reduced or absent reflex action

General systems theory: theory that explains how parts of whole things work together in systems, including relationships between wholes and parts as they function, behave, and react

Generativity/self-absorption: middle adulthood stage of life according to Erikson which centers around the ages of 30 to 60, but also continues into older adulthood. The stage is characterized by a desire to establish and guide the next generation or by a sense of stagnation and concentration on oneself.

Generic name: name assigned by the manufacturer who first develops a drug

Gerontic nursing: nursing specialty concerned with the care of the well and ill older adult

Gerontology: study of all aspects of the aging process and their consequences

Gingiva: tissue surrounding the teeth. Gingivae (plural) are often called the gums of the mouth.

Gingivitis: inflammation of the gingivae or gums

Glycosuria: presence of sugar in the urine; if due to an unusually large intake of sugar or to marked emotional disturbances and is temporary, there is little cause for alarm

Goal: an aim or an end; an expected outcome

Gonorrhea: highly contagious, sexually transmitted bacterial infection of the genitourinary system caused by the organism *Neisseria gonorrhoea.*

Good-samaritan law: law that holds certain health practitioners harm-

less when undertaking to aid a person in emergency situations

Granulation tissue: new tissue composed of fibroblasts and small blood vessels

Grief: emotional response to loss. *Dysfunctional grief:* distorted or abnormal grief response, including *inhibited grief* (suppression of grief reaction), and *unresolved grief* (lengthy or denied grief reaction). *Abbreviated grief:* short but genuine grief reaction. *Anticipatory grief:* grief reaction before actual loss.

Ground: conducting connection between a source of electricity and the earth

Group process: study of a group's characteristics and ways of functioning

Growth: increase in physical size of an organism or any of its structural organs

Gustatory: pertaining to taste

Halitosis: offensive breath

Health: state of optimal functioning or well-being

Health-belief model: what people believe to be true about themselves in relation to health

Health maintenance organization (HMO): a broad term encompassing a variety of health-care delivery systems that use group practice and provide an incentive to use a prepaid comprehensive health-care system

Health problem: condition related to health requiring intervention if disease or illness is to be prevented or resolved and coping and wellness are to be promoted

Health-risk appraisal: assessment of the total person, identifying both healthy and unhealthy practices

Heat: energy of the motion of molecules of a material

Heave: upward lift or rising of the chest, particularly of the precordial chest area

Helping relationship: interaction that sets the climate of movement of the participants toward common goals

Hematuria: blood in the urine; if present in large enough quantities, urine may be bright red or reddish brown in color

Hemiplegia: paralysis of one half of the body

Hemolysis: process of freeing a red blood cell of its hemoglobin by destruction of the cell membrane

Hemoptysis: sputum containing blood

Hemorrhage: excessive blood loss owing to the escape of blood from blood vessels

Hemorrhoids: abnormally distended rectal veins

Heparin lock: IV needle or catheter with an injection pad attached at the end

Herpes simplex II (genital herpes): highly contagious viral infection caused by the type 2 strain of the herpes simplex virus (HSV) and transmitted by direct person-to-person contact, particularly sexual

Hesitancy: delay or difficulty in initiating voiding

Heterosexuality: having sexual feelings for a person of the opposite sex

Hiccups: involuntary spasmodic contractions of the diaphragm; synonym for singultus

Hierarchy of needs: as defined by Maslow, certain needs are more basic than others; a person strives to at least minimally meet certain needs before attending to others

High-level wellness: functioning to one's maximum potential while maintaining balance and purposeful direction in the environment

Hirsutism: excessive growth of body hair

Holism: concept that views a person as more than the total sum of parts and shows concern and interest in all aspects of the person

Holistic health care: health care that takes into account the whole person interacting in the environment

Holistic nursing care: care given with regard for all the components and human dimensions of a person ("the whole person")

Home health agency: an agency, eligible to receive Federal funds, that provides home-based care; may be independent, hospital operated, or health department managed

Home health care: that component of a continuum of comprehensive health care whereby health services are provided to persons and families in their places of residency for the purpose of promoting, maintaining, or restoring

health or of maximizing the level of independence while minimizing the effects of disability and illness

Homeostasis: various physiologic and psychologic mechanisms respond to changes in the internal and external environment to maintain a balanced state

Homeothermic: ability to regulate and maintain body temperature, regardless of environmental temperature

Homosexuality: having sexual feelings for a person of the same sex

Hospice care: provision of care and support to dying clients and their families through spiritual, emotional, and physical interventions

Host: animal or person on which or within which microorganisms live

Hot–cold theory: theory that asserts that many diseases, foods, and herbs can be categorized as hot or cold. When there is an imbalance in the body, the proper foods must be taken to rebalance the body.

Human dimension: physical, emotional, intellectual, environmental, sociocultural, and spiritual components of a person

Human sexuality: integration of the physical, mental, emotional, and social aspects of a person that denote maleness or femaleness

Humanism: concern and understanding of others which attests to the dignity and worth of all persons

Hydration: union of a substance with water. The term is often used as the opposite of dehydration, in which case it means that there is normal intracellular and extracellular water volume.

Hydrolytic: substance capable of a reaction that takes up water

Hydrometer: instrument used to determine the specific gravity of urine

Hydrostatic pressure: force exerted by a fluid against the container wall

Hygiene: science dealing with the preservation of health and well-being

Hyperalimentation: intravenous infusion of solution that contains sufficient nutrients to support life and maintain normal growth and development; synonym for total parenteral nutrition (TPN)

Hypercalcemia: excess of calcium in the extracellular fluid

Hyperextension: state of exaggerated extension

Hyperkalemia: excess of potassium in the extracellular fluid

Hypermagnesemia: excess of magnesium in the extracellular fluid

Hypernatremia: excess of sodium in the extracellular fluid

Hyperperistalsis: bowel sounds greater than 34 per minute

Hyperphosphatemia: above normal serum concentration of inorganic phosphorus

Hyperpyrexia: high fever, above 41°C (105.8°F)

Hypersomnia: condition characterized by excessive sleeping, especially daytime sleeping

Hypertension: blood pressure elevated above the upper limit of normal

Hypertonic: having a greater concentration than the solution with which it is being compared

Hyperventilation: condition in which there is more than the normal amount of air entering and leaving lungs

Hypervolemia: excess of plasma

Hypnosis: technique that produces a subconscious condition accomplished by suggestions made by a hypnotist

Hypnotic: pharmaceutical agent used to induce sleep

Hypocalcemia: insufficient amount of calcium in the extracellular fluid

Hypokalemia: insufficient amount of potassium in the extracellular fluid

Hypomagnesemia: insufficient amount of magnesium in the extracellular fluid

Hyponatremia: insufficient amount of sodium in the extracellular fluid

Hypophosphatemia: below normal serum concentration of inorganic phosphorus

Hypoproteinemia: insufficient amount of protein substances in the extracellular fluid

Hypospadias: developmental anomaly in male infants in which the urethral opening is on the underside of the penis or on the perineum

Hypotension: blood pressure below the lower limit of normal

Hypothermia: body temperature below the lower limit of normal

Hypotonic: having a lesser concentration than the solution with which it is being compared

Hypovolemia: deficiency of plasma

Hypovolemic shock: shock owing to a decrease in blood volume

Hypoxemia: deficient oxygenation of blood

Hypoxia: inadequate amounts of oxygen available to the cells

Iatrogenic disease: disease caused unintentionally by drug therapy

Iatrogenic infection: infection that occurs as a result of a treatment or diagnostic procedure

Ideal self: self a person would like to be or feels he should be; includes aspirations, moral ideals, and values

Idiosyncratic reaction: unusual, unexpected response to a drug

Ileal conduit: urinary diversion in which the ureters are connected to the ileum with a stoma created on the abdominal wall

Illness: abnormal process in which any aspect of the person's functioning is altered (in comparison to the previous condition of health)

Imagery: pain relief modality which uses mind body interaction; the imaging of the eradication of the source of the pain or its healing in a pleasurable environment

Immune response: specific reactions in the body as it responds to an invading foreign protein such as bacteria, or even in some case, the body's own proteins

Immunization: process of rendering a person immune or resistant to particular antigenic agents or bacteria

Immunoglobulin: animal protein found in body fluids with known antibody activity and characteristics

Impaction (fecal): collection of hardened feces in the rectum which cannot be passed

Implementing: carrying out the plan of care

Impotence: condition in which a man is unable to attain or maintain an erection to such an extent that he cannot have satisfactory sexual intercourse; synonym for erectile failure

Incentive spirometer: equipment to help maximize lung inflation

Incest: practicing sexual behavior between persons who are so closely related that marriage between them is legally or culturally not allowed

Incident report: documentation that describes any injury or potential for injury suffered by a client in a health-care agency

Incision: wound made with a sharp, cutting instrument

Incomplete proteins: proteins that lack or contain insufficient amounts of all the essential amino acids necessary for protein synthesis; also termed low biological value proteins

Incontinence: inability to voluntarily control the discharge of urine or feces

Incubation period: stage of infection that includes the interval between the invasion of the body by the pathogen and the appearance of symptoms of infection

Independent intervention: nursing action carried out at the instruction or order of a nurse; actions within the legal scope of nursing's independent domain

Independent variables: factors in a research study that differ

Indirect transfusion: infusion of blood from a container in which the donor's blood was received

Individual supply: system of supplying a client's medications for a period of time

Inductive reasoning: pattern of reasoning in which a specific idea or action is identified, and then conclusions are made about general ideas

Indwelling catheter: catheter that remains in place for continuous urinary drainage; Foley catheter

Infection: disease state resulting from pathogens in or on the body

Infiltration: escape of fluid into subcutaneous tissue

Inflammatory response: localized response of the body to injury or infection; protective mechanism that eliminates invading pathogens and allows for tissue repair to occur

Informal teaching: unplanned teaching sessions dealing with the client's immediate learning needs and concerns

Informed consent:

Inguinal hernia: abnormal protrusion of the intestine and/or omentum through a weak point in the abdominal wall or downward at an angle into the inguinal canal

Inhalation: (1) act of breathing in;

synonym for inspiration. (2) administration of a drug in solution by way of the respiratory tract.

Injection: introduction of medication into the body by a syringe attached to a needle

Inner canthus: angle of the eye where the upper and lower lids meet

Insensible water loss: nonperceptible water lost from the body as moisture through the breath and by evaporation from the skin

Insomnia: difficulty in falling asleep, intermittent sleep, or early awakening from sleep

Inspection: purposeful and systematic observation

Inspiration: act of breathing in; synonym for inhalation.

Inspiratory reserve volume (IRV): additional amount of air that can be inspired beyond the tidal volume

Instillation: pouring or dropping a liquid into a body cavity or onto a surface

Insulator: poor conductor of heat

Integument: skin

Integumentary system: skin and its appendages (*i.e.*, hair, glands in the skin, and nails)

Intellectualization: defense mechanism which separates the emotion of an event from the facts because the emotion is too painful to be acknowledged. By using rational explanation for the occurrence of the event, the person is able to divest the event of any personal significance.

Intensive level care: care warranting close observation, monitoring, or treatment requiring skilled care; reimbursed by insurance

Interdependent (collaborative) intervention: nursing action performed by the nurse in collaboration with other members of the health-care team

Intermediate level care: care warranting skilled services for a client in which an improvement in function is expected; reimbursed by insurance; synonym for rehabilitative level care.

Intermittent fever: body temperature that alternates between a period of fever and a period of normal or subnormal temperature

Intermittent pulse: period of normal pulse rhythm broken by periods of irregular rhythm

Internal respiration: act of using oxygen by body cells; synonym for tissue respiration

Internal rotation: body part turning on its axis toward the midline of the body

Interpersonal skills: elements required for positive relationships to exist between persons

Interstitial fluid: fluid between the cells

Interview: planned communication for a specific purpose (*e.g.,* data collection)

Interviewing techniques: communication skills specifically designed to gather and to validate information

Intracellular fluid (ICF): fluid within the cell; synonym for cellular fluid

Intractable pain: severe pain that is extremely resistant to relief measures

Intradermal injection: injection made under the epidermis

Intramuscular injection: injection into the muscle tissue

Intraoperative phase: time period lasting from admission to the operating room area to transfer to the postanesthesia recovery area after surgery is completed

Intravascular fluid: fluid within the vascular system; synonym for plasma

Intravenous infusion: injection of relatively large quantities of solution into a vein

Intravenous injection: injection into the vein

Intravenous pyelogram (IVP): x-ray examination of the kidneys and ureters after a contrast material is injected intravenously to determine the kidney's ability to excrete urine

Introjection: person internalizes some aspect of the external world and keeps it intact in his psyche

Intuitive problem solving: direct understanding of a situation based on a background of experience, knowledge, and skill, which makes expert decision making possible

Inunction: rubbing substances into the skin

Invasion of privacy: action that invades the right of a person to be left alone

Ion: atom or molecule carrying an electric charge in solution

Ionization: process by which substances dissociate to form ions

Irrigation: flushing of a tube, canal, or area with solution

Ischemia: deficiency of blood in a particular area

Isokinetic exercise: exercise involving muscle contractions with resistance varying at a constant rate

Isolation: protective procedure designed to prevent the transmission of specific microorganisms; also called protective aseptic techniques and barrier techniques

Isometric exercise: exercise in which muscle tension occurs without a significant change in muscle length

Isotonic: (1) having approximately the same concentration as the solution with which it is being compared; (2) exercise in which muscles shorten (contract) and move

Jaundice: yellow appearance of the skin

Kardex nursing care plan: trade name for a care plan documentation system which generally encompasses (1) prescriptions for nursing care related to activities of daily living, (2) nursing diagnoses and related client goals and nursing orders, and (3) the nursing care related to diagnostic measures and the medical regimen

Kegel exercises: repetitious contraction and relaxation of the pubococcygeal muscle to improve vaginal tone and urinary continence

Kinesthesia: awareness of positioning of body parts and body movement

Knee–chest position: position in which the client rests his knees and chest with body flexed approximately 90 degrees at the hips

Korotkoff sounds: series of sounds that correspond to changes in blood flow through an artery as pressure is released

Kussmaul's respiration breathing: an extreme rate and depth of breathing

Laceration: wound caused by a blunt instrument or object that tears tissue

Laissez-faire leadership: leadership style in which the leader relinquishes all power to the group

Language: prescribed way of using words; a means to express thoughts and feelings

Lanugo: fine hair that covers the fetus and decreases as full gestation approaches

Laryngoscope: lighted, tubular instrument used for visual examination of the larynx

Laryngoscopy: visual examination of the larynx

Lateral: pertaining to the side

Law: rule of conduct established and enforced by the government of a society

Lawsuit: legal action in a court of law

Laxative: drug used to induce emptying of the intestinal tract

Lead: placement pattern of electrodes used in electrocardiography

Leadership: ability to direct or motivate others toward the achievement of predetermined goals

Learning: increasing one's knowledge; having one's behavior changed in a measurable way as a result of an experience

Lesbian: term used to describe a female homosexual

Liability: legal responsibility for one's acts (and failure to act); includes responsibility for financial restitution of harms resulting from negligent acts

Libel: untruthful, written statement about a person that subjects him to ridicule or contempt

Licensure: to be given a license to practice nursing in a state or province after successfully meeting requirements

Life review/reminiscence: universal phenomenon identified by Butler as a review of one's life through one's recollections

Lift: see *heave.*

Line of gravity: vertical line that passes through the center of gravity

Linguistic: speech designed to convey meaning

Lipid: group name for fatty substances, including fats, oils, waxes, and related compounds

Liter: metric standard of measurement for liquids. One liter contains 1000 milliliters.

Lithotomy position: same as the dorsal recumbent position except the feet are placed in stirrups and the buttocks are at the edge of the examining table

Litigation: process of lawsuit

Liver biopsy: needle aspiration of a sample of liver tissue

Living will: nonbinding document expressing a client's desire not to have life sustained by artificial life support systems or heroic efforts

Local adaptation syndrome (LAS): localized response of the body to stress, precipitated by trauma or pathology

Localized symptoms: symptoms that are limited or restricted to a discrete area

Long-term care facilities: nursing homes

Loss: inaccessibility or change in a valued person, object, or situation. *Actual loss:* loss tangible to both the person sustaining the loss and to others; *perceived loss:* loss tangible only to the person sustaining it; *physical loss:* loss of life, limb, an object, person, pet, or job; *psychologic loss:* loss that affects a person's self-image; and *anticipatory loss:* loss behaviors displayed before the actual loss occurs.

Love and belonging needs: understanding and acceptance of others in giving and receiving love

Lozenge: small, solid medication intended to be held in the mouth until it dissolves

Lumbar puncture: insertion of a needle into the subarachnoid space; synonym for spinal tap

Lysis: gradual return of an elevated body temperature to normal

Macroshock: electric current passing through a relatively large area of a person

Magnetic resonance imaging (MRI): use of magnetism and radio waves to produce cross-sectional images of body tissues on a computer screen

Maintenance level care: care warranting assistance with personal care and homemaker services for a client for whom there is no expected change of condition; not reimbursed by Medicare or other insurance

Malnutrition: literally "bad nutrition." May be related to dietary excesses or deficiencies, or may occur secondary to illness or treatments.

Malpractice: act of negligence as applied to a professional person, such as a physician, nurse, or dentist

Manslaughter: second-degree murder

Many-tailed binder: type of bandage with multiple tails; synonym for scultetus binder

Masochism: practice of inflicting discomfort on oneself for sexual stimulation

Mastectomy: surgical excision of the breast, used as a treatment for breast cancer; surrounding tissue and lymph nodes may also be removed

Masturbation: self-stimulation for sexual satisfaction

Maturation: physical developmental changes influenced by genetic and environmental factors

Mechanism: patterns of action performed by different parts of the body to serve a common goal

Meconium: first stool of a newborn

Medicaid: Title XIX (Social Security Act, 1965) to make health care available to those persons with less than the minimum income, and not qualifying for Medicare

Medical asepsis: practices designed to reduce the number and transfer of pathogens; synonym for clean technique

Medical diagnosis: statement about a specific disease process using terminology from a well-developed classification system accepted by the medical profession

Medicare: Title XVIII (Social Security Act, 1965) to provide a measure of health coverage to all Social Security recipients

Medication: substance that modifies body functions when taken into the living organism; synonym for drug

Menarche: initiation of the menstrual cycle

Meniscus: curved surface at the top of a column of liquid in a tube

Menopause: decrease of cyclic hormonal production and cessation of menses in females, usually between the ages of 45 and 60

Menses: monthly menstrual period

Mentorship: relationship in which an experienced person (the mentor) advises and assists a less experienced person

Metabolic acidosis: proportionate deficiency of bicarbonate ions in the extracellular fluid

Metabolic alkalosis: proportionate excess of bicarbonate ions in the extracellular fluid

Metabolism: breakdown of a drug to an inactive form; also referred to as biotransformation

Microshock: electric current passing through a relatively small area of a person, generally a part of the heart

Micturition: process of emptying the bladder; urination; voiding

Midlife crisis: realization that the halfway point in life has been reached, and youthful goals may not have been achieved

Mild pain: pain that could be described as being between 1 and 3 on a scale of 1 to 10; synonym for slight pain

Milia: tiny, pearly white bumps across the nose, cheeks, or forehead of an infant, caused by accumulation of sebum in the ducts of the sebaceous glands

Milliequivalent: unit of measurement to describe electrolyte chemical activity; abbreviated mEq. One milliequivalent is equivalent to the activity of 1 milligram of hydrogen.

Milliliter: one thousandth of a liter; abbreviated ml

Minerals: inorganic elements found in nature

Misdemeanor: crime of lesser offense than a felony and punishable by fines, imprisonment (usually for less than 1 year) or both

Model: abstract outline or visual representation of a complex state or occurrence

Moderate pain: pain that could be described as being between 4 and 7 on a scale of 1 to 10; between pain that is described as mild or severe

Molding: shaping of the fetal head that occurs at birth to accommodate to the size and shape of the birth canal

Mongolian spot: smooth, brown to gray-blue nevus typically found in the sacral region in Orientals, Blacks, Native (North) Americans, and some southern Europeans. It usually disappears during early childhood.

Monilian infection: infection by the parasitic fungus *Monilia* (*Candida*); usually sexually transmitted

Monosaccharides: simple sugars containing one sugar molecule. Glucose (blood sugar) and fructose (fruit sugar) are the most common monosaccharides. Monosaccharides are also the end products of carbohydrate digestion.

Morality: judgment regarding justice in personal and social situations

Morals: like ethics, concerned with what constitutes right action; more informal and personal than the term ethics

Moratorium: identity state in which a person is considering various alternatives prior to making a commitment

Mourning: period during which a person learns to accept grief

Murder: illegal killing of another person. *First-degree murder:* murder with malice aforethought. *Second-degree murder:* murder without previous deliberation; sometimes called manslaughter.

Mutual aid self-help groups (MASH): member-organized and run self-help groups offering emotional support and education to assist members in coping with personal and health problems

Myelination: production of myelin, a lipid substance that forms a sheath around the axon of certain nerve fibers

Narcolepsy: condition characterized by an uncontrolled desire to sleep

Narrative: descriptive record of the client's condition; includes client's response to interventions by health professionals and client's progress toward goal achievement

Nasal speculum: instrument used for inspection of the internal nares

Nasogastric feeding: feeding a client through a tube inserted into the nares and down to the stomach

Necrosis: death of cells

Negligence: performing an act that a reasonably prudent person under similar circumstances would not do, or failing to perform an act that a reasonably prudent person under similar circumstances would do

Neurologic hammer: instrument used to test reflexes

Nitrogen balance: comparison between nitrogen intake (protein eaten) and nitrogen output (protein excreted in the urine, feces, hair, nails, and skin)

Nits: lice eggs

Nocturia: frequency of urination during the night

Nocturnal emission: ejaculation due to erotic dreams while sleeping; synonym for wet dream.

Nocturnal enuresis: involuntary urination while a person is sleeping

Nocturnal myoclonus: condition characterized by marked muscle contraction which results in the jerking of one or both legs during sleep

Noncompliance: disregard of orders or not completing what is expected

Nonelectrolyte: molecules that remain intact and do not ionize

Nonmaleficence: principle of avoiding evil

Nonproductive cough: forceful expiratory effort without production of mucus; also called a dry cough

Nonverbal communication: exchange of information without the use of words

Normal flora: microorganisms that normally inhabit various body sites and are part of the body's natural defense system

Nosocomial infection: hospital-acquired infection

NREM: nonrapid eye movement that characterizes four stages of sleep

Nuclear family: family unit, family of marriage, parenthood, or procreation, and their immediate children

Nurse practice act: laws established to regulate nursing practice

Nursing: profession focusing on the holistic person receiving health-care services and providing a unique contribution to the prevention of illness and maintenance of health

Nursing actions: any action performed by a nurse to assist clients to meet health goals: promote wellness, prevent disease/illness, restore health, facilitate coping with altered functioning

Nursing audit: method of evaluating care the outcomes of nursing care or the process by which these outcomes are achieved using a review of client records

Nursing care conference: formal meeting of nurses to discuss some aspect of a client's care

Nursing care plan: written guide to direct the efforts of the nursing team as they work with clients to meet health goals; specifies prioritized nursing diagnoses, client goals, and nursing orders

Nursing care rounds: procedure in which a group of nurses visit clients individually at their bedside to gather information that helps to plan and evaluate nursing care

Nursing diagnosis: actual or potential health problem that independent nursing intervention can prevent or resolve. *Actual problem* is present. *Possible problem* may be present, but more data are needed to confirm or disconfirm the problem. *Potential problem* may occur; defining characteristics are present as risk factors.

Nursing examination: systematic physical examination of the client for objective data to better define the client's condition and help the nurse in planning care; usually performed in a head-to-toe format

Nursing history: assessment of the client by interview to identify the client's health status, strengths, health problems, health risks, and need for nursing

Nursing order: prescribes the nursing care to be given to assist clients to meet health goals

Nursing process: five-step systematic method for giving client care; involves assessing, diagnosing, planning, implementing, and evaluating

Nursing theory: attempts to describe or explain the phenomenon (process, occurrence, or event) called nursing; includes the concepts of person, health, environment, and nursing

Nutrition: study of the nutrients and how they are handled by the body, as well as the impact of human behavior and environment on the process of nourishment

Obesity: weight greater than 20% above ideal body weight

Object permanence: awareness that an object or person does not cease to exist when out of sight

Objective data: information perceptible to the senses; may be verified by another person

Objectivity: remaining neutral while applying research criteria

Observation: conscious and deliberate use of the five senses to gather data

Occult blood: blood present in such minute quantities that it cannot be detected with the unassisted eye

Official name: name by which a drug is identified in official publications

Old-old: term used to describe older adults over the age of 75, sometimes referred to as frail-old

Older adult: after middle age; refers to adults over the age of 65

Olfactory: pertaining to smell

Oliguria: scanty or greatly diminished amount of urine voided in a given time; 24-hour urine output is 100 ml to 400 ml

Oncotic pressure: pressure exerted by plasma proteins on permeable membranes in the body; synonym for colloid osmotic pressure

Open wound: injury characterized by a break in the continuity of the skin so that there is exposure of underlying tissue to the atmosphere

Ophthalmoscope: lighted instrument used for examination of the interior eye

Organism: apex of sexual activity where rhythmic contractions of the genital organs and many other physiologic changes occur

Orgasmic dysfunction: condition in which a woman is unable to reach orgasm

Orthopedics: correction or prevention of disorders of the locomotion of the body

Orthopnea: type of dyspnea in which breathing is easier when the client sits or stands

Orthostatic hypotension: temporary fall in blood pressure associated with assuming an upright position; synonym for postural hypotension

Osmolality: property of a solution that describes the total number of dissolved particles in a solution; the concentration of solutes in a solvent

Osmoreceptors: special neurons that are sensitive to changes in osmotic pressure of surrounding fluids

Osmosis: passage of a solvent through a semipermeable membrane from an area of lesser concentration to an area of greater concentration until equilibrium is established

Osmotic pressure: drawing power for water or the attraction for water exerted by solute particles

Ossification: formation of or conversion into bone or a bony substance

Osteomalacia: softening of the bones owing usually to a deficiency or loss of calcium salts from the body

Osteoporosis: condition characterized by loss of calcium from bone tissue

Ostomy: general term referring to an artificial opening; usually used to refer to an opening created for the excretion of body wastes

Otoscope: lighted instrument used for examination of the external ear canal and the tympanic membrane (eardrum)

Outcome: end product of nursing care; client outcomes are measurable changes in client behavior or state of health

Outer canthus: lateral angle of the eye where the upper and lower lids meet

Overhydration: above-normal amounts of water in extracellular spaces

Overweight: weight between 10% and 20% above ideal body weight

Ovulation: discharge of ovum from the female ovary at approximately the midpoint of each menstrual cycle

Ovum: female reproductive cell, often called an egg

Pack: moist cloths or dressings applied to a large body area

Pain: sensation of physical or mental suffering or hurt which usually causes distress or agony to the one experiencing it

Pain threshold: amount of stimulation required before a person experiences the sensation of pain

Pain tolerance: point beyond which a person is no longer willing to endure pain (*i.e.,* pain of greater duration or intensity)

Pallor: paleness of the skin

Palpation: method of examining by feeling a part with the fingers or hand

Palpitation: perception of one's own heartbeat

Paracentesis: withdrawal of fluid from a body cavity, usually from the abdominal cavity

Parainsomnia: patterns of waking behavior that appear during sleep

(*e.g.,* sleep walking, sleep talking, nocturnal erections, and so forth)

Parallax: apparent change of position of an object when observed from two different angles

Paralytic ileus: paralysis of intestinal peristalsis

Paraplegia: paralysis of the legs

Parenteral: outside of intestines or alimentary canal; popularly used to refer to injection routes

Paresthesia: numbness and tingling

Passive exercise: manual or mechanical means of moving the joints

Passive immunity: antibodies against harmful effects of microorganisms or toxins are produced by other persons/animals and passed on to an individual. Two common examples are: passive immunity is acquired by a fetus from its mother in utero or by an infant from its mother through breastfeeding.

Pathogen: disease-producing microorganism

Pediculicide: preparation for destroying lice

Pediculosis: infestation with lice

Perception: conscious process of organizing and interpreting data from the senses into meaningful information

Percussion: technique in the physical examination which involves striking the finger of one hand into the finger of the other hand to evaluate some organ

Percussion hammer: instrument with a rubber head used for tapping a body surface

Perfusion: passing of fluid through body tissue

Periodontitis: extensive inflammation of the gums and alveolar tissues; synonym for pyorrhea

Perioperative nursing: wide variety of nursing activities carried out before, during, and after surgery

Perioperative period: entire time period from the decision to do or have surgery through recovery from the surgery

Periorbital edema: edema or swelling around the orbit of the eye

Peripheral resistance: restraint to blood flow created by arteriole walls in an partial state of contraction

Peristalsis: involuntary, progressive wavelike movement of the musculature of the gastrointestinal tract

Person: a living human being, with all the characteristics that make up an individual personality

Personal hygiene: measures of personal cleaning and grooming which promote physical and psychologic well-being

Petechiae: small, purplish, hemorrhagic spots on the skin which do not blanch with applied pressure

*p*H: expression of hydrogen ion concentration and resulting acidity of a substance

Phagocytosis: engulfing of microorganisms, foreign particles, or other cells by phagocytes

Phantom limb pain: sensation of pain without demonstrable physiologic or pathologic substance; commonly observed after the amputation of a limb

Pharmacodynamics: study of drug activity at the cellular level

Pharmacokinetics: study of the movement of drug molecules in the body in relation to its absorption, distribution, metabolism, and excretion

Pharmacology: study of actions of chemicals on living organisms

Pharmacopeia: official drug document

Philosophy: study of wisdom, of fundamental knowledge, and of the process used to develop and construct our own perception of life

Phlebitis: inflammation of a vein

Phlegm: thick, respiratory secretions

Physiologic jaundice: yellowness of the skin, sclera, mucous membranes due to excessive bilirubin in the blood of a newborn. It is caused by immature liver function at birth. As the liver function matures, the jaundice disappears, usually within a few days.

Physiologic needs: need for oxygen, food, water, temperature, elimination, sexuality, activity, and rest. These needs have the highest priority and are essential to survival.

Piggyback: intermittent IV administration of medications through a primary IV line

Placebo: Latin word meaning "I shall please"; an inactive substance that gives satisfaction to the person using it

Plaintiff: person or government bringing a lawsuit against another

Planned change: process of effecting change by purposeful and systematic efforts

Planning: establishment of client goals to prevent, reduce, or resolve the problems identified in the nursing diagnoses and determination of related nursing interventions

Plantarflexion: flexion of the foot so that the foot is in a dropped position

Plaque: transparent, adhesive coating on teeth consisting of mucin, carbohydrate, and bacteria

Plasma: liquid constituent of blood; synonym for intravascular fluid

Pleural friction rub: coarse, crackling, grating sound heard over the thoracic area

Pneumonia: inflammation and/or infection of the lungs

Podiatrist: one who treats foot disorders; synonym for chiropodist.

Podiatry: health discipline that deals with the treatment of foot disorders; synonym for chiropody

Poikilothermic: maintenance of body temperature at or near the temperature of the environment

Polarity: presence of electrically charged particles

Polyp: tumor on a stem that bleeds easily and may become malignant

Polypharmacy: dispensing or use of multiple drugs for one or more health problems

Polypnea: fast respiration rate; synonym for tachypnea

Polysaccharides: complex CHO compounds composed of ten or more glucose units. Starch, dextrins, and cellulose are common polysaccharides.

Polyuria: excessive output of urine (diuresis)

Portal of entry: point at which organisms enter a host

Postanesthesia recovery (PAR) room: area to which clients are taken after surgery is completed for assessment of recovery from anesthesia and monitoring of potential complications

Posterior fontanelle: triangular-shaped, membrane-covered space remaining at the junction of the occipital and parietal bone sutures in a fetus or an infant

Postoperative phase: time period lasting from admission to the postanesthesia recovery area through recovery and convalescence

Postural hypotension: temporary fall in blood pressure associated with assuming an upright position; synonym for orthostatic hypotension

Power: extent to which a person is able to influence his own and others' lives

Precordium: anterior surface of the chest wall overlying the heart and its related structures

Preferred provider arrangement (PPA): any arrangement whereby clients are channeled to specific individual providers of health plans

Preferred provider organization (PPO): any arrangement whereby clients are channeled to specific organizations as providers of health plans

Prefilled cartridge: previously prepared single dose of medication inserted into a holder for injection

Preformed water: water in food

Pregnancy: condition resulting from union of a sperm and an egg; period of time from fertilization of the ovum to delivery of the newborn; approximately 9½ lunar months in humans

PreLinguistic: sounds that precede speech in infancy

Premature beat: irregular rhythm in which a heartbeat occurs sooner than the pace at which previous ones were noted

Premature ejaculation: condition in which a man consistently reaches orgasm and ejaculation during sexual activity before or soon after coitus begins

Preoperative phase: time period lasting from the decision that surgery is necessary until the client is transferred to the operating room area

Presbycusis: normal loss of hearing as a result of the aging process

Presbyopia: normal loss of visual accommodation for close work as a result of the aging process

Prescription: used by physician to convey medication plans for a client

Pressure sore: area of cellular necrosis caused by a lack of circulation to the involved area; synonym for bedsore and decubitus ulcer

Primary hypertension: abnormally elevated blood pressure with no known cause; synonym for essential hypertension

Priority setting: process of ranking client problems in terms of the threat they pose to client well-being

Private law: rule that regulates relationships among people; synonym for civil law

Privileged communication: information that cannot be revealed in court by the person receiving it

Problem-oriented record (POR): documentation system organized according to the person's specific health problems; includes data base, problem list, plan of care, and progress notes

Process: series of actions, changes, or functions to bring about a result

Proctosigmoidoscopy: visual examination of the rectum, rectosigmoid junction, and lower sigmoid colon

Prodromal stage: stage of an infection when a person is most infectious. Early signs and symptoms of disease are present but are vague and nonspecific.

Productive cough: cough that produces respiratory tract secretions

Projection: a person attributes his own undesirable or unacceptable impulses to another person or object

Pronation: assumption of the prone position, such as when the patient is lying on his abdomen

Prone position: lying horizontal, with face downward; palms turned downward

Prospective payment: under this plan, clients are classified by major diagnostic related groups (DRGs), with a rate or payment amount assigned prospectively to each DRG for reimbursement of health-care providers

Proteinuria: albumin in the urine; indication of kidney disease

Protocol: written plan that details the nursing activities to be executed in specific situations

Protrusion: state or condition of being forward or projecting

Pseudomenstruation: slight, bloody, mucous discharge from the vagina of a female infant in response to maternal hormonal influences

Psychiatric hospital: institution that provides in-hospital mental health services for clients with acute or chronic alternations

Psychiatric nurse specialist: community health nurse with a specialty in psychiatric nursing

Psychogenic pain: pain for which no physical cause can be identified

Psychomotor learning: acquisition of physical skills

Psychosocial development: development governed by social, cultural, and emotional variables

Psychosomatic disorder: physiologic alterations and illness believed to be due to psychologic influences

Puberty: period of time during which primary and secondary sexual characteristics develop and the capability of sexual reproduction is attained

Public health service: local, state, or national official agency that provides community services for the promotion of health and prevention of illness

Public law: rule that regulates relationships between people and their government

Pulmonary embolism: embolism carried to the lungs

Pulse: wave produced in the wall of an artery with each beat of the heart

Pulse deficit: difference between the apical and radial pulse rates

Pulse pressure: difference between systolic and diastolic pressures

Puncture wound: injury caused by a pointed object that penetrates the skin; synonym for stab wound

Purkinje system: interlacing network in the heart that carries electric currents through the ventricles

Purulent: containing pus

Pyorrhea: extensive inflammation of the gums and alveolar tissues; synonym for periodontitis

Pyrexia: elevation above the upper limit of normal body temperature; synonym for fever

Pyuria: pus in the urine; urine appears cloudy

Quality assurance program: ongoing evaluation program designed and implemented to secure the excellence of health care; may involve an assessment of structure, process, and outcome standards

Quickening: first perceptible movement of the fetus in utero

Race: division of human beings based on distinct physical characteristics

Radiation: diffusion or dissemination of heat by electromagnetic waves

Radiography: examination by x-ray film

Radioisotope: radioactive chemical

Radiopaque: substance that x-rays cannot penetrate

Rales: abnormal lung sound described as crackling in nature

Range of motion: complete extent of movement of which a joint is normally capable

Rape: sexual violation of a person by someone who uses forces, threats, and abuse

Rapport: feeling of mutual trust experienced by persons in a satisfactory relationship

Rationalization: giving questionable behavior a logical or socially acceptable explanation; behavior justification

Reaction formation: giving a reason for behavior that is opposite from its true cause

Reactive hyperemia: body's flooding of an area with blood after the area has suffered from poor circulation for a period of time

Readiness: condition of possessing the ability to change

Reality orientation: method of care used to promote awareness of reality in confused or disoriented clients

Reception: process of receiving data about the internal or external environment through the senses

Receptor: specialized structures within a cell that interact with a drug

Recipient: person who receives another person's blood

Recommended dietary allowance (RDA): recommendations for average daily amounts of essential nutrients that healthy population groups should consume over time

Reconstitution: addition of fluid to a powdered drug to create a solution for administration

Record (medical record, chart): legal document consisting of a compilation of a person's health care information

Referred pain: pain in an area removed from that in which stimulation has its origin

Reflex: unconscious effecting of a particular automatic response mediated by the nervous stem

Reflex incontinence: state in which a person experiences an involuntary loss of urine, occurring at somewhat predictable intervals when a specific bladder volume is reached

Reflex pain response: automatic response of the central nervous system to the stimulus of pain

Regional anesthesia: anesthetic drug is injected or applied topically to inhibit transmission of sensory stimuli

Registration: official listing of the names and qualifications of persons who meet minimum requirements to practice in the occupation or profession of their choice

Regression: returning to an earlier method of behaving

Rehabilitation: process of restoring a person's highest level of possible wellness and returning that person's ability to live and work as normally as possible after a disabling illness or injury

Rehabilitation center: community center providing rehabilitation services

Rehabilitative level care: care warranting skilled services for a client in whom an improvement of function is expected; reimbursed by insurance; synonym for intermediate level care

Relapsing fever: body temperature that returns to normal for at least a day after which fever returns

Relationship: interaction of persons over a period of time

Relax: to become less rigid, to slacken effort, and to decrease tension

Religion: organized system of beliefs about a higher power; often includes set forms of worship, spiritual practices, and codes of conduct

REM: rapid eye movement that characterizes the dream state of sleep

Remittent fever: body temperature that fluctuates several degrees above normal but does not reach normal between fluctuations

Repolarization: process of restoring polarity

Repression: exclusion of an anxiety-producing event from conscious awareness

Reservoir: natural habitat for the growth and multiplication of microorganisms

Resident flora or bacteria: microorganisms that normally live on a person's skin

Residual urine: urine that remains in the bladder after the act of micturition

Residual volume (RV): air remaining in the lungs after maximal exhalation

Resonance: quality of the sound heard on percussion of a hollow structure such as the chest

Respiration: act of breathing and using oxygen in body cells

Respiratory acidosis: proportionate excess of carbonic acid in the extracellular fluid

Respiratory alkalosis: proportionate deficiency of carbonic acid in the extracellular fluid

Respiratory distress syndrome: condition of the newborn marked by dyspnea, cyanosis, expiratory grunt and intercostal in drawing. It is usually caused by immaturity of lung function and occurs most frequently in premature infants.

Respite care: care in which someone comes into the house for a few hours to relieve the caregiver. Sometimes the client is sent to a nursing home for a short period of time to give the caregiver a rest.

Respondeat superior: master–servant rule that states that an employer is legally liable for his employee's acts

Responsibility: obligation to perform some act for which one can be held accountable

Rest: condition in which the body is in a decreased state of activity with the consequent feeling of being refreshed

Restraint: device used to limit movement or immobilize a client

Retarded ejaculation: condition in which a man is unable to ejaculate into the vagina or has delayed intravaginal ejaculation

Retention: inability to void although urine is produced by the kidneys

and enters the bladder; excessive storage of urine in the bladder

Retention sutures: sutures used to provide extra support in wounds in obese clients, or in wounds with increased risk of dehiscence

Reticular activating system: network of neurons in the core of the brain stem with ascending and descending tracts to other areas of the brain which monitors and regulates incoming sensory stimuli and level of arousal

Retrograde pyelogram: x-ray examination of the kidney and ureters after a contrast material is injected into the renal pelvis through the ureter

Retrospective audit: evaluation of nursing care/client outcomes after the client has been discharged (may use postdischarge questionnaires, client interviews, or chart review)

Rh: an inherited antigen

Rhonchi: abnormal, continuous sound characterized by a sonorous, dry, coarse sound heard over the large airways. This sound may clear with a cough.

Right: claim to a particular privilege

Risk factor: something that increases a person's chance for illness or injury

Risk management: process of identifying, analyzing, and treating risks to improve client care and reduce malpractice claims

Roentgen ray: high-energy electromagnetic wave capable of penetrating solid matter and acting on photographic film; synonym for x-ray

Rotation: turning on an axis

Sadism: practice of inflicting harm on another person for sexual stimulation

Sadomasochism (SM): practice of using sadism and masochism simultaneously

Safety and security needs: a person's need to be protected from actual or potential harm and to have freedom from fear

Sanguineous: containing or mixed with blood

Scar: connective tissue that fills a wound area

Schemata: mental representation of familiar experiences or events

School phobia: unrealistic fear of attending school, possibly reflecting severe, abnormal separation anxiety

Scientific knowledge: knowledge arrived at by applying scientific methods

Scientific method: systematic problem-solving process which involves (1) problem identification, (2) data collection, (3) hypothesis formulation, (4) plan of action, (5) hypothesis testing, (6) interpretation of results, and (7) evaluation resulting in conclusion or revision of the study

Scrub nurse: nurse who assists the surgeon during surgery, maintaining surgical asepsis while draping, handling instruments, and handling supplies

Scultetus binder: type of bandage with multiple tails; synonym for many-tailed binder

Sebaceous gland: gland found in the skin that secretes an oily substance called sebum

Sebum: fatty secretion of the sebaceous glands

Secondary hypertension: abnormally elevated blood pressure caused by known pathology

Sedative hypnotic: pharmaceutical agent used to induce sleep

Self-actualization needs: need to reach one's potential through full development of one's unique capabilities. This is the highest level need.

Self-concept: mental image or picture of self; includes body image, subjective self, ideal self, and social self

Self-esteem: a person's perception of his total being, including self-worth and body image

Self-esteem needs: need to feel good about oneself and to believe others hold one in high regard

Self-identity: person's sense of who he is, including present status and future direction

Semantics: study of the meaning of words

Semen: seminal plasma containing sperm

Semi-Fowler's position: low, semi-sitting position with the head of the bed raised 15 to 30 degrees

Semipermeable membrane: selectively permeable membrane which allows water to pass through it but is either impermeable or very selectively permeable to solutes

Sensoristasis: arousal state of the reticular activating system; general drive state

Sensory deficit: impaired functioning of one or more senses: visual, auditory, olfactory, gustatory, tactile, kinesthetic, visceral

Sensory deprivation: condition resulting from decreased sensory input or input that is monotonous, unpatterned, or meaningless

Sensory overload: condition resulting from excessive sensory input to which the brain is unable to meaningfully respond

Sensory-perceptual alteration: disturbance in the body's ability to receive or process data from its internal or external environment; NANDA approved nursing diagnosis

Serous: resembling blood serum, clear and watery in appearance

Set point: level at which the hypothalamus attempts to maintain body temperature

Severe pain: pain that could be described as being between 8 and 10 on a scale of 1 to 10; synonym for excruciating pain

Sexual dysfunction: condition that prevents a person or couple from engaging in or obtaining satisfaction from sexual activity

Sexual intercourse: sexual activity in which the penis is placed in the vagina; synonym for coitus

Sexuality: degree to which a person exhibits and experiences maleness and femaleness physically, emotionally, and mentally

Sexually transmitted disease: pathologic condition spread by sexual activity and intimate genital contact

Sharp pain: quick, sticking, and intense discomfort

Shearing force: force created when layers of tissue move upon each other

Shifting pain: discomfort that moves from one area to another

Shock: body's reaction to acute peripheral circulatory failure owing to an abnormality of circulatory control or to a loss of circulating fluid

Significance: way a person feels he is loved and approved of by the persons important in his life

Sims' position (right and left): position in which the client is on his side with the top knee flexed sharply into the abdomen and lower knee less sharply flexed

Single-parent family: family with only one parent, predominantly female

Singultus: involuntary spasmodic contractions of the diaphragm; synonym for hiccups

Sinoatrial node (S-A node): tissue in the right atrium where the heartbeat originates; also called the heart's pacemaker

Situational crisis: change that results when a person faces an event or situation that causes a disruption in his life

Situational stress: changing events or situations occurring in day-to-day life

Sitz bath: special type of bath that applies heated water to the pelvic or rectal area

Skin sutures: used to approximate wound tissues and skin, may be silk, synthetic, wire, or metal staples

Skin tests: tests to determine antigen–antibody reaction

Slander: untruthful oral statement about a person that subjects him to ridicule or contempt

Sleep: state of altered consciousness throughout which varying degrees of stimuli preclude wakefulness

Sleep apnea: periods of no breathing during sleep which may last from 15 seconds to 2 minutes

Sleep cycle: passage through the four states of NREM sleep (I, II, III, IV), then reversal (IV, III, II), and then, instead or reentering stage I and awakening, entering REM sleep and returning to stage II

Sleep deprivation: condition resulting from decreased REM sleep, NREM sleep, or total sleep, characterized by progressive symptoms: irritableness or complete personality disintegration

Slight pain: pain that could be described as being between 1 and 3 on a scale of 1 to 10; synonym for mild pain

Smegma: thick secretion of sebaceous glands found under the labia minora and around the clitoris in the female and under the male prepuce

SOAP format: method of charging narrative progress notes; organizes data according to subjective information (S), objective information (O), assessment (A), and plan (P).

Social isolation: sense of aloneness because of decreasing relationships with others, resulting from attitudinal, geographic, financial, or illness-related factors

Social self: way a person feels others see him

Socialization: integration of behavior patterns, attitudes, motivations, and values deemed important by a person's culture

Sodomy: term used to describe sexual activity of placing the penis in the rectum; synonym for anal sex

Soixante-neuf: French word meaning 69; refers to a couple engaging in cunnilingus and fellatio simultaneously while assuming a position resembling the number 69

Solute: substance dissolved in a solution

Solvent: liquid holding a substance in solution

Somatic pain: pain originating in structures in the body's external wall

Somnambulism: sleep walking

Sordes: accumulation of mucous and crust formation on the teeth and around the lips

Source-oriented record: documentation system in which each healthcare group records data on its own separate form

Spasticity: increased muscle tone

Specific dynamic action: caloric cost of digesting, absorbing, and metabolizing food; represents about 10% of total calorie intake

Speed shock: body's reaction to a rapid injection of a substance into the circulatory system

Sperm: male reproductive cell; synonym for spermatozoon

Spermatogenesis: development of mature sperm in the male testes

Spermicide: chemical agent used to destroy sperm

Sphincter: circular muscle that constricts a passage or closes a natural orifice

Sphygmomanometer: instrument used for the indirect measurement of blood pressure

Spina bifida: congenital anomaly in which there is a defective closure of the bony encasement of the spinal cord. The spinal cord and meninges may protrude through the defective closure.

Spinal tap: insertion of a needle into the subarachnoid space; synonym for lumbar puncture

Spiritual distress: nursing diagnosis describing an alteration in spiritual health (*e.g.,* spiritual pain, alienation, anxiety, guilt, anger, loss, despair)

Spiritual need: lack of anything necessary for spiritual health (*e.g.,* meaning and purpose, love and relatedness, forgiveness)

Spirituality: anything that pertains to a person's relationship with a nonmaterial life force or higher power

Spirometer: instrument used to measure lung capacities and volumes. One type is used to encourage deep breathing (incentive spirometry).

Spooning: nail having a concave outer surface

Stab wound: injury caused by a pointed object that penetrates the skin; synonym for puncture wound

Standard: acceptable, expected, level of performance established by authority, custom, or consent

Standard of care: description of conduct that illustrates what a reasonably prudent person would have done, or would not have done, under similar circumstances

Standardized care plan: prepared plan of care that identifies the nursing diagnoses, client goals, and related nursing orders common to a population (*e.g.,* newborn) or problem

Standards of nursing: optimum levels of nursing care used for comparison of actual performance

Standing order: document that details the nursing care to be implemented in specific nursing situations, frequently when a physician is not present; may expand scope of nursing responsibilities

Stare decisis: Latin phrase meaning "Let the decision stand." *Stare decisis* is the basis for common law.

Stereotyping: assigning characteristics to a group of people without considering specific individuality

Sterilization: (1) the process by which all microorganisms, including spores, are destroyed; (2) surgical procedure performed to render a person infertile

Stertorous breathing: noisy respirations

Stethoscope: instrument used in auscultation to convey to the ear sounds produced in the body

Stimulus: agent, act, or other influence capable of initiating a response by the nervous system

Stock supply: system of supplying large quantities of medication on a nursing unit

Stoma: artificial opening for waste excretion located on the body surface

Stool: excreted feces

Strength (muscle): ability of the muscle to move actively against resistance

Stress: condition in which the human system responds to change in its normal balanced state

Stress incontinence: state in which a person experiences a loss of urine of less than 50 ml occurring with increased abdominal pressure

Stressor: anything causing a person to experience stress; the change in the balanced state

Stretching exercises: exercises that allow muscles and joints to be stretched gently through their full range of motion and that promote flexibility

Striae: line or band elevated above or depressed below surrounding tissue; or difference in color and texture

Stridor: harsh, high-pitched sound usually heard on inspiration when upper airways become narrowed

Stroke volume: quantity of blood forced out of the left ventricle with each contraction

Subconjunctival hemorrhage: bleeding under the conjunctiva into the sclera of the eyeball as a result of increased vascular tension during birth

Subculture: group of persons with different interests or goals than the primary culture

Subcutaneous injection: injection into the subcutaneous tissue that lies between the epidermis and the muscle

Subjective data (symptoms, covert data): information perceived only by the affected person

Subjective self: a person's perception of himself; who he thinks he is

Sublimation: conscious expression of an unacceptable impulse or feeling in a more acceptable way

Sublingual: area in the mouth under the tongue

Suffocation: stoppage of breathing or the lack of air reaching the lungs; asphyxiation

Sundowning syndrome: describes a phenomenon when a person habitually becomes confused or disoriented with darkness

Supination: assumption of the supine position, such as when the client is lying on his back

Supine position: position in which the client lies flat on his back with legs together (dorsal position)

Suppository: oval- or cone-shaped substance which is inserted into a body cavity and which melts at body temperature

Suppressant: drug that depresses a body function

Suppression: person consciously turns his attention away from a perceived treat

Suprapubic catheter: catheter inserted into the bladder through a small abdominal incision above the pubic area

Surgical asepsis: practices that render and keep objects and areas free from microorganisms; synonym for sterile technique

Surgical risk: classification of surgery as major or minor; major surgery has the potential for significant client risk and postoperative complications

Susceptibility: degree of resistance of a host to a pathogen

Suture: line of union between adjoining bones of the skull

Symmetry: correspondence in shape, size, and relative position of parts on opposite sides of the body

Sympathomimetic agent: drug that produces effects that mimic the action of the sympathetic nervous system

Symptom: abnormal indication of an illness

Synergistic effect: combined effect of two or more drugs is greater than the effect of each drug alone

Synovial joint: freely movable joint in which there is a space between the articulating bones

Syphilis: sexually transmitted disease caused by the bacterium *Treponema pallidum*

Systemic symptoms: symptoms manifested throughout the entire body

Systolic pressure: highest point of pressure on arterial walls when the ventricles contract

Tachycardia: rapid heart rate

Tachypnea: abnormally rapid rate of breathing

Tactile: pertaining to touch

Target heart range: between 70% and 85% of the maximum heart rate (*i.e.,* the greatest number of beats per minute of which the heart is capable)

Tartar: hard deposit on the teeth near the gum line formed by plaque build-up and dead bacteria

Teaching: planned method, or series of methods, used to help someone learn

Temperament: a person's style of approaching people, situations, or events

Temperature: refers to the hotness or coldness of a substance

Terminal illness: illness from which there is no reasonable expectation of recovery or cure

Theory: statement that explains or characterizes a process, an occurrence, or an event based on observed facts but lacking absolute or direct proof

Therapeutic touch: "unruffling" or unblocking of congested areas of energy in the body and redirecting the energy for the promotion of comfort, relaxation, healing, and a sense of well-being

Third space fluid shift: distributional shift and trapping of body fluids into body spaces such as the pleural, peritoneal, or pericardial, or into the interstitial space (plasma-to-interstitial shift)

Thoracentesis: aspiration of fluid or air from the pleural space

Thrill: abnormal tremor accompanying a vascular or cardiac murmur felt on palpation

Thrombophlebitis: inflammation in a vein associated with thrombus formation

Thrombus: blood clot. The plural form is thrombi.

Tidal volume (TV): amount of air inspired and expired in a normal respiration

Tissue respiration: act of using oxygen by body cells; synonym for internal respiration

Tonus: normal, partially steady state of muscle contraction

Topical: application of a substance directly to a body site

Tort: wrong committed by a person against another person or his property

Total body water (TBW): total amount of water in the body, expressed as a percentage of body weight. The term total body fluid (TBF) is also used; fluids are usually considered to include water and electrolytes.

Total incontinence: state in which a person experiences a continuous and unpredictable loss of urine

Total lung capacity (TLC): amount of air equal to the tidal volume plus the residual volume

Total parenteral nutrition (TPN): feeding a nutritionally complete hypertonic solution through a major central vein; synonym for hyperalimentation

Trace elements: minerals found in the body in quantities less than 5 g and needed in only very small amounts (18 mg or less)

Trade name: drug name selected by the company selling the drug, also called brand name, proprietary name

Traditional family: composed of a husband, wife, and their children, who live together in one house

Traditional knowledge: knowledge passed down from generation to generation

Tranquilizer: pharmaceutical agent used primarily to reduce anxiety

Transducer: instrument that converts energy from one form to another

Transient flora or bacteria: microorganisms picked up on the skin as a result of normal activities which can be removed readily

Transient pain: pain that passes quickly; synonym for brief pain

Transsexuality: condition in which the person feels trapped within the wrong sex body

Transvestism: practice of arousing sexual desire by wearing clothing of the opposite sex

Trauma: injury

Tremor: involuntary facial movements

Trendelenburg's position: elevating the feet and legs while keeping the trunk flat on the bed; the head may rest on a small pillow

Trial: hearing of evidence in a legal

case before a judge (and jury) with the intent of reaching a decision or verdict

Trichomonal infection: sexually transmitted disease caused by the parasitic protozoa *Trichomonas vaginalis*

Triglycerides: predominant form of fat in food and the major storage form of fat in the body; composed of one glyceride molecule and three fatty acids

Trimester: one of the three periods of approximately 3 months into which pregnancy is divided

Tuning fork: instrument that sets up vibrations; used primarily for testing hearing

Turgor: tension of a cell determined by its hydration

Tympany: drumlike sound on percussion resulting from the presence of air or gas

Typing: determining a person's blood type

Ultrasonography: use of ultrasound to produce an image or photograph of an organ or tissue

Ultrasound waves: extremely high-frequency and inaudible sound waves

Unilateral: affecting or occurring on one side only

Unit dose: separate packaging and labeling of individual drug doses

United States dietary guidelines: general recommendations for choosing a healthy diet made by the U.S. Department of Agriculture and the U.S. Department of Health and Human Services

Upper GI series: x-ray film visualization of the esophagus, stomach, and duodenum

Urge incontinence: state in which a person experiences involuntary passage of urine occurring soon after a strong sense of urgency to void

Urgency: strong desire to void

Urinalysis: laboratory examination of a urine specimen

Urination: process of emptying the bladder; micturition; voiding

Urinometer: instrument used to measure the specific gravity of urine

Utilitarianism: ethical theory which states that those acts that produce

the greatest overall balance of good for the greatest number of people are right

Vaginal speculum: two-bladed instrument used to examine the vaginal canal and cervix

Vaginismus: condition in which the muscles of the vagina contract tightly to prevent penile penetration

Validation: act of confirming or verifying

Valsalva's maneuver: forcible exhalation against a closed glottis, resulting in increased intrathoracic pressure

Value system: organization of values ranked along a continuum of importance

Values: set of beliefs that are meaningful in life and that influence relationships with others

Variables: factors in a research study

Varicosity: swollen, twisted vein

Vector: nonhuman carrier, usually an arthropod, that transfers pathogens from one host to another

Vehicle: means for transmitting organisms

Ventilation: exchange of gases

Veracity: truth telling

Verbal communication: exchange of information using words

Verdict: decision reached by a jury in a legal proceeding

Vernix caseosa: cheeselike substance made of sebum and epithelial cells. It acts in utero as a protective covering for the skin of the fetus.

Vesicular: pertaining to vesicles or small blisters

Vesicular breathing: normal sound of respirations heard on auscultation over peripheral lung areas

Vial: glass bottles with self-sealing stoppers through which medication is removed; may be single or multiple dose

Vibration: rhythmic contraction and relaxation of the arms and shoulders while holding the hands flat on the client's chest wall

Virginity: state of a person who has never engaged in sexual activity, particularly sexual intercourse

Virtue: attainment of moral-ethical standards

Virulence: ability to produce disease

Visceral: pertaining to inner organs

Visceral pain: pain originating in the internal organs in the thorax, cranium, or abdomen

Visual: pertaining to sight

Visual recognition memory: remembering that occurs as a result of a visual stimulus

Vital capacity (VC): maximal amount of air that can be exhaled following maximal inhalation

Vital signs: body temperature, pulse and respiratory rates, and blood pressure; synonym for cardinal signs

Vitamins: organic substances needed by the body in very small amounts to help regulate body processes; are susceptible to oxidation and destruction

Voiding: process of emptying the bladder; micturition; urination.

Voluntary agency: nonprofit organizations that provide health care for communities; usually dealing with a particular segment or aspect

Waiver: legal provision that gives up a right or claim

Wheeze: continuous, high-pitched sound heard over the small bronchial tubes

Widowhood: status change resulting from the death of a husband or wife

Wound: injury that results in a disruption in the normal continuity of a body structure

X-ray: high-energy electromagnetic wave capable of penetrating solid matter and acting on photographic film; synonym for roentgen ray

Yin-yang: energy forces in Chinese teaching which must be in balance for good health: Expression of strong emotions will result in disharmony and imbalance between these forces.

Z-track: zig-zag technique used to administer irritating medications intramuscularly

Index

The letter *f* after a page number indicates a figure; *t* following a page number indicates tabular material.

in health-illness status, 23
Sociocultural needs
    health-illness status and, 24
    preoperative assessment of, 1251
Socioeconomic factors
    in grief reactions, 230
    health care provision and, 115–117
    learning ability and, 363
    nutrition and, 781, 782t
    in personal hygiene, 559
Sodium
    dietary, 770t, 946
    as electrolyte, 946, 957–958, 959–960t
Sodium bicarbonate for intravenous therapy,
        composition of, 984
Sodium lactate solution for intravenous ther-
        apy, composition of, 984
Sodomy, definition of, 1067
Soft diet, 785
Soil as pathogen reservoir, 502
Solutions
    definition of, 1124t
    for intravenous therapy
        changing of, 992
            procedure for, 993–995
        composition of, 983–984t
        sterile, handling of, 515, 519, 519f
Somatic pain, definition of, 720
Somnambulism, definition of, 701, 703t
Sounds
    adventitious, 415, 458, 462t, 905–906
    bowel, 817–818
    breath, 415, 415t, 905–906
        developmental level and, 902, 902t
    heart, 459–460, 464f, 465t
    in joints, 471
    percussion, 438, 439t
Source-oriented record, 312, 313t, 314–
        315f
Spastic hemiparesis, gait in, 641f
Spasticity of muscle, definition of, 642
Specialists
    certification of, 80, 82
    health care fragmentation and, 43
    nurse, 9t
Specific dynamic action, calorie requirements
        for, 758
Specific gravity of urine, 856t
    determination of, 861
    in fluid balance assessment, 977
Specimen collection
    blood, 1194–1195
    from isolated client, 527
    secretions, 1195
    urine, 857, 859–860, 860–861f, 1195
Speculum
    nasal, 433f, 434
    vaginal, 433f, 434
        use of, 465, 467, 471f
Speech. *See also* Language; Verbal
        communication
    disorders of, in preschool children, 190
Speech therapist, services of, 44
Speed shock in intravenous therapy, 1000t
Sperm, production of, 1064
Spermicides, 1086, 1086f

Sphincters
    of anal canal, function of, 812, 812f
    control of, in toddlers, 182, 184
    of urinary system, 851
Sphygmomanometer, 419–420, 419–420f,
        419t
    care of, 427
Spica bandage, application of, 1214
Spinal accessory nerve, assessment of, 475,
        475t
Spinal anesthesia, 1247
Spinal cord
    disorders of, mobility and, 629
    injury of, sexuality and, 1072
Spinal tap, 1189–1190, 1189f
Spiral-reverse turn in bandage application,
        1214
Spiral turn in bandage application, 1214
Spiritual beliefs, 1101–1103
Spiritual dimension in health-illness status,
        23
Spiritual distress, 1113–1114
    case study of, 1114–1117
    definition of, 1109
    nursing diagnosis of, 1109, 1110–1111t
Spirituality, 1100–1118. *See also* Religious
        values
    assessment of, 1108–1109
    counseling in, 1112
    cultural differences in, 119
    definition of, 1100–1101
    development of, 162–163, 162f, 163t
        in adolescents, 202
        in middle adults, 211
        in preschool children, 189
        in school-age children, 194–195
        in young adults, 208
    everyday living and, 1101
    factors affecting, 1106–1107
    health and, 1101
    illness and, 1101
    implementing in, 1109, 1111–1113
    nurse as role model in, 1107–1108
    nursing diagnosis of, 1109, 1110–1111t
    nurturing of, 1111–1112
    planning in, 1109
    religious faiths and, 1101–1106
        Christianity, 1102–1106, 1104–1105f
        Judaism, 1102–1104, 1104f
    in terminal illness, 1106
Spiritual needs, 1100
    of dying patient, 234–235
    health-illness status and, 24
Spirometry
    incentive
        as breathing exercise, 911, 911f
        postoperative, 1257
    in respiratory function assessment, 907t
Splint, hand-wrist, body alignment and, 648,
        648f
Sponge, vaginal, as contraceptive method,
        1086, 1086f
Sponge bath for temperature reduction,
        1231, 1237–1238
Spoon nails, 443f
Sprain of joint, mobility in, 629

Sputum, analysis of, 907–908t
Stab wound for drainage tube, 1209
Standard orders for nursing activities, 306
Standards
    comparison of, to data, in diagnosing,
        276–277
    for nursing education, 80–81
    for nursing evaluation, 322–323
        identification of, 322–323
    for nursing practice, 14–15, 80, 81f
Standards of care
    in meeting client goals, 308
    in negligence cases, 85
    student nurses' responsibility for, 92
Standing order for medications, 1127
Standing position, 435, 436f
    body alignment in, 640, 642, 642f
Staples in wound closure, 1209–1210, 1209f
    removal of, 1217, 1220
Stat order for medications, 1127
Statutory law, 79–80
Steam in sterilization/disinfection, 513
Steppage gait, 641f
Stepping reflex, 172t
Stereotyping of groups of people, 113–114,
        114f
Sterile technique. *See* Surgical asepsis
Sterile urine specimen, collection of, 860,
        861f
Sterilization (aseptic procedure), 512–514
    cleaning of items before, 512–513, 513f
    definition of, 505–506, 506t
    methods for, 513–514
        selection of, 512
Sterilization (contraception), 1086f, 1087
    spiritual beliefs on, 1103
Stertorous breathing, definition of, 415
Stethoscope
    in auscultation, 439
    in blood pressure assessment, 420–421,
        421f, 422t
    in heart examination, 459–460, 464f, 465t
    in thorax assessment, 458
Stimulants as laxatives, 829–839
Stimulation
    of appetite, 785
    in pain management
        contralateral, 741, 743
        cutaneous, 741, 743
        electrical, 748
        sensory. *See* Sensation
    of urination, 864–865
Stimulus
    adaptation to, 1040
    definition of, 1040
Stockings, antiembolism, assistance with, 566,
        575
    procedure for, 573–575
Stoma, definition of, 837, 883
Stomatitis, 588
Stool
    characteristics of, 818, 819t
    collection of, for laboratory examination,
        818, 820
    definition of, 811
Stool softeners, use of, 829–839

Photo credits

Cover photos

(from left back cover to right front cover)

Gates Rhodes, courtesy of the School of Nursing, University of Pennsylvania: first, third, fifth, sixth through tenth

© *Ken Kasper:* eleventh

Lippincott Learning Systems: second and fourth

Unit and Chapter opener photos

D. Atkinson: Chapter 13

Tracy Baldwin: Chapter 8

Karen Baldwin: Unit III, right

Jane Barry: Chapter 36

Robert Coldwell, courtesy of Community Home Health Services of Philadelphia: Chapter 26, bottom

GE Medical Systems: Chapter 41

© *Ken Kasper:* Chapters 23, 24, and 40

Robert Neroni, courtesy of Thomas Jefferson University: Chapters 5, 7, 17, 20, and 22

Patrick O'Kane: Unit III, left

Gates Rhodes, courtesy of the School of Nursing, University of Pennsylvania: Units I, II, IV, V, VI, VII, VIII, and IX; Chapters 1, 2, 3, 4, 6, 9, 10, 11, 12, 14, 15, 16, 18, 19, 21, 30, 33, 34, 37, 38, 39, and 43

Art Siegel: Chapter 35

All Photographers are gratefully acknowledged for the reuse of their photographs in the marginal applications in the front of the book and on the verso pages of the Unit openers.